The Dictionary of MODERN MEDICINE

The Dictionary of MODERN MEDICINE

Compiled and edited by

JC SEGEN, MD

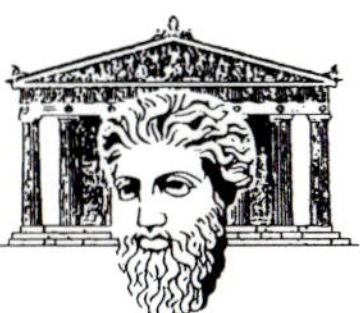

The Parthenon Publishing Group
International Publishers in Medicine, Science & Technology

Casterton Hall, Carnforth,
Lancs, LA6 2LA, UK

120 Mill Road, Park Ridge,
New Jersey 07656, USA

An impossibility does not disturb us until its accomplishment shows us what fools we are--Henry S Haskins

For Susan,
Joseph ,
Monica and
David

In the memory of Gilbert Beltran Garcia, MD
1951-1988

Published in the UK by
The Parthenon Publishing Group Limited, Casterton Hall, Carnforth, Lancs LA6 2LA, England

Published in the USA by
The Parthenon Publishing Group Inc., 120 Mill Road, Park Ridge, New Jersey 07656, USA

British Library Cataloguing-in-Publication Data

Segen, J.C.
The dictionary of modern medicine: A sourcebook of currently used medical expressions, jargon and technical terms. – (Dictionary series)
I. Title II. Series
610.3
ISBN 1-85070-321-3

Library of Congress Cataloging-in-Publication Data

Segen, J.C.
The dictionary of modern medicine : a sourcebook of currently used medical expressions, jargon, and technical terms / edited and compiled by J.C. Segen.
p. cm.
Includes bibliographical references.
ISBN 1-85070-321-3
1. Medicine--Dictionaries. I. Title.
[DNLM: 1. Dictionaries, Medical. W 13 S4545d]
R121.S429 1992
610'.3--dc20
DNLM/DLC
for Library of Congress 91-39484
CIP

First published 1992

Printed and bound by Butler & Tanner Ltd, Frome & London, UK

Foreword

I believe that the Golden Age of Medicine is at hand for patients (not necessarily for doctors), and only for those patients in developed countries who have good comprehensive health insurance. Salient achievements have included huge advances in science, abundant technology, excellent facilities, enough physicians, generally adequate medical care funding, pluralism in the delivery of care in most countries, rapid communications and computers, constructive entrepreneurialism, an era of preventive medicine, and the application of scientific management principles to all of medicine.

In fact, William Foege of the Carter Presidential Center in Atlanta tells us that for every one day that has passed since the year 1900, we have added seven hours to the average expected life span at birth of an American--an incredible modern achievement--seven hours of life added for every 24 hours lived since 1900. And yet much stands between us in any country and any ideal medical system. In fact, virtually every country in the world seems to be searching for that ideal system and changing their existing system, no matter what it currently is.

"*...and the times they are a-changing*"--Bob Dylan. And with those changes, extraordinary changes in language, especially in medical science.

Would you believe a medical dictionary that includes such diverse and heretofore undefined terms as: A-64077, advance directives, Ayur-Veda, Baltimore Affair, the Chinese lantern sign, EMS, hyperendemnicity, monopsony in medical economics, Orphan Annie (eye) nuclei, pimping, rule of nine, Slutsky affair, teat and udder sign, "unbundling" of health care reimbursement and Zero population growth?

When I use a word, I may mean it to say exactly what I may mean it to mean. Okay. But how will anyone else know what I mean? That is the reason for dictionaries. There are dictionaries and then there are dictionaries. But I don't think there has ever been another dictionary like 'The Dictionary of Modern Medicine'. Certainly there has been no such in medicine. Language experts and even ordinary readers interested in what really happens in modern medicine will adore this book. It is super-helpful.

Surely no one but a pathologist would have had the visual perception and sensitivity to recognize that a book such as this is needed and the conceptual creativity to include so many interesting terms and concepts. And to have had the patience and persistence to tabulate and define all of these, more than ten thousand, terms is a monumental achievement.

Wordsmiths of the world, enjoy.

George D Lundberg, MD, *Editor*
Journal of the American Medical Association
Chicago

INTRODUCTION

Much has changed in the world and in medicine since the standard medical dictionaries were compiled at the beginning of the 20th century. A well-educated physician was conversant in the classics, specialization in medicine consisted of a one-to-three year apprenticeship in one of a handful of disciplines, and subspecialization was virtually unknown. The diagnostic armamentarium consisted of a microscope, a stethoscope and X-rays; virology, genetics, immunology and other disciplines were primitive; molecular biology and computers were decades in the future. Disease mechanisms were poorly understood, bacterial infections were often fatal; other diseases either did not exist or were not recognized and little therapy was available. The average person's life span was less than 55 years.

The world, medicine, physicians and their patients have changed considerably in the intervening decades. Specialization and subspecialization are expected of today's physicians and require six to nine years after medical school. English has become the lingua franca in medicine and the world at large. Diagnostic modalities and therapeutic options are seemingly endless; patients have become 'clients' and have life spans of more than 75 years. Disease mechanisms are being dissected by molecular biologists and immunologists using a bewildering array of techniques; medical information doubles every seven to ten years; computers have become standard tools. Physicians now share many decisions with patients, lawyers, bureaucrats and ethicists. The changes in medicine have engendered a new vocabulary and a medical dictionary should have its finger on the pulse of those changes.

This work is not designed to replace traditional dictionaries, but rather to complement them. This is a compilation of terms, many of recent vintage that are integral to the language of modern medicine, a language replete with acronyms, jargon, neologisms and the argot of new disciplines, diseases, their diagnosis and therapies. The Dictionary of Modern Medicine has categorically avoided terms from classic anatomy and biochemistry, common usage terms (eg hand, teeth), eponyms and pronunciation guidelines, having as its major raison d'etre, the provision of details that complement and supplement the information available in standard references.

Joseph C Segen, MD
Manhasset, New York
November, 1991

Key to symbols and features

thyroid hormone in patients with hypothyroidism of hypothalamic or pituitary origin who have an underlying mild ACTH deficiency CLINICAL Hypotension, shock, fever, dehydration, anorexia, weakness, apathy LABORATORY Hyponatremia, hyperkalemia, lymphocytosis, hypoglycemia TREATMENT Pharmacologic doses of glucocorticoids

'Addressin' A homing protein, peptide or other molecule that provides a

Adoptive immunotherapy An experimental therapy for terminal cancer consisting in the transfer of 'activated' anti-tumor cells, eg combining lymphokine-activated killer (LAK) cells or tumor-infiltrating lymphocytes (TIL) with IL-2 into patients with metastatic malignancy (Science 1989; 244:1430n&v); about 10% patients with terminal renal cell carcinoma and melanoma have achieved partial or complete remission with the LAK/IL-2 regimen

Adverse event (AE) LEGAL MEDICINE An injury caused by medical management (rather than the underlying disease), which prolongs hospitalization, produces a disability at the time of discharge, or both; *AEs OCCUR IN 0.2 TO 7.9% OF HOSPITALIZATIONS*, 1 to 60% of which are due to negligence; 70% had a disability of less than six months, 14% resulted in death (N Engl J Med 1991; 324:370, J Am Med Assoc 1991; 265:3265); AEs are caused by drug complications, wound infections and technical complications and those due to negligence due to diagnostic mishaps, therapeutic mishaps and events occurring in the emergency room; one-half of AEs were related to an operation and are more common in older patients (ibid, 324:377) see **Malpractice**

Term

Relevant patient details

Field of Medicine or Biology

Relevant emphases

References and nature of the article
- br Book review
- c Correspondence
- cr Case report
- ed Editorial
- n&v News and views
- rv Review article

Cross-references

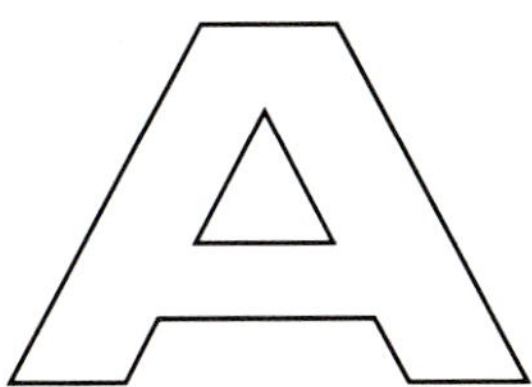

A Symbol for: Absorbance; radioactivity; adenosine; admittance (Electricity); Alanine; alveolar gas; Ampere; area; mass number

a Symbol for: Absorptivity; acceleration; activity (chemical activity); arterial blood gas; atto-

a/A ratio PHYSIOLOGY The ratio between the oxygen in the arterial blood and the alveoli, which serves as an estimate of the pulmonary gas exchange; in normal subjects, the ratio is relatively constant (> 0.75) for 21% to 100% oxygen in the inspired air, and becomes increasingly variable in those with pulmonary disease

A_1AT see α_1-antitrypsin

A4 see Amyloid β peptide

A68 A neuronal antigen (recognized by a monoclonal antibody Alz-50), present in the developing fetus by 32 weeks of development, disappearing by age two; A68 is present in brain tissue and cerebrospinal fluid and is a major subunit of paired helical filaments of Alzheimer's dementia and is derived from low molecular weight tau protein (possibly Tau 69, Nature 1990; 346:22c), but is more phosphorylated

A-64077 An experimental therapeutic agent under development which inhibits the 5-lipoxygenase pathway of arachidonic acid metabolism that attenuates the bronchoconstrictive response by asthmatics to cold air and allergen-induced nasal constriction, a response largely due to the eicosanoids produced by 5-lipoxygenase, including sulfidopeptide leukotrienes, 5-HETE and leukotriene B4 (N Engl J Med 1990; 323:1740, 1745)

AABB American Association of Blood Banks A professional, non-profit organization established in 1947 and dedicated to education, delineation of standards, policy and other facets of transfusion medicine and is responsible for collecting one-half of the blood supply in the US and transfusing 80%; the AABB is involved in accreditation of transfusion facilities, maintains a rare donor supply and serves as a reference laboratory

Abandonment LEGAL MEDICINE Negligent termination of a physician-patient relationship either without the patient's consent or without giving adequate notification, so that the patient may continue his/her care with another physician; abandonment may be broadened to include infrequent visits by the physician to the patient while hospitalized; see Malpractice

Abbreviated new drug application CLINICAL PHARMACOLOGY An application made in the US by a pharmaceutical company requesting authority to market a 'new' drug for which both its therapeutic indications and formulation have been previously approved by the FDA in another similar drug; if the previous drug is deemed safe and effective, the Office of Health and Human Services is required to approve or disapprove the new drug within 180 days

A-B-C sequence EMERGENCY MEDICINE The first level of life support measures used in cardiopulmonary resuscitation according to the 'American school' of cardiology, is the simple mnemonic of 'airway, breathing and circulation'; advanced life support then continues as the D-E-F for 'drugs, electrocardiogram, fibrillation'; see C-A-B

ABC method see Avidin biotinylated horseradish-peroxidase complex

A-B-C/D-E-F sequence

Airway	Ensure airway patency (clear bronchotracheal tree)
Breathing	Ensure breathing by intermittent positive pressure ventilation
Circulation	Compress chest at 60/minute
Drugs/Fluids	Place intravenous line
EKG*	Monitor cardiac rhythms
Fibrillation	Defibrillate

*Electrocardiogram

ABC see Aneurysmal bone cyst

ABCD A simple mnemonic for the clinical features of early malignant melanomas, where A refers to asymmetry, B to border irregularity, C to variegation of color and D to a diameter greater than 6 mm (CA-A Cancer Journal for Clinicians 1985; 35:4)

ABC superfamily ATP-binding cassette transporters A family of oligopeptide permease proteins, which includes the multi-drug resistance protein and a series of bacterial and eukaryotic transporters that are selective for a wide range of substrates including short oligopeptides, transporting them across membranes; the PSF (peptide supply factor) gene product has structural homology with the ABC transport proteins and the gene has been identified within the class II MHC (major histocompatibility complex) on chromosome 6, where it is thought to play a key role in antigen presentation (Nature 1990; 348:744, 741, Science 1990; 250:1723)

Abdominal angina Intermittent severe ischemia resulting in colicky abdominal pain beginning 15-30 minutes postprandially 1-2 hours in duration, which appears when two or all three (superior and inferior mesenteric and celiac) major abdominal arteries have severe atherosclerosis; since the intestine's oxygen demand increases with meals, the patients avoid the pain by not eating and thus lose weight; malabsorption may occur since absorption is oxygen-dependent Treatment Bypass, endarterectomy, reimplantation, percutaneous transluminal angioplasty

Abdominal apoplexy Acute hemoperitoneum; small amounts of blood in the peritoneal cavity produce minimal (hyperosmolar) irritation as the erythrocytes lyse; when a visceral artery ruptures (splenic artery more commonly than the hepatic); the hyperosmolar irritation takes on clinical importance, causing acute 'peritonitis', abdominal pain, diminished bowel sounds and an increased leukocyte count

Abdominal bath RADIOTHERAPY A treatment field extending from the diaphragm to the pelvis, used to treat abdominal lymphomas or ovarian carcinoma; lead blocks are used to shield the right hepatic lobe during the initial 15 Gy whole abdominal dose, given by antero-posterior opposed fields; horizontal decubitus (cross-table) lateral fields are then used to bring the para-aortic and mesenteric lymph node radiation dose to 30 Gy, followed by another 14 Gy through antero-posterior ports, thus totalling 4400 (Cancer 1975; 36:796)

Abdominal cocoon Idiopathic sclerosing peritonitis A condition that is considered to be a sequel to peritonitis, said to be common in those treated with a LeVeen shunt where reactive fibrosis encases the small intestine Treatment Surgical lysis of adhesions

Abelson leukemia virus A retrovirus carrying the v-*abl* oncogene that is capable of transforming immature B lymphocytes to pre-B lymphocytes (class switching), causing B cell leukemias in mice

ABER Auditory brainstem evoked response An expensive and time-consuming method for evaluating infants at high risk for hearing loss that partially depends on the infant's maturity; ABER yields a low false negative rate when screening for early deafness

abl A proto-oncogene located on chromosome 9, which, in chronic myelogenous leukemia (CML), translocates to chromosome 22 adjacent to the 'breakpoint cluster region', bcr, forming the Philadelphia chromosome; this hybrid gene encodes a protein with tyrosine kinase activity; the normal (non-mutated) c-*abl* proto-oncogene is apparently critical in normal myelopoiesis as it inhibits myeloid colony formation; contrariwise it is mutated in 90% of those with CML (Science 1989; 245:1107), implying that c-abl is an active inhibitor of myeloid clonal expansion

abl**p210** see P210$^{bcr/abl}$

Abnutzung pigment German, worn away The brownish, 'wear and tear' pigment, ceroid that is deposited with aging in cardiac muscle, liver, brain and other organs

Abortion Although the term abortion is generic and implies a premature termination of pregnancy for any reason, the lay public better understands the word 'miscarriage' for involuntary fetal loss or fetal wastage Glossary **COMPLETE ABORTION** An abortion is considered complete only if a curettage has been performed, given the possibility of necrotizing decidual tissue remaining in the uterus, which may act as a nidus for infection **CRIMINAL ABORTION** Deliberate termination of pregnancy under illegal circumstances; although prior to the Roe *vs.* Wade decision, see there, physicians regularly performed 'criminal' abortions, in the usual parlance, criminal abortion implies a clandestine termination of pregnancy under non-sterile and unsuitable conditions, predisposing the mother to sepsis and death by exsanguination through mutilation of the uterus and perineum **EARLY ABORTION** An abortion performed before the 12th week of gestation **HABITUAL ABORTION** A third (or more) consecutive abortion, related to stress, nutritional status, an event occurring in up to 1:200 women, many of whom may eventually have successful gestations **INCOMPLETE ABORTION** Partial expulsion of fetus and placenta with pain and bleeding, which is potentially fatal for the mother, treated with curettage **INDUCED ABORTION** The voluntary termination of pregnancy, which can be either a dilatation and curettage when performed in the first trimester or a saline abortion when performed later **INEVITABLE ABORTION** The 'terminal' stage of threatened abortion where there is dilatation of the cervix and rupture of membranes, treated with curettage **LATE ABORTION** An abortion performed after the 12th week of gestation **MISSED ABORTION** The retention of a fetus known to be dead for four or more weeks, the interventional approach is expectancy as spontaneous delivery occurs usually by the sixth post-mortem week **SALINE ABORTION** Voluntary termination of pregnancy during the second trimester by replacing 200 ml of amniotic fluid with 200 ml of 20% saline solution, stimulating uterine contraction, followed by fetal delivery within 12-24 hours **SEPTIC ABORTION** Fetal loss due to a bacterial infection of the uterus, which is 50 times more common in intrauterine device-users; bacteria implicated include the native vaginal flora, including, *Clostridium perfringens*, aerobic and anaerobic streptococci and gram-negative bacilli **SPONTANEOUS ABORTION** A term equivalent to 'miscarriage' as used by the lay; spontaneous abortions occur at any time and for a wide variety of reasons; it is estimated that 20-50% of all conceptuses spontaneously abort, half of which are attributed to aneuploidy, especially loss of a sex chromosome and trisomy, especially 16 **THREATENED ABORTION** Vaginal bleeding at any time within the first 20 weeks of pregnancy, accompanied by colicky pain, backache and a bright red to brownish discharge, occurring in up to 20% of early pregnancies of which one-half progress to inevitable abortion, no therapy is consistently effective, although bed rest, analgesics and sedatives are advised

A box D loop MOLECULAR BIOLOGY A highly conserved (ie DNA nucleotide sequence similarity among many eukaryotic species) region located between base pairs +10 and +20 'upstream' on the tRNA gene, having the dual role of encoding functional tRNA and promoting tRNA transcription, acting as a site of receptive protein binding

ABPA Allergic bronchopulmonary aspergillosis

'Abracadabra therapy' A therapeutic modality that may effect a cure in certain conditions in mentally-impressionable subjects; it is not known why warts in children may occasionally regress with the physician simply touching the wart and murmuring 'abracadabra', the classic incantation uttered by magicians (prestidigitators)

Absence attack see Petit mal epilepsy

Absinthism Intoxication with an alcoholic beverage popular in fin-de-siècle France; the active toxin, thujone, is extracted from wormwood (***Artemisia pontica***, a plant used for de-worming, hence the trivial name); Absinthe's neurological effects (mental deterioration, loss of time/space orientation and hallucinations) eventually led to its ban in 1915 (J Am Med Assoc 1988; 260:3042)

Absorption IMMUNOLOGY A laboratory technique that consists in either a) Removal of antibody from serum by adding an antigen or b) Removal of an antigen by adding an antibody; absorption allows an antiserum to be purified by removingm unwanted immunoglobulins or may be used to 'fish' for an antigen or antibody of interest

Abstract The leading paragraph(s) that introduces a report of scientific information; the New England Journal of Medicine has adopted a structured format that includes: a) Background b) Methods c) Results and d) Conclusions; the purpose of the abstract is to enable the reader to efficiently grasp the essence of the article

Abstract 'creep' SCIENTIFIC JOURNALISM Growth in the length of abstracts, especially those longer than that stated in a journal's instructions for authors, some 'creep' occurs when authors attempt to provide as much information as possible, under the assumption that only the abstract will be read; a second, major cause of abstract 'creep' results from the advance of medical science, where the complexity of the physiology, molecular pathology, experimental design or procedure requires greater details for the reader to grasp the question being addressed (N Engl J Med 1990; 323:488c)

Abtröpfeln Abtröpfung German, dropping off DERMATOPATHOLOGY A term used by histopathologists referring to the 'falling off' of epithelioid cells in a junctional nevus as they 'penetrate' the superficial dermis

Abzymes Hybrid catalytic molecules designed to have a certain specificity, which is carried out by combining an antibody with an enzyme; although these two molecules have different functions, both bind molecules in a relatively specific manner and thus the 'marriage' of the two functions is logical; the 'Ab-' portion corresponds to the highly specific binding sequence, analogous to an immunoglobulin's variable region and the '-zyme' portion incorporates catalytic machinery; the spin-off will be 'custom-made' catalysts for use in biology and medicine (Science 1988; 240:426); two general types of 'abzymes' a) Catalytic antibody that takes advantage of an antibody's ability to selectively stabilize transitional state configurations or overcome entropic barriers by aligning reaction partners, accomplished by adding a catalyst that is either synthesized or a polypeptide with enzymatic activity, eg lipolytic abzymes (Science 1989; 244:437) and b) Hybrid enzymes that exploit a natural receptor to a designated specificity, accomplished by either redesigning an existing active site of enzyme action (Method: oligonucleotide-directed mutagenesis) or by adding or replacing an entire catalytic domain, thereby generating a hybrid enzyme, eg selective fusion of nucleic acid-specific binding domains to the non-specific phosphodiesterase enzyme, resulting in sequence-specific DNA (analogous to that of restriction enzymes) or RNA-cleaving molecules (Science 1989; 243:1184, Nature 1990; 348:482n&v)

Academic boycott A concerted political effort by physicians and/or scientists that indicates their displeasure with a country's prevailing policy regarding fundamental human rights, eg the academic boycott of South Africa, which developed in the wake of the death of Steve Biko or the boycott of the International conference on AIDS originally scheduled to meet in Boston in 1992 due to the US government's policy about not allowing visas to HIV-positive individuals; such efforts may prove instrumental in causing a change in policy, although the academicians in the boycotted country may suffer considerably therefrom (J Am Med Assoc 1991; 266:501); see Biko

ACAT Acyl-coenzyme A:cholesterol transferase The enzyme responsible for forming cholesteryl esters from cholesterol

Acatalasia Takahara's disease A hereditary condition first described in the Japanese, caused by a deficiency in tissue and erythrocyte catalase, the enzyme responsible for reducing peroxide to water and oxygen; as peroxide accumulates, malignant alveolar pyorrhea and oral gangrene ensue, requiring removal of all teeth

Acceleration-deceleration injury A major cause of cerebral morbidity, related to abrupt movement and deformation of the brain within the cranial cavity **ACCELERATION** The head suddenly accelerates, eg a blow to the head and the stationary brain is struck by the accelerated cranium at the site of the blow **DECELERATION** A rapidly moving skull is abruptly stopped, eg an auto accident, while the brain continues forward and impacts directly below the site where the skull stops; the immediate loss of consciousness is thought to be due to deformation of the brainstem and reticular activating system, with concomitant shearing, stretching, diffuse neuronal and axonal injury; tissue destruction is most marked in the inferior frontal gyri and anterior temporal lobes; the mechanism of acceleration-deceleration injury is the same as Contrecoup lesions, but the former term addresses the clinical aspects of the kinetics, while the latter addresses the pathological effects of abrupt movements on the brain

'Access' The ability of a person or group to obtain health care, which is a function of a) Geographic or logistical factors, eg rural communities have poor access to medical attention, due to a relative lack of providers, b) Finances or ability to pay for services and c) Other factors including ethnic, social and psychiatric aspects of the individual(s) seeking health care

Accessory cell A macrophage that aids in immune recognition by binding circulating antigens Note: Binding of an antigen to a self cell is a sine qua non for T cell response to an antigen, as the T cell receptor requires a self major histocompatability complex class II molecule with a bound foreign antigen before it can respond to an antigen; see Antigen-presenting cell

Accordion sign A periodic 'crumpling' of 2 distinct radiologic densities EMERGENCY RADIOLOGY Compression and medial displacement of a calcified splenic artery, which, when seen on the plain abdominal film of trauma victims, has been fancifully likened to an accordion and is suggestive of splenic rupture or hematoma formation (Am J Radiol 1972; 116:423) GASTROINTESTINAL RADIOLOGY A finding in upper gastrointestinal radiocontrast studies, described in advanced progressive systemic sclerosis (PSS), where the jejunum is dilated and foreshortened with mural fibrosis and the valvulae conniventes are of normal thickness, thus imparting an accordion-like corrugated appearance to the contrast column (Am J Roentgenol 1973; 119:332) Note: Other radiologic findings in the gastrointestinal tract in PSS include pneumatosis intestinalis, pseudo-obstruction, intussusception, sacculations and volvulus of the small intestine PEDIATRIC RADIOLOGY Crumpling and shortening of long bones, especially the femurs, seen in type II osteogenesis imperfecta, a disease accompanied by low birth weight, beading of the ribs, early death due to respiratory insufficiency resulting from a defective thoracic cage, softened skull, fragile skin with defective type I collagen; heredity is variable, affecting 1:60 000 live births; one-half are stillborn

Accountability MEDICAL ETHICS The extent to which individual(s) are answerable to a higher authority; physicians are held accountable before the law, the Hippocratic oath and their patients; scientists are accountable before the law, their peers and grant-giving agencies

Accountability 'fever' see 'Dingellization'

Accreditation HOSPITAL ADMINISTRATION The process of validating that a body or facility, eg a hospital, meets a series of standards in terms of physical plant, administration and professional staffing; most hospitals in the USA are accredited by non-profit, professional 'policing' organizations, eg the Joint Commission on Accreditation of Hospitals (see JCAH) created to assure the public that a facility has met the accrediting organization's standards

Accumulation theory see 'Garbage can' hypothesis

Accuracy LABORATORY MEDICINE The extent to which a value obtained from a test reflects or agrees with the true value of the analyte being tested, measured statistically by standard deviations Note: Precision The degree of reproducibility of test results, regardless of whether or not they are accurate, measured statistically by the Coefficient of variation

Ace of spades appearance GASTROINTESTINAL RADIOLOGY 1) The normal appearance of the duodenal bulb in a radiocontrast study of the upper gastrointestinal series; Cf Cloverleaf appearance 2) see Bird's beak appearance

Ace of clubs appearance see Cloverleaf appearance

ACE inhibitors Angiotensin converting enzyme inhibitors A group of drugs, eg captopril, enalapril that supplant β-blockers and diuretics in the treatment of hypertension

Acetowhite lesions GYNECOLOGY A whitish patch seen on the uterine cervix when it is 'painted' with 5% acetic acid (vinegar); most condylomatous lesions of the uterine cervix are white, the whiter the lesion, the greater the hyperkeratosis; given their premalignant potential, especially when positive for human papilloma viruses types 16, 18 and 33, all acetowhite lesions warrant biopsy; see HPV

Acetylcholine receptor antibodies AChR antibodies A group of antibodies that are reactive with epitopes other than the binding site for acetylcholine or α-bungarotoxin; AChR binding antibodies are present in up to 88% of patients with active myasthenia gravis, which wax and wane as a function of disease severity; AChR

Achilles' heel cleavage MOLECULAR BIOLOGY A method that allows a segment of DNA to be cut precisely at the desired location and nowhere else Background: Restriction endonucleases have been and continue to be the workhorses of molecular biology; they cleave DNA at specific recognition sites, ie each time a specific 4-to-6 oligonucleotide sequence appears, a restriction endonuclease clips the DNA into pieces ranging from 2.5 (or smaller) to 35 kD; 45 kD is near the limit of resolution of conventional electrophoretic gels; restriction endonucleases have been vital workhorses in gene cloning and sequencing *PROBLEM:* Even the most selective of restriction endonucleases ('rare choppers') cut the DNA into too many small pieces, a major obstacle in handling large DNA segments required for the Human genome project (see there) *SOLUTION:* Use a bacterial DNA-binding protein, the lac repressor, which recognizes a 20 base sequence, the lac operator (synthesized according to the needs of the investigator, containing the recogition sites for two commonly used restriction endonucleases; when the lac repressor is added to the yeast cell, the repressor finds the operator and binds it, covering up the two restriction sites (like Thetis' hand over Achilles' heel, see below note); then a methyltransferase is added, inactivating the restriction sites, except for the two 'hidden' below the lac repressor; removal of the lac repressor then leaves the genome with one recognition site for each of two enzymes; thus like Achilles' heel, a genome is vulnerable to cutting in only one site (Science 1990; 249:271, 217n&v); Cf Triplex DNA; Achilles' heel has been used in other contexts: a) The terminus of a DNA helix is likened to Achilles' heel, given its lability when it is not 'capped' by a telomere (J Theor Biol 1973; 41:181) and b) Psychological vulnerability to a degree sufficient to undermine a subject's character development; Achilles' mother, Thetis, dipped him into the River Styx which made him invulnerable to arrows except at the one place on the heel where she had held him

Achoo 'syndrome' Photic sneeze An autosomal dominant 'condition' affecting an estimated 25% of the population causing sneezing upon passing from dark to bright light, also known as the helico-cilio-sternutatogenic reflex

Acid aerosol ENVIRONMENT Colloidal suspensions of hydrogen ion-containing particles that form the so-called 'summer haze' and are generated by sulfur dioxide and nitrogen dioxide emissions from coal-burning electrical power plants; acid aerosols are transformed into ammonium bisulfate, sulfuric and nitric acids and coupled to low level ozone, where they are inculpated in pulmonary dysfunction in those who exercise during the warm weather (J Am Med Assoc 1990; 264:561) Note: Acid 'rain' derives from the same sources

'Acid blob' activation domain A structural motif that has been identified in various transcription factors that function by stimulating either RNA polymerase II or another general transcription factor

Acid-fast stain(s) Special histological stains (Ziehl-Neelsen, Kinyoun and others), used to identify ***Mycobacterium*** species, which are acid-fast due to the mycolic acid content in the outer capsule; at an increased temperature, the basic fuchsin in phenol penetrates the capsular wax, hardens and retains the dye during treatment with acid alcohol; acid-fast stains may adhere to free hydroxy and carboxi- group of mycolic acid, explaining the acid fastness of pine pollen, keratohyaline, lead inclusions, histoplasmosis and lipofuchsin, as well as ***Nocardia*** species and certain propionic bacteria; the Fite acid-fast uses a xylene-oil combination to partially 'restore' the acid-fastness lost in routine processing and is used to identify lepra

Acidophilic body Any densely acidophilic, eosinophilic (ie pink), often 5-15 μm in diameter mass seen by light microscopy with the hematoxylin & eosin stain GYNECOLOGIC PATHOLOGY Dense pink, rounded, periodic acid Schiff positive (PAS-positive) 2-8 μm in diameter masses, also known as hyaline globules, composed of basement membrane material seen intra- and extracellularly in tumor cells in the ovarian endodermal sinus tumor HEPATOPATHOLOGY Individual condensed and necrotic hepatocytes with dense pink cytoplasm and a pyknotic nucleus, often multiple with periportal distribution, partially surrounded by a 'round cell' infiltrate, a finding characteristic of acute viral hepatitis RENAL PATHOLOGY Rounded intranuclear and intracytoplasmic inclusions with ragged edges composed of protein, lead and occasionally iron, seen in the renal tubular cells and hepatocytes of those with chronic lead exposure, often accompanied by aminoaciduria and glycosuria

Acid phosphatase stain A histochemical stain used in hematology, to identify enzymes that hydrolyze organic phosphate esters at pH 5.0; acid phosphatase is present in normal lymphoblasts, neutrophils, mast cells, and pathologically in Gaucher's disease, histiocytosis X, hairy cell and acute lymphocytic leukemias,

Acid vesicle system PHYSIOLOGY Subcellular structures in all nucleated mammalian cells formed as a result of either Receptor-mediated endocytosis, in which the ligand (molecule being internalized) is bound to receptors that cluster in specialized submembranous regions known as coated pits, ie 'coated' by the protein clathrin; once internalized, the vesicles are acidified; at pH 5-5.6, the ligand dissociates from its receptor; subcellular structures may also form as a result of lysosomal enzyme targeting is similar to process receptor-mediated endocytosis, but is poorly understood; intracellular acid vesicles include: Coated vesicles (receptor-mediated macromolecule transport from the cell surface), endosomes (macromolecule sorting), lysosomes (degradation of internalized macromolecules) and the Golgi complex; defects in the acid vesicle system are implicated in: Familial hypercholesterolemia, myotonic dystrophy, I-cell disease, type III mucolipidosis and infections, including chlamydial, Legionella species, nocardiosis, toxoplasmosis and chloroquine-resistant malaria (N Engl J Med 1987; 317:542rv); see Clathrin, Coated pits, CURL

Acid rain ENVIRONMENT Precipitation laced with the detritus of developed nations' profligacy, produced predominantly by power plants that burn coal of variable purity, generating sulfur dioxide and nitrous oxide, which lower the pH of precipitation; the summary report from the National Acid Precipitation Assessment Program (NAPAP) on the effects of acid rain in the US (which cost $570 million, required 10 years and accumulated 6000 pages of data), concluded that acid rain a) Adversely affects aquatic life in 10% of lakes and streams in the eastern US b) Contributes to the decline of certain trees at high elevations by reducing their tolerance to the cold weather and c) Contributes to soil erosion and corrosion of buildings and materials (Science 1991; 251:1303)

Acorn deformity Spinning top deformity A descriptor for the radiocontrast findings in distal urethral stenosis, in which there is pre-stenotic widening of the urethra, fixation and narrowing of the bladder neck, forcing of large volumes of urine through a thin-walled urethra; the deformity is seen by voiding cystourethrography and is most commonly symptomatic in young males

Acoustic coupler see Modem

Acridine orange An immunological fluorochrome that non-specifically binds to RNA (red fluorescence), DNA (green fluorescence), proteins, polysaccharides and glycosaminoglycans; acridine orange also acts as a non-specific tissue stain which a) Detects increased mitotic activity (implying cancer in the proper setting) or b) Is more sensitive (but less specific) than the gram stain in wound swabs (Arch Pathol Lab Med 1988; 112:529); because it is carcinogenic, intercalating itself within replicating DNA causing insertional or deletional mutations, acridine orange is not routinely used in most histological laboratories

Actin A major muscle protein, which with myosin, is responsible for muscle contraction; actin is an ATPase that binds to adenine nucleotides and appears to have an active mechanicochemical role in cell function; it is a thin filament protein of muscle that is divisible into a monomeric form, G-actin and a mature contractile form, F-actin, formed from G-actin polymers, capable of functioning in absence of myosin (Nature 1990; 347:37, 44, 21)

Acting out PEDIATRIC PSYCHIATRY A manifestation of masked adolescent depression, where desperation is denied or somatized, indicating a need for psychiatric intervention; acting-out behaviors include school truancy, substance abuse and somatization (headaches or abdominal pain)

'Actinic' cancer Any cutaneous malignancy that is attributed to excess exposure to solar radiation, most commonly appearing in the head and neck region, followed by the legs and trunk; in one study, the incidence of squamous cell carcinoma in men rose from 42 to $106/10^5$ between 1960 and 1986 and in women from 10 to $30/10^5$; the incidence of malignant melanoma in men rose from 5 to $20/10^5$ between 1960 and 1986 and in women from 5 to $17/10^5$ (J Am Med Assoc 1989; 262:2097); see Melanoma

Activated charcoal CLINICAL TOXICOLOGY An agent used in early management of oral intoxications, effective against most toxic substances except mercury, iron, lithium and cyanide; if the drug has an enterohepatic cycle, as do barbiturates, glutethimide, morphine and other narcotics and tricyclic antidepressants, charcoal administration may be repeated for up to 24 hours; usual adult dose 50-100 g

Activated macrophage IMMUNOLOGY A mononuclear phagocyte that has been 'turned on' by lymphokines; activated macrophages are twice the size of resting macrophages, have increased lysozymes and surface expression of MHC class II antigens and are pivotal in defending against microorganisms that grow well in histiocytes and other cells

Activation The conversion, often enzymatic, of a molecule to a functionally reactive form, eg activation of the complement or coagulation cascades

Activin A member of the transforming growth factor β protein family with diverse biological roles, including differentiation of erythroid precursors, stimulation of insulin and anterior pituitary hormone secretion, modulation of granulosa cell differentiation (activin binds to follistatin, an FSH release inhibitor, Science 1990; 247:836), differentiation of certain erythroleukemia cell lines and may act in early mesodermal development, triggering tissue transition from a blastula to mesoderm, ectoderm and endoderm (Nature 1990; 347:391, 337); see Mesoderm-inducing factors

Active noise control The use of energy-consumptive systems to reduce 'white' noise, through application of new algorithms and computer controlled digital processors, generating sounds that are opposite that of the undesired noise(s), effectively cancelling their effects (Science 1991; 252:508rv)

Activin A peptide growth factor related to tumor growth factor-β, first identified in ***Xenopus*** species, that acts on the mesoderm (notochord and segmented myo-tomes), either inducing the development of a rudimentary axial pattern with anteroposterior polarity at high concentrations and dorsoventral polarity at low concentration (Nature 1991; 349:17n&v) or by revealing a preexisting pattern (Nature 1991; 351:409)

Actomyosin A G actin-like contractile protein complex found in platelets that has an actin:myosin ratio of 100:1 (muscle has a ratio of 7:1), which appears with platelet activation

Acumentin A motility protein present in neutrophils and macrophages that regulates the length of actin filaments by binding to the slow-assembly end of the actin molecule

Acupuncture A method of healing practiced in China for more than 2000 years, in which fine needles are placed in one or more of 800 sites on the skin; acupuncture has been used for conditions as diverse as analgesia, arthritis, hypertension and gastric ulcers; when genuine acupuncture is compared to sham acupuncture in the control of moderate stable angina, there is no significant difference (J Intern Med 1990; 227:25)

Acute disseminated encephalitis An acute complication of viral infection (1:1000 cases of measles) or vaccination ($1:10^6$ measles vaccinations), involving the entire brain and spinal cord or focally affecting a nerve or cord root Pathogenesis Unclear, but may be an immune reaction to cerebral proteins (eg myelin basic protein), and is considered to be the human equivalent of experimental allergic encephalomyelitis Clinical Meningial signs and, if serious, coma and death Treatment None

Acute fatty liver of preg-

ACUTE ABDOMEN, ETIOLOGY

INFECTION Amebiasis, hepatitis, falciparum malaria, pneumococcal pneumonia, rheumatic fever, salmonella gastroenteritis, staphylococcal toxemia, syphilis in 'tabetic crisis', trichinosis, tuberculosis, typhoid fever, viral enteritides, Herpes zoster, infectious mononucleosis, Whipple's disease

INFLAMMATION Appendicitis, cholangitis, cholecystitis, Crohn's disease, diverticulitis, gastroenteritis, hepatitis, lupus erythematosus, mesenteric lymphadenitis, pancreatitis, peritonitis due to organ perforation, perinephric abscesses, pyelonephritis, ulcerative colitis, intestinal obstruction, rheumatoid arthritis, polyarteritis nodosa, Hennoch-Schoenlein disease

INTOXICATION Black widow spider bites, heavy metals, mushrooms

ISCHEMIA Renal infarction, mesenteric arterial thrombosis

MALIGNANCY Pain due to organ infarction, Hodgkin's disease ('classically' with alcohol ingestion), leukemia, lympho-proliferative disorders

METABOLIC DISEASE Adrenal insufficiency (Addisonian crisis), diabetic ketoacidosis, familial hyperlipoproteinemia, familial mediterranean fever, hemochromatosis, hereditary angioneurotic edema, hyperparathyroidism, hyperthyroidism, acute intermittent porphyria, uremia, withdrawal from drug abuse

OBSTETRICS/GYNECOLOGY Twisted ovarian cyst, ectopic pregnancy, endometriosis, pelvic inflammatory disease

REFERRED PAIN Pneumonia, myocardial infarct, pleuritis, pericarditis, myocarditis, hematomata of the rectal muscle, renal colic, peptic ulcer, nerve root compression

TRAUMA Perforation, ruptured aortic aneurysm, ruptured spleen, ruptured bladder

nancy see Fatty liver of pregnancy, acute

Acute mountain sickness see Mountain sickness, acute

Acute necrotizing ulcerative gingivitis (ANUG) A condition characterized by progressive necrosis of intraoral tissues, seen in those with poor oral hygiene and suboptimal nutrition Clinical Pain, edema, punched-out oral ulceration, pseudomembrane formation, halitosis; anaerobic oral flora (***Fusobacterium*** species and oral spirochetes) that also cause Vincent's angina (which affects the soft palate and tonsils), cancorum oris and upper respiratory abscesses Treatment H_2O_2, antibiotics, eg tetracycline, if fever or lymphadenopathy is present, saline rinse and local anesthetics; non-response may indicate presence of another condition, eg erythema multiforme, lichen planus, pemphigus and pemphigoid Note: 'Trench mouth' is a coinage of World War I vintage which attributed ANUG to living in close quarters, ie trenches

Acute phase reactants (APR) Proteins that migrate in the α_1 and α_2 regions of a serum electrophoresis gel, rising and falling with acute inflammation; APRs traditionally include: α_1-antitrypsin, α_1 acid glycoprotein, amyloid A and P, anti-thrombin III, C-reactive protein, C1-esterase inhibitor, C3 complement, ceruloplasmin, fibrinogen, haptoglobin, orosomucoid, plasminogen, transferrin Note: Some of the above do not meet the criteria defined by the French Society for Clinical Chemistry (Lab Manage 1983; 21:48) but are retained as APRs for convenience

Acute phase response (APR) The constellation of non-specific host responses induced by interleukin-1, interleukin-6 and tumor necrosis factor and interferons; the APR is associated with tissue injury, infection, inflammation and rarely malignancy, eg Hodgkin's disease and renal cell carcinoma, and causes functional changes in the liver (increased synthesis of acute phase proteins), endocrine system (abnormal glucose tolerance, increased gluconeogenesis, thyroid dysfunction, altered lipid metabolism), immune system (left shift leukocytosis, hypergammaglobulinemia), metabolic system (decreased albumin synthesis, energy consumption, increased ceruloplasmin, decreased iron and zinc levels) and nervous system (lethargy); the most measured molecule in the response is the highly nonspecific C-reactive protein, which may rise 10- to 1000-fold within hours from a normal of 100 μg/L

Acute radiation injury syndrome Atomic bomb disease A complex described in highly exposed victims of the Hiroshima and Nagasaki bomb blasts (J Am Med Assoc 1946; 131:504), as well as nuclear reactor accidents Clinical 5-25 centiGray (cGy); the symptoms are a function of level of exposure Less than 75 cGy Asymptomatic with chromosomal aberrations Less than 125 cGy Asymptomatic with a mild decrease in leukocytes and platelets Less than 200 cGy Anorectic with anorexia, nausea, vomiting, fatigue, leukopenia and thrombocytopenia and transient symptoms; leukopenia occurs in 50% of those exposed to less than 350 cGy, who experience a 50% mortality with severe marrow depression; at exposure levels above 500 cGy, gastrointestinal complications of hemorrhagic gastroenteritis occur within two weeks, causing death in most of those exposed Hyperacute radiation disease is extremely rare and the doses may be in excess of 5000 cGy, causing fulminant cardiovascular, gastrointestinal and central nervous system collapse with death in 24-48 hours

Acute salicysm see Aspirin

Acute tubular necrosis (ATN) The histopathological finding in acute renal failure and seen in shock, crush injuries, hemoglobinuria, toxic nephrosis, ischemic injury of transplanted kidneys (cold ischemia is tolerated for up to 48 hours, warm ischemia, only several hours) Histopathology Relatively scant morphological changes, ranging from hydropic changes to frank actual tubular necrosis; ATN in transplanted kidneys is managed in an expectant fashion as renal function may resume spontaneously within 2-4 weeks

Acute tumor lysis syndrome (ATLS) A group of biochemical derangements seen at the onset of cytotoxic therapy for malignancy, where rapid cell death causes hyperkalemia, hyperphosphatemia, hyperuricemia and hypocalcemia Note: Cytolysis of large, mitotically active tumors causes metabolic imbalances themselves severe enough to cause death by renal failure; the serum level of lactate dehydrogenase (LD, especially isoenzymes LD_3 and LD_4) provides a crude estimate of tumor-load; by extension, an elevated LD may indicate an increased risk for ATLS; ATLS occurs in breast and oat cell carcinoma (of the lungs), metastatic adenocarcinoma, lymphosarcoma, non-Hodgkin lymphomas, eg lymphoblastic and Burkitt's lymphomas, chronic myeloid leukemia, acute lymphoblastic leukemia, multiple myeloma and metastatic medulloblastoma

METABOLIC DERANGEMENTS IN ACUTE TUMOR LYSIS SYNDROME

HYPERURICEMIA Release of uric and nucleic acid precursors (by massive cytolysis), aggravated by acid urine, renal dysfunction, dehydration and edema, possibly causing renal shutdown through massive tubular precipitation of uric acid crystals

HYPERKALEMIA Release of intracellular potassium, worsened by acidosis, renal dysfunction, potassium-sparing diuretics, adrenal insufficiency,diabetes mellitus, hypocalcemia or hyponatremia appearing as muscular weakness and cardiac arrhythmias, including atrioventricular block, tachyarrhythmia or cardiac arrest

HYPERPHOSPHATEMIA/HYPOCALCEMIA Minerals released by lysing cells, cause soft tissue mineralization, exacerbating renal failure by intratubular crystallization and may cause neuromuscular irritability, with tetany, convulsions

Acyclovir 9[2-Hydroxyethoxy-methyl]guanine A nucleoside analogue with antiviral activity that inhibits Herpes simplex virus-2 (HSV-2, genital herpes); acyclovir is activated by HSV thymidine kinase by monophosphorylation and then triple phosphorylated by host enzymes, producing a potent inhibitor of HSV-2's DNA polymerase; HSV-2 resistance to acyclovir is increasingly reported, frustrating HSV-2 ulcer therapy; foscarnet (trisodium phosphormate), a pyrophosphate analogue, inhibits DNA polymerase and may circumvent resistance (N Engl J Med 1989; 320:297); acyclovir is used as suppressive therapy for genital Herpes simplex infection, reducing the recurrence rate from 12/year to 1/year (J Am Med Assoc 1991; 265:747); acyclovir is more effective than vidarabine in reducing viral shedding by HSV-infected infants, but equally effective as a therapeutic agent (N Engl J Med 1991; 324:444); Cf Gancyclovir

ADA see Adenosine deaminase

Adam XTC/Ecstasy, MDM, MDMA, 3,4-Methylene-dioxymethamphetamine A 'schedule I' controlled substance analogue ('designer drug') of amphetamine, potentially causing fatal overdose, which is selectively neurotoxic to the serotonergic nerve fibers (J Am Med Assoc 1988; 260:51) and manufactured in clandestine laboratories; the drug was developed but never marketed in 1914 as a dietary suppressant and languished until the 1970s, when a small group of psychiatrists used it as an adjunct to insight-oriented psychotherapy, during which time the drug enjoyed a 6-month legalized hiatus so that the psychiatric community could use it experimentally; by 1983 it had become a recreational drug on college campuses (cost: $10-40 per 100 mg 'hit'), producing a pleasant nonhallucinogenic 'high' in low doses (J Am Med Assoc 1987; 257:1615), with sensory components of amphetamine, mescaline and amphetamine (Science 1988; 239:864), but is hallucinogenic above 150 mg; Cf Eve Toxicity At high levels, MDMA causes serotonin neurotoxicity, agitation, hallucinations, sweating, dilated pupils, tachycardia, fever, spasticity, hypotension, bronchospasm and acidosis; see Designer drugs, 'Ice'

Adam complex PSYCHIATRY A guilt complex that a person who breaks a parental 'law' that the subject, often a child, did not previously know was forbidden; eg incestuous relations; this form of guilt is likened to Adam and Eves' 'fall from grace' in the garden of Eden

ADAM complex OBSTETRICS A heterogeneous acquired complex that develops in utero; the ADAM complex, ie amniotic deformity, adhesions (Streeter bands) and mutilations, may be considered a 'sequence' and is associated with craniofacial defects, eg clefts, distortions, dislocations, limb deformities, amputations and secondary syndactyly (Am J Med Gen 1978; 2:81)

ADAMHA Alcohol, Drug Abuse and Mental Health Admini-stration

Adam's apple Anterior prominence of the thyroid cartilage, immediately inferior to the superior thyroid notch and most prominent in males, which is used as a landmark in performing the now-rare emergency tracheostomy; in the tradition of folk physiology, the body of the first man, Adam, was wiser than his soul; when Adam took a piece of the forbidden fruit from Eve it stuck in his throat, as his 'wise' throat was telling him not to swallow the apple

ADAP see Alzheimer's disease-associated protein

Adaptin(s) A family of proteins that is critical to clathrin-coated vesicle-mediated intracellular transport of proteins; Cf COP(s)

ADC see AIDS dementia complex

ADCC Antibody-dependent cell-mediated cytotoxicity A mechanism for eliminating bacteria, viruses, tumor and foreign cells, mediated by T cells, NK cells, large granular lymphocytes, macrophages and neutrophils; ADCC is a model of the relationship between antibody, usually IgG and thymus-independent lymphocytes, where target cells with attached specific antibodies are lysed by 'killer' cells having Fc receptors for the attachment of IgG, triggering target cell lysis; see CD 16

ADD Attention deficit disorder see Attention deficit-hyperactivity disorder

Addict SUBSTANCE ABUSE A person who is vulnerable to the compulsive heavy consumption of substances with abuse potential; in order of risk of addiction, cocaine and amphetamines have greater abuse potential than opiates and nicotine, which in turn have greater addictive potential than alcohol and related drugs (benzodiazepine, barbiturates), which are greater than cannabis, hallucinogens and caffeine; see Substance abuse

Addisonian crisis A state of acute adrenal insufficiency, induced by the stress of infections, trauma, surgery, dehydration with salt deprivation or evoked by replacing thyroid hormone in patients with hypothyroidism of hypothalamic or pituitary origin who have an underlying mild ACTH deficiency Clinical Hypotension, shock, fever, dehydration, anorexia, weakness, apathy, depressed mentation Laboratory Hyponatremia, hyperkalemia, lymphocytosis, eosinophilia, hypoglycemia Treatment Pharmacologic doses of glucocorticoids

'Addressin' A homing protein, peptide or other molecule that provides a form of message indicating a molecule's destination, eg ELAM-1

ADE see Acute disseminated encephalomyelitis

Adenoma malignum A rare, very well-differentiated adenocarcinoma arising in the endocervical columnar epithelium that is remarkable for its bland histology; although the prognosis is similar to that of the usual type of endocervical adenocarcinoma when correctly diagnosed, in actuality, adenoma malignum has a relatively poor prognosis due to its verisimilitude to benign endocervical glands, and underdiagnosis by the uninitiated

Adenosine deaminase (ADA) The ADA gene is located on chromosome 20q13-ter and encodes a 38 kD deaminating enzyme, without which there is accumulation of adenosine, deoxyadenosine, adenosine triphosphate (ATP), S-adenosyl homocysteine and deoxyATP; deoxyATP is a potent inhibitor of ribonucleoside-diphosphate reductase, an enzyme involved in purine synthesis; excess adenosine also inhibits intracellular DNA-methylation (called 'suicide inactivation' as this causes cell death); ADA deficiency is a uniformly fatal autosomal recessive disease, comprising 40% of patients with severe combined immunodeficiency Mechanism dATP inhibits ribonucleotide reductase in S phase of growth cycle, aborting DNA synthesis and incorporation of dATP into polyadenylated RNA; dATP accumulation inhibits RNA synthesis and single-strand separation of DNA; the lymphocytes are also relatively deficient in 5'-nucleotidase; increasing ADA levels inhibit the synthesis of S-adenosylmethionine which donates methyl groups to DNA; ADA is defective or absent in AIDS, anemia and lymphoproliferative disorders Note: ADA's structure is intimately linked to its function, with a pivotal role being played by theGlu and Asp residues, which fold ADA into an α/β-barrel motif with a zinc atom in the active site (Science 1991; 252:1278) Clinical Cellular immune dysfunction, oral candidiasis, intractable diarrhea, failure to thrive, severe diaper rash, pseudoachondrodysplasia, death before age two Laboratory Marked decrease of lymphocytes < 0.5 X 10^9/L (US: < 500 mm^3), especially of T cells, cells, eosinophilia; increased adenosine and deoxyadenosine in serum and urine Treatment ADA deficiency rarely responds to bone marrow transplantation and is a prime candidate for gene therapy, where the absent gene is inserted with a retroviral vector; see Cartilage-hair syndrome

Adenylyl cyclase An enzyme intimately linked to the G proteins on the cytoplasmic face of the cell membrane, which generates the second messenger, cAMP (cyclic adenosine monophosphate) when stimulated by an extracellular message in the form of receptor binding of a hormone or other ligand, light or odors (Science 1990; 250:1403)

ADFR therapy Activate, depress, free and repeat A therapeutic modality (phosphorus, followed by calcitonin and calcium, administered in three month cycles), used to attenuate post-menopausal bone loss in women for whom estrogen therapy is contraindicated or unacceptable (Clin Rheumatol 1989; 8 Suppl 2:56)

ADHD see Attention deficit-hyperactivity disorder

Adhesin Protein ligating components of bacteria (pili in *Pseudomonas aeruginosa*, lipotechoic acid in group A streptococcus) which bind to glycoprotein or glycolipid receptors on human epithelial cells (Infect & Immunol 1989; 57:3720), explaining the pulmonary morbidity due to *P aeruginosa* seen in intubated ICU patients

Adhesions SURGERY Collagen-rich fibrous bands that form after any intervention in the peritoneal cavity, thought to be related to a focal decrease in the plasminogen activator within the mesothelial lining; gentle manipulation of the organs and removal of blood minimizes adhesive band formation, which may be severe enough to cause intestinal obstruction, but nothing effectively prevents adhesions

Adhesion proteins MOLECULAR BIOLOGY A group of 'sticky' proteins found in the extracellular matrix that facilitate vascular egress of circulating leukocytes, eg ELAM-1 Endothelial leukocyte adhesion molecule 1, located on vascular endothelium stimulated by inflammatory lymphokines (eg IL-1 and tumor necrosis factor), attracting neutrophils to sites of inflammation (Science 1989; 243:1160), lymph node homing receptor (Science 1989; 243:1165) found on the membranes of B and T cells, which transmigrate in the high endothelial venules and the 140 kD GMP-140 granule membrane protein; adhesion proteins have a 'mosaic' structure, composed of tandem arrays of sequences adopted from other proteins, incorporating functional domains into 'homing' molecules; dissection of these functions may determine the susceptibility of certain sites to metastases and 'engineering' of the receptors may direct neutrophils to, or away from inflammatory targets

Adhesion receptors A group of membrane-bound proteins responsible for interaction of cells and matrix molecules that regulate adherence and chemoattractant gradients directing cell migration; there are three groups of adhesion receptors: 1) The immunoglobulin superfamily of adhesion receptors, including T cell receptor/CD3, CD4, CD8, MHC class I, MHC class II, sCD2/LFA-2, LFA-3/CD58, ICAM-1, ICAM-2 and V-CAM, 2) The Integrin family, including LFA-1, Mac-1, p150,95, VLA-5, VLA4/LPAM-1, LPAM-2 and 3) The selectin family, including Mel-14/LAM-1, ELAM-1 and CD62

Ad hoc committee A committee formed with the purpose of addressing a specific issue or issues that theoretically is disbanded once it fulfills its raison d'etre

Adipocere 'Gravewax' Hardened waxy adipose tissue seen in an unembalmed body lying a year or more in cold wet ground (or cold acidic water, which inhibits tissue hydrolysis); see Bog bodies

Adipsin A serine protease secreted by adipocytes into the circulation that is deficient in some animal models of obesity; adipsin has activities similar to and 61% sequence homology with complement factor D (Science 1989; 244:1483)

Adjectival eponym An eponym that has been so long in common usage that it has passed into public 'domain' and in so doing, is most commonly written in lower case (a convention apparently borrowed from German); thus fallopian tubes, gram stain, mendelian genetics and müllerian ducts are no longer capitalized; see Eponym; Cf Autoeponym

Adjunct Something joined or added to another thing but which is not an essential part thereof, eg radiotherapy is an important adjunct to surgery and may represent appropriate adjuvant therapy

Adjunctive therapy ONCOLOGY A treatment modality used in malignancy after one or more of the conventional therapeutic arms (surgery, chemotherapy and radiotherapy) has failed; adjunctive modalities include immunotherapy (BCG, interleukin-2-stimulated lymphokine-activated killer cells, α-interferon) and regional hyperthermia with chemotherapy; see IL-2/LAK cells

Adjuvant IMMUNOLOGY A non-specific immune enhancer, eg Freund's adjuvant, composed of particulate-containing oily substances that promote protein aggregation, which when mixed with an antigen, acts as a tissue depot, slowly releasing antigen and activating the immune system

Adjuvant disease An animal model for rheumatoid arthritis, consisting of an acute aseptic synovitis, induced in rats by injection of Freund's complete adjuvant, which consists of an oil-water emulsion containing killed *Mycobacterium tuberculosis*

Adjuvant therapy ONCOLOGY Treatment given after surgical resection of a tumor, in an effort to prevent recurrence at distal sites, or when residual malignancy is thought to remain after excision; it is recommended for women with axillary lymph node-positive breast cancer, eg hormonal manipulation and chemotherapy; but does not improve survival in lymph node-negative women; a gain of four months of life costs $5-7000 (N Engl J Med 1991; 324:160) Colon cancer Adjuvant therapy for stage III adenocarcinoma, using 5-FU and levamisole (side effects: Nausea, diarrhea, leukopenia), has a reported 32% improvement in 5-year survival (J Clin Oncol 1989; 7:1447), and may be appropriate also for stage II carcinoma (J Am Med Assoc 1990; 264:1444) Lung cancer Adjuvant therapy may decrease survival

Administration The sum total of management and direction of health care organizations (personnel, budgets and logistics) and the implementation of health care policy; management requires a chain of command, proper organization, assignment of responsibility, positive worker interaction and feedback; administration is an ever-increasing component of physician activities and includes responsibilities in quality assurance, and record keeping; in laboratory medicine, administration requires management of physical and human resources

Administrative costs The costs incurred by the 'business' component of health care facilities or universities, which includes staffing and personnel costs, nursing home and hospital administration, insurance overhead and overhead expenses; the per capita health care administration cost in the US of $400-500 contrasts to a per capita cost in Canada of $100-150; it has been noted that if the US were as efficient as the Canadian health care bureaucracy, the $70 billion of annual savings would fund health care for the estimated 35 million Americans who are uninsured and underinsured (N Engl J Med 1991; 324:1253); see Indirect costs

Admissible evidence FORENSIC MEDICINE Any item, exhibit, object or materials which a local, district or federal court will accept as linking a person(s) with the commitment of an act; eg a) A knife embedded in the victim, belonging to the accused, covered with the victim's blood b) The killer's name uttered by a dying victim is admissible evidence in: Michigan, California, Washington DC and the State of Washington

Adoptive immunity The transfer of immunity from one organism to another by either injection of immune-competent cells, as in granulocyte transfusions or 'humors', as in passive immunity in neonates resulting from placental transfer of IgG across the placenta

Adoptive immunotherapy An experimental therapeutic modality used to treat terminal malignancy consisting of the transfer of 'activated' anti-tumor cells, eg combining lymphokine-activated killer (LAK) cells or tumor-infiltrating lymphocytes (TIL) with IL-2 into patients with metastatic malignancy (Science 1989; 244:1430n&v); about 10% of patients with terminal renal cell carcinoma and melanoma have achieved partial or complete remission with the LAK/IL-2 regimen

ADPKD see Autosomal dominant polycystic kidney disease

ADR Adverse drug reaction

Adsorption Removal of non-specific agglutinins by incubation in serum that does not contain the antigens to be measured

Adsorption chromatography A technique in which molecules are separated according to their adsorptive properties, where a mobile (fluid) phase is passed over an immobile (solid) adsorptive stationary phase; Cf Affinity chromatography

Adult respiratory distress syndrome (ARDS) Adult hyaline membrane disease, Bronchopulmonary dysplasia, DaNang lung, Pump lung, Stiff lung syndrome, Wet lung, White lung syndrome, Transplant lung A clinical complex characterized by acute pulmonary edema and respiratory failure accompanying a wide range of medical and surgical conditions that do not initially involve the lungs and are unrelated to cardiac failure, often associated with interstitial pneumonitides (usual, desquamative and lymphoid types), which occurs as frequently as 150 000 cases/year Clinical A 6-24 hour latency period is followed by hypoxia, decreased aeration, dyspnea and 'stiff' lungs, ie decreased pulmonary compliance Radiology Extensive, bilateral fluffy infiltrates Pathology Atelectatic, heavy (> 1000 g, normal <400g) congested lungs filled with proteinaceous material, erythrocytes and occasionally, hyaline membranes Etiology Gram-negative sepsis, pneumonia, shock, aspiration (of gastric content), trauma, drug overdose Pathogenesis Abundant fibrin and fibronectin in the exudative phase results in hyaline membrane formation and alveolar fibrosis, due to local urokinase deficiency or presence of urokinase inhibitors, eg plasminogen-activator inhibitor, PAI-1 (N Engl J Med 1990; 322:890) Treatment PEEP, prayer Prognosis is a function of the underlying etiology

Adult T-cell leukemia-lymphoma (ATLL) A rapidly-progressive lymphoproliferative malignancy of mature T lymphocytes, commonly associated with infection by the retrovirus, HTLV-I, first described in southeastern Japan, also seen in the Caribbean, Africa and among blacks in the southeastern USA, in whom the disease is aggressive with skin lesions, hypercalcemia, rapid enlargement of hilar, retroperitoneal and peripheral lymph nodes with mediastinal sparing, invasion of central nervous system, lungs, gastrointestinal tract and opportunistic infections, eg *Pneumocystis carinii*; ATLL has been subdivided into five clinical forms: 1) Acute Median age 52, lymphadenopathy, hepatosplenomegaly, cutaneous lesions, up to a 20-year latency, often resistant to chemotherapy with poor prognosis following disease onset Laboratory Increased calcium ions, white cells 10 to 500 × 10^9 (US: 10 to 500 000/mm^3), Sezary-like cells with CD3, CD4, CD2 (T11) and Tac+ surface antigens, causing a chronic, smoldering lymphoma 2) Chronic Clinically between acute and smoldering disease 3) Smoldering Characterized by erythematous skin nodules filled with lymphocytes that may undergo 'blast transformation' to the typical acute T cell leukemia (ATL) 4) Crisis When either 2) or 3) transform to ATL 5) Lymphoma Most common in US Blacks with hypercalcemia, leukemia, hepatosplenomegaly, erythematous skin lesions and lytic bone lesions; see T-cell lymphoma

Advance directive Self determination MEDICAL ETHICS Instruction(s) providing competent persons the means by which they can influence their own treatment in the event of serious illness and/or loss of mental abilities; a person may clearly indicate in advance how treatment decisions are to be made regarding the use of artificial life support by either written directions (ie a living will) and/or by appointing a proxy to make the health care decisions (J Am Med Assoc 1990; 263:2365); nursing homes are four times more likely than hospitals to override advance directives, as they may be simply ignored or prioritized by other considerations (N Engl J Med 1991; 324:882, 889); see DNR orders, Durable powers of attorney, Euthanasia, Living will

Advanced glycosylation endproducts (AGEs) A group of glycoproteins are derived from the Amadori reaction induced by hyperglycemia and held responsible for the various manifestations of diabetes mellitus, including vasculopathy that causes leakage of proteins across vessels and progressive stenosis of small and large vessels; in diabetics, hyperglycemia causes proteins to combine with glycosylation endproducts in a reversible (early glycosylation endproducts) or irreversible (AGEs) fashion; hemoglobin (Hb) A is one of the AGEs formed in hyperglycemia and measurement of Hb A1c correlates well with adequate glucose control in diabetics Pathophysiology AGEs accumulate in vessels, forming covalent bonds with amino groups of vessel-based proteins (collagen IV, laminin and heparan sulfate proteoglycan), trapping transmigrating low-density lipoproteins, enzymes, growth factors and other proteins, destroying the orderly self-assembled basement membrane system; a macrophage receptor for the AGE-protein complex has been identified that induces secretion of TNF and IL-1, both of which release collagenases and proteases, stimulate proteoglycan degradation and induce proliferation resulting in 'sloppy' basement membrane synthesis; thus, the vessels are thicker than normal, but 'leaky'; AGEs are also inculpated in diabetic cataracts and the increased incidence of atherosclerosis in diabetes mellitus; plaque formation may be initiated by lipoprotein deposition in a process of protein trapping and cross-linking; knowledge of AGE levels is useful in long-term control of diabetes mellitus, as they require less hospitalization as they are recognized to be out of control earlier and treated more aggressively (N Engl J Med 1990; 323:1021) Treatment Aminoguanidine may have currency in preventing the conversion of Amadori products to AGEs; more theoretical is the goal of stimulating the macrophage removal system

Adverse event (AE) FORENSIC MEDICINE An injury caused by medical management (rather than the underlying disease), which prolongs hospitalization, produces a disability at the time of discharge, or both; AEs occur in 0.2 to 7.9% of hospitalizations, 1 to 60% of which are due to negligence; 70% had a disability of less than six months, 2.6% were permanent and 14% resulted in death (N Engl J Med 1991; 324:370, J Am Med Assoc 1991; 265:3265); AEs are caused by drug complications, wound infections and technical complications and those due to negligence due to diagnostic mishaps, therapeutic mishaps and events occurring in the emergency room; one-half of AEs were related to an operation and are more common in older patients (ibid, 324:377) see Malpractice, Misadventure, Negligence

Advertising The public notification of a product's availability and related activities for its promotion; in medicine, two forms of advertising have undergone ethical scrutinization, that of 1) Physician advertising, which, although traditionally considered beneath the dignity of the healing professions, which is being done with increasing frequency, see 'Yellow professionalism' and 2) Prescription drug advertising; in the US, the Food and Drug Administration is responsible for regulating the use of drugs and promotion for their use by the pharmaceutical industry and requires a 'fair balance' in advertising, such that all activities must present a balanced account of the clinically relevant information, ie the risks and benefits, that would influence the physician's prescribing decision; types of drug-related advertising **'COMING SOON' ADVERTISING** A form of 'Teaser' advertising that indicates the name of a drug without claims for potentialindications, safety or effectiveness **DIRECT-TO-CONSUMER ADVERTISING** The use of mass media, eg television, magazines, to publicly promote drugs that by law require a physician's prescription; the intent of such advertising is have patients and/or the lay public request their physician to prescribe drug 'X' **INSTITUTIONAL ADVERTISING** A form of 'Teaser' advertising in which a drug company is linked to a field of research **INTRODUCTORY ADVERTISING** Promotional activities for a drug that has not yet been released **PREAPPROVAL ADVERTISING** see 'Teaser' advertising **REMEDIAL ADVERTISING** Advertising that attempts to rectify a situation in which a company has falsely misrepresented the drug's efficacy or approved uses **REMINDER ADVERTISING** Advertising that calls attention to a drug's existence in the market; any claims of efficacy in reminder activities requires that the promotional activities meet 'fair balance' and brief summary requirements **'TEASER' ADVERTISING** Advertising for a product that has not yet come to market; under US regulations, a drug company must choose between either 'Institutional' or 'Coming soon' forms of 'teaser' advertising (J Am Med Assoc 1990; 264:2409rv)

A end SUBCELLULAR PHYSIOLOGY One of two ends of microtubules that polymerize from α- and β- tubulin dimers; the rate of assembly at the A (net assembly) end is greater than the rate assembly at the D (net disassembly) end, thus microtubule formation and metabolism are analogous to a treadmill

Aerobic exercise Intense exercise in which re-synthesis of high energy compounds occurs in the presence of oxygen, this being the form of exercise which boasts the greatest health benefits as the energy expenditure is maximized while performing rhythmic contractions of large muscles over distance, eg jogging or against gravity, eg jazz-dancing, both of which are types of 'endurance' training, causing physiological cardiac hypertrophy and with time, a desirable physiologic bradycardia; see Exercise

Affiliation The association of one institution or organization with another, which in US hospital parlance, is the close tie of a health care institution to a medical school or university; in a typical symbiotic affiliation, the hospital gains prestige and a supply of resident physicians who provide patient care, while the medical school gains a clinical teaching facility

Affinity IMMUNOLOGY The strength of the sum of the multiple binding sites between an antibody and an antigen, which increase the stability of the linkage, as measured by the association or affinity constant; the antibody recognizes the three dimensional configuration of an epitope rather than a single specific binding site; low-affinity complexes may persist in the circulation, localize in the glomerular basement membrane and compromise renal function; see Avidity, Immune complexes

Affinity chromatography A technique for isolating pure antigen or antibody, based on the fact that antibodies bind to their corresponding antigen; a fluid with an antigen of interest is poured through a column containing the corresponding antibody bound to a plastic bead (the solid phase); all non-binding molecules will flow through the column; in the second step, an elution buffer, eg acetate at pH 3.0 or diethylamine at pH 11.5, is poured through the column to remove the substance or ligand of interest

Affinity maturation IMMUNOLOGY The increase in the average affinity of antibodies (to an antigen) produced after immunization, due to an increase of more specific and less heterogeneous IgG antibodies, after the more heterogeneous early response by IgM molecules

Affirmative action A phrase popularized in the 1960s, meaning the removal of artificial barriers to the employment of women and minorities; with time, the phrase has come to mean any effort to recruit and hire members of previously disadvantaged groups in an effort to erase past inequities; see Reverse discrimination

AFIP see Armed Forces Institute of Pathology

Aflatoxin B1 A mold toxin derived from ***Aspergillus flavus*** that may contaminate grains and is both mutagenic and a liver-specific co-carcinogen; dietary exposure to aflatoxin B1 in grains is inculpated in the high incidence of hepatocellular carcinomas in Africa and China and is thought to act by causing G→T and G→C transversions (substitutions) in the p53 tumor suppressor gene, especially affecting codon 249, facilitating the development of various tumors (Nature 1991; 350:427, 429); see p53

AFP see α-fetoprotein

Africa connection A catch phrase used before HIV-1 was implicated in AIDS, coined in an attempt to explain why the same disease that predominantly afflicted male homosexuals and drug abusers in the USA was also afflicting heterosexual Africans; Cf Monkey connection, Mosquito connection

Africanized bee 'Killer bee' A honey bee strain from Africa (***Apis mellifera*** L) that has certain behaviors with adaptive value in the tropics, including swarming, absconding tendencies, defensive behavior and opportunistic use of resources; the africanized bee has slowly migrated north and south from its tropical site of introduction in Brazil in the1950s and has supplanted the European honey bee, although there is mixture of the races at the 'frontier' zones in both South America (Nature 1991; 349:782) and the northern hemisphere (Science 1991; 253:309, ibid, 1991; 252:1435br)

Agent Orange ENVIRONMENT A 50:50 mixture of 2,4-D n-butyl ester or 2,4-dichlorophenoxyacetic and 2,4,5-T n-butyl ester or trichlorophenoxyacetic acids in a diesel oil vehicle; Agent Orange was used as a general defoliant for forest, brush, broad-leafed crops, used in Southeast Asia by the American forces, as a tactic of warfare, for the purpose of destroying the jungle cover used by the Viet Cong guerilla forces during the Vietnam conflict as camouflage; experiments with defoliant chemicals as herbicides began during World War II and four agents of potential military use were weeded out of the 12 000 chemicals tested; the US defoliation effort in Vietnam began in late 1961 and by the time the aerial defoliation program (see operation Ranch Hand) ended in 1968, 6603 square miles (17 300 km^2) had been sprayed with defoliant, predominantly Agent Orange (J Am Med Assoc 1988; 260:1249), mostly from fixed wing aircraft; see Times Beach Note: Agent Orange was contaminated with 1 to 20 ppm of 2,3,7,8-tetrachlorodibenzo-p-dioxin (TCDD) that causes chloracne, cancer, affecting enzyme levels, porphyrin metabolism and immune dysfunction; because TCDD stores in adipose tissue, its long-term effects are currently unknown; the lawsuit brought by the exposed Vietnam veterans resulted in a $180 million settlement (Sci News 1988; 134:325) **AGENT PURPLE** A (50:30:20 mixture of 2,4-D n-butyl ester, 2,4,5-T n-butyl ester and 2,4,5-T Isobutyl ester) was used as a general defoliant for forest, brush, broad-leafed crops on an interim basis in exchange with Agent Orange **AGENT WHITE** (Tordon 101, Tri-isopropanolamine) was used for long-term jungle control and brush suppression **AGENT BLUE** (Phytar 560-G, sodium cacodolyte and cacodylic acid) was used as a rapid defoliant of short duration and for rice destruction

'Age pigment' see Ceroid, Lipofuscin

Agnogenic myeloid metaplasia HEMATOLOGY A chronic progressive panmyelosis characterized by variable fibrosis of the bone marrow, massive splenomegaly secondary to extramedullary hematopoiesis and a leukoerythroblastic anemia with dysmorphic red cells, circulating normoblasts, immature white cells and typical platelets Clinical Patients are commonly older than 50 and present with an insidious onset of weight loss, anemia, abdominal discomfort due to splenomegaly, often accompanied by hepatomegaly; 80% of cases are accompanied by non-specific chromosome abnormalities Prognosis Average survival 5 years, often ending in acute leukemia; see Pseudonym syndrome

A/G syndrome A disease complex characterized by amenorrhea and galactorrhea, seen in females with hyperprolactinemia caused by a microadenoma within the sella turcica

Ague cake spleen A descriptor for any organ (liver, pancreas, spleen) that is blackened, brittle, dry and enlarged; the spleen may be 1000+g in P falciparum malaria Ague (Middle English, malarial fever with shaking chills, Chaucer, 1388)

'Aguecheek's disease' A fanciful synonym for the dementia seen in hepatic encephalopathy, coined after Sir Andrew Aguecheek, a timorous minor character in Shakespeare's Twelth night

AH_{50} An assay that measures activity of the alternate pathway of complement-mediated hemolysis; the AH_{50} serves as a screen for homozygous deficiencies of complement factors C3, factor I and factor H

Ahasuerus syndrome see 'Wandering Jew syndrome'

AI Artificial intelligence A system in computer sciences which simulates human 'intelligence'; philosopher JR Searle divides the AI community into a) Those who feel computers think, ie human thought is equivalent to a complex computer program and b) Those who feel computers can't think but programs can be designed to contain dynamics with components of intelligence (Scientific American 1990; 262/1:26, 32); see Expert system, Neural networking

AID Artificial insemination by donor; see Artificial reproduction

AIDS Acquired immunodeficiency syndrome A condition intimately linked to the retrovirus, human immunodeficiency virus (HIV-1); although long-term survival of HIV-infected subjects is possible, once clinical AIDS develops, it responds only temporarily to therapy Incubation period In homosexual and bisexual men infected with HIV is estimated to be 11.0 years before clinical AIDS develops (J Am Med Assoc 1990; 263:1497); 162 073 cases have been diagnosed in the US, as of December 1990; 5 million are infected in Africa (WHO estimates, 1991) and 10 million are positive worldwide; in the US and most other developed nations, *AIDS pattern I* prevails, which is more common in male homosexuals and bisexuals, intravenous drug abusers, hemophiliacs and sexual partners or the progeny of any of these groups ; in Africa and Asia, *AIDS pattern II*, ie that of heterosexual promiscuity is most prevalent; AIDS is defined by the 'Revision of the CDC Surveillance case definition of AIDS' (J Am Med Assoc 1987; 258:143); see ARC, Hairy leukoplakia, HIV-1, HIV-2, Patient zero, VLIA (Virus-like infectious agent)

Acute AIDS syndrome A transient flu-like syndrome representing an early response to HIV-1, occurring 1-6 weeks after exposure to HIV-1 Clinical Sore throat, lymphadenopathy, anorexia, nausea, vomiting and a maculopapular rash, less commonly, diarrhea, lightening-like pain, major weight loss, abdominal cramping, palmoplantar desquamation Laboratory Mild leukopenia, occasionally inversion of the CD4:CD8 ratio (see Flow cytometry), antibodies to HIV products (gp120, gp160, p24 and p41) first appear six months or more after infection; the acute syndrome affects one-third of previously healthy subjects but is distinctly uncommon in homosexuals

AIDS-belt A now-defunct term that referred to a group of tropical African nations reporting more than 1000 cases of AIDS, where the disease affected heterosexuals and related to sexual promiscuity; the 'belt' countries were: Burundi, Central African Republic, the Congo, Kenya, Malawi, Rwanda, Tanzania, Uganda and Zambia

AIDS-'case zero' see Patient zero

AIDS dementia complex An insidious (30% of asymptomatic HIV-positive subjects have electroencephalographic abnormalities, N Engl J Med 1990; 323:864) condition characterized by progressive cognitive, motor and behavioral dysfunction, affecting up to two-thirds of AIDS patients, as HIV-1 has specific tropism for microglial cells (Science 1990; 249:549), possibly related to the gp120's structural similarity to neuroleukin Clinical Poor ability to concentrate, loss of memory, gait incoordination, dysgraphia, slowing of psychomotor functions and eventually, apathy Histopathology Degeneration in the subcortical white matter and deep gray matter, white matter vacuolization in the lateral and posterior columns of the spinal cord; HIV envelope glycoprotein, gp120, blocks the calcium channel, increasing intraneuronal calcium to toxic levels (Science 1990; 248:364), suggesting possible response of the dementia to calcium channel manipulation with nimodipine

AIDS embryopathy An HIV-induced complex in children born to intravenous drug-abusing mothers, characterized by craniofacial defects including microcephaly, hypertelorism, box-like head, saddle nose, long palpebral fissures with blue sclera, a triangular philtrum and patulous lips

AIDS encephalopathy see AIDS dementia

AIDS enteropathy An AIDS-related condition, which when seen in the AIDS-related complex, may presage clinical AIDS and is defined by the absence of a microorganism Clinical Diarrhea, often worse at night, weight loss, occasionally fever and possibly malnutrition with impaired D-xylose absorption Histopathology Partial villous atrophy with crypthyperplasia in the small intestine, viral inclusions, decreased plasma cells and increased intraepithelial lymphocytes in the large and small intestine

'AIDS-gate' An 'affair' in which French authorities, allegedly delayed the approval of the American enzyme-linked immunosorbent assay (ELISA) for detecting antibodies to the human immunodeficiency virus (HIV-1) for a period of months, at which time an equivalent French test was available; it has been suggested that the delay may have caused exposure of hemophiliacs to HIV, an unknown number of whom became infected during this period (Nature 1991; 353:197n); the term derives from the Watergate scandal that occurred during Nixon's presidency, which resulted in his resignation from the White House

AIDS litigation For a comprehensive review of the impact of AIDS in the US legal system, see J Am Med Assoc 1990; 263:1961, 2086; in a landmark legal decision, the US State of Florida has labelled AIDS a sexually-transmitted disease, which then implies that HIV testing may be carried out without consent (Am Med News 14/Dec/90)

AIDS and malaria Despite the association that had been

assumed by some models, malaria is not more frequent or severe in children with progressive HIV-1 infection nor does malarial infection appear to accelerate the rate of progression of AIDS (N Engl J Med 1991; 325:105)

AIDS precautions Those activities intended to minimize exposure to contaminated blood (and potentially bloody fluids, including extreme care, hand washing, use of face masks, double-gloving Note: Since early 1988, labeling of specimens as potentially contaminated with HIV is discouraged by the CDC, allegedly as it introduces a false sense of security that unlabeled specimens do not contain HIV-1; see Universal precautions

ARC AIDS-related complex Prodromal manifestations of AIDS where the criteria for defining a case as AIDS are not yet present; ARC is a 'Chinese menu disease', requiring two or more clinical features and two or more abnormal laboratory results; the patients may also have non-specific lymphadenopathy (Am J Surg Path 1985; 11:94), see AIDS, Follicle lysis, HIV-1

AIDS-related complex (ARC)

Clinical features	Laboratory
Temp. > 38° C	CD4 T-cells < 0.4 X 10^9
Weight loss > 10%	CD4:CD8 T-cell ratio < 1.0
Lymphadenopathy > 3 months	Anemia, leukopenia Thrombocytopenia
Diarrhea > 3 months	Polyclonal gammopathy
Night sweats > 3 months	Anergy (to skin testing)
Fatigue	Decreased mitogenic response (PHA)

AIDS statistics 1989, USA: 35 000 new cases 1988, 32 000; Incidence, USA: 14/10^5, higher in Blacks and Hispanics Groups affected: Homosexuals, 56%; IVDAs, 23% Annual incidence (per 100 000) US: Washington DC 81; New York 39; New Jersey 28; Florida 27; California 23 (MMWR 1990; 39:81, 39:279); in the US, 100 777 people have died of AIDS from 1981-1990, nearly one-third in 1990 and is the most common cause of death in young US adults, surpassing heart disease, cancer, suicide and homicide; 3/4 of the deaths have affected the 25-44 age group, 59% of the deaths have occurred in male homosexuals, 21% in female drug abusers; death rate (per 100 000) 29 Blacks, 22 Hispanics, 9 Whites, 3 Asians and American Indians (MMWR 1991; 40:41) *New cases per 100 000 in US* 1990: Washington 121, New York State 47, New Jersey 32, Florida 31, California 25 (MMWR 1991; 40:55) AIDS is the leading cause of male death in the Ivory Coast (1447 deaths/10^6) and is second in women (340/106) after pregnancy-related disease; 41% of male, and 32% of female cadavers were infected (Science 1990; 249:793)

AIDS therapy Various therapeutic modalities have been used to treat HIV-positive individuals, some of which are successful in temporarily halting the disease's inexhorable progression *Effective (FDA-approved)* AIDS drugs: Zidovudine Effective (not-yet FDA-approved) AIDS drugs: ddC (dideoxycytidine), ddI (dideoxyionsine) *Experimental substances* DAB/486IL-2 An IL-2 receptor-specific 'fusion' cytotoxin that selectively eliminates HIV-infected cells bearing high-affinity IL-2 receptors (Science 1991; 252:1703) *Ineffective substances* Compound Q (GLQ 223), dextran sulfate, isoprinosine, lentinan (an extract of shiitake mushrooms), peptide T, TIBO derivatives

AIDS vaccine The intense research in this arena has yet to produce a viable vaccine; promising results have been obtained in animal models, eg administration of intact live HIV-2 to cynomolgus monkeys who did not manifest SAIDS (simian AIDS) after exposure to SIV (Science 1990; 248:1180) and in in vitro systems; despite HIV's extreme mutability and the previously bleak prediction that a vaccine might prove impossible to surmount, researchers are hoping to have a viable vaccine by 1995 (Science 1991; 254:647n); see gp160 vaccine, HGP-30, Zagury

AIL Angiocentric immunoproliferative lesions

AILA Angioimmunoblastic lymphadenopathy

AIN Anal intraepithelial neoplasia, see Intraepithelial neoplasia

Ainhum Black toe disease Dactylosis spontanea Tropical medicine A possibly autosomal dominant condition affecting young black males of Africa and Central America, in whom broad fibrous bands cause annular digitoplantar constriction, especially of the fifth toe, resulting in autoamputation; pseudoainhum is caused by neurologic disease and ectodermal dysplasia

Air ambulance Emergency medicine A vehicle, often a helicopter, used to evacuate a person who requires immediate medical attention that cannot be provided in their current location; air ambulances, unlike their terrestrial counterparts, cannot be viewed as flying critical care units, as the most fundamental components of patient evaluation, eg assessment of breath, bowel and cardiac sounds are impossible because of the high noise levels (90-110 dB), which when accompanied by the vibrations and extreme space limitations, make air transport of patients in critical condition a 'scoop and run' operation (J Am Med Assoc 1991; 266:515c)

Air meniscus sign A crescent-shaped radiolucency bordering a mass lesion, characteristic of pulmonary hydatid cysts, where air enters the cyst forming a radiolucency between the outer layer (host) and the inner layer (hydatid membrane of ***Echinococcus granulosus***), in the USA, the most common air meniscus sign is due to ***Aspergillus fumigatus***

AIS Abbreviated injury scale A classification of severity of injury formulated in 1985 by the American Association of Automotive Medicine; see Injury severity score

AKA Above the knee amputation An 'elective' procedure used for severe (gangrenous) peripheral vascular disease, an operation commonly required in older diabetics; the AKA is preferred to a below the knee amputation in treating peripheral vascular disease if the gangrene extends above the malleoli, as the AKA has a higher healing rate (85-100%), better rehabilitation with a prosthesis and fewer complications

Alar Daminozide ENVIRONMENT A pesticide extensively used by apple producers in the US with the added advantage of inducing a 'natural' red color and increasing shelf life; one of Alar's metabolic products, UDMH is carcinogenic with an estimated increased cancer risk of 1 to 4 per million exposed (Science 1989; 244:755c); when the data generated by the Natural Resources Defense Council was published, estimating the cancer risk in children at 24 cancer deaths/10^5, a public outcry forced a temporary ban on its use, as 20-50% of apples tested were contaminated; in subsequent re-evaluation of Alar, the US Environmental Protection Agency concluded that the carcinogenic effect is about one-half of the previous estimate (Science 1991; 254:20n&v)

Albatross 'syndrome' Postgastrectomy-personality disorder A complex described in patients who continue to have abdominal pain, nausea, vomiting, drug dependency and poor food intake, despite successful surgery for upper gastrointestinal ulcers; the complex has been likened to the Albatross of *THE RIME OF THE ANCIENT MARINER*, as the patients incessantly demand that the surgeon do something to alleviate their suffering Note: This 'syndrome' was described two decades ago (Can Med Assoc J 1967; 96:1559) prior to the availability of the H_2-blocking agents (Cimetidine, ranitidine) and is of largely historic interest

Albinism A group of diseases that share a metabolic defect in the production of mature melanin; Albinism has been subdivided into three major groups: 1) Generalized or oculocutaneous albinism All six subtypes of this group are autosomal recessive and the most common is that due to tyrosinase deficiency, also Chediak-Higashi, Hermansky-Pudlak and Cross syndromes 2) Partial albinism An autosomal dominant condition with a focal white patch, similar to Waardenburg syndrome 3) Ocular albinism An X-linked recessive condition

ALC Alternate level of care

Alcian blue stain A proprietary water-soluble phthalocyanin dye (CI 74240) used in histology, which can be modified at different pHs for identifying specific mucopolysaccharide families; at pH 2.5, the stain identifies sialomucins produced by gastric and small intestinal glands; at pH 1.0, the sulfomucins produced in the large intestinal glands are more prominent

Alcoholism A chronic disease characterized by the regular intake of 75 or more grams of alcohol per day Chronic effects In addition to the well-described co-morbidity associated with portal hypertension, hepatic failure, hyperestrogenemia and psycho-social disruption, there is transient hyperparathyroidism that induces hypocalcemia, hypomagnesemia and osteoporosis (N Engl J Med 1991; 324:721); restriction fragment length polymorphism (RFLP) analysis of cerebral tissue in alcoholics suggested an association of some forms of alcoholism with the D_2 receptor gene, located on C-11q22-q23 (J Am Med Assoc 1990; 263:2055), although the association is controversial (ibid, 264:3156); see Standard drink

Alcoholic cardiomyopathy A clinicopathologic state induced by chronic ethanolism, a major cause of dilated cardiomyopathy, characterized by severe left ventricular dysfunction and a 40-80% three-year mortality, presenting as sudden death or ventricular fibrillation; alcohol is directly cardiotoxic, decreasing inotropism or force of myocardial contraction due to decreased calcium and impaired excitability, resulting in mitochondrial damage with decreased oxidative enzyme activity and energy production and swelling of the endoplasmic reticulum; alcohol also interferes with myocardial lipid metabolism, protein synthesis and ATPase activity; acetaldehyde, alcohol's major metabolite stimulates the release of norepinephrine (J Am Med Assoc 1990; 264:377); alcoholic cardiomyopathy may be associated with other overlapping conditions, related either to other substances of abuse, eg tobacco-related cardiac disease or to alcohol's effect on other organ systems, eg cerebrovascular accidents and hypertension

Alcoholic fatty liver A liver demonstrating acute and subacute, ie precirrhotic, changes induced by alcohol, a toxin that interferes with fatty acid oxidation, impairing the tricarboxylic acid cycle, resulting in incomplete β-oxidation products from fatty acids Pathology Liver weighs 2500 g or more (normal 1500 g), and is yellow and greasy Histopathology see Fatty liver Ultrastructure Enlarged and distorted mitochondria, dilated smooth endoplasmic reticulum; see Fatty liver

Alcohol flush syndrome A vasoactive phenomenon common among Orientals; restriction fragment length polymorphism (RFLP) analysis reveals a defective aldehyde dehydrogenase gene with inability of these subjects to metabolize acetaldehyde

Alcoholic neuropathy Pseudotabes A nutritional neuropathy described in alcoholics, characterized by burning pain in the lower extremities, paresthesia, especially acral in distribution, decreased tactile and position sensation, ataxia and weakness of the legs with atrophy and fasciculations, ulcerations of immobile parts Treatment Dietary

Alcoholic paranoia see Othello syndrome

Alcoholic rose gardener 'syndrome' Subacute and chronic mycosis due to the low-grade dimorphous fungal pathogen, ***Sporotrichosis schenckii***, is reportedly more common in alcoholics employed as gardeners; the association, if true, is probably related to the lesser caution exercised by alcoholics who have increased skin abrasions and lesser concern for early infections

Alcoholic, type I 'Maintenance-type' alcoholic An anxiety-prone or passive-dependent person who drinks to alleviate problems; the onset in either sex is after age 25; type I alcoholics have a high reward dependence and avoid harmful or novel situations; most 'have minimal (if at all) antisocial tendencies;

Alcoholic, type II 'Binge' drinker The thrill-seeking alcoholic who enjoys the novelty of drinking; type II alcoholics may be antisocial, have a history of early violence, and be the biological sons of alcoholic fathers, becoming alcoholics by age 25

Aleukemic leukemia A clinical variant of acute leukemia

where the peripheral blood reveals pancytopenia and few discernible blast cells on peripheral blood smears; leukemic cells are seen only by a bone marrow biopsy

Aleutian mink disease A chronic fatal parvoviral infection of minks causing a polyclonal expansion of B lymphocytes

A-level An educational 'track' in Britain that focuses a student at circa age sixteen into one of several subjects in preparation for the material he plans on 'reading' while in the university

Alexin Obsolete for Complement

Alglucerase An 'orphan drug' used to treat type I Gaucher's disease, indicated for those patients with symptomatic anemia, hemorrhagic diathesis, bone disease or hepatosplenomegaly (J Am Med Assoc 1991; 265:2934/FDA)

Algorithm A logical set of rules for solving problems of a specified type that assumes that all of the data is objective and there are a finite number of solutions to the problem; algorithms form the basis of traditional computing, defined by the parameters used in programming, eg the 'and' and 'or' gates that allow a sequence to proceed or to 'loop'; the use of algorithms in solving complex clinical problems is inherently attractive, but often fails as disease causes subjective signs and symptoms and thus 'logical' algorithms cannot substitute for clinical experience; see Back-propagation

'Alice in Wonderland' changes A fanciful coinage for the cyclical, radiologically observed increases and decreases in the size of a prolactin-secreting pituitary adenoma, described in a patient receiving an ergot compound with dopaminic activity

Alice in Wonderland syndrome Bizarre perceptual distortions of the body image, space and size that may occur in 1) NEUROLOGY As a pre-epileptic aura or as a symptom preceding a migraine 2) PEDIATRICS Perceptual distortions as a presenting symptom of infectious mononucleosis that may be accompanied by convulsions, ataxia, nuchal rigidity, meningitis with mononuclear cells in the cerebrospinal fluid, encephalitis, transverse myelitis, Bell's palsy and Guillain-Barre syndrome 3) SUBSTANCE ABUSE Distortions of time, space and sensation associated with hallucinogens Note: There is little reason to subdivide this 'syndrome' into types I and II as per AE Rodin and JD Key, 1989

Alkaline tide PHYSIOLOGY A transient postcibal rise of the blood's pH, related to the sequestration of hydrogen ions by the stomach during early digestion

Alkylating agents Chemotherapeutic drugs with unstable, highly reactive electrophilic rings that combine with tertiary nitrogens in purines and pyrimidines, as well as -NH_2, -COOH, -SH and PO_3H_2 groups forming stable covalent bonds; DNA, RNA and proteins each have one or more of these groups, but DNA damage at the N-7 position of the guanine ring is the most crippling to the proliferating, ie neoplastic cells; alkylating agents include busulfan, chlorambucil, cyclophosphamide, melphalan, nitrogen mustard and nitrosourea, administered intravenously or per os

'All-American operation' A coinage from Dr Brunchwig's pelvic surgery service at Memorial Sloan-Kettering Cancer Institution (New York City), referring to radical surgery for a 'Frozen pelvis', consisting of total pelvic exenteration with radical en bloc resection of the rectum, uterus and urinary bladder; see Heroic surgery; Cf 'North American', 'South American' operations

Allele One of two or more variations of a gene located at a particular site on a chromosome; in eukaryotic cells, alleles exist in pairs and one allele is contributed by each parent; the particular phenotypic expression is a function of whether the gene is dominant, in which case, only one allele is needed for phenotypic expression, or recessive, requiring that both alleles be the same for the phenotypic expression of a trait

Allelic dropout A phenomenon may occur in the polymerase chain reaction, in which there is a failure to amplify one of the alleles and the specimen is interpreted as being negative for the presence of a segment of DNA of interest; allelic dropout occurs at specific temperatures (88-90°C) in the thermoregulator device

Allelic exclusion GENETICS A phenomenon whereby one of the two genes for which an individual is a heterozygote is expressed, while the gene is excluded or not expressed, typically seen in the expression of immunoglobulin genes; this expression of one allele at a locus is characteristic of cells of the immunoglobulin 'superfamily', eg B and T cells, and is a mechanism that explains how a cell can express only one immunoglobulin or one specific T cell receptor

Allergen immunotherapy see Desensitization therapy

Allergic polyp see 'Inflammatory polyp'

Allergic 'salute' Frequent upward rubbing of the nose by the dorsal surface of a fisted hand, in an attempt to relieve itching, most often seen in children with allergies, which with time causes a central nasal groove

Allergic 'shiners' Dark, discolored circles under the eyes, often accompanied by mouth breathing in children with allergic rhinitis which causes venous stasis due to impeded blood flow through the edematous nasal mucosa, while obstruction of the nasal passages obliges mouth breathing Diagnosis Presence of eosinophils in the mucus Note: 'Shiner' is an Americanism for a trauma-induced, often fisticuff-related, unilateral periorbital hemorrhage, also known as a 'Black eye'

Allied health personnel All health care personnel who are a) Not physicians, dentists, podiatrists and registered nurses and b) Have received specialized training and require special licensure; these workers include dieticians, laboratory technologists, medical technicians, medical transcriptionists, phlebotomists, physicians' assistants and practical nurses

Allograft Homograft A graft (organ, tissues or cells) donated from genetically distinct individual of the same species; Cf Xenograft

Allostery The cooperative interaction of two or more functional sites on a protein, or two or more proteins that results in ligand binding; allostery depends on dynamic interaction with a substrate or other molecule, eg heme-heme interactions

Allotype A set of determinants or sequence of amino

acids on immunoglobulin chains (and other proteins demonstrating heterogeneity) that is relatively specific for the individual and frequently more common in a racial group; Cf Idiotype, Isotype

α Symbol for: A band in serum electrophoresis

α-amanitin A bicyclic 8-residue polypeptide derived from *Amanita phalloides* that inhibits transcription by RNA polymerase II and other RNA polymerases

3-α-androstanediol glucuronide 3-α-diol G A metabolite of dihydrotestosterone, the levels of which in blood and urine reflect peripheral androgen action and which are decreased in androgen deficiency or testicular hypofunction

α_1-antitrypsin (A1AT) A circulating glycoprotein that inhibits proteolytic enzymes, including trypsin, chymotrypsin, elastase and others, which is inherited in a co-dominant fashion; the gene is located on chromosome 14 and encodes 25 different allelic forms classified according to electrophoretic mobility, of which the PiMM phenotype is normal; the most common A1AT deficiency phenotype is PiZZ, characterized by early-onset emphysema and cholestasis, cirrhosis, hepatic failure and a marked increase in hepatocellular carcinoma Treatment Prolastin in the face of chronic obstructive pulmonary disease, intravenous or nebulized for direct delivery to the lungs; the gene for A1AT may be transferred via adenoviruses to the lung epithelium; following transfer, A1AT mRNA is expressed as is functioning A1AT, a feat that has broad implications in treating this and other enzyme deficiency conditions (Science 1991; 252:431)

α_2-antiplasmin deficiency A rare autosomal recessive condition characterized by premature fibrinolysis with early hemorrhages beginning at birth Treatment Antifibrinolysis, eg tranexamic acid

α **band** see α rhythm

α **chain disease** see Heavy chain disease

α **decay** RADIATION PHYSICS High energy, ie in the million electron volt range, radioactive decay products caused by the emission of α particles, which themselves are products of a disintegrating nucleus; see α particles

α **effect** ENDOCRINOLOGY The metabolic, hemodynamic and modulatory effects of epinephrine and norepinephrine are a function of the concentration of adrenergic receptors on the α and β cells of the pancreatic islets; α effects (epinephrine acting on β islet cells) include: Glycogenolysis, gluconeogenesis, inhibition of insulin-stimulated glucose uptake in skeletal muscle and arteriovenous vasoconstriction

α-fetoprotein (AFP) A 70 kD protein, first synthesized by the embryonic yolk sac, later by the fetal gastrointestinal tract and liver which has 40% homology with albumin; AFP's role in fetal development remains unclear; measurement of AFP levels in pregnant women serves to screen for open neural tube defects (incidence 1-2/1000 births); AFP levels in the fetal serum are 150-fold greater than in amniotic fluid, which in turn are 200-fold greater than that of maternal serum; maternal serum levels are 3-400 µg/L in the third trimester; the levels in the fetal serum and amniotic fluid peak at 13 weeks, while the maternal levels peak at 30 weeks; increased AFP during pregnancy may be due to central nervous system defects (spina bifida and other open neural tube defects, hydrocephaly, cyclopia, microcephaly, sacrococcygeal teratoma), gastrointestinal anomalies (esophageal and duodenal atresia with impaired fetal swallowing, omphalocele, due to transudation, gastroschisis, pseudoobstruction and short bowel), hematology (fetomaternal hemorrhage, hydrops fetalis), immunodeficiency syndromes (severe combined immune deficiency and/or adenosine deaminase deficiency, combined T and B-cell defects, ataxia telangiectasia), cardiovascular (Fallot's tetralogy) and other causes including cystic hygroma, Turner syndrome, fetal demise, twin gestation, congenital nephrotic syndrome; AFP are increased in adults in hepatocellular carcinoma, endodermal sinus tumors, Sertoli-Leydig cell tumor, pancreatic and gastric malignancies, teratomas, alcoholic and viral hepatitis, hypertyrosinosis; AFP elevation is also present in infants at risk of subsequent fetal death, up to four to five months after the screening, regardless of the presence of neural tube defects or multiple gestations (N Engl J Med 1991; 325:6, 55)

α **heavy chain disease** see Heavy chain disease

α-helix A structural protein motif deduced by Pauling and Corey, where there are 3.6 amino acid residues per turn; the α helix of proteins has a right-handed 'screw' sense and is stabilized by intrachain hydrogen bonds between NH and CO groups; bundled together, α helices are found in keratin, myosin, fibrin and epidermin

α-interferon see Interferon

α **particle** A radioactive decay product, ^{4}He nucleus, composed of 2 protons and 2 neutrons with marked ionizing capacity (3-9 million electron-volts) but a short range (3-9 cm in air, 25-40 µm in water/soft tissue) derived from α decay, see there; α particles arising from radon, uranium and plutonium 'daughters' are implicated in inhalation-induced neoplasia of the respiratory tract; while α particles are highly tissue-destructive, they travel only short distances and are blocked by a thick piece of paper or skin

α **rhythm** ELECTROENCEPHALOGRAPHY A type of electrical activity in adults, recorded from the posterior regions, which may be abolished with visual stimulation and attenuated by thinking and is typically seen in relaxed adults with closed eyes; α rhythm occurs at 8-13 Hz, and has bihemispheric asynchrony, where the non-dominant hemisphere has a greater wave amplitude; focal central nervous system disease is accompanied by focally altered α rhythm, which becomes diffuse in coma; non-invasive diagnostic modalities of computed tomography and magnetic resonance imaging have relegated electroencephalography to a diagnostic modality of lesser importance in localizing cerebral masses

ALT 1)Alanine aminotransferase (glutamate pyruvate transaminase, GPT) 2) see Antilymphocyte therapy

Alternate complement pathway Properdin pathway IMMUNOLOGY A route of complement activation that occurs independently of complement-fixing antibodies; complement is a non-specific arm of the immune system, encharged with lysis of target organisms; the alternate pathway is more complex than the classic pathway, requiring a 'priming' C3 convertase (C3,Bb) and an 'amplification' C3 convertase (C3b,Bb); in the presence of properdin, C3 convertase is stabilized, activating later complement components, leading to opsonization, leukocyte chemotaxis, increased vascular permeability and cytolysis; the alternate pathway is activated by: Properdin, IgA, IgG, lipopolysaccharide and snake venom; both pathways are stimulated by trypsin-like enzymes Note: C3b is continuously degraded when in contact with particulate activators; the surface provides protection from breakdown; C3b and factor B interact with serum protein factor D, cleaving factor B producing C3bBb, forming a positive feedback loop generating C3b; C3b + Bb + properdin form C5 convertase

Alternative birthing center An obstetrical unit or facility that provides a pleasant, 'friendly' atmosphere for women who are expected to have an uncomplicated vaginal delivery; these centers are staffed by obstetricians or midwives and located either within a hospital or are free-standing units; see Lamaze, Natural childbirth

Alternative medicine see Holistic medicine

Alternative splicing (AS) MOLECULAR BIOLOGY The removal of varying lengths of DNA from precursor messenger RNA (mRNA), a mechanism for generating different proteins from the same DNA transcript and effecting gene control by serving as an on-off switch for variable expression of one gene in different organs (Science 1991; 251:33); in the basic splicing process, noncoding, intervening sequences of RNA are removed and exons are joined by two cleavage-ligand events requiring precise recognition of the 5' and the 3' splice junctions and assembly of a 'spliceosome' complex, involving interactions between the pre-mRNA and the small nuclear ribonucleoprotein particles (sNURPs) U1, U2, U5 and the U4/U6 particle; it is thought that the U1 sNRNP plays a critical role in selection of the 5' and 3' splice sites (Science 1991; 251:1045); AS is tissue-specific and related to the presence of stable double-stranded intron-exon (secondary structure) regions, the repression of which allows expression of the non-expressed exon, as in the alternative splicing of chicken tropomyosin, depending on whether the myogenic cells are in the myoblast (pre-differentiation) or myotubule (post-differentiation) stage (Science 1991; 252:1823, 1842); see Spliceosome

Alu family MOLECULAR BIOLOGY A family of 150-300 base pair sequences of DNA intermediate repeats (dispersed blocks of related non-identical) that are often associated with introns, contain a recognition sequence for the restriction endonuclease Alu I, cap regions and a poly-A tail; about fifty of the highly homologous Alu regions have been identified and are thought to play a role in initiating DNA synthesis; see Tandem repeats

Alveolar-capillary block syndrome A 'syndrome' of historical interest that was based on a concept that the distance that oxygen had to travel was increased in pulmonary interstitial disease and required extra diffusion time to reach equilibrium, thus explaining the hypoxia typical of these conditions, a value that is widely recognized as overestimated

Alveolar soft part sarcoma A malignant tumor most commonly occurring in the soft deep tissues of the legs of young adults, especially females **Pathology** Circumscribed firm, yellow-gray masses with areas of necrosis and hemorrhage; the fibrous tissue separates the tumor into nests composed of large cells with vesicular nuclei and prominent nucleoli **Histogenesis** Cell of origin is uncertain **Prognosis** Larger tumors are more aggressive **Treatment** Wide excision

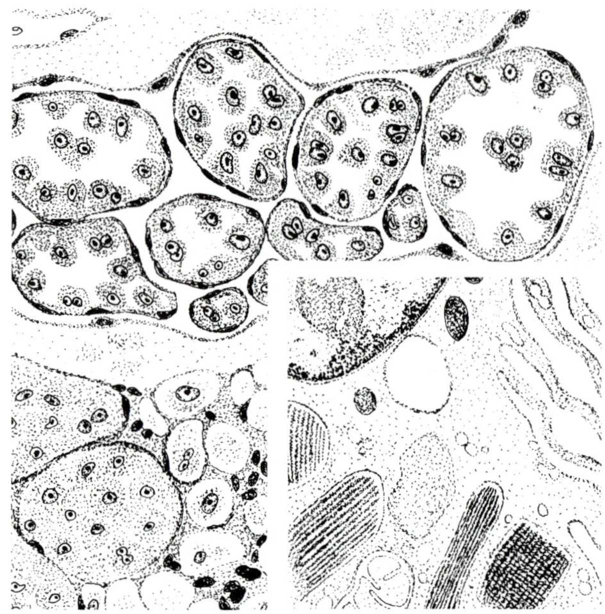

Alveolar soft part sarcoma

Alzheimer's disease (Alois, Psychiatrist, Breslau, 1864-1915) Despite the virtually diagnostic clinical manifestations, this remains a "pathologist's" disease, characterized by generalized frontal and parietotemporal cerebral atrophy (basal ganglia and reticular formation are less commonly affected) and a histopathological triad *1) SENILE (NEURITIC) PLAQUES*, which consist of dilated, tortuous, presynaptic axon terminals, most common in the cortex *2) NEUROFIBRILLARY TANGLES*, appearing as twisted fascicles of neurofilaments, commonly surrounding the nucleus in a neuron and *3) GRANULOVACUOLAR DEGENERATION*, consisting of intracytoplasmic vacuoles within the neurons containing argyrophilic 'dots' of unknown origin; Hirano bodies, consisting of glassy eosinophilic inclusions composed of actin filaments located in the proximal dendrites are distinctly less common **Molecular biology** Alzheimer's disease is not caused by a single genetically homogeneous gene (Nature 1991; 347:194); major molecules involved in Alzheimer's disease include 1) A 4.2 kD polypeptide (β-amyloid polypeptide, A4) isolated from senile plaques and neurofibrillary tangles of Alzheimer's brains is encoded by a gene on chromosome 21; APP had been linked to Down syndrome and associated with duplication of proto-oncogene *ets*-2, although this relation proved to be weak, given the heterogeneity at 21q21; A68 protein is present in homogenates of Alzheimer brains, and implicated in the formation of neuritic plaques and neurofibrillary tangles (68 kD); a protein-precursor for Alzheimer's type amyloid may contain structures capable of inhibiting serine proteases, possibly explaining the deposition of these fibrils in Alzheimer brains Treatment Tetrahydroaminoacridine (THA, an inhibitor of acetylcholinesterase), was claimed to improve the quality of life in Alzheimer's patients, see THA

Alzheimer's disease-associated proteins A group of proteins, eg A-68, considered specific for Alzheimer's disease, identified by the ALZ-50 antibody (J Am Med Assoc 1990; 263:2907)

ALZ-50 A monoclonal antibody that reacts against brain tissue from patients with Alzheimer's disease, that selectively binds to protein A-68 and is an early marker of Alzheimer's disease (J Am Med Assoc 1990; 263:2907)

ama Against medical advice A phrase referring to a patient's self-discharge from a health care facility, contrary to what the physician(s) perceive to be in the patient's best interests; a discharge 'ama' must be documented by the patient's signature, given the potential for lawsuit if the discharged patient dies before admission to another facility

Amadori reaction A reaction that links the aldehyde group of a glucose and the amine group of a protein, eg Maillard reaction

Amadori products Amadori rearrangement A step in non-enzymatic 'glycosylation' of collagen, see Maillard reaction, Browning reaction, which begins when a glucose's aldehyde combines with a protein's amino group forming the unstable 'Schiff base' later undergoing an 'Amadori rearrangement' forming a stable, but still reversible Amadori product, eg hemoglobin A1c, which with time, dehydrate and rearrange themselves into advanced glycosylation endproducts; free amino groups of proteins react with glucose aldehydes to form a Schiff base, resulting in an Amadori rearrangement; the resultant ketoamine structure is cyclized to form a hemiketal, forming the chemical basis of glycosylated hemoglobin (HbA_{1c}), see Advanced glycosylation endproducts

Amalgam Dental amalgam A mixture of silver and mercury used to fill teeth; although amalgam has been used by dentists for 150 years, it is unclear whether prolonged exposure to 'inert' amalgam mercury is innocuous (J Am Med Assoc 1991; 265:2934/FDA); see Fluoridation

Amber codon UAG One of three 'nonsense' codons (a triplet of DNA nucleotides, the others are ochre, UAA and opal, UGA) that terminates protein synthesis; amber suppressors are mutants that encode tRNAs, the anticodons of which respond to both UAG and to their usual codons

Ambiguity MOLECULAR BIOLOGY The occurrence of errors in protein synthesis that is more common in vitro, where an incorrect amino acid is incorporated into a growing protein chain in response to a nucleotide triplet or codon for another amino acid; ambiguity represents a true error and thus contrasts to 'wobble', in which the degeneracy of the DNA code has only 20 different amino acids for 61 possible codons, where 'sloppy' translation is not uncommon event in the translation of messenger RNA from the DNA template; Cf Ambiquity

Ambiguous genitalia Male or female external genitalia that is indistinct or discordant with the genotype, where the sex assigned to the infant is chromosomally incorrect, usually in the form of a male-to-female phenotype 'conversion', where the children adapt to their assigned sex

Ambiguous genitalia Ambiguous sexuality Acquired sexual discordance in which the phenotype and genotype are correct, but the 'psychotype' is incorrect, requiring transsexual conversion; see Transsexuality

Ambiquity A property of enzymes, where they exist, either bound to a carrier protein or are free in the circulation; Cf Ambiguity

Ambulatory care center Walk-in clinic A free-standing facility that provides non-emergent medical, or less commonly, dental services; most visits to these centers occur outside of the regular work hours by patients who feel that their particular problem cannot wait until their private physician is available (Can Med Assoc J 1990; 143:740); because many such centers often have short waiting times, may not require appointments and have a non-permanent or rotating medical staff, ambulatory care centers have been likened to 'fast food' restaurants, receiving facetious sobriquets, eg 'Doc-in-the-Box', 'McStitch'

'Ambu' bag EMERGENCY MEDICINE A self-refilling bag-valve-mask unit with a 1-1.5 liter capacity, used for artificial respiration which, although suboptimal for the non-intubated patient, is effective for ventilating and oxygenating intubated patients, allowing both spontaneous and artificial respiration

Ames test TOXICOLOGY A bioassay that detects mutagenesis, used to detect and screen for toxic compounds with carcinogenic potential Technique *Salmonella typhimurium*, TA100, which cannot synthesize histidine (and therefore requires histidine in the growth medium) is incubated in a histidine-poor medium with the compound of interest; if the chemical is mutagenic, then TA100 reverts to a form that can synthesize its own histidine

AMF see Autocrine motility factor

AMI Acute myocardial infarction

Amiloride An aerosolized sodium channel blocker that may slow the progression of pulmonary dysfunction in cystic fibrosis, a disease of excess sodium reabsorption, thickening of the mucus and decreased secretion clearance (N Engl J Med 1990; 322:1189)

Amino acid The essential building block for polypeptides and proteins, which is abbreviated in a three letter code, or for even more efficient communication by a single letter designation, a convention of particular use among molecular biologists (Table, below)

Amino acid residue see Residue

2-Aminopurine A specific protein kinase inhibitor that blocks the induction of the genes for β-interferon, c-*fos* and c-*myc* by virus or poly(I)-poly(C) at the level of transcription

Amino acid abbreviations

Alanine	Ala	A	
Arginine	Arg	R	†
Asparganine	Asn	N	
Aspartic acid	Asp	D	
Arginine *or* Aspartic acid	Asx	B	
Cysteine	Cys	C	†
Glutamine	Gln	Q	
Glutamic acid	Glu	E	
Glutamine *or* Glutamic acid	Glx	Z	
Glycine	Gly	G	
Histidine	His	H	†
Isoleucine	Ile	I	▲
Leucine	Leu	L	▲
Lysine	Lys	K	▲
Methionine	Met	M	▲
Phenylalanine	Phe	F	▲
Proline	Pro	P	
Serine	Ser	S	
Threonine	Thr	T	▲
Tryptophan	Typ	W	▲
Tyrosine	Tyr	Y	
Valine	Val	V	▲

▲Essential amino acids

†Amino acids that are essential during growth periods

Amnesty International An organization that works for the release of persons detained (anywhere) for their consciously held beliefs, color, ethnic origin, sex, religion, or language, provided they have neither used nor advocated violence, opposing torture and the death penalty and was recipient of the 1977 Nobel Peace for Peace; 400 000 members; 7 networks include one for health professionals; see IPPNW, Red Cross, Médicins sans Frontières

Amniotic band 'syndrome' Idiopathic in utero formation of fibrous adhesion bands that encircle the fetus' fingers, limbs or head, causing autoamputation of the constricted part

Amniotic fluid embolism A syndrome that results from a traumatic delivery and 'injection' of amniotic fluid into the maternal circulation Incidence 1:80 000 deliveries; maternal mortality approaches 80% Etiology Idiopathic, predisposed to by the high intrauterine pressure that allows amniotic fluid to pass into the maternal venous circulation, where the meconium is especially toxic to the mother; the use of prostaglandin E_2 may facilitate amniotic fluid embolism (J Am Med Assoc 1990; 263:3259c)

'Amok' 'Latah' A psychotic reaction described in the native populations of Malaysia and Africa in which the subject goes on a homicidal rampage, indiscriminately stabbing, shooting or killing anyone within reach of his weapon until he is overpowered or is himself killed; Cf Piblokto

Amorph GENETICS A 'silent' mutated allele with no effect on the phenotypic expression of a trait

Amotivational syndrome SUBSTANCE ABUSE A condition induced by chronic marijuana abuse, affecting predisposed individuals who are often young, learning disabled and emotionally immature; in this psychologic background, marijuana, a drug that reinforces passivity and social withdrawal, causes a loss of interest in the environment, generalized apathy and passivity, loss of desire to work or perform adequately, loss of energy and generalized lassitude, moodiness, emotional lability, impairment of ability to concentrate and process new information, slovenly appearance and habits and a lifestyle that revolves in part around procurement of marijuana and other drugs; see 'Gateway' drugs

AMPA receptor α-amino-3-hydroxy-5-methyl-4-isoxazoleproprionate receptor A glutamate receptor that mediates the fast component of excitatory post-synaptic potentials

Amphipathic molecule A molecule that has hydrophobic and hydrophilic characters with positive, negative or no net charge at pH 7

Amplification systems Groups of proteins that function in coordinated sequences, forming positive feedback loops for expansion of the response to a signal of relatively low intensity; Amplification loops include a) Coagulation, the best-described is factor Xa activating factor 'X' in the presence of factor VIII, Ca^{++} and phospholipid b) Complement which augments the B cell response, see Alternate and Classic pathways and c) Cytokines, responsible for amplifying the T cell response, interleukins, kinins, lipid mediators and mast cell products; see Gene amplification

Amputation sign RADIOLOGY The descriptor for the sharp cut-off seen on air bronchograms, most commonly due to pulmonary thromboembolism, less commonly, carcinoma, tumor emboli, myxoma and intravascular sarcoma

Amsterdam dwarf see Dwarf

Amsterdam strategy POPULATION CONTROL The Amsterdam Forum world stabilization strategy A blueprint for limiting world population growth that was developed in 1989 and signed by 79 countries, which calls for developed nations to contribute 4% of their foreign aid budgets to international population programs (Science 1991; 252:1247n&v); see Contraceptives; Cf Mexico City policy, ZPG

Amygdalin A β-cyanogenic glycoside that is structurally related to the semisynthetic laetrile, which is derived from the pits of certain fruits; see Laetrile

Amyl nitrate 'Poppers' A substance of abuse that is similar in action to nitroglycerin, available in glass ampules; amyl nitrate decreases the blood to the brain, acting to enhance an orgasm Note: In the early days of the AIDS epidemic, amyl nitrate was briefly inculpated in the pathogenesis of the disease

Amylin A 37 residue polypeptide that has a 45% sequence homology with calcitonin; it is present in normal and diabetic pancreas and is a major component of islet amyloid in patients with non-insulin-dependent diabetes mellitus, in whom it is reported to be increased in the serum (Lancet 1990; 1:854)

Classification (3rd Intl Symp. Amyloidosis)
Familial
1) Amyloid polyneuropathy Fiber type: AFp (prealbumin)
2) Familial mediterranean fever Fiber type: AA
3) Familial amyloid syndrome Östertag's disease
Generalized
1) 'Primary' amyloidosis (the variable end of immunoglobulin light chains), affecting the tongue, gastrointestinal tract, heart, kidneys, muscle, skin, nerves, ligaments and seminal vesicles: AL Fiber
2) Associated with plasma cell dyscrasia; most patients have an M component (amyloid deposits in the liver, spleen, kidneys and adrenal glands) and rarely, myeloma; survival is less than two years; AL fiber
3) Secondary to inflammation or infection Deposition of amyloid protein A (AA fibers) fibrils; in the pre-antibiotic era, secondary amyloidosis was most commonly associated with chronic infection, eg tuberculosis, chronic osteomyelitis and leprosy; in the current setting, secondary deposits occur in chronic inflammation, eg Crohn's disease, ulcerative colitis and familial mediterranean fever, connective tissue disease, eg dermatomyositis, lupus erythematosus, rheumatoid arthritis and Sjögren syndrome, tissue destruction, eg bronchiectasis, malignancy, eg alpha heavy chain disease, Hodgkin's disease, leukemia, myeloma and Waldenström syndrome and heroin abuse, presenting with proteinuria and nephrotic syndrome
Localized
1) Lichen amyloidosis Fiber type: AD
2) Endocrine-related Fiber type: AEt Amyloid may occur with endocrine neoplasms, including pancreatic islet cell tumors, medullary thyroid carcinoma and parathyroid hyperplasia and adenomata seen in the MEN (Multiple endocrine neoplasia) syndrome
Senile types: Heart Fiber type: ASc
Brain Fiber: ASb
3) β_2-microglobulin derived amyloid cannot traverse the dialysis membrane, in patients on chronic dialysis, causing cystic bony lesions and carpal tunnel syndrome
Note: Reclassification of amyloidoses using a biochemically valid system is possibly of greater utility than classifications based on ethnic and clinical differences, which have considerable overlap

Amyloid β-fibrillosis A term coined in 1838 by Schleiden to describe starch-like constituents of normal plants, a term later used by von Rokitansky for a peculiar material in the liver and spleen that Virchow thought was polysaccharide; the various amyloids are unified by a common molecular theme, that of the β-pleated protein sheet, demonstrable by X-ray crystallography and responsible for amyloid's Congo red staining and its resistance to proteolytic digestion; a 28-residue polypeptide similar to β-amyloid enhances neuron survival in vitro, implying that amyloidosis is a defense reaction (Science 1989; 243:1488)

Amyloid β protein (ABP) A4 β-amyloid A 4 kD polypeptide derived from altered processing of amyloid precursor protein (APP), an integral membrane glycoprotein secreted as a carboxyl-terminal truncated molecule that is deposited in small vessels of the leptomeninges and cerebral cortex in Alzheimer's disease, representing a major component of the neurofibrillary tangles and senile plaques (Science 1990; 248:492, 1122), which may be of vascular origin (Nature 1990 344:497c); ABP may also accumulate in Down syndrome, infectious encephalopathy and cerebral amyloid angiopathy **Ultrastructure** Haphazardly arranged fibrils 8-10 nm in diameter by 30-100 nm length; crystallographic analysis demonstrates β-pleating; ABP may be found in skin, intestine and adrenal gland (J Am Med Assoc 1991; 265:309n&v); it is unclear whether ABP causes Alzheimer's disease or is a 'passenger' protein produced by damaged neurons; a transgenic mouse with the amyloid precursor has been generated (Science 1991; 253:323, 266n&v)

Amyloidosis Systemic amyloidosis is divided into 1) AL amyloidosis Primary amyloidosis A condition associated with plasma cell dyscrasias, where the accumulated amyloid fibers correspond to fragments of immunoglobulin light chains and 2) AA amyloidosis Reactive or secondary amyloidosis A group of conditions seen in patients with chronic inflammation, see amyloid, where the accumulated fibers derive from a circulating acute-phase lipoprotein, known as serum protein A; both types of amyloidosis contain amyloid P component, a non-fibrillary glycoprotein also found in the circulation; Scintigraphy after injection of ^{123}I-labelled serum amyloid P component can locate tissue deposition of amyloidosis and if the deposition is active, cytotoxic therapy may be instituted (N Engl J Med 1990; 323:508)

Amyotrophic lateral sclerosis Lou Gehrig disease A 'motor neuron disease', characterized by upper limb weakness, atrophy and focal neurological signs; the gene defect is heterogeneous and located distal to the centromere on chromosome 21 (N Engl J Med 1991; 324:1381) Note: Only 5% of the cases are familial; see Motor neuron disease

Amytal interview An interview carried out under the influence of Amytal, a sedative, which by causing full relaxation, with minimal sedation, attempts to elicit information from a subject who is voluntarily 'guarding' against its revelation

ANA see Anti-nuclear antibodies

Anabolic-androgenic steroids A group of 17-α-alkylated testosterone analogs, commonly abused by athletes (especially body builders) at many professional levels, abused by international athletes 1-2%, college athletes 5%, 12th grade male athletes, 6% and professional football players 7-8% (J Am Med Assoc 1988; 260:3441; Science 1988; 242:184) Lipid profile with abuse (most marked with oral stanazol than with IV testosterone (J Am Med Assoc 1989; 261:1165) marked decrease in

HDL-cholesterol (especially HDL_2) and mild increase in hepatic triglyceride lipase (HDL catabolism) Therapeutic indications for anabolic steroids: Children and adolescents with delayed puberty, growth promotion, small penis and hypogonadism (J Am Med Assoc 1988; 260:3484) Other indications include the management of osteoporosis, aplastic anemia, endometriosis, angioedema and deficiency of testosterone (J Am Med Assoc 1989; 261:1165) **Adverse effects, male** Breast enlargement, testicular atrophy, sterility, sperm abnormalities, impotence and prostatic hypertrophy **Adverse effects, female** Clitoral hypertrophy, beard growth, baldness, deepened voice, decreased breast size **Adverse effects, both sexes** Aggression and antisocial behavior, 'roid rage, see below; increased risk of cardiovascular disease, liver tumors, peliosis hepatis, jaundice, acne, accelerated bone maturation, resulting in short stature, liver tumors (hepatic adenomas and carcinoma) that may regress with steroid abstinence (J Am Med Assoc 1989; 261:1857); high-doses are thought to be physically addicting, as abrupt reduction in dose results in acute hyperadrenergic withdrawal symptoms (tachycardia, hypertension, nausea, vomiting, headaches, vertigo, diaphoresis and piloerection), paralleling other withdrawal syndromes, including those related to sedative, hypnotic and cocaine withdrawal (J Am Med Assoc 1989; 262:3166); anabolic steroids act at the benzodiazepine/GABA receptor and may respond to benzodiazepine (J Am Med Assoc 1990; 263:2049c); the use of stanozolol (manufactured for horses, J Am Med Assoc 1990; 263:1699), an oral anabolic steroid, resulted in forfeiture of a gold medal in the men's 100-meter sprint (world record of 9.79 sec) in the 1988 Seoul Summer Olympics; the athlete in question's testosterone levels were 15% normal, indicating significant short-term hormonal suppression **Laboratory** Androgen analogs are detectable to levels 1 part per billion, four days after last use if the hormone is water-soluble, or 14 days after use in lipid-soluble compounds; one analog, nandrolone was detected up to 13 months after its alleged last use; see review J Am Med Assoc 1990; 264:2923; anabolic steroids have been conferred 'schedule III' drug status in the US under the Controlled Substances Act, thus prescriptions may be scrutinized according to registration, reporting, record keeping and prescribing practices; anabolic steroid prescriptions may be refilled no more often than 5 times within six months (J Am Med Assoc 1991; 265:1229) Note: The most flagrant abuse of anabolic steroids allegedly occurred in East Germany, where they were administered to Olympic athletes without regard to the potential effects; scientists became adept at creating formulations and delivery systems, eg intranasal spray, that eluded detection by Olympic drug-testing laboratories (Science 1991; 254:26n&v); see 'Roid rage, 'Stacking'

Anaclitic depression PEDIATRICS The result of disruption of the mother-child dyad; by six months, infants are strongly attached to the mother figure; if the children are separated from the mother figure after this point by the mother's death or incarceration and a substitute mother figure is provided, the initial panic and searching reactions give way to anxiety, ending with apathy and withdrawal, accompanied by hypotonia and inactivity, a saddened facial expression, profound disturbances in motor, social and language development and, when the reaction is extreme, death

Anaerobes Bacteria that grow optimally without oxygen; bacteria require from normal atmospheric pressure (21%) to less than 0.5% oxygen for optimal growth; Obligate or strict aerobes require molecular oxygen as a terminal electron acceptor, resulting in the formation of water and do not obtain energy by fermentative pathways, eg ***Micococcus*** and ***Pseudomonas*** species; Microaerophiles require oxygen as terminal electron acceptors but grow in neither atmospheric nor in anerobic environments, eg ***Campylobacter jejuni*** grows optimally in 5% O_2, 10% CO_2 and 85% N_2; facultative anaerobes grow in either environments, using oxygen as the terminal electron acceptor, yielding 38 ATP molecules when catabolizing a molecule of glucose, or in a 'pinch', utilizing glucose by the less energy-efficient fermentative metabolic pathway, yielding 2 ATP molecules, eg ***Escherichia coli***, ***Staphylococcus aureus***; aerotolerant anaerobes grow poorly in O_2 or CO_2 environments and are clearly happier under anaerobic conditions, eg ***Clostridium carnis, C histolyticum, C tertium***; Obligate anaerobes are divided into a) Moderate anaerobes capable of growth in reduced oxygen (2-8%) environment, eg ***Bacteroides fragilis, B melaninogenicus, Fusobacterium nucleatum, Clostridium perfringens*** and b) Strict aerobes that are incapable of growth in O_2 levels above 0.5%, eg ***Clostridium haemolyticum, C novyi B, Selenomonas ruminantium, Treponema denticola***; see Oxygen toxicity

Analgesic drug 'ladder' CLINICAL PHARMACOLOGY An algorithm for managing cancer pain, ie the levels of intensity of therapy: *FIRST STEP* Non-opioids with/without adjuvants (neurolytic blockage, cordotomy, chemical hypophysectomy and others) *SECOND STEP* Weak opioids, with/without non-opioids and/or adjuvants *THIRD STEP* Strong opioids, with/without non-opioids and/or adjuvants

Analgesic nephropathy Tubulointerstitial inflammation associated with papillary necrosis caused by ingestion of combinations of analgesics, including acetaminophen, aspirin and phenacetin which result in hematuria, renal colic and pyelonephritis; intravenous pyelogram reveals 'ring' shadows and multiple cavitations characteristic of papillary necrosis **Complications** Increased risk of future transitional cell carcinoma

Analog PHARMACOLOGY A drug or therapeutic substance whose effect mimics that of another, but which has a dissimilar chemical structure COMPUTERS (adjective) The mode in which most laboratory instruments produce information, where data is generated as non-discrete signals, as AC or DC current, voltage changes or pulse amplitudes; the analog data must be converted into a digital form before it can be manipulated by a computer, which, being a digital device, performs discrete mathematical operations

Analog computer LABORATORY MEDICINE A computer in

which the data is acquired in the form of continuous electrical variables across a continuum of temperature, pressure or flow; patient specimens evaluated by automated instruments in clinical chemistry and hematology yield analog data that must be converted into digital (discrete) information prior to its transfer to other sites in the hospital

'Anal-retentive' A colloquial term for a person with an 'anal personality', who, according to classic freudian psychoanalysis, has traits that arose in the anal phase of psychosexual development, in which defecation constituted the primary source of pleasure, and retention of feces is held to represent defiance to the parent; the typical 'anal-retentive' is obstinant, rigid, meticulous, compulsive and overconscientious, which is a behavioral profile typical of many physicians and scientists

Anal tag Swollen skin at the peripheral end of an anal fissure, often accompanied by pain on defecation and fresh bleeding

Analysis of variance see ANOVA STATISTICS A statistical method which determines whether the source of variability among data sets is due to true differences in the sets or due to random variations or 'statistical noise'; ANOVA compares the means of several random variables, assuming that each has a normal distribution with the same variance; these algorithms are quite complex and are usually computer-based

Anaphylactoid reaction An anaphylaxis-like reaction occurring without an allergen-IgE antibody event, caused by a nonimmune release, eg reaction to radiocontrast, chymopapain, aspirin of vasoactive and inflammatory mediators, including release of histamine

Anaphylaxis A hypersensitivity (Gel and Coombs type I) reaction that occurs upon exposure to an antigen to which the body has previously formed an IgE antibody; within seconds of exposure to the antigen, IgE molecules cross link on the surface of mast cells and basophils, stimulating the release of low molecular weight mediators of anaphylaxis; in the primary response, preformed molecules are released, including eosinophil chemotactic factor, heparin, histamine, serotonin and various enzymes; in the secondary response, acute phase reactants (see there) are produced and released

Anchor disease CD11/CD18 leukocyte glycoprotein deficiency A rare disease of neonatal onset with delayed umbilical cord separation, leukocytosis and poor wound healing, accompanied by defects in neutrophil adherence, chemotaxis, secretion, phagocytosis and particle-stimulated respiratory burst, resulting in severe recurring bacterial infections of mucocutaneous regions that become systemic; anchor disease is due to defective 180 kD membrane glycoprotein, the α subunit of the heterodimeric protein Mo1, the C3bi receptor of neutrophils and monocytes (Hem/Onc Clin N Am 1988; 2:13)

Anchorage TISSUE CULTURE Adherence by cells, usually fibroblasts to a solid or semisolid support medium, which is required for optimal growth; the loss of anchorage dependence is a hallmark of cell (malignant) transformation that may be induced by oncogenic viruses; see Cadherin, CAM (cell adhesion molecule); Cf Cell senescence

Anchovy paste appearance A descriptor for the olive-brown (less commonly, creamy white) grumous material seen in hepatic and cerebral amebiasis (***Entamoeba histolytica***), composed of autolyzed necrotic debris and hemorrhage (a lesion of middle-aged men)

Ancient schwannoma Degenerated neurilemmoma A benign, potentially large tumor of peripheral nerve that is most common in the retroperitoneal space characterized by cyst formation, calcification, hyalinization and hemorrhage Treatment Simple excision; see Peripheral nerve sheath tumor(s)

ANDA see Abbreviated new drug application

Andes' disease Mondor's disease see Mountain sickness

'Andy Gump' A descriptor for a patient with a diminutive mandible, which may be *A) CONGENITAL* and seen in Pierre-Robin deformity and in otocephaly; in the latter, the mandibular hypoplasia and associated deformities are incompatible with extra-uterine life *B) POST-SURGICAL* Resection of the upper mandible as part of aggressive surgery in cancer of the floor of the mouth and *C) POST-TRAUMATIC* A fracture unique to elderly edentulous subjects, in which there is posterior mandibular displacement and airway obstruction, thus known as an 'Andy Gump fracture' Note: Andy Gump was a syndicated comic strip character lacking a mandible

'Anecdotal' Unsubstantiated, as in anecdotal patient response to unproven cancer therapy, or anecdotal cause-and-effect relationship between a noxious environmental element and clinical disease; Cf Blinding

Anemia panel A group of laboratory parameters that have been determined to be the most cost-efficient, sensitive, specific in evaluating a patient with anemia; the anemia panel includes the CBC (complete blood count) with indices, reticulocyte count; if the anemia is hypochromic and microcytic, the panel should include iron levels, iron-binding capacity, measurement of the levels and percent saturation of ferritin; if the anemia is macrocytic, then vitamin B_{12} and folate levels are measured; see Organ panel

Anemone cell villiform tumor A heterogeneous group of large cell malignancies with numerous circumferential or polar microvilli, an ultrastructural finding that usually implies epithelial origin; the lack of tonofilaments and intercellular junctions implies that some of these tumors may actually be large cell lymphomas (Ultrastruc Path 1984; 7:143)

Anencephaly The congenital absence of a major portion of the brain, skull and scalp, an anomaly occurring in the first month of gestation, at a frequency of 0.14 to 0.7/1000 live births; the primary abnormality is failure of cranial neurulation, the embryologic process separating the forebrain precursors from the amniotic fluid; since the neural tissue is exposed, the cerebral tissue is hemorrhagic, fibrotic and gliotic without functional cortex Etiology Usually idiopathic, possibly multifactorial or polygenic in origin; most anencephalics die within the first week and are of use as potential organ donors (N

Engl J Med 1990; 322:669)

Anergy IMMUNOLOGY A state in which viable T cells have a diminished or absent lymphokine secretion when the T cell receptor is engaged by an antigen, which can be induced in mature and differentiated CD4+ T cells by exposure to complexes of antigen and appropriate (self) major histocompatibility complex in absence of certain uncharacterized co-stimulatory signals on the antigen-presenting cells (Science 1991; 251:1228); see Deletion

Aneuploid GENETICS A congenital or acquired alteration in the number of chromosomes that deviates from multiples of a haploid set of chromosomes, which in humans is 23 (normally present as a diploid complement, ie 23 + 23); the degree of aneuploidy in a dividing population of cells can be analyzed by flow cytometry and carries a negative prognostic significance in epithelial malignancies including breast carcinoma and endometrial carcinoma; Cf Polyploidy

Aneurysmal bone cyst (ABC) A metaphyseal lesion of the long bones of young patients, seen as a physalliferous osteolytic cortical expansion, likened to a soap bubble; the term aneurysmal bone cyst is, like pyogenic granuloma and ganglion cyst, a misnomer that has withstood the sands of time and the dint of logic, since it is neither an aneurysm nor a cyst **Histopathology** Blood-filled space partially lined by fibrous tissue, mixed with osteocytes, fibroblasts, histiocytes and giant cells **Treatment** Curettage, optional filling with bone chips

'Angel dust' see PCP

'Angel of death' J Mengele, a Nazi who committed medically Auschwitz concentration camp, who eluded authorities and drowned in Brazil in 1979; Cf 'Death angel'

Angel wing sign A pattern of symmetrical perihilar 'soft' radiodensities seen on a plain chest film in patients with simple silicosis, due to massive fibrosis where large masses are most prominent in the upper lobes; the term 'Angel wings' has also been used as descriptor for the findings of neonatal pneumomediastinum, see Spinnaker sail sign

Angina, recurrent Sharp precordial pain directly related to cardiac ischemia, occurring in 3-5% of patients with coronary artery bypass surgery, due either to progressive stenosis or occlusion of a bypass graft or progressive stenosis in a previously ungrafted artery **UNSTABLE ANGINA** Acute (less than 6 months in duration) coronary insufficiency in which the symptoms are intermediate in severity between stable angina pectoris and myocardial infarction, *SUBDIVIDED INTO: 1) SEVERE, FREQUENT ANGINA PECTORIS OF NEW ONSET*, 1-2 months in duration and anginal pain occurring at low or no workload *2) CRESCENDO ANGINA* Confirmed coronary artery disease and a well-established pattern of stable angina with recent diminution of exercise tolerance and blunting of response to sublingual nitroglycerin and *3) ANGINA AT REST* The group at greatest risk for subsequent myocardial infarction with frequent and prolonged at-rest anginal attacks, see Silent ischemia (Mayo Clin Proc 1990; 65:384) **VARIANT ANGINA** A form of angina attributed to a focal magnesium deficiency; although the serum levels are the same as normal subjects, those with coronary spasm retained more magnesium after infusion (Am J Cardiol 1990; 65:709)

Angiogenic factors A group of substances present in the circulation, most of which are polypeptides, including angiogenin, fibroblast growth factor, transforming growth factors as well as some lipids

Angiogenin A 14 kD polypeptide that induces vascularization in normal fetal development and wound healing as well as in cancer and in diabetes; angiogenin's presence in the liver implies physiologic roles other than angiogenesis

Angioid streaks Peripapillary, gray in non-Caucasians to red-brown in Caucasians linear striations radiating from the optic fundus along stress lines or toward the equator in an abnormal Bruch's membrane; one-half of cases of angioid streaks occur in patients with pseudoxanthoma elasticum; angioid streaks also occur in fundi rendered brittle by calcium (tumor-related calcinosis), heavy metal, eg lead intoxication and may be seen in acromegaly, a-β-lipoproteinemia, diabetes mellitus, hemochromatosis, hemolytic anemia, hypercalcinosis, hyperphosphatasia, idiopathic thrombocytopenic purpura, myopia, neurofibromatosis, Paget's disease of the bone, senile elastosis, sickle cell anemia, Sturge-Weber syndrome and tuberous sclerosis

Angioimmunoblastic lymphadenopathy (AILA) A condition first described in 1975 by Lukes (N Engl J Med 1975; 292:1) as a hyperimmune B-cell proliferation, characterized by a triad of histopathologic changes: 1) Pleomorphic infiltrate of small and large immunoblasts and plasma cells with effacement of nodal architecture 2) Arborizing vascular proliferation with endothelial cell hyperplasia and 3) Interstitial deposits of amorphous eosinophilic PAS-positive, presumably cellular debris **Clinical** Polyclonal gammopathy, middle aged to elderly patients, hemolytic anemia, fever, night sweats, weight loss, generalized lymphadenopathy, hepatosplenomegaly, skin rashes **Median survival** 15 months; some cases evolve to immunoblastic lymphoma or monoclonal gammopathy **Differential diagnosis** AIDS, angiofollicular lymphoid hyperplasia, drug reaction, histiocytosis X, Hodgkin's disease, immunoblastic lymphoma, malignant histiocytosis, atypical or reactive lymphoid hyperplasia

Angiotensin II (A-II) A molecule derived from angiotensin I that elicits varying responses in the cardiovascular system, neurons and electrolyte transport regulation; the cognate receptor is unstable, present in low concentrations, has a transmembrane topology similar to G protein-coupled receptors and is highly concentrated in the adrenal medulla, cortex and in the kidneys (Nature 1991; 351:230); the A-II receptor is divided into two forms, of which the AT1 receptor is held responsible for controlling blood pressure and volume (Nature 1991; 351:233)

Angiotropic (malignant) lymphoma Malignant angioendotheliomatosis A lesion first described as a neoplastic vascular proliferation that was later shown to be either a B-cell, or less commonly, a T-cell lymphoma with a predilection for intravascular spaces **Clinical** Onset with multiple indurated and erythematous plaques or papules mimicking erythema nodosum, fever, neurological signs, minimal involvement of lymph nodes, bone marrow and spleen; see Lymphoma

Angle du mort A common site of leakage in gastroenterostomy, specifically where the residual gastric pouch of a Hofmeister closure meets the anastomotic line with the small intestine

Animalcule Anton van Leuwenhoek's term for the first microorganisms he saw with his microscope

'Animal House fever' A limited outbreak of organic dust syndrome; the index report occurred in a college fraternity 'rush' party, which in the USA is an exercise in bacchanalian revelry; those who consumed more than ten drinks (see 'Standard drink') had more acute symptoms of pulmonary mycotoxicosis related to the fresh fungus-laden straw spread on the party floor which caused the air to be visibly thick with organic dust composed of fungal hyphae and spores Clinical Shaking chills or sweats, cough or shortness of breath and myalgia; the term Animal House fever was coined after a motion picture about a college fraternity, entitled 'Animal House' (J Am Med Assoc 1987; 258:1219ed) and is distinct from Silo-filler's disease, a chemical pneumonitis due to NO_2 exposure and Farmer's lung, an acute hypersensitivity pneumonitis, in which repeated exposure to organic dusts containing thermophilic fungi may progress to interstitial lung disease

Animals rights activism A movement that believes in and fights for the humane treatment of animals; the organizations include ALF (Animal Liberation Front), a group listed as a terrorist organization by US Federal Bureau of Investigation and by Scotland Yard, Nature 1991; 349:13c), PAWS (Performing Animal Welfare Society) and PETA (People for Ethical Treatment of Animals); researchers have become victims of acts ranging from destruction of records and equipment to extreme violence; scientists have responded to this movement by reducing the number of animals used, refining procedures and replacement of animals, where possible, with alternate experimental models (J Am Med Assoc 1990; 263:936, ibid, 262:2716, N Engl J Med 1991; 324:1640ed) Note: 20 million animals are used in biomedical research in the US (the US Department of Agriculture, the responsible regulatory agency, considers dogs, cats and monkeys as animals, and mice, rats and birds as something else, Nature 1991; 350:642n); see Silver Springs monkeys, Toxicity testing

Animal Welfare Act A legislative act by the US Congress in 1985 and re-written in early 1991 with the purpose that animals not be subjected to senseless pain and suffering; the Act required $800 million for the construction of newer facilities and an additional $200 million/year in operating expenses for improved sanitation and requiring humane treatment with 30 minutes of exercise and socialization and 60 minutes of 'positive physical contact with a human' (Science 1989; 243:17); compliance was re-estimated to cost $537 million (Nature 1991; 349:641ed)

Anion gap The urinary anion gap is calculated as sodium plus potassium minus chloride and is a crude index of the levels of urinary ammonium and used to evaluate hyperchloremic metabolic acidosis; a negative anion gap implies gastrointestinal loss of bicarbonate; a positive anion gap suggests defective renal tubular acidification (N Engl J Med 1988; 318:594)

ANLL Acute nonlymphocytic leukemia

Ann Arbor classification A system for staging Hodgkin's disease, thereby guiding therapy; clinical data is added based on A (absence) or B (presence) of associated symptoms, eg night sweats, fever or weight loss of > 10%; other symptoms of Hodgkin's disease include lethargy, fatigability, anorexia and pruritus

ANN ARBOR CLASSIFICATION

- I Single involved lymphoid region, organ or site
- II Two or more involved lymphoid regions, or one extralymphoid site and a lymphoid region on the same side of the diaphragm
- III Lymphoid regions involved on both sides of the diaphragm, variably accompanied by localized involvement of extralymphatic organs or spleen
- IV Disseminated involvement of one or more extralymphatic organs or tissues, with or without associated lymphadenopathy

Anneal see Reanneal

Anniversary phenomenon Sudden death related to psychological trauma that elicits an exaggerated autonomic nervous system response and fatal arrhythmia, inexplicably occurring on the anniversary of a past event; see Voodoo death; Cf Harvest Moon phenomenon

Anomalad A dysmorphogenic complex characterized by a primary malformation and its derived structural defects (eg Pierre-Robin syndrome with cleft palate, glossoptosis and micrognathia); Cf Sequence

ANOVA see Analysis of variance

ANP see Atrionatriuretic peptide

Anterior cleavage syndrome Mesodermal dysgenesis OPHTHALMOLOGY Anomalous development of the anterior segment of the eye with corneal opacification, abnormal anterior chamber angle, potentially glaucoma and abnormalities of the iris

Anterior cord syndrome A spinal cord injury complex with loss of voluntary motor function, pain and temperature sensation and intact distal position, vibratory and light touch sensation, dysfunctional anterior and lateral columns and intact posterior columns; the anterior cervical cord syndrome is a variation on this theme, caused by trauma to the relatively mobile cervical vertebrae, common in whiplash-type injury (spinal hyperextension)

Anterior horn disease NEUROLOGY A group of conditions that predominantly affect the anterior horns of the spinal cord, including Werdnig-Hoffmann disease or infantile spinal muscle atrophy, the classic 'floppy infant' syndrome, characterized by hypotonia, symmetrical areflexic weakness with death by age two, amyotrophic lateral sclerosis, a distal disease of adults with fasciculations and wasting of 'bulbar' muscles and poliomyelitis, which is characterized by fever, asymmetric distal involvement, later becoming generalized, with muscle weakness of respiratory and bulbar muscles

Anthropology Time-table of the development of ***Homo sapiens*** 36 000 000 YEARS BC ***Dryopithecus*** The hairy, tree-climbing herbivorous ancestor of all primates with a 200 cc cranial capacity (CC) **15 000 000** BC Orangutans and gorillas dropped out of the competition to become Earth's intelligent life and stopped evolving; ***Ramapithecus***, the oldest hominid, with a 350 cc CC, was a vegetarian, walked on all fours with less dependence on the upper extremities, and spread from Africa to Southeast Asia **4 000 000** BC ***Australopithecus*** had a 450 cc CC, measured 1.2 meters with bipedal locomotion, but had yet to figure out how to make and use tools **2 500 000 BC** Australopithecus split, one branch died, the other had by **1 500 000 BC** begun to kill for meals Note: The 2-8 000 000 year period is important as man began to walk fully erect, had formed the primitive family unit of male breadwinner and female homemaker and women had developed continuous sexual availability, which was hormone-dependent,rather than seasonal, ie estrus cycling **2 000 000** BC ***Homo habilis*** had a 500-750 cc CC, was slightly under 1.5 meters tall, had an ape-like jaw, used tools, killed and ate raw meat and used iron-based pigments for painting **1 500 000** BC ***H erectus*** had a 1100 cc CC, was the first known human ancestor to walk fully erect, used and made tools, invented fire, wandered off to Southeast Asia into Indonesia, the Java man and into China the Peking man **100 000** BC ***H sapiens*** had a 1400 cc CC, lived in caves; some of his paintings survive; at the time, the planet's population was 2 million; neanderthals lived from **250 000** TO **30 000** BC Note: Man's evolution is thought to have been that of australopithicene ape-men and/or ***H habilis***, who evolved into ***H erectus,*** an arguably distinct species, who then developed into ***H sapiens*** (GP Rightmire, The Evolution of Homo erectus, Cambridge University Press, 1990); see Lucy, Mitochondrial 'Eve'

Antibiotic bonding A technique that pretreats plastics to be used for indwelling devices, eg intravascular catheters, in order to prevent coating by bacterial glycocalyx, which counteracts opsonization, rendering systemic antibiotics ineffective **Method** Catheters are pretreated with a cationic surfactant material, tridodecylmethylammonium chloride, which enables subsequent bonding of anionic antibiotics, eg cephalosporins, penicillins (J Am Med Assoc 1991; 265:2364)

Antibody see Immunoglobulin

Antibody-dependent cell cytotoxicity see ADCC

Antibody titer The level of a specific antibody that is present in the circulation, usually as a result of an acquired infection; titers usually rise abruptly at the time of infection and fall slowly; meaningful evaluation of a subject's exposure to an infection requires that the specimen be drawn at two different time intervals, as one 'draw' merely indicates exposure

Anticardiolipin (antibody) syndrome 'Circulating lupus anticoagulant syndrome' (CLAS) A clinical condition characterized by the presence of circulating anticardiolipin antibodies (which overlap with lupus anticoagulants) that may be seen in lupus patients in association with a) Thromboembolic phenomena, associated with habitual abortion, due to thrombosis of placental vessels, recurrent myocardial infarction, pulmonary hypertension, occasionally also cerebral and renal infarction; the thrombosis may be related to the antibodies which inhibit PGI_2 (prostacyclin) production and interfere with the release of arachidonic acid from the cell membrane b) Neurologic dysfunction (myelopathy, chorea, epilepsy, transient ischemic attacks, migraines, amaurosis fugax) and others, eg livido reticularis, labile hypertension, thrombocytopenia, Coombs' positivity and hemolytic anemia; the antibody is thought to cause disease by acting on platelet membranes or vascular endothelia; high titers (> 7 standard deviations) of IgG anti-cardiolipin antibodies are reported to be 80% specific for this condition Note: In absence of previous spontaneous fetal loss, elevation of the anticardiolipin antibody is not a risk factor for fetal wastage (N Engl J Med 1991; 325:1063); anti-cardiolipin antibodies cross-react with DNA, explaining the biological false positive serological test for syphilis commonly seen in lupus patients; Cf Lupus anticoagulant

Anticytoplasmic antibody Neutrophil cytoplasm antibody A circulating antibody that is present in 84-100% of patients with active generalized Wegener's disease (Mayo Clin Proc 1990; 65:1110) and when elevated in HIV-1 infections, is regarded as biologically false positive; anti-NCA are quantified by flow cytometry and indirect fluorescent microscopy

'Anti-dumping' laws Legislation that has been enacted in the USA to prevent the inappropriate transferral of patients, who are medically unstable, eg in early labor or impending rupture of aortic aneurysm, to other health care facilities; these laws were enacted in the wake of a case in Texas, where an indigent pregnant woman was transferred 240 km to another hospital, allegedly motivated by a financial decision (Am Med News 23/Sep/91); see Dumping

Antifolate chemotherapy The use of an antimetabolite, methotrexate to compete with folate, inhibiting dihydrofolate reductase, the enzyme responsible for reducing inactive dihydrofolate into the active tetrahydrofolate form; this block causes a buildup of toxic dihydrofolate, shutting down synthesis of purine nucleotides and thymidylate; antifolate therapy is used to treat malignancy; see Leukovorin rescue

Antigen-antibody complex see Immune complex

Antigen capture assay An assay designed to detect low levels of antigen in sera or supernatants **Method** A solid surface is coated with purified high-titer antibodies to an antigen of interest; a fluid presumed to contain the antigen of interest is washed over the solid surface and the antigen, if present, is 'captured'; a second antibody with an attached 'marker', eg an enzyme, is then used to detect the presence of the captured antigen; this technique found temporary use for detecting HIV positivity, but is far less sensitive than the polymerase chain reaction

Antigenic drift A relatively minor change that occurs

every year or every several years in the genome of a virus, classically occurring in subtypes of influenza A, which are named based on the three different hemagglutinins (H1, H2, H3) and two different neuraminidases (N1, N2), and result from point mutations of the DNA encoding these proteins; see Influenza A

Antigenic shift A major change in a genome due to gene rearrangement(s) between two related organisms, eg that which occurs when two subtypes of influenza A simultaneously infect one cell; antigenic shift is rare but results in completely new antigens for which a population is immunologically 'naive', resulting in a potential for major epidemics; see Influenza A

Antigen-presenting cells (APC) A heterogeneous group of immune cells that present antigen (usually a peptide) to immune-responsive lymphocytes, eg CD4 helper T cells, an activity that is thought to be mediated by a peptide supply factor encoded by a transporter gene in the major histocompatability complex (Nature 1991; 351:323, 271); 'traditional' APCs include macrophages, Langerhans cells or dendritic reticulum cells that actively 'process' antigen; 'facultative' APCs include B cells, keratinocytes, endothelial cells and Kupffer cells, which are more passsive antigen carriers; APCs are divided into: a) APCs presenting exogenous antigen found in the extracellular fluid; these antigens are processed in the endosomal compartment of the APCs and displayed in association with MHC class II molecules, b) APCs presenting endogenously synthesized antigen produced by all self cells which are processed in a distinct intracellular compartment and displayed in association with MHC class I molcules and c) APCs presenting exogenous antigen that is internalized, processed and presented in association with MHC class I molecules (Science 1990; 249:918); see MHC restriction

Antiglobulin test Coombs' test A test used to detect the presence of incomplete antibodies, eg anti-Rh_0 to red cell antigens; after washing away other serum proteins, the anti-Rh_0 IgG remains attached to the red cell surface; these erythrocytes may then be agglutinated by the addition of rabbit anti-human IgG raised in the direct antiglobulin test (DAT or direct Coombs' test); red cell antigens are either IgM (causing direct in vitro agglutination—due to the multiple binding sites on IgM) or IgG (which due to its small size and few binding sites is incapable of bridging the gap between two erythrocytes, due to the repulsive electrostatic forces); true positive DAT occurs in hemolytic anemia, non-specific uptake of protein on the red cell surfaces and transfusion reactions; false positive DAT occurs with insufficiently washed cells, absence of the antibody in the Coombs serum, high dissociation due to loss of antigen from the red cell membranes and low levels of IgG coating the red cells; the indirect antiglobulin test (IAT) is performed on commercial (reagent) group O cells to detect antibodies in the serum capable of causing a transfusion reaction; IAT is also used in crossmatching, antibody screening and identification, red cell typing, determining antibody titers and D^u testing

Antilymphocyte serum An antiserum 'raised' in one species against the lymphocytes of another species, which, upon injection, causes profound lymphopenia; Antilymphocyte serum formerly had currency in immunosuppression for ameliorating graft rejection

Antimongoloid slant Antimongolic fissures A descriptor for a downward slant of the eyelid in the horizontal plane that is opposite that of mongoloids; the finding is non-specific and may be seen in various congenital syndromes, including: Franceschetti or oculomandibulofacial syndrome, accompanied by a bird facies and in Treacher-Collins syndrome

Antimongoloid syndrome An inherited disease caused by a partial deletion of chromosome 21 characterized by mental retardation, antimongoloid palpebral slant, craniofacial dysmorphia, pyloric stenosis, retarded skeletal growth, cryptorchidism and hypospadias

Antineoplastons Two substances purportedly isolated from urinary peptides that are alleged to have antineoplastic activity and claimed to inhibit the growth of osteosarcoma and myeloblastic leukemia; the National Cancer Institute (USA) has concluded that this agent has no effect in treating malignancy

Antinuclear antibodies (ANA) Any of a group of circulating antibodies that are directed against a variety of antigens in the nucleus, including histone, double- and single-stranded DNA and ribonucleoprotein, commonly seen in connective tissue diseases; in the usual test for anti-nuclear antibodies, the patient's serum is incubated with a standard tissue, eg Hep-2 cells, and the presence of ANA is detected by fluorescence microscopy (see figure page 28); the homogeneous pattern is characteristic of ANA against ribonucleoprotein, seen in lupus erythematosus (SLE), rheumatoid arthritis, progressive systemic sclerosis (PSS) and others; the 'rim' or 'shaggy' pattern of staining is associated with antibodies to ribonucleoprotein and DNA and is most typical of SLE; the nucleolar pattern is typical of the anti-RNA ANA seen in PSS; the speckled pattern may be seen in all forms of connective tissue disease and thus is highly non-specific; see Speckled pattern

Anti-phospholipid antibodies see Anticardiolipin antibodies, Lupus anticoagulants

Antiporter see Na^+/H^+ antiporter

Antipromoter ONCOLOGY Any substance that blocks the action of a promoter molecule in carcinogenesis, potentially acting at any stage in the transformation sequence; these substances include dietary fiber, vitamins A, C and E, selenium, indoles, flavones and isothiocyanates; see Tumor promoter

Anti-Purkinje cell antibody A circulating antibody that has been associated with subacute cerebellar degeneration and gynecologic, especially ovarian malignancy (Mayo Clin Proc 1990; 64:1558)

Antisense DNA DNA is composed of two nucleotide helices; when a gene transcribes information, encoding a chain of mRNA that is translated into a protein; the helix opens, revealing a 'sense' strand and an 'antisense' strand of DNA; the antisense strand of DNA acts as a template, yielding a sense mRNA; the other, *SENSE* strand of DNA encodes an *ANTISENSE* mRNA, which con-

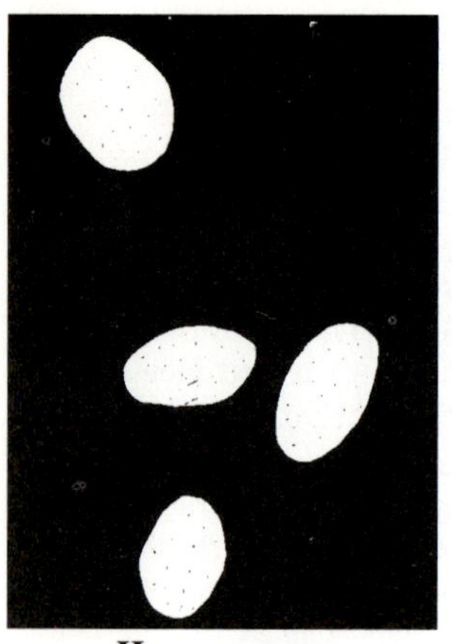
Homogenous

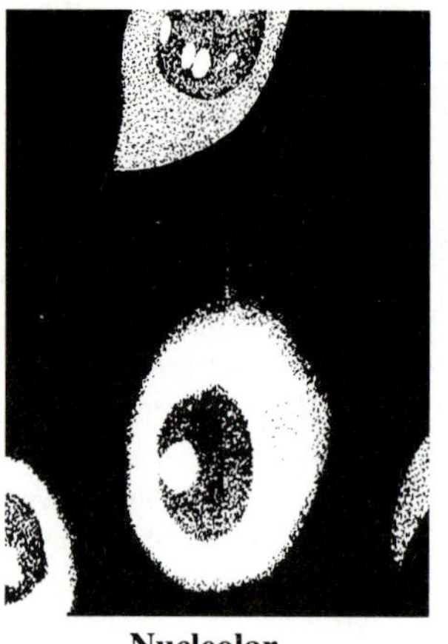
Nucleolar

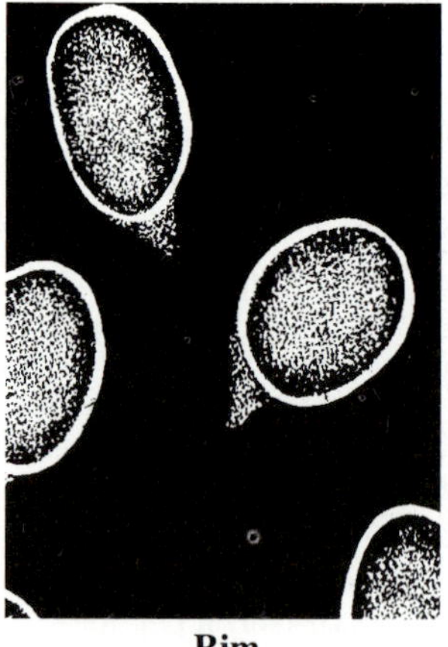
Rim

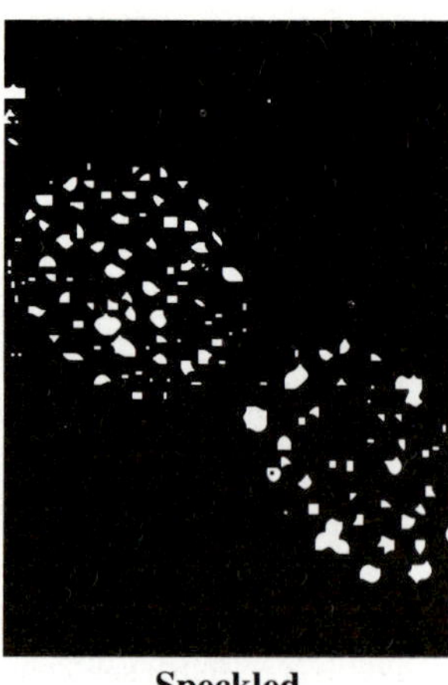
Speckled

trols the production of certain enzymes; antisense mRNA can link to its mirror image sense mRNA, preventing translation; the possibilities for this technology, potentially representing a new therapeutic tool, direct antisense oligonucleotides against viral sequences and activated oncogenes; see Triple helix (Sci Am 1990; 262/1:40)

Antisense RNA An RNA molecule produced from altered DNA that is an exact mirror image of the packaging sequence of retroviral RNA, which prevents it from binding with the packaging protein, thus yielding new (but empty) viral particles without the genetic information needed to infect other cells; an antisense strategy might be of use in protecting patients infected with HIV, possibly introducing the antisense message into stem cells (Proc Natl Acad Sci 1991; May 15, 1991 Lei Han

Anti-sense therapy An as-yet hypothetical therapeutic modality for treating tumor and viruses that would be based on antisense RNA, where complementary strands of nucleotides are used to turn off defective genes; antisense therapy would consist of administering an antisense DNA or an RNA strand mirror-image of an oncogene's mRNA 'sense' strand; since the mRNA can only act in a single-stranded state, the oncogene cannot 'drive' tumor proliferation; interference with a regulatory gene could potentially evoke translational arrest, a goal being actively pursued in AIDS research, targeting HIV-1's rev (art/trs), using antisense phosphorothioate oligodeoxynucleotides (Proc Natl Acad Sci 1989; 86:4244)

Anti-sperm antibody Any of a group of antibodies produced against various components of the sperm; low titers (< 1:8) of anti-sperm antibody are present in 90% of prepubertal boys and are of no significance; 50% of infertile female have levels of 1:16 or greater, most commonly anti-sperm (immobilizing) tail IgG or IgA antibodies, while male homosexuals tend to develop anti-sperm head (agglutinating) IgM antibodies

Antitampering Act A US federal law (PL 98-127) that criminalizes tampering (changing the labeling or content) of non-prescription ingestible consumer products; the legislature was enacted on the heels of an 'incident' in the early 1980s, in which a cyanide-bearing compound was placed by an unknown perpetrator in bottles containing a proprietary, over-the-counter acetaminophen-based analgesic, resulting in seven deaths in the Chicago area Note: Tampering with pharmaceuticals carries a fine of $25-100 000 and imprisonment of up to 20 years

Antithymocyte globulin (ATG) A therapeutic agent that has currency in treating aplastic anemia, especially in older patients and/or in those who lack a HLA-matched sibling donor; ATG is pooled monomeric horse IgG prepared from the plasma or serum of several healthy horses hyperimmunized with human thymic lymphocytes; commercial ATG contains 50 mg/ml of equine immunoglobulin and its therapeutic use is associated with 50% marrow recovery compared to no recovery without therapy Side effects Serum sickness occurs in most of those treated, rarely, anaphylaxis

Antitrust laws Legislation and statutes that limit the ability of an organization or group of individuals to monopolize a service (or product), thereby controlling and restricting free trade; in the US, physicians may be prevented from certain vehicles of professional organization by antitrust laws, reducing the art of medicine to the equations of commerce

Antler pattern see Staghorn pattern

ANUG see Acute necrotizing ulcerative gingivitis

Aortic arches EMBRYOLOGY An array of six paired arteries that arise from the aortic sac in conjunction with the branchial arches formed in the fourth and fifth weeks of embryologic development, the vast bulk of which disappears shortly thereafter; the residuum of the first arch corresponds to the adult maxillary artery, the second arch gives rise to the hyoid and stapedial arteries; the third aortic arch forms the common carotid and the first segment of the internal carotid artery; the fourth arch persists on both sides of the embryo, forming part of the adult aortic arch on the left and the most proximal segment of the right subclavian artery on the right; the fifth arch is transient; the sixth arch gives rise to the proximal segment of the right pulmonary artery on the right and the ductus arteriosus on the left side; Cf Pharyngeal arches

Aortic arch syndrome Takayasu's disease

Aortic nipple sign RADIOLOGY A normal variation of the

cardiac shadow seen on a plain chest film at the aortic arch, causing the unwary to misdiagnose a tumor or lymphadenopathy; the 'nipple' corresponds to the left superior intercostal vein, enlarged when it serves as collateral circulation (Radiology 1970; 95:533)

AP-1 family MOLECULAR BIOLOGY A protein that binds to the DNA binding site TGACTCA, an 'enhancer' region, a site incriminated in tumor induction by tumor promoters; AP-1 may be an intermediate in transmitting information from the cell surface via protein kinase C to the nucleus; homodimeric cJun can bind directly to the AP-1 recognition site, but the homodimeric cFos only participates in the binding as heterodimeric cFos/cJun (joined by a leucine zipper motif, explaining how heterologous proto-oncogenes function (Science 1989; 243:1689, 1695); see Leucine zipper

AP-2 A mammalian transcription factor, ie a DNA-binding protein, that when dimerized, binds to cAMP and the phorbol ester inducible sequence motif found in the cis-regulatory regions of various viral and cellular genes (Science 1991; 251:1067)

APACHE II INTENSIVE CARE MEDICINE An acronym for acute physiology and chronic health evaluation, second generation evaluation, a system of objective criteria for predicting the outcome of critically ill patients in an ICU based on age, physiologic status and underlying health; it acts as a tool for scoring the severity of illness in patients admitted in an intensive care unit; the APACHE II scores total 71 points and are derived from age (maximum, 6 points), physiologic status based on 12 physiologic parameters (maximum, 60 points), chronic health problems (maximum, 5 points) and reasons for admission to the intensive care unit, yielding a weighted diagnostic component (Mayo Clin Proc 1990; 65:1549); according to one study, APACHE II offers little advantage over the simple 'eyeballing' of patients by ICU residents (physicians in training) and attendings in predicting patients' outcome (J Am Med Assoc 1988; 260:1739); see Medisgroups, Prognostic scoring systems

Apartheid medicine	Black	White
Per capita health care expenditure	$51	$201
Hospitals	Overcrowded	Underutilized
Infant mortality	5.6-fold greater than whites	
Life expectancy	13 years less than white males	
Tuberculosis	15-fold greater than whites	
Cause of death	Infections Parasites	Cancer Cardiovascular

Apartheid medicine The health care system practiced until recently in the Republic of South Africa, which was historically a 'soft' some extension of the government's racial discrimination policies; health care professionals who protested about the tortures or treated former detainees were regularly harassed or inexplicably committed suicide while in police custody (J Am Med Assoc 1990; 264:2097); see Academic boycott, Biko, Torture

Apathetic hyperthyroidism A masked hyperthyroidism, most commonly seen in depressed older patients, where the hypermetabolic state is manifested by weight loss and congestive heart failure, complicated by supraventricular tachyarrhythmias

APC see Antigen-presenting cells

APC gene A gene located on chromosome 5q reported to encode a protein with tumor suppressor activity; see Tumor suppressor genes

APECED Autoimmune polyendocrinopathy-candidiasis-ectodermal dystrophy An autosomal recessive disorder characterized by a variable combination of failure of a) Parathyroid and thyroid glands, adrenal cortex, gonads, pancreatic β cells, gastric parietal cells and hepatitis, b) Chronic mucocutaneous candidiasis and c) Dystrophy of the dental enamel, nails, alopecia, vitiligo and keratopathy Clinical Hypoparathyroidism, adrenocortical failure, gonadal failure, candidiasis, malabsorption (N Engl J Med 1990; 322:1829)

APGAR score A bedside test to evaluate a neonate's post-partum status and potential for survival in the neonatal period, based on an acronym of Virginia Apgar's name, where each of five parameters: Appearance or color, Pulse, Grimace-reflex, Activity or muscle tone and Respiratory effort, is give a value of 0 to 2, the higher the score, the better the infant will fare during the neonatal period (Anesth Analg 1953; 32:260)

Apheresis see Hemapheresis

Aphrodisiac Any agent, eg rhinocerous horn, that is alleged to increase libido or the duration of sexual activity, none of which has survived scientific scrutiny; agents that have a 'positive' effect on libido, eg testosterone, yohimbine and bupropion, have side effects that make any amorous gain a Pyrrhic victory; see Spanish fly, Yohimbine

Apical cap sign RADIOLOGY 1) A subtle blush or shadow on a plain chest film in the left lung apex caused by blood leaking from a traumatically ruptured aorta into the pleura, indicating a need for emergency aortic aortography and surgery 2) Dunce cap sign A finding on a plain abdominal film in pheochromocytomas; the enlarged rounded tumor located in the adrenal medulla forms the 'head' and the triangular dunce-cap representing the normal residual cortex which may be pushed superiorly

apo- A prefix indicating the protein component of a conjugated molecule, eg apoferritin, apolipoprotein

Apolipoproteins A family of molecules that comprise the protein moiety of lipoproteins; the ABC designation for apolipoproteins was first used in 1971 and subsequently popularized; coronary artery disease is associated with decreased ApoA-I, ApoA-II and HDL-cholesterol or increased ApoB, cholesterol and triglycerides APOA ApoA is the major protein (60% total) component of HDL; both ApoA subtypes are synthesized in the liver and intestine and catabolized in the liver and kidney APOA-I A 28.3 kD single chain protein that activates lecithin:cholesterol acyltransferase and comprises 75% of the ApoA in HDL APOA-II A 17 kD protein of unknown function composed of two identical disulfide

Apolipoproteins

Type	Serum level*	MW‡	Component of:
A-I	40/110	28 kD	HDL, band 1.21, chylomicrons)
A-II	25/40	17 kD	HDL
B-100	1.7/90	250 kD	LDL, VLDL
B-48	Trace	120 kD	Chylomicrons
C-I	8.5/5.5	6 kD	Chylomicrons, VLDL, HDL, LDL
C-II	6/5.5	9 kD	Chylomicrons, VLDL, HDL, LDL
C-III	13 /13	9 kD	HDL, VLDL, chylomicrons, LDL
E	1.2/4.5	37 kD	VLDL, chylomicrons, HDL, LDL

*SI (μmol/L)/US (mg/dl)

‡Molecular weight in kilodaltons

bond-linked polypeptides that constitutes 20% of HDL **ApoB** A protein that is the major component (95%) of LDL and comprises 40% of chylomicrons and VLDL; ApoB is divided into ApoB-100 and ApoB-48, which share the amino terminal sequences and 'kringle' domains **ApoB-100** A 550 kD protein synthesized in the liver that is the major component in lipoproteins of endogenous origin (LDL, VLDL, IDL), provides the recognition signal targeting LDL to the LDL (apoB, E) receptor and is considered l'enfant terrible of atherosclerosis; ApoB-100's sequence is similar to plasminogen, thereby linking thrombosis with atherosclerosis **ApoB-48** A 250 kD protein that is a major chylomicron component synthesized in the intestine that terminates shortly after an organ-specific RNA stop codon (UAA; a certain amount translates beyond UAA, producing a protein similar to hepatic Apo B-100); ApoB-48 has an obligatory role in the synthesis of chylomicrons and is essential for the intestinal absorption of dietary fats and fat-soluble vitamins **ApoC** A major component of VLDL and a minor component of HDL and LDL, divided into **ApoC-I** A 6.5 kD protein that is a minor component of VLDL, HDL and LDL **ApoC-II** A 8.8 kD protein that is minor constituent of VLDL and HDL, which activates lipoprotein lipase and is essential for the clearance of chylomicrons and VLDL; congenital ApoC-II deficiency (Breckenridge syndrome) is an autosomal recessive condition characterized by recurring pancreatitis; with time, diabetes mellitus Laboratory Hypertriglyceridemia, increased cholesterol; absent Apo C-II, 50% decreased apo A-I, A-II and B, marked decrease in LDL and HDL, marked increase in chylomicrons and VLDL, mild increase in apolipoprotein E (N Engl J Med 1978; 298:1265) Treatment Dietary **ApoC-III** A 8.7 kD protein inhibitor of lipoprotein lipase, a major constituent of chylomicrons and VLDL; ApoC-III over-expression induced in transgenic mice, results in hypertriglyceridemia (Science 1990; 249:790) **ApoE** A 34 kD protein encoded on chromosome 19, secreted by macrophages that mediates the uptake of lipoproteins (VLDL, HDL, LDL and cholesterol esters) into cells by virtue of different binding domains for the each receptor; the LDL receptor has a leucine zipper motif (Science 1991; 252:1817) Note: Defective ApoE binds poorly to the LDL-receptor and causes type III hyperlipoproteinemia

Apoptosis An intrinsic 'program' of cell death characterized by chromatin condensation and DNA degradation; apoptosis is a mechanism used by the immune system for antigen-induced clonal deletion of cortical thymocytes, ie immune tolerance (Science 1990; 250:1721), and is the most common form of eukaryotic cell death in embryogenesis, metamorphosis, tissue atrophy and tumor regression, induced by cytotoxic T-lymphocytes, killer and natural killer cells, lymphotoxins and glucocorticoids, withdrawal of interleukins or by targeting with the potentially therapeutic monoclonal antibody, APO-1 (Science 1989; 245:301)

Apoptotic cells Dense, eosinophilic, pyknotic cells surrounded by a thin clear space, often lying within epithelium

APP Amyloid β protein precursor A membrane-spanning glycoprotein expressed in many mammalian tissues, encoded by a gene located on chromosome 21 Note: A 40-amino acid fragment of APP, known as A4 is a major component of amyloid and accumulates in Alzheimer's diseased brains; of the possible alternately spliced APP transcripts, the most commonly expressed APP contains exons of 56- and 19- residues; the 56-residue exon has 50% homology to the Kunitz serine proteinase inhibitors (KPI), and like KPI, inhibits trypsin

Apparent volume of distribution (aVD) CLINICAL PHARMACOLOGY The ratio of the total amount of drug in the body to the concentration of the drug in the plasma, or the 'apparent' volume necessary to contain the entire amount of the drug if the drug in the entire body were in the same concentration as in the plasma; the aVD doesn't correspond to any fluid volume per se and in the case of those drugs stored in adipose tissues, the aVD may be hundreds of times larger than the body's volume! thus a large aVD would indicate that most of a drug is stored in tissue; the aVD for any one drug is a constant which allows correlation of the plasma to tissue levels

Apple core appearance see Napkin ring lesion

Apple core erosions Circumferential narrowing of the femoral neck caused by erosion initiated by extrinsic pathological processes in the hip joint, seen in synovial osteochondromatosis, pigmented villonodular synovitis, rheumatoid arthritis, amyloidosis and multicentric reticulohistiocytosis (Am J Radiol 1983; 141:107)

Apple jelly nodule A finding classically associated with tuberculosis or 'Lupus vulgaris', which may also be seen in sarcoidosis and other granulomatous processes, consisting of a small, soft yellow-brown 'glassy' cutaneous papule which, when compressed with a glass slide (a bedside test known as diascopy) oozes to one side (likened to apple jelly); the lesions heal with a central scar as the lesion extends outward and are thought to be sites at risk for future squamous cell carcinoma

'Apple peel' syndrome Autosomal recessive jejunal atresia which becomes symptomatic at birth with vomiting of bile, thought to be related to in utero obstruction of the superior mesenteric artery Pathology Twisting of the stenosed distal small intestine around the marginal artery has been fancifully likened to an apple peel Treatment Resection of the stenosed intestine

Applesauce sign PEDIATRIC RADIOLOGY A finding in infants with cystic fibrosis; the sticky meconium admixed with gas produces 'lumpy' or granular masses likened to applesauce visualized by plain abdominal films

Applique red cells Marginal form A virtually pathognomonic morphology of the early ring form of the *Plasmodium falciparum* trophozoite which appears 'plastered' on the surface of the erythrocyte, Cf Banana form, Ring form

Approach-avoidance (conflict) Any situation in which there is both an attraction towards something and repulsion therefrom, eg a compelling attraction towards a strongly disliked person, or a strong desire to view a horrifying automobile accident

'Approved but not funded' A research proposal or grant application that is considered technically feasible by the major US grant-giving body, the National Institutes of Health, but which, given the current budgetary constraints, cannot be funded (less than 25% of grants in the US are funded, although 95% are considered technically feasible); approved but unfunded proposals are often excellent, innovative and performable (Science 1991; 250:1198n&v)

A protein A protein located on the U1 small nuclear ribonucleoprotein particle (snRNP) that harbors an 80-amino acid RNA-recognition motif (RRM) required for sequence-specific RNA binding

A/P ratio The ratio of actual to predicted mortality, a parameter that some authors feel is related in an inverse fashion to the quality of care provided by a health care facility, a posture that may be more a function of a populations' degree of sickness (Mayo Clin Proc 1990; 65:1549)

Aprotes PHYSIOLOGY Elementary ions that are either positively-charged cations (sodium, potassium, calcium and magnesium) or negatively-charged anions (chloride and sulfate), which neither donate nor accept protons; since they are neither acids, nor bases, they cannot act as buffers

Aprotonin A bovine protease inhibitor with antifibrinolytic activity, is added to fibrinogen in 'Fibrin glue', theoretically enhancing the persistence of the fibrin seal, although this effect is controversial; see Fibrin glue

APUD system Amine precursor uptake and decarboxylation system A morphological and functional subgroup (Nature 1966; 211:598) of the endocrine system, encompassing the C cells of the thyroid and ultimobranchial body, type I cells of the carotid body and paraganglia, norepinephrine and epinephrine-producing cells of the adrenal medulla, melanoblasts, pineal gland and posterior pituitary cells: APUD cells take up tryptophan, converting it to 5-HT (serotonin), which is later converted to MAO, 5HIAA; 'APUD' tissue is visualized with: Silver stains (Fontana-Masson, an argentaffin stain or Bodian, an argyrophilic stain), bichromate, diazo salts, formaldehyde-induced autofluorescence, immunoperoxidase, electron microscopy (dense-core neurosecretory granules)

APUDoma A tumor producing small peptide hormones originating from the APUD system, including small (oat) cell carcinoma of the lung, carcinoid tumors of the lung, thymus, gastrointestinal tract and prostate, medullary carcinoma of the thyroid, pancreatic islet cell tumors, malignant melanomas and ganglioneuroma Clinical Heterogeneous, reflecting the functional nature of the tumor and/or metastases Pathology APUDomas are tumors which have a 'neuroendocrine' appearance characterized by sheets of intermediate and relatively monotonous 'blue cells', and which by electron microscopy demonstrate dense core or neurosecretory granules; see MEN

Aquifer ENVIRONMENT A generic term for a body of water located in the ground; see Plumes

Ara-C Cytosine arabinoside An antimetabolite analog of deoxycytidine, used synergistically with antifolates, alkylating agents and cis-platinum for treating leukemia, causes nausea, vomiting, myelosuppression and in high doses, cerebral dysfunction and ataxia

ARAT Acyl coenzyme A:retinol acyltransferase An intestinal enzyme that esterifies retinol (vitamin A) that is absorbed in chylomicrons

Arbor vitae uterus A descriptor for a developmental anomaly of the uterus characterized by two longitudinal ridges in the endocervical mucosa, oriented antero-posteriorly with complex secondary branches

ARC see AIDS-related complex

ARDS see Adult respiratory distress syndrome

ARESLD Alcohol-related end-stage liver disease

ARF Acute respiratory failure An acute decrease in PaO_2 to < 50 mm Hg or an acute increase in $PaCO_2$ with a resultant fall in arterial pH to < 7.30, due to hypoventilation, shunting or a ventilation/perfusion mismatch

Argentine hemorrhagic fever Caused by the Junin arenavirus, named in 1953 after its city of isolation, related to contact with rodent urine; 23 epidemic outbreaks have been recorded, occurring in the maize-producing region of Argentina; the high (15-45%) mortality may be reduced to 1-4% by using convalescent serum Rodent vectors ***Akodon arenicola, Calomys laucha and C musculinus*** Clinical After a 1-2 week incubation, the patients present with mucocutaneous hemorrhage, fever, anorexia, nausea and vomiting, fluid losses (causing oliguria, hypotension and shock), severe myalgia, leukopenia, thrombocytopenia and transient hypocomplementemia Treatment Rehydration and specific Junin virus immune plasma that reduces the mortality

Argentaffin reaction A histological staining reaction based on the reduction of ammonical silver to metallic silver, which while relatively nonspecific, is of use in identifying APUD cells, producers of polypeptides, classically, serotonin

Argentophil reaction similar to above in principle, but with pretreatment by a reducer (which makes it more sensitive (and less specific)

Arginine fork An arginine-rich structural motif present on RNA-binding proteins, eg Tat protein from human immunodeficiency virus that binds to a bulged region of

RNA, an interaction required for RNA transcription; it is thought that the electrostatic charge provided by the arginine is more critical to RNA binding and activation than the actual protein sequence (Science 1991; 252:1167)

Arizona A gram-negative bacillus of the ***Salmonella*** tribe, itself part of the Enterobacteriaceae family; infection therewith is uncommon, usually gastrointestinal with nausea and diarrhea

Armed Forces Institute of Pathology (AFIP) A section of the US military that opened in 1862 as the Army Medical Museum, and now comprises a collection of 2.2 million pathological specimens; the AFIP currently employs 125 pathologists and 575 ancillary staff, generates 350 publications per year, handles 350 consults/day, spends an estimated 60 000 hours/year training pathologists and has an operating budget of $35 million (J Am Med Assoc 1989; 261:2807)

Armed macrophages Macrophages capable of antigen-specific cytotoxicity, 'armed' by cytophilic antibodies (IgG or IgM) or arming factors, ie cytokines from T-cells

ARP-1 Apolipoprotein AI (apoAI) regulatory protein-1 A member of the steroid receptor superfamily that has various effects on lipid metabolism and cholesterol homeostasis; ARP-1 binds to DNA, down-regulating the apoAI gene and in addition binds to the thyroid hormone-responsive element and the regulatory regions of apoB, apoCIII and insulin gene (Science 1991; 251:561)

Arrestin A vision-related protein, maximally activated by high levels of light, eg midday sun; arrestin binds to opsonin, blocking activation of transducin, shutting down rod-cell activity

Arrowhead body An organelle seen by ultrastructure, the presence of which serves to mark the transition of a *Babesia* trophozoite to gametocyte

Arrowhead complex A structure seen by electron microscopy formed from heavy meromyosin that has ATPase activity and actin filaments, which are normal components of fibroblasts, chondrocytes, nerve and epithelial cells

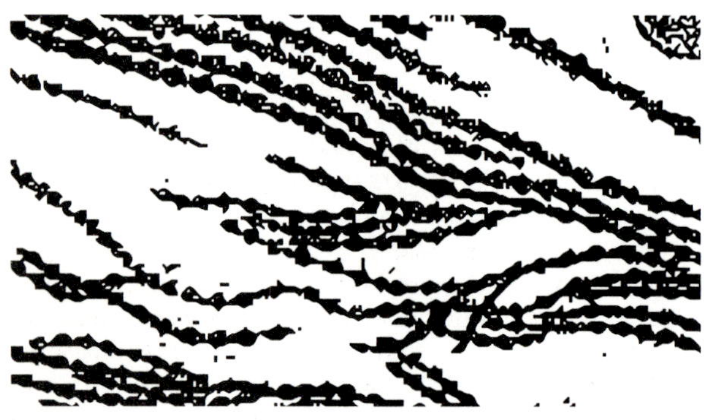

Arrowhead complexes

Arrowhead sign Radiology Segmental dilatation of bile ducts, with sharp, conical tapering; first described in Chinese immigrants with relapsing pyogenic cholangitis (Am J Radiol 1974; 122:368)

ARS see Autonomously repeating sequence

Arterial switch operation The surgical corrective procedure of choice for the relatively common (5-8% of all congenital cardiac malformations) transposition of the great vessels, a condition accounting for 25% of deaths due to cardiac malformations occurring in the first year of life; the 'switch' operation should be performed early to prevent development of pulmonary vascular disease (J Thorac Cardiovasc Surg 1986; 92:361)

Arteriosclerosis A generic term for arterial hardening (calcium deposition, thickening by fibrous tissue deposition), equated by the lay public with atherosclerosis; see Atherosclerosis

Forms of arteriosclerosis

Arteriolosclerosis, which may be a) Benign, associated with hyaline arteriolosclerosis or b) Malignant, associated with myofibroblast hyperplasia, 'onion-skinning' of the endothelial basement membrane and deposit of fibrinoid material in the vascular wall

Atherosclerosis Formed by cholesterol and cholesterol esters, covered by a fibrous plaque which, with time becomes calcified, ulcerated and causes thromboembolism of the coronary artery (cerebral 'strokes', myocardial infarcts, lower leg ischemia—especially in diabetics, ischemia of the large intestine)

Mönckeberg's sclerosis Idiopathic and often asymptomatic annular calcified bands occurring in the muscular media of medium to small blood vessels of the extremities that have been fancifully likened to a goose's neck

Artifact A substance or signal that interferes with or obscures the interpretation of a study; a structure that is not representative of a specimen's in vivo state or which does not reflect the original sample but which is rather the result of the isolation procedure, its handling or other factors; artifacts occur in electronic readout devices, eg EEG, EKG and EMG due to loose leads or electrical contacts Histology Tissue processing artifacts see 'Floaters' Radiology The artifact seen depends on the procedure, eg Barium enema, where zones of inconstant segmental contractions of the colon may be confused with organic constrictions or anatomic variations, due to mucosal or intramural tumors

Artificial blood Artificial oxygen carrier While blood, ie the erythrocyte is the ideal vehicle for transporting oxygen, it is: a) Immunologically foreign to the recipient, potentially eliciting an immune reaction b) May transmit infection, eg human immunodeficiency virus (HIV), hepatitis and others and c) Is unacceptable to certain religious groups eg Christian Scientists, Jehovah's Witnesses Note: Transfusion without permission in the US risks a felonious charge of assault and battery; in most situations, a blood loss of 20-25% is well tolerated and crystalloids, eg dextrose, are adequate to raise the blood volume to acceptable levels; the ideal artificial

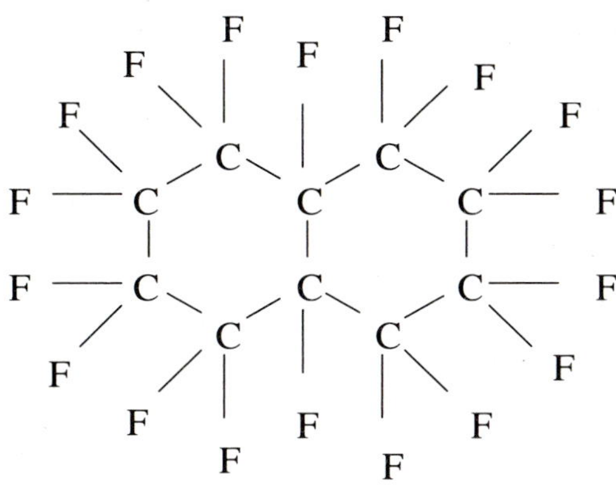

Perfluorocarbon

blood should be: a) Nontoxic b) have an oxygen on- and off-loading or P_{50} similar to red cells c) Have a reasonable serum half-life d) Maintain adequate oncotic pressure; Few substances have these properties and none have FDA approval; some candidates include: Perfluorochemicals (Fluosol, Green Cross, Osaka Japan, see Figure); synthetic chelaters of oxygen and polymerized, stroma-free pyridoxylated hemoglobin (Poly SFH-P, Northfield, Northfield, Illinois); the major impediment to the use of hemoglobin is that removal of the whole molecule from the erythrocyte causes dissolution of the polypeptide tetramer, resulting in molecules that filter through the kidneys, causing renal failure

Artificial dermis see Artificial skin

Artificial heart see Jarvik-7, Penn State heart, Ventricular assist device

Artifical pancreas see Biohybrid artifical pancreas

Artificial reproduction Non-coital and/or non-natural manipulation of the reproductive processes such that one (or rarely both) of the child's genetic parents is not the rearing parent(s); the term artificial reproduction (AR) includes: Artificial insemination of the natural, the gestational or the rearing mother by the husband or a donor, ovum donation into a gestational and rearing mother, in vitro fertilization, surrogate motherhood, cryopreserved embryo transplantation and permutations of the above; in addition to the issues of anonymity of donors, donor screening (as a form of eugenics) and possible commercialization of surrogacy, the legal, ethical, social and psychological ramifications of AR are extraordinarily complex as a child may theoretically have up to five (six) parents—a genetic mother and father, a gestational mother (and her husband) and a rearing mother and father; see Baby M, in vitro fertilization, Surrogate motherhood

Artificial 'skin' A synthetic material designed to have the fundamental physicochemical properties of skin, including optimal 'wetting' and 'draping', leading to adherence, control of bacterial invasion and fluid loss, while eliciting cellular and vascular invasion which would synthesize a dermal matrix while biodegrading the artificial graft; artificial dermis is composed of a porous mat of collagen-chondroitin 6-sulfate strands covered by a thin skin of silastic; burn sites covered with artificial dermis heal more rapidly and have better cosmetic results than the usual grafts (Ann Surg 1988; 208:313); Cf Split-thickness graft, Spray-on-skin

Artificial sweeteners A group of substances that have a taste similar to the usual dietary sugars, glucose and sucrose, but are metabolized incompletely or not at all, resulting in a minimal net gain of calories; given the known, albeit minimal, potential for the induction of bladder cancer in the saccharine and cyclamates, aspartame is recommended for use in pregnant women; see Aspartame, Cyclamates, Sugar substitutes

Artificial tears A solution containing 0.5% carboxymethyl cellulose or 5% polyvinyl alcohol, used to treat xerophthalmia, classically associated with Sjögren syndrome, which may also be due to sarcoidosis, senile lacrimal gland atrophy, acute or chronic infectious dacryoadenitis, eg gonococcal and trachoma or tumors, including lymphomas, pseudolymphoma, primary or metastatic carcinoma

Asbestos A generic commercial name for finished products containing a type of mineral fiber; the USA has used 30 billion (10^9)tons of asbestos since 1900 and asbestos is a component of an estimated 3000 manufactured products; maximum exposure levels by 1976 OSHA standards are 2 fibers/cc^3/8 hour period **Clinical** disease is graded according to the severity of peribronchial fibrosis, although fibers may not be found

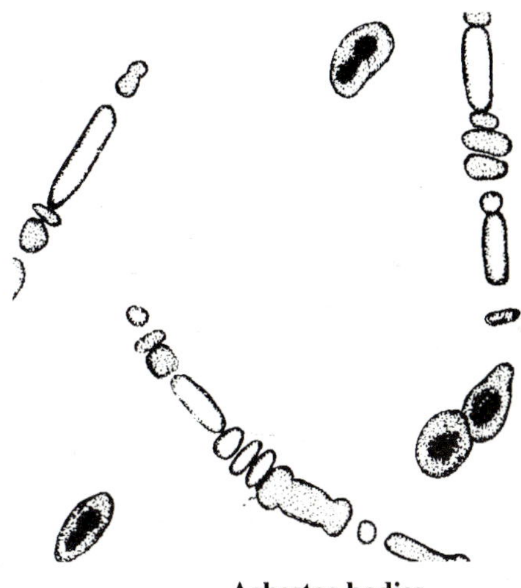

Asbestos bodies

within the plaques **Pathology** Calcified fibrous plaques on serosal surfaces, benign or malignant mesotheliomas Note: Mesotheliomas, although characteristic of asbestos exposure, may also be induced in experimental models by nickel, viruses and radiation; asbestos may induce gastrointestinal, hematopoietic, kidney and ovarian neoplasia, pleural calcification and non-malignant respiratory disease and peritoneal mesotheliomas (Br J Ind Med 1987;44:396); at highest relative risk for mesothelioma are workers exposed to fibers with the greatest length-to-diameter ratio, eg crocidolite which affects miners in South Africa and western Australia Note: These fibers were once used in a cigarette filter-making process and the exposed workers had an 8-fold increase in cancer and 14-fold increase in non-malignant respiratory disease (N Engl J Med 1989; 321:1220); amosite fibers are known high-risk fibers, causing mesothelioma in miners, insulators and factory workers; tremolite fibers mined in Greece and inculpated in the 'Metsovo lung', are associated with a moderate risk for future mesothelioma and chrysotile fibers; 'Canadian' (white) asbestos, which have a low risk of malignancy; anthophyllite fibers and serpentine fibers have no known malignant potential; fibers are quantified based on bleach digestion of wet formaldehyde-fixed tissue, which reveals a broad range of asbestos fibers and related ferruginous bodies; control subjects have less than 10 bodies per gram of tissue; patients with asbestosis and mesothelioma have from 0 to 2000/gram

Ascertainment A method by which people are selected for inclusion in a genetic study, where certain factors, eg whether or not a proband has a smoking spouse, are considered as criteria for inclusion or exclusion

ASCII American Standard Code for Information Exchange COMPUTERS A standardized set of characters, including the upper and lower case letters of the English and other alphabets, various special, numeric and control characters and symbols used by most computer systems for transmission of computer data

Ash leaf lesion DERMATOLOGY An oblong hypopigmented cutaneous macule, simulating the leaf of the green ash (*Fraxinus lanceolata*), seen by a Wood lamp in children with tuberous sclerosis or Pringle-Bourneville disease, where the presence of three or more such lesions is considered diagnostic; Cf Oak leaf configuration, neurofibromatosis

ASIA motor score American Spinal Injury Association motor score A clinical tool used to evaluate neuromuscular dysfunction in patients with spinal cord injury, in which the strength of 20 specific muscles in the body is assigned a value from 1 to 5 for a total of 100 in absence of motor dysfunction to 0 in complete quadriplegia (N Engl J Med 1991; 324:1849)

'Asian esophageal cancer belt' A region of Central Asia extending from the Caspian littoral region in Iran to the northern provinces of China with a very high (prevalence/100 000) 110 males, 184 females (Mazandaran province of Iran) incidence of esophageal carcinoma; in contrast, the US prevalence ranges from 1.2 in white females to 15.6 in black males (Proc Nutr Soc 1985; 44:101)

ASO Anti-streptolysin O A serologic test that monitors group A β-hemolytic streptococcal infection, ie 'strep throat' (90% positive) and acute streptococcal glomerulonephritis (± 25% positive); untreated patients have a 4-fold increase in IgM antibody titers (measured in Todd units, TU) within 3 weeks of onset; early penicillin suppresses and/or delays the ASO response, < 166 TU is the usual cutoff for 'normal'; > 250 TU in adults and > 333 TU in children is evidence of recent infection; ASO levels may also increase in acute rheumatic fever; the test is based on the principle of hemolysis inhibition; 1 unit of streptolysin O is added to serial dilutions of the patient's blood and incubated; the highest dilution that inhibits red cell lysis forms the basis for Todd units, the reciprocal of endpoint dilution Note: Cholesterol interference may occur and must be eliminated from the test sample

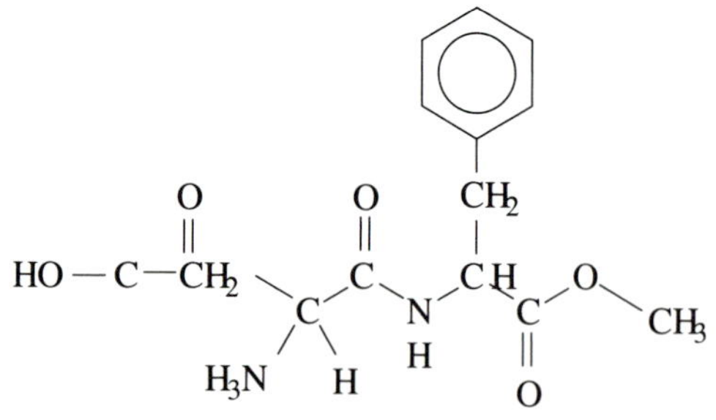

Aspartame

Aspartame An artificial sweetener that is a dipeptide of aspartic acid and phenylalanine, discovered in 1965, approved by the US Food and Drug Administration in 1983, which appears to be safer than saccharin (with the notable exception of patients with phenylketonuria), although some 'soft' experimental data has indicated an association with brain tumors; see Artificial sweeteners

Aspiration pneumonia Inhalation of highly acidic gastric content is a clinical event that most often occurs in the comatose or obtunded, and has a mortality of up to 70%; after the insult, there is progressive respiratory depression, hypoxia, tachypnea and tachycardia; the tracheobronchial tree 'sweats' thin frothy fluid while the parenchyma is acutely inflamed, hemorrhagic and edematous with atelectasis and necrosis

Assassin bug Cone-nosed arthropod of the order Hymenoptera (true bugs), vector for *Trypanosoma cruzi* (Chaga's disease)

Assault and battery FORENSIC MEDICINE *ASSAULT* The unlawful placing of an individual in apprehension of immediate bodily harm without his consent *BATTERY* The unlawful touching of another individual without his consent; one incident of assault and battery may elicit two lawsuits 1) A criminal action by the state against the assailant and 2) A civil action for monetary compensation by the plaintiff claiming injury; Documentation of informed consent prevents routine accusation of assault and battery

Assigned risk A risk that insurance companies are required by law to take; eg insuring cigarette smokers; assigned risk insurance, eg malpractice insurance for physicians, is written by an insurance company only because it is compelled to do so by law

Assignment The transfer by an insurance beneficiary (ie, the patient) to the provider (ie, the physician) of the right to receive payment from a 'third party' (ie, the insurance company); in assignment, the patient is still liable for physician fees that are in excess of that provided (usually 80%) by the insurance company; see Participation

Association constant A value that describes the equilibrium state of a reversible reaction, eg an enzyme-substrate or antigen-antibody reaction

Assumption-of-risk doctrine A legal concept that those individuals who knowingly expose themselves to hazards with potential for bodily harm cannot hold others liable if harm occurs; this doctrine may be invoked when a hospital employee is injured in the normal performance of his duties or when a blood recipient becomes infected with HIV, if the blood was properly tested (and the donor was in the 'Window period'), the indications for transfusion were correct and the recipient knew of the potential risk for infection; see 'Blood shield' statutes

AST Aspartate aminotransferase, formerly glutamate oxaloacetate transaminase (GOT) A cytoplasmic and mitochondrial transaminase enzyme that is increased in myocardial, renal and cerebral infarction, hepatic and skeletal muscle disease

Asterisk sign An early finding by computed tomography of ischemic necrosis of the femoral head (Legg-Perthes' disease), where a star-shaped structure is formed by thickened bony trabeculae

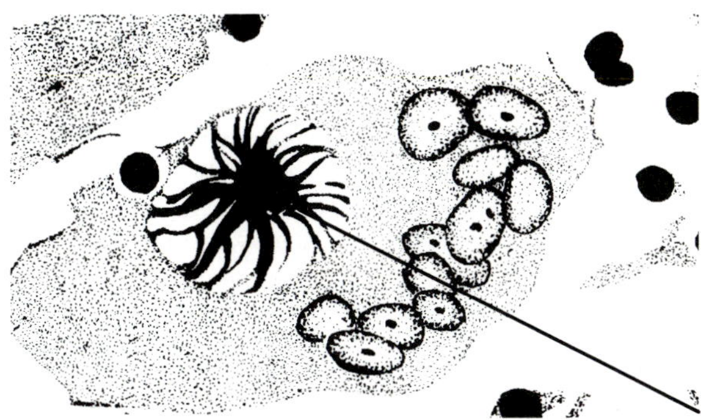

Asteroid body, sarcoidosis

Asteroid body A term applied to any structure with a stellate appearance MICROBIOLOGY A descriptor applied to the centrally located chlamydospores of *Sporotrichum schenckii* that are surrounded by a stellate eosinophilic material thought to be represent antigen-antibody complexes SURGICAL PATHOLOGY Nonspecific delicate, acidophilic and stellate cytoplasmic striations of intermediate filaments seen in multi-nucleated giant cells of sarcoid granulomas, berylliosis, necrobiosis lipoidica and rarely in granular cell tumors

Asteroid hyalinosis OPHTHALMOLOGY A form of vitreous humor degeneration characterized by multiple whitish 'dots' floating in the vitreous humor corresponding to particulate calcium-lipid complexes

Asthma triad Bronchospasm, nasal polyps and increased sensitivity to aspirin (acetylsalicylic acid, but not sodium salicylate), to indomethacin, aminopyrine and yellow food additives, eg tartrazine yellow, FD&C yellow, #5; the triad is described in 10% of typical asthmatics and the accompanying reaction (severe bronchospasm, urticaria and hypotension) is attributed to defective prostaglandin metabolism, unmasked by these agents, some of which inhibit cyclo-oxygenase, perhaps diverting arachidonic acid metabolism towards production of spasmogenic leukotrienes; the triad may be inherited or due to environmental factors

Astral fibers MOLECULAR BIOLOGY Microtubules arising from the centrioles during mitosis, radiating from the mitotic poles toward the periphery of a dividing cell

Astrovirus A small, non-enveloped (28-30 nm in diameter) RNA virus with a cubic symmetry, that is less pathogenic than the Norwalk agent; it most often infects children, in whom it is more common than enteroviruses and one half as common as rotaviruses as a cause of gastroenteritis (N Engl J Med 1991; 324:1757) Clinical Diarrhea, headache, malaise, nauses and vomiting

ATA 'box' Adenine-thymine-adenine A triplet of nucleotides identified as having promoter activity in transcribing the β-hemoglobin gene; single nucleotide substitutions in the ATA box result in decreased β-hemoglobin production and these mutations may appear in some patients with β-thalassemia

Ataxia-telangiectasia Louis-Bar syndrome An autosomal recessive condition that causes sinopulmonary infections, choreoathetosis, slurring of speech and muscular atrophy Laboratory Decreased IgG4 and IgA2, occasionally also decreased IgE Clinical Progressive cerebellar ataxia, oculocutaneous telangiectasia, thymic aplasia or hypoplasia (cellular defect), increased susceptibility to radiation-induced chromosomal damage and carcinoma and rearrangements due to defective DNA repair; immune complexes deposit in glomeruli, choroid plexus, heart valves and synovium; vasoactive amines (histamine, serotonin), IgE, platelets; presence of macrophages; antigen and antibody valences, class of antibody, antibody:antigen ratio, affinity of antibody:antigen, types of vasculature through which the ICs are passing, response of the reticuloendothelial system to the ICs; see phakomatosis

ATCC American Type Culture Collection The oldest repository of cell lines in the USA (Rockville, Maryland) that contains 50 000 strains of biologicals in its regular collection, 2800 cell lines from 75 animal species; the ATCC is an invaluable resource for biomedical researchers who purchase the cells for use in toxicity assays, recombinant DNA experiments and production of human proteins Budget $12 000 000 Annual shipments 35 000 Note: The proprietary rights over ownership of cell lines with commercial potential have become an issue since the 'Mo' cell line, derived from a patient whose HTLV-2-infected cells (obtained from his spleen, removed as part of the treatment protocol for hairy cell leukemia) produce GM-CSF in large quantities; the ATCC has been called the 'Swiss bank' of biology as it is a repository of biological material, including cell lines and DNA probes from researchers seeking patents and who are required to submit a sample and yet still want those secrets protected (ATCC will not release material unless explicitly instructed to do so by the researcher once a patent is issued, and then charges a small handling fee); ATCC is a center for standardization and exchange, it accepts US patent deposits and is recognized under the 1981 Budapest treaty as an international agency; the ATCC has 10 000 items in its protected inventory

ATF Activating transcription factor A cellular protein that stimulates transcription of the adenovirus E4 transcription unit, acting early in infection at any of several 'enhancer' binding sites

ATG see Antithymocyte globulin

Atherosclerosis A condition caused by intramural deposition of LDL, secondary to exposure of smooth muscle to lipid, resulting in platelet-induced smooth muscle proliferation, see Atherosclerotic plaque; 'hard' risk factors: Hypertension (> 160/95 mm Hg), increased LDL-cholesterol (total cholesterol > 265 mg/dl), smoking (> one pack/day), diabetes mellitus; 'soft' risk factors include maleness, family history of previous atherosclerotic heart disease, increased apolipoprotein B, apolipoprotein C-III, total cholesterol, triglycerides, decreased HDL-cholesterol, as well as hyperhomocysteinemia, as high levels of homocysteine, a highly reactive amino acid, are toxic to vascular endothelium and may potentiate the auto-oxidation of the low-density lipoprotein cholesterol, promoting thrombosis (N Engl J Med 1991; 324:1149) **Pathology, early** Fatty streaks, common in children, flat, lipid-rich lesions consisting of foamy macrophages and smooth muscle **Pathology, late** Fibrous plaque, calcification, increased intimal smooth-muscle cells, in a connective tissue matrix, containing intracellular and extracellular cholesterol Complications within atheromatous lesions: Aneurysms (dissecting and fusiform) of arterial wall subjacent to atheroma, bleeding into plaque, calcifications and thrombosis Note: The degree of atherosclerosis may be reduced by regular exercise, a vegetarian diet, fish substituted for meat and eggs, one alcoholic drink a day, and possibly various bio-feedback modalities, eg yoga **Treatment: Medical** see Cholesterol-lowering drugs **Treatment: Interventional (conservative)** Balloon angioplasty, plaque scraping and plaque 'grinding' **Treatment: Interventional (conventional)** Bypass surgery

Atherosclerotic plaque The histologic lesion that comprises the initial lesion of atherosclerosis and which is composed of lipid, leukocytes, smooth muscle cells and extracellular matrix in the intima of the large arteries; the plaque stage is preceded by the adherence of circulating monocytes and lymphocytes to the endothelium, with accumulation of foam cells (lipid-laden macrophages); the adhesion is thought to be mediated by a protein highly homologous to VCAM-1, a cell adhesion molecule (Science 1991; 251:788); smooth muscle cells isolated from plaques in culture, produce platelet-derived growth factor (PDGF)-like mitogens, which are thought to act as autocrine stimulators of atherosclerosis; chemically reactive lipids, eg malondialdehyde, are released from peroxidation, altering low-density lipoprotein, resulting in receptor-mediated deposition of a cholesteryl ester in the foamy macrophages of incipient atheromatous plaques (Science 1988; 241:215)

Athlete diseases see Sports medicine

Athlete's foot Tinea pedis A malodorous dermatophytosis of the toe webs and soles of the feet of athletes, most common in adolescent males resulting in maceration, erosion and pruritus due to *Trichophyton rubrum, T mentagrophytes and Epidermophyton floccosum* **Treatment** Drying, if recalcitrant, haloprogin and tolnaftate, if refractory, griseofulvin

Athletic heart Athlete's heart A heart typical of highly trained athletes characterized by an increased left ventricular diastolic volume and increased thickness of the left ventricular wall, as seen by two-dimensional echocardiography; the upper limit of 'physiologic' ventricular hypertrophy is 16 mm for canoeists and rowers (and 13 mm for other athletes); ventricular walls greater than 16 mm indicate concomitant pathologic hypertrophy, eg hypertrophic cardiomyopathy (N Engl J Med 1991; 324:295); arrhythmias seen in athletic hearts are usually benign and include sinus bradycardia, wandering pacemaker, cardiac blockages, nodal rhythm, atrial fibrillation, ST segment and T-wave changes, increased P wave amplitude and right ventricular hypertrophy

Atomic absorption spectrophotometry LABORATORY MEDICINE A highly sensitive (to 1 ng/L) technique used to analyze various elements, especially metals, including aluminum, arsenic, beryllium, calcium, copper, iron, lead and lithium, which are present in trace amounts **Principle** Atoms are excited above a ground state by flame vaporization, and the radiation emitted as the molecules return to a ground state is measured in unexcited non-ionized molecules

Atrial 'kick' CARDIOLOGY An abrupt notch in the pressure curve in the ventricular outflow tract that is typical of idiopathic hypertrophic subaortic stenosis

Atrionatriuretic peptides Peptide hormones derived from atriopeptigen, released from cardiac myocyte storage granules that alter 1) The electrical activity at cell membranes, suppressing ion flow at the sodium channel and increasing calcium channel permeability, a change attributed to conformational change in the channels (Science 1990; 247:899) and 2) The contractile activity of the heart; when vascular volume is increased, atriopeptin is released, increasing the glomerular filtration rate, renal blood flow, urine volume and sodium excretion, while decreasing the plasma renin activity; when the vascular volume is decreased, a negative feedback loop suppresses atriopeptin release; ANP acts through cGMP as a second messenger, inhibiting sodium absorption across the inner-medullary collecting duct and cGMP-kinase inhibits the channel via a G protein pathway (Nature 1990; 344:336)

'At risk' pregnancy A pregnancy at risk for spontaneous abortion (an event occurring in 20-60% of all pregnancies); various factors weigh in 'at-risk' gestation including maternal factors, age, anticardiolipin antibodies and increased levels of thyroid autoantibodies (J Am Med Assoc 1990; 264:1422)

Attending physician The physician who is on the medical staff of a hospital or health care facility who is legally responsible for the care given to a patient while he or she is in the hospital; a patient's 'attending' is also regarded as a person's private physician if that physician cares for the person on an individual and/or outpatient basis; see Private physician

Attention deficit hyperactivity disorder ADHD The most common neurobehavioral disorder of childhood, affecting 2-6% of school children, characterized by impulsiveness, distractibility, variably accompanied by hyperactivity and/or aggressiveness, immaturity and emotional lability; although ADHD is considered idiopathic, neurochemistry and genetics may play a role Note: Family stresses, eg divorce, parental death, depression and sickness must be evaluated prior to diagnosing a child as 'hyperactive' **Diagnosis** PET imaging, the glucose metabolism of adults diagnosed in childhood as having ADHD is lower, especially in the premotor cortex and the superior prefrontal cortex, cerebral regions involved in control of attention and motor activity (N Engl J Med 1990; 323:161); phenylethylamine excretion may serve as a diagnostic marker **Treatment** Stimulants, primarily methylphenidate HCl (Ritalin) as well as dextroamphetamine and magnesium pemoline (J Am Med Assoc 1988; 260:2256); see Breuning affair

Attenuation Diminution of an effect MICROBIOLOGY Decreased virulence of a microorganism, eg that of bacille Calmette-Guerin (BCG), a strain of *Mycobacterium bovis* that has been attenuated by multiple subcultures on a bile-glycerine medium; the resulting bacterium is immunogenic, ie capable of eliciting antibody formation, but is non-virulent; live attenuated organisms are used to produce the poliomyelitis vaccine but may occasionally revert to a wild type RADIOLOGY Attenuation is the reduction of the intensity of a beam by either absorption or scattering

Attestation HEALTH CARE REIMBURSEMENT A document signed by a physician stating that he or she performed the diagnostic or therapeutic procedures on a patient for which a bill is being submitted

Atypical lymphocyte Downey cell A dysmorphic lymphocyte that occurs in various non-neoplastic conditions, classically seen in toxoplasmosis (<20% of circulating leukocytes are atypical), infectious mononucleosis, cytomegalovirus infection and viral hepatitis; these cells have abundant cytoplasm with basophilic condensations where they abut erythrocytes; Atypical lymphocytes, have been divided into *TYPE I* Monocyoid or prolymphocytic Kidney-shaped or lobulated nuclei, with densely homogeneous hypergranular chromatin, more similar to mature lymphocytes than plasma cells; the cytoplasm is bubbly, pushed to one side and basophilic *TYPE II* Cytoplasmic radiations from the nucleus ('ballerina skirt' cells); the cells have one or more nucleoli, the nuclear chromatin is less dense and the cytoplasm is less foamy than type I, containing occasional azurophilic granules, and has basophilic 'scallops' around adjacent red cells *TYPE III* The nuclei are coarse, spanning the cell's breadth, have clumped red-to-purple chromatin with 1-4 nucleoli; the cytoplasm is abundant, basophilic and 'scallops' around adjacent erythrocytes (H Downey, Arch Int Med 1923; 32:82)

Atypical measles A virulent form of measles affecting children vaccinated with an inactivated measles vaccine (available between 1963 and 1967), which followed exposure to natural measles, characterized by high fever, pneumonia, pleural effusion, obtundation and an atypical maculopapular, petechial and vesicular rash with very high measles antibody titers; atypical measles is due to the inability to form antibodies to the F protein of the virus, which is responsible for viral penetration, cell fusion (syncytium formation), and hemolysis, resulting in cell-to-cell spread of the virus

Atypical mycobacterium Any Mycobacterium exclusive of ***M lepra***, ***M tuberculosum*** or ***M bovis*** (the latter two of which cause 'typical' tuberculosis); atypical Mycobacterium are so designated because they grow more rapidly, produce no niacin, fail to reduce nitrates, produce heat-stable catalase and are highly resistant to isoniazid; of interest is ***M avium-intracellulare***, which is associated with AIDS and ***M marinum***, seen in the Chesapeake bay, affecting fishermen and aquarium keepers and ***M ulcerans***, endemic to the banks of the upper Nile

'Aunt Millie' approach Pattern recognition CLINICAL DECISION-MAKING An unsound (albeit usually correct) sequence of clinical logic (N Engl J Med 1987; 316:738cpc), from the quip:

> 'How do I know it is Aunt Millie?
> Because it looks like Aunt Millie'

Pattern recognition is the traditional model for teaching pathology and radiology, both of which are visual 'arts'; although it allows molding of future generations in an accepted paradigm, exceptions to any 'rules' are generally relegated to wastepaper basket categories, as exceptions cannot be explained or understood in an arbitrarily-defined context; Cf Heuristic method, Stochastic process

Aura NEUROLOGY A subjective (illusionary or hallucinatory) or objective (motor) event marking the onset of an epileptic attack or a migraine

Australia antigen Hepatitis B viral antigen, first isolated from an Australian aborigine, which locates in the hepatocyte cytoplasm and in scattered mesenchymal cells; early stages of hepatitis B are characterized by sublobular involvement of all cells, later stages by scattered antigen-positive hepatocytes; the presence of hepatitis B antigen within a population's livers correlates epidemiologically with an increased incidence of hepatocellular carcinoma in that population; Cf Dane particles

Australian X syndrome see Murray Valley encephalitis

Austrian syndrome A subgroup of patients (usually alcoholics) with pneumococcal pneumonia, meningitis and endocarditis with rupture of the aortic valve who present with bacteremia and despite adequate antibiotic therapy have a high (80%) mortality (Med Clin North Am 1984; 68:179)

Author 'inflation' The growth in number of people receiving authorship credit on published reports in biomedical sciences Note: Scientific advances require multiple expertises, and credit may be shared by clinicians, molecular biologists, laboratorians and statisticians, thus single-author papers in science are increasingly anachronistic (N Engl J Med 1990; 323:488c)

Authorship The credits for a publication in the sciences are problematic; the advantages of being an author on published reports in the literature are considerable, and include peer respect, conferral of 'expert' status and career advancement, which is often a function of how many publications a person has generated, see CV-weighing; sharing authorship credits has the potential disadvantage of being the co-author on a report later deemed fraudulent; Dr A Relman, emeritus editor of the New England Journal of Medicine, delineated four criteria (table), at least two of which must be met to legitimately share authorship credits (Science 1988; 242:658)

AUTHORSHIP *('Relman's criteria')*
1. Conception of idea and design of experiment
2. Actual execution of the experiment; hands-on experience
3. Analysis and interpretation of data
4. Writing the manuscript

Autocrine motility factor (AMF) MOLECULAR BIOLOGY A cytokine that stimulates random and directed tumor cell motility and generation of inositol triphosphate, both of these activities are inhibited by pertussis toxin, implying that AMF acts by a guanine nucleotide-binding protein (G protein) pathway (J Natl Cancer Inst 1990; 82:54); a 78 kD glycoprotein acts as an AMF receptor on melanomas and may have a role in melanocyte locomotion (Cancer Res 1990; 50:409); see also Scatter factor

Autoeponym A term reserved for a condition affecting the author who described it and/or who died of the disease named in his honor **CARRION'S DISEASE** DA Carrion, a medical student who inoculated himself with a skin lesion from verruca peruana (*Bartonella bacilliformis*) to prove that the agent was both infectious and the agent of Oroya fever that killed 7000 of those who built the railroad from Lima to La Oroya; he died within 23 days (Am J Surg Path 1986; 10:595) **HUNTINGTON'S DISEASE** George Huntington, his father and his father's father all studied their own disease that was traced back to an index case in 1649 in Bures, England Lewis syndrome Autosomal dominant synostosis of the first metacarpophalangeal joint of the thumb or stiff thumb 'syndrome' **JONES FRACTURE** A diaphyseal fracture of the fifth metatarsal, which Jones incurred '...whilst 1dancing...' and who considered it a stress fracture **PRAUSNITZ-KÜSTNER (PASSIVE TRANSFER) TEST** A clinical assay that measures allergic response to foreign proteins that was identified by Küstner who was allergic to fish, injected his serum into Prausnitz's skin, which, when followed by a 'challenge' fish extract injection into Prausnitz's skin, causing a typical wheal and flare reaction **RICKETTSIA SPECIES** Named for Howard Ricketts, who in 1906 identified the organism responsible for Rocky mountain spotted fever (*Rickettsia rickettsii*); Ricketts died in 1910 in Mexico City while investigating typhus (*Rickettsia prowazekii*) **THOMSEN'S DISEASE** A benign autosomal dominant myopathy, described by Julius Thomsen (who had it), which is first seen in childhood, characterized by tonic rigidity and spasticity, which is overcome by repeated voluntary contraction of the muscles to reduce the clinical and muscular 'stiffness' of these patients (the 'warm-up' effect) **TROUSSEAU SIGN** Superficial petechial hemorrhage and thrombophlebitis, occurring secondary to visceral malignancy, described by Trousseau prior to his own death from gastrointestinal malignancy

Autoimmunity Reaction of an organism's immune system to self antigens as if they were non-self; autoantibody production increases with age and is intimately linked to connective tissue disease; in one autoimmune model, experimental allergic encephalitis of mice, there is a trimolecular complex formed from myelin basic protein (BP), the major histocompatibility complex (MHC) and the T cell receptor; the autoimmune proliferative response may be blocked by an antibody raised against the BP-MHC complex, implying that autoimmunity may ultimately respond to specific 'magic bullet' therapy (Nature 1991; 351:147); see Clonal anergy, Superantigen

Autologous blood transfusion (ABT) Collection and reinfusion of the patient's own blood and/or blood products, which despite a slight inconvenience of surgical delay and vasovagal reactions, is the preferred transfusion option for appropriately-selected patients; the blood volume available for ABT can be increased using recombinant erythropoietin and iron supplements (N Engl J Med 1989; 321:1163); although in principle, ABT can be used for any elective surgical procedure, blood is most often needed for orthopedic (total hip replacement) and cardiovascular surgery; ABT represents 5-15% of the blood used in elective surgical procedures and reduces the use of homologous transfusion in cardiac surgery from a peak of 82% to as low as 27% (J Am Med Assoc 1991; 265:86); ABT may also be considered in selected pediatric, geriatric or occasionally obstetric surgery; although most surgery does not require transfusions, some procedures are especially 'bloody', and place an enormous strain on a blood bank's resources, eg an average of 13 units of packed red cells are used in a liver transplantation, one-third of which may be provided by blood salvaged from the operative field (Mayo Clin Proc 1989; 64:340); see Intraoperative 'autologous' blood transfusion

Autologous unit A unit of red blood cells that is to be transfused into a donor at the time of elective or anticipated surgery; *CATEGORIES OF AUTOLOGOUS DONATION:* **1) PREOPERATIVE PHLEBOTOMY** Drawing of blood prior to an elective or anticipated surgical procedure; up to 5 units can be made available in the 20 days preceding surgery, using a 'piggie-back' method **2) IMMEDIATE PREOPERATIVE PHLEBOTOMY** or acute normovolemic hemodilution ***3) INTRAOPERATIVE SALVAGE*** and **4) POSTOPERATIVE SALVAGE** Autologous transfusion reduces the risk of most types of transfusion reactions, except clerical errors, contamination and low transfusion temperatures, and is increasing popular as it substantially reduces the number of homologous (ie, non-autologous) units transfused; up to 60% of all blood products required in elective surgical procedures can be fulfilled by the patient's own blood; 50% of those who donate autologous units for specific medical indications (rare blood types or presence of multiple blood cell alloantibodies) utilize the blood; 21% of those who donate autologous units without specific medical indications utilize that blood (Arch Pathol Lab Med 1990; 114:516)

Autologous bone marrow transplantation (ABMT) A therapeutic modality for leukemic patients who are in relapse, and thus likely to die of their disease in which a suitable (HLA-matched) donor cannot be found; the bone marrow is removed during the second remission, treated in vitro to remove the leukemic cells and is then cryopreserved; the patient then receives supralethal chemoradiotherapy and the marrow is reinfused; autologous bone marrow transplantation in acute lymphocytic leukemia yields a 20-30% survival rate

Autolymphocyte therapy (ALT) An immunotherapy for treating metastatic renal carcinoma, in which a patient's leukocytes are removed, stimulated by monoclonal antibodies, causing the leukocytes to produce and secrete cytokines; the cytokine supernatant is then removed and readministered with an aliquot of the patient's own leukocytes; despite an early report of success (April 1990, Lancet) with this modality, conservative oncologists are awaiting further, more definitive reports of success

Autonomic triad Dilated pupils, moist palms and tachycardia, a characteristic finding in schizophrenics that may be accompanied by increased systolic pressure of 10-20 mm Hg Note: Schizophrenics appear to be hypersensitive to all stimuli: noise, odor, touch and light

Autonomously replicating sequence MOLECULAR BIOLOGY A sequence of DNA that serves as an initiation site on a gene for replication; Cf Transcription unit

Autopoietic Gaia ENVIRONMENT A theory advanced by L Margulis that organisms evolve in symbiotic systems, eg humans filled with ***Escherichia coli*** evolved through mutually driven ('symbiotic') mutations rather than by random mutation of either organism, in a 'vacuum'; autopoietic (self-maintaining) systems can range from the size of bacteria to that of the entire planet and are composed of living organisms and environments that are codependent and interactive; Gaia analyses requires integration of data and concepts from fields that have not traditionally overlapped or interacted (Science 1991; 252:378); see Gaia; Cf Neo-darwinism

Autoradiography A technique that detects the presence of radioisotopes, usually immobilized on a nylon or nitrocellulose membrane when exposed to a radiation-sensitive medium, eg unexposed radiologic film; autoradiography is used in molecular biology to detect radioactive probes which have bound to segments of DNA or RNA of interest; autoradiography allows visualization of Southern and Northern blot hybridizations

Autosomal dominant polycystic kidney disease (ADPKD) A relatively common (1:400-1:1000) condition, held responsible for 6-9% of end-stage renal disease in the USA and Europe, caused by the defective gene, PKD1, on the short arm of chromosome 16, close to the α-hemoglobin complex; a second defective gene with identical clinical features is responsible for 4% of cases, but is thought to cause a milder disease **Clinical** Acute or subacute onset of azotemia and hypertension, related to increased activity of the renin-angiotensin-aldosterone system, possibly related to the ischemic pressure induced by the expanding cysts (N Engl J Med 1990; 323:1091); ADPKD first appears in adults with upper quadrant tenderness; extrarenal disease is due to defective extracellular matrix, with hepatic cysts, diverticulosis, berry and abdominal aneurysms, annuloaortic ectasia, valvular regurgitation, anemia, very high erythrocyte sedimentation rate and leukocytosis **Diagnosis** Ultrasonography (ibid; 323:1085); see Polycystic kidneys

A-V block Atrioventricular block Any delay in conduction or failure of the electrical impulse to reach the ventricular conducting system, which may arise in the atrium, at the A-V node, in the bundle of His or in the bundle branches; A-V blocks are of 3 types: **1) FIRST DEGREE A-V BLOCK** P-R intervals are > 0.20 seconds but all the P waves are conducted to the ventricle **2) SECOND DEGREE A-V BLOCK** A) MOBITZ I P-R intervals increase in length until a beat is 'dropped' B) MOBITZ II P-R intervals are constant but occasionally the P fails to conduct an impulse; Mobitz II blocks have potentially serious clinical implications **3) THIRD-DEGREE A-V BLOCK** No atrial beats conduct to the ventricle

A-V dissociation Atrioventricular dissociation The independent depolarization of the atria and ventricles where the rate of the ventricular pacemaker is faster than that of the atrial pacemaker; in contrast to a pathologic A-V or third-degree block, normal conduction may occur once the electrical conditions return to normal

AVEC microscopy Allen video-enhanced contrast or Dynamic microscopy A television camera that distinguishes weak contrasts by amplifying differences in brightness; AVEC microscopy studies the direction of transportation of materials along microtubules, which are packaged in vesicles and 'walked' along the microtubule by projections in the axons (Science 1990; 250:1204n&v); see Kinesin

Aviation medicine In-flight emergencies US Federal Aviation Agency regulations require that an 'enhanced' medical kit (stethoscope, sphygmomanometer, airway tube, syringes, epinephrine, nitroglycerin, 50 ml 50% dextrose, diphenhydramine injectable) be carried on any airplane with more than 30 seats; types of in-flight emergencies: Syncope 29%, cardiac/chest pain 16%, asthma/shortness of breath 10% and allergic reaction 5% (J Am Med Assoc 1989; 262:1653) In-flight deaths (J Am Med Assoc 1988;259:1983) Statistics 0.31 deaths/million passengers—regardless of flight length; 125 deaths/billion passenger kilometers; 25 deaths per million departures; the average victim was male, age 53.8, physicians were available in 43% of cases Cause of death Cardiac 56%, terminal cancer 8%, respiratory 6%, miscellaneous and no cause remainder Alcohol abuse, pilots see N Engl J Med 1990; 323:455rv

Aviator's astralagus ORTHOPEDICS A generic term referring to various permutations of fracture and fracture-dislocations of the talus; the term was coined in 1919 when the fracture was related to aviation accidents in pilots whose aircraft had been descending too rapidly and which had a rudder bar which caused the above fracture at the time of the airplane's impact

Avidin A 68 kD tetrameric glycoprotein found in egg-white that has an high affinity for biotin, an association used in immunology for the avidin-biotinylated immunoperoxidase method, see ABC; when eggs are eaten in excess, the avidin-biotin avidity may cause biotin deficiency

Avidin biotinylated horseradish-peroxidase complex method A commercial method for detecting antigen or antibody in tissues; avidin, a 68 000 egg-white glycoprotein with a very high natural affinity (and multiple binding sites) for biotin, a vitamin readily bound covalently to an antibody; the ABC system (Figure) allows amplification of antigen 'signal' obtained by the multiple binding sites available on the avidin; the avidin:biotin linkage can be used for gene mapping, double label studies, DNA in situ hybridization, hybridoma screening, Southern blotting, radioimmunoassay, solid phase ELISA, immune electron microscopy, studies of neuronal transport and as a means of controlling enzymatic reactions (Biochemistry 1990; 29:11274) Method The tissue containing the antigen of interest is frozen, air-dried and acetone fixed, incubated with a primary antibody, washed, then incubated with a secondary antibody bearing attached biotin, washed, re-incubated with fluorescently or enzyme-tagged avidin and finally counterstained

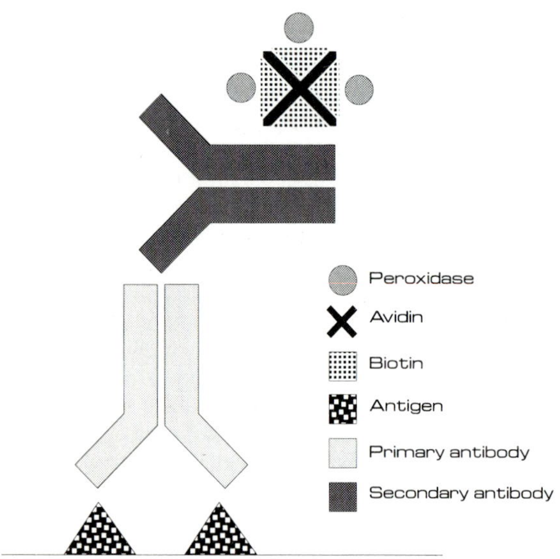

Avidity IMMUNOLOGY The degree of stability of an antibody with its antigen, a function of the number of shared binding sites; Cf Affinity

AVM Arteriovenous malformation A potentially fatal congenital intracranial anomaly with large arteries feeding in a mass of communicating vessels which empty into large draining veins filled with 'arterialized' blood; AVMs present as subarachnoid hemorrhage and mass effects potentially producing hydrocephalus; 7% of subarachnoid hemorrhages are due to cerebrovascular malformations, including capillary and venous angiomas and capillary telangiectasias

a wave A positive a wave is a component of a normal jugular phlebogram produced by retrograde transmission of the pressure pulse, corresponding to atrial systole; the a wave begins before the first heart sound peaking at the moment the first sound begins; abnormalites of the a wave indicate cardiopulmonary disease; it may disappear in atrial fibrillation, be 'swallowed' in the v-y descent of a prolonged P-Q interval, it may be very large (giant) when the atrium is contracting against resistance (eg tricuspid valve stenosis or atresia, pulmonary hypertension or pulmonary edema) or bear a presystolic 'notch' (pulmonary edema); Cf Cannon wave

Axillary tail Axillary fat pad The fibroadipose tissue in the axilla that contains the lymph nodes (numbering from 12 to 25) and lymphoid drainage from the breast and arm; in carcinoma of the breast, the number of positive lymph nodes in the axillary tail constitutes the single most important prognostic indicator of survival, where a breast carcinoma with no positive lymph nodes is associated with a greater than 80% five-year survival, while a patient with 20 or more positive lymph nodes is associated with a less than 20% five-year survival

Ayur-Veda Sanskrit Life knowledge The oldest existing medical system, practiced primarily in the subcontinent of India; Ayur-Veda holds that disease is caused by an imbalance of homeostatic and immune mechanisms related to three physiological principles known as 'doshas'; Vata dosha represents fluid and motion, corresponding to the Western concepts of circulation and neuromuscular activity; Pitta dosha directs all metabolic activities, energy exchange and digestion; Kapha dosha represents structure, cohesion and fluid balance and when deranged, predisposes toward respiratory disease, diabetes mellitus, atherosclerosis and tumors; the therapeutic modalities include transcendental meditation, a 'healthy' life style, herbal compounds and behavior modification (J Am Med Assoc 1991; 265:2633; 266:1749ed, 266:1769c)

Azo dye A group of dyes produced from amino compounds by diazotization and coupling the reactants; the reactions are a function of the number of -N=N- groups in the molecule; the dyes are used for plastics, rubber and in the cattle industry; the carcinogenicity of these substances is related to the ortho-hydroxylated metabolites complexed with sulfates and glucuronic acid

Azorean neurologic syndrome Machado-Joseph spinopontine atrophy syndrome

AZT 3'-azido-3'-deoxythimidine see Zidovudine

Azurophilic granules Primary granules Primary lysosomes Membrane-bound organelles in neutrophils that act as reservoirs for digestive and hydrolytic enzymes prior to their delivery to a phagosome, appearing as large, coarse non-specific blue-purple granules within progranulocytes, myelocytes and neutrophils containing myeloperoxidase (causing oxygen-dependent bacteriolysis), lysozyme (which destroys the bacterial wall), neutral proteases (cathepsins C and G and elastase which destroy inflamed tissue), acid hydrolases (glycosidases, phospholipases, acid proteases, β-glucuronidase, α-mannosidase, N acetylglucosaminidase, which degrade material ingested), α-naphthyl acetate, α-butyrate esterase, naphthol ASD chloracetate esterase, cationic proteins, defensins, bactericidal or permeability-increasing protein (BFI), C5a inactivating factor and sulfated mucosubstances Note: The other major granulocytic granules are secondary or specific granules, which contain alkaline phosphatase, aminopeptidases, lysozyme and basic proteins and tertiary granules

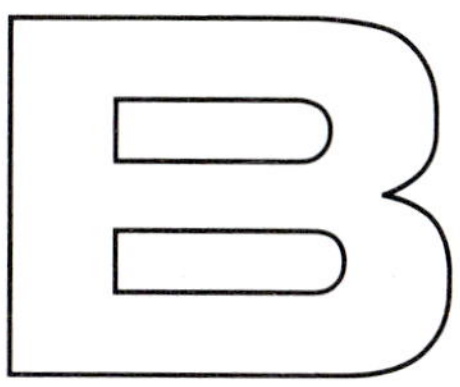

B Symbol for: Bel; blood; boron; 5-bromouridine; magnetic induction

b Symbol for: base; inconvertible enzyme

33B3.1 A monoclonal antibody raised against the interleukin-2 receptor, which is as effective in preventing graft-versus-host disease in renal transplantation as rabbit antithymocyte globulin with fewer side effects and infections (N Engl J Med 1990; 322:1175)

B19 parvovirus The virus inculpated in erythema infectiosum which may affect about 40% of teachers and day-care workers (J Am Med Assoc 1990; 263:2061); see Fifth disease

Babbling Quasi-random vocalizations in infants that precede language acquisition; babbling is intimately linked to the abstract structure of language and not (contrary to prevailing opinion) a concrete specific linguistic structure, as language acquisition in the profoundly deaf is not hindered by the lack of auditory and verbal signals, indeed deaf infants born to deaf parents produce a manual version of vocalizations ('man-bling'), in which similar ('phonology', morphology, syntax and semantics) language structures are acquired in the manual form (Science 1991; 251:1493)

Baby Doe An infant born in April, 1982 in Indiana who was diagnosed as having Down syndrome and a tracheoesophageal fistula that required surgery for the infant's prolonged survival; given the infant's anticipated poor quality of life; the parents decided to withhold treatment with the approval of the local court and the child died within six days; the ensuing ethical debate resulted in an interpretation of section 504 of the Rehabilitation Act of 1973 that contends it is unlawful to withhold nutritional support or necessary medical treatment from handicapped infants

Baby (Jane) Doe An infant born in October, 1983 on Long Island, New York, with multiple birth defects, including spina bifida, microcephaly and hydrocephalus; the parents decided to withhold treatment; a complaint by an unidentified person designated as a 'private citizen', forced the US federal government to become involved via the Health and Human Services, which questioned whether a parent has the right to initiate or terminate the life-support for infants and children with overwhelming disease or conditions for a party that is underage and is unprotected; the two Baby Doe cases resulted in 1) The **BABY DOE LAW** Public Law 98-457 A legislative act in 1984, requiring states to establish mechanisms in their child-protection services responsive to reported medical neglect of disabled children and 2) The **BABY DOE REGULATIONS** Federal regulations promulgated in 1985 for implementing the 'Baby Doe Law', requiring that disabled infants with life-threatening conditions receive the '...appropriate nutrition, hydration and medication, which in the treating physician's....reasonable medical judgement will be most likely to be effective in ameliorating or correcting all such conditions' Treatment (but not nutritional support or necessary medication) may be withheld if the infant is a) In an irreversible coma or b) If the treatment is unlikely to prevent death in the near future

Baby Fae heart Hypoplastic left heart syndrome (HLHS) Pediatric cardiology A condition characterized by hypo- or agenesis of the left ventricle, aortic and mitral valves; the ascending and transverse aorta is narrowed with a diaphragm-like aortic coarctation at the preductal aortic isthmus; postnatal life hinges on adequate blood supply, ie is ductus dependent, unrestricted atrial shunting and a balance between the pulmonary and systemic vascular resistances (N Engl J Med 1986; 315:949); HLHS surgery is difficult as there are extensive malformations and thus carries a high mortality (J Am Med Assoc 1985; 254:3321) Note: Baby Fae was a 2-week-old premature infant with HLHS who survived for 20 days in October 1984 when she received a walnut-sized heart from a 71/2 month old baboon, in an operation performed by L Baily in Loma Linda, California

Baby L A 36 week, 1970g baby girl, born in the mid 1980s to a young mother of 3 healthy live children, who developed oligohydramnios and hydronephrosis during the last trimester; decelerations in the fetal heart rate and thick meconium below the umbilical cord were noted at delivery; APGAR scores were low and resuscitation efforts allowed weaning of an infant responsive only to pain; consultation among members of the nursing and medical staff and nearly two years of intensive care led to the unanimous opinion that the child's condition was hopeless and the medical team declined further efforts to salvage a child who was deaf, blind, quadriplegic, in a permanent vegetative state and required 16 hours/day of intensive nursing care, contrary to the wishes of the mother (although physicians usually abide by the wishes of patients, family members or guardians in resuscitation efforts); the Baby L case is a 'charged' issue in which both parents and a health care system must resolve the ethical dilemma of whether to allow one child to die and spend those resources elsewhere; Baby L was transferred to another facility and has the mental status of a 3 month-old (N Engl J Med 1990; 322:1012; 323:1148c)

Baby Lance The 'Minnesota Baby Doe' A 7 month-old baby boy who was the first major legal test of the 'Baby Doe regulations' see there; Baby Lance was beaten to unconsciousness and an irreversible coma by a caregiver; the higher Minnesota court ruled that heroic measures were not required, given his hopeless condition (Am Med News 24/Oct/86)

Baby M A female infant born in mid-1980s in New Jersey by a surrogate mother contract; at the time of birth, the gestational and natural mother decided to renege on the contract and the ensuing court battle became a cause celebre on the issue of surrogate parenthood; on one side was the natural father, a biochemist and his wife, a pediatrician with multiple sclerosis; on the other side was a woman who was the gestational and natural (genetic) mother, receiving $10 000 in expenses for providing use of her uterus in a surrogate contract; at the close of the case, the court ruled for the natural father who was allowed to retain the child Note: The Baby M case was not true surrogacy, as the gestational mother was also the genetic mother; see Artificial reproduction, Surrogate motherhood

Baby bottle syndrome Severe caries of deciduous dentition, due to prolonged use of milk or juice bottles as a sleeping aid for infants

'Babysitter' A person, often an intelligent family member, who stays by the bedside of a patient respirating by mechanical ventilation, ensuring that no malfunctions or other problems arise

BAC Blood alcohol content

Bacillary angiomatosis Epithelioid angiomatosis A distinct vascular proliferative disorder of the skin and lymph nodes seen in subjects seropositive for human immunodeficiency virus (HIV), potentially causing disseminated visceral disease, eg bacillary peliosis hepatis Clinical Erythematous papules and nodules, fever and bacteremia Histopathology Lobular capillary proliferation composed of protuberant atypical endothelial cells containing clusters of curved Warthin-Starry positive curved bacilli which may also be gram-negative Treatment Erythromycin, other antibiotics; tissue analysis with an oligonucleotide primer complementary to the 16S ribosomal RNA genes of eubacteria and DNA sequence by the polymerase chain reaction amplification, reveals that bacillary angiomatosis is due to a previously uncharacterized rickettsia-like organism, most (98.3% sequence homology) related to *Rochalimaea quintana* (N Engl J Med 1990; 323:1573, 1581, 1587); see Peliosis hepatitis

Bacillary bodies Iron-containing cytoplasmic inclusions in bone marrow precursors of the erythroid series that are increased in hemolytic anemia or after splenectomy

Back bleeding CARDIOVASCULAR SURGERY An unreliable test to determine the completeness of thrombectomy of an occluded artery (unreliable in that it gives a false sense of security since back bleeding may occur through the nearest arterial branch while a major arterial 'distad' remains occluded); for an operation to be considered successful, a test of arterial integrity, eg intraoperative angiography, is required

Back calculation EPIDEMIOLOGY An approach used to quantify the magnitude of the AIDS epidemic and forecast future trends, which requires only AIDS incidence data and an estimate of the incubation period distribution; although this technique suffers from such features as the limited knowledge of the incubation period, the effects of therapy on the incubation period, errors in the AIDS incidence data, it is more attractive than alternate approaches including simple extrapolation of the AIDS incidence curve, surveys of HIV prevalence and a mathematical model, which requires an enormous amount of often uncertain data (Science 1991; 253:37); see 'Look-back' programs

Back extensor strength (BES) A parameter used to evaluate elderly patients with lower back pain and osteoporosis that may be measured by using a back isometric dynamometer (Mayo Clin Proc 1991; 66:39)

Background A baseline of minimal 'chaos' in any study, eg radioactivity in sample that may be due to cosmic radiation, instrument noise and radioactive contamination

Back-propagation COMPUTERS A learning algorithm used in a three layer (inner, middle correctional and outer) neural network (a computer simulation of neurological connections), which allows the system to 'learn' from errors by altering the strength of neural connections, ie allowing the system to teach itself; some workers consider the brain to be the biological correlate of back-propagation (Science 1990; 247:524)

Backscatter One of two parameters measured in flow cytometry, detected at a 90° angle to the laser's light beam which corresponds to the fluorescence of individual cells or intracellular components stained with rhodamine- or isothiocyanate-labelled monoclonal antibodies Note: The other parameter is forward scatter, measured at 180° angle to the light, ie directly in front of the laser, and is a function of the cell's size; see FALS, Flow cytometry

Back-to-back pattern A 'soft' histologic criterion seen in well-differentiated adenocarcinomas that separates malignant lesions from premalignant hyperplasia or atypical lesions; when glands are arranged in a back-to-back fashion, the intervening stroma (and by extension, the basement membrane) disappears, a finding characteristic of gastrointestinal, endometrial and ovarian adenocarcinomas

Back typing Reverse typing TRANSFUSION MEDICINE A 'cross-match' in which a person's serum, which may contain antibodies, is tested against a panel of commercially available erythrocytes (the antigens of which are well characterized) to determine whether a person has antibodies to any red cell antigens; Cf Front typing,

Major cross-match, Minor cross-match

Backward failure Cardiac failure attributed to elevated filling pressure of the ventricles, due to obstruction, as occurs with mitral ortricuspid stenosis, which causes increased venous pressure with congestion, ie backward failure; the term is a physiologic concept of dubious importance and thus has decreasing clinical currency; Cf Forward failure

Backwash ileitis The contiguous mucosal involvement of the terminal ileum, extending proximally, seen in 10-15% of cases of ulcerative colitis as a 'spillover' phenomenon; unlike Crohn's disease which may involve the entire gastrointestinal tract, ulcerative colitis is usually confined to the colon and rectum and occasionally, a 'backwashed' segment of ileum

Baclofen A γ-aminobutyric acid (GABA) antagonist that may be administered per os or intrathecally to reduce recalcitrant spinal spasticity in patients with multiple sclerosis or spinal-cord injury (N Engl J Med 1989; 320:1517)

Bacteriophage A virus that infects bacteria; of interest in the study of human disease are the temperate phages of *Escherichia coli*, in particular the lambda bacteriophage, a double-stranded 48 500 base pair DNA virus that is commonly used as a vector for molecular cloning; upon entry into the bacterial host, it replicates either by a) Lysis The phage's circular DNA replicates many times, independently of the bacterium, causing the cell to burst or by b) Lysogeny The phage DNA integrates itself within the bacterial chromosome per se and is carried to future generations of the bacterium

BAD operon MOLECULAR BIOLOGY A group of 3 genes (B, A and D) that encode three enzymes, an isomerase, a kinase and an epimerase, respectively, requiring in addition the presence of the positively-acting protein AraC for transcription of the ara operon into BAD mRNA

BADS Black locks, albinism and deafness, sensorineural type A condition with certain features of oculocutaneous albinism but is not true albinism as the melanocytes in BADS are reduced or absent

'Bad trip' SUBSTANCE ABUSE A hallucinogenic drug-induced experience in which the desired pattern of time-space disorientation causes a varying amount of anxiety on the person taking the 'trip'; see Flashbacks, 'High'

BAER Brainstem auditory evoked response A clinical method for evaluating hearing by using scalp electrodes; the early responses reflect electrical activity at the cochlea, cranial nerve VIII and brainstem; late responses are due to cortical activity

Bagassosis A hypersensitivity pneumonitis seen in cane sugar workers, who are sensitive to *Thermoactinomyces sacchari*, a fungus that grows well in sugar cane pressings; the term derives from the cellulose-rich olive husks, bagasse, remaining after olives are pressed to extract oil, and is generic for various 'pressings'; see Farmer's lung

Bag cell neuron A neuron of the gastropod mollusk, *Aplysia californica*'s nervous system that serves as a model for studying the neuroendocrine system

Bag of worms A lesion or density imparting a polyvermiform pattern or one in which the activity is fancifully likened to a quivering mass of live elongate organisms CEREBRAL ANGIOGRAPHY The appearance of arteriovenous malformations in which there is little interposed cerebral tissue; this finding may also be mimicked by intracranial tumors, although the irregular and bizarre vessels may be separated by a mass GASTROINTESTINAL DISEASE An uncommon descriptor for the gross appearance of the stomach in Menetrier's disease in which the stomach is soft, smooth and enlarged and the mucosa has large, swollen inelastic worm-like rugal folds, separated by deep valleys NEUROLOGY Asynchronous, involuntary quivering and squirming of multiple skeletal muscle fascicles of the tongue, which disappear during sleep and may be suppressed with rest, sedation or volition, characteristically seen as a manifestation of Sydenham's chorea SURGICAL PATHOLOGY The quasi-pathognomonic gross appearance of a plexiform neurofibroma seen in von Recklinghausen's disease, where a major nerve trunk is transformed into a redundant convoluted serpentine mass of tumorous nerves UROLOGY The tactile sensation of a varicocele lying within the scrotal sac

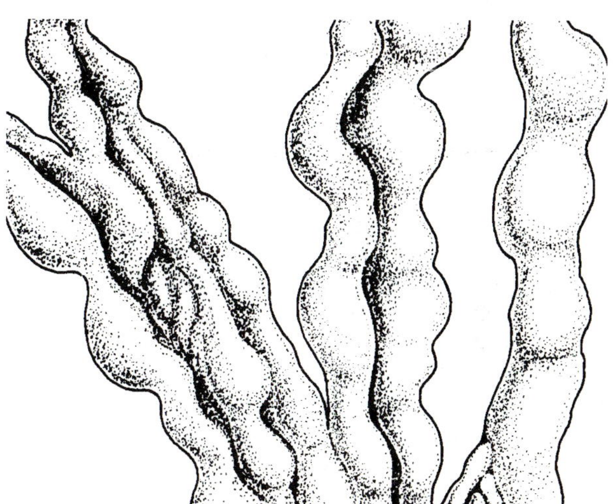

Bag of worms appearance, plexiform neurofibroma

'Bags' Loose suborbital skin caused by inflammation and edema, associated with vasodilation (the prominence of the blood vessels impart the dark color); bags occur with lack of sleep, smoking, and other aerosolized irritants; 'bags' occur in allergic 'shiners', various dermatitides and in aging

Baghdad button An indurated lesion of cutaneous leishmaniasis caused by *Leishmania tropica*

Bairnesdale ulcer A necrotizing skin ulcer due to *Mycobacterium ulcerans*, first described in Australia; see Buruli ulcer

Bak^a An antigen found on the platelets of most normal subjects; immune-mediated neonatal thrombocytopenia may be due to an IgG anti-Bak^a antibody, produced in women who are Bak^a negative and passively transferred to the fetus

BAL 1) Blood alcohol level; useful values > 100 mg/dl, legal intoxication, most states in the US; > 200 mg/dl narcosis, > 300 mg/dl, stupor and coma 2) Broncho-alveolar lavage A 'wash' of the upper respiratory tract to obtain cells representative of any inflammatory or neoplastic process in the lungs; BAL material is used for a) Cytopathologic analysis b) Analysis of the CD4:CD8 ratio and (rarely) c) To obtain cells for gene rearrangement, ie Southern blot hybridization, to diagnosis lymphoma (Mayo Clin Proc 1990; 65:651); like acetylcholinesterase levels and gallium scans, flow cytometry of the BAL is useless in diagnosing hilar sarcoidosis (Am Rev Resp Dis 1987; 135:747), although increased CD4 T cells and decreased neutrophils in a BAL may be suggestive of sarcoidosis in certain patients; Flow cytometry has a relatively low diagnostic value in hypersensitivity (increased CD8 T cells and normal to increased neutrophils) and idiopathic pulmonary fibrosis (increased neutrophils)

Balance billing HEALTH CARE REIMBURSEMENT A bill submitted to a patient whose insurance only pays for part of the service(s) rendered by the physician or hospital, dunning him for the unpaid portion

BALB/c mouse IMMUNOLOGY A strain of inbred white mice that develops a myeloproliferative response to intraperitoneal injection of mineral oil and complete Freund's adjuvant

Bald sac sign A myelographic finding caused by lateral migration of nerve roots to the periphery of and adherence to the dural sac occurs in a background of arachnoiditis with clumping of nerve roots

Bald spot MOLECULAR BIOLOGY An area on a hybridization blot (Southern, Northern, Western) that does not hybridize and which represents a technical artefact due to inadequate bathing of hybridization fluid in the bag containing the radiolabelled or biotinylated probe

Bald tongue Complete atrophy of lingual papillae, seen in pernicious or iron-deficiency anemias, pellagra (specifically known as the bald tongue of Sandwith), syphilis Clinical Pain, burning and a beefy red color

Balkan nephropathy An tubulointerstitial nephropathy endemic to the littoral regions of the Danube river, affecting the Balkan countries of Bulgaria, Romania and Yugoslavia Etiology Although uncertain, the environmental effects of Eastern Bloc progress make the recently implicated aromatic hydrocarbon leachate out of the low-grade coal, lignite, into local water supplies more likely than the previously suggested possibility of fungal nephrotoxins (which had been related to high regional rainfall or genetic factors) Clinical Most patients die within 10 years of onset Histopathology Prominent cortical involvement with interstitial fibrosis, amyloid deposits, chronic inflammation, marked loss of renal tubules and atrophy

Ballerina skirt cell Downy type II cell HEMATOPATHOLOGY A descriptor for the morphology of one of the three types of atypical lymphocytes seen in infectious mononucleosis, here demonstrating cytoplasmic radiations extending from the nuclear membrane

Ball-and-chain model NEUROPHYSIOLOGY A model first proposed in 1977 for the physical conformation of the potassium ion channel; this ion channel is constructed of a 19-20 residue peptide (ball) domain tethered by a 17 residue (chain) to the cytoplasmic face of the cell and 'pops out' of a transmembrane pore upon electrical activation, allowing the channel to gate for potassium in either a resting, an open and an inactivated state (Science 1991; 252:1092; 250:533); the model was corroborated using a combination of site-specific mutagenesis and patch-clamping (Science 1990; 250:533, 568, 506); see Voltage-gated channels

Ball-and-socket Ball in socket An adjectival descriptor for a morphology in which there is a sharply circumscribed round mass surrounded by a clear or lucent space followed by a density similar to the first central 'ball' Bone radiology A sequel of epiphyseal fractures with a primary fusion of the central portion of the epiphysis, appearing as a ball within a relatively radiolucent 'socket', seen in infantile scurvy, battered child syndrome, and acromelic dwarfism PARASITOLOGY A 'ball-and-socket appearance is typical of the trophozoites and occasionally the cysts of *Endolimax nana* and *Ioda-moeba buetschlii* (figure) where there is a large, deeply staining karyosome lying in an empty space; the nuclear membrane is not visualized as the chromatin is not peripheral RHEUMA-TOLOGY A descriptor for the compressive erosions in the interphalangeal joint of rheumatic diseases, where a central sclerotic zone is surrounded by an osteoporotic 'ring'

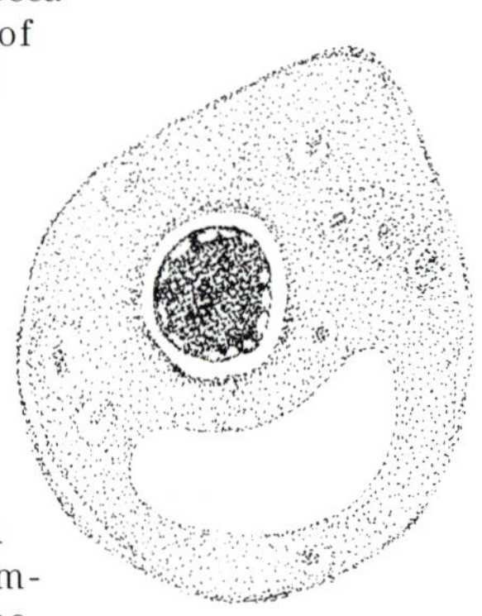

Ball-and-socket

Ball in claw pattern DERMATOPATHOLOGY A descriptor for the histopathological appearance of the dermal-epidermal junction in lichen nitidus, characterized by epidermal flattening, hydropic degeneration or absence of basal cell layer, varying degrees of epidermal detachment, abundant lympho-histiocytic infiltration in the upper dermis, occasional multinucleated giant cells; the lateral margins (rete ridges) form a pincer around the infiltrate; see Collarette Clinical Flat-topped, flesh-colored papules located on the penis, arms and abdomen Note: The ball and claw or ball in talon is an ending to the cabriole leg where a bird of prey's or lion's claw grasps a ball, a style thought to have developed between 1690-1730 in the English school of furniture design, inspired by the Dragon's claw grasping a pearl, a motif originating in China

Ballistics FORENSIC MEDICINE The energy imparted to tissue is calculated as $E = mv^2$ (m = mass; v = velocity); one study (J Am Med Assoc 1988; 259:2730) corrects several popular misconceptions and warrants review;

relevant terms **CAVITY** The permanent cavity along a bullet's trajectory is caused by the bullet per se, the temporary cavity is related to tissue stretching 11 times the diameter of the bullet, not the 30- to 40-fold increased diameter as stated in older literature; however the kinetic energy transferred during the short life of the temporary cavity is more destructive to parenchymal tissues, eg spleen, liver than deformable tissue, eg muscle, lung and fat; the explosion-related pressure generated in the temporary cavity is about 4 atmospheres, not the previously stated 100 atmospheres **VELOCITY** The difference in tissue destruction between high or low velocity projectiles is likely caused by the fragmentation of the bullet itself (as in the M-16 semiautomatic weapon) **YAW** The angle between line of flight and the bullet's long axis; bullets enter tissue and tumble once they are inside, rotating 180°, exiting with the base forward, explaining the large size of some exit wounds

Balloon angioplasty see Percutaneous transluminal coronary angioplasty

Balloon cell A non-specific descriptor for any cell with abundant clear cytoplasm, which may be benign or malignant, of any embryologic origin and store any histologically clear material in the cytoplasm; Ballooned cells include carcinoid cells, ependymal cells (myxopapillary ependymoma), hepatocytes, see Ballooning degeneration, histiocytes storing glycosaminoglycans and mucopolysaccharides, neurons (Farber's disease, lipogranulomatosis, mannosidosis) and pigmented cells either benign (balloon cell nevus) or malignant (balloon cell melanoma); Cf Signet ring cell

Balloon form A morphologic variant of *Trichophyton rubrum* and *T mentagrophyte microaleuriospores*, causing superficial dermatoses, tinea pedis and tinea corporis

Ballooning BONE RADIOLOGY Biconcave compression of the end-plate of the vertebral body by pressure arising in the intervertebral discs, most commonly in the lumbar spine, characteristic of osteoporosis; Cf Fish vertebrae

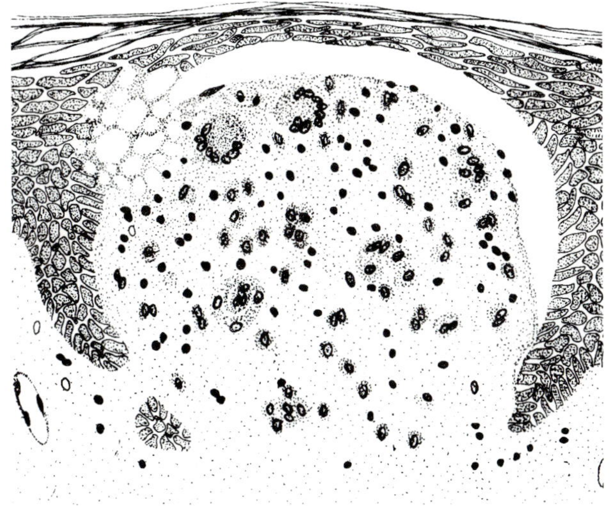

Ball in Claw

Ballooning degeneration HEPATIC PATHOLOGY A histopathologic change seen within ballooned infected hepatocytes in acute viral hepatitis A and acute stage of hepatitis B; the cells have abundant pale granular cytoplasm; the 'ground-glass' granularity of the cells is due to the accumulation of viral particles NEUROPATHOLOGY A descriptor for the changes seen in vincristine therapy-induced peripheral neuropathy, enhanced by VP-16 HISTOPATHOLOGY Vacuolization, vesicle formation, unraveling of the myelin lamellae and electron-opaque material within and adjacent to the axon (Cancer 1982; 49:859)

Balloon tamponade EMERGENCY MEDICINE A hemostatic procedure for upper gastrointestinal bleeding using a Sengstaken-Blakemore tube (a rubber tube surrounded by a long inflatable balloon that places gentle pressure on the esophageal lumen, usually quenching the bleeding) and a larger round tube, inflated in the stomach, 'anchoring' the device to the desired location; balloon tamponade is indicated for bleeding esophageal varices or persistent hemorrhage of the esophagus for any reason

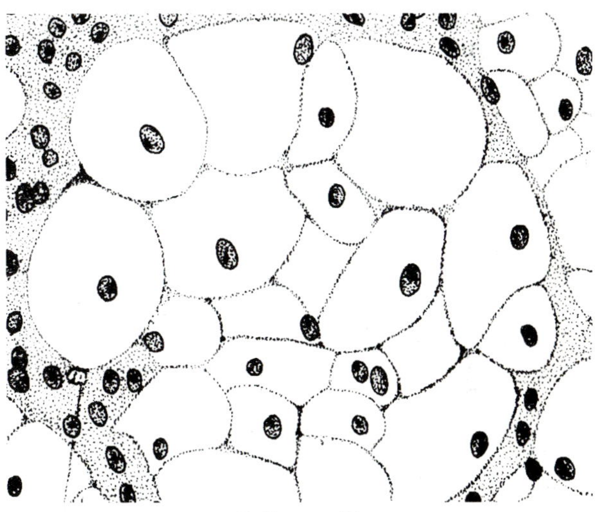

Balloon cells

Balloon valvoplasty, percutaneous A method used to treat stenotic cardiac valves, including 1) Pulmonic valve, where balloon valvoplasty is considered the optimal therapeutic modality 2) Mitral valve The results may be suboptimal if the valve ring is extensively calcified, but good if the valve is pliable or 3) Aortic valve Valvoplasty is considered the optimal therapy only for frail, elderly patients who are otherwise poor surgical candidates (Mayo Clin Proc 1990; 65:198rv); recurrence of symptoms, restenosis and death occur in 50%; see Inoue balloon

Ball valve obstruction A partial endobronchial obstruction allowing facile entry but not free egress of air, resulting in the build-up of pressure in the terminal airways and potential rupture of alveoli; air percolates into soft tissues causing interstitial emphysema; if extreme, ball-valve air leaks may cause a tension pneumothorax with increased positive pressure in the hemithorax, shifting the mediastinum and compromising the circulation

BALT Bronchiole associated lymphoid tissue see MALT

Baltic myoclonus An autosomal recessive form of light-sensitive myoclonic epilepsy which at autopsy reveals loss of Purkinje cells Treatment Valproic acid

Baltimore affair A full-scale investigation by the US Congress, headed by representative Dingell that was initiated when a Nobel Laureate (discoverer of reverse transcriptase) at the Massachusetts Institute of Technology was one of a number of co-authors, but not the main author, on a report (*ALTERED REPERTOIRE OF ENDOGENOUS IMMUNOGLOBULIN GENE EXPRESSION IN TRANSGENIC MICE CONTAINING A REARRANGED MU HEAVY CHAIN GENE* Cell 1986; 45:247), in which irregularities of data were alleged (Science 1991; 251:1552); Dr Baltimore was exonerated (Science 1989; 244:413), requested that the paper be retracted and apologized for his role, albeit quite peripheral to the events (Nature 1991; 351:94-95); it is unclear whether scientifically unsophisticated juries and politicians should be allowed to evaluate complex data Time table of the events: Nature 1991; 351:95n&v; Bottom lines: Science 1991; 253:24 n&v; see 'Dingellization', qui tam lawsuit, 'Whistle blowing'

Bamboo hair Trichorrhexis invaginata Dry fragile, poorly growing hair with a 'ball-in-cup' invagination of the distal into the proximal hair shaft, related to a transient defect in keratinization, which improves by puberty, a finding central to Netherton syndrome

Bamboo vertebrae Universal syndesmophytosis that may be associated with osteoporosis and bony ankylosis, a finding typical of ankylosing spondylitis

Banana form Crescent form The morphology of the macrogametocyte that corresponds to the female sexual intraerythrocytic form of ***Plasmodium falciparum*** which also has compact chromatin

Banana sign An ultrasonographic finding when a major neural tube defect accompanies the Arnold-Chiari malformation with herniation of the cerebellar tonsils and midbrain structures into the foramen magnum, causing ventriculomegaly due to compression of the outflow from the third and fourth ventricles; the 'banana' corresponds to the compressed cerebral hemisphere

Band HEMATOLOGY A region on an SDS-PAGE gel electrophoresis of the 'ghost' (membrane devoid of hemoglobin) of red blood cells, when subjected to a hypoosmolar (low-ionic strength) solution; electrophoresis divides the membrane into bands 1 and 2 (spectrins), bands 2.1 and 2.2 (ankyrin), band 3 (a 90 kD glycoprotein dimer forming part of the erythrocyte ion channel, which is involved in anion transport, band 4.5 (a glucose transporter) and band 5 (actin) MOLECULAR BIOLOGY Any 'spot' on an electrophoretic gel, corresponding to the distance of migration of a molecule of interest (DNA, RNA or protein) which is the combined function of molecular weight and ionic charge (pI); bands are detected by a radioactive or biotinylated complementary probe of DNA (Southern blot), RNA (Northern blot) or protein (Western blot)

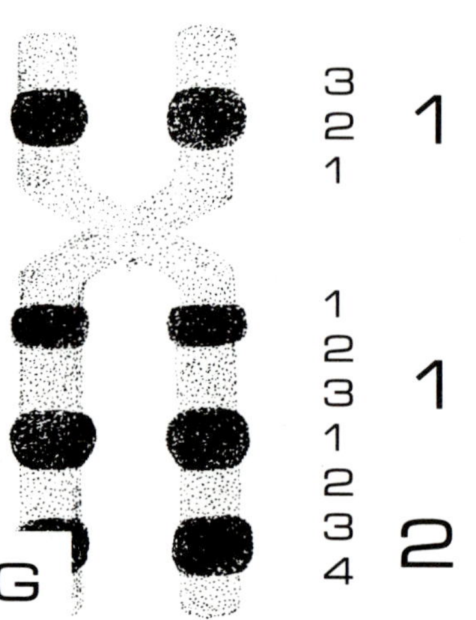

Band cell Band, Band form An immature neutrophil with a nucleus lacking the segmentation typical of mature polymorphonuclear leukocytes, having one continuous nuclear membrane 'band'; more than 5% of the neutrophils in the peripheral blood implies increased neutrophil production; see Left shift

Band form A mature trophozoite intraerythrocytic form of ***Plasmodium malariae***; see Applique form, Ring form; Cf Band form

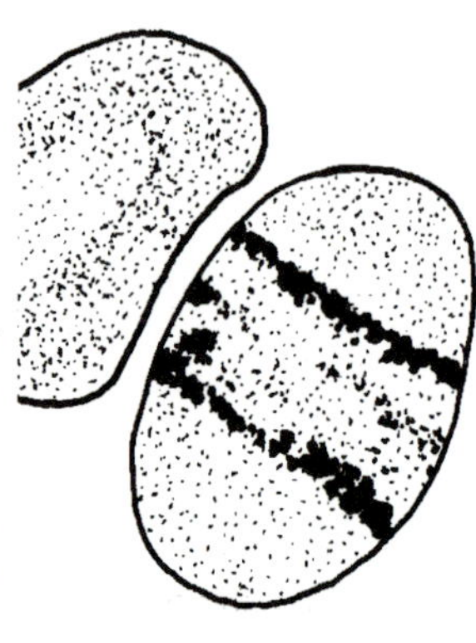

Band form

Banding CARDIAC PATHOLOGY Zonal changes of cardiac muscle due to myocardial ischemia, characterized by opaque transverse bands within myocytes adjacent to an intercalated disc, accompanied by shortening and scalloping of the sarcomere, fragmentation of Z bands, distortion of myofibrils and displacement of mitochondria away from intercalated disc; see Contraction band necrosis; Cf Wavy changes

Banding CYTOGENETICS A group of techniques for evaluating chromosomal 'landmarks', which allows identification of gross chromosomal defects that are regularly associated with either congenital conditions, eg trisomies, monosomies, aneuploidies or with acquired

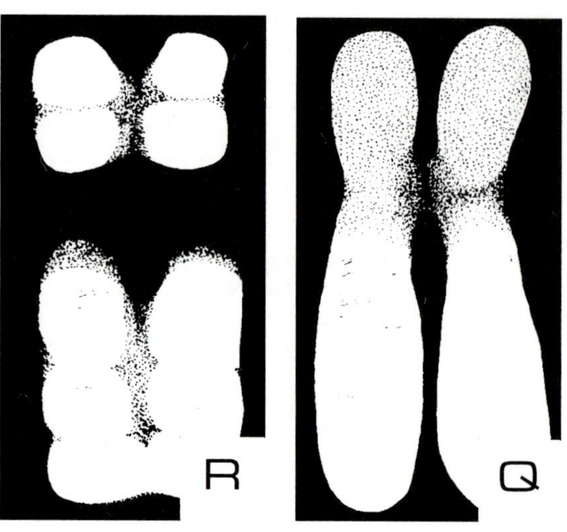

CHROMOSOMAL BANDING

C Centromere banding The chromosomes are pretreated with strong bases, eg NaOH or strong acids, eg HCl, followed by Giemsa staining, which selectively highlights the centromeres

G Giemsa banding The chromosomes are pretreat ed with either concentrated salt, eg NaCl at high temperature or with proteolytic enzymes and then Giemsa stained

Q Quidine banding The chromosomes are stained with fluorescent dyes and then Giemsa stained

R Reverse banding The chromosomes are pretreated with alkaline solutions and analyzed at high temperature with controlled pH; the image seen is opposite that of G and Q anding

disease, or translocations in lymphoproliferative disorders

Band keratopathy A broad deposit of opaque calcium phosphate in vertical lines parallel to, within and often lateral to the limbus, on Bowman's membrane, seen by slit lamp examination; bands in absence of phosphate elevation may presage the onset of renal failure; although band keratopathy is classically associated with hyperparathyroidism, it may occur in any hypercalcemia, eg in subcorneal calcium deposition in chronically inflamed eyes (chronic iridocyclitis of juvenile rheumatoid arthritis or Still's disease), increased vitamin D absorption, uveitis, pilocarpine therapy, glaucoma and laser-induced injury; non-calcific band keratopathy occurs with elastotic degeneration

Band ligation A therapeutic modality used to treat potentially fatal esophageal varices associated with portal hypertension, which may be more effective than the widely accepted sclerotherapy used to obliterate varices (J Am Med Assoc 1991; 266:187n&v)

Bandpass width LABORATORY INSTRUMENTATION The range of wavelengths between two points used by a spectrophotometer or colorimeter, at which point the transmittance is 1/2 the peak value, where the remaining wavelengths were blocked by a bandpass filter

Band regularity CYTOGENETICS A term that connotes constancy of DNA-protein interactions; chromosomal bands are presumed due to folding of the chromosomes, where each band represents approximately 5% of any one chromosome

Bandshifting MOLECULAR BIOLOGY A difference in the rate in DNA band migration in gel electrophoresis that occurs despite equal size of the fragment or band of DNA; the amount of bandshifting migration is relatively small, in the range 1-4%, which may become significant in forensic DNA analysis; the faster migration is corrected for by running a 'monomorphic' probe that attaches to a fragment of DNA similar in all persons (Science 1989; 246:1556); bandshifting is a function of the actual size (in number of nucleotides) of the band, the concentration of the gel (ie concentration of the agarose) and the actual running time (speed of the run); one way to eliminate this problem is to run a sequencing gel, in which the actual 'signature' of the entire hypervariable (unique to the individual in question) has been previously amplified by a PCR technique (Science 1990; 247:1018); see DNA fingerprinting

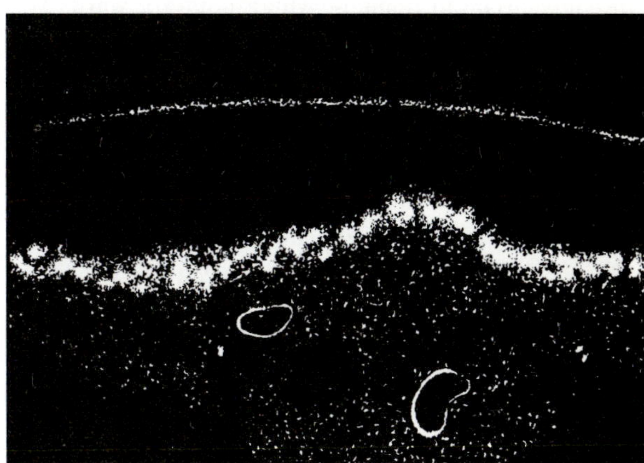

Band test

Band test Lupus band test IMMUNOPATHOLOGY Immune deposition of IgG,with varying amounts of IgM, IgA, C3 at the dermal-epidermal junction in discoid (DLE) and systemic lupus erythematosus (SLE); the band test is negative in the uninvolved areas of DLE; 90-95% of lupus erythematosus patients have bands in clinical lesions, 80% have bands in sun-exposed skin and 50% of non-sun-exposed skin; the presence of dermal bands is poorly reflective of renal disease, although DLE and SLE patients with a negative band test or IgM deposits alone may have a better prognosis or less intense renal involvement, hypocomplementemia and anti-DNA antibodies; 'bands' also appear in acne rosacea, anaphylactoid purpura, atopic and contact dermatitides, autoimmune thyroiditis, early bullous pemphigoid, cold agglutinin syndrome, dermatomyositis, facial telangiectasia, hypocomplementemic vasculitis, lepromatous leprosy, polymorphous light eruption, primary biliary cirrhosis, procainamide and hydralazine-induced lupus erythematosus, pyoderma gangrenosum, rheumatoid arthritis and scleroderma; a band is also seen in NZB/NZW mice, the animal model for lupus erythematosus; Cf Antinuclear antibodies

BANF Bilateral acoustic neurofibromatosis see Neurofibromatosis, type II

Bangungut see Sudden unexplained nocturnal death

B-antigen, acquired TRANSFUSION MEDICINE A modified antigen found on the membranes of A1 red blood cells that agglutinates as though it were a group B erythrocyte, due to enzymatic modification of the normal A1 into a B-like antigen, caused by bacteria, including *Escherichia coli*, *Clostridium tertium* and *Bacteroides fragilis*, associated with gastrointestinal pathology, eg carcinoma or severe infection

BAO Basal Acid Output Production of gastric H+ under baseline conditions, normal: 0-10 mmol/hr; BAO serves to measure the completeness of vagotomy; patients with Zollinger-Ellison syndrome have a ratio of basal to maximal acid output (BAO/MAO) of greater than 60%; BAO is also increased in pernicious anemia, gastric carcinoma, myxedema and rheumatoid arthritis; Cf MAO, PAO

Barbed ends MEMBRANE PHYSIOLOGY The portion of the nonmuscle actin filament which points towards the membrane or sites of attachment

Barber pole pattern A descriptor of the angiographic appearance of the 'supercoiled' superior mesenteric artery and vein as seen in a midgut malrotation with volvulus (Radiol 1973; 109: 555)

Barbell tumor see Dumb-bell

Bar code Machine-readable identifier A rectangle with a series of lines of varying thickness, each corresponding to the numbers 0-9 that may be 'scanned' by a device detecting variations in light patterns, allowing the symbols to be recognized directly by a computer's central processing unit; in the hospital, bar coding may be used to provide the patient with a unique identifier, eg for laboratory specimens, X-rays and medical records, preventing incorrect transferral of data and to facilitate documentation

Barefoot doctor A term originating in and being phased out of the Republic of China, referring to countryside health-aides who were neither barefoot nor doctors (J Am Med Assoc 1988; 259:3561)

Bare lymphocyte syndrome An autosomal recessive immune deficency disorder described in several North African kindreds due to non-expression of HLA-A, -B or -C (Class I) major histocompatibility complex, caused by a defect in surface expression of β_2-microglobulin; in some cases, the HLA-Dr determinant is also not expressed Clinical Variable, from asymptomatic to mucocutaneous candidiasis, respiratory tract infections, opportunistic infections, chronic diarrhea and malabsorption, poor response to antigens, aplastic anemia and leukopenia with normal or increased B cells with decreased T cells (N Engl J Med 1985; 313:757) MOLECULAR BIOLOGY The condition is thought to be due to a defect in gene activation and/or a defect in accessibility of the promoter protein (Science 1991; 252:709)

Barium burger test A method for evaluating increased gastric retention of food as occurs in the gastric outlet obstruction (GOO), where the 'burger' is 'flavored' with barium contrast; GOO is diagnosed if barium is retained for more than 6 hours in an intact stomach or for more than 3 hours in a resected stomach (Am J Gastroenterol 1972; 58:411)

Barium enema A barium-rich fluid used to visualize the colonic lumen, of greatest utility in delineating colonic neoplasia

Barium peritonitis A rare complication of a barium enema, in which there is a high (50%) mortality, due to intraperitoneal perforation with leakage or spillage of radiocontrast material, variably accompanied by feces, release of histamine and vasoactive substances into the peritoneum with activation of coagulation pathways causing fibrinous peritonitis

Barium 'sandwich' A mixture of solid food and barium contrast used to evaluate esophageal deglutition by fluoroscopy, obtaining information beyond the capabilities of the plain 'barium swallow'

BARK β-Adrenergic receptor kinase A membrane protein that down-regulates (desensitizes) cellular sensitivity to sensory, neurotransmitter and hormonal stimulation, mediating stimulatory effects of catecholamines on the adenylyl cyclase system and by extension regulating intracellular cAMP levels; the β-ARK gene sequence is similar to protein kinase C and cAMP-dependent protein kinase(Science 1989; 246:235)

BARN Bilateral acute retinal necrosis A herpes virus-induced anterior and posterior uveitis, papillitis with retinal detachment occurring 1-3 months after onset, of which only 50% are bilateral

Barney Clark see Clark, Barney

Barrel A descriptor occasionally used in medicine referring a morphology or pattern likened to a barrel Rounded bulging vessel constructed of wooden staves, bound with metal hoops with flattened ends, designed to hold liquid or grains, whose length is slightly greater than its diameter

Barrel cervix GYNECOLOGY A descriptor for the rounded thickening seen in the rare lymphoma of the uterine cervix

Barrel chest RESPIRATORY MEDICINE A broad chest with hyperinflated, poorly aerated lungs, typical of emphysema; a similar short, but broadened chest of a different etiology occurs in Morquio syndrome or mucopolysaccharidosis, type IV

Barrel staves pattern An ultrastructural finding in clear cell sarcoma (malignant melanoma of soft parts) that simulates flattened and curved barrel staves, corresponding to the internal structures of premelanosomes

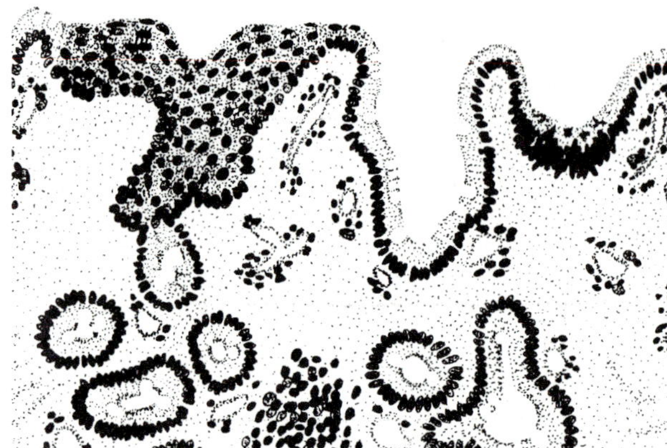

Barrett's esophagus

Barrett's esophagus The occurrence of columnar epithelium lining a segment of the distal esophagus, occasionally accompanied by peptic ulceration; although most patients are adults, it may affect children, leading to speculation that the condition has a congenital component; Barrett's esophagus places a patient at an estimated 35-40-fold increased risk of suffering adenocarcinoma of the esophagus, which is almost invariably accompanied by dysplasia, and has a prognosis similar to that of epidermoid carcinoma of the region (14.5% five-year survival) **Histopathology** Barrett's epithelium is of three broad types: atrophic gastric fundus with parietal and chief cells, cardiac (junctional type), consisting of mucus glands and specialized columnar glands, possibly representing a form of intestinal metaplasia

Barrier method Contraceptives (condom or diaphragm) that attempt to prevent the boy-meets-girl-make-baby sequence; the theoretical effectiveness of barrier methods is 2.5 pregnancies/100 woman-years, the actual effectiveness is closer to 15/100; see Pearl index

Barrier precautions INFECTION CONTROL Any method or device used to reduce the contact with potentially infectious body fluids, including facial masks, doubled gloves and fluid-resistant gowns

Basal cell carcinoma syndrome see Nevoid-basal cell carcinoma syndrome

Basaloid carcinoma Cloacogenic carcinoma A histologic variant ofepidermal carcinoma arising at the anorectal transition zone and comprising 20% of all carcinomas of this region; although this tumor histologically mimics basal cell carcinoma (from whence its name), it often displays mucin production and squamous differentiation and behaves clinically like a 'garden variety' anal carinoma, the distinction appears to be unwarranted Note: Anal carcinoma has been associated with independent carcinomas of partners, eg of the uterine cervix, condyloma acuminatum and with the practice of receptive anal intercourse in the male homosexuals, thus indirectly inculpating human papillomaviruses

Basal metabolic rate (BMR) A calculated value that allows a crude calculation of a person's proteo-caloric requirements; the most commonly used formula is that of Harris and Benedict:

BMR, men: 66 + (13.7 X weight) + 5 X height) - (6.8 X age)

BMR, women: 655 + (9.6 X weight) + 1.8 X height) - (4.7 X age)

Baseball finger Mallet finger A flexion deformity at a 30 angle of the distal phalanx, produced by a blow to the tip of the finger, in US most often associated with catching a baseball thrown at high speed, with forced flexion of the distal phalanx and separation (by rupture or avulsion fracture) of the common extensor tendon from its insertion in the base of the distal phalanx; accompanied by inability to extend the fingertip

Baseball stitch A type of surgical repair used to close the uterus in the classic Cesarian section incision, an incision more cephalad than the now-preferred lower uterine segment incision as it is associated with greater immediate and remote morbidity; the baseball stitch closure is continuous, not locked, with 2-0 chromic and each needle 'bite' begins on the raw surface of the wound, exiting through the serosa a few millimeters from the cut edge, infolding the cut edge, bringing the serosal surface over to cover the uterus

Basement membrane An organized multi-molecular layer composed of collagens, predominantly type IV, glycoproteins, eg laminin and fibronectin and proteoglycans, eg dermatan sulfate, which is subjacent to epithelium and endothelium; basement membranes are dynamic structures involved in cell growth, adhesion and differentiation; dissolution of the basement membrane is a final step in the development of metastasizing carcinoma

Base pair A pair of hydrogen-bonded bases that link to each other; in the DNA double helix, purines (adenine and guanine) or pyrimidines (cytosine and thymine) link to each other

Base pairing The complementary binding of the bases in a nucleic acid, between two strands of DNA or a strand of DNA and RNA; see Hybridization

BASIC Beginners' All-purpose Symbolic Instruction Code A high-level symbolic computer programming language that is commonly used to write programs for mini- and microcomputers

Basket cell NEUROHISTOLOGY A cell of the cerebellar cortex, the axons of which give off splays of fine branches which enclose the Purkinje cells in a basket-like fashion HEMATOLOGY A fragmented and degenerated leukocyte in a peripheral blood smear with a bare nucleus partially surrounded by a coarse network of splayed, red-purple nucleoplasm that may be seen in a normal subjects and increased in atypical lymphocytosis, chronic lymphocytic and acute leukemias, thus being similar in origin to 'Smudge' cells

Basophil A granular leukocyte bearing distinctly basophilic secondary granules containing heparin, histamine, platelet-activating factor and other mediators of the immediate hypersensitivity, released when IgE cross-links to the high affinity Fc receptors on the cell's surface

Basophilic stippling Punctate stippling HEMATOLOGY A finding in Wright-Giemsa-stained erythrocytes that appears as 'blue' dots, spots and blots within erythrocytes consisting of a) RNA granules (coarse stippling) due to RNA instability in young red cells, seen in lead poisoning (lead inhibits ALA dehydrogenase and ferrochetolase, impairing heme incorporation and inhibiting nucleotidase), defective hemoglobin C or hemoglobin E synthesis, sideroblastic or megaloblastic anemia, thalassemia major and minor, preleukemic states, pyrimidine 5'nucleotidase deficiency b) Aggregates of precipitated ribosomes (fine stippling), resulting in diffuse polychromasia secondary to increased erythrocyte production in thalassemia, malabsorption and pernicious anemia

BAT Blunt abdominal trauma

Bathing suit distribution A pattern of truncal skin involvement in rheumatic heart disease (erythema marginatum), characterized by flattened, slowly enlarging maculopapules that undergo central healing, a pattern also seen in X-linked lipidosis, Fabry's disease (angiokeratoma corporis diffusa, punctate to macular, non-blanching telangiectasia), glycosphingolipidosis, fucosidosis and sialidosis

Bathing trunk nevus Giant congenital melanocytic nevus A congenital pigmented skin nevus covering any large area, thus also designated as 'stocking', 'cap' or 'coat sleeve' nevi; these nevi may be 20 cm or larger in greatest dimension with satellite lesions, deeply pigmented with moderate growth of hair, require multiple operations for excision and about 12% undergo malignant degeneration; Histologic patterns: Compound or intradermal nevus, neural nevus and blue nevus; involvement of the head and neck region may be associated with epilepsy, mental retardation and leptomeningeal malignant melanoma; the draining lymph nodes are often pigmented, corresponding to benign nevus cell aggregates within lymphoid tissue Note: A bathing trunk pattern also occurs in the neurocutaneous melanosis complex, or in lower 'girdle' mongolian spots, which may be extensive if the patient also has a bilateral nevus of Ota

Battered buttock 'syndrome' A rare complex described in females consisting of fracturing of fat or traumatic lipomas, in which tissue is sheared between the dermal anchorage of the skin and the deep fascia

Battered child syndrome Trauma 'X', Child abuse A tragedy that claims 2-5000 lives/year in the USA, often first recognized radiologically by certain characteristic findings, consisting of metaphyseal fragmentation, due to repeated subperiosteal contusions with hemorrhage, which heals with a thickened cortex, incomplete 'bucket handles' (avulsed metaphyseal fragments torn from the periphery of the cartilage-shaft junction), old fractures, sub-periosteal hematomas due to 'wringing' of extremities with epiphyseal dislocations, metaphyseal cupping, shortening of the shaft and a ball-and-socket configuration); pelvic fractures (which rarely occur by falling, as the child's caretakers may claim, and are always of a suspicious nature); fractures of posterior ribs (often at the articulation between the transverse process and the rib tubercle), spine and sternum (Am J Radiol 1986; 146:895), a post-mortem radiological survey may be indicated in order to convict the caretaker/parent of manslaughter (N Engl J Med 1989; 320:507, 531ed); Cf Child abuse

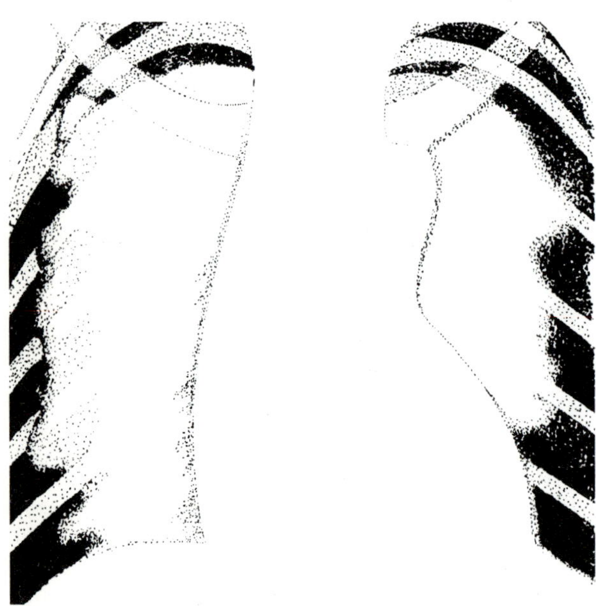

Batwing distribution

Battered prize fighter face A descriptor of the facies seen in the X-linked or autosomal dominant otopalatodigital syndrome of Taybi, which is characterized by frontal bossing, a broad nasal bridge, flattened facies, accompanied by a cleft palate and micrognathia, deafness, mental and growth retardation, deformities of the hands and feet and pectus excavatum

Battle-axe appearance see Halberd bone

Battledore placenta A morphological placenta variant where the umbilical cord is placed at the margin, not thought to have clinical significance Battledore: Old English, a flat, wooden paddle used in the game of battledore, an ancestor of badminton

Batwing distribution Butterfly distribution RADIOLOGY A descriptor for shaggy, bilateral perihilar lung opacifications, seen on an antero-posterior chest film, due to intraalveolar fluid exudation, first described in uremia, but more typical of pulmonary edema and may occur in pulmonary alveolar proteinosis

Baud A unit of velocity of electronic transferral of data, where one baud is equal to 1 bit/second; standardized transmissions are 300, 1200, 2400 and 9600 baud; see Computers, Modem

Bayonet hairs A developmental defect of the hairshaft with excess keratinization of the upper third, thought to be common in ichthyosis and seborrhea and occasionally seen in normal scalps

Bayonet hand A deformity described in hereditary multiple exostosis (diaphyseal aclasis) characterized by ulnar deviation of the carpus and subluxation of the radius

Bayonet incision An elongated S-shaped incision used to treat lacerations and for providing access in reconstructive surgery to the wrist bones; the bayonet incision is not indicated in the rheumatoid wrist where the distal skin flap may slough, requiring an abdominal pedicle flap

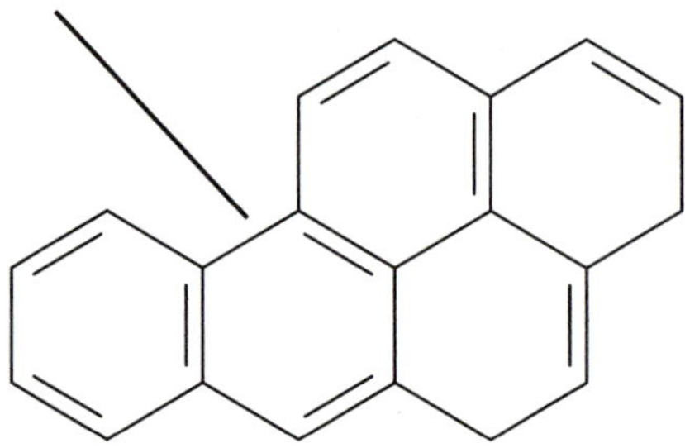

Bay region EXPERIMENTAL ONCOLOGY The site on benzo(a)pyrene (Figure), an indirect carcinogen that is metabolically activated by the P-450 system at the 7, 8 double bond, leading to a 7, 8 oxide, which is rapidly

converted to a 7, 8 dihydrodiol and later epoxidated near the bay region at the 9, 10 double bond; the resulting product, a diol-epoxide is a poor substrate for epoxide hydratase and is released from the mitochondria into the cell as a highly reactive electrophil, becoming an 'ultimate' carcinogen, as it reacts with negative charges in DNA; P-450 reactions at the K region (see there) yield a non-reactive non-carcinogenic inert molecule

BBB syndrome see Hypertelorism-hypospadias syndrome

B cell see B lymphocyte

B-cell lymphoproliferative syndrome (BLS) An uncommon, life-threatening complication of bone marrow or organ transplantation caused by profound immunosuppression, which may be induced by Epstein-Barr virus; BLS occurs in 0.23 to 0.45% of the recipients of HLA-identical bone marrow, especially in those patients who suffered severe graft-versus-host disease and were treated with anti-CD3 antibodies Clinical Ranges from self-limited, spontaneously-resolving infectious mononucleosis to oliclonal or monoclonal proliferations and aggressive lymphomas Prognosis 80-90% mortality in bone marrow recipients; 60% survival in those receiving other organs; one 'magic bullet' modality uses anti-B cell antibodies (monoclonal antibodies to CD21 and CD24 antigens) to suppress the B-cell lymphoproliferative syndrome and is well-tolerated, although its efficacy remains unproven (N Engl J Med 1991; 324:1451)

BCG bacille Calmette-Guerin A strain of ***Mycobacterium bovis*** that has been grown for multiple generations on potato, bile glycerine agar to a point where it has retained its immunogenicity but lost its virulence; BCG is an effective vaccine for tuberculosis and has been used to non-specifically stimulate the immune response in patients with certain malignancies, eg melanoma; because of its long-term persistance in the body, it has potential use as a vector for genes encoding HIV proteins including Gag, Pol, Env, reverse transcriptase, gp20, gp40 and tetanus toxin (Nature 1991; 351:479, 442); extrachromosomal and integrative expression vectors carrying the regulatory sequences for major BCG heat-shock proteins (hsp60 and hsp70) allow the expression of foreign antigens present in BCG (Nature 1991; 351:456), and may be used as a live recombinant vaccine vehicle to induce immune response to the pathogen's protein

B chromosome GENETICS Supernumerary segments of DNA that are present in many species, which appear to be driven to self-duplication, as they are transmitted at higher rates than otherwise expected from classic Mendelian genetics

***bcl*-2** MOLECULAR BIOLOGY The B-cell leukemia/lymphoma gene, an altered protooncogene associated with follicular lymphoma, mapping to chromosome 18q21, the site of t(14;18) translocations; increased expression of bcl-2 is an early event in certain lymphomas, and when present in diffuse or nodular large cell lymphomas, indicates a poor prognosis (those with a *bcl*-2 rearrangement survive less than 3 years; those with a duplication of chromosome 2 survive less than 1 year (N Engl J Med 1989; 320:1047)

Bcl-2 A 25 kD protein encoded by the ***bcl***-2 miniproto-oncogene and located on the inner mitochondrial membrane, which blocks programmed cell death (Science 1990; 348:334), an event that occurs by apoptosis

BCNU see Carmustine

B complex IMMUNOLOGY A designation for the major histocompatibility complex (MHC) in chickens with loci encoding class I and II MHC antigens as well as red blood cell antigens

B complex NUTRITION An obsolete and incorrect term for the water-soluble vitamin B1 and B2 isoforms

bcr Breakpoint cluster region A 5.8 kilobase DNA segment on chromosome 22 that is related to malignant transformation of pluripotent hematopoietic stem cells in chronic myelogenous leukemia (CML); in CML there is a reciprocal translocation between chromosome 9, band q34 (a site containing the human homolog of the Abelson viral oncogene, c-*abl*) and chromosome 22 band q11 (the location of the breakpoint cluster region); this translocation results in formation of the 'Philadelphia' chromosome (named after the city of its discovery), which transcribes a hybrid mRNA encoding a protein with tyrosine kinase activity

BDNF Brain-derived neurotrophic factor A member of the nerve growth factor family, which selectively elicits growth in the retinal ganglion, evokes increased secretion of dopamine in the substantia nigra and GABA in the forebrain; in the MPTP-induced model of Parkinson's disease, 75% of dopamine neurons are lost, an effect prevented by addition of BDNF, implying that loss of this trophic factor may have a role in Parkinson's disease (Nature 1991; 350:230, 195); see MPTP, Neurotropin-3, Nerve growth factor

B-DNA A sequence-dependent local variation in the structure of the DNA helix, seen in states of high hydration, which influences groove width, helical twist, mechanical rigidity, bending and resistance to bending; each segment of DNA has its own molecular surface 'signature', critical for specific recognition by proteins that repress and enhance DNA transcription; see DNA forms

Beaded hair disease Monilethrix An autosomal dominant condition characterized by short brittle hair that may evolve to alopecia and a high incidence of cataract formation

Beaded ureter see Corkscrew ureter

Beading CARDIOVASCULAR PATHOLOGY Luminal irregularity of arteries supplying regions affected by electrical injury; beaded vessels are at risk for subsequent thromboses RADIOLOGY Diffusely distributed dilated divisions and diverticular outpouchings (figure, page 52) of the common bile duct punctuated by short annular fibrotic strictures seen by direct cholangiography in primary sclerosing cholangitis (N Engl J Med 1984; 310:900cpc) ORTHOPEDICS Multiple post-fracture tumefactions of the ribs, characteristic of osteogenesis imperfecta, type II, see Accordion, Rosary

'Beads on a string' see Solenoid structure

Beak sign UROLOGIC RADIOLOGY A gently curved outward bulging of renal cortex adjacent to a well-circumscribed renal mass in the late or nephrogram phase of selective renal angiography, indicating the presence of a slowly expanding, usually benign avascular renal cyst with smooth inner walls, seen in arterionephrosclerosis, but also seen with renal cell carcinoma

Beaking PEDIATRIC RADIOLOGY A finding in lateral films of the spine in mucopolysaccharidoses and mucolipidoses where there is a bird-beak-like tapering of the anteroinferior or anterosuperior margin of the lumbar vertebrae; a 'beak' is also described in the medial aspect of the proximaltibia at the epiphyseal plate in Blount's disease or coxa vara, the functional correction of which may require osteotomy

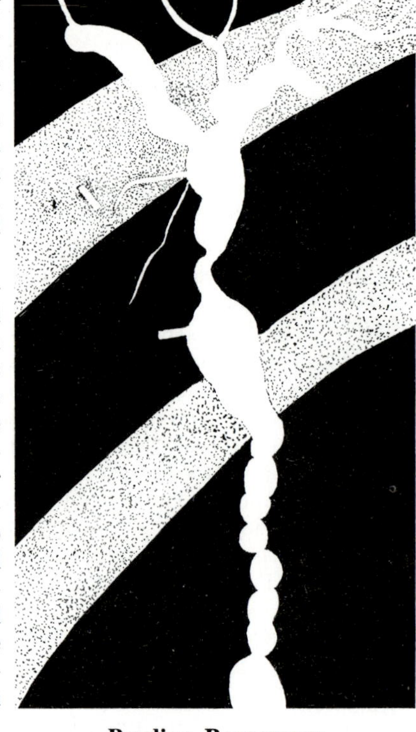

Beading, RADIOLOGY

Bean bag cells Histiocytes filled with phagocytosed leukocytes, erythrocytes, and cellular debris, seen in histiocytic phagocytic panniculitis

'Bean counter' A colloquial expression for an administrator or functionary in any institution's finance department, who 'counts beans', an ancient form of exchange

Bearskin rug appearance A descriptor for the gross pathology of the small intestinal mucosa in Whipple's disease, in which the villi are distended with macrophages; the serosa is dull, the intestinal wall is thickened and the mesentery indurated

'Bear tracks' OPHTHALMOLOGY A descriptor for blotchy congenital pigmentation seen in the ocular fundus, without known clinical significance

Beaten brass/silver RADIOLOGY Variably-sized rounded zones of bony attenuation of the cranial bones caused by pressure from the cerebral cortical gyri, resulting from premature closure of the cranial sutures and by extension, increased intracranial pressure

Beat knee Coal miner's knee Prepatellar bursitis caused by prolonged kneeling often associated with trauma and/or infection, either acute, associated with serous effusions or chronic with hemorrhage, loose bodies and calcifications

Beaver body MICROBIOLOGY A stool contaminant confused by the inexperienced with helminth eggs, corresponding to an alga, ***Psorospermium haeckelii***, found in crayfish tissues and in the stool following a typical Creole meal

Bed HOSPITAL ADMINISTRATION A unit of 24-hour patient occupancy in a hospital or other inpatient health care facility, which is a measure of the hospital's size; licensure and certificates-of-need are based on the number of beds, allocated according to intended use or duration of stay and designated as an obstetric bed, oncology bed, outpatient bed, ie less than 24-hour use, resident bed, ie long-term stay for persons requiring custodial and personal, but not medical or nursing care and temporary bed, ie that which is allowed when a hospital temporarily exceeds its legally allowed capacitysee Certified bed, 'Swing' bed

Bed bug A blood-sucking arthropod that is either cosmopolitan (***Cimex lectularius***) or tropical (***C hemipterus***) in distribution; the bedbug elicits pruritus and in sensitive individuals, urticaria, vesiculo-bullous lesions arthalgia and asthmatic symptoms

Bedside testing LABORATORY MEDICINE Evaluation of analytes in the immediate vicinity of a patient, often in a relatively critical state; devices used are often less accurate than the machines used in a hospital's laboratory, but have the advantage of short 'turn-around' time, eg two minutes, facilitating therapy, using minimal volumes, eg 250-500 µl; bedside testing may be used for pH, PO_2, PCO_2, sodium, potassium, hematocrit, glucose, calcium and chloride (J Am Med Assoc 1991; 266:382); Cf Stat testing

Bedsore see Pressure ulcer

BEE Basal energy expenditure The amount of oxygen consumed while resting and fasting, extrapolated to 24 hours, roughly equivalent to 25 kcal/kg; see Basal metabolic rate

Beef growth hormone An anabolic steroid used by the cattle industry to increase the muscle mass, the safety of which has been seriously questioned, to the point that some countries have banned importation of such meat (Science 1990; 249:875rv); Cf Bovine somatotropin

Beef tapeworm ***Tenia saginata***

Beehive on the bladder RADIOLOGY A descriptive term for a biconvex triangular deformity, the apex of which corresponds to the bladder end of a colovesicular fistula; the colon becomes fixed to the peritoneal surface of the bladder, resulting in restricted bladder contraction, stasis and focal cystitis with necrosis of the fibromuscular tissue between the bladder and the colon, causing a fistula (Ann R Col Surg Eng 1982; 63:195)

Beer drinker syndrome A disease complex of historical interest that occurred when cobalt was added to the malt as a 'frothing' agent, affecting those consuming two or more liters of cobalt-treated beer/day Clinical Cardiomegaly, congestive heart failure, tachycardia, hypotension, hepatomegaly, dyspnea Prognosis: 50% fatality

Behavior modification PSYCHOLOGY The use of operant conditioning models, ie positive and negative reinforcement as espoused by BF Skinner to modify behavior

Behavioral teratology A postulated form of teratogenesis in which drugs or toxins induce permanent behavioral 'damage'; it is difficult to verify behavioral changes given the subtlety of teratogenic effects and the subjectivity of interpretation; functional neurotransmitters appear early in fetal development and may be vulnerable to teratogenic agents during periods of fetal or postnatal immaturity

Beige mice A mutant murine model for Chediak-Higashi disease characterized by pigmentary abnormalities, defective natural killer cell activity and an increased incidence of malignancy

BEIR studies Biological effects of exposure to low levels of ionizing radiation A series of studies from the National Research Council (UK) that periodically analyze the cancer data from Japanese atomic bomb blast survivors and from those with long-term exposure to low levels of radiation BEIR IV studied the long-term effects of short-range α radiation, primarily from radon gas in the home and in uranium mines; BEIR V was released in 1989 (Science 1990; 247:22) and indicated that those with low-level exposure were 3-4 times more likely to get cancer

Bejel An non-venereal infection by a strain of *Treponema pallidum* that is virtually indistinguishable from venereal *T pallidum* (syphilis); bejel affects children in Saharan Africa and the Middle East Clinical, early Lymphadenitis, condyloma-like oropharyngeal and anogenital lesions Clinical, late Lesions mimic those of tertiary syphilis, including gumma, bony deformities and nodular skin ulcers Treatment Penicillin, erythromycin and tetracycline

Bell clapper testicle Congenital lengthening of the tunica vaginalis or mesorchium; the testicle lies horizontally in the scrotum, predisposed to torsion and infarction, the testicle has been likened to the clapper of a bell

la Belle indifference see Conversion disorders

'Belly' tap Abdominal tap CRITICAL CARE MEDICINE A rapid method for differentiating the 'surgical' abdomen, ie that requiring surgery from a 'non-surgical' abdomen, avoiding an unnecessary laparotomy; the tap consists in either a bilateral flank or four-quadrant cytologic sampling along the peritoneal gutter with a 20- or 18-gauge spinal needle; the yield is about 80%, demonstrating unclotted blood or if delayed, florid acute inflammation, both requiring immediate intervention; 'belly' taps are indicated in: Blunt abdominal trauma alone or in combination with injuries to the head, thorax or the extremities or with concomitant substance abuse, acute pancreatitis, post-operative peritonitis or peritonitis in children with a second disease process

Belt Any broad geographical region boasting an increased incidence of a particular disease process; see AIDS belt, Asian esophageal cancer belt, Lymphoma belt

Bench A long worktable; a colloquial term for the site where hands-on experimental research, ie 'benchwork', is performed

Bends, the see Caisson's disease

Benign lymphadenopathy Any non-malignant regional or generalized enlargement of lymph nodes, which may be divided into histological patterns (table)

BENIGN LYMPHADENOPATHY PATTERNS

NODULAR AIDS, giant lymph node hyperplasia (Castleman's disease), reactive hyperplasia, rheumatoid arthritis and in secondary syphilis

PARACORTICAL Dermatopathic lymphadenitis, nodular paracortical hyperplasia, immunoblastic response to viruses and drugs

SINUSOIDAL Sinusoidal hyperplasias, histiocytic medullary reticulosis, histiocytosis X, sinus histiocytosis with massive lymphadenopathy (Rosai-Dorfman disease), sinusoidal lipogranulomas and as a reactive pattern in certain malignancies, eg Kaposi sarcoma, metastatic carcinoma, melanoma

DIFFUSE OR OBLITERATIVE Post-vaccinial or other viral lymphadenitis, eg Herpes zoster, phenytoin hypersensitivity, dermatopathic lymphadenopathy, atypical reactions to metastatic carcinoma and melanoma, lupus erythematosus, angioimmunoblastic lymphadenopathy, infectious mononucleosis

GRANULOMATOUS Lymph nodes draining joint and breast (silicon) prostheses, intravenous drug-abuse, yersinia, lymphogranuloma venereum, tularemia, tuberculosis and atypical mycobacteria, cat-scratch disease, sarcoidosis, sarcoid-like changes seen in lymph nodes draining tumors, fungal, brucellosis, toxoplasmosis, syphilis and leshmaniasis

MIXED Metastatic carcinoma, allergic eosinophilic granulomatosis; Cat scratch disease, granulomas, infectious mononucleosis, lymphogranuloma venereum, sarcoidosis, toxoplasmosis and

DEPLETED AIDS-related complex; see Follicle lysis, Lymph node necrosis

Benign lymphoepithelial lesion Mikulicz disease A lesion of the salivary and lacrimal glands, clinically related to Sjögren's syndrome and thought to be autoimmune in nature Histopathology Clusters of epithelial cells (epimyoepithelial cells) and abundant lymphocytic infiltration with occasional germinal centers; BLEL may demonstrate transition to carcinoma, implying that the lesion arises in the epithelium (Am J Clin Path 1989; 92:808); Cf 'Eskimoma'

Benign 'metastasis' Presence of non-malignant non-lymphoid tissue in lymph nodes, eg thyroid follicles in regional lymph nodes of the neck, potentially confused with carcinoma (Cancer 1969; 24:309); when thyroid follicles are seen, microscopic size, lack of stromal proliferation or psamomma bodies, presence of round-to-oval follicles that are not papillary or crowded, bland, uncrowded nuclei with fine chromatin and small nucleoli militate against malignancy; see Lymph node inclusions

Benign neglect Certain lesions and clinical conditions are well known for their tendency to be either stable over time, eg verruca vulgaris or to actually regress, eg capillary hemangioma; because these lesions do not undergo malignant degeneration and at most, represent cosmetic problems, an appropriate 'therapy' is that of benign neglect

Benign triton tumor Neuromuscular choristoma; see Triton tumor

Benzodiazepine receptors BZ-1, BZ-2 Two different receptors for benzodiazepine have been tentatively identified in the brain; BZ-1 receptors may affect neural pathways involved in normal sleep patterns, while BZ-2 receptors are involved in memory and motor functions

Benzoylecgonine The major metabolite of cocaine, which is the molecule most often measured in the toxicology laboratory; see Cocaine

Bergalis, Kimberly A young woman who became infected with HIV-1 by her dentist (J Am Med Assoc 1990; 264:2018), the first case of this route of transmission known to AIDS epidemiologists; the 'Bergalis case' has heightened the debate on whether a) HIV-infected health care workers should provide 'hands-on' health care, potentially endangering the lives of patients and b) Whether physicians and other health care workers should be regularly tested for HIV-1, and whether the results of those tests should be available to the public

Beri-beri A disease caused by deficiency of thiamine (vitamin B_1), phosphorylated into thiamine pyrophosphate, a coenzyme in carbohydrate metabolism, required for synthesis of acetylcholine, a neurotransmitter; beri-beri affects the heart (cardiac dilatation and fatty degeneration), peripheral nerves (myelinolysis and axonal degeneration), subcutaneous tissues (edema and vascular congestion) and serosal linings (effusions) **Clinical** Fatigue, apathy, irritability, depression, muscular atrophy, paresthesias, abdominal pain and if extreme, increased intracranial pressure and coma **Dry beri-beri** affects the central and peripheral nervous system **Clinical, children** Plethoric with pallor, hoarseness due to nerve paralysis, apathy, dyspnea, tachycardia and hepatomegaly **Wet beri-beri** is more cardiocentric **Clinical** The afflicted children are malnourished with pallor, edema, tachycardia, dyspnea, renal failure, right-sided cardiac failure **Treatment** Thiamine-rich foods, eg milk, vegetables, cereals, fruits

Berry aneurysm A 0.2-0.5 cm saccular dilatation of arteries at the base of the brain, at or adjacent to the circle of Willis (95% of berry aneurysms) or at the vertebrobasilar arteries (5%), due to a developmental or congenital weakness in the medial muscle layer of the cerebral arteries; 30% of the aneurysms are multiple, located at bifurcations, often anterior (figure) and appear in 1-2% of all autopsies; most berry aneurysms rupture when they surpass 1 cm in diameter and are more likely to rupture under stress, due to acutely increased systemic blood pressure, eg coitus, athletic competition, but is not related to trauma; berry aneurysms may be associated with aortic coarctation, polycystic renal disease, collagen disorders, eg Ehlers-Danlos and Marfan syndromes, arteriovenous malformation and fibromuscular dysplasia

BES see Back extensor strength

BEST A T1-weighted inversion recovery sequence, a variant of the echo-planar technique of MRI, developed by P Mansfield of Nottingham, used for ultra-high-speed imaging of the brain; Cf MBEST, MRI

BESWL Biliary extracorporeal shock-wave lithotripsy

β decay Low-level radioactive decay in which β particles (usually an electron with an antineutrino, less commonly a positron with an antineutrino) are emitted; Cf α decay, Electron capture

β effect Hormonal action of epinephrine and norepinephrine resulting in metabolic, hemodynamic and modulatory changes, a function of the concentration of adrenergic receptors on the α and β cells of the pancreatic islets; βeffects (epinephrine acting on α islet cells) include: lipolysis, ketogenesis, stimulation of glucagon secretion, β_2 arterial vasodilatation and β_1 increases in myocardial rate, contractility and conductivity

β emitter A radioisotope that decays with the emission of an electron (β particle), designated as 'soft' if the electron emitted is of low energy and has a short distance of penetration, or 'hard' if the electron is high-energy with a great penetrating distance

β-enolase An enzyme, two forms of which are present in skeletal and cardiac muscle, that catalyzes glycolysis of 2-phosphoglycerate to phosphoenolpyruvate; in acute myocardial infarction, the rapid peak of β-enolase at 12 hours is potentially more specific and of more use than that of creatine kinase (Br Heart J 1987; 58:29); Cf Cardiac enzymes

Beta-gamma bridge IMMUNOLOGY A 'spanning' of the usually well-defined peaks in the β and γ regions in serum protein electrophoresis (figure), seen in chronic hepatopathies, classically in alcoholic liver disease; the

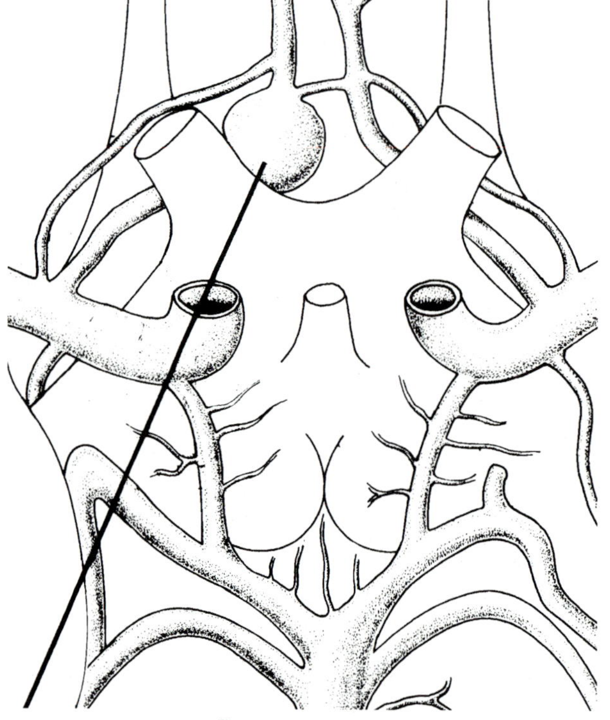

Berry aneurysm

β-γ bridge also occurs in chronic infections and connective tissue disease and is due to polyclonal production of proteins that migrate in the region, which may 'bury' small monoclonal expansions or the clone may produce polymeric forms of the protein resulting in differences in electrophoretic mobility, causing a 'pseudo-polyclonal' expansion Normal β migrating proteins: Transferrin and β-lipoprotein Normal γ migrating proteins: IgG, IgA, IgM

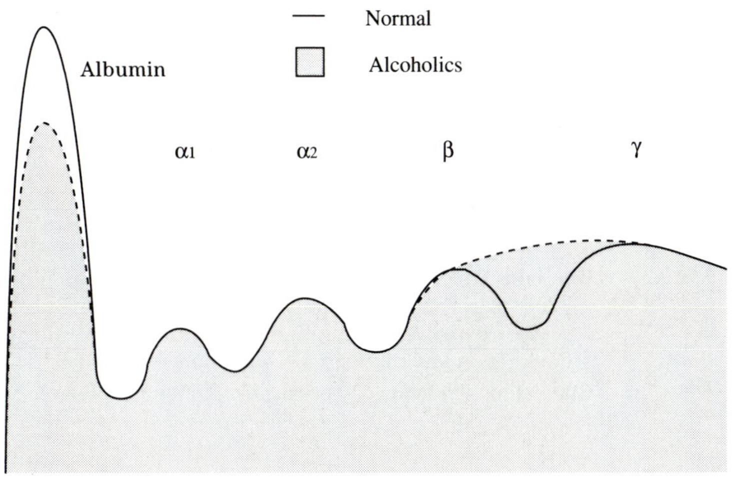

Beat-gamma bridge

β-glucuronidase A lysosomal hydrolase that is increased in the cerebrospinal fluid of 75% of patients with metastatic intracranial carcinoma and in 25% of patients with intracranial myelogenous leukemia

β hemolysis see γ 'hemolysis'

β-lipotropin β-LPH A 91-residue peptide derived from the carboxy-terminal portion of pro-opiomelanocortin (POMC), the precursor molecule for corticotropin-related peptides, eg ACTH, MSH and others which arrive through the mechanism of alternative slicing; see POMC

β_2 microglobulin (β2M) Thymotaxin A 11.8 kD polypeptide produced by the thymic epithelium and expressed on the surface of antigen-presenting cells, providing one of two immunoglobulin-like domains, in part participating in the selection of MHC I peptides (Nature 1990; 346:751), and which, by ensuring the proper folding of class I molecules, is a key non-antibody member of the immunoglobulin superfamily; β2M is non-covalently linked to the major histocompatability complex (MHC) class I proteins, and is a component of the class I trimer (peptide antigen/class I/β_2-microglobulin) and that presents antigens to cytotoxic T cells; while the highly polymorphic class I MHC proteins determine the immune response, β2M is chemotactic and stimulates T cell maturation; as a free molecule, β-2M markedly increases the generation of antigenic complexes capable of T cell stimulation (Nature 1991; 349:74); β-2M is co-expressed with CD1 thymocyte glycoproteins and intestinal IgG receptor; disruption of the gene in a mouse embryonal stem cell line through homologous recombination with a nonfunctional β2M generesults in an unexpectedly healthy mouse that lacks $CD4^-8^+$ T cells with defective T cell mediated cytotoxicity and thus β2M is not critical to survival (Nature 1990; 344:742; Science 1990; 248:1227)

β-pleated sheet A protein structural motif elucidated by Pauling and Corey, so called as they had previously delineated the α-helix; the polypeptide chains in β sheets are almost completely extended, with an axial distance of 35 nm, versus an axial distance of 15 nm in the α helix); the β-pleated sheet is stabilized by hydrogen bonds between NH and CO groups of different polypeptide strands; adjacent molecules may run in the same direction (parallel) or in the opposite (antiparallel) direction, eg silk fibroin; the β-pleated sheet is a tertiary structure elucidated by X-ray crystallography and seen by electron microscopy, which can be produced experimentally by treating Bence-Jones proteins with enzymes and is a structure typical of amyloidosis Histopathology The β-pleated structure may be appreciated by the Congo red stain using polarizing light to reveal the characteristic apple-green birefringence Ultrastructure Extracellular 700-1000 nm in diameter, fine complex non-branching fibrils

beta testing The on-site testing of a device, equipment, hardware or software under the same working conditions for which it was designed, in order to identify potential problems associated with its use, colloquially known as 'working out the bugs'

Betel nut chewing A habit popular among Javanese, Malayan and Indian men; the 'chew' is composed of ground betel nut, slaked lime, ground spices including ginger and pepper wrapped in a betel leaf; the Indians add tobacco to their chew and have a high incidence of oral cancer (comprising 36% of all cancers in this group), whereas the Javanese and Malayans who don't add tobacco have a very low incidence of cancer, exonerating betel nuts; see Khaini cancer

Bethesda unit BU HEMATOLOGY A unit measuring factor VIII (F8) inhibitory activity in plasma; 1.0 BU reduces F8 in 1.0 ml of plasma from 1.0 to 0.5 units; BUs are measured when F8-dependent hemophiliacs become refractory to F8 therapy, caused by a circulating inhibitor or a F8 antibody

Bezoar Any concretion or conglomerate mass of foreign material in the stomach, facilitated by partial or complete gastrectomy, as acid hydrolysis of gastric content is diminished; bezoars remains undigested in stomach, causing discomfort or frank pain, halitosis, gastric wall erosion or ulceration and potentially peritonitis, hemorrhage, obstruction, nausea, vomiting, a palpable mass, more easily palpable in tricho- than in phyto-bezoars; vegetable (phyto-) bezoar may result from ingesting the persimmon ***Disopyros virginiana***, which contains phlobantanin, a substance that coagulates on contact with dilute acid, the dissolution of which requires per os enzyme treatment, a low-fiber diet and decreased intake of high-fiber fruits (persimmons, pears, citrus) in bezoars due to gastrectomies; trichobezoars are seen in trichophagic neurotics; anecdotal association with gastric carcinoma is probably a statistical artefact Note: Aggregates of *Candida* species within the renal collecting ducts have also been termed bezoars Note: Bezoar is a translation of the Arabic 'Badzehr' for antidote or anti-poison; bezoars from the Middle East were from the stomachs of goats and gazelles, those from South America, the vicuna, each thought to have medicinal value in the treatment of aging, snakebites, evil spirits and the plague

BFP Biological false positive A laboratory result that is positive in a subject known to be a true negative for the substance being measured; the classic BFP is a positive result with the VDRL (venereal disease research laboratory) serological test for syphilis, seen in 10-20% of patients with lupus erythematosus; BFPs are common cause of the 'Ulysses' syndrome, see there

BFU Burst-forming unit Erythron A self-renewing cell giving rise to a cluster of erythroid clones, known as the burst unit, which in turn gives rise to the colony-forming units (CFU); 'bipolar' BFUs have either erythroid or megakaryocytic differentiation

BH_4 Tetrahydrobiopterin cofactor Synthesized from GTP, BH_4 is a cofactor for tyrosine and tryptophan hydroxylase, both of which are required for dopamine and serotonin synthesis; deficiency of BH_4 may result from three different enzyme defects; without BH_4, phenylalanine cannot convert to tyrosine and thus accumulates, accounting for 2% of cases of phenylketonuria

Bhopal ENVIRONMENT An ecodisaster occurring in India in late 1984, caused by leakage of methyl isothiocyanate (MIC) gas, used in the production of carbaril pesticides , which caused the deaths of (according to various estimates) 1800 to 5000 people, injuring up to 300 000 Note: In 1978, the US National Institute for Occupational Safety and Health (NIOSH) indicated MIC had poor warning properties, eg smell, and thus had been considered a dangerous chemical **Clinical** Acute toxicity consisting of respiratory distress, attributed to cyanide toxicity, including dyspnea, cough, throat irritation, chest pain and hemoptysis; with time the lesions evolved to interstitial pulmonary fibrosis; ocular effects include burning, edema, erythema, tearing, pain, photophobia and corneal ulceration; negative impact of MIC is reported in gestation, in the immune, neuromuscular and other systems, although some effects did not reach statistical significance (Indian J Med Res 1990; 91:28, J Am Med Assoc 1990; 264:2781rv); see Disaster; Cf Chemical warfare

Biclonality A generic term for the rare occurrence of an uncontrolled expansion of two (or more) clones of neoplastic cells, as would be biclonal expansion of two B cell lines or B and T cell lines (Am J Clin Path 1989; 92:362); this contrasts to the more common, uncontrolled clonal expansion of a single, often hematopoietic progenitor cell line; Cf Composite lymphoma

BIDS syndrome Brittle hair (and fingernails), intellectual impairment, mild decreased fertility and short stature An autosomal recessive condition affecting the Amish kindred of Pennsylvania

'Big science' A term that refers to large long-term, multicenter and often multinational research efforts that are goal-oriented, initiated by consensus committees, rather than an individual investigator and costly, ie multiples of billions ($, US), eg Human genome project, the 'War on Cancer', the Space station and Superconducting super collider; Cf 'Little science'

'Big spleen disease of Africa' see Tropical splenomegaly

Biko, Steve A black activist from the Republic of South Africa (RSA) who was tortured to death while in prison and under medical supervision, six days after being detained by police for questioning; although torture and murder by police in RSA was common before and after Biko's death in 1977, the case brought to fore issues of apartheid medicine and physician involvement in activities clearly against the tenets of the Hippocratic Oath, one of the physicians involved in the Biko case lost his license to practice medicine; see Academic boycott, Apartheid medicine

Bile lake HEPATIC PATHOLOGY An extravasated pool of bile (figure) lying outside of partially necrotic liver cell plates, caused by peripheral (extrahepatic) biliary obstruction and rupture of the bile canaliculi

Bile reflux syndrome A post-gastrectomy complex characterized by retrosternal pain, anorexia, nausea, bilious vomiting **Treatment** Roux-en-Y anastomosis

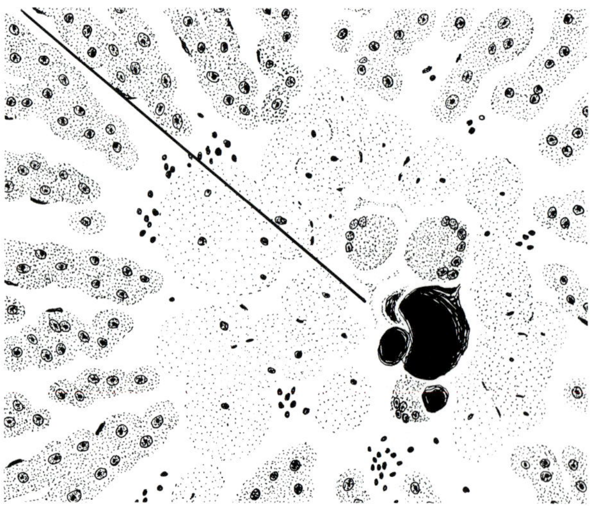

Bile lake

Billiard ball effect FORENSIC PATHOLOGY That which occurs after a second shotgun blast to the same body site, where the original shotgun pellets are struck from the rear by the incoming pellets, splaying deeper into the body at multiple angles, likened to the opening shot or 'breaking' in a game of billiards

Bill of patient rights A statement of the ethical principles used by a health care facility that obligates all members of the professional, operational and voluntary staff working in that facility to respect a patient's dignity and rights

Binder Granulator CLINICAL PHARMACOLOGY An inert agent used to impart cohesive qualities to a powdered drug or other material, ensuring that a drug tablet will remain intact after compression; binders include starch, gelatin, gums, methylcellulose and sugars including sucrose, dextrose, molasses and lactose; see Inactive ingredient

Binding domains MOLECULAR BIOLOGY Structural motifs present on DNA-binding regulatory proteins that govern gene expression, either enhancing or repressing mRNA synthesis; 'binding proteins' recognize sequence specific sites 'binding domains' on the DNA and often share sequence homology with each other, eg Leucine zipper motif and protein products of the myc, fos and jun proto-oncogenes; see DNA-binding proteins, Transcription factors

Binding protein Carrier protein A generic term for a circulating protein that reversibly binds a variety of small molecules, including amino acids, sugars, inorganic ions, vitamins and others

Binge A component of bulemia, which consists of a 'session' of hyperpolyphagia, in which up to 15 000 calories may be consumed in one hour; binges are commonly followed by self-induced emesis or 'purging' Complications Gastric rupture (Mallory-Weiss syndrome), vascular compression, pancreatitis, aspiration pneumonia, ipecac-induced myocarditis, cardiac failure, refeeding edema, metabolic alkalosis, hypokalemia and hypochloremia, see Binge-purge syndrome

Binge drinking An early phase of chronic alcoholism, characterized by episodic 'flirtation' with the bottle by binges of drinking to the point of stupor, followed by periods of abstinence; bouts of heavy alcohol consumption are accompanied by alcoholic ketoacidosis (accelerated lipolysis and β-hydroxybutyric acid production due to impaired insulin secretion), decreased food consumption and recurrent vomiting

Binge-purge syndrome Bulemia (Greek, to eat like an ox) is a compulsive eating disorder, usually afecting women that is of later (age 17-25) onset than anorexia nervosa, but similar in its preoccupation with food; bulemics may consume enormous quantities of food, a 'binge', followed by self-induced emesis, a 'purge'; bulemics may have concomitant impulsive behavior (alcohol and drug abuse), poor peer and parental relations; sexual promiscuity and stealing may be required to financially support the eating 'addiction; see Binge; Cf Scarlet O'Hara 'syndrome'

Binging SUBSTANCE ABUSE A phenomenon described in intravenous cocaine abuse, where the subject may inject the cocaine up to five times per hour for up to 48 hours without sleeping or eating, since in cocaine, the 'high' (burst of euphoria) is shorter and the craving for more cocaine is very intense (J Am Med Assoc 1989; 262:1467c); cocaine 'bingers' are often too paranoid to share their needles and thus less likely to spread HIV; the animal model of cocaine abuse correlates closely with 'binging', as given unlimited access, the rats 'binge' to death within two weeks, dying of cardiorespiratory failure; with 'Ice', a substance of abuse of recent vintage, binging occurs cyclically, with 4-5 days of binging, followed by a 2-3 day period of rest; see Ice

Bioassay Any test that measures the functional or effective amount of a substance in an in vivo system, either within a cell or an organism, eg infectivity or hormonal stimulation

Bioavailability The in vivo presence of a substance in a form that allows it to be metabolized, serve as a substrate, bind a specific molecule or participate in biochemical reactions; bioavailability depends on the pI or ionic form, presence of side chains or the conformation of the epitope; bioavailability is affected by the route of administration, rate of metabolism, lipid solubility and binding proteins

Biochemical convergence A series of 'simplification' events seen in cells evolving toward malignancy; the cells lose such features of differentiation and organ-specificity as microvilli, desmosomes, intermediate filaments and suffer down-regulation of 'differentiated' enzymes

Biocomputing A somewhat nebulous term referring to computing activities and research on biochemical or biological phenomena, eg neural networking, biosensors and molecular design (*BIOCOMPUTERS,* Kaminuma and Matsumoto, Chapman and Hall 1991); Cf Computers, Medical informatics

Biocontrol ENVIRONMENT The use of natural products or engineered microorganisms to protect food crops against insects, circumventing the use of chemical pesticides; biopesticides include ***Bacillus thuringiensis*** (Bt), an organism that has been endowed with a wide range of activity thanks to recombinant engineering of a gene that encodes a chimeric Bt protein toxic to a wide range of insects, or by splicing the Bt toxin gene into other organisms; other biocontrol products include baculovirus-derived toxins and pheromones (Science 1991; 252:211n&v)

Biodegradable ENVIRONMENT Any molecule or substance that can be degraded by the enzyme system of a living organism; see Bioremediation

Biodiversity ENVIRONMENT The existence of multiple flora and fauna in an ecosystem; it is widely accepted that the loss of biodiversity, ie a reduction in the number of species, subspecies and strains is dangerous and could have diasastrous consequences for humans, as well as the planet's ecosystem; an example would be growing a crop food, eg corn or rice from only one highly productive, rapid growing, spoil-resistant strain; while seemingly having all the desirable features, should the strain then become susceptable to a particular pathogen, all those dependent on the crop could face famine

Biofeedback A form of operant conditioning in which the patient learns to control certain deranged physiologic functions; the patient is made aware of nature of the dysfunction by watching or listening to aninstrument which records or measures the deranged process, eg Control of fecal incontinence by watching the recorder of a balloon manometer, control of constipation in the elderly by watching an anal-plug electrode, reduction of pulse rate by listening to amplified pulse sounds; biofeedback may be successful in controlling hypertension, Raynaud's phenomenon, seizures and pain

Biohazardous waste Waste products including body fluids and tissues that may carry dangerous human pathogens; these waste products often originate from health care facilities and/or research laboratories, and place a relatively small or confined group of people at risk for infection during the time necessary for the infectious agent to desiccate or otherwise become inactive; biohazardous waste became a 'media epidemic' in the 1980s when vials of blood with HIV-1 washed up on beaches in metropolitan New York; these materials are indicated by an internationally recognized biohazard symbol (figure); see Biosafety, Regulated waste

Biohybrid artificial pancreas A therapeutic device currently being developed as an optimal insulin delivery system, which is constructed of a selectively permeable tubular membrane containing xenogeneic pancreatic islets that locks out molecules larger than 50 kD, which is coiled in a protective housing and connected to the vascular system; the low kD of the membrane prevents access of the immune system to the foreign islets; six of ten pancreatectomized dogs maintained good control of the fasting glucose with long-term implantation of the biohybrid (Science 1991; 252:718); see Organoid; Cf Insulin pump, Islet cell transplantation

'Biolistics' CELL BIOLOGY A technique that 'shoots' DNA of interest at a high speed directly into organelles, using a 1 μm tungsten projectile coated with a nucleic acid of interest, shot from a specialized 'gun'; biolistics developed as a solution to the problem of directly transforming, ie introducing foreign DNA into chloroplasts and mitochondria, which is difficult as these organelles are invested with a double membrane envelope that prevents nucleic acid entry (Science 1988; 240:1533, 1538; Nature 1987; 327:90)

Biologicals Therapeutic agents that derive directly from the pools of various living organisms (usually mammals or other humans); biologicals are thus not amenable to chemical or physical standardization steps required of pharmaceuticals, are potentially impure chemically and their safety cannot be assumed; biologicals are regulated by the Food and Drug Administration and include vaccines, anti-toxins and blood plasma products prepared from donor pools Note: 'Drugs' prepared by recombinant DNA technology, eg lymphokines and other biological response modifiers are also biologicals and regulated by the Food and Drug Administration, but are considered safe as they derive from non-pathogenic recombinant viruses and their doses can be standardized

Biological clock see Circadian rhythm

Biological response modifiers (BRM) A broad family of molecules that modulate the immune response; BRMs include interferons, interleukins, (hematopoietic) colony-stimulating factors and tumor necrosis factor, B cell growth factor and differentiating factors, eosinophil chemotactic factor, lymphotoxin, macrophage chemotactic factor, macrophage activating factor, macrophage inhibiting factor, osteoclast-activating factor and others, many of which are generated after a T-cell recognizes an antigen present on the surface of a self antigen-presenting cell), which, once activated, produces a 'catalog' of lymphokines (cytokines); many BRMs are commercially available, produced by recombinant DNA technology; the first FDA-approved agent was α-interferon, used to treat hairy cell leukemia, and although BRMs have already been called the 'fourth therapy' in the anti-cancer armamentarium (the first being surgery, radiotherapy and chemotherapy), BRM therapy is in its infancy and most of the agents are not fully characterized or available for clinical use, although many are in early stages of the drug development process; ; the therapeutic effects of BRMs include 1) Regulation and/or increased immune response 2) Cytotoxic or cytostatic activity against tumor cells 3) Inhibition of metastasis, or cell maturation and 4) Stimulation of marrow stem cells, required for recuperation from cytotoxic insult secondary to chemotherapy; the adverse reactions vary according to the agent, dose schedule and route of administration **Side effects** Flu-like with fever, chills, malaise, arthralgia, myalgia, anorexia, headache, symptoms that often decrease with time, despite a continued high dose (a phenomenon known as tachyphylaxis); the optimal route of administration for each BRM is at present empirical COLONY-STIMULATING FACTORS Five myelopoietic cytokines bind to specific cell receptors and orchestrate growth and differentiation of hematopoietic cells; granulocyte-macrophage colony-stimulating factor (GM-CSF) is produced by activated T cells and NK cells; erythropoietin, granulocyte-CSF and macrophage-CSF are produced by monocytes and other cells; CSFs have a role in recuperation of hematopoiesis after bone marrow transplantation or toxic chemotherapy, mitigating the effects of chemotherapy, allowing higher than usual doses of chemotherapeutic agents to be given and/or stimulating the phagocytic activities of macrophages and granulocytes **Side effects** are similar to, but less intense than those of other BRMs, eg flu-like and gastrointestinal symptoms, dyspnea and hemorrhage INTERFERONS (IFNs) were the first BRMs to be delineated (in 1957, the 'dark ages' of immunology) and are divided into α-IFN (20 subtypes) and β-IFN (2 subtypes), both produced by macrophages and bind to a type I membrane receptor and γ-IFN, produced by T and NK lymphocytes, which binds to a different receptor; IFNs are 1) Antiviral, causing those cells playing host to certain viruses (eg rhinovirus, papillomavirus and retrovirus) to produce proteins capable of interfering with intracellular viral replication, 2) Antiproliferative, acting by unknown mechanisms, possibly decreasing the translation of certain proteins, slowing the cell cycle and 3) Immunomodulation, stimulating or increasing certain immune effects (T cell activation, maturation of pre-NK cells and increased phagocytosis and cytotoxicity by macrophages **Side effects** Flu-like symptoms, gastrointestinal (nausea, vomiting, anorexia, diarrhea, dysgeusia, xerostomia), neurological (confusion, somnolence, poor concentration, seizures, transient aphasia, hallucinations, paranoia, psychoses), cardiopulmonary (tachycardia, dyspnea, orthostatic hypotension, cyanosis), hepatorenal (increased transaminases, increased BUN, proteinuria) and hematological (neutropenia, thrombocytopenia); α-IFN has FDA approval for treating hairy cell leukemia, AIDS-related Kaposi sarcoma and condylomas, and is active in other hematopoietic malignancies, as well as malignant melanomas, renal and transitional cell carcinomas **Interleukin** The best studied in clinical applications is Interleukin-2 (IL-2), which is not directly cytotoxic, acting rather as an immune modulator and immune regulator; IL-2 is produced by activated T cells in response to macrophage-processed antigen and IL-1 in the medium, and 1) Facilitates T cell proliferation by binding to 'high-affinity' receptors on activated T cells, enhancing T cell cytotoxicity, 2) Facilitates the secretion of and enhances the functions of other cytokines (interleukins, suppressor factors and colony-stimulating factors), increased B cell production via T helper cells, facilitates proliferation and activation of NK cells; IL-2 and LAK (lymphokine-activated killer) cell combination may induce partial or (rarely) complete remissions in metastatic renal cell carcinoma, malignant melanoma and colonic adenocarcinoma **Side effects** Flu-like, gastrointestinal and neurological symptoms (as above), cardiovascular (capillary leak syndrome, peripheral edema, ascites, arrhythmias, orthostatic hypotension), bronchopulmonary (nasal congestion, cough, dyspnea, tachypnea, pulmonary edema), hepatorenal (increased transaminases, increased BUN, proteinuria, oliguria) and hematological (anemia, thrombocytopenia) **Monoclonal antibodies** Immunoglobulins produced by fusing an immortal mouse cell line (eg myeloma) with a mouse plasma cell that produces antibody against an antigen of interest, forming a mouse 'hybridoma' that is an immortal antibody-producing factory; theoretically, monoclonal antibodies (MoAbs) could target a specific antigen on a tumor cell's surface, initiating an immune-mediated tumor-lysis or toxins linked to the constant end of a MoAbs heavy chain, being directly toxic to tumor cells; viable anti-tumoral products for use in human malignancy have been hindered because the human recipients of MoAbs react immunologically against various epitopes on the mouse immunoglobulin, producing human anti-mouse antibodies, see HAMA; one solution is to 'humanize' the antibodies, using only the portion of the mouse immunoglobulin absolutely required for immune recognition **Tumor necrosis factor** TNF Cachectin TNF is produced by macrophages and other cells and is directly toxic to tumor cells or may cause vascular endothelial damage, causing necrosis in the vessels supplying tumors; TNF may increase production of immune cells (natural killer or NK and B cells, neutrophils), increasing NK cytolytic activity; TNF side effects are similar to other BRNs; see also Colony-stimulating factors, Interferons, Interleukins, T-cells and Tumor necrosis factor

Biological thyroid hormone (BTH) Thyroid hormone preparations that derive from slaughterhouse animals, which contain both thyroxine (T_4) and triiodothyronine (T_3), in proportions that differ according to the animal species, iodine content in the diet of the animal, season of the year and other factors; BTH is available as either crude desiccated thyroid or thyroglobulin; endocrinologists do not use these preparations as their potency and bioavailability is uncertain, making them difficult to measure and titrate; BTH still has considerable currency for 'nutritionists' and 'holistic health' practitioners who reason that the more 'natural' the product, the safer it is (J Am Med Assoc 1989; 261:2694ed)

Biological warfare The use of infectious agents as a weapon of war; the known deployment of biological weapons was in 1347 by the Tartars who catapulted their dead (from bubonic fever) into the beseiged city of Caffa, spreading the disease to the Genovese defenders; a similar result was obtained by the British who gave smallpox-infected blankets to the American Indians; during World War II, the British experimented with (but never deployed) biological weapons, detonating bombs filled with ***Bacillus anthrax***-laced cattle cakes on the uninhabited Gruinard Island in 1942, an island declared habitable in 1988; agents of potential use as biological weapons include, in addition to anthrax, botulinum toxin and the agents for Argentine hemorrhagic fever, Q fever, Rift Valley fever and tularemia; deployment of such weapons is prohibited by the Biological and Toxin Weapons Convention (1972), supplementing the Geneva Protocol of 1925 (J Am Med Assoc 1989; 262:644); biological warfare research was alleged to have been responsible for an anthrax outbreak due to an explosion in a weapons plant in Sverdlovsk; the 'Yellow rain' incident is equally unclear, alleged to have been due to deployment of biological weapons, alternately explained as having been induced by bee pollen

Bioluminescence see Chemiluminescence

Biomagnetism The study of magnetic fields associated with life functions is a new 'discipline' of biomedicine, the boundaries of which are not yet delineated; it potentially offers a new tool for localizing electrical activity seen in normal and abnormal cortical and cardiac functions; the EEG and EKG 'average' the impulse throughout large regions of measured organ's electrical activity, magnetocardiogram and magnetoencephalogram sample the magnetic field produced by the ion flow inside the cell itself; biomagnetism is an intradisciplinary 'hybrid' with roots in quantum mechanics, superconductivity and bioelectricity

Biomass Environment The sum total of living and dead organisms and organic detritus in an ecosystem or on the planet

Biomaterials Any synthetic or synthetic device that is intended to replace an aging or malfunctioning (or cosmetically unacceptable) native organ, in the form of an implant or prosthesis; see Breast implants, Hybrid artificial pancreas, Shiley valve, Teflon, Total hip replacement

Biopesticides see Biocontrol

Biophysical profile Obstetrics Measurement of five fetal activities that usually identify a fetus at risk for potentially poor outcome, except for the non-stress test, the other parameters may be measured simultaneously by dynamic ultrasound imaging: Fetal breathing movement, a non-stress test, fetal muscle tone, fetal movement and amniotic fluid volume

Bioremediation ENVIRONMENT The addition of microorganisms and/or nutrients to supplement a process of biodegradation, as may occur in an oil spill Note: The release of organic chemicals to water and soil may have dire and long-term consequences to the integrity of an ecosystem; assessment of the extent of biotic remediation of soil contaminated by polyaromatic hydrocarbons, eg mineralization of naphthalene and phenanthrene by bacteria requires that abiotic attenuating processes (chemical dilution, migration, volatilization and sorption) be considered in the model (Science 1991; 252:830); see Iron hypothesis

Biosafety Any activity related to safeguarding a population from the biologically untoward effects of exogenous (usually infectious) agents, while minimizing the environmenal impact of that agent; because of the legal ramifications of exposure to these agents, biosafety has generated a new administrative bureacracy in hospitals, academic and research facilities, the function of which includes risk assessment and waste management; see Biohazardous waste

Biosafety levels A classification for the degree of caution that must be exercised when working with infectious agents **BIOSAFETY LEVEL 1** organisms are relatively innocuous and are not known to cause infection in healthy human adults, eg *Bacillus subtilis* and *Naegleria gruberi* **BIOSAFETY LEVEL 2** organisms are 'moderate risk' agents that may cause human disease of varying severity, potentially affecting healthy adults; often good microbiologic technique, such as minimizing exposure to aerosols is a sufficient precaution for these agents, eg Creutzfelt-Jakob agent, hepatitis B, *Salmonella* spp and *Toxoplasma* spp **BIOSAFETY LEVEL 3** organisms are indigenous or exotic and may infect personnel by aerosols, autoinoculation or ingestion, resulting in disease with potentially serious or lethal consequences, eg human immunodeficiency virus, *Mycobacterium tuberculosa*, St Louis encephalitis virus and *Coxiella burnetii* **BIOSAFETY LEVEL 4** organisms are dangerous and exotic, require a maximum containment facility and pose a high individual risk of exposure and risk to laboratory personnel, eg Lassa fever virus (US Dept Health and Human Services Publication [NIH] 88-8395, May 1988); see Maximum containment facility

Biotechnology GENETIC ENGINEERING The methodological component of molecular and cell biology that consists of the application and modification of biological systems and reactions, eg fermentation, monoclonal antibody production and agritechnology, providing the tools and framework for dissecting cellular and subcellular function and dysfunction, immunologic mechanisms, membrane physiology, cell signalling, oncogenesis, virology and others; the tools of biotechnology include recombinant DNA and monoclonal antibody techniques

Biotin deficiency syndrome A nutritional deficiency syndrome which may be induced by excess consumption of raw egg whites which contain avidin that chelates biotin, resulting in enteritis and dermatitis; biotin is a coenzyme in carboxylation reactions; sources include egg yolks, milk, tomatoes and yeast

Biotrodes Food-based electrodes Many plants contain enzymes that can be integrated directly into an electrode, thereby measuring molecules of interest, eg bananas contain polyphenol oxidase and can measure dopamine; corn kernels contain pyruvate decarboxylase and can be used to measure pyruvate, sugar beets contain tyrosine and jack beans contain urease

Biphenotypic leukemia A dual clonal expansion of two or more leukocyte populations may occur in 21-35% of adult leukemias having both lymphoid and myeloid markers; a finding associated with fewer complete remissions (29% for biphenotypic and 71% for pure lymphocytic leukemias) and decreased survival (8 months vs 26 months); acute lymphocytic leukemias that co-express myeloid antigens have a poor prognosis (N Eng J Med 1991; 324:800)

Bipolar cells HEMATOPATHOLOGY Primitive or 'early' cells found in the bone marrow that have yet to terminally differentiate and are thus capable of giving rise to erythroid and megakaryocytic daughter cells, depending upon the type of locally produced cytokines NEUROPATHOLOGY Elongated, well-differentiated cells, thought to be a feature dictated by the pre-existing fibers; bipolar cells are seen in the pilocytic astrocytoma (bipolar spongioblastoma), a relatively common pediatric tumor found in the third ventricle and cerebellum; in adults, the tumor most commonly affects the temporal lobe DERMATOPATHOLOGY Elongated, wavy, slender melanocytes filled with fine melanin granules, having long branching dendritic processes, grouped in irregular bundles, often located in the superficial dermis, characteristic of the common type of blue nevus

Bipolar disorder Manic-depressive disease A psychiatric disorder affecting 1% of the US population, first appearing by age 30; about one-half of patients have two or three episodes during their lives, each from 4-13 months in duration; an autosomal dominant form was linked to chromosome 11 (Nature 1987; 325:783) Treatment Lithium salts prevent or attenuate manic and depressive episodes, maintained at 0.8-1.0 mmol/L (N Engl J Med 1989; 321:1489); if a manic episode is unresponsive to therapy, electroconvulsive therapy may be effective

Bipolar traits Personality traits that represent extreme opposites of expression, eg dominance-submission, extraversion-introversion, passive-aggression

Bird's beak sign A radiologic descriptor for gastrointestinal tract findings by barium studies COLON 'Ace of spades' appearance A sharply delineated, voluptuously-curved, cut-off of the enema column in a volvulus of the sigmoid colon; if the barium passes proximally, 2 kissing 'bird beaks' are seen, known as an Omega loop ESOPHAGUS The over-distended esophagus of achalasia tapers into a pointed beak corresponding to the non-relaxing lower esophageal sphincter, seen by an upper gastrointestinal radiocontrast study (barium 'swallow'), also known as a 'sigmoid' esophagus ILEOCECAL VALVE The contour of the normal ileocecal valve seen by radiocontrast studies of the lower gastrointestinal tract

Bird breeder's disease/lung A hypersensitivity reaction to aspirated avian feather and proteins, occurring in those raising budgerigars, chickens, ducks, parakeets, pigeons and turkeys

Bird facies A facial dysmorphia characteristic of the Pierre- Robin anomalad, consisting of high-arched, cleft palate, micrognathia and glossoptosis resulting in a bird-like face (the mandibular growth may normalize with time); similar facies may appear alone or associated with Franceschetti (oculomandibulofacial), Hallermann-Streiff, Seckel ('bird-head') and Strickler (cerebrocostomandibular) syndromes

Bird fancier's lung see Parrot fever

Bird-headed dwarfism Seckel syndrome An autosomal recessive complex characterized by growth and mental retardation, a beak-like nose, micrognathism, microcephaly, prominent maxilla and eyes, hypertelorism, strabismus, antimongoloid slant of the palpebral fissures, premature balding, short trunk, variable musculoskeletal changes, eg kyphoscoliosis, joint dislocations, clubbing of fingers and genitourinary anomalies eg cryptorchidism; see Parrot beak syndrome

Birdshot calcification see Buckshot calcification

Birdshot retinopathy Vitiliginous chorioretinitis, see DISC

BI-RG-587 AIDS PHARMACOPOEIA A dipyridodiazepinone that is a potent inhibitor of human reverse transcriptase, capable of in vitro inhibition of HIV-1 replication; BI-RG-587 may be of use as an adjunct to nucleoside analogs, eg zidovudine, ddC, ddI or when HIV-1 becomes refractory to them (Science 1990; 250:1411); see AIDS

Birefringence see Polarization

BIRRU Benign idiopathic recurrent rectal ulceration see Solitary rectal ulcer syndrome

Birth cushion OBSTETRICS A prepartum pillow provided to parturients allowing them to assume a partially squatting, au naturelle position for delivery; 'squat' deliveries appear to require fewer forceps deliveries and shorter second stages of labor (Lancet 1989; 2:74)

Birthing room see Alternate birthing center

Bisferiens pulse A double-beat pulse palpated over the carotid or brachial arteries, characteristic of idiopathic hypertrophic subaortic stenosis (obstructive cardiomyopathy) and aortic regurgitation; the ascending limb (percussion wave) initially arises rapidly and forcefully, producing a systolic pulse peak, followed by a dip or trough and a second slower and broader positive (tidal) wave; in some patients, the pulse is intermittent, and may be evoked by mechanical (Valsalva) or pharmacologic (nitroglycerin or catecholamines) maneuvers; Cf Spike-and-dome Note: The other double beat pulses are dicrotic and anacrotic pulses

Bit COMPUTERS The basic linguistic unit of the binary system, corresponding to an 'on-off' in a computer's memory or logic circuit

Bite cell HEMATOLOGY When hemoglobin denatures (as in α-thalassemia or G6PD deficiency), it precipitates into clumps (Heinz bodies) that stick to the red cell membrane; the spleen 'pits out' a fragment of membrane with precipitated hemoglobin as the cells pass through the splenic sinusoids and the cells appear as if a central piece had been removed and are then called Blister cells; when the blister(s) rupture, the erythrocytes are called keratinocytes or horn cells

Bitterfeld ENVIRONMENT An industrial city in East Germany considered by some to be 'Europe's dirtiest city', a title suggested by a combination of a) The lack of treatment of industrial waste water containing aluminum, zinc, copper, mercury, chlorine, phenols and insecticides b) Air pollution caused by use of low-quality brown coal as an energy source and by untreated pollutants from 80 factories manufacturing film, dyes, pesticides, polyvinyl chlorides and other chemicals and c) Soil erosion due to strip mining; a secret (pre-unification) study commissioned by Communist authorities found that Bitterfeld's children were immune compromised, suffered retardation of bone growth and respiratory disease; the clean-up of Bitterfeld is projected to cost DM 20×10^9

BKA Below the knee amputation An 'elective' procedure often required for peripheral vascular disease; while preferred by the patient (since their sense of loss is lessened), the BKA often requires re-amputation, an important factor related to mortality; furthermore, the prosthetic device fits less satisfactorily to the BKA than the AKA, see there

B-K mole syndrome see Dysplastic nevus syndrome

BK virus A small human polyomavirus which, like the JC virus, is capable of transforming infected cells in culture; primary BK virus infection is usually subclinical, occurs most commonly in early childhood, persists in the renal epithelium and may be reactivated in the face of immune compromise, potentially causing severe tubulo-interstitial nephritis and cystitis in recipients of bone marrow transplants, or in the immunocompromised patients, eg those with hyperimmunoglobulin M immunodeficiency syndrome; Cf JC virus

Black adenoma An extremely rare, often nonfunctional tumor of the adrenal cortex (associated with Cushing syndrome) arising between the reticular and fasciculate zones; the color is due to lysosomal accumulation of lipofuscin Histopathology Polygonal cells with microvilli and desmosomes Differential diagnosis Hematoma, hemangioma, melanoma and myelolipoma

Black cardiac disease of Ayerza A condition characterized by asthma, bronchitis, cyanosis (hence the name), causing secondary polycythemia, dyspnea, emphysema, fibrosis, pulmonary arterial sclerosis, right cardiac ventricular dilatation and hypertrophy, clubbing of the fingers, congestive hepatosplenomegaly and a reactive bone marrow

Black's classification of cavities (see table, page 62)

Black death/bubonic plague The bubonic plague is a infection that in the full-blown fulminant form with explosive *Yersinia pestis* growth may be fatal in 24 hours, destroying normal tissue architecture; after 3

Black's classification

I Those that began as structural defects (pits and fissures)
II Proximal surfaces of bicuspids and molars
III Proximal surfaces of cuspids and incisors, not involving the incisal angle
IV As in III, requiring work on the incisal angle
V Cavities on the gingival 1/3 of the labial, buccal or lingual surfaces of the teeth
VI Cavities on the incisal edges and cusp tips
Note: class VI is not a true Black group

days of incubation, patients suffer high fever, black blotchy rashes (disseminated intravascular coagulation plus petechial hemorrhage) and become delirious; the bursting of a bubo (a massively enlarged, painful lymph node) is excruciatingly painful enough to 'raise the dead' Epidemiology ***Y pestis*** is transmitted by the oriental rat flea (***Xenopsylla cheopis***), which bites the rat, ingesting ***Y pestis*** that rapidly reproduces in the flea's gut forming a 'plug' of obstructing bacteria in the flea's gastrointestinal tract, whereupon the flea becomes ravenously hungry, goes into a feeding frenzy, repeatingly biting the host and regurgitating ***Y pestis***, as the usual hosts (the rats) start dropping like flies, the flea becomes less discriminating and attacks any warm-blooded animal; once in the human population, aerosol becomes the most common mode of transmission, the bacteria's fraction I glycoprotein is antiphagocytic, the endotoxin is responsible for the disseminated intravascular coagulation and shock, and thus is well-armed against the host's counterattack Note: The black plague arrived with the Tartars in Sicily in late 1347, reaching Paris by the following winter, and within 3-4 years of its debut, 25 million had died, 20-35% of Europe's population at the time (J Infect Dis 1984;149:335; Scientific American 1988; 2:118)

'Black diaper' disease see Black urine disease

Black disease see Black fever

Black dot ringworm A non-inflammatory endothrix form of tinea capitis involving the hair shaft, with minimal folliculitis; the 'black dot' designation refers to the patchy baldness where the hair breaks at the surface of the scalp resulting in black ('polka') dots; the spores in the hair shaft measure 5-8 μm and do not fluoresce with Wood's light; fungi implicated include ***Trichophyton tonsurans, T violaceum***, and the African dermatophytic fungi, ***T yaoundei***; Cf Ectothrix

Black dot UROLOGY An early transillumination finding seen in the scrotum in torsion of the testicular appendix, which is a normal persistant embryologic remnant; the black dot may be visualized before major edema appears

'Black eye' 1) see Raccoon eyes 2) A blackened conjuntival nodule in patients using norepinephrine eye drops caused by an adrenochrome pigmented metabolite; other causes of black eyes include choroidal melanoma and melanocytoma of the optic disc and other drugs, eg Atabrine, minocycline

Blackfan-Diamond see Diamond-Blackfan syndrome

Black fever Hindi, Kala azar Invasion of the reticuloendothelial system by ***Leishmania donovanii***, with accumulation of histiocytes in the spleen, lymph nodes, bone marrow, lungs, gastrointestinal tract, kidneys and testes; when fulminant, accompanied by hepatosplenomegaly, lymphadenopathy, pancytopenia, fever, weight loss, hemorrhage and hyperpigmented skin

Black fly Buffalo gnats ***Simulidium*** species flies that measure 1-5 mm, suck blood and cause hemorrhagic oozing papules accompanied by edema and lymphadenopathy, which in tropical Africa, Central and South America; black flies are vectors for ***Onchocerca volvulus***, see River blindness

Black hairy tongue An anglican term equivalent to the American 'Hairy tongue'; Cf Black tongue, 'Hairy tongue'

Black heel Talon noire A disease of athletic adolescents whose sports require considerable 'footwork', eg lacrosse, tennis, football, tennis; the lesion is the result of a shear-stress rupture of papillary capillaries during violent sports in which there are sudden stops and twists on the heels

Black light A lamp that emits electromagnetic radiation invisible to the human eye, commonly understood to be ultraviolet radiation, Cf Wood's lamp

Black lipid membrane A lipid bilayer that is constructed from either natural or artificial lipids, with holes small enough to force the membrane to remain flat (which would otherwise spontaneously form rounded liposomes), as flattened membranes are necessary to study lipid membrane and partition characteristics (J Memb Biol 1989; 109:221)

'Black liver disease' A blackened liver characteristic of the rare autosomal recessive asymptomatic Dubin-Johnson disease, due to defective conjugated bilirubin excretion; bilirubin levels are usually ≤ 120 μmol/L (US ≤ 7 mg/dl), 60% conjugated (direct); estrogens should be avoided as they may intensify the jaundice

Black lung disease Anthracosis is present in the lungs of all urban dwellers and these minimal deposits of carbon dust have no clinical significance; in coal miners, early and significant peribronchiolar deposition of aggregates of pigmented macrophages ('coal dust macules'), are diagnostic for 'coal workers' pneumoconiosis (CWP), and with time, convert to firm blackened 'miliary' nodules with scarring, emphysema, especially in smokers, fibrosis and thickening of the pulmonary arteries, causing obliterative vasculitis, the end stage of which is termed progressive massive fibrosis; the conversion of pneumoconiosis to massive fibrosis may be related to the burden of dust, presence of concomitant silica, underlying tuberculosis, obliterative vascular disease and immune mechanisms; in the USA, certain medical benefits are available (Public Law 92-303) to those with black lung disease

'Black measles' A descriptor for the darkened hemorrhagic cutaneous spots seen in Rocky mountain spotted fever, likened to the rash of hemorrhagic measles (rubeola)

Blackout A sign of early chronic alcoholism (or substance abuse) characterized as an episode of amnesia totalis lasting from hours to days after a period of intense drinking or alcoholic binge; blackout may be due to alterations in central serotoninergic neurotransmission, as these patients also have decreased plasma levels of tryptophan Treatment Zimelidine (a serotonin-reuptake inhibitor) may improve the memory in moderate intoxication (J Am Med Assoc 1990; 263:2683)

Black pain disease see Black urine disease

Black patch delirium A transient clinical complex most common in the elderly who had both eyes patched after eye surgery; the patients are restless, anxious, disoriented in time and space, suffer persecutory delusions, hallucinations and suicidal ideation Treatment Time

Black piedra A superficial phaeohyphomycosis of the tropical Americas and Indonesia, affecting the stratum corneum with little or no deep tissue response Clinical Fragile hair with hardened and gritty nodules of *Piedraia hortae*, often affecting the scalp hairs; Tinea nigra is another form of superficial phaeomycosis, due to *Exophiala wernickii* and *Stenella araguata*; Cf White piedra

Black plague see Black death

Black rain ENVIRONMENT Precipitation colored by soot, incompletely combusted petroleum products and other industrial pollutants; the health effects of drinking intensely 'black' rain water, eg from the burning Kuwait oils is uncertain

Black spot Tache noir, seen at the tick or mite bite sites of Spotted fevers

Black stool A clinical finding often caused by malignancy-related 'occult' hemorrhage; tar-colored or 'tarry' stools appear with as little as 50-75 cc of blood, usually above the ligament of Treitz (as oxidation of the heme by the combined action of enzymes and bacteria requires a number of hours), but may also be due to drugs, eg salicylates, steroids, rauwolfia, phenylbutazone, indomethacin, all known to cause gastrointestinal blood loss in normal subjects and even more in those with underlying digestive tract anomalies; black stool may also be iatrogenic (Charcoal, iron and bismuth) Note: The further 'south' the initial point of bleeding, the more likely there will be fresh blood (hematochezia) versus melena (partially metabolized blood); melena evokes a clinical work-up for the source of bleeding to include upper gastrointestinal tract radiocontrast studies (upper 'GI'), barium enema, endoscopy and biopsies

Black stone A gall bladder concrement that, unlike a brownstone, is composed of a mucin glycoprotein matrix; black stones comprise from 10-90% of all gallstones, depending on the population being studied, and have more calcium, carbonate and unmeasured residue, but less cholesterol and fat

Black sunburst pattern OPHTHALMOLOGY A darkened stellate 'lesion' seen in the optic fundus of patients with sickle cell-hemoglobin C (SC) retinopathy due to the high rate of glycolysis in the end arteriolar system

Black thyroid gland syndrome Intense black pigmentation of the thyroid gland which is benign and associated with minocycline therapy (Arch Otolaryngol Head Neck Surg 1990; 116:735)

Black tobacco The flue-cured blond or Virginian tobacco differs from the pungent, cruder air-cured black tobacco; black tobacco was formerly thought to be less carcinogenic as the incidence of lung cancer in countries consuming black tobacco was once lower, a finding that is now thought to have been a statistical artefact due to slowly increasing exposure; indeed, black tobacco may be even more malicious, as the incidence of bladder cancer in black tobacco smokers is 2.5-fold greater than in blond tobacco smokers and the urine of black tobacco smokers contains twice the mutagenic activity (see Ames assay) as blond tobacco (Carcinogenesis 1989; 10:577); when skin surfaces are painted with the two tars, the latency prior to cancer formation in the black tobacco was shorter; in the lungs there is no difference in the incidence of cancer between blond and black tobacco

Black toe disease see Ainhum; Cf Blue toe disease

Black (hairy) tongue Lingua nigra A variant of hairy tongue, characterized by hyperkeratosis of the filiform papilla and secondary hemosiderin deposition; the lesion is anterior to the circumvallate papillae, related to prolonged antibiotic therapy, resulting in overgrowth of chromogenic bacteria on the papillae, or due to oral bismuth therapy; see Hairy tongue; Cf Hairy leukoplakia

Black tongue A hyperpigmented tongue seen in canines with niacin deficiency, equivalent to pellagra

Black urine A clinical finding due to pathologic excess of various pigments, including homogentisic acid, see Black urine disease, methemoglobin, hemoglobin; Nonpathologic causes of black urine include cascara, iron-sorbitol-citric acid complexes, levodopa, radiocontrast media, methocarbamol, naphthol, phenols, pyrogallol, salicylates, diatrizoates

Black urine disease Alcaptonuric ochronosis An autosomal recessive defect in tyrosine metabolism, more common in males that is due to homogentisic acid oxidase (HAO) deficiency; metabolic pathway of phenylalanine and tyrosine ➔ ring opening of homogentisic acid ➔ malylacetoacetic acid; without HAO, HA polymerizes into a blackened, oxidized, poorly soluble polymer, concentrating in the liver and kidney; the condition is first recognized by the mother who cannot clean the children's diaper since the urine oxidizes to pitch black upon exposure to air Clinical Arthritis due to homogentisic acid deposition in cartilage, tendons, as well as in the sclera, viscera and skin; when severe, pigment deposition can compromise cardiac, renal or pulmonary function, spilling into the urine as a melanin-like product; Cf Blue diaper syndrome

Black vomit The 'vomito negro' typical of the 'intoxication' period of group B arboviral yellow fever may be intense, recurrent and fatal; the darkened color is from altered blood, accompanied by hiccupping, tarry stools, anuria, wild delirium, coma and death

Blackwater fever A rare, often fatal complication of *Plasmodium falciparum* malaria Clinical Fever, severe hemolysis with hemoglobinuria, marked jaundice, thrombosis as the parasitized red cells agglutinate, adhering to the vascular endothelium causing occlusive thrombi and local ischemia, a sequence facilitated by concomitant disseminated intravascular coagulation or related to a drug-dependent, eg quinine, hypersensitivity reaction; renal thrombosis may beget renal failure, with parasitized erythrocytes plugging glomerular capillaries and red cell and epithelial cell casts in the urine

Black widow spider ***Lactrodectus mactans*** A venomous spider indigenous to North America, measuring 13 mm in length with a leg spread of 40 mm that bites with anterior fangs and is potentially fatal in the very young or old; the bites are more common in summer in those using an outdoor privy (WC), explaining why most bites are on the buttocks and genitalia Clinical Immediate sharp, cramping and/or burning pain, dizziness, weakness, spreading to the entire body, activation of the autonomic nervous system (nausea, vomiting, sweating, salivation, tremors, muscle cramping, muscle spasms, twitching, paresthesias) if severe, accompanied by rapid shallow breathing, tachycardia and systolic hypertension, acute nephritis and hemoglobinuria in small children

Blacky pictures PSYCHIATRY A series of 12 pictures in the family life of a dog named Blacky, developed in 1946 for analyzing psychosexual development of children; while the validity has been questioned, they continue to have some analytic currency

Bladder training A biofeedback technique used to treat urinary incontinence, an affliction affecting one-third of women age sixty or older based on a combination of behavior modification, a schedule of voluntary micturition, and patient education that emphasizes neurological control of lower urinary tract function; bladder training reduces the episodes of incontinence by 57% and the volume loss by 54% in women with urinary incontinence who had been urodynamically classified as having either urethral sphincteric incompetence and those with detrusor instability (J Am Med Assoc 1991; 265:609)

Blade of grass sign An elongated, radiolucency extending over a long bone, ending in a sharply demarcated curvilinear 'margin', seen in the destructive phase of Paget's disease of the bone

Blanks LABORATORY MEDICINE A negative control specimen required for immunoassays and quality assurance in many laboratory tests; a blank is processed in tandem with the test serum or tissue, differing therefrom in that a primary antibody is not added in the first step; blanks assure a true negative result, allowing comparison of a possibly positive result with a known negative

BLARS β-lactam antibiotic-resistant staphylococci A term that correctly refers to the mechanism of antibiotic resistance, ie β–lactamase production by Staphylococcus), rather than to the antibiotic (methicillin) in which this resistance was first recognized; nevertheless, 'methicillin-aminoglycoside-resistant ***Staphylococcus aureus***' (see there), has more currency in the literature Note: Bacteria resistant to methicillin are often also resistant to nafcillin and oxacillin and respond poorly to cephalosporins

Blasts Blast cells Relatively large, primitive or early hematopoietic (erythroblast, lymphoblast, megakaryoblast and myeloblast) cells that are actively synthesizing DNA, have a prominent nucleolus and abundant RNA

Blast crisis Blast transformation HEMATOLOGY The abrupt transition of a chronic, relatively indolent but malignant lymphoproliferation, often chronic myelogenous leukemia into an accelerated aggressive phase, with a marked increase in blast cells, where > 30% of the circulating cells are blasts; blast crises are usually refractory to therapy Clinical Progressive leukocytosis, thrombocytosis or thrombocytopenia, anemia, lymphadenopathy, hepatosplenomegaly, splenic and bone pain, fever and thromboses Treatment Response to the accelerated blast phase of leukemia is usually short-lived; myeloid blastic transformations are commonly treated with hydroxyurea; 25% of lymphoblastic transformations respond to prednisone with vincristine; Cf Relapse

Blast injury An injury due to explosions or rapid decompression, the severity of which is a direct function of the intensity of the blast wave; death is caused by exsanguination from ruptured pulmonary vessels with hemorrhage, hemoptysis, air embolism, hypoxia and respiratory failure; other lesions include cardiac contusion, causing arrhythmia, rupture of hollow organs, cerebral injuries (parenchymal hemorrhage and air embolism) and rupture of the tympanic membranes Treatment Supportive; if air embolism is present, hyperbaric oxygen is indicated; other facets of blast injuries include impinging flying objects and whether the subject was submerged or free-standing at the time of the explosion; Cf Nuclear war

Blast transformation see Blast crisis

Bleed Traditionally used as a verb, 'bleed' has acquired nominative status in the highly colloquial synonym for an 'episode of hemorrhage'; an extension of the neologism is a 'bleeder', which may refer either to a) A patient who is hemorrhaging from acute trauma, or one whose marrow has been virtually destroyed by the miraculous vicissitudes of chemotherapy or to b) A blood vessel in an operative or endoscopic field that is overtly hemorrhaging; Cf 'Clotter'

BLEL see Benign lymphoepithelial lesion

Blepharoplasts Fine, dark, occasionally argentophilic dots characteristic of normal ependymal epithelial cells that are positive with PTAH, iron hematoxylin and glial stains, which correspond to the basal bodies of ependymal cilia; when ependymal cells are displaced from the ventricles, blepharoplasts aggregate around the nucleus

Blighted ovum A grossly abnormal or anembryonic pregnancy with inevitable spontaneous abortion; these gestational products have villous edema, hydropic swelling and an absence of villous blood vessels, causing confusion with gestational trophoblast disease; see 'Grapes on a plate', Mole

Blinding CLINICAL PHARMACOLOGY The process of making patients unware of whether a drug (or therapeutic modality) being administered is a placebo/sham treatment, ie control group or the drug or treatment being investigated; studies are blinded with the intention of removing patient subjectivity; double blinding is when the clinical investigator(s) are also unaware of the drug's identity, removing interpretive subjectivity; triple blinding is when the patients, the clinical investigators and those encharged with interpreting the data are unaware of the 'therapeutic arm' in their data set; see Double blinded studies, 'Nocebo', Placebo, Triple blinded studies; Cf Control

Blind loop syndrome Stagnant or Afferent loop syndrome A complication of Billroth II subtotal gastroenterostomy (end-to-side enteroenteric anastomosis) that may be seen years after the surgery; the afferent loop consists of duodenum and a variable portion of jejunum, a loop that is a temporary reservoir for 1-1.5 liters of biliary and pancreatic secretions; after a fatty meal, the contents of a partially obstructed afferent loop may build up, 'explosively' enter the stomach and be regurgitated as greenish bilious fluid Note: In the rare complete obstruction, the vomitus is free of bile; blind loopness may be accompanied by gastric atrophy, hypochlorhydria and the clinical manifestations of bacterial overgrowth, commonly anaerobes, eg ***Bacteroides*** species and anaerobic lactobacilli, as well as enterobacteriaceae, enterococci, clostridia and diphtheroides, accompanied by cobalamin (vitamin B_{12}) malabsorption, the result of bacterial competition for B_{12}; other symptoms include intermittent diarrhea due to disaccharidase deficiency, abdominal 'colic', hemorrhage vitamin deficiencies and neurologic symptoms; with prolonged partial obstruction, the stool becomes steatorrheic (bulky, gray and greasy) accompanied by weight loss; complete blind loop obstruction may be a medical emergency with rapid deterioration, shock and perforation peritonitis Treatment Antibiotics Trimethoprim-sulfamethoxazole, loop shortening, afferent-to-efferent or Roux-en-Y anastomoses or gastrojejunostomy

Blind spot 'syndrome' of Swan A periodic compensatory diplopia or squint that is not a syndrome per se, has no cliniccal significance and responds to simple optical correction

Blister beetle see Spanish fly

Blister cells see Bite cells

Blobs NEUROPHYSIOLOGY Clusters of cells measuring 0.2 mm in diameter that are located in layers II and III of the visual cortex that have a high content of mitochondrial cytochrome oxidase and are involved in color perception

Block OBSTETRICS Regional anesthesia to ameliorate parturitional pain, not associated with compromise in uterine contractility **CAUDAL BLOCK** Extradural, given as a single injection or continuous drip; caudal blocks are technically demanding and require more anesthetic **EPIDURAL BLOCK** The most popular method, given as a single injection or intrathecal 'drip', inserted in the L2-L3 or L3-L4 interspaces; little local anesthetic is used and the bearing-down reflex is not abolished **PARACERVICAL BLOCK** Used in the first stage of labor, consists of injecting a local (less than 2 hour in duration of action) anesthetic in the lateral paracervical region; one-half of infants experience post-anesthetic bradycardia and paracervical blocks are ill-advised if the placental circulation is already compromised **PUDENDAL BLOCK** Used in the second stage to relieve episiotomy-related pain, by transvaginally injectiong local anesthetics into the pudendal nerve **SPINAL BLOCK** Subarachnoid block Anesthesia is rapid and complete with very low doses, but it is rarely used as it abolishes the bearing-down reflex and the mother cannot cooperate

Blocking antibody Any immunoglobulin that competes with another for an antigenic binding site; blocking antibodies may appear in malignancy, preventing a tumor's destruction by cytotoxic T cells

'Blocked pipe' appearance A descriptor for the eosinophilic casts within distal renal tubules and collecting ducts, characteristic of 'myeloma kidney', a finding thought to be more common in lambda light chain myeloma; see Myeloma kidney; Cf Tubular 'thyroidization'

Blocking IMMUNOLOGY Reduction or elimination of nonspecific binding of an antibody to an epitope, accomplished by washing with the serum of a mammal other than one used in the assay system; blocking is the first step in enzyme-linked immunosorbent assay, see ELISA

Blocking antibody CLINICAL IMMUNOLOGY A protective venom- or allergen-specific immunoglobulin G present in high titers in those exposed to anaphylaxis-producing substances; the IgG successfully competes with IgE, blocking the allergenic epitope, preventing mast cell degranulation TRANSFUSION MEDICINE An often incomplete antibody, usually an immunoglobulin G that when diluted, adheres to erythrocyte antigens, blocking agglutination; since agglutination is used to detect red cell antigens, blocking antibodies may cause incorrect blood group typing, appearing in Rh, -K and -k blood groups; their presence may be corrected for by pre-treating test erythrocytes with enzymes or suspending them in colloid solutions when performing the agglutination reaction

Blood and thunder OPHTHALMOLOGY Fundoscopic appearance of retinal central vein occlusion; the veins are dilated and tortuous, the nerve head is hyperemic, accompanied by superficial retinal hemorrhages and soft exudates with only slightly impaired visual acuity

Blood brain barrier (BBB) PHYSIOLOGY A structural and functional barrier that exists between the capillaries and the brain; water, O_2 and CO_2 readily cross the BBB, glucose is slower, Na^+, K^+, Mg^{++}, Cl^-, $HCO3^-$ and $HPO4^{--}$ require 3-30-fold more time to equilibrate with the cerebrospinal fluid than with other interstitial fluids; urea penetrates very slowly; catecholamines and bile salts essentially do not cross the BBB (kernicterus is due to accumulation of bile salts in the brains of neonates whose BBB is yet immature); integrity of the BBB is impaired in hepatic encephalopathy

Blood 'doping' SPORTS MEDICINE Induced erythrocythemia, where an athlete places a unit of autologous blood in storage to be transfused immediately prior to an endurance event, eg long-distance running, resulting in increased athletic performance due to better oxygen delivery to the tissues (J Am Med Assoc 1987; 257:2765) Note: Long distance runners have physiological anemia, which allows an elevated velocity of circulation, dissipating the heat generated while running and rapidly delivering oxygen to the tissues; blood doping results in polycythemia, sluggish red cell circulation and predisposition towards thrombosis, and has been inculpated in at least one race-related fatality

Blood filter A device attached to a unit of blood or components designed to retain blood clots and debris; the standard blood filters have pore sizes ranging from 170-260 μm, allowing them to trap the most clinically significant particles; for platelet concentrates and cryoprecipitates, the so-called microaggregate filters (pore size, 20-40 μm) are preferred as they trap degenerated platelets, leukocytes and fibrin; routine use of micropore filters to reduce the incidence of transfusion-related adult respiratory distress syndrome is controversial and slows the rate of flow, making them unpopular in urgent care

Bloodgood syndrome see Blue domed cyst

Bloodhound face A descriptor for the facies characteristic of cutis laxis, where the infant has an 'aged' face, sagging jowls, accompanied by a hooked nose, everted nostrils, a short columella, a long upper lip and everted lower eyelid; the entire cutis is loose, resembling a poorly-fitted suit

Blood mole The retained blood-covered product of a missed abortion that forms a firm, nodular fleshy mass

'Blood shield' statutes TRANSFUSION MEDICINE Those laws that protect the health care team from liability for transfusing blood products that subsequently prove to be from an individual infected with hepatitis B, HIV-1 or other pathogen, when the indications for transfusion were appropriate for the patient's condition and the unit was tested to be negative for infections by widely-used tests in accordance with the blood bank's own standard operating procedures and 'industry standards'; *THESE LAWS REGARD BLOOD AS A SERVICE*, in the widely accepted landmark case of Perlmutter *vs.* Beth David Hospital, *RATHER THAN A PRODUCT*, as in the earlier Cunningham *vs.* MacNeal Memorial Hospital decision, which would therefore be subject to product liability, based on warranty theory

Blood storage lesions TRANSFUSION MEDICINE Those reversible changes that occur in a unit of packed red cells while stored at 4°C until time of transfusion: Increased potassium, inorganic phosphate; decreased pH, sodium, 2,3 DPG

Blood warmers Devices that warm blood stored at 4° C to body temperature and indicated for a) Rapid infusion of cold blood at rates in excess of 50 ml/kg/hour in adults and at rates in excess of 15 ml/kg/hour in children, b) Exchange transfusion in children, c) Massive transfusion directly into a central venous line and d) Transfusion into patients with cold agglutinins

Bloody show OBSTETRICS Cervical discharges of prelabor and early labor, consisting of pink nonhemorrhagic discharge preceding the onset of labor by hours to days, but is not itself an indication for admission to the labor and delivery unit

'Blooming' see Virilization

Blot Blotting MOLECULAR BIOLOGY A nitrocellulose or nylon membrane bearing a molecule of interest, eg DNA, RNA or protein, transferred to the membrane from an electrophoretic gel by either osmosis or vacuum; following transfer of the molecule of interest, the membrane is bathed in a solution that contains a 'mirror-image' molecule to the one that is already on the membrane, producing a 'hybridization blot' **SOUTHERN BLOT** A technique for identifying the presence (or absence) of a segment of DNA in a sample; the procedure begins by partial enzymatic digestion of nucleic acids, cutting the DNA at specific sites by a restriction endonuclease, each of which recognizes and cuts at a five or six nucleotide sequence; for example, ***Hin*dIII**, from ***Haemophilus influenzae*** cuts DNA at all sites bearing the nucleotide sequence A/AGCTT (at the mirror image sites on the two DNA chains between the two adenines A/A), resulting in a mixture of DNA fragments of varying lengths measuring up to 30 kD that is then electrophoresed in an agarose gel and transferred to a membrane; because the DNA on the membrane is single-stranded, it has a high affinity for its complementary strand; the final step in the blot is to radioactively 'tag' the complementary DNA (a Southern blot after Dr E Southern) or RNA (Northern blot) or protein (Western blot) Note: Northwestern blots are combined RNA-protein hybridizations (Science 1984; 224:506 Lancet 1984;1:1438); the various blots were named by molecular biologists who thought it droll to base the names of further, non-DNA blots on directions of the compass, and thus these techiques were not described by Drs Northern or Western; see Southern blot, Western blot

Blowback phenomenon FORENSIC PATHOLOGY A finding in close-contact, often 'execution-type' gunshot wounds where the muzzle of the weapon is in direct contact with the victim's skin; the gases accompanying the explosion expand within the victim and push some of the subcutaneous tissue back outside of the wound; the blowback pressure plus the heat of the muzzle itself burns the muzzle's 'signature' onto the victim's flesh if no clothing is worn at the point of contact, aiding in identification of the weapon

Blow-out fracture A fracture of the floor and medial walls of the orbit caused by a blunt object, eg baseball, fist, rock) with herniation of the orbital contents (fat, inferior oblique and inferior rectus into the maxillary sinus), accompanied by diplopia, enophthalmos and limitation of the upward gaze

Blow-out fracture of the hip see Dashboard fracture

Blow-out metastases An osteolytic bone metastasis, seen as an expansile, marginated, trabeculated lesion, characteristic of metastatic thyroid and renal carcinomas and also seen in liposarcoma, melanoma, pheochromocytomas, lung and breast carcinoma

Blue The color corresponding to wavelengths 455-492 nm

Blue baby A neonate with cyanosis of any etiology

Blue belly Cullen's sign Periumbilical bluish discoloration due to intraperitoneal hemorrhage, seen in acute pancreatitis

Blueberry muffin appearance PEDIATRICS Multiple blue-brown cutaneous nodules, corresponding to aggregates of leukocytes, seen in infants with cytomegalovirus infections, as well as in other 'TORCH' (toxoplasmosis, rubeola, CMV and herpes) infections, in the rare congenital leukemia and in neonates with multiple blue-brown nodular metastases of neuroblastoma to the skin Note: Given the neuroblastoma's tendency to regress in very young children, tumor extension to lymph nodes, liver and skin is not a harbinger of death or disaster, unlike bone metastases which carries a poor prognosis; 'blueberry infants' under age six months have a good prognosis even without therapy; a useful clinical sign is to press lightly on the skin, causing them to blanch, surrounded by an erythematous halo, probably due to the release of catecholamines

Blueberry muffin baby Dermal erythropoiesis A generalized rash characterized by multiple raised 2-7 mm in diameter dark blue-magenta nodules corresponding to foci of erythropoiesis which regress within 3-4 weeks after birth (Pediatrics 1967; 40:627) due to the presence of generalized hemorrhagic-purpuric eruptions

'Blue bloater' A patient with chronic obstructive lung disease (COPD) who has the symptoms of chronic bronchitis, a normal to decreased lung capacity, increased residual volume with air-trapping, decreased expiratory flow, and characteristic arterial blood gas parameters (decreased PO_2, increased PCO_2, despite normal diffusing capacity), cyanosis and right-sided congestive heart failure, due to sleep apnea and inexorably progressive chronic pulmonary hypertension; with time, it may be impossible to distinguish this from other forms of COPD; see 'Pink puffer'

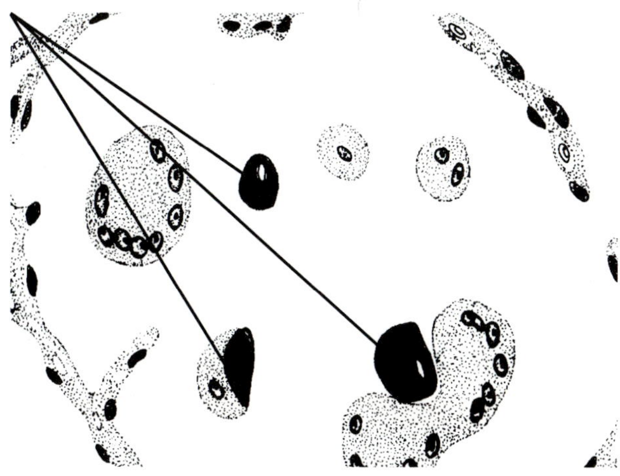

Blue bodies

Blue bodies PULMONARY CYTOLOGY Laminated, extracellular, birefringent and ovoid 15-20 µm structures composed of calcium carbonate found adjacent to or surrounded by macrophages; by hematoxylin and eosin staining, they are blue-gray, by periodic acid Schiff staining, red-purple; blue bodies were described in diffuse interstitial pneumonia but may occur in any accumulation of alveolar macrophages (Am J Clin Path 1984; 81:675)

Blue bone An early lesion of otosclerosis characterized by repeated cycles of lacunar resorption and replacement of the otic capsular bone in a background of immature vascularized spongy neo-osteogenesis with basophilic (bluish) cementum, which with time, evolve to bony mosaics

'Blue book' see TTAPS

'Blue cell' tumor(s) SURGICAL PATHOLOGY Any neoplastic, usually malignant tumor, the cells of which share several histologic features in common; they are arranged in nests, sheets and masses and composed of relatively monotonous, round to oval, 8-15 µm in diameter cells with poorly defined cytoplasmic borders and strongly basophilic (blue by hematoxylin staining) nuclei; the embryologic origin of the cells may not be recognizable by conventional light microscopy, but is required information for guiding therapy and thus requires ancillary information that may be provided by histological pattern, immunohistochemistry, immunoperoxidase for presence of intermediate filaments and electron microscopy Blue cell tumors, children: Neuroblastoma, Ewing sarcoma, non-Hodgkin's lymphoma, embryonal rhabdomyosarcoma Blue cell tumors of adults: APUDoma, mesenchymal chondrosarcoma, hemangiopericytoma, large cell lymphomas, Merkel cell tumor, small cell type osteosarcoma, Small/oat cell carcinoma, alveolar rhabdomyosarcoma

Blue Cross and Blue Shield Association (BCBSA) The largest health insurance association in the US; the BCBSA is a non-profit fiscal intermediary for the government (under contract with the Health Care and Financing Administration) for payment of Medicare costs; the BCBSA administers and approves BCBS health care plans, provides services related to the bureaucracy of providing health care and represents the BCBS plans in issues of national interest; Blue Cross is the bureaucracy involved in hospital reimbursement, while Blue Shield is the reimbursement intermediary for physicians; see 'Major medical', Wrap-around policy

Blue diaper syndrome Tryptophan malabsorption syndrome An autosomal recessive condition characterized by impaired growth, hypercalcemia and nephrocalcinosis, recurrent infections, renal abnormalities and indicanuria; the blue color results from oxidation of indican to indican blue upon exposure to air; Cf Black urine disease

Blue domed cyst Bloodgood disease Schimmelbusch syndrome A form of fibrocystic breast disease affecting perimenopausal women, characterized by cysts filled with light brown (post-hemorrhagic) fluid with benign stromal and epithelial hyperplasia; tenderness is exacerbated prior to menstruation Note: The blue color of the cysts is due to the Tyndall effect, see there

'Blue dot' tumor Acinic cell carcinoma of salivary glands, so designated given the abundance of clear cells with basophilic cytoplasmic granularity (due to glycogen and hormones, Cancer 1987; 60:1706); it comprises 1-3% of all salivary gland tumors, is more common in young males and men, located in the parotid gland Treatment Complete surgical excision is paramount Prognosis Relatively low-grade 12% recur, 8% metastasize

Blue ear A consequence of external ear trauma, where the green-brown hemosiderin coupled with the Tindall effect imparts a bluish tinge to the ear

Blue eye OPHTHALMOLOGY An ocular infection seen in Australian aborigines due to conjunctival granulomata from infection by the equine gastric nematode Habronema; Cf Red eye

Bluefish see Scombroid poisoning

Blue globules GYNECOLOGIC CYTOLOGY Round to oval masses of blue-staining mucus, measuring about the size of an epithelial cell seen in late menopausal vaginal smears, which may simulate a hyperchromatic (ergo malignant) nucleus; an alternate view is that the globules represent degenerated parabasal cells; either way, they are benign

Blue masses Mercury masses An obsolete term for an obsolete therapyused to eradicate Pediculus pubis composed of mercury oleate, mercury, honey, glycerin, glycyrrhiza, a compound of relatively significant toxicity, as mercury comprised 35% of the compound's weight; P pubis is currently treated with lindane (γ benzene HCl) and malthion lotions and pyrethrins with piperonyl butoxide

Blue nevus of Jadassohn-Tieche A nevus characterized by solitary lesions presenting at birth or which develop with time, more common on the acral parts and buttocks of females, appearing as elevated sebaceous yellow, smooth plaques on the scalp, face, < 1 cm in diameter that may appear in the oral cavity, uterine cervix and prostate Histopathology Aggregates of deeply pigmented, spindled bipolar dendritic melanocytes in the deep dermis and skin appendages and islands of large closely-packed cells with oval nuclei and abundant cytoplasm filled with finely granular melanin; a variant, the cellular blue nevus, is more common on the buttocks, often pigment-poor, may undergo malignant transformation and, if the cell clusters penetrate lymph nodes, may be confused with melanoma

'Blue people' A colloquial expression for the clinical appearance of subjects who have been exposed to high levels of sodium nitrite, which oxidizes hemoglobin to methemoglobin, resulting in a dusky blue-gray appearance of the skin surface; those persons with congenital methemoglobinemia are at particular risk for hemoglobin oxidation by nitrites; other risk groups include dynamite workers, amyl nitrite 'poppers', cardiac patients being treated with nitroglycerin, newborns (erythrocyte cytochrome b5 reductase is low, N Engl J Med 1986; 314:757) Note: Up to 40% of hemoglobin can be methemoglobin with minimal symptoms of mild fatigue and dyspnea (Eleven blue men, Little Brown, Boston, 1953)

Blue-ringed octopus *Hapalochlaena maculosa* and *H lunulata*; both produce tetrodotoxin, an inhibitor of action potentials by sodium channel blockage, with the potential for respiratory shut-down; Cf Puffer fish

Blue rubber bleb nevus syndrome Bean syndrome An autosomal dominant condition characterized by multiple compressible cavernous hemangiomas of the skin, mucosal membranes, gastrointestinal tract and liver that are blue-purple and rubbery, measuring up to several centimeters in diameter with a bleeding tendency, rarely, painful and disfiguring, producing hypochromic anemia; the hemangiomas may also be located in the spleen, adrenal gland, central nervous system, penis, liver and lung (Trans Path Soc Lond 1860; 11:267) Diagnosis Angiography

'Blues', the A colloquial expression for a) Blue Cross and Blue Shield and b) Transient depression

Blue sclera Sclera of variable thickness that retain the normal fetal transparency so that the blue uvea is visible; blue sclera occur alone or with brittle bones and deafness, many of which are autosomal dominant; variants of blue sclera/brittle bone diseases include Eddowes-Lobstein syndrome (ELS), osteogenesis imperfecta tarda, characterized by brittle bones, multiple fractures, dislocation and hypermotility of joints, onset in late childhood or adolescence, with blue sclera, keratoconus, cataracts, dysodontogenesis, van der Hoeve syndrome, which is similar to ELS with osteosclerosis and deafness, Vrolik syndrome, which is similar to the van der Hoeve syndrome, but which lacks blue sclera and the Blegvad-Haxthausen syndrome, which is similar to the van der Hoeve syndrome and has cutaneous atrophy and zonular cataract; blue sclera may also be seen in AIDS embryopathy, Bloch-Sulzberger syndrome, Crouzon syndrome, Cornelia de Lange syndrome, Ehlers-Danlos syndrome, Foelling syndrome, in the Loja form of Laron dwarfism, in Lowe syndrome, Marfan's disease, pseudohypoparathyroidism, Turner syndrome and Werner syndrome

Blue skin Bluish discoloration of the skin is abnormal and the result of various toxins, including cyanide, gold (therapeutic), or silver-based drugs, amiodarone or photosensitivity to tetracycline, sulfonamides, phenothiazines or exposure to blue dyes (J Am Med Assoc 1987; 257:3229c)

'Blue spell' A bout of hypoxia, cyanosis, dyspnea, restlessness and syncope with acutely decreased arterial PO_2 and decrease of an already compromised pulmonary blood flow, characteristic of Fallot's tetralogy, but which also appears in other cyanotic congenital heart disease; see Shunts (right-to-left)

Blue stroma PATHOLOGY A low-power microscopic morphology of any inflamed tissue, first described in endometrial stroma

Blue tags TRANSFUSION MEDICINE Given the significance of transfusing an incorrect blood unit in the ABO blood group system, California state law requires color coding of ABO units, where O units are blue (group A is yellow, group B is pink and group AB is white)

Blue toe syndrome Atherothrombotic microembolism of the lower extremities due to recurrent cholesterol embolic 'showers' with painful cyanotic discoloration of the toes and embolism to other sites that completely resolve between attacks; despite the gangrene-like appearance, blue toes may respond to conservative therapy without amputation Diagnosis Arteriography Medical treatment Dypyridamole plus aspirin Surgical treatment Thromboendarterectomy of aorta (J Cardiovasc Surg 1990; 31:87); see Black toe disease

Blue tongue sign A strikingly blue tongue due to selective D_2 dopamine antagonism, as seen in metoclopramide therapy, causing a dystonic reaction, accompanied by trismus, torticollis, facial spasms, opisthotonus and oculogyric crises, a reaction occurring in 1:500 young women treated with metoclopramide; blue tongue has been anecdotally associated with haloperidol (Med J Aust 1989; 150:724c)

Blue top tubes CLINICAL CHEMISTRY 4.5 ml tubes containing sodium citrate as an anticoagulant, used to collect specimens for coagulation factor assays, fibrinogen, glucose-6-phosphate dehydrogenase, partial thromboplastin time, prothrombin time, thrombin time

Blue valve syndrome A descriptor for the bluish, vaguely translucent and hypermobile (floppy) cardiac (most prominently the mitral) valves that have been removed from patients with Marfan disease(s), which demonstrate mucoid degeneration

'Blue velvet' SUBSTANCE ABUSE The 'street' name for an intravenous drug of abuse, consisting of paregoric and triphenamine-HCl mixed with talc **Desired effects** Euphoria, excitement **Untoward effects** Depression, tachycardia, systolic murmur, rales, hepatomegaly with centrilobular hepatic necrosis, sudden death

B lymphocyte An immune cell derived from bursa (a site which has proven difficult to identify in humans); B cells comprise 30% of the circulating lymphocytes and are concentrated in the follicular zones of lymphoid tissue, while the T cells are located in the deep cortex; B cells are responsible for antibody production, immune defense against viruses and bacteria, surveillance (cytolysis of potentially malignant 'self' cells), mediation of antibody-dependent cell cytotoxicity, allergic reactions, formation of antigen-antibody complexes and production of cytokines; surface and cytoplasmic antigens indicate the degree of B cell maturation and function; cytoplasmic IgM is present in pre-B cells and surface immunoglobulin and complement receptors are seen in mature cells B cell markers include CD9, CD10, CD19, CD20, CD24, the Fc receptor, B1, BA-1, B4 and Ia (N Engl J Med 1987; 317:1452)

BMI see Body mass index

B-mode see Ultrasound

BMR Basal metabolic rate

Board certified An adjective for a US or Canadian physician who has both a) Completed the minimum years (ranging from four to eight years) of post-medical school residency training, ie a physician who is 'Board-eligible' and b) Passed an examination, commonly called the 'Boards' that tests his theoretical knowledge in the area of specialization; Board certification is commonly required for acceptance to a hospital's medical staff; approximately 250 000 physicians in the US are certified by one of 23 specialty boards and 12 000 are certified by more than one specialty board

Board-like rigidity Spastic rigidity of the abdominal wall muscles induced by acute peritonitis, classically elicited by a perforated peptic ulcer although any fulminant peritonitis may elicit the same reaction; see Hippocratic facies

Board of medical examiners A body that is recognized by a state's government, which may if necessary, exercise its authority to place a physician on probation, to suspend or to revoke his license to practice medicine; the infractions which would cause a state board to initiate punitive actions against a physician include drug abuse, irregular subscription practices regarding 'controlled drugs', ie those drugs with addictive potential and various other major deviations from the tenets of the Hippocratic Oath

'Bobble-headed doll syndrome' A neurologic symptom complex described in children with a cyst in the third ventricle, characterized by bobbing of the head in three-second cycles and rhythmic flexion and extension of the extremities that may be controlled voluntarily and which ceases during sleep, accompanied by mental retardation, generalized fine tremor, hydrocephalus, obesity and visual impairment

Body mass index A clinical parameter used to determine obesity, where a BMI of less than 25 is considered obese

'Body packing' SUBSTANCE ABUSE A method for smuggling narcotics in which a 'courier' swallows condoms or other impermeable containers filled with pure cocaine or heroin in order to escape detection by customs agents and specially-trained dogs; the Body packer 'syndrome' consists of a constellation of medical complaints including intestinal obstruction and rupture of the bags, the latter almost invariably fatal (Br Med J 1988; 296;1035) Note: Body packing began in the mid-1980s with cocaine (pretax street value $18 000/kg), originating from South America; more recently, the couriers are from Africa, carrying heroin (street value $200 000/kg) originating from Afghanistan, Pakistan, and the 'Golden Triangle' (Thailand, Laos and Burma), these 'sherpas' swallow between 55 and 100 doubly-wrapped 'balloons', totalling 700-1.5 kg, making as many as 3 'runs' per month, for $5-10 000 per shipment (Personal communications, Lt JB, NYPD Organized Crime; SS, DEA, New York field office, JFK Intl Airport) **Diagnosis, ultrasonography** Sickle-shaped echo with a dorsal echo deficit; most 'packs' are in the stomach at the time of examination (Dtsch Med Wochenschr 1990; 114:1865) **Diagnosis, scout films**, see 'Double condom' sign

Body rocking NEUROLOGY Repetitive flexion and extension of the trunk due to tardive dyskinesia, a complication of antipsychotic therapy, most common in the elderly and in women, which may persist indefinitely; body rocking may also be seen in autistic children

Bog body ANTHROPOLOGY A human body that has been 'pickled' by the acidic water in bogs and marshes, nearly 700 of which have been catalogued from Scandinavia and Britain, and who died 10-1000 years prior to their discovery; most were victims of violent death; the best studied of bog bodies is the Lindow man, 'Pete Marsh'

Boiled lobster appearance Erythema neonatorum A brilliant red vasomotor flush of no clinical significance that may transiently (up to 24 hours) cover the entire infant mimicking inflammation; Cf Harlequin changes

Bolivian hemorrhagic fever An infection endemic to the grain-producing province of Beni in Amazonian Bolivia, caused by an arenavirus excreted in the urine of the rodent vector, *Calomys callosus* Clinical High pediatric mortality, with early fever, anorexia, nausea, vomiting, myalgia, neurologic signs (50% have intention tremor, 25% develop convulsive encephalopathy); Cf Haverhill fever

Bombay phenotype TRANSFUSION MEDICINE The O_h phenotype is a variant of the ABO antigens on red cells; for A or B antigens to be expressed on red blood cells, the cells must have a precursor substance (H antigen) encoded by the H gene; O_h type red cells do not agglutinate with antisera containing anti-A, anti-B or anti-H type antibodies as these erythrocytes lack the H gene, and therefore H substance; these subjects do have anti-A, anti-B and anti-H antibodies in their serum, which may cause problems when cross-matching donors and recipients Note: The condition was described in Bombay (Lancet 1952; 1:903)

Bombesin A 14-residue neuropeptide that is analogous to gastrin-releasing peptide, which is produced in the gastrointestinal tract, stimulating gastrointestinal smooth muscle contraction, release of gastric acid and most gastrointestinal hormones except secretin, with which bombesin has a yin-yang effect, see Secretin; when administered into the cerebral cisterna, bombesin elicits hypothermia, analgesia, hyperglucagonemia and hyperglycemia; bombesin also stimulates proliferation of bronchial epithelial cells, pancreas (Digestion 1990; 46 supp2:202) and small cell carcinoma; anti-bombesin antibodies have theoretical potential for treating small cell carcinoma of the lung, since these tumors both secrete bombesin and have bombesin-like receptors (J Am Med Assoc 1988; 259:957)

Bond The 'glue' that maintains the molecules in their three-dimensional configuration **COVALENT BOND** Electron pair bond Electrons are shared between two atoms, classified as polar or nonpolar when the sharing is uneven; covalent are the strongest bond in biological systems; the bond strength of a single covalent bond is 50-110 kcal/mol, a double bond, 120-170 kcal/mol and a triple, 195 kcal/mol; the molecular structure is stabilized by weaker bonds **ELECTROSTATIC BOND** Ionic bond The attractive force that exists between an anion and cation **HYDROGEN BOND** A weak association between an electronegative atom (the acceptor atom) and a hydrogen atom covalently bound to a donor atom; the greater the length between atoms, the weaker the bond strength (4-5 kcal/mol) **HYDROPHOBIC INTERACTION** The attractive force between nonpolar or polar molecules in an aqueous solution **NONCOVALENT BOND** Any bond between molecules that don't share pairs of electrons, eg electrostatic bond, hydrogen bond, hydrophobic interaction **VAN DER WAALS BOND** A weak attraction when two atoms approach each other, the result of fluctuating dipoles, occurring in both polar and non-polar atoms (1 kcal/mol)

Bonding NEONATOLOGY The emotional ties formed between the infant and mother that occur in the early post-partum period, considered analogous to imprinting in animals; Cf Anaclitic depression

Bone and stone disease see Stone, bone and groan disease

Bone densitometry The measurement of bone mass or density; all of the current methods (single-photon absorptiometry, dual-energy photon absorptiometry, dual-energy X-ray absorptiometry) are based on a tissue's absorption of photons derived from either a radionuclide or an X-ray tube, the latter of which have an increased accuracy and shorter scan time; bone densitometry objectively determines the risk of suffering fractures, by quantifying osteoporosis, which with dementia, constitute the two most common morbid conditions of the elderly; other methods to evaluate osteopenia include 'eye-balling' of a plain film of a bone requires a bone loss of at least 30% before osteoporosis can be diagnosed with certainty and the 'feel' of the bone when it is drilled by the surgeon at the time of joint replacement is even cruder; other indications for performing bone densitometry analyses include indirect evaluation of estrogen deficiency, osteopenia, long-term glucocorticoid therapy and primary asymptomatic hyperparathyroidism (N Engl J Med 1991; 324:1105rv); see Osteoporosis

Bone hunger see Hungry bone(s) disease

Bone/joint panel A group of laboratory parameters that have been determined to be the most cost-effective, sensitive, specific (and 'efficient') in evaluating a patient with bone and joint complaints; the B/J panel includes measurement of uric acid, calcium, phosphorous, alkaline phosphatase, total protein and albumin; see Organ panel

Bone marrow transplantation A modality used to treat aplastic anemia (5-year survival, 80%), acute nonlymphocytic leukemia (ANLL, 50%) and acute lymphocytic leukemia (ALL, 25%); the 750 ml of marrow required for bone marrow transplantation (BMT) is 'harvested' from the iliac crests, a painful procedure; in ALL, BMT of an HLA-matched or preferably, an identical donor is an option generally reserved for those in second or subsequent remissions, or used to induce first remissions in 'high-risk' ALL; see Autologous BMT; in ANLL, BMT may induce first remissions in 50-60% of younger (< 20 year old) patients; see Chemotherapy, Relapse, Remission; BMT survival in leukemia 32-48%, depending upon chronicity and cell type; BMT survival in non-neoplastic conditions 63-75+%; minor HLA mismatching does not ensure failure (N Engl J Med 1990; 322:485, 417) Complications Acute or chronic graft-versus-host disease (35-60%), interstitial pneumonia, idiopathic or viral (Cytomegalovirus, Herpes simplex, varicella-zoster), rarely, post-BMT leukemic relapse or acute myeloid leukemia from donor into an HLA-identical sib for chronic myelocytic leukemia (N Engl J Med 1990; 322:1794cr) Cause of death Opportunistic infections 17% of BMTs suffer CMV-associated interstitial pneumonia with an 85% mortality; prophylactic gancyclovir reduces the incidence of this complication (N Engl J Med 1991; 324:1005); these infections are due to immune defects; other causes of interstitial pneumonia include *Pneumocystis carinii* or radiation Clinica Graft-versus-host disease Skin rash, hepatic defects, diarrhea, infections and autoimmune phenomena Cost $75-150 000 (1990 dollars) Indications BMT is appropriate and often successful therapy for leukemia and aplastic anemia, but less successful in treating lymphoma, thalassemia major, osteopetrosis, inborn errors of metabolism, congenital immune deficiencies, eg Wiscott-Aldrich disease and severe combined immune deficiency Note: 75% of post-BMT leukemic relapses occur in the first two years; in ANLL, 50-60% of those transplanted in the first remission survive, 25% survive in the second remission; adjuvant therapy includes cyclophosphamide and busulfan

Bone pearls Small rounded osseous masses seen in electrical injury, due to actual melting of the bone by intense heat, eg lightening; adjacent bone may have rarefaction, periostitis and fractures

Bone pointing 'syndrome' Hexing phenomenon A reaction described in primitive aboriginal societies where a witch doctor points a bone at someone during a ritual and that person becomes ill and dies shortly thereafter; an analagous situation in modern society is a subject being told he/she has little time to live from a terminal disease upon which they lapse into a state of apathy and die; see Anniversary phenomenon, Voodoo death; Cf Harvest Moon phenomenon

Bone-within-a-bone pattern PEDIATRIC RADIOLOGY A descriptor for a morphology seen under different circumstances a) Normal A 'double bone' appearance in the infant vertebral body, seen at 1-2 months of age, with peripheral decrease of bone density and retention of a sharp cortical outline, thought to represent post-natal bone remodelling b) Pathological A symmetrical increase in bone density accompanied by a lack of 'tubulation'; when limited to the end-plates of the vertebrae, the radiological appearance results in a Sandwich vertebra (see there) or if more extensive, a miniature 'Vertebra within a vertebra', classically associated with osteopetrosis, but also seen in osteomyelitis, sickle cell infarction with periosteal elevation, osteolysis, endosteal absorption and neo-osteogenesis along the inner cortex of the medullary space, Gaucher's disease, cleidocranial dysostosis, late post-irradiation changes in young children, or Thorotrast-related

Bone spicule appearance OPHTHALMOLOGY Fundoscopic appearance of retinitis pigmentosa seen as jagged, jet-black pigmented patches at the equator, often accompanied by bilateral nyctalopia

BOOP Bronchiolitis obliterans organizing pneumonia A disease formerly considered a form of interstitial pneumonia **Etiology** Obscure, but may be associated with toxic fumes, infection, connective tissue disease **Clinical** Cough, dyspnea, 'flu' symptoms, 50% recovery, 12% BOOPs eventually die of the disease, many develop usual interstitial pneumonia; obstructive symptoms are limited to smokers, most of whom have restriction disease and impaired diffusing capacity, remission may follow use of corticosteroids **Radiology** Patchy ground-glass appearance on a plain antero-posterior chest film **Histopathology** Patchy, polypoid masses of intraalveolar granulation tissue in small airway lumina and alveolar ducts with preservation of the alveolar architecture and uniform intrabronchiolar fibrosis (N Engl J Med 1991; 324:1195cpc)

Booster Re-exposure to an antigen usually as a deliberate, often iatrogenic attempt to induce a secondary immune response months to years after a primary response to an antigen, 'boosting' the response

Booster phenomenon An increase in the size of the tuberculin reaction (> 6 mm, or from less than to greater than 10 mm) after a second PPD skin test for tuberculosis; persons with a booster phenomenon are thought to have enhanced immunologic 'recall', due to either a) Previous infection with ***M tuberculosis*** or b) Infection with a non-tuberculous mycobacteria; this phenomenon is most common in the elderly previously infected with ***M tuberculosis***, who usually do not convert to active disease

Booster 'shot' A second immunization dose, administered after an appropriate time interval, allowing the body to mount an immune response; when a person is exposed, eg to 'dirty' wounds or plans potential exposure, eg travel to regions endemic for certain infectious agents, the booster shot provides a rapid anamnestic response that outpaces the development of disease, eg tetanus

Borderline An adjectival expediency widely use in medicine for any condition that cannot be neatly placed in one of usually two categories, each of which has a distinct clinical significance, therapy and prognosis

Borderline hypertension That range of systolic and diastolic blood pressures in which there is no unequivocal benefit obtained by therapy

Borderline leprosy Dimorphous leprosy The spectrum of leprosy is broad: in tuberculous leprosy, there are adequate host defenses resulting in reactive granulomatous disease with scattered large, sharply demarcated, hairless anesthetic plaques; lepromatous leprosy carries a relatively poor prognosis, in which there are multiple skin nodules filled with innumerable bacilli; between these two extremes are the borderline lesions, borderline tuberculous leprosy and borderline lepromatous leprosy

Borderline personality PSYCHIATRY A personality disturbance that may be defined in terms of constitution, ie one that lies between a neurotic, who is capable of coping with his environment and a psychotic, who has lost contact with reality, or a person who is neither clear-cut schizophrenic nor non-schizophrenic; the borderline personality may be also be defined in adaptability, ie one who is not clearly beyond the reach of classical analytic techniques, but who responds poorly thereto, ie neither analyzable nor nonanalyzable

Borderline tumor SURGICAL PATHOLOGY A term of considerable use in evaluating neoplasms with many (but not all) of the histological criteria of malignancy, as the future behavior of these tumors cannot be reliably predicted; the borderline concept has currency in epithelial tumors of the ovary and stromal tumors of the uterus (see below); the Virchowian paradigm of morphological changes predicting the true nature of disease is problematic as some borderline lesions may evolve toward frank malignancy, while other morphologically identical lesions are stable or regress; the borderline dilemma is relatively common in the 'borderline tumor' or 'cystadenocarcinoma of low malignant potential' of the ovary,which has a behavior between an innocuous cystadenoma and a frankly malignant cystadenocarcinoma; these tumors may display serous, mucinous or endometrioid differentiation, and are characterized by complex oligocellular piling-up ('tufting') of the superficial cells Serous 'borderline' tumors comprise 15% of serous tumors of the ovary, one-half of which are unilateral; 20% are extraovarian; 5-year survival is 100%; 10-year survival is 75% versus 50% and 13% for malignant serous cystadenocarcinomas Mucinous 'borderline' tumors comprise 6-13% of all mucinous tumors of the ovary; 90% are unilateral; 10-year survival is 68% versus 34% for mucinous cystadenocarcinomas; endometrioid 'borderline' tumors are rare; other tumors of 'borderline' malignant potential affect 1) Epithelium, eg adenomatous hyperplasia of the endometrium with atypia, adenomatous colonic polyps with atypia 2) Mesenchymal cells, eg 'smooth muscle tumors of uncertain malignant potential' (STUMP), tumors that affect the uterus and the stomach; other mesenchymal tumors with 'borderline' behavior include epithelioid hemangioendothelioma and low-grade chondrosarcomas 3) Hematopoietic cells, eg pseudolymphomas, monoclonal gammopathies of uncertain significance, refractory anemia/myelofibrosis, lymphomatoid papulosis and cells of uncertain lineage, eg giant cell tumors of bone

Borna disease virus An agent that causes disease of domestic horses and sheep in Central Europe, characterized by neurological disease in the form of behavioral disorders (aggression, eating disorders, hyperactivity, disrupted social and sexual activity) (Science 1990; 250:1278)

Bornholm disease Devil's grip, Epidemic pleurodynia, Silvest's disease An acute viral infection, most commonly caused by coxsackievirus (usually B1-6, but also A4, A6, A10 and enteroviruses 1, 6, 9, 19); a summer, early fall disease first described on the Danish island of Bornholm Clinical Paroxysms of crushing, 'vise-like' pain, in the chest of adults or upper abdomen of children, shortness of breath Complications Septic meningitis 5%, orchitis

Borrowed servant An employee (eg a nurse) who is paid by one person or organization (eg a hospital) and who is temporarily employed by another person (eg a surgeon); in the usual medico-legal context, the temporary employer is responsible for the actions of the 'borrowed servant'; see Respondeat superior

Bossing Frontal bossing Rounded prominence of the frontal and parietal bones in an infant's cranial vault, due to various etiologies, eg a) Untreated vitamin D-induced rickets, causing a thickened outer table (alternately, Boxhead, Caput quadratum) with permanent enlargment of the head b) Congenital anemia, eg thalassemia with massive hematopoiesis in an expanded marrow space, also known as 'hot cross bun skull' and c) Others, including conditions associated with 'gargoyle' facies, acromesomelic dysplasia of Maroteaux, anhydrotic ectodermal dysplasia, craniometaphyseal dysplasia of Pyle, frontodigital syndrome, Kenney's tubular stenosis syndrome, nevoid-basal carcinoma syndrome, Taybi syndrome, thanatophoric dwarfism and, recently, AIDS embyropathy

Boston exanthem An exanthematous roseoliform salmon-colored maculo-papular face and chest rash caused by echovirus 16, preceded by a high 1-2 day fever which subsides with the onset of the rash; both last a week, more common in children in the late summer; epidemic or sporadic

Bota see Linitis plastica

Bottlenecks GENETICS A marked qualitative reduction in gene pool diversity due to low number of genetically distinct individuals in the population, ie a population bred from two individuals has far fewer variables on the allelic loci (a bottleneck) than a second population bred from hundreds of individuals; the variability of allelic loci in bottlenecks increases, a finding that is discordant with theoretical models (Science 1987; 235:1325); despite the presumed advantage to species survival of increased variability of genetic loci at such bottlenecks, inbred populations are less fit, having increased juvenile mortality (ibid, 237:963c); see Consanguinity, Inbreeding; Cf Biodiversity

Botulinum toxin One of several toxins produced by *Clostridium botulinum*, of which type A toxin, a 150 kD molecule has been purified and is being used to treat neuromuscular junction disease, including dystonias, eg blepharospasm, spasmodic torticollis, hemifacial spasm, tremors, task-specific dystonia and spasmodic dysphonia, a speech disorder with loss of voice, pitch breaks and hoarseness Mechanism of action Botulinum toxin binds to presynaptic cholinergic nerve terminals; the toxin is then internalized and inhibits exocytosis of acetylcholine; sprouting later occurs, forming new terminals that re-innervate the muscle fibers (N Engl J Med 1991; 324:1186rv)

Bougienage A technique introduced 60 years ago for treatment of corrosive burns of the esophagus; following stabilization, an intraluminal silicon splint is left in place for 2-3 weeks, followed by daily bougienage, tapered to once every two days and finally once/week for many months; early bougienage increases complications

Bouttonneuse fever see Fièvre Bouttonneuse

Boutonnier deformity RHEUMATOLOGY Flexion of the proximal interphalangeal PIP joint and hyperextension of the DIP, caused by the detachment of the extensor tendon from the middle phalanx, volar displacement and resultant action as a flexor, associated with lupus erythematosus, Jaccoud's (post-rheumatic fever) arthritis, rheumatoid arthritis and camptodactyly; likened to a carnation secured in a lapel

Bovarism PSYCHIATRY A condition with sexual overtones, that appears to most commonly affect older single women, in which the fantasized world overlaps and becomes confused in the patient's mind with the real world; the term derives from the principal character in Gustav Flaubert's Madame Bovary

Bovine growth hormone see Bovine somatotropin

Bovine somatotropin (BST) A 190-amino acid protein produced by the bovine pituitary gland that evokes somatic growth (partially mediated by insulin-like growth factor) and increased milk production, for which

BST use in cows is approved by the US Food and Drug Administration; recombinant or genetically engineered BST is regarded as completely safe (J Am Med Assoc 1990; 264: 1003) and is distinct from 'beef growth hormone', an anabolic steroid used in the cattle industry, the safety of which is being seriously questioned (some countries are moving to ban importation of such meat) Science 1990; 249:875rv); the bioengineered product was approved by the US FDA for use in boosting milk production in cows; there are some reports that some cows so treated may suffer reproductive losses, chronic mastitis and other chronic toxic effects (J Am Med Assoc 1991; 265:1391c, 1423)

Bovine spongiform encephalopathy (BSE) A recently described disease of cattle, popularly known as 'mad cow' disease for the presentation of the cows with high-stepping or staggering gait, anxiety, increased sensitivity and kicking while being milked, less commonly exhibiting frenzy and aggression; BSE was first described in the UK in cows fed with sheep offal and is a 'prion' disease and therefore similar to kuru and Creutzfeldt-Jakob disease in that there are prominent vacuolar (spongiform) lesions in the brain and disease-specific fibrils derived from the normal glycoprotein PrP and is related to transmissible mink encephalopathy, which similarly results from infected feed; the BSE brouhaha resulted in a British beef ban by the rest of the European community (Nature 1990; 345:763); see Prions

Bowlegs Genu varum External deviation of the knee(s), a certain degree of which in normally present in infants and which corrects itself by 12-18 months, coinciding with bipedal ambulation; when the degree of bowing falls outside of a standardized curve, rickets must be considered as vitamin D-induced osteomalacia allows bending of the femoral shaft that bears the mechanical brunt of ambulatory kinetics; when combined with anterior curvature of the tibia and fibula, the children may have a 'saddle-sore' stance; anterior or antero-lateral bowing of the tibia may occur in neurofibromatosis as a prelude to fractures, which are commonly complicated by pseudoarthrosis

Bowler hat sign GASTROINTESTINAL RADIOLOGY Spreading of barium contrast material around an adenomatous or villotubular colonic polyp, at the base of which there is a recess between the stalk and the polyp 'body', forming the 'crown' of the bowler hat; the sign cannot differentiate between benign (leiomyomas, lipomas, 'garden variety' polyps) and malignant (leiomyosarcomas, lymphomas, metastatic melanomas), but merely signals their presence

Bowel 'prep' A preoperative enema, often used in conjunction with prophylactic oral and parental antibiotics to purge the large intestine of food and feces prior to intestinal surgery; the most popular agent for preparing the large intestine for surgery is polyethylene glycol for mechanical cleansing; the remaining surgeons use conventional enemas, dietary restriction and cathartics (Dis Col & Rect 1990; 33:154)

Box MOLECULAR BIOLOGY A repeated oligonucleotide 'motif' that appears in multiple sites along the DNA and which functions as a signal for gene transcription or gene regulation; see Homeobox

Boxcar An adjectival descriptor used for any periodically interrupted series of elongated objects with parallel lateral sides CARDIOVASCULAR PATHOLOGY Boxcar nuclei are typical of hypoxic myocytes, following ischemic insult of any kind FORENSIC MEDICINE Columns of intravascular blood interrupted by air in the small blood vessels and capillaries of the brains in scuba divers who died of air embolism due to rapid ascent and intravascular expansion of gases; see Caissons' disease MICROBIOLOGY 'Boxcar'-like organisms are arranged in long parallel chains of bacteria in an end-to-end arrangement, characteristic of ***Clostridium perfringens*** and ***Bacillus anthracis*** MYCOLOGY Arrangement of arthrospores of ***Geotrichum*** and ***Trichosporon*** species and ***Coccidioides immitis*** (alternating bands of pigmentation frequently cause rudimentary bodies arthroderma, described in ***Fusarium solani*** hyphae stained by safranin; ***Geotrichum*** species have a morphology of hockey sticks OPHTHALMOLOGY Boxcar pattern is seen in vascular stasis with segmentation of the venous column (of blood) in the retinal vein, a sequela of central retinal artery occlusion

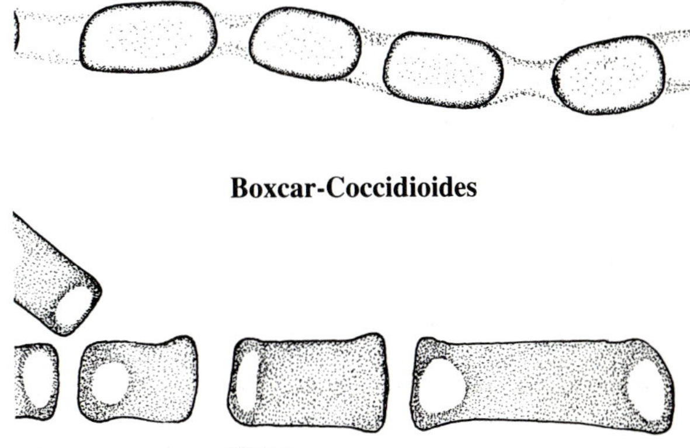

Boxcar-Coccidioides

Boxcar-Geotrichum

Boxer fracture A fracture of the fifth metacarpal neck following a direct blow impacting on the fifth metacarpal head with the fist clenched, causing dorsal angulation of the fracture line and volar displacement of the head

Box-head see Bossing

Boxing SPORTS MEDICINE A contact sport that causes major neuropsychological defects in its long-term practitioners when tested by the Wechsler and Bender Gestalt test, causing variable organic mental disease with impaired recent memory, dysarthria, nystagmus, computed tomographic evidence of cortical atrophy and a cavum septum pellucidum (J Am Med Assoc 1984; 251:2663, 2676) *ACUTE BOXING INJURIES* Cerebral edema, ischemia and (temporal or uncal) herniation Note: The 'knock-out' punch causes generalized flaccidness, apnea, bradycardia, dilated pupils, unresponsiveness to light, rarely accompanied by a seizure; recovery occurs within 30-60 seconds; magnetic resonance imaging is better able than computed tomography to evaluate boxing injuries as it excels in detecting hematomas, white lesions, ie atrophy, contusion and early hydrocephaly (J Am Med Assoc 1990; 263:1670); see 'Punch-drunk' syndrome

BOXING: MECHANISMS OF SEQUELAE

Rotational (angular) acceleration Subdural hematomas, intracerebral hemorrhage and diffuse axonal injury (rupture of individual axons)

Linear acceleration Focal ischemia and retinal detachment

Carotid injury Potential dissection of arteries, thrombosis or initiation of hypotensive or bradycardic reflexes

Impact deceleration Hitting the mats or ropes results in 'contrecoup' injuries and subdural hemorrhage

Box jellyfish *Chironex fleckeri* and the related *Chiropsolmus quadrigatus* are lethal coelenterates, responsible for 74 documented deaths (countless unconfirmed), due to a high molecular weight dermatonecrotic venom, the nature of which is as yet unknown

B protein A 25 kDal protein contained within snRNPs (small ribonuceloprotein particles); the variability of this and other (A and C) proteins may explain the differential splicing and polyadenylation as variations in pre-mRNA processing machinery

Brachytherapy A modality of radiation therapy in which implanted beads or seeds containing iridium-192, radium-226 and other radioisotopes are used to treated certain carcinomas with high amounts of local radiation, eg as in invasive carcinoma of the uterine cervix

Brady-tachy syndrome see Sick sinus syndrome

Brain-bone-fat syndrome An autosomal dominant condition with progressive neurological disease leading to death, accompanied by developmental cysts on the acral parts and bones Histopathology Narrowed cerebral blood vessels, gliosis, calcified basal ganglia, demyelinization and senile plaqe formation

Brain death see Multiorgan donation

Brain-derived growth factor see BDGF

'Brain drain' A colloquialism for the migration of highly trained and/or skilled workers, especially physicians and scientists from underdeveloped countries to countries offering better working conditions and/or life styles Note: While the USA has been a favored mecca for drained brains, there is increasing emigration to Europe and Japan, as the US budget deficit reduces the funding of innovative research

Brainerd diarrhea An epidemic of diarrhea in Minnesota that immortalized the town and immobilized the population, beginning in 1984, presumably due to an infectious agent, although none was identified; 2-3 weeks after ingestion of raw milk from one of the local dairies in this community of 14 000, 8% of those exposed had diarrhea which slowly improved with time (J Am Med Assoc 1986; 256:469, 484, 510)

Brain-graft surgery A neurosurgical procedure for treating Parkinson's disease, in which chromaffin adrenal cells are transplanted into the caudate nucleus; the early Swedish cases were discouraging, but in the animal model, the MPTP-treated monkey, promising results were reported by grafting fetal substantia nigra into the caudate; the success reported by the Mexican team in 1987 has not been reproduced elsewhere and the neurosurgical community has taken a 'wait-and-see' policy (J Am Med Assoc 1989; 262:449; N Engl J Med 1989; 320:337); of one small series (Mayo Clin Proc 1989; 64:282), one patient had significant improvement, one-half of the remainder required less levodopa and dopaminic agonists Technique Implant fetal mesencephalic cells unilaterally into the putamen of one patient, resulting in focal dopamine production, replacing that missing in parkinsonism, verified by PET scanning; clinical improvement was most marked contralateral to the implantation side, evidence of a positive benefit from the surgery (Science 1990; 247:574)

'Brake' drugs SPORTS MEDICINE Steroid hormones used by female athletes to delay body growth and minimize body fat, thereby preventing the center of gravity from shifting, giving them a competitive 'edge', allowing a 15-to-18-year old to compete as a prepubertal gymnast; medroxyprogesterone (estrogen) and cyproterone (antiestrogen) delaying puberty by suppressing ovulation and menstruation Side effects Premature closure of the epiphyseal plate, resulting in short stature as adults

Bran A product derived from grain that contains a water-soluble fiber with a high content of β-glycan, a substance which, by an unknown mechanism, reduces LDL-cholesterol by 5-15% (J Am Med Assoc 1991; 265:1833) Note: Rice bran may be more effective in reducing cholesterol than oat bran as it may be defatted, further reducing cholesterol by 25%; see Dietary fiber

Branched chain amino acids Valine, leucine, isoleucine The amino acids that accumulate in maple syrup urine disease, which is due to a deficit in oxidative decarboxylation of the keto-acid derivatives of these amino acids

Branched chain ketonuria see Maple syrup urine disease

Brancher enzyme Any enzyme that catalyzes the addition of branches and side chains to a polymer, eg amylo-1,4 →1,6 transglucosidase, which packs sugar molecules onto starch, the enzyme that is defective in type IV glycogen storage disease, Cf Debrancher enzyme

Brancher disease Amylopectinosis An inborn error of metabolism related to a deficiency of the 'brancher' enzyme, the deficiency of which causes type IV glycogen storage (Anderson's) disease, with muscular weakness especially of the tongue, hepatosplenomegaly, hepatic fibrosis, followed by cirrhosis, ascites and early death in the face of normal mental development; brancher disease responds to liver transplantation with decreased deposition of amylopectin in the liver and freedom from neuromuscular or cardiac morbidity associated with extrahepatic amylopectin deposits (N Engl J Med 1991; 324:39); Cf Debranching enzyme

Branching snowflake test A crude but useful bedside test using a glass microscopic slide for differentiating amniotic fluid (positive) from maternal urine (negative), based on the radiating 'fern-like' pattern of amniotic fluid

Brassy cough A descriptor for the non-productive 'metallic' cough heard in children with acute bacterial or viral laryngotracheitis, often accompanied by inspiratory stridor and respiratory distress

BRAT diet Bananas, rice, apples, toast A bland diet prescribed for viral gastroenteritis that, with water, replenishes liquids and electrolytes lost in pediatric diarrhea; other foods appropriate for diarrhea include plain chicken, crackers and potatoes Brat (noun) A spoiled, tedious, ill-mannered child

Bravo The code-name for an atmospheric nuclear test in which a 15-megaton thermonuclear device was detonated on March 1, 1954 on the Bikini Atoll of the northern Marshall Islands; in Bravo, most of the 253 inhabitants of the Rongelap and Utrik Atolls suffered from acute radiation sickness and many later developed neoplasia of the thyroid in the form of nodules or carcinoma, due to exposure to β radiation from radioiodines (J Am Med Assoc 1987; 258:629); Cf Smoky

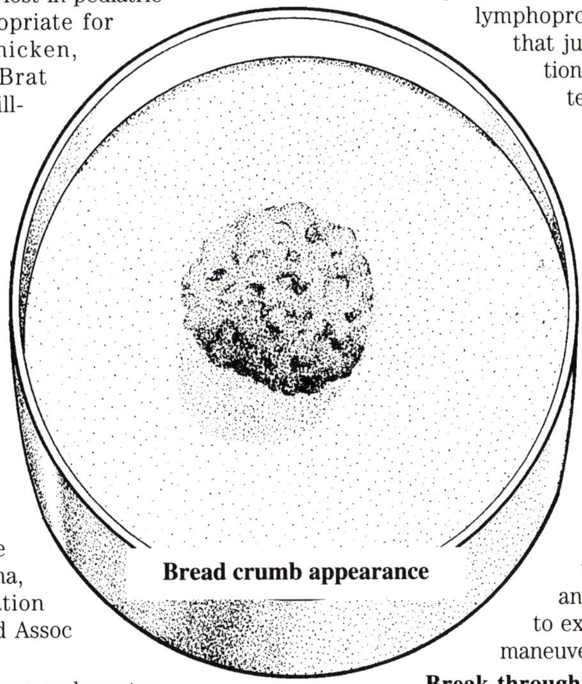

Bread crumb appearance

Brawny edema Cutaneous changes characteristic of chronic venous insufficiency with thickening, induration, liposclerosis and non-pitting edema; the brawny color is due to hemosiderin from lysed erythrocytes; with chronic ischemia, the skin undergoes atrophy, necrosis and stasis ulceration, surrounded by a rim of dry, scaling and pruritic skin

'Bread and butter' disease A catch-phrase for routine maladies treated by each specialty that comprise a large part of the physician's work-load and present little intellectual challenge; 'bread and butter' surgical pathology includes routine specimens, eg hernia sacs, gall bladders, appendices, cataracts and tonsils

Bread and butter lesion CARDIAC PATHOLOGY Diffuse fibrinous and serofibrinous 'stringy' adhesions or plaque-like thickening on the chronically inflamed pericardium of rheumatic heart disease; similar lesions occur in connective tissue disease, eg lupus erythematosus, viral pericarditis, post-acute myocardial infarction, neoplasia, uremia, trauma, radiation and fusobacterium infection; the end-result may be restrictive pericardial fibrosis, which compromises the inflow of blood to the ventricle

Bread crumb appearance MICROBIOLOGY A descriptor for the gross morphology of cultures of *Blastomyces dermatitidis* grown at 37°C, *Streptomyces madurae, Fusobacterium nucleatum* and *M tuberculosis*, which have been fancifully likened to broken pieces of French or Italian bread OPHTHALMOLOGY see Granular dystrophy

Breakage syndromes GENETICS A group of autosomal recessive disorders characterized by congenital chromosomal breaks and rearrangements that increase the risk for malignancy, including Bloom and Fanconi syndromes, ataxia-telangiectasia and xeroderma pigmentosum; Cf Fragile X Note: Acquired diseases may also have chromosomal breakages, structural rearrangement and aneuploidy caused by viral infections, eg chickenpox, hepatitis, measles and malignancy, often lymphoproliferative, with translocations that juxtapose oncogenes with functional genes, encoding hybrid proteins that 'drive' expansions and leaving the cells locked in a 'turned-on' position, eg acute myelogenous leukemia t(8;21) and chronic myeloid leukemia t(9;22)

'Breaking' EMERGENCY MEDICINE A maneuver used in drowning and near-drowning victims to clear the pharynx of water and vomitus; the victim is turned prone (on his stomach), the hands of the person rendering cardiopulmonary resuscitation are locked together under the abdomen and the fluid-filled body is lifted to expel the water and gas; Cf Flake maneuver, Heimlich maneuver

Break-through bleeding GYNECOLOGY A nebulous term applied to various types of gynecologic bleeding, usually referring to mid-cycle bleeding in oral contraceptive users, thought to be the result of insufficient estrogenic stimulation; the term is not applicable to abnormal bleeding in oral contraceptive users

'Breakthrough organism' see Progenote

Breast implant An inert sac filled with silicone, some of which are covered by polyurethane foam, used to augment cosmetically the female contour; with time, the implants covered by polyurethane (composed of long chains of isocyanate monomers joined together in ester linkages), are hydrolyzed in vivo, yielding various degradation products, including 2-toluene diamine, a known carcinogen, present in concentrations of up to 6 μg/g of tissue around the breast, conferring up to a 1 in 50 (estimated) chance of suffering cancer (Science 1991; 252:1060); see Biomaterials, Silicone

Breast milk NEONATOLOGY Human milk is similar to cow milk in the water content (88%, specific gravity, 1.030), fat content (3.5%), energy value (0.67 kcal/ml) and type of sugar (lactose); mom's milk has less protein (1.0-1.5% vs. 3.3% cow's milk, the latter due to a 6-fold increase in casein), more carbohydrate (6.5-7.0% vs 4.5%), less minerals and different vitamins (more vitamins C and D, less thiamine and riboflavin and equivalent amounts of vitamins A and B and niacin); maternal milk is usually sterile, provides IgA and is more easily digestible, as reflected in rapid transit time; breast-fed infants have a better response to vaccines than formula-fed infants (Acta Paediatr Scand 1990; 79:1137); Cf Necrotizing enterocolitis, White beverages

'Breathing' BIOCHEMISTRY A local unfolding of a polypeptide to allow the exchange of one isotopic molecule for another **MOLECULAR BIOLOGY** A local unwinding of the DNA double helix to allow formation of transcription bubbles; alternately, the 'chaotic' transient rupture and reforming of interchain hydrogen bonds that facilitates the interaction with the regulatory DNA-binding proteins; Cf Premelting

Breath tests Clinical tests used to evaluate malabsorption, in which a food containing a substance emitting low levels of radioactivity is ingested and, if malabsorbed, is exhaled through the lungs **^{2}H-lactose test** A test to detect lactase deficiency Method: 1.0 g of lactose/kg body weight is given per os; an increase of breath ^{2}H of > 20 ppm above basal levels of ^{2}H indicates lactose malabsorption, the release of which depends on release of the ^{2}H from unabsorbed lactose through bacterial metabolism **^{14}C-xylose test** A test for general malabsorption Method: 1.0 g (5-10 µCi) of 'hot' xylose is administered per os; increased breath radioactivity at 30 min indicates overgrowth in the small intestine by gram-negative anaerobes

Breech position OBSTETRICS Buttocks presentation at the time of delivery, a position that carries a 3-6-fold increased mortality due to complications, including umbilical cord prolapse, tentorial tearing and cerebral hemorrhage of the after-coming head; in the US breeches are usually delivered by cesarian section; types of breech **FRANK BREECH** Thighs are flexed over the abdomen and the legs extended COMPLETE BREECH legs are flexed on the thighs and the fetus sits like Buddha Incomplete breech SINGLE OR DOUBLE FOOTLING One or both feet are the presenting parts

Bremsstrahlung German, braking radiation A broad spectrum (rather than an energy peak) of electromagnetic radiation that is generated by the rapid deceleration of a photon or electron when it hits the electron cloud of the atomic nucleus; most X-rays generate a significant amount of bremstrahlung, which deeply penetrates organic tissues, as these are formed of molecules with low atomic weights

Brick dust appearance LABORATORY MEDICINE Granular red-brown crystalline material corresponding to amorphous urates seen in a normal acid urine, composed of calcium urate, magnesium urate, sodium and potassium urates which crystallize when the urine is acidified

Brick-red sputum A thickened mixture of blood, bacteria, necrotic lung tissue and mucus, characteristic of *Klebsiella pneumonia*

Bridging CARDIOLOGY A designation for systolic narrowing of the left anterior descending coronary artery seen by angiography as an isolated finding during cardiac catheterization or in patients with coronary artery disease, left ventricular hypertrophy or hypertrophic cardiomyopathy; Cf Rat-tail, Sawfish patterns

'Bridging' TRAUMATOLOGY The 'spanning' of breaks in the skin by blood vessels, seen after a blunt object strikes tightened skin' rupturing the epidermis and dermis whilst the blood vessels (being more mobile) remain intact, 'bridging' the gap

Bridging fibrosis HEPATOPATHOLOGY The loose spanning of hepatic lobules by broad bands of fibrous tissue and collagen, seen by light microscopy in the healing phase of cirrhosis

Bridging necrosis HEPATOPATHOLOGY A finding seen by low-power light microscopy, consisting in spanning of hepatic vessels by confluent necrosis, linking portal tracts to centrilobular veins and to each other; the 'bridge' is necrotic, with broad bands of apoptotic hepatocytes and fibrotic condensation of 'stroma'; presence of bridging necrosis is considered to be the only reliable criterion for establishing the diagnosis of chronic active hepatitis, a disease which may evolve to cirrhosis or be a precursor of hepatocellular carcinoma

Bright plaque An optic fundoscopy finding consisting of a light-reflecting fragment of atherosclerotic plaque lodged in a retinal arteriole that may be associated with amaurosis fugax

Brilliant cresyl blue A high pH histological dye with affinity for nucleic acids used to delineate platelets, immature red cells and Heinz bodies

Brim Thickening of the iliopectineal line in the pelvic bone, a radiologic finding suggestive of Paget's disease of the bone that may also be seen in osteoporosis and osteoblastic metastases

British anti-Lewisite Dimercaprol 2,3-dimercaptopropanol A sulfhydryl compound that was developed in World War II as an antidote to the vesicant arsenical war gas, which may be used as a therapeutic chelator for arsenic and mercury

British fetal hemoglobin A congenital hemoglobinopathy due to a regulatory defect in postnatal γ chain synthesis; hemoglobin F in these subjects comprises 20% in homozygotes and 3.5-10% in heterozygotes and is of clinical importance as it may mimic massive feto-maternal hemorrhage and thereby possible overdosage of Rh immune globulin

'Brittle and shallow' A descriptor for the sleep of the elderly who are easily aroused (brittle) and do not fall into a deep sleep (shallow); see REM, Sleep disorders

Brittle bones Bones with increased osseous fragility, a phenomenon seen in Osteogenesis imperfecta, caused by various genetic defects, eg point mutation in collagen, type I

Brittle cornea syndrome An uncommon disease reported among Tunisian Jews characterized by red hair, blue sclera and brittle corneas with spontaneous perforation

Brittle diabetes Insulin-dependent diabetes mellitus in which the blood glucose fluctuates widely, swinging rapidly from the hypoglycemia to hyperglycemia despite frequent 'titration' of the insulin dose

Brittle hair syndrome Trichothiodystrophy A condition characterized by brittle, sulfur-poor hair, mental and physical retardation, onychodystrophy and ichthyotic skin, which is caused by an inherited defect in the 'excision repair' pathway; see Excision repair syndromes, Xeroderma pigmentosum; Cf Kinky hair syndrome

BRMs see Biological response modifiers

Broken ring sign A finding by magnetic resonance imaging (figure) that consists in disruption of the lateral wall of the superior vena caval 'ring', seen in anomalous pulmonary venous connection to the superior vena cava (MayoClin Proc 1985; 60:874)

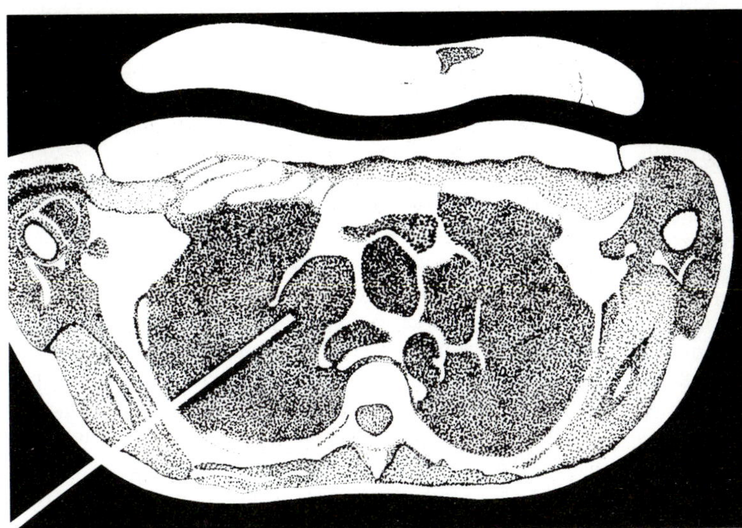

Broken ring sign

Broken straw sign SURGICAL PATHOLOGY Bent, elongated eosinophilic cells with occasional cross-striations seen by light microscopy in embryonal rhabdomyosarcoma

Brompton mixture An oral analgesic 'cocktail' of morphine, cocaine, chloroform water, alcohol and flavored syrup first formulated at the Brompton Chest Hospital; 'Brompton' mixture is currently is a generic term for an alcoholic solution containing an opioid (heroin or morphine) and either cocaine and/or a phenothiazine and is used to treat the pain of terminal cancer

Bronchopulmonary dysplasia A chronic lung disease affecting an estimated 7000 premature infants/year in the USA treated for respiratory distress syndrome with supplemental oxygen and mechanical ventilation; the diagnosis is clinical and is made at one month of age in premature infants who have undergone mechanical ventilation for at least one week, who have symptoms of persistent respiratory distress, who are dependent on supplemental oxygen and who have rounded radiolucencies on a plain film of the chest Laboratory Increased leukotrienes C4, D4 and E4 in the lavage fluid (Am J Dis Child 1990; 144:160) Histopathology 40% of the infants die and microscopy of the lungs reveals necrotizing bronchiolitis, alveolar fibrosis, emphysema and arterial changes of pulmonary hypertension Prognosis Those who survive infancy have pulmonary dysfunction in later life, in the form of airway obstruction, airway hyperreactivity and hyperinflation (N Engl J Med 1990; 323:1793)

Bronze baby syndrome A complication of phototherapy (used for infants with clinical jaundice and indirect hyperbilirubinemia) characterized by dark gray-brown skin discoloration (which may be many months in duration), significant elevation of direct bilirubin, mixed hyperbilirubinemia and evidence of obstructive liver disease; other complications of phototherapy include; loose stools, rashes, overheating, overcooling and dehydration

Bronze diabetes A clinically (but not pathologically) distinct form of diabetes mellitus that occurs in association with hemochromatosis, in which there are yellow-red hemosiderin deposits in the skin

Brown oculocutaneous albinism An autosomal defect in pigment production seen in Africa and New Guinea characterized by hyperkeratosis, photophobia, pachydermia and a relatively low amount of pigment

Brown atrophy ANATOMIC PATHOLOGY A change described in the hearts, livers and other organs of older subjects; the organs are smaller and flabby; by light microscopy there is extensive accumulation of lipofuscin ('aging' pigment)

Brown bowel syndrome Melanosis coli Accumulation of lipofuscin (ceroid) pigment in the intestinal wall, which is positive by periodic acid-Schiff, Fontana-Masson, modified acid-fast and oil red-O stains Clinical Chronic abdominal pain, pancreatitis, biliary atresia, cirrhosis, peptic ulcer disease and mucoviscidosis

Brown-Brenn stain A variant of the gram stain used to identify bacteria in histological sections

Brown fat A tissue designed to generate heat with abundant mitochondria that imbue the tissue with a pardous hue; although human adults essentially lack this 'superfat', thermogenesis from brown fat is crucial to infant survival as well as hibernating animals; in brown fat mitochondria, an inner-membrane protein acts as a natural uncoupler of oxidative phosphorylation, causing transmembrane transportation of H+, short-circuiting the membrane's usual proton gradient, directly converting the energy released by NADH into heat; the glucose utilization index in brown fat is a function of the amount of available food (Biochemistry 1991; 273:233)

Brown heroin A contaminated substance of abuse first described in heroin imported from Mexico in 1974 that caused folliculitis and subcutaneous nodules, noninfectious musculoskeletal hypersensitivity, fever, paraspinal myalgias, arthralgias, periarticular tenderness; the color was due to 'additives', including procaine and opium-processing contaminants (noscapine, papaverine) imparting a brown tinge and a viscid consistency to the heroin (Ann Int Med 1977; 87:22) Side effects Hyperyglobulinemia, biological false positive serological reaction for syphilis

Brown induration Chronic passive pulmonary congestion A gross finding in any chronic condition with long-standing transalveolar leakage of blood, often accompanied by increased pulmonary venous pressure **Etiology** Congestive heart failure, Goodpasture's disease, hemosiderosis, mechanical obstruction of pulmonary vein, mitral valve stenosis **Pathogenesis** Chronic hemorrhage and edema within thickened alveolar walls results in fibrotic induration accompanied by brawny discoloration of the soggy lungs

Browning reactions Any of a group of complex enzymatic (eg oxidization) and non-enzymatic (eg caramelization, degradation of ascorbic acid and Maillard reaction) reactions that affect foods when processed or stored

Brown lung disease see Byssinosis

Brown journal A colloquialism of little utility for the American Journal of Kidney Disease

Brown-Pearce tumor A transplantable anaplastic carcinoma originating in a syphilitic scar in the rabbit scrotum; the tumor metastasizes to spermatic cord and the peritoneum

Brown-Sequard syndrome A clinical complex characterized by hemiparaplegia caused by hemilateral compression or destruction of the spinal cord associated with homo-/ipsilateral motor paralysis, loss of vibratory, joint and tendon sensatiion and diminished tactile discrimination with contralateral anesthesia and loss of temperature sensation; the syndrome occurs with traumatic spinal cord injuries, tumors, as a complication of spinal irradiation or Herpes zoster

Brown spider *Loxosceles reclusa* and *L laeta* are secretive spiders that seek secluded sites and bite when bothered **Local symptoms** Cyanosis, necrosis, pustule or bullae, rimmed by ischemia and erythema expanding to 20 cm over weeks and months **Systemic symptoms** Fever, chills, nausea, vomiting, dizziness, myalgia, arthralgia and potentially fatal intravascular hemolysis with hemoglobulinuria and acute renal failure

'Brown stains' SURGICAL PATHOLOGY A colloquial term for immunoperoxidase (special) stains, which are used to detect antigens, eg leukocyte common antigen, cytokeratin(s), S-100, in tissues by linking monoclonal antibodies raised against the antigen(s) of interest to an enzyme in the last of several antigen-antibody linking steps; if the antigen X is present, the enzyme digests a colorless substrate into a a brown pigmented product

Brown stool The normal fecal color is due to the content of mesobilifuscin dipyrrole, a byproduct of heme synthesis which does not react as either bilirubin or blood

Brown-Symmers disease Acute fulminant, often post-viral encephalitis in children, accompanied by fever, vomiting, irritability, eventuating in bulbar and cerebral disturbances with respiratory difficulties, strabismus, nystagmus, hemiplegia; the condition may be fatal within days

Brown syndrome NEUROLOGY Neural crest syndrome Congenital analgesia with neurogenic anhidrosis, loss of deep and superficial pain sensation, dental dysplasia, meningeal thickening with cystic degeneration, hyperreflexia, mild mental retardation **Laboratory** Abnormal homovanillic acid and vanilmandellic acid assays (Arch Neurol 1966; 15:294) OPHTHALMOLOGY Restriction or loss of ability to elevate the eye in adduction, often associated with down-turning of the affected eye, a compensatory tilt of the head associated with congenital fibrosis and shortening of the anterior sheath of the superior oblique tendon sheath of the trochlear muscle **Etiology** Idiopathic or associated with inflammation, possibly related to forceps delivery **Treatment** Surgical

Brown teeth of Capdepont An autosomal dominant dysodontogenesis characterized by small, yellow-brown teeth **Treatment** Remove teeth, replace with prostheses

Brown tonic see Hoxsey method

Brown tumor Osteitis fibrosa cystica A hyperparathyroidism-induced tumor-like mass of bony tissue characterized by fibrosis, cyst formation, marked osteoclastic resorption, multinucleated giant cells and hemosiderin (which imparts the brown color) deposits and rounded, cyst-like radiological defects; brown tumors also occur in secondary hyperparathyroidism and may be the first sign of renal osteodystrophy in patients with end-stage renal disease who are maintained alive by renal dialysis and have sufficient time to develop the osseous reaction

Brown-Vialetto-van Laere sydrome see Bulbar palsy

Brueghel syndrome Grotesque involuntary facial movements seen in later adult life, most common in women, characterized by forceful opening of the jaw, retraction of the lips, spasm of the platysma and protrusion of the tongue (alternately, the jaw may be clamped shut and the lips may purse); the name derives from Brueghel's painting, *DE GAPER*

Bruit CARDIOLOGY An arterial 'thrill' caused by atherosclerosis; when auscultated over the carotid arteries, bruits predict future cerebrovascular accidents; it is unclear whether surgical correction actually helps, as the ischemic event often occurs at a distance from the identified 'danger zone'

Brush border PHYSIOLOGY A specialized portion of the free or apical aspect of certain epithelial cells, especially of the intestine, which contain absorptive microvilli and glycocalyx, which is rich in hydrolytic enzymes; brush border antibodies were first described in rodents with Heymann nephritis and occur in 50% of patients with ulcerative colitis and in 20% of patients with Yersinia enterocolitis

Brutal beginning INFECTIOUS DISEASE A descriptor for the abrupt onset of disease (often within 1-2 hours) seen in half of the cases of leptospirosis **Clinical** Fever, headache, myalgia, nausea, vomiting, pain, hepatomegaly

'B' symptoms ONCOLOGY Systemic disease associated with leukemia and lymphoma, including significant fever (in Hodgkin's disease, the classic, but uncommon Pel-Ebstein fever), night sweats and unintentional weight loss of > 10%; 'A' symptoms represent the absence of clinical manifestations of malignancy

BSE 1) Breast self-examination, 2) see Bovine spongiform encephalopathy

BSL see Biosafety level

B-type virus A virus enzootic to macaques and Old World monkeys that is closely related to Herpes simplex and displays a similar clinical pattern characterized by intermittent shedding and reactivation during periods of stress and immunosuppression, occasionally proving fatal to human handlers of monkeys (MMWR; J Am Med Assoc 1987; 257:3193); B-type viruses are oncogenic and have an eccentric core of nuclear material, similar to MMTV (mouse mammary tumor virus; see C-type virus

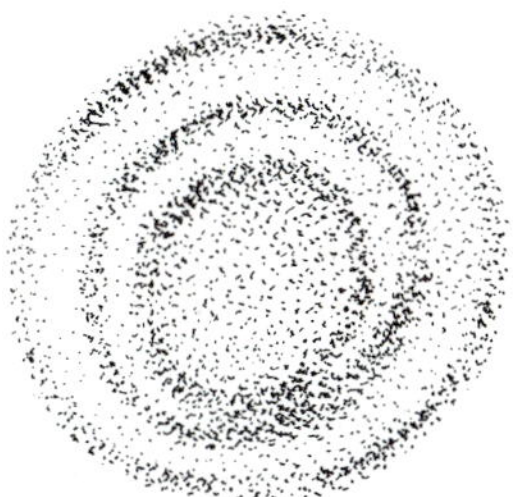
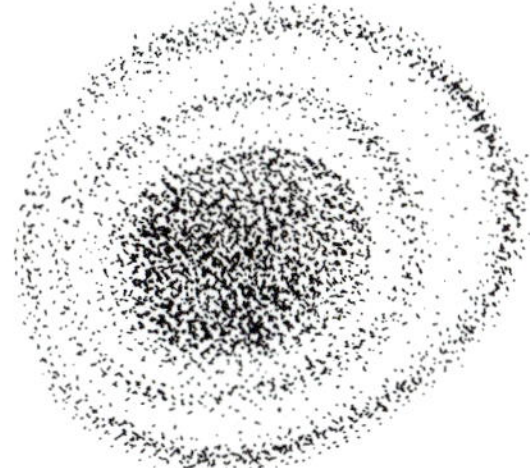

Early form B-type virus Late form

'Bubble and hole disease' Subacute spongiform encephalopathy Creutzfeldt-Jakob disease A colloquial descriptor for the spongiform changes seen by light microscopy in the cerebral cortex and basal ganglia, resulting in neuronal loss and fibrillary gliosis Ultrastructure The 'holes' correspond to intracytoplasmic membrane-bound vacuoles within neuronal and glial processes

'Bubble boy' David X, a child with severe combined immunodeficiency who had been kept alive in a gnotobiotic environment at the University of Texas since birth; at the age of 12 he received a bone marrow transplant from a histoincompatible sibling to reconstitute his immune system; to prevent graft-versus-host disease, the donor marrow was treated with monoclonal antibodies and complement to reduce alloreactive T-cells; the child died of an Epstein-Barr-induced polyclonal gammopathy that evolved into a monoclonal proliferation, ie a lymphoma (N Engl J Med 1985; 312:1151)

Bubble gum cytoplasm A fanciful descriptor for massive cytoplasmic vacuole(s) that may be seen in endocervical cells obtained from a routine papanicolaou-stained smear in a subject with an intrauterine device

Bubble signs Three radiologic signs related to accumulated gas in the upper gastrointestinal tract in neonates secondary to atresias at different levels SINGLE BUBBLE A gas pocket in the upper left quadrant, seen in complete stenosis at or proximal to the pyloris, or in complete gastric atresia DOUBLE BUBBLES Two upper abdominal gas pockets in neonates with duodenal atresia, annular pancreas (which wraps around the duodenum causing luminal stenosis) or the ultrarare midgut volvulus; the smaller bubble on the right corresponds to the duodenum and the larger to the left, the stomach Note: In atresia, there is no passage of gas to the intestine; thus intestinal gas militates against atresia TRIPLE BUBBLES A trio of upper abdominal gas pockets considered pathognomonic for jejunal atresia, where the upper right bubble corresponds to gas in the stomach, the left bubble corresponds to gas in the duodenal bulb and the lower right bubble corresponds to gas in the pre-atretic jejunum

Bubble stability test see Foam stability test

'Bubbly' lung PEDIATRIC RADIOLOGY A vaguely vacuolated pattern seen on a plain chest film in infants with hyaline membrane disease or in Wilson-Mikity syndrome

Bubbly vacuolization SURGICAL PATHOLOGY A Swiss cheese-like appearance of the cytoplasm of lipoblasts, malignant melanoma, Burkitt's lymphoma and malignant fibrous histiocytosis

Bubo Soft matted plum-colored lymph nodes measuring 4-5 cm in diameter, seen in lymphogranuloma venereum

Bubonic plague see Black death

'Bucket handle' fracture FORENSIC RADIOLOGY Fragmentation of the distal end of one or both femurs, seen at the bone margins as a crescent-shaped osseous density paralleling the metaphysis, seen radiologically when the growth plate is tipped at an obliquity to the radiographic beam; incomplete 'bucket handles' are characteristic of child abuse-related injuries, which may also be associated with subperiosteal neoosteogenesis (trauma of recent origin), distal transverse dense lines (previous growth disturbance) and cortical thickening (evidence of remote trauma), see Battered infant syndrome, Child abuse

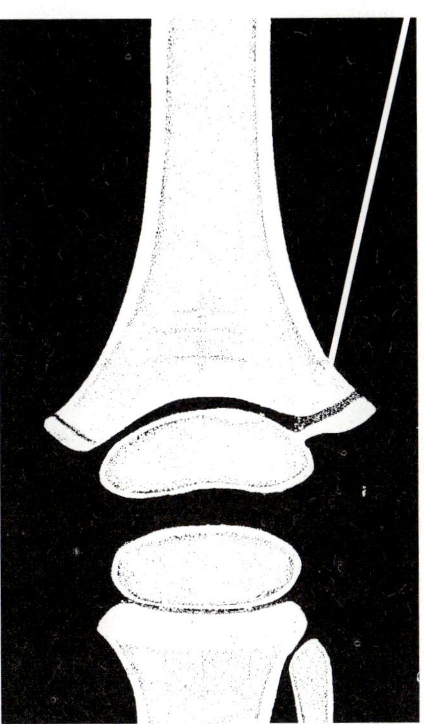

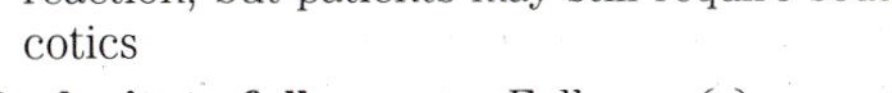
Bucket handle fracture

Bucket handles Folds of the skin of undetermined significance that may occur in low (anal agenesis, stenosis or incomplete rupture of the anal membrane) or high (complete failure of invagination of the proctodeum) obstructions of the terminal large intestine

'Bucking' RESPIRATORY THERAPY Violent resistance by a patient to intubated ventilation that may cause asynchronous breathing, ergo ventilation:perfusion (V/Q) mismatching and risk of barotrauma, cardiac arrhythmia and increased intracranial pressure; the newer ventilatory support devices rarely evoke this reaction, but patients may still require sedation, or narcotics

Buckminsterfullerene see Fullerene(s)

Buckshot pattern A pattern of multiple minute lesions, radiodensities or cell clusters, likened to the innumerable pellets from a shotgun blast HEMATOLOGY

Scattered subcutaneous aggregates of lymphocytes seen in nodular lymphoid hyperplasia

Buckshot (birdshot) calcifications RADIOLOGY Widely spread and minute ('miliary') calcifications that correspond to partially calcified (healing) granulomas in pulmonary, splenic and lymphoid histoplasmosis; in the lungs the granulomas may erode into the bronchi and be expectorated as broncholiths: Cf Miliary calcification

Buckyballs see Fullerene(s)

'Buddy' taping TRAUMATOLOGY Immobilization of fingers or toes adjacent to one that is fractured or otherwise injured; buddy taping is used for injuries of the proximal interphalangeal joint with incomplete collateral ligament tearing, where the affected finger is taped to an adjacent 'buddy' and immobilized for two weeks, or more if there is also distal dislocation

Buffalo hump Gibbus A mass of adipose tissue present at the lower cervical and upper thoracic vertebrae, characteristically seen in long-standing Cushing's disease/syndrome; a gibbus may also accumulate in the thoracolumbar regions of black South Africans with achondroplasia (possibly related to their practice of carrying infants on their backs), mucopolysaccharidoses and chronic osteomyelitis induced by coccidioidomycosis and ***Mycobacterium tuberculosis***

Buffer CHEMISTRY A chemical system that minimizes the effects, in particular the pH, of changes in the concentration of a substance COMPUTERS A storage zone, that 'resides' temporarily in the random access memory and contains either input or output data, remaining there while waiting for an output (less commonly an input) device, eg a printer, to allow it access to perform a function Note: Buffer sizes can be increased with 'spooling' software or by increasing the printer's random access capacity

Buffer theory CLINICAL NUTRITION A theory on the regulation of food intake and weight autoregulation that holds that only changes in the original equilibrium or rapid fluctuations in the food intake or body weight are opposed; the set point is easily disturbed, with rapid weight loss when food is not available, or rapid gain when ingestion is acutely increased

'Buffy' coat LABORATORY MEDICINE The flavescent band of cells and cellular debris that forms between the upper layer of plasma and the lower layer of red cells when whole blood is spun at 5000 RPM, corresponding to leukocytes; the 'buffy-crit' is usually 1-2% and is often increased in leukemia and leukocytoses

'Bug' COMPUTERS A bug is any defect in a system, often a software problem MICROBIOLOGY A highly colloquial term that is used interchangeably with bacteria

'Bugeyes' ENDOCRINOLOGY A colloquialism for marked bilateral exophthalmos with proptosis, caused by the infiltrative ophthalmopathy, which is seen in more than one-half of Graves' thyrotoxicosis, but which is less common in non-Grave's hyperthyroidism; other ocular signs in Grave's disease include upper lid spasm and lid retraction, external ophthalmoplegia, easy tearing with a gritty sensation of the eyes, supra- and infra-orbital swelling, congestion, edema and weakness of the extrinsic ocular muscles; when severe chemosis and inflammation are present, it is designated as malignant exophthalmos Pathogenesis Hypersecretion of a LATS-like (long-acting thyroid stimulator-like) substance

Bulimia An eating disorder that is either primary (bulimia nervosa) or a component of other diseases, eg schizophrenia, oral contraceptives, Kluever-Bucy and Kleine-Levin syndromes

Bulldog scalp see Cutis verticis gyrata

Bulldog syndrome An X-linked dysmorphia complex described by Simpson, characterized by a large, square protruding jaw, a broad nasal bridge, an upturned nose tip, macroglossia and broad short limbs, resulting in a physiognomy fancifully likened to that of a bulldog

'Bulldozing' invasion SURGICAL PATHOLOGY A colloquialism for a broad elephant-foot-like front of tissue invasion characteristic of a) Squamous cell carcinomas of low aggressiveness, eg verrucous carcinoma of the oral cavity and external female genitalia, a relatively 'bland' malignancy that evokes little inflammatory response, which may be underdiagnosed as verrucous or pseudoepitheliomatous hyperplasia and b) Hepatocellular carcinoma as it invades into the diaphragm and lungs, usually seen in a terminal stage of disease; Cf 'Stabbing' invasion

'Bull's eye' appearance Targetoid appearance A common descriptor for a rounded lesion or mass that is circumferentially rimmed by two or more distinct densities or colors; the inner cicle is often dark (or radiopaque), rimmed by a lighter (or radiolucent) ring that in turn is surrounded by a third, dark or radiopaque circle; the opposite (light-dark-light) has been called a Doughnut pattern

Bull's eye granules HEMATOLOGY Dense core (α) granules of platelets

Bull's eye lesion DERMATOLOGY Morphology of erythema multiforme, a lesion mediated by circulating immune complexes, elicited by infections, drugs, collagen vascular disease; in addition, the skin may have erythematous plaques and vesiculo-bullous lesions; bull's-eye lesions are also a classic lesion of Lyme's disease that is seen 1-3 weeks before the onset of the arthritic symptoms; mucosal involvement has been designated as Stevens-Johnson syndrome ENDOSCOPY A finding within the gastrointestinal lumen, in which edematous folds surround a central depression (mass lesion with a central ulcer), non-specific finding seen in solitary amebomas, actinomycosis, amyloidosis, appendiceal disease, tuberculosis; single endoscopic 'bull's-eyes' include submucosal carcinoid, primary carcinoma, Kaposi sarcoma, leiomyoma, leiomyosarcoma, lipoma and lymphoma; multiple 'bull's-eyes' occur in neoplasia: metastases from primary breast, lung and renal carcinoma, Kaposi sarcoma, lymphoma and mastocytosis (N Engl J Med 1990; 322:1298cpc) OPHTHALMOLOGY A fundoscopic finding described in chloroquine-induced retinopathy, where a depigmented lesion surrounds the macula, surrounded by another ring of relative hyperpigmentation, with possible permanent loss of visual acuity GASTROINTESTINAL RADIOLOGY The bull's-eye lesions are similar to those seen by endoscopy, are caused by centrally ulcerated lesions, suggestive of malignancy, where the central zone is hypodense, ie necrotic, implying a rapidly growing lesion that has outgrown its vascular supply; multifocal bull's eyes are suggestive of malignant melanoma; unifocal bull's eyes occur in carcinoma metastatic to the gastrointestinal tract, benign or malignant smooth muscle tumors of the intestinal wall, Kaposi and other sarcomas, eosinophilic granuloma and ectopic pancreatic tissue SURGICAL PATHOLOGY An uncommon histological finding in breast carcinoma, where vacuoles have a central spot that variably stains with Giemsa, eosin or periodic acid Schiff, possibly a processing artifact (J Clin Pathol 1975; 28:929)

Bull neck INFECTIOUS DISEASE Prominent and acute cervical lymphadenopathy associated with soft tissue edema that has a brawny color, demonstrates 'pitting', is warm and tender and affects children over age 6; the change may be so extensive as to cover the sternocleidomastoid muscle's border; the 'bull neck' is seen in children with epiglottitis who present with agitation, a muffled cry, labored respiration, cyanosis, drooling and dysphagia, due to ***Hemophilus influenzae*** type B, ***Corynebacteria diphtheriae*** and rarely, ***Streptococcus pneumoniae*** and ***Staphylococcus aureus***

Bullet nose deformity, see Canoe paddle

Bullis fever Camp Bullis fever An epidemic illness related to a bite from the Lone Star tick, Amblyomma americanum that occurred in a military 'boot' camp in 1942 Clinical Fever, headache, nausea, rash, neutropenia, thrombocytopenia and persistent lymphadenitis; although historically attributed to ***R rickettsia***, it may have been caused by ***Ehrlichia canis*** (J Am Med Assoc 1988; 260:3006c)

Bumper fracture(s) FORENSIC MEDICINE Compression fracture of the lateral tibial plateau with separation of the plateau's margin or depression of the central articular surface, due to abduction of the leg caused by an automobile bumper striking the lateral aspect of an extended leg and fixed foot, where the valgus stress forces the two bones into a close contact; bumper fractures are often bilateral and involve both the tibia and fibula; while the height of the bumper fracture on the victim's leg may determine the intensity of the driver's braking effort at the time of impact but the amount of bony and soft tissue destruction is a poor determinant of vehicular speed at impact

BUN Blood urea nitrogen In the US, urea concentrations in the blood are expressed as BUN (Normal adults, 8-26mg/dl); the International system or SI expresses nitrogen as urea (Normal adults, 2.9-8.2 mmol/L); BUN/Creatine ratio normally is 20:1; increased BUN or azotemia is divided into prerenal (due to poor perfusion with decreased glomerular filtration rate, seen in dehydration, shock, decreased blood volume and congestive heart failure), renal azotemia (decreased glomerular filtration caused by acute or chronic renal failure, see Uremia) and postrenal (rare, due to urinary tract obstruction or perforation with extravasation of urine; decreased BUN occurs in pregnancy (due to increased GFR), malnutrition, high fluid intake, severe liver disease (decreased protein production)

'Bundling' An attempt by one pharmaceutical company to link the availability of a drug to a mandatory (and for-profit) monitoring system, in order to reduce the liability from a well-known and potentially fatal side effect of the drug; the only drug that has been thus far 'bundled' is clozapine, an agent that has proven more effective than other neuroleptic agents in treating schizophrenia, as it offers better control of psychotic symptoms and is used when patients don't respond to usual therapies neuroleptics; because 1-2% of clozapine-treated patients develop potentially fatal agranulocytosis, its manufacturer, had made the drug available at a cost of $9000/year in one-week supplies, to be released only after blood had been drawn from the patient, in order to closely monitor the white cell count (N Engl J Med 1990; 323:827); an obvious concern with 'bundling' is that the practice would spread to other drugs, increasing the price of therapeutics Note: In response to protests from the American Medical Association, the manufacturer unbundled itself from the monitoring system and reduced the price, which is three-fold more expensive in the US than Europe (J Am Med Assoc 1991; 265:837n&v)

Bundling HEALTH CARE FINANCING The combining of multiple surgical procedures under one fee schedule, such that the sum of the fees is less than each individual fee alone, eg excision of a lipoma, hernia sac repair and scar removal would be combined under one fee schedule and the surgeon paid less than for each individual procedure; Cf Unbundling INFORMATION SCIENCE The practice of combining a number of 'electronic journals', usually produced by one publisher for one reduced price; see Electronic journal

Bungarotoxin NEUROPHYSIOLOGY An anticholinergic neurotoxin derived from venom of the snakes of the genus ***Bungarus***, which binds in a non-covalent fashion to nicotinic-type acetylcholine receptors, preventing depolarization at the postsynaptic membrane of the neuromuscular junction

Buprenorphine An opiate analog that substitutes for methadone in heroin addicts Side effects Sedation, constipation

Burgundy red urine A deep red urine produced in porphyria caused by uroporphyrin in the urine, a consistent finding in those with congenital erythropoietic porphyria, intermittently so in those with hepatic porphyria

Burkitt's lymphoma see Lymphoma, Burkitt's

Burking FORENSIC MEDICINE Homicidal suffocation, accomplished by sitting on the victims' chest with a hand placed over the mouth and nose; in pre-Victorian Scotland, bodies for the study of anatomy were supplied by grave-robbing at a price of 10 guineas; W Hare who ran a boarding house in Edinburgh's Tanner Row and W Burke formed a partnership circumventing the unpleasantries of grave-robbing, for which they stood trial for 'burking' 15 victims; Burke was hanged

Burn cancer A malignancy, usually squamous cell carcinoma that arises in a background of burns (especially in radiant energy induced burns) Note: A healing wound, when examined by light microscopy may perfectly mimic the malignant fibrosarcoma, as it is characterized by markedly atypical fibroblasts, nuclear hyperchromatism and bizarre mitotic figures

'Burned out' germinal centers see Germinal centers

'Burned out' mucosa A gross anatomic finding in severe, long-standing cases of ulcerative colitis, with virtually complete mucosal denudation and scattered residual pseudopolyps

'Burned-out' phase 'Spent' phase HEMATOLOGY A desirable end-stage of polycythemia vera, where hyperproduction of erythrocytes settles down and much of the bone marrow is replaced by reactive fibroblasts which produce the collagen typical of myelofibrosis

Burning feet syndrome Causalgia with excessive perspiration, slight weakness and changes in the reflexes

Burning tongue 'syndrome' Transient glossodynia related to eating Hot foods, see there

'Burnout' A feeling of hopeless frustration often accompanied by depression, experienced by workers in certain fields; in the health care field, without an active, self-renewing support group, nurses and social workers assigned to AIDS units, oncology and geriatrics, in which there is an endless parade of dementia, deterioration and death, tend towards callousness and desire to change fields

Burnout syndrome Compassion fatigue A form of chronic stress in which the subject gives of himself or herself 'until it hurts', described as a sensation of depletion without time for psychological 'replenishment'; these subjects (usually health care givers) suffer chronic fatigue, have muscle tension, may engage in substance abuse, usually alcohol also Old Soldier syndrome

Burr cells Echinocytes Greek Echino, sea urchin HEMATOPATHOLOGY Erythrocytes with regular spines or bumps on the surface, seen after venomous snake (crotalids/pit viper) bites, uremia, pyrokinase deficiency (mechanism: decrease of cellular ATP), erythrocytes low in potassium (as may occur after transfusion of very old blood which may be close to its 42 day maximum shelf limit), gastric ulcers and carcinoma; similar cells (with longer spines) may be seen in acanthocytosis typical of a-β-lipoproteinemia; more attenuated spines are designated as 'created' erythrocytes with an undulating cellular membrane associated with exposure to hypertonic saline

Burt affair Sir Cyril Burt, a British mathematician cum psychologist credited with accumulating data on a group of identical twins raised separately; although Burt had been considered the greatest British psychologist, after his death in 1971, it become apparent that some of the studies probably had not been performed at all, and many of the research associates named in publications were probably fictitious; Cf Breuning case

Buruli ulcer A deeply penetrating ulcer caused by *Mycobac-terium ulcerans* seen in Central Africa, New Guinea, Malaysia and Australia Treatment None is consistently effective

Burst BIOCHEMISTRY An abrupt onset of a reaction Virology The rupture of cell filled with viral progeny

Burst-forming activity see Interleukin-3

Burst-forming unit (BFU) HEMATOLOGY A small, partially-differentiated lymphocyte-like progenitor cell that arises from a pluripotent stem cell, the CFU-GEMM (colony-forming unit for granulocytes, erythrocytes, megakaryocytes and monocytes) in the bone marrow, giving rise to either erythrocytes (BFU-E) or megakaryocytes (BFU-Meg)

Burst therapy A relatively high dose (administered over a short period) of a drug which has untoward side effects when therapy with the agent is prolonged; burst therapy is used for corticosteroids, in which a typical 'burst' dose consists of 50-150 mg/day of prednisone for several days, followed by a rapid drop to 10-20 mg/day, followed by discontinuation if the patient can be 'weaned'

Buserelin A gonadotropin-releasing hormone analogue that down-regulates the pituitary-gonadal axis, used to treat metastatic prostatic carcinoma; see Disease flare

Bush tea see Jamaican vomiting sickness

'Butterfly drug' CI-911 A drug whose distinct molecular structure has earned it this interesting appellation

Butterfly fragment ORTHOPEDICS A wedge-shaped fragment of bone which is split off the main fragments, seen in a comminuted (more than two fragments) fracture, usually of long bone

Butterfly needle A short needle with flexible plastic handles that fold for insertion and lay flat for stabilization with tape; alternately known as scalp vein needles as they are the most practical and commonly used intravenous needles for infants

Butterfly pattern RADIOLOGY The fine diffuse infiltrates seen by a plain chest film that radiates bilaterally from the hilum to the lung periphery, characteristic of pulmonary alveolar proteinosis Note: The 'Bat wing' pattern is more radiodense, sharply defined, prominent in the hilum and associated with pulmonary edema Bat wing and Butterfly wings Some authors have considered the two patterns synonymous

Butterfly rash An often photosensitive facial rash typical of lupus erythematosus, consisting in an erythematous blush or scaly reddish patches on the malar region, extending over the nasal bridge (the facial 'seborrheic' region), potentially becoming bullous and/or secondarily infected; 'butterfly' region rashes have been described in AIDS (N Engl J Med 1984; 311:189), ataxia-telangiectasia, Bloom syndrome, Cockayne syndrome, dermatomyositis, erysipelas (St Anthony's fire, accompanied by waxy guttate indurations of the nose and cheeks that are red, hot, tender and painful with raised borders, a streptococcal skin infection of warm climates, often due to β-streptococcus group A (rarely also group C), pemphigus foliaceus, pemphigus erythematosus (an autoimmune vesiculobullous disorder with immune deposition of IgG and C3), riboflavin deficiency, tuberous sclerosis with smooth, red-yellow papules (adenoma sebaceum), appearing by age four at the nasolabial fold

Butterfly scheme A graphic representation of control loops found in regulation of serum calcium under physiological and pathological conditions and the potential for adaption in each situation

Butterfly-shaped pigment dystrophy of the fovea Ophthalmology An autosomal recessive dystrophy of the retinal pigment epithelium that is bilateral, symmetrical and asymptomatic

'Butterfly' tumor The trivial name for the aggressive bilateral, oftenbifrontal and symmetrical growth pattern of grade III and IV astrocytomas (glioblastoma multiforme), in which there is leaf-like tumor growth on both sides of the corpus callosum with extension along the white tracts, mixed with hemorrhage and necrosis Clinical More common in men with a vague familial tendency, accompanied by hemorrhage causing a stroke-like clinical picture and potentially, sudden death Pathology Butterfly gliomas are poorly demarcated macro- and microscopically

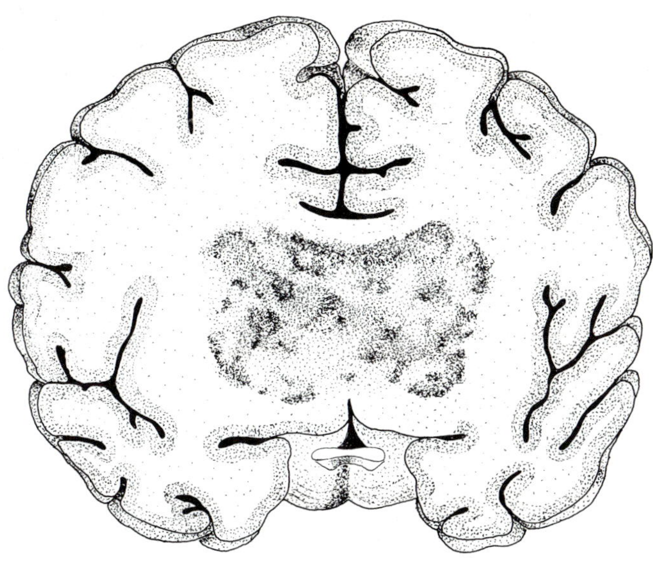

Butterfly tumor

Butterfly vertebra A congenital anomaly of a vertebra with persistence of the fetal notocord remnant due to incomplete embryologic notocord regression, or chorda dorsalis; sagittal clefts appear, causing a characteristic 'pinching' of the superior and inferior aspects of the body and compensatory overgrowth of the vertebral bodies above and below the affected bone

Buttock cell Hematopathology A small lymphocyte with deep central nuclear cleavage, seen in lymphosarcoma cell leukemia, mixed cell malignant lymphoma or nodular or diffuse poorly differentiated lymphocytic lymphoma; Cf Cerebriform nuclei

Button TRANSFUSION MEDICINE An aggregate of erythrocytes adherent to the bottom of a test tube after centrifugation, if with gentle shaking of the test tube, the cells remain adherent, agglutination is assumed to have occurred, implying presence of both an antigen (on the erythrocyte) and a specific antibody (immunoglobulin in the serum)

Button hole stenosis see Fishmouth stenosis

'Buttonholing' A clinical finding in cutaneous neurofibromatosis in which compressed tumors seem to 'pop' through an opening in the deep dermis, likened to a button; other skin tumors (eg lipomas and fibroepithelial polyps) generally do not 'button-hole'

Button sequestrum A preserved island of bone (sequestrum) lying within a 'punched-out' osteolytic lesion of the skull, well-described in eosinophilic granuloma of the diploâ (skull), also be seen in infections (*M tuberculosis*, staphylococcal infection), metastatic carcinoma, multiple myeloma, radiation necrosis, meningioma, benign osseous tumors and secondary to a ventriculoatrial shunt

B-virus see B-type virus

Bypass obstruction A partial occlusion of the mainstem bronchus resulting in hyperdistension of an entire lobe, with potential for interstitial emphysema and rupture, in a fashion identical to that of the ball-valve phenomenon

Bypass surgery see Coronary artery bypass graft

Byssinosis Brown lung An occupational lung disease, secondary to inhalation of airborne cotton, hemp, linen; the early stages of disease are attributed to endotoxin (N Engl J Med 1987; 317:605), characterized by coughing, wheezing, airway obstruction; the later stages by chronic bronchitis, emphysema and interstitial lung disease; see Farmer's lungs

Byte COMPUTERS Eight binary bits, a unit for measuring computer memory and storage capacity; in perspective, two kilobytes is roughly equivalent to one type-written page; the current generation of personal (desktop) microcomputers built around Intel's 80386 microprocessor (chip) or Motorola's 68030 chip have 1-16 Megabytes of random access memory and 40-300 megabytes of hard drive storage capacity; see Computers, RAM

BZ-1, BZ-2 receptors see Benzodiazepine receptors

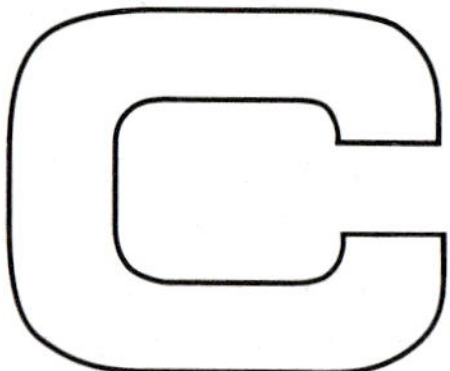

C Symbol for: Carbon; Centigrade; complement; cysteine; cytidine; cytosine

c Symbol for: centi-; complementary (molecular biology) molar concentration; speed of light

CAA see Cerebral amyloid angiopathy

CAAT box MOLECULAR HEMATOLOGY A semi-conserved 'box' of DNA with the 'consensus' sequence GG(T/C)CAATCT, located approximately 80 nucleotides upstream (in the 5' direction) from the start site for transcription of α and β globin genes, forming part of the promoter site for RNA polymerase II

CA 15-3 A proprietary antibody raised against an antigen in the serum that is often elevated in metastatic carcinoma of the breast

CA 19-9 A tumor-associated antigen that is present in tissue associated with mucin or in the circulation located on the sialylated Lewis A blood group antigen (subjects who are genotypically Lewis a-b- comprise 5% of the population and cannot synthesize the antigen); pancreatic carcinoma is present in 72% of those with serum levels above 37 U/ml and 97% of those with levels above 1000 U/ml; although the monoclonal antibody to CA 19-9 cannot be used to screen for pancreatic cancer, it can be used to detect post-surgical recurrence and to differentiate between benign and malignant disease of the pancreas (Am J Gastroenterol 1990; 85:350rv)

CA-125 A cell surface glycoprotein first identified in mucinous ovarian carcinomas that is also expressed on adenocarcinomas of the uterine cervix, endometrium, gastrointestinal tract and breast, measured in the serum, where rising levels indicate a poor prognosis, but low levels are of little clinical utility (Gynecol Oncol 1987; 26:284)

C-A-B sequence The order of emergency life support, where C Chest compression is followed by A Airway maintenance and B Breathing; CAB is preferred by the Dutch school of cardiology, while the 'American' school-prefers the A-B-C sequence, see there

CABG see Coronary arterial bypass graft

Cabin fever see Relapsing fever

CACA box MOLECULAR BIOLOGY The DNA oligonucleotide, CCACACCC contains CACA, a conserved sequence or 'box' located 93 residues upstream from the the β globin gene; base pair substitutions in the ACA box 31 residues upstream, the CAT box 76 residues upstream or the duplicated CACA box cause inaccurate and inefficient transcription by RNA polymerase, resulting in thalassemia

Cachectin see Tumor necrosis factor (TNF)

CAD 1) see Cold agglutinin disease 2) Coronary artery disease

Cadherins A family of 118-135 kD membrane glycoproteins that are specific Ca^{++}-dependent cell-cell adhesion molecules crucial for tissue differentiation, structure and cell sorting; cadherins are divided into neural cadherin (N-CAM), which binds to neurons, epithelial cadherin (E-cadherin) or uvomodulin, liver cadherin (L-CAM) and placental cadherin (P-cadherin) which have 50-60% sequence homology with each other; cadherins are key regulators of morphogenesis; they form a complex with the cytoskeleton, colocate with the tyrosine kinases of the ***src*** family and thus cadherin-mediated cell-cell junctions may play a role in intercellular signalling; cadherin down-regulation is associated with tumor cell invasion (Science 1991; 251:1451); see also CAM (Cell Adhesion Molecule)

Caenorhabditis elegans A small nematode that has proven to be a major 'workhorse' model in experimental biology, providing key information in embryology, as the exact lineage of each of the worm's adult cells is known and neurology, where the connections of each of the *C elegans'* 302 neurons has been determined; it has provided the basis for key discoveries in programmed cell death, heterochronic genes, sex determination and neuronal guidance; the goal of the nearly 100 research groups that are studying ***C elegans*** is to map its 100 million DNA (the human genome has 3×10^9) base pairs by the year 2000, an effort known as the 'worm project' (Science 1990; 248:1310rv)

Cafe-au-lait spots Large smooth ('coast of California'), sharply-demarcated cutaneous macules which are light brown in caucasians, dark-brown in blacks, due to increased epidermal melanocytes and melanin; while up to 10% of the population has these spots, six or more spots larger than 1.5 cm is virtually diagnostic of von Recklinghausen's disease; cafe-au-laits spots also occur in Albright's disease (see Coast of Maine), Russel-Silver syndrome, congenital syphilis and Jaffee-Campanacci disease

Cafe coronary Complete upper airway obstruction by a bolus of food, often meat, with occlusion of both the esophagus and larynx, so named as the sudden onset of symptoms simulates a myocardial infarct; the victims are speechless, breathless and without help, eg Heimlich maneuver, lifeless; cafe coronaries occur in the inebriated, bedentured, mentally retarded, demented, or in those who simply like to eat Clinical Violent coughing, cyanosis, collapse and death Note: Although a cafe coronary was the alleged cause of death at age 33 of the corpulent siren of the 60s, Elliot (Mama) Cass, according to Dr K Simpson, forensic pathologist and G Thurston, Coroner of London, she in fact died of atherosclerotic heart disease; Cf Steakhouse syndrome, Sushi syncope

Cafeteria diet Snack diet, 'Trash' diet An experimental system for studying obesity that allows rats free or cafeteria-style access to cookies, candy, cake ('junk-food'); if the diet is begun in prepubertal animals, they remain lean despite excess intake; if the diet is begun as adults, they become obese, due to insufficient thermogenesis; this serves as a non-genetic animal model for obesity of the pure over-feeding type, in which adipsin levels (a serine protease analog synthesized by adipocyte), are normal; genetically obese rats have low adipsin levels

Caged ATP EXPERIMENTAL BIOLOGY An ATP molecule bound to $CH_7(CO)NO$, which in this form, can neither serve as a substrate for myosin ATPase, nor bind to myosin headpieces

CAGUGX A loop of nucleotides corresponding to the iron-responsive element in the messenger RNA for ferritin; CAGUGX is located in the 5' direction (upstream) and is not translated into protein but is sensitive either to iron or to an iron-induced protein-linked substance that binds to the CAGUGX stem-and-loop structure, increasing ferritin synthesis

Cain complex PSYCHIATRY A destructive sibling rivalry, in which one of the sibs resents the other for perceived favoritism from a parental figure; so named after the biblical Cain, son of Adam and Eve, who killed his brother Abel

'caine family PHARMACOLOGY An essentially interchangeable group of local anesthetics including carbocaine (Mepivacaine) and xylocain (Lidocaine)

20(S)-Camptothecin A chemotherapeutic plant alkaloid isolated from ***Camptotheca acuminata*** that targets DNA topoisomerase I (a 100 kD protein, that relaxes supercoiled DNA, acting in semiconservative replication of double-stranded DNA), which is responsible for the breakage-reunion reaction of coiled DNA; since there are increased levels of topoisomerase I in colonic carcinoma, camptothecin has potential in otherwise recalcitrant metastatic colonic carcinoma (Science 1989; 246:1046)

Caissons' disease the Bends, the Chokes A clinical complex caused by rapid whole body decompression, with intravascular 'boiling' of nitrogen and resultant morbidity or mortality in scuba divers and high-altitude pilots or workers in high-pressure environments **Clinical, acute** Headache, nausea, vomiting, vertigo, tinnitus, dyspnea, tachypnea, convulsions and shock, joint and abdominal pain; nitrogen gas in the brain causes 'boxcar' air bubbles in leptomeningeal vessels separating the blood 'column', potentially causing death **Clinical, chronic** Dysbaric (ischemic) osteonecrosis with medullary infarcts of the femoral and humoral heads and rarely, malignancy (malignant fibrous histiocytoma) arising in the site of bone infarction (Undersea Biomed Res 1984; 11:305) Note: Caissons are air compression chambers used for underwater construction; Roebling, engineer of the Brooklyn Bridge (an engineering 'triumph' of the 19th century) was among the first to suffer from the late deforming arthritic effects of Caissons' disease

Cake kidney Clump kidney Congenital fusion of both renal anlage at the midline into a solid, irregularly lobed mass located caudad to the usual site or as far south as the pelvic floor; the blood is supplied by the lower aorta or common iliac arteries; the ureters are anterior and short, but may enter the bladder normally **Clinical** Lower abdominal pain, caused by stretching of the vascular pedicle, obstruction, infection, calculus formation and nephritis; Cf Horseshoe kidney

'Cake' omentum The exceedingly rare diffuse omental involvement by malignancy, usually of epithelial origin, including carcinomas of the colon, stomach, pancreas and ovary

Calabar swelling A transient, one week in duration allergic response to microfilarial infestation by ***Loa Loa*** as well as ***Dipetalonema perstans***, described in West and Central Africa; Vector ***Cryosops silacea*** and ***C dimidiata***, biting flies of the rain forest

Calciferol A molecule with vitamin D activity, derived from steroids by breaking the B ring's 9-10 bond, eg cholecalciferol and ergocalciferol

Calcineurin A protein present in highest concentrations in the central nervous system, which binds both Ca^{++} and calmodulin, inhibiting the latter's activity

Calcisome A subcellular organelle involved in pumping Ca^{++} in permeabilized neutrophils (J Clin Invest 1987; 80:107)

Calcitonin A 32 residue polypeptide (plasma levels 100 pg/ml) produced by the parafollicular or 'C' (ultimobranchial) cells, cleaved from the larger molecule, katacalcin, circulating as polymers joined by disulfide bonds; calcitonin is rapidly secreted in response to small increases of plasma Ca^{++}, pentagastrin, glucagon, β-adrenergics and alcohol and is the physiological antagonist of PTH; although excess or deficient PTH and vitamin D cause clinical disease, fluctuation of calcitonin levels is asymptomatic; see C cells

Calcium channel blocker CARDIOLOGY Background: The extra- to intracellular calcium ratio is usually 10 000:1, a ratio crucial to normal neuromuscular function; during hypoxia, calcium accumulates in the cytoplasm and mitochondria, causing post-insult vasospasm (possibly also lipid peroxidation and free radical damage); thus in the early re-perfusion stages after a hypoxic event, calcium is moleculum non gratum and it is philosophically sound to administer calcium channel blocking agents; although it is unclear whether this strategy actually works, most customers swear by verapamil for preventing post-ischemic vasospasm of the coronary and cerebral arteries

Calcium hypothesis A hypothesis that explains neuronal release of neurotransmitters, positing that membrane depolarization is required only to open the calcium channels and increase internal calcium concentration near the membrane transmitter release sites (Nature 1991; 350:153)

Calcium paradox A phenomenon in chronically ischemic (and hypocalcemic) smooth and cardiac muscles which, when re-exposed to normal calcium levels, become overloaded with calcium, enter a sustained contracted state and die, thought the result of a) Calcium loading by hypoxic mitochondria and b) Exacerbation of ischemia by hypercalcemia-induced vasospasm, triggering thromboxane and prostaglandin release; a similar but less understood event is known as the oxygen paradox

Calcium shock EXPERIMENTAL BIOLOGY A 'trick' used at the research bench to facilitate passage of substances into cells and bacteria; excess calcium in a cell culture medium causes cells to enlarge and membranes to become 'leaky', allowing transmembranous passage of relatively large molecules, eg plasmids

Calcium 'soap' Numerous greasy, millet seed-sized masses, classically described on peritoneal surfaces in acute pancreatitis, caused by lipase-induced fat necrosis where the free fatty acids complex with calcium, producing opaque chalky-white deposits ('soap')

Caldesmon An 83 kD protein that binds both actin and calmodulin inhibiting actomyosin ATPase, preventing the binding of myosin; myosin dissociates from microfilaments during mitosis, an action thought to be mediated by transient caldesmon phosphorylation, possibly explaining the profound changes in the cell shape during mitosis (Nature 1990; 344:675)

Calicheamicin/esperamicin ONCOLOGY A family of antitumor antibiotics derived from ***Micromonospora calichensis*** and ***Actinomadura verrucosospora***, respectively that have 4000-fold greater antitumoral activity than adriamycin and which share a molecular motif of a double-triple-double carbon bond, known as an enediyene; this motif rearranges to form two chemically active radical sites which extract critical hydrogen atoms from DNA's sugar-phosphate backbone, resulting in double strand breakage; this new class of anti-tumoral agents is in phase I trials (Nature 1991; 349:566n&v)

California disease A trivial name for coccidioidomycosis

California encephalitis (CE) A viral infection by any of four California Bunyaviridae; most CE is by the LaCrosse virotype, occurring in the summer in north central USA; in endemic regions, CE causes 20% of acute childhood meningitides with a very low mortality rate; the infectious cycle is maintained in the mosquito vector, ***Aedes triseriatus*** Clinical Non-specific viral prodrome, followed by a 3-8 day meningismus with spontaneous resolution, excellent prognosis with possible psychological residua

California relative value studies (scale) HEALTH CARE REIMBURSEMENT A numerical coding system for all diagnostic and therapeutic procedures performed by or directly under the supervision of a physician; the system is used by physicians to determine a procedure's level of difficulty, which in part determines the fee; Cf RBRVS (Resource-based relative value scale)

cALLA common acute lymphocytic leukemia antigen CD10 antigen A marker for non E-rosette-forming pre-B lymphoblasts that comprise the most common cell type (65%) of childhood acute lymphocytic leukemia (ALL), which when accompanied by the Ia antigen indicates a relatively good prognosis; cALLA is also positive in B cell lymphomas, Burkitt's lymphoma and 40% of T cell lymphoblastic lymphomas; ALL affects both adults and children, with a pronounced peak between ages two and six; ALL blasts are often cALLA, TdT and Ia positive; white cell count is often $< 100 \times 10^9$/L (US: < 100 000/mm^3) Prognosis With treatment, 90% achieve complete remission and have a prolonged survival

Calmodulin A ubiquitous 148-residue protein subunit of erythrocyte and other plasma membrane calcium channel ATPases, which reversibly binds calcium in response to various stimuli, eg contraction and relaxation of smooth muscle; when complexed to Ca^{++}, calmodulin binds cAMP phosphodiesterase, hydrolyzing it, acting on protein kinases, releasing hormones, catalyzing biochemical reactions, triggering microtubule catabolism; calmodulin is also involved in DNA repair, activating synthase-phosphorylase kinase, catalyzing activation of phosphorylase b, mediating the degradation of glycogen to glucose

Caloric test A clinical test for evaluating vestibular function, using thermic stimuli to induce endolymphatic flow in the horizontal semicircular canal and horizontal nystagmus by creating a temperature gradient between the two sides of the canal

Calpain A proteolytic enzyme present in red cells and platelets that is activated by high intracellular concentrations of calcium, which in the platelets cleaves calmodulin-binding proteins during platelet activation, serving to terminate Ca^{++}-dependent signal transduction

Calpain II A calcium-activated protease (EC 3.4.22.17) involved in mitosis (Science 1988; 240:911) that changes its intracellular location during various phases of mitosis: it is plasma membrane-bound during interphase, migrating with the dividing chromosomes, perinuclear in anaphase and mid-cell in telophase

Calsequestrin A soluble, acidic Ca^{++}-binding glycoprotein in sarcoplasmic reticulum vesicles with 43 calcium ions, serving as a reservoir for intracellular calcium when the cytoplasm is overloaded

CAM Cell adhesion molecules A family of calcium-independent intercellular adhesion proteins (Science 1989; 245:631) that are cell selective; the three forms of (Neuronal) N-CAMs are produced by alternative splicing, modified by different polysaccharide groups and are presumed to direct cellular traffic during embryonal development, appearing during neuroepithelial morphogenesis, disappearing during migration and reappearing during ganglionogenesis; see Selectin

Cambium layer ANATOMIC PATHOLOGY A dense zone of primitive undifferentiated mesenchymal cells immediately below a mucosal lining, seen in a) Botryoid rhabdomyosarcoma, where the cambium cells are malignant and the tissue below the cambium layer is loose and myxoid andin (see figure, page 87) b) Mesenchymal cystic hamartoma where the cells are benign, the layer averages 1-2 mm in thickness and is separated from the respiratory epithelium by a collagen layer of < 0.2 mm (N Engl J Med 1986; 315:1255)

Camel back curve Double quotidian febrile 'spikes', ranging from 38-40° C; infections with a characteristic twice daily peak in fever, include gonococcal endo-

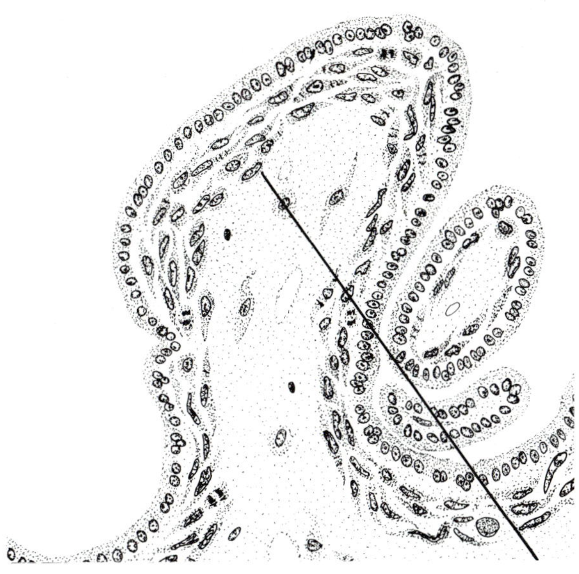

Cambium layer

carditis, measles, visceral leishmaniasis and Rift Valley fever; Cf 'Saddleback' curve

Camel nose see Tapir nose

CAMP Continuous air monitoring program A system of monitoring air pollution in the US

cAMP see cyclic adenosine monophosphate

CAMP test MICROBIOLOGY A culture plate test used for presumptive identification of group B streptococci, which exhibit a cleared zone when grown adjacent to β-lysin-producing staphylococci Technique *Streptococcus agalactiae*, a group B streptococcus that produces the CAMP factor is streaked on a sheep blood agar plate perpendicular to a streak of β-lysin-producing *Staphylococcus* forming an 'arrowhead' of hemolysis pointing towards the *Staphylococcus* Note: CAMP is an acronym of Christie, Adkinson and Munch-Peterson, three Australian public health workers who recognized the reaction on agar plates while investigating an outbreak of scarlet fever; see Reverse CAMP test

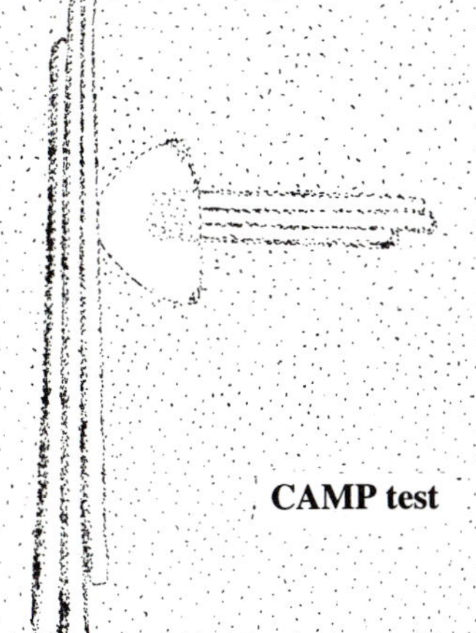

CAMP test

Campath-1 antigen CDw52 An antigen present on most lymphocytes and monocytes but not on other cells; Campath-1H is a 'humanized' antibody raised against this antigen (Tissue antigens 1990; 35:118)

Campylobacter A genus of gently-curved gram-negative rods that are common zoonotic commensal organisms found in the gastrointestinal tracts of a wide variety of wild and domesticated animals, and cause three types of human disease-enteric, eg diarrhea, typically by *C jejuni*, extraintestinal, most often by *C fetus* and gastric, due to *C pylori*, recently re-classified as *Helicobacter pylori*; most human infections have been attributed to consumption of contaminated water or food, and it has been suggested that some cases of human *C jejuni* infection may be due to magpie and jackdaw (bird) attacks on milk bottles (Lancet 1990; 336:1425); see *Helicobacter pylori*

Cancer A generic term for malignancy of any embryologic origin Note: The lay public and, unfortunately also many health professionals use the term 'cancer' interchangeably with 'carcinoma', a malignancy of epithelial and occasionally neuroepithelial origin

Cancer clusters see Clusters

Cancer families Malignancy occurs with greater frequency in certain families; when the cancer occurs in older subjects, the investigation may suggest exposure to an environmental agent that all family members have in common with a minimal genetic contribution; when family members develop malignancy while young, a significant genetic component is presumed to act with minimal environmental contribution and are known as 'cancer families'; family members of patients with early-onset malignancy, especially of the colon and breast, may have a 20- to 30-fold increased risk of malignancy, the cancer often being of one or at most a few 'restricted' histological types, eg an association of colonic and endometrial adenocarcinoma, or ovarian and breast carcinomas; analysis of heredity and the potential contributions by environmental (dietary, viral, electromagnetic radiation and other) exposures is complex; see Dysplastic nevus syndrome, Li-Fraumeni syndrome

Cancerization 'Carcinogenesis' ONCOLOGY A series of genotypic and phenotypic changes that occur in cells ultimately considered malignant, by virtue of having metastatic potential; the cancerization process is difficult to dissect as the genomic events, eg gene amplification, chromosome translocations, deletions and point mutations, don't always translate into phenotypic changes reflective of the *in vivo* realities of malignancy; an accepted cancerization model holds that cancer results from inducers and promoters in the form of chemicals, toxins, radiation and unknown environmental influences that impact on a genome that develops increasing susceptibility to environmental 'hits', responding with decreased production of tumor suppressor proteins and increased production of proteins that 'drive' cell proliferation, often derived from proto-oncogenes; this multistep or multi-'hit' process requires genetic alterations in the form of activated proto-oncogenes (dominant alterations) and inactivated tumor suppressor genes (recessive alterations), requiring up to ten distinct genomic mutations before malignant degeneration occurs (Science 1989; 246:1386); in the well-characterized cancerization cascade for familial adenomatous polyposis, the first step involves a mutation of the MCC (mutated in colorectal cancer) gene on chromosome 5q21 (Science 1991; 251:1366), resulting in increased cell growth, followed by the loss of methylated sites, a mutation of the c-*ras* gene, loss of the DCC gene on chromosome 18 and the p53 gene on chromosome 17, during which time the cell morphology is transforming from an increasingly aggressive adenoma, carcinoma *in situ* to eventually become malignant; see Inducer, One-hit/two-hit model, Proto-oncogenes, Tumor promoter, tumor suppressor

'Cancerization' SURGICAL PATHOLOGY A relatively specific term that traditionally refers to extension of a ductal carcinoma-in-situ into lobules ('lobular cancerization'), although this may represent a morphological variant of ductal carcinoma in situ; the term has been used by some surgical pathologists for a visible transition zone between an epithelial lesion with marked atypia and well-differentiated carcinoma, as in 'cancerization' of a villous adenoma of the colon

Cancer phobia An excessive fear of suffering the ravages of malignancy, a 'condition' that more commonly affects those who have directly cared for a loved one who suffered marked pain or disfigurement for a protracted period before death; cancer phobia is considered an appropriate indication for a simple mastectomy in patients with a diagnosis of carcinoma-in-situ, which may be treated more conservatively by close observation and periodic mammograms and breast examination

Cancer-prone personality A person who is at an increased risk of suffering malignancy due to ill-defined and nebulous internal conflicts; it is unclear whether this state actually exists as evaluation of 'proneness' is based on non-objective personal data (Prof Ed Pub, Am Cancer Soc); Cf Psychoneuroimmunology

Cancer screen Any measurable clinical or laboratory parameter that can be used to detect early malignancy; although these tests are relatively non-specific, they are highly sensitive, and detect the vast majority of subjects who are 'abnormal' in the parameter being measured; the most common cancer screens are those that detect occult blood in the stool as a screen for colon cancer and mammography for identifying microcalcifications and geographic densities for detecting breast carcinoma; logistically viable cancer screens must be viewed in the context of a cost-benefit ratio, and are not available for many of the more common malignancies, eg lung cancer, which theoretically could be detected by annual chest films, although this has not been recommended; Japan has responded to its 'epidemic' levels of gastric carcinoma by recommending periodic gastroscopy for its population

Cancer screening The testing of a large group of people for malignancies that are common to the group; screening tests must be inexpensive and, in order to detect all people who are abnormal for the analyte, highly sensitive

Cancer screening guidelines *BREAST CANCER* Self-breast examination on a monthly basis, a baseline mammogram at age 40 and mammography every 1-2 years thereafter, depending on risk factors *COLON CANCER* Recommendation by the National Cancer Institute, American Cancer Society and Americal College of Physicians for colorectal carcinoma is annual fecal occult blood test after age 40 and flexible sigmoidoscopy every three-to-five years after age 50 (N Engl J Med 1991; 325:37) *PROSTATE CANCER* Annual digital rectal examination after age 40, and measurement of prostate-specific antigen or acid phosphatase in the serum *UTERINE CERVIX CANCER* Annual papanicolaou test and pelvic examination after initiation of sexual activity; after three normal years, the test may be reduced in frequency at the discretion of the patient's physician

Cancer surgery Surgical treatment of a malignancy, a relatively routine procedure in most body sites; not all malignancies are amenable to surgical therapy, as a) Some tumors respond better to non-surgical treatment, eg lymphoma, which often responds to multiagent chemotherapy, choriocarcinoma, which responds to a single agent, methotrexate or seminoma, which responds to radiotherapy b) The lesion may have extended to or beyond vital structures, eg intracranial glioma or pericardial involvement c) The site is a surgical 'danger zone'; eg, esophagus and tail of the pancreas, associated with poor surgical salvage; see Operable cancer, Resectable cancer

Cancer-to-cancer metastasis A rare event in which there is metastatic penetration of one malignancy into another (Cancer 1968; 22:635); 'donor' cancers include bronchogenic 33%, breast 10%, gastrointestinal 10%, prostate 10%, thyroid 10%; 'recipient' cancers include hypernephroma 60%, lymphoproliferative 12% and others

Candida balls A bezoar composed of fungi; see Bezoar

Candida enolase A 48 kD antigen present in the serum of many patients with invasive candidal infection, an event usually associated with terminal cancer; detection of candida enolase complements blood cultures, but does not replace them (N Engl J Med 1991; 324:1026)

Candida krusei A *Candida* species that has recently emerged as a major systemic pathogen in patients with bone marrow transplantation who have received prophylactic fluconazole therapy, administered to prevent infection by *Candida albicans* and *C tropicalis* (N Engl J Med 1991; 325:1274); see Bone marrow transplantation

Candidate gene method MOLECULAR BIOLOGY A technique used to identify a gene possibly involved in a disease process by picking a cloned gene known to have a physiologic role in the diseased tissue; one then searches for mutations in the gene (often point mutations) in patients who have the disease in question; this method is considered more scientific than the 'serendipitous' technique of finding a mutated gene by 'reverse genetics'

Candidate hormone An incompletely studied substance

with hormone-like activity, eg enteroglucagon, urogastrone

Candidiasis see Mucocutaneous candidiasis

Candidiasis hypersensitivity syndrome Yeast connection A complex, the very existence of which is controversial, said to occur in women, due to an overgrowth of *Candida albicans* on mucosae, especially the vagina and gastrointestinal tract Etiology Broad-spectrum antibiotics, oral contraceptives and pregnancy Clinical Chronic gastrointestinal symptoms, eg bloating, heartburn, constipation and diarrhea, as wells as depression, loss of concentration, poor memory, fatigue, irritability, nasal congestion Treatment Nystatin had been recommended by certain health professionals; in a randomized study of oral and/or vaginal nystatin versus placebo, there was no difference in response of symptoms (N Engl J Med 1990; 323:1717)

Candle flame appearance CARDIOLOGY A finding by Doppler color flow imaging consisting of a central blue color, corresponding to a zone of high velocity, surrounded by a yellow-orange blush, corresponding to a turbulent, zone of lower blood flow; the 'candle flame' sign is typical of mitral stenosis, other morphological permutations in mitral stenosis have been described as having scimitar, mushroom and bifid jet shapes (Mayo Clin Proc 1986; 61:623)

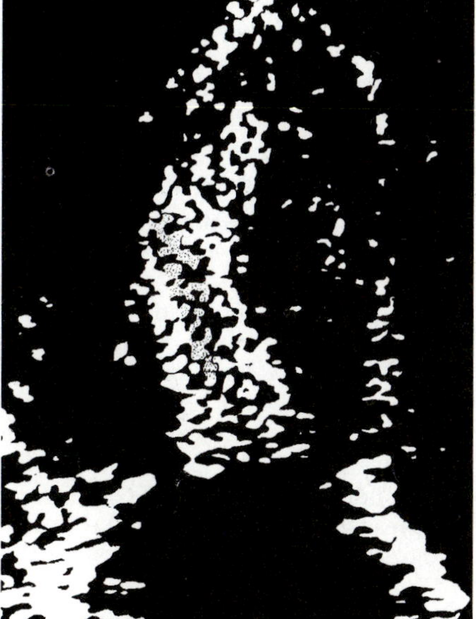

Candle flame appearance

Candlestick appearance BONE RADIOLOGY A sharply marginated 'cut-off' of the terminal phalanges with a central depression, seen in burns, diabetes mellitus, gout, leprosy, malabsorption, occlusive vascular disease, porphyria, psoriasis (Cf Pencilling), Raynaud's disease, rheumatoid arthritis, scleroderma

Candle wax bone see Melorheostosis

Candle wax drippings A descriptor for a morphology likened to the pearlescent gutterings of melted candle wax NEUROPATHOLOGY Smooth pinpoint-to-thumbnail-sized rounded elevations on the lateral ventricular walls or cerebral cortex in patients with tuberous sclerosis HISTOPATHOLOGY Architectural distortion, gliosis and bizarre, often enlarged neurons OPHTHALMOLOGY Fundoscopic changes in which the vascular sheath is surrounded by preretinal inflammatory exudates, appearing as bulbous perivascular dilatations, a finding suggestive of sarcoidosis

C & S Culture and sensitivity MICROBIOLOGY A set of tests performed on a clinical specimen, where isolation of a potentially-pathogenic bacterium is followed by antibiotic susceptibility testing; see MIC

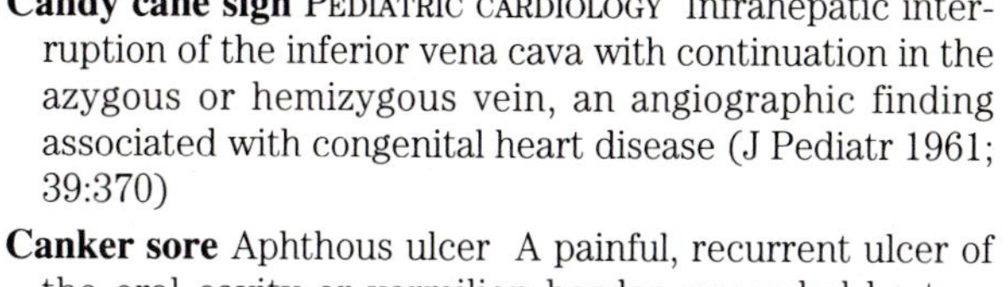

Candy cane sign PEDIATRIC CARDIOLOGY Infrahepatic interruption of the inferior vena cava with continuation in the azygous or hemizygous vein, an angiographic finding associated with congenital heart disease (J Pediatr 1961; 39:370)

Canker sore Aphthous ulcer A painful, recurrent ulcer of the oral cavity or vermilion border, preceded by tenderness and pruritus, beginning as an erythematous indurated papule that rapidly erodes, leaving an ulcerated base, covered with grayish exudate; although associated with Behçet syndrome and inflammatory bowel, the condition is idiopathic and may be of allergic, autoimmune, drug-related, endocrine, hypersensitive, infectious (viral), stress-related or traumatic origin, with secondary bacterial infections that respond to topical tetracycline; the ulcer itself responds poorly to treatment, eg oral rinses with benadryl, xylocaine and corticosteroids

Cannabinoid see Marijuana

Cannabinoid receptor see THC receptor

Cannon 'a' wave (CAW) An abnormal jugular venous pressure curve with an accentuated a wave, of sufficient intensity to cause the earlobes to 'flap', due to reduced right ventricular compliance, tricuspid stenosis or an arrhythmia in which the atrium contracts against a closed or stenosed tricuspid valve; a less 'explosive' but still prominent 'a' wave may by associated with pulmonary hypertension; CAWs may be regular, as are atrioventricular junctional rhythms, where a CAW occurs every second beat in a 2:1 block, or irregular, which are more common and may occur in complete heart blocks without atrial fibrillation, ventricular tachycardia and atrioventricular dissociation

Cannonball metastases One or several large, well-circumscribed metastatic nodules within the lungs, classically seen in renal cell carcinoma, also seen in choriocarcinoma

Canoe paddle rib A rib deformity described in Hurler and Hunter types of mucopolysaccharidoses, with a spatula-like narrowing at the vertebral origin and widening of the middle of the ribs, ending in a 'bullet-nose' broadening at the anterior end; canoe paddles also occur in craniocarpotarsal dysplasia or Freeman-Sheldon syndrome, or may refer to the distal femur in Pyle's disease

Canthaxanthin B,B-carotene-4,4'-dione A highly lipid-soluble synthetic carotenoid that in humans cannot be converted to vitamin A, used as a food coloring and added to animal feed to 'enhance' the color of chicken skin and egg yolks and the flesh of rainbow trout; it is not approved for prescription nor as an over-the-counter drug, but is marketed as an oral tablet for skin tanning under various names, is available in combination with β-carotene and has been implicated in aplastic anemia (J Am Med Assoc 1990; 264:1141)

Canyon hypothesis VIROLOGY A possible site for virus-receptor binding that is present in rhinoviruses and picornaviruses, in which the target is bound while prohibiting anti-viral antibody interaction as the narrowness of the 'canyon' renders the pathogen inaccessible to the immune system (Science 1991; 251:1456)

C'ao Gio A Vietnamese folk therapy consisting of rubbing coins over warm, oiled skin to draw out fever, appearing as darkened erythematous zones, which when seen in feverish children in the emergency room, erroneously raise the question of child abuse

Cap MOLECULAR BIOLOGY A complex methylated structure at the 5' end of mRNA and hnRNA, consisting of a terminal 7-methylguanylate nucleotide in a 5'-5' linkage to the initial mRNA molecule, possibly having a role in mRNA synthesis after translation

CAP Catabolite activator protein MOLECULAR BIOLOGY A cAMP-binding molecule responsible for positive feedback control of the lac (gene cluster in ***Escherichia coli*** required for lactose metabolism) and ara (gene cluster in ***E coli*** required for arabinose metabolism) operons, that attracts RNA polymerase, facilitating the initiation of transcription; CAP is required for the transcription of many genes; see BAD operon

CAP College of American Pathologists, see CAP Survey

CAPD Continuous ambulatory peritoneal dialysis; see Peritoneal dialysis

Capillary electrophoresis A highly-sensitive (in the picomolar range, which is 10 000-fold more sensitive than conventional electrophoresis) and efficient technique that allows separation of proteins, nucleic acids and carbohydrates

Capillary leakage syndrome A toxic effect that may occur in therapy with GM-CSF (granulocyte-macrophage colony-stimulating factor), consisting of progressive dyspnea and pericarditis, used to treat progressive metastatic solid tumors (Br J Cancer 1989; 59:142); a similar response may occur in interleukin-2 therapy, where large amounts of fluid (10-20 liters) are held hostage in peripheral tissues, accompanied by high fever, confusion and disorientation

Capital budget HOSPITAL ADMINISTRATION Any financial allocation for the purchase of fixed and durable goods; in hospitals, capital includes beds, buildings, equipment and other items that are not operating expenses

Capitation Capping HEALTH CARE FINANCING A form of payment for health care services in the US in which physician(s) are paid a fixed fee per person (ie per capita) served, regardless of how often the services might be used, in exchange for which the physician takes complete responsibility for the patients' physician services; 'Capitated' care is typical of health maintenance organizations and of some preferred provider organizations

Capping IMMUNOLOGY An energy-consuming contractile filament (actin and myosin)-mediated process occurring on the lymphocyte surface that 'strips' the cells of immunoglobulin receptors, functions as the initial signal for activation of the lymphocyte; after antigens are bound by surface, often divalent immunoglobulins, there is initial focal coalescence (patching; see figure, left), followed by migration of the cross-linked antigen-immunoglobulin complexes towards one pole, forming a 'cap' that is internalized by the B cell; an analogous phenomenon also occurs in T cells and in prolymphocytic leukemic cells; cross-linking is the mitogenic signal that triggers cell differentiation MOLECULAR BIOLOGY Addition of a methylation cap to eukaryotic mRNA; Cf Methylation

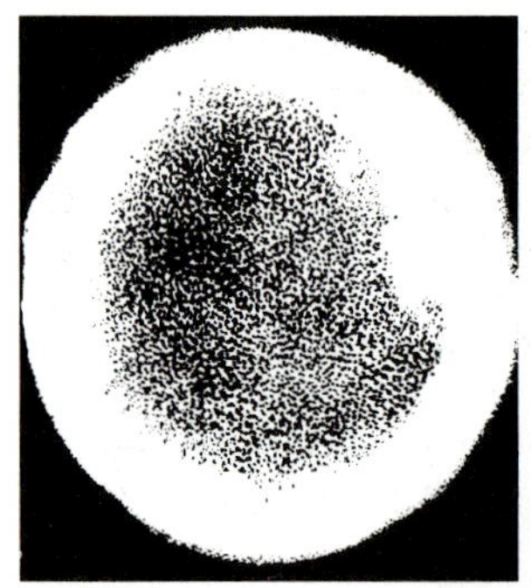
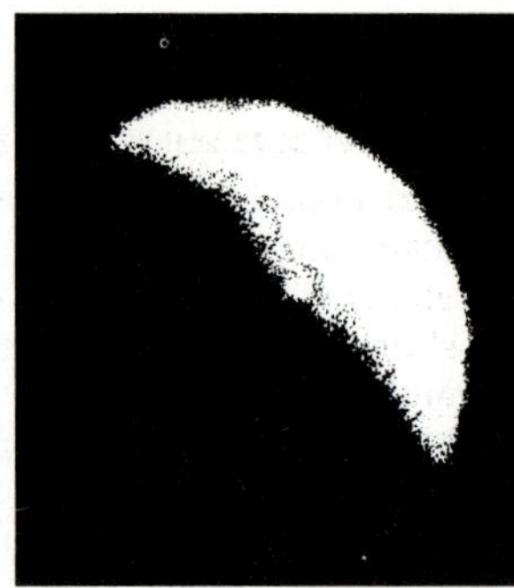

Capping

CAPS Coronary arrhythmia pilot study (Am J Cardiol 1988; 61:704)

Capsaicin A chemical derived from hot peppers that may be used to treat painful dysesthesias of herpes and diabetes; topical capsaicin triggers release of the neuropeptide substance P from the type C nociceptive fibers, opens the calcium and sodium channels causing the initial pain associated with 'hot' foods; substance P is not replenished (due to a combination of early sodium channel inactivation and later calcium buildup that inactivates voltage-gated channels and/or mediates degradation of neurofilaments, preventing axonal transport of substance P), thus pain sensation is reduced after the initial pain; capsaicin's effectiveness as a topical agent for painful peripheral neuropathy is unclear and requires up to a month of use before the reduction of pain occurs (J Am Med Assoc 1990; 264:13); see Spicy foods

Capsular drops RENAL PATHOLOGY Exudative glomerular lesions in end-stage diabetic glomerulosclerosis, consisting of PAS-positive focal thickenings of Bowman's capsule that 'hang' into the urinary spaces

CAP survey College of American Pathologists survey An organized program from the CAP survey that provides information on proficiency and productivity among clinical laboratories, comparing techniques and instruments, the work load performed per technician, the total number of tests performed and the cost per test; CAP's interlaboratory comparison program is the largest in the world and serves to satisfy the regulatory requirements of most accrediting agencies

Capsid VIROLOGY The protein envelope of a virus that is composed of protein subunits known as capsomers

'Captain of the ship' The legal doctrine arising from McConnel *v.* Williams (Pennsylvania, 1949) that holds a person in charge, eg a surgeon, ultimately responsible for all those under his supervision or command, regardless of whether the 'captain' is directly responsible for an alleged error or act of negligence; see also 'Borrowed servant', Respondeat superior

Caput medusae see Medusa head

Cap Z protein PHYSIOLOGY A heterodimeric protein located in the Z line of skeletal muscle, composed of 2 subunits (32 kD and 36 kD) that selectively binds to the '+' ends of actin filaments, stabilizing them and preventing depolymerization

Carapace pattern NEUROLOGY A pattern of sensory loss affecting the very short nerves of the upper body (trunk and thorax)

Carcinogenesis see Cancerization

Carcinoid syndrome A symptom complex caused by carcinoids arising from the enterochromaffin system, most concentrated in midgut that release vasoactive substances, including bradykinin, histamine, prostaglandin, substance P and serotonin; serotonin and its metabolite, 5-HIAA, cause most of a carcinoid's symptoms, which usually arise in metastases, often from a primary ileal carcinoid metastatic to the liver Clinical Episodic cutaneous flushing beginning on the face, spreading to the trunk, later becoming telangiectatic; these symptoms are precipitated by alcohol, food, stress or liver palpation; other findings include diarrhea or obstructive symptoms, bronchospasms, pleural, peritoneal, retroperitoneal and endocardial fibrosis, the last involving the right valves and right ventricular wall, potentially evoking cardiac failure Laboratory 5-HIAA in urine as high as 1000 mg/24 hours (normal, 2-8 mg/24hours)

Carcinoma A malignancy of epithelial and occasionally neuroepithelial origin, a term that is often incorrectly equated to the more encompassing term 'cancer', which is used by the lay public for malignancy; carcinomas are subdivided according to the type of tissue in which they arise, eg glands, ergo adeno(-carcinoma), squamous epithelium, ergo squamous cell carcinoma and renal and bladder epithelium, eg transitional cell carcinoma; Cf Cancer

Carcinoma-associated antigens Antigenic alterations that result from the direct or indirect effects of certain malignancies on native antigens, transforming the epitopes to a form that is no longer recognized as self, eg a) T antigen The precursor molecule of the blood group MN, enzymatically unmasked by sialidase-producing bacteria which do not occur in vivo and b) Tn antigen The result of somatic mutation at the pluripotent hematopoietic stem cell level due to the blockage of the transfer of galactose to N-acetyl-D-galactosamine Note: Most subjects have naturally occurring antibodies directed against T and Tn antigens that may be exposed in carcinomas as well as T-cell lymphomas

Carcinoma en cuirasse A markedly indurated carcinoma, involving a broad expanse of skin and subcutaneous breast tissue that is covered by papules and nodules evolving into morphea-like plaques Histopathology Exuberant desmoplasia and few tumor cells; the cuirasse pattern is usually associated with carcinoma of the breast, but may also occur with carcinoma of the stomach, prostate, lung, uterus and pancreas Cuirasse, French, Breast plates used in suits of armor during the Middle Ages

Carcinoma in situ SURGICAL PATHOLOGY A carcinoma in which all of the cytological and pathological criteria used to define malignancy have been met, but which has not yet invaded; the term carcinoma in situ (CIS) allows the pathologist to skirt the issue of appropriate treatment, since CIS may regress or may be stable for a long period of time; although the cervix was one of the first locations where CIS was recognized, most other epithelia in the human economy have CIS lesions; in sexual epithelia, the term 'intraepithelial neoplasia' (IN), the least severe of which, grade I, corresponds to the formerly popular term, mild dysplasia, which is followed by grade II IN (moderate dysplasia) and grade III IN (severe dysplasia), which is generally equated to carcinoma in situ; CIS is widely regarded as the lesion that immediately precedes microinvasive carcinoma; see Intraepithelial neoplasia, Microinvasive carcinoma; Cf Borderline tumors

Carcinomatosis A preterminal condition characterized by the presence of disseminated, fulminant extension of multiple metastatic carcinomas

Carcinosarcoma A malignancy of dual, ie epithelial and mesenchymal embryologic origin; although the term is firmly entrenched in the medical literature, the vast majority of these highly aggressive tumors are carcinomas and the cells display marked sarcoma-like spindling, thus the terms sarcomatoid carcinoma or spindle cell carcinoma are more appropriate; the epithelial nature of the cells can be confirmed by immunoperoxidase or by electron microscopy; see Spindle cell carcinoma; Cf Pseudosarcoma

Cardiac 'cirrhosis' A hepatopathy characterized by hepatocellular atrophy, centrilobular necrosis and extensive fibrosis (the end-stage is virtually identical to posthepatitis cirrhosis), caused by repeated and/or prolonged congestive heart failure with increased venous pressure and reduced hepatic blood flow

Cardiac concussion see Steering wheel injury

Cardiac 'cripple' A person who had an innocent cardiac murmur or normal physiologic variant of an electrocardiogram that is misinterpreted as indicating cardiac failure, whose physical activity is subsequently restricted and/or who receives various cardiac medications; see Innocent murmurs

'Cardiac' enzymes A group of three enzymes (figure, page 92) used to monitor suspected myocardial ischemia, including creatine phosphokinase (CPK), for which the isoenzyme CK-MB has the greatest clinical import, although β-enolase may be equally useful; the rise in CPK is followed by aspartate aminotransferase (AST, formerly glutamate-oxaloacetate transaminase) and lactate dehydrogenase (LDH); following myocardial infarction, these three enzymes rise and fall in the same order over a period of a week; see β enolase, CK-MB, Flipped pattern

Cardiac injury panel A cost-effective, abbreviated battery of parameters for evaluating patients who may have suffered an acute myocardial infarct, measuring

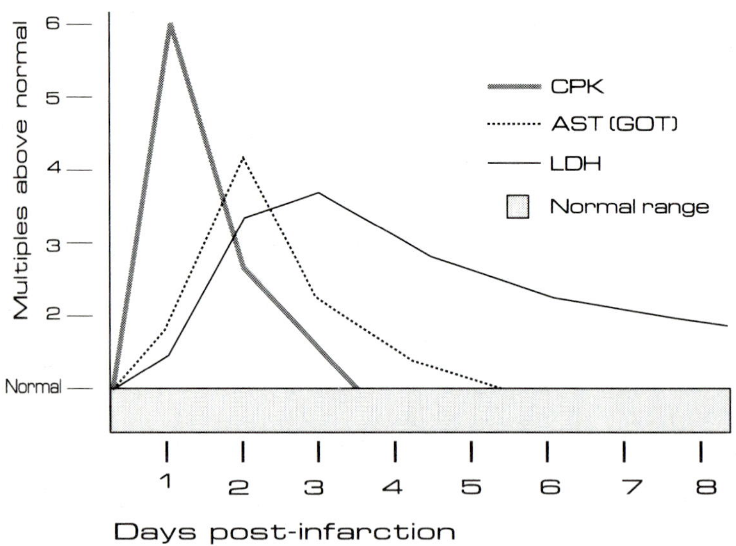

lactate dehydrogenase, creatine kinase and creatine kinase isoenzymes; see Organ panel

Cardiac risk evaluation panel A group of tests determined to be cost-effective in stratifying a subject according to his risk for suffering atherosclerosis-related morbidity that measure serum levels of cholesterol, triglycerides, HDL-cholesterol and glucose; see Organ panel

Cardiac series RADIOLOGY A group of four plain chest films (Postero-anterior, lateral, right and left anterior oblique views) obtained after a 'barium swallow', used to evaluate the relative contribution of the chambers and vascular structures to the cardiac boundaries per se

Cardiolipin Diphosphatidyl glycerol A phospholipid that comprises the major antigen component of the Wasserman reaction for syphilis; see Anticardiolipin antibodies

Cardiovocal syndrome of Ortner Hoarseness due to compression of the left laryngeal nerve between the aorta and dilated pulmonary artery, often first seen in infancy Clinical Symptoms are those of the underlying cardiac conditions including lesions of the aortic arch and congenital cardiac defects, mitral valve stenosis, coronary artery disease and hypertension

Caries A destructive disease affecting the enamel and dentine linked to infection by ***Streptococcus mutans*** and microaerophilic organisms that thrive when protected by a layer of hardened dental plaque; caries is most common in the young who have refined carbohydrate-rich diets, especially when they 'snack' excessively (as this increases the oral pH); caries affects specific older population groups, including those with diabetes mellitus, cancer or other form of immunocompromise; see Fluoridation, Periodontal disease, Plaque

Carmustine (BCNU) A member of the nitrosurea family of chemotherapeutic agents (related compounds include lomustine (CCNU) and semustine) that partially overlap the range of activity and toxicity of alkylating chemotherapeutic agents, which is of particular use in Hodgkin's disease; BCNU crosses the blood-brain barrier and is thus useful in treating both meningeal leukemia and brain tumors

L-Carnitine β-hydroxy-γ-N trimethylammonium butyrate An amino acid required for the transport of long-chain fatty acids across the mitochondrial membrane for catabolism to CO_2 or ketone bodies, acting as an acyl (fatty acid) carrier; carnitine is endogenous (synthesized in the liver and kidney) or exogenous (red meat and dairy products) in origin; carnitine deficiency may be caused by absence of carnitine palmityl transferase, or may occur in cobalamin deficiency, electron transfer flavoprotein deficiency, renal Fanconi syndrome, isovaleric acidemia, medium chain acylCoA dehydrogenase deficiency, methylmalonic and propionic acidemias and valproate therapy for seizure disorders may develop a toxicity syndrome with associated carnitine deficiency Clinical Myoglobinuria, and potentially renal failure, hypoglycemia, hypotonia, hepatomegaly, hepatic coma, congestive heart failure, neurologic changes (progressive myasthenia, lethargy, encephalopathy, coma, death), cardiomegaly, cardiac arrest, impaired growth and development

Carnosinase The enzyme that hydrolyzes carnosine to histidine and β-alanine, without which there is toxic accumulation of carnosine; carnosinase deficiency is characterized by severe psychomotor retardation, accompanied by myotonic and grand mal seizures Treatment Low-protein diet

Carnosine A dipeptide composed of β-alanine and histidine that is concentrated in skeletal muscle with unknown function that may act as a buffer, stabilizing the pH of anaerobically contracting muscles

Carotid endarterectomy A surgical technique for relieving carotid artery stenosis with the purpose of reducing the morbidity and mortality of cerebral ischemia; in the USA, 500 000 new strokes occur annually, with a total of 1.8 million long-term survivors, 60% of whom require assistance; 40% of first stroke victims remain permanently dependent; carotid endarterectomy is a procedure of scientific and cognitive uncertainty as to its ultimate benefit (Mayo Clin Proc 1990; 65:625, 756ed)

Carpal tunnel An anatomic region on the volar surface of the wrist, where the carpal bones form a concavity bridged by the flexor retinaculum

Carpal tunnel syndrome A clinical complex with median nerve neurapraxia, most common in post-menopausal women, either as a chronic idiopathic flexor tenosynovitis or as part of systemic conditions, eg acromegaly, amyloidosis, diabetes mellitus, granulomatous disease, hypothyroidism, mucopolysaccharidosis type I-S, myxedema, obesity, pregnancy, or local processes (ganglia, bone dislocations, lipoma,exuberant callus formation in wrist fractures, eg Colles or Smith fractures, gout, pseudogout and rheumatoid arthritis causing flexor tenosynovitis Clinical Most symptomatic at night, with hypesthesia of the median nerve region, thenar muscle atrophy, attenuation of response by nerve conduction and EMG studies; the median nerve is a 'mixed' nerve and sensory loss precedes motor dysfunction, affecting sensation in the palmar aspect of the radial 3 1/2 fingers Differential diagnosis Proximal sites of nerve entrapment, eg Pancoast tumor, pronator teres syndrome Treatment, early Steroid injection Treatment, late Longitudinal section of the epineurium in the face of thenar atrophy (Mayo Clin Proc 1989; 64:829rv)

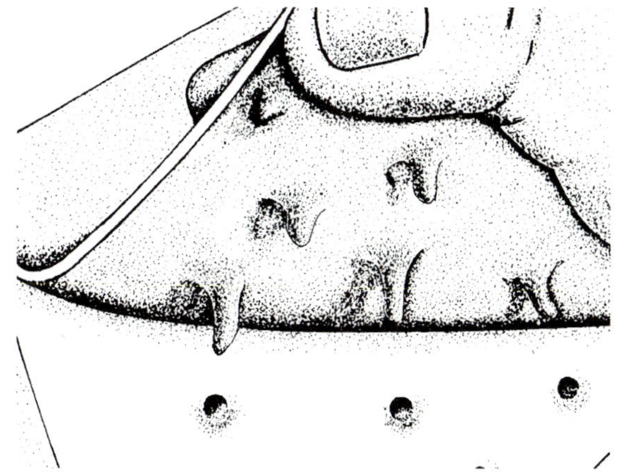

Carpet tack appearance

Carpet tack appearance DERMA-TOLOGY A descriptor for the multiple small keratin plugs (corresponding to the follicular openings) attached to the underside of scales removed from skin affected by discoid lupus erythematosus, or pemphigus foliaceus (Br J Dermatol 1987; 116:127)

Carrot cells A colloquial term for the elongated angulated cells seen in granulosa cell tumors of the ovary, a 'soft' criterion differentiating these tumors from the far less common ovarian lymphoma

CAR syndrome Cancer-associated retinopathy A paraneoplastic complex due to autoantibodies reactive against retinal components, in particular, a 23 kD protein, the CAR antigen, with loss of visual acuity due to retinal nerve demyelinization, described in pulmonary small cell carcinoma (N Engl J Med 1989; 321:1589)

Cartilage-hair hypoplasia syndrome Autosomal recessive short-limbed dwarfism, common in the Amish, an ethnic group of German descent located in Pennsylvania Clinical Bone dysplasia, bradycarpia, redundant skin, sparse hair, defective pigment, malabsorption and death by age 20 Immune defects Neutropenia with defective T cell-mediated immunity, potentially fatal vaccinia, progressive vaccine-related poliomyelitis, defective antibody production and severe combined immunodeficiency, related to defective adenosine deaminase activity Treatment Antibiotics, leukocyte interferon, bone marrow transplantation; see Adenosine deaminase deficiency

Cartoon Any schematic, usually in color, representation of a biological process or molecule, presented either in a journal or in a lecture; Cf 'Nettergram' Note: Cartoon is traditionally defined in the US as either a panel in a comic strip, or a satirical drawing with a caption commenting on public or political matters or an animated 'short' film with such characters as Elmer Fudd, Popeye and Tom and Jerry

Cartwheel pattern A pattern that has a vague roundness, from which short curved radiations appear to emanate Cartwheel nucleus Peripheral chromatin clumping, characteristic of plasma cell nuclei CARTWHEEL PATTERN 'Whorled' cellular arrangement described in neurogenic tumors, less commonly in astroblastomas Note: The cartwheel pattern is virtually identical to the 'pinwheel' and 'storiform' patterns; separation of tumors based on these highly subjective criteria is academically unsatisfactory, see Pinwheel pattern, Storiform pattern CARTWHEEL PIGMENTATION Ocular fundus A non-specific 'whorling' of pigment in the fundus, seen in tyrosinase positive albinism, yellow-mutant albinism, Chediak-Higashi syndrome and Hermansky-Pudlak syndromes

Cascades Molecular systems capable of self-propagation or amplification; once a cascade is initiated, it may continue to be amplified through positive feedback loops and pathways until it is downregulated by local mechanisms often in the form of proteolytic enzymes; cascades in humans include the coagulation, complement, kinase and electron transport (mediated within the mitochondria via cytochrome oxidases) cascades

Case-control study EPIDEMIOLOGY A study that begins with a disease and searches for past differences in exposure (or other characteristics) between groups of affected and non-affected individuals; this retrospective study method is useful when few clues exist as to causation or when the evidence implicating a particular agent is strong but the actual number of patients is too small to allow a prospective study; see Epidemiology

Case-fatality ratio EPIDEMIOLOGY A value calculated as 100 cases of a disease 'X', divided by the number of persons with the disease who died in a given period of time; the resulting ratio is equal to the rate of a disease's occurrance; see Cause-fatality ratio

Case mix The characteristics of a health care facility's patient population for a given period of time, classified by disease, diagnostic or therapeutic procedures performed, method of payment, duration of hospitalization, intensity and type of services provided; in the USA, a hospital's case mix is based on the diagnosis-related groups, see DRGs

Case-mix index (CMI) HEALTH CARE REIMBURSEMENT A hospital's CMI is the average of the relative weights assigned to its patients' diagnosis-related groups and is a measure of the complexity of illness in a hospital's discharged patients; hospital populations with more complex illnesses have higher case mixes and thus receive higher Medicare reimbursement; see 'Creep', DRGs and 'Optimization'

Caseous debris Caseation Cheesy, dry yellow-white grumous material, resulting from combined coagulation and liquefactive necrosis, classically associated with tuberculosis, but also seen in histoplasmosis Note: The

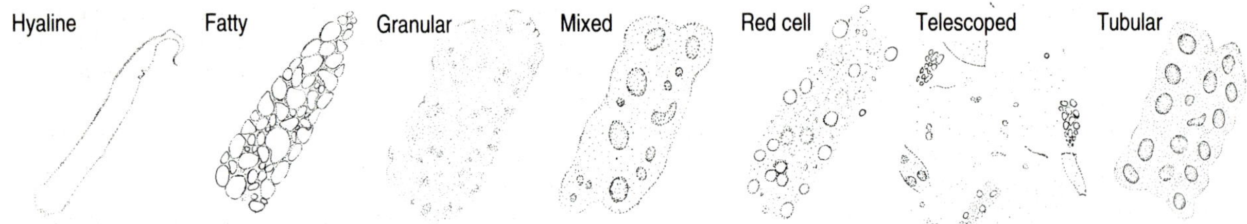

keratinaceous debris within epidermal inclusion cysts has a similar consistency

Cassette A segment of eukaryotic DNA that can be substituted for by another sequence by transposition; the cassette model serves to explain the expression of various mating types of primitive organisms

Cassette mutagenesis MOLECULAR BIOLOGY A technique where point mutations are induced in oligonucleotide segments of DNA or tRNA that are then analyzed for loss or gain of functional properties (generally with repressor or enhancer proteins) to determine 'allowable' substitutions in the nucleotide structure Note: Three-dimensional analysis (Science 1988; 241:53) of molecular surfaces is crucial for understanding biological interactions; the protein sequence bears the information needed to determine its three-dimensional structure

CAST Cardiac arrhythmia suppression trial A long-term multicenter study which examined whether suppression of asymptomatic or mildly symptomatic post-myocardial infarction ventricular ectopia and arrhythmia reduces the incidence of sudden death; preliminary results indicate that the class I-C antiarrhythmic agents, encainide and flecainide actually increase post-myocardial infarction mortality (N Engl J Med 1989; 321:406)

Casts Translucent proteinaceous 'castings' of the renal tubules seen in the urine (figure), which are markedly increased in renal disease, the nature of which are crude indicators of the type of renal disease; the protein matrix of all casts is composed of albumin, small (< 50 kD) globulins and glycoprotein secreted by Henle's ascending loop and the distal tubule together forming Tamm-Horsfall protein, uromodulin; casts are classified according to type of a) Matrix, eg hyaline or waxy b) Inclusions, eg crystals, fat, granules, hemosiderin and melanin c) Pigments, eg bilirubin, drugs, hemoglobin, myoglobin and d) Cells, eg bacteria, red cells, leukocytes, tubular epithelial cells; in general, red cell casts are associated with glomerular injury, white cell casts with parenchymal injury and broad casts with dilated collecting ducts, as occurs in chronic pyelonephritis

Cast syndrome see Superior mesenteric artery syndrome

CAT 1) Children's apperception test; see Psychologic testing 2) Chloramphenicol acetyl transferase, a 'reporter' gene 3) Cholesterol acyl transferase 4) Computerized axial tomography 5) ***Felis catus*** A mammal of medical interest that is a) A model for certain human diseases, eg dermatosparasix, a defect in the conversion of type I procollagen to collagen, or mannosidosis, a condition affecting the shorthair cat and Niemann-Pick, type I, which affects Siamese cats b) A vector for i) Parasites, eg ***Ancylostoma braziliense, A caninum, Brugia pahangi*, Clonorchis sinensis, Cryptosporidium*** species, ***Dipylidium caninum, Dracunculiasis medinensis*, Echinococcus vogeli, E multilocularis, Gnathostoma spinigerum, Isospora belli, Leptospira*** species, ***Opistorchis felineus, Sarcoptes scabiei, Toxoplasma gondii, Trypanosoma cruzi*, Wuchereria bancrofti***) Bacteria, eg ***Pasteurella multocida, Yersinia pestis, Campylobacter jejuni, Francisella tularensis*** and iii) Fungi, eg ***Microsporum canis, Sporothrix schenckii***; see Cat scratch disease

*Parasites that have part of their life cycle in humans

Catalytic antibody A biologically selective enzyme in which catalytic activity is introduced into the highly selective binding site of a monoclonal antibody, allowing enzymatic catalysis of pre-determined specificity (Science 1988; 240:427); the specificity is achieved by site-directed mutagenesis (ie substitution of an amino acid into a combining site thereby introducing a catalytic residue, Science 1989; 245:1104); other strategies for producing specific catalysts include genetic modification of active enzyme sites and chemical modification of biological or synthetic receptors bearing catalytic groups; see Abzymes

Catalytic motif One of a family of oligopeptides, eg Asp-His-Ser and Asp-His-Zn that correspond to specific catalytic sites in an enzyme, which can be studied by site-directed mutagenesis to probe the chemical functionof the amino acid residues or by transplanting the catalytic motifs into antibody combining sites (Nature 1990; 348:589c)

Catalytic RNA An RNA molecule that can act as its own enzyme, ie a 'ribozyme', cutting out introns, splicing and assembling itself without the aid of protein enzymes; the discovery of this unexpected mechanism of RNA action netted its discoverers (T Cech, U of Colorado and S Altman, Yale) the 1989 Nobel prize in Chemistry (Science 1989; 246:325)

Catastrophic benefits HEALTH CARE INDUSTRY The second tier of health insurance or a health care plan, where the basic (usually non-hospitalization) medical services form a first tier of coverage; once the benefits have been exhausted from the first tier, coverage is provided under the catastrophic portion of the policy or plan, where 'deductible' fees must be paid and co-payment requirements met; see Wrap-around policy

Catastrophic health insurance A health insurance plan proposed by US Congressman Pepper that would include all the coverage provided in the Pepper Commission plan (see there) as well as providing long-term care and medical coverage for all US citizens who are currently uninsured; while the plan is noble, the cost would be very high

Catastrophic illness Any morbid condition that results in health care costs exceeding a person's income and/or compromising his financial independence, reducing him to subsistence or near-poverty levels; such illnesses are usually life-threatening and may leave significant residual disability, eg AIDS, major burns, trauma with residual paralysis or coma and preterminal malignancy

Cat-bite fever An infection by ***Pasteurella multocida***, an oral saprobe of felines, forming an abscess at the inoculation site, potentially causing focal arthralgia (other complications are rare); Cf Cat scratch disease

CAT box see CACA box

Catchment area HEALTH CARE INDUSTRY A region served by a health care facility or health care plan that is delineated by population distribution, geographic boundaries or transportation patterns Note: A facility's catchment demographics is modified by whether it provides secondary (in which case the traditional boundary definitions are valid) or tertiary care where referral patterns often define the catchment area

Cat-cry disease see Cri du chat

Category X drug CLINICAL PHARMACOLOGY A therapeutic agent that has a confirmed teratogenic effect that is contraindicated for use during pregnancy, eg vitamin A congeners used for severe recalcitrant acne, which causes a characteristic clinical complex in neonates; see Retinoic acid embryopathy

Caterpillar cell A descriptor for a cell with an elongated vesicular nucleus, central wavy chromatin and finger-like projections to the nuclear membrane, a morphological variant of the Anitschkow cardiac histiocyte, 'owl eye' cell, aggregates of which are known as Aschoff nodules

Caterpillar dermatitis An allergic reaction evoked by contact with the urticariogenic hairs of the larvae of the brown-tail, flannel, Io or tussock moths

Caterpillar hump artery A fanciful descriptor for a variant of the right hepatic artery that may be mistaken surgically for the cystic artery

Cat eye syndrome Anal atresia-coloboma of iris syndrome An autosomal dominant condition characterized by vertical iris coloboma (hence, 'cat eye'), microphthalmia, pale optic discs, ocular hypertelorism, downward slanting of palpebral fissures, preauricular fistula, anal atresia, umbilical hernia, mental retardation and variable cardiac and renal defects; most cases have one or more extra copies of chromosome fragment 22q11

Cathartic colon A colon affected by long-term abuse of cathartics and laxatives **Clinical** Intractable diarrhea with hypokalemia, protein-losing enteropathy, cachexia, hypoγglobulinemia, finger-clubbing and potentially increased constipation, resulting in a vicious cycle of increased use of purgatives by the patient **Pathology** Loss of haustra, a mucosa likened to shark skin (as well as snake, lizard and toad skin) and melanosis coli if the agent is of the anthracene group, eg cascara, senna **Radiology** Barium studies may be normal or have complete loss of haustral markings, or mimic ulcerative colitis **Histopathology** Flattening of the mucosa without epithelial destruction, chronic inflammation and fatty infiltration of the submucosa, hypertrophy of the muscularis mucosa, occasionally, degeneration of Auerbach's plexus and lipofuscin deposits

Cathepsin(s) A group of lysosomal proteinases or endopeptidases that function optimally at an acidic pH, stored within the azurophilic granules of neutrophils; cathepsin B functions at an acidic pH and degrades matrix glycoproteins; cathepsin D functions at acidic pH and is a heterodimeric 34 kD and 14 kD estrogen-induced lysosomal protease produced in breast tissue; a 52 kD cathepsin D precursor molecule is increased in hormone-dependent breast carcinoma, the serum levels of which are predictive of early recurrence and death in node-negative cases; high levels have an increased risk of 2.6 for recurrence and a relative risk of 3.9 for death (N Engl J Med 1990; 322:297); Cf Metastasis

Cathode ray tube see Video display terminal

Cat scratch disease A self-limited regional lymphadenitis of children and adolescents, caused by close contact with or being scratched by household pets; 95% are due to cats, 5% to dogs **Clinical** Erythematous papules at the inoculation sites including the hands and forearms, anorexia, malaise, fever, parotid swelling, maculopapular rashes, regional or generalized lymphadenopathy, splenomegaly, encephalopathy; the agent was identified at the Armed Forces Institute of Pathology (Science 1983; 221:1403) as a small, pleomorphic gram-negative bacillus and later cultured (J Am Med Assoc 1988; 259:1347) in a biphasic (broth then agar) Brain-Heart infusion medium at 30-32°C **Histopathology** Lymphoid hyperplasia, granuloma and abscess formation **Diagnosis** History, Skin-test **Treatment** Gentamycin, ciprofloxacin (J Am Med Assoc 1991; 265:1563); Cf Cat bite fever

Cat's elbow see Katzenellenbogen

Cat's-eye reflex Leukocoria A white reflection seen through the pupil in a) Retinoblastoma (due to the tumoral deformity of the fundus) b) End-stage retrolental fibroplasia (caused by a flattened to nodular scarred white retrolental membrane that is nonreactive to light; salvage of vision in either is rare with a persistent anterior persistent hyperplastic primary vitreous humor, due to non-involution of the fetal hyaloid artery and accompanying fibrovascular tissue; leukocoria also occurs in visceral larva migrans due to ***Toxocara*** species

CAT-signal bioassay VIROLOGY An assay in which an indicator cell contains long terminal repeats (LTR) of a retrovirus, eg HIV-1, linked to chloramphenicol acetyltransferase (CAT); when HIV-1 is added, CAT increases in the medium (Science 1988; 239:184)

Cat's paw sign A fanciful term for the radiocontrast findings of intramural hemorrhage of the small intestine, in which there is short length of splaying in the radiocontrast column; see Stacked coin sign; Cf Coiled spring

Cauliflower ear An external ear deformity caused by inadequate treatment, ie through-and-through stitches, of an otohematoma, commonly due to contact sport-related trauma in adolescents or falls in the elderly and children, which occurs as the natural evolution of hematomas in this site is towards granulation tissue and exuberant fibrosis; primary cauliflower ear occurs in polychondritis

Cauliflower lesion A descriptor for any broad-based pedunculated polypoid mass that freely grows into a lumen or hollow viscus, including: Sclerosing stromal tumor of the uterus, colonic adenocarcinoma, papillary transitional cell carcinoma of the urinary bladder, villous adenoma of the colon

Cause-facility rate EPIDEMIOLOGY The number of deaths due to a disease per unit of time (usually one year) divided by either 1000 or 10 000 people with the disease; see Case-fatality rate

Cause of death FORENSIC MEDICINE **PROXIMATE CAUSE OF DEATH** The most important, immediate, direct or actual cause, or last event or act that occurred prior to the chain of events leading to death **IMMEDIATE CAUSE OF DEATH** The concluding or final event that actually produces death; see Death

Cavalry fracture A crushing plantar-flexion fracture of the tarso-metatarsal joint that occurs when a violent force is applied to the heel along the axis of the foot when the toe is fixed; such fractures were common in the battlefield when a cavalryman was thrown from and then had his foot pinned under his fallen horse; tarsometatarsal fractures are now more commonly associated with automobiles, stepladders or in misguided steps (J of Bone and Joint Surgery 1971; 53B:474)

Cave disease A trivial name for pulmonary histoplasmosis that affects explorers of bat-infested caves, as bat dung is an ideal growth medium for ***Histoplasma capsulatum***

'Cayenne pepper' lesion A descriptor for the hyperpigmented and petechial lesions of the lower legs, arms and trunk, due to idiopathic capillaritis, seen in Schamberg's disease (pigmented purpuric dermatitis) or secondary to drug reactions

CBC Complete blood count LABORATORY MEDICINE The automated analysis of certain parameters of the cells in the circulation, often performed by a Coulter counter; the CBC includes a count of the red cells, white cells and platelets, hemoglobin, hematocrit, mean corpuscular hematocrit, hemoglobin and volume in the red cells and a differential count of white cells, dividing them into lymphocytes, monocytes, granulocytes, basophils and eosinophils

CCAAT Box MOLECULAR BIOLOGY One of the cis-regulatory elements that mediates transcription; the CCAAT and GGGCG ('promoter-proximal') sequences are located 60-120 nucleotides upstream from the transcription start site and necessary for optimal promoter activity; a family of proteins bind to the CCAAT and the SP1 protein binds to the GGGCG (Science 1988; 241:582)

C cells Neuroectodermal calcitonin-secreting cells that are derived from the APUD system, located laterally in the thyroid; in submammalian beasts, C-cells (figure) are in a separate organ, the ultimobranchial body; see Calcitonin

CCHF see Crimean-Congo hemorrhagic fever

CCK Cholecystokinin

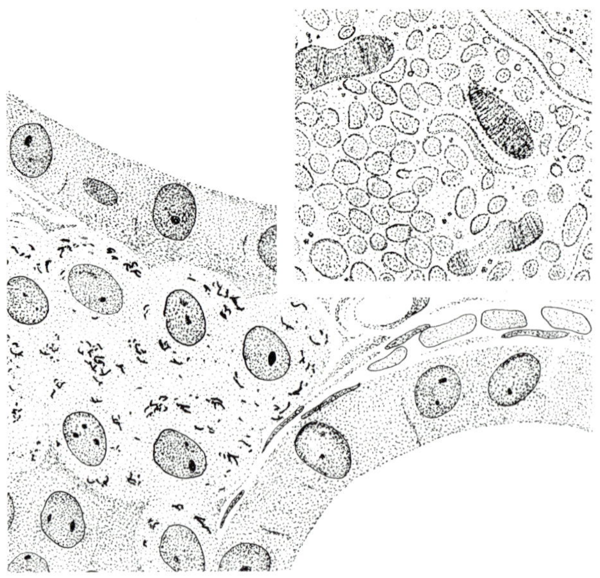

C cells

CCNU Cyclonexyl-chloroethyl-nitrosourea A highly toxic chemotherapeutic agent that is used in adjunctive therapy of high-grade astrocytomas; see Nitrogen mustards

CD Cluster of differentiation A system of nomenclature of the surface antigens of human leukocytes, characterized by monoclonal antibodies, allowing leukocytes and other hematopoietic cells to be categorized the expression on the cell surface of one or more to be classified according to lineage, where most cells express more than one surface antigen Note: the 'w' (workshop) designation that follows some CDs indicates an incompletely characterized antigen

CD1 A family of major histocompatibility complex class I-like molecules expressed on the surface of immature thymocytes, Langerhans cells and certain B cells; CD1 is a ligand for T cell subpopulation, is present in the intestinal epithelium adjacent to the gut-associated lymphoid tissue (GALT) and may be involved in epithelial immunity (Science 1990; 250:679)

CD2 T11 A 50 kD molecule involved in cell adhesion, which is the receptor that binds to the leukocyte function associated antigen-3 (LFA-3) or CD58; CD2 is a 'pan-T' cell marker, ie is present on most T lymphocytes and corresponds to the E-rosette receptor

CD3 T3, OKT3 A 'pan-T' cell antigen, ie an antigen present on virtually all T cells, consisting of multiple 16 to 28 kD in length polypeptide chains, designated gamma sigma, epsilon and eta, which are closely associated with each other and the T cell receptor (CD4); most antibodies against the CD3 antigen are directed against the 20 kD epsilon chain; see Pan-T cell markers

CD4 A surface glycoprotein that participates in adhesion of T cells to target cells and is involved in thymic maturation and transmission of intracellular signals during T cell activation by the class II major histocompatibility complex; CD4 has inducer or helper activity for T cell, B cell and macrophage interactions and evokes T cell proliferation in response to soluble antigens or autologous non-T cells, providing appropriate signals for B cell proliferation and differentiation into immunoglobulin-secreting cells; CD4 is also a high-affinity receptor for HIV-1's gp120, binding at amino acid residues 42 to 55 of the NH_2 terminal domain, which has an immunoglobulin-like fold similar to the complementarity-determining region of the kappa light chain; CD4 also binds immunoglobulins independently of the Fc receptor (Science 1990; 248:1639), and is an accessory to the T cell receptor and a receptor for p56lck, a cellular tyrosine kinase receptor with immunoglobulin-like domains (Nature 1990; 348:411, 419)

CD4/CD8 ratio The ratio of circulating T lymphocytes with 'helper cell' determinants (CD4 antigen) on the cell surface to T lymphocytes with 'suppressor cell' determinants (CD8 antigen); the partition between CD4 and CD8 cell lines is regarded as irreversible, although a small percentage of circulating CD3 cells coexpress both CD4 and CD8 molecules); the explanation for this coexpression is that in most CD8 T cells the CD4 genes are methylated and therefore 'terminally' repressed, while in the CD4 and CD8 coexpressing cells, the CD4 genes are not methylated and CD4 expression is inducible by interleukin-4 (Nature 1991; 349:533)

CD4 cell A circulating T lymphocyte with a 'helper' phenotype; in AIDS patients, the levels of CD4+ cells is a crude indicator of immune status and susceptibility to certain AIDS-related conditions, and these patients may suffer Kaposi sarcoma as the CD4+ cells fall below 0.3 x 10^9/L (US: 300/mm^3), non-Hodgkin's lymphoma below 0.15 x 10^9/L (US: 150/mm^3), *Pneumocystis carinii* below 0.1 x 10^9/L (US: 100/mm^3) and MAIS (*Mycobacterium avium-intercellulare*) below 0.05 x 10^9/L (US: 50/mm^3)(N Engl J Med 1991; 324:1332)

CD4 immunoadhesin A molecule formed by fusing CD4 (the receptor for HIV) with an immunoglobulin that both binds gp120 and blocks HIV; this synthetic molecule has therapeutic potential as it mediates ADCC towards HIV-infected but not uninfected cells and is easily transported across the primate placenta (Nature 1990; 344:667)

CD4 T cells see Helper T cells

CD4(178)-PE40 A recombinant protein that consists of the HIV envelope glycoprotein-binding region of CD4 linked to the translocation and ADP-ribosylation domains of *Pseudomonas aeruginosa* exotoxin A; this hybrid toxin ('magic bullet') selectively binds to and destroys HIV-1-infected human T cells (in vitro) after productive infection of T cells has occurred, an event signaled by the presence of viral gp120 at the cell surface, and thus has potential currency as an HIV-virostatic agent (Proc Natl Acad Sci 1990; 87:8889; J Am Med Assoc 1990; 263:345)

CD5 T1 antigen A 67 kD glycoprotein with receptor activity that is present on most T cells and on a subpopulation of B cells, as well as in chronic lymphocytic leukemia, which binds to the B-cell surface protein CD72/Lyb-2 (Nature 1991; 351:662)

CD6 T12 antigen A 100 kD antigen present on most T cells, similar in distribution to CD3

CD7 A 40 kD antigen present on most T cells, which may correspond to the Fc receptor for IgM

CD8 T8 antigen A 33 kD heterodimeric protein that binds to class I MHC antigens on antigen-presenting cells; CD8 is physically associated with a p56 tyrosine kinase that phosphorylates adjacent proteins and is a marker for T cells with suppressor and cytotoxic activity; see Cytotoxic T cells

CD8 cells T lymphocytes with a CD8 antigen on the cell surface, which are suppressive, lack inducer functions and are responsible for suppressing mitogen-induced and antigen-specific antibody production, requiring CD4 cooperation for this activity

CD9 A 24 kD protein present on pre-B cells, monocytes, granulocytes and platelets, which has protein kinase activity

CD10/Neutral endopeptidase 24.11 cALLA (common acute lymphoblastic leukemia antigen) A zinc metalloproteinase expressed in acute lymphoblastic leukemia, normal lymphoid precursors, neutrophils and other cells; CD10/NEP mediates the enkephalin-mediated inflammatory response (Nature 1990; 347:394)

CD11 A group of three different α chains CD11a (180 kD), CD11b (170 kD) and CD11c (150 kD) leukocyte adhesive antigens (LFA/Mac-1) that are associated with an invariant 95 kD β–glycoprotein (CD18); this group, the CD11/CD18 family (Leu-CAM integrin family) of leukocyte adhesive glycoproteins are present on neutrophils and monocytes, eg Mo1 (CR3:iC3b), LeuM5 (p150,95) and LFA-1; CD11 requires the associated CD18 β chain, without which neutrophils fail to migrate to sites of infections, and cannot adhere in vitro to endothelial cell monolayers; see CD18, Leukocyte adhesion deficiency

CD13 Aminopeptidase-N A 150 kD glycoprotein present on monocytes, granulocytes, some macrophages and connective tissue

CD14 My23 A 55 kD glycoprotein expressed by monocytes and macrophages that is a cell surface receptor, which when it binds its ligand, lipopolysaccharide binding protein-soluble lipopolysaccharide (LBP-LPS), releases tumor necrosis factor (Science 1991; 252:1321)

CD15 LeuM1 Hapten X A carbohydrate antigen present in the secondary granules of granulocytic leukocytes, which is present on Reed-Sternberg and Hodgkin cells; see CD30

CD16 Low-affinity Fc receptor A receptor that is expressed in a variety of forms on natural killer (NK) cells, granulocytes and macrophages, which participates in antibody-dependent cell cytotoxicity

CD18 A 95 kD glycoprotein β chain that is non-covalently linked to specific α chains of the CD11 family of molecules; a genetic defect in the CD18 gene results in Leukocyte adhesion deficiency syndrome, see there

CD19 A 95kD transmembrane polypeptide with two immunoglobulin domains, which is expressed on B cells from earliest pre-B cells to plasma cells

CD20 A 35 kD transmembrane ion channel, the gene for which is located on chromosome 11q12-13, expressed on B cells late in ontogeny

CD21 A 140 kD protein encoded by chromosome 1q32 that is a receptor for C3d component of complement and Epstein-Barr virus, which is expressed in early B cells and dendritic reticulum cells

CD22 A 130 kD protein with five extracellular immunoglobulin-like domains that has significant sequence homology with neural cell adhesion molecule (N-CAM), which is expressed in the cytoplasm of early B cells and on the cell surface of mature B cells with surface immunoglobulins

CD23 Low-affinity IgE receptor A 45-50 kD receptor for B cell growth factor, which is expressed in increased amounts on B cells that have been stimulated with interleukin-4

CD24 A 42 kD glycoprotein present on B cells and granulocytes, an expression that is lost following activation; CD24 is expressed on the surface of many B cell leukemias and lymphomas

CD25 Tac antigen A 55 kD glycoprotein that is the α chain of the interleukin-2 receptor, which complexes to the β chain, both of which are encoded on chromosome 10, and is expressed on activated B and T cells and activated macrophages

CD28 A 44 kD glycoprotein expressed as a homodimer on the surface of most T cells; CD28 is the initial point in a signal transduction cascade, which when stimulated, increases IL-2 enhancer activity with secretion of IL-2 as well as tumor necrosis factor-α, granulocyte-macrophage colony-stimulating factor (GM-CSF), interferon-γ and lymphotoxin (Science 1991; 251:313)

CD30 Ki-1 antigen A 105 kD glycoprotein that is present on activated T cells, B cells, embryonal carcinoma cells and Reed-Sternberg cells and anaplastic large cell lymphoma (Histopathology 1990; 16:409); see CD31

CD31 Ki-1 antigen A 140 kD glycoprotein that is present in granulocytes, monocytes, platelets and endothelial cells; see CD30

CD33 A 67 kD transmembrane glycoprotein present on myeloid cells, monocytes and myeloid leukemias

CD34 A 105-120 kD transmembrane glycoprotein expressed on immature hematopoietic cells and endothelial cells

CD35 CR1, Complement C3b receptor A 160-220 kD group of antigens expressed on erythrocytes, B cells, monocytes, granulocytes, some natural killer cells and dendritic cells

CD36 gpIIIb, gpIV A 90 kD membrane glycoprotein that acts as the receptor for thrombospondin and collagen, as well as for *Plasmodium falciparum*; CD36 is expressed on monocytes, platelets, endothelial cells and weakly on B cells

CD37 A 40-45 kD glycoprotein expressed on mature B cells

CD38 A 45 kD antigen present on the surface of progenitor B cells, T cells and plasma cells

CD39 An 80 kD antigen present on the surface of B cells, T cells and macrophages, but not on pre-B cells or plasma cells

CD40 A 45-50-kD transmembrane glycoprotein that is expressed on B cells, epithelial cells and some carcinoma cell lines; cross-linking of CD40 to a monoclonal anti-CD40 antibody in the presence of IL-4 results in the production of a long-lived human B cell line, previously achieved only when the B cells are transfected with the Epstein-Barr virus (Science 1991; 251:70)

CD41 Platelet glycoprotein IIb/IIIa A glycoprotein that is a Ca^{++}-dependent complex between the 110 kD gpIIIa or CD61 antigen and the heterodimeric 135 kD gpIIb; CD41 is the receptor for fibrinogen, von Willebrand factor, collagen and fibronectin, which is present on the surface of platelets and megakaryocytes and absent in Glanzmann's thrombasthenia syndrome

CD42 A surface antigen on platelets and megakaryocytes that is divided into CD42a or glycoprotein IX, a 23 kD antigen and CD42b or glycoprotein Ib, a 170 kD heterodimeric antigen, either of which may be reduced or absent in Bernard-Soulier disease

CD44 A widely distributed surface receptor for hyaluronic acid (Cell 1990; 61:1303), which binds to cell adhesion glycoproteins

CD45 Leukocyte common antigen T-200 A transmembrane glycoprotein receptor expressed on most hematopoietic cells which is structurally similar to tyrosine phosphatase and has phosphotyrosine phosphatase activity; T lymphocytes express various forms of the CD45 antigen, resulting from the use of different CD45 exons during transcription, eg the CD45R+ T cell subset is involved in graft-versus-host reactions and interleukin-2 activity, which may interconvert into the CD45RO+ T cell subset that responds to recall antigens (Nature 1990; 348:163); CD45 may also regulate signal transduction by modulating the phosphorylation state of B cell antigen receptors (Science 1991; 252:1839)

CDw52 see CAMPATH-1 antigen

CD56 Natural killer cell

CD61 Platelet glycoprotein IIIa see CD41

CD62 GMP140 PADGEM A member of the recently designated selectin family of cell adhesion molecules, which is a granule-associated glycoprotein present in platelets and endothelial cells that is brought to the cell surface when these cells are stimulated by thrombogenic agents, allowing these cells to bind neutrophils and monocytes at the site of tissue injury (Nature 1991; 349:196n&v)

CD71 Transferrin receptor

CD72/Lyt-2 A cell surface protein that is only expressed on B cells which serves as a ligand for CD5 receptor; see CD5

CDC 1) Calculated date of confinement 2) Cancer detection center 3) Capillary diffusion capacity 4) Cell division cycle 5) Centers for Disease Control, see below 6) Chenodeoxycholate 7) Crohn's disease of the colon

CDC Center(s) for Disease Control The pre-eminent epidemiologic agency of the world, located in Atlanta, Georgia, established in 1946 from the Office of Malaria Control in War Areas (at the time, CDC meant Communicable Disease Center); the Epidemic Intelligence Services was established in 1951; the CDCs' successes have included the description of Lassa fever (1969), proof of sexual transmissibility of HBV (1971), documentation of an epidemic of Reye syndrome (1973), identification of Legionnaire's disease (1976), playing a pivotal role in the eradication of smallpox (1977) and the first reports of AIDS (1981); CDC future directions include: Adolescent health, chronic disease and epidemiology of violence; see May 16, 1990 issue of the Journal of the American Medical Association

cdc25 protein A protein required to dephosphorylate a specific tyrosine residue in p34cdc2, a key protein in the biochemical engine that controls the eukaryotic cell cycle, which activates p34cdc2/cyclin B kinase, triggering the onset of mitosis (Nature 1991; 351:194c)

CDE diet A Choline-deficient, ethionine-supplemented diet used to produce experimental pancreatitis in rodents; in this diet, the normally discrete lysosome and zymogen granules fuse (a process called crinophagy) into bodies which extrude across the basolateral wall of the acinar cell, delivering digestive and lysosomal enzymes to the interstitial and peripancreatic adipose tissue; cathepsin B is also recruited, activating trypsinogen and trypsin, which in turn activate other protease precursors

CDI Cartilage-derived inhibitor A peptide isolated from stromal tissue that inhibits angiogenesis (proliferation and migration of capillary endothelial cells), explaining why cartilage is resistant to ingrowth of capillaries (Science 1990; 247:1408)

cDNA DNA that is complementary to a messenger RNA actively translating various proteins; cDNA fragments are inserted into a viral gene coding for the β-galactosidase enzyme; by extension, bacteria containing the virus with an altered β-galactosidase will contain the protein fragment encoded by the cDNA, which is identified on a cell culture plate by radioactively 'tagging' a monoclonal antibody to the desired protein and performing autoradiography

cDNA library MOLECULAR BIOLOGY A living repository of genetic material raised in a bacteriophage-infected *Escherichia coli* (or, less commonly, other bacteria) that contains only inserted segments of DNA, ie introns, which is created by making complementary DNA (cDNA) from a full set (hence, the term library) of mRNAs in a cell, using reverse transcriptase (RNA-dependent DNA polymerase) that converts single-stranded cDNA to double-stranded DNA, then carrying out the steps required to establish a gene library

CD-ROM Compact disk-read only memory

CDS see Controlled Drug Substances

CEA Carcinoembryonic antigen A glycoprotein present in the circulation in nanogram amounts first described as relatively specific for detecting occult primary adenocarcinomas; CEA is increased in up to 30% of colorectal, lung, liver, pancreas, breast, head and neck, bladder, cervix, prostatic and medullary thyroid carcinomas, and may be increased in lymphoproliferative disorders, malignant melanoma and in heavy smokers; although elevation is not a reliable cancer screen, it is useful for monitoring recurrent colon cancer; a 35% increase of CEA above a patient's post-resective surgery baseline, may indicate need for a 'second look' operation to rule out metastases; CEA is increased in 60-90% of metastatic lung cancer

C/EBP A DNA-binding protein, first thought to bind to the **C**CAAT boxes, later shown to act as a viral **E**nhancer **B**inding **P**rotein; C/EBP is present at high levels in hepatocytes, adipocytes, intestinal mucosal cells and in neurons, binding to DNA as a dimer, joined by a leucine 'zipper' motif; see DNA-binding, Helix-turn-helix, Zinc finger

Celery stick sign PEDIATRIC RADIOLOGY A descriptor for a disorganized diaphysis and metaphysis with osteitis of long bones, seen in the distal femur and proximal tibia, where longitudinal radiolucent striations alternate with sclerotic bands; 'celery stick' changes are typical of children with rubella embryopathy, infected during the first trimester (Am J Radiol 1966; 97:82,92), but also occur with other transplacental infections, including cytomegalovirus, herpes simplex, syphilis, toxoplasmosis (see TORCH), malignancy, eg leukemia, neuroblastoma, systemic disease, scurvy, hypervitaminosis D, osteogenesis imperfecta, osteoporosis

Celiac sprue Gluten-sensitive enteropathy A malabsorptive syndrome resulting from hypersensitivity of intestinal mucosa to α-gliadin, a gluten extract composed of glutamine and proline-rich proteins, present in wheat, barley, rye and to a lesser degree, oats **Pathogenesis** Uncertain, although some data implicates viral infection, eg the α-gliadin peptide of gluten has considerable homology with the E1B protein of human adenovirus 12; antibodies to E1B cross-react with α-gliadin and celiac disease is more common in those previously exposed to adenovirus 12 **Clinical** Diarrhea, weight loss, anemia, hemorrhage, osteopenia, muscular atrophy, peripheral neuropathy, central nervous system and spinal cord demyelination (sensory loss, ataxia), amenorrhea, infertility, edema, petechiae, dermatitis herpetiformis, especially if the patient has an HLA B27 haplotype **Histopathology** Mucosal flattening, lengthening of the crypt with crypt hyperplasia, loss of villi and nuclear polarity, causing local and systemic changes Note: Crypt hyperplasia and villous atrophy may transiently occur in gastrointestinal hypersensitivity reactions to milk, fish, rice and chicken and should be ruled out **Treatment** Eliminate gliadin from diet; poor response is due either to non-compliance or incorrect diagnosis Without treatment, 10-15% develop lymphoma (immunoblastic lymphoma, less commonly, T cell lymphoma), a risk that increases with disease duration; the otherwise rare small intestinal adenocarcinoma is up to 80-fold more common in sprue patients; Cf Tropical sprue

Cell adhesion molecules see CAM

Cell block CYTOLOGY A paraffin-embedded specimen derived from dried mucus, sputum or debris found in clear fluids of pleural, pericardial, endobronchial and other sites that cannot be processed in the usual fashion for cytological analysis; cell blocks are suspended in formaldehyde, centrifuged at 2500 rpm and processed as per routine for histological specimens

Cell-in-cell pattern Partial molding of one cell into another, a cytopathological feature of small (oat) cell carcinoma of the lung; usually the nuclei of pulmonary small cell carcinomas are hyperchromatic and fragile and some have a morphology likened to pulled taffy candy; confusion arises if the dense nuclei are surrounded by eosinophilic cytoplasm, thus mimicking the squamous pearls of epidermoid carcinoma of the lungs; this distinction is of practical importance as small cell carcinomas may respond to radiotherapy, while squamous cell carcinomas are unsalvageable if surgically unresectable

Cell junction PHYSIOLOGY An intercellular zone of adherence between and contributed by two cells, functionally divided into Adhering junction A mechanical junction that holds cells in place, eg spot desmosome, belt desmosome, hemidesmosome Communicating junction A junction that mediates the passage of small molecules between cells, eg gap junction, synaptic 'junction' Impermeable junction A tight impermeable junction that seals two cells allowing no leakage, eg septate junction, tight junction

Cell-mediated immunity (CMI) The arm of the immune system that acts through the 'direct' cell action, commonly equated to T-cell immunity (humoral or B cell immunity is 'indirect', mediated by antibodies) Postulated route of CMI An antigen arrives on the 'scene' and is processed by a specialized macrophage, the antigen presenting cell (APC), which presents the antigen to a T cell within the self MHC (major histocompatibility complex) class II protein complex present on the APC surface; antigen is then presented to T cells, activating various T cells having helper, suppressor and cytotoxic functions; the 'activated' T cells then produce cytokines that a) Autoamplify T cell reactivity, b) Activate macrophages or c) Facilitate immunoglobulin production, thus facilitating the action of killer cells; CMI is pivotal in host defense against tuberculosis, fungi, tumor cells and plays a key role in allograft rejection; see ADCC, APC

Cellular oncogene see Protooncogene

'Cellulite' A term used by the lay public for cosmetically undesirable subcutaneous layer(s) of adipose tissue that causes peau d'orange-like dimpling of the skin surface; cellulite is not an accepted medical term, either clinically or pathologically, as histologic examination reveals nothing more than 'garden variety' adipocytes, although billions of dollars are spent annually in the US alone to rid the body of this physical manifestations of dietary excess

centiGray see Gray

Census The number of inpatients (ie occupied beds) in a health care facility, exclusive of newborns; see Bed

Centers for Disease Control see CDC

centiMorgan GENETICS A unit of physical map distance on a human chromosome, equivalent to a 1% crossover frequency

Central cord syndrome A post-traumatic condition affecting the spinal cord, in which a lesion spreads from the central gray matter peripherally to the myelin; voluntary myelinated motor fibers to the arms are more central and those to the legs more peripheral; in the central cord syndrome, lower motor neuron changes occur in the arms and are accompanied by leg spasticity; sensory defects are a function of the degree of anterolateral and posterior column destruction, often accompanied by altered pain and temperature sensation in hands; cases of acute onset may be accompanied by urinary retention and incontinence

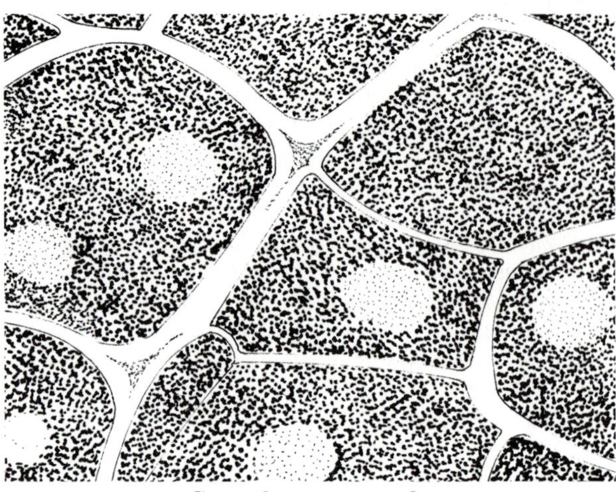

Central core myopathy

Central core myopathy Shy-Magee disease An autosomal dominant myopathy causing hypotonia in infancy and non-progressive proximal weakness, with sparing of the cranial muscles **Histopathology** Central muscle fiber zone lacking oxidative or glycolytic enzyme activity **Ultrastructure** Decreased numbers of mitochondria with disorganized myofibrils

Central dogma MOLECULAR BIOLOGY The pedagogical tenet held in the infancy (circa 1960s) of molecular biology that translation of a protein invariably follows a chain of molecular command, where DNA acts as the template for both its own replication and for the transcription to RNA (and with subsequent maturation, to messenger RNA), which then serves as a template for translation into a protein; although this represents the usual flow of

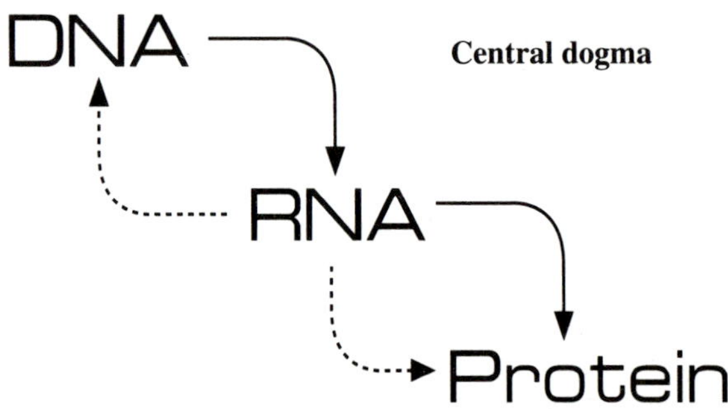

Central dogma

molecular information, it is now well-established that RNA may also act as its own RNA polymerase (Science 1988; 239:1412) and may serve as a template (via reverse transcriptase and formation of a complementary DNA strand) for its own replication Note: The recognition of the prion, an infectious particle composed only of protein will further complicate this once simple scheme; see Prion

Central (reparative) giant cell granuloma ORAL PATHOLOGY A predominantly osteodestructive lesion of uncertain pathogenesis that is most common in the young female mandible, and more osteodestructive than the peripheral giant cell granuloma Radiology Radiolucent destructivelesion with faint trabeculation and loculation Histopathology Loose fibrillar connective tissue, fibroblast proliferation, hemosiderin pigmentation and variably-sized giant cells Differential diagnosis Giant cell tumor of bone, parathyroid hormone-induced 'brown' tumor (hyperparathyroidism) Treatment Curettage Note: It is unclear whether this condition is neoplastic or reactive

Central pontine myelinolysis (CPM) Neuropathology A condition characterized by softening of the base of the brain at the pons, related to aggressive correction of hyponatremia, and first identified in alcoholics; CPM has also been described in AIDS, infection, lymphoproliferative disorders, malnutrition, myeloid leukemia and local venous obstruction Prevention consists of slow correction of the electrolytic imbalance

Central supply The department in a health care facility that stores, distributes and assures the availability of sterile materials, equipment, instruments, reusable and disposable items

Centrosome see MTOC (microtubule organizing body)

Centronuclear myopathy see Myotubular myopathy

CEOT Calcifying epithelial odontogenic tumor of Pindborg A slow-growing lesion of the oral cavity, mandible and maxilla, that affects any age group, population and sex; although the CEOT is locally invasive, radical therapy is not required Histopathology Polyhedral epithelial cells with minimal stroma; the cells may demonstrate nuclear pleomorphism; intracellular degeneration results in amyloid-like eosinophilic material that may with time become calcified

Cephalad march CRITICAL CARE MEDICINE The slow progression of weakness and loss of sensory perception seen in an acute epidural hematoma

Cephalosporin see Third generation cephalosporin

Cerebral amyloid angiopathy (CAA) A sporadic disease that is present in an estimated 5-10% of primary non-traumatic cerebral hemorrhage, in which extensive vascular deposition of amyloid β protein is inculpated in recurrent and extensive intracerebral hemorrhages, resulting in neurotrophic and neurotoxic effects that are reversed by tachykinin-type neuropeptides; CAA is idiopathic or may be associated with human hereditary cerebral hemorrhage with amyloidosis, Dutch type, see HCHWA-D

Cerebral gigantism Sotos syndrome An autosomal dominant disease with rapid early growth without endocrinopathy, accelerated bone maturation or precocious puberty Clinical Enlarged hands and feet, thickened subcutaneous tissues, mild mental retardation, EEG abnormalities, dilated ventricles, dolichocephaly, antimongolic slanting of the palpebral fissures, macrognathy, hypertelorism, poor coordination and an increased risk for malignancy, including Wilm's tumor, hepatic, parotid and ovarian carcinomas

Cerebral palsy A symptom complex affecting 0.4% of all term births; 75% of quadriplegic cerebral palsy has a known etiology—53% are congenital, 14% due to intrapartum asphyxia and 8% are due to other identified causes; 40% of non-quadriplegic cerebral palsy have known causes—35% are congenital, 5% are due to other causes (Am J Dis Child 1989; 143:1154)

Cerebriform nuclei Twisted, convoluted nuclei with a cerebral gyri-like appearance, classically seen in the atypical T cells of mycosis fungoides, Sezary syndrome and lymphomatoid papulosis; although cerebriform cells are usually T lymphocytes, they may also be B lymphocytes

Ceredase An orphan drug (Genzyme Corp, Boston) product that is available under a treatment IND protocol for Gaucher's disease, which acts to replace the missing glucocerebrosidase

Ceride A wax ester formed from a long-chain fatty acid and a long-chain aliphatic alcohol

Ceroid Alcohol-insoluble, oxidized polyunsaturated lipid pigment(s) that results from the peroxidation of unsaturated lipids, which are similar or identical to lipofuscin; ceroid accumulates in the liver, heart and gut macrophages in the elderly and is thus termed 'wear and tear' pigment and has been inculpated in age-related organ dysfunction, see 'Garbage can' hypothesis, in hypovitaminosis E, in cathartic colon and in hereditary conditions, eg Batten's disease and sea-blue histiocytosis

Ceroid 'granuloma' A finding in chronic cholecystitis, in which there are focal aggregates of neutral fat and lipofuscin-laden macrophages, contrasting with cholesterosis, which also occurs in chronic cholecystitis and is a diffuse process with cholesterol-laden macrophages accumulating immediately subjacent to the mucosa, imparting a macroscopic appearance, fancifully termed 'strawberry' gall bladder

Certificate of need (CON) A document often required by state law in the US and issued by a governmental body to an individual or organization proposing to a) Construct or modify a health care facility b) Make major capital equipment purchases or c) Offer a new health care service; CONs can be used by government to prevent duplication of services or excess regional development of facilities or services; if a major purchase, eg a magnetic resonance imager (MRI), is made by a health care facility without an approved CON, the sponsoring institute's 'part A' costs may not be reimbursed

Certified bed A 'legal' bed in a health care facilitythat has been approved for use by patients on a permanent basis, which the governing body (usually the state board of health) has deemed to have sufficient staffing to support its unqualified use; see Bed; Cf 'Swing' bed

Cerumen see Wet cerumen

Cervical 'collar' An erythematous rash affecting the second and third cervical nerve roots in reactivated varicella-zoster

Cervical rib A uni- or bilateral congenital anomaly of the first thoracic rib, affecting up to 1% of the population, 15% of whom have an associated thoracic outlet syndrome (see there); cervical ribs range from type I, a short bar extending from the transverse process to type IV, which is a complete extra rib articulating with the sternum

Cervix mark NEONATOLOGY A fluid-filled vesicle of no clinical significance, that lies atop the caput succedaneum, the edematous 'mass' at the presenting aspect of the head in a vaginally delivered infant

Cesarian section C-section OBSTETRICS Surgical extraction of a product of conception, which has become the single most commonly performed invasive procedure in many nations **Statistics** Brazil has the world's highest rate of C-sections at 32/100 hospital deliveries; Japan and Czechoslovakia have the lowest at 7/100 (J Am Med Assoc 1990; 263:3286); USA, non-Hispanic Caucasians, 20.6/1000, Hispanics, 13.9/1000 (N Engl J Med 1989; 321:233); frequency, post-C-section vaginal delivery, 5% in USA, 43% in Norway; private patients are more likely to have C-sections than clinic patients (N Engl J Med 1989; 320:706); the C-section is the oldest of all surgical operations; royal law (lex regia) by Numa Pompilius (715-672 BC) decreed that children be excised from any woman dying late in pregnancy, later known as lex caesarea under the rule of the Caesars; some scholars maintain that the name derives from the Latin caedere, to cut, an abdominal birth would thus be partus caesareus

CETP see Cholesteryl-ester transfer protein

CFCs Chlorofluorocarbons ENVIRONMENT A family of stable non-toxic, non-flammable, non-corrosive chemicals used as coolants, foaming and cleaning agents and aerosol propellants; in 1988, 1 million metric tons of CFCs were consumed on the planet, 730 000 metric tons of CFC-11 and CFC-12, resulting in a net addition of 100% to the atmospheric gases, since this last group requires many decades to naturally disappear; CFC-related goods and services generate $\$28 \times 10^9$/year and employ 700 000 workers in the US, where refrigerants comprise 30% of CFC use; foam-blowing agents for polystyrene and polyurethane 28% (rigid foam is used for insulation; non-rigid for cushions) and industrial solvents and cleaning agents 19% (in 1978, aerosol CFCs were banned in the USA); CFCs are largely responsible for depleting the ozone layer and are minor contributors to the greenhouse effect; CFC-12 (CF_2Cl_2) is the most widely used coolant which is targeted for replacement by the less ozone-depleting HCFC-134a; international treaties plan to reduce CFC use to one-half the current levels by 1999; industry retooling to less ozone-depleting CFCs will cost $10 billion; the Montreal protocol assumes that certain substitutes, eg HCFC-22, for 'hard' CFCs (CFC-11, -12, -113, -114, -115) are less damaging, although the terms 'ozone-depleting potential' and 'halocarbon global warming potential' are not equivalent (Nature 1990; 344:508, 513, 493); potential CFC substitutes for refrigerant, CFC-12: HCFC-134a (CF_3CFH_2), HCFC-22 (CHF_2Cl); potential CFC replacements, blowing agent, CFC-11 ($CFCl_3$): HCFC-141b (CH_3CFCl_2), HCFC-123 (CF_3CFCl_2), HCFC-22 (CHF_2Cl); potential CFC replacements for cleaning agents, CFC-113 ($CF_2ClCFCl_2$), see Science 1990; 249:31 Note: Bromocarbons (halons) CF_3Br and CF_2ClBr fire-extinguishers have an atmospheric half-life of 10- and 2-fold greater than that of a proposed substitute, CHF_2Br, which has a seven year half-life (Science 1991; 252:693); see Greenhouse effect, Ozone layer

CFS see Chronic fatigue syndrome

CFTR Cystic fibrosis transmembrane conductance regulator, see Cystic fibrosis

CFU-GEMM A colony-stimulating factor for all cell lines (granulocytes, erythroid, megakaryocytes and macrophages); complete absence of CFU-GEMM is implicated in the pancytopenia of Fanconi's disease and myelodysplasia and its production can be suppressed by chemicals, drugs, radiation, malnutrition, viral and bacterial infections

CFU-S Colony-forming units, spleen A heterogeneous population of cells that are thought to contain the ultimate stem cell, as the putative cells have the key capabilities of proliferation, pluripotentiality and self-renewal

CGD see Chronic granulomatous disease

CGRP Calcitonin gene-related peptide A 37-residue polypeptide produced by alternate splicing of pre-mRNA from the calcitonin gene; CGRP is a potent vasodilator that functions by activation of K/ATP channel (Nature 1990; 344:770), acting as a positive feedback signal for acetylcholine synthesis, increasing the number of acetylcholine receptors in cultured cells; it is secreted by the thyroid C cells and by the sensory nerve endings at the same site of secondary and tertiary calcification in bone, increasing the cAMP levels in osteoblasts; CGRP is structurally related to N-proCT, see there

CHAD Cold hemagglutinin disease(s) see Cold agglutinins

Chain growth and synthesis MOLECULAR BIOLOGY DNA synthesis in vivo occurs in the 5' to 3' direction; in vitro (chemical) synthesis of DNA occurs in the 5' to 3' direction; peptide synthesis in vivo occurs from amino terminus towards the carboxy terminus; in vitro (chemical) peptide synthesis starts at the carboxyl terminus, working toward the amino terminal

Chain-like thickening NEPHROPATHOLOGY A histopathologic feature of stage III membranous glomerulonephritis, best seen with a PAS stain, a finding that follows the 'spike stage' and corresponds to a variable corrugated pattern of thickened glomerular basement membrane with a few recognizable projections

Chain of custody Chain of evidence FORENSIC MEDICINE The path that objects, eg bullets, knives or clinical specimens, eg semen specimen in alleged rape, must take for these materials to be legally accepted as evidence in a court of law; emergency room physicians and pathologists often find themselves part of the chain and have a responsibility to doc ument all pertinent details regarding the specimen and to turn these materials into the appropriate authorities

Chain of lakes appearance A finding by endoscopic retrograde cholangiopancreatography (ERCP), which is described in chronic pancreatitis where the main pancreatic duct measures 1.0 cm in average diameter and is 'punctuated' by scattered focal obstructions; other ERCP features of chronic pancreatitis include strictures, cysts and ductal calculi

Chair see Endowed professorship

'Chair' A non-sexist sobriquet for the chairman, -woman or -person, ie the presiding officer in an organization; in academics, the 'chair' is often a full professor who is responsible for the academic, clinical, administrative and research activities of the department; Cf Endowed chair, Professor

Chairman The head of an academic department; see 'Chair', Cf Chief

Chair rung appearance A microscopic morphology consisting of periodic constrictions in asbestos fibers that are focally surrounded by protein-mineral complexes

Chalasia chair A device formerly used to treat gastrointestinal reflux in young children; in infants less than 6 months of age, the device may exacerbate reflux

'Chalk bone' disease Osteopetrosis or Albers-Schönberg disease

Chalk streaks Verkalkung Short whitish striations seen on gross examination of intraductal carcinomas of the breast, tumors that are often 'gritty' to cutting, the result of desmoplasia with microcalcifications; chalk streaks are rarely seen in other epithelial malignancies

Challenge stock IMMUNOLOGY A precisely calibrated dose of an antigen that is administered after previous exposure to an infectious agent, eg HIV-1 that is used to test a vaccine's efficacy

Chalone A target organ or tissue-specific (but not species-specific) inhibitor of cell proliferation or other activity, which, unlike true hormones are not produced by a specific organ

Champagne bottle legs NEUROLOGY Marked distal peroneal muscle atrophy with tapering of the distal extremities and hypertrophy of the proximal muscles ('stork leg' appearance), characteristic of advanced Charcot-Marie-Tooth type of chronic familial peripheral neuropathy; pes cavus may be the only early finding, which is followed by foot drop (leading to a high 'steppage' gait); walking is difficult given the combination of sensory ataxia and muscular weakness; electromyography reveals slow conduction velocity and increased distal latency; see Onion bulb, Piano playing

Champagne glass appearance RADIOLOGY A fanciful descriptor for the inner pelvic contour with narrowed sacrosciatic notches typical of achondroplasia, where the pelvic width exceeds the depth due to an increased iliac base; in contrast, the 'brandy snifter' contour is normal and 'wine glass' contour occurs in Morquio syndrome

Chancroid A shallow, painful ulcer caused by ***Haemophilus ducreyi***, that clinically mimics the painless syphilitic chancre

'Chandelier' sign GYNECOLOGY A highly colloquial term for the extreme hypersensitivity to pain in women with pelvic inflammatory disease; an internal examination in afflicted women evokes pain of such intensity that the patient seemingly leaps out of the examination stirrups 'for the chandelier'

Chaos Non-linear analysis THEORETICAL BIOLOGY A complex, non-linear, yet completely deterministic order that is present in all living systems, which is extremely sensitive to initial conditions and perturbations, such that minute changes impact on a ground state, potentially leading to large differences in an end state; all healthy physiological systems have innate variability or chaos, the loss or reduction of which leads to a less complicated and more ordered state, signaling an impaired system; although the mathematics of non-linear dynamics is arcane, it is present in biological systems by design (Science 1989; 243:604), appearing in normal fluctuations of the heart rate, blood flow and blood pressure; the chaos phenomenon has been studied in cardiology, epidemiology, immunology, neurology, psychiatry and other fields (J Am Med Assoc 1991; 266:12rv)

Chaperones A class of proteins that facilitate the correct assembly or disassembly of oligomeric protein complexes, participating in the transmembrane targeting of certain proteins; chaperones include nucleoplasmins, chaperonins (see below), heat shock protein 70 and 90 classes, signal recognition particle, trigger factor and BiP, an immunoglobulin heavy chain-binding protein (Science 1990; 250:956)

Chaperonins A group of 60 kD cytosolic proteins, eg heat shock protein 60, hsp60, that use the energy from ATP hydrolysis to maintain proteins in the necessary folded configuration for proper function, thus having 'foldase' activity; other postulated roles for chaperonins include protein transport, oligomer assembly, DNA replication, mRNA turnover and protection of the cell from various stresses; some chaperones have auto-foldase activities (Nature 1990; 348:339); Cf Chaperones, Heat shock, hsp70

CHARGE complex A disease complex of probable neural crest origin, diagnosed when infants have four of the seven components of the CHARGE acronym: Coloboma, Heart defects (conotruncal or septal), Atresia of the nasal choanae, Retarded growth and development, Genital hypoplasia and Ear anomalies and/or deafness; other findings in the CHARGE complex include facial palsy, renal anomalies and cleft lip/palate (J Med Genetics 1988; 25:147)

'Charley horse' The result of a contusion injury to the thigh involving the quadriceps muscle; without immediate compression, the ensuing hematoma and pain can be substantial; the origin of this American colloquialism for muscle stiffness is unknown, but it is anecdotally related to a horse named Charley who walked with a limp, drawing a roller to flatten the playing field in the Chicago White Sox baseball park in Chicago during the 1890s

'Charlie Chaplin' gait A gait that occurs in bilateral external torsion of the tibia, caused by faulty sitting or sleeping habits, as in prolonged maintenance of the 'spread-eagle' or frogleg position Treatment early, change sleeping habits, brace and if too late, osteotomy

Chase A term that can be either a noun or verb, which refers to the halting of a chemical or dynamic reaction, in which a so-called 'pulse' incorporation of a labelled or radioactive compound is 'chased' by a non-labelled compound; this sequence of events allows evaluation of the kinetics of a reaction; Cf Pulse-chase experiment

'Chatterbox' syndrome see Cocktail party syndrome

Chauffeur fracture An oblique fracture of the distal radius extending radially from the articular margin with separation of both the styloid process and a triangular portion of attached bone; these fractures were seen forty or more years ago when all automobile engines were started mechanically by a crank and the engine 'backfired', and therefore is an injury likely to occur in antique car enthusiasts Note: The last production automobile to have a hand crank (for emergency starting) was Citroen's venerable 2CV, produced until July 1990

'Checkerboard' nucleus see Tortoise shell nucleus

Checkerboard pattern HISTOLOGY A normal interspersion of dark (type I) and light (type II) skeletal muscle fibers which develops by the 30th fetal week, a pattern that is directly controlled by the nervous system and which is lost in many myopathic diseases, as may occur in proliferative myositis, mitochondrial myopathies and neurogenic atrophy

Checkerboard titration A laboratory method used to study the effect of varying any one parameter on the sensitivity and specificity of, eg a staining system while the other parameters of the system are held constant; the equilibrium is called the plateau titer

Check valve see Ball valve obstruction

Cheese disease see Tyramine hypertension

Chemical colitis An acute inflammatory colitis that develops hours after self-administration of a 'cleansing' enema containing soap or other inappropriate agents, eg hydrogen peroxide, vinegar and potassium permanganate, resulting in hypertonic, detergent or directly toxic effects Clinical Effects range from vague pain to cramping, anaphylaxis, serosanguinous diarrhea, hypovolemia and acute hemoconcentration; when the mucosal damage is severe, bacteria may penetrate the mucosa, causing sepsis, hypokalemia, pseudomembrane formation, hemorrhagic necrosis, intestinal gangrene and acute renal failure; see Soap colitis

Chemical diabetes mellitus A subclinical or preclinical form of diabetes mellitus characterized by diabetes mellitus-like response curves to glucose tolerance tests or other provocative tests; it is controversial whether therapy is beneficial for these patients

'Chemical McCarthyism' A phrase coined in reference to the US government-sponsored drug abuse testing of employee urine, which in the USA, smacks of infringement of constitutional rights, and to be reliable, would require trained micturition observers, represents an invasion of privacy (Science 1987; 237:744); the phrase was coined after US Senator Joe McCarthy who during the early 1950s led zealous and often unfounded defamation campaigns against suspected communists

Chemical 'mumps' see 'Iodine mumps'

Chemical peel DERMATOLOGY A technique in which trichloroacetic acid (TCA) is 'painted' on elderly sun-exposed skin with extensive actinic keratoses (a pre-malignant condition); TCA causes chemically-induced exfoliation of the epidermis and upper dermis, reducing future incidence of basal and squamous cell carcinoma in the treated region as well as removing fine wrinkles (Mayo Clin Proc 1988; 63:887)

Chemical pollutant ENVIRONMENT A chemical substance that enters the environment through industrial, agricultural or other human activities, which poses an immediate or potential hazard to plant, animal or human life; the major chemical pollutants are heavy metals, eg mercury and lead, aromatic hydrocarbons, eg benzene and other petrochemicals, organic solvents, eg toluene and xylene, organo-halogens, eg polychlorinated biphenyls (PCBs) and polybrominated biphenyls (PBBs), dioxins and others including nitrogen and sulfur dioxides

Chemical shift to the left see Neuroblastoma

Chemical 'splenectomy' Therapeutic immune paralysis A method that inhibits splenic endocytosis of opsonized, ie immunoglobulin or complement-coated cells or microorganisms by blocking Fc receptors; the targets are thus bound, but not endocytosed; chemical splenectomy is a state inducible by high-dose (1 mg/kg/day) corticosteroids or IV immunoglobulin (0.4 g/kg/day); the effect lasts as long as the therapy and is an alternative to surgery in immune-related hypersplenism, eg autoimmune hemolytic anemia, autoimmune neutropenia and Felty syndrome

Chemical warfare The use of chemicals as weapons of war, usually deployed as gases; these weapons were used in World War I against an estimated 1.3 million soldiers and the tremendous morbidity of these substances led to their ban under the 'Geneva Protocol' of 1925; despite the ban, in World War II, it has been all reported that the Italians used poison gas against the Ethiopians, the Japanese used them against the Chinese in Manchuria and the Germans developed tabun and sarin, and although they had packaged these potent cholinesterase inhibitors into bombs, they were never deployed; because of the relatively transient nature of the injuries, the remoteness or difficulty of access to a site of an attack, language barriers between the victims and the interviewers and the deterioration of the chemicals themselves with time, allegations of the use of chemical weapons may be difficult to corroborate; chemical weapons were allegedly deployed in a) The 'Yellow rain' incident in the 1970s, in which the Laotian and Kampuchean governments attacked Hmong villages with trichothecane and b) In August 1988 by Iraqi troops under Saddam Hussein against the Kurds in northern Iraq Agents Phosgene, nerve agents (sarin, soman, tabun), which are chemical mixtures, including diisopropylfluorophosphate that react with the serine hydroxyl group of acetylcholinesterase, inhibiting neural transmission, hydrogen cyanide, blistering agents (mustard gas) and thionyl chloride, which are gases that are intended be fired from long range artillery see Nature 1990; 344:482, 341:271 Clinical Mustard gas, the prototypic chemical weapon, causes marked irritation of the skin, eyes, upper respiratory and gastrointestinal tracts; the skin lesions heal in 'geographic' waves, leaving residual hyperpigmentation or induration (J Am Med Assoc 1989; 262:640, 644); at the time of Glasnost, the US stockpile had global overkill of 4000 (in contrast, the overkill for nuclear weapons is estimated at 10-20); one-half of the US chemical agents are in the form of nerve agents; although the Soviets have declared 45 000 tonnes of chemical weapons, the actual amount is estimated to be 270-360 000 tons; see Biological warfare; Zyklon B

Chemiluminescence LABORATORY MEDICINE A reaction in which chemical energy is converted into light by an oxidation reaction, where a precursor molecule reacts in the presence of peroxide and an alkali to form a high-energy peroxide intermediate (luminol, lophine, lucigenin); when specially designed peroxides, eg AMPPD, AMPGD are used, very low molar amounts, 10^{-18} of a substance of interest, eg DNA and RNA probes, oligonucleotides and immune molecules may be detected

Chemonucleolysis NEUROSURGERY Injection of chymopapain as an alternative to laminectomy in certain cases of intervertebral disc rupture, 10-40% meet the criteria; the stated advantages of chemonucleolysis include earlier ambulation and ability to perform the procedure on an outpatient basis

Chemoprevention The use of diet or drugs to reduce the incidence of cancer; use of vitamin A or β carotene does not prevent secondary non-melanoma skin cancer (N Engl J Med 1990; 323:789); high doses of the vitamin A analog, isoretinoin prevent second primary malignancies in the head and neck region (N Engl J Med 1990; 323:795); among the agents with chemopreventive effects (as supported by 'soft' data) are vitamins C, vitamin E, bran and other dietary fibers, and cruciferous vegetables

Chemoreceptor trigger zone Area postrema NEUROANATOMY The emetic center is located in the floor of the fourth ventricle, receiving vagal afferents or stimulated directly by apomorphine, cardiac glycosides, ergot compounds, chemotherapeutic agents, staphylococcal enterotoxin, salicylate and nicotine and other circulating chemicals; in contrast to the adjacent but distinct vomiting center, the CTZ does not respond to electrical stimulation

Chemosurgery Mohs micrographic technique A technique used in plastic surgery for excising superficial, locally invasive, tumor microfingerlets of primary skin cancers, yielding a cure rate of more than 98% for these tumors (Mayo Clin Proc 1988; 63:175); the technique is of use in treating skin tumors that are broad, but not deep, eg basal and squamous cell carcinomas, but not malignant melanomas, optimally designed for lesions > 1-2 cm, recurrent skin tumors, cancer recurrence-prone sites (nose, eyes, ears) and aggressive histologic subtypes, eg morphea-like or metatypical basal cell carcinoma **Technique** The surface of the lesion plus 3-5 mm margin of normal tissue is coagulated with dichloroacetic acid, overlaid with a 20% zinc chloride paste and covered with an occlusive dressing; the $ZnCl_2$ fixes the tissue similar to formaldehyde; after from 1 to 48 hours, a 'saucer' of tissue is removed and submitted for frozen section analysis to determine sites, if any, of deep tumor extension; although tedious in short-term, the Mohs' procedure reduces future recurrences while preserving uninvolved tissue

Chemotaxis IMMUNOLOGY A stimulus that is exerted along a chemical's concentration gradient; chemotaxins are usually small molecules and in vivo act to attact macrophages and other cells along a concentration gradient

Chemotherapy The use of various agents, most of which are toxic to cells undergoing division, to induce tumor cell lysis; successful chemotherapy is a function of tumor responsiveness, which most predictably occurs in lymphoproliferative malignancies, eg leukemias and lymphomas as well as in small cell carcinoma, an undifferentiated carcinoma; because these agents are most effective against rapidly proliferating cells, 'collateral damage' to the dividing cells in skin and hair, bone marrow and gastrointestinal tract are predictable, causing reversible hair loss, myelosuppression, nausea and vomiting is the norm; the most feared late effect of chemotherapeutics, especially in successfully treated pediatric leukemias is the induction of a second malignancy, which is usually refractory to therapy, see Damocles' syndrome; popular therapeutic acronyms BACOD (bleomycin, adriamycin, cyclophosphamide, oncovorin*, prednisone), BA-COP (bleomycin, adriamycin-cyclophosphamide, oncovorin*, prednisone, CAF (cyclophosphamide, adriamycin, 5-fluouracil), CHOP (cyclophosphamide, hydroxydaunomycin#, oncovorin*, prednisone), COMP (cyclophosphamide, oncovorin, methotrexate, prednisone), COP (cyclophosphamide, oncovorin*, prednisone), COPP (chloramphenicol, oncovorin*, procarbazine, prednisone), M-BACOD (methotrexate + citrovorin rescue, bleomycin, doxorubicin, cyclophosphamide, vincristine, decadron), MOPP (methchlorethamine or nitrogen mustard, oncovorin*, procarbenzine, prednisone), MOP-BAP (MOPP-bleomycin, adriamycin, prednisone), PROMACE (prednisone, methotrexate, citrovorin rescue, doxorubicin, cyclophosphamide, etoposide), SCAB (streptozocin, CCNU, ie lomustine,adriamycin, bleomycin), TRAMPCOL (*Vincristine, #Doxorubicin); see Combined modality therapy

Chemotherapy-induced leukemia see Secondary malignancy

Chemzymes A group of small, soluble organic molecules that catalyze chemical reactions in a fashion similar to that of natural enzymes catalyzing biochemical reactions; chemzymes copiously produce innumerable copies of the same three-dimensional and chiral form of a desired molecule; chirality is a feature essential to biological systems, since the incorrect isomeric, ie dextro- or levo- form is not recognized by the body and cannot be metabolized; chirality has plagued drug companies, as separation of a biologically useful chiral form from the afunctional chiral form may be tedious or impossible and often the drug is packaged as a 1:1 mixture of right- and left-handed forms; Corey (Nobelist, 1990) et al of

Harvard modified a boron-containing organic compound, resulting in the first chemzyme, dubbed the 'CBS' (Corey, Bakshi, Shibata) enzyme that favors production of one chiral form over the other in a 20:1 ratio; 20 chemzymes have been described (Science 1989; 245:354); see Chirality

Chernobyl The site of an nuclear reactor accident occurring in April 1986 at a power plant near Kiev in the Ukraine, caused by a steam explosion, exposing 200 people to significant total-body doses of radiation; A team performed bone marrow transplants in 13 people exposed to doses of 5.6-13.4 Gy; two survived with recovery of endogenous hematopoiesis; the others died of burns, interstitial pneumonitis, graft-versus-host disease and combined acute renal and respiratory failure (N Engl J Med 1989; 321:203); Although two critical populations (the emergency clean-up crews and the 10^5 residents evacuated from the 30 km zone around the reactor) were not studied epidemiologically, a five-year post-blast study revealed little excess cancer in those exposed to the radiation; the Hiroshima studies revealed 700 excess cancers in a 110 000 exposed survivors over a period of 45 years (Nature 1991; 351:335n); see Acute radiation injury, Goiana, Pilgrim plant, Sellafield, Three Mile Island

Cherry angioma Senile angioma De Morgan spot A ruby red, 1-3 mm in diameter papule surrounded by a pale halo, common on the trunk and extremities of older adults, located in the superficial corium, consisting of dilated, thinned capillaries, causing superficial bumps

Cherry blossom appearance Branchless fruit-laden tree A descriptor for punctate cavitary radiocontrast-filled defects that percolate directly through the ducts, a sialologic appearance described in Sjögren's disease; the contrast material may persist for up to a month

Cherry hemangioma see Cherry angioma

Cherry red color Mucocutaneous discoloration classically associated with carbon monoxide poisoning; 'cherry red' also refers to oropharyngeal discoloration in acute epiglottitis

Cherry red spot myoclonus syndrome Sialidosis, type I An inherited deficiency of α-N-Acetylneuraminidase, most common in the Japanese of preadolescent onset Clinical Coarse facies, dysostosis multiplex, hearing loss, mental deterioration, cherry red colored macules in the optic fundus, lenticular opacification, gradual visual failure, myoclonus and tonic-clonic seizures, peripheral neuropathy with burning feet (N Engl J Med 1986; 315:296)

Cherry spots Bright red macules in the optic fundus of patients with Tay-Sachs syndrome (GM2-gangliosidosis type 1), Niemann-Pick diseases, Sandhoff's disease (GM2-gangliosidosis type 2), generalized gangliosidosis (GM1-gangliosidosis type 1), cherry red spot myoclonus syndrome or sialidosis, type 1, sialidosis type 2, Goldberg syndrome, mucolipidosis type 1, metachromatic leukodystrophy and retinal vasculopathy PATHOGENESIS a) Storage disease type cherry red spots Ganglion cell lysosomes are engorged with lipid, the retina is pale and the central vascularized fovea is prominently red b) Vascular type cherry red spots are caused by central retinal arterial occlusion or microaneurysms, the retina is edematous and the ganglion cells are swollen from hydropic degeneration, causing retinal opacification; the central fovea being free from ganglion cells, appears bright red against the background

Cherubism An autosomal dominant condition, 100% penetration in males, with a cherub-like physiognomy, first recognized by age 5 with puffed-out cheeks, agenesis of permanent teeth, dental dysgenesis, exophthalmos and progressive bilateral soap-bubble expansile lesions at the angle of the mandible, submandibular lymphadenopathy Histopathology Giant cell reparative granuloma onset

Cheshire cat 'syndrome' A name that dignifies one of two clinical dilemmas, where either the patient a) Has the 'classic' signs and symptoms of a well-defined and often treatable disease that cannot be confirmed by histologic or laboratory criteria or b) Has the disease with few of the characteristic findings; in either event, the clinician is left with an 'animal' fancifully likened to that seen by Alice in Wonderland, who saw the Cheshire cat's grin without the cat, making it difficult to convince others of the cat's existence

Chevron pattern see Christmas tree pattern

'Chew' Chewing tobacco; see Smokeless tobacco

Chewing gum diarrhea An osmotic diarrhea caused by excessive intraluminal sorbitol in 'sugarless' chewing gum Note: The hexitol type sugar alcohols, sorbitol and mannitol, are major constituents of sugar-free dietary foods, which are not used by bacteria as substrates and thus by remaining in the intestinal lumen may cause osmotic diarrhea; the amount consumed may be large, eg 50-100 sticks of gum/day, translating into 85-170 g sorbitol/day (Am J Dig Dis 1978; 23:568)

Chewing tobacco see Smokeless tobacco

CHH syndrome see Cartilage-hair hypoplasia syndrome

Chicago disease North American Blastomycosis

Chicken breast deformity An asymptomatic, asymmetric deep depression of the costal cartilage along each side of the sternum, most apparent below the nipple level, involving the 4th to 7-8th costal cartilages, comprising the most common type of protrusion deformity of the sternum (pectus carinatum); Cf Pouter-pigeon

Chicken fat clot A descriptor for a slowly formed post-mortem blood clot, composed mainly of leukocytes that settled to dependent parts of the vasculature Pathology Yellow, rubbery and non-adherent to vascular walls Histopathology Polymorphous cell population with abundant neutrophils, few red cells and fibrin; chicken fat clots may occur in fulminant bacterial endocarditis; Cf Currant jelly clots

Chicken footprint eggs A descriptor applied to the eggs of *Taenia* species (*T solium* and *T saginatum*) that have a thick, bile-stained, radially striated shell enclosing a six-hooked embryo (oncosphere); these eggs are indistinguishable from each other, from the eggs of *Echinococcus granulosus* and from those of other animal taeniid tapeworms; absolute identification requires that the embryo's six hooks be seen; Cf Prince Charles looking to the left

Chicken footprint nucleus A large nucleus with radiating striations, seen in the convoluted T-cell lymphoma of Lukes and Collins, a tumor of adolescents and young adults that is thought to be of thymic origin as 50-75% are mediastinal and often display markers typical of primitive intrathymic T-cells; these tumors are mitotically active and have a 'starry sky' pattern

'Chicken liver era' A facetious term for the 'new age' in the study of gastric physiology, which began in 1976 (Am J Dig Dis 1976; 21:296); ^{99m}Tc is bound to sulfur colloid, injected into a chicken where it concentrates in the Kupffer cells; the chickens are then killed, the liver resected, diced up and served in the stew as part of a radionuclide meal; gastric emptying is then studied by scintiscans of the supine patient

Chickenpox Varicella, Human Herpesvirus type 3 An acute HHV-3 infection, most common before age 10 Clinical 2 week incubation, followed by a scarlatiform prodromal rash, low-grade fever, anorexia, malaise, crops of reddish papules that become intensely pruritic vesicles, increasing in number for 3-4 days, the itching and excoriation of which causes extensive scarring Complications Secondary bacterial infection, viral pneumonia (1:400 require pneumonia-related hospitalization), thrombocytopenia, purpura fulminans, encephalitis (5-15% mortality, 15% with permanent neurological sequelae), myocarditis, glomerulonephritis, hepatitis, myositis; after resolution of clinical disease, HHV-3 becomes latent, integrating its DNA into the dorsal root ganglion cells Note: Chronic HHV-3 infection is the recrudescence form of herpes zoster or shingles

Chicken wing appendage A descriptor for a form of phocomelia with foreshortened arms and forearms, flexion contraction at the elbows, a proximal thumb and short, tapered fingers, a finding typical of the Cornelia de Lange syndrome, which may be accompanied by a low hairline, hirsutism, bushy eyebrows, an antimongoloid slant of the eyes and various cardiac defects, eg ventricular septal defect

Chicken wire pattern A descriptor applied to a delicate plexiform or reticulated pattern imposed on that of another density LIVER PATHOLOGY A pattern of fibrosis associated with alcoholic hepatitis; Cf Bridging fibrosis SOFT TISSUE PATHOLOGY The arrangement of the capillaries in myxoid liposarcoma RADIOLOGY A descriptor for the pattern of calcification in chondroblastoma, a pediatric tumor, pattern also used for chondroblastoma is 'Fluffy cotton wool'

Chief Chief of service The head of a department or section of a clinically-oriented service in a health care facility Note: The term has various uses, although perhaps the most common use equates a 'chief' to the department head of a non-academic institution, or when used in the context of academic medicine, the director of a service, who is subordinate to the chairman

Chief cell hyperplasia A pathologic state of primary or secondary increase in the production of parathyroid hormone; the primary form is a constant feature of MEA types I and IIa (but not type IIb) Pathology All glands are enlarged; the cells are arranged in nodular aggregates; the secondary form is caused by peripheral disease, eg renal dysfunction, chronic malabsorption; the glands display from minimal to florid hyperplasia, weighing up to 5 g, where small uniform cells with finely granular and transparent cytoplasm completely replace the fat typical of a normal parathyroid gland

Chief 'syndrome' A condition that most often occurs after the admission of a 'very important person' (V.I.P.) to a major medical center or university hospital; since the chief of a service may be more involved in administration than in 'hands-on' practice of his specialty, he may be unfamiliar with the location of where essential equipment is located and be out of practice with routine procedures; because a V.I.P. is deemed worthy of nothing less than the best, the chief is pressed into service with potentially less-than-felicitous results; see V.I.P. 'syndrome'

Chilblains Pernio A cutaneous inflammation due to cold, damp climates, ie in the UK; presumed due to prolonged arteriolar vasoconstriction Clinical, early Pallor and coolness of acral parts, often due to 'underdressing' Clinical, late The skin displays patches of painful pruritic erythema, variably accompanied by blistering, swelling and encrusted ulceration; light microscopy reveals acute, occasionally necrotizing angiitis in a background of chronic inflammation; the term Chyll blayne is of Welsh origin, where the treatment for prolonged exposure to cold was warm wine; the current armamentarium includes proper clothing, cessation of smoking and corticosteroids

Child abuse see Battered child syndrome

CHILD syndrome Congenital Hemidysplasia-Ichthyosiform erythroderma-Limb Deformity An X-linked congenital lethal complex that is uniformly fatal in males; male:female 19:1 Clinical Unilateral ichthyosis, limb malformation, accompanied by ipsilateral hypoplasia of paired organs, eg lung, thyroid, psoas muscle, central nervous system and cranial nerves

Childhood trauma The mental result of a sudden external blow or series of blows, rendering the child temporarily helpless and breaking past ordinary coping and defensive operations (Am Med News 27/May/1991); see Battered child syndrome

Chikungunya An acute alpha-virus infection of the Sahara, tropics and subtropics, afflicting children in the rainy months, with fever, arthralgia and rash, likely a 'spillover' from the cycle maintained in wild primates; Vectors *Aedes aegypti, A africanus, A furcifer*

Chimera Any individual or molecule that derives from two or more species CLINICAL GENETICS An organism with two or more cell lines/genotypes/karyotypes descended from at least two zygotes (a very rare phenomenon seen only in twins), resulting from chorionic vascular anastomoses, transplantation, or double fertilization and subsequent participation of both fertilized meiotic products in one developing embryo; all hermaphrodites should be karyotyped to evaluate possible chimerism, a finding confirmed by the presence of two distinct blood groups, due to an exchange of primordial blood cells between non-identical twins early in fetal development, prior to development of an immune system capable of rejection; Cf Freemartin, Mosaics Note: The chimera of Greek mythology was a female monster that breathed fire, had the head of a lion, the tail of a serpent and the body of a goat (Iliad 6.181-82, Theogony 319ff)

China paralytic syndrome An acute flaccid paralysis of unknown etiology affecting children in northern China every summer, which has been recently described in epidemic proportions among Latin American children; the condition shares certain features of polio and, like polio attacks the motor neurons of the spinal cord (Science 1991; 253:26n&v)

'China white' 3-Methylfentanyl A synthetic ('designer') drug of abuse derived from the anesthetic, fentanyl, which has opiate properties and is 1000-fold more potent than morphine; it has been held responsible for more than 100 overdose deaths in California since 1979, and recently caused an 'epidemic' of overdosage in Pennsylvania (J Am Med Assoc 1991; 265:1011) Note: China white is a generic 'street' term for white powdered agents, either natural, eg heroin or synthetic, eg above that have opiate effects Analysis Solid-phase radioimmunoassay (J Anal Toxicol 1990; 14:172); Cf Adam, 'Ice'

Chinese character appearance Any visual pattern that to the occidental eye simulates Chinese ideographs or kanji, where a relatively monotonous background is punctuated by short, curved well-circumscribed and complexly-arranged densities BONE PATHOLOGY Haphazardly arranged trabeculae in woven and immature bone, a light microscopic finding characteristic of fibrous dysplasia MICROBIOLOGY Loosely cohesive clustering of *Corynebacterium* colonies seen by light microscopy, also known as a 'picket fence' arrangement PEDIATRIC DERMATOLOGY A pattern of blisters seen in incontinentia pigmenti (Bloch-Sulzberger and Goltz-Gorlin syndromes), appearing at birth in bizarre linear arrays, almost exclusive to females, associated with congenital ocular anomalies, cerebral malformations and severe neurological defects; the skin lesions heal by crusting, leaving a 'splashed' appearance in their wake

Chinese hamster ovary cell A cell line isolated in 1958 used in research that grows well in culture and spontaneously transforms to a malignant morphology, due to cytoskeletal disorganization; this cell line can be induced to revert to a normal morphology, and CHO's resistance to DNAse I can be reverted to normal with the addition of cyclic AMP (Mutat Res 1980; 74:21)

Chinese hamster ovary cell assay A tissue culture assay to detect a bacterium's production of enterotoxin, where exposure to a toxin-bearing fluid results in cell damage causing the cells to form round clusters (syncytia)

Chinese lantern sign PEDIATRICS A finding in hydranencephaly and poroencephaly seen by transillumination of the infant skull, consisting in a lack of opacification as there are no cerebral hemispheres, although the brain stem and basal ganglia are well-formed; intellectual or voluntary motor development is impossible and most infants die by age 1

'Chinese menu' diseases A highly colloquial term for conditions, the diagnosis of which is based on the presence of major and minor criteria in the patient; these diseases include AIDS-related complex, Behcet disease, Carney syndrome, chronic fatigue syndrome, polymyositis (proximal muscle weakness, electromyographic findings with myopathic changes, muscle biopsy demonstrates necrosis, increased creatinine phosphokinase, dermal lesions); acute rheumatic fever (Jones' criteria), rheumatoid arthritis, lupus erythematosus and tuberous sclerosis (Gomez classification) Note: The coinage refers to a type of menu that was formerly popular in Chinese restaurants where the meals were selected based on one choice of dish from column A and one from column B

Chinese restaurant syndrome An abrupt allergic reaction, the susceptibility to which is an autosomal recessive trait, caused by sensitivity to monosodium glutamate (MSG, a seasoning used in Chinese restaurants and soy sauce) Clinical Severe headaches, numbness, palpitations, vertigo (especially with chronic MSG exposure), thirst, abdominal and chest pains, sweating and flushing Onset: One-half hour postcibum, lasting up to 12 hours

Chip COMPUTERS An integrated circuit that contains a million or more microscopic components etched on a silicon wafer; the term may be considered a generic synonym for microprocessor and is the key component of computers

Chipmunk face A descriptor for the expanded globular maxilla with marrow hyperexpansion into facial bones, combined with prominent epicanthal folds, a physiognomy characteristic of severe β thalassemia of Cooley; Chipmunk facies may also refer to soft tissue swelling, eg diffuse parotid gland swelling, accompanied by xerostomia and reddened eyes, described in Sjoegren syndrome

Chirality Handedness The three-dimensional conformation of a molecule, referring to whether the molecule has a left-handed, levo- or L- orientation, as do most molecules in functioning biological systems or a right-handed, dextro- or D- orientation; chirality is a property integral to the existence of all members of the physical universe, from elementary particles, eg electrons and molecules to higher organisms, chirality was first discovered by Pasteur in 1848 in tartaric acid salts (Sci Am 1990; 262/1:108); see Chemzymes, Thalidomide

Chiropodist see Podiatrist

Chiropractic A system of health care founded in 1895 based on the concept that the nervous system is the single most important determinant of a person's state of health; abnormal nerve function may result in musculoskeletal derangements and aggravate pathological processes in other body regions or organ systems; chiropractic treatment consists of adjustment and manipulation of the vertebral column and extremities, which some chiropractors supplement with physiotherapy, nutritional support and radiography (for diagnostic purposes only), but do not perform surgery or prescribe drugs; there are 30 000 licensed chiropractors in the USA who attend a four-year post-secondary school education in one of 16 schools of chiropractice; Cf Osteopathic medicine

Chisel fracture An incomplete fracture of the head of the radius where the fracture line extends distally from the center of the articular surface

Chi-squared distribution STATISTICS A theoretical frequency distribution representing the sum of the squares of number n (the degrees of freedom), where the normally distributed variables have a mean of zero and a standard deviation of one, thus assuming a Gaussian distribution

Chitterlings An ethnic food popular especially among the Blacks in the American South which, if improperly prepared may result in infections by ***Yersinia enterocolitica*** O:3 (N Engl J Med 1990; 322:984); Chitterlings consist of the external seromuscular layer of the large intestine of the pig, prepared by boiling several times in spices and finally baked to a crisp consistency and served

Chloasma see Melasma

Chloride channel An ion channel in the plasma membrane of most cells with roles in regulating cell volume, transepithelial transport and stabilization of membrane potential in muscle; there is a wide diversity of chloride channels and their importance most evident when the channels are defective, as in cystic fibrosis, where the gene defect translates into a block in cAMP activation of the chloride channel or in certain forms of myotonia (Nature 1990; 348:510)

Chloroquine-resistant malaria Backgound *Plasmodium falciparum*, the parasite responsible for the malignant tertian form of malaria is increasingly resistant to the previously effective chloroquine, a pharmacologic 'staple' used as malaria prophylaxis in visitors to highly endemic regions of western Africa; the exact incidence of chloroquine-resistant ***P falciparum*** malaria is unknown, but may exceed 25% which may be prevented by 250 mg/week of mefloquine (J Am Med Assoc 1991; 265:361)

Chloroma Chloro, Greek, green A variant of granulocytic leukemia, remarkable for the greenish color (due to neutrophil myelo- or verdoperoxidase) seen in freshly sectioned tissue; notably, a 'green tumor' may precede marrow and peripheral blood involvement by years; first described in 1811 as a retro-orbital, paranasal and lacrimal tumor composed of masses of immature (primitive) granulocytes; since the color is not always present, the term granulocytic sarcoma is preferred, often occurring in acute myelocytic leukemia (2.5-8.0% of which have granulocytic sarcoma); some data suggest the granulocytic sarcoma may be two-fold more common in chronic myeloid leukemia and associated with: Polycythemia vera and myelofibrosis with myeloid metaplasia **Clinical, childhood form** Acute, often presenting as an orbital tumor mass with ocular proptosis with intracranial, soft tissue, gastrointestinal tract, gonadal, mammary, cutaneous, nodal, paranasal sinusoidal masses; axial bones, eg skull and paranasal may be involved with subperi- and periosteal tumefactions and local bone destruction **Clinical, adult form** Chronic, often painful due to cranial and spinal cord compression, followed by motor dysfunction; male:female, 2:1; a leukemic phase may develop 1-49 months after the onset of chloroma symptomatology **Laboratory** Sheets of myeloblasts that are positive for naphthyl ASD and chloroacetate esterase enzymes

Chlorosis Virgin's disease, Green sickness A term first used in 1681 for iron deficiency anemia, named for the yellow-green skin pallor of its young female victims; other findings included: Koilonychia and increased jugular venous pressure; in adult women, iron deficiency is associated with hypochlorhydria and premature graying

CHO cell see Chinese hamster ovary cell

Chocolate A comestible prepared from ground and roasted beans of the cacao plant, native to South America, ***Theobroma cacao*** and composed of cocoa butter, a substance high in stearic acid, converted in vivo to oleic acid, possibly lowering cholesterol levels; one-third of cocoa butter is palmitic acid, which evokes elevation of cholesterol Note: Carob, the sweet pulp of a Mediterranean evergreen leguminous tree, ***Ceratonia siliquia*** is a chocolate surrogate (produced for those who are either truly allergic to chocolate or who adhere to the tenet that chocolate is inherently evil) is high in palm kernel oil, ie a 'tropical oil', thus considered to be atherogenic and is high in sodium, ergo associated with hypertension; chocolate craving is regarded as more intense in females and may be associated with increased progesterone levels and theobromine may be the chemical in chocolate responsible for the intense cravings in those people who are facetiously known as 'choco-holics' Note: Chocolate was the ceremonial brew of Aztecs, Mayas and Toltecs and returned with Columbus to the Royal Court of Spain, where it remained a state secret until it was stolen by the Italians in 1606; chocolate was first consumed in the solid form in 1847

Chocolate agar Chocolatized agar Blood agar that has been heated to open the pyrrole ring, forming hemin, a required growth medium for bacteria not possessing hemolysins, usually grown in a microaerophilic (3-10% CO_2) environment, providing an ideal growth medium for ***Haemophilus influenzae, Neisseria*** species and fastidious anaerobes

Chocolate cyst Endometrioma GYNECOLOGY A periadnexal or ovarian cyst filled with thick inspissated, old and unclotted blood, seen in endometriosis that grossly is likened to chocolate Note: Carcinoma occurs in approximately 0.5% of ovarian endometriosis and is usually of the endometrioid or clear cell types, more often seen in women younger than those with 'garden variety' ovarian carcinomas

'Chokes' The 'chokes' Sudden onset of respiratory distress occurring in Caisson's disease which is associated with pulmonary edema, hemorrhage, atelectasis and emphysema, thought due to an increase in platelet adhesion to gas bubbles that release vasoconstrictors and platelet factor 3, causing coagulopathy

Choked disc Papilledema with swelling of the nerve head, caused by increased intracranial pressure with edema-induced blurring of the disc margins and obliteration of the optic cup, elevation of the nerve head, capillary congestion, hyperemia, venous engorgement, loss of venous pulse, peripapillary exudates, retinal wrinkling and punctate nerve fiber layer hemorrhage; if the pressure is reduced, the fundus returns to normal without loss of vision; increased intracranial pressure is due to meningoencephalitis, hemorrhage, metabolic disease, toxins, trauma and tumors; see also Pseudotumor cerebri

Cholecystokinin (CCK) A 33-residue peptide, the activity of which resides in the 8 N-terminal amino acids (CCK-8), CCK is released from the small intestinal mucosa by certain amino acids, eg tryptophan and phenylalanine and medium- to long-chain fatty acids; CCK stimulates gall bladder contraction, pancreatic acinar cell secretion, relaxes the sphincter of Oddi and induces satiety in food-deprived rats; see hormone Families

Cholera cot Hybrid hospital equipment, consisting of a combination cama-commode, required in *Vibrio cholera* infection, as the victims are flat on their backs with no place to go Note: In the late 20th century, cholera epidemics have become vanishingly rare, with the notable exception of the recent South American epidemic (MMWR 1991; 40:108)

Cholera toxin A heat-sensitive enterotoxin produced by *Vibrio cholera* composed of five 11.6 kD cell-binding B subunits forming a ring around a finger-like 27 kD (Nature 1991; 351:371, 351) catalase that transfers ADP-ribose to a G protein, locking adenyl cyclase in the 'on' position; cholera toxin's functional properties are shared by pertussis toxin, diphtheria toxin and exotoxin A

Cholesterol BIOCHEMISTRY Cholesterol levels are closely linked to atherosclerosis and thus incriminated in cardio- and cerebrovascular disease; total cholesterol > 6.21 mmol/L (US: > 240 mg/dl) is associated with a high risk, 5.17-6.18 mmol/L (US: 200-239 mg/dl) is associated with a 'borderline' risk and < 5.17 mmol/L (US: 200 mg/dl) is associated with a low risk for atherosclerotic heart disease; other high risks include: LDL-cholesterol > 160 mg/dl, HDL-cholesterol < 35 mg/dl; Low risks LDL-cholesterol < 130 mg/dl, HDL-cholesterol > 55 mg/dl Note: All subjects in high and borderline groups should have LDL-cholesterol levels measured and other atherosclerosis risk factors determined; LDL-cholesterol > 130 mg/dl, requires dietary control; LDL-cholesterol that remains > 160 mg/dl after 3-6 months of diet, requires drug therapy, especially in those with HDL-cholesterol < 35 mg/dl (Am J Cardiol 1990; 65:7F) Note: Cholesterol levels undergo a slow decline in evolving colonic carcinoma, thus serving as a 'soft' criterion for cancer (J Am Med Assoc 1990; 263: 2083) Note: transgenic mice that overexpress LDL-receptors have reduced cholesterol levels (Science 1990; 250:1273); see Hypercholesterolemia

Cholesterol-lowering drugs *PRESCRIBING PRACTICES, USA* (J Am Med Assoc 1990; 263:2185); the most cost-efficient in reducing low-density lipoprotein are niacin and lovastatin; the most efficient in increasing high-density lipoprotein levels are niacin and gemfibrozil (J Am Med Assoc 1990; 264:3025) *TYPES OF DRUGS AVAILABLE 1) BILE ACID SEQUESTRANTS* Colestyramine, cholestipol are used to treat hypercholesterolemia, enhancing hepatic catabolism of cholesterol to bile acids *2) NICOTINIC ACID* suppresses hepatic synthesis of lipoprotein Note: Both niacin and bile acid sequestrants are poorly tolerated and may cause hepatitis (Mayo Clin Proc1991; 66:23) *3) FIBRIC ACIDS* Clofibrate, gemfibrozil, fenofibrate; fibric acid's mechanism of action is unknown; these agents cause a modest (10-20%) reduction in serum cholesterol *4) PROBUCOL* reduces cholesterol by enhancing the clearance of LDLs, but also reduces serum HDL, an undesired effect; long-term probucol therapy delays the onset of atherosclerosis in Watanabe rabbits, an animal model of atherosclerosis *5) INHIBITORS OF 3-HYDROXY-3-METHYGLUTARYL-COENZYME A (HMG-COA) REDUCTASE,* a rate-limiting step in cholesterol synthesis; this family of compounds was isolated in 1976 from ***Penicillium citrinum*** (Compactin or mevastatin, Lovastatin) and first approved by the FDA (1987); lovastatin with gemfibrozil may cause severe myopathy and life-threatening rhabdomyolysis with renal failure and is a combination discouraged by the US Food & Drug Administration (J Am Med Assoc 1990; 264:71)

CHOLESTEROL THERAPY	C	L20	L40
Total cholesterol	-17%	- 27%	- 37%
LDL Cholesterol	-23%	- 32%	- 42%
VLDL Cholesterol	—	- 34%	- 31%
Apolipoprotein B	-21%	- 28%	- 33%
Apolipoprotein A-II	—	+ 8%	+13%
HDL Cholesterol	+ 8%	+ 9%	+ 8%
Apolipoprotein A-I	+ 7%	+ 6%	+ 11%
Triglycerides	+11%	- 21%	- 27%
GI side effects*	58%	13%	14%

*Dyspepsia, myopathy and increased alanine transferase (J Am Med Asso 1988; 260:359); Cholestyramine, 12 g/day (C); lovastatin, 20 mg/d (L20); 40 mg/d (L40) tid:

Cholesterol pneumonia see Lipoid pneumonia

Cholesterol-raising fatty acids Exogenous dietary lipids that increase total and/or LDL-cholesterol, eg palmitic acid, myristic acid, trans-monounsaturated fatty acids and probably also lauric acid (N Engl J Med 1990; 323:481ed); see Tropical oils

Cholesteryl-ester transfer protein (CETP) A 74 kD hydrophobic plasma glycoprotein that facilitates the transfer of cholesteryl esters from their site of synthesis in HDL to lipoproteins containing apolipoprotein B; CETP deficiency has only been described in Japanese cohorts, possibly due to a 'founder effect' as the mutation is the same in all the identified persons with the defect which is associated with increased longevity, possibly related to the antiatherogenic effect of CETP deficiency (N Engl J Med 1990; 323:1234)

Cholestyramine resin A bile acid sequestering drug used as a first-line LDL-cholesterol-reducing drug, which acts by increasing hepatic catabolism of cholesterol Note: Some 'soft' data suggest that long-term therapy is associated with a two-fold increase in malignancies of the gastrointestinal tract

Cholinergic crisis see Myasthenic crisis

CHOP A chemotherapeutic regimen used for low and intermediate-grade lymphomas; Cyclophosphamide (750

mg/m2, IV, day 1), Adriamycin (doxorubicin, 50 mg/m^2, IV, day 1), Oncovin (1.4 mg/m^2, to a maximum dose of 2 mg, IV, day 1), Prednisone (100 mg, PO, days 1-5, repeat every 3 days); CHOP produces remission in 65% of previously untreated low-grade lymphomas and 35-45% remission in the intermediate-grade lymphomas Note: a second 'generation' of combinations of these agents demonstrates up to 60% remission in early reports; see Chemotherapy, Remission

Chorea gravidarum Choreiform movement that may appear in the first trimester of pregnancy, occasionally reappearing with subsequent pregnancy Treatment None (given the teratogenic potential of anticonvulsants); if severe, terminate pregnancy

Chordoma A malignant tumor derived from the fetal notochord that appears most commonly in fifth and sixth decade, arising in the sacrococcygeal region and spheno-occipital regions, the latter more common in younger patients Pathology Chordomas are soft, gelatinous and hemorrhagic, having a microscopic appearance fancifully likened to soap bubbles (physaliferous cells) with cleared glycogen-filled cytoplasmic vacuoles Treatment Surgery, radiotherapy Prognosis Recurrence is common, often years after adequate therapy

Chorionic villus biopsy (CVB) A method for early (first trimester) prenatal diagnosis of fetal chromosomal anomalies and other disease; tissue is obtained at 9-11 weeks (vs 16th week for amniotic fluid analysis) from the developing placenta by ultrasound-guided transcervical catheter aspiration biopsy; the tissue obtained is from the chorion frondosum, the layer which develops chorionic villi; the diagnostic yield of CVB is 97.8%; the yield of amniocentesis performed at 16 gestational weeks is 99.4%, CVB has a 30% greater (7.2 % loss vs 5.7%) wastage of normal fetuses; the unanticipated fetal wastage attributed to CVB is 6-8/1000 (N Engl J Med 1989; 320:609)

Choristoma Non-specialized tissue that develops in utero corresponding to microscopically normal cells and tissues located in abnormal sites, eg ectopic breast tissue

Choroideremia Tapetochoidal dystrophy A form of X-linked hereditary retinal degeneration (Other hereditary retinal degenerations include Refsum's disease, gyrate atrophy and a-β–lipoproteinemia), characterized by centripetal loss of visual fields due to a gene mutation localized to chromosome Xq21 (Nature 1990; 347:674)

Christchurch albumin A congenitally altered form of proalbumin (Science 1987; 235:348, Nature 1978; 274:384)

Christchurch chromosome A defective chromosome 1 with loss of the short arm in the cultured cells of a New Zealand family, associated with lymphoproliferative disorders, eg chronic lymphocytic leukemia

Christian Science A religious doctrine established in 1879 by MB Eddy in which therapy, in the form of so-called 'healings', which consist of 'heartfelt yet disciplined prayer' by members of the Christian Scientist Church are administered to the sick in lieu of drugs or most standard measures normally used to alleviate pain; while anecdotal 'healing' testimonials available from the Christian Science Church imply that their form of therapy is better for the care of children than conventional medical therapy, some peer-reviewed reports, eg J Am Med Assoc 1989; 262:1657, suggest the contrary; Christian Scientists do not smoke or drink; Christian Science has major impacts on American medicine: 1) Christian Scientist parents may override the physician'in the care of underage minor children 2) Christian Scientists may be difficult to treat (especially as unconscious victims of trauma), as they may refuse the therapy deemed appropriate by conventional medical thinking, which when administered, may possibly result in civil action 3) Religious exemption statutes allow healers to perform their services ('healing') without liability and at standards of practice that are variance for those expected of physicians and 4) 'Healing' therapy can be billed to an insurance company, Medicare or Medicaid (J Am Med Assoc 1990; 264:1379)

Christiansen-Krabbe disease Krabbe disease Progressive infantile poliodystrophy associated with blindness, seizures, deafness, with onset by age in the first year of life

Christian's triad A classic but rarely observed trio of symptoms in histiocytosis X, consisting of lytic bony lesions, diabetes insipidus and exophthalmos

Christian syndrome An autosomal dominant digital dysmorphia characterized by shortened thumbs and distal phalanxes

Christian-Weber disease Relapsing non-suppurative panniculitis Focal painful aggregates of subcutaneous fat necrosis with erythematous, ulcerating and eventually atrophic skin, seen in corpulent middle-aged women Clinical Fever and the condition may be acute or chronic, fulminating or transient, systemic or confined to the skin and variably associated with polyserositis Etiology Unknown, possibly related to trauma, cold, drugs, chemicals and may occur in patients with lupus erythematosus, rheumatoid arthritis, diabetes mellitus, sarcoidosis, after corticosteroid withdrawal, in acute and chronic pancreatitis and in pancreatic carcinoma Laboratory Increased lipase, amylase

Christmas disease Hemophilia B, Factor IX deficiency

Christmas tree bladder Pine cone bladder A broad, flat and smooth-walled atonic bladder with a flaccid base and a jagged superior funneling into the posterior urethra, described as characteristic of spastic neurogenic bladder, a finding by cystography that may be mimicked by outlet obstruction with superimposed urinary tract infection; diagnosis of neurogenic bladder based on radiologic findings may therefore prove difficult Pathology The bladder is markedly trabeculated, with a peaked dome and attenuated epithelium

Christmas tree deformity PEDIATRIC SURGERY A severe form of jejunoileal atresia in which only a single branch of the superior mesenteric artery fully develops, supplying in a retrograde fashion, a markedly shortened ileum arranged in pattern fancifully likened to a reversed 'christmas tree'

Christmas tree pattern Chevron pattern DERMATOLOGY A clinical finding in pityriasis rosea; the lesions are oval, 1 cm pink-brown papules covered by fine keratinaceous scales, corresponding to parakeratosis, which are aligned parallel to the skin cleavage lines of the trunk; the lesions lasting 2-12 weeks before fading MOLECULAR BIOLOGY A descriptor for appearance seen when a complex of multiple transcribing pre-mRNA molecules arise from a single chain of DNA, see Feather pattern

Christ-Siemens-Touraine syndrome An ectodermal dysplasia with anhidrosis, heat intolerance, hypoplasia of sebaceous and sweat glands causing dry smooth and glossy skin, gonadal hypoplasia, ageusia, anosmia, upper respiratory tract infections, mental retardation, absent nipples, partial anodontia or peg-teeth, hypotrichosis, saddle nose, dysphagia, physical and mental retardation, feminine appearance and cleft palate, predominantly affecting males

Chromatin puff see Chromosome puff

Chromatography A laboratory technique in which mixtures of complex molecules are separated along a gradient of pressure or solubility between a mobile (either liquid or gas) and stationary (solid or liquid) phase; the molecules are separated by absorption, gel filtration, ion exchange or partitioning or a combination of these priciples; see Gas-liquid chromatography, High-performance liquid chromatography, Ion exchange chromatography, Partition chromatography, Thin-layer chromatography

Chromatoid bodies Darkly staining, elongated, relatively well-circumscribed masses, 1-4 in number that are located in amoebic cysts in ***Entamoeba histolytica, E hartmanni, Entamoeba coli*** and ***Endolimax nana***

Chromogranins A family of 20-100 kD acidic glycoproteins present in the soluble fraction of neurosecretory granules, serving as a 'pan-endocrine' marker for neuroendocrine tumors, eg small cell carcinoma; Chromogranins A, B and C have been characterized; the latter two are also known as secretogranin I and II

Chromosomal RNA Oligonucleotide segments of RNA that serve to 'prime' the growth fork of DNA in the lagging strand after DNA duplication; Cf Okazaki fragment

Chromosome A structure present in the eukaryotic nucleus that consists of one or more (23 in humans), usually paired, very long (100 to 300 million base pairs each in humans) DNA molecules that are associated with RNA and histones; the complete complement of chromosomes contain the complete genetic information present in a living organism; chromosomes are classified into groups sharing structural similarity in terms of length from the centromere, divided into group A (chromosomes 1-3), group B (chromosomes 4 and 5), group C (chromosomes 6 to 12 and the X chromosome), group D (chromosomes 13 to 15), group E (chromosomes 16 to 18); group F (chromosomes 19 and 20); group G (chromosomes 21, 22 and the Y chromosome); see Banding, Flow cytometry, Human genome project, Ploidy analysis

Chromosome analysis Karyotyping GENETICS A laboratory procedure in which cells of fetal origin are obtained either in the first trimester by chorionic villus biopsy or later in pregnancy by amniocentesis and grown in a tissue culture medium to detect major chromosomal defects (terminology, table); the technique is indicated for mixed congenital anomalies with mental or growth retardation, infertility, in cryptorchidic testes, ambiguous genitalia, repeated neonatal death, advanced maternal age and in analysis of neoplasia; see Banding; Cf DNA hybridization, Polymerase chain reaction

CHROMOSOMES: KARYOTYPING TERMS

:	Break without union
::	Break and join
cen	Centromere
chi	Chimerism
del	Deletion
der	Unbalanced karyosome
dic	Dicentric
dmin	Double minute
dup	Duplication
i	Isochromosome
inv	Inversion
mos	Mosaicism
p	Short arm (petit)
q	Long arm (the letter ifter p)
r	Ring
ter	
+	A gained chromosome or segment thereof
-	A lost chromosome or segment thereof
→	Site of origin of transfer of a segment of chromosome to another

Chromosome breakage syndromes A group of inherited diseases in which the chromosomes have an increased fragility, eg ataxia-telangiectasia, Bloom, Fanconi, Louis-Bar syndromes and xeroderma pigmentosum, resulting in a marked increase in susceptibility to certain malignancies

Chromosome 'jumping' MOLECULAR BIOLOGY Cloning and mapping of large segments of DNA; see Jumping library

Chromosome puff A localized separation of polytene chromosomes, eg chromosomes of ***Drosophila melanogaster***, which represents a site of active RNA synthesis, ie transcription, which when very large, is known as a Balbiani ring

Chromosome 'walking' MOLECULAR BIOLOGY A time-consuming method that sequences (ie, determines the sequence of) segments of DNA located on either side of a region of a fully characterized (ie, 'sequenced') segment of DNA, 'walking' out in overlapping short fragments of DNA, each 15-20 000 bases in length, from a point of known sequence, enabling one to sequence (ie, determine the sequence of) DNA that is far removed from the marker gene; see Cystic fibrosis gene, Chromosome jumping

Chronic fatigue syndrome (CFS) Akureyri, Yuppie disease, Chronic Epstein-Barr (see below) syndrome, Postviral syndrome A condition first described in the mid-1980s in California, which shares clinical features with epidemic neuromyasthenia, Iceland or Royal Free Hospital disease (N Engl J Med 1988; 319:1726ed); CFS often follows viral infections, eg herpes, hepatitis, cytomegalovirus, or may be induced by an unrecognized virus; the polymerase chain reaction reveals enteroviral RNA sequences in muscle, possibly also in the brain in 53% of CFS, in contrast to 15% of controls (Br Med J 1991; 302:692); the Centers for Disease Control (CDC) case definition requires the presence of Major criteria 1) Recent onset of debilitating or recurring fatigue of > 6 months duration and 2) Exclusion of clinically similar conditions, as well as the presence of eight of ten minor criteria 1) Low-grade fever (< 38.6° C) or chills 2) Sore throat (or pharyngitis) 3) Painful anterior and/or posterior cervical and axillary lymphadenopathy 4) Unexplained muscular weakness 5) Myalgia 6) Generalized fatigue of > 24 hours for previously tolerated exercise 7) Severe generalized headache 8) Migratory arthralgia 9) Neuropsychological complaints, eg photophobia, irritability, inability to concentrate, depression and 10) Sleep disturbance Note: Although CFS had been associated with Epstein-Barr virus infection, more than half of those with the chronic fatigue syndrome improved without a change in EBV titers (J Am Med Assoc 1990; 264:48) Treatment None; the 'cures' reported are thought to be due to placebo effect or spontaneous remission (N Engl J Med 1988; 319:1692);

Chronic granulomatous disease(s) (CGD) A heterogeneous group of immune system defects characterized by recurrent and potentially fatal pyogenic infections of early onset; two-thirds of CGD are X-linked and the remainder autosomal recessive; the neutrophils ingest pathogens, but fail to produce superoxide and related microbicidal oxygen intermediates (the respiratory 'burst') due to defective NADPH oxidase, resulting in recurrent bacterial, eg *Staphylococcus aureus* and *Enterobacteriaceae* and fungal, eg *Aspergillus* species infections with sinusitis, pneumonia and abscess formation; male:female ratio 4:1 Diagnosis Nitrotetrazolium blue test Incubation of patient neutrophils with nitrotetrazolium blue (NTB); normal NADPH oxidase digests NTB to a toxic product, causing cell lysis, which appears as blue blobs on the peripheral smear; in CGD, the NBT is negative due to defective NADPH oxidase, a multicomponent complex of a membrane-bound heterodimeric cytochrome b, composed of glycosylated heavy 91 kD (gp91-phox) and light 22 kD (gp22-phox) components of the enzyme and two or more cytosolic proteins (p47-phox and p67-phox); the mutation in the X-linked CGD lies in the gp91-phox gene and in the autosomal recessive CGD in the p47-phox gene Treatment Interferon-γ may be used on a maintenance basis in these patients to reduce the incidence of serious infection (N Engl J Med 1991; 324:509), the mechanism of which may be related to a 'boost' in other components of the immune system

Chronic mucocutaneous candidiasis see APECED

Chronic obstructive pulmonary (or lung) disease (COPD, COLD) An umbrella term for pulmonary diseases with partially overlapping signs and symptoms, including asthma, bronchiectasis, chronic bronchitis and emphysema; COPD, usually associated with a long history of cigarette smoking, is the fifth most common cause of death (65 000 annual deaths), the third most common (after heart diseases and schizophrenia) cause of chronic disability of older individuals and the most common cause of pulmonary hypertension and cor pulmonale in the USA; the major COPD lesions, chronic bronchitis and emphysema commonly coexist; the former is responsible for the alveolar hypoxia, low PO_2, high CO_2 and low pH that lead to pulmonary hypertension; the latter is seen in 65% of males at autopsy and 15% of females and is due to the unopposed effect of elastases within the lungs; patients with COPD have been divided into type A, ie those with emphysema, fancifully known as a Pink puffer and type B, ie chronic bronchitis, known as a Blue bloater; respiratory function and dyspnea in severe COPD may improve with theophylline therapy, which improves respiratory-muscle function (N Engl J Med 1989; 320:1521)

Chubby puffer syndrome A sleep apnea complex affecting obese, prepubescent males resembling those with Pickwick syndrome, caused by primary alveolar hypoventilation; although temporarily ameliorated by tonsillectomy, the condition is more central, possibly arising in the reticular activating system Treatment Weight loss or tricyclic antidepressants; Cf Pink puffer

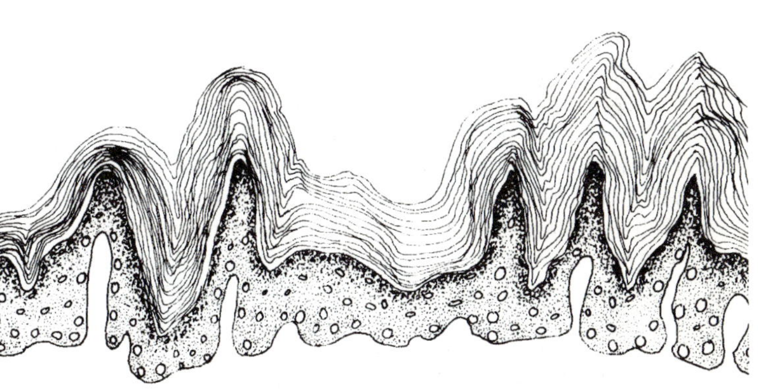

Church spire pattern

Church spire pattern DERMATOPATHOLOGY Irregular epidermal acanthosis and hyperkeratosis simulating church spires; classically seen in seborrheic keratosis, but also occurs in: Acanthosis nigricans, actinic keratosis, papillary intradermal nevi, 'stucco' keratosis, verruca vulgaris and erythrokeratoderma variabilis

Chylomicronemia syndrome A clinical complex characterized by marked chylomicronemia with plasma triglyceride levels in excess of 225 mmol/L (US: 2000 mg/dl) Clinical Abdominal and chest pain, pancreatitis, memory defects, carpal tunnel-like paresthesiae, hepatospleno-megaly,chronic eruptive xanthomata and insulin resistant diabetes, possibly related to marked hypertriglyceridemia; symptoms are exacerbated by alcohol, β-adrenergic blockers, diuretics, estrogens and glucocorticoids

CIC Circulating immune complexes see Immune complexes

CID Cytomegalic inclusion disease see CMV

CIE 1) see Counterimmunoelectrophoresis, 2) Cross immunoelectrophoresis

Cigar bodies A descriptor for short, finger-like structures MICROBIOLOGY A descriptor for the morphology of the yeast form of ***Sporo-thrix schenckii***, seen microscopically with a lactophenol cotton blue stain; see Alcoholic gardener syndrome VETERINARY PATHOLOGY A descriptor for the ultrastructural morphology of insulin granules in the β cells of the canine pancreas

Cigarette paper scales A descriptor for the flattened, flaked keratotic scales found on the trunk in pityriasis rosea, which are round to oval, salmon-colored and peripherally attached patches that follow the lines of cleavage, likened to a christmas tree

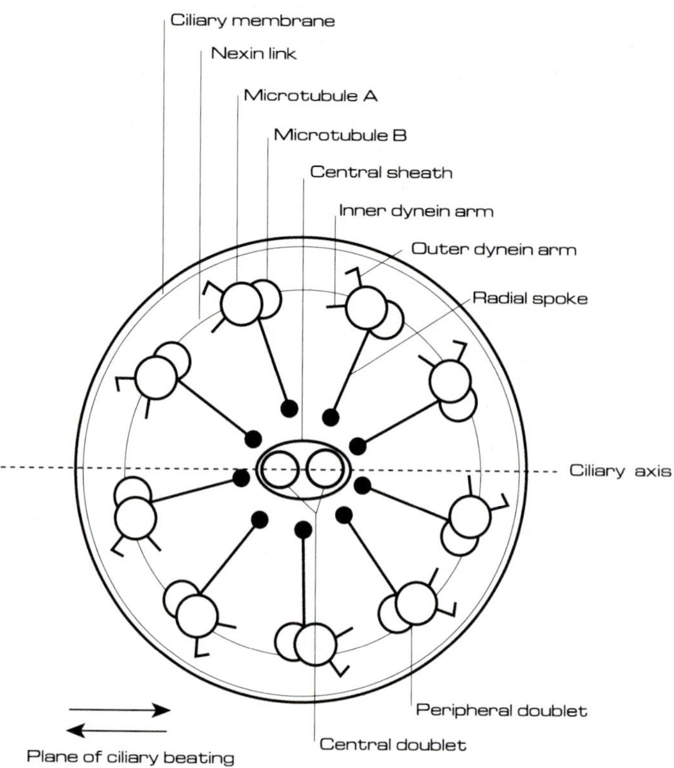

Cigarette-paper skin A descriptor for the markedly attenuated skin with a shiny, velvety surface seen in Ehlers-Danlos syndrome, type I (less commonly also in type II), caused by defective synthesis, processing or stability of types I and III collagen **Clinical** Premature rupture of membranes, tearing out of sutures and poor wound healing Ultrastructure Irregular and enlarged collagen fibers

Cigarettes see Fetal tobacco syndrome, Passive smoking, Smoking

Ciguatera poisoning The ciguatera, a coral reef fish, in his battle to remain a coral reef inhabitant, secretes ichthyosarcotoxin (ciguatoxin, a lipid-soluble, heat-stable substance isolated from bottom-dwelling fish in temperate and tropical zones), which is produced by the reef dinoflagellate, ***Gambierdiscus toxicus*** and concentrated, unchanged up the food chain by herbivores and carnivores; ciguatera poisoning is the most common marine intoxication in the USA, 400 species are implicated, including barracuda, grouper, red snapper, amberjack, surgeonfish, sea bass and (unlike scombroid poisoning) may cause morbidity regardless of the form of preparation **Clinical** Onset 6-12 hours after ingestion with nausea, vomiting, cramping, diarrhea, paresthesias, reversal of temperature sense, arthralgias, myalgias, cranial nerve palsies, pruritus with alcohol ingestion, chills, hypotension, bradycardia, respiratory paralysis or death, average duration 8 days **Diagnosis** RIA or ELISA **Treatment** IV mannitol completely and rapidly reverses symptoms (J Am Med Assoc 1988; 259:2740); Cf Scombroid poisoning

Cilia Whiplike, motile structures that extend from the plasma membranes, comprising a major structural 'motif' in eukaryotes consisting of a 9 + 2 pattern (see illustration) of nine peripherally-placed doublets and a centrally-placed doublet of microtubular filaments; in contrast, centrioles and basal bodies have a 9 + 3 motif; the ciliary motif is found at all phylogenic levels, from bacterial flagella to the human cilia of the upper respiratory tract, choroid plexus, axial thread of the chromosome, spermatozoa and fallopian tubes; cilia movement occurs in either a metachronous or isochronous fashion; human diseases affecting the cilia include a) Choroid plexus carcinoma and papillomas, which have a 9 + 0 configuration b) Immotile cilia syndrome, in which the dynein arms are absent **Clinical** Recurrent sinopulmonary infections, decreased female fertility and sperm motility c) Kartagener syndrome, which is similar to the immotile cilia syndrome, but has in addition, situs inversus, sinusitis and bronchiectasis and d) Young syndrome

Ciliary neurotrophic factor (CNTF) A small polypeptide of neuronal origin that promotes in vivo survival of motoneurons (Science 1991; 251:1616)

CIN Cervical intraepithelial neoplasia A malignancy arising in uterine cervical epithelium and confined thereto, representing a continuum of histological changes ranging from well-differentiated CIN 1, (formerly, mild dysplasia) to severe dysplasia/carcinoma in situ, CIN 3; the lesion arises at the squamocolumnar cell junction at the transformation zone of the endocervical canal, with a variable tendency to develop invasive epidermoid carcinoma, a tendency that is enhanced by concomitant human papillomaviral infection, of which HPV 6 and 11 are associated with the 'garden variety', ie benign condylomas; HPV types 16, 18 occur in CIN 3, while types 31, 33, 35, 52, 56 may appear in CIN; see Carcinoma in situ, Intraepithelial neoplasia

Cinchonism A mild toxic state that develops when the plasma levels of the antimalarial agent, quinine exceed 10-12 mg/L **Clinical** Flushed and sweaty skin, tinnitus, blurred vision, dizziness, nausea, vomiting and diarrhea; truly toxic levels are associated with skin rashes, somnolence, blindness and profound hypotension

'Cinderella' A colloquialism of minimal utility for a relatively neglected area of medicine, a 'forgotten' disease or organism; Cinderella is the rag-beclad heroine in the children's story from Perault's Mother Goose tales

'Cinderella dermatosis' A fanciful synonym for erythema dyschronicum perstans (ashy dermatosis), a term originating from its analogy to Cinderella, who was covered in ashes while she carried out menial tasks

Circadian rhythm Zeitgeber The diurnal cadence; without cyclical cues provided by light, man's daily rhythm is 25.4 hours; the internal clock may reside in the pineal gland, derived embryologically from the ependyma at the roof of the third ventricle, an aggregate of parenchymal cells surrounded by a neuroglial network, weighing 100-180 mg, with direct retinal innervation (retinohypothalamic tract), which is thought to act by secreting melatonin; in rats, the 'biogenic oscillator' resides in the ventral hypothalamus, in hamsters, in the suprachiasmatic nucleus (Science 1990; 247:95); biological clocks affect drug metabolism, production of substances measured to detect and monitor disease, myocardial ischemia and oxygen demand (J Am Med Assoc 1991; 265:386), psychosomatic disease and sleep disorders, which may be thrown out of synchronization by shiftwork, and may be reset or completely suppressed by a light stimulus at a critical time and at a critical strength (Nature 1991; 350:59, 18); daily peaks are described for hormonal secretion, eg adrenal gland, drug metabolism, eg antacids, halothane, physiologic activities, eg blood pressure, cell division, hematopoiesis, natural killer cell activity; see Insomnia, Jet lag, Melatonin, Shift work

Circular A-21 A document generated by the US Office of Management and Bureau that prescribes the general guidelines for the (indirect) costs, eg 'overhead' that may be cahrged to the recipients of federally-funded grants and contracts by educational institutions (Science 1991; 252:636n&v); see Indirect costs

Circular DNA A 65-200 kilobase fragment of DNA formed by a process of 'looping out and deletion', containing a constant region of the μ heavy chain (Cμ) and the 3' part of the u 'switch' region joined to the 5' part of the switch segment for the class to which the cell has switched; circular DNA is a normal product of rearrangement among gene segments encoding the variable regions of immunoglobulin light and heavy chains, as well as the T cell receptor (Nature 1990; 345:452)

Circulating lupus anticoagulant syndrome (CLAS) The association of recurrent thromboses (including cerebral), repeated spontaneous abortions and renal disease frequently in ANA-negative lupus patients has been termed the circulating lupus anticoagulant syndrome with repeated fetal wastage and an IgM gammopathy (J Am Med Assoc 1985; 253:3278)

Circulating nurse A nurse who participates in a surgical procedure, coordinating, planning and implementing all the nurse-related activities during an operation, who has not scrubbed with surgical team itself; see Scrub nurse

Circumcision Surgical removal of the foreskin, either by an obstetrician, or as a part of a religious rite (the Bris), by a rabbi; the American Academy of PEDIATRICS recommends (Pediatrics 1989; 84:388) circumcision as it reduces the incidence of balanitis (Arch Dermatol 1990; 126:1046), balanoposthitis, phimosis, colonization by fimbriated pyelonephritogenic ***Escherichia coli*** and other bacteria, urinary tract infection (urinary tract infections are 10-20 times more common in uncircumcised boys); the lifetime risk for penile cancer in uncircumcised males is 600-fold greater than circumcised males; the risk for cancer of the uterine cervix is closely linked to human papillomavirus infections (HPV 16 in 50% and HPV 18 in 10%) in uncircumcised male partners; the incidence of sexually-transmitted diseases, eg genital herpes, syphilis, gonorrhea, chancroid and HIV-1 is lower in the circumspect and circumcised (N Engl J Med 1990; 322:1308, 1312)

'Circumcision', female see Female circumcision

Circumoral pallor A rim of pale perioral skin seen in scarlet fever

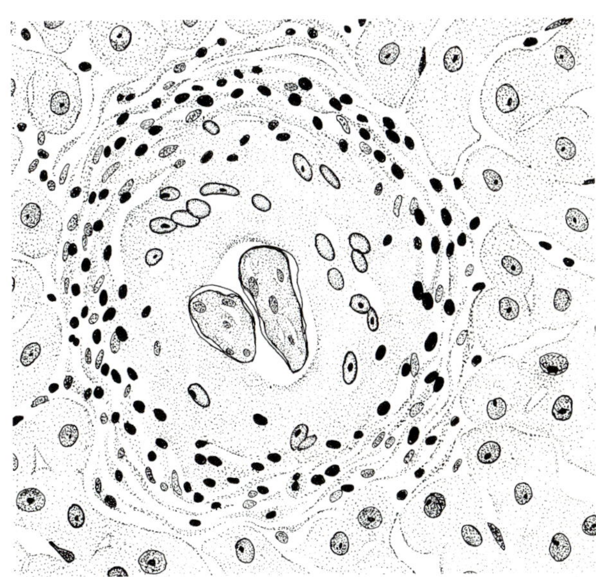

Circumoval body

Circumoval bodies Granulomas in schistosomal infections that surround the eggs (or ova, hence the name); circumoval bodies are found histologically in the bladder, caused by *S haematobium* or in the liver (see above figure) due to *S mansoni* **Histopathology** Schistosomal egg partially or completely rimmed by a foreign-body giant cell reaction with concentric fibrosis and a lymphocyte and plasma cell response; with time, the liver develops marked fibrosis, whereupon it is termed 'pipestem fibrosis'

Circumstantial homosexuality The practice of homosexual acts when there are no opportunities for heterosexual activity, most commonly occurring in adolescents in detention centers, youth prisons and residential treatment centers, which may be accompanied by sadism and sexual exploitation Note: Homosexual experimentation is not thought to predict future homosexual behavior

Circus movement Reentry or reciprocal movement CARDIOLOGY Circus movement forms the basis for some (if not all) supraventricular tachycardia and requires that there be a) An available circuit of conducting tissue b) A difference in refractoriness in the two limbs of the circuit and c) A rate of conduction through the tissue that is slow enough in the less refractory limb so that the more refractory limb has had time to recover when the circus impulse approaches a second time; Supraventricular flutter and fibrillation are likely due to an ectopic pacemaker

Cirrhotic glomerulonephritis Renal disease related to liver failure; subendothelial and mesangial thickening of glomerular basement membrane, with fusion of the epithelial foot processes seen in patients with micro- or macronodular cirrhosis; Cf Hepatorenal syndrome

CIS see Carcinoma-in-situ

cis MOLECULAR BIOLOGY A mutation that is active only when it is on the same chromosome, but not when it is on the opposite chain is said to be cis-active, if the mutation is active at another chromosome site or on another chain, it is trans-active

***cis*-activation** cis-acting locus A region of the DNA molecule affecting genes located on the same, ie not opposite or trans molecule; Cf trans-activation

cis-platinum diaminedichloride A chemotherapeutic agent that forms covalant bonds and crosslinks with DNA, used to treat head and neck, ovarian, testicular and bladder cancer **Side effects** Nephrotoxicity, requiring adequate hydration to maintain renal flow and high chloride concentration; nausea is a constant feature of cisplatinum therapy, which responds to Ondansetron, a selective antagonist of serotonin S_3 receptors

Cistron Structural gene MOLECULAR BIOLOGY A unit of genetic information or an independent transactive complementation unit of DNA that was thought to encode one polypeptide; the term is no longer used as it lends to confusion, as it is defined by techniques that have fallen into disuse

Citation classic An article or abstract in a scientific journal that has been cited in the subsequent biomedical literature more than four hundred times, an objective criterion specified by the Institute for Scientific Information (J Lab Clin Med 1990; 116:755); Citation classics are often examined by the Nobel committee as a benchmark of original work; see Landmark article; Cf Uncitedness index

Citation impact (CI) A major parameter for measuring the importance of a scientific report is the frequency with which it is cited in subsequent scientific literature; CI is a datum generated by the ISI (Institute of Scientific Information, Philadelphia) from their science indicators database, which generally ignores laboratory techniques; the highest citation impact is produced by the workers at Harvard, where each paper was cited an average of 24.63 times (Science 1990; 247:1183) discounting-methodology papers, the CI is used by the Nobel institute for evaluating future candidates for Nobel prizes Note: Of the 894 most cited papers in biology identified by the ISI, the 220 researchers sponsored by the Howard Hughes Medical Institute accounted for 82, while the 3000 scientists of the National Institute of Health (USA) accounted for 84; the disadvantage of the CI is that some papers may win a high citation score because they are erroneous or use poorly designed studies, attracting critical citations, as occurred with cold fusion (Science 1991; 252:639n&v)

Cited scientist Most cited scientist A scientist whose research is considered by his peers to be of sufficient merit to cite in bibliographies of their own research reports; for the decade from 1981-90, the 35 papers from J Messing (molecular biology, Rutgers) were cited 18 229 times; the 93 papers of MJ Berridge (biochemistry, Cambridge) were cited 16 004 times and the 81 papers of T Maniatis (molecular biology, Harvard) were cited 11 167 times (Science 1991; 254:28n); Note: Techniques that represent major advances in methodology may be reason for frequent citation, and unless it is coupled with a major theoretical advance, may not be considered of Nobel prize-winning potential

CJD Creutzfeldt-Jakob disease, see Prions, Spongiform encephalopathy

CJM Cell junction molecule A protein, similar in function to cell adhesion molcules and surface adhesion molecules (SAMs) but which is a component of complex intercellular junctions, including belt, gap, spot and tight junctions

CK-MB Creatinine phosphokinase, MB isoenzyme LABORATORY MEDICINE An isoform of CK that is typically increased in myocardial infarction, which may also be increased in muscular dystrophy, polymyositis, myoglobinuria, occasionally in malignancy, eg lung cancer, all possibilities that must be considered in the face of an elevated CK-MB without myocardial infarction

CLA A conjugated dienoic derivative of linoleic acid (an 18-carbon essential polyunsaturated fatty acid), in which the two pairs of double bonds are separated by a single carbon instead of a pair of carbons (like normal linoleic acid); the double bond position shift may be induced by heating, free-radical oxidation and enzymatic reaction; CLA is present in cheese and cooked meat and may be anti-carcinogenic, incorporating itself directly into the protected cells, quenching oxygen free radicals and singlet oxygen (Med Oncol Tumor Pharmacol 1990; 7:169); Cf PUFAs

'Clap' Sexually-transmitted disease A colloquial sobriquet for gonorrhea, derived from either a) Provencal, clap, a heap of stones, from which rabbits made their homes, evolving in Old French to rabbit's burrow, arriving in Middle English as clap(er) a brothel or b) Middle French, clapoir, a bubo Note: Since buboes are not seen in gonorrhea, the latter origin is unlikely

Clark, Barney A dentist who was the first patient to receive a completely artificial heart, the Jarvik 7, in an operation performed by cardiovascular surgeon, William de Vries at the University Hospital in Salt Lake City; Clark later died of renal failure and on postmortem examination had pseudomembranous colitis (N Engl J Med 1984; 310:273); see Artificial heart, Jarvik 7

CLAS 1) Cholesterol-Lowering Atherosclerosis Study A randomized, placebo-controlled trial using colestipol and niacin in men with previous coronary artery bypass surgery; in treated subjects, elevated triglyceride-rich lipoproteins have a major role in atherogenesis (Circulation 1990; 81:470); CLAS/CLAS-II at the four-year mark continue to demonstrate the benefits of this regimen on blood lipids, lipoprotein-cholesterol and apoprotein and nonprogression of atherosclerotic lesions and/or regression (J Am Med Assoc 1990; 264:3013) 2) Circulating lupus anticoagulant syndrome see Anticardiolipin antibody syndrome, Lupus anticoagulant

Clasp knife phenomenon NEUROLOGY A manifestation of corticospinal spasticity in which there is increased tone in either flexion or extension with sudden relaxation as the muscle continues to be stretched, imparting a sensation fancifully likened to that of an opening clasp knife; this effect is often accompanied by weakness of the affected extremity, increased tendon reflexes and a Babinski sign; Cf Cogwheel phenomenon, Gegenhalten

Class action (lawsuit) A legal action undertaken by one or more plaintiffs on the behalf of themselves and all other persons with an identical interest in an alleged wrong; in the US, a number of medically-related class action suits have appeared, resulting in prolonged legal battles with settlements by the product manufacturer(s) allegedly at fault costing hundreds of millions of dollars to settle the claims; see Agent Orange, Dalkon shield, Shiley valve

Classic pathway IMMUNOLOGY The usual route of activation of the complement cascade (the non-specific arm of the immune system, which is responsible for lysis of target organisms and cells); the classic pathway is initiated by C1q binding to either IgM or to two adjacent IgG molecules; the resulting conformational change of C1q autoactivates C1r2, in turn activating C1s2, cleaving C4 (C4b) followed by C2 (C2a); C4b,2a, the C3 convertase of the classic complement pathway, initiates opsonization, leukocyte chemotaxis, increased vascular permeability and finally cytolysis; the classic complement pathway is activated by IgG, IgM, DNA, staphylococcal protein A and C-reactive protein; both the classic and alternate pathways are stimulated by trypsin-like enzymes; see Common pathway; Cf Alternate pathwat

Class switching Physiology A step in the normal maturation of hemoglobin during fetal development requires switching from embryonal zeta chain, which is structurally similar to the α chain, and occurs on chromosome 16 to mature α chain production; β chain production is a two stage maturation process with early loss of the ε chain, the presence during fetal and early post-natal life of a γ chain, the decrease of which coincides with increased expression of the β chain

Clathrin MEMBRANE PHYSIOLOGY A heterodimeric membrane transport protein, composed of one heavy (80 kD) and several light (20-40 kD)chains that polymerize three-legged protein complexes, termed triskelions, which aggregate into 'patches' at the internal face of the cell membrane forming a cage-like polyhedral lattice around the coated pits and vesicles and mediate selective transport events; clathrin is pivotal in transport vesicle biogenesis, facilitating receptor transport by concentrating and sorting the receptors into specific intracellular compartments, eg Golgi apparatus and endosomes (Science 1988; 242:1396), while retaining Golgi membrane protein within the cell (Science 1989; 245:1358); clathrin thus acts as a shuttle molecule, endlessly cycling between the membrane and lysosome; Cf Golgi-derived coated vesicle

Claw finger A deformity that results from combined paralysis of the median and ulnar nerves, characterized by hyperextension of the metacarpophalangeal joint and hyperflexion of the proximal interphalangeal joints Treatment Tenodesis, capsulodesis or arthrodesis

Claw foot Pied en griffe A foot deformity due to atrophic paralysis of the intrinsic foot muscles, allowing the long extensors of the toes to dorsiflex the proximal phalanges and the long flexors to shorten the foot, heighten the arch and flex the distal phalanges, pulling the foot into talipes equinus; claw foot occurs in chronic polyneuropathies and is characteristic of Charcot-Marie-Tooth disease; Cf Lobster claw deformity

Claw hand Main en griffe The hand deformity may follow the claw foot deformity of Charcot-Marie-Tooth disease, where the atrophy is usually confined to the distal arm and may occur in Dejerine-Sottas' hypertrophic polyneuropathy and Refsum's disease; a similar 'stiff hand' occurs in mucopolysaccharidosis, type I-S; Cf Lobster claw deformity

Claw toes A deformity characterized by metatarsophalangeal joint hyperextension and interphalangeal joint flexion, usually associated with neuropathic conditions, eg Friedrich's ataxia, poliomyelitis and spinal cord injury, which may occur in a familial setting Pathogenesis Although paralysis of the intrinsic muscles of the foot is a commonly evoked explanation, the muscles are functionally and histologically normal Clinical Incapacitating and painful callosities at the 'new' pressure points, especially of the great toe Treatment Conservative, tendon resection, joint resection

Clean (adjective) Free of dirt or pollution; clean is used colloquially for an organ or tissue lacking pathological findings, eg 'clean' coronary arteries and aorta are typically seen at autopsy in persons dying with terminal cancer or alcoholism

Clean wound A superficial wound produced by uncontaminated sharp objects, either electively, eg surgical procedure or by accident, being cut by sharp glass or metal, eg broken glass; clean wounds theoretically do not require antibiotic coverage or tetanus prophylaxis (although it is commonly administered, often as an act of 'defensive' medicine; see Dirty wound

Clearance The theoretical volume from which the drug is totally removed in a unit time; see Therapeutic drug monitoring

Clear (light) cells HISTOLOGY Finely vacuolated, cholesterol-filled cells with central dark nuclei arranged in clusters and located in the midzone or zona fasciculata of the adrenal cortex; these cells are thought to be the major reserve for glucocorticoid and sex hormone production when the adrenal gland is stressed; see Compact (dark) cells

Clear cell acanthoma DERMATOLOGY A sharply demarcated, solitary lesion of the legs that mimics seborrheic keratosis and pyogenic granuloma **Histopathology** Enlarged clear, glycogen-filled basal cells, mild spongiosis, elongated intertwining rete ridges, parakeratosis with few granular cells and weak DOPA positivity; it is unclear whether this is a tumor or a hyperplasia

Clear cell adenocarcinoma A malignancy of the vagina and uterine cervix, two-thirds of which cases have occurred in young women who were exposed in utero to estrogen analogues, especially diethylstilbestrol (DES) as well as hexestrol or dienestrol; relative risk for those exposed, 0.014; 5-year survival, 80+% with local recurrence **Histopathology** Tubes and cysts lined by clear cells, admixed with solid areas and papillary formations

Clear cell carcinoma 1) ENDOMETRIUM A tumor of elderly women, of presumed müllerian origin **Histopathology** Solid, papillary, tubular and cystic arrangement of glycogen-filled 'hobnail' cells, once described as 'mesonephric carcinomas', histologically similar to DES-induced clear cell adenocarcinoma of the vagina, but not asoociated with DES **Prognosis** Poor; 5-year survival of 0% if the lesion is greater than stage I 2) LIVER A tumor comprising 5% of hepatocellular carcinomas, cytologically mimicking metastatic renal cell and adrenal cortical carcinomas **Histopathology** 'Alveolar' pattern of clear cells **Prognosis** Similar to usual hepatocellular carcinoma 3) OVARY A tumor of presumed müllerian origin that may be associated with endometriosis, comprising up to 10% of primary ovarian carcinomas, affecting women circa age 55 Pathology Yellow with cystic degeneration **Histopathology** Tubules lined by 'hobnail' cells **Prognosis** Five-year survival, 40%

Clear cell chondrosarcoma A radiolucent low-grade sarcoma of the epiphysis of long bones, especially of the proximal femur, affecting all ages; male:female ratio, 2.5:1, metastases occur to other bones and lungs **Treatment** en bloc resection and wide margin Prognosis 15-20% mortality

Clear cell myeloma A monoclonal plasma cell expansion, clinically similar to the 'garden variety' of myeloma, which has vacuolated cytoplasm and clonally increased IgA and kappa chains and lytic bone lesions (Am J Surg Pathol 1985; 9:149)

Clear cell sarcoma Malignant melanoma of soft parts A sarcoma of young, often female adults, of the lower extremities and acral regions, intimately bound to tendons as circumscribed but unencapsulated melanin-bearing tumors of neuroectodermal origin Prognosis 45-60% mortality, late recurrence; see Barrel-staves appearance

Clear cell tumor A neoplasm composed of clear cells that may be of any embryologic (endo-, ecto-, meso- or neuroectodermal) origin; the cytoplasmic clearing may be real (lipid, mucopolysaccharide and mucosubstance) or artifactual due to post-fixation shrinkage of cytoplasmic content away from an intact and rigid cell membrane; clear cell tumors include balloon cell melanoma, carcinoma, eg signet ring cells, seen in carcinomas of the stomach as well as in renal cell, adrenal, ovary, parathyroid and thyroid, clear cell tumors of tendons and aponeuroses, germ cell tumors (seminomas, dysgerminoma), histiocytosis X, lymphoma (B- and T-cell clear cell lymphomas), myeloma, clear cell type, myxoid lesions (benign and malignant), paraganglioma, xanthoma; see Clear cell carcinoma

Clear-glass appearance RADIOLOGY A descriptor for the 'empty' holes, spaces and clefts seen in osteoporosis, compared to the ground-glass graininess characteristic of osteomalacia

Cleaved cell A malignant lymphocyte that has one or more deep clefts, linear infoldings of the nucleus, condensed chromatin and indistinct nucleoli, typicaly seen in the follicular small cleaved cell lymphoma, an Intermediate grade lymphoma, which despite widespread disease at the time of diagnosis follows a relatively prolonged and non-aggressive course; large cleaved cells are typical of immunoblastic (Rappaport's diffuse histiocytic) lymphoma, in which the cells are slightly larger than the small cleaved cells and somewhat more mitotically active, having a slightly more aggressive clinical course, falling between an intermediate and a high grade lymphoma by the Working formulation, see there

Clenched fist syndrome A cutaneous abscess most often infected by ***Eikenella corrodens*** due to a traumatic laceration, typically over the 3rd and 4th metacarpophalangeal joints, the result of striking someone in the teeth; with improper management, local osteomyelitis may develop **Treatment** Debridement and broad-spectrum antibiotics to 'cover' for the often-present anaerobes

CLIA '88 Clinical and Laboratory Improvement Amendment of 1988; Legislation passed by the US Congress bringing physician office laboratories (POLs) under strict federal regulation with the purpose of improving the reliability of physician office testing; although the details have not been finalized, the regulations took effect 1 July 1991; see POLs

Climacteric The perimenopausal period of functional ovarian involution, characterized by vasomotor lability, eg Hot flashes, dysmenorrhea, redistribution of fat, dyspareunia, hormonal changes, eg increased FSH and LH, decreased PGE2, estrogen and progesterone; postmenopausal ovaries continue to secrete androgens, which are peripherally converted into postmenopausal estrogens, incipient osteoporosis and decreased skin elasticity

'Climbing up on oneself' Gower sign NEUROLOGY A clinical sign referring to the manner in which children with well-developed Duchenne's muscular dystrophy arise from a sitting to a standing position; ambulation is often lost by age 12; 75% die by age 20 secondary to respiratory paralysis

Clinical alert Clinical update Prepublication release of information from publicly-funded research that may have an immediate effect on patient care; the format and criteria for clinical alerts was pending consensus as of early 1991, but have included alerts on the use of immunoglobulins to reduce the incidence and severity of bacterial infections in children with AIDS and the benefits of performing carotid endarterectomy on symptomatic patients with 70-99% occlusion of one or both carotid arteries (Am Med News 11/Mar/91); see Ingelfinger rule; Cf Embargo arrangement

Clinical ecologist A non-traditional practitioner of medicine who claims to have special expertise in the diagnosis and treatment of 'environmental illness', a condition that is not thought to exist by many mainstream medical practitioners; see Environmental hypersensitivity, Yeast connection

Clinical faculty An unpaid member of a medical school staff who regularly practices his specialty in a private setting privately, and devotes less than 50% of his time to the institution; the responsibilities of 'voluntary track' faculty include participation in teaching efforts, administrative functions and/or research efforts; clinical faculty members receive the titles of clinical instructor, clinical assistant professor, clinical associate professor and professor, in increasing rank of accomplishments

Clinicopathological conference (CPC) A formal discussion of a patient's clinical, radiological, laboratory data, in front a large group of junior and senior colleagues; the CPC is often presented as an 'unknown' problem case, and in the first portion of the presentation does not include (for the sake of didactics) the confirmed histopathological diagnosis; the presentation of the patient's baseline data is then followed by discussion of the case as an unknown by an expert, to view the steps he would have taken in arriving at a diagnosis; the final stage of the CPC is discussion by the pathologist who usually is the ultimate arbiter regarding the diagnosis; Cf Professorial rounds

CLIP Corticotropin-like intermediate lobe peptide One of the peptides released from Pro-opiomelanocortin (POMC); CLIP's precursor is the 39 residue ACTH that splits into two peptides, α-MSH (residues 1-13) and CLIP (residues 18-39); see POMC

Clipase Intracellular proteolytic enzyme(s) that remove the pre- and pro- portions of hormones, eg for parathyroid hormone (PTH), a 25-residue polypeptide is 'clipased' from the 115-residue pre-pro-parent, yielding a 90-residue pre-PTH; a 6-residue segment is then removed by tryptic 'clipase' from the pre-PTH yielding the mature 84-residue PTH

Cloacogenic carcinoma see Basaloid carcinoma

Cloasma Melasma A rash caused by the hormonal effects of pregnancy or birth control pills, exacerbated by the sunlight Clinical Irregular flat symmetrical light brown areas on the malar region, cheeks and forehead; the 'pregnancy mask' tends to fade with delivery or discontinuation of birth control pills

Clock theory A hypothetical explanation for the events involved in somatic cell duplication, which holds that the production of mitotic progeny are the work of an oscillating biological metronome that alternately swings between mitosis and interphase, a concept championed by marine biologists; research data supports a merging of the Clock theory with the Domino theory (Science 1989; 246:614); Cf Domino theory

Clonal anergy IMMUNOLOGY Inactivation of immune cells encountering an antigen in absence of a second antigenic signal; since a second signal is normally required for response to an infectious agent (or other antigen); clonal anergy can be reversed by incubating the anergic cells in IL-2

Clonal deletion Negative selection IMMUNOLOGY A maturation process occurring in the context of the major histocompatibility complex (MHC) in which the T cells that recognize self antigens are eliminated in the thymus; clonal deletion is a normal component of the natural self-tolerance; self antigens expressed in the thymus result in physical elimination of autoreactive thymocytes prior to complete maturation; most peripheral circulating CD4+ T cells (which survived intrathymic clonal deletion) are unresponsive to any stimulus, indicating that suppression of autoimmunity also involves clonal anergy (Nature 1990; 345:540); clonal deletion is an important mechanism for eliminating autoreactive T cells, effected by the minor lymphocyte stimulation (Mls) family of antigens, which by interacting with the Vβ portion of the T cell receptor, mimic bacterial superantigens; clonal deletion and functional inactivation of self-reactive cells explains intrathymic as well as peripheral tolerance in T cells, the latter explaining clonal anergy (Nature 1991; 349:245); see Superantigen

Clonal expansion Proliferation of cells arising from a single cell that are virtually identical in structure and function to the progenitor cell; clonal expansions can be a) Physiological or defensive if the expanding clone is capable of responding to down-regulatory mechanisms, ie can be turned off or b) Non-physiologic as they don't respond to down-regulating mechanisms; although often malignant, clonal expansions may be clinically benign (eg, lymphomatoid papulosis, composed of large atypical histologically malignant T lymphocytes with clonal rearrangement of T-γ or T-β receptor genes); B cell clonality is detected by gene rearrangements with Southern blot hybridization or by the polymerase chain reaction

Clonal selection IMMUNOLOGY A theoretical model that holds that antigenic stimulation of preexisting clones of lymphocytes accounts for the main characteristics of the humoral immune response; antigen X interacts with several clones, initiating antigen-dependent differentiation leading to clones of memory cells and plasma cells; clonal selection occurs in two phases a) The antigen-independent phase in which innumerable B cells 'mindlessly' proliferate and b) The antigen-dependent phase where a circulating B cell encounters a recognized antigen, becomes activated, divides and secretes antibody

Clone An organism or cell arising from a single parent that is an exact genotypic (and phenotypic) duplicate thereof; clones occur in nature in the production of multiple daughter cells in a monoclonal gammopathy, or can be created in the laboratory as an 'engineered' process using the methods of recombinant DNA technology

Cloning MOLECULAR BIOLOGY Synthesis of multiple copies of a segment of DNA Principle: A sequence of DNA of interest is inserted by recombinant techniques into a 'vector', a circular fragment of DNA capable of independent or autoreplication within a bacterium, eg bacteriophages, cosmids and plasmids, which are introduced into ***Escherichia coli***, grown within the bacteria in culture media and after the appropriate growth,vectors removed and the segments of DNA of interest are isolated; cloning of genes for a human disease is usually based on chromosomal assignment by 'reverse genetics', where the first step is the labor-intensive identification of DNA probes close, ie within several hundred kilobases, to the gene of interest, followed by the construction of a restriction map surrounding the probe's sequence which is followed by a search for mRNA transcripts derived from the region, often by finding a probe sequence in the 'mapped' region that has been conserved during evolution; genes that are defective in human disease and identified by this method include the genes responsible for chronic granulomatous disease, cystic fibrosis, retinoblastoma and Wilm's tumor Note: DNA amplification by the polymerase chain reaction is an updated and more sensitive method for producing multiple copies of segments of DNA of interest; see cDNA library

Closed loop systems CRITICAL CARE MEDICINE 'State of the art' electronic systems used in intensive care units that monitor multiple patient parameters, eg pulse and respiratory rate and regulate controllable everything via computer, including the rate of infusion of intravenous drugs and fluids

'Clotter' A colloquial term for a hematologist specialized in disorders of coagulation

Cloudy swelling A descriptor for the histopathological changes seen in dilated, flabby beri-beri myopathic hearts, where myocytes are pale and swollen due to hypoxia-induced hydropic degneration of mitochondria resulting in uncoupling of oxidative phosphorylation, decreased ATPase activity, sodium-potassium pump failure and intracellular accumulation of potassium

Clove cigarettes A cigarette made of a mixture of tobacco leaves and cloves, spice prepared from the dried flowers of the tropical tree, ***Eugenia aromatica***, produced in Indonesia, where they are the preferred smoking product, 30-40% of which is shredded clove buds, the remainder, tobacco; importation to the US began in 1970, peaked in the mid 1980s and is on the decline; eugenol is the main (85%) constituent of clove oil; while not carcinogenic or mutagenic in test animals, clove cigarettes cause respiratory depression, atelectasis, alveolar edema, bronchopneumonia and may exacerbate asthma (J Am Med Assoc 1988; 260:3641)

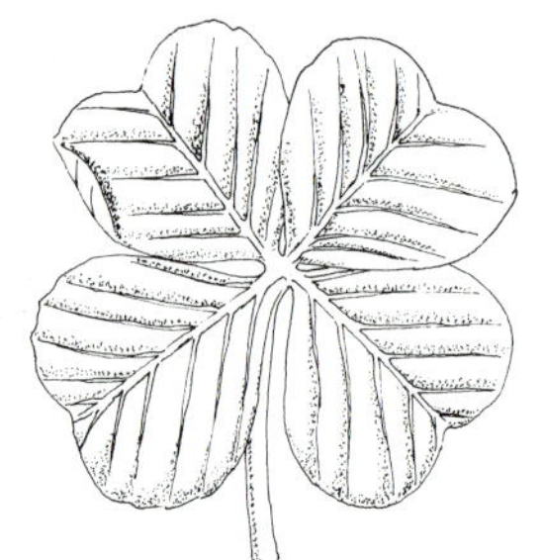

Cloverleaf A morphological descriptor for a multilobed pattern that appears to emanate in a two-dimensional plane from a single point, likened to the low leguminous herb of the genus, ***Trifolium*** (figure) Note: When the same pattern is seen in three dimensions, it is termed 'popcorn'

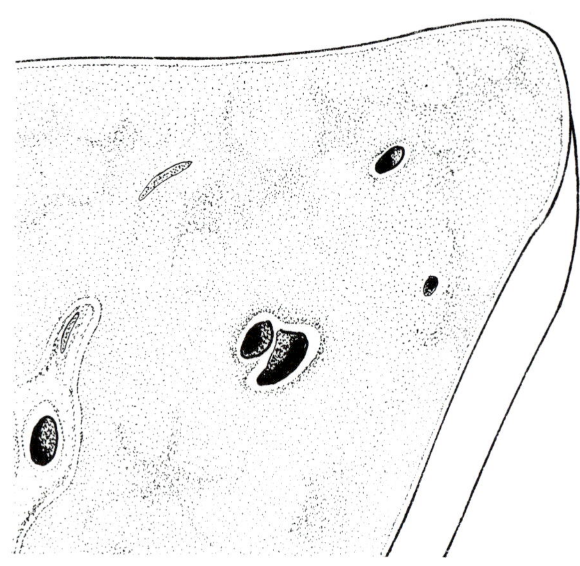

Cloverleaf appearance

Cloverleaf anemia German, Kleeblattanämie, 'neurocirculatory edema'of liver A pattern of patchy paleness admixed with hyperemia due to irregular transhepatic blood flow; the edematous Disse's spaces are pale, compromising the hyperemic capillary circulation, classically associated with cranial injuries

Cloverleaf cells Hyperconvoluted lymphocytes seen in diffuse large cell lymphoma, similar to the 'Popcorn cells' of Hodgkin's disease

Cloverleaf duodenal bulb 'Ace of clubs' sign RADIOLOGY A finding in upper gastrointestinal barium studies, where the duodenal bulb is extensively scarred by multiple previous ulcers with central pinching of the duodenal bulb; Cf Ace of spades

Cloverleaf pigmentation Variegated pigmentation of the iris seen in the Nail-patella syndrome

Cloverleaf skull Kleeblattschädel PEDIATRIC RADIOLOGY Severe deformation of the cranial vault in which a frontal film demonstrates a tri-lobed appearance caused by premature closure of the sutures accompanied by hydrocephaly, seen in thanatophoric dwarfism and accompanied by a prominent forehead, depressed nasal bridge, shortened limbs, bowing of the femora, epiphyseal cupping, flattening of the vertebral bodies, an achondroplasia-like pelvis and mental retardation

Cloverleaf structure Cloverleaf diagram MOLECULAR BIOLOGY The normal planar representation of transfer RNA which folds back upon itself to allow the maximum stability through formation of multiple hydrogen intrachain bonds at the 'arms' of the cloverleaf; the segments of RNA that are not hydrogen bonded are termed 'loops'

Clozapine A first-line drug for treating schizophrenia, which causes potentially fatal agranulocytosis in 1-2% of those treated; the drug became the center of controversy regarding its manufacturer's practice of Bundling, see there

Clubbing Terminal expansion of a relatively short cylindrical object, simulating the tip of a drumstick or a caveman's club

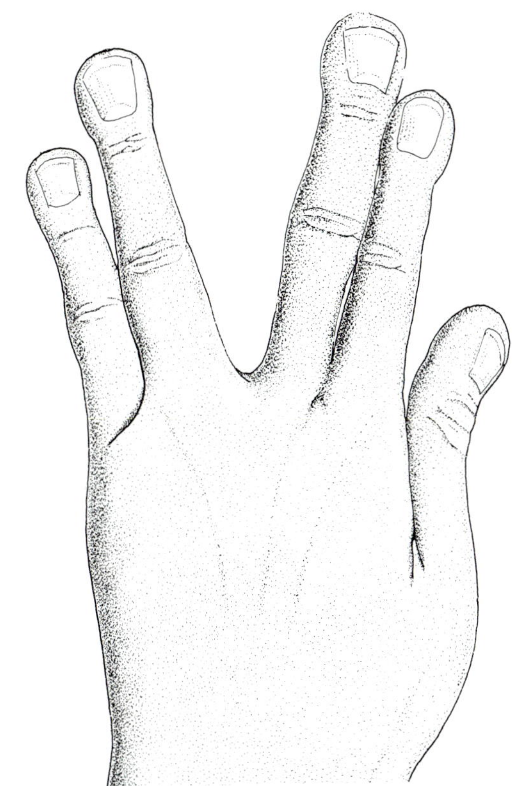

Finger clubbing

Clubbing of the fingers Expansion of the fingertips, often accompanied by underlying hypertrophic osteitis, associated with chronic 'central' (pulmonary origin) hypoxia due to infection, congenital heart disease, cystic fibrosis, bronchogenic carcinoma, bronchiectasis, pneumoconiosis, interstitial pulmonary fibrosis; clubbing may rarely occur in nonpulmonary disease including Crohn's disease, ulcerative colitis, cirrhosis, thyroid acropachy, Grave's disease

Clubbing of the hand PEDIATRIC ORTHOPEDICS Absent radius or less commonly, the ulna, resulting from soft tissues acting as tension bands, pulling the wrist entirely off the end of the ulna; the defect may be associated with congenital heart disease and blood dyscrasia, eg Fanconi's anemia; Cf TAR syndrome

Clubbing of kidneys Focal, finger-like expansion of the renal calices, accompanied by cortical scarring, seen by tomography during intravenous urography, a finding characteristic of chronic pyelonephritis; see 'Thyroidization'

Clubfeet Talipes varus A congenital deformity of the foot, formed from a combination of equinus (plantar flexion of the forefoot), calcaneus (dorsiflexion of the forefoot, the cacaneus forms the plantar prominence), varus (the heel and forefoot are inverted, the plantar surfaces medially) and valgus (eversion of the forefoot and lateral facing of the plantar surface) **Etiology** Unknown, possibly related to muscular dysplasia, anomalous insertion of tendons, arthrogriposis, congenital constriction bands, in utero compression, central nervous system disease (spina bifida, poliomyelitis, Friedrich's ataxia), in the 'whistling face' syndrome of Sheldon-Freeman and in the Moebius syndrome

'Club Med' dermatitis A photodermatitis consisting in linear, mirror-image, hyperpigmented tender patches with scalloped edges, located on the inner thighs; this entity arose in a subject who played a 'drinking game' in which participants rolled limes up and down their thighs: furocoumarin (citrus, celery, parsley) elicits erythema and vesiculation if the exposed skin is subsequently exposed to light Note: This phototoxic reaction was first described in 1916 in women wearing oil of bergamot (N Engl J Med 1986; 314:319c)

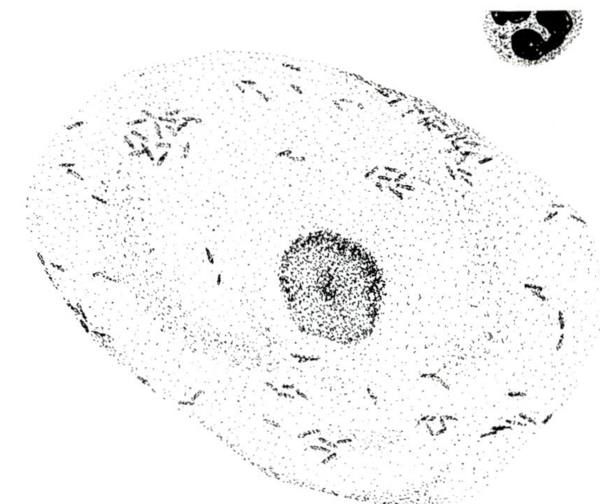

Clue cell

Clue cells GYNECOLOGICAL CYTOLOGY A superficial squamous epithelial cells with peripheral clumps of gram-negative ***Gard-nerella (Haemophilus) vaginalis***, which imparts a stippled, granular appear-ance on a 'wet mount' of a cervical smear, figure, above **Treatment** Metronidazole

Cluster EPIDEMIOLOGY A disease process occurring in a group of people living or working within one stratum (physical, social or economic) of society, who appear to share one or more environmental factors in common, as in cancer 'clusters'; while cluster studies occasionally bear the fruit of a legitimate cause-and-effect relation (DES and vaginal adenocarcinoma, PVC production and the packing industry and angiosarcoma, thalidomide and phocomelia), the ratio of reports to actual associations is very low (100:1) in terms of proving a relation between a putative cause and the effect and the Centers for Disease Control has relegated the study of clusters to state departments of health (J Am Med Assoc 1989; 261:2297)

Cluster headache A short-lived (30 minutes to two hours) intense unilateral cephalalgia that has a 'clock-setting'

predictability, often occurring with spring to fall seasonality, of 3-8 weeks duration, later disappearing for months to years; the headaches cause a knife-like intranasal or retrobulbar pain; unlike migraines (in which the patients prefer to lie still in a darkened room), cluster victims restlessly pace, bang their heads against the wall and have suicidal ideation; cluster headaches are thought to be of vascular origin **Treatment** Prevention (ergotamine tartrate, methysergide) is more effective than analgesia of an acute attack

Cluster of grapes A descriptor for a pattern in which there are multiple rounded, variably-sized vesicular masses

Cluster of grapes appearance PATHOLOGY The gross morphology of a hydatidiform mole, a trophoblastic disease in which the chorionic villi undergo massive swelling ranging from 1-30 mm in diameter (total weight, 200 g) with hydropic degeneration; a complete mole usually occurs without identifiable embryonal tissue; choriogonadotropin levels are markedly increased

Cluster of grapes sign Septation sign PEDIATRIC RADIOLOGY A finding in infants with congenital polycystic kidney disease; the excretory urogram reveals an afunctional non-visualized kidney, the walls of which contain viable vessels visualized in the vascular or opacification phase of urography RADIOLOGY A finding consisting of multiple round-to-oval radiological shadows seen by a plain chest film in mucoid impaction of the bronchi in bronchiectasis

CME Continuing medical education Professional education that physicians participate in on a part-time basis following completion of formal post-medical school specialty training, eg residencies and fellowships; CME may be required for maintaining state licensure, eg New York State requires 150 hours of accredited CME every two years and takes the form of lectures, seminars, refresher courses, workshops, audio- and video-tapes and may be sponsored by medical schools, professional organizations and hospitals Note: It was increasingly common for the pharmaceutical industry to sponsor CME and symposia; according to the ethical guidelines adopted by the American Medical Association (J Am Med Assoc 1991; 265:501), these companies can no longer directly or indirectly provide for travel, lodging, honoraria, or personal expenses incurred during continuing medical education

CMO I, II Corticosterone mixed (function) oxidases CMO II deficiency is an autosomal recessive enzymopathy accompanied by a marked decrease in aldosterone and its metabolites, increased plasma renin activity and 18-hydroxicorticosterone with hyponatremia, hyperkalemia, early onset metabolic acidosis, growth retardation and occasionally spontaneous amelioration with maturation

c-*myc* A cellular oncogene that translocates in Burkitt's lymphoma from its normal site on chromosome 8 to chromosome 14 within the immunoglobulin heavy chain gene, at different sites, either in the switch region or within the variable region; this translocation leads to oncogene activation at a transcriptionally active site and lymphoma-genesis; see *myc*

CNRS Centre National de la Recherche Scientifique A French government-based research organization created in 1939, whose stated purpose is to conduct and encourage basic research in the whole of science; life science is one of its seven subdivisions; over 40% of the 26 000 employees are researchers 1990 BUDGET FF10 330 million DIRECTOR F Kourilsky (Nature 1990; 346:127n&v); see SERC; Cf INSERM

CNTF see Ciliary neurotrophic factor

Coagulation panel A group of assays designed to efficiently identify a probable cause of hemorrhage in a patient who is bleeding, including prothrombin time, activated partial thromboplastic time, platelet count and bleeding time; see Organ panel

COAGULATION FACTORS

I	Fibrinogen
II	Prothrombin
III	Thromboplastin
IV	Calcium (obsolete term)
V	Proaccelerin (obsolete term)
VI	Accelerin (obsolete for Factor Va)
VII	Proconvertin (obsolete term)
VIII	A composite of three separate proteins
VIII:C	Low weight component with coagulant activity, deficient in classic hemophilia
VIII:Ag	Antigenic portion of molecule
VIIIR:RCo	Supports ristocetin-initiated platelet aggregation
VIII:vWF	von Willebrand factor, platelet adhesion
IX	Christmas factor, plasma thromboplastin
X	Stewart-Prowel factor
XI	Plasma thromboplastin antecedent
XII	Hageman factor
XIII	Laki-Lorand factor; fibrinoligane

Coal miner's elbow Student's elbow Olecranon bursitis caused by prolonged pressure, friction or trauma to the elbow; Cf Beat knee

Coal workers' pneumoconiosis An occupational lung disease affecting those with prolonged exposure to carbon dust, which accumulates in the macrophages of peribronchiolar tissues **Clinical** Early pneumoconiosis is often a 'pathologist's disease', ie the diagnosis can only be established by histological examination; with time, dyspnea, pulmonary hypertension and respiratory failure develop **Histopathology** The early lesion is the 'coal macule', a pigmented parenchymal nodule that undergoes massive fibrosis, producing stellate contracted lesions **Treatment** None; see Anthracosis

Coast of California pattern DERMATOLOGY Smooth, gently curved borders of the macular cafe-au-lait skin lesions seen in patients with neurofibromatosis, likened to the smoothly contoured Pacific coastline of the US state of California

Coast of Maine pattern DERMATOLOGY Jagged contours of the macular (Cafe-au-lait color) skin lesions in McCune-

Albright disease (polyostotic fibrous dysplasia, precocious puberty and multiple endocrine dysfunctions), usually 3-4 in number, often unilateral, located on the buttocks or neck, likened to the convoluted and craggy contoured Atlantic coastline of the US state of Maine

Coatamer A cytosolic complex containing the same coat proteins (COPs) as those of the Golgi transport vesicles, one of which, β-COP, resides exclusively within complex (Nature 1991; 349:248); Cf GERL

Coated pit A specialized depression in the cytoplasmic face of the cell membrane that is lined by the scaffolding protein, clathrin, which is pivotal in down-regulating hormonal activity, as the coated pits internalize and degrade receptors for vasoactive intestinal polypeptide, insulin and other hormones, playing a role in hormone receptor-mediated endocytosis; see Clathrin

Cobblestone A widely used descriptor for multiple, equally-sized rounded densities that project from a single linear surface, when the image is two-dimensional or that rise above a flattened plane when viewed in three dimensions, a pattern likened to pre-infernal combustion engine roadways, paved by multiple similarly-sized 'cobbled' stones GASTROINTESTINAL DISEASE Characteristic radiologic and gross appearance (figure) of the intestinal mucosa in Crohn's disease due to submucosal involvement; to the endoscopist, cobblestoning refers to the uniform nodules (due to the submucosal edema), while the pathologist refers to severe ulcerative disease with crisscrossing of the ulcers through inflamed but intact mucosa; intestinal 'cobblestoning' may also occur in ulcerative colitis (where ulcers alternate with regenerating mucosa), ischemic colitis, lymphoid hyperplasia of common variable immunodeficiency, amyloidosis, mucoviscidosis, pneumatosis cystoides intestinalis, multiple lymphangiomas and polyposis coli; in the intestine, the mucosal rugosities may correspond to polyps or be filled with air, lymphoid tissue and amyloid GYNECOLOGY A roughened appearance rarely seen by colposcopy of the uterine cervix infected with ***Neisseria gonorrhoeae*** OPHTHALMOLOGY Multiple sharply demarcated non-elevated, lesions with prominent choroidal vessels, located between the ora serrata and the equator, seen in peripheral chorioretinal atrophy, a common aging phenomenon, seen in one-fourth of all autopsies, one-third of which are bilateral ORAL DISEASE Multiple, closely-set intraoral papilloma-like fibromas that impart a pebbly tactile sensation in Cowden's premalignant multiple hamartoma syndrome SOFT TISSUE PATHOLOGY Multiple 'hobnail' projections of malignant endothelial cells into the vascular lumina seen in angiosarcoma, a pattern mimicked by Kaposi sarcoma and spindle cell hemangioendothelioma

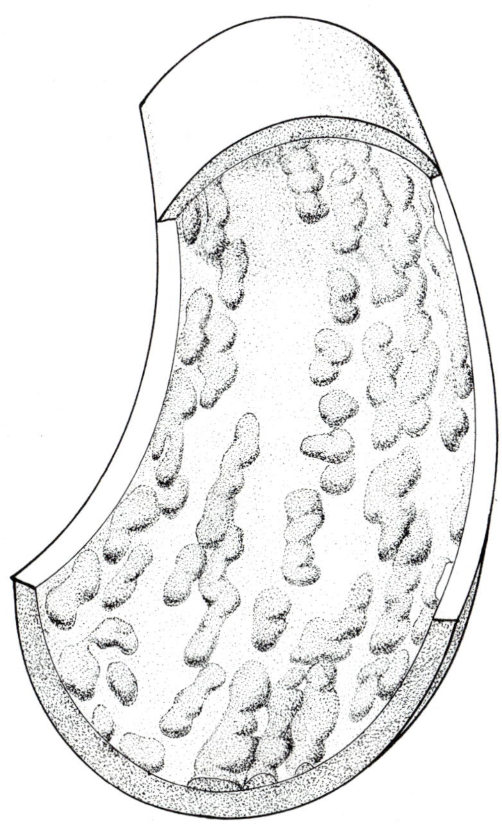

Cobblestoning, colon

Cobrahead sign The pattern seen by an excretory urogram of the ureterovesicular junction, in a urinary bladder ureterocele; a thin outer membrane corresponding to the ureteral walls, seen as a dark halo, encloses a cystically-dilated distal intravesicular ureter that protrudes into the bladder, where opacified urine collects in both the dilated segment and the bladder; simple ureteroceles of adults are associated with stenosis of the ureteral orifice and prolapse of the distal ureter into the bladder, possibly due to the persistence of Chiralla's membrane and blockage of the ureteral orifice

Cobweb pattern Lacy neurofibrillary material present in the center of the rosettes of neuroblastomas, ganglioneuroblastomas and benign ganglioneuromas which ultrastructurally corresponds to 6-10 nm cytoplasmic filaments, cell processes with microtubules, rare dense core granules, synaptic vesicles and cell junction material

Coby H A seven year-old boy with acute lymphocytic leukemia who died while awaiting a potentially life-saving bone marrow transplantation, a procedure that was not at the time funded by public monies in the state of Oregon; see Health care rationing, Oregon plan, 'Rule of rescue'

Cocaethylene A cocaine metabolite produced by an alternate metabolic pathway in the presence of alcohol, which is associated with a marked increase in coronary artery spasm and commonly present in post-mortem body fluids from those who have died while simultaneously abusing cocaine and alcohol

Cocaine SUBSTANCE ABUSE A powder (Benzoylmethylecgonine $C_{17}H_{21}NO_4$) derived from ***Erythoxylon coca*** that evokes intense physical and psychological addiction **Clinical** Cardiovascular symptoms are most prominent, with dysrhythmia, eg ventricular tachycardia and fibrillation, myocarditis, myocardial infarction, sudden death, convulsions, hyperpyrexia, cerebral vasculitis, loss of sense of smell and (due to collapse of nasal mucosa and matrix) a nose to smell with, decreased oxygen diffusing capacity, spontaneous pneumomediastinum, eating disorders, eg bulimia and anorexia; with chronic abuse, there is increased sensitivity ('reverse tolerance') to the non-euphorigenic effects of cocaine, including hyperactivity and anesthesia, see Kindling **Binge** A session of cocaine snorting that is repeated as often as every 10 minutes over a period from 12 hours to an entire week; with time, cocaine-induced euphoria deteriorates to neuropharmacological dependence and compulsive abuse ensues in up to 20% and actual addiction occurs in 5% which may reach the point of excluding all else but obtention of more drug **Cause of death** Arrhythmia due to ventricular fibrillation and cardiovascular collapse, respiratory arrest with pulmonary edema, cerebrovascular insults associated with hypertension **Clinical detection of cocaine abuse** Chronic rhinitis, rhinorrhea, ulceration of nose, perforation of the nasal septum and madarosis (singeing of eyebrows and eyelashes due to hot vapors associated with smoking crack) **Chronic abuse** Seizures are common in habitual abusers, who have diffuse cortical atrophy, seen by computed tomography and diffuse slowing of waves, seen by electroencephalography (Neurology 1990; 40:404) **Drug testing** Urine and serum may be screened for benzoylecgonine, cocaine's major metabolite, by enzyme-labelled competitive immunoassay, see EMIT and confirmed for legal purposes by the 'gold standard' method, gas chromatography-mass spectrometry, see GC-MS; cocaine's plasma $T_{1/2}$ is 90 minutes; cocaine-induced euphoria lasts 45 minutes **Pathology Brain** Subarachnoid hemorrhage, cortical atrophy **Gastrointestinal tract** Intestinal ischemia due to α adrenergic vasoconstriction **Heart** Mononuclear cell inflammation of the myocardium with myocytic necrosis **Lungs** Congestion, spontaneous pneumothorax **Nose** see below, Cocaine nose **Oral cavity** Cocaine's pH of 4.5 causes dental erosion, and has been implicated in increased caries in cocaine abusers, although this may be related to a change in eating habits **Pharmacology** Cocaine's presumed site of action is the nucleus accumbens and the 'high', like that of amphetamine, is attributed to cerebral 'flooding' with dopamine, where it blocks the re-uptake of dopamine by the cell producing it; the increased dopamine in the synaptic cleft is also held responsible for cocaine's addictive properties (N Engl J Med 1988; 318:1173rv) Cocaine receptors are located on dopamine transporters

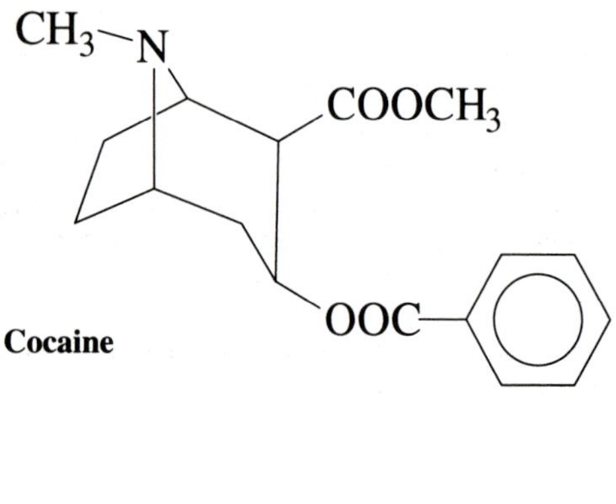

CH_3—N $COOCH_3$ OOC

Cocaine

Pregnancy Abruptio placentae, premature onset of labor, vaginal bleeding after intravenous injection, placental vasoconstriction, spontaneous abortion, congenital malformation, perinatal mortality, neurologic and behavior defects, tachycardia and hypertension **Psychiatric disorders** Dysphoria, paranoid psychosis, severe depression **Rehabilitation** Experimental drugs for treating cocaine addiction include buprenorphine (a mixed opiate agonist-antagonist), desipramine and flupenthixol (both antidepressant), carbamazepine (antiseizure), buspirone (anxiolytic) bromocriptine (dopamine antagonist) and mazindol (dopamine blocker) Science 1989; 246:1379 **Sexual dysfunction** Cocaine's myth as an aphrodisiac derives from its ability to delay ejaculation and orgasm, causing temporary mood elevation and heightened sensory awareness; one subject inserted cocaine intraurethrally for this purpose and developed priapism, paraphimosis, disseminated intravascular coagulation, gangrene, massive necrosis of the extremities, resulting in the loss of nine fingers, the penis and both legs below the knees (J Am Med Assoc 1988; 259:3126/8); chronic cocaine abuse evokes impotence, subfertility, eg low sperm counts, low motility and increased abnormal sperm forms (Fertil Steril 1990; 53:315) **Statistics** Three million US citizens use cocaine regularly (600 000 use heroin), 10-15% of the entire US population has tried cocaine (40% of those between age 25-30) and 10-15% of experimenters eventually become addicted; cocaine is implicated in 5/1000 deaths in ages 25-30; up to 25% of motor vehicle accident fatalities in drivers aged 15-45 in New York City had cocaine in their system (J Am Med Assoc 1990; 263:250) **Street names** Bolivian marching powder, Coke, Flake, Snow, Toot **Treatment** Cocaine-induced acute rhabdomyolysis may potentially respond to dantrolene, a drug used in malignant hyperthermia (N Engl J Med 1989; 321:1271c) **Withdrawal** Abstinence from cocaine results in a triphasic response consisting of a) 'Crash' Paranoia, hypersomnia followed by hyperphagia b) Withdrawal with prolonged anhedonia and cocaine craving and c) Extinction (Science 1991; 251:1580rv) Notes: Cocaine was found in the tombs of Western Hemisphere Indians circa 600 AD; Sigmund Freud was major supporter of cocaine's beneficial effects, and later became addicted thereto; one half of the US supply is from Peru's Huallaga Valley; several 'epidemics' of cocaine and stimulant abuse have occurred in the USA, in the 1890s, the 1920s ('drug madness'), early 1950s and late 1960s (amphetamines) and now in the 1980s; patients with pseudocholinesterase deficiency are at increased risk of sudden death as this enzyme is part of cocaine's metabolic route ; see Binge, Crack, Freebase, Kindling

'Cocaine nose' A constellation of findings in chronic intranasal abusers of cocaine **Clinical** Frequent rubbing of nose Rhinoscopy Unremarkable mucosa or visible perforation **Histopathology** Granulomas, inflammation, massive mucosal edema, erosion and necrosis of the nasal mucosa Surgical complications Localized septal collapse, poor mucosal healing, inadequate correction of septal deflection **Treatment** Rhinoplasty may be performed on highly selected patients, although the results are often poor; submucosal resection and septoplasty should be avoided (Plast Reconstr Surg 1990; 86:436)

Cocarcinogen see Tumor promoter

Coccal lesions OPTIC FUNDOSCOPY A descriptor for the black hemorrhagic dots that float in the vitreous humor, caused by small hypertension-induced leakage of blood

Coccoon A descriptor for the fibrotic encasement of the entire small intestine seen in sclerosing peritonitis, a spontaneous idiopathic process in young women, following peritoneovenous shunting, practolol therapy, peritoneal dialysis and chemotherapy, in which unknown toxins may stimulate fibroblastic proliferation and reactive fibrosis

Cockroach A largely nocturnal insect of the order Blattaria that ranges from 5 mm (***Attaphila***) to 10 cm (***Megaloblatta***) in length of which 3500 have been catalogued; in the US, the most familiar roaches include ***Periplaneta americana, Blattella germanica, Blattella orientalis*** and are of medical interest as they are potential vectors for bacteria, especially ***Salmonella*** species; other organisms cultured from cockroaches include ***Shigella, Proteus*** and ***Mycobacterium*** species, ***Escherichia coli, Klebsiella pneumoniae*** and ***Pseudomonas aeruginosa***, but their relative contribution as vectors for infections is unknown and difficult to study, but they have been implicated in hepatitis; 97.5% of low income housing has them, with an average of 33 600/dwelling and thus their presence in an environment is associated with poor sanitation

Cockscomb cervix Collar, Hood, Pseudopolyp formation A transverse ridging of uterine cervix and upper vagina, described in one-fourth of females exposed in utero to diethylstilbestrol (DES), a finding of no known pathological significance Histopathology Core of fibrous tissue, lined by metaplastic squamous epithelium, or occasionally tubal or endometrial epithelium; see Clear cell adenocarcinoma, DES

Cocktail Any mixture of partially-related substances that may be touted as having complementary activities towards the same goal, eg analgesic cocktails (Brompton's mixture), fluor cocktail (liquid scintillation counting), immunosuppressive cocktail (a Gemisch of agents used to suppress graft-versus-host disease) or a keratin 'cocktail', a mixture of antibodies to a two or more of the 19 different well-defined subclasses of keratins with molecular weights between 40 and 68 kD

Cocktail party 'syndrome' Chatter-box 'syndrome' A descriptor for the behavior of children with arrested hydrocephalus, who are highly sociable, hyperloquacious, pseudointelligent (speaking in a seemingly erudite fashion on subjects about which they have no true understanding), scanning dysrhythmic speech; Cocktail party chatter is also a symptom of Williams 'elfin face' syndrome with mild mental retardation, congenital cardiac defects (valvular stenoses and septal defects) and, due to hypercalcemia, nephrosclerosis and bony sclerosis; see Elfin face syndrome

Cocktail purpura An unusual form of thrombocytopenic purpura, induced by the quinine in tonic water, due to ingestion of 'gin & tonic(s)'

Cocktail sausage appearance Diffuse periosteal swelling of a toe, a rare radiological finding seen in rheumatoid arthritis

'Cocktail' therapy Any mixture of drugs to produce a therapeutic effect may be considered a 'cocktail', eg antibiotic or chemotherapeutic agents administered in combination; the term has had most currency in immunology as a mixture of immunosuppressive agents for controlling rejection; one early immune cocktail had azathioprine and steroids, and was used to counter early renal transplant rejection, having various side effects, including osteoporosis, anemia, diabetes, cataracts, hearing loss, gout and reduced growth in younger transplant victims; when cyclosporine was added to the cocktail in 1983, the one-year survival for transplanted kidneys rose to 90%, for transplanted hearts to 80% and for transplanted livers to 70%; despite this improvement, 20% require a second transplant due to graft failure, rejection or drug-related complications; FK-506, a new immunosuppressive promises further improvement in graft survival

'Code blue' Code EMERGENCY MEDICINE A message announced over a hospital's public address system indicating that a cardiac arrest requiring medical attention is in progress; in a similar context, to be 'coded' is to undergo cardiopulmonary resuscitation

Code of ethics see Hippocratic Oath

Code of Hammurabi A code of laws promulgated by Hammurabi, the great Amorite king of Babylon in Mesopotamia; specifically the physicians in this culture which flourished circa 2000 BC were known as asu, skilled in herbal medicine, mineral cures, snakebites, fractures and visible sores; the asu were under strict government regulation; the scale of fees was fixed by law, based on the patients ability to pay and the seriousness of the disease; payment was made only upon recovery of the patient and the physican was severely punished for failure; loss of a nobleman's sight would translate into loss of the physician's hand, and so on

Co-dominance CLINICAL GENETICS A clinical state in which each allele of a gene expresses an effect in a heterozygous individual; eg α-1 antitrypsin deficiency, which has 25 different allelic forms or the red cell blood group MN(Ss), where there are 3 possible expressions: M, MN and N

Codon A triplet of RNA nucleotides derived from DNA that symbolizes each amino acid; because there are four possible nucleotides in each of the three positions, there are 4 x 4 x 4 = 64 possible combinations of RNA triplets, which translate into one start codon, three stop codons and 20 amino acids, resulting in redundancy or 'degeneracy' of the genetic code and many amino acids have more than one codon and some have up to six codons; this redundancy allows for considerable error to occur in translation while still encoding functional proteins

Coefficient of variation (CV) STATISTICS A calculation that compares two different analytic methods, which assumes a Gaussian distribution of data, quantitating the 'between-run' precision of an analytic procedure when a stable control product is analyzed with each run of patient sample, defined by formula as 100 x standard deviation divided by the mean

Coffee A beverage made from dried, roasted beans of the coffee tree (*Coffea arabica*), a moderate stimulant causing mild physical dependence; annual US consumption: 1 million metric tons (33 million gallons/day) Note: Regular coffee is made from arabica beans, decaffeinated coffee from robusta beans; coffee is of medical interest for its postulated negative impact on the cardiovascular system and for an increased risk of malignancy reported in heavy coffee drinkers Note: When each 'association' is rigorously examined with properly designed studies of large populations, the relative risks often fall below the levels of statistical significance Cardiovascular system More than five cups/day was associated with a 2.5-fold increase in coronary artery disease (N Engl J Med 1986; 316:977), arrhythmia, increased LDL-cholesterol and apolipoprotein-B; a later study of the relation of coffee to myocardial infarct and strokes revealed a relative risk (RR) of 1.04 (not significant), in 4+ cups/day and a RR of 1.63 (marginally significant), for decaffeinated coffee, a beverage known to increase the LDL-cholesterol (NEJM 1990; 323:1026); Coffee's role as a carcinogen is heuristically logical as coffee derivatives can be used in thymidine-poor culture media to increase breaks or gaps in certain 'fragile sites' of the chromosomes, in particular, 3p14.2, 6q25.3, 16q23.2, an effect attributed to caffeine's inhibition of DNA repair in replicating cells, 20 of the sites cited in one study (Science 1984; 226:1199) are associated with human malignancy and caffeine may be used to enhance the expression of chromosomal damage in the 'Fragile X' (Xq27) syndrome (N Engl J Med 1987; 316:483); in one small cohort, there was a marked increase in pancreatic cancer in heavy coffee drinkers, a conclusion repeatedly refuted by subsequent studies; the risk for colorectal carcinoma may be decreased (RR, 0.6-0.8) in heavy (> 5 cups/day) coffee consumption; the increase in pancreatic carcinoma (RR: 1.03) is not statistically significant (Am J Epidemiol 1989; 130:895, Cancer Res 1989; 49:1049)

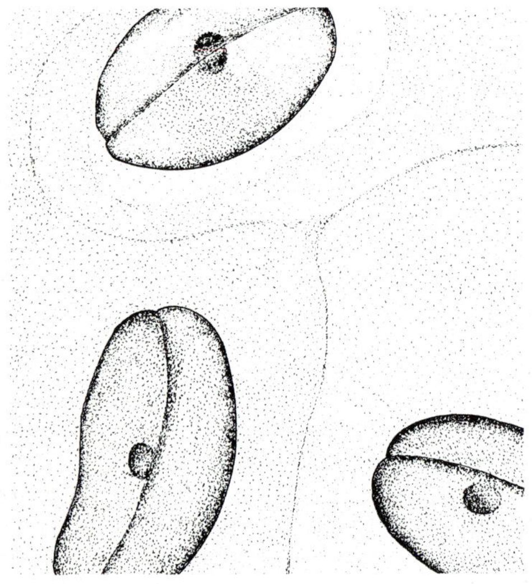

Coffee bean cells

Coffee bean appearance A descriptor for an oval cell often invested with a linear groove GYNECOLOGIC PATHOLOGY A descriptive term for coelomic epithelial cells often seen in Brenner tumor of the ovary (figure); similar cells are described in granulosa cell tumors which, when multi-nucleated, may appear as 'florettes', considered a degenerative phenomenon MICRO-BIOLOGY A descriptor for ***Pneumocystis carinii*** trophozoites, which have also been likened to a 'Folded envelope'

Coffee grounds appearance A descriptor for the color and consistency of gastric hemorrhage that is associated with both benign or malignant ulcers; 'coffee grounds vomitus' is characteristic of yellow fever

Coffin A heavily-leaded container used to transport relatively large amounts of radioactive material, eg from the manufacturer; see Pig

Coffin lid crystals A descriptor for the three- to six-sided colorless prism-shaped crystals that may be seen in a) Synovial fluid, associated with acromegaly, hyperparathyroidism, hemochromatosis, hypomagnesemia, hypophosphatasia, myxedema, ochronosis and Wilson's disease; the crystals may complicate other arthritic conditions eg gout, osteoarthritis, rheumatoid arthritis, chondrocalcinosis b) Urine Ammonium magnesium phosphate (triple phosphate) crystals in neutral or alkaline urine, associated with urinary tract infections; see Struvite concrements

Cogwheel phenomenon NEUROLOGY Circular jerking rigidity in flexion and extension in a background of a tremor that continues throughout the entire range of movement, a finding characteristic of parkinsonism; this jerky movement is due to an underlying tremor rhythm; it is less commonly 'smoothly' rigid, fancifully termed lead pipe rigidity; Cf Clasp knife phenomenon, Gegenhalten

Coherence therapy see ADFR therapy

Cohort A group of persons with a defined disorder

Cohort effect ADOLESCENT PSYCHIATRY Those influences that a peer(s) exercises on an individual, including drug abuse, sexual mores and suicide

Cohorting EPIDEMIOLOGY Separating of patients, eg infants in a neonatal unit, into small groups, such that the patients are treated by a limited number of health care workers; in infants, cohorting and frequent hand-washing results in a reduced incidence of respiratory syncytial virus infection (Arch Dis Child 1991; 66:227)

Cohort study EPIDEMIOLOGY A longitudinal study of a specific group or cohort sharing a selected, often morbid condition, with the purpose of identifying features unique to the cohort that may be related to the morbid condition; see Epidemiology

Coiled coil MOLECULAR BIOLOGY A structural motif in proteins formed by two or three α helices in parallel and in register that cross at a 20° angle, are strongly amphipathic with hydrophobic and hydrophilic residues that repeat every seventh residue; coiled-coil domains are thought to be critical for a number of as-yet unkown biological activities and may be found in flagellins, β chains of G proteins, heat shock proteins, keratins, myosins, tropomyosins and in α and β tubulins, and may coexist with other structural motifs, including leucine zippers and zinc finger domains (Science 1991; 252:1162)

Coiled spring appearance Posttraumatic intramural hematoma of the third segment of the duodenum, seen in barium studies, where the folds over the mass are stretched; a similar finding may be seen inintussusception; see Stacked coin appearance

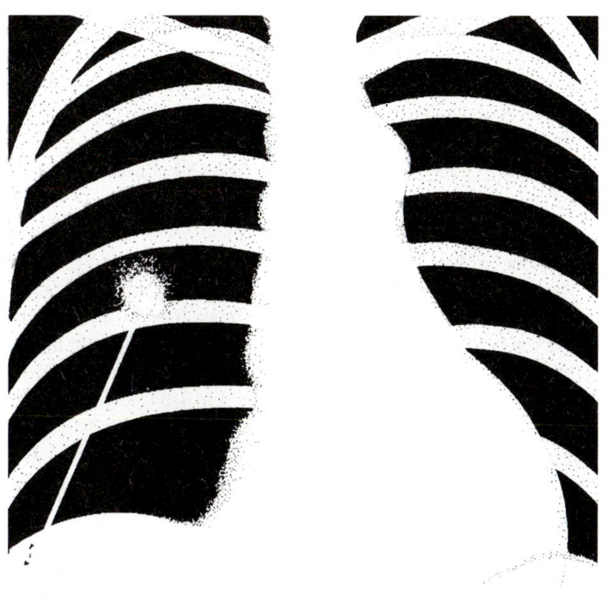

Coin lesion

Coin lesion RADIOLOGY A rounded, circumscribed nodule measuring less than 4 cm that may be surrounded by well-aerated pulmonary parenchyma, appearing as an incidental finding in an otherwise unremarkable plain chest film; in the US, coin lesions are often malignant and details of importance include age, smoking history, geography and previous malignancy **Etiology** Infection (abscesses, aspergilloma, bacteria, coccidioidomycosis, echinococcal cysts, ***Dirofilaria immitis***, histoplasmosis, tuberculosis), benign masses (bronchial adenoma, chondroma, diaphragmatic hernia, benign mesothelioma, neurogenic tumor, sarcoidosis, sclerosing hemangioma, Wegener's granulomatosis, rheumatoid nodules); malignant masses (primary lung carcinomas, which comprise 35% or more, metastases approximately 10%, sarcoma, myeloma, Hodgkin's disease and choriocarcinoma)

COLA Commission of Office Laboratory Assessment A coalition group formed by the American Medical Association, College of American Pathologists and the American Association of Family Practitioners for the purpose of accrediting physician office laboratories, see POLs; also, Cost of living adjustment An increase in salary given to those who move to a more expensive region of the country

COLD Chronic obstructive lung disease, see COPD

Cold abscess Focal, well-circumscribed acute inflammation without the usual signs of a 'hot' abscess, eg dolor, calor, rubor and functio laesa; cold abscesses may occur in normal individuals infected by an attenuated organism or as a result of inadequate antibiotic therapy, classically a paravertebral tuberculotic cold abscess; cold abscesses are also characteristic of the hyperimmunoglobulin E syndrome; see Job syndrome

Cold agglutinin disease Cold agglutinin syndrome An immune disorder characterized by IgM autoantibodies that optimally agglutinate red cells at very low temperatures, eg 4°C; low titers (< 1:32) of cold agglutinins are detectable in many normal subjects; polyclonal cold agglutinins increase after certain infections, eg mycoplasma, cytomegalovirus, Epstein-Barr virus, trypanosomiasis and malaria, peaking within 2-3 weeks and are of no significance if non-hemolytic; cold agglutinins should be ruled out in all patients with acquired hemolytic anemia and a positive direct Coomb's test and certain antibodies have been implicated, eg anti-I, -i, -Pr, -Gd, Sd^a; Cold agglutinin syndrome occurs in 1) Elderly patients with a monoclonal kappa proliferation or concomitant lymphoma, often large cell (Rappaport's 'histiocytic') type or 2) Younger patients with a polyclonal proliferation induced by ***Mycoplasma pneumoniae*** infection (anti-I antibodies) or infectious mononucleosis (anti-i antibodies); the cells are coated with C3d (C3d is also increased in up to 40% of patients with ***Mycoplasma*** infections, 20% of adenovirus infections); cooling of acral parts results in intravascular agglutination and complement fixation; elevation of the complement-bearing red cells to body temperature evokes mild, self-limited hemolysis; Cf 'Room temps'

Cold hemoglobinuria see Paroxysmal cold hemoglobinuria

Cold hypersensitivity Excess autonomic system reaction to low environmental temperature, characterized by bradycardia and a local wheal-and-flare reaction; when familial in nature, the reaction is dignified as 'Cold urticaria'

Cold laser see Excimer laser

Cold nodule Radioisotopic imaging THYROID A focus of reduced radioisotope uptake on a ^{123}I or ^{99m}Tc scintillation scan of the thyroid, seen in either cystic (seen in follicular adenomas that have outgrown their vascular supply resulting in cystic degeneration) or solid, often nonfunctional lesions; when the mass is solid by ultrasound, a biopsy is warranted as most carcinomas are cold nodules Note: Benign lesions, eg non-functional follicular adenomas are usually 'cold' as well; hepatic lesions that may be 'hot' or 'cold' include abscesses and tumor nodules; each warrants a biopsy, best visualized by ^{198}Au and ^{99m}Tc; Cf Hot nodules, Warm nodules

Cold Spring Harbor laboratory One of the premier institutes of molecular biology in the world, located on Long Island, New York; it is home to 3 Nobel Laureates: JD Watson, A Hershey, B McClintock; 120 scientists from 18 countries work in the CSHL; on-going research projects include tumor viruses, eukaryotic genetics, cell biology, ultrastructure, protein chemistry, X-ray crystallography, yeast genetics, neuroscience, HIV gene regulation; CSHL is involved in education from grade-school to the post-graduate level (35 annual conferences) and publications (two journals, 140 titles in print) Budget: $26 million (Science 1990; 250:496)

'Cold turkey' SUBSTANCE ABUSE A colloquialism for the

acute opiate withdrawal syndrome, usually referring to heroin withdrawal Clinical Rhinorrhea, lacrimation, perspiration, yawning, followed by restlessness, anxiety and irritability, dilated pupils, anorexia, nausea, vomiting, abdominal cramps, tremors, convulsions and shock if severe; the reaction may be precipitated by naloxone, a pure opiate antagonist

'Cold turkey' method SUBSTANCE ABUSE A cessation technique used for narcotic or nicotine addiction, where the symptoms of withdrawal are treated as little as possible, with the hope that once the addict has passed through the 'cathartic' trauma of withdrawal, he would be unwilling to re-initiate drug abuse

Cold-(induced) urticaria-angioedema Autonomic nervous system reactivity to low temperatures Clinical forms, Acquired After cold exposure, the patient suffers a pruritic urticarial eruption, potentially evolving into angioedema, accompanied by headaches and wheezing; if the whole body is cooled (swimming in winter), hypotension, collapse and death may ensue Hereditary, Immediate-type Erythematous maculopapules accompanied by a burning sensation, pyrexia, arthralgias, and leukocytosis Hereditary, Delayed-type Erythematous swelling 9-18 hours after a cold 'challenge'

Coley's toxin IMMUNOLOGY A 'cocktail' of bacterial products, including hemolytic streptococcal proteins, eg streptokinase and streptodornase formulated by Wm Coley, New York in 1893, that was occasionally successful in treating cancer or evoking tumor regression; the first case was an inoperable head and neck sarcoma that regressed with each attack of erysipelas; the toxin caused high fevers related to endogenous tumor necrosis factor production

Colic PEDIATRICS A symptom complex affecting young infants, in which paroxysmal abdominal pain of presumed intestinal origin is accompanied by severe crying, lasting until the infant is completely exhausted; in absence of organic causes (strangulated hernia, intussusception, pyelonephritis and others), no therapy gives consistent relief and parents are often obliged to wait until the infant outgrows it, often by six months of age

Colipase A trypsin-activated proenzyme secreted by the exocrine pancreas that acts on fat droplets, binding at the bile salt-triglyceride-water interface, providing a recognition site for lipase

Collagen diet see Liquid diet

Collagen disease and arthritis panel LABORATORY MEDICINE A group of tests that are designed to establish the diagnosis of rheumatic disease in the most cost-effective manner possible, which entails measurement of the erythrocyte sedimentation rate, rheumatoid factor (by latex agglutination), uric acid levels, antinuclear antibody and C-reactive protein; see Organ panel

Collagen disease/lupus erythematosus diagnostic panel An abbreviated group of serum assays that serve to diagnose collagen vascular disease in the most cost-effective way possible

Collagenous stalk motif Collagen is characterized by the repeating triple helix of amino acid residues, Gly-X-Y, a motif also found in secretory proteins, eg complement C1q, pulmonary surfactant apoprotein, asymmetric acetylcholinesterase and serum mannose-binding protein and non-secretory proteins, eg macrophage scavenger receptor (Nature 1990; 343:570)

Collagen vascular diseases A group of 'rheumatic' diseases characterized by arthropathies, immune complex deposition, renal involvement, and partial or complete temporary response to corticosteroids, including dermatomyositis, mixed connective tissue disease, polyarteritis nodosa, rheumatoid arthritis and systemic lupus erythematosus

Collar sign RADIOLOGY A radiolucent band of edema surrounding a benign peptic ulcer, seen by barium studies of the upper gastrointestinal tract

Collar button abscess An advanced abscess of the finger that forms on the palmar and dorsal surfaces, commonly located at the metacarpophalangeal joint; the infection tends to spread beneath the palmar fascia or into the dorsal compartment opposite the web space, later filling the web space, extending along the synovial tendon sheath into the midpalmar or thenar spaces Treatment Palmar and dorsal incision and drainage

Collar button lesions Numerous small deep ulcers with narrow necks, paralleling a barium-filled large intestinal lumen affected by ulcerative colitis; the 'button' surface corresponds to the eroded ulcer base and the 'button neck' corresponds to the sides of the islands of preserved mucosa; a similar phenomenon occurs in colonic amebiasis ulcers; see Flask lesion

Collarette A rim of thickened epidermis in pyogenic granuloma, morphologically similar to the pincer-like surrounding epidermis of lichen nitidus, Cf Ball in claw lesion

Collar-stud abscess An abscess of the ocular orbit present beneath the skin and constricted in a 'collar stud'-like fashion by the orbital septum Treatment Enlarge the septum with an artery forceps to provide effective drainage (DK Sen, Int Surg 1970; 54:379)

'Collateral damage' The undesired but unavoidable comorbidity associated with a therapeutic modality, eg chemotherapy-induced collateral damage to the bone marrow and gastrointestinal tract; the term was first popularized during the Iraq-Kuwait conflict in reference to unintentional, but inevitable loss of life and destruction of civilian property and non-military facilities, when these are adjacent to military targets; the term is applicable to medicine (N Engl J Med 1991; 324:1746c), eg 'collateral damage' to the bone marrow in chemotherapy

Collision tumor The extremely rare merging of two originally separate (primary) tumors from two organs, most often seen clinically at the esophago-gastric junction, where a squamous cell carcinoma of esophageal origin merges with an adenocarcinoma of gastric origin; diagnosis of a 'collision' tumor requires that the colliding tumors be histologically distinct; Cf Composite tumor, Mixed tumor

Collodion baby An infant covered with thickened, taut, parchment paper-like skin that is cyclically shed as a manifestation of lamellar type ichthyosis; the tightened skin results in a flattened nose, ectropion, fixation of the lips into an O-shape, 'cracking' of the skin with respiratory effort; hair may be absent or may penetrate the membrane **Prognosis** Uncertain **Treatment** High humidity and high hopes Note: Collodion was a solution of gun-cotton, a highly explosive compound prepared by steeping cotton in nitric and sulfuric acids in ether that was supplanted by dynamite; collodion formed a colorless gummy liquid that dried in air, used in photography for covering plates and in surgery for covering wounds

Colloidal gold curve see Gold curve

Colloid bodies Hyaline, cytoid or Civatte bodies DERMATOPATHOLOGY Densely eosinophilic, dyskeratotic cells that are often surrounded by a cleared space due to retraction of viable squamous epithelium away from the dead cells, a finding characteristic of lichen planus

Colloid carcinoma Mucinous carcinoma SURGICAL PATHOLOGY A gelatinous subtype of secretory adenocarcinoma, histologically appearing as clusters of tumor cells floating in pools of pale mucin; colloid carcinomas occur in a) Breast Although focal colloid features may occur in 'garden variety' breast carcinomas of ductal and lobular types, tumors with predominantly colloid features comprise only 2% of all cases; colloid carcinomas of the breast occurs in slightly older women, has a lower incidence of lymph node metastases, an excellent short-term prognosis (most deaths 12 years or more after diagnosis) and may have neuroendocrine features Note: Juan Rosai feels the benign behavior is related to its status of being a form of in situ ductal carcinoma b) Colon Colloid type adenocarcinoma comprises about 5-15% of colonic carcinoma and is thought to have a slightly worse prognosis; see Mucin lakes

Colloid droplets Homogeneous masses of eosinophilic debris seen in the renal tubules in bismuth and mercury poisoning

Colloid solution TRANSFUSION MEDICINE A suspension of particles that are so small (1 nm to 1 µm in diameter) that they do not settle out of solution in absence of external force, eg centrifugation; colloid solutions are used to provide prolonged volume expansion and include 5% albumin, 25% albumin, plasma protein fraction (which contains 83% albumin and 17% globulins, less commonly used as rapid infusion may induce hypotension), Dextran 40 (Rheomacrodex), dextran 70 (Macrodex) and hydroxyethyl starch (HESPAN) a polymer synthesized from amylopectin Note: The albumin-containing solutions are heated for 10 hours at 60°C, which inactivates any viral contaminants; Cf Crystalloid solutions

Colon cut-off sign RADIOLOGY Gaseous distension of the right and transverse colon with decreased or absent air beyond the splenic flexure, characteristic of acute pancreatitis; the inflamed transverse mesocolon (which is attached to the anterior pancreas) 'cuts off' the barium flow, causing mesenteric arterial thrombosis and ischemic colitis (RADIOLOGY 1962; 79:763)

Colonic irrigation ALTERNATIVE MEDICINE A controversial procedure in which a series of enemas are administered over a short period by a gravity-dependent device; the technique is practiced by chiropractors, 'colon therapists', 'nutrition therapists', naturopaths and 'homeopaths' with the nebulous purpose of 'detoxification'; the use of a wide variety of detoxifying enemas is an integral component of 'metabolic therapy'; see 'Holistic' medicine, Unproven treatments for cancer SURGERY An intraoperative procedure for antegrade cleansing of the large intestine in an emergency colon resection, which can be used in elective left-sided colonic surgery in patients who are clinically stable, circumventing the need for a temporary colostomy (Dis Col Rect 1990; 33:245); see Bowel prep(aration)

Colony bank obsolete for Gene library

Colony forming unit (CFU) HEMATOLOGY The complex of the hematopoietic stem cell and its progeny; the most likely candidate cell with potential for giving rise to all hematopoietic lineages has been regarded as the CFU-S (spleen) that forms undifferentiated heterogeneous colonies containing pluripotent stem cells; all terminally differentiated or end-stage hematopoietic cells in the circulation theoretically arise from one CFU, although the role of CFU-S as the most primitive hematopoietic stem cell has been challenged, other contenders for the most primitive title include CFU-Blast, CFU-D (CFU, Diffusing chamber), CFU-GEMM (CFU, granulocyte-erythroid-macrophage-megakaryocyte) and CFU-LM (CFU, lymphoid-myeloid)

Colony stimulating factors (CSF) Glycoproteins that control the production, differentiation and function of granulocytes and mono-macrophage systems (table, page 130); see Biological response modifiers

Colorado tick fever An acute tick-born (Vector *Dermacentor andersoni*) RNA reoviral infection occurring in the early spring in the Rocky mountains **Clinical** Chills, biphasic ('saddleback') fever, myalgias of the back and legs, headache, retro-orbital pain, photophobia, malaise and nausea Prognosis Excellent with little residua

Color blindness Most color blindness is X-linked; it is tested by using the Ishihara pseudoisochromic charts; more than 90% occur in males; color blindness is subdivided into: 1) Incomplete achromatopsia, defective vision of blue color which worsens with age 2) Deuteranopia or daltonism, defective vision of blue and green 3) Partial protanopia, defective red vision (uncertain heredity pattern) and 4) Partial tritanopia

'Columbus theory' The theory that syphilis originated in the New World and was brought back to Europe by Columbus' crew from venereal contacts with natives of Hispaniola, causing the 'great pox' epidemics among the sexually promiscuous in the 16th and 17th centuries

Column chromatography A technique for separating a variety of different sized molecules, in which the mobile phase is poured through a glass or plastic column containing a stationary phase, which is a solid, commonly Sephadex beads of different porosities, which will retain molecules with certain characteristics; the molecule of interest is then washed out or eluted using a solvent

Coma depassé A long-standing coma in which there is no sign of higher cerebral activity or cortical function, ie

Colony Stimulating Factors

Granulocyte-CSF Chromosome 17, produced by endothelial cells, fibroblasts and macrophages that stimulates granulocyte formation and act synergistically with IL-3 to form megakaryocytes, granulocyte-macrophages and colonies with a high proliferative potential; G-CSF may successfully 'drive' myeloid leukemia into terminal differentiation, forcing it into a less aggressive disease

Granulocyte-macrophage-CSF Chromosome 5, produced by endothelial cells, fibroblasts and T cells that stimulates formation of granulocyte and macrophage colonies, acting synergistically with other factors to stimulate megakaryocytie blast cell and BFU-E colonies

Colony-stimulating factor-1 Chromosome 5, produced by endothelial cells, fibroblasts and macrophages that stimulates formation of macrophage colonies and acts synergistically with other factors

Multi-CSF Interleukin-3 Chromosome 5, produced by T cells that stimulates formation of granulocyte, macrophage, eosinophil and mast cell colonies and acts synergistically with other factor s to stimulate BFU-E colonies and hematopoietic precursor colonies

Erythropoietin Chromosome 7, produced by renal interstitial cells that stimulates formation of erythroid colonies, acting synergistically with IL-3 to form BFU-E colonies; see Erythropoietin

Brain dead NEUROPATHOLOGY 'Respirator brain' reveals global softening of noble tissue, microscopically corresponding to autolysis and/or necrosis

Coma panel LABORATORY MEDICINE A group of tests that have been determined to be the most cost-effective under the diagnosis-related group (DRG) system for health care reimbursement in the US, which includes assays for alcohol, ammonium, calcium, creatinine, glucose, lactic acid, osmolality, phenobarbital and a general toxicology screen in the blood and urine; see Organ panel

Coma vigil NEUROLOGY Extreme dementia with degeneration of the cerebral white matter that may accompany apparently uncomplicated head injuries Histopathology Petechial hemorrhages, especially in the corpus callosum, ventricular dilatation, chalky white discoloration in the spinal cord and extensive wallerian degeneration

Combat fatigue Battle fatigue Old soldier/sergeant syndrome An affliction of soldiers occurring after long periods of combat duty without respite, consisting of loss of self-esteem, anxiety, tremulousness, depression, extreme emotional lability, dyspepsia and dyspnea; see 'Burn-out syndrome', Old soldier's heart, Post-trauma stress disorder

Combination therapy REPRODUCTIVE PHARMACOLOGY The most common form of steroid contraception, where the tablets contain both an estrogen (ethinyl estradiol, 30-35 μg) and a progesterone analog, (norethindrone, norgestrel or levonorgestrel, 0.5-1.5 mg) taken for three weeks with a one week 'rest' period to allow 'breakthrough' bleeding

Combined modality therapy The use of more than one broad class of therapeutics, eg radiotherapy and chemotherapy to treat a disease, usually malignant; the use of combined therapies is a function of the stage of a disease; lower stage malignancies respond to single modalities, eg early carcinomas respond to surgery and localized lymphoproliferative disease responds to chemosurgery, while more advanced or extensive disease requires multimodality therapy; combination chemotherapy may be of use in treating AIDS as the commonly-used agents, eg zidovudine and ddI attack different sites in HIV viruses (Science 1991; 253:1557)

Comet cell Comma cell Decoy cell An atypical transitional epithelial cell with elongated cytoplasmic wisps or tails seen in bacterially-infected urine; the nucleus is normal in size, without nuclear atypia and filled with dense degenerated chromatin, mimicking a cell with transitional cell carcinoma in situ

Comet tail sign RADIOLOGY A curvilinear soft tissue density extending from the lateral pleura to the hilum, caused by contracted fibrous scarring, seen in the Folded lung syndrome, see there

Comma cell CYTOLOGY see Comet cell SURGICAL PATHOLOGY A morphological variant cell of unknown significance seen in neurofibromas

Commando operation A term first used by Hayes Martin, a pioneer in head and neck surgery, referring to the en bloc removal of an advanced primary malignancy of the oral cavity, usually squamous cell carcinoma (lymphoma is amenable to radio- or chemotherapy); the 'commando' is one of the most aggressive surgical procedures, which entails partial removal of the mandible, floor of the mouth and/or tongue accompanied by a radical neck dissection; the operation was named after the British Commandos, a special strike force that crossed the English channel carrying out raids against the German U-boats; the analogy is apropos given the high risk of not safely returning home by either the commandos or the patient; see also Heroic surgery, Radical neck dissection

'Commitment' HEMATOLOGY An irreversible maturation step by plasma cells which have terminally differentiated, ie have undergone heavy chain rearrangement and thus are 'clonal' and capable of producing only one specific immunoglobulin; cell specificity or idiotype is conferred by the heavy and light variable regions

Committed step A point of no return in a synthetic reaction or in cellular differentiation, after which a cascade of reactions occurs or a cell undergoes terminal and irreversible 'specialization'

Common cold Acute nasopharyngitis Rhinitis and coryza that is usually spread by aerosol, caused by any of a number of viruses: Rhinovirus has 111 serotypes and is inculpated in 15-40% of common colds, coronavirus in 10-20%; other viral causes of the common cold include influenza A, B, C, parainfluenza, respiratory syncytial virus, adenovirus, rarely coxsackie and enterovirus; group A β-hemolytic streptococci cause 2-10%; in 30-50% no etiologic agent is identified Incidence, common cold 41/100 annual cases, USA **Clinical** Influenza-like syndrome Note: When the symptoms are protracted, antibiotics may be indicated to 'cover' for bacterial infections including Group A streptococcus, ***Haemophilus influenzae, Corynebacterium diphtheriae, Mycoplasma pneumoniae, S pneumoniae, Staphylococcus aureus*** and ***Neisseria meningitidis***

Common pathway PHYSIOLOGY The final route in a molecular 'cascade' in which there is a complex interplay among enzymes, substrates, activators and inactivators, and a relatively small signal is 'amplified' by a positive feedback loop to produce an effect; the common pathway of coagulation is initiated by either the extrinsic or intrinsic pathway, either of which activates factor X (Xa), which in turn activates factor II, converting it into thrombin in the presence of factor V, Ca^{++} and membrane phospholipid, activates prothrombinase producing thrombin from prothrombin; prothrombin then converts fibrinogen into fibrin, forming a blood clot that becomes irreversible when factor XIII is activated; the common pathway of complement is initiated by either the alternate or the classic pathways, either of which activates C3 convertase; see Amplification, Cf Cascades

Common variable immunodeficiency (CVID) A heterogeneous, often autosomal recessive group of immune dysfunctions characterized by a decrease in most immunoglobulin isotypes (B cell precursors are present but don't differentiate into plasma cells) and T cell defects without major defects in cell-mediated immunity; CVID affects 20-90/10^6 live births **Clinical** Average age at the time of diagnosis is 12 years, by which time, the patients have suffered recurrent bacterial infections, chronic otitis, sinusitis, bronchiectasis, bronchiectasia, pneumonitis, diarrhea, malabsorption, sprue-like enteritis, achlorhydria, pernicious anemia, cholestasis and giardiasis, affecting up to 50% of patients are well established **Pathogenesis** CVID is caused by various blocks in B-cell maturation, possibly induced by Epstein-Barr virus infection, which may turn off B cells, reduce immunoglobulin production or cause nonglycosylation of the secreted antibodies or T cell suppression of immunoglobulin production **Laboratory** Marked hypo-gammaglobulinemia, impaired antibody response to antigens, decreased 5'-nucleotidase in lymphocytes these patients have a 50-fold increased risk for gastric cancer, 70% of whom have decreased gastrin secretion in response to bombesin (a clinical marker for CVID patients at risk for gastric carcinoma N Engl J Med 1988; 318:1563) **Treatment** Intravenous gammaglobulins (Mayo Clin Proc 1991; 66:83cr/rv)

Communicating hydrocephalus Enlargement of cerebral ventricles due to an imbalance between production and absorption of cerebrospinal fluid, where the ventricular pathway is open and the fluid moves freely into the spinal subarachnoid space, but is blocked by obliteration of the subarachnoid cisterns around the brainstem or subarachnoid spaces over the cerebral convexities **Etiology** Arnold-Chiari malformation, infections, eg bacterial meningitis, toxoplasmosis, cytomegaloviral or other viral meningitides, subarachnoid hemorrhage, increased production of cerebrospinal fluid, eg choroid plexus papilloma, Hurler syndrome due to fibrosis in the subarachnoid space, hypervitaminosis A

Community cell borders CYTOLOGY Cell borders shared in common by clusters of malignant epithelial cells, a 'soft' criterion for cytological diagnosis of malignancy

Comorbidity The presence of two or more morbid conditions or diseases that may complicate a patient's hospital stay; in the US health care environment, comorbidity is a term of considerable importance when determining the length of reasonable hospitalization under the diagnosis-related group system of classification, see DRGs

Compact (dark) cells HISTOLOGY Clusters of non-vacuolated, darkly acidophilic, lipochrome-laden cells, located in the inner zone (zona reticularis) of the adrenal cortex; Compact cells are thought to be the major source of glucocorticoid and sex hormone production under normal circumstances; Cf Clear (light) cells

Compartment syndrome The result of ischemia, trauma or infection of the forearm's deep flexor compartment, with increased tissue pressure due to venous occlusion followed by arterial occlusion of the anterior interosseous artery (which has little collateral reserve space); when untreated, chronic ischemia converts the forearm musculature into fibrous tissue, causing Volkmann's ischemic contraction with a severe flexion deformity of the wrist and fingers; early therapy (fasciotomy) is crucial as end-stage disease requires major reconstructive surgery for salvage of function

'Compassion fatigue' see Burn-out syndrome

Compassionate investigational new drug (IND) protocol A protocol that allows physicians to obtain experimental drugs (or drugs in development) from a manufacturer to treat patients for whom conventional therapies have failed or for whom no other drug exists; although these protocols cannot generate data regarding drug efficacy, they can generate data regarding dosage and potential side effects; see IND

Competency IMMUNOLOGY The ability of the immune system to mount a response to an antigen; Cf Anergy MEDICAL MALPRACTICE The ability of a trained physician or other health care professional (who may also be certified by a corresponding specialty board) to perform procedure(s) and practice his specialty in a skilled fashion; see Board certification, Malpractice; Cf Impaired health care provider PSYCHOLOGY A set of abilities in a person needed for adequate decision-making, which is a measure of a person's autonomy and ability to give permission for either diagnostic tests or for dangerous, but potentially life-saving procedures; the difficulty in legally defining competency is the subjectivity that enters in trying to determine whether a person is too rigid or is flexible enough to evaluate the advantages and disadvantages of his options; Cf Autonomy

Complement activation The initiation of one of the non-specific arms of the immune system that follows assembly of a molecular complex on the cell surface, ultimately leading to lysis of the target cells; complement activation may result in tissue injury including immune-complex-mediated vasculitis, glomerulonephritis, hemolytic anemia, type II collagen-induced arthritis, myasthenia gravis and non-immune-mediated forms of tissue damage, burns and ischemia

Complementarity BIOCHEMISTRY The matching and mutual compliance of two surfaces or molecules to each other, eg the adaption of an enzyme's active site to its substrate, ie the 'induced fit' model or the adherence of two complementary strands of nucleic acids to each other, as in hybridization; see Hybridization, Induced fit model

Complement cascade IMMUNOLOGY A complex, multimolecular biological system involving more than 20 different proteins that self-assemble on cell surfaces functioning in concert with the specific immune defenses to mediate host defense reactions and antimicrobial defense; the coup d'grace to the hapless target cell is the polymerization of C9 on its surface forming a transmembrane 'doughnut' that facilitates the egress of ions, resulting in cell death; Cf Alternate pathway, Classic pathway, Common pathway

Complement multimer see Complement cascade, Doughnut structure

Complete carcinogen A carcinogenic substance or agent, eg ultraviolet-B light, that acts as both an initiator and promoter

Compliance see Patient compliance

Composite tumor A tumor, eg a lymphoma that involves the sequential emergence of different chromosomal rearrangements (heuristically implying a worsened prognosis with each transition, as predicted in the multistage carcinogenesis model); a composite lymphoma present with one histological form, eg follicular lymphoma and a chromosomal rearrangement, eg t(14;18), which juxtaposes the *bcl*-2 oncogene on chromosome 18 with the immunoglobulin heavy chain genes on chromosome; this may then be followed by a second translocation, eg t(8;14) which results in the activation of the c-myc oncogene, which may be accompanied by an aggressive lymphoblastic lymphoma (N Engl J Med 1988; 318:1373); Cf Biclonal lymphoma, Collision tumor, Compound tumor, Mixed tumor

Compound A 11-Dehydroxicorticosterone **COMPOUND B** Corticosterone **COMPOUND E** Cortisone **COMPOUND F** Cortisol **COMPOUND Q** A purified form of the plant protein tricosanthin, derived from Chinese cucumber root and imported from China as an unproven therapy for AIDS; compound Q has also had currency as an underground agent for inducing second trimester abortions and treating choriocarcinoma

Compound tumor A neoplasm in which two or more histologically (and embryologically) distinct components, eg follicular and medullary (parafollicular) carcinomas of the thyroid merge, such that future clinical behavior cannot be determined (Cancer 1983; 52:1053); Cf Biclonal lymphoma, Collision tumor, Composite tumor, Mixed tumor

Computed (axial) tomography imaging CT scanning A diagnostic technique in which multiple X-rays are taken from different angles in a single plane and a series of three-dimensional images ('slices') of the different tissue densities are constructed by computer; see Spiral CT; Cf Magnetic resonance imaging

Computer An electronic device that follows programmed instructions written in a logical language and processes the information in binary code; there are three levels of computer complexity a) Mainframe computers, capable of simultaneously manipulating large blocks of data, b) Minicomputer which is capable of performing several logical 'conversations' virtually simultaneously and c) Microcomputer, traditionally the slowest, with the storage and memory capabilities Note: The advances in technology and design have erased may of the differences between the microcomputer and the minicomputer, leaving the divisions nebulous and of little utility; see AI (artificial intelligence), Buffer, Dumb terminal, Electronic publishing, Icon-driven, Menu, Modem, Mouse, RAM, ROM, RISC chip, SIMM, Smart terminal, Video display terminal Glossary **AND** A word used in programming that restricts the available logical choices, as both of two conditions must be met for a sequence of logic to be allowed **BAUD** A unit of data transmission equalling 1 bit/sec, named after the French inventor, JME Baudot **BIT** Binary digit A unit of binary system measurement, in which all information is based on the logic of a switch being 'on' or 'off' **BOOT** To load the software into the computer's random access memory **BYTE** 8 bits, equivalent to one typed character **CAD** Computer-assisted design **CHIP** see Microprocessor **COMPILER** A computer program that translates high-level (people) language into bits (machine language) **CPU** Central processing unit; the 'thinking' part of a computer, in microcomputers, the CPU is incorrectly equated to the 'box', which also contains the logic board, the hard and floppy drives **CURSOR** The flashing point on a computer monitor, located at the point of data entry **DATABASE** A 'universe' of information that allows information to be accessed in any of a number of ways, eg by patient name, diagnosis, date of admission or discharge **DOS** Disk operating system Programmed information that is loaded into the computer's random access memory at start-up, which tells the machine what it can and cannot do **IBM 'CLONE'** Any microcomputer that is fully capable of writing and reading software written for the three generations of microcomputers based on Intel's 80C88, 80C286 and 80C386 microprocessors using Microsoft Corporation's disk operating system Integrated circuit An electronic circuit mounted on a silicon crystal (chip), which forms the basic unit of a microprocessor **INIT** Any small software program that is 'loaded' into the random access memory (RAM) prior to the disk operating system, bypassing the microcomputer's 'resource manager', which is responsible for directing the flow of information through the computer; INITs are not recognized by the resource manager and thus are 'invisible', but may cause problems in an often unpredictable fashion; INITs in the MacIntosh environment include Dayna's DOS-mounter, Pyro!, Virex, Suitcase and Adobe's Type Manager **I/O DEVICE** In/Out device Hardware that allows both data input and output, eg modems, disk drives; input only devices include the mouse, keyboard or scanning devices; output only devices include printers and dummy terminals **Macro** see Programmable key **Magnetic core memory** The earliest form of computerized data storage, in which each bit of information was represented by a change in the direction (clock- or counterclockwise) of a magnetic field, memory that has long been replaced by semiconductors which are several orders of magnitude smaller **Monitor** The video display unit for a computer's activity **MS/DOS** Microsoft's disk operating system, the standard disk operating system used in IBM microcomputer models PC, PC/XT and AT and IBM 'clones' **Number 'crunching'** A colloquial term for intense and complex mathematical computations, eg three-dimensional rotation of complex molecules and images **Operating system** The internal system that oversees movement of information between the CPU and the input-output devices **OR** A word used in programming that expands the available logical choices, such that either of two conditions may be met for a sequence of data flow or processing to be allowed **Parallel interface** A port that sends or receives 8 bits at a time **Peripherals** Accessory hardware components including printer, modem, flat-bed scanner, mouse **Port** The computer gate to the outside world **Programmable key** One of the keys, usually an 'F' key, on a microcomputer's standard keyboard, that has been defined or modified to suit the needs of the user, alternately called a 'Macro' **Prompt** The carrot on its side (>) that indicates the drive being accessed **Serial interface** A port that sends out information one bit at a time, as do modems **Spreadsheet** A software program which provides a flexible format of rows and columns of numerical values for various calculations **Virtual memory** Open-ended random access memory **WYSIWYG** What you see is what you get (pronounced, wissy-wig) A 'hard' or paper copy that corresponds exactly to what is viewed on a computer's visual display, the cathode ray tube; a wysiwyg display in a microcomputer requires a high-resolution monitor, the appropriate graphics card and newer generation of microprocessor

Computer languages **BASIC** Beginners' all-purpose symbolic instruction code A high-level symbolic computer programming language well-suited for writing programs for mini- and microcomputers; BASIC is a compiled or interpreted language which is both user-friendly and relatively high level **COBOL** Common business-oriented language a slower language, standard in the industry **FORTRAN** Formula Translation language A fast, high-level computer language, used for science and math, but less user-friendly than BASIC **MUMPS** Massachusetts general hospital utility multiprogramming system High level language program designed to handle large, complex databases

Computer virus A short, self-replicating computer program that 'infects' other programs by insinuating its own logic into existing programs, known as a 'Trojan horse' virus, then forcing the host program to bear the 'offspring'; a computer virus modifies host programs to include a version of itself, carrying its 'genetic code' in the form of machine language and telling the 'host' system to insert the 'virus' into its main logic—the hard memory; computer viruses can consume memory, execute unwanted operations or delete material ranging from a small file in a microcomputer to wreaking havoc in a mainframe; such viruses may 'infect' corporate, military and hospital networks, destroying vital information; some viruses have been implanted as 'time bombs' destroying information when a sequence of specific commands is given on or after a certain date (Science 1988; 240:133)

Computer worm A computer program which is self-contained, living off weaknesses in the computer host's logic; the worm may do nothing more than reproduce, ie consume memory and slow the processing of data, but is incapable of 'reinfection'

CON see Certificate of need

Conantokins Antokin, Tagalog, sleepy A family of pepides isolated from cone snails that induce local anesthesia and which may be specific for the NMDA receptor; see Conotoxins, 'King-Kong' peptide

Concanavalin A Immunology A lectin that stimulates the proliferation of certain subsets of T lymphocytes; Cf PHA and PWM

Concentration camp syndrome A psychological complex representing the residual effects of persecution, mental and physical stress, most specifically referring to the survivors of the Nazi concentration camps, although the complex may also be seen in the survivors under the dictatorships of the Khmer Rouge, Pinochet, Idi Amin and others Clinical Chronic tension, vigilance, irritability, depression, fear, disordered sleep, nightmares, headaches, fatigue, excess sweating and potentially, complete withdrawal from human contact; see Post-traumatic stress disorder, Survivor syndrome, Torture

Concerted evolution Molecular biology The production and maintenance of homogeneity or loss of heterogeneity within repeated multi-gene families that occurs in the genes of individuals and populations, resulting from 'biased' gene conversion, switching genes to a dominant form, rather than having a 'permanent hybrid' genome (Science 1991; 251:308)

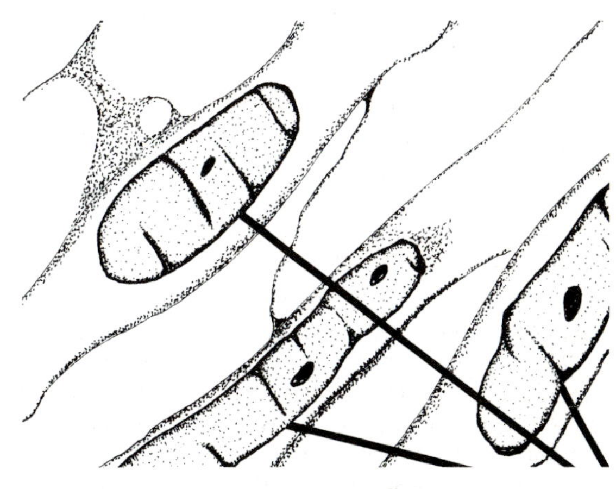

Concertina nuclei

Concertina nucleus A fanciful descriptor for the large, oval nucleus (figure, page 133) with multiple sharp, transverse lines punctuating the cleared nucleoplasm, which is highly characteristic of nuclei in smooth muscle tumors, ie leiomyomas of the gastrointestinal tract and uterine, less commonly described in diverticulosis coli

Condom A diaphanous device for reducing sexually-transmitted disease, which is relatively effective in reducing the heterosexual transmission of the human immunodeficiency virus Note: The term was first dignified in English in 1705 by the Duke of Argyll who used a 'Quondam for debauching ladies', although earlier history is murky, as it is unclear whether a Dr Condom existed, nor, despite the Gallic 'amour d'amour' and the ville de Condom in southern France, is there evidence linking the appliance, also known as a 'French letter' with a Norman origin

Condyloma acuminatum 'Cauliflower' excrescence An epithelial proliferation induced by human papilloma viruses of low malignant potential, eg types 6, 11; condylomata may be precursors to malignancy, especially types 16, 18, 31, are at a high risk for future squamous cell carcinoma, but are uncommon in the usual vulvar condylomata **Treatment** Interferon α-2a (J Am Med Assoc 1991; 265:2684)

Coned cecum A concentric fibrotic tapering of the cecum with a grossly patent ileocecal valve, a radiocontrast finding in chronic amebiasis

'Confetti' lesions DERMATOPATHOLOGY A descriptor for the innumerable, small, scattered hypopigmented macules seen in 96% of patients with tuberous sclerosis, best seen in a darkened room by Wood's ultraviolet light Note: The hypopigmented macules have amounts of melanocytes, decreased melanosomes and melanin (N Engl J Med 1986; 315:1018)

Confidence limits STATISTICS The endpoints of the confidence interval, a range over which it can be stated with a given probability or 'degree of confidence', that a parameter of interest, eg a mean or standard deviation will be present

Confidentiality The right a person has to not have information about his personal circumstances revealed publicly by professionals whose advice and aid he has sought in confidence; the legal aspects of this issue are quite complex, as often the physician has the ethical dilemma of reporting a disease that may harm a greater public, while compromising the confidentiality of an individual patient, as occurs in AIDS or in a seriously psychotic person with homicidal tendencies

Conflict of interest That which occurs when a person is presumed to be unduly compromised in his objectivity as he has a vested interest or bias in the analysis of data that might affect him financially Note: When a researcher has commercial ties with a business that would benefit from his research, the potential for bias is significant; Harvard University's guidelines (Science 1990; 248:154) are the most stringent, delineating both the conflict of interest and conflict of commitment, where no more than 20% of a working week should be dedicated to an outside interest; see Harvard's guidelines, Krimsky index

Conformation MOLECULAR BIOLOGY The three-dimensional configuration of a molecule in space, which is a function of the molecule(s), whether they are arranged in a chain, the types of bonds, the energy of the system and the presence of other molecules in the system; see Protein folding

Confounding variable Confounder A factor that distorts the true relationship of the variables being examined in a study with the end-point changes in those same variables, by virtue of being related in a nonlinear fashion to those variables, extraneous to the study question and unequally distributed between the study groups

Confronting cisternae An ultrastructural finding consisting of lamellar layering of Golgi-related structures, described as specific for AIDS, but which is also found in herpes-infected tissue, sarcomas, hepatomas, giant cell tumor of bone and multiple sclerosis; Cf Tubular reticular structures

Congener Any member of a family of related molecules

Congenic mice Inbred strains of mice that are genetically identical except at one locus or well-defined group of loci; a line of congeneic mice is produced by eliminating those mice with background genes of less interest while at the same time backcrossing the progeny bearing the characteristics and by extension, the gene(s) of interest

Congenital diabetes see Fetal diabetic 'syndrome'

Congenital malignancy Neoplasia that appears at or shortly after birth; as spontaneous remission is not uncommon in these tumors, some of these 'malignancies' may represent hyperplastic reactive albeit monotonous proliferations; examples: Leukemia (often an aggressive disease), sarcoma (although histologically malignant, clinically benign), melanoma (potentially transplacental) and neuroblastoma

Congenital rubella syndrome Gregg syndrome A malformation complex in a fetus infected in vitro by a mother with active rubella ('German measles'); the malformations are consonant with the embryologic stage at the time of infection, with developmental arrest affecting all 3 embryonal layers, inhibiting mitosis, causing delayed and defective organogenesis of involved tissues; maternal infection in the first eight weeks of pregnancy causes embryopathy in 50-70% of fetuses; the susceptible period extends to about the 20th week; infection in late pregnancy is associated with little fetal morbidity **Clinical** Cardiac malformations, eg patent ductus arteriosus, pulmonary valve stenosis, ventricular septal defect, hepatosplenomegaly, interstitial pneumonia, low birth weight, congenital cataracts, deafness, microcephaly, petechia and purpura and central nervous system symptoms including mental retardation, lethargy, irritability, dystonia, bulging fontanelles and ataxia **Laboratory** Viral isolation, detection of specific IgM antibodies in the fetus by hemagglutination inhibition **Vaccination** Attenuated live virus vaccine is administered to all children between the ages of 15 months and puberty; effective antibodies develop after immunization in 95% of patients; in 1986, 11 cases of congenital rubella were reported in the US; see Extended rubella syndrome

Congo-Crimean hemorrhagic fever (CCHF) A tick-borne infection by Bunyaviridiae, seen in Eastern Europe, Central Asia, Middle East, Africa Clinical After a 3-6 day incubation, abrupt headache, myalgia, fever, chills, nausea, watery stools, anorexia; conjunctivitis, leukemia, severe thrombocytopenia Prognosis 10-50% mortality

Conicotine A metabolite of nicotine that may remain at detectable levels in the circulation for up to a week after a last cigarette; measurement of urinary conicotine is used by insurance companies to determine whether subjects applying for health and/or life insurance are indeed non-smokers and entitled to lower premium costs, as non-smokers are in general healthier; see Nicotine, Smoking

Conjugal malignancy Neoplasia affecting marriage partners is low; the risk of suffering rare malignancy, eg glioma in non-related persons living together is extremely low $1/10^8$; in the face of such events and the absence of consanguity, environmental factors, eg carcinogens and/or viruses weigh heavily in the etiologic 'equation' (Cancer 1985; 55:864)

Connectin see Titin

Connexon see Gap junction

Conotoxins A mixture of 10-30 residue in length toxic peptides that act as high affinity ligands for various receptors and ion channels, produced by cone snails (*Conus* species, of which there are 500 known species, each producing a unique assortment of toxins); conotoxins have a wide variety of effects, including inhibition of acetylcholine receptors, local anesthesia and blockage of ion channels that regulate the flow of potassium, sodium and calcium ions; the diverse spectrum of venomous peptides may result from a 'Fold-lock-cut' synthetic pathway, one toxin binds a type of glutamate receptor (NMDA receptor, see there); the snails appear to have evolved a battery of toxins as a necessity to simultaneously act on multiple subclasses of ion channels in order toquickly stop their prey (Science 1990; 249:257)

Consanguinity A state of close genetic relationship, affecting the progeny of a mating and marriage between close blood relatives, eg first cousins, an event accounting for 20-50% of marriages from Asia and Africa, which is associated with increased gross fertility due to younger maternal age at first live birth, and increased morbidity and mortality in the offspring; adverse effects of inbreeding are uncommon (Science 1991; 252:789); see Bottleneck, Inbreeding

Consent A document or verbal agreement by the patient that gives permission to perform a therapeutic or diagnostic procedure; any operation or intervention performed without consent constitutes assault and battery, see 'Ghost surgery'; even if an operation is successful, punitive damages may be awarded, as lack of consent constitutes an intentional invasion of another's rights; thus all elective diagnostic or therapeutic procedures require an 'informed consent' document

Conservative therapy The management of a clinical nosology with the least aggressive of therapeutic options, often equated with 'medical' as opposed to 'surgical' treatment, eg drug, diet and lifestyle management of severe but asymptomatic coronary atherosclerosis, in contrast to aggressive management of the same condition with coronary artery bypass surgery; see Benign neglect, Palliative therapy; Cf 'Heroic' therapy

Consolidation chemotherapy ONCOLOGY A phase of chemotherapy for leukemia or other lymphoproliferative malignancies that follows the initial 'intensification' phase of chemotherapy, in which a patient is given (for example), several cycles of 3 days of daunorubicin followed by 7 days of Ara-C, separated by a resting period of two to three weeks; objective response is then 'consolidated' by one or two more identical cycles of chemotherapy, which in turn is followed by the maintenance phase

Constant region The highly conserved portion of an immunoglobulin molecule that can be separated from the whole molecule by partial digestion with either papain or pepsin, forming a crystallizable fragment (Fc), for which certain cells, eg macrophages have a specific Fc receptor; see Fc, Variable region

Contact inhibition The inhibitory effect of normal cells on each others' growth, such that lateral contact prevents further cellular expansion, a feature of normal cells grown in tissue culture medium

Contact inhibiting factor (CIF) A factor that induces reversion of certain growth characteristics of cancer cells to a more 'normal' appearance in tissue culture media; CIF induces contact inhibition (once normal cells have spread out in a monolayer, further growth is inhibited),anchorage dependence (normal cells will not grow in a suspension) and dependence on serum-based 'growth factors'; CIF may induce tumor regression in hamsters with melanomas

Contact lenses 18.2 million people in the USA (FDA estimate) wear contact lenses, 50% wear soft contacts, 25% hard contacts and 25% use extended-wear soft lenses that cause a 4-fold increase in ulcerative keratitis (N Engl J Med 1989; 321:773, 779)

Contact ring FORENSIC PATHOLOGY A funnel-shaped depression of the skin with marginal abrasion and bruising of the epidermis caused by a zero range or 'execution' type gunshot wound that leaves a 'fingerprint' of the firearm's muzzle

Containment The confining or prevention of further dissemination of a potentially hazardous, eg biologic, radioactive or toxic, agent(s) Primary containment Protection of personnel and immediate environment from the agent, use of proper safety equipment and for some biologic agents, the use of vaccines Secondary containment Protection of the environment external to the 'contained' area which is provided by a combination of facility design and operational practices see Biosafety levels, Regulated waste

Contamination The presence of any foreign or undesired material in a system, eg toxic contamination of the ground water in an ecosystem or viral contamination of a tissue culture plate

Contiguity theory A theory that attempts to answer why the spread of malignancy in the lymph nodes of

Hodgkin's disease occurs in a distinctly nonrandom fashion; it is postulated that the lymphoma spreads from an initial focus to adjacent lymph nodes, transmigrating to more distal organs, leaving no trace in the initial sites of spread; this theory is tenuous as 1) The often-involved spleen has no lymphatic vessels and 2) All peripheral nodes may be involved without intervening mediastinal involvement

Continuing medical education see CME

Continuous ambulatory peritoneal dialysis see Peritoneal dialysis

Contraceptive Any method for preventing a fertilized, term product of conception, including barrier methods (condoms, diaphragm), hormone combinations, spermicides, implantable hormonal contraceptives, RU 486 and others (Science 1989; 245:356); population growth is having an increasing impact on the health of society and its control is being addressed on international fora, see Amsterdam strategy, although not all governments believe this is a problem, see Mexico City policy; contraceptives under development include spermicides with antiviral properties, a reliable ovulation predictor, reliable and reversible male sterilization, male contraception, an antifertility vaccine once-a-month pill, designed to induce menses at a designated time, without disturbing subsequent menstrual periods Note: The US litigation system is considered by some to be the primary impediment to development of anything beyond well-intentioned rhetoric, given the claims of unforeseen embryopathy, see 'Litogen', Pearl index, Wrongful birth

Contraction alkalosis A reduced extracellular fluid compartment with increased extracellular bicarbonate and increased bicarbonate resorption in the renal tubules, a finding characteristic of chronic furosemide therapy **Treatment** Discontinue therapy and substitute acetazolamide (carbonic anhydrase inhibitor) until metabolic derangement is corrected

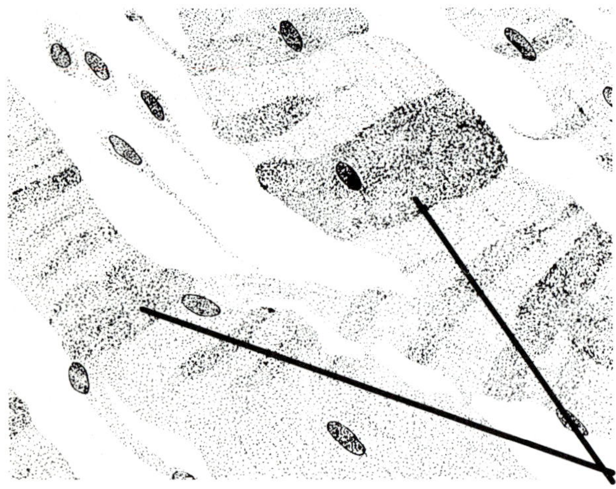

Contraction band necrosis

Contraction band necrosis A nonspecific finding in irreversibly ischemic myocytes, which is often the only, albeit unreliable histologic change seen in hyperacute myocardial infarction, where central coagulated cells are arrested in the relaxed state and reperfusion around the infarct results in cell death 'frozen' in a hypercontracted state, spanning the cell's width (figure) **Histopathology** Hypercontracted, structureless masses of contractile protein and transverse eosinophilic bands span the myocyte in ischemic zones, early mononuclear inflammation is followed by acute inflammation **Ultrastructure** Thickened and 'compacted' Z bands **Pathogenesis** Increased intracellular calcium due to increased sarcolemmal permeability with irreversible anoxia and shock, probably catecholamine-mediated Note: Contraction bands also occur in cardiac muscle in selenium deficiency in Keshan disease and in skeletal muscle in Duchenne and Becker types of muscular dystrophy

Contragestion Any contraceptive method that specifically prevents the gestation of a fertilized egg, eg the 'morning after' pill or RU-486, either by making viable implantation uninhabitable or by promoting the fertilized product's expulsion; see Contraceptive

Contrast-induced nephropathy Acute renal failure that occurs in 2-16% of those who have had radiocontrast studies of the kidney; diabetics do not appear to be at higher risk than other subjects; (N Engl J Med 1989; 320:143,149,179), although those with diabetic nephropathy, pre-existing renal insufficiency and congestive heart failure are at higher risk for nephropathy and studies suggest that the incidence of this condition would be reduced by use of non-ionic, low-osmolality contrast agents

Contrecoup TRAUMATOLOGY A cerebral 'bruise' diametrically opposite the site of the impinging blow to the cranium; the head is in motion and the brain lags behind by a split-second; a blow to the back of the head results in lesions of the frontal lobes and horns of the temporal lobes; a blow to the top of the skull results in contrecoup lesions to the hippocampus and the corpus callosum; in 'COUP' LESIONS, the head is stationary and receives a blow; the brain lesion is directly below the site of the injury Note: Contrecoup is also described in blunt pulmonary trauma with subpleural capillary disruption, hemorrhage, edema, infiltration by leukocytes, protein and fluid obstruction of the small airways

Contreras method An unproven cancer therapy using laetrile and administered in a private clinica in Tijuana, Mexico; see Laetrile, Tijuana

Control LABORATORY MEDICINE A specimen having known or standardized values for an analyte that is processed in tandem with an unknown specimen; the 'control' specimen is either known to have the substance being analyzed, ie 'positive' control or known to lack a substance of interest, ie 'negative' control CLINICAL RESEARCH A group of subjects with features similar to an experimental or treatment group, in whom no intervention is undertaken; a control population is required in order to assure validity of the results; see Double blinding, Zelen design

Controlled drug substances Drugs with potential for abuse or substances with potential for addiction, held under strict governmental control, delineated by the Comprehensive Drug Abuse Prevention and Control Act and passed by the US Congress in 1970, requiring that such substances be prescribed only by a licensed physician, with stringent control of registration, reporting, record keeping, prescribing these substances; misuse or questionable practices of prescribing controlled substances may lead to investigation, penalties and potential punitive action(s) Note: The Drug Enforcement Administration, a branch of the Department of Justice was created to enforce the Controlled Substances Act, gather intelligence and conduct research in the area of dangerous drugs and drug abuse; the Act classified these potentially addicting drugs into five groups or 'schedules' (table) that differ on the stringency of control, conditions of record keeping and order forms required for their use

CONTROLLED DRUG SUBSTANCES

Schedule I drugs High abuse potential, no accepted medical use in the US, eg Acetorphine, bufotenine, dextromoramide, etorphine, hashish, heroin, LSD (N,N-diethyl-D-lysergamide or lysergic acid diethylamide), marihuana, mescaline, PCP (Phencyclidine), peyote, phenampromide

Schedule II drugs High abuse potential, potentially leading to severe psychologic or physical dependence, a currently acceptable medical use, eg narcotics (cocaine, codeine, hydromorphone, meperidine, methadone, morphine and oxymorphone) and non-narcotics (amphetamine, amobarbital, methaqualone, nalorphine, paregoric, pentobarbital, percodan phencyclidine and secobarbital)

Schedule III drugs High abuse potential, moderate to low physical dependence and high psychologic dependence potentials, with acceptable medical uses, eg amphetamines, barbiturates, codeine formulations, doriden, paregoric, Noludar

Schedule IV drugs Minimal abuse potential, limited physical or psychological dependence, potential eg Chloral hydrate, Dalmane, Equanil, Librium, Miltown, paraldehyde, phenobarbital

Schedule V drugs Very low abuse or dependence potential, eg Lomotil, some formulations of Robitussin, diazepam

Conversion disorders Hysteria A group of psychiatric reactions in which the patient 'converts' mental problems into a physical manifestation, including the sensation of something being stuck in the throat, 'globus hystericus', recurrent abdominal pain without physical findings, hysterical blindness, gait disturbances, paralysis, sensory loss, seizures and urinary retention, often reporting disturbing symptoms with indifference, 'la belle indifference'; see Factitious diseases

Convertase see Prohormone convertase

Cookie bite cells see Bite cells

Cookie cutter An adjectival descriptor for a sharply circumscribed or punched out lesion with minimal complexity of the scalloped, vertical margins

Cookie cutter borders DERMATOLOGY A descriptor for the gross morphology of the scalloped ulcerated margins of squamous cell carcinoma

Cookie cutter etching FORENSIC PATHOLOGY A descriptor for the sharply demarcated but ragged or scalloped edges of a wound in a close range (4-5 feet) shotgun wound, where the charge enters the body in a conglomerate mass

Cookie cutter technique EXPERIMENTAL BIOLOGY A proprietary process for selecting subpopulations of cells growing on film-lined culture dishes by cutting around the cell(s) of interest using an ACAS interactive laser cytometer that 'welds' the plastic film to a dish allowing one to strip away the unwanted cells and film, permitting isolated cells to proliferate (Meridian Instruments, Okemos MI)

Cooking A 'soft' method of altering scientific data, consisting in selection of data to achieve agreement (C Babbage, Reflections on the decline of Science, London, 1830); example: 7 runs of a particular experiment are performed; 3 or 4 are inconclusive, while the remainder are vaguely suggestive of a trend; the equivocal results are 'cooked' out; while not blatently fraudulent, such tampering with data is unethical; see Fraud in science, Trimming

Coombs' test see Antiglobulin test

Cooties Colloquial for body lice (***Pediculus humanus***), thought to have derived from the Malay, koot for louse Note: 'Cooties' is most commonly used by the layperson for any disagreeable substance, eg sputum or organism, eg 'germs' in the environment, and is thus of little utility

COP Colloid oncotic pressure

COP(s) Coat proteins A family of proteins that are present in Golgi-derived coated vesicles, including α-COP (160 kD), β-COP (110 kD), γ-COP (98 kD), δ-COP (61 kD), at least one of which, β-COP has sequence similarity to β-adaptin proteins of clathrin-coated vesicles (Nature 1991; 349:215); see Coatamer; Cf Adaptin(s)

Cop-1 Copolymer I A mixture of 14-23 kD myelin-like polymers synthesized from L-alanine, L-glutamic acid, L-lysine, and L-tyrosine, which suppresses experimental allergic encephalomyelitis, the animal model of multiple sclerosis, and reported (N Engl J Med 1987; 317:408) to be useful in treating multiple sclerosis; see Myelin basic protein

COP-BLAM III A 'third-generation' chemotherapeutic regimen (cyclophosphamide, Oncovin (vincristine), prednisone with bleomycin, Adriamycin (doxorubicin) and methotrexate) used for advanced lymphoma; although 5% of patients die from COP-BLAM's toxicity, 60-70% have a prolonged disease-free survival, methotrexate decreases tumor spread to the central nervous system Note: The use of multiple non-cross-resistant drugs circumvents the tumor's anti-chemotherapeutic 'defense' mechanisms, which include amplification of the MDR (multi-drug resistance) gene

COPD see Chronic obstructive pulmonary disease

Copper penny appearance see Sclerotic bodies

Copper-7 An intrauterine device (IUD) that was withdrawn from the US market in 1986 by its manufacturer, when the 'trickle-down' phenomenon of lawsuits (see Dalkon shield) threatened to make the product an economic liability; see Litogen

Copper sulfate test A rapid test for determining the specific gravity of blood that serves as an indirect measurement of hematocrit and used in transfusion medicine to determine blood donor acceptability; specific gravity of 1.053, which corresponds to a hematocrit of 125 g/L (US: 12.5g/dl), a level adequate for blood donation in females, specific gravity of 1.055, which corresponds to a hematocrit of 135 g/L (US: 13.5g/dl), adequate for male donation

Copper wire appearance A descriptor for the fundoscopic appearance in grade III arteriolosclerotic retinopathy, in which the arterial wall is opacified to a degreee that the blood column is only seen perpendicularly, ie through the vessel wall, yielding a burnished copper wire appearance due to light reflection; Cf Silver wire appearance

Copy editing see Proof-reading

Coral reef lesion A macroscopic descriptor for tortuous, ectatic submucosal veins that may rupture in colonic angiodysplasia, a disease so difficult for the surgeon to document in vivo and the pathologist to verify ex vivo that it has been called the 'Emperor's new clothes' syndrome

Cor bovinum Cor taurinum CARDIOLOGY A heart affected by tertiary syphilis, in which aortitis and consequent aortic valve insufficiency results in circumferential stretching of the valvular leaflets and rolling of the free margin, causing massive cardiomegaly, with weights of 600-1000 g being recorded (normal 275g female, 325g male); see Tree barking

Cord cells TRANSFUSION MEDICINE Red blood cells obtained from the neonatal circulation via the umbilical cord; the potency of the antigens expressed on the fetal erythrocytes can be very weak (I, Le^a, Le^b, Sd^a, Ch, Rg, Gy^a, Hy), weak (A, B, P1, Lu^a, Lub, Yt^a, Xg^a, Vel) or very strong (Rh, K, Fy, Jk, MNSs, Di, Do, Co^a, Au^a)

Corduroy cloth appearance RADIOLOGY A fanciful descriptor for the vertically oriented, finely reticulated loss of bony density seen in vertebrae affected by hemangiomas, best seen on a lateral film

Core window That timespan in which a hepatitis B infected patient has detectable hepatitis core antigen (HBc) in the serum but has yet to produce detectable levels of hepatitis B surface antibody; thus 'core window' period in hepatitis B differs from the 'window' period; see hepatitis serology, Window period

Corkscrew esophagus The radiocontrast image of an esophagus with periodically spaced, high amplitude spastic peristaltic contractions of the lower esophagus, attributed to increased responsiveness to neurotransmitters or hormones, clinically characterized by the 'corkscrew esophagus triad', which consists of retrosternal pain, increased intraluminal pressure and uncoordinated muscle contractions, as well as dysphagia and weight loss, but it may also be asymptomatic; in the lower esophagus, the contractions may increase the intraluminal pressure, producing transient pseudodiverticuli, thus the aliases of 'Rosary bead', nutcracker and 'supersqueezer' esophagus

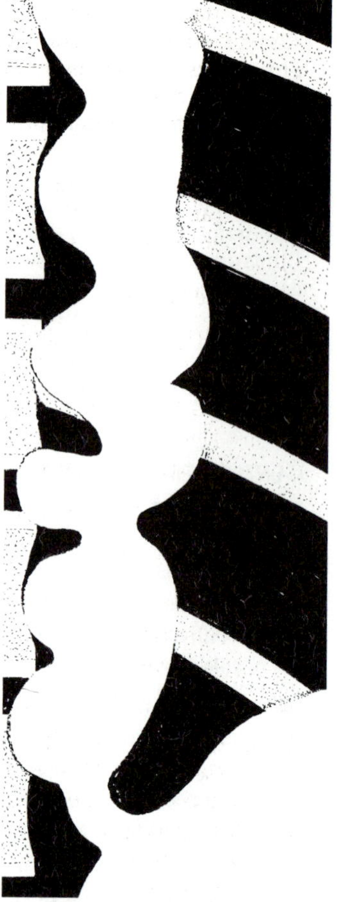

Corkscrew esophagus

Corkscrew hairs Kinking of the individual hairs, a 'classic' clinical finding in vitamin C deficiency that may be associated with perifollicular hemorrhages; Cf Kinky hair, Wooly hair

Corkscrew mesentery Twisted taper mesentery A descriptor for the mesenteric arteriographic appearance of a volvulus in which the main vessel is twisted upon itself

Corkscrew metaplasia A term for the micrsocopic findings in bile reflux-induced gastritis; although erythema, friability and bleeding may be seen at endoscopy, the correlation of clinical disease with histology is poor

Corkscrew (distal) ureter A 'curlicue' appearance of the ureters due to extrinsic compression as in the uncommon ureteral varices

Corkscrew vessels Tight tortuosity of blood vessels seen in the liver of patients with advanced micronodular, often alcoholic cirrhosis, a logical result of collapse of the hepatic parenchyma without loss of vascular length, resulting in 'crimping' of the vessels; this appearance may be seen by hepatic arteriography via the hepatic coeliac or superior mesenteric artery; corkscrew vessels are now a radiologic curiosity as hepatic arteriography has been largely supplanted by computed tomography (CT) and magnetic resonance imaging (MRI) and is only rarely indicated, eg in the rare vascular tumors

Cork worker's syndrome A form of hypersensitivity pneumoconiosis due to exposure to moldy cork dust; see Farmer's lung

Corneal ring An annular superficial ulcer of the corneal limbus, which is a coalescence of several marginal ulcers in a background of marginal keratitis **Etiology** Systemic diseases including infections (bacillary dysentery, brucellosis, dengue, gonorrhea, hookworms, influenza, tuberculosis), connective tissue disease (Gold intoxication, lupus erythematosus, periarteritis nodosa, rheumatoid arthritis, scleroderma, Sjögren syndrome) and others, eg ischemia, lethal midline granuloma, leukemia, porphyria, ulcerative colitis, Wegener's disease **Histopathology** Neutrophils, eosinophils and plasma cells

Corn flake appearance MICROBIOLOGY A descriptor for the yellow-tan, bread crumb-like colonies of the scotochrome (Runyon group II) ***Mycobacterium szulgai*** when grown on a Lowenstein-Jensen agar slant, fancifully likened to a breakfast cereal

Coronary arterial bypass graft (CABG) A procedure in which vascular grafts, usually saphenous, less commonly cephalic veins are anastomosed end-to-side to the internal mammary arteries, bypassing atherosclerotically stenosed coronary arteries; some work suggests that the internal mammary artery is a better donor conduit, given its relative resistance to collapse; internal mammary procedures are associated with longer survival, better long-term patency and lower rate of reoperation; it is unclear whether medical therapy (diet, exercise and cholesterol-lowering drugs) is more beneficial than surgery, although the so-called 'triple bypass' is indicated in unstable angina **Statistics** In the US, each year 800 000 survive an acute myocardial infarct, another 200 000 do not; 175 000 undergo CABG, two-thirds of whom are thought to benefit from the procedure (see below, Medical therapy); CABG is indicated in patients with chronic stable angina who are medical 'failures', patients with two-vessel disease and left anterior descending coronary arterial stenosis; CABG is also indicated in patients with two- or three-vessel disease and ischemia detected by an exercise stress test; in one study, the annual mortality in surgically-treated patients with single, double and triple vessel disease was 0.8%, 0.8% and 1.2% and for medically treated patients, 1.1%, 0.6% and 1.2%, respectively; medical therapy is preferred in those without evidence of myocardial ischemia and in those with one- or two-vessel disease without significant left anterior descending coronary arterial stenosis Note: Moderate alcohol consumption reduces the serum cholesterol, raises HDL-cholesterol and may reduce the risk of coronary athersclerosis (Am J Cardiol 1990; 65:287) Complications, CABG Progression of atherosclerosis, recurrent angina (see Angina), arrhythmia, sudden death, which is reported to occur in 2% of surgically- and 6% of medically-treated patients followed for 5 years; Cf Percutaneous transluminal angioplasty; Thallium imaging, Treadmill exercise test

Coronary artery steal Like all arterial steal syndromes, in which relatively oxygenated blood is 'stolen' or shunted from a potentially critical area of low perfusion to an area of higher perfusion; the 'coronary steal' is unique in that it may be iatrogenic and occur in pharmacologic-stress imaging (see there) using dipyridamole to induce vasoconstriction, causing a fall in the blood flow to the subendocardium distal to the site of the stenosed coronary artery

Coronary perfusion pressure (CPP) A pressure gradient that exists between aortic and right atrial pressures during the relaxation phase in cardiopulmonary resuscitation; CPP correlates well with myocardial blood flow and serves to predict outcome during cardiac arrest; a minimum pressure of 15 mm Hg is required for spontaneous return of circulation; in evolving myocardial infarcts, multiple 1-mg doses (high dose regimen) of epinephrine (adrenalin) improve survival when arrested patients do not respond to low dose regimens (J Am Med Assoc 1991; 265:1139)

Coroner FORENSIC MEDICINE An elected or appointed public official whose chief responsibility is to investigate and provide official interpretation regarding the manner and possible cause(s) of deaths occurring a) Suddenly, b) Violently, c) Without explanation or natural cause, d) for which the stated causes conflict with the findings at the scene of death or at postmortem examination and e) Due or potentially due to foul play Note: The office of the coroner in the US is a political appointment, a custom that dates to English common law, where the representative of the crown (coroner) determined whether the king would share in the deceased's worldly goods; in the USA, because of the political aspects of the office, the pathologist is often a victim of the machinations of an elected government and may be forced to choose between ethics and his own continued employment Note: Politics were responsible for the dismissal of forensic pathologists of international renown in Los Angeles, New York City and Michigan

Corpora amylacea Ovoid, lamellated and sharply-circumscribed masses of pale to darkly eosinophilic structures, likened to starch granules, have been described in the brain, prostatic duct lumina and lungs which have no known clinical significance

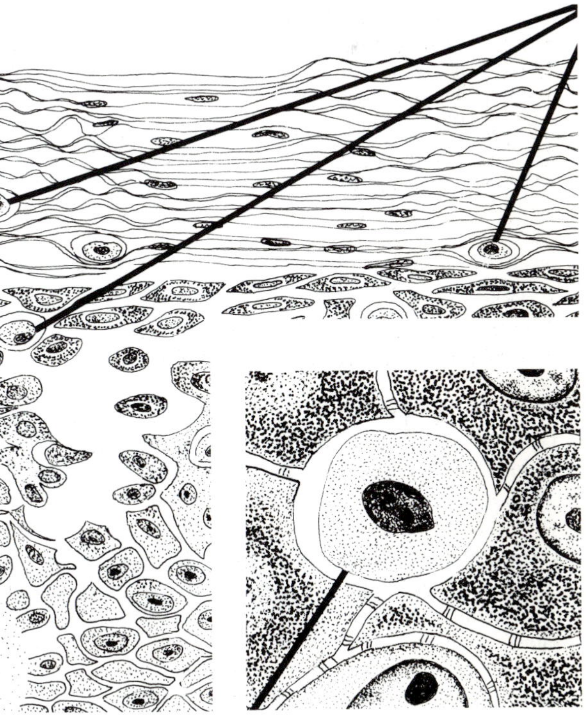

Corps ronds

Corpora arenaceus Brain dust, Valentin's corpuscles NEUROPATHOLOGY Basophilic intra- and extracellular, PAS (periodic acid Schiff)-positive masses seen by light microscopy in the cerebral white matter, thought to be an aging phenomenon, representing axonal degradation endproducts, composed of glycoproteins and mucopolysaccharides, which have been described in Huntington's and Parkinson's diseases and Herpes simplex-induced encephalopathy

Corps ronds DERMATOPATHOLOGY Double-contoured dyskeratotic squamous cells (figure, page 139) with large, round basophilic masses surrounded by a clear halo, located in the spinous layer of the epidermis, classically described in Darier's disease, also found in: benign familial pemphigus, keratosis follicularis and warty dyskeratoma; Cf Colloid bodies

Corpus delecti FORENSIC MEDICINE The substantial and fundamental fact(s) and material evidence necessary to prove the commission of a crime; since the vast majority of cases of medical malpractice do not imply deliberate acts or criminal intent, these cases are tried in civil and not in criminal court

Cor pulmonale A heart affected secondarily to pulmonary disease, resulting in right ventricular hypertrophy (ventricular wall thicker than 5mm or autopsy weight greater than 65 g); primary lung diseases evoking cor pulmonale include pulmonary vascular disease, parenchymal defects, an abnormal ventilatory drive, defects in the thoracic cage or defective pumping mechanism; in chronic cor pulmonale, there is a combination of cardiac hypertrophy and dilatation, while in acute cor pulmonale, there has only been time sufficient for cardiac dilatation; in the older population, chronic cor pulmonale is the third most common cardiac disorder after atherosclerotic and hypertensive heart disease; because of its relation to cigarette smoking, cor pulmonale was formerly more common in males **Medical treatment** Supplementary oxygen, corticosteroids, anticoagulants, vasodilators and other therapy to address underlying lung disease **Surgical treatment** Selected patients are candidates for lung and heart-lung transplantation (J Am Med Assoc 1990; 263:2347)

Cortical oscillations NEUROLOGY Cortical rhythms that range from 4-7 Hz theta waves during sleep to 14-60 Hz waves while aroused are generated and synchronized by layer 5 pyramidal neurons from the neocortex (Science 1991; 251:432); see Chaos

Corticotropin-releasing factor see CRF

COS cell COS-1 cell An altered African green monkey kidney cell line that has been transformed by the SV40 virus and used in transfection experiments for efficient vector expression

Co-sleeping PEDIATRICS, SOCIAL MEDICINE The habit by a young child of sleeping in the parents' bed for all or part of the night, a custom that occurs in 20% of Hispanic households in the US versus 6% of white households and is more common in single parent families and in those living in multiple households; regular co-sleeping is associated with increased sleep disorders (Pediatrics 1989; 84:522)

Cosmid MOLECULAR BIOLOGY A large recombinant plasmid which has an inserted lambda phage cos site that allows the plasmid to be packaged in vitro in a phage coat and efficiently introduced into bacteria; cosmids are designed to carry 35-45 kilobase 'inserts' of DNA and are used to clone large DNA fragments and construct genomic libraries; see Plasmid, Cf YAC cloning

cot curve COT curve analysis MOLECULAR BIOLOGY That relation defined by the equation $Ct = 1/(1 + K C_0t)$, which quantifies the rate of reassociation of DNA as a function of an organism's genomic complexity and when plotted, yields a sigmoid-shaped curve; 10-15% of mammalian genomic DNA reassociates immediately and is regarded as simple sequence DNA as it is composed largely of different sets of repeated oligonucleotides arranged in long tandem repeats; Cf Zoo blot

Cot-sides 'syndrome' Hospital bed 'syndrome' An event with medicolegal implications that occurs in brain-damaged patients (who often are, in addition, elderly and suffer osteoporosis), who have fallen out of a hospital bed with the sides up, which is a fall from a greater height than that which occurs with the sides down Prognosis Poor; coma and death are common

Cotton An adjectival descriptor for a pattern characterized by wispy radioopacities or whitish patches

Cotton ball patches A descriptor for multiple rounded fluffy nodules seen on a plain chest film in patients with pulmonary histoplasmosis

Cotton balls Cotton wool Irregular, rounded, 'fluffy' patches of sclerotic bone seen by a plain skull film in the thickened diploe of advanced Paget's disease, associated with exuberant chaotic bone formation in a background of osteosclerosis; cotton wool patches may also occur in metastases, hereditary hypophosphatasia and chondroblastomas

Cotton candy lung PULMONARY PATHOLOGY A descriptor for the gross findings of endstage panlobular or panacinar emphysema, in which residual fibrosed septae have been likened to cotton candy, a wispy, sugar-based snack traditionally consumed in county fairs, carnivals and circuses

Cotton wool exudates Retinitis angiospastica OPHTHALMOLOGY A descriptor for the fluffy exudates and axoplasmic debris seen in the retinal nerve fiber layer, that accumulate after microinfarcts in the retinal nerve fiber layer, typical of grade III hypertensive retinopathy, but also occurs in collagen vascular disease, diabetes mellitus (nonproliferative retinopathy), immune suppression, infections (***Babesia microti***, cytomegalovirus, ***Pneumocystis carinii***), ischemia, pheochromocytoma and bone marrow transplant recipients **Histopathology**, see Cytoid bodies

'Couch potato' A facetious American colloquialism for sedentary individuals, usually males, whose predominant non-work activity consists in lying on a couch, watching television; anecdotal evidence suggests that these subjects may represent an evolving clinical entity; typical of the couch potato 'syndrome' is a diet of high-carbohydrate, salt-laden foods, eg pretzels, potato chips (potato 'crisps'), popcorn and other forms of 'junk' food, decreased physical activity and a psychological state of suggestibility and decreased environmental interaction; whether this lifestyle predisposes to increased atherosclerotic heart disease, hypertension and other nosologies has yet to be formerly studied, although preliminary data suggests that children who spend prolonged periods of time watching television have higher cholesterol levels, related to a combination of snacking on high calorie foods and inactivity (J Am Med Assoc 1990; 264:2976)

'Cough CPR' EMERGENCY MEDICINE Subjects who develop sudden ventricular fibrillation can maintain consciousness for over 90 seconds with an arterial pulse by vigorous coughing in rapid sequence with a physiological staccato rhythm; cough cardiopulmonary resuscitation (CPR) has two components: a) Vigorous inhalation, causing negative intrathoracic pressure ('thoracic diastole' or Mueller's maneuver) and b) Explosive coughing, causing positive intrathoracic pressure ('thoracic systole' or Valsalva maneuver)

Coulter A proprietary cell counter that functions on the principle of the electrical impedance of particles; the Coulter counter (Hialeah, Florida) has become an 'industry standard' instrument used in clinical hematology laboratories to determine a wide range of parameters of the cells in the circulation, allowing automated loading of specimens and electronic classification of broad categories of conditions, including the relative increase or decrease of erythrocytes, leukocytes and platelets in the circulation

Counterimmunoelectrophoresis (CIE) LABORATORY MEDICINE A rapid immunoassay capable of detecting nanogram quantities of an antigen by the formation of a precipitin line in a gel between an antibody and antigen of different electrophoretic mobilities, CIE is of use in the early diagnosis of bacterial meningitis, for identifying ***Streptococcus pneumococcal*** serotypes, ***Haemophilus influenza*** type b and ***Neisseria meningitidis*** groups A, C, D, W135, X, Y and Z

Coup see Contrecoup

Coup de sabre appearance A curved, sharply demarcated, depressed and hyperpigmented linear groove, often seen on the frontoparietal scalp, accompanied by linear alopecia and dermal atrophy, which is seen in localized scleroderma, an appearance fancifully likened to that of a saber blow

Couplet CARDIOLOGY A pair of successive premature ventricular contractions (PVC); sporadic PVC may occur in young subjects, increase with age and are of no clinical significance unless there is underlying cardiac disease, in which PVC are a risk factor for sudden cardiac death; PVC may result from medication (digitalis, quinidine and tricyclic antidepressants) and are ample indication for discontinuing the drugs Note: The term 'ventricular premature depolarization' is more semantically and physiologically correct than 'premature ventricular contraction'

Couvade see Sympathy pregnancy

'Cover' To prophylactically treat a patient with antibiotics who is at risk for a bacterial infection after surgery or open trauma

'Coverage' 1) The extent of insurance or benefits afforded by an insurance policy, eg typical 'coverage' for medical malpractice insurance ranges from $1-3 million per incident and $3-5 million for complete liability coverage; these values depend on the state (of the US) where the physician is practicing medicine; for individual health insurance, coverage is the amount and type of benefits that would be paid by the policy 2) The provision of medical services by one physician for another, who is usually board certified in the same specialty as the physician for whom he is 'covering'; in the US, a physician is compelled to ensure that 'coverage' is provided should he take a vacation, otherwise he may be legally liable for 'abandonment', should one of his patients need his services in his absence

'Cow method' TRANSFUSION MEDICINE A highly colloquial term of occasional currency which refers to the Sub-subdivision of a unit of blood, such that one unit can be processed either into a 'quad' pack of 125 ml each, which have a normal shelf-life or transferred into two to four smaller aliquots with a 24-hour shelf-life or apportioned at the time of use into pediatric transfer packs that outdate in 24 hours, providing 12 20 ml aliquots of blood and four 'mini-units' of fresh frozen plasma; see Quad pack

Coxsackie A family of picornaviruses from Enteroviridiae, named for a city in New York State where they were first identified; there are 23 virotypes of Coxsackie A viruses types based on pathogenicity in newborn mice and 6 types of Coxsackie B Clinical syndromes Herpangina (Coxsackie A), hand, foot and mouth disease (group A16), summer grippe, aseptic meningitis (both A and B), Epidemic pleurodynia, acute nonspecific pericarditis and myocarditis (group B)

CP-96,345 A potent highly-selective nonapeptide antagonist of substance P's NK1 receptor, a receptor that in the guinea pig is concentrated in the locus ceruleus (Science 1991; 251:435, 437); see NK receptors, Substance P

CPC Chronic passive congestion, see Nutmeg liver; Clinicopathologic conference

CPD Citrate phosphate dextrose TRANSFUSION MEDICINE A storage medium that allows preservation of packed red cells for up to 21 days at 4°C **CPDA-1** Citrate phosphate dextrose-adenine, which supplies ATP, extending the shelf life of blood to 35 days, yielding a higher ATP level CPDA + ADDITIVE SOLUTIONS In addition to the substances provided in the CPDA preservation fluid, additive solutions containing saline, dextrose, adenine and other additives allow a maximum shelf life of packed red cells of 42 days

CPE see Cytopathologic effect

C-peptide A biologically inactive moiety of proinsulin stored within secretory granules in a 1:1 ratio with insulin; C peptide measurement is of use in detecting fictitious insulin injection and in diagnosing insulin-secreting tumors in diabetics, where > 7 ng/ml of C-peptide after induced hypoglycemia supports a diagnosis of insulinoma

CPFs N-carbomethoxycarbonyl-prolyl-phenylalanyl benzylester(s) A family of molecules derived from the dipeptide prolyphenylalanine that bind to gp120, the envelope protein of HIV-1, which is involved in the pivotal first step in HIV-1 infection, binding directly to the host cell's CD4 receptor; the CPF(DD) isomer is highly specific for gp120 and in an in vitro model system, prevents the spread of infection (Science 1990; 249:287) by binding to gp120, preventing HIV's binding to the CD4 receptor, while still preserving CD4's ability to function in the class II major histocompatibility complex

CpG island MOLECULAR ONCOLOGY One of multiple cytosine-guanine dinucleotides on double stranded DNA that are the site of frequent mutations (a mutational 'hot spot') in the p53 gene (Science 1991; 253:49); see p53; these sites are susceptible to methylation, which represses the expression of a structural gene; CpG islands may exist in clusters, fancifully termed a 'CpG archipelago' as in the transcripts of Wilms tumor, which are variably expressed and explain the pathogenic heterogeneity characteristic of Wilms tumorigenesis (Science 1990; 250:991, 994)

cpm Counts per minute NUCLEAR MEDICINE A unit of measurement indicating the energy released by a γ ray emitting isotope, eg 125I, detected by a scintillation counter; see RIA; Cf ELISA

CPM see Central pontine myelinolysis

CPPT Calcium pyrophosphate dihydrate see 'Coffin lids'

CPR Cardiopulmonary resuscitation Those activities performed on a person in order to revive him from apparent death, ie one whose heart and/or lungs are apparently not functioning; as a facet of DNR orders, CPR in the elderly may be considered a futile exercise, as septuagenarians subjected to CPR rarely survive to hospital discharge, despite 'successful' CPR (J Am Med Assoc 1988; 260:2069); see A-B-C sequence, C-A-B sequence, Cough CPR

C protein HISTOLOGY A minor muscle protein of unknown function MOLECULAR BIOLOGY A protein that associates with hnRNA (heterogeneous nuclear RNA) that may be involved in spliceosome assembly; Cf C-peptide, C-reactive protein, Protein C

CPT Current procedural terminology HEALTH CARE REIMBURSEMENT A systemic listing and coding of procedures and services performed by physicians in the USA, each of which is identified by a five-digit number: 00100-01999 and 99100-99140 are anesthesiology services; 10000-69999 are surgical procedures; 70000-79999 are radiology (nuclear medicine and diagnostic ultrasound) services; 80000-89999 are pathology and laboratory medicine services; 90000-99999 are medical services; CPT terminology was developed to serve as free-standing descriptions of medical procedures, eg 25105 corresponds to an arthrotomy of the wrist joint for synovectomy

CPU Central processing unit COMPUTERS The hardware that comprises the 'thinking' part of a computer; although the CPU is one microprocessing chip on the logic or 'mother' board, for microcomputers, the simple-minded often equate the CPU to the entirety of the electronic circuitry in the box containing the hard and floppy drives; thus defined, the *CPU CONTAINS* various components including *1) THE ROM BIOS*, which stores all the information programmmed into the computer on 'read-only memory' chips and circuits; the ROM bios sets the CPU's limits in terms of RAM memory, eg 640 kilobytes and hard drive capacity, eg 40 Megabytes *2) TIMER CHIP*, which places the commands or activities of the microprocessor in a sequence so that they can be carried out in order *3) MATH-COPROCESSOR* and *4) CACHE MEMORY* A memory-containing circuit built into the mother board that accelerates accession of information more quickly than is possible with the floppy or hard drive, acting in a sense as a fast access hard drive; see Computer

CR1 A 30 kD receptor on the surface of B cells that binds to complement C3b with high affinity, and with lesser affinity to complement C4b, ligands which, once bound, modulate B cell activity

CR2 A 140 kD receptor on the surface of B cells that binds to complement C3d and modulates B cell activity

CR3 A heterodimeric receptor for complement C3bi, which is a composite of CD11a (α chain) and CD18 (β chain)

CR3 deficiency syndrome see Leukocyte adhesion deficiency syndrome

Crabtree effect An anomalous response observed in malignant cells in tissue culture; when a glucose-containing substrate is added to a cell-culture medium, normal cells respond by an increase in both glycolysis and respiration, while malignant cells respond with increased glycolysis and inhibition of respiration

Crack SUBSTANCE ABUSE A 'free-base' form of cocaine, prepared by sodium bicarbonate extraction of cocaine-HCl, resulting in inexpensive yellowish crystals, which when smoked in a pipe produce a brief, very intense 'high'; crack is considered the most addicting substance of abuse in existence and may cause addiction within one week; crack appeared on the drug scene in the USA, circa 1985 and already out-competes other drugs of abuse in producing human tragedy in the form of loss of family structure and 'crack' babies Note: For crack ethnography, see Science 1989; 246:1377; see Binging, Cocaine, Crack 'smile', Free base cocaine

Crack babies The infants born to crack-addicted mothers are at a high risk for prematurity, low birth weight, birth defects, respiratory and neurological defects; up to 30% of babies admitted to neonatal ICUs in some US inner city hospitals have crack-abusing mothers and these infants are feared to fare far worse than 'cocaine babies' and have a characteristic trembling likened to a delicately shaking cup of tea; they are four times more likely to be premature, more commonly suffer SIDS, and given the high mortality and morbidity of the mothers, are often in foster care; in 1980, 19% of children in certain zones of the urban US had foster parents; by 1990, this figure had risen to 50%, largely attributed to crack; see Neonatal withdrawal syndrome

'Cracked dermis' DERMATOPATHOLOGY A soft histologic

criterion seen in Kaposi sarcoma where the dermal collagen is dissected, forming bizarre clefted spaces

Cracked ice pattern BONE RADIOLOGY Poorly defined, patchy, mottled appearance due to tumoral replacement of medullary bone, characteristic of Ewing sarcoma; the preferred descriptor is 'moth-eaten'

Cracked pot sign of MacEwen A finding of late hydrocephalus, where increased intracranial pressure leads to palpable separation of the cranial sutures; percussion of the skull evokes a 'jagged' sound, unlike the clear sound when a normal noggin is knocked, a noise likened to a 'cracked vessel' Clinical The skin is thin and shiny, the veins prominent and the cry high-pitched; see Hydrocephalus, Setting sun sign

Cracker sign RHEUMATOLOGY Extreme difficulty in eating dry foods, eg salted crackers, a clinical finding typical of xerostomia, a component of Sjögren syndrome

Cracking artifact HEMATOPATHOLOGY A cleared space seen by low-power light microscopy, which surrounds germinal centers or nodules in lymph nodes; it is a 'soft' criterion supporting the diagnosis of nodular lymphoma and is related to the differences in density between the compact nodule of the homogeneous tumor cells in lymphoma and the surrounding uninvolved tissues; the difference in density between the nodules and surrounding tissue in benign reactive hyperplasia, which may mimic nodular lymphoma is less marked and thus 'cracking' is less common in benign lymphadenopathies

Crack 'smile' 'Life mark' Traumatic lacerations inflicted by a razor or knife extending from the tragus to the oral commisure, often involving the facial nerve and less commonly the parotid duct, that are inflicted on drug pushers or other addicts who have been responsible for a 'bad deal' Treatment End-to-end anastomosis of facial nerve, cannulation with stent if the parotid gland is affected (J Am Med Assoc 1991; 265:1528c)

CRADA Cooperative Research And Development Agreement A component of the US Federal Technology and Transfer Act of 1986, that allows business to invest in ongoing government-funded research, eg National Institute of Health activities, providing extra capital with the hope that the businesses will be able to transfer any technology 'spun off' into commercially viable products, patents or inventions (Science 1989; 245:1034); see 'Krimsky index'

Cradle cap NEONATOLOGY Diffuse or focal, greasy encrustation of the scalp in infants that occurs at about six months of age that may be the presenting or only manifestation of seborrheic dermatitis; the lesions may contiguously involve other 'seborrheic' regions, ie ears, nasal alae, eyebrows and eyelids

Cranial vault OBSTETRICS Those bones that form the movable part of the fetal skull (two frontal, two parietal and occipital bones), and mold themselves to the female birth canal, allowing passage of the cephalic-presenting infant

Craniotabes NEONATOLOGY Softening of the cranial bones to such degree as to allow them to be indented by digital pressure, most often at the vertex of the parietal bone near the sagittal suture; craniotabes occurs in neonates, especially in premature infants and in those exposed to abnormal intrauterine pressures and is usually of no clinical significance, although persistence beyond the first few months of life warrants investigation; occipital bone softening is of more concern, as the irregular calcifications typical of craniotabes may also be seen in osteogenesis imperfecta, cleidocranial dysostosis, lacunar skull, congenital hypothyroidism, Down syndrome and rickets

CRAO Central retinal artery occlusion OPHTHALMOLOGY A fundoscopic finding often due to embolization, appearing as arteriolar narrowing and stasis with segmentation of the venous blood column, resulting in a 'boxcar' appearance; regional infarction of the superficial retina and accompanying edema results in a cherry red appearance; with time, the edema resolves and the fundoscopic findings mimic the usual type of retinal atrophy

Crash COMPUTERS The abrupt malfunction of a computer, due either to a) A software crash, in which a software malfunctions for any of a number of reasons, eg opening a 'system' file and changing the program's instructions; these crashes are often resolved by simple exercises, including rememorizing the system software or by using a 'utility' program, eg Norton utilities to circumvent the problem b) A hardware crash is usually far more serious and can be due to wear or 'trauma' to the machinery, eg dropping; the lost data may be recuperated in hard-disk crashes, if the magnetic storage disk is intact and can be opened in a 'safe' (clean and dust-free) environment CRITICAL CARE MEDICINE An abrupt decompensation of a patient's clinical status

Crashcart CAC cart EMERGENCY MEDICINE A cart that is readily accessible to health care workers and strategically placed in sites in a hospital where patients most commonly 'crash', ie undergo acute cardiovascular decompensation, including the recovery and emergency rooms and intensive care units; a crashcart contains both equipment, eg syringes, gloves, tongue depressors, tubes and airways, as well as medications, eg aminophylline, calcium chloride, digoxin, ferosemide, heparin, naloxone, phenytoin, propranolol and verapamil, required for resuscitation of a person who has 'arrested'

'Crazy pavement' appearance A descriptor for mottled zones of pigmented and depigmented skin, reminiscent of cobblestone pavement, seen in the children suffering from the kwashiorkor-marasmus disease 'complex'

C-reactive protein (CRP) A 120 kD polypeptide produced in the liver that is a biological marker for inflammation and necrosis, so named for its ability to bind the C polysaccharide of the ***Streptococcus pneumoniae*** cell wall; CRP is an acute phase reactant, whose functions include complement activation, binding of T cells, inhibition of clot retraction, suppression of platelet and lymphocyte function and enhancement of phagocytosis by neutrophils Quantification Latex agglutination, rate nephelometry

'Cream cheese' appearance GYNECOLOGY Thickened, whitish caseous or tree bark-like exudate that adheres in plaques to the vaginal mucosa, a colposcopic appearance seen in vaginal candidiasis

CREB protein Cyclic AMP response element binding protein A 43 kD protein which, after phosphorylation, activates nuclear transcription, binding as a dimer to consensus cAMP response elements (CRIe 5'TGACGTCA3') by a 'leucine zipper' motif Note: Transcription of some genes is activated by second messengers, eg cAMP that act through specific protein kinases and requires both the cAMP response element and the 'A' kinase (EMBO Journal 1990; 9:225); see Leucine zipper motif

Creationism EVOLUTIONARY BIOLOGY The philosophy based on the Judeo-Christian concept that all forms of life, in particular, the human were created out of 'nothingness', ie de novo, a theory that is diametrically opposite that of darwinism or evolution, in which all organisms evolved from a previous ancestor; despite the lack of valid scientific evidence supporting creationist theories, creationist 'science' has accrued wide-spread sympathy in some states of the Southeastern USA; Cf Darwinism, Gaia hypothesis

'Creep' see DRG creep

Creeping fat GASTROENTEROLOGY The delicate circumferential extension of the mesenteric fat around the small and large intestinal serosa, characteristic of Crohn's disease, but also described in renal transplant patients

Crenation artefact HEMATOLOGY Distortion of erythrocytes, appearing as echinocytes in peripheral blood smears due to hyperosmolar fixative, or water contamination of the Wright-Giemsa stain

Crepitation 'Crunching' of tissue caused by the presence of gas, due to a) Spontaneous rupture of small pulmonary blebs (most common in young men, causing mediastinal or apical emphysema, of little clinical significance) and b) Gas-producing microaerobic or anaerobic bacteria (requiring a low red-ox potential, eg ***Clostridia perfringens, C sporogenes, C tertium, Bacteroides*** species, peptostreptococci and peptococci), potential inoculums in open trauma, causing cellulitis, myonecrosis, foul odor and abundant gas production with minimal systemic disease

Crescendo angina see Angina, unstable

Crescent A commonly-used adjectival descriptor (alternately termed 'Quarter moon') for a sharply circumscribed, smoothly curved radiolucent or light-colored mass in a dark background, which converges at both ends

Crescent BONE RADIOLOGY A curvilinear subcortical radiolucency corresponding to a fracture line and bony collapse, seen in early ischemic necrosis of the epiphysis of the femoral head, a finding that may also be seen in the humoral head, and may be accentuated by traction (Radiol 1970; 94:505) RENAL PATHOLOGY Epithelial crescents are curved, semilunar lesions seen by low-power light microscopy, which correspond to extracapillary proliferation of Bowman's (glomerular) capsule epithelium, acquiring a fibroblast-like spindled morphology, possibly stimulated by release of fibrinogen from basement membrane; crescents may be accompanied by collagen and fibrin deposition, mononuclear cell proliferation; crescents may be seen in primary and secondary glomerular disease RENAL RADIOLOGY A scalloped curvilinear radiolucency seen in the kidneys secondary to chronic lower urinary tract obstruction, eg concrement-induced obstruction, seen in the early phases of urography; the crescent is due to accumulation of radiocontrast material within flattened collecting tubules and thus indicates residual renal function in contrast to the rim sign, in which there is no renal function, best seen by angiography

Crescentic glomerulonephritis (CGN) A glomerulopathy that may be associated with diabetes mellitus, characterized by heavy proteinuria, microaneurysms and hypertension; without therapy, 80-90% eventually require regular dialysis; CGN may be a) Idiopathic or primary, a condition which, in absence of an infection, multisystem disease or other primary glomerulopathy reveals extensive (greater than 50% of glomeruli are involved) crescents, divided into Type I Anti-glomerular basement membrane antibody without pulmonary hemorrhage Type II Immune complex crescentic glomerulonephritis and Type III Idiopathic; CGN may also be superimposed on other primary glomerulopathies, including membranoproliferative (mesangiocapillary) glomerulonephritis, membranous, IgA nephropathy and focal and segmental glomerulosclerosis; CGN may be secondary to infection, eg Post-streptococcal GN, infective endocarditis, sepsis, hepatitis, multisystem diseas, cryoglobulinemia, Goodpasture's disease, relapsing polychondritis, Henoch-Schönlein purpura, lupus erythematosus, disseminated vasculitis, polyarteritis nodosa, Wegener's disease, lung cancer, lymphoma and other malignancy (idiopathic diffuse)

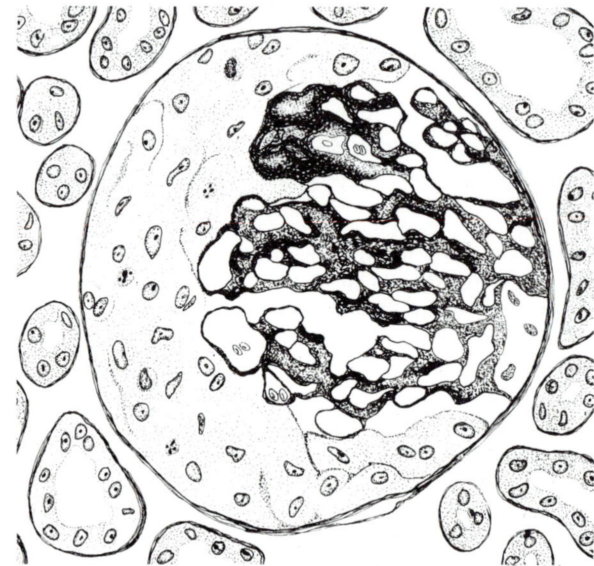

Glomerular crescent

CREST complex An acronym for the pentad of clinical signs seen with mixed connective tissue disease, including Calcinosis, Raynaud's phenomenon, Esophageal dysmotility with eventual stricture, Sclerodactyly and Telangiectasia; CREST has a slightly better prognosis than other connective tissue disorders, but is susceptible to the late complications of biliary cirrhosis and pulmonary hypertension Laboratory Anticentomere antibodies are characteristic of CREST, but may also seen in progressive systemic sclerosis, older women or in those with HLA-DR1

Cretin Congenital hypothyroidism A condition caused by defective thyroxine or thyroglobulin synthesis, associated with a goiter, iodine deficiency or thyroid gland defects (aplasia, hypoplasia or dysgenesis) Clinical Cold intolerance, serosal effusions, myxedema, low metabolic rate, increased cholesterol and profound mental retardation (hypothyroid idiocy); when detected in neonatal screening and treated early, these children have normal school performance at age 10 (J Pediatr 1990; 116:27) Note: Cretin is from French for Christian, as these children are so profoundly retarded that they were considered to be incapable of sinning and therefore the purest of God's creatures, ergo the most perfect Christians

Crewcut appearance Hair on end appearance Outward radiations perpendicular to the surface, Neoosteogenesis of the outer table of the skull characteristically seen in children and young adults with thalassemia, as well as in sickle cell anemia, hereditary spherocytosis, cyanotic congenital heart disease, polycythemia vera and metastatic neuroblastoma; the 'crewcut' appearance may occur in the periostitis of long bones in congenital syphilis, which when in the tibia, gives rise to Saber shins

CRF Corticotropin releasing factor A potent neuropeptide that stimulates synthesis and secretion of proopiomelanocortin-derived peptides, which is released in the median eminence of hypothalamus into the portal circulation of the pituitary gland, regulating (via cAMP and Ca^{++} as intracellular messengers) ACTH secretion; CRF injection evokes hormonal, metabolic, circulatory and behavioral biological stress response; CRF is markedly increased in pregnancy and its activity is turned off by a 37 kD binding protein (Nature 1991; 349:423)

CRH Corticotropin releasing hormone; see CRF

Crib death A synonym used by lay persons for Sudden infant death syndrome, see SIDS

Cribriform An adjective for a sieve-like histological pattern, in which sheets of epithelial cells are punctuated by gland-like spaces; the cribriform pattern is highly suggestive of adenoid cystic carcinoma

Cri-du-chat syndrome Lejeune syndrome An embryopathic complex that is more common in females due to the loss of the short arm of chromosome 5, occasionally due to a ring chromosome Clinical High-pitched feline mewing which often diminishes with age, low birth weight, mental and physical retardation, hypertelorism, hypotonia, microcephaly, micrognathia, epicanthal folds, a moon-like facies, low-set ears, congenital cardiac defects, short metacarpals and metatarsals, pes planus and partial syndactyly Prognosis The lifespan relatively normal

Criminal homicide see Murder

Criminal insanity see Insanity

'Criminal' nerve of Grassi A branch of the right posterior vagus which passes to the left behind the esophagus, terminating in the cardia; the sobriquet 'criminal' derives from the significant potential for ulcer recurrence if the nerve is not severed during surgery

Criminal victimization SOCIAL MEDICINE A social condition most common in women who are single mothers, who suffer physical and mental abuse from boyfriends, having in general more stress, less well-being and 2.5-fold greater inpatient costs than non-victims (Arch Int Med 1991; 151:342)

Crisis INFECTIOUS DISEASE Abrupt improvement ('breaking' of a fever) of untreated lobar pneumonia, most often due to *Streptococcus pneumoniae*, occurring at the end of the first week, at the time when the production of antibodies rises and successful phagocytosis of the bacteria occurs, a clinical finding common in the pre-antibiotic era MEDICINE Any acute exacerbation of a clinical condition, eg Addisonian crisis TISSUE CULTURE The self-imposed limit on the growth of cultured, non-neoplastic fibroblasts and other cell lines; after 50-100 generations, these cells undergo a series of agonal changes in the genome, including the shortening of telomers, lose their ability to divide and die

Crisscross heart 'Upstairs downstairs' heart, Superoinferior heart A rare cardiac malformation in which the atrioventricular spatial relation places each ventricle in a position contralateral to its corresponding atrium, characterized by a horizontal interventricular septum, with complex cardiac plumbing; one-third have atrioventricular discordance Clinical Cyanosis and heart failure Treatment Palliative rather than corrective surgery

Crithidia assay From *Crithidia luciliae*, a hemoflagellate, the kinetoplast of which is a modified mitochondrion containing abundant double-stranded DNA; the crithidia assay has been used to quantify anti-DNA antibodies in the serum of patients with lupus erythematosus by direct immunofluoresence

CRNA Certified registered nurse anesthetist

Crocodile tear 'syndrome' A clinical analog of gustatory hyperhidrosis, in which the peripheral autonomic pathways for lacrimation and salivation are misdirected or short-circuited, usually following facial nerve injury, where food or chewing induce unilateral or inappropriately abundant tearing, due to faulty regeneration of nerve fibers which originally supplied the salivary glands are routed to the lacrimal gland via the petrossal nerve

'Crock' A derogatory colloquialism for a hypochondriac

Cross bite ODONTOLOGY A form of malocclusion in which there is a reversal of the normal relation of the mandibular with the maxillary teeth; in normal dentition, the mandibular teeth lie inside the maxillary teeth and the outside mandibular cusps (incisal edges) meet the central portion of the opposing maxillary teeth

'Cross country' fashion SURGICAL PATHOLOGY A descriptor for the manner in which the polymorphic infiltrates of pulmonary lymphomatoid granulomatosis destroys the lung, 'spilling over' into the interstitium Note: Originally described as benign, lymphomatoid granulomatosis is clearly premalignant or frankly malignant, as the average patient survives 14 months and often involves extrapulmonary sites, eg skin, central nervous system and kidney, extending in a lymphoma-like fashion, often causing a septic death

Crossed eyes Convergent strabismus A process affecting 3% of all children; once recognized, strabismus should be treated immediately to allow maximum development of visual accuity, binocular function and cosmetic results Note: In general, children do not outgrow strabismus

Crossed syndrome(s) NEUROLOGY Cranial nerve lesions that are opposite to the side of a hemiplegia, which may occur in transient occlusion of the basilar artery

Cross-feeding MICROBIOLOGY The growth of two or more organisms in the region, as each is dependent on the waste or synthetic products of the other organism; see CAMP test

Cross infection Person A has microorganism A; person B has microorganism B; upon person-to-person contact, microorganism B infects person A, microorganism A infects person B; both patients must be treated with the appropriate antimicrobial agent for both infections, otherwise a 'ping-pong' infectious sequence may develop

Cross-linkage theory A biologic model for aging that assumes that post-translation cross-linking of normally translated intra- and extracellular proteins is responsible for aging, eg glycosylation end-products causing cataracts and collagen degeneration causing atherosclerosis; while not central to the pathogenesis of aging, the cross-linkage theory provides a valid framework for aging process; see Garbage can theory

Cross match TRANSFUSION MEDICINE An agglutination test that determines donor-recipient blood compatibility; cross matches are of two types: 1) Major Crossmatch Patient serum (which may contain antibodies) is cross-reacted against the donor's red cells and 2) Minor cross-match Patient erythrocytes are incubated with donor serum, this is of lesser clinical significance and reveals donor antibodies against low incidence antigens (eg C^w, -Wr^a, -Li^a)

Cross-match/transfusion ratio TRANSFUSION MEDICINE The C/T ratio is the ratio of units of packed red blood cells that are cross-matched (in the blood bank for potential infusion during surgical procedures) to the number of units actually transfused; under optimal conditions, this ratio is 2.5 or less for general surgery and somewhat higher for obstetrics and gynecology; a high C/T ratio may indicate excess caution by the surgeon or overordering, while low ratios indicate effective prediction of actual usage

'Crossover' unit TRANSFUSION MEDICINE A unit of autologous blood product(s) that is made available for general use after the donor's surgery and potential need for the blood has passed; the FDA has recommended against using cross-over units, reasoning that a) Donor criteria are less stringently applied when accepting a donor for transfusion of his own blood and b) The unit has a greater potential for being infected

Cross-reaction IMMUNOLOGY A partial reaction or 'recognition' of an epitope by an antibody which was generated in response to another antigen

Cross-sectional study EPIDEMIOLOGY A survey that determines the difference in the prevalence of disease among various segments of the population at a particular time, which may be used to infer a causitive relation; Cf Epidemiology

Croup PEDIATRICS A generic term for a heterogeneous group of relatively acute, often infectious conditions characterized by a brassy, seal-like barking or 'croupy' cough accompanied by inspiratory stridor and hoarseness, resulting from intense edema, laryngeal mucus, subglottic stenosis, accompanied by dyspnea, tachypnea, cyanosis, sternal and intercostal retractions; a common form is viral laryngotracheitis with progressive subglottic edema, affecting children age 3 months to 3 years, commonly due to respiratory syncytial virus and parainfluenza virus; bacterial laryngotracheitis predominantly affects those ages 3 to 7 and is due to ***Haemophilus influenzae*** and ***Corynebacterium diphtheriae*** Clinical Progressive dyspnea, dysphagia, low-grade fever, chills and an upper respiratory tract infection in the recent past RADIOLOGY see Gothic arch Treatment Mist tents, antibiotics; 'croup'-like coughs may occur with upper airway obstruction due to aspiration of a foreign body, retropharyngeal abscess, intraluminal masses (angioedema, hemangioma), extrinsic compression, eg hematoma secondary to neck trauma, spasms initiated by endotracheal intubation, hypocalcemic tetany and asthma

Crowding SOCIAL MEDICINE Excess population density; under long-term crowding conditions, the behavior of individual mice in colonies of mice begins to 'autodestruct' two-to-four generations after passing twice the optimal population density; maternal instincts fail, juvenile behavior extends into adulthood, younger animals become aggressive and males huddle together in small 'gangs' Note: Correlating rodent data to the human social fabric is fraught with error, despite the disturbing implications

Crowing PEDIATRICS Noisy respiratory 'cawing', stridor and severe respiratory distress, heard in infants with a) Congenital laryngeal stridor Crowing may be the first sign of congenital epiglottic and superglottic deformity or flabbiness (laryngomalacia and tracheomalacia) with collapse and partial inspiratory airway obstruction, a condition more common in males; during the paroxysms, the children are hoarse, aphonic,dyspneic, have inspiratory muscle retractions and if prolonged, fail to thrive, b) Double aortic arch and c) Others, including branchial cleft cysts, chondromalacia, congenital goiter, croup, intraluminal webs, laryngeal masses, lymphangioma, macroglossia, mandibular hypoplasia, mucus retention cysts, Pierre-Robin syndrome and thyroglossal duct remnants

Crow's feet appearance A fanciful descriptor for short linear striations radiating from one point or a short line NEURORADIOLOGY Angiographic morphology of cerebellopontine angle hemorrhages RADIOLOGY Vague linear opacifications radiating from the pleura into the pulmonary parenchyma, seen on a plain chest film in pleural asbestosis (N Engl J Med 1987; 316:198cpc)

Note: Crow's feet on a chest film are usually benign, but may also appear in malignant mesotheliomas and other tumors SURGICAL ANATOMY A fanciful synonym for the terminal branches of the left (anterior) vagus nerve, which are preserved in highly selective vagotomy for surgical therapy of peptic ulcer disease

CRT Cathode ray tube see Video display terminals

Cruciferous vegetables CLINICAL NUTRITION A group of indole-rich vegetables, eg broccoli, brussels sprouts, cabbage, cauliflower and mustard that have anti-tumor promoting activity in laboratory animals; crucifer consumption is decreased in patients with colonic cancer; see Tumor promoter

Cruciform DNA Foldback DNA An unstable, non-double helix form of DNA, consisting of a pair of hairpin oligonucleotide palindromes, generated either as an intermediate in homologous genetic recombination, resulting in a transient 'Holliday' junction or as a supercoiled palindromic sequence; the binding protein that recognizes cruciform DNA is an evolutionally conserved nuclear protein, the non-histone high mobility group protein 1, HMG-1 (Science 1989; 143:1055); cruciform DNA is useful for in vitro studies of DNA kinetics and structural analysis, but is thought to be a 'forbidden' structure under natural conditions

Crumbled bone disease Osteogenesis imperfecta, type II An autosomal recessive, often lethal condition (50% are stillborn), with low birthweight, beading of ribs with multiple fractures and an accordion-like collapse of shortened, bent and deformed long bones with potentially fatal neonatal respiratory insufficiency in those who survive birth

Crumpled tissue paper appearance A descriptor for the faintly striated eosinophilic cytoplasm in the foamy 20-80 μm Gaucher histiocytes, best seen by a PAS (periodic acid Schiff) stain; the striations are due to bilayered stacks of glucosyl ceramide within lysosomes Ultrastructure Twisted tubules arranged in rod-shaped, 125 nm in diameter membrane-bound fascicles; cytoplasmic striation may be seen in the pseudo-Gaucher cells of thalassemia, lymphomas and type II dyserythropoietic anemia

Crush syndrome Traumatic rhabdomyolysis A condition that results from prolonged and continuous pressure on the limbs, which reflects the disintegration of muscle and influx of myolytic products into the circulation; the crush syndrome was first described during the Battle of Britain (Br J Med 1941; 1:427), when it was induced by massive trauma resulting from air-raid and rocket (V-1 and V-2) bombings; the victims went into shock only after they had been released from entrapment by crushing objects, despite initial response to wound care and intravenous therapy Laboratory Increased potassium, purines, phophates, lactic acid, myoglobin, thromboplastin, creatine kinase, creatine and BUN, hemoglobinuria and myoglobinuria Pathophysiology Crush syndrome was attributed by the early workers to blockage of the distal convoluted renal tubules by myoglobin, but later shown to result from post-anoxic acute tubular necrosis with local renal vasoconstriction due to stimulation of the autonomic nervous system, a pathogenic 'cascade' that also occurs in drug-induced (eg heroin) coma; also implicated in the syndrome is the so-called reperfusion injury (N Engl J Med 1990; 322:825; ibid, 1991; 324:1417) Note: Rhabdomyolysis, myoglobinuria and renal failure with hypocalcemia due to a shift of extracellular calcium into injured muscle, impaired Na^+-K^+-ATPase activity; intramuscular pressure in patients with compressed limb injuries may increase to 240 mm Hg, resulting in rhabdomyolysis independent of ischemia and anterior compartment syndrome

'Crushed cranberry' appearance A fanciful descriptor for the gross appearance of *Actinomadura pelletieri*, where the colonies are blood red and glistening

Cruzan, Nancy Beth A 32-year-old woman who was in a prolonged unconscious (vegetative) state since an automobile accident in 1983, despite her parents' efforts to disconnect her life support; according to the Supreme Court of Missouri, *'THE STATE'S INTEREST IS NOT IN QUALITY OF LIFE, BUT RATHER IN LIFE ITSELF, AN INTEREST THAT IS UNQUALIFIED'*; in the USA, 10 000 patients are in a persistent vegetative state, each at an annual cost of $130 000 (N Engl J Med 1990; 322:1226) Note: This 'right-to-life' case ended in December 1990 with the removal of life support and Ms Cruzan's death; see Persistant vegetative state

Cruzin A highly specific neuraminidase inhibitor isolated from *Trypanosoma cruzi* which is identical both functionally and molecularly to high-density lipoprotein (HDL); when *T cruzi* epimastigotes are grown in a lipoprotein-depleted medium, addition of HDL and cruzin restores multiplication; cruzin binds to *T cruzi*, inhibiting neuraminidase produced in the infective trypomastigote (Mol Bio Parasitol 1988; 28:257)

CRYO see Cryoprecipitate

CRYOGLOBULINEMIA

Type I Monoclonal cryoglobulinemia The underlying disease is often malignant; IgG (Malignant myeloma), IgM macroglobulinemia or lymphoma/chronic lymphocytic leukemia, rarely others (IgA nephropathy) and benign monoclonal gammopathy

Type II Poly-monoclonal cryoglobulinemia A complex of immunoglobulins including mixed IgM-IgG, G-G, A-G or other combinations that may be associated with lymphoreticular disease or connective tissue disease (rheumatoid arthritis, Sjögren syndrome, mixed essential cryoglobulinemia)

Type III Mixed polyclonal-polyclonal cryoglobulinemia Mixtures of IgG and IgM, occasionally also IgA, associated infections; rheumatoid arthritis, lupus erythematosus, Sjögren syndrome, Epstein-Barr and cytomegalovirus inclusion viruses, subacute bacterial infections, poststreptococcal, crescentic and membranoproliferative glomerulonephritides, diabetes mellitus, chronic active hepatitis, biliary cirrhosis

Cryoglobulinemia A clinical condition caused by proteins, especially polymeric IgG3 that precipitate in vivo on cooling of acral parts, often associated with immune complex-related disease, which has been divided into three clinical forms, table, page 147 Clinical Arthralgias, vascular purpuras, cold intolerance, hypertension, congestive heart failure Laboratory Decreased C4 and other complement proteins

Cryocrit A crude, rapid method for quantifying cryoglobulin; a hematocrit tube of serum is cold-incubated, spun and the percentage of precipitate determined

Cryoprecipitate 'CRYO' TRANSFUSION MEDICINE A product derived from a unit of whole blood, which has a volume of 15 ml and provides a minimum of 80 units of factor VIII:C procoagulant (for hemophilia A), factor VIII:vWF (for von Willebrand's disease), factor XIII, fibronectin and fibrinogen (for disseminated intravascular coagulation, dysfibrinogenemia)

Cryopreservation Freezing of tissue Certain human tissues, eg packed red cells and pre- and post-fertilization products can be reversibly frozen by using glycerol, which a) Lowers the freezing point of fluids by increasing the number of molecules in solution and b) Transforming water into a glass-like solid instead of ice crystals which would rupture the cells; in animals, hyperglycemia allows subfreezing survival Note: In California, whole body cryopreservation has been offered commercially , although no body has been successfully thawed; see Frozen cells, in vitro fertilization

Cryopreservatives TRANSFUSION MEDICINE Agents that allow long-term storage of packed red cells for up to a projected 40 years, with 85% viability of erythrocytes 24 hours after transfusion; the agent of choice is 40% glycerol, which is stored at -80°C, requires post-thaw washing to reduce the glycerol to 1% and which tolerate wide fluctuations of temperature during transportation; other cryopreservatives include 20% glycerol which is stored at -150°C and is therefore difficult to transport, 14% hydroxyethyl starch and 15% DMSO-dimethylsulfoxide; see Frozen blood, HES

Cryostat SURGICAL PATHOLOGY A device that houses a microtome, maintaining it at -20°C to -30°C, for the purpose of providing the surgeonrelevant information, eg an intraoperative diagnosis of malignancy for a breast lesion, or whether the margins are involved in a basal cell carcinoma of the skin, on how to best continue a procedure, while the patient is under anesthesia; see Frozen section

Crypt abscess GASTROINTESTINAL PATHOLOGY Aggregates of neutrophils, eosinophils, fibrin and sloughed epithelial cells within a partially ruptured colonic glandular lumen; this histologic finding (figure) is highly characteristic of ulcerative colitis, but may be seen in Crohn's disease, inflammatory bowel disease, radiation colitis and infection by ***Helicobacter*** species

Crystallin(s) A large family of homologous water-soluble proteins that form the major structural component of the ocular lens, divided into α, β and γ crystallins, ranging from the 28 kD monomeric γ crystallin to the larger oligomeric and polymeric crystallins (Nature 1990; 347:776); crystallins are diverse and taxon-specific; while some crystallins are specialized for the lens, others have been found to be identical to enzymes found in other tissues, which are structurally related to heat shock proteins (Science 1991; 252:1078ed)

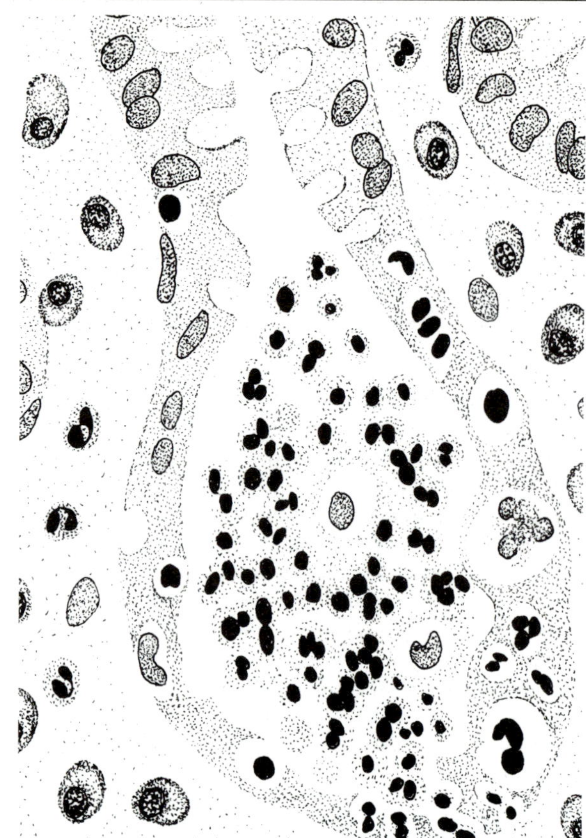

Crypt abscess

Crystalloid solution A balanced isotonic solution, eg Ringer's lactate or saline fluid solution which may be used for volume expansion; because of the low osmotic pressure of these solutions, within minutes of administration, 80% of the crystalloid migrates to the interstitial space, while 20% remains in the vessels; there is thus a controversy in transfusion medicine whether blood volume should be expanded with colloid solutions (which are composed of high molecular weight substances, and therefore retained within the vessels and not associated with peripheral edema) or crystalloid solutions (which are less expensive, easily excreted and do not induce allergic reactions; Cf Colloid solutions

CSF see Colony-stimulating factors

CSI Cholesterol/saturated fat index NUTRITION Wild game is lean and has cholesterol levels of 5/100 g versus > 15/100 g for today's meat, a finding that may explain why the Neanderthal did not suffer from cardiovascular disease

CSIF Cytokine synthesis inhibitory factor; see Interleukin-10

CTCL Cutaneous T cell lymphoma

CTL see Cytotoxic T lymphocyte

C/T ratio see Cross-match/transfusion ratio

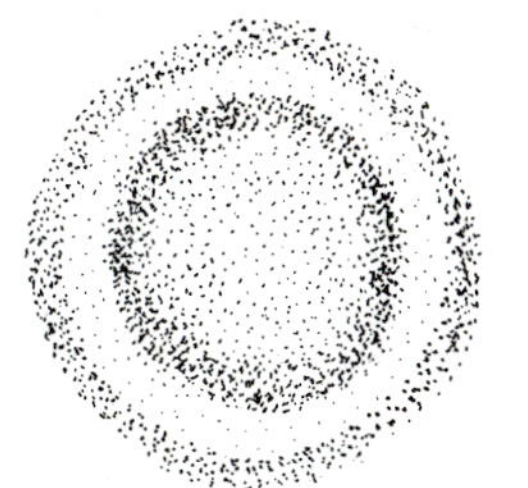
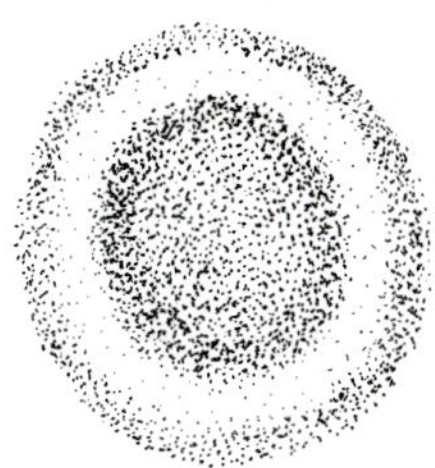

Early form **Type C virus** **Late form**

C-type virus A single-stranded RNA retrovirus with a central nucleoid, which has oncogenic potential, ie capable of acting as a proto-oncogene, first appearing in the infected cells as immature 'A' particles; see B-type-virus, Retrovirus

CTZ see Chemoreceptor trigger zone

Cul-de-sac French, blind pouch An anatomic 'blind alley', seen in a) Pouch of Douglas, the most dependent (ie lowest) extension of the free peritoneal cavity, located between the anterior rectal serosa and posterior uterine serosa, gravity makes this a favored site for accumulation of acute inflammatory debris and tumor aggregates b) Conjunctiva The reflexion of the cornea and conjunctiva c) Dura The end of the spinal canal and d) Colonic cecum, Latin for cul-de-sac

Culex A globally-distributed genus of mosquitoes (family Culicidae) with over 2000 species, including the common mosquito of temperate climates, mosquitoes that are vectors for Togavirus, Bunyavirus, eastern equine encephalitis, St Louis encephalitis, microfilariases, eg ***Wuchereria bancrofti, Dirofilaria immitis*** and avian, but not human malaria; the genus ***Aedes*** has intermediate hosts for ***Wuchereria bancrofti***, and vectors for togaviral infections, including dengue and yellow fever; ***Anopheles*** is the only genus of mosquitoes that is a vector for human malaria

Culling HEMATOLOGY Removal of abnormal, aged or damaged cells from the circulation by the spleen due to its unique circulation, which allows selective 'harvesting' of antibody-coated red cells and platelets as well as removal of deformed or defective erythrocytes; Cf Pitting

Cultural psychoses Acting-out behaviors that are unique to certain, often primitive societies, often accompanied by a strong component of superstition; one classification divides these reactions into 'taxa' which appear to have some validity; see Amok, Latah, Piblokto, Zombies

Cupid's bow shape A morphology with two convex curves joined at the midpoint, likened to the mythical Cupid's bow ORAL DISEASE A descriptor for a double lip anomaly, characterized by redundancy of tissue on the inner mucosal aspect of, usually the upper, lip, that is either congenital or acquired through trauma or in a background of nontoxic thyroid enlargement (Ascher syndrome), the bow is seen when the lips are 'pursed' RADIOLOGY The normal smooth parasagittal biconcavity of the caudal face of the 3rd, 4th and 5th lumbar vertebrae, with the bow pointing anteriorly

Cupping PEDIATRIC RADIOLOGY A widened, metaphyseal concavity caused by muscular and ligamentous pulling on softened bone, which may occur at the sternal ends of the ribs, the proximal tibia and humerus and the distal radius and ulna; cupping was first described as radiological evidence of repeated trauma to the growth plates of long bones and thus is suggestive of child abuse, but also occurs in achondrogenesis, cretinism, congenital syphilis, diastrophic and thanatophoric dwarfism, hypervitaminosis A, homocystinuria, hypophosphatasia, infarction, infection, leukemia, metaphyseal dysostosis, phenylketonuria, scurvy, sickle cell anemia, thermal injury, trauma, vitamin D rickets

CUPS Carcinoma of unknown primary site, see Occult primary malignancy

Curare A generic term for a quaternary neuromuscular-blocking alkaloid first used as an arrow poison by the Indians on the Amazon and Orinoco rivers, obtained from plants of the ***Strychnos*** species; curare and related compounds are used as adjuvants in surgical anesthesia for relaxation of skeletal muscle and to prevent trauma in electroconvulsive therapy

Curbstone sign UROLOGY Sharp intravesicular pain occurring as a patient with urinary calculi descends a staircase or steps down from a curbstone/kerbstone, a pain caused by calculi bouncing on the trigone

Cure ONCOLOGY Restoration to one's usual state of health; although this is the ideal goal of all fields of health care, oncologists are often reluctant to use the term in reference to malignancy, especially lymphoproliferative disorders, given the known tendency of these tumors to recur ten or more years after therapy; it is thus common practice by oncologists to substitute the more guarded terms, 'no evidence of disease' or 'remission' for what non-cognoscenti call 'cure'; Cf Remission

curie A unit of radioactivity equivalent to 3.7×10^{10} disintegrations/second of a radioactive nuclide

CURL Compartment of uncoupling of receptor and ligand MEMBRANE PHYSIOLOGY A fusion vesicle in the cell characterized by a low (circa 5) pH that facilitates the separation of LDL and other ligands from their respective receptors, allowing the recycling of the receptor to the cell surface

Curlicue ureter A ureter that has herniated either into the inguinal region (male) or sciatic region (female); the horizontal loops imply loop herniations with development of a hydrocele (J Am Med Assoc 1952; 149:441)

Curly toe A congenital deformity in which one or more toes are deviated plantarward, medially and rotated laterally at the distal interphalangeal joint; the twisting of the terminal pulp may cause the toe to curl under the adjacent toe; curly toes are often bilateral and symmetrical with familial tendencies Treatment Surgery

Currant jelly An adjectival descriptor for a tissue or material with a rubbery, elastic consistency, usually replete with erthrocytes, which impart a deep violet or magenta hue, fancifully likened to jelly

Currant jelly clot Red-black, gelatinous and non-adherent coagulum composed of red cells with scattered leukocytes, a type of postmortem intravascular blood clot, that develops more rapidly than the slowly sedimenting Chicken fat clot

Currant jelly sputum An endobronchial secretion composed of blood admixed with sputum, mucus and scattered debris, 'classically' described in untreated *Klebsiella pneumoniae* pneumonia

Currant jelly stools Dark red, gelatinous stools composed of blood and mucus, passed by 60% of children with intussusception; similar stools are passed in those with juvenile 'retention' polyps RADIOLOGY Contrast studies reveal a Coiled spring appearance

Current procedural coding see CPT coding

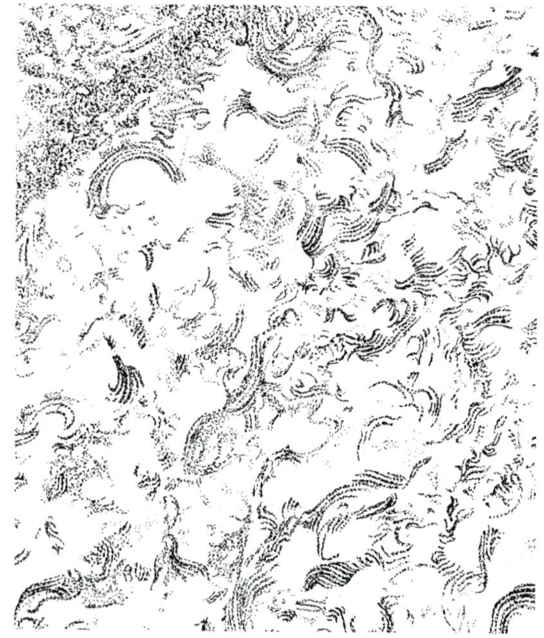

Curvilinear profiles

Curvilinear profiles Farber bodies A pathognomonic finding (figure) of Farber's disease, a glycosphingolipidosis that consists of comma-shaped rods within vacuoles, seen by electron microscopy (N Engl J Med 1991; 324:395) Histopathology Wispy, PAS-positive material; similar (if not identical) material occurs in the cytoplasmic inclusions in peripheral lymphocytes or skin fibroblasts in juvenile lipofuscinosis (Batten-Mayou-Spielmeyer-Vogt disease, amaurotic familial idiocy, Batten's disease, Kufs disease, Jansky-Bielschowsky syndrome and Spiel-meyer-Vogt disease), Cf Fingerprint profiles Clinical Intellectual deterioration, progressive loss of motor function, ataxia and retinal pigmentary degeneration; death commonly occurs in the teens to twenties

Custodial care Non-medical care provided to a person who is able to function in a relatively independent fashion, but who needs environmental protection or who needs to have medical attention readily accessible; individuals requiring custodial care include the elderly, the moderately handicapped and those with later stages of malignancy or AIDS; see Hospice; Cf Home health care industry

Cusum statistics Cumulative **sum**mation statistics are used to quality control laboratory values, calculated by adding the observed values to the assumed values based on an idealized Gaussian distribution, serving to compare two different analytic methods; see Westgard's multirule

Cut and patch repair see Patch and cut repair

Cutaneous horn A focal hyperproduction of keratin seen in various keratoses (solar, seborrheic or inverted follicular keratoses), in marsupialized tricholemmal or epidermoid cysts and verruca vulgaris; cutaneous horns are very rarely seen in squamous cell or sebaceous gland carcinoma

Cut-corner configuration PEDIATRIC RADIOLOGY A rounding of the 90° angle at the distal metacarpals of Hurler syndrome

'Cut-down' A surgically-created venous access for situations where a) percutaneous placement of a venous cannula is not possible, there is no 'good vein', emergent situations or global venous sclerosis (as in intravenous drug abuse); any peripheral vein can be used, the most commonly used include the cephalic vein at the shoulder, the basilic vein above the elbow, the saphenous vein at the ankle or when extremely urgent, the external jugular vein

Cutie-pie A type of handheld Geiger-Mueller radioactivity detector that measures α and β radiation energetic enough to pass through the mica window; the drawbacks of these radiation detectors are that they a) Do not distinguish between types of particles or energy levels b) Lose their sensitivity above 10 000 cpm and c) Detect a minuscule fraction of γ radiation

Cutis anserina see Goose-flesh

Cutis marmorata Skin with a lacy reticulated red-to-bluish vascular pattern extending over most of the body, a vasomotor reaction to low ambient temperature, occurring either transiently in neonates or as a persistent change, seen in Cornelia de Lange, Down or trisomy 18 syndromes; in Cutis marmorata telangiectatica congenita (van Lohuizen's disease), the skin findings are similar but more intense and restricted to one limb; the lesion becomes more pronounced with changes in the ambient temperature or with physical activity and may spontaneously involute during adolescence

Cutis verticis gyrata Bulldog or washboard scalp An alteration of the scalp, more common in males that often develops in adolescence as redundant 1-2 cm folds of scalp skin which cannot be flattened by traction; when primary (idiopathic), cutis gyrata is associated with mental retardation, ocular defects, seizures, spasticity and cranial dysmorphia; cutis verticis gyrata may be secondary to chronic inflammatory diseases, tumors (eg cylindromas, see Turban tumor), giant congenital pigmented nevus, melanocytic nevi, acromegaly and pachydermoperiostosis

'Cut-off' ANESTHESIOLOGY The point at which elongation of the carbon chain of the 1-alkanol family of anesthetics results in a precipitous drop in the anesthetic potential of these agents, eg at greater than 12 carbons in length, there is little anesthetic activity, beyond 14 carbons, none; this phenomenon was studied by Fourier transform IR spectroscopy and shown to be due to a change in the hydrogen bond-breaking activity (Science 1990; 248:583) LABORATORY MEDICINE The term cut-off most commonly refers to either a) A time after which a specimen cannot be processed due to logistics or the necessity for 'batching' specimens to reduce the labor in performing certain assays and b) A critical value for an analyte which is two or more standard deviations above or below a mean or 'cut-off' and therefore is abnormal

Cut-off sign Colonic cut-off sign RADIOLOGY An abrupt 'amputation' of the colonic gas column occurring at the splenic flexure, characteristic of acute pancreatitis but also seen in ischemic colitis or thrombosis of the mesenteric vasculature

'Cutting edge' A highly colloquial adjective, equivalent to 'state of the art', as in 'cutting edge research'

CV see Coefficient of variation

C value paradox EVOLUTIONARY BIOLOGY The heuristically incongruous finding that the mass of DNA or 'C value' does not reflect the evolutionary complexity of the organism, thus some small primitive organisms have a high C value, while other relatively 'sophisticated' organisms have a low C value; the paradox is partially resolved by the presence in the latter of abundant redundant or functionless DNA, the latter which is known as 'junk DNA'

CVID see Common variable immune deficiency

C-virus see C-type virus

c-v wave CARDIOLOGY An abnormally prominent pulsation of the jugular vein in tricuspid valve insufficiency, variably accompanied by systolic pulsations of the liver and a blowing systolic murmur in the 4th and 5th left parasternal spaces, which is more intense with inspiration

c wave The wave in the normal jugular phlebogram corresponding to early ventricular systole caused by bulging of the tricuspid valve into the right atrium

'CV-weighing' ACADEMIA The evaluation of a candidate for an academic appointment, based on the thickness ('weight') of his curriculum vitae (CV); 'CV-weighing' equates quality with quantity and may pressure a researcher to either 1) 'Unbundle' the research, ie separate various aspects of the experimental question(s) and report them individually, in order to 'fatten' his CV's or 2) Compromise the scientific ethic, which ranges in degree from the seemingly innocuous 'fixing' of data, to the extremely rare overt fabrication of data; to resolve this dilemma, some academic centers are evolving towards using the Institute of Scientific Information's 'Citation impact', or evaluating a researcher's innovativeness to determine whether an appointment and promotion is merited Note: A creative report in a 'cutting edge' journal eg, Cell, Nature or Science outweighs many reports in highly specialized (often a euphemism for 'second-string') journals; see Authorship, Citation impact, Uncitedness index; Cf 'Hot' paper

CWP see Coal Workers Pneumoconiosis

'CYA' see Defensive Medicine

Cyclamates A family (calcium cyclamate and its metabolites, cyclohexylamine, cyclamic acid, sodium cyclamate) of artificial sweeteners banned by the US Food and Drug Administration in 1970, when a study revealed increased bladder carcinoma in rats given extremely high doses; subsequent studies (Env & Mol Mutagen 1989; 14:188) have failed to reveal direct, intrinsic genotoxicity of cyclamate, although when added to saccharin (another artificial sweetener), there is an additive tumorigenic effect, causing increased growth potential of focal areas of bladder epithelium; see Artificial sweeteners

Cyclic AMP

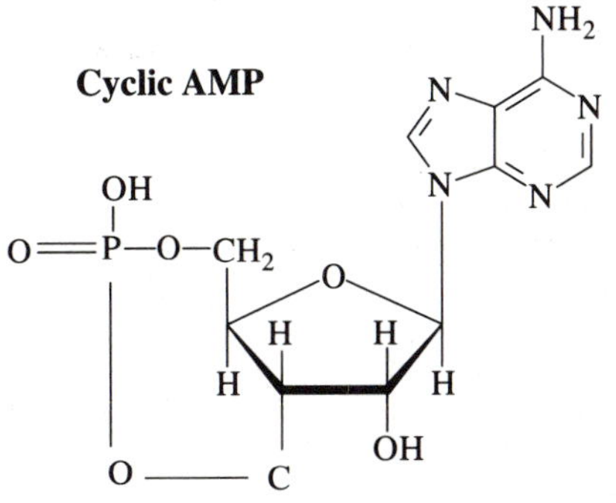

OH | O=P—O—CH_2 ... O —— C (structure: NH_2, N, N, N, N, O, H, H, H, H, OH)

Cyclic AMP Cyclic adenosine monophosphate An intracellular mediator (second messenger) of hormonal action, produced from ATP by adenylate cyclase; cAMP acts on a) Hormone receptors b) The guanine nucleotide regulatory system c) The catalytic unit of the cyclase itself and d) Ion channels, modulating their activity by phosphorylation or by direct interaction with the channels on the cytoplasmic face (Nature 1991; 351:145); binding of a hormone to its cognate receptor induces a conformational change in the regulatory G (guanosine) protein, binding GTP, forming cAMP from ATP by adenylate cyclase, either increasing (ACTH, β-adrenergic agonists, calcitonin, corticotropin-releasing factor, dopamine, follicle-stimulating hormone, glucagon, luteinizing hormone, prostaglandin E1, parathyroid hormone, serotonin-5HT, thyroid-stimulating hormone and vasopressin V1) or decreasing (acetylcholine, α_2-adrenergic agonists, angiotensin II, insulin, opiates, oxytocin, somatostatin) intracellular substances; cAMP action is terminated by degradation to 5'AMP through phosphodiesterase, which in turn may be inhibited by various drugs, eg theophylline, and is regulated by Ca^{++}; cAMP modulates protein kinase activity, regulates synaptic transmission, hormonal secretion, urinary osmolality, phosphate excretion, osteolysis, glycogenolysis and synthesis, lipolysis, activation of cAMP-dependent smooth muscle protein kinase phosphorylates target proteins throughout the cell; see Second messengers

Cyclic edema A transient condition affecting women who work on their feet, possibly of psychogenic origin, as it occurs in the emotionally labile; cyclic edema is a diagnosis of exclusion, to be considered after ruling out angioneurotic edema, IgE-dependent or complement mediated urticaria and other immune-related nosologies

Cyclosporin A

Cyclic neutropenia A disorder characterized by periodic episodes of severe neutropenia occurring in 3-4 week cycles, accompanied by maturational arrest of myeloid precursors in the bone marrow **Clinical** Fever, oral ulceration, cervical lymphadenopathy and multiple acute local infections that, while severe are rarely fatal **Treatment** If symptomatic, antibiotics, eg aminoglycosides and penicillin Note: Cyclic neutropenia occurs in the collie dog

Cyclin(s) A family of cell cycle control proteins synthesized during each cell cycle, controlled by a serine-threonine protein kinase $p34^{cdc2}$; cdc2 encodes the catalytic subunit of maturation promoting factor, inducing the transition of G2 to M phases of the cell cycle; cyclin A is a 33 kD protein identical to an adenovirus-associated protein (E1A p60); cyclin B is a 58 kD protein that is regulated post-transcriptionally and post-translationally in the cell cycle (Nature 1990; 346:760); cyclins regulate the cell cycle and fluctuate according to the phase of the cycle; cyclin catabolism marks a cell's exit from mitosis, an event that occurs when cyclin is recognized by the ubiquitin-conjugating system (Nature 1991; 349:132)

Cyclooxygenase pathway A major pathway of arachidonic acid metabolism, giving rise to prostaglandins (PG); the first product is the unstable PGG_2, which absorbs oxygen and kicks out a free radical forming PGH, which is then metabolized in the individual cells forming PGE_2, $PGF_{2\alpha}$ PGD_2, PGI_2 (prostacyclin) and thromboxane A_2; other arachidonic acid metabolic pathways include lipooxygenase (forming HETE and leukotrienes) and the epoxygenase pathways (cytochrome P450 microsomal enzyme pathway); the pathway is involved in the early, non-specific response to trauma and injury (vasoconstriction and platelet aggregation)

Cyclopia Fraser syndrome An extreme form of holoprosencephaly characterized by fusion of the ocular globe and doubling of the normal ocular structures and arhinia **Genetics** Chromosome defects described in cyclopia include 3p duplication, 2p deletion, balanced 3/7 translocation, anomalies of chromosome 7 and the most common defect, trisomy 18

Cyclophilin An abundant and ubiquitous 18 kD cytoplasmic protein withpeptidyl-prolyl isomerase activity, catalyzing the interconversion of *cis*- and *trans*-rotamers; cyclophilin's high-affinity binding to the cyclosporin A explains cyclosporin's immunosuppressant activity (Science 1990; 250:1406); Cf Immunophilins

Cyclosporin A A cyclic endecapeptide, extracted from certain fungi that induces potent T cell suppression (possibly in the G_0 or G_1 phase of mitosis) by binding to calmodulin, blocking gene activation and mRNA transcription, inhibiting cytotoxic T cell production of IL-2 and other T lymphocyte-activating cytokines; cyclosporin has ushered in a new era of transplantation, without which the success rate in liver, heart-lung (see Domino-donor), kidney and bone marrow (given the high incidence of graft-versus-host disease) transplantation would be much lower; cyclosporin is of potential use in other immune-related disorders, eg Crohn's disease, although diseases with autoimmune underpinnings, eg insulin-dependent diabetes mellitus, do not respond (Pediatrics 1990; 85:241); cyclosporin mouthwash is effective therapy for oral lichen planus, markedly reducing erythema, erosion, reticulation (whitish lesions) and pain (N Engl J Med 1990; 323:290); cyclosporin may be of use in aplastic anemia, in combination with antilymphocyte globulin and methylprednisone (N Engl J Med 1991; 324:1297) or for treating psoriasis (N Engl J Med 1991; 324:277) **Toxicity** Kidney (atrophy, sclerosing glomerulonephritis, tubulointerstitial fibrosis and reduced glomerular filtration rate), hypertension, anemia, anaphylaxis, nausea, tremor, paresthesias, increased Epstein-Barr virus infections, lymphoma and pseudolymphoma production, fluid retention, thromboses, encephalopathy, seizures, coma, hirsutism and liver toxicity **Laboratory** Increased creatinine, uric acid, bilirubin and cholesterol

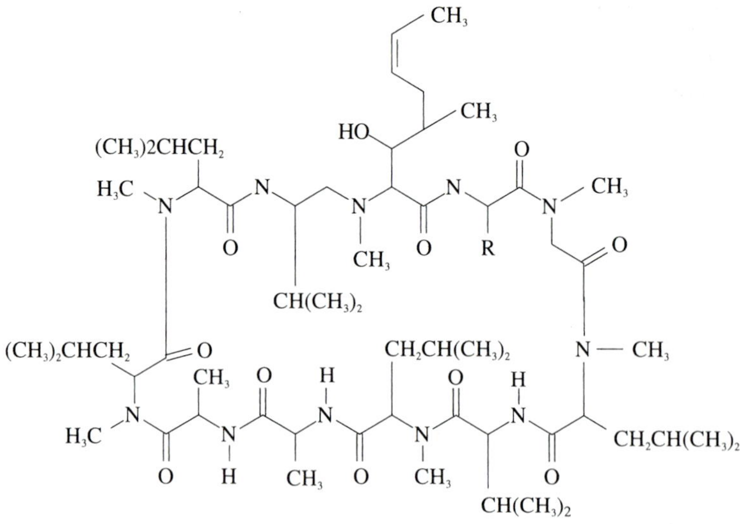

Cylindroma A generic term for a tumor that forms well-circumscribed nests of epithelial cells with internal 'blobs' of hyaline, surrounded by a myxoid stroma, often with a high content of mucin, surrounded by hyaline-like sheath **Dermal cylindroma** A tumor with apocrine differentiation, which may be solitary or multiple (with a hereditary component, often associated with trichoepitheliomas) that most commonly occurs on the scalp, see Turban tumor, which begins in adolescence and rarely undergoes malignant degeneration; low-power light microscopy reveals jigsaw puzzle-like islands of cells, separated from each other by a hyaline sheath and a narrow band of collagen, composed of two cell types: small dark peripheral cells arranged in a palisaded pattern and larger, centrally placed lighter-staining cells

Note: the term was formerly used for adenoid cystic carcinoma of the salivary glands (named for its typical 'Swiss cheese' pattern of growth)

***Cynomolgus* monkeys** A primate that is imported for use in many areas of research from AIDS vaccine development to behavioral sciences; the shipments to the US were strictly reduced in late 1989, when the CDC in Atlanta isolated filovirus (a virus related to the potentially devastating Ebola virus) in some of the monkey shipments, which to date has proven to be of no human consequence; see AIDS vaccine

CYP1A1 The major polycyclic aromatic hydrocarbon (PAH) inducible-cytochrome P4501A1 gene, which is thought to have a role in pulmonary carcinogenesis and toxicology, the product of which, CYP1A1-dependent monooxygenase, transforms certain xenobiotics, eg PAH procarcinogens in tobacco smoke to potent carcinogenic metabolites; active cigarette smoking causes the gene to remain in a 'turned-on' state and its expression is increased in certain lung cancers (J Natl Cancer Inst 1990; 82:1333)

***CYP*21** The gene that encodes a microsomal cytochrome P-450 responsible for steroid 21-hydroxylation (adrenal 21-hydroxylase P-450c21); mutation of the CYP21 gene in the form of deletions or transfers of the deleterious sequences from the adjacent pseudogene CYP21P resulting in gene conversion, is usually responsible for 21-hydroxylase deficiency (N Engl J Med 1991; 324:145)

Cystic fibrosis An autosomal recessive disease that is most common in those of celtic stock (1:2000 births, US; carriers 1:25 caucasians, 1:250 blacks) in which excessive chloride and sodium in secretions causes thickening of mucus and decreased clearance of secretions (N Engl J Med 1990; 322:1189), in part related to defective cAMP-dependent phosphorylation of a chloride selective channel of both epithelial cells and lymphocytes Physiology Both the cAMP-dependent protein kinase and protein kinase C fail to activate otherwise normal chloride channels Clinical Progressive lung disease, pneumonia (*Pseudomonas aeruginosa* or *P cepacia*), exocrine pancreatic insufficiency, impaired growth, increased sweat electrolytes, especially chloride, as well as meconium ileus, nasal polyposis and hepatobiliary disease Screening The ΔF508 deletion is present in 68% of all cases of CF (76% of US caucasians but less common in other races, eg 30% in Ashkenazic Jews); more than 20 different gene mutations cause cystic fibrosis; the sensitivity of a CF test in the average white couple in the US is a mere 56% (76% X 76%), every successfully avoided case of cystic fibrosis would cost an estimated $2.2 million (J Am Med Assoc 1990; 263:2777), assuming that all parents informed of a cystic fibrosis gestational product would opt for an abortion; screening is not thought to be cost-effective Diagnosis Sweat chloride test, see there Treatment Pancrease, a porcine-derived enzyme concentrated within microspherules, coated by an acid-resistant polymer (McNeil), designed to reduce the degree of malabsorption (J Am Med Assoc 1990; 263:2450); aerosolized α_1-antitrypsin to counteract the excess production of neutrophil elastase and aerosolized DNAse, which digests the partially degraded neutrophils that accumulate in the alveoli; see Passive smoking; a potential therapeutic modality would involve the activation of chloride channels by a multifunctional calcium/calmodulin protein kinase (Nature 1991; 349:793)

Cystic fibrosis transmembrane conductance regulator MOLECULAR BIOLOGY A 1480-residue protein involved in chloride transport in the lungs, pancreas and sweat glands that is encoded within the J3.11 and met oncogene markers, which has a deleted phenylalanine at position 508; CFTCR was identified by chromosome 'walking' and 'jumping' by LC Tsui (Children's Hospital, Toronto) and F Collins (U of Michigan), locating the defective 250 kilobase gene on the long arm of chromosome 7 (Science 1989; 245:1073), CFTCR has five functional domains, two transmembrane domains, two nucleotide binding domains and a regulatory domain; the 508 deletion induces changes in the nucleotide binding domain (Science 1991; 251:555)

Cystosarcoma phylloides see Phylloides tumor

Cytapheresis TRANSFUSION MEDICINE The collection of cells for therapeutic transfusion; although by definition, cytapheresis could refer to any collected cells, it is understood in the more restricted sense of a procedure for 'harvesting' either platelets, or less commonly, granulocytes; in each, the donor is often a friend or family member of a patient requiring the cells on a regular basis; the frequency of donation is limited by loss of erythrocytes (ideally, less than 25 ml/week), plasma loss (less than 1000 ml/week) and in granulocytapheresis, the accumulation of hydroxyethyl starch, see there; the most common indication for platelet apheresis is transient thrombocytopenia caused by chemotherapy for malignancy when the patient's platelet count fall below 10×10^9/L; the indications for granulocytapheresis are less clearly defined

Cytoid bodies Cell-like bodies OPHTHALMOLOGY Swollen ganglion cell axons, appearing in the optic fundus as globular, acidophilic masses with a deep red or blue 10-20 µm in diameter nucleoid, seen in microinfarcts of the inner retinal layer, the histological translation of Cotton-wool patches, seen in grade III hypertensive retinopathy

Cytokines Proteins of the immune system, known as biological response modifiers which 1) Coordinate the interaction between the humoral and cellular immune 'systems' and 2) augment the immune response; by convention, cytokines are divided into a) Monokines, produced by macrophages eg α and β interferons, interleukin-1, tumor necrosis factor and several colony-stimulating factors and b) Lymphokines, produced predominantly by activated T cells and natural killer cells eg γ-interferon, interleukins (IL-2 to IL-6), granulocyte-macrophage colony-stimulating factor and lymphotoxin; see also Biological response modifiers, Colony stimulating factor(s), Fibroblast growth factor, Interferons, Interleukins, Platelet-derived growth factor, Transforming growth factor β, Tumor necrosis factor

Cytokine synthesis inhibitory factor see IL-10

Cytomegalovirus A member of the herpes (DNA) virus group, which is global in distribution and in developing nations, universally acquired in infancy CMV is trans-

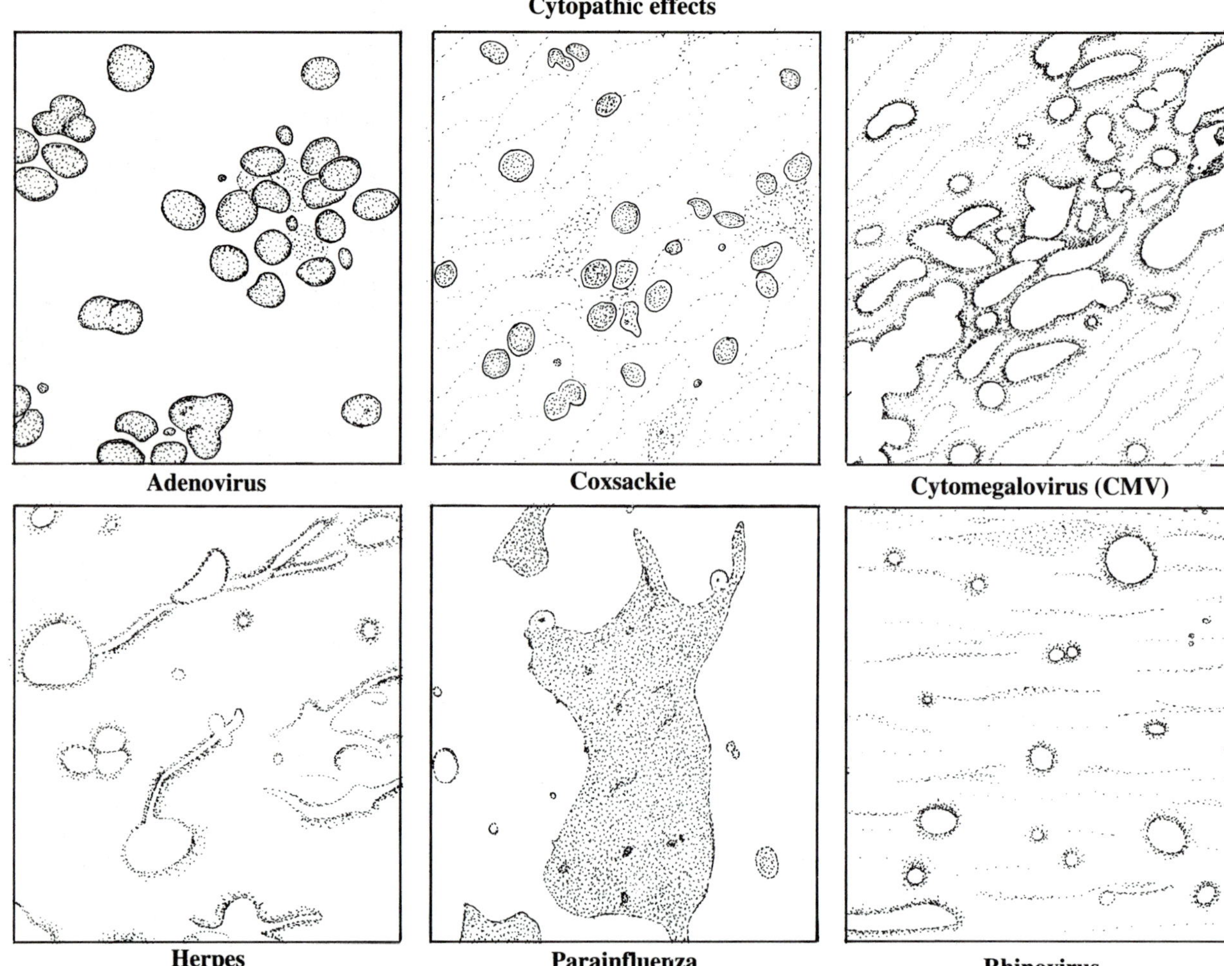

missid in blood; it is rarely a serious infection unless the host is previously (immuno)compromised, eg as in AIDS, or secondary to bone marrow transplantation **Histopathology** Classic 'owl's eye'-like inclusion bodies have been described in virtually all tissues; see TORCH panel for in utero effects

Cytopathologic effect VIROLOGY The characteristic cytologic changes that occur in virally-infected cells in tissue culture (see above figures); the CPE is a means of presumptive identification of a virus obtained from a clinical specimen, eg Adenovirus produces grape-like clusters in HEK cells; rhinovirus produces irregular, rounded 'dewdrop' changes in culture cells; rubella is diagnosed by exclusion, as it interferes with the CPE of other viruses

Cytotoxic T lymphocyte (CTL) A T cell with a CD8 receptor on the surface that recognizes (via the T cell receptor), interacts with and lyses malignant or virally-infected native cells bearing self, ie 'haplotype restricted', class I major histocompatibility complex (MHC) molecules; once recognition occurs, CTLs react to the MHC class I 'restricted', antigen-bearing cell, by secreting a) lymphokines, recruiting other lymphocytes to the region and b) proteinases and proteins (perforins) that form nonspecific ion channels in the target cell membrane,
cause a rapid loss of osmotic pressure and bursting of the target; CTLs downregulate the immune response and one CTL may attack many targets; see Helper cells, Perforin, Suppressor cells

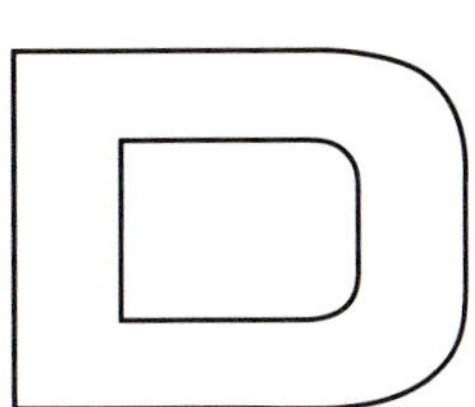

D Symbol for: Aspartic acid; Deuterium; diopter

d Symbol for: Deci-; Deoxyribose; Dextrorotary

D_1, D_2, D_3 receptors see Dopamine receptors

D17S74 A highly polymorphic gene located on the long arm of chromosome 17 (17q21) that is closely linked to an early-onset form of familial breast cancer which is accompanied by proliferative breast disease (Science 1990; 250:1684)

Dachau hypothermia experiments see Unethical medical research

DAD Diffuse alveolar damage The histological findings in adult respiratory distress syndrome, see there RADIOLOGY Acute onset of diffuse pulmonary infiltrates Histopathology The acute exudative phase with edema and hyaline membrane formation is followed by a subacute proliferative phase at one week, ending with fibrosis by the second or third week Etiology AIDS, air embolism, cardiopulmonary bypass, connective tissue disease (lupus erythematosus, rheumatoid arthritis, scleroderma), drugs (therapeutic or of abuse), eosinophilic granuloma, heat injury, hemosiderosis, high altitude, iatrogenic (PEEP), infections, molar pregnancy, noxious inhalants and gases, acute pancreatitis, shock, uremia; see Adult respiratory distress syndrome

DAF Decay accelerating factor A complement-regulating glycoprotein that is covalently anchored to the cell membrane by a glycophospholipid at the protein's COOH terminus, (Science 1989; 243:1196), binding activated C3b and C4b, inhibiting the assembly of C3 convertase (C3bBb) at cell surfaces, thereby preventing amplification of the classic pathway of the complement cascade on the host cell membrane; DAF is defective in paroxysmal nocturnal hemoglobinuria, see there

DAG see Diacylglycerol

Dagger sign Ossi-fication of the posterior longitudinal ligament (OPLL) with spinal cord compression due to a dense, vertical ossified 1-5 mm wide strip or plaque at the posterior margin of the vertebral body and intervertebral disks; although usually located in the cervical spine, the ossification may appear at T4 to T7 Diagnosis Tomography, CT-imaging or myelography Note: OPLL may be a disorder, distinct from spondylosis deformans and ankylosing spondylitis or merely a permutation of the DISH complex, see there

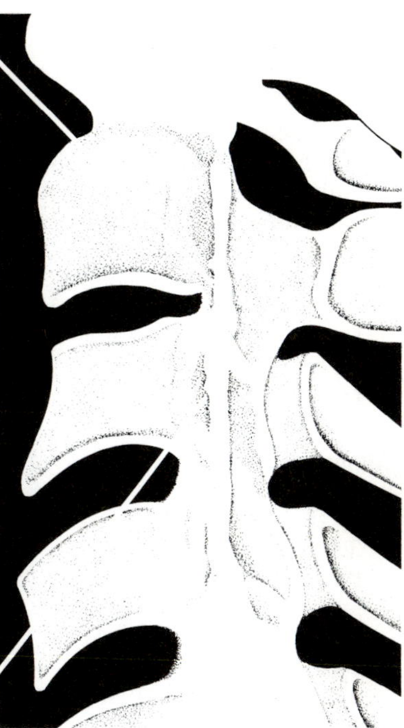

Dagger sign

Daily census see Census

Daisy An adjectival descriptor for a pattern in which a central mass is surrounded in a rosette-like fashion with oval structures that abut the central mass at one end Daisy flower pattern Histopathology Radiating stellate fibrillary forms, corresponding to tyrosine crystals seen in pleomorphic adenoma when stained with Mayer's hemalum and tartrazine

Daisy form HEMATOLOGY A rosette-like intraerythrocytic pattern of mature schizonts of *Plasmodium malariae*

Daisy pattern MYCOLOGY A descriptor for the light microscopic morphology of Sporothrix schenckii when cultured at 20°C, the hyphae of which simulate the petals of a daisy, a pattern that may also be seen in Candida species

Dallas criteria Those criteria established by a group of internationally renowned cardiac pathologists in Dallas in 1984 and 1987 that set standards for the diagnosis of myocarditis (as obtained in an endomyocardial biopsy), subdividing them into: No myocarditis, borderline myocarditis or lymphocytic myocarditis (Human Pathol 1987; 18:619)

Dalkon shield An intrauterine device (see figure, page 156) produced by AH Robins that was withdrawn from the market in 1974 after it was associated with seven maternal deaths, 110 cases of septic abortion, increased pelvic inflammatory disease and salpingitis; it was found that minute breaks in the shield allowed ascending bacteria continuous access from the vagina into the endometrial cavity; as a direct result of the mounting costs of settling the lawsuits, in 1989, the manufacturer filed for bankruptcy, setting aside a trust fund of $2.5 billion (US) to settle the claims of those alleged to have been damaged by the Dalkon shield (Wall Street Journal 70:A3, Nov 7, 1989); Cf Copper-7, intrauterine devices, Pelvic inflammatory disease

DALM Dysplasia-associated lesion or mass An acronym indicating an increased incidence of adenocarcinoma in a colon with ulcerative colitis when the pathologist finds dysplasia and the endoscopist finds a tumor mass; DALM alone may be a sufficient criterion for performing a proctocolectomy (Gastroenterol 1981; 80:366)

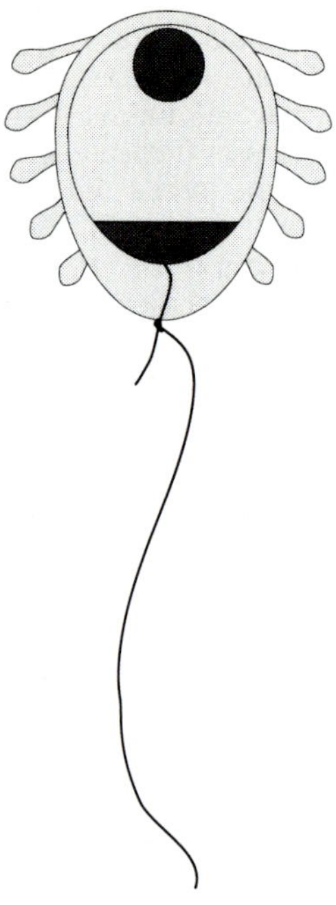

Dalkon shield

Damocles' syndrome Stress and anxiety experienced by the patients and families of those 'successfully' treated for childhood leukemia, as a) the cure rate averages 50% and b) 2-10% of treated patients with leukemia suffer future (often lymphoproliferative) malignancy; this state of long-term uncertainty is likened to that of Damocles Note According to Cicero, Damocles was a courtier under Dionysius I, tyrant of Syracuse who lavished praise on his king in order to ensure his own survival; Dionysius invited him as guest of honor at a magnificent banquet, at which Damocles was seated directly beneath a naked sword suspended by a single horsehair; a sword of Damocles therefore implies imminent danger

DAN Diabetic autonomic neuropathy A neuronal dysfunction seen in long-standing insulin-dependent diabetes mellitus, thought to be the result of various insults including ischemia, impaired neuronal protein synthesis, abnormal axoplasmic transport, polyol or myo-inositol metabolism and microangiopathy

Danazol A non-virilizing androgen that increases the resistance of erythrocytes to osmotic lysis; danazol is the most effective agent available for treating endometriosis, and may be of use in treating autoimmune hemolytic anemia and autoimmune thrombocytopenia (Acta Haematol 1990; 44:286), although it may itself mediate immune thrombocytopenia (Prog Clin Biol Res 1990; 323:241)

Dancing eyes Prominent nystagmus with rapid changes in all directions (rotary, vertical, horizontal and diagonal); dancing eyes was first described in glycogen storage disease, type VIII, but may occur in normal subjects; there is no demonstrable enzymopathy, although inactived hepatic phosphorylase is implicated Clinical Central nervous system accumulation of α-granular glycogen in the axons and in the synaptic spaces causing truncal ataxia, nystagmus, 'dancing eyes', neurologic deterioration, spasticity, swallowing difficulties and possibly aspiration pneumonia Prognosis Hypotonia, decerebration and death

Dancing eyes-dancing feet syndrome of Kinsbourne A rare idiopathic (or due to occult retinoblastoma) encephalopathy of early childhood onset Clinical Irregular, rapid jerking spasms of the trunk and limbs (myoclonus) and eye (opsoclonus) with gait ataxia, intention tremor and nystagmus Treatment ACTH and cortisone may induce remissions

Dander A mixture of microorganisms, desquamated epithelium, hair and sebum from domestic animals (dogs and cats) that evokes allergic reactions in atopic individuals

Dane particles A particle seen by electron microscopy in the acute infective stage of hepatitis B, which measures 42 nm and has an inner icosahedral 27 nm in diameter core, composed of DNA polymerase (Lancet 1970; 1:695); see Hepatitis B

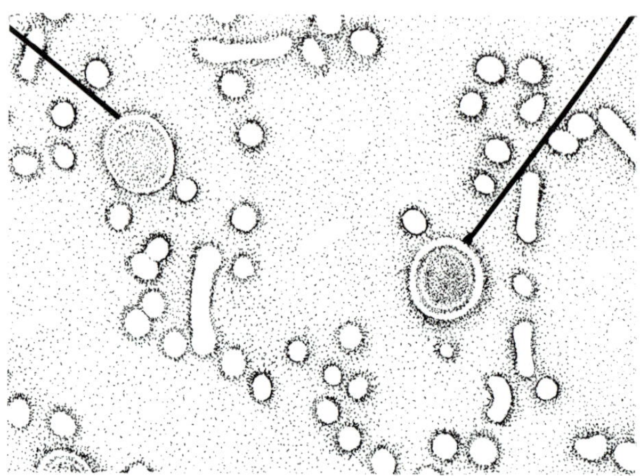

Dane particles

'Danger' space A region of surgical anatomy that lies posterior to the retropharyngeal space, descending in the posterior mediastinum directly to the diaphragm

Danger space infection A potentially life-threatening infection of the 'danger' space by extension from the retropharynx, causing dysphagia, dyspnea, high fever, nuchal rigidity and esophageal regurgitation Treatment Immediate open drainage

Dapsone Diaminodiphenyl sulfone A sulfa drug classically used for leprosy, which has therapeutic currency for treating dermatitis herpetiformis and for malaria prophylaxis; Cf Thalidomide

Dark adaption The time required for the retina to become fully responsive to low illumination after exposure to bright light

Dark (basal) epithelial cells Dedifferentiated cells seen in preneoplastic epithelia (skin, respiratory tract) as electron-dense cells with large nuclei, prominent nucleoli, scant cytoplasm and abundant free ribosomes (Cancer 1982; 50:107)

Dark cells see Compact cells

Darkfield microscopy A technique ofHistopathology in which an object is illuminated at an oblique angle and appears bright against a dark background (all light reaching the eye is reflected); darkfield microscopy is the preferred method for identifying spirochetes; Cf Serological tests for syphilis

Dark reactivation MOLECULAR BIOLOGY The enzymatic repair of DNA damaged by ultraviolet light, which causes thymine dimerization; repair occurs via excision, recombination or SOS repair mechanisms

Darmbrand German, burning bowel Enteritis necroticans A lesion that is similar or identical to pigbel, consisting in severe, necrotizing and hemorrhagic intestinal, often jejunal necrosis due to the β toxin of ***Clostridium perfringens***, type C, resulting in massive release of hemoglobin, shock, bloody diarrhea and abdominal pain Darmbrand was first described in Europe in the malnourished survivors of World War II; see Pigbel

Darsee affair A major affair that affected the departments of internal medicine and cardiology at two major US universities, which among other 'casualties' in the medical literature, invalidated a multicenter study on cardiovascular disease; the physician allegedly responsible began alleged manipulation of data as a university undergraduate, later generating multiple published reports and abstracts at Emory University and at Harvard University, generating 116 publications between 1978 and 1982; many of the publications shared authorship with researchers of renown, who were compelled to retract the papers once they were aware of the allegations (N Engl J Med 1983; 308:1415; J Am Med Assoc 1983; 2867); see Authorship, Fraud in science, Honorary authorship, Slutsky affair

Darting motility The characteristic 'falling leaf' pattern of movement of flagellated parasites, eg ***Trichomonas vaginalis;*** Cf Tumbling motility

Darwinism The currently-accepted paradigm of evolution, which holds that the cumulative changes in successive generations of organisms, ie the evolution of species, results from mutation and selection of organisms that are best adapted phenotypically to survive in their environment, ie 'survival of the fittest'; see Autopoietic Gaia, Neo-darwinism; Cf Creationism, Lysenkoism

Dashboard fracture A shear fracture with hip dislocation that occurs when a seated (usually front seat) passenger is thrown forward, striking his knee against the dashboard transmitting axial force to a flexed and adducted femur, with dislocation of the hip through a rent in the posterior capsule or where posterior rim of the acetabulum is sheared off by the femoral head

Dashboard perineum A descriptor for the appearance of an elongated perineum, resulting from an overzealous perineal repair at the time of delivery or during posterior colpoplasty; the dashboard defect may be surgically corrected by transverse repair of a longitudinal incision made through the mucosa and underlying perineal body

DAT Direct antiglobulin test, see Coomb's test, direct

Data Factual information in the form of measurements or statistics **FRAGILE DATA** Unexpected or unusual results obtained from a study, which because of either the small size of the cohort studied and therefore low statistical power or the unexpected results, may reach conclusions that do not withstand the rigors of scientific scrutiny **HARD DATA** Tangible data of any nature, eg blood levels of an analyte, persons in a defined region with a certain type malignancy **INCONCLUSIVE DATA** Results from the study of a phenomenon that fall far below that required for statistical significance, eg $p > 0.05$; alternately, data from multiple studies that consistently reach opposite conclusions of low statistical power **SOFT DATA** Those results from a study or series of studies that demonstrate a consistent trend, eg the risk of suffering a morbid condition, but which falls short of statistical significance

Data bank see National Practitioner Data Bank

Database A pool of computer-stored information, organized in such a way that the information can be retrieved by any of the parameters or 'fields' used for the data's entry, eg patient name, medical record number, date of admission, date of surgery; for MS/DOS-based microcomputers, dBASE III and its daughter, dBASE IV continue to be 'gold standard' software programs

DATTA Diagnostic and therapeutic technology assessment A program sponsored by the American Medical Association that polls opinions on issues of clinical interest that are rendered by consultants selected from a panel of 1700 experts, nominated by their respective medical specialty societies Note: DATTA data is usually at the end of each issue of the Journal of the American Medical Association

Daughter NUCLEAR MEDICINE A nuclide that is formed from the radioactive decay of a parent molecule; see Radon

Davis *v.* Davis A legal dispute over the custody of frozen embryos that had been conceived by in vitro fertilization, which arose when the parents got a divorce; the court designated the embryos as 'children in vitro', providing them with legal protection (N Engl J Med 1990; 323:1200)

Dawn phenomenon DIABETOLOGY Early morning hyperglycemia, which is not preceded by hypoglycemia, related to increased insulin requirements in insulin-dependent diabetes, possibly the result of nocturnal pulses of growth hormone; the phenomenon also occurs in 'insulin-pump' users receiving continuous subcutaneous insulin infusion who are supposed to be euglycemic and thus is an effect attributed to residual endogenous insulin or insulin-like molecules Note: In contrast, the Somogyi phenomenon is a 'counter-regulatory' hyperglycemia, where insulin therapy causes hypoglycemia, stimulating the release of counter-regulating hormones to increase the glucose levels; the two phenomena are responsible for 'brittle diabetes'; Cf Subcutaneous insulin resistance syndrome

Day care PEDIATRICS SOCIAL MEDICINE A facility in which infants and pre-school children are supervised and their needs attended to while the parent works; because of the childrens' proximity to each other, miniepidemics of gastrointestinal and respiratory tract infections are common in these centers (J Am Med Assoc 1991; 265:2212); see 'Quality time

DCB1 A unique bacterium capable of detoxifying highly

chlorinated aromatic compounds, including toxic polychorinated biphenyls PCBs; in the detoxification scheme formulated by J Tiedje at Michigan State University; DCB1 removes chlorine from chlorobenzoate, producing benzoate, then a benzoate-oxidizing bacterium transforms benzoate to acetate; finally a methanogen finishes the process by converting the end-products into methane (Science 1987; 237:975rv); see PCBs

DCC gene A gene deleted in colorectal cancer (hence the name) and located on chromosome 18 that was the first identified tumor suppressor gene

dDAVP 1-deamino, 8-D-arginine vasopressin A long-acting antidiuretic analog of vasopressin, administered as a nasal spray, which is the current drug of choice in treating diabetes insipidus

ddC dideoxycytidine A reverse transcriptase inhibitor that is being used in an AIDS therapeutic trial, which is similar in most aspects to ddI, below

ddI 2',3'-dideoxyinosine A purine analog that inhibits HIV-1 in vivo and is converted by a complex metabolic pathway to a triphosphorylated moiety, ddA-TP, which inhibits HIV reverse transcriptase and suppresses HIV replication by blocking the synthesis of viral DNA; ddI is associated with an increase in CD4 (T-helper) cells, and a marked reduction in p24 antigen (an indicator of HIV activity) in the blood; ddI is better tolerated than zidovudine and causes less myelosuppression than AZT **Side effects** Painful peripheral neuropathy, pancreatitis **Laboratory** Hyperuricemia, asymptomatic elevations of serum aminotransferase **Phase I results** Weight gain of two+ kg and/or clinical improvement (N Engl J Med 1990; 322:1333, 1340) and promising anti-retroviral activity in children with AIDS (ibid 1991; 324:137); see AIDS, Zidovudine

DDDR pacing Dual-chamber, rate modulated pacing An optimized rhythm for an implantable cardiac pacemaker, which requires periodic reprogramming as a function of a patient's activities (Mayo Clin Proc 1989; 64:495)

DDS syndrome A hypersensitivity reaction seen in 1:5000 leprosy patients treated with dapsone (DDS, 4,4'-diaminodiphenylsulfone, that blocks the p-aminobenzoic acid condensation reaction required for folate synthesis) **Clinical** Hemolysis, hypoalbuminemia, agranulocytosis and a potentially fatal combination of hepatitis and exfoliative dermatitis **Treatment** Discontinue dapsone, high dose steroids, eg > 100 mg/day of prednisone

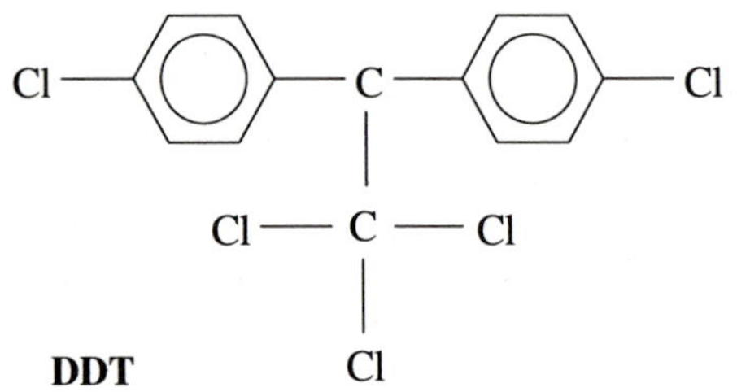

Cl—C₆H₄—C—C₆H₄—Cl
Cl—C—Cl
Cl

DDT

DDT Dichloro-diphenyl-trichloroethane ENVIRONMENT A highly hepatotoxic and potentially neurotoxic insecticide that accumulates in adipose tissue; DDT is non-biodegradable and concentrates up the food chain; because of its genotoxicity to wildlife and unknown effects on humans, its use as a pesticide was banned in the USA in 1971, but continues to be used elsewhere for control of arthropods, including body lice and vectors of typhus fever and malaria

'DEAD box' proteins A family of proteins that share the tetrapeptide, Asp-Glu-Ala-Asp, abbreviated DEAD (in the single letter code of amino acids) and DEAH (H for Histidine) and have roles in splicing, translation, development and cell growth; the prototypic DEAD-box protein is eIF4A, which uses the energy generated from ATP hydrolysis to unwind mRNA secondary upstream, facilitating the attachment of 40S ribosome (Nature 1991; 349:487ed); see Spliceosome; Cf RGD superfamily

Dead fetus 'syndrome' Macerated 'fetus syndrome' The clinical complex due to intrauterine death with retention of the fetus for greater than 48 hours (missed labor), which occurs after the 20th gestational week; the philosophy in the USA is to await spontaneous onset of labor for up to two weeks, then induce labor (barring fetal or maternal dystocia), using either prostaglandin E_2 in a vaginal or cervical gel, or oxytocin; intraamniotic saline injection is no longer recommended Complication Disseminated intravascular coagulation

Dead space CLINICAL THERAPEUTICS That portion of a syringe's tip and needle that contains medication that cannot be administered; dead space is of considerable importance in insulin therapy and in those medications where the syringe has < 0.5 cc capacity PULMONARY PHYSIOLOGY All non-air exchanging spaces of the upper respiratory tract, roughly equivalent to two ml of 'dead space' per kilogram of body weight, therefore a 70 kg person has 140-150 ml of 'dead space' in the oronasopharynx, bronchi and bronchioles Note: Anatomic dead space (respiratory system volume exclusive of alveoli) and physiologic dead space ('wasted ventilation' or volume of gas not equilibrating with blood) are the same in healthy subjects, clinically measured by single breath nitrogen curve; the relation of ventilation (V) to blood flow (Q), V/Q ratio may be substantially altered in disease states; see Lung, physiological volumes, V/Q ratio

'Dear Doctor' letter A remedial communication required by the Food and Drug Administration (USA), when a pharmaceutical company has advertised a drug with incomplete or misleading information about a product's effectiveness or safety; see Advertising

Death The Uniform Determination of Death Act passed by the US Congress, 1981 states that an individual is dead if there is 1) Irreversible cessation of circulatory and respiratory functions or 2) Irreversible cessation of all functions of brain, including the brain stem, a concept endorsed by the American Medical Association and the American Bar Association; see Cause of death, Harvard criteria

'Death Angel' A nurse in Nevada accused of killing patients on her service and running a 'book-making' operation, allegedly placing odds (and bets) on a patient's potential for survival; the patient around whom the accusations hovered was an elderly man dying of the complications of alcoholic cirrhosis; none of the allegations were verified, the nurse was exonerated and the sobriquet was considered an example of news media malpractice; Cf Angel of death

Death rattle A sound characteristic of end-stage lung disease, eg terminal lung cancer or pulmonary edema that occurs when the clearance of large airway secretions becomes nearly impossible; as air moves to and fro in the bronchi, the sound acquires a gurgling or rattling quality, often presaging death

Death Star CYTOLOGY A fanciful descriptor for the morphology of the rounded aggregates of malignant cells obtained from fine needle aspiration biopsies from breast carcinoma, which often connote a poor prognosis; 'death stars' may occur in various forms of ductal carcinomas of the breast, deriving name (and significance) from a secret weapon used in the science fiction film, Star Wars

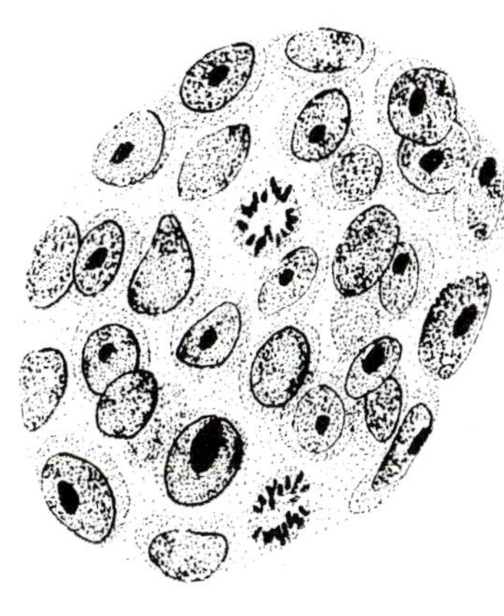

Death star

Debrancher disease Glycogen storage disease type III Forbe's disease An autosomal recessive disease of adult onset affecting Jews of north African descent caused by a deficiency of amylo-1,6-glucosidase (debrancher enzyme, which removes side chains from storage forms of glycogen and the glycogen can only be degraded to within 4 units of a branch point; such 'closely-shaved' glycogen is known as 'limit dextrin' Clinical Massive hepatomegaly and biventricular cardiac hypertrophy, slowly progressive weakness and wasting of muscles, protuberant abdomen, hypoglycemia in childhood, hypoglycemic response to epinephrine and glucagon Electromyography Myopathic changes, abnormal electrical irritation

Debridement Surgical cleansing of wounds, which consists of wide excision of potentially unclean wounds, making fresh margins, removing necrotic tissue and foreign debris Note: Although debridement has been credited with a decreased incidence of clostridial myositis in dirty wounds (5% in World War I vs 0.08% in the Korean conflict), this decrease is more likely the result of antibiotic therapy (J Am Med Assoc 1988; 259:2730)

Debrisoquin CLINICAL PHARMACOLOGY A drug used to evaluate a major pathway for the metabolism of wide variety of drugs, including tricyclic antidepressants; 7% of the population is deficient in the debrisoquin enzyme and thus have high or even toxic levels of certain drugs

Debulking operation SURGICAL ONCOLOGY Excisional reduction of large malignant tumor masses; debulking serves three purposes a) Reduction of tumor 'load' (bulk) b) Oxygenation of tissues (malignant cells often survive well in low oxygen environments and oxygen may be toxic to them) and c) Allows malignant cells the 'space' necessary to freely proliferate, at which time they become susceptible to chemotherapeutic agents that act optimally at various steps in the cell growth cycle, eg only 10% of the cells in larger tumor masses are actively proliferating and quiescent cells are not susceptible to chemotherapy; in gynecologic oncology, debulking is performed in extensive metastatic ovarian carcinoma, a tumor in which implants may virtually cover the peritoneum; debulking attempts to excise all tumor implants greater than one centimeter in diameter, followed by radiation and chemotherapy, after which, if the tumor has 'melted' sufficiently, a second, hopefully definitive operation may be performed; this combined modality approach yields a 50% five-year survival; the patient is then 'followed' with serial measurements of CA-125, a serum marker for recurrent malignancy Note: Debulking procedures may be of use in aggressive high-grade lymphomas; see Second-look operation

Decavitamin A multivitamin preparation containing the ten most 'common' vitamins, vitamins A, B_1, B_2, B_6, B_{12}, C, D, E, folic acid, niacinamide and calcium pantothenate; see Multivitamins

Decay-accelerating factor see DAF

Decay disaster Decay catastrophe NUCLEAR MEDICINE The radioactive disintegration of an atom, eg ^{125}I, in a sample that results in radiolabeled molecular fragments of free iodide with decreased immunoreactivity in the remaining iodine when measured by radioimmunoassay; see RIA (radioimmunoassay)

Deceleration injury EMERGENCY MEDICINE A motor vehicle accident-related injury, where the freely-mobile heart in the pericardial cavity is thrown forward and either tears the fixed ligamentum arteriosum or if the deceleration is extreme, ruptures the aorta, causing massive fatal hemopericardium

Deceleration Dip OBSTETRICS The periodic and transient slowing of the fetal heart rate in response to uterine contractions, ie stress **UNIFORM DECELERATION** The fetal heart rate response to uterine contractions is symmetrical and has a uniform temporal relation thereto; uniform decelerations are DIVIDED INTO A) EARLY DECELERATION TYPE I DIP Due to vagal stimulation elicited in the first stage of labor by fetal head compression and B) LATE DECELERATION TYPE II DIP Due to uteroplacental insufficiency, potentially associated with a less favorable outcome and may signal early vasomotor lability **VARIABLE DECELERATION** The fetal heart response is asynchronous with respect to uterine contractions; the curves on the fetal heart monitor are more angulated and saw-toothed and may be related to compromise in placental blood flow, eg umbilical cord compression, and like late decelerations may signify parturition-related difficulties; see Fetal heart monitor

Decentralization ADMINISTRATION A process in which specific duties are assigned to each worker, defining areas of responsibility but not autonomy

Decerebrate rigidity **NEUROLOGY** A rarely-evoked clinical condition characterized by hyperextension of extremities, pronation of the arms and hyperflexion of the hands; decerebrate rigidity is evoked in experimental animals by transection of the brain at the superior border of the pons; decerebrate posturing in humans implies tentorial herniation, often associated with paralysis of the contralateral third cranial nerve; Cf Decorticate posturing

Decibel 10 $\log_{10}$ (P/P_o) a measurement of relative auditory power intensity Note: Loudest human sounds according to the Guiness' book of world records: Loudest snore 87.5 dB; loudest whistle 122.5 dB; loudest shout 123.2 dB; other loud sounds: Race cars 125 dB; rock & roll concerts 130 dB, toy guns, up to 170 dB; whales 188 dB; prolonged levels above 150 cause hearing loss or deafness; see Noise-induced hearing loss

Decidua GYNECOLOGY Uterine endometrial tissue that has been transformed by pregnancy; 'decidualization' begins at the inception of conception and is complete by the end of the first month **DECIDUA BASALIS** The layer immediately external to the embryo, forming a compact layer adherent to the chorion frondosum, constituting the maternal vascular 'socket' in which the placenta is plugged **DECIDUA CAPSULARIS** The layer that covers the endometrium around the remainder or non-basalis portion of the embryonic sac, covering the chorion laeve, eventually expanding to fuse with the **DECIDUA PARIETALIS** That portion of the decidua seen at the fallopian tube junction with the endometrium, or 'corners' of the endometrium

Decidual cast The en tirety of the decidual components with some hypersecretory endometrium that is characterized by Arias-Stella changes

'Deciduous tree in winter' sign RENAL PATHOLOGY A fanciful descriptor for the discrete granules and clumped deposits of IgA, seen by immunofluorescence microscopy in the glomerular mesangium in Berger's disease (IgA nephropathy), in which there may be subsequent deposition of IgG and IgM; the vasculocentric deposits also appear in the dermis, supporting an immune complex origin of this condition

Decision level(s) LABORATORY MEDICINE An alternative to reference values, representing values for laboratory test results, which when exceeded, require a response by the clinician, eg a total serum calcium level above 2.55 mmol/L (US: 10.2 mg/dl) or below 1.75 mmol/L (US: 7.0 mg/dl); Statland, the principal champion of decision levels, delineated a list of 100 commonly ordered analytes (Clinical Decision Levels for Lab tests, Medical Economics, Oradell, New Jersey, 1988) Note: 'Panic values' are conceptually similar but more extreme in degree of the deviation of the value from the norm, and require that the laboratory report the results immediately to the clinician, given the pernicious portent of the results; see Panic values

'Decorate' IMMUNOLOGY A verb for positive staining of cells or tissue by the immunoperoxidase method (IPM); when a tissue, eg epithelium has an antigen of interest, eg cytokeratin is said to be 'decorated' when stained with (usually) monoclonal antibodies to cytokeratin; the substrate for most IPMs yields a red-brown color and thus these techniques are drolly known as Brown stain methods; see Avidin-biotinylated complex, Immunoperoxidase

Decorin A small chondroitin-dermatan sulfate proteoglycan consisting of a single glycosaminoglycan chain and a core protein containing 10 repeats of a leucine-rich 24 amino acid sequence (repeats that also occur in other proteoglycans including biglycan and fibromodulin); decorin binds TGF-β and is involved in down-regulating TGF-β's autocrine functions (Nature 1990; 346:281)

Decorticate posture A clinical sign elicited in deep coma, indicating severe diffuse cortical dysfunction, as may occur in a deep coma, where primitive reflex posturing prevails after loss of higher cortical control, characterized by fisted hands, arms flexed on the chest, extended legs, often in response to painful stimuli, a sign of midbrain dysfunction; Cf Decerebrate posture

Decoy cells Comet cells URINARY CYTOLOGY Small, exfoliated epithelial cells with scant cytoplasm, large dense, degenerated nuclei and coarse chromatin; decoy cells mimic those of bladder carcinoma but lack nuclear detail and structure (Acta Cytologica 1971; 15:303)

Decubitus ulcer see Pressure ulcer

Deductible HEALTH CARE INDUSTRY The amount of money an insured individual must pay before the benefits of a insurance policy or a health care plan begin; after the deductible has been paid, the insurer assumes any further costs

Deepers HISTOTECHNOLOGY A colloquial term for additional tissue that is cut from a paraffin block, usually requested by the histopathologist when light microscopic examination of the original stained tissue fails to demonstrate the anticipated pathology or architectural landmarks

'Deepest pockets' MEDICAL MALPRACTICE A colloquial adjective referring to the party that will ultimately be responsible for paying an injured plaintiff when multiple parties, eg the physician(s), health care facility, manufacturer of an allegedly defective device or dangerous or teratogenic drug, are named in a successful lawsuit for malpractice, ie the party with the 'deepest pockets'

Deep vein thrombosis (DVT) A postoperative condition seen in one-half of those undergoing total hip replacement who have not received prophylaxis, 2-3% of which evolve to fatal pulmonary thromboembolism; acute DVT occurs in 1:1000 of the general population; 92% are idiopathic, approximately 8% are due to isolated deficiencies of protein C, protein S, antithrombin III and plasminogen (N Engl J Med 1990; 323:1512)

DEET N,N-diethyl-m-toluamide An insect repellent that reduces exposure to ticks, carriers of Lyme disease and Rocky Mountain spotted fever Note: DEET may cause seizures and should be used with caution in children

Defensive medicine A style of patient management practiced by physicians in order to protect themselves from the whims of a litigious society, eg in the USA, where anything less than a perfect outcome is unacceptable to the consumer, for whom the threshold for litigation appears to decrease as medical technology increases, despite the known risks for certain procedures;

defensive practice is designed to minimize lawsuits and includes such 'devices' as a) Informed consent A document that indicates that a patient should understand the intended outcome and potential risks of a procedure Note: The disadvantage of providing a list of potential complications (each of which may be extremely rare) may overwhelm the patient, causing him to forego a needed procedure b) Documentation The paperwork generated and signed by a physician when managing a patient, which is considered to be 'unreasonably excessive' and c) Medical workup Over-ordering of diagnostic tests to rule out 'zebras' (unusual diseases that are not seriously considered as diagnoses, but have been known to occur in rare circumstances), as a form of the highly prevalent CYA (Cover your ass)*; although defensive medicine is virtually a standard of practice in the US, its financial impact is difficult to quantify, and is estimated by some to increase the cost of the health care system by 20-40%* This highly colloquial and vulgar American abbreviation is commonly used at all levels of medical practice and training, and has appeared in at least one major medical journal; 'CYA', ie diagnostic 'overkill', has acquired a mystical overtone, in that the physician may be advised to 'CYA' to ward off the evil humors of litigation

Deficiency disease Any clinical condition that results from the inadequate availability of an essential nutrient, including protein, minerals or vitamins

Degeneracy The presence of two or more 'synonym' codons for a single amino acid, ie redundancy

Degenerate code MOLECULAR BIOLOGY Although there are 64 RNA nucleotide triplets or codons, there are only 20 amino acids and three stop codons; there is therefore, redundancy or 'degeneracy', indeed, three amino acids, leucine, serine, arginine may be translated from six different RNA codons; the survival advantage to this redundancy is that it allows a wide margin of error to occur, where 'sloppy' translation of an incorrect base pair will nevertheless encode a normal protein; thus point mutations may exist without yielding a defective protein, although a point mutation in a situation of 'alternative splicing' may yield stop codons; see Wobble

Degenerin(s) An as-yet poorly characterized class of proteins that have been associated with late-onset neuronal deterioration, acting either as membrane receptors or transmembrane channels (Nature 1991; 349:588)

Degmacytes see Bite cells

Degrees of freedom STATISTICS The total number of ways in which a data set, observations and means can vary independently, given the number of independent measurements minus the number of restrictions

DEHP bis(2-ethyhexyl)phthalate A plasticizing agent that is responsible for the toxic effects of polyvinyl chloride (PVC), see there

'Dehydration fever' Increased temperature in a neonate due to inadequate fluid intake, most severe in high ambient temperatures or when the infant is overclothed

Deja French, already PSYCHIATRY A group of paramnesias in which there is a perception of being familiar or having had previous experiences which have not occurred (deja) or complete absence of memory (jamais) for events known to have been experienced by the subject, each of which has been associated with neurotic depersonalization and temporal lobe epilepsy **DÉJÀ ENTENDU** Intense feeling of having previously heard something **DÉJÀ EPROUVÉ** Intense feeling of having previously experienced something **DÉJÀ FAIT** Intense feeling of having previously done something **DÉJÀ PENSÉE** Intense feeling of having previously thought something **DÉJÀ RACONTÉE** Intense feeling of having previously related, ie having told someone something **DÉJÀ VÉCU** Intense feeling of having previously lived-through something **DÉJÀ VOULU** Intense feeling of having previously wished something **DÉJÀ VU** Intense feeling of having previously seen something; see Jamais

Delaney clause A legislative addition to the US Food, Drug and Cosmetics Act, proposed by JJ Delaney (NY-Democrat) in 1958 prohibiting use of food additives that are known to be carcinogenic in experimental animals or in humans; in 1986, the US Congress recognized that state-of-the-art techniques could detect nano- and picogram amounts of potential carcinogens, posing little risk for malignancy (1:10 000 000), and reasoned that 'risk assessment' is the best way to determine the likelihood for malignancy (N Engl J Med 1988; 319:1262); see Alar, Ames test, Risk assessment

Deletion IMMUNOLOGY One of two mechanisms of T cell tolerance, which occurs during intrathymic maturation of T cells, resulting from programmed cell death; see Anergy MOLECULAR BIOLOGY The loss of genetic material ranging from a single base for RNA or base pair for DNA to a large portion of a chromosome

Deletion syndromes CLINICAL GENETICS Hereditary disease complexes due to the loss of major chromosome segments; all are rare, often have microcephaly and an IQ < 50 **4P- DELETION SYNDROME** Wolf-Hirshhorn syndrome Low birth weight, hypertelorism, cleft palate, micrognathia, hypospadia, cryptorchism **5P- DELETION SYNDROME** see Cri du chat syndrome **9Q- DELETION SYNDROME** Antimongolic palpebral slanting, epicanthal folds, low-set ears, micrognathia, short and webbed neck, mammary hypertelorism, arachnodactyly **11Q-DELETION SYNDROME** Growth retardation, aniridia, Wilm's tumor, gonadoblastoma, ambiguous genitalia in males **13Q- DELETION SYNDROME** Rare, low birth weight, failure to thrive, holoprosencephaly, large deformed ears, microphthalmia, retinoblastoma, hypertelorism, broad protuberant nose without bridge, hypoplasia of the hands, syndactyly, atrial and ventricular septal defects; ambiguous genitalia, cryptorchism, hypo- and epispadias, hypoplastic kidneys and anal atresia **18Q-DELETION SYNDROME** Rare, seizures, hypotonia, midfacial hypoplasia, deep-set eyes, visual abnormalities, (glaucoma, strabismus, nystagmus, optic atrophy), external auditory canal atresia, fish-shaped mouth, cleft lip or palate, patellar dimples, supernumerary ribs, arachnodactyly, talipes equinovarus, cardiac malformations, cryptorchism, hypoplastic external genitalia, survival to adolescence **18P- DELETION SYNDROME** Rare, low birth weight, Turner syndrome-like features, holoprosencephaly, low-set floppy ears, hypertelorism, epicanthal folds, strabismus, ptosis, hypotonia, stubby hands, partial webbing of toes, normal lifespan **21Q DELETION SYNDROME** Rare, growth retardation, skeletal malformation, large low-set ears, prominent nasal bridge, micrognathia, downward slanting palpebral fissures, high-arched cleft palate or lip, hypotonia, pyloric stenosis, hypospadias and cryptorchism **22Q- DELETION SYNDROME** Rare, hypotonia, high arched palate, large low-set ears, epicanthal folds, syndactyly of the toes

Delilah syndrome PSYCHIATRY A clinical complex seen in the daughters of domineering aggressive men, characterized by marked sexual promiscuity, related to fear and dislike of the father and an unconscious switching of roles with the father figure, such that they seduce and overcome men, allegorically as the biblical Delilah seduced and overcame the powerful Samson; Cf Don Juan syndrome

Delirium An acute defect in cognate functions, due to toxins, substance abuse, acute psychosis and metabolic disease states, a state which can either progress or regress, Cf Dementia

Dell HEMATOLOGY The central cleared area of an erythrocyte

Dellen OPHTHALMOLOGY Foci of stromal degeneration with reversible corneal attenuation, caused by a break in the tear film layer due to a local elevation of the cornea, eg pterygium, filtering blebs, suture granuloma or limbal tumor

Delphi method A multi-stage survey technique intended to produce a consensus from a target group of experts regarding therapy for a particular nosology or other-point of clinical interest Method Published data and unpublished information are obtained, integrated then submitted anonymously to the experts and feedback is obtained; the data is then reevaluated and re-submitted to the experts, conclusions are reached, the data is then re-re-evaluated, re-re-submitted to the experts and so on until either their stamina is exhausted or a consensus is reached

Delta agent Hepatitis D virus (HDV) A virus causing a form of hepatitis that was first described in southern Italy (Gut 1977; 18:997); the delta agent is a 1.7 kilobase, circular single-stranded non-enveloped incomplete RNA virus similar to virioids and the satellite RNA of plants; HDV has a small and highly conserved domain with replicational features and a larger, less conserved domain, bearing antigenic determinants; although HDV has little sequence homology with hepatitis B virus (HBV), it is a subviral satellite of HBV, and is dependent on HBV for packaging its genome into viral particles; thus HDV requires that the patient be previously infected by HBV, as HDV is ensconced in HBV surface antigen or HBsAg; patients with delta viremia are positive for HBsAg, anti-HBc and usually HBe; HDV is found in IV drug abusers (73% in Los Angeles are positive for HDV), hemophiliacs and AIDS patients; HDV is often associated with fulminant hepatitis and is endemic in many parts of the world; see Hepatitis

Delta bilirubin Biliprotein A bilirubin fraction tightly bound to albumin with a serum $T_{1/2}$ of 17 days, detected only in patients with conjugated hyperbilirubinemia in whom it is a substantial fraction of the direct-reacting bilirubin; the existence of this fraction explains the slow resolution of hyperbilirubinemia after hepatitis or after surgical correction of biliary obstruction

Delta cell tumor see Somatostatinoma

Delta check LABORATORY MEDICINE A technique for quality control of clinical specimens in which patient results are compared to his previous values; the delta check is easier in theory than in practice, as it is cumbersome, requires a great amount of computer time and increases the rate of false positivity for analytes

ΔF508 see Cystic fibrosis

Delta osmolality LABORATORY MEDICINE That value representing the difference between the calculated and the measured (by freezing point depression) osmolality; greater than 40 mosmol/kg often presages a poor clinical course, indicating accumulation of osmotically active metabolites or toxins including: ethanol, ethylene glycol, isopropanolol, ketoacids, lactic acid, azotemia, methanol

Delta sign NEURORADIOLOGY A descriptor for a filling defect in cerebral venous sinus thrombosis, seen by computed tomography, accompanied by hemorrhage, hyperdensity along the straight sinus and linear hyperdensity corresponding to the thrombosed veins

Delta wave CARDIOLOGY An EKG finding in the Wolff-Parkinson-White (WPW or pre-excitation) syndrome, characterized as a slow upstroke of the QRS wave in a background of short P-R intervals Note: WPW syndrome pre-disposes patients to re-entrant tachycardia and occurs in normal hearts, Ebstein's anomaly, corrected transposition (ventricular 'inversion') and in cardiomyopathy

Dematiaceous fungi A group of environmental saprobic fungi (about 20 species) that produce a melanin-like pigment and may cause clinical conditions, including chromoblastomycosis and phaeohypomycosis; phaeohypomycosis results in diseases ranging from the benign tinea nigra, caused by ***Exophiala werneckii*** and ***Stenella araguata***, to the pernicious fungal sepsis, caused by ***Cladosporium, Curvularia, Exophiala, Mycocentrospora*** species

Dementia The end stage of mental deterioration, often idiopathic and/or seen in Alzheimer's disease and in repeated trauma ('Punch-drunk' syndrome, torture victims) Note: Dementia is a component of senility that should be, but rarely is, separated from 'Alzheimer's disease', a term that has long lost its original specificity, which was described (Zbl Nervenkh 1906; 25:1134; 1907; 30:177) as idiopathic early or pre-senile dementia

Demic diffusion ANTHROPOLOGY A theory of the spread of ancient culture, which modifies the more general diffusion theory by postulating that the farmers advanced at a rate of one kilometer per year, assimilating the hunter-gatherers' gene pool (Nature 1991; 351:143, 97); see Diffusion; Cf Migration

'De minimis' rule A maxim of ancient common law, '*de minimis non curat lex*', the law does not concern itself with trifles; the 'de minimis' rule seeks to avoid overburdening the legal system with lawsuits of little merit, eg a lawsuit against a pathologist who opens the cranial cavity (without specific permission) in a medically indicated autopsy; see Malpractice--Frivolous lawsuit

Demographics The objective characteristics of a population, including age, racial origin, religion, income and education, often referring to the patient population served by a health care facility, eg Patient demographics; Cf Epidemiology

Denaturation A process in which non-covalent, eg hydrogen bonds and covalent, eg disulfide bonds are broken, either reversibly or irreversibly, resulting in a change in the native conformation of a protein or a nucleic acid, leaving the primary structure intact

Dendritic keratitis Linear, arborescent lesions on the anterior corneal surface seen in the relatively mild keratitis caused by Herpes simplex; Cf Geographic ulcer

Dendritic reticular cells Cells of the mononuclear phagocytic system (MPS) located in the skin (Langerhans cells), lymph nodes (interdigitating cells of the paracortex), in the marginal sinus of afferent lymphatics (veiled cells) and spleen that present antigen to T cells; these cells are characterized by nonspecific esterase, endogenous peroxidase, Birbeck granules, a tennis racquet-like structure seen by electron microscopy, a 15 kD antigen recognized by the M1-8 monoclonal antibody (Lab Invest 1989; 61:98), and depending on their maturation, may have CD1 surface antigen, Fc receptors and complement receptors CR1 and CR3; the Langerhans cells express class MHC I as well as abundant MHC class II HLA-DR determinants, and are thought to migrate in a 'veiled' fashion via the afferent vessels into the paracortical regions of the draining lymph nodes and into the thymus where the cell processes interdigitate with T cells, coercing them into maturation

Dendritic reticulum cell sarcoma A nonlymphoid neoplasm, thought to arise from reticulum cells native to the lymph nodes Histopathology Interfollicular storiform proliferation of oval or spindled tumor cells with bland nuclei Prognosis Unknown, given this tumor's rarity, although it may recur and metastasize to the liver

Dendritic ulcers Herpetiform corneal ulcers seen in the autosomal recessive tyrosinemia (Richner-Hanhart syndrome) Clinical Self-mutilation, mental retardation, punctate palmoplantar hyperkeratosis, multiple lipomas Treatment Early dietary restriction of tyrosine and phenylalanine prevents mental retardation

Dengue Spanish, via Swahili, kadingapepo ka, a kind of; dinga, sudden cramp-like seizure; pepo, evil spirit, plague A flavivirus infection caused by the flavivirus, a group B arbovirus, transmitted by the mosquito, *Stegomyia Aedes aegypti* Clinical forms Benign dengue fever, seen in the African and American tropics and Malignant dengue hemorrhage shock syndrome (Science 1988; 239:476), causing severe bone pain or 'break bone fever', accompanied by a biphasic or 'saddleback' fever curve, prostration, headache, myalgia, lymphadenopathy, a morbilliform maculopapular truncal rash that spares the palmoplantar regions Laboratory Lymphocytopenia, thrombocytopenia

Dengue shock syndrome (DSS) A dengue-induced hemorrhagic fever Clinical Prolonged high fever, petechiae, hepatomegaly, severe hypotension and a narrow pulse pressure Laboratory Elevated hematocrit, thrombocytopenia; DSS is a medical emergency requiring rapid fluid expansion, heparin, sodium bicarbonate, sedation and oxygen

Denial PSYCHIATRY An ego defense mechanism used by a person to consciously or unconsciously negate the existence of a disease or other stress-producing factor in his environment

Dense core granule see Neurosecretory granules

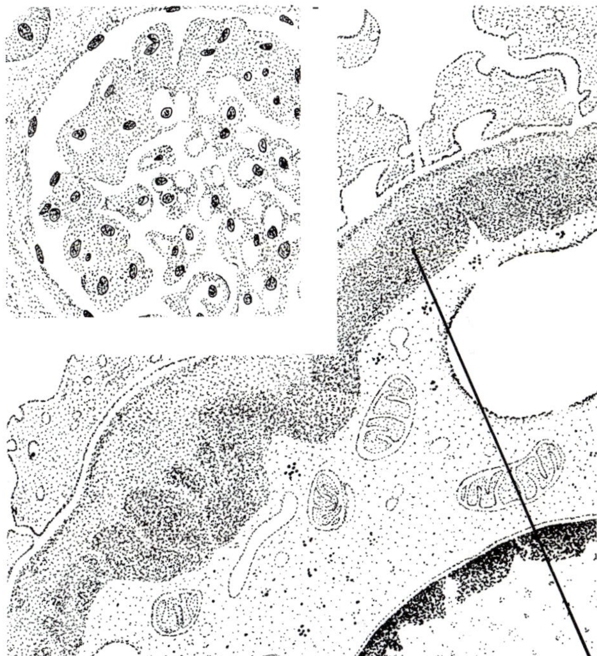

Dense deposits, glomerulus

Dense deposit disease Type II membranoproliferative glomerulonephritis A glomerulopathy in which electron-dense material (usually complement C3) is deposited in the glomerular capillary basement membrane, with decreased serum C3 due to alternate complement pathway activation in the face of normal C4; there is patchy mesangial proliferation in Bowman's capsule, and accumulation of basement membrane material in the peritubular capillaries and arterioles Prognosis Poor; see 'Tramtrack' appearance

Dense granule A round storage site in platelets that houses ADP, ATP, calcium, pyrophosphate and serotonin Note: ADP is considered the key player in platelet activity and held responsible for propagating the primary platelet response and enlargement of the hemostatic plug; Cf α granules, Storage pool disease

Dens in dente Dens invaginatus ORAL PATHOLOGY A malformed tooth with invaginated outer enamel epithelium of the odontogenic germ layer; in its mildest form occurs in 5% of the population; the tooth is grossly and radiologically malformed appearing as a tooth within a tooth

Density gradient centrifugation IMMUNOLOGY see Ficoll-

Hypaque MOLECULAR BIOLOGY Centrifugation of large molecules, eg RNA and DNA in a solution with a density gradient molecule, eg cesium chloride, a commonly used medium for ultracentrifugation

Dental amalgam see Amalgam

Denver developmental screening test A psychological screening test for assessing a child's neurodevelopmental maturation

Denver shunt A peritoneo-venous shunt that relieves ascites and improves renal function

Deoxyribonucleic acid see DNA

Dependence SUBSTANCE ABUSE A psychological or physiological compulsion for a person to use a substance (usually a narcotic) on a chronic and repeated basis; the dependence on the drug may become overwhelming, compelling the abuser to sacrifice his quality of life in exchange for the drug

Dependent Adjective The lower-most aspect of a body part or cavity; decubital ulcers occur on the dependent parts, eg sacrum and abscesses and tumor masses tend to collect in the most dependent regions of a cavity, eg in the cul-de-sac in acute peritonitis

Dependents Noun Individuals, eg wife, children, and occasionally, grandparents and others, who rely on someone else for a significant portion of their financial support; see Extended family, Most significant other, Nuclear family

Depersonalization syndromes PSYCHIATRY A group of personality disorders in which the patient thinks that either he or those in his environment have been changed into other people or life-forms, eg Phantom double syndrome of Capgas A delusion that impostors have replaced friends and relatives, most often in women who deny knowing their spouse Clerambault-Kandinsky syndrome A delusion in which a person thinks that his mind is controlled by outside influences Presenile dermatozoon psychosis of Ekbom A delusion that parasites are crawling over the body

Depolarizing bipolar cells Retinal neurons that are hyperpolarized by glutamate and L-2-amino-4-phosphonobutyrate, decreasing membrane conductance by increasing the rate of cGMP hydrolysis by a G protein-mediated process (Nature 1990; 346:269)

Depraved FORENSIC PSYCHIATRY An inherent deficiency of moral sense and rectitude, equivalent to the statutory term, 'depravity of heart', defined as the highest grade of malice, or with indifference to the lives of others, a requirement (in the USA) for a person's conviction of second-degree murder

Depraved heart murder FORENSIC MEDICINE Killing of a person by extreme atrocity, with malicious intent inferred by the nature of the act; a depraved heart murder may also be defined as one in which there was extremely negligent and unjustifiable conduct carrying a high degree of risk of bodily harm or death to others, which may be unaccompanied by any intent to kill, but nevertheless result in death; see Manslaughter, Murder, Serial murder

Deprenyl Selegiline A drug that is believed to slow the progression of Parkinson's disease Mechanism Unknown but the drug may increase the dopamine levels by inhibiting monoamine oxidase, thereby preventing Parkinson's disease, given that dopaminergic regions of the substantia nigra are destroyed in this condition (N Engl J Med 1989; 321:1364); see MPTP

Derived protein A protein derived from a larger molecule by digestion, changing the pH or heating

Dermatoglyphics The study of the combined patterns of skin ridges on the fingers and toes, palms and soles; dermatoglyphic patterns have been studied in conditions as diverse as autism, celiac disease, congenital cataracts and dislocation of the hip, Prader-Willi syndrome, systemic lupus erythematosus and von Recklinghausen disease, to name a few, and used to differentiate among various races, although its main, albeit uncommon use, is in the study of trisomies, 13, 18 and 21; see Simian crease, Triradius

DES Diethylstilbestrol A synthetic estrogen that is several times more potent than natural estrogens; DES's use during pregnancy was banned in 1972 as in utero exposure before the 18th gestational week caused vaginal wall adenosis in 35-70% of female infants exposed, see Cockscomb cervix and vagina; 0.14% of cases progress to vaginal adenocarcinoma, and are thought to have a better prognosis that non-DES clear cell adenocarcinoma, which may be a function of increased surveillance, rather than due to a difference in tumor biology; DES acts as a carcinogen by forming transient covalent bonds to the DNA of rapidly dividing cells, having a five-fold greater affinity for female DNA than male DNA (J Biol Chem 1989; 264:16847); other DES changes include obliteration of vaginal fornices, microglandular hyperplasia of the cervix (cervical ectropion, and transverse ridging (cock's-comb appearance) and a 2.5-fold increase in primary infertility (Am J Obstet Gynecol 1988; 158:493) Treatment Surgery for the carcinoma is aggressive, including vaginectomy, hysterectomy and lymphadenectomy; a postulated relation between prenatal DES exposure and neoplasia of müllerian remnants of males remains undetermined

Desalting LABORATORY MEDICINE The removal of inorganic salt ions from a sample by dialysis, ion-exchange chromatography and electrophoresis, without which the assay may be significantly affected

Desensitization ALLERGY MEDICINE IMMUNOLOGY A therapeutic modality that attempts to reduce IgE-mediated hypersensitivity to various substances by administering ever-increasing amounts of an antigen, eg urushiol in poison ivy, sumac and pollen, with the purpose of eliciting the formation of blocking antibodies

Desert rheumatism San Joaquin fever A clinical condition caused by coccidioidomycosis, a pathogenic fungus endemic to the arid Southwestern USA Clinical Subclinical disease during childhood exposure with malaise, fever, chills, headache, backache, chest pain, dry cough, fine macular erythema and rarely, meningitis

DESI drug Drug Efficacy Study Implementation The 1962 Kefauver-Harris amendment to the Food and Drug Act that required drug manufacturers to prove both safety and efficacy of a marketed drug; with the aid of the

National Academy of Science and the National Research Council, thousands of drugs were reviewed for thousands of indications, 40% of which had equivocal effects and were considered to be 'less-than-effective'; in 1982, the HCFA stopped reimbursement for less-than-effective agents that had been recommended for various acute and chronic conditions, eg peripheral or cerebral vasodilators, combinations of asthma therapies with sedatives, gastrointestinal antispasmodics with sedative, steroid with antibiotic creams, diuretics with potassium, phenylbutazone with antacids, cerebral 'stimulants' and others (J Am Med Assoc 1990; 263:831)

Designer antibody A generic term for an immunoglobulin that has been genetically engineered for a specific purpose, forming chimeric antibodies by combining for example, the gene segments encoding a mouse immunoglobulin's variable region with a human constant region, reducing the hybrid molecule's antigenicity, since the 'mousier' the molecule, the more likely its various epitopes will elicit an immune response in humans; see Humanized antibody

'Designer' drug An abuse substance produced in clandestine laboratories, eg analogs of fentanyl (a short-acting narcotic analgesic used in surgery that is 1000-fold more potent than morphine), that are methylated, escape detection by standard drug screens, and which, in a sense, is not illegal; other designer agents of high analgesic potential include sufentanil and alfentanil, which are up to 2000-fold more potent than morphine; designer drugs include analogs of meperidine (MPPP, PEPAP, PCP) and amphetamine (phenylethamine); these drugs are most popular in California, where they comprise up to 20% of that state's substances of abuse (J Am Med Assoc 1986; 256:3061); see Adam, 'Ice'

'Designer' lymphocytes A lymphocyte containing inserted genes that enhance the cells' tumorlytic activity, endowing it with desirable characteristics, eg tumor-infiltrating lymphocytes, resulting in 'adoptive immunotherapy'

'Desktop' hypoglycemia Erroneous diagnosis of hypoglycemia due to errors in collection or handling of a blood specimen Note: If a prolonged delay between time of collection and analysis of glucose levels is anticipated, the specimen should be collected in sodium fluoride, which in the US are often 'grey top' blood collection tubes, as NaF paralyses the red cells' glycolytic system, preventing falsely low levels of glucose

Desmin A 55 kD muscle-type intermediate filament present in mesenchymal cells, including vascular endothelial cells, smooth and skeletal muscle cells and possibly also myofibroblasts; desmin is of greatest use in identification of muscle tumors Note: Malignant tumor cells often forget their embryological lineage and display more than one intermediate filament; see also Intermediate filaments

Desmoid Aggressive fibromatosis A nonencapsulated mass on the anterior abdominal wall of postpartum females, often related to trauma,which according to some anecdotal reports, may regress with local progesterone injection

Desmolase 17,20-desmolase An enzyme complex of the mixed function oxidase and cytochrome P-450 systems that removes a hydroxyl side chain from cholesterol yielding delta5-pregnenolone; desmolase deficiency is a very rare ezyme defect described in 46 XY male pseudohermaphrodites with ambiguous genitalia, who should be raised as females and receive hormonal supplementation

Desmoplakin(s) Two membrane-bound proteins, desmoplakin I (250 kD) and desmoplakin II (215 kD) that are found in the desmosomes of all epithelia, thus serving as markers for the presence of cell junctions, and which have homology with the bullous pemphigoid antigen

Desmoplasia Desmoplastic response SURGICAL PATHOLOGY A dense stromal reaction in which malignant epithelial cells are compressed into single cell layers ('indians in a file'), a pattern that is highly characteristic of infiltrating ductal carcinoma of the breast, which may be due to stromalysin-3, a secreted matrix metalloprotein; see Stromalysin-3

Desquamative interstitial pneumonia (DIP) A form of interstitial pneumonia that is most common in adults and characterized by the filling of alveoli with large mononuclear macrophages, minimal interstitial changes and no necrosis, hyaline membrane formation and fibrin deposition RADIOLOGY Bilateral ground-glass opacifications Treatment Corticosteroids

Detailing HEALTH CARE INDUSTRY An activity of sales representatives ('detail men'), eg from pharmaceutical companies or manufacturers of medical devices, where legitimate attempts are made to provide details or scientific information on the product's potential uses, benefits, side effects and adverse effects; detailing information is often packaged with a subtle bias towards the product's good results

Detector INSTRUMENTATION Any component of a device that recognizes an incoming signal, eg a detector of organic compound eluted from a column in gas-liquid chromatography or a detector of radiation in Geiger counter

Detergent MOLECULAR BIOLOGY A surface-active emulsifying agent used to lyse cells and solubilize membranes

Detoxification INTERNAL MEDICINE A generic term for the removal of a toxic excess of any agent, including overdosage of a therapeutic agent, drug of abuse or toxic agent, eg pesticides and heavy metals from the body by induction of vomiting, administration of activated charcoal, hemodialysis, peritoneal dialysis or use of metabolic interference, eg treating methanol intoxication with ethanol overloading; the term often refers to medically supervised withdrawal from a substance of abuse and treatment of the symptoms of the withdrawal syndrome; see 'Cold turkey' method 'HOLISTIC' MEDICINE A poorly-defined process of ridding the body of various 'toxins' in the form of food preservatives and additives that practitioners of 'Metabolic therapy' (see there) consider a major cause of malignancy, where 'detoxification' is carried out in the form of enemas with coffee, soapsuds, herbs and hydrogen peroxide, often accompanied by wheat grass and ethylene diamine tetraacetic acid (EDTA) chelation

Detroit case Biomedical ethics A secretly planned (but never implemented) project to perform experimental amygdalotomies with destruction or removal of temporal-lobe brain tissue on mentally ill patients who had been imprisoned for various violent crimes (N Engl J Med 1987; 316:114c); see Tuskagee study, Willowbrook State School

Detroit fibrinogen A congenital defect in fibrinogen, first described in a city well known for acquired bleeding disorders; fibrinopeptide A is structurally normal and released normally by thrombin; an amino acid substitution close to the point of bond splitting prevents a conformational change necessary to expose the terminal domain, resulting in a prolonged thrombin time; see Dysfibrinogenemia

Developmental milestone Pediatrics Any of a series of activities, eg, raising the head, rolling over, walking or other significant points in a child's physical and/or mental development that may be used to assess maturation and detect developmental delay

Developmental noise Evolutionary biology Random events in development of an individual organism that results in uncontrolled phenotypic variation, eg color of eyes in Drosophila or the morphology of facial features

Devil's grip see Bornholm's disease

Devil's nips Petechial and ecchymotic patches seen on easily traumatized sites of the body, seen in purpura simplex, a heterogeneous disease of older women, possibly representing milder forms of vascular, platelet or platelet factor disorders, a reaction enhanced by aspirin

Dewdrop appearance Minute rounded nodules of amyloid seen by gross examination of the heart, occasionally seen in cardiac amyloidosis

Dewlap jowls Wattles Bilateral median, hanging folds of loose tissue on the ventral aspect of the neck seen in cutis laxa, which may be accompanied by a bloodhound-like face

Dexamethasone suppression test (DST) A clinical test that measures the ability of dexamethasone (a potent synthetic glucocorticoid) to suppress ACTH and cortisol secretion; the test is performed in two stages: the low-dose DST (1.0 mg of dexamethasone per os is followed by plasma cortisol measurement, where > 5.0 µg/dl) confirms increased corticosteroid production; the high-dose test locates the site of hyperproduction in the 'steroid axis' and is suggestive of Cushing's syndrome (false positives range from 5% in the ambulatory subjects to 25% in the chronically ill, anorectics, alcoholics, uremics and others); in the high-dose DST, having established the presence of a Cushing's syndrome, 8 mg of dexamethasone is given per os; suppression of cortisol to < 50% of baseline values is consistent with either an adrenal tumor that is not under pituitary control or an ectopic ACTH-producing tumor; the DST was reported to have moderate sensitivity (40-50%) and high specificity (90-95%) for the diagnosis of depression, a claim later proven incorrect (J Am Med Assoc 1988; 259:1699); see Metapyrone test

Dextran A high molecular weight, branched-chain polysaccharide polymer of D-glucose that is permeable to water and forms a viscid gelatinous material, that is synthesized commercially or naturally by glycosyl transferases on the surface of certain bacteria AIDS Dextran sulfate was reported to inhibit HIV-1 and HIV-2 binding to CD4+ cells (Science 1988; 240:646); therapeutic trials proved disappointing Dentistry Dextrans formed from sucrose by ***Streptococcus mutans*** are intimately linked to dental plaque and caries, as they form a 'shell' trapping lactic acid adjacent to teeth Microbiology Dextran is abundantly present in yeasts and bacteria, serving as a source of energy and a component of the bacterial capsule Molecular biology Dextrans form the solid phase, eg Sephadex, for molecular sieve chromatography, which separates molecules according to size, based on the number of cross-links formed in the dextran Transfusion medicine Various weights of dextrans are produced by ***Leuconostoc mesenteroides*** in preparing commercial colloid substances, dextran 40 (40 kD) and dextran 70 (70 kD); these substance have the desired properties of being sticky, viscid and gelatinous, exerting oncotic pressure to retain fluids within vessels and are widely used as replacement fluids and volume expanders; see Colloid solutions, Crystalloids

Dextrin A partial lysate of intermediate lengths of polysaccharide (starch) by hydrochloric acid or amylase, which is composed of glucose, maltose and short dextrin polymers

Dextrocardia A heart misplaced into the right chest, with the apex in the left; the cardiac function is normal if there is concomitant situs inversus of the abdominal organs (mirror-image dextrocardia); if the dextrocardia is due to immotile cilia, sinusitis and bronchiectasis (Kartagener syndrome) may also be present; the EKG demonstrates mirror-image electrical activity with P, QRS and T waves in leads I, aVR and aVL that are the reverse of normal and the right activity resembles that normally seen in the left side of the chest; if the abdominal organs are not reversed, dextrocardia may be associated with ventricular inversion, single-chamber ventricle, pulmonary valve stenosis and anomalies of the venous return

Dextrose Obsolete for D-glucose

DF-2 Dysgonic fermenter-2 Infectious disease A fastidious gram-negative bacillus (native to the canine oral flora) that causes infections of dog-bite wounds, resulting in cellulitis, septicemia (potentially serious with Waterhouse-Friderichsen-type adrenal cortical collapse), endocarditis, gangrene, malar purpura (a finding that is quasi-pathognomonic of generalized Schwartzman reaction); the patients are weakened or have had splenectomies, some of whom (3/17 of the initial cohort) die with disseminated intravascular coagulation

DHFR Dihydrofolate reductase An enzyme essential for DNA synthesis as it catalyzes reactions involving one-carbon transfers from a donor X-C to an acceptor Y; Methotrexate owes its chemotherapeutic effect to paralysis of DHFR

'Diabesity' A common clinical association of adult-onset diabetes mellitus and obesity, a subgroup of which has been dignified as 'Syndrome X', see there

Diabetes-dermatitis syndrome Dermatopathy accompanying α-cell tumors (glucagonomas) of the pancreatic islet cells Clinical Necrotizing migratory erythema; glucagon inhibits intestinal motility, causing ileus, constipation or diarrhea and may have associated glossitis, angular cheilitis, venous thrombosis, black-outs Note: The syndrome may rarely be caused by insulinoma

Diabetic embryopathy A complex of major congenital anomalies affecting 8-12% of children born to diabetic mothers; these changes occur early (between the 5th and 8th week of gestation) in embryologic development, eg sacral agenesis, holoprosencephaly, atrioventricular septal defects, tetralogy of Fallot and other cardiac, genitourinary and gastrointestinal defects and can be reduced to the normal 'background' levels (1-2%) by prenatal counselling and aggressive maintenance of normoglycemic levels during gestation (J Am Med Assoc 1991; 265:731); see Honeybee syndrome

Diabetic ketoacidosis A hyperglycemia-induced clinical crisis most common in juvenile-onset diabetics Clinical Vomiting, nausea, thirst, diaphoresis, hyperpnea, drowsiness, fever and potentially coma Laboratory Marked elevation of glucose, usually > 33.6 mmol/L (US: > 600 mg/dl), increased ketone bodies, acidosis, dehydration, decreased potassium, sodium and phosphate, relative increases in protein, albumin, calcium, bilirubin, alkaline phosphatase, aspartate aminotransferase and creatine kinase and increased anion gap Treatment Insulin, fluid and electrolyte replacement, treatment of initiating factors, eg leukocytosis or hypothermia, avoidance of complications, eg hypokalemia, late hypoglycemia, rebound CNS acidosis and CNS deterioration

Diabetic nephropathy A clinical disease caused by the renal changes in diabetes mellitus, which include the Armanni-Ebstein lesion, arterionephrosclerosis, chronic interstitial nephritis, fatty changes in the renal tubules, glomerulonephritis, Kimmelstiel-Wilson disease (focal and segmental glomerulosclerosis), nephrotic syndrome, papillary necrosis, pyelonephritis and tubulointerstitial nephritis Treatment If renal failure is in an early stage, the patients are good transplant candidates, while terminal renal failure requires dialysis

Diabetic panel A battery of cost-efficient laboratory tests that are used to evaluate patients with a 'working diagnosis' of diabetes mellitus, determine the level of long-term glucose control and co-morbid conditions; the panel includes carbon dioxide, cholesterol, chloride, creatinine, fasting glucose, hemoglobin A_{1c}, potassium, sodium, triglycerides; see Organ panel

Diabetic retinopathy GRADE I Generalized arterial narrowing due to vasoconstriction and hyaline deposition in blood vessels GRADE II As above with arterial thickening and arteriovenous 'nicking' known as copper or silver wiring due to vascular thickening GRADE III As above with hemorrhage, exudation or cotton wool changes; diabetic retinopathy is related to poor diabetic control, as measured by glycosylated hemoglobin (J Am Med Assoc 1988; 260:2864)

1,2-Diacylglycerol (DAG) An intracellular 'second messenger' that is released from the cytoplasmic face of a cell membrane after a ligand, eg a hormone interacts with a cognate receptor on the cell's external surface and activates a G protein; DAG acts on protein kinase C, increasing the secretion or production of hormones, enzymes, neurotransmitters, vasoactive compounds and other molecules; see PIP2, Second messenger

Diagnosis of exclusion A disease or clinical nosology that is extremely rare, and often unresponsive to therapy, the diagnosis of which should only be entertained when all other possible (potentially treatable) conditions have been completely ruled out, eg 'growing pains' or idiopathic midline granuloma

Diagnosis-related groups see DRGs

Diagnostic 'overkill' The use of excess or overlapping tests that merely confirm a diagnosis, eg the ordering of a magnetic imaging study of the brain when a previous computed tomography has already identified an intracranial mass (J Am Med Assoc 1991; 265:2229); this form of overkill is thought to be more common in academic medicine, where tests can be ordered 'out of curiosity', with relative disregard for cost-efficiency; Cf Defensive medicine

Dialysis Separation of macromolecules from low molecular weight molecules by use of a semipermeable membrane; see Hemodialysis, Peritoneal dialysis

Dialysis ascites Exudative peritonitis related to chronic dialysis Pathogenesis Unknown, but related to infections, stress or protein catabolism in a background of fluid overload and poor nutrition Treatment Some success has been reported with a LeVeen shunt

Dialysis dementia Dialysis encephalopathy Aluminum toxicity affecting those with terminal renal failure requiring long-term dialysis; aluminum is present in the dialysate solutions and in the oral $AL(OH)_3$ required to control terminal renal failure and accumulates in the brain and serum in these patients Clinical Speech disturbances, myoclonus, apraxia, seizures, mental deterioration, bone pain, osteolysis (fractures, pseudofractures), microcytic anemia, porphyria cutanea tarda and delta wave patterns by EEG similar to those of metabolic encephalopathy Treatment Chelation (desferroxamine); recognition of the association has led to decline of the disease

Diamond-Blackfan syndrome An autosomal recessive, occasionally consanguinous condition associated with pure red cell aplasia of early infancy onset with anemia, pallor and failure to thrive, accompanied in 30% of cases by minor physical abnormalities, including short stature, thumb deformities and ocular changes Pathogenesis Possibly related to a stem-cell defect, given the marked decrease of colony-forming units (CFU-E) and the burst-forming units (BFU-E); steroids may stimulate the proliferation of the structurally and functionally abnormal erythroblasts, resulting in 'immature' erythrocytes (fetal hemoglobin, presence of the 'i' surface antigen and a fetal enzyme 'profile') Treatment Transfusion, corticosteroids, bone marrow transplantation, growth factor therapy

Diamond skin A rhomboid urticarial skin reaction described in swine infected by ***Erysipelothrix rhu-***

siopathiae, a zoopathic infection of those occupationally exposed by cuts and superficial abrasions (butchers, fish-mongers); other human disease induced by ***E rhusiopathiae*** includes septicemia and endocarditis (with high mortality)

Diana complex PSYCHIATRY A reversal of roles by a woman, such that she affects the mien, appearance and dress of a man; the name derives from Diana, the virgin Greek goddess of the hunt, sister of Apollo who was known as a huntress and for her vigor or 'male' qualities

Diaper dermatitis Jacquet's erythema A dermatopathy of early infancy due to prolonged contact with soiled diapers, soaps or topical lotions, resulting in secondary maceration of a skin that is scaly and erythematous with papulovesicular or bullous lesions, which may be extensive, often sparing the crural folds; secondary bacterial and yeast infections may complicate recalcitrant cases; chronic diaper dermatitis may undergo papular induration

Diaphragmatic flutter Rapid, rhythmic diaphragmatic contractions that have a cogwheel pattern of respiration, likened to hiccups, lasting for a period of seconds to weeks and if intense, interfere with gas exchange Treatment Empirical, as with hiccups

Diaphragmatic hernia of Bochdalek A common (1:2000 live births) congenital malformation, due to a defective closure of the pleuroperitoneal membrane (posterolateral), resulting in a common cavity, with the abdominal organs (usually left-sided) prolapsing into the chest cavity, compromising respiration; morphological permutations may be discovered later in life, eg parasternal hernias or membranous defects; with peri- and postoperative ventilatory support and bicarbonates, the formerly reported 90% mortality has been reduced to 40%

Diazo reaction A method described in 1883 by Ehrlich that continues to be widely used for measuring bilirubin, which consists in mixing bilirubin with diazotized sulfanilic acid (the diazo reagent) to produce reddish-purple azodipyrroles; the diazotization reaction of unconjugated bilirubin can be accelerated using alcohol (the van der Bergh reaction), which measures the so-called indirect bilirubin

Diazo salt Diazonium salt A salt with a diazonium group (figure) that is prepared from an arylamine by diazotization

$-N^{+}{\equiv}N$

Diazo stain A histochemical stain that uses stables salts of a diazonium salt of a dye, eg fast red B or fast red GG to detect enterochromaffin granules as seen in carcinoid tumors within formalin-fixed paraffin-embedded tissues

Dibucaine number ANESTHESIOLOGY Background Succinylcholine (SC) is a potent muscle relaxant, used in anesthesiology for tracheal intubation that has a rapid onset of action (30-45 seconds post-IV injection) with a short (5-10 minutes) duration of action, given its rapid metabolism by plasma cholinesterase; prolonged apnea following IV SC may be due to an inherited (frequency 1:2500) or acquired deficiency of cholinesterase caused by liver dysfunction, pregnancy, neostigmine, IMAOs and organophosphate pesticides; given the importance of identifying these subjects, several assays were devised, of which the dibucaine test has proven the most useful; dibucaine inhibits PC, which in turn inhibits the normal cholinesterase by 80%, but atypical cholinesterase by only 20%; the percent of cholinesterase inhibition is calculated by a formula, yielding the Dibucaine number

DIC see Disseminated intravascular coagulation

Dicing FORENSIC MEDICINE Multiple 0.5-1.0 cm, cube-like lacerations of the skin seen in motor vehicle accident victims who strike shattered tempered glass car windows

Dicumerol A polycyclic aromatic compound derived from sweet clover that is an anticoagulant analog of vitamin K which uncouples oxidative phosphorylation; see Warfarin

DIDMOAD syndrome Wolfram syndrome An autosomal recessive condition characterized by the acronym's symptoms diabetes insipidus, diabetes mellitus, optic atrophy and neural deafness (DIDMOAD), which may be accompanied by ischemic muscle contractures, autonomic dysfunction, neurogenic bladder and hypertension

Diener German Dienen, to serve PATHOLOGY An attendent who maintains and cleans the hospital morgue and who may assist in performing autopsies

Diet To eat and drink sparingly or according to a prescribed regimen; diets are either for supplementation, ie weight gain or restriction, ie weight loss; in restrictive diets, the intent is to limit one or more dietary components eg gluten or oxalate, or to globally reduce caloric intake Diet types **BLAND DIET** A mechanically soft diet that is commonly prescribed in peptic ulcer disease as it has no spices or gastric irritants, although it is of dubious efficacy; see Histamine (H2) receptor, Spicy foods **BRAT DIET** see there **'CRASH' DIET** A semi-starvation type of fad diet which has a wide variety of formulations that is followed for a short period time by a person wishing to rapidly lose weight; such radical approaches to rarely result in the desired permanent loss of weight **ELIMINATION DIET** A regimen used in individuals, especially children with atopy, suspected of being allergic to certain foods, where one food or major food group is eliminated at a time to determine whether there is reduction of the symptoms attributed to allergy; Cf Desensitization diet **FAD DIET** Any of a number of diets that either eliminate one or more of the essential food groups or recommend consumption of one type of food in enormous excess, often reducing the consumption of other foods; fad diets rarely follow modern dietetic principles of weight loss, which hinge on the combination of a) Eating less or b) Consuming more energy through exercise, and are thus rarely endorsed by the medical profession **LIQUID DIET** A variant of the very low calorie diet that fulfils the daily fluid requirements and places little functional demand on the gastrointestinal tract; liquid diets have little fiber and do not provide adequate protein or calories, circa 1000 kcal/day **MACROBIOTIC DIET** see Macrobiotics **NOVELTY DIET** see Fad diet, above **ORNISH REGIMEN** Beans, bean curd, grains, maximum of two ounces of alcohol, fruits, vegetables, weekly sessions of 'meditation' and stress management **Prohibited** Meat, poultry, fish, egg yolks, caffeine and all dairy products (except one cup of fat-free); no fat or oil added to foods) **Result** Weight loss; 39% decrease in total cholesterol, 59% drop in LDL-cholesterol **PRITIKIN DIET** see Pritikin **RESTRICTION DIET** A diet intended to reduce the incidence of various conditions, eg a) Atherosclerosis Reduction of body weight, decreased consumption of saturated fat, cholesterol and increased consumption of bran b) Hypertension Salt restriction, although only one-half of patients have a pressor response to salt restriction c) Cancer Fat is epidemiologically linked to cancer of the breast, colon, prostate and possibly also ovaries; polyunsaturated fats are a substrate for peroxidative reactions and thus should be reduced; increased fiber and cruciferous vegetables in the diet is linked to decreased colonic carcinoma, an effect thought to be due to decreased contact of the colonic mucosa with carcinogens; alcohol consumption is associated with hepatoma, oropharyngeal and esophageal cancer with very low cholesterol d) Renal failure A low protein regimen that slows the progression of renal failure **STARVATION DIET** see Very low calorie diet **VERY LOW CALORIE DIET** A potentially dangerous diet that provides 300-700 kcal/day, which must be supplemented with high quality protein given the risk of death through intractable cardiac arrhythmias and which should be limited to 3-6 months; side effects of this form of crash diet include orthostatic hypotension, due to loss of sodium and decreased norepinephrine secretion, fatigue, hypothermia and cold intolerance, xeroderma, hair loss, dysmenorrhea; see Elemental diet, TPN

Dietary fiber Indigestible material of plant origin, including cellulose and cell wall polymers, eg pectin, which provides stool 'bulk'; dietary fiber is of use in slowing the intestinal transit in those with diarrhea and accelerating the transit in those with chronic constipation; see Bran,Water-soluble fiber

'Diet pills' Therapeutic agents that either suppress appetite or increase the basal metabolic rate, including amphetamines, available only by prescription and over-the counter dietary aids, including phenylpropanolamine, ephedrine and caffeine, which in high doses may cause marked agitation, hypertension, seizures and potentially death due to cerebral hemorrhage; see Artificial sweeteners, Diet

'Diff' White blood cell differential (count) HEMATOLOGY A colloquial term for the differential count of circulating leukocytes, which is usually generated by 'Coulter counter'-type multichannel instrument; the results are provided qualitatively, where 42-75% of circulating white cells are granulocytes, 20-50% are lymphocytes and 2-10% are monocytes, as well as quantitatively, where the absolute count of granulocytes is 1.4-6.5 X 10^9/L, that of lymphocytes is 1.2-3.4 X 10^9/L and monocytes is 0.1-0.6 X 10^9/L

Differential (growth) medium MICROBIOLOGY A bacterial growth medium that has a variety of integrated organic compounds and salts that favor the growth of certain organisms

Differential pivot CLINICAL DECISION MAKING A key step in arriving at a patient's diagnosis, which consists in finding a 'pivot' or the key finding that is at the center of the patient's disease; once a pivot is found, a list of viable or reasonable differential diagnoses is created from which most likely causes are considered and either validated or discarded (N Engl J Med 1982; 306:1263); Cf Artificial intelligence, Expert systems

Differential splicing see Alternative splicing

Differentiation antigens see Oncofetal antigens

Differentiation therapy The use of various agents to force a malignancy to mature into a normal morphology, resulting in remission of clinical disease, a modality that has proven effective in treating acute promyelocytic leukemia, using triretinoin to cause reversion of the 15;17(q22;q12-21) translocation; the breakpoint on chromosome 17 occurs in the region that encodes the retinoic acid receptor-α, a receptor involved in the growth and differentiation of myeloid cells (N Engl J Med 1991; 324:1385)

'Difficult' patient LEGAL MEDICINE A patient who is troublesome, paranoid, or refuses to follow instructions; termination of a relationship with such patients requires that they be given reasonable advance notice, often an open-ended length of time, a list of competent board-certified physicians who treat the same condition; all communications with difficult patients must be documented in a legally acceptable form; see ama; Cf 'Good' patient

Diffusion ANTHROPOLOGY A general theory of the spread of ancient culture that holds that social, economic and political change occurred by learning, ie by slow diffusion of cultural parameters; see Demic diffusion; Cf Migration

Digest (noun) A mixture of molecules obtained by chemical or enzymatic hydrolysis of larger molecules, eg DNA digest obtained from restriction endonuclease hydrolysis of a DNA macromolecule

Digital computer A computer that performs mathematical and logical operations on discrete blocks of data in the form of bits; Cf Analog computer

Digital subtraction angiography (DSA) RADIOLOGY A computerized enhancement of images obtained with conventional angiography, used primarily to study the carotid, aortic arch and vertebral circulation, as well as that of the lower extremity; DSA uses less contrast, reduces radiation exposure, enhancing the contrast image at a sacrifice of the spatial resolution

'Dilapidated brick wall' DERMATOPATHOLOGY A fanciful descriptor for marked acantholysis, with scattered preserved intracellular bridges, seen in the overlying epithelium in benign familial chronic pemphigus or Hailey-Hailey disease, that may occasionally be seen in other acantholytic processes including pemphigus vulgaris

Diluent CLINICAL PHARMACOLOGY An inert substance added to a drug formulation, increasing its bulk in order to make the tablet a practical size for use; diluents include dicalcium phosphate, calcium sulfate, lactose, cellulose, kaolin, dry starch and powdered sugar; see Inactive ingredient

Dilution end point IMMUNOLOGY A value, measured in titers, that corresponds to the minimum amount (titer) of an antibody in a system of interest, determined by serial dilution of a serum or other fluid with the antibody, while holding the antigen constant

Dimethyl sulfate protection MOLECULAR BIOLOGY A method used to identify protein-binding regions of DNA regions, which do not allow methylation of adenine and guanine nucleotides in the presence of a bound protein; subsequent digestion of a treated DNA molecule by a restriction endonuclease will not be allowed in sites that have been 'protected' by dimethyl sulfate; see Footprinting

Dimorphism MYCOLOGY A property of fungi that may produce two different forms depending on whether the organism is being cultured (25°C) or is at body temperature (37°C) a) Yeasts at 37°C, mycelia at 25°C ***Blastomyces dermatiditis, Histoplasma capsulatum, Paracoccidioides brasiliensis, Sporotrichum schenckii,*** b) Spherules at 37°C, mycelia at 25°C ***Coccidioides immitis*** c) Yeasts and hyphae at both 37°C and 25°C, ***Candida*** species

Dimorphic anemia A dual population of erythrocytes in the peripheral blood smear, in which there are both microcytic hypochromic and normocytic macrocytic red cells, a finding in combined iron deficiency and B12/folic acid deficiency, as well as idiopathic acquired sideroblastic anemia with B_{12}/folic acid deficiency

Dimple sign Pinching of a subcutaneous lesion results in a central dell or dimple, seen in well-circumscribed, often benign superficial dermal tumors, including dermatofibromas, inclusion cysts, lipomas and neurofibromas; Cf 'Tent' sign

Dinner fork appearance ORTHOPEDICS A descriptor for the clinical deformity seen in fractures of the distal radius with dorsal angulation (Colles fracture), a fracture common in osteoporotic post-menopausal women who fall on outstretched hands, where the distal fractured ends of the radius and ulna (and hand) are deviated in a palmar direction

'Dingellization' ACCOUNTABILITY FEVER A colloquial term for zealous investigation of purported cases of scientific misconduct and/or fraud, coined in reference to a US legislator who has chaired 'fraud in science' committees that have investigated alleged research-related improprieties of several key scientists who had received federal grant monies (Science 1991; 251:508n&v); see Baltimore affair, Gallo probe, 'Whistle blowing'

Diogenes syndrome Senile neglect GERONTOLOGY A dementia-related lassitude in which a subject allows his home and personal environment to deteriorate, and may begin to collect objects of little value, eg milk cartons, string; Diogenes (412-323 BC) was a Greek philosopher who taught that a virtuous life was a simple one, proving his point by living in a bathtub; he condemned the excesses of his contemporaries and wandered about Athens with a candle, looking for an honest man

Dioxin ENVIRONMENT Any member of a family of highly-toxic compounds in which two benzene rings are linked by two oxygen atoms; the prototypic dioxin is 2,3,7,8-Tetrachlorodibenzo-p-dioxin (TCDD), a chemical byproduct of the herbicide, 2,4,5-trichloro-phenoxy-acetic acid, Agent Orange; other dioxins include polychlorinated dibenzo-p-dioxins (PCDD) and polychlorinated dibenzofuran (PCDF); dioxin came to public attention in the late 1970s in Times Beach, Missouri, where dioxin-contaminated waste oil had been sprayed on the ground since 1971 to control dust, and associated with the deaths of horses and a general deterioration of the local human population's health; the clean-up of Times Beach has cost mega-millions and its residents were forced permanently to evacuate; dioxin and Agent Orange have been implicated in soft tissue sarcomas (Lancet 1981; 1:268) and lymphomas; the liver (acute toxicity and hepatoma) and immune system (thymic atrophy and defective cell-mediated immunity) are the most severely involved in animal studies; in humans, intense chronic exposure causes weight loss, myalgias, insomnia, dyspnea, cold intolerance, irritability, peripheral neuritis, hepatomegaly, hemorrhagic cystitis, chloracne, actinic elastosis, loss of libido and impotence **Laboratory** Increased prothrombin time and lipid levels; dioxin was released in an industrial accident in Seveso, Italy, 1976 at a factory producing 2,4,5-trichlorophenol; the total TCDD released was less than 1.3 kg; there were no fatalities; some suffered chloracne; the levels of TCDD may rise to four times baseline levels (8 pg/g of plasma lipid) in those who eat contaminated fish, eg in the Baltics (N Engl J Med 1991; 324:8); dioxin exposure of greater than one year with a latency of greater than 20 years is associated with a 46% increase of all cancers and 42% increase in cancers of the respiratory tract (N Engl J Med 1991; 324:212); dioxin's toxic and carcinogenic effects may be due to membrane receptor binding (Science 1991; 251:524n&v); see Agent Orange; Cf Bitterfeld

Cl Cl O O Cl Cl

Dioxin (TCDD)

Dip see Deceleration

DIP see Desquamative interstitial pneumonia

Dip/peak pattern see Harvest Moon festival

Dipstick Reagent strip LABORATORY MEDICINE A blotting paper impregnated with enzymes or chemicals sensitive to various parameters of clinical interest, which when dipped in urine, undergoes a color change allowing a substance to be semiquantitatively measured, including bilirubin, glucose and reducing substances, hemoglobin, nitrates, ketones, pH, protein, hemoglobin, specific gravity and urobilinogen; reagent strip methodology was born in part out of the relatively low diagnostic yield of routine urinalysis Note: Some interfering substances may alter the strip's reactivity for a particular analyte (strip manufacturers provide lists of substances most likely to cause interference); if the clinical suspicion is strong for the presence of a disease, a proper quantitative analysis of the specimen should be performed

Diphtheria toxin A highly toxic 62 kD protein produced by ***Corynebacterium diphtheriae*** that inhibits eukaryotic protein synthesis by inactivation of elongation factor-2

Dipole moment see Magnetic resonance imaging

Direct costs HEALTH CARE ADMINISTRATION Those costs that are incurred as a direct result of patient management, including salaries, reagents and supplies, equipment costs, heating, lighting and water; Cf Indirect costs

Direct diagnosis MOLECULAR BIOLOGY The diagnosis of a disease state based on well-established and relatively constant mutations that are directly detectable in the DNA molecule, eg sickle cell anemia and α_1-antitrypsin, both of which have point mutations that are identical in all patients; direct diagnosis can be used when there are large gene deletions, insertions or nonsense mutations

Directed donation TRANSFUSION MEDICINE The donation of blood products intended for use by one specified recipient; pre-AIDS directed donations were carried out in the context of a) Donor-specific transfusions prior to renal transplantation b) Platelet pheresis transfusions and c) Transfusions of rare blood types; directed donation has increased in the recent past due to public concern about the safety of the blood supply and the general feeling that a friend or family member is less likely be infected by the HIV virus than an anonymous donor (although the available data does not support this conclusion); Cf Autologous donation, Intraoperative autologous donation

Direct fluorescent antibody method IMMUNOLOGY A technique in which a molecule of interest is detected directly by an antibody labelled or tagged with a fluorochrome, eg FITC (fluorescein-isothiocyanate); the direct test is most often used for detecting the presence of immune depositions in a histologic section, eg IgG or C3 complement deposits in an epithelial basement membrane or in glomeruli; Cf Indirect immunofluorescence

Director of laboratories A physician who is a licensed doctor of medicine or osteopathy (MD or DO) and who is acceptable to an accrediting agency, eg the JCAH (Joint Commission of Accredited Hospitals); a person with a PhD may act as director of one section of the clinical laboratories but may not render opinions regarding patient management

Direct-to-consumer advertising see Advertising

'Dirty background' A finding in Papanicolaou-stained smears of uterine cervical cytology consisting in cell debris and necrosis often associated with inflammation, due to Gardnerella or Trichomonas species, pregnancy, post-partum, post-menopause, in oral contraceptive users and cervical carcinoma; a 'dirty background', then has no specific clinical significance

'Dirty' chest of Simon RADIOLOGY Patchy radiopacities on a plain chest film due to mucous gland hyperplasia, seen in bronchiectasis, which is often associated with bronchitis

Disappearing bone disease Progressive massive disease of unknown pathogenesis, that most often affects subjects older than age 30 after suffering trauma, characterized by extensive bone resorption variably associated with hemangiomas or lymphangiomas, pain, progressive weakness and elevated alkaline phosphatase

Disaster see Decay disaster

Disaster Any usually unanticipated event that requires urgent response, bringing people and/or property out of harms way in order to minimize loss of life or destruction; disasters are described by certain parameters a) Natural, eg geophysical (earthquakes, volcanoes) and weather-related (floods, hurricanes) or man-made origin (transportation-related, structural collapse, war, hazardous materials, explosions, fires) b) Location single site, eg explosion or multiple sites, eg hurricanes c) Predictability, eg hurricane 'season' vs toxic spill d) Onset, ie gradual vs acute e) Duration, ie brief vs extended f) Frequency, eg hurricanes vs mass intoxication (N Engl J Med 1991; 324:815rv)

Disaster 'syndrome' PSYCHOLOGY A response in survivors of major natural or man-made disasters that has been subdivided into four chronologic stages: MINUTES TO HOURS Stunned apathy, disorientation DAYS Inefficiency while attempting to help other victims in worse condition than self, onset of guilt at having survived WEEKS Euphoria and enthusiasm at rebuilding and renewing activities, sense of communality with co-victims MONTHS Resolution; Cf Concentration camp syndrome

DISC Diffuse inflammatory salmon-patch choroidopathy Birdshot retinopathy An idiopathic condition characterized by a 'quiet eye' in children and adolescents due to posterior segment inflammation, symmetrical retinal vascular leakage, macular edema and multiple depigmented spotting with narrowing of retinal arterioles

Discharge summary A document prepared by the attending physician of a hospitalized patient that summarizes the admitting diagnosis, therapy received while hospitalized, prognosis and plan of action upon the patient's discharge

'Discovery rule' LEGAL MEDICINE A rule that expands the Statute of limitations (which usually limits a plaintiff's right to initiate a lawsuit to 2-3 years after an alleged tort occurred), such that the time period during which a lawsuit may be initiated begins from the moment the victim of the tort or plaintiff becomes aware of the act of malpractice

Disease flare-up see Flare

Disease of regulation Any clinical nosology, the symptoms of which are attributed to the loss of homeostatic mechanisms responsible for maintaining in balance a hormone, eg parathyroid hormone or the autonomic nervous system, eg blood pressure

Disease of the week 'syndrome' A hypochondriacal complex described in medical students, who, as they learn about a disease, discover that they, too, have all of the symptoms of the disorder being described

Disenfranchized population SOCIAL MEDICINE Any group of people who are without a home or a political voice and who live at the whims of their host; disenfranchized populations include the homeless or refugees of war and natural disasters and suffer from a wide variety of illness, low-grade malnutrition and inability to educate themselves and integrate themselves into the host population; see Refugee

DISH Diffuse idiopathic skeletal hyperostosis of Forester RHEUMATOLOGY A disease complex affecting the middle-aged and elderly, characterized by florid neo-osteogenesis (bone spurs and potentially spinal fusion) at ligamentous insertions in numerous sites; serious problems may arise if the cervical spine is involved, potentially causing dysphagia; the process appears to be more prominent on the right side; DISH may be associated with impaired glucose tolerance, diabetes mellitus and obesity

Dishface deformity Facies scaphoidea A concave face that occurs in an unrepaired midface fracture, characterized by a protruding forehead, prominent jaw, depressed nose and malar prominences seen in the LeFort III fracture, which extends bilaterally through the frontozygomatic suture lines, the base of the nose and the ethmoid region; the lateral rims of the orbits are separated and the infraorbital rim may be fractured; in this most severe type of LeFort fracture, cerebrospinal rhinorrhea may occur, indicating 'violation' of the cranial vault and there is loss of direct contact with the anterior teeth

Dishwater pus A fanciful descriptor for the seropurulent discharge typical of synergistic necrotizing cellulitis due to an anaerobic bacterial infection, which is most commonly associated with cardiorenal dysfunction, diabetes mellitus, obesity and perirectal infections **Clinical** After a 3-14 day incubation, there is abrupt development of a malodorous lesion with sloughing of skin, gas production in the wound, muscle involvement and marked systemic toxicity **Treatment** Opening and aeration of the wound kills bacteria through oxygen toxicity

Disinfection Elimination of the ability of a surface or material to act as a vector for an infectious agent; objects may be disinfected by a variety of methods including chemicals (alcohol, chlorine, hexachlorophenes, iodines, phenols or quaternary ammonium compounds), high dry heat or 'wet' autoclaved heat; 'high-level' disinfectants are used for instruments that will penetrate the body cavities, eg surgical instruments and include ethylene oxide, glutaraldehyde (2%), formaldehyde (8%), alcohol (70-90%), stabilized hydrogen peroxide (6%), phenolic compounds (3%), iodophors (500 ppm), bleach (1000 ppm) and pasteurization at 75°C Note: The Creutzfeldt-Jakob disease agent, a prion is extremely resistant to disinfection in the form of boiling, chemicals (alcohol, β-propiolactone, formalin) and irradiation and requires Biosafety Level 2 practices; see Biosafety level

Disk kidney see Cake kidney

Diskectomy see Laminectomy

Disomy The inheritance of both haploid chromosomes from one parent, either the father, paternal disomy or mother, maternal disomy

Disruption OBSTETRICS The in utero destruction of a previously formed normal fetal body part, caused either by a) 'amputation', the result of pressure-induced strangulation by an amniotic band or b) interruption of regional blood supply, causing ischemia, necrosis and sloughing of the dead part; see Dysmorphology

Disseminated intravascular coagulation (DIC) A pernicious clinical event in which the balance between coagulation and fibrinolysis tips toward coagulation; 30-65% of DIC is caused by infection; DIC is divided into a 'fast' DIC, which presents as an acute, fulminant, uncompensated consumptive coagulopathy with clinical manifestations of bleeding due, for example, to abruptio placentae, septic abortion, amniotic fluid embolism, toxemia, massive tissue injury, as occurs in burns, surgery, trauma, infections, gram-negative sepsis, meningococcemia, Rocky Mountain spotted fever, incompatible blood transfusion and purpura fulminans; 'fast' DIC requires replacement of deficient or consumed factors; 'Slow' DIC occurs in diseases that are chronic, indolent and compensated, for which there is little overt manifestation of bleeding; the clinical picture is rather painted by thrombosis, microcirculatory ischemia and end-organ infarction, due for example, to acute promyelocytic leukemia, dead fetus syndrome, transfusion of coagulation factor concentrates, neoplasia (adenocarcinoma of the pancreas, prostate, lung, stomach), aortic aneurysm, cocaine, monoamine oxidase inhibitors, giant hemangioma (Kasabach-Merritt syndrome), liver disease, vasculitis, chronic and/or low-grade infections, eg histoplasmosis, aspergillosis, malaria and compensated obstetric conditions, (eg, hemolysis, eclampsia, infection, hypoxia, acidosis, respiratory distress); 'slow' DIC may respond to heparinization **Pathogenesis** 1) Endothelial cell damage by endotoxins, hypoxia and acidosis or immune complexes; endothelial damage results in a thrombogenic surface that activates platelets and the intrinsic coagulation pathway 2) Release of factor III (tissue thromboplastin) by neoplasia, trauma or complications of pregnancy (leading to extrinsic pathway activation) **Laboratory** Increased prothrombin time, partial thromboplastin time, fibrinogen degradation products (FDPs) and fibrinopeptide A; decreased fibrinogen, platelets, factor V, factor VIII, antithrombin III and plasminogen **Histopathology** Kidneys demonstrates diffuse cortical necrosis, necrotic columns of Bertini with acute ischemic infarct

DIT 3,5-diiodotyrosine Iodinated precursor for either T_3 or T_4

Dithiocarb Dithiocarbamate A drug with potent antioxidant capacity and chelating activities that improves the depressed immune responses of newborn and aging mice, mice immunosuppressed through chemotherapy of radiotherapy or those with a murine retrovirus-induced immunodeficiency; dithiocarb has a similar effect in AIDS and appears to improve survival (J Am Med Assoc 1991; 265:1538)

Divalent metal ions Divalent cations Metal ions that have major roles in metabolic functions, including Ca^{++}, Mg^{++}, Cu^{++}, Mn^{++}, Co^{++} and Zn^{++}, the physiologic levels of which in the human economy range from gram to trace quantities

Dive bomber sound An adjectival descriptor for the sound heard by electromyography corresponding to the myotonic response (delayed relaxation of the muscle following a maintained contraction or twitch), elicited by movement of the needle electrode within the muscle as well as percussion; in the myotonias (dystrophia myotonica, paramyotonia and myotonia congenita), prolonged trains of potentials occur in great profusion in response to movement of the electrode, producing a sound likened to that of the Junkers Ju-87 (Stuka) bomber when diving

Diversity see Gene diversity

Diversion colitis Inflammation in the bypassed segments of the colorectum after surgical diversion of the fecal stream; diversion colitis may be asymptomatic or appear as a bloody discharge, colicky anorectal pain, tenesmus, purulent or hemorrhagic discharge and occurs in the majority of diverted colons from one month to years after the procedure Endoscopy Friable, erythematous and granular mucosa that mimicks both Crohn's disease and ulcerative colitis Histopathology Acute superficial inflammation, crypt abscesses, edema, ulceration and increased lymphoid follicles Pathogenesis Possibly due to local nutritional deficiency of the mucosa Treatment Local application of short-chain fatty acids (N Engl J Med 1989; 320:23)

DKA see Diabetic ketoacidosis

DMSO Dimethylsulfoxide A substance that occurs naturally in minute amounts in certain foods, and which has been used as an industrial solvent for making paper since the 1940s DMSO is of potential use for treating familial amyloidotic polyneuropathy, acetaminophen hepatotoxicity; human trials suggest it may have analgesic and anti-inflammatory properties; DMSO reduces the ice crystals formed in frozen section tissues from the operating suite, and may be an effective cryopreservative medium Note: DMSO has been used (without proven efficacy) to treat arthritis, mental illness, emphysema and cancer

DNA Deoxyribonucleic acid

DNA amplification see Gene amplification

DNA analysis A vast array of techniques are used to analyze genes and DNA and include Chromosome walking, Fingerprinting, Footprinting, Hybridization, Jeffries' probe, Jumping libraries, PCR (polymerase chain reaction), RFLP (restriction fragment length polymorphism) analysis and Southern blot hybridization

DNA binding protein Any of a group of proteins that form dimers and bind at specific sites on DNA, often located near highly-positively charged regions of amino acids interacting with negatively-charged DNA, either activating or quenching gene expression, acting during cell growth and differentiation or during normal cell function; three structural motifs capable of binding DNA have been recognized a) Helix-turn-helix motif, seen in MyoD protein b) Leucine zipper motif, see in the protein products of the *fos, jun* and *myc* oncogenes and c) Zinc finger motif, seen in growth signal-regulating proteins; see Helix-turn-helix motif, Leucine zipper motif, Zinc finger motif

DNA clock MOLECULAR PHYLOGENY The use of DNA hybridization studies to infer relatedness of organisms and their points of evolutionary divergence from each other Method DNA is melted and hybrids are allowed to form, comparing the degree of hybridization from homoduplexes, which are duplexes of DNA strands from the same species and heteroduplexes, duplexes of DNA strands from different species (Science 1988; 240:1598, 241:1756); see 'Homology', Mitochondrial 'Eve'

DNA conformation The three-dimensional configuration of DNA with respect to coiling and supercoiling, which is classified as Form I Native DNA in its supercoiled form Form II DNA subjected to partial DNAse digestion, which introduces a single nick and thus has a relaxed conformation Form III DNA that has been incubated with DNAse and because both of DNA's helices have been broken, ie, double 'nicked', has a linear form; see Cruciform DNA; Cf DNA structural types, DNA supercoiling

DNA fingerprinting see Fingerprinting

DNA folding Folded DNA The native DNA configuration that results from the interplay between the DNA itself (the 'internal message') and its regulatory proteins (the 'external message'); this dynamic conformation is pivotal in understanding the effects of DNA; establishment of 'ground rules' for DNA-protein interactions requires knowledge of DNA's 'surface morphology', obtained by complex mathematical and biophysical modeling (Science 1988; 241:323); see DNA-binding proteins

DNA forms DNA's conformation is a function of a) The types of bonds and the stacking of the nucleotides, which is deduced by diffraction analysis and b) The medium, in particular, the state of hydration, which can facilitate or hinder certain three-dimensional configurations **A-DNA** Right-handed, double-stranded, stable at intermediate relative hydration of the medium, 11 bases per turn of the double helix, contains major and minor grooves; the phosphate groups face each other across the major groove; A-DNA is less common than B-DNA **B-DNA** The most common form of DNA in living cells, also known as Watson-Crick DNA, which is right-handed, double-stranded, stable at high relative hydration of the medium, contains 10.6 bases per turn of the double helix and has major and minor grooves; the twist improves the stacking of the bases along each backbone chain **cDNA** Complemenatry DNA, see cDNA **C-DNA** Right-handed, double-stranded, stable at low relative hydration of the medium, 9.3 bases per turn of the double helix **H-DNA** A convoluted configuration of DNA that contains adjacent triple-stranded and single stranded regions with sharply-angled hinging and kinking; H-DNA requires intense supercoiling to maintain this structure, which is a function of the acidity of the pH of the medium; it is unknown whether the H-DNA configuration exists in vivo **J-DNA** A unique and convoluted configuration of DNA that exists in mildly alkaline solutions; it is unknown whether the J-DNA configuration exists in vivo (Science 1988; 241:1791) **k-**

DNA Extranuclear DNA contained within kinetoplasts, which exists in the form of maxicircles and minicircles; analysis of k-DNA by buoyant density, DNA hybridization or polymerase chain reaction is of use in speciating organisms with kinetoplasts, eg ***Leishmania*** species (N Engl J Med 1991; 324:476cpc) **mtDNA** see Mitochondrial DNA **rDNA** Any segment of DNA that encodes ribosomal RNA **Z-DNA** DNA that is expressed in vivo as a regulator of function; it is left-handed, has a zig-zag (hence Z-DNA) configuration and contains multiple CGCGCG nucleotides; a configuration in which the phosphate groups face each other across a deep minor groove; see Left-handed DNA

DNA gyrase A type II prokaryotic topoisomerase that catalyzes the negative supercoiling of DNA ahead or downstream from the advancing replicating fork (structure, Nature 1991; 351:624); see DNA supercoil

DNA hybridization A technique for determining the presence of a target DNA in a sample of tissue or cells Method A sample of cells is lysed, the protein is removed by digestion with proteinase K and the DNA extracted using phenol, chloroform and isoamyl alcohol; the DNA is then denatured with a salt, sodium hydroxide, separating one of DNA's chains; the single-stranded or denatured DNA may be immobilized on a blotting paper as in Southern blot hybridization or present in a tissue as in in situ hybridization; the final step adds a ^{32}P-labeled probe or a biotinylated probe that is visualized by either autoradiography, as in the ^{32}P-labelled probe or by adding avidin-biotin acid phosphatase, which evokes a color change in the substrate upon digestion Applications of DNA hybridization Rapid diagnosis of infection, eg in tissue, using in situ hybridization a) Virus, eg cytomegalic inclusion virus, Epstein-Barr virus, human papillomavirus, Herpes simplex virus, adenovirus, HIV-1 b) Bacteria, eg enterotoxin-producing ***Escherichia coli*** and gonococcus and detection of neoplasia a) Specific DNA mutations (point mutations, deletions, translocations), clonal expansions of rearranged immunoglobulins (B-cell lymphomas) or T-cell receptors (T-cell lymphomas) and other specific mutations associated with various neoplasms b) Detection of integrated viral DNA and c) Detection of oncogenes Diagnosis of genetic diseases; see HLA analysis, Paternity testing, RFLP analysis

DNA instability syndromes see DNA repair syndromes

DNA library see Library

DNA ligase An enzyme that links strands of DNA during repair and replication, catalyzing the formation of phosphodiester bond between the 3'-OH and the 5'-PO_4 of DNA's phosphate backbone

DNA methylation see Methylation

DNA ploidy see Flow cytometry, Ploidy analysis

DNA polymerases A group of enzymes involved in DNA replication, forming two distinct complexes acting in sequence a) DNA-polymerase α-primase complex, which first initiates DNA synthesis at the replication origin, acting as the polymerase for the lagging strand, opposite the Okazaki fragments, followed by b) DNA polymerase sigma complex, which initiates replication on the leading strand template Note: Some prokaryotic DNA polymerase complexes can replace the DNA polymerase sigma complex (Nature 1990; 346:534); prokaryotic DNA polymerases I, II and III (pol I, pol II, pol III) correspond to the eukaryotic DNA polymerases α, β and γ, designated as pol α, pol β and pol γ; see Replication

DNA polymorphism A condition where more than one normal but different nucleotide sequences exist at a particular site in DNA; these inherited differences in DNA sequences are normal variations of an individual's DNA, also known as restriction length polymorphisms and can be exploited to document the pattern of inheritance of genes associated with certain diseases; the term polymorphism requires that the less frequent of two loci be found in more than 1% of the population; see RFLP (restriction fragment length polymorphism) analysis

DNA probe A small single-stranded fragment of cloned, biotin-labelled or radiolabelled DNA that is complementary to a DNA molecule of interest; this complementary can be detected a) Semiquantitatively by the Dot-blot technique, b) When located in a tissue of interest by in situ hybridization and c) Immobilized on a nitrocellulose or nylon membrane, see Southern blot hybridization

DNA repair syndromes DNA instability syndromes A heterogeneous group of diseases with damaged genomes, chromosomal 'instability', hypersensitivity to irradiation and mutagenic chemicals and an increased risk of suffering malignancy, including ataxia-telangiectasia, Bloom syndrome, dyskeratosis congenita, Fanconi's anemia, progeria and xeroderma pigmentosum

DNA restriction site polymorphism see DNA polymorphism, RFLP (restriction fragment length polymorphism) analysis

DNAse protection assay Any method for studying DNA, in which the parent double-stranded DNA is 'protected' from DNase digestion by virtue of being bound by a protein Technique A segment of DNA is subjected to digestion by a restriction endonuclease (a DNase), which will reduce the entire DNA chain to mono- and dinucleotides, except for the segment of DNA protected by a bound protein; the protein is then removed from the DNA and the sequence is determined by either the Maxam-Gilbert or Sanger technique; see Achilles heel cleavage, Dimethyl sulfate protection assay, Footprinting

DNA structures see DNA forms

DNA supercoil A circular double helix of DNA that has been twisted into a supercoil by a DNA gyrase, rendering it more compact, resulting in rapid sedimentation by ultracentrifugation and rapid migration by gel electrophoresis; reversal of the supercoil is accomplished by topoisomerase, which 'nicks', opens and closes the strands; see Topoisomerase

DNA topology The surface properties of a DNA molecule, which are a function of **Linking number** The number of times one strand of the double helix crosses over the other **Twist** The periodicity of winding of one strand around another, ideally, one per 10.4 base pairs, intracellularly however, probably much less due to protein binding and crowding and **WRITHE** The supercoiling of the overall helical structure in space

DNCB Dinitrochlorobenzene A compound used to measure a person's ability to mount a de novo cell-mediated reaction; the skin of a subject not previously exposed to DNCB is 'painted' with DNCB, a substance that acts as a hapten; in normal subjects, re-exposure to DNCB 2 weeks later elicits a type IV hypersensitivity reaction

DNR Do not resuscitate MEDICAL ETHICS An order written in a patient's chart that explicitly and unequivocally states that cardiopulmonary resuscitation should not be initiated if a patient is found in cardiac arrest; DNR orders may be written at the request of the patient, or if incompetent, at the request of the patient's family; although in theory, DNR or 'No code' orders may be written by the physician if he feels that CPR will not be successful in restoring meaningful life to the patient, see Baby L, most physicians are disinclined to 'play God'; DNR orders do not preclude treating airway obstruction, congestive heart failure, arrhythmias and metabolic derangements, although it is a fine line between this type of 'supportive care' and resuscitation DNR generally is understood to mean not intubating not using a defibrillator or minimal efforts at resuscitation; 22% of patients participate in DNR decisions and the family, 86% of the time (J Am Med Assoc 1986; 256:233); Cf Advanced directives, Euthanasia, Living will

DOA Date of admission, Dead on arrival

DOB Date of birth

DOC Date of confinement or delivery

'Doc-in-a-box' A deprecative sobriquet for a physician who provides primary health care, usually at an hourly rate and in the setting of a free-standing ambulatory care clinic

Docking protein see Signal recognition particle

'Doctor Death' A retired pathologist and self-proclaimed 'obitiatrist' (a physician who assists patients wishing to commit suicide), who invented a 'self-execution machine' allowing a patient to switch an intravenous saline line to thiopental and from there to potassium chloride, thereby causing a painless and fatal arrhythmia (Am Med News 22/May/90); the first client to use the device was a middle-aged woman suffering from Alzheimer's dementia (N Engl J Med 1990; 323:750), who preferred death to the slow inexhorable deterioration of mental function; 'Dr Death' was barred by court injunction from allowing others to use the device; in October, 1991, the same physician provided the expertise and equipment for two assisted suicides (NY Newsday 25/Oct/91; see Euthanasia; Cf Angel of death; Dr 'X'

'Doctor-nurse game' The complex 'pas de deux' between physician and nurse(s); in the US, nurses have begun to demand complete equality and the autonomy to make decisions about patient management, the wisdom of which is questionable (N Engl J Med 1990; 323:201c) as the education differs substantially (3-5 years for a nurse, 11-14 years for a physician) and the medico-legal responsibility is ultimately born by the physician

Doctor-patient interaction The doctor-patient 'game' comprises the social aspects of a confidential relationship shared by the physician and his patient; several models of this relation have been described and each 'player' in the dyad has an appropriate role: a) **ENGINEERING MODEL** The physician distances himself from the moral dilemmas of the relation per se, merely providing all the facts, allowing the patient to make his own decisions b) **PRIESTLY (PATERNALISTIC) MODEL** The physician guides the patient through both various disease processes and the moral dilemmas of his life and c) **CONTRACTUAL MODEL** The physician and the patient each share in the moral responsibilities of the medical decisions; see 'High touch'

DOD Dead of disease

DOE Dyspnea on exertion

Dogs The canine is the vector for many microorganisms capable of causing human disease (N Engl J Med 1985; 313:985), including Arthropods and mites (*Cheyletiella yasguri*, *Sarcoptes scabei*, var hominis, var canis), bacteria (*Brucella abortus, B suis, B melitensis, B canis, Campylobacter jejuni*, CDC-designated bacteria, including DF-2, IIj, EF-4, M-5, *Francisella tularensis, Leptospira canicola, Pasteurella multocida, Yersinia pestis*), parasites (*Ancylostoma brasiliense, A caninum, Babesia microti, Dirofilaria immitis, Dipetallonema perstans, Dipylidium canum, Echinococcus granulosa, E multilocularis, Giardia lamblia, Gnathostoma spinigera, Multiceps multocida, M senilis, Spirometra (Diphyllobotrium)) mansonoides*, (sparganosis), *Toxocara canis, Toxoplasma gondii*), rickettsia, eg *Ehrlichia canis* (J Am Med Assoc 1987; 257:3100, N Engl J Med 1987; 316:853), virus (rabies)

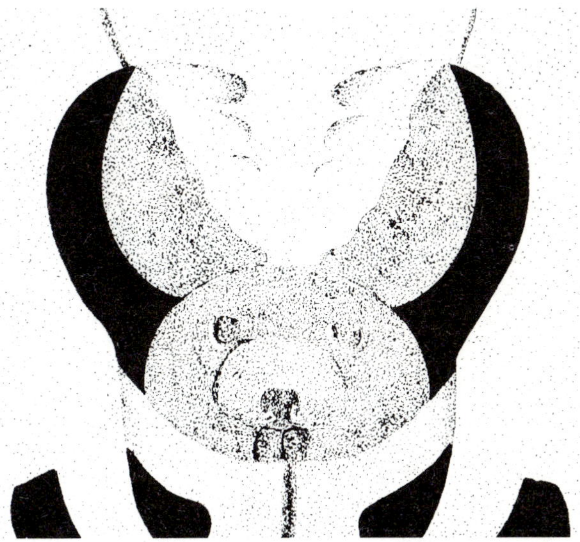

Dog ear appearance, radiology

'Dog ear' appearance PLASTIC SURGERY A one-sided mound of excess tissue, appearing after the repair of certain skin lesions and defects; 'dog ears' may be inevitable in complex wounds, occurring when the long axis of an elliptical incision is too short (the general rule being a 4:1 length-to-width ratio) and may appear at both ends of the surgical incision; excision requires either lengthening of the wound, creating an oblique limb at the incision or loosening with a Y-shaped incision, repairing by shortening (excising) the long side and lengthening the short side RADIOLOGY A fanciful descriptor for the symmetrical settling of free blood or fluid on either side of the bladder at the posterior pelvic floor, visualized in the supine victim of massive trauma to organs, fractures and rupture of organs, illustration, page 175

Doigt-en-lorgnette French, telescoped finger A finger in which there is concentric osteolysis and bony collapse, classically seen in yaws (*Treponema pertinue*)-induced osteitis; see Yaws

Doll face PEDIATRICS A face with chubby cheeks and prominent chin, described as typical of glycogen storage disease type Ia or von Gierke's disease, further characterized by hepatomegaly, enlarged kidneys, growth retardation Laboratory Hypoglycemia, lactic acidosis, increased uric acid and hyperlipidemia Prognosis Good; Cf Cherubism

Doll's head maneuver NEUROLOGY A clinical sign for evaluating brainstem function in a comatose patient; in the normal subject, as the head is turned rapidly to one side, the eyes conjugately deviate in the direction opposite to the head's movement; loss of this reflex implies dysfunction of the brainstem or of the oculomotor nerves; infero-lateral deviation of the eyes in combination with pupillary dilatation and implies dysfunction of the third cranial nerve, possibly due to tentorial herniation

Dolomite A generic term for calcium-magnesium carbonate that may be self-administered as a calcium supplement to ensure healthy bones, which is mined in the Dolomite mountains of Northern Italy (and elsewhere); some of the mineral deposits may be contaminated with heavy metals (lead, cadmium and others), for which there is a maximum ceiling of 5 parts per million allowed by the US Food and Drug Administration Note: Dolomite has been claimed by some advocates of 'holistic' health, to be the most natural (and therefore 'healthiest') calcium supplement available; one of the most vocal of these advocates ironically died of a malignant bone tumor

Domain MOLECULAR BIOLOGY A folded, relatively globular, 40-400 amino acid residue in length region of a protein or polypeptide chain that may present a spatially distinct 'signature', often allowing it to interact in a specific fashion with other proteins or receptors; the term 'domain' is also used for a) The functional disulfide bond-linked polypeptide loops on the constant and variable regions of both the light and heavy chains of the immunoglobulin molecule b) A chromosome region in which the supercoiling is independent of the rest of the molecule and c) A long segment of DNA bearing a functional gene that is highly-susceptible to DNAse degradation; Cf Motif

Domino donation Transplantation of heart and lungs of cadaveric origin into patient A, who has suffered from long standing lung disease, eg cystic fibrosis, but who has a heart suitable for donation, while transplanting patient A's heart into patient B; it is estimated that optimal domino-donation in the USA would free an extra 50-75 hearts for transplantation

Domino theory A hypothetical explanation of cell duplication that holds that the daughter of a somatic division is produced by a series of linear metabolic pathways where the initiation of a new pathway hinges on completion of a previous pathway, a concept championed by yeast biologists, in contrast to the Clock theory that postulates the existence of a series of 'switches'; accumulated data supports a merging of the two theories (Science 1989; 246:614)

Domoic acid An excitatory neurotransmitting kainic acid analog that is a neurotoxic glutamate agonist that causes increased firing of neurons; domoic acid is produced by marine vegetation (***Nitzschia pungens***) that may be concentrated in mussels and cause envenonation in seafood restaurants; an outbreak in Prince Edward Island in 1987 was clinically characterized by vomiting, abdominal cramps, diarrhea, incapacitating headache, seizures, hemiparesis, ophthalmoplegia and loss of short-term memory (N Engl J Med 1990; 322:1775, 1781), which may prove useful in developing a model for Alzheimer's disease

Don Juan syndrome Satyrism PSYCHIATRY A form of male sexual deviancy in which the subject masks his feelings of insecurity regarding his own masculinity and/or latent homosexuality by myriad sexual liaisons with the opposite sex; to the Freudians, this represents an Oedipus complex in which the sexual promiscuity represents a search for maternal love; Male hypersexuality is considered a sociopathy, as there is no emotion attached to the relations and up to 50% of subjects are impotent; Cf Delilah syndrome

Donor One who donates tissue(s), an organ, blood or blood products; in the usual parlance, a donor is an altruistic individual who contributes blood products, often on a regular basis; formerly, a 'two-tier' system of quality of blood products existed in North America, where the 'better' blood was from voluntary donation in non-urban environments, while the less-desirable blood, ie more commonly infected with hepatitis virus and other pathogens, came from paid donation (often from a 'disenfranchized' population, eg drug addicts or the homeless, who exchange blood for money) in urban regions DONOR REQUIREMENTS The donor must have a corporal temperature of < 37.5°C, pulse 50-100, blood pressure of 100 to 180 mm Hg systolic, and 50 to 100 mm Hg diastolic, hematocrit of > 41% for men and 38% for women, no skin lesions, 48 hours passed since last plasmapheresis or platelet donation, more than 12 months passed since receiving hepatitis B immunoglobulin DONOR REJECTION A donor rejected if he has received therapy for malaria within the past 3 years (or travelled to a malaria endemic area within last 6 months), has ever had hepatitis B surface antigenemia, or lives with a hepatitis B carrier, has a 'high-risk' life style, has donated blood within the last 8 weeks, has a temperature > 37.5°C, or has, within the last six months: Delivered a term-infant, received Rho-GAM or blood products, had surgery or a tattoo, is being treated with antihistamines, steroids, tetracycline, barbiturates; there are four-week deferrals for tetanus, smallpox and oral polio vaccines DONOR BLOOD TESTS Alanine aminotransferase, hepatitis B surface antigen, hepatitis B core antigen, hepatitis C antibody, HIV-1, HTLV-I, serological test for syphilis

Do not resuscitate see DNR

DOOR Deafness, onycho-osteodystrophy, mental retardation A rare autosomal condition in which sensorineural deafness is accompanied by aplasia or hypoplasia of finger and toenails and digital anomalies and epilepsy **Laboratory** Increased plasma and urinary 2-oxoglutarate (Am J Med Genet 1987; 26:207)

Dopamine receptors Dopamine's diverse physiological activities are mediated by G protein receptors D_1 and D_2 receptors are considered together, as they are both located in the brain and endocrine tissues and have a variable response to neuroleptics agents that are used to treat schizophrenia; D_1 receptors have a viable response to neuroleptics, and when stimulated, increase the levels of adenylyl cyclase, while D_2 receptors respond to low (nanomolar) doses of these agents by decreasing adenylyl cyclase activity; the reported association between the D_2 receptor gene and alcoholism (J Am Med Assoc 1991; 265:2667c) has not withstood rigorous scrutiny; D_1 receptor mRNA is most abundant in the caudate, nucleus accumbens and olfactory tubercle and D_1 receptors may mediate behavioral changes, modulate D_2 receptor activity and regulate neuron growth and differentiation; the D_1 receptor is encoded by a long intronless gene on chromosome 5 (Nature 1990; 347:72,76,80); both D_1 and D_2 receptors are potential therapeutic targets for psychomotor disorders, eg Parkinsonism, schizophrenia and drug and alcohol abuse D_3 receptor is a recently characterized receptor that is both autoreceptor and post-synaptic receptor, located in the limbic system and associated with cognitive, emotional and endocrine functions; the D_3 receptor appears to mediate some of the effects of antipsychotic and anti-Parkinson's disease drugs that had been previously attributed to D_2 receptors (Nature 1990; 347:146)

Doppler effect A physical principle based on the decrease in oscillation frequency of an object emitting sound or energy waves as it passes a point of measurement; this principle is applied in the Doppler flowmeter used to evaluate blood velocities, which are distinctly abnormal in atherosclerotic arteries

Doppler color flow imaging CARDIOLOGY A noninvasive two-dimensional Doppler technique which provides a real-time image of the blood flow 'jet', allowing the severity of valvular stenosis to be determined, see Candle Flame, Mushroom, and Scimitar signs (Mayo Clin Proc 1986; 61:623)

Doppler sonographic imaging Any of a group of imaging modalities that takes advantage of the Doppler shift, a change in pitch resulting from the relative motion between an ultrasound source and an observer, which is directly related to the velocity of the moving object (red cells) and the cosine of the angle (Doppler angle) between the direction of blood flow and the ultrasound beam (the ideal Doppler angle is the rarely achievable 0°; it usually ranges from 45° to 60°)

DORA Directory of rare analyses A book published by the American Chemical Society listing uncommonly ordered clinical tests and details on the laboratories performing them (AACC press 1725 K St NW Suite 1010, Washington DC 20006)

Dosage effect TRANSFUSION MEDICINE The presence of different quantities of an antigen on the red cell surface depending on whether the allele encoding the antigen is homo- or heterozygous, resulting in variability in the agglutination reaction in certain red cell antigens, including Kidd, MNS (but not s), Kell, Jk^a, Xg^a, Rh-C, Rh-c, Rh-E, Rh-e

Dot and blot hemorrhages OPHTHALMOLOGY Relatively small hemorrhages seen in the inner nuclear layer that extend to the outer plexiform layer, typical of the retinal fundi of patients with diabetic retinopathy, which when seen in three dimensions, are anointed as 'serpiginous' hemorrhages

Dot blot A rapid ('quick and dirty'), hybridization technique for semiquantifying a specific RNA and DNA fragment in a specimen without performing the more time-consuming Northern and Southern blots **Method** The DNA is serially diluted and 'spotted' on a nitrocellulose or nylon membrane, denatured (ie one of the DNA strands is separated) with NaOH, then bathed in a solution containing a heat-denatured, presumably complementary DNA fragment (a 'probe') that is 'tagged' with a radiolabel, eg ^{32}P or ^{35}S, or a non-radioactive label, 2-acetyl-aminofluorene, which attaches to the guanine nucleotides; complementarity between the two single strands results in 'hybridization' that is detected by virtue of the probe's radiolabel through autoradiography or if biotinylated, by enzymatic digestion of a substrate, resulting in a color change detectable by spectrophotometry; see 'Quick and dirty'

Dot-DAT Dot blot-direct antiglobulin test A variant of the Coombs test(Am J Clin Path 1987; 88:733), in which IgG is immobilized on a nitrocellulose membrane or solid phase; the patient's red cells are co-incubated on the membrane; subjective interpretation is essentially eliminated as the test need not be placed on a scale (1+ to 4+) as for the usual DAT, thereby reducing false positivity and negativity to a minimum

Dot dystrophy OPHTHALMOLOGY A pattern of microcystic dystrophy occurring in healthy individuals, characterized macroscopically by groups of tiny, round or comma-shaped, gray-white opacities in the pupillary zones, uni- or bilaterally, corresponding to minute cystoid spaces

Dot plot diagram Depiction of test results as a special type of scattergram in which the horizontal axis represents discrete categories rather than a continuous scale and the vertical axis is assigned values falling in a range; dot plots can depict many clinical states over a wide spectrum of health and disease (J Am Med Assoc 1988; 260:3309), allowing projection of disease-positive and disease-negatives states, forming a basis from which multiple studies of diagnostic performance may be compared

Double-barrelled aorta An aorta with a second vascular lumen formed in the media of the aortic wall connecting the proximal and distal intimal tears in an aorta with a dissecting aneurysm

Double blinded studies Clinical studies in which both the patients and researchers are unaware of whether a patient is in the treatment or experimental drug arm or in the placebo arm of the study; see Blinding, Triple blinding; Cf Anecdotal

Double bubble sign RADIOLOGY Two distinct gas pockets seen in an upper gastrointestinal radiocontrast study in atresia of the second segment of the duodenum, 20-30% of whom have Down syndrome; the larger left bubble corresponds to gastric gas; the smaller right corresponds to gas in the duodenal bulb; the double bubble may also occur in an annular pancreas with or without duodenal atresia, duodenal stenosis, peritoneal bands and volvulus Note: The duodenal bubble is correspondingly smaller if there is passage of air; see Bubble

Double condom sign SUBSTANCE ABUSE A finding seen by barium enema in Body packers, who swallow doubly and triply-wrapped condoms filled with heroin and cocaine in order to escape detection by the US customs when deplaning from Nigeria, Colombia and elsewhere; the condoms at the time of packaging, trap annular air pockets, revealing the 'double condom'; see 'Body packing'

Double contrast studies RADIOLOGY A technique used to enhance visualization of the intestinal mucosa; after a cleansing enema of tap water, administered with atropine to prevent potential volume overload-induced vaso-vagal syncope, the patient ingests a suspension of a milkshake-like radiocontrast solution, eg 1g of Barosperse, Intropaque or others per 2 ml water; the contrast is allowed to flow to the splenic flexure in the prone patient and followed by insufflation of air and rotation of the patient to his back, maintaining the left side elevated; further manipulation of the patient occurs under fluoroscopic control and spot films are taken to monitor the study (Radiology 1976; 118:1); single contrast studies identify 77% of colonic lesions > 1.0 cm and 18% of those < 1.0 cm, compared to 98% in > 1.0 cm lesions by double contrast and 78% in lesions < 1.0 cm; it is less commonly used for colitis, given the high correlation with endoscopy and facile access of the endoscope

Double diffusion IMMUNOPATHOLOGY A semiquantitative method for detecting an antibody (or antigen) in a system; a known antigen is placed in a well cut in a block of agar; a test serum which may have the antibody is placed in a second well; the two molecules migrate in a centrifugal fashion; if an antibody and its antigen are present in the system, eg Ouchterlony technique a precipitation line occurs that is detectable by Coomassie Blue staining; see

Double discordance PEDIATRIC CARDIOLOGY Corrected transposition of the pulmonary arteries and aorta The major cardiac arteries are in a mirror-image of their normal location, ie the aorta arises from the anterior left heart and the pulmonary artery from the right posterior heart, the blood from the morphologic right atrium reaches the pulmonary trunk by traversing a mitral valve and morphologic left ventricle; blood from the morphologic left atrium traverses the tricuspid valve and morphologic right ventricle reaching the aorta; the coronary arteries are similarly reversed, ie the right is anterior, the left, posterior; many of those with this complex have other cardiac malformations including conduction and ventricular septal defects, requiring surgical repair and carrying an operative mortality of 25% and a 60% ten-year survival

Double duct sign Irregular, nodular, 'rat-tailed' obstruction or interruption of both the common bile duct and pancreatic duct, seen by endoscopic retrograde cholangiopancreatography (ERCP), a finding suggestive of pancreatic adenocarcinoma, especially if the remaining pancreatic duct is normal

Double minutes MOLECULAR BIOLOGY Redundant doublet and tetrad fragments (minutes) of chromosomes that may be seen when normal cells are exposed to methotrexate or which appear in malignant cells as localized reduplications of DNA, see HSR (homogenously staining regions) or as independent paired chromosomal fragments seen in a quinacrine-stained chromosome preparation

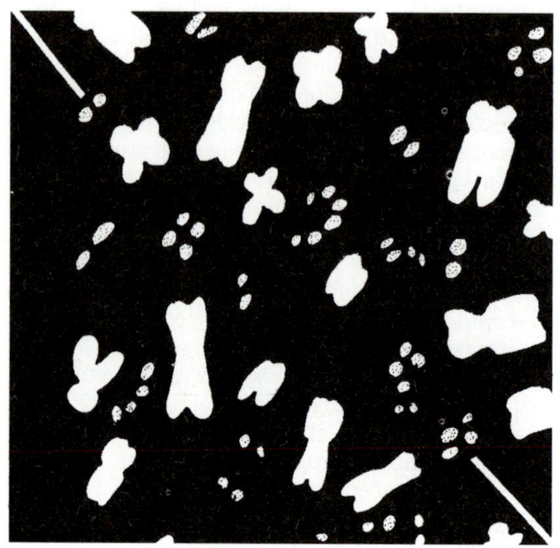

Double minutes

Double pneumonia An obsolete term for bilateral lobar pneumonia, a vanishingly rare condition; double pneumonia also refers to combined viral-bacterial pneumonias which may follow each other, eg an initial *Staphylococcus aureus* infection, causing a one hundred-fold enhancement of infectivity and increased multiplication rate of influenza viruses through production of a hemagglutinin-cleaving enzyme

Double ring appearance OPHTHALMOLOGY A small pale double-contoured spot corresponding to the retinal nerve head surrounded by a pigmented or pale ring, seen in optic nerve hypoplasia, attributed to a primary defect in retinal ganglion cell or axonal differentiation, resulting in visual field defects varying in severity from blindness to virtually normal vision; asymmetrical hypoplasia presents as deviation (strabismus) towards the good eye, not often recognized early enough to reverse the commonly associated visual loss

Double set-up examination OBSTETRICS A two-team approach for a high-risk, eg placenta previa, vaginal delivery, where the first team is prepared for a normal, ie uneventful, vaginal delivery, while the second team, including an anesthesiologist and gynecologist, is on alert should the delivery 'go sour', ready to perform an immediate cesarean section; see Cesarian section

Double wall sign EMERGENCY MEDICINE A radiological finding on a plain supine abdominal film caused by rupture of a hollow gastrointestinal viscus, eg stomach, duodenum or colon, where free air (pneumoperitoneum) outlines the falciform ligament and enhances visualization of loops of small intestine; see inverted 'V' sign

Double whammy 'syndrome' The ability to propulse the eyeball out of its socket, performed by simultaneously contracting the superior and inferior oblique external ocular muscles and orbicularis while relaxing the rectus muscles (Am J Ophthmol 1960; 67:583), with some assistance by external digital pressure; this 'condition' is not associated with pathology and may be performed as a parlor trick

Double zone of hemolysis MICROBIOLOGY A finding on a blood culture plate consisting of an inner zone of complete β-hemolysis and an outer zone of partial hemolysis, a finding characteristic of ***Clostridium perfringens***, see Hemolysis

Doubling time (of tumors) A parameter used to determine tumor aggressiveness, serving to prognosticate, objectively measure therapeutic success, quantify growth kinetics and growth rate of a malignancy; tumor doubling time tends to be characteristic for a particular tumor: 1.5-5 days for Burkitt's lymphoma, 4 days for acute lymphocytic leukemia, 25 days for early breast cancer, 125 days for late breast cancer Note: The growth rate is slower due to the central necrosis; 135 days for pulmonary adenocarcinoma; often by the time a tumor reaches a clinically detectable size of about one cm, it comprises a mass containing 10^9 cells and has undergone 30 doublings; 10 further doublings result in a one kg tumor mass, which, given the hypermetabolism of most malignancies, may be sufficient to make most patients very sick or cause death; the tumor doubling rate does not truly reflect tumor growth since an increasing proportion of daughter cells enter the G_0 or resting phase of the growth cycle; in large malignancies, only 10% of the tumor's cells may be proliferating at any one time; successful chemotherapy hinges on the proportion of cells actively proliferating and therefore susceptible to these agents; Cf Gompertzian growth curve

Doughnut GENERAL SURGERY A sleeve of tissue that is excised after a major gastrointestinal tract resection, often of the distal colon, when a carcinoma extends close to the margin of the original segment Note: Doughnut excisions are most commonly used for infiltrating adenocarcinomas of the lower rectum, where salvage of sphincter function is a function of the length of the tissue available for anastomosis

Doughnut A commonly used adjectival descriptor for a targetoid lesion or radiodensity in which the central and peripheral fields are relatively more radiodense or darker that the middle field Note: Today's doughnuts originated from sweet breads in 16th century Holland and acquired the hole in the early 1800s, an innovation claimed by both the Pennsylvania Dutch and a sea captain, Hanson Gregory

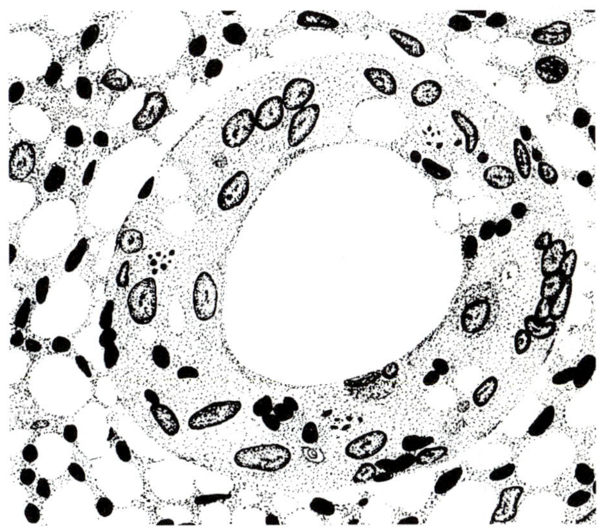

Doughnut granuloma

Doughnut granuloma 'Fibrin ring' A lipid granuloma composed of epithelioid histiocytes, neutrophils, mononuclear or 'round' inflammatory cells, giant cells and a central cleared lipid vacuole; while a characteristic finding in Q fever (***Coxiella burnetii***), it occurs in less than one-half of cases and is located in the bone marrow and liver

Doughnut kidney A rare congenital renal malformation, formed by the fusion of the renal anlagen prior to its rotation and caudal migration; the kidneys are located on the sacral prominence or in the pelvic floor; the ureteropelvic junctions emerge anteriorly and the blood vessels enter posteriorly; Cf Disk and Horseshoe kidneys

Doughnut sign CARDIOVASCULAR IMAGING A descriptor for the radionuclide image of a large anterior wall myocardial infarction in which there is decreased uptake of ^{99m}Technetium stannous pyrophospate in the central infarcted zone, surrounded by a zone of intermediate uptake; the doughnut sign is seen in larger infarcts and is associated with a poor prognosis GASTROINTESTINAL ENDOSCOPY see Bull's-eye sign PULMONARY RADIOLOGY A well-circumscribed mass (coin lesion) with a central, rounded hypodense area corresponding to central tumor necrosis, usually associated with bronchogenic carcinoma, less commonly also seen in abscesses but these are often accompanied by a fluid level

Doughnut structure IMMUNOLOGY A multimeric assembly of C9 complement protein monomers that are inserted into cells, forming a transmembranous pore through which a cell targeted by the complement cascade disintegrates, an event that follows the common pathway of the complement activation and the previous reversible assembly of a leaky patch MEMBRANE PHYSIOLOGY A homopolymeric protein contained within the outer wall of gram-negative bacteria and the outer membrane of mitochondria that is freely permeable to small, < 10 kD molecules

Dough sign HEMATOLOGY A morphological descriptor suggestive of monocytes, where the 'dough' represents the nuclei of blasts and promonocytes which have been squashed in the middle

Doula OBSTETRICS According to the original Greek usage, a doula is an experienced woman who guides and assists a new mother in her infant-care tasks; in an early study in the US, the term doula was defined as a woman who provides emotional support to primiparous women during labor and delivery; adding a doula to the obstetric team is believed by some to reduce the need for a cesarean section, epidural anesthesia, use of oxytocin and duration of labor (J Am Med Assoc 1991; 265:2197)

Dowager's hump Dorsal kyphosis caused by multiple wedge fractures of the vertebral bodies as seen in type II (age-related) osteoporosis Note: Dowager is old French for a widow with a title or property from her husband

Downgrading reaction A subacute deterioration in the clinical and immune status in patients with leprosy accompanied by increased load of organisms, due either to poor drug compliance or to the emergence of a drug-resistant strain of ***Mycobacterium leprae***; Cf Upgrading reaction

Downregulation PHYSIOLOGY The reduction of a cell's response to a hormone or other ligand by internalization of its cognate receptor and degradation within a coated pit; see Clathrin, Coated pit

Downstream MOLECULAR BIOLOGY A descriptor for a location on a molecule of interest, eg protein or DNA that is 'before' or in front of a reference point DNA transcription Downstream refers to nucleotides located on the transcribed DNA strand from the 3' to 5' direction DNA translation: Downstream refers to the nucleotides on the messenger RNA strand from the 5' to the 3' direction Electron transport system: Downstream is the direction from the highest to the lowest level of energy Replication: Downstream is in the direction of the replicating fork Polypeptide chain: Downstream is the direction of the linkage of the amino acids from the N-terminal to the C- terminal

Doxorubicin An anthracycline that is a highly effective antileukemic agent, which impairs cardiac growth in a dose-dependent fashion, where those receiving more than 228 mg/m^2 had a greater incidence of ventricular failure (N Engl J Med 1991; 324:808)

'Downward' negotiations The practice by grant-giving bodies of reducing the number of grants after they have been approved with the purpose of saving money; see 'Approved, but not funded'

Doxorubicin Adriamycin An anthracycline antibiotic used to treat lymphoproliferative malignancy and solid tumors and associated with dose-dependent cardiotoxicity, due to either free radicals or uncoiling of DNA secondary to DNA-binding by drug; see Chemotherapy

2,3 DPG Diphosphoglycerate An inorganic phosphate produced in red cells by the Rapoport-Luebering shunt; 2,3 DPG binds to the β chain of reduced hemoglobin, lowering hemoglobin's affinity for oxygen and by extension, facilitating oxygen release to the tissues, causing a 'right shift' of the oxygen dissociation curve; DPG further shifts the curve to the right by lowering the erythrocyte's pH; when transfused, red cells regain 50% of the 2,3 DPG within 3-8 hours and 100% within 24 hours; see Storage lesion

dpm Disintegrations per minute

DPT 1) An analgesic/sedative 'cocktail' of Demerol, Phenergan and Thorazine 2) see DTP vaccination

D receptors see Dopamine receptors

Dragged disc phenomenon A finding seen in advanced retrolental fibrodysplasia (retinopathy of prematurity), in which the scar in the optic fundus 'drags' the disc and retinal vessels, displacing the macula; when severe, a 'V'-shaped or funnel-shaped detachment of the retina may occur; see also Cat's-eye reflex

Dr Death see 'Doctor Death'

Dread disease rider A clause in a health insurance policy that pays additional benefits for certain diseases known to incur high financial costs, eg extensive burns or cancer or which are known to cause significant and permanent residual morbidity, ie loss of eyes or limbs

DREZ Dorsal root end zone One of the central nervous system pathways that may be surgically sectioned to relieve chronic pain (other sites include the anterolateral cord and the trigeminal tract); DREZ lesions are produced by thermal coagulation or laser and relieve 65-70% of the intractable pain associated with brachial and lumbar plexus avulsion and spinal cord trauma

DRGs Diagnosis-related groups A system of classifying patients according to diagnosis, length of hospital stay and therapy received that was developed in the US in the 1970s by a group at Yale University as a mechanism of utilization review; the DRGs are derived from all of the possible diagnoses in the International Classification of Disease (ICD-9-CM) system, classifying them into 23 major diagnostic categories based on organ systems, then further breaking them down into 470 distinct groups; DRGs are used as a form of cost containment intended to limit the wastage of medical services and were adopted in 1983 by Medicare as a mechanism of paying hospitals, changing from a cost-based, retrospective-reimbursement system to a prospective payment system, giving hospitals a financial incentive for reducing health care costs (N Engl J Med 1988; 318:352); numerical coding and accuracy have become crucial for both the hospital and reimbursement agencies; the coding error rate is about 20% and approximately 60% of these errors favor the hospital; Cf CPT coding

DRG creep 'Creep' HEALTH CARE REIMBURSEMENT A method of coding of diagnosis-related groups (DRGs) under Medicare's prospective payment plan in a fashion that does not conform to the 'optimization' rules governing coding DRGs, usually erring in favor of the hospital, ie paying the hospital more than it is entitled to; causes of 'creep' include mis-specification, miscoding and resequencing (N Engl J Med 1988; 318:352); see Case-mix index, DRGs, Optimization

Drift see Antigenic drift

Drinking water see Maximum contaminant levels, Tapwater

'Drip' A colloquial term for the purulent penile discharge beginning 2-5 days after *Neisseria gonorrhoeae* infection, caused by neisserial endotoxins, and seen in other neisserial infections, including *N meningitidis, N catarrhalis,* as well as *N flava, Mima polymorpha, M polymorpha* var *oxidans* and *Chlamydia trachomatis*; chronic thin mucopurulent discharges are colloquially known as 'gleet'

Drooping lily sign RADIOLOGY A descriptor for a pattern seen in intravenous pyelography, caused by obstruction with eventual development of hydronephrosis of the superior pelvis in renal duplication (not visualized), causing inferior and lateral displacement of the renal pelvis; the normal renal pelvis has an oblique line paralleling the psoas muscle—here the renal pelvis runs inferior and medially)

Drop attacks NEUROLOGY Episodic and precipitous loss of motor function, where the victim is either standing or walking and suddenly the legs give way and the subject plummets, fully conscious to the floor; the idiopathic form is most common in middle-aged to elderly women, attributed to age-related defects in reflexes; drop attacks may also occur in vertibrobasilar ischemia, acute labyrinthine vertigo, cataplexy, 'plateau waves'; drop attacks with loss of consciousness occur in syncope and seizures

Droplet nuclei EPIDEMIOLOGY 1-3 µg in diameter particles of liquid that contain single or small clumps of bacteria; droplet nuclei are considered the infective unit for airborne respiratory infections

Drowning A mechanism of death that claims 7000 lives annually in the US, comprising 15% of the non-motor vehicle-related accidental deaths Pathophysiology **'DRY' DROWNING** Asphyxiation secondary to prolonged glottic spasm that persists beyond apnea; the lungs demonstrate little water **IMMERSION SYNDROME** Cardiac arrest due to an intense vasovagal discharge, the 'diving' reflex 'Secondary' drowning Death occurs 15 minutes to 72 hours after rescue, caused by intense pulmonary edema and adult respiratory distress syndrome **'WET' DROWNING** Laryngospasm followed by relaxation and aspiration of copious amounts of fluid (the most common form); the site of drowning death may be determined by analysis of the lung fluids, eg in brackish water, microscopy reveals diatoms; the mechanism of death is a function of the type of water FRESH WATER DROWNING DEATH is due to ventricular fibrillation with a rapid increase in potassium (> 8 mg/dl) secondary to osmotic hemolysis of red cells in the lungs, with death occurring 2-4 minutes after submersion ICE COLD WATER 'DROWNING' DEATH is due to vaso-vagal cardiac arrest, and thus does not per se represent drowning SALTWATER DROWNING DEATH is due to myocardial ischemia, and occurs 6-7 minutes after submersion SWIMMING POOL DROWNING DEATH is due to massive pulmonary edema related to chlorinated water

Drug abuse see Substance abuse

Drug development Small phase I trials to evaluate safety and dosage, randomized phase II clinical studies of effectiveness and large phase III trials to compare the drugs to others

Drug holiday A period of prescribed abstinence from a drug, considered to be a way in which the total dose of antipsychotic drugs can be reduced, decreasing the incidence of tardive dyskinesia; it is unknown whether drug holidays actually achieve this goal

'Drug lag' CLINICAL THERAPEUTICS A term analogous to the 'missile gap' of the Cold War, coined by the pharmaceutical industry indicating its disapproval of the prolonged delays that occur before a new pharmaceutical agent is allowed in the US drug marketplace (J Am Med Assoc 1978; 239:423); see NDA (New drug application)

Drug monograph A document promulgated by the US Food and Drug Administration specifying the ingredients and composition a prescription drug may contain, the conditions for which it may be prescribed, directions for its use, warnings concerning potential side effects and other relevant information; once a drug monograph is released, any company that meets the drug's monograph requirements may produce and market the drug under its own name without seeking special approval from the FDA, as long as there are no current applicable patents on the drug's formula

Drumstick appendages CYTOGENETICS A mass of X chromatin that is attached to one of the lobes of a polymorphonuclear leukocyte; in accord with the Lyon hypothesis, cells demonstrate one 'drumstick' (or Barr body) less than the karyotype number, characteristic of sexual dimorphism, ie normal; thus an XY male has none, an XX female or XXY Klinefelter syndrome each have one, an XXX 'superfemale' has two and so on

Drumstick fingers see Clubbing, Trommelschläger fingers

Drumstick spores see Tennis racquet spores

Drusen OPHTHALMOLOGY Yellow-white, occasionally confluent nodules composed of aggregated abnormal glycoproteins and glycolipids produced by and adjacent to the basal cells of the retinal pigment epithelium; drusen are the earliest stage of senile degeneration of the macula and is a finding suggestive of retinitis pigmentosa; by low-power light microscopy, drusen appear as nodules filled with homogeneous wispy debris, corresponding to basement membrane material

'Dr X' A surgeon suspected of causing the untimely demise of 30-40 patients from 1963 to 1968 at a now-defunct hospital in New Jersey, who was indicted on five counts of murder, allegedly administering curare as part of his modus operandi; after losing his medical license in the US, he returned to Mar de la Plata, Argentina, where he died in 1984

Dry gangrene see Gangrene

Dry socket Alveolitis sicca dolorosa ODONTOLOGY A complication seen in 1-2% of all tooth extractions, most commonly in molar tooth extraction wounds consisting of focal osteomyelitis in which the clot in the socket disintegrates prematurely and becomes a nidus for oral bacteria, characterized by severe pain and foul odor without purulence; once established, the condition responds poorly to therapy and must be aggressively prevented and treated with tetracycline, either locally or systemically at the time of extraction

Dry pleurisy Plastic pleuritis A complication of acute bacterial pneumonia, tuberculosis or rheumatic fever Clinical Pain and guarding on inspiration, with patients lying on the affected side to 'splint' Histopathology Multiple sero-fibrinous adhesions on the visceral pleura, which may, if intense, cause a fibrothorax

'Dry tap' HEMATOLOGY A needle biopsy of bone marrow, usually obtained from the iliac crests, in which either only blood without clot or no material at all is obtained (a true 'dry tap'); dry taps are due to reticulum fibrosis, marrow necrosis or an extremely packed marrow, occurring in 5-10% of all marrow biopsies; at least 60% of dry taps are malignant; most are lymphoproliferative disorders, including hairy cell leukemia, acute myelocytic leukemia, myelofibrosis, lymphoma and myeloma, the remainder are metastatic carcinomas, with benign disease accounting for the remainder, eg iron deficiency, marrow hypoplasia, hemosiderosis, granulomas and pernicious anemia of dry taps

DSM Diagnostic and Statistic Manual of mental disorders A document produced by the American Psychiatric Association that standardizes the criteria required for establishing the diagnosis of psychiatric nosologies

DTAA di-tryptophan aminal acetaldehyde; see Eosinophilic myalgia syndrome

DTPA ^{99m}Tc diethylenetriamine pentaacetic acid A radionuclide used to evaluate renal perfusion for bilateral comparison of blood flow

DTP vaccine An immunization preparation composed of diphtheria and tetanus toxoids and pertussis vaccine; the recommended schedule for administration is at 2, 4, 6 and 15 months, a booster at 4-6 years and a repeat of the tetanus and diphtheria toxoids at ages 14-16; Contraindications Acute febrile or during suspected evolving neurological illness or when a previous DTP resulted in an allergic reaction; although lifelong protection is not conferred by natural disease or immunization, most cases are prevented by the DTP vaccine Note: The pertussis component of the DTP vaccine may cause neurologic complications, which are uncommon (Pediatrics 1988; 81:345); a genetically engineered mutant for use in a vaccine is under development (Science 1989; 246:497)

DUB see Dysfunctional uterine bleeding

Duesberg, P A well-respected molecular biologist from the University of California who has taken the unusual position that the cause-and-effect relation between AIDS and infection by human immunodeficiency virus (HIV), remains unproven (Proc Natl Acad Sci 1989; 86:755; Nature 1990; 345:659ed, Nature 1991; 350:10c)

Dugas, Gaetan see Patient 'Zero'

Dukes classification A system for prognosticating colorectal carcinoma (table) that has been modified with time: Dukes' original classification of intestinal wall invasion (J Pathol 1932; 35:323) recognized only three categories: A Limited to the bowel wall, B Through the bowel wall and C Regional lymph node involvement by tumor; the most widely used permutation of the 'Dukes' is that of Astler and Coller, in which the carcinoma is divided into depth of invasion of the mucosa, muscularis propria and serosa (Ann Surg 1954; 139:846), with addition of a D (distal metastasis group, Ann Surgery 1967; 166:4290) and tallying of involved lymph nodes (N Engl J Med 1984; 310:737) Note: The TNM classification of colonic adenocarcinoma is increasingly preferred by surgical pathologists; see TNM classification

Dukes classification

Class	Depth of invasion	5-year survival
A	Limited to the mucosa	100.0%
B1	Muscularis propria, negative nodes	66.4%
B2	Penetrating muscularis propria, negative nodes	53.9%
C1	Limited to wall , positive nodes	42.8%
C2	Through wall, positive nodes	22.4%
(D)	Non-Dukes designation for distal metastases	3.0%

Dumbbell Barbell An adjectival descriptor applied to a tubular structure with terminal bulbous enlargement and central constriction

Dumbbell bones A descriptor for the shortened and terminally enlarged long bones seen in the hyperplastic metaphysis in metatropic dwarfism; the descriptor has also been applied to the end-stage of subperiosteal hemorrhages with calcification of the periosteum as may occur in resolving scurvy

Dumbbell gallbladder see Hourglass gall bladder

Dumbbell tumors A non-specific term for any of a variety of tumors, most of which are benign, all of which have a central constriction a) Carcinoid 'Iceberg' tumor A submucosal tumor located in the large bronchi, 15% of which metastasize b) Ganglioneuroma A tumor located in a vertebral body that may cause bony resorption or erosion of the pedicles c) Leiomyoma A tumor of the gastrointestinal tract with both intra- and extraluminal components d) Neurofibroma A tumor located on either side of the intervertebral foramina impinging on the spinal cord, usually thoracic with central constriction or 'pinching' of the tumor by the thick fibers of the intervertebral discs e) Paraspinal neuroblastoma A tumor with intraspinal extension that has a central constriction by the spinal ligaments f) Pleomorphic adenoma A tumor that extends through the gap between the ascending ramus of the jaw and the styloid process and stylomandibular ligament, entering the parapharyngeal space interfering with phonation, obstructing the nasal choanae and eustachian tube in the deep tissue, seen in 10% of pleomorphic adenomas

Dum-dum FORENSIC PATHOLOGY An irregularly weighted bullet that tumbles upon entry into the body, causing massive tissue destruction as it adds a rotational component to a bullet's trajectory

Dummy terminal Dumb terminal A peripheral unit connected to a mini- or mainframe computer that consists of a keyboard, a monitor and cables to allow accession of a database without the option to input data, alter the database or interact with the computer's central processing unit; see Computers; Hospital information system

Dumping Patient dumping The practice, often by private, for-profit hospitals, of transferring indigent, uninsured patients to other, usually public hospitals for economic reasons; patient-transfer guidelines and laws are generally limited to cases of 'unstable' emergencies and women in active labor (N Engl J Med 1988; 319:643); Cf 'Anti-dumping' laws

'Dumping' FORENSIC MEDICINE A term used in two contexts regarding a subject's untimely demise and disposal of a body a) Homicide Dumping is an expedient for removing the bodies of execution victim(s), often in the context of organized crime or drug wars; in New York City, favored 'dumping grounds' include the long-term parking lot of JFK International Airport and the marshes off the West Shore expressway in Staten Island, where the victims are often found in the trunk (boot) of an abandoned automobile b) Accidental death When a drug abuser overdoses and dies, his friend(s), fearing the legal consequences of acknowledging drug abuse per se, or the potential accusations of homicide, may remove (dump) the body after having first attempted resuscitation, resulting in changes to the body which themselves may mimic 'injuries' of a homicidal nature

Dumping syndrome A disease complex confusing to both those who read about it and to those who write about it, seen in about 20% of those subjected to gastric surgery, including resection, gastroenterostomy with total gastric vagotomy and gastric bypass; most inculpated in 'dumping' are pyloric ablation and bypass Clinical Diaphoresis, palpitations, colicky abdominal pain and diarrhea, due to rapid movement (dumping) of gastric contents into the small intestine **Early dumping, synonyms** Afferent loop, bilious vomiting, early postprandial postgastrectomy and small stomach syndromes A condition affecting 5-10% of those with sub-total gastrectomies, caused by the release of vasoactive substances, eg serotonin, bradykinin, glucagon Clinical Onset 20-30 minutes after meals with early satiety, upper gastric discomfort and vasomotor phenomena (flushing, diaphoresis, palpitations, tachycardia and hypotension), resolving in one hour, weakness, nausea, diarrhea, cramping and borborygmi, flatulence, aerophagia, vomiting, anemia; when prolonged malabsorption, steatorrhea, weight loss and osteomalacia may ensue Laboratory Increased glucose (worse with high carbohydrate meals), increased hematocrit and decreased blood volume, related to dehydration, decreased serum K^+ **Late dumping** A less common condition that is more polymorphous clinically; most symptoms are due to reactive postcibal hypoglycemia, as the rapid entry of glucose releases GIP (gastroactive intestinal polypeptide), inhibiting the hyperglycemic response to glucagon; spontaneous remission may occur 3-12 months after surgery Treatment, medical Decrease carbohydrate intake, smaller meals, pectin (a dietary-fiber), acarbose, anticholinergics, L-dopa and opiates Treatment, surgical 2-5% are medical failures, requiring surgical conversion to a Roux-en-Y Note: Other post-gastrectomy syndromes include the small capacity, afferent and efferent loop syndromes, bile gastritis, anemia, postvagotomy diarrhea and metabolic bone disease

Dunce mutation Uder normal circumstances fleas, eg *Drosophila melanogaster*, can be trained to avoid noxious stimuli; fleas bearing the dunce mutation cannot, due to a defective cAMP phosphodiesterase gene; the mechanism is unclear

Duodenal 'sweep' GASTROENTEROLOGY A term used by both radiologists and endoscopists that refers to the first and second segments of the duodenum as it sweeps superiorly and posteriorly past the gastric antrum

Duplication (9p) syndrome A rare condition of which about 60 cases have been reported, normal birth weight, circa 50 IQ, microcephaly, flappy ears, 'beady' eyes, bulbous nose, 'worried' look, unilateral grin, clinodactyly, long carpal bones with short metacarpal bones

Durable power of attorney An 'advance directive' document that allows patients to appoint a substitute decision maker to implement their preferences for continued life support in the event of incapacitation; see Advanced directive, Living will

Dust, nuclear Leukocytoclasis Abundant scattered basophilic granularity seen in acutely inflamed and necrotic tissue due to karyolytic nuclear debris

DVT see Deep vein thrombosis

Dwarfism Nanosomia A generic term for excessively short stature; the term 'dwarf' is less preferred than dysplasia, dysostosis, eponyms and others; 35% of nanosomia is familial, 25% is idiopathic, 10% is due to pituitary failure, 10% to hypothyroidism, 10% to congenital gonadal aplasia and the remainder due to various causes; proper classification of the more than 55 congenital conditions associated with nanosomia, allows determination of the likelihood of conceiving a second similarly afflicted child **LETHAL DWARFISM** Any form of nanosomy accompanied by premature death, including achondrogenesis, eg Fraccaro-Parenti and Houston-Harris syndromes, homozygous achondroplasia, chondrodysplasia calcificans congenita punctata, campomelic syndrome, hypophosphatasia, osteogenesis imperfecta, thanatophoric dwarfism **NONLETHAL DWARFISM** Achondroplasia, diastrophic dwarfism, fibrous dysplasia, spondyloepiphyseal dysplasia congenita, metatrophic dwarfism, chondroectodermal dysplasia (Ellis-van Crevald syndrome), asphyxiating thoracic dysplasia, Laron dwarfism, metaphyseal chondrodysplasia (cartilage-hair hypoplasia), mesomelic dwarfism (Langer and Reinhard-Pfeiffer type); see Bird-headed dwarfism (Seckel syndrome), Bird face, Cherubism, Elfin face syndrome, Leprechaunism, Progeria, 'Walt Disney' dwarf

Dwarf megakaryocyte Micromegakaryocyte A small platelet precursor with agranular cytoplasm and hyalinoplasmic zones (pseudopods), associated with large atypical platelets, often indicating abnormal megakaryopoiesis, often associated with myeloproliferative disorders, eg myelofibrosis with myeloid metaplasia

Dwarf tapeworm *Hymenolepsis nana* The only human tapeworm that has no intermediate host; it is most common in warm, dry climates; infection is by direct subject-to-subject transmission, often among children, families and in institutions; the eggs hatch in the stomach and small intestine, penetrate the villi and metamorphose into cercocysts; recalcitrant infections are maintained by autoinfection Clinical Irritability, headache, convulsions, vertigo, anorexia, abdominal pain, weight loss, nasopharyngeal and anal pruritus and intermittent diarrhea Treatment Praziquantel or niclosamide

Dyad symmetry see Palindrome

Dying-back neuropathy A pattern of neuropathy seen in 'toxic' damage to large diameter peripheral sensorimotor nerves, affecting the long axons, eg lower extremities, before the short, eg cranial nerves; the condition, also known as distal axonopathy is a generic reaction to beriberi, pontocerebellar atrophy, spastic paraplegia and thallium intoxication

Dynamin A microtubule-bundling protein

Dynein A 500 kD ATPase that forms the arms of the axoneme in cilia and flagella, which requires a divalent cation, eg Ca^{++} or Mg^{++} for its action; dynein is responsible for movement of cilia, located on the subfiber A of the ciliary microtubules; according to the 'dynein-walking' model, the dynein arms on the A subfiber of one doublet push the B subfiber on the adjacent doublet toward the tip of the axoneme; the force produced by the sliding of adjacent doublets is the result of repeated formation and breaking of the cross-bridges between the dynein arm of one doublet and the subfiber of the adjacent doublet; see Cilia

Dynorphin One of three opioid neuropeptides (endorphins) in the gastrointestinal tract (the others are met-enkephalin and leu-enkephalin), which are antisecretory, inhibiting plexus neurons, causing constipation and eating disorders in rats and possibly also in humans

Dyserythropoiesis Congenital dyserythropoietic anemia (CDA) A group of inherited conditions characterized by multinuclearity of erythroblasts, nuclear budding, karyorrhexis, mitotic abnormalities, premature extrusion of nucleus, internuclear bridging, nuclear-cytoplasmic maturational dyssynchrony, cytoplasmic vacuolization, basophilic stippling and siderotic granules Clinical Lifelong familial mild-to-moderate anemia and ineffective erythropoiesis **CDA, type I** Megaloblastosis, Cabot type Autosomal recessive condition characterized by macrocytic anemia, binuclearity, internuclear bridging, Cabot rings and anti-I antibodies **CDA, type II** HEMPAS, Degas type Autosomal recessive condition that comprises 65% of CDA characterized by normocytic anemia, bi- and multi-nuclearity of erythroblasts, pluripolar mitoses with karyorrhexis, anti-I antiantibodies; see HEMPAS **CDA, type III** Swedish or Bjoekman type Autosomal dominant condition characterized by erythroid gigantoblasts, less than 12 nuclei and macrocytic anemia '**CDA, type IV**' Inherited dyserythropoiesis that does not fall into neat categories

Dysfibrinogenemia(s) Qualitative, usually autosomal dominant fibrinogen defects, first described in 1958 that now includes 140 different families; disease severity ranges from innocuous to hemorrhagic diathesis; most are asymptomatic and detected by presurgical screens, given the abnormalities in coagulation parameters; these subjects suffer frequent spontaneous abortion, bleeding, poor wound healing, arterial and venous thromboses Laboratory Fibrin levels and clotting times are normal; increased prothrombin time, thrombin time, reptilase time Note: Each type is designated by its city of origin, followed by a Roman numeral; five cities have four types each, Baltimore-IV, London-IV, Oslo-IV, New York-IV, Paris-IV

Dysfunctional uterine bleeding (DUB) Excess menstrual hemorrhage of hormonal origin, related to 'breakthrough bleeding' or estrogen withdrawal, often occurring in anovulatory cycles; no organic genital or extra-genital cause can be found in 75% of cases, although adolescent DUB is attributed to immaturity of the hypothalamic-pituitary-ovarian axis; peri- and post-menopausal DUB often occurs in endometria that are deaf to the ovary's curtain call; DUB in the elderly requires curettage to rule out malignancy

Dysgenic gonadoma Gonadoblastoma

Dysmorphology The systemic study of structural defects of prenatal onset, a complex field in which single or multiple primary malformations are idiopathic or related to chromosome defects (recurrence rate of 2-5%), drugs, chemicals, toxins or radiation; the most common single primary defects are congenital hip dislocation, talipes equinovarus, cleft lip and/or palate, septal defects, pyloric stenosis and neural tube defects Relevant definitions **Deformation** An alteration in the shape or structure of a part that differentiates normally, but cannot develop fully due to in utero constraints, eg compression, or oligohydramnios **Disruption** Destruction of a previously normal part, either through interruption of a vascular supply or by entanglement and/or tearing of the structure (often a digit) by floating amniotic bands **Malformation** An isolated defect which, if surgical correction is possible, has an excellent prognosis Sequence An array of multiple congenital anomalies resulting from an early single primary defect of morphogenesis that unleashes a 'cascade' of secondary and tertiary defects see Multiple malformation syndrome, Sequence

Dysmyelopoietic syndromes A group of hematologic malignancies and premalignancies: Idiopathic sideroblastic anemia, Refractory anemia with excess 'blasts (RAEB), subacute and oligoblastic leukemia, chronic myelomonocytic leukemia, preleukemias, for which there is considerable overlap; most predictive of the lesion's future behavior is the presence of excess blasts in the bone marrow and circulation, neutropenia and thrombocytopenia

Dysplasia A term that signifies defective growth, used by pediatricians for the altered growth of tissues or an extremity and by pathologists for a histologic lesion that has premalignant potential PEDIATRICS The more common dysplastic syndromes include anhidrotic ectodermal dysplasia (Christ-Siemans syndrome), atridigital dysplasia (Holt-Oram syndrome), chondro-ectodermal dysplasia (Ellis-van Creveld syndrome), hidrotic ectodermal dysplsia (Clouston syndrome), metaphyseal dysplasia (Pyle's disease), oculoauriculovertebral dysplasia (Goldenhar syndrome), oculodentaldigital dysplasia (ODD syndrome), olfactogenital syndrome (Kallmann syndrome) and progressive diaphyseal dysplasia (Camurati-Engelmann syndrome) SURGICAL PATHOLOGY A histological lesion with pre-malignant portent, affecting epithelial linings, in particular squamous epithelium of the uterine cervix, oral cavity, upper respiratory tract, penis, anus and elsewhere; epithelial dysplasia may be induced by human papilloma viruses (HPV), especially types 16, 18, 31 and 33 and is similar (if not identical) to intraepithelial neoplasia, a term that has become increasingly popular among pathologists

Classification, Dysplastic nevi

Type A Sporadic dysplastic nevus without melanoma

Type B Familial dysplastic nevi without melanom

Type C Sporadic dysplastic nevi with melanoma

Type D1 Familial dysplastic nevi with 1 case of melanoma in family

Type D2 Familial dysplastic nevi with two or more melanomas in family (relative risk, 150 if the family member has dysplastic nevi or 500 if they have had a previous melanoma but no risk if he/she has no dysplastic nevi

(N Engl J Med 1986; 315:1615)

Dysplastic nevus A skin lesion that is generaly regarded as premalignant, which is characterized by irregular, greater than 5 mm in diameter macules numbering from a few to hundreds with a central papule, variegated dark color and lenticular changes Histopathology A 'motheaten' Malpighian layer with features ofdysplastic nevus superimposed on a junctional or compound nevus and 1) Basilar melanocytic hyperplasia with elongation of rete ridges 2) Cytologic atypia with enlarged hyperchromatic melanocytic nuclei 3) Spindled or epithelioid, horizontally arranged melanocytes, aggregated in variably-sized nests, fusing with adjacent rete ridges ('bridging') 4) Lamellar or concentric dermal fibroplasia and 5) Patchy or diffuse superficial dermal lymphocytosis Clinical classification (of congenital nevi): Small (< 1.5 cm diameter), medium (1.5 to 20 cm), both of which lack hair, but have homogeneous pigmentation and a smooth surface and large (> 20 cm in diameter), eg garment nevi, which have grossly irregular surface, hypertrichous and variegated pigmentation, 10% of which evolve toward malignancy; congenital nevi are either located in the lower dermis or reticular dermis, associated with appendages, nerves and vessels or appear as single or single-file cells between collagen fibrils Note: At least one authority on pigmented lesions has rejected the term 'dysplastic' nevus, as pathologists often disagree on the term dysplasia, the clinical presentation of common, dysplastic nevi and frank melanomas overlap considerably, only 10-20% of melanomas arise from preexisting neval clusters and it is thought that any melanocyte is capable of giving rise to a melanoma

Dysraphism Cinercephaly, cephalocele, spina bifida and myelodysplasia; failure to close neural tube at 4-5th fetal week

Dyssomnology The study of sleep disorders, see Sleep disorders

Dystrophic calcification The combination of fat necrosis and caseating necrosis, as seen in damaged heart valves and atherosclerotic blood vessels (arising in mitochondria), calcification in hyperparathyroidism which develops in the basement membrane of the renal tubules

Dystrophin A 400 kD protein, found in low amounts (0.002% of the total muscular protein) as an intracellular component of the transverse tubular system in normal muscle, which is markedly decreased in Duchenne's and Becker's myotonic dystrophies; dystrophin is most abundant in the neurons of the cerebral and cerebellar cortices, concentrated at post-synaptic membrane specialization; it is postulated that in Duchenne's muscular dystrophy, the role in neurons differs from that of muscle and the cognitive impairment may be due to an alteration of dystrophin at the synaptic level (Nature 1990; 348:725); dystrophin may stabilize cultured myotubes and isolated mature muscle fibers (ibid, 1991; 349:69), where it is located in the cell membrane (Nature 1991; 349:335); it is detected by immunoblotting and immunofluorescence; see Nebulin

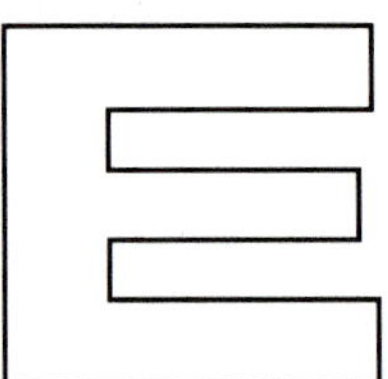

E Symbol for: Glutamic acid; redox potential

e Symbol for: Natural logarithm (2.7187818285); electron

E1a protein A 289-residue promotion and transcription activating protein required for the efficient expression of early viral, eg adenovirus genes; E1a's activating region is structurally distinct from other transcription activators and may interact directly with the cell's transcription 'machinery' (Nature 1990; 346:147)

E26 virus An avian acute leukemia virus that induces a mixed erythromyelocytic leukemia in chickens and carries two oncogenes, v-*myb* and v-*ets* that are structurally related to the human oncogene, **erg**

EAE see Experimental allergic encephalomyelitis

EAEC Enteroadherent ***Escherichia coli*** An agent causing a rare chronic diarrhea in infants with failure to thrive; EAEC serotypes implicated in Traveller's diarrhea include O55, O111, O119, O125-128, O142

Earlobe crease It had been reported that the number of creases in the earlobe correlates with the incidence of coronary artery disease; both increase with age and are probably unrelated (Ann Int Med 1987; 147:65);

Early gene VIROLOGY A gene produced by a host cell shortly after integration of a virus into the host's genome, which encodes enzymes of interest to the virus; see Late genes

'Earmarking' see 'Pork-barrel' awards

Ears Bladder ears UROLOGY Transient, bilateral extraperitoneal herniation of the bladder, occurring in a reported 10% of infants, often less than 6 months of age; bladder ears are of clinical interest, as these children may also have inguinal hernias

Eastern equine encephalitis A rare, sporadic and aggressive enzootic infection by a single-stranded RNA Toga family virus that primarily affects birds Vector The ornithophilic mosquito, ***Culiseta melanura*** is largely confined to the Northeastern US, especially Massachusetts; infection of horses and humans is an accidental 'dead-end' occurring when the virus is transmitted to other mosquitos, eg ***Aedes vexans, Aedes sollicitans*** and ***Coquillitidia perturbans***; about five human cases occur per year in the USA, carrying a 30-70% mortality and severe neurological sequelae in humans (MMWR 1989; 28:619) Clinical Presents with-meningismus, lethargy, stupor, high fever and spinal pleocytosis; Cf St Louis equine encephalitis, Western equine encephalitis

EBNA Epstein-Barr nuclear antigen

Ebola disease A hemorrhagic fever syndrome caused by an RNA virus that is similar to that of Marburg disease; the Ebola virus was first isolated in 1976 in a devastating epidemic in Zaire and Sudan Clinical Onset with gastrointestinal symptoms, arthralgias, intractable diarrhea and high mortality; infection is by direct contact rather than aerosol Treatment Interferon, Convalescent serum

Ebullism Air embolism at high altitude where the total ambient pressure is 47 mm Hg or less (> 20 000 meters); in addition to acute hypoxia, the body fluids boil/evaporate causing widespread air bubble formation in vessels and tissue; in experimental mammals at high altitudes, vaporization occurs at the entrance of the great veins into the heart, blocking venous return, which is rapidly fatal due to abrupt cardiac failure

Eburnation A marbled appearance of weight-bearing joints with complete cartilaginous erosion, leaving polished, sclerotic bone as the new articular surface; cross-section of the articulation reveals a narrowed joint space, osteosclerosis and cystic changes overlying the affected bone, which is surrounded by bony and cartilaginous overgrowths (osteophytes/exostoses)

EBV see Epstein-Barr virus

EC see Enzyme Commission

ECFMG Educational Commission for Foreign Medical Graduates An organization formed by the American Hospital Association, American Medical Association, American Board of Medical Specialties, Association of American Medical Colleges and others for the purpose of establishing standards and evaluating the qualifications of graduates of foreign medical schools

ECHO virus Enteric cytopathogenic human orphan virus A virus with 30 types, belonging to the picornavirus (small single-strand RNA) family; ECHO virus produces a characteristic cytopathic effect in cell culture Clinical Upper respiratory tract infections, exanthema, diarrhea, viremia and less commonly, viral meningitis and poliomyelitis

Echocardiography A noninvasive group of two-dimensional imaging techniques using Doppler ultrasonography that provide information on pressure differences and blood flow in the heart and great vessels; the principle common to these methods is that blood flowing to (and through) the heart produces sound, some of which is reflected back by each acoustic interface the blood encounters, ie the Doppler effect, which is received by a transducer; the time elapsed between the sound's transmission to the time that the echo is received is converted to a display; when a number of depth samples are taken in sequence, an imaging plane is created, allowing construction of a two-dimensional echocardiogram, a procedure of considerable use in evaluating pericardial and myocardial disease, ischemic and congenital heart diseases and infectious endocarditis (N Engl J Med 1990; 323:101rv, 165rv)

Eclampsia, pre-eclampsia Greek, 'to shine forth' A clinical complex most common in late pregnancy or the immediate puerperium, characterized by hypertension, albuminuria, proteinuria, hypoproteinemia, increased nitrogen (BUN), hemoconcentration and sodium retention with resultant edema Pathology Patchy, subcapsular hepatic hemorrhage, capillary fibrin deposition in the liver and glomerular tufts with placental aging and infarcts; pre-eclampsia is most common in primigravidas, after the 24th gestational week, but may occur as soon as trophoblastic tissue is present Treatment If mild, bed rest and sedation; if severe, antihypertensive therapy, eg vasodilators, α methyldopa; if convulsions, magnesium sulfate; see HELLP syndrome

'Eclipse' The period between the time a cell is infected by a virus and the production of intracellular viral progeny

'Eclipsed' antigen IMMUNOLOGY Any non-self antigen, eg that of a parasite, which so closely mimics the host antigen that it doesn't elicit an immune response

ECMO see Extracorporal membrane oxygenation

ECOG Eastern Cooperative Oncology Group

E coli O157:H7 see *Escherichia coli* O157:H7

Eco*RI, *Eco*RII** MOLECULAR BIOLOGY Restriction endonucleases from ***Escherichia coli that are used to cut double stranded DNA at specific sites on the DNA double strand, G*AATTC (G*CCTGG for EcoR II); EcoR I is a major 'workhorse' used in DNA analysis to cut the DNA down to size

Ecstasy see Adam

ECT see Electroconvulsive therapy

Ectoderm EMBRYOLOGY The most external layer of the embryo that gives rise to epidermis, the teeth, tongue, palate, salivary glands, anogenital region, hypophysis, nervous system and sensory organs, eg eyes, ears and nose

Ectopic hormone A hormone is considered ectopic if there is a) Biochemical or clinical evidence of abnormal endocrine function, eg increased hormone levels or an endocrine 'syndrome' b) Disappearance of the endocrine abnormality with tumor resection or persistence of the syndrome despite resection of the gland normally responsible for that hormone's production and c) Presence of hormone in greater than normal amounts and/or presence of an arteriovenous gradient of the hormone and/or hormone synthesis by the tumor in tissue culture Note: Ectopic hormone production is most common in malignancy and may cause a paraneoplastic syndrome Mechanism Unknown, possibly due to amplification of genes that are not expressed under the usual circumstances, de-repression of previously inactive genes or dysdifferentiation, ie abortive attempts towards differentiation

Ectopic pregnancy The implantation of an embryo in sites not designed to accommodate the massive vascular supply required by a growing fetus, an event that cost the US health care system an estimated $462 million in 1985, and has increased in incidence from 4.5/1000 pregnancies in 1970 to 15/1000 in 1985, and is most common in fallopian tubes scarred by gonococcal salpingitis, with a recurrence rate of 10-30%; relative risk (RR) factors (J Am Med Assoc 1988; 259:1823) for suffering an ectopic pregnancy include current intrauterine device use (RR, 13.7), prior tubal surgery (RR, 4.5), history of pelvic inflammatory disease (RR, 3.3), a history of infertility (RR, 2.6), douching and infection with ***Chlamydia trachomatis*** (J Am Med Assoc 1990; 263:3164), or douching with an infected douche solutions (J Am Med Assoc 1991; 265:2670c); hCG levels are often lower in ectopic than in intrauterine pregnancy, a fact complicating early management of ectopic pregnancy Histopathology Endometrial curettings demonstrate the 'classic' Arias-Stella phenomenon, a histologic mimic of endometrial carcinoma

Ectothrix A form of tinea capitis involving the hair shaft, which may be inflammatory or non-inflammatory; the spores surrounding the hair shaft are small (2-3 μm) and fluoresce bright green with Wood's light, as with ***Microsporum canis, M audouinii, M distortum, M ferrugineum*** or are large (5-10 μm) and do not fluoresce, as with ***Trichophyton verrucosum, T mentagrophytes, T megninii, T gallinae, M gypseum, M fulvum,*** and ***M nanum***; Cf Endothrix

EDC/EDL Expected date of confinement or labor An estimate of the 'usual' duration of pregnancy; gestational or menstrual age is estimated from the first day of the last menstrual period (ie 2 weeks before ovulation and fertilization); in general, about 280 days (40 weeks) elapse between the first day of the last menstrual period and delivery of the infant, ie 9 1/3 or 10 lunar months; obstetricians calculate gestational age; embryologists are more correct as they calculate the ovulation or fertilization age (280 days minus roughly two weeks)

Edge artifact IMMUNOPATHOLOGY Nonspecific peripheral coloration of paraffin-embedded tissue by immunoperoxidase stain, caused by tissue drying artifact

Editing see Proofreading

Edman digestion MOLECULAR BIOLOGY A technique used to determine the sequence of a protein's amino acids; a peptide of interest is treated with phenylisothiocyanate (Edman reagent), which attaches at the N-terminal residue, making the first peptide bond in the protein labile to digestion by a mild acid; the first amino acid is removed and determined by chemical means; repetition up to 20-30 amino acids can be accomplished automatically by the sequenators; see Sequencing

EDRF Endothelium-dependent relaxing factor A substance produced by endothelium, now known to be nitric oxide (Nature 1990, 346:69) that causes hyperpolarization and relaxation of arterial smooth muscle; see Myocardial infarction; see Nitric oxide

EDTA Ethylenediaminetetraacetic acid Edetic acid A chelating agent that binds divalent, eg arsenic, calcium, lead and magnesium and trivalent cations and is used to treat lead and other heavy metal intoxication; EDTA is added to specimen tubes to transport specimens in laboratory medicine for analysis in a) Chemistry, eg carcinoembryonic antigen, lead, renin b) Hematology where it is the preferred anticoagulant for blood cell counts, coagulation studies, hemoglobin electrophoresis and sedimentation rate and c) Transfusion medicine where it prevents hemolysis by inhibiting complement binding

EEC syndrome An often autosomal dominant dysplastic syndrome characterized by ectrodactyly, ectodermal dysplasia and cleft lip and/or palate, variably accompanied by attenuated, dry, poorly pigmented skin, sparse hair, eyebrows, defective skin adnexae, eg nail hypoplasia, poor dentition, syndactyly and/or 'clawing' of hands and feet, urinary tract and ocular (blepharophimosis, atretic lacrimal punctata, strabismus) anomalies, granulomatous perleche and candidiasis; see Tabby mutation

EEE see Eastern equine encephalitis

EEO Equal employment opportunity A job that is not subject to adverse exclusion based on a candidate's, race, sex, religion or national origin; theoretically, in the US, all publically-offered positions, especially in academics are based on the principle of equality of opportunity

EF-1 and **EF-2** see Elongation factors

EF13 *Vibrio hollisae*, CDC Enteric Group 42 An organism that inhabits the US Gulf coast and the Chesapeake Bay, which has been isolated from some patients with diarrhea and gastroenteritis who had eaten raw seafood

E-ferol syndrome see Vitamin E overdose

Efficiency LABORATORY MEDICINE The relative ability of a test to detect a person with a disease, while maintaining the rate of false positive results to a minimum; the efficiency of a test is defined as the number of true positives and true negatives multiplied by one hundred, divided by the sum of true positives, true negatives, false positives and false negatives

Effort syndrome see Neurasthenia

EF hand PHYSIOLOGY A secondary protein structural motif (α-helix-loop-α-helix) that is typical of sites that bind ions, eg Ca^{++}, which is derived from aspartic and glutamic acid side chains and carbonyl groups and contains six-to-eight oxygen molecules; EF hands are present in calmodulin and diacylglycerol kinase (Nature 1990; 344:345); see Recoverin

EGF see Epidermal growth factor

Egg-shaped heart 'Pumpkin' heart PEDIATRIC CARDIOLOGY A descriptor for the globoid cardiac shadow on a plain chest film of young children with transposition of the great vessels where there is a large ventricular silhouette and a small 'waist' due to the abnormal location of the aorta directly in front of the pulmonary artery, associated (by physiological necessity) with a ventricular septal defect Note: A similar radiologic finding is seen in the hypoplastic left heart syndrome, especially in the face of congestive heart failure Note: A globoid cardiac enlargement is common in children with congenitally defective hearts in congestive failure

Egg white injury 'syndrome' see Biotin deficiency syndrome

Eggshell calcification Fine peripheral rimming of calcium in the enlarged hilar and peribronchial lymph nodes, characteristic of silicosis

EHEC Enterohemorrhagic ***Escherichia coli***(s) A group of ***E coli*** serotypes (implicated are O29, O39, O145) that produce shiga-like toxins resulting in bloody inflammatory diarrhea, evoking a hemolytic uremic syndrome; see Escherichia coli O157:H7

Ehrlichiosis A rare tick-borne infection of humans caused by ***Ehrlichia canis***, that usually affects dogs Clinical Fever, chills, rigors, malaise, nausea, myalgia, anorexia, acute respiratory failure with infiltrates, acute renal failure with increased creatinine and encephalopathy Laboratory Leukopenia, thrombocytopenia, increased transaminases Treatment Chloramphenicol, tetracycline (J Am Med Assoc 1990; 264:2251)

EHS tumor Engelbreth-Holm-Swarm tumor A tumor of experimental rodents that prolifically produces basement membrane material, serving as a source for laminin, fibronectin and proteoglycans

EIA Enzyme immunoassay see ELISA, EMIT

EIA see Exercise induced anaphylaxis

Eicosanoid A 20-carbon, cyclic fatty acid derived from arachidonic acid, synthesized from membrane phospholipids; eicosanoids and other arachidonic acid metabolites, eg HETE, HPETE, leukotrienes, prostaglandins and thromboxanes are site-specific, increased during shock and after injury, and have diverse functions, including bronchoconstriction, bronchodilation, vasodilation and vasoconstriction

EIEC Enteroinvasive ***Escherichia coli*** A group of relatively uncommon ***E coli*** serotypes, including O28ac, O29, O42, O112a and others that produce a Shiga-like toxin Clinical Inflammatory dysentery

eIF-4F A specific initiation factor mediating the activity of the 5' cap structure (m7GpppX), located on eukaryotic mRNA, required for efficient translation; one of eIF-4F's subunits, eIF-4E, is present in limiting amounts and is regulated by phosphorylation; decreased eIF-4E phosphorylation results in decreased DNA translation; overexpression of eIF-4E in some tumor cell lines may evoke tumor transformation (Nature 1990; 345:544)

Einstein sign EMERGENCY MEDICINE A ruptured aortic aneurysm mimicking biliary colic; Albert Einstein was admitted to a New Jersey hospital in 1955 with a diagnosis of acute cholecystitis, despite a 10-year history of aortic aneurysm and pulsations typical of impending rupture; he died three days later (N Engl J Med 1984; 310:1538c)

Ejection click A cardiac sound heard in early systole, related to cardiac dilatation or hypertension in the aorta and pulmonary artery; ejection clicks may be so close to the first heart sound that they simulate a splitting thereof; aortic clicks are constant and best appreciated at the left lower sternal border, occurring in aortic dilatation (aortic stenosis, Fallot's tetralogy, truncus arteriosus); pulmonary ejection clicks occur with pulmonary stenosis, are best heard at the left midsternum and disappear with inspiration; a midsystolic ejection click heard at the apex, preceding a late systolic murmur is suggestive of mitral valve prolapse

Ejection fraction CARDIOLOGY The volume of blood in the

ventricles that is effectively propulsed forward during systole; the ejection fraction is measured dynamically by injecting a bolus of 99mTc and is heard as a high-pitched click

ELAM-1 Endothelial leukocyte adhesion molecule An endothelial glycoprotein that mediates neutrophil adhesion; ELAM-1's primary structure has a lectin-like domain, an epidermal growth factor-like domain, 6 tandem-repeated motifs and amino acid homology shared by complement-regulating proteins; ELAM-1's production is induced by interleukin-1, tumor necrosis factor and substance P and is immune-regulatory, recruiting neutrophils to sites of inflammation, mediating cell adhesion by a carbohydrate ligand, sialyl-Lewis X (Science 1990; 250:1130) and serves as an adhesion molecule ('addressin') for skin-homing T cells, acting in addition to the VLA-4 and LFA-1 integrins (Nature 1991; 349:796, 799)

Elastin A fibrous protein similar to collagen, ie one-third of the amino acids are glycine with abundant proline, valine and arginine and is formed by cross-linking small globular subunits to the lysine residues; elastin's rubbery nature makes it well-suited for its prominence in arterial walls, vocal cords, alveolar septa and ligaments, having an amorphous wavy appearance by light microscopy; defects in the cross-linking in elastin's unique β spiral as well as increases or decreases in elastin are implicated in atherosclerosis, emphysema, Ehlers-Danlos, type V, Menke's kinky hair syndrome, pseudoxanthoma elasticum and X-linked cutis laxa

'Elderly primigravida' A woman who delivers her first child after age 35; these women are often professionals who delay childbearing to pursue a career; there is no increased risk to the pregnancy per se, although the medical risks due to increased age may cause increased pregnancy-induced complications (N Engl J Med 1990; 322:659)

Elective surgery Any surgical procedure that can be performed with advanced planning, eg cholecystectomy, hernia repair, colonic resection, coronary artery bypass, in contrast to emergency surgery that is required by trauma or impending organ rupture, eg appendicitis or rupture of an aortic aneurysm

Electra complex PSYCHIATRY The female equivalent of the Oedipus complex in which the daughter perceives the mother as a rival, while the father is the psychosexual source of nourishment; Electra of Greek mythology killed both her mother and her mother's lover in retaliation for their murder of Electra's father

Electrical alternans CARDIOLOGY Marked swings in the amplitude of the QRS complex that occur every 2 to 3 beats, caused by 'circus movement' in the myocardium, due to various causes, including tamponade, pericardial effusion, pneumopericardium, cardiac muscle dysfunction and paroxysmal supraventricular tachycardia

Electrocerebral inactivity see Brain death

Electroconvulsive therapy (ECT) Electroshock PSYCHIATRY Iatrogenic induction of generalized tonic-clonic seizures, a technique formulated in the 1930s by the Hungarian psychiatrist Meduna, who observed that some schizophrenic patients improved after insulin-induced comas Method Succinylcholine is used during anesthesia to attenuate seizure activity, utilizing a sine wave shock pattern or a brief pulse; 5-10 sessions are often sufficient for treating depression (85-95% of cases of severe depression are effectively ameliorated), bipolar disease, manic type, schizo-affective disorders or catatonic schizophrenia; chronic disease requires longer therapy; why ECT works is unclear, although evidence points to an answer from neurochemistry, neuroendocrinology and neurophysiology; contraindications are few, although patients with intracranial masses, tumors, hematomas and evolving strokes respond poorly, due to the transient breakdown in the blood brain barrier and the increased intracranial pressure; the relation of long-term ECT to cerebral atrophy remains unresolved; an uncommon and feared complication is ECT psychosis, which is characterized by loss of memory, attenuation of affect and hallucinations

Electroimmunodiffusion see Rocket electrophoresis

Electrolyte/fluid balance panel A group of assays used to detect and diagnose, in the most cost-efficient way possible, the most common imbalances of electrolytes and fluid, including measurement of sodium, potassium, chloride, pH, PCO_2, CO_2 content, osmolality in the plasma and urine and BUN; see Organ panel

Electromagnetic field (EMF) PUBLIC HEALTH An invisible field of electromagnetic radiation of the spectrum of energetic particles that move as quanta (radiowaves, infrared, visible light, ultraviolet and γ radiation); EMFs are generated by moving electrical charges that propagate outward from any object carrying electrical current and result from an electric field that pushes or pulls charged particles or ions in the direction of the field; electric fields are stopped by most objects from skin to concrete having a strength of 1 mV/m^2 (similar to the strength of cells' intrinsic electrical activity; the second component of EMF is a magnetic field that acts on moving particles, pushing them perpendicularly to their direction of motion, passing through most matter without losing strength; the actual power generated by a magnetic field is a few milligauss (1% of the strength of the earth's magnetic field); tumor cells exposed in vitro to extremely low electromagnetic fields (ELF) of 60 Hz electomagnetic radiation from electrical distribution systems (powerlines, video display terminals, household appliances) have increased mitotic activity; some reports have suggested that ELF radiation may be associated with a 1.5-2.5-fold increase in leukemia, lymphoma and intracranial malignancy, especially in children living close to either 765 kV power lines or 15 kV distribution lines (US Environmental Protection Agency, 1990, Science 1990; 249:1096n&v; 250:23n&v) Note: ELF increases ornithine decarboxylase activity or cell membrane resistance to spontaneous lysis

Electromechanical dissociation CARDIOLOGY Mechanical failure with adequate, albeit occasionally bizarre electrical activity; while the pathogenesis is unknown, pump failure may be due to depletion of high-energy phosphates, acidosis and cytoplasmic accumulation of calcium; two-thirds of sudden cardiac deaths are attributed to electromechanical dissociation (Circulation 1981; 64:18)

Electron capture NUCLEAR MEDICINE A type of radioactive decay; the radioisotope captures an inner shell electron, converting a proton to a neutron (decreasing the atomic number, without changing the atomic mass); a neutrino is emitted as well as (depending on the isotope's energy) either γ radiation or an Auger electron

Electronic journal publishing An 'on line' journal; the availability of the latest scientific information is close to reality; as of 1991, most of the technology exists; erasable CD-ROM devices and an electronic 'book' containing 256 megabytes of information are already available; it is probable that the first users of electronic journals will be medical libraries, responding to consolidation or 'bundling' of major and minor journals

Electronic data publishing A type of formal scientific communication in which data, eg DNA sequences by GenBank, are gathered, processed and distributed electronically, serving to complement and support printed publications; in contrast to electronic journal publishing, scientific conclusions that are supported by the data are published in the 'hard copy' or paper journal, while the data itself is published via a network-accessible database (Science 1991; 252:1273)

Electron microscopy see Microscopy, Scanning electron microscope, Scanning tunneling microscope

Electron spin resonance spectrometry (ESR) A technique for measuring the mobility of cell membrane lipids in which synthetic phospholipids containing a nitrogen group are introduced into an otherwise normal phospholipid membrane; ESR measures the energy absorbed by the unpaired electron of the nitroxide group; these studies have demonstrated that natural membranes have a low viscosity and are fluid-like; see Photobleaching (Nature 1990; 345:485)

Elemental diet A basic diet composed of oligopeptides and amino acids, disaccharides or partially hydrolyzed starch and minimal fat; these diets provide proton neutralization sufficient to maintain gastric pH above pH 3.5; in patients with severe burn injury, only 3% of patients maintained on an elemental diet had major upper gastrointestinal hemorrhage compared to 30% fed with a regular diet; commercial elemental diets include Precision, Travasorb and Vivonex (Am J Surg 1980; 140:761)

Elementary body The 300-nm extracellular and infective form of ***Chlamydia*** species, which is uniform, acidophilic, coccoid and once within the cell, perinuclear; elementary bodies attach to specific membrane receptors on the host cell and are endocytosed; after six hours in a phagosome, the elementary body reorganizes into larger (800-1000 nm) particles known as reticulate bodies

Elephant ear appearance PEDIATRIC RADIOLOGY A descriptor for flaring of the iliac wings, flattening of the acetabular roofs and ischial tapering; the iliac index, which is one-half the sum of the iliac and acetabular angles, is characteristically reduced in Down syndrome

Elephant feet invasion see Bulldozing

Elephantiasis Pachydermic cutaneous induration elicited by chronic lymphatic blockage, a clinical event that may occur in a) The legs, causing edema, chronic inflammation and eventually pachydermia, due to lymphatic plugging by microfilaria, eg ***Wuchereria bancrofti, Brugia malayi, Onchocerca volvulus***; the scrotal lymphedema may extend cranially to the renal lymphatics and rupture into the renal pelvis, causing chyluria b) The penis and scrotum due to lymphogranuloma venereum (Durand-Lefevre-Nicholas disease c) The arm, often secondary to axillary lymph node dissection in a modified radical mastectomy

Elephantiasis neuromatosa A clinical variant of von Recklinghausen's neurofibromatosis in which the lesions are deep, diffuse and massive, causing broad-based hanging of tissue filled with neurofibromas; Cf Bag of worms appearance

Elephantiasis nostra Pseudoelephantiasis A disease of temperate climates, caused by inflammation, edema or obstruction of the scrotal lymphatics, due to acquired non-filarial infections, including ***Streptococcus*** species, granuloma inguinale, lymphogranuloma venereum, syphilis and tuberculosis

Elephant man, the Joseph Merrick A 19th century Londoner who suffered from a severe deforming disease that had been diagnosed by medical historians as von Recklinghausen's disease, which was subsequently rediagnosed as Proteus syndrome, see there (Br Med J 1986; 293:683)

'Elephant policy' see Trolley car policy

Elephant skin Subcutaneous edema with redundancy of the skin and dermal thickening with elephantiasis, seen in *Onchocerca volvulus*

Elevator testicle see Migrating testicle

ELF see Electromagnetic radiation

Elfin face syndrome of Williams An idiopathic hypercalcemic disease complex, possibly associated with hypovitaminosis D, with a characteristic facies, ie small mandible, prominent maxilla, an upturned nose, depressed nasal bridge, anteverted nares, medial eyebrow flare, a 'Cupid's bow' upper lip, short palpebral fissures, carious peg teeth, as well as feeding difficulties, failure to thrive, supravalvular aortic stenosis and septal defectsClinical Angina, syncope and occasionally sudden death, onychodysplasia, mild mental retardation, classically associated with an adeptness at vacuous 'cocktail party chatter', nephrosclerosis and bony sclerosis induced by hypercalcemia; Cf Cocktail party 'syndrome'

ELISA Enzyme-linked immunosorbent assay A heterogeneous immunoenzymatic assay that approaches the sensitivity of radioimmunoassay and has the advantage of lower cost, simpler equipment, faster 'turn-around time' and none of the problems and inconvenience that is inherent in handling radioactive substances; ELISA may be used to measure virtually any antigen and antibody, although radioimmunoassay continues to be preferred in research, given its ease of performance Principle An antigen of interest is incubated in a medium containing an antibody (usually monoclonal) raised against the antigen and bound to a 'solid' phase, ie either attached to a bead or to the wall of plastic plate with multiple wells; a second incubation is carried out with a detector antibody raised against the monoclonal antibody, often with an attached indicator enzyme, eg peroxidase or alkaline phosphatase; Note: The detector antibody is linked to an enzyme, eg peroxidase; a final step is addition of a substrate that is digested by the detector's enzyme, producing a color measured by spectrophotometry; ELISA is used in the clinical laboratory to detect viral antigens including cytomegalovirus, various hepatitis A and B viral antigens and antibodies, human immunodeficiency virus' gp120, as well as *Neisseria gonorrhoeae*, choriogonadotropic hormone, thyroid-stimulating hormone and others, see ABC, EMIT, PAP

'Elisha method' Mouth-to-mouth artificial respiration

ELK Ears (nose and throat), lungs, kidneys An acronym for the organs involved in Wegener's disease; limited Wegener's disease spares the kidneys and lacks signs of systemic vasculitis, whereas generalized Wegener's disease involves the kidneys and/or has signs of systemic vasculitis; disease exacerbation is best monitored by measuring titers of anticytoplasmic antibodies by indirect immunofluorescence (Mayo Clin Proc 1989; 64:28)

Ellipse sign An oblong 'mass' seen in an upper gastrointestinal radiocontrast study corresponding to simple (non-malignant) pooling of contrast material in an ulcer base

Elliptocytosis An autosomal dominant condition, affecting up to 1:2500 of the general population, in which 15% of the erythrocytes are ovoid; hemolysis is relatively uncommon, although it may be severe in 5%

Elongation MOLECULAR BIOLOGY Any synthetic reaction which proceeds by adding one component per synthetic cycle, as in elongation of a protein chain; see Translation

Elongation factors MOLECULAR BIOLOGY Proteins that have been found in eukaryotes, eg eEF-1, eEF-2 that are similar to the TuTs complex of prokaryotes, which facilitate the binding of the amino-acyl-tRNA to ribosomes and subsequent transfer to the peptidyl-tRNA complex Note: For the growth of a peptide chain, two sites on the ribosome are required, the A site, which accommodates the incoming Amino-acyl-tRNA, holding the tRNA until the next codon has arrived and the P site, containing the Peptidyl-tRNA complex, the tRNA linked to the amino acids added to a nascent peptide chain

'Emasculated' hormone CLINICAL PHARMACOLOGY A drug designed to simulate a target hormone molecule involved in a receptor-hormonal ligand interaction, which may be partial agonists or antagonists of the target hormone; these substances include propranolol, a β-adrenergic receptor antagonist, an 'emasculated' adrenaline and cimetidine, a histamine H2-receptor antagonist, which might be regarded as an 'emasculated' histamine (Science 1989; 245:486)

EMB agar MICROBIOLOGY A bacterial growth medium containing eosin and methylene blue, as well as peptones and lactose, used as a differential growth medium for enterobacteriaceae

Embargo arrangement MEDICAL JOURNALISM An unwritten agreement between the news media (Newspapers, television, radio) and scientific and medical journals, in which 'newsworthy' stories about major therapeutic advances or diseases are not publicly disseminated until physicians or scientists receive the journal(s) and have had sufficient time to evaluate the results of the trial; once a member of the media breaks the silence, as occurred in the 'Reuters News Agency/aspirin' case (N Engl J Med 1988; 318:918ed), the rest of the media 'breaks herd', and 'stampedes' with the story; see Ingelfinger rule

EMBO European Molecular Biology Organization

Embolism The presence of extraneous material within vessels **AIR EMBOLISM** The presence of gas is of greatest importance when it is in the coronary and cerebral arteries; although difficult to quantify, 100 cc is considered sufficient to cause death; to document its presence at autopsy, the organ must be opened underwater (to detect bubbling) **AMNIOTIC FLUID EMBOLISM** An embolus containing lanugo, squames, mucus and debris which occurs when the opened maternal circulation communicates with amniotic fluids **FAT EMBOLISM** An embolic event that follows long bone fractures, and less commonly hepatic trauma; embolic fat 'metastasizes' to the lungs, causing dyspnea, shock, to the brain causing coma, to the kidneys causing lipiduria **NITROGEN EMBOLISM** An embolic event that shares certain features in common with air embolism, which is directly responsible for the 'bends' or Caisson's disease, occurring in divers who surface too rapidly, where the nitrogen 'boils' in the vessels, causing joint and abdominal pain, or if it affects the brain, may prove fatal **PARADOXICAL EMBOLUS** An embolus that migrates in the direction opposite, ie 'paradoxical', to the blood flow, a potential complication of right-to-left shunt in congenital heart disease where septic or other vegetations from the right side of heart (or from peripheral veins) pass through a patent foramen ovale to the systemic circulation

Embryoid body A histological component of a germ cell tumor containing an embryonal disk, an amniotic sac and an amniotic cavity; rare germ cell tumors with abundant embryoid bodies are known as 'polyembryoma'; occasionally, the semantically incorrect 'embryonal' body or the distinct 'glomerular' body is used interchangeably with embryoid body, which may be partially mimicked by cellular aggregates seen in the neuroectodermal tumor of infancy, Wilm's tumor or the Schiller-Duval bodies of the yolk sac tumor; see Glomeruloid body

'Embryoma' An outmoded, imprecise term implying a structure that recapitulates an undifferentiated primitive, often mesenchymal tumor; although embryoma is still used by some pathologists, the preferred term is blastoma, as in pulmonary blastoma, neuroblastoma or nephroblastoma Note: Embryoma is still an accepted term when referring to the ultra-rare parotid embryoma

EMD see Electromechanical dissociation

Emergency doctrine A guiding principle that grants permission to health care providers to perform a procedure under circumstances where it is impossible or impractical to obtain consent; this allows the surgeon to repair other potentially life-threatening situations at the same time he is performing a procedure for which there is appropriately documented consent; the emergency doctrine is a component of fully informed consent; see Informed consent; see Good Samaritan laws; Cf 'Rule of rescue'

Emergency medical service (EMS) An organized system, created by the US government in 1973 (Public law 93-154) that provides emergency care, intimately linked to the universal emergency telephone number, 911; the care is provided from vehicles, ie ambulance or helicopter, by certified and licensed personnel, eg emergency medical technicians, in restricted geographic regions; services provided by the EMS system include: Emergency medical communications, transportation, disaster plans and consumer training programs; see Air ambulance

Emergency response see Fight-or-flight response

EMIT Enzyme-multiplied immunoassay technique A proprietary immunoassay (Syva Corp, Palo Alto), consisting of a homogeneous (one phase) enzyme-labeled competitive immunoassay, used for therapeutic drug monitoring, eg antiepileptic, antiasthmatic, antineoplastic and cardioactive agents, detection of 'abuse' drugs, eg cannabinoids and cocaine metabolites and hormones, eg thyroxine

Emperipolesis Active intrusion of viable hematopoietic cells in the cytoplasm of histiocytes, a histological finding typical of sinus histiocytosis with massive lymphadenopathy, that may also be seen in histoplasmosis, rhinoscleroma and salmonellosis

'Emperor's new clothes' syndrome A facetious sobriquet for angiodysplasia of the right colon, which consists of a convoluted mesh of dilated, tortuous submucosal veins seen by the radiologist with selective mesenteric angiography, but which is invisible to both the surgeon and the pathologist, as the dilated vessels collapse upon resection (N Engl J Med 1974; 291:569, 573cpc); post-resection injection of silicon rubber into the arteries is required to visualize angiodysplasia, a disease of the elderly, which may be congenital or neoplastic or secondary to fecal impaction Note: gastric angiodysplasia causes a 'Watermelon appearance', see there

'Empty calorie' CLINICAL NUTRITION A unit of food-derived energy, usually in the form of carbohydrates, which is essentially devoid of nutritive value, ie lacking protein, vitamins, dietary fibers; empty calories are typical of 'junk' or snack foods, including potato chips (potato crisps), pastries, cakes and soft drinks; see Cafeteria diet, Couch potato, Junk food

Empty scrotum syndrome Functional prepubertal castrate syndrome Bilateral absence of functional testicular tissue in a genotypically and phenotypically normal male; the absence of muellerian-derived tissue implies that functional testicular tissue was present in the fetus, which was followed by prepubertal atrophy Clinical Eunuchoid habitus, delayed puberty, but in marked contrast to true eunuchs, subjects with this syndrome are short in stature Treatment Androgen to induce secondary sex characteristics and a penile prosthesis

Empty sella syndrome NEURORADIOLOGY The finding of a moderately enlarged sella turcica that may not translate into clinical findings, caused by a partial or complete absence of the sellar diaphragma, most commonly seen in obese, middle-aged women; the compression of the hypophysis against the floor and posterior wall by the extended suprasellar cisterns in not invariably accompanied by pituitary hypofunction, although thyroid-stimulating hormone, gonadotropin and prolactin levels may be diminished and/or accompanied by diabetes insipidus; Primary empty sella syndrome is due to chronically elevated intracranial pressure or secondary to regional surgery or irradiation Clinical The patients may complain of vague headaches, systemic hypertension, pseudotumor cerebri and if secondary, cerebrospinal fluid rhinorrhea, but is most often asymptomatic

EMS see Emergency medical service

ENA see Extractable nuclear antigens

Enalapril An angiotensin-converting enzyme inhibitor with vasodilating activity that improves hemodynamic indexes and the symptoms of congestive heart failure, resulting in reduced mortality and hospitalization in patients with low ejection fraction; added benefit may result in regimens that include hydralazine-isosorbide dinitrate (N Engl J Med 1991; 325:293, 303)

en bloc French, entirety Surgical en bloc resection is performed in certain malignancies with the hope of removing the entire primary lesion, the contiguous draining lymph nodes and everything lying between, as in a modified radical mastectomy; in necropsies, en bloc refers to complete evisceration of the thoraco-abdominal cavity

Encainide MJ 9067 An analog of lysergic acid with antiarrhythmic activity, which with flecainide, was entered in the CAST (Cardiac Arrhythmia Suppression Trial) study evaluating the effect of such agents in patients with asymptomatic or mildly symptomatic arrhythmia; the treated group mortality had a 3.5-fold greater incidence of death with arrhythmia than with the placebo-treated group; encainide is not thought to be an appropriate prophylactic agent for arrhythmia (N Engl J Med 1991; 324:781); Cf CAST, Flecainide

Encode MOLECULAR BIOLOGY The process of reading a message from a segment of DNA nucleotides, transcribing that message into code for a messenger RNA from a structural gene, with the ultimate step being a mature protein

en coup de sabre see Coup de sabre appearance

Endod Soapberry plant PARASITOLOGY A plant, the dried berries of which are used in Ethiopia as a laundry detergent, which contains a group of oleanic acid glucosides known as lemmatoxin, which make endod toxic to schistosome-bearing snails (J Am Med Assoc 1991; 265:2650)

Endoderm The innermost of the embryo's primary germ layers, which gives rise to the lining of the mouth, pharynx, gastrointestinal and respiratory tracts, liver, gall bladder and pancreas

Endodermal sinus tumor Yolk sac tumor An ovarian tumor of female children and adolescents, characterized by elevated α-fetoprotein levels, a large tumor mass (average 15 cm in diameter) composed of a meshwork of cuboidal cells arranged in pseudopapillary structures that recapitulate the embryonal yolk sac Prognosis Untreated, three year survival 13%; with multidrug regimen, 50%; see Germ cell tumor

Endolymphatic stromal myosis see 'Spaghetti tumor'

Endometrioid cancer An adenocarcinoma that histologically mimics that of primary endometrial carcinoma, which occurs in a) The ovary, where it comprises 10-25% of epithelial malignancies and in 10-20% of cases is accompanied by endometriosis, a condition which may precede the tumor; the prognosis is two-fold better than that of serous or mucinous cystadenocarcinomas of the ovaries b) The prostate A histologic variant of the usual type of prostatic adenocarcinoma that has a similar clinical behavior and prognosis

Endomyocardial biopsy A biopsy of the endocardium and subjacent myocardium, a procedure used to detect inflammation, anthracycline cardiotoxicity or the rare presence of cardiac tumors (Mayo Clin Proc 1990; 65:1415); see Dallas criteria

Endomyocardial fibrosis (EMF) A restrictive cardiomyopathy that affects relatively young patients and causes the death of 15-25% of those in equatorial Africa, which is less common elsewhere; EMF is characterized by dense fibrotic thickening of the inflow tracts of both the right and left ventricles, causing tricuspid and mitral valve regurgitation, while sparing the outflow tracts, resulting in a defect in diastolic filling with intact systolic function, which often progresses decreased cardiac output and congestive heart failure Pathogenesis Uncertain, although fruits rich in serotonin (plantain) are implicated as EMF resembles the lesions of carcinoid syndrome; althernately, carnitine deficiency Treatment Surgical excision of the fibrosed area and valve replacement may be effective; Cf Fibroelastosis

Endonuclease A generic term for any of a group of hydrolytic enzymes that attack specific internal DNA and RNA oligonucleotide sequences; bacterial restriction endonucleases are major tools in molecular biology and used for hybridization and probe analysis; see ***Eco***R I, ***Hind***III

Endorphin A generic term for endogenous opioid peptides that include endorphin, leu-enkephalin, met-enkephalin and dynorphin, each of which binds to a cognate receptor; endorphin is divided into α-, β- and γ-endorphins, which have the same N-terminal amino acid sequences but are cleaved at different C-terminal sites from the precursor protein β-lipotropin; β-endorphin is linked to hypophyseal secretion and possibly also the perception of pain Note: Endorphins are providing answers to the pathogenesis of addiction disorders and the perception of pain; see Enkephalin and POMC

Endothelin A 21-residue peptide encoded by a gene on chromosome 6, derived from a 203 residue preprohormone and first isolated from aortic endothelial cells; endothelin is the most potent known vasoconstrictor, causing prolonged pressor response, stimulating aldosterone release, impairing renal hemodynamics and excretory functions and inhibiting renin release; endothelin is increased in cardiogenic shock and myocardial infarction, pulmonary hypertension, major abdominal surgery, liver transplantation, uremia and hypertension and may play a role in the pathogenesis of congestive heart failure, vasospasm, vasculitis, sepsis, cyclosporine nephrotoxicity and toxemia of pregnancy (Mayo Clin Proc 1990; 65:1441); endothelin excretion is increased in patients treated with cisplatin, due to renal tubular damage (J Am Med Assoc 1991; 265:1391c); three endothelins (ET-1, ET-2 and ET-3) have been identified and are secreted by different cells; two distinct G protein-linked endothelin receptors exist, one of which is highly specific for ET-1, the other binds all three; various drug companies are targeting the therapeutic potential of an endothelin antagonist, the first of which is phospharamidon, a neutral protease inhibitor (Nature 1990; 348:673n&v) Note: The endothelin receptor cDNA has been cloned and expressed (Nature 1990; 348:730, 732)

Endothelium-derived growth factor see Nitric oxide

Endothrix see Black dot ringworm

Endotoxin 'Lipid A' A heat-stable lipopolysaccharide derived from gram-negative bacterial cell walls, which induces the release of pyrogens from neutrophils, potentially causing hemorrhagic shock and altering resistance to infection

Endowed professorship Chair An academic appointment that is supported fully or partially by the income of an endowment, which is usually awarded to an individual who is already a fully-tenured professor; see Professor; Cf 'Chair'

Endoxin Endogenous digoxin A low weight molecule, ie < 500 kD that is antigenically related to and cross-reactive with digoxin; endoxin is a physiologic inhibitor of ATPase, causing contraction of vascular smooth muscle and is increased in states of chronic volume expansion, renal failure, essential hypertension and acromegaly

End-stage renal disease (ESRD) The decompensated stage of chronic renal failure, 30% of cases are directly related to diabetes mellitus (J Am Med Assoc 1990; 263:1954) and ESRD may be seen in kidneys subjected to chronic dialysis; 27% of ESRD in the USA occurs in blacks (who have an increased incidence of diabetes mellitus, glomerulopathies and hypertension); in the US, blacks have a reduced rate of transplantation of kidneys (and other organs) and a reduced rate of survival when transplanted (N Engl J Med 1991; 324:302) Histopathology Intravascular smooth muscle proliferation, evoked by ischemia, venous thrombosis, proliferation of arterial granular cells and Bowman's epithelium

Enema see Barium enema, Colonic irrigation

Engel's phenomenon PUBLIC HEALTH '*AS INCOME FALLS, FOODS CHARACTERISTIC OF HIGHER EARNINGS DISAPPEAR UNTIL THE POOREST HAVE TO SUPPORT LIFE ON FOODS PROVIDING THE MOST CALORIES* (low protein) *FOR THE LEAST MONEY*' (J Am Med Assoc 1985; 254:3178c), a phenomenon that occurs wherever there is poverty

Engrailed A homeobox gene that was first discovered in

Drosophila melanogaster, and thought to be 600 million years old, having been found in most organisms, from worms to humans; 'engrailed' controls formation of the nervous system in all animals and segmentation in the lower animals (arthropods) but not in higher animals (annelids, vertebrates) Note: A homeobox is a gene triggering a cascade of structural and developmental changes in embryos

Engrailed protein(s) A group of homeodomain proteins that are conserved in mice and other vertebrates and which play a role in establishing muscle identity during embryogenesis and in enabling neuromuscular target recognition (Science 1990; 250:802, ibid, 1991; 251:1239)

Enhancer MOLECULAR BIOLOGY A sequence of DNA, which, regardless of orientation (either in the 3' or the 5' direction) or position (ie, up to thousands of base pairs distant from), is capable of increasing the amount of RNA produced (transcribed) in a cell

Enkephalin(s) A family of endogenous pentameric opioids that are produced in the central nervous system and gastrointestinal tract, first isolated in 1975, which share amino acid homology with each other, having in common the first 4 amino acids (H-Tyr-Gly-Gly-Phe-); see Endorphin, POMC

Enkephalinase see CD10

Enolase A 90 kD neuroendocrine enzyme that catalyzes the formation of high-energy phosphoenolpyruvic acid during glycolysis, which is composed of dimeric combinations of α, β and γ chains, yielding five isoenzymes; see Neuron-specific enolase

en plaque A generic term for a flattened lesion that is often whitish and fibrous in consistency, which is located on an organ's surface, as in 'en plaque' meningioma, 'en plaque' mesothelioma and so on; since the term is a descriptor of gross morphology that may not correlate with histological findings, when used alone it is non-specific and of little diagnostic utility

Enriched food A comestible to which various nutrients, eg vitamins and minerals, have been added to compensate for those essential nutrients removed by the rigors of refinement; see Fortified food, Refined food

ENT Ears, nose and throat An American colloquialism for the surgical specialty, otorhinolaryngology

Enteritis necroticans see Pigbel

Enteroclysis A small bowel radiocontrast study, administered as an enema, which specifically studies the post-duodenal small intestine, requires greater interpretive skills and increased radiation exposure without improving the diagnostic yield

Enthesopathy Inflammation at the enthesis (zone of a ligament's insertion into the bone), seen in certain rheumatic diseases, typically, HLA-B27-linked ankylosing spondylitis Treatment Non-steroid anti-inflammatory drugs

Entrapment syndromes A group of neuromuscular disorders caused by anatomic restriction or compression of peripheral nerve(s) Clinical Pain, especially at night, paresthesia, muscle weakness which if not relieved, evolves into atrophy of the innervated muscle group; the most common of the entrapment syndromes is that affecting the carpal tunnel; others include the obturator canal and tarsal tunnel syndromes

Envelope appearance see Sealed envelope appearance

env A retroviral gene that encodes envelope glycoprotein, ENV; see HIV-1, HTLV(s), Retrovirus

Environmental hypersensitivity Environmental illness Total allergy syndrome Immune dysregulation syndrome A polysymptomatic condition believed by 'clinical ecologists' to result from immune dysregulation induced by common foods, allergens and chemicals, resulting in various physical and mental disorders; the medical community has remained largely sceptical of the existence of this 'disease', given the plethora of symptoms attributed to environmental illness, the lack of reproducible laboratory abnormalities and the use of unproven therapies to treat the condition; the incidence of psychiatric disorders, eg depression, anxiety and somatization is 2.5-fold greater in those with environmental illness (J Am Med Assoc 1990; 264:3166); see Clinical ecologist, Candidiasis hypersensitivity syndrome

Enviromental protection agency (EPA) A US federal agency created to facilitate coordinated and effective government action on the part of the environment; the EPA's current priorities include health risk assessment, air pollution, both 'criteria' type, eg smog and particulate and 'toxic' type, eg benzene, drinking water contamination, indoor air pollution, occupational exposure to chemicals, pesticide exposure, radon, ecological risks, global climate change, habitat alteration, ozone depletion, species extinction and loss of biodiversity (Science 1990; 249:616n&v); see Superfund, Toxic dump; Cf Bitterfeld, OSHA

Environmental terrorism Deliberate and wanton destruction of natural resources and the environment to serve a political or military end; the term was coined during the '100-hour war', in which Iraqi forces a) Caused the largest oil spill on record, jeopardizing water-desalination facilities and b) Used high-explosives to ignite 600 or more oil wells in Kuwait, which released major amounts of sulfur dioxide and partially combusted hydrocarbons (Nature 1991; 350:11c), and required nearly nine months to extinguish; see Greenhouse effect

Enzyme Commission A body of the International Union of

ENZYMES MAJOR CLASSES

EC 1 Oxidoreductase Catalyzes oxidation/reduction reactions

EC 2 Transferase Catalyzes the transfer of one molecular species to another

EC 3 Hydrolase Catalyzes hydrolytic cleavage

EC 4 Lyase Catalyzes the removal or addition of a group to a double bond, or other cleavages involving electron rearrangement

EC 5 Isomerase Catalyzes intramolecular rearrangement

EC 6 Ligase Catalyzes a reaction that joins two molecules

Biochemistry (IUB) that periodically convenes and makes recommendations on classification and nomenclature of enzymes and definitions of units; natural enzymes are designated 'EC' followed by four digits, separated by periods that serves to classify an enzyme according to main division (table), subclass, sub-subclass and serial number within the sub-subclass eg EC 3.1.21-31.X, an enzyme that corresponds to a family of hydrolases

Enzyme induction The stimulation of the increased production of an enzyme by a drug or other compound, a process in which the inducing substance combines with the repressor, preventing its continued blockage of the gene by its operator

Enzyme-linked immunosorbent assay see ELISA

Enzyme-multiplied immunoassay technique see EMIT/TM

Enzyme replacement therapy A generic term for any therapeutic modality in which a congenitally defective or absent enzyme is administered, either a) Directly, by coupling the enzyme to a carrier molecule or by organ transplantation or b) Indirectly, by introducing the gene into the recipient; see Adenosine deaminase deficiency

Enzyme therapy A generic term for a therapeutic modality in which an enzyme that is present in adequate amounts under normal conditions, is supplemented with a related or identical enzyme to perform a specific task, eg rapid lysis of blood clots in evolving myocardial infarction by streptokinase, tissue plasminogen activator or urokinase

EOE Equal opportunity employer, see EEO

Eosinophilic fasciitis of Shulman A disorder with sclerodermoid changes in the trunk and extremities, peripheral eosinophilia and hyperγglobulinemia **Histopathology** Inflammation of the skin, subcutaneous tissue, fascia, and muscle, reflective of the length of clinical disease **Treatment** Corticosteroids

Eosinophilic major ('basic') basement membrane protein An abundant 14 kD arginine residue-rich protein that is a major cationic (from whence, 'basic') constitutent of eosinophils, which, while devoid of enzymatic activity, displays non-specific toxicity to helminths, tumor and 'tagged' host cells

Eosinophilic-myalgia syndrome (EMS) An 'epidemic' intoxication that occurred in North America, and which has been attributed by some workers to a form of L-tryptophan; this essential amino acid is ingested in adequate amounts in the diet, but it is believed by some to be of use in treating insomnia, neurasthenia and premenstrual syndrome, and thus may be self-administered by 'health advocates'; tryptophan's subsequent metabolism to serotonin, gave rise to some claims that it could ameliorate obsessive-compulsive disorders and depression **Epidemiology** 1500 cases of EMS were described in 1990 in subjects who had allegedly ingested this particular form of L-trytophan; EMS was linked to a new strain of *Bacillus amyloliquefaciens* used to produce high-dose tryptophan, while reducing the amount of powdered charcoal used in purification (N Engl J Med 1990; 323:357); interleukin-5 was implicated in the tissue injury by altering the blood eosinophilia (Proc Natl Acad Sci 1990; 87:8647) **Clinical** Myalgia, myopathy, arthralgia, alopecia, angioedema, dermatoglyphism, morbilliform rash, sclerodermoid lesions, oral ulcers, restrictive lung disease, dyspnea, fever, lymphadenopathy and edema of the extremities **Laboratory** Eosinophilia greater than 1 x 10^9/L (US: > 1000/mm^3), mild increase in creatinine phosphokinase and myopathy **Histopathology** Sclerosing dermatopathy, arteriolitis (N Engl J Med 1990; 322:869); the most responsible agent was determined to be an altered amino acid, DTAA (di-tryptophan aminal acetaldehyde) a contaminant that was introduced in the manufacturing process of tryptophan (Nature 1991;349:5n); see 'peak E'; Cf Eosinophilic fasciitis; see also, Ann Int Med 1990; 112:85; high-dose L-tryptophan was recalled by the FDA in April 1990

EPA 1) Eicosapentaenoic acid, see Omega-3 fatty acids 2) see Environmental Protection Agency

EPEC Enteropathic ***Escherichia coli*** An agent causing epidemic diarrhea Note: the serotype system is based on the Kaufman-White O, H and K antigen system, of the 140 O serotypes of ***E coli***, 055, 0111, 0119 are most often associated with EPEC, a more often sporadic than epidemic condition **Treatment** Symptomatic; see EAEC, EHEC, EIEC

Ephelis Freckle The most common pigmented lesion of young light-skinned Caucasians, often of Celtic stock, consisting in light brown 1-10 mm macules that fade in winter and become accentuated in summer Pathology The melanocytes are normal in number but contain hyperplastic and elongated melanosomes

Epibolin see Vitronectin

Epidemiologic necropsy EPIDEMIOLOGY A method for studying the incidence of a morbid condition in a population that is designed to minimize the bias introduced by selection for autopsy (necropsy); criteria for eliminating the selection bias include a) Exclusion of patients who did not die in the hospital b) Standardization of the population being autopsied and the population being compared and c) Reduction of the clinical selection bias (J Am Med Assoc 1991; 265:2085)

EPIDEMIOLOGY The study of factors that influence the health and disease of populations rather than individuals; 'types' of epidemiology **ANALYTIC EPIDEMIOLOGY** Causative epidemiology The study of diseases distributed in a seemingly non-random fashion, attempting to identify factors in the disease-bearing population A that differ from the non-diseased population B; analytic epidemiology is divided into cross-sectional, prospective and retrospective forms **CASE-CONTROL EPIDEMIOLOGY** see Retrospective epidemiology **CLINICAL EPIDEMIOLOGY** A decision-making process applied by an individual practicing physician, where decisions are based on the likelihood of a patient having disease process X or Y, given a patient's age, previous state of health, family history, the season, the previous appearance of similar diseases in the community and other parameters **CROSS-SECTIONAL** Study of 'slices' of the population and disease prevalence in each over time **DESCRIPTIVE EPIDEMIOLOGY** An epidemiological study that tabulates the incidence of various types of disease process, providing details on mortality, morbidity, demographics and other relevant information **EXPERIMENTAL EPIDEMIOLOGY** Clinical trials in which a preventive or therapeutic measure is compared to the usual negative control population in order to determine or compare response rates **PROSPECTIVE EPIDEMIOLOGY** A study over time of a cohort of individuals having a feature of clinical or other interest, eg hypertension, exposure to an environmental toxin and so on; this population is compared in a parallel population of individuals presumed not to be exposed to the same factor **RETROSPECTIVE EPIDEMIOLOGY** Case-control study An epidemiological study that begins with a disease process in a population and searches for differences in exposures or features of that population which might have put it at risk for the disease in question

Epidemiology intelligence service A branch of the Centers for Disease Control (CDC) that was founded in 1951 to: a) Train field epidemiologists b) Assist the CDC in preventing and controlling communicable diseases and c) Provide public health services to state and local heath departments, thereby improving national (USA) disease surveillance; see CDC

Epidermal growth factor (EGF) A 53-residue trisulfated polypeptide of the tyrosine kinase family of growth stimulators, related to the ***erb*** oncogene that acts on the membrane receptor; EGF serum levels are 0.016 nmol/L (US: 100 pg/ml); EGF stimulates the mitogenic response, increasing transportation, phosphatidyl inositol turnover, bulk endocytosis, ruffling of the plasma membrane, glycolysis, activity of ornithine decarboxylase, synthesis of DNA, RNA, proteins, macromolecules; S Cohen shared the 1986 Nobel prize for his work on EGF with R Montalcini-Levi who worked on neuronal growth factor Note: EGF accelerates wound healing (N Engl J Med 1989; 321:76) and is found in abundance in rodent saliva; the phrase 'licking of one's wounds' thus becomes a logical activity after trauma (ibid, 1990; 322:134c)

Epidermal growth factor-like domain Calcium 'two finger' domain A calcium-binding polypeptide motif present within epidermal growth factor-like domains of various proteins including coagulation factors IX and X, which contains a consensus region, Asp/Asn, Asp/Asn, Asp*/Asn*, Tyr/Phe (the asterisk denotes β-hydroxylated residues), that is critical to ligand binding (Nature 1991; 351:164)

Epidermal growth factor receptor (EGFR) A 400 amino acid protein having significant amino acid homology with the low-density lipoprotein receptor and coagulation factors, which is present in carcinomas, cornea, fibroblasts, glia, neurons, T cells, vascular endothelium, liver and placenta; measurement of EGFR may be useful in prognosticating malignancy, as breast cancer is more aggressive in EGFR-positive than EGFR-negative patients (Cancer Cells 1989; 7:353)

Epidermoid pearl see Squamous pearl

Epigenetic defects Alterations that are present at certain sites or epigenetic 'switch regions' along the DNA molecule that control gene expression in higher organisms; a gene's expression is related to the pattern of cytosine nucleotide methylation and may be altered when the DNA is damaged, resulting in defective gene expression, related to oncogenesis and aging; demethylation defects may be repaired by recombination during meiosis or transmitted to the offspring Note: Methyl groups act as recognition sites for regulatory proteins; see CpG Island, Methylation

Epithelial collarette A rim of crusted epidermis partially or completely surrounding the raised, red, pedunculated nodule in pyoderma gangrenosum; Cf Ball in claw appearance

Epithelioid Latin, like epithelial An adjective applied to cells, in particular histiocytes, whose morphology mimics large epithelial cells; epithelioid histiocytes are negative by immunoperoxidase stains for cytokeratin, a marker for epithelial differentiation and positive for the Mac-387 antigen, a histicyte marker

Epithelioid angiomatosis see Bacillary angiomatosis

Epithelioid granuloma A granuloma in which multiple histiocytes fuse into giant cells in a background of mononucleated histiocytes and chronic inflammatory cells; the granuloma may be accompanied by caseating necrosis, as in tuberculosis, or may be 'naked' as in sarcoidosis; granulomas occur in a) Non-malignant conditions including angioimmunoblastic lymphadenopathy, cat scratch disease, histiocytosis X, sarcoidosis, sinus histiocytosis, atypical lupus erythematosus, toxoplasmosis, tuberculosis and b) Malignant conditions including Hodgkin's disease and Lennert's lymphoma (diffuse lymphoma with high content of epithelioid histiocytes)

Epithelioid hemangioendothelioma A tumor of medium-to-large veins, composed of plump-to-spindled endothelial cells that bulge into vascular spaces in a tombstone-like fashion; these tumors are thought to have 'borderline' aggression, where one-third develop local recurrences, but only rarely metastasize; it is unclear whether the epithelioid hemangioendothelioma is truly neoplastic or an exuberant tissue reaction, nor is it clear if this is equivalent to Kimura's disease

Epithelioid sarcoma A low-grade, albeit treatable soft tissue sarcoma affecting the upper extremity of males (male:female ratio, 2:1) affecting those aged 10-35, commonly related to previous trauma **Histopathology** Central geographic necrosis, positive staining for cytokeratin, epithelial membrane antigen and vimentin **Prognosis** Recurrence is common; 45% metastasize to various sites including the lung, regional lymph nodes and scalp **Treatment** Adequate local excision or amputation **Differential diagnosis** includes benign lesions, eg fibromatosis, fibrous histiocytoma, nodular fasciitis, infectious granuloma, necrobiosis lipoidica, rheumatoid nodule and malignant lesions, eg synovial sarcoma, fibrosarcoma, malignant melanoma

Epitope IMMUNOLOGY Any site on a molecule (an antigenic determinant) that is capable of eliciting antibody formation; the minimum size of a molecule capable of evoking antibody formation is approximately 1 kD; if the molecule is smaller, as in haptens, it may evoke an immune response by virtue of its association with a carrier protein; large non-polymeric molecules may have many epitopes; when the van der Waals surfaces of proteins are constructed by X-ray crystallography, epitopic sites appear to require prominently exposed regions ('hills' and 'ridges') with surface rigidity; the more flexible sites being less antigenic; see Idiotype, Immunogenicity

EPO see Erythropoietin

Eponym Any syndrome, lesion, surgical procedure or clinical sign that bears the name of the author who first described the entity, or less commonly, the name of the index patient(s) in whom the lesion was first described; despite a movement toward eliminating the possessive 's for eponyms, the author prefers the 'McKusick rule' (J Am Med Assoc 1984; 252:1041), in which the 's is eliminated if it occurs in a) A hyphenated eponym, eg Blackfan-Diamond and Lesch-Nyhan syndromes b) Precedes a sibilant, eg Hodgkin cell or Cushing syndrome, which would then acquire the 's, should the eponym then modify a non-sibilant noun, as Hodgkin's disease and Cushing's disease or c) Itself ends in a sibilant, eg Wilms tumor; this rule allows retention of commonly used nomenclature without sacrifice of euphony as would occur in His and Her's diseases Note: Other spoken languages resolve the possessive dilemma more gracefully, with 'da', 'de' and 'di' in the Romance languages, 'no' in Japanese and 'sche' in German (J Am Med Assoc 1986; 255:1879c, 256:1295c); Cf Adjectival eponym, 'Autoeponym'

Epoxygenase pathway An arachidonic acid metabolic route with omega and omega-1 oxidation by cytochrome P450 microsomal enzymes with formation of EETs (epoxy-eicosatetraenoic acids), vasotonic effectors and inhibitors of platelet aggregation in experimental models, although it is unclear whether EETs are produced in humans

ε (epsilon) Symbol for: Immunoglobulin E heavy chain; molar absorptivity

Epstein-Barr immunodeficiency syndrome X-linked immunodeficiency of Duncan A variable X-linked (or autosomal recessive) condition accompanied by congenital cardiovascular and central nervous system defects associated with fatal infectious mononucleosis Immunology Poor response to EBV infection with bone marrow aplasia, agranulocytosis, agammaglobulinemia, poor B-cell response to antigens and mitogens, decreased natural killer cell activity, T cell subset abnormalities Cause of death Hepatitis, immune suppression and B-cell lymphomas

Epstein-Barr nuclear antigen A molecule that is the earliest indicator of Epstein-Barr virus infection, appearing in B lymphocytes before the detection of virus-directed protein is detectable within the infected cells' nuclei

Epstein-Barr virus (EBV) A DNA herpesvirus associated with aplastic anemia, Burkitt's lymphoma (usually African type), chronic fatigue syndrome (J Am Med Assoc 1988; 260:971, although the connection between EBV and the chronic fatigue syndrome is being increasingly questioned), hairy cell leukemia, histiocytic sarcoma in renal transplantation and immune compromise; EBV may facilitate development of various lymphoproliferative disorders including Hodgkin's and non-Hodgkin lymphoma, infectious mononucleosis, Izumi fever, undifferentiated nasopharyngeal carcinoma, which occurs in mainland China, and thymic carcinoma; in model systems, expression of EBV's latent membrane protein elicits cell changes similar to those seen histologically in nasopharyngeal carcinoma, representing a block in terminal differentiation

Epulis see Giant cell reparative granuloma

Equilibrium constant (K) A value (constant) that reflects the concentrations of the reactants and products of a chemical reaction when it has reached a steady state (equilibrium), which varies with the temperature and is related to the free energy in the reaction; the 'K' value of a reaction equals the mathematical product of the concentrations of the chemical reactants, each raised to a power (usually 2) equal to the coefficient of the product in the equation, divided by the product of the concentrations of the reactants, each raised to its coefficient

Equipoise Biomedical ethics A state of genuine uncertainty of the ultimate benefits or disadvantages of both therapeutic arms in a clinical trial; because the clinical investigator may become biased as a study progresses, due to the perceived benefit of one of the therapeutic regimens being evaluated, he may enroll fewer and fewer patients in the perceived less beneficial arm, due to ethical considerations, and may ultimately defeat the very purpose of the study for lack of patients in the control arm; a moral exit to this dilemma, known as 'clinical equipoise' is possible, since genuine uncertainty exists in the 'expert' medical community at large; the investigator may thus continue to enroll control patients 'blindly', despite his bias (N Engl J Med 1987; 317:141)

***erb*A, *erb*B** Oncogenes with tyrosine kinase activity that have structural homology to the avian erythroblastosis retrovirus, which encode proteins located at the cell membrane; erbB is an NH_2-terminal truncated form of epidermal growth factor receptor expressed in various malignancies, eg breast and salivary gland carcinomas; gene amplification (increased copy numbers) of the c-*erb*B-2 (HER-2/neu) gene may indicate poor prognosis in breast carcinoma due to a lower disease-free interval and lower survival rates (J Clin Oncol 1990; 8:1)

ERCP Endoscopic retrograde cholangiopancreatography A clinical procedure in which an endoscope is inserted through the ampulla of Vater with the injection of radiocontrast material to delineate the bile and pancreatic ducts; ERCP is used to detect bile stones, seen as a frank blockage of the duct(s) or findings suggestive of pancreatic adenocarcinoma, see Rat tail tapering

Erethism A clinical condition of historic interest that was most common in children caused by mercuric vapor characterized by hostility, loss of memory and self confidence; see Mad Hatter syndrome, Minamata disease, Pink disease

erg A human oncogene located on chromosome 21, first identified in a colonic tumor cell line that is closely related to the v-*myb* and v-*ets* oncogenes of the chicken E26 virus

Ergotype A T cell in the process of activation; the development of autoimmunity in animal models, eg experimental autoimmune encephalitis (EAE) can be circumvented by injecting anti-ergotype T-lymphocytes to prevent full-scale T cell activation (Science 1989; 244:820); see EAE

Erlenmeyer flask deformity A morphological descriptor for a deformity, lesion or mass that is broad-based and tapers to a relatively narrow neck, likened to the flask used in organic chemistry BONE RADIOLOGY The Erlenmeyer flask change corresponds to undertubulization of the distal femur and a loss of the usual constriction, due to ischemic necrosis; this non-specific finding may be seen in healing fractures, rickets, scurvy, cystic fibrosis, extra- and intrahepatic biliary atresia, enchondromatosis, chronic lead poisoning, Gaucher's disease, adult hypophosphatasia, osteopetrosis, diffuse osteosclerosis, Pyle's disease (craniometaphyseal dysplasia or dysostosis), dysosteosclerosis, thalassemia major, von Gierke's disease GASTROENTEROLOGY The Erlenmeyer flask appearance refers to the colonic pathology seen in patients with fulminant *Entamoeba histolytica*-induced amebiasis; gross examination reveals mucosal ulcerations with a narrow neck and a flask-like broad base; the extensive submucosal lesion may be covered by a relatively intact-in-appearance mucosa; the organisms invade the crypts, spread laterally in a background of necrosis and are best seen by a diastase-resistant periodic acid Schiff stain

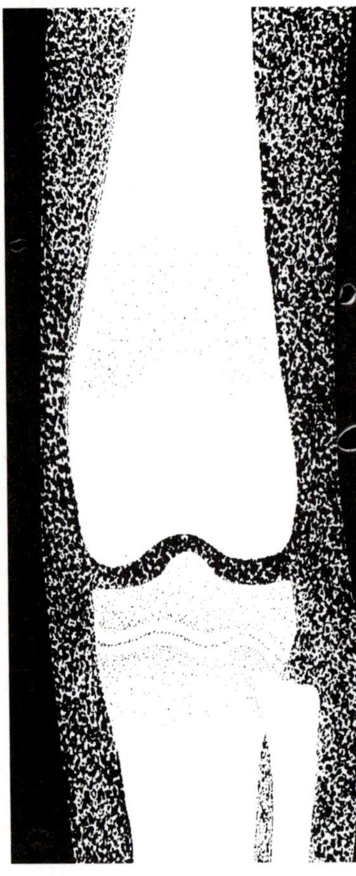

Erlenmeyer flask deformity, bone

Error LABORATORY MEDICINE An erroneous result from a patient sample, the frequency of which reflects the laboratory's quality control procedures and adherence to well-designed procedure manuals **ALLOWABLE (ANALYTICAL) ERROR** A level of systemic error that is 'acceptable', both statistically and analytically, eg 95% limit of error **PRESYSTEMIC ERROR** An error that occurs prior to the specimens' analysis, eg specimen mislabeling, operator-related inconsistencies in performing tests, different volume 'draws' into a blood collection tube, varying the concentration of anticoagulant, altering coagulation studies **RANDOM ERROR** An error that cannot be corrected, which is intrinsic to a properly designed analytical system, eg anything beyond two standard deviations of a statistical mean **SYSTEMIC ERROR** A defective statistical analysis or equipment-related problem that consistently yields erroneous results, which is detectable and correctable by quality assurance and quality control procedures MALPRACTICE see Misadventure STATISTICS see Type I error, Type II error

Error catastrophe GERONTOLOGY A theoretical explanation of the process of aging, which holds that the decline of bodily function typical of later life is due to an increased 'sloppiness' in protein synthesis, resulting in the accumulation of defective and non-functioning products that eventually prove to be incapable of maintaining normal cell function; see 'Garbage can' hypothesis

Error-prone repair see SOS repair

Erysichthon syndrome A condition characterized by overeating, insatiable hunger and indiscriminate dietary indulgence, despite repeated warnings of the dangers by cardiologists and other health care providers, eg a patient who has suffered myocardial infarction; Erysichthon of Greek mythology angered the gods who instilled in him an insatiable hunger that ultimately caused him to eat himself

Erysipelas St Anthony's fire A superficial infection of the very old or very young, caused by β-hemolytic group A streptococci, group C streptococci, staphylococci, pneumococci Clinical Abrupt onset of fever, malaise, vomiting, characteristic skin lesions with cellulitis, brawny induration, geographic discoloration and a butterfly rash on the face with minimal necrosis Laboratory Increased erythrocyte sedimentation rate, leukocytosis Treatment Rest, hot packs, penicillin Note: Erysipelas is a disease of Hippocratic antiquity; the term arrived in Middle English in 1398 with the writings of Trevisa

Erysipeloid An infection by the microaerophilic gram-positive *Erysipelothrix rhusiopathiae*, which is almost exclusive to those who occupationally handle animal products, manifested as sharply-demarcated red maculopapular lesions of the hands, which may spontaneously heal Complications Arthritis, Endocarditis

Erythroid differentiation factor see Activin

Erythromelia A clinical condition more commonly affecting older women, characterized by episodic, vasodilation-induced erythema of the acral parts, accompanied by burning pain; erythromelia may be idiopathic or secondary to hypertension, obstructive vascular disease or polycythemia Treatment Most cases respond to aspirin, methysergide or epinephrine

Erythropoietin A 46 kD glycoprotein growth factor produced predominantly by cells adjacent to the proximal renal tubules in response to signals from an oxygen-sensitive substances in the kidneys, eg heme; erythropoietin binds to receptors in erythroid precursors that mature into red cells; it is increased by hypoxia or by ectopic production from tumors, eg cerebellar hemangioblastoma, hepatoma, pheochromocytoma, uterine leiomyoma and renal cell carcinoma; it may not be increased in anemic premature infants and is decreased in secondary anemia, chronic inflammation, polycythemia vera and certain cancers (N Engl J Med 1990;

322:1689) and may be useful in myeloma-related (ibid, 322:1693) anemia; the erythropoietin gene is regulated by a carbon monoxide-inhibitable heme protein that acts as the oxygen sensor; erythropoietin production is modulated by adenosine that is increased in renal transplants and is inculpated in the erythrocytosis seen in 10-15% of these transplants; theophylline, a non-specific adenosine antagonist, attenuates both the production of erythropoietin and the erythrocytosis (N Engl J Med 1990; 323:86); recombinant erythropoietin improves the anemia and quality of life parameters, ie energy, functional abilities, sexual activity and happiness in patients on hemodialysis (J Am Med Assoc 1990; 263:825), and ameliorates zidovudine-induced anemia in AIDS patients if the endogenous eythropoietin is less than 500 U (N Engl J Med 1990; 322:1488); Erythropoietin therapy is indicated for anemia of renal failure and prematurity, and may be beneficial for increasing the number of units of autologous red cells that may be donated prior to surgery, for increasing the number of units that may be phlebotomized in patients with hemochromatosis and in increasing the units that may be drawn from a person with a rare blood type (N Engl J Med 1991; 324:1339rv)

Escalation situations PSYCHOLOGY A set of circumstances in which the individuals or organizations involved in a project tend to persist in 'failing courses of action'; escalation situations are due to variables of the project itself, as well as psychological, social and organizational variables (Science 1989; 246:216)

Escape beat CARDIOLOGY An automatic beat occurring after an interval longer than the dominant cycle length, ie a normal ventricular contraction occurring when the usual cardiac pacemaker, the sinoatrial node, defaults Note: The atrioventricular node, which has an intrinsic rhythm of 35-60 beats/min, allows a slower pacemaker to take over, thus acting as a safety mechanism; since escape beats are a defense mechanism, they should not be pharmacologically suppressed

'Escapees' Older relatives of those at risk for Huntington's disease (see there) who did not develop the disease

***Escherichia coli* 0157:H7** A shiga-like verotoxin-producing serotype of *E coli* inculpated in outbreaks of hemorrhagic diarrhea, linked to eating undercooked meat in 'fast-food' restaurants; the 0157:H7 agent is a relatively common stool isolate; of pathogens in one series in Minnesota, O157:H7 was the fourth most common isolate after, in order, *Campylobacter* species, *Salmonella* species, *Aeromonas* species and it was more common than *Yersinia* species (Mayo Clin Proc 1990; 65:787) Clinical Colicky pain, bloody diarrhea RADIOLOGY Submucosal edema and 'thumbprinting'

Escutcheon The patch of pubic hair; the normal female escutcheon is a triangle pointing downward, sharply cut off at the level of the pubic symphysis; the male escutcheon is diamond-shaped with both downward and upward angles; a male pattern in a female may indicate pathological excess of androgen or be a familial trait without significance Note: An escutcheon is a heraldic shield on which a coat of arms is depicted and in a broader sense, the shield itself

E sign see Figure 3 sign

'Eskimoma' Lymphoepithelioma-like carcinoma Malignant lymphoepithelial lesion A poorly differentiated squamous cell carcinoma admixed with non-malignant lymphoid stroma, formerly affecting the salivary glands and esophagus of Eskimo women, related to the manner in which these women prepare mukluks, ie by chewing sealskins covered by ashes (a source of lye and potential co-carcinogen (Cancer 1964; 17:1187)

Esophageal rings/webs Overhanging folds of mucosa that constrict the esophageal lumen, causing dysphagia; the upper esophageal constriction is known as a web, the lower esophageal constriction is a ring Treatment Surgery is usually neither indicated nor successful

Esperamicin see Calicheamicin

Espundia Mucocutaneous leishmaniasis caused by *L braziliensis*, a natural infection of large rodents that may be transmitted to humans by the sandfly, causing severe ulcerating lesions of the nasal cavities, see Tapir nose, with scarring and secondary bacterial infections, accompanied by fever, anemia and weight loss; in advanced cases, the prognosis is poor

ESR Erythrocyte sedimentation rate A simple laboratory test that measures the rate at which red cells in well-mixed venous blood settle to the bottom of a special test tube, which serves as a non-specific indicator of inflammation (Acta Med Scand 1921; 55:23) and is elevated in collagen vascular disease, neoplasia, pregnancy, anemia and hyperproteinemia and decreased in polycythemia, microcytosis and in sickle cell anemia

ESR see Electron spin resonance spectroscopy

ESRD see End-stage renal disease

Essential amino acids A group of eight amino acids, isoleucine, leucine, lysine, methionine, phenylalanine, threonine, tryptophan and valine that are essential for normal growth and development of humans; the absence of an essential amino acid results in a negative nitrogen balance; in premature infants, histidine, arginine and cystine are also required; see Amino acids

Essential dietary component CLINICAL NUTRITION A requirement in the diet, without which a deficiency state or syndrome will develop, including water (1-2 liters/day), calories (2000 to 3500 kcal/d) carbohydrates, fat, protein, vitamins, minerals and fiber; see Essential amino acids, Essential Fatty acids, Fiber, Trace minerals, Vitamins

Essential fatty acids Fatty acids (FAs) that humans cannot synthesize, which contain double bonds more distal than the COOH end of the 9th carbon atom; esential FAs include a) Linoleic acid (18:2 *cis*-delta 9, delta 12), which has two unsaturated carbon bonds, the first of which is attached at the methyl end to the 6th carbon (hence, n-6 or omega-6) and b) Linolenic acid (18:3 *cis*-delta 9, delta 12, delta 15)

Essential hematuria A condition that causes symptomatic episodic gross hematuria, most commonly affecting male children between age 2 and 11, often in a background of chronic glomerulopathy, 'nil' disease or Berger syndrome Prognosis Spontaneous resolution

Essential hypernatremia A disease complex characterized by increased secretion of anti-diuretic hormone

(ADH) in response to volume contraction, but lack of response of ADH to hyperosmalarity, which may be seen in sodium retention and in burn patients with central pontine myelinolysis

Essential hypertension Primary hypertension A condition comprising 95% of hypertension, which is associated with impaired endothelium-mediated vasodilation, an impairment that may play an important role in the functional abnormalities of resistance vessels (N Engl J Med 1990; 3223:22); essential hypertension requires long term drug therapy, in contrast to secondary hypertension, eg that due to unilateral renal artery stenosis (Goldblatt kidney), pheochromocytoma and primary aldosteronism, which may respond to surgery

Essential nutrient see Essential dietary component

Essential thrombocythemia A primary myeloproliferative disorder in which the platelet count is consistently > 1000 X 109/L; the condition has many clinical features of polycythemia vera, affecting the same age group, splenomegaly, similar bone marrow findings and intensity of leukocytosis; the Polycythemia Vera Study Group has delineated criteria to establish the diagnosis of essential thrombocythemia: 1) Platelets > 1 x 10^9/L (US: < 1000/mm^3) 2) Hemoglobin < 2.05 mmol/L (US < 13g/dl) 3) Iron in the marrow or if absent, little increase in hemoglobin after one-month of oraliron therapy, 4) Absent marrow fibrosis by biopsy and 5) Absence of Philadelphia chromosome

Essential thrombocytopenia A condition affecting young adults with thrombotic complications occurring in less than one-half of cases, associated with vasocclusion-induced cephalgias and erythromelalgia **Treatment** Conservative, anegrelide if symptomatic (Mayo Clin Proc 1991; 66:149)

Esthiomene A pre-antibiotic era complication of lymphogranuloma venereum with chronic vulvar ulceration and labial lymphedema

Esthesioneuroblastoma Olfactory neuroblastoma A tumor arising in the nasal cavity, retrobulbar region or the middle cranial fossa that affects those between ages 3 and 79 **Pathology** The tumor is red-gray, hemorrhagic and composed of uniform small cells arranged in Homer-Wright rosettes **Differential diagnosis** Lymphoma, plasmacytoma, embryonal rhabdomyosarcoma **Prognosis** Five-year survival 50-60%; late recurrence is common

Estrogen receptor assay (ERA) The estrogen receptor is a protein found in high concentrations in the cytoplasm of breast, uterus, hypothalamus and anterior hypophysis cells; the ER levels are measured by oncologists to determine a breast cancer patient's potential for response to hormonal manipulation (60% of breast cancers are 'estrogen positive'); one-half of ER-positive patients respond favorably to anti-estrogen (tamoxifen citrate) therapy, in contrast to less than one-third of ER-negative patients respond to tamoxifen; see 'Flare' phenomenon Note: Breast carcinoma induced by the ras oncogene is not hormonally-dependent, implying a multistep progression from benign to dysplastic to malignant **Laboratory** ER levels > 10 fmol/mg of protein are positive; the estrogen receptor levels may be quantified by biochemical means and semiquantified by immunocytochemical, immunohistochemical (Cancer Res 1989; 49:1052) methods, gel electrophoresis and protamine sulfate precipitation

Estrogen (replacement) therapy (ERT) Estrogen administered to postmenopausal women, often in the form of a vaginal cream, which ameliorates the effects of lost ovarian function, reducing the progression of osteoporosis, asserting a cardiovascular protective effect (decreased LDL-cholesterol and increased HDL-cholesterol), reducing hot flashes, urogenital symptoms, including vaginal dryness, burning, itching, dyspareunia, bleeding and skin changes as well as depression; the increased risk of endometrial cancer is partially offset by adding progestational agents to the regimen Note: By meta-analysis, ERT is associated with a 3.4-fold increased risk in women with a family history of breast cancer (J Am Med Assoc 1991; 265:1985)

État glacé A neuropathological finding characterized by cerebellar pallor with conglutination of the granular cell layer neurons, occurring without a gliotic reaction, possibly representing postmortem autolysis

État lacunaire see Lacunar state

État marbré Status marmoratus A neuropathological con-

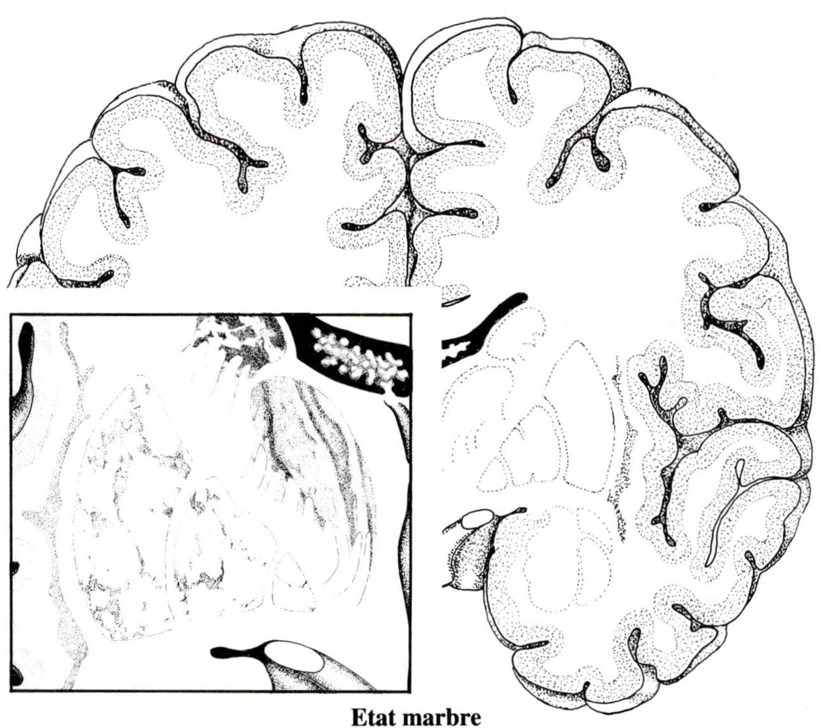

Etat marbre

dition associated with the athetoid form of cerebral palsy or Little's disease **Pathology** Hypermyelination of the striatum and basal ganglia, figure; the myelin is arranged in coarse perivascular bundles, fancifully likened to veined marble, which by light microscopy corresponds to moderate fibrillary gliosis

ETEC Enterotoxic ***Escherichia coli*** A group of ***E coli*** serotypes (implicated are O6, O8, O15, O20, O25 and others) which, like ***Vibrio cholerae*** and ***Yersinia*** species, cause secretory or 'traveller's' diarrhea, due to a 80 kD heat-labile toxin that 'locks' the adenylate cyclase into the 'on' position; other ETECs produce diarrhea by a heat-stable toxin which locks guanylate cyclase in the 'on' position, produced by serotypes O20, O27, O63 and others

ETF syndrome(s) A rare and polymorphous group of clinical conditions characterized by a defect in electron transfer flavoprotein or related enzymes, resulting in sarcosinemia, variably accompanied by mental and growth retardation and acute metabolic dysfunction, including vomiting, hepatic enlargement and hypertension

Ethanolaminosis A disease complex characterized by decreased ethanolamine kinase activity and increased phosphatidyl ethanolamine in the liver and urine, with cardiomegaly, hypotonia, cerebral dysfunction, and a gamut of clinical findings similar to type II glycogen storage disease, with death occurring by age two

Ethics committee A multidisciplinary committee in a health care facility that is composed of a broad spectrum of personnel, eg physicians, nurses, social workers, priests and others, which addresses the moral and ethical issues within the hospital, eg forming policies regarding the institution's obligations for care of the indigent, developing 'do not resuscitate' protocols and resolving on-going moral conflicts; see DNR, Institutional review board

Ethidium bromide (EB) A planar molecule that is a 'workhorse' reagent in molecular biology; EB introduces itself (intercalates) between base pairs on a 'closed' circular double-stranded DNA molecule, generating positive superhelical coils; since natural closed DNA is negatively supercoiled, the amount of ethidium bromide required to achieve zero supercoiling is a measure of the density of the DNA's original negative supercoils; since EB fluoresces in ultraviolet light, it has the added advantage that is facilitates 'tracking' of bands of DNA during gel electrophoresis; see Intercalation

Ethnomedicine Folk medicine Any of a number of 'traditional', often aboriginal, medical systems that combine the use of native plants and herbs administered by a medicine man, witch doctor, curandero or shaman who recieves his education through a long apprenticeship and who may administer the therapy by a ritual, verbally evoking the help of a deity; ethnomedicine is practiced with decreasing frequencies in cultures ravaged by 'civilization', despite the finding that a number of medications have been shown to have therapeutic value in the context of Western medicine; see Hot-cold syndrome, Shaman; Cf 'Folk' medicines

Ethylene glycol A chemical used as an antifreeze, as ink and paint solvents and in polyester manufacture; antifreeze is an inebriating and highly toxic (50-100 ml may be fatal) ethanol surrogate occasionally used by alcoholics **Mechanism of toxicity** Ethylene glycol is converted by alcohol dehydrogenase to glycolic acid (causing metabolic acidosis and the glycolate is further metabolized to oxalate (causing renal toxicity); 4-methylpyrazole inhibits alcohol dehydrogenase, forming a basis for therapy (N Engl J Med 1988; 319:97); clinical intoxication with ethylene glycol develops in three stages 1) Central nervous system symptoms, occurring within the first 24 hours 2) Cardiovascular symptoms, up to 72 hours in duration 3) Respiratory arrest and renal failure with anuria **Laboratory** Anion-gap metabolic acidosis, increased measured serum osmolality and osmolar gap, hypocalcemia; urinalysis reveals double-refractile envelope-shaped calcium oxalate dihydrate or needle-shaped calcium oxalate monohydrate crystals in the urine or proximal convoluted tubules, protein, erythrocytes and epithelial casts **Diagnosis** Gas-liquid chromatography, fluorometric, colorimetric methodologies **Treatment** Gastric lavage, emesis, charcoal and catharsis, calcium gluconate for symptomatic hypocalcemia

Ethylene oxide OCCUPATIONAL MEDICINE A gas used to sterilize medical supplies and other materials; approximately 270 000 workers in the USA are exposed to ethylene oxide, with high levels of exposure occurring in 96 000 hospital workers and 21 000 workers in commercial sterilization of medical supplies, pharmaceuticals and for spices (NIOSH data); exposed workers are at increased risk for hematopoietic malignancy (N Engl J Med 1991; 324:1402), as well as renal and gastric malignancy

Etidronate An organic biphosphonate that inhibits osteoclast-mediated bone resorption; when administered cyclically, it increases spinal bone density and decreases the incidence of new vertebral fractures in the elderly (N Engl J Med 1990; 323:73); see also Coherence therapy, Osteoporosis

EtOH Ethanol

Etoposide VP-16-213 A semisynthetic chemotherapeutic agent that derives from podophyllotoxin, extracted from the root of the American mandrake ***Podophyllum pelatatum***, which blocks cells in the late S-G2 phase of mitosis, possibly by its effect on topoisomerase (DNA degradation), inhibiting nucleoside transport and mitochondrial electron transport; it is active against monocytic leukemia, lymphoma, small cell carcinoma, testicular cancer and Kaposi sarcoma and may be administered in a combination with cyclophosphamide and doxorubicin (Cancer 1991; 67:215)

Eucalyptus oil Steam-distilled oil from ***Eucalyptus globulus***, used as an expectorant and antiseptic; an overdose of as little as 3.5 ml may be fatal **Clinical** Epigastric pain, nausea, vomiting, vertigo, ataxia, myasthenia, pallor, cyanosis, stridor, delirium, convulsions, stupor, transient coma or death

Euchromatin Nuclear chromatin that is maximally uncoiled, seen in interphase as a ground-glass clearing of the nucleoplasm

Eumelanin The pigment that is native to skin and hair, which is composed of cross-linked tyrosine polymers

Eunuchoidism A condition characterized by androgen insufficiency of pre-pubertal onset with infantile genitalia and secondary sexual characteristics, aspermia, lack of male hair pattern, high-pitched voice, infertility, lack of libido, poor muscular development, 'female' fat pattern, increased long bone growth with an arm span 4 cm > height, small testes, < 2 cm in length (normally about 4 cm); see 'Fertile' eunuch syndrome, Hypogonadotropic eunuchoidism

Euroblood Packed red cells, which in certain regions of the US comprise a significant minority (up to 30% in metropolitan New York) of the units transfused; Euroblood is in a sense, a 'waste' product, as the blood is collected for the serum, in order to purify various plasma proteins, including coagulation factors and fibrinogen

Euthanasia '*...INDUCING (DEATH OR)...PAINLESSLY PUTTING TO DEATH PERSONS SUFFERING FROM INCURABLE CONDITIONS OR DISEASES.*' On the heels of publishing a story by a Gynecology resident who 'killed' a young terminally ill woman with ovarian cancer (It's Over, Debbie, Anonymous J Am Med Assoc 1988; 259:272) and the ensuing debate about euthanasia, George Lundberg, editor of the Journal of the American Medical Association offered a classification of the types of **VOLUNTARY EUTHANASIA** PASSIVE EUTHANASIA The physician chooses not to treat a condition, eg pneumonia in a terminal cancer or Alzheimer's patient or treat the condition in a non-aggressive fashion; see Slow code SEMIPASSIVE EUTHANASIA Nutritive support is withheld in a comatose patient; see Cruzan, Nancy SEMIACTIVE EUTHANASIA A life support 'line' from a comatose patient is disconnected, see Quinlan 'ACCIDENTAL' EUTHANASIA Double effect A narcotic intended to relieve pain depresses respiration enough to cause either immediate death or secondarily induces a fatal pneumonia; see It's over, Debbie SUICIDAL EUTHANASIA Intentional overdose by alcohol or barbiturates by the terminally ill patient, facilitated by the physician who makes the lethal dose available; see Dr Death ACTIVE EUTHANASIA Administra-tion of a fatal overdose of morphine or potassium by the physician, see following; it has been suggested that in the Netherlands, 2% of the population dies by euthanasia, which is defined as the active killing of a patient by a physician at the patient's own request; to be legally acceptable by Dutch law, three conditions must be met: 1) The act must be voluntary and initiated by the patient 2) The life situation must be hopeless, where both the physician and patient recognize that recovery is impossible and 3) The decision must be corroborated by a colleague who agrees with the appropriateness of the request (J Am Med Assoc 1989; 262:3316); passive euthanasia is the foregoing of life-sustaining therapy, which corresponds to any of the first five above delineated forms of euthanasia; see Advance directive, DNR orders **INVOLUNTARY EUTHANASIA** takes several forms CRYPTEUTHANASIA Without patient consent ENCOURAGED EUTHANASIA Chronically ill are pressured into choosing death to spare their families the emotional and financial strain SURROGATE EUTHANASIA The patient is incompetent to make such a decision and DISCRIMINATORY EUTHANASIA Vulnerable groups, eg the elderly, poor, disabled and racial minorities are assisted more than others(N Engl J Med 1990; 322:1881)

Euthyroid sick syndrome LABORATORY MEDICINE A complex of deranged laboratory parameters found in patients who are critically ill with nonthyroid diseases that alter the serum levels of thyroid hormones and which in absence of the underlying nonthyroid illness would be correctly interpreted as indicative of disease of the thyroid 'axis' Laboratory Peripheral decrease or inhibition of 5'-deiodinase, the deiodination enzyme, resulting in decreased peripheral 5'-monodeiodination of thyroxine (T_4), reversed, free and total T_3; TSH, TRH and (usually) the free thyroxine levels are normal; in absence of suggestive thyroid symptomatology, thyroid function tests in sick patients may prove fruitless and not require treatment for hypothyroidism, but rather for their underlying condition, eg Anorexia nervosa, chronic obstructive pulmonary disease, fever of unknown origin, infection, malignancy, myocardial infarction and trauma

Eutrophication ENVIRONMENT The release of excess nitrogen-based nutrients into the ocean, the mouths of major rivers and into lakes, eg Lake Okeechobee, Florida, which are the result of 'run-offs' of fertilizers from farming and treated sewage products, causing massive overgrowth of vegetation and algae that consume the oxygen dissolved in the water, asphyxiating the lowest organisms in the food chain, causing major alteration of the local estuarial ecosystems and loss of higher organisms; see Nitrates, Red tide

Eve 3,4 Methylenedioxyethamphetamine; see Adam

'Event' see Misadventure

Evoked potential Electroencephalography EEG Any stimulus-evoked response potential recorded by EEG, which varies according to intensity, modality, location and level of consciousness

Evolution Any time-related change in the genetic composition of a population, described in terms of allelic frequencies that change in response to a) Mutations There are an estimated 10^{-4} mutations per gene per generation b) Selection Survival to reproductive age of the 'fittest', ie those best adapted to their environment c) Genetic drift Gene frequencies of progeny differ from their parents and d) Migration Shift of populations causes allelic 'drift'

Evolutionary clock see Molecular clock

Exchange proteins see Phospholipid-transfer proteins

Exchange plasmapheresis see Plasmapheresis

Exchange transfusion NEONATOLOGY A therapeutic procedure for reducing 'immunotoxins' in the neonate; exchange transfusion is appropriate in a) Hemolytic disease of the newborn, caused by maternal IgG antibodies against fetal antigens b) Neonatal hyperbilirubinemia, due to red cell and bilirubin metabolic defects c) Lesser indications, including, hematomas, prematurity, perinatal infection, respiratory distress syndrome, hyaline membrane disease, disseminated intravascular coagulation, marked (often iatrogenic), hypermagnesemia, adenosine deaminase deficiency with SCID, congenital idiopathic thrombocytopenic purpura, hypovolemia or anemia, cardiovascular surgery and necrotizing enterocolitis Complications Thrombocytopenia, iron-deficiency

Excimer laser Cold laser CARDIOLOGY A laser used in coronary artery angioplasty that delivers pulsating ultraviolet light to excise atherosclerotic plaques within stenosed arteries; in contrast, balloon coronary angioplasty has a 30-40% restenosis rate, while 'hot-tip' lasers (constant pulse infrared radiation) have been abandoned as there is a 20-30% incidence of vessel perforation, the 'bed' left after hot laser therapy is roughened and charred, and forms a nidus for future atherosclerotic lesions, creating a false intramural channel rather than a true lumen; in one report, 90% of patients treated with excimer lasers had reduction of the stenosis from 81% to 37%; 20% had complications in the form of restenosis that was required a conventional semi-invasive procedure, eg balloon angioplasty (Circulation 1990; 81:1849, 2018ed); Cf Percutaneous transluminal coronary angioplasty

Excision repair Cut-and-patch repair MOLECULAR BIOLOGY A mechanism by which damaged DNA is repaired, involving removal of the damaged nucleotide(s), either through nuclease-catalyzed single nucleotide base excision (short patch) or segmental excision (long patch) of the damaged region, followed by DNA synthesis with a DNA polymerase, which uses the intact DNA strand as a template, followed by joining to the intact strand with a DNA ligase; mutagens affect each pathway differently, eg methotrexate inhibits the short patch repair system (Cancer Res 1990; 50:1786)

Excision repair syndrome(s) A group of conditions characterized by a defect in the excision repair pathway, eg xeroderma pigmentosum, Cockayne syndrome and trichothiodystrophy (Nature 1991; 350:190n&v); see Brittle-hair syndrome, Xeroderma pigmentosum

Excitability proteins Membrane proteins, including membrane receptors, ion channels and ion pumps that are activated by electrical activity and are the sites of action of many therapeutic agents; these groups have been exploited therapeutically, as non-specific 'ligands' and include β-adrenergic receptor blockers, eg propranolol, an anti-hypertensive, dihydropyridine, calcium channel blockers, nifedipine for angina pectoris, GABA receptor potentiator, eg benzodiazepine for status epilepticus, dopamine receptor blockers, phenothiazine, Na+, K+-ATPase blockers and digoxin for congestive heart failure; since all drugs have undesirable side effects and the expression of these proteins varies according the tissue, it is theoretically possible to identify mRNAs specific for a target tissue, producing more specific drugs with have fewer side effects

Exclamation mark hairs Short (3 mm in length) irregularly thickened and terminally dilated hairs with tapered proximal ends, seen in alopeciaareata

Exclusion colitis see Diversion colitis

Exclusion map GENETICS A schematic representation of each of a haploid complement of chromosomes, which is formed by pooling negative data from linkages analyses for a particular disease, which allows 'unsuccessful' studies to provide useful information where a particular will not be found (J Med Genet 1990; 27:73)

'Execution' wounds FORENSIC MEDICINE Homicidal gunshot wounds intended to kill the victim, carrying the legal implication of first-degree manslaughter; in close-range executions, hand-guns are used, the entrance wound is often in the parieto-occipital region and the gun's muzzle is in direct contact with the victim's head; when the victim is mobile, other weapons are preferred by the 'executioner', eg a 'sawed-off' shotgun; the crime-scene at an 'execution' differs from that of gun-related crimes of passion and suicides; in the former, multiple erratic shots may have been fired throughout the scene or into the victim (executions tend to be more 'efficient') and the scene may show more signs of struggle and violence which crescendo into homicide; in suicides, the crime-scene is often quite neat (except for pieces of the tissue adjacent to the exit wound), the angle of the entrance wound implies complete knowledge of the act and only one fatal shot can possibly be fired; see Murder one

Executive monkey A stress-producing situation in which monkeys were forced to decide whether a nearby monkey would receive an electric shock; these primates developed stress ulcers occasionally resulting in fatal perforation (Psychosom Med 1958; 20:379) Note: Although the concept that non-human primates (which are phylogenically and physically proximous to man) should react like humans when placed in related situations, subsequent studies only weakly corroborated the original 'executive monkey' studies

Executive profile A broad battery of laboratory parameters that may be measured annually on specimens from quasi-important people, ie 'executives', in order to detect any potentially morbid condition that may require early intervention; one commercially available executive profile measures the A/G ratio, albumin, alkaline phosphatase, direct and indirect bilirubin, BUN, BUN/creatinine ratio, calcium, chloride, cholesterol (HDL-, LDL- and total), triglycerides, creatinine, glucose, iron, lactate dehydrogenase, 'liver' enzymes (alanine aminotransferase, aspartate aminotransferase, γ-glutamyl transferase), phophorous, potassium, total protein and immunoglobulins, sodium, uric acid, STS-RPR, thyroxine (T_4), urinalysis, CBC with differential count of leukocytes and platelet count; see Organ panel

Exercise Substantial literature supports the benefits of exercise; although it is heuristically logical that exercise would reduce the incidence of ischemia, poor adherence to exercise regimens, the number of subjects required to achieve statistical significance and other factors make it difficult to confirm these benefits **Carbohydrate metabolism** Exercise increases removal of glucose from the circulation by replenishing depleted glycogen in the muscles and increasing the sensitivity of insulin receptors, allowing more efficient glucose metabolism **Cardiovascular system** Exercise increases coronary artery collateralization, oxygenation of the heart, enlarges the diameter of the proximal coronaries and, in addition, decreases the myocardium oxygen demand by

Exercises: kcal consumed/hour	
Distance running (15 km/hour)	1000
Contact sports (wrestling, karate)	900
Bicycling (25 km/hour)	800
Swimming, freestyle	800
Basketball, volleyball	700
Jogging (9 km/hour)	600
Tennis	500
Coitus	450
Walking	400

decreasing the heart rate and systolic blood pressure Cancer and cardiovascular mortality (J Am Med Assoc 1989; 262:2395) Metabolic 'cost' of various activities, see table Coagulation Increased fibrinolytic activity with increased platelet factor 4, β-thromboglobulin and increased sensitivity of platelets to prostaglandin I_2 (inhibitory to ADP-induced platelet aggregation) Laboratory Med 1989; 1:29) Hypertension Exercise is more effective than drug therapy in lowering the blood pressure (J Am Med Assoc 1990; 263: 2766) Lipid profiles Increase in high density lipoprotein and decreased cholesterol are seen only when exercise occurs 75% or above the maximal heart rate (Am Heart J 1990; 119:277) Osteoporosis Exercise reduces bone mineral loss Psychology Exercise is widely thought to promote a sense of well-being, help people to cope better and be mentally healthier Note: It is difficult to separate the benefits of exercise from the lifestyles of 'healthy' people, in that those who exercise regularly tend to have a more balanced diet and, if they abuse drugs and tobacco and drink alcohol at all, do so in extreme moderation

Exercise-associated amenorrhea A finding described in female long-distance runners; in prospective studies, although menstrual irregularities occur in the form of anovulatory cycles, irregular cycles and decreased endogenous production of progesterone with shortened luteal phases, true amenorrhea does not occur (N Engl J Med 1990; 323:1221); the menstrual dysfunction may be accompanied by osteopenia, osteoporosis and hypoestrogenic amenorrhea (J Am Med Assoc 1990; 263:1665); see Running

Exercise-induced anaphylaxis A distinct form of allergy manifest by a sensation of cutaneous warmth, pruritis and secondary erythema, urticaria, hypotension and upper airway obstruction Differential diagnosis Cholinergic urticaria and anaphylaxis; see MK-571

Exfoliatin An exotoxin produced by *Staphylococcus aureus* strains that carry a group II phage

Exodus ball GYNECOLOGICAL CYTOLOGY A rounded cluster of endometrial cells (figure) seen in a vaginal from 6-10 days after menstruation, which has no pathological significance

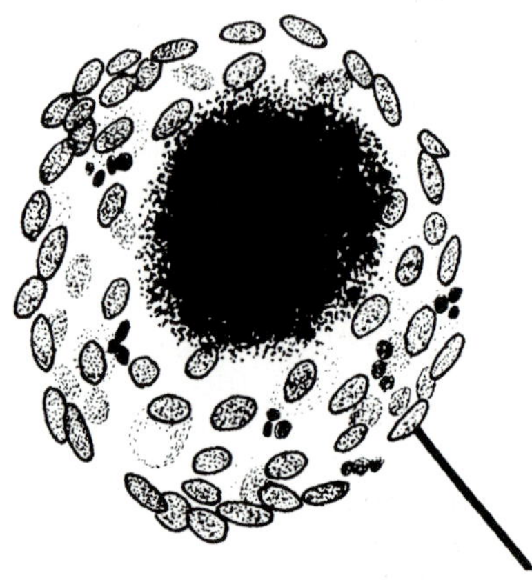

Exodus ball

Exon MOLECULAR BIOLOGY A coding sequence of DNA that is transcribed into mature mRNA and later translated into proteins; exons form functional and folding regions, domains and subdomains; introns (unused or 'junk' DNA) are spliced out DNA segments marking the turns or edges of secondary structures; the DNA contained in the 46 chromosomes is sufficient to produce approximately 3 million proteins; that there are only 30-100 000 proteins begs the question whether all of the remaining is 'junk' and how is it accounted for in the genome; the tens of thousands of proteins are derived from a finite number, possibly from 1000 to 7000 exon motifs, which have existed for about two billion years (Science 1990; 250:1377; 1342)

Exonuclease An enzyme that catalyzes the hydrolysis of the nucleotides, beginning at either the 3' end or the 5' end of the DNA molecule; 3' to 5' exonuclease activity is present in DNA polymerases I, II and III, removes mismatched nucleotides from the 3'-end of a growing strand of DNA, thus having a proof-reading or editing role; 5' to 3' exonuclease activity is present in DNA polymerase I and III and removes RNA priming molecules

Exotoxin A bacteria toxin, prototypically, *Vibrio cholera* that causes increased cAMP production by intestinal mucosal cells and increased flow of water and ions into intestinal lumen ie diarrhea Mechanism Cholera exotoxin transfers the ADP-ribose moiety from NAD to the α subunit of the Guanine-nucleotide membrane-bound (G) protein, reducing GTPase activity, leaving adenylate cyclase in the 'on' position; ***Escherichia coli*** enterotoxin, inculpated in traveler's diarrhea may act similarly; see Endotoxin, Traveler's diarrhea

Expanded rubella syndrome A complex of symptoms that may affect infants with the congenital rubella syndrome in addition to the 'classic' findings of congenital heart disease, corneal clouding, microcephaly, mental retardation and deafness; the 'expanded' symptoms include hepatosplenomegaly, thrombocytopenic purpura, intrauterine growth retardation, interstitial pneumonia, myocarditis and metaphyseal bone lesions; see Congenital rubella syndrome, TORCH

Experimental allergic encephalomyelitis An acute neurological disease of mice that is an ideal model system for studying autoimmune phenomena of the central nervous system, which are mediated by CD4+ T lymphocytes reactive against myelin basic protein, in which the immune reaction causes myelinolysis, wasting and paralysis; see Autoimmunity

'Experiments of nature' see 'Inborn errors of metabolism'; Cf Natural experiment

Expert system An artificial intelligence system that is designed to help in a particular decision-making process; the key component of such a system is a knowledge base, which combines a database of facts, beliefs and an algorithm based on heuristic logic, eg expert systems of internal medicine, CADUCEUS, INTERNIST; see Artificial intelligence, Neural networking

Expert witness see Physician expert witness

Explosive syndrome PSYCHIATRY Episodic outbursts of verbal abuse and physical violence in response to minor provocation, which occurs in organic brain disease, after cerebral trauma, related to psychiatric disease, metabolic dysfunctions, including hypoglycemia, Wilson's disease, uremia, hyperammonemia, increased androgens ('roid rage'), premenstrual syndrome, Cushing's disease; the patients are usually pleasant between outbursts and apologetic for the explosions Treatment Some patients respond to propranolol (Mayo Clin Proc 1988; 62:204)

Expression cloning A technique of molecular biology in which pools of clones from a cell line's complementary DNA (cDNA) library are transfected into another cell that is capable of expressing a protein of interest, eg the noradrenaline transporter (Nature 1991; 350:351)

Expression vector MOLECULAR BIOLOGY A vector that directs programmed protein synthesis, allowing an experimenter to utilize the bacterial genes to increase the production of mRNA synthesis to produce 'industrial' quantities of a protein of interest; expression vectors are used to synthesize hormones, eg insulin and enzymes, eg tissue plasminogen activator by the biotechnology industry

Extern A student in his third or fourth year of medical school (in North America), who attends ward rounds of a university hospital, and learns clinical medicine by example and quasi-active participation in patient management; a common complaint of externs is their common role as a gofer' (as in 'go for this...', go for that...'), performing menial 'scut' duties, and other subtle forms of psychological abuse; see Pimping; Cf Intern

External cranioplasty see Head shaping

Extended family SOCIAL MEDICINE A family composed of a core nuclear family unit of mother/father/children, and any other blood relative who lives either in the same household or closely proximous thereto, including in-laws, cousins and grandparents and provide an interactive system of moral, and often economic support; dissolution of the extended family 'unit', like the disintegration of the nuclear family, through the forces of divorces and economics, has been held responsible for loss of moral cohesion and increase in certain forms of mental illness in advanced societies; see 'Significant other'

Extended haplotypes HLA associations with allelic loci that exist in linkage disequilibrium, eg B8/DR3/SC01/GL02 is associated with membranoproliferative glomerulonephritis and A25/B18/DR2 is associated with complement C2 deficiency; extended haplotypes may be the result of crossover suppression by environmental factors in conjunction with certain HLA types, producing autoimmune phenomena, eg B-27 associated with ***Klebsiella***, DR2 associated with lepra and increased cellular immune response

External version OBSTETRICS An active intervention consisting of gentle external rotation of the fetus from the undesirable breech position to the more easily deliverable cephalic position; the potential procedure must be weighed against the danger of premature separation of the placenta, rupture of membranes or of the uterus and potential litigation; such a risk often proves too great; in the US, most breech presentations are delivered by cesarean section; see Cesarian section

Extracellular matrix A complex, self-assembling network of proteins and glycoproteins which interact with cell surfaces, consisting of two major components: interstitial stroma and basement membranes; components of the extracellular matrix, includes collagens, types IV and VII, heparan sulfate proteoglycan and glycoproteins, the most abundant of which is laminin

Extracorporeal membrane oxygenation ECMO A form of artificial oxygenation of blood, in which a cannula in the jugular vein is connected to a small reservoir, into which the blood drains by gravity; the blood is then pumped from the reservoir through a membrane oxygenator and heat exchanger and returned to the patient via the right carotid artery cannula; ECMO is considered a vital part of the surgical repair of congenital diaphragmatic hernia in infants (Surgery 1989; 106:611)

Extracorporeal shock-wave lithotripsy see Lithotripsy

Extractable nuclear antigens (ENA) A group of antibodies that react against the Sm antigen, a nonhistone nucleoprotein devoid of nucleic acid (after Smith, a propositus with the antigen) and ribonucleoprotein (RNP), an antibody now known as anti-U1 small nuclear RNP; anti-Sm antibodies are relatively specific for lupus erythematosus, RNP are common in mixed connective tissue disease, demonstrating a 'speckled' pattern of immunofluorescence

Extrinsic pathway The arm of coagulation activation that, like the intrinsic pathway converges on the common pathway, ie factor X activation; the extrinsic pathway is activatedby exposure of blood to tissue factor, circulating factor VII, Ca^{++} and phospholipid; Cf Common and Intrinsic pathway

Eye rolling Rhythmic eye movements which accompany rotation of thehead, seen in the Pelizaeus-Merzbacher form of leukodystrophy

'Eye structure' see Replication bubble

Eye teeth Colloquial for the maxillary canine teeth

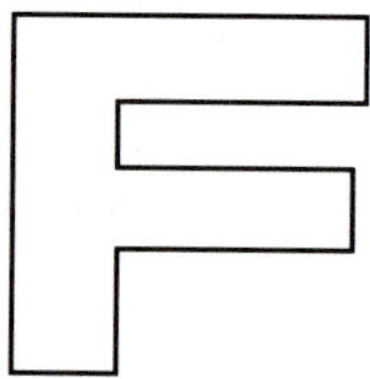

F Symbol for: degrees Fahrenheit; farad; Faraday constant; fertility factor (bacteriology); fluorine; force; fragment (of an antibody); inbreeding coefficient; phenylalanine; ratio of variances

f Symbol for: Breathing frequency (Pulmonary function testing); femto-; frequency; friction coefficient

F_1 hybrid RESEARCH The progeny that result from mating two different inbred strains of the same species; the F_1 hybrid is capable of accepting allografts from either of the inbred parents, but cannot accept an allograft from a non-self F_0 generation, since the entire complement of the MHC (major histocompatibility complex) is distinct and thus capable of evoking an immune reaction in the graft recipient

F508 see Cystic fibrosis

Fab Fragment IMMUNOLOGY The papain-digested fragment of an immunoglobulin molecule that is cleaved at the hinge region and bears the variable domains of the light and heavy chains (V_L and V_H) and the constant domain of the light chain and the first constant domain of the heavy chain (C_L and C_H1), a cleavage that occurs at residue 224 in IgG1 and near this site in the other immunoglobulins and yields two Fab fragments and an Fc fragment

F(ab')$_2$ fragment Fab" fragment A pepsin-digested fragment of the immunoglobulin molecule, which in IgG1 is cleaved between residues 234 and 233, yielding a Fab" fragment containing the heavy and light chain variable domains (V_H and V_L) and the light chain constant domains, as well as the first domain of the heavy chain's constant region (C_L and C_H1), as well as an Fc' fragment

FAB classification French American British classification for acute leukemias (table) which are divided into cells with lymphoid (ALL) or myeloid (AML) differentiation; of childhood ALL, 70% are predominantly L1, 27% are L2 and 3% (or less) are L3 or Burkitt cell type (N Engl J Med 1991; 324:800); in adults with ALL, 30% are L1, 65% are L2 and 5% are L3

Fabian Bridges An indigent male homosexual who, despite his diagnosis of AIDS, continued to have anonymous sex, nomadically migrating to various cities in the US, presumably infecting multiple others; health officials were unable to quarantine him, arrest him on any vice charges or institutionalize him on the grounds of incompetency; eventually, the gay community charitably provided him with shelter and supervision until he died (J Am Med Assoc 1987; 257:344); see High disseminator, Patient zero; Cf Typhoid Mary

Facioscapulohumeral dystrophy An autosomal dominant limb-girdle dystrophy of childhood onset and variable presentation **Clinical** The dystrophic changes begin in the face with hypomimia and pouting lips, later extending to the shoulder girdle; other disorders with a major 'limb-girdle' component include: Emery-Dreifuss dystrophy, endocrine myopathies, congenital myopathies (central core, myotubular and nemaline types), mitochondrial myopathies, polymyositis, progressive muscular atrophy, scapuloperoneal syndrome and 'slow-channel' myasthenia

FACS 1) Fellow, American College of Surgeons 2) Fluorescence-activated cell sorter A device attached to a flow cytometer that allows separation of a relatively pure population of cells by 'tagging' them with a monoclonal antibody raised against a component in the cell of interest; the monoclonal antibody and therefore the desired cell is stained with a fluorescent dye; the cells are then sent through the flow cytometer, a device that allows only one cell to pass at a time; the stained cells fluoresce and the machine's computer then sends every cell with fluorescence greater than a 'gated' cut-off level of scattered light down chute A, the remaining cells are diverted to chute B which may have defined a second parameter of interest or may be waste; see Flow cytometry

FAB classification

Acute lymphocytic leukemia (ALL)

L1	Small monotonous lymphocytes
L2	Mixed L1 and L3-type lymphocytes
L3	Large homogeneous blast cells

Acute myeloid leukemia (AML)

M1	Myeloblasts without maturation
M2	Myeloblasts with maturation(best AML prognosis)
M3	Hypergranular promyelocytic leukemia (Faggot cells) M3V variant, microgranular promyelocytic leukemia
M4	Myelomonocytic leukocytes
M5	Monocytic, subtype a) Poorly differentiated monocytic leukemia b) Well differentiated monocytic leukemia
M6	Erythroleukemia or DiGugliermo syndrome
M7	Megakaryocytic leukemia Pleomorphic undifferentiated cells with cytoplasmic blebs; myelofibrosis or increased marrow reticulin; positive for platelet peroxidase antifactor VIII

F-actin A two-stranded helical polymer of actin molecules which, with the tropomyosin-troponin regulatory complex, forms the thin filaments of skeletal muscle, see Nature 1990; 348:217)

Factitious 'diseases' PSYCHIATRY Self-produced lesions or biochemical changes produced by psychoneurotics, gratifying various self-motivated needs, including sympathy and narcotics; these conditions share the same raison d'etre, differing only in the site of injury and the agent used to produce the lesions; see Munchausen syndrome, Self-mutilation **FACTITIOUS DERMATITIS** A skin condition produced by sharp objects, thermal or chemical agents with an appearance by gross and histologic examination that reflects the damaging agent **FACTITIOUS DIARRHEA** A condition almost exclusive to women due to excessive and inappropriate use of laxatives, occurring in a) Anorexics, who are often women age 18-40 with an altered self image, for whom weight control is a central focus and laxatives are an alternative to vomiting or b) Older women, who are perimenopausal and emphatically deny the abuse, where the motives for laxative abuse are complex and may be related to secondary gain of attention or may be a component of hysteria; side effects of prolonged laxative abuse include chronic diarrhea, colicky abdominal pain, nausea,vomiting, weight loss, weakness, hypokalemia, skin pigmentation, arthralgia, cyclic edema, nephrolithiasis (ammonium urates); see Cathartic colon **FACTITIOUS FEVER** A fever of unknown origin described in either young female health professionals, following a legitimate disease or in older neurotic women who are prone to self-mutilation **FACTITIOUS HYPOGLYCEMIA** Surreptitious ingestion of hypoglycemic agents, eg sulfonylureas or insulin; often by women ages 30-40, employed in the health professions who have highly variable levels of glucose Diagnosis Measurement of oral hypoglycemics, insulin antibodies and C-peptide; the C-fragment of the insulin molecule is present in the serum of normal subjects at a ratio of 5-15:1 and is substantially reduced in those who inject insulin **FACTITIOUS PANNICULITIS** A condition characterized by diffuse indurated subcutaneous nodules, due to auto-injection of mineral and cotton seed oil, liquid silicones (see Sexual reassignment), drugs, eg meperidine, morphine, pentazocine, tetanus toxoid, milk and feces Clinical Acute inflammation evolving into end-stage fibrosis, avascular necrosis and when infected, ulceration **FACTITIOUS PURPURA** Devil's pinches Patchy self-inflicted lesions that may be produced by pinching flesh; see Conversion disorders

Factor A molecule or group of molecules that are known to exist in a system, but which are poorly characterized when the system is first described; with time, the molecules are characterized and/or sequenced, such that the 'factor' designation falls into disfavor and retains historic interest

Non-coagulation factors **FACTOR A** Factor C3 (obsolete) **FACTOR B** Complement C3 proactivator, a protein of the alternate complement pathway **FACTOR C** Cytoplasmic component that causes mitochondrial contraction (obsolete) **FACTOR D** Protein activator of factor B of the alternate pathway of complement activation **FACTOR F** Fertility-bearing plasmid; see Factor IF **FACTOR G** Translocase (obsolete) **FACTOR H** A complement protein that inactivates C3b (alternate pathway) **FACTOR I** A protein that degrades C3b (alternate pathway) **FACTOR IF** Initiation factor for protein synthesis (obsolete) **FACTOR P** Properdin (obsolete) **FACTOR R** Antibiotic resistance-bearing plasmid; Release factor (proteins that release a polypeptide chain from the ribosome) **FACTOR S** A component produced with serotonin by sleep-deprived experimental models, which induces non-REM or slow-wave sleep, composed of muramyl peptide, a normal component of bacterial walls, possibly serving to explain why bacterially 'naive' newborns don't have slow-wave sleep; Cf S factor **FACTOR T** Elongation factor, a protein that participates in the elongation of prokaryote polypeptides **FACTOR V** Nicotinamide adenine dinucleotide (NAD) or NADP MICROBIOLOGY A requirement for growth of certain bacteria (eg most *Haemophilus* species); NAD is supplied by the co-cultured *Staphylococcus aureus* **FACTOR X** Hemin MICROBIOLOGY A group of heat-stable tetrapyrrole compounds provided by several iron-containing molecules, eg heme and hematin, which are required for synthesis of catalase, peroxidase and the cytochrome electron transport system; bacteria dependent upon factor X include *Hemophilus influenzae, H haemolyticus, H aegyptius, H ducreyi* cannot synthesize protoporphyrin from delta-aminolevulinic acid, a reaction that aids in speciating *Haemophilus* Note: *H influenzae, H hemolyticus* and *H aegyptius* require both factors V and X; 'Factor X' was once used for vitamin B_{12} and biotin **FACTOR Y** Pyridoxine (obsolete)

'Fad' diet see Diet

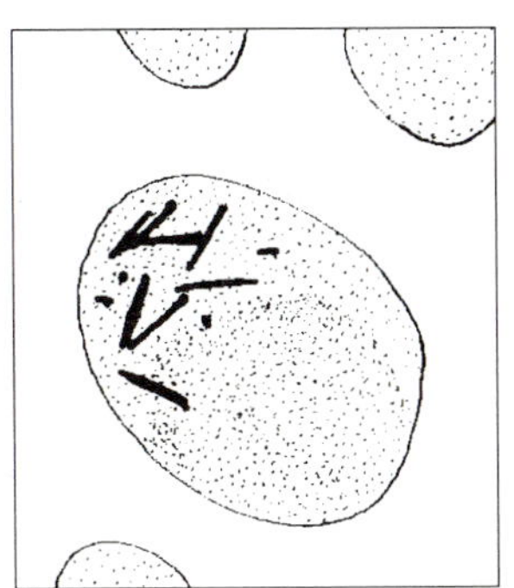
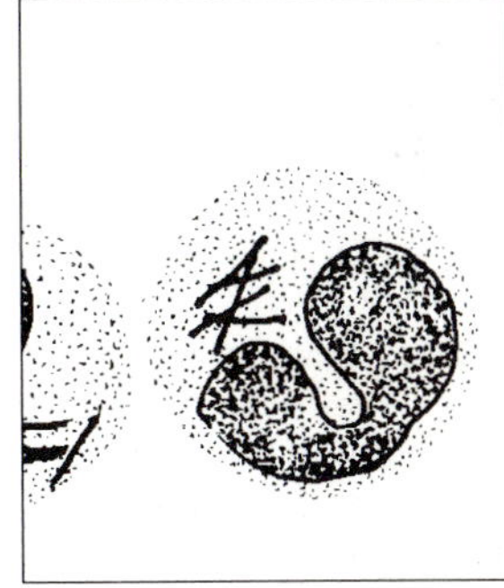

Faggot cells

Faggot cells HEMATOPATHOLOGY Leukemic cells of the French-American-British class M3 (acute promyelocytic leukemia), characterized by bundles of Auer rods, hence the name; the trans-Atlantic translation has transformed the adjectival 'faggot' into the bulkier, but less confusing, 'bundle of kindling wood' cell; a faggot or fagot is a bundle of sticks, twigs or small branches, to be used as kindling wood, or a bundle of iron or steel rods

Failed disk syndrome see Laminectomy

Failure to thrive PEDIATRICS The inability of a child to gain weight or one who loses weight without discernable cause, due to: a) Environmental deprivation, the more common cause of failure to thrive, in which children have poor appetites, are apathetic and withdrawn; this constellation of findings is typical of abused children, offspring of schizophrenics or in children with physical deformities or secondary problems causing the parents to subconsciously reject them or b) Organic diseases, which include ill-defined cerebral lesions, chromosome defects, chronic infection or inflammation, cystic fibrosis, eclampsia, endocrinopathy, heart disease, idiopathic hypercalcemia, malabsorption, malignancy, renal insufficiency or tubular defects and the TORCH complex; see Battered child syndrome; Cf Infanticide

Faith healing An alternate form of health care lying outside of the mainstream of medical practice, in which the therapy consists of trusting in a 'higher' or other power(s) without active medical or surgical intervention; Cf Christian science, Psychic surgery

'Falling leaf' motility see Darting motility

Fallout Radiation that settles out of the atmosphere following a nuclear explosion, see Nuclear war; more colloquially, 'fallout' refers to the broad consequences of an error or action

FALS Forward angle light scatter Determination of a particle's size by flow cytometry by the amount of light scattered when the detector is at 180° or directly in front of the laser beam, known as forward scatter; see Backscatter, Flow cytometry

False aneurysm A blood-filled pseudo-vascular space that parallels the native vessel lumen and which may carry blood if there is a site of exit and re-entry; the 'vessel' wall is formed by reactive connective tissue; false aneurysms are secondary to trauma

F protein see Atypical measles

Falstaff snore A loud snore heard in the sleeping obese, named after the portly Falstaff, a minor character in Henry IV, part I, Act II, who was a '...fat-kidneyed rascal...fast asleep and snorting like a horse'; the snore may occur in the sleep apnea syndrome (Br Med J 1987; 294:371c)

FAM 5-Fluorouracil, adriamycin (doxorubicin) and mitomycin C A chemotherapeutic regimen used with varying degrees of failure in gastric carcinoma

Familial combined hyperlipidemia A common (1:100) autosomal dominant disorder in which there is increased triglyceride and/or cholesterol, where the common denominator is increased hepatic synthesis of apolipoprotein-B with a mild decrease in HDL-cholesterol and apo-A1 and an increase of LDL and/or VLDL Clinical Early coronary atherosclerosis with a first myocardial infarction occurring as early as age 40; the patients are often overweight and hypertensive; smoking is forbidden as it exacerbates the arteriosclerosis

Familial dysautonomia Riley-Day syndrome An autosomal recessive condition of Jews, affecting neurons of the peripheral sensorimotor autonomic and central nervous system Clinical Failure to thrive, episodic vomiting, upper respiratory tract infection, autonomic dysfunction (skin blotching, lacrimation, defective temperature control, diaphoresis, hypertension and postural hypotension) and early demise

Familial dysβ-lipoproteinemia An uncommon (1:10 000) autosomal recessive condition with defective apolipoprotein-E, poor 'remnant' catabolism and overproduction of triglyceride-rich lipoproteins, eg very low-density lipoprotein Clinical Palmoplantar tuberoeruptive xanthomas, atherosclerosis at or before age 50 with peripheral vascular and coronary vessel disease Treatment Diet, exercise, drugs, eg bile acid-binding resins and nicotinic acid and in post-menopausal women, low-dose estrogens

Familial dyslipemic hypertension Williams-Hunt-Hopkins syndrome A complex that affects two or more siblings in a family, which may comprise up to 12% of all hypertensives and 25% of hypertensives diagnosed before age 60 Laboratory HDL-cholesterol is < 10th percentile, LDL-cholesterol and triglyceride levels are > 90th percentile (J Am Med Assoc 1988; 259:3579)

Familial hypercholesterolemia A common (1:500) congenital autosomal defect in the LDL receptor gene, resulting in dysfunctional or absent receptor Clinical Early coronary atherosclerosis in men and first myocardial infarctions by age 40 (women may remain asymptomatic throughout life), tendinous xanthomas, corneal arcus and xanthelasma Laboratory Elevated LDL-cholesterol, circa 300-500 mg/dl (20% of cholesterol in this range is due to familial hypercholesterolemia) Treatment Smoking cessation, diet, exercise, drugs (bile-acid binding resins, eg cholestipol, cholestyramine and nicotinic acid, a low cholesterol and low saturated fat diet, liver transplant may provide LDL receptors Note: Acquired hypercholesterolemia may be transient, due to dietary excess or related to acute intermittent porphyria and anorexia nervosa; congenital hypercholesterolemia is relatively common, often autosomal recessive and polygenic, different alleles being affected in each cohort; in a French-Canadian cohort, a 10 kilobase deletion in the LDL receptor gene causes the loss of the promoter and the first exon, abolishing production of the LDL-receptor mRNA; see Cholesterol-lowering drugs

Familial hypertriglyceridemia A common (1:200) autosomal dominant disorder, due to increased hepatic triglyceride, cholesterol and cholic acid synthesis, with increased very low-density lipoprotein and transportation of triglycerides by high density lipoprotein Clinical Increased triglycerides in obesity, alcohol consumption, drug therapy (β-adrenergics, diuretics, estrogens and steroid therapy) Treatment Diet, exercise, drugs, eg clofibrate, gemfibrozil

Familial multiple hamartoma syndrome see Multiple hamartoma syndrome

Familial mediterranean fever (FMF) Familial paroxysmal polyserositis An autosomal recessive disease affecting eastern Mediterranean rim Jews, Armenian and Sephardic, the latter which comprise one-half of cases, as well as Arabs, Greeks, Turks, and other 'rim' inhabitants, causing episodic serosal (especially peritoneal) inflammation, more common in men Pathogenesis Unclear, possibly due to a deficiency of an inflammatory inhibitor (of neutrophil chemotaxis by complement C5a) with abnormalities of suppressor T cells or defective arachidonic acid metabolism Clinical Onset by adolescence as recurring peritonitis, arthritis and pleuritis, with acute febrile attacks, diffuse abdominal pain, muscle 'guarding', leukocytosis and malabsorption that resolve within 24 hours; long-term prognosis is good in absence of renal amyloidosis which causes terminal nephropathy, an event preventable by colchicine therapy

Family 'ganging' A form of health care provision that may be practiced by some physicians in less financially-advantaged regions in the USA, eg inner cities, in which a patient is encouraged to bring his entire family along for a check-up or other evaluation at the time of his return visit, regardless of whether it is indicated; 'ganging' is most commonly practiced when providing services to Medicaid patients, for whom the level of reimbursement to the physician is very low; see Medicaid

Family cancer syndromes see Fetal overgrowth syndrome of Beckwith Wiedeman

Farcy An accidental infection of humans, resulting from contact with domestic animals, especially horses, infected by ***Pseudomonas mallei***, a strict aerobic gram-negative bacillus, a condition known as glanders Clinical Epithelioid granulomas in the skin and lymphatics ('farcy buds') with induration of the connective tissue of the head and neck; see Glanders

Farmer's lung Farm worker's lung An IgG1-mediated form of extrinsic allergic alveolitis or hypersensitivity pneumonitis that occurs in non-atopic individuals, who after repeated exposure to organic dust and fungi, eg ***Aspergillus*** species, become allergic to thermophilic actinomycotic organisms; 90% of patients have antibodies to moldy hay, an ideal growth medium for the fungi implicated (***Microspora vulgaris, Thermoactinomyces vulgaris*** and ***Micropolyspora faeni***) Pathogenesis Unknown, possibly due to an immune complex deposition in the lungs causing a type III hypersensitivity reaction Clinical Attacks may last several days and occur between May and October (the growing season in the Northern Hemisphere), causing rales, cyanosis, fever, dry cough, rhonchi and dyspnea, beginning 4-8 hours after exposure to stored corn, barley and tobacco; with time, weight loss Pulmonary function tests Reduced volumes and impaired gas exchange Radiology Normal or diffuse interstitial reticular pattern, occasionally with fine nodular shadows Histopathology Chronic inflammation, peribronchiolar granulomatous response and foreign-body-type giant cell reaction, eventually developing fibrosis Treatment Corticosteroids Complications Pulmonary hypertension, right ventricular hypertrophy and failure; Cf Silo filler's lung

Faroe Islands A small archipelago between Norway and Iceland (capital Torshavn, population 46 000, major industry, fishing), with an isolated population that is of medical interest as a) The first cases of multiple sclerosis coincided with the landing of British troops in 1943, lending support to a slow viral etiology (Ann Neurol 1979; 5:6) and b) The population had been devastated in 1846 when measles killed one-fourth of the population of 8000

Farr's law of epidemics William Farr, an English statistician, who analyzed the mortality of a waning smallpox epidemic (1838-39) and demonstrated mathematically that the fall in mortality of an epidemic occurs at a uniformly accelerated rate; when applied to the current AIDS epidemic, some data suggest that the rate of increase in new cases may be slowing (at least in some developed nations) and a 'crest' in AIDS might arrive by 1993 (J Am Med Assoc 1990; 263:1522)

FARS Fatal accident reporting system

Fasciculin II A glycoprotein expressed on axonal subsets in the grasshopper that mediates selective fasciculation (a form of neuronal recognition), belongs to the immunoglobulin superfamily, is homologous in structure and function to N-CAM (neuronal cell adhesion molecule), myelin-associated glycoprotein and other cell adhesion molecules (Science 1988; 242:700)

FASEB Federation of American Societies for Experimental Medicine

Fast CT imaging A technique using the same computed tomographic principle delineated by EMI in 1972; fast CT scanners are of greatest use in cardiac imaging, as the scan requires less than a fraction of a second, allowing the scanning of multiple slices, which can be repeated at frequent intervals for a specified period; fast CT provides information about cardiac anatomy, pulmonary and coronary arteries, myocardial perfusion and microcirculation (Mayo Clin Proc 1990; 65:1336rv)

Fast food Prepared food from a restaurant that specializes in providing a full 'meal', often consisting of a form of hamburger or permutation of the chicken 'theme', French fries and a soft drink or a milk shake, in less than two minutes; one-fifth of the US population of 230 million purchases at least one 'fast-food' meal daily; a diet consisting solely of fast food overloads the body with protein, fat and calories and be low in vitamins, mineral and fibers (Consumer Reports 1988; 54:355)

'Fast' hemoglobins A hemoglobin (Hb) with an electrophoretic mobility greater or faster than HbA on a pH 8.6 gel, including HbBart, HbI, HbH, HbA_{1a}, HbA_{1b} and HbA_{1c}, based on their order of elution from a column containing cation-exchange resin; see Glycosylated hemoglobin

Fastidious organism MICROBIOLOGY A term that is theoretically applicable to any living organism, as each has specific growth requirements, and therefore is 'fastidious'; in the clinical laboratory, although it is a fact that parasites and viruses have highly specific (and therefore, fastidious) growth requirements, 'fastidious' has come to be applied to bacteria that grow poorly or not at all on the usual growth media, under the usual conditions; such organisms may a) Grow optimally at room temperature (25°C) or at 4°C b) Grow very slowly, ie over the space of several weeks, whereas culture plates are generally discarded as 'no-growths' after one week of incubation c) Require a microaerophilic or strictly anaerobic atmosphere d) Require special growth media or e)

Require a combination of the above

Fasting specimen LABORATORY MEDICINE A blood specimen that is drawn from a patient who has not eaten for 12 hours; fasting is an absolute requirement for a limited number of tests, eg glucose tolerance test; prolonged fasting causes a marked (240%) increase in bilirubin, a marked(50%) decrease in blood glucose and significant increases in plasma triglycerides, glycerol and free fatty acids, without affecting the cholesterol levels

'Fast track' paper SCIENTIFIC JOURNALISM A publication in the sciences that is of such 'newsworthiness' that the journal, eg Cell, Nature, Science may choose to either bypass or accelerate the usual review and typesetting processes so that it will appear as little as two weeks after the manuscript's submission; the advantage to the journal is that it maintains a reputation for quality reporting, as the papers may have Nobel prize-winning potential; the disadvantage is that some 'hot' papers, eg 'cold fusion' (J Elect Chem, 1989), may ultimately prove to be inaccurate, causing the journal to lose credibility (Science 1991; 251:260n&v); Cf Citation impact, 'Hot paper'

Fast twitch fibers see White fibers

Fat, dietary see Fatty acids, Fish oil, Olive oil and Tropical oil

DIETARY FATS (saturation)	A	B	C
Safflower Oil	9%	13%	72%
Sunflower Oil	11%	20%	69%
Corn Oil	13%	25%	62%
Olive Oil	14%	77%	9%
Soybean Oil	15%	24%	61%
Peanut Oil	18%	48%	34%
Cottonseed Oil	27%	19%	54%
Lard	41%	47%	12%
Palm Oil	51%	39%	10%
Beef Tallow	52%	44%	4%
Butterfat	66%	30%	4%
Palm-kernel Oil	86%	12%	2%
Coconut Oil	92%	6%	2%

A % Saturated fatty acids B % Monounsaturated fatty acids C % Polyunsaturated fatty acids

Fat distribution There are two patterns of distribution of corporal adipose tissue, as measured by the ratio of the corporal diameter at the hips and waist, waist:hip ratio, normal: 0.7-0.8; these patterns differ significantly in co-morbidity of obesity; in the 'gynecoid' or female pattern, fat deposits in the lower body (abdomen, buttocks, hips, thighs) by means of mesenchymal differentiation or hyperplasia; in the 'android' or male pattern, the fat is predominantly upper body, depositing around the abdomen, the adipocytes are more sensitive to insulin and catecholamines and the fat accumulates by hypertrophy, possibly a function of membrane receptor density; the android pattern has greater lipolytic and lipogenic potential, and thus carries a greater risk for hypertension, cardiovascular disease, diabetes mellitus and hyperinsulinemia; see Obesity; Cf Morbid obesity

Fat embolism Emboli composed of fat are common, relatively innocuous and may occur in alcoholism, bone marrow biopsy, cardiopulmonary bypass, compression injury, diabetes, lymphangiography, pancreatitis, sickle cell anemia and steroid therapy; contrarily, the fat embolism 'syndrome' is neither common nor a trivial condition; clinically significant fat emboli may be endogenous or exogenous and most are due to major fractures and trauma to parenchymal organs (most deaths in the immediate post-trauma period have significant fat embolism), burns, blast injury, severe infections, especially α-toxin-producing ***Clostridium*** species Pathogenesis Coalesced fat globules of up to 20 μm in diameter may circulate in the 'embolic' phase, possibly causing sudden death on entering the pulmonary microcirculation (the lung is the only site of embolism in most patients); the subsequent or 'ameboid' phase is characterized by emboli in the cardiac, cerebral, renal and other arteries, causing hypoperfusion due to mechanical obstruction by fat globules, platelets, erythrocytes and early non-specific immune mediators, eg serotonin and kinins; in the final or enzymatic phase, lipase enters the circulation, catabolizing the neutral fats into highly toxic free fatty acids, evoking inflammation, hemorrhage and chemical pneumonitis due to lipolysis and disruption of the surfactant Clinical Hypoxia (50% of femoral shaft fractures have reduced arterial PO_2 within the first few days), acute onset of dyspnea, tachypnea, cyanosis, tachycardia with sudden onset of right-sided cardiac failure, showers of petechiae, thrombocytopenia, cerebral embolism (with changes in personality, confusion, drowsiness, weakness, agitation, spasticity, defects of the visual field and rarely, extreme pyrexia) Treatment No therapy is consistently effective

Fatigue fracture A stress fracture that occurs in the feet of otherwise fit foot soldiers, caused by repeated, relatively 'trivial' trauma to normal bone, resulting in local bone resorption; among civilians, stress fractures are either occupational or afflict the so-called 'week-end warrior', who strenuously exercises an often untrained or sedentary skeleto-muscular system

Fatigue syndrome see Chronic fatigue syndrome; Cf Compassion fatigue syndrome

'Fat-mobilizing hormone' A fanciful term for a non-existant 'factor', the production of which has been claimed to be induced by the Atkin's diet; see Diets, Cf Starch blocker

Fat necrosis Liquefactive necrosis that is initiated by trauma and effected by lipolytic enzymes; fat necrosis is relatively common in a) The breast, where it is often well-circumscribed and by light microscopy demonstrates large epithelioid and bizarre cells, causing both clinical and(occasionally) histological confusion with carcinoma and b) Pancreas, where blockage of the ducts by concrements facilitates the breakdown of normal barriers, causing focal leakage of lipases and subsequent calcium 'soap' formation; see Soap

Fat sickle cells A descriptor for plump variant drepanocytes, which are typical of hemoglobin SC that may be associated with target cells and 'Washington monument' crystals

'Fat spurt' PEDIATRICS A temporary relative increase in subcutaneous adipose tissue occurring in preadolescence

Fatty acids, diet The relative importance of saturation of the bonds in fatty acids remains unclear, although saturated animal-derived and 'tropical' oils are thought to have the greatest atherogenic potential, while the literature suggests that those high in monounsaturated fats, in particular olive oil have the least atherogenic potential Note: The table from the US Department of Agriculture is provided to place these studies in context as they are reported

Fatty degeneration Accumulation of fat globules due to deterioration of lipid storage and metabolic pathways of intracellular origin; Cf Fatty infiltration

'Fatty food attack' Severe transient colicky abdominal pain that occurs in response to ingestion of fried or fat-laden foods, which is considered a common clinical sign of cholelithiasis

Fatty infiltration Intracellular accumulation of fat that is of extracellular origin; Cf Fatty degeneration

Fatty liver A lipid-laden liver due to the accumulation of triglycerides of both intra- and extrahepatic origin; fatty change is the single most common biopsy finding in alcoholics and may be divided according to the size of the fat droplets **LARGE FAT DROPLET FATTY LIVER** The nucleus is displaced to the side and the cytoplasm is replete with large fat vacuoles, appearing in chronic alcoholics (see Alcoholic fatty liver), choline deficiency, obesity, steatosis, protein-calorie malnutrition (kwashiorkor, jejuno-ileal bypass), diabetes mellitus and steroid therapy **SMALL FAT DROPLET FATTY LIVER** The nucleus is central and surrounded by mutiple bubbly vacuoles filled with globules of fat that may be seen in alcoholics as well, and occurs in acute fatty liver of pregnancy, eclampsia/pre-eclampsia, Reye syndrome, Jamaican vomiting sickness, intravenous tetracycline, toxic shock syndrome and valproic acid therapy

Fatty liver of pregnancy Acute fatty liver of pregnancy A rare (1:10-15 000) idiopathic complication of pregnancy, most commonly affecting primiparas with male infants or twin gestation, occasionally associated with pre-eclampsia **Clinical** Onset after 35th week, possibly progressing to fulminant hepatic failure with jaundice, encephalopathy, disseminated intravascular coagulation and death Prognosis When this condition was first recognized in the 1970s, the reported mortality was 85%; more recently, fetal mortality is reported to be 23%, maternal, 18%, possibly representing recognition of earlier or milder cases **Pathogenesis** Estrogens are implicated and may act by altering the membrane fluidity **Histopathology** Fine droplet fat deposition in the hepatocytes and cholestasis **Treatment** Terminate pregnancy; the condition may respond to S-adenosyl-L-methionine (Adv Intern Med 1990; 35:289, Hepatology 1990; 11:59)

Fatty streak A defect confined to the vascular lumen that is the earliest lesion of atherosclerosis, which has no respect for age, race, sex or social status, and occurs as early as one year of age **Histopathology** Intimal lipid and foam cell (fat-laden histiocytes filled with cholesteryl esters) accumulation at the ostia of branches of the aorta and aortic valve rings; in advanced lesions, smooth muscle appears in the streak, later giving rise to fibrous plaques; fatty streaks are most prominent and extensive in those exposed to a westernized diet

Faust complex The obsessive desire for knowledge to the exclusion of virtually all else; the legend of Faustus was first related in a play by Marlowe in 1592 and has been retold in various forms by Goethe, Thomas Mann and others; the essential feature is that of a scholar who sinfully trades his soul for knowledge and power; academic physicians often subconsciously feel they will be granted the power, knowledge (and health) and, like the later versions of the Faustus theme, their sins will ultimately be forgiven (J Am Med Assoc 1966; 196:156); Cf Physician invincibility syndrome

Favism A condition characterized by episodic hemolysis affecting subjects with glucose-6-phosphate dehydrogenase deficiency, type Gd/Med that occurs after ingesting fava beans (Italian broad beans), which are high in oxidating pyrimidine derivatives, divicine and isouramil, which are capable of destroying erythrocyte glutathione, an antioxidant

Favus A disfiguring scalp dermatophytosis caused by ***Trichophyton violaceum*** and ***Microsporum gypseum*** resulting in destruction of the hair follicles and alopecia

FBI sign Fat-blood interface ORTHOPEDICS A semi-lunar soft tissue effusion, seen radiologically by a 'horizontal' beam in post-traumatic lipohemarthrosis; the FBI sign is most commonly seen in the knee and in the shoulder (because of increased marrow fat and blood in the joint space)

F body A fluorescent structure corresponding to the distal Y chromosome, seen in male interphase cells and spermatozoa when stained with quinacrine mustard dihydrochloride

FBS Fasting blood sugar levels Normal values in an adult: 3.9-5.8 mmol/L (US: 70-105 mg/dl); diabetes mellitus > 7.8 mmol/L (US: > 140 mg/dl)

F cell A red blood cell in adults containing (persistent) hemoglobin F, which is of no pathological significance, Cf Fetal erythrocyte

F^+ cell A 'male' bacterium that donates an F plasmid to the F^- or 'female' bacterium and has the pilus to enact the exchange

Fc Fragment, crystallizable The portion of an immunoglobulin heavy chain's constant region remaining after papain digestion; prolonged papain digestion of Fc results in the smaller Fc' fragment; incubation with pepsin results in low molecular weight peptides and the pFc' fragment, which has a region for the Fc receptor on macrophages and monocytes

Fc receptor A cation permease receptor that is activated by binding of the immunoglobulin Fc fragment; binding of the Fc fragment is followed by an influx of Na^+ or K^+ which activates macrophage functions including phagocytosis, cell movement and generation of H_2O_2

FDA Food and Drug Administration An agency of the US government established by the Federal Food, Drug and Cosmetic Act in 1938, charged with determining the safety of drugs before marketing and assuring that certain labeling specifications and advertising standards be met while marketing the product; the Durham-Humphrey Amendment of 1952 increased governmental control of drugs by restricting the refilling of perscriptions; the Kefauver-Harris Amendment of 1962, following in the wake of the thalidomide disaster, added that a product must be proven both effective and safe, requiring a series of clinical testing phase prior to marketing; see Investigational new drug

FD&C yellow #5 Tartrazine, a ubiquitous colorant used in foods and drugs that cross-reacts with aspirin, exacerbates asthma and may cause a life-threatening anaphylactic reaction Note: In the USA, the approved colorants are designated by numbers under the Food, Drug and Cosmetic Act, abbreviated as FD&C

Fd fragment(s) That portion of the IgG molecule that remains after papain digestion, consisting of two separate fragments of heavy chain joined to an intact light chain

Fd' fragment That portion of the IgG molecule that remains after pepsin digestion, consisting of two separate fragments of heavy chain joined to an intact light chain

FDP Fibrin degradation products, Fibrin 'splits' polypeptide fragments that result from wild and unchecked primary fibrinolysis occurring in a) Intravascular pathology, associated with disseminated intravascular coagulation, deep vein thrombosis and pulmonary embolism (ie, pathological fibrinolysis) or in b) Extravascular conditions, eg hematomas, neoplasia, sepsis, allograft rejection, glomerular and severe liver diseases and obstetric complications, eg abruptio placentae, eclampsia, retained dead fetus

Feather pattern Christmas tree pattern MOLECULAR BIOLOGY A descriptor for the ultrastructural pattern seen by the technique of rotary shadowing (foigure) after gene activation by DNA-polymerase, when multiple pre-rRNAs simultaneously initiate transcription on a single DNA molecule, where each of the feather's 'branches' corresponds to lengths of nascent rRNA, the chains of which are progressively shorter towards the initiation site

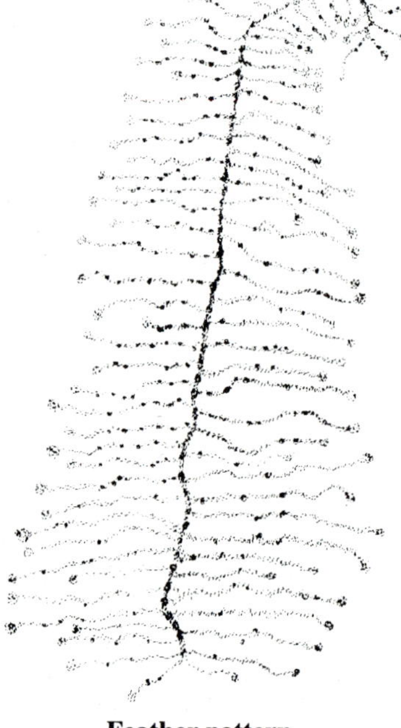

Feather pattern

Feathery degeneration HEPATIC PATHOLOGY A descriptor for the hepatocytic changes due to chronic cholestasis secondary to extrahepatic biliary destruction; the 'feathers' may represent phospholipids and bile acid crystals, which may be accompanied by an intracellular triad consisting of hydropic swelling, aggregation and reticulation of bile pigment and feathery cytoplasm, possibly related to the toxic effect of bile salts Figure: The solid lines indicate the 'feathers', the dashed lines, the often associated (and non-specific) Mallory bodies

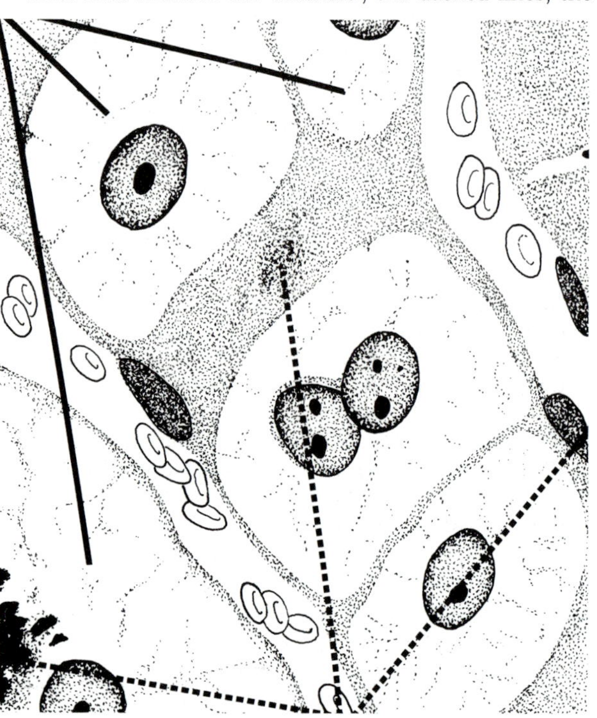

Feathery degeneration

Feather-stitched pattern A closely packed arrangement of connective tissue and stromal cells arranged in 'stitched' lines, characteristic of ovarian fibromas, often accompanied by hyaline bands (as seen in the related ovarian thecoma) and edema, seen by low-power light microscopy; Cf Herringbone Note: The feather-stitch is a modified 'mattress' stitch

Febrile lumbago Dull, ill-defined lower dorsal and lumbar pain occurring in spinal osteomyelitis, accompanied by low-grade fever and hematogenous 'seeding' of bacteria

Febrile torticollis A neck spasm accompanied by dull, ill-defined pain, low-grade fever and bacteremia seen in osteomyelitis of the cervical spine

FEBS Federation of European Biochemical Societies

Federal Register An official daily publication produced by the US federal government that serves to notify the public of any changes of federal regulations, rulings, legal notices, proclamations and documents generated by the executive branch of the government; the range of material published in the Federal Registry includes activities regarding safety of products, occupational health, standards of foods and drugs; proposed changes in policies or rules published in the Register are accompanied by an invitation to citizens or others to participate in the decision-making process by submitting data or arguments regarding the proposal

Feedback loop PHYSIOLOGY Any control system, in particular those involving hormonal and receptor-ligand interactions, in which the output signal or effect, eg increase of the production of a hormone by an end-organ, is received by the early components of the system, causing an alteration in the subsequent output, either decreasing (negative feedback) or increasing (positive feedback) the production of an early-stage component of the system

Fee-splitting MEDICAL REIMBURSEMENT A practice that is considered frankly unethical, in which physician A refers a patient to physician B and shares a portion of fee received by physician B Note: This contrasts sharply with concept of a 'Finder's fee' that compensates a referring physician for locating a certain type of patient for participation in clinical research protocols

Fehldiagnose German, Unclear diagnosis The inability to establish a diagnosis in a patient who is ill, despite an extensive work-up, and who is ultimately discharged without a primary diagnosis; in one study (Dtsch Med Wschr 1989; 114:1431), 1.5% of all hospitalized patients were discharged without a diagnosis, ie had Fehldiagnose, having presented with fever of unknown origin, syncope, chronic pain, non-specific inflammation or hematological changes

FEIBA Factor VIII inhibitor by-passing activity; see Prothrombin complex concentrate

'Felinization' Transverse ridging of the esophagus occasionally seen by a barium 'swallow' in patients with long-standing reflux esophagitis, simulating the morphology of a normal feline esophagus; see Water brash appearance; Cf Leopard spotting

Fellowship A term that when defined in the usual context of US medical academics, a fellowship is a post-residency training period of one to two years in a subspecialty, eg interventional radiology, immunopathology and microsurgery of the hand, that allows a candidate to develop a particular expertise that may have a related subspecialty board; the time period of a fellowship is often used to prepare for the specialty boards examinations

Felon Whitlow A purulent infection within the tight fascial plane adjacent to the terminal intraphalangeal joint of the fingers or toes, secondary to an open wound; as the inflammatory mass expands within the confined space, the vascular supply is compromised and a scenario is created that predisposes the site to osteomyelitis (most often, streptococcal or staphylococcal), pulp necrosis and sloughing of tissue; the pain is very intense and seemingly disproportionate with the scant amount of swelling and erythema clinically evident **Treatment** Drainage by an incision directly over the site of maximum swelling; the term has also been applied to a localized painful herpetic skin infection 'seeded' in an open abrasion by contact exposure

Female circumcision A group of disfiguring procedures performed on the female genitalia in many Central and West African countries, which are required for tribal identity; three types of 'circumcision are described: the simplest and least commonly used consists of slitting the hood of the clitoris; more common is complete excision of the clitoris and labia minora; the most extreme form, infibulation or pharonic circumcision, consists of excision of the entire vulva (clitoris, labia minora and majora), sewing the vaginal wall closed with thread and thorns to a small tubular channel, allowing only the passage of urine and menstrual flow; the operation is considered a prerequisite for marriage, and may be performed by local women who are 'specialized' in the procedure and who use old razors or broken glass and are often complicated by shock, infection and hemorrhage (Am Med News 27/Apr/90); Cf 'Love surgery'

Female 'prostate' RADIOLOGY A filling defect occasionally seen in women where the levator ani muscle is more prominent than usual; associated with urethritis, and best visualized in the prone position, while the real prostate is less pronounced in prone position UROLOGY Paraurethral glands seen rarely in female humans, but are well-studied in rodents, homologous to the male prostate; the female prostate may contain psammoma bodies, and if enlarged, require transurethral resection

Fenoldopan An investigational antihypertensive agent that is a dopamine (D_1) receptor antagonist with renal vasodilatory activity, administered by intravenous drip and has been reported to be as effective as nitroprusside with renoprotective effect (Circulation 1990; 81:970)

FEP Free erythrocytic porphyrin

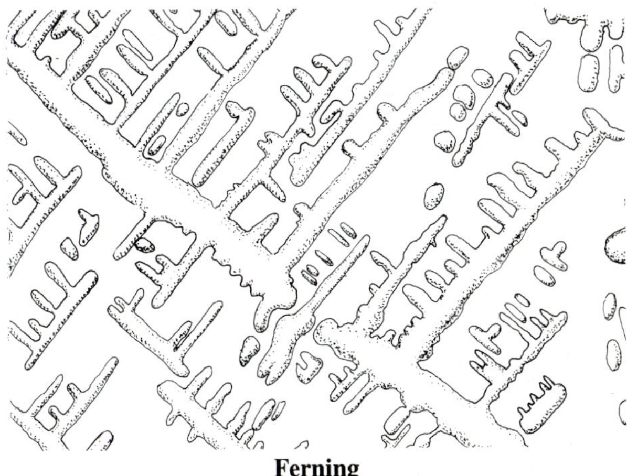

Ferning

Ferning A term for two light microscopic patterns (figure) related to normal gynecologic physiology, in a) Cytology Ferning is a palm leaf-like pattern seen in dried endocervical mucus, consisting of a branched heterogeneous network of crystallized glycoprotein, sodium and potassium chloride salts that forms a parallel canalicular system facilitating sperm penetration; the ferning reaction is induced by estrogen and seen from days 7-18, peaking on day 14 of the menstrual cycle, and b) Endometrium Ferning corresponds to complex branching of endometrial glands, which is histological evidence that ovulation has occurred; other parameters corroborating ovulation include subnucleolar vacuolization with palisading of the gland cells, stromal 'decidualization', glandular necrosis, vascular thrombosis; inflammation and aggregates of stromal cells; see Spinnbarkeit

Ferruginous body A generic term for asbestos fibers clad in iron, protein and mucopolysaccharides; the definition has been expanded to include any iron-covered elongated fiber that can't be digested by macrophages, including fiberglass, aluminum silicates and diatomaceous earth (Arch Pathol Lab Med 1985; 109:849); Cf Asbestos body

'Fertile' eunuch syndrome A variant of Kallmann syndrome with selective luteinizing hormone deficiency and intact FSH production (ie normal 'equipment' with aspermatogenesis, thus, despite the name, these patients are infertile but may be rendered fertile with hormonal support) Treatment Chorionic gonadotropin, the luteinizing hormone-like activity of which stimulates spermatogenesis

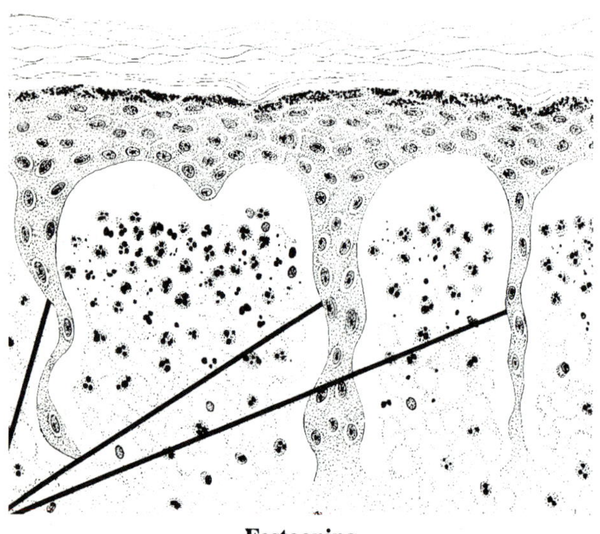

Festooning

Festooning DERMATOPATHOLOGY A descriptor for the ribbon-like strands of epithelial cells (figure) that extend vertically from the basal cell layer to the epidermal canopy, periodically tethering the fluid-filled bullae to the dermis; festooning is a histologic finding characteristic of dermatitis herpetiformis, likened to festoons or party streamers

Fetal alcohol syndrome (FAS) A disease complex due to in utero exposure to alcohol, representing the most common cause of mental retardation in pregnancy (surpassing Down syndrome and spina bifida), affecting at least one-third of the infants born to women who are defined as alcoholics, ie those who consume greater than 50 grams of alcohol/day; FAS affects 1-2 per 1000 live births in the USA and is thought to be related to the toxic effects of acetaldehyde, produced by both the mother and fetus (Science 1988; 242:273); the alcohol may interfere with the placenta's ability to transfer amino acids and zinc, essential for normal growth, explaining the associated intrauterine growth retardation Clinical Prematurity, perinatal asphyxia, intrauterine growth retardation that may persist into adulthood, mild to profound developmental delays, mental dysfunction, microcephaly, cranial defects, atrial septal defect and facial dysmorphogenesis (short palpebral fissure, epicanthal folds, short up-turned nose, thin upper lip, long smooth filtrum, micrognathia, maxillary hypoplasia), muscular hypotonia, bone anomalies (vertebral malformation and spina bifida) with joint contraction; when FAS children are re-examined as adolescents and adults, their IQ averages 68, with academic functioning at the second to fourth grade levels, poor mathematical abilities, maladaptive behavior, including poor judgement, distractibility and difficulty in perceiving social cues; the subjects tend to be short and microcephalic (J Am Med Assoc 1991; 265:1961) Note: The 50% decrease in alcohol consumption during pregnancy reported from 1985-88 is attributed to educational efforts (J Am Med Assoc 1991; 265:876)

Fetal-brain tissue grafting The engraftment of fetal ventral mesencephalon, adrenal gland or other tissues to the caudate nucleus of the brain in patients with Parkinson's disease as a therapeutic modality; the best thus far reported response occurs with mesencephalic tissue, which is reported to ameliorate rigidity, bradykinesia, postural imbalance, gait disturbance and facial expression (Arch Neurol 1990; 47:1281); see Parkinson's disease

Fetal diabetic 'syndrome' A complex seen in the children born to diabetic mothers, who have a 3- to 5-fold increased incidence of various congenital and acquired anomalies, including visceromegaly, increased body fat, respiratory distress, and hyaline membrane disease, cardiomegaly, ventricular septal hypertrophy, skeletal anomalies, hypoplastic left colon syndrome (aganglionosis-like presentation), hypocalcemia and immaturity

Fetal distress syndrome Intrauterine fetal hypoxia caused by prematurity or antepartum maternal infection, diabetes mellitus, eclampsia, hemolytic disease of the newborn, hemorrhage and others Clinical Tachycardia (>160/min) or bradycardia (<100/min, which carries a worse prognosis) and decreased pH

'Fetal' erythrocyte Prolonged presence of hemoglobin F in neonatal erythrocytes, which is thought to have no pathological significance Note: At birth, red cells contain 53-95% HbF that usually completely disappears by 45-70th day of life; Cf F cell

Fetal heart rate (FHR) OBSTETRICS In the non-stressed fetus, the FHR is a reflection of cardioaccelerator and cardiodecelerator reflexes; proper analysis of the FHR requires evaluation of a baseline FHR occurring between uterine contractions or periodic changes in the FHR and non-periodic, short-term fluctuations in the FHR; see Deceleration

Fetal hemoglobin An 'immature' hemoglobin composed of two α and two γ chains that usually disappears in the neonatal period Fetal-to-adult hemoglobin 'switch' The β

globin locus is comprised of five different genes expressed in embryonic, fetal and adult erythrocytes as a function of the LAR (locus activation region), located 6-20 kilobases upstream of the genes, which turns the genes on, one at a time in predetermined sequence (Nature 1990; 344:309) Note: β hemoglobin is not expressed in fetal erythrocytes, explaining why these cells, circulating in the fetus' 'hypoxic' environment, are not susceptible to sickling; hydroxurea may evoke an increase in hemoglobin F levels and a decrease in sickle cell hemolysis (N Engl J Med 1990; 322:1037); normally, the finding of red cells with fetal hemoglobin in the maternal circulation implies fetal-maternal hemorrhage, measured by the Kleihauer-Betke test (a test that determines the number of erythrocytes with fetal hemoglobin, a value of importance if the infant is Rh-postive and the mother is Rh-negative and requires Rh immune globulin to prevent sensitization against the fetal red cell antigens); in hereditary persistence of fetal hemoglobin (HPFH), the number of cells with hemoglobin F in the maternal circulation is greater than the baby's total blood volume, and therefore the condition's presence may be suspected by mere calculations of maternal and fetal volumes; HPFH may be a) Type I where there is uniform distribution of hemoglobin F in all red cells, as in the Greek, Kenyan and Black American forms and b) Type II where there is heterogeneous distribution of hemoglobin F in all red cells, as in the British and Swiss forms

Fetal hydantoin syndrome A congenital complex caused by in utero exposure to anticonvulsants, affecting the infants of pregnant women being treated with these agents Clinical Growth retardation, microcephaly, midfacial hypo- or dysplasia, hypertelorism, short nose, broad depressed nasal bridge, cleft lip and palate, onychodigital dysplasia, cardiac malformations, mental retardation and rarely neuroblastoma Note: in utero exposure to carbamazepine affects the same organs and to a similar degree as hydantoin, causing craniofacial defects 11%, developmental delay 20% and fingernail hypoplasia 26% (N Engl J Med 1989; 320:1661), which is not unexpected, given that both agents are metabolized by the arene oxide pathway, yielding an intermediate epoxide that may be a direct teratogen Note: Another anticonvulsant, valproic acid in the first trimester is associated with spina bifida; see Fetal trimethadione syndrome

Fetal overgrowth syndrome of Beckwith-Wiedemann A congenital complex related to paternal disomy/maternal deficiency of the chromosome fragment, 11p15.5 (a region that also contains the gene for insulin-like growth factor-2), characterized by gigantism, visceromegaly, macroglossia, exomphalos and hypoglycemia; 12.5% of these subjects suffer tumors associated with a defective chromosome 11p15.5, including Wilm's tumor, hepatoblastoma and rhabdomyosarcoma (Nature 1991; 351:665, 609); see Imprinting

Fetal rubella syndrome see Congenital rubella syndrome

Fetal tissue transplantation BIOMEDICAL ETHICS Fetal tissues are attractive as transplantation 'donors'; they grow readily, are capable of multilineage differentiation and have reduced antigenicity; fetal tissues have been used in experimental protocols for treating immunodeficiency states, metabolic diseases, Parkinson's disease and diabetes mellitus, although the latter two have shown no clear long-term benefits Note: The use of human fetal tissues in research is ethically charged and has been hotly debated in Parliament, the US Congress, Germany and the governing bodies of other nations (Science 1989; 246:775, J Am Med Assoc 1990; 263:565); see Fetal-brain tissue grafting

Fetal tobacco syndrome A malformation complex affecting infants born to women smoking more than one pack of cigarettes/day during pregnancy; the neonates are 200 g lighter, the infant mortality is 40% greater (and is indirectly responsible for 4000 excess infant deaths, in the form of increased spontaneous abortion, fetal wastage, perinatal mortality, sudden infant death syndrome) and the children have impaired cognitive and emotional development; by age 10, children born to actively smoking (as well as 2/3 of infants born to passively 'smoking') mothers are one centimeter shorter, with decreased adult height and are 3-6 months behind peers in measurable parameters of intelligence and have a decreased height as adults; tobacco is synergistic with other environmental toxins impacting on the fetus, eg benzene exposure to infants in utero or in early infancy is implicated in excess leukemia in later life, if one parent also smokes, there is a two-fold increase, if both parents smoke, there is a five-fold increase in leukemias Note: Tobacco smoke contains 4720 different compounds and is the most highly concentrated aerosol known to man and is the most powerful determinant of poor fetal growth in the developed world (J Am Med Assoc 1985; 253:2998); see Passive smoking, Smoking

Fetal trimethadione syndrome A fetal dysmorphia complex described in 1970, affecting two-thirds of pregnancies in which the anti-convulsant, trimethadione was administered Clinical Brachycephaly, midfacial hypoplasia, upslanting eyebrows, saddle nose, prominent forehead, cleft lip and palate, cardiac (eg tetralogy of Fallot, septal defects), genital (eg hypospadias), simian crease, growth and mental retardation and other malformations; Cf Fetal hydantoin syndrome

Fetal Warfarin syndrome A fetal dysmorphia complex caused by in utero exposure to dicumarol (Warfarin) Clinical Developmental defects causing optic atrophy and affecting the central nervous system with fatal fetal bleeding, hypoplasia of the nose and extremities and diffuse epiphyseal 'stippling', similar to Conradi-Huenermann chondrodysplasia punctata Note: Heparin is not teratogenic but may cause stillbirth

FETI Fluorescence excitation transfer immunofluorescence IMMUNOLOGY A laboratory method for measuring the serum levels of various substances, eg morphine, albumin, thyroxin-binding globulin and IgG, in which two fluorescent labels are used, one that fluoresces at a maximum at 525 nm and the other that fluoresces at a minimum at 525 nm; when the antigen is absent in the serum, fluorescence is quenched, as the two cancel each others' effect; when present, the antigen causes a proportionate increase in fluorescence

Fetor hepaticus A sweet, musty odor on the breath of those with hepatic encephalopathy, due to mercaptans, the degradation products of sulfur-containing molecules

Fever The sacred disease Hippocrates considered fever the body's way of burning off toxins, which has proven conceptually correct; Sydenham, the 'English Hippocrates' called fever 'a mighty engine which Nature brings into the world for the conquest of her enemies' (J Infect Dis 1984; 149:339); modern appreciation of hyperpyrexia comes from the desert lizard (***Dipsosaurus dorsalis***), an ectotherm that controls its temperature by moving to hotter places in the cage; animals that are infected but unable to move to warmer areas of a cage, have a higher mortality, lending credence to fever's role in immune defense; when corporal temperature is raised by endogenous pyrogen, T-cell production increases 20-fold; endogenous pyrogen also shifts iron (needed by bacteria) away from plasma; hyperthermia (up to 40°C) has been associated with regression of malignancy, see Coley's toxin

Fever blister(s) Multiple minute perioral vesicles caused by Herpes simplex

Fever of unknown origin (FUO) A febrile state with temperature of 37°C or more of at least two, preferably three weeks in duration, for which a cause cannot be identified despite thorough physical examination and aggressive and relevant laboratory work-up; the etiology ultimately proves infectious in 30-40%, collagen vascular in 15-20% for both children and adults; in adults, 20-30% of the remainder are due to malignancy, which comprises 10% of the remainder in children; other rare causes include sarcoidosis and colitis; hereditary FUOs are rare and appear in Fabry's disease, familial mediterranian fever, type 1 hyperlipidemia and cyclic neutropenia

Fever therapy A therapeutic modality that continues to intrigue cancer biologists, in that hyperthermia is associated with an enhancement of immune function, related to the release of a wide variety of pyrogenic (and nonpyrogenic) cytokines; controlled hyperthermia may be used to enhance tumor cell lysis, and is most successful when combined with chemotherapy and radiotherapy; Cf BCG therapy

F_0F_1 ATPase ATPase synthase membrane protein complex MOLECULAR BIOLOGY A group of 15 proteins that form the enzyme system required to generate ATP from ADP + Pi; the complex is present at all levels of phylogenetic sophistication, from plant and animal; in higher eukaryotes, it is seen as knobby protuberances on the inner membrane of the mitochondrium

FFP Fresh frozen plasma CLINICAL THERAPEUTICS A blood component separated from whole blood at 5°C by centrifugation at 4100 rpm (5000G, a so-called 'hard' spin) and frozen to -18°C within 6 hours of collection; FFP provides 80-120 mg of fibrinogen and at least 80 units each of factors VIII and XIII; FFP is indicated for prothrombin time > 16 seconds, acute hepatic decompensation, massive hemorrhage, massive transfusions where more than 10 units of packed red cells causes coagulation factor depletion; FFP is administered pre-operatively in patients with known coagulopathies, eg hemophilia B, in therapeutic apheresis, disseminated intravascular coagulation, idiopathic thrombocytopenic purpura and hemolytic disease of the newborn

FGF see Fibroblast growth factor

FHR see Fetal heart rate

Fiber Dietary fiber Indigestible plant-derived residues composed predominantly of cellulose; dietary fiber, eg bran, increases the transit time for nutrients in (surgically) shortened gastrointestinal tracts and decreases the transit time in long or constipated gastrointestinal tracts; increased dietary intake of fiber is associated with decreased colonic malignancy and with tumor regression in the premalignant familial adenomatous polyposis (Proc Nat Acad Sci 1989; 81:1290) and diverticulosis; fiber improves the plasma lipid ratios, evoking a 10-17% reduction in cholesterol (including reduced HDL-cholesterol) as well as a reduced dietary intake of energy, fat and cholesterol-rich foods (J Am Diet Assoc 1990; 90:223); see Bran

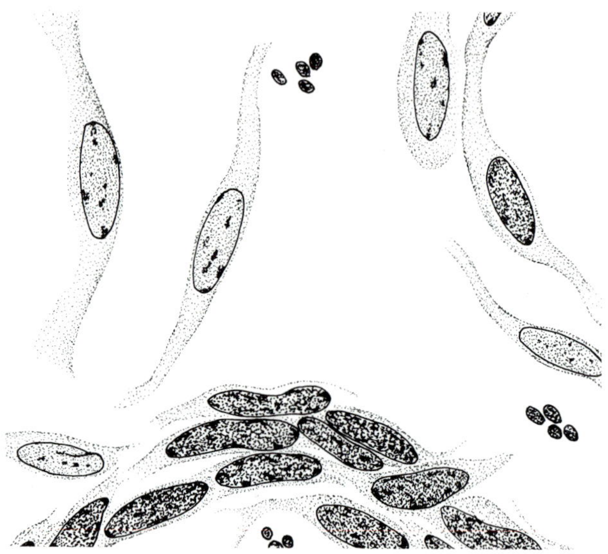

Fiber cells

Fiber cells GYNECOLOGIC CYTOLOGY An elongated malignant epithelial cell (figure) with hyperchromatic nuclei and irregularly clumped chromatin that may be seen in papanicolaou-stained smears of carcinoma-in-situ of the uterine cervix(figure); Cf Tissue culture appearance PULMONARY CYTOLOGY Elongated, twisted keratin-filled malignant cells seen in well-differentiated bronchogenic carcinoma cells, derived from the peripheral 'husks' of squamous pearls ; Cf Tissue culture appearance

Fibrillin A 350 kD glycoprotein that is the main component of microfibrils, which is markedly reduced in Marfan syndrome (N Engl J Med 1990; 323:152)

Fibrin caps Exudative glomerular lesions (figure, page 217) seen in later stages of diabetic glomerulosclerosis composed of aggregates of plasma protein suspended between endothelial or epithelial basement membrane

Fibrin glue A commercial product used to seal operative wounds, by partially re-enacting the final stage of the

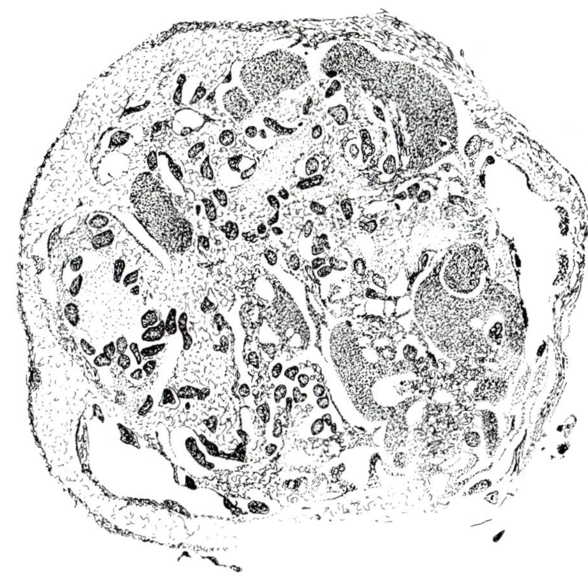

Fibrin caps

coagulation cascade in which fibrinogen is converted to fibrin in the presence of thrombin, factor XIII, fibronectin and calcium ions; lyophilized and concentrated fibrinogen is reconstituted with aprotonin, a proteinase that theoretically enhances the persistence of fibrin, warmed to 37°C; thrombin and calcium chloride are mixed separately and then both are applied with a double-barreled syringe; fibrin sealants are of greatest use in cardiothoracic and general vascular surgery in controlling focal slow bleeding, diffuse oozing, puncture wounds, lymphatic leaks and diffuse parenchymal organ hemorrhage (Transfusion 1990; 30:741rv)

Fibrinoid necrosis 'Smudgy' eosinophilic fibrin-like deposits corresponding to degeneration of collagen or ground substance that may be seen in arterial walls in malignant accelerated hypertension and periarteritis nodosa, but which may also be seen in the Arthus reaction, acute rheumatic fever, subacute bacterial endocarditis, adjacent to peptic ulcers, rheumatoid arthritis, immune complex disease, hepatitis B, malignancy, complement C2 deficiency, Henoch-Schönlein purpura, lupus erythematosus and other collagen vascular disease

Fibrinoligane Coagulation factor XIII (obsolete)

Fibrinolysin Plasmin (obsolete)

Fibroblast growth factor (FGF) Either of two 13.5 kD endothelial cell factors that bind heparin and promote angiogenesis Note: FGF receptor serves as a portal of entry for Herpes Simplex virus-1 (Science 1990; 248:1410)

Fibrocystic disease (FCD) SURGICAL PATHOLOGY A relatively common disease of the female breast, first appearing circa age forty, presenting as a diffusely indurated breast; there appears to be a) No potential for future malignancy in FCD with adenosis (sclerosing or florid), apocrine metaplasia, cysts (macro- or microscopic), ductal ectasia, fibroadenoma, fibrosis, hyperplasia b) Minimal risk for future malignancy with glandular 'crowding', ie 2-4 epithelial cells in depth, mastitis, especially periductal, squamous metaplasia c) 1.5-2-fold increased risk of future malignancy with hyperplasia (moderate or florid, solid or papillary) or in a papilloma with a fibrovascular core d) 2-5-fold increased risk of future malignancy with atypical hyperplasia (borderline lesion), either ductal or lobular Note: Carcinoma-in-situ of the breast carries an 8-10-fold increased risk of future cancer development

Fibroelastosis, endocardial A rare idiopathic condition of early childhood onset with focal or global cartilage-like fibroelastic endocardial thickening, most prominently affecting the left ventricle; the heart may be dilated, hypertrophic or both **Pathogenesis** Uncertain; postulated mechanisms include hypoxia, hemodynamic pressure overload (one-third of cases have congenital cardiac malformations), lymphatic obstruction, fetal endomyocarditis of viral origin, metabolic or enzymatic defects or autoimmune phenomena **Pathology** Increase in collagen and elastic fibers parallel to the surface **Prognosis** Fibroelastosis may cause sudden cardiac arrest in children or slow congestive heart failure in adolescent or adult survivors; Cf Endomyocardial fibrosis

Fibrolamellar carcinoma Polygonal cell hepatocellular carcinoma A rare low-grade hepatocellular carcinoma variant most common in acirrhotic young (age 5-35) females, possibly associated with use of oral contraceptives; 50% are resectable and 50% of the resectable cases are curable **Prognosis** Excellent; the average survival is 32 months, while the usual hepatocellular carcinoma is fatal within 6 months Pathology Nests of deeply eosinophilic neoplastic hepatocytes with cytoplasmic hyalin droplets or pale bodies, surrounded by broad lamellar fibrotic bands

Fibromatoses A family of benign fibrous tissue proliferations that have similar microscopic features and aggressiveness intermediate between benign fibrous lesions and low-grade fibrosarcoma, differing from the former in their marked tendency to recur, and from the latter as they do not metastasize; these lesions are either a) Superficial (fascial), affecting the palm (Dupuytren's contracture), penis (Peyronie's disease) and knuckles or b) Deep (aponeurotic), associated with desmoid tumors

Fibronectin(s) A class of large dimeric glycoproteins that are abundant in the extracellular matrix and basement membrane and mediate the adhesion of cells (through a tetrapeptide, Arg-Gly-Asp-Ser) to fibrin, sulfated proteoglycans and collagens type I, II, III, V and VI; at least 20 different fibronectin chains have been identified, all of which are generated by alternative splicing of the RNA transcript from the fibronectin gene; fibronectin plays a major role in contact inhibition, in cell-substrate adhesion, migration of cells during embryogenesis, inflammation and in wound healing; malignantly transformed cells do not express fibronectin

Fibrous dysplasia A non-neoplastic process affecting the bone that is divisible into a) Monostotic fibrous dysplasia, a condition more common in the femur, tibia and ribs of children and older adolescents and b) Polyostotic fibrous dysplasia, which is less common and associated with endocrinopathy, precocious puberty and cutaneous hyperpigmentation (cafe au lait spots),the triad that defines Albright syndrome Note: Cafe-au-lait spots and fibrous dysplasia without precocious puberty corresponds to Jaffe syndrome **Radiology** Long bones demonstrate a fusiform expansion with multiple loculations **Pathology** The tissue is gray-yellow and gritty to cutting and by light microscopy, demonstrates curved attenuated bony spicules, fancifully likened to fishhooks or Chinese characters (see there) lying in a fibroblastic background **Treatment** Curettage

Fibrous plaque The advanced lesion of atherosclerosis, composed of proliferated smooth muscle fibers, macrophages (foam cells or lipid-laden histiocytes) and lymphocytes; the plaque surface is covered by Pancake cells overlying a dense connective tissue matrix that may 'prolapse' into the vascular lumen, deforming blood flow; calcium deposition in the plaque, cracking and ulceration, results in a 'complicated' plaque; Cf Fatty streak

FICA Fluoroimmunocytoadherence IMMUNOLOGY A technique in which column chromatography is used to isolate antigen-binding cells

Ficin A thiol proteinase used in transfusion medicine to remove the sialic acid, thereby reducing the zeta potential and by extension, increasing the immunologic 'signal' and therefore the detection of weak or non-agglutinating antibodies; ficin treatment enhances Ii, Kidd, Lewis and Rh agglutination and destroys Duffy, MNSs, Lutheran, Chido, Rogers, Tn and others

Ficoll IMMUNOLOGY A synthetic 400 kD, water soluble sucrose and epichlorohydrin polymer used to prepare Ficoll-Hypaque, a proprietary density gradient medium used to separate and purify leukocytes by centrifugation, after the 'buffy coat' has been removed by pipetting from blood diluted in saline or Hanks medium; Ficoll-Hypaque separation provides optimal preparation of leukocytes and platelets for flow cytometric analysis

Fiddleback spider see Brown spider

Fidelity MOLECULAR BIOLOGY The accuracy with which any molecule is copied (replicated), translated or transcribed

Field effect The action of an agent on an entire organ system EMBRYOLOGY The field effect refers to a combination of specific multisystem defects, eg in a renal/supermammary nipple defect (Am J Dis Child 1987; 141:989) ONCOLOGY The field effect is the constellation of loco-regional changes resulting from carcinogenic toxin(s) that induce frankly malignant changes in one site and concomitantly cause premalignant dysplasia or carcinoma-in-situ in the remaining organ, tissue or 'field'; thus despite adequate resection, the remaining field may be 'cancerized', despite a normal appearance, thus making it more susceptible to future malignancy; the effect occurs in tissue of any embryologic origin, and is easily recognized in epithelia of the colon, breast ducts, bladder, bronchial and laryngeal epithelium; in one classic study (Cancer 1967; 20:699), 38 000 sections were obtained from 250 patients with bronchial carcinoma; using strict histologic criteria, 3.5% had a second primary carcinoma; in contrast, a field effect is difficult to prove in non-epithelial tissues and its existence is implied by such terms as 'pseudolymphoma' and 'smooth muscle tumor of uncertain malignant potential'; Cf 'Cancerization'

Field inversion electrophoresis (FIE) MOLECULAR BIOLOGY A gel electrophoresis technique that allows separation of large DNA molecules, which migrate at similar rates, despite large differences in length, due to 'reptation'; in FIE, the electric field is periodically inverted, such that the DNA makes large movements forward and small movements backward

Fiery agent of the Israelites Filariasis

Fièvre boutonneuse A benign rickettsial spotted fever caused by ***Rickettsia coronii***, affecting visitors to the Mediterranean rim countries (natives develop permanent immunity) Vector Dog tick, ***Rhipicephalus sanguineus*** **Clinical** Initial lesion is a tache noire or primary eschar, followed by a diffuse maculopapular, later petechial rash with little systemic illness; agglutinin reactions to OX19 and OX2 are positive in the second week **Treatment** Doxycycline, tetracycline, chloramphenicol

Fifth disease Erythema infectiosum A childhood exanthema caused by the moderately contagious B19 parvovirus; the condition was so named as it was the fifth childhood disease typically accompanied by a rash; the other nosologies classically associated with rashes in childhood are rubella, measles, scarlet fever and a mild, atypical variant of scarlet fever (Filatov-Dukes disease); Cf Fourth disease, Sixth disease

Fifth pathway GRADUATE MEDICAL EDUCATION A route by which foreign, ie non-North American medical graduates may become eligible to begin internship or residency, ie specialty training in the USA, consisting of a year of supervised clinical training; the fifth pathway was created in response to one country's withholding of the medical school diplomas from the graduates until they had provided a year of rural service

Fifth plague of Egypt An epidemic of ancient Egypt described in the Bible's Old Testament (Exodus 9:3); although the agent of the fifth plague is unknown, medical historians postulated various nosologies including plague (***Yersinia pestis***), foot and mouth disease (picornavirus), rinderpest, anthrax and Rift Valley fever (J Am Med Assoc 1986; 256:1444c)

Fight bite A jagged laceration on the dorsum of the hand, often over the knuckles, seen when belligerent A's fist strikes belligerent B's teeth, causing abrasions, deep lacerations, puncture wounds and a sizeable inoculum of mixed oral flora, including staphylococci, 50% of which produce penicillinase, also β-hemolytic streptococci, ***Eikenella corrodens***; without treatment, a fight bite may become complicated, resulting in the clenched fist 'syndrome'

Fight-or-flight response General adaption 'syndrome' A generalized 'physiological' reaction displayed by most mammals in the face of imminent danger or anticipated pain; this emergency response evokes a full-scale activation of the central nervous system and the release of 'stressors' by the adrenal medulla, eg epinephrine and norepinephrine and cortex, eg corticosteroids, mineralocorticoids, as well as renin and insulin **Clinical** Tachycardia, diaphoresis, tremor, pallor, increased inotropism, vasoconstriction, mydriasis, bronchodilation and hyperglycemia

FIGLU Formiminoglutamic acid A breakdown product of histidine that is increased in the urine in folic acid deficiency (which diminishes purine biosynthesis and is partially offset by the ability of accumulated 5-amino-4-imidazole carboxamide ribotide to slow purine degradation); elevated urinary FIGLU after oral histidine ingestion favors a diagnosis of folic acid deficiency as the cause of a megaloblastic anemia Note: two-thirds of patients with vitamin B_{12} deficiency also have increased FIGLU excretion

FIGO International Federation of Gynecologists and Obstetricians A major contribution of this international body of experts has been to stage gynecologic malignancy, in particular, carcinomas of the ovary (table)

FIGO Staging, ovarian carcinoma

Stage I Malignancy of one (Ia) or both (Ib) ovaries, without ascites Five-year survival: 60%

Stage II Malignancy of one (IIa) or both (IIb) ovaries, with pelvic extension and ascites Five-year survival: 40%

Stage III Malignancy involves one or both ovaries, intraperitoneal metastases outside pelvis and/or positive retroperitoneal lymph nodes Five-year survival: 5%

Stage IV Involvement of one/both ovaries with metastases and histologically confirmed extension to pleural cavity or liver Five-year survival, 3%

Figure 3 sign Pediatrics A combination of pre- and post-stenotic aortic dilation seen on a plain chest film of patients with postductal coarctation of the aorta; when this same finding is viewed by a barium 'swallow' study, it is known as the 'letter E' signs due to two vertical indentations in a barium-filled esophagus; the higher indentation corresponds to the left subclavian artery and the aortic knob, the lower indentation corresponds to post-stenotic aortic dilatation; Cf Reverse 3 sign

Figure 8 appearance Molecular biology A descriptor for the 'cartoon' model of two circles of DNA partially linked by a recombination event in progress

Figure 8 sign see Snowman sign

Filaggrin A structural protein that specifically binds to intermediate filaments

Filaments see Intermediate filaments

Filamin Cell physiology A flexible homodimeric protein produced by smooth muscle cells and fibroblasts, composed of two 270 kD chains, which is involved in sol-gel transitions in vertebrate cells and links actin fibers, enabling them to form a three-dimensional network, which in solution, forms a semisolid gel

Filaria A generic term for nematodal worms of the superfamily Filarioidea that cause human disease, including ***Wuchereria bancrofti, Brugia malayi, Loa loa***, microfilaria of ***Mansonella*** (formerly, ***Dipetalonema***) ***perstans***, ***Mansonella ozzardi*** and ***Onchocirca volvulus***; filarial vectors include the mosquito (***Aedes, Culex, Mansonia***), black fly (***Simulium***), midge (***Culicoides***) and tabanid fly (***Chryosops***)

Filarial fever Acute, recurring, episodes of high-grade fever, often with shaking chills, edema, lymphadenitis with retrograde progression, caused by filarial permeation of lymphatic channels, by ***Wuchereria bancrofti***, ***Brugia malayi*** and ***Loa loa***; filarial fever occurs 5-10 times/year and each 'attack' lasts about a week; microfilariasis per se is asymptomatic

Filgrastim see G-CSF

Film badge Nuclear medicine A device that holds a photographic film capable of absorbing radiation, which is used to quantify a person's exposure to occupation-related X-rays and gamma-radiation; the maximum radiation exposure allowed by the NIOSH is 5000 mRad/year or 1500 mRad for any one quarter

Fimbrin An actin-binding protein that cross-links adjacent filaments, forming parallel actin filaments

Finder's fee Compensatory remuneration for a service rendered, eg locating or finding a client; this practice derives from the world of business and when used in a medical context, is a fee offered to a physician for his help in locating subjects for participation in clinical trials of diagnostic or therapeutic modalities, as an attempt to reduce the chronic problem of finding an adequate number of appropriate subjects for such trials (N Engl J Med 1990; 323:192); Cf Fee splitting

Fine droplet fatty liver see Fatty liver

Finger motif Molecular biology see Zinc-finger motif

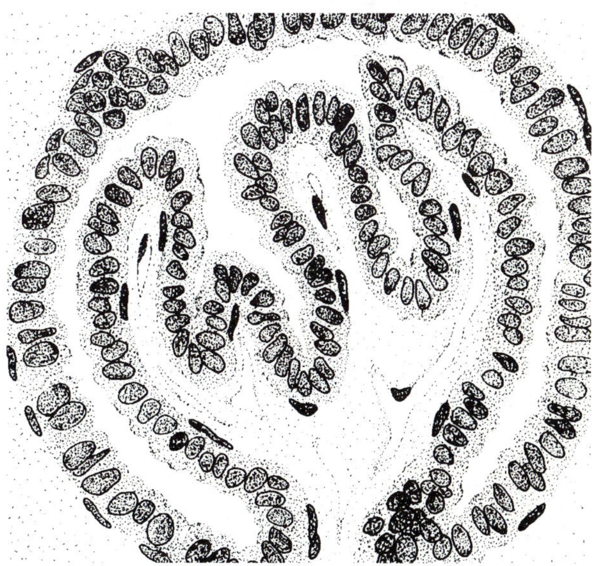

Finger-in-glove appearance

Finger fracturing A crude post-mortem technique for evaluating an organ's consistency, where increases or decreases in firmness, determined by simple 'pinching'

of a 1-2 cm in thickness slice of tissue is suggestive of certain pathological nosologies; under normal circumstances, the liver fractures readily; in cirrhosis, the liver is markedly indurated due to intense fibrosis; contrarily, normal lung is resistant to fracturing and in acute necrotizing pneumonia, it may be pinched, shredded or easily torn

Finger-in-glove appearance SURGICAL PATHOLOGY Focal glandular outpouchings seen within glands in mild endometrial hyperplasia (figure, page 219), which may be secondary to chronic anovulation and/or associated with Stein-Leventhal syndrome and infertility RADIOLOGY 'Gloved finger' shadow of Simon A descriptor for a mucoid plug within a bronchiectatic segment of a fibrotically thickened bronchus or bronchiole, as seen on a plain film of the chest

Finger nucleases Those enzymes secreted by the skin of the digits that are capable of digesting ribonucleic acid, especially RNA, thus requiring special precaution by molecular biologists who do 'RNA work'

Fingerprint DERMATOGLYPHICS Increased ulnar loops and decreased whorls and arches are seen in Alzheimer's disease (Arch 1985; 42:50), a pattern similar to that seen in Down syndrome; see Dermatoglyphics

Fingerprint appearance RENAL PATHOLOGY A descriptor for the layered epithelial crescents, thrombi and hematoxylin material, accompanied by granular deposition of IgG, C3 and fibrin in diffuse glomerulonephritis **Ultrastructure** Reticular aggregates in capillary endothelium, which in lupus erythematosus may represent a reaction of the endoplasmic reticulum to injury

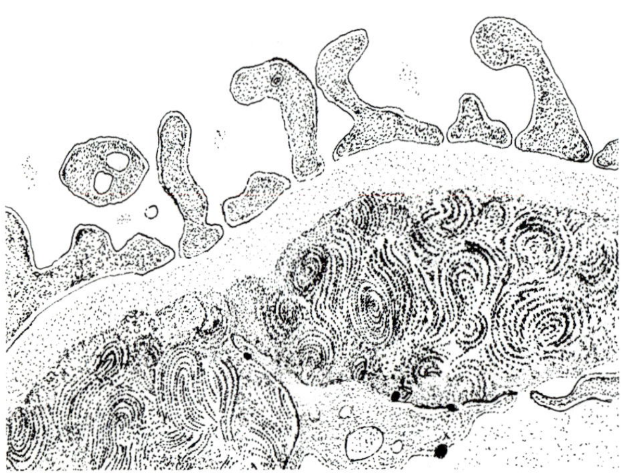

Fingerprint appearance

Fingerprint, chemical The 'signature(s)' that a chemical compound and its metabolites have, when analyzed by a highly sensitive technique, eg HPLC or GC-MS, which may be stored on a computer's hard disk and electronically matched ('fingerprinted') with an unknown specimen for the purpose of identification

Fingerprint pattern OPHTHALMOLOGY A horizontally-oriented, whorled filagreed layering with apposition and separation of linear densities of vacuolated ground substance, seen in corneal dystrophy; the pleomorphic gray opacities are slightly basophilic, amorphous intraepithelial material under the corneal basement membrane, composed of a protein-polysaccharide matrix, seen in microcystic or map-dot dystrophy **Ultrastructure** Amorphous fibrillogranular material

Fingerprint profile A type of 'mixed' or irregular cytoplasmic inclusions composed of ceroid/lipofuscin, appearing as short curved lamellations, seen by electron microscopy in juvenile lipofuscinosis (Batten-Spielmeyer-Vogt disease) **Clinical** Intellectual deterioration, progressive loss of motor function, ataxia and retinal pigmentary degeneration; death commonly by early adulthood **Treatment** None; see Curvilinear profiles; Fingerprint profiles may also be seen in peripheral lymphocytes or skin fibroblasts in amaurotic familial idiocy, fucosidosis, Hermansky-Pudlak disease, Jansky-Bielschowsky syndrome and Kufs' disease

Fingerprint, protein A highly characteristic pattern of spots that identifies a protein in a relatively specific fashion **Technique** A protease, eg trypsin, digests a relatively pure protein, eg hemoglobin for detecting a β chain of interest; the digestion cuts the protein after every arginine and after every lysine residue; the resulting fragments are electrophoresed, then turned at 90° and chromatographed, producing a two-dimensional 'fingerprint' that is visualized by spraying with ninhydrin, turning the paper with the polypeptide fragments purple (Biochim Biophys Acta 1958; 28:543)

Fingerprinting, DNA MOLECULAR BIOLOGY DNA fingerprinting may be defined in terms similar to that of RNA fingerprinting, ie oligonucleotide sequence pattern-matching; DNA fingerprinting currently refers to a technique based on short, tandem-repeated (or hypervariable) genomic sequences (minisatellites) that are highly specific; the likelihood that two individuals have the same DNA fingerprint is approximately 1:30 billion, and thus is more specific than RFLP (restriction fragment length polymorphism) analysis; the insert-free wild-type M13 bacteriophage detects these hypervariable minisatellites, which have an accordion-like length since the number of 'repeats' varies with each person; the DNA sequence that detects these differences is located to two clusters of 15 base pair repeats translating to (Glu, Gly, Gly, Gly, Ser)n in the bacteriophage's protein III gene; this probe's (Jeffries probe, Nature 1985; 314/316:67) specificity makes it useful in paternity testing, in human genome mapping and forensic medicine, where it is being increasingly used in criminal law (J Am Med Assoc 1988; 259:2193, Science 1989; 244:1033, ibid 246:1558); see Bandshift

Fingerprinting, RNA A method used to identify specific RNA molecules **Principle** RNAse T1 is used to cut RNA at the 3' end of each guanylate residue, resulting in short 2-20 base pair oligonucleotide sequences, allowing a matching of two RNAs by length, without the need to sequence the RNA

Finnish congenital nephrotic syndrome An autosomal recessive form of proliferative mesangial glomerulosclerosis that is frequent in Finns, often fatal, associated with eclampsia and low birth weight **Pathogenesis**

Absence of heparin sulfate anionic sites in the glomerular basement membrane with alteration of type IV collagen **Histopathology** Microcystic changes in the tubules at the corticomedullary junction and arteriolar hypertrophy **Treatment** None; Cf French congenital nephrotic syndrome

Fire ant An arthropod that is acquiring increasing importance in clinical medicine; the black imported fire ant, ***Solenopsis saevissima richteri*** and the red imported fire ant, ***S invicta*** are originally native to South America and have spread extensively in the southeastern USA as they have no natural enemies; they are omnivorous, attacking livestock, crops and electrical insulation; the fire ant sting injects a venom causing intense burning and pruritus, due to the presence of necrotoxin or solenamine; the reactions range from a wheal-and-flare response, a sterile pustule to anaphylaxis-related death (32 have been reported); fire ant venom is 95% alkaloid with a small aqueous fraction containing soluble proteins Note: In contrast, hymenopteran (wasps, bees and hornets) venom is an aqueous solution containing proteins (N Engl J Med 1990; 323:462)

First arch syndrome A sequence type of developmental embryopathy with anomalous development of the first branchial arch due to inadequacy of the stapedial artery, a function of maternal nutrition during early pregnancy **Clinical** Facial bone hypoplasia, including macrostomia, hemignathia and mandibular deformity Note: These changes may be accompanied by hypertelorism, cleft lip and palate, deformities of the middle and inner ear or may accompany well-described clinical syndromes, including Franceschetti-Klein, Goldenhar, Pierre-Robin and Treacher-Collin syndromes; see Sequence

First order kinetics A reaction system in which the rate of an enzyme reaction is determined by substrate concentration; this is difficult to define in closed systems since the rate changes as more substrate is consumed; see Michaelis-Menten equation; Cf Zero order kinetics

First pass elimination Presystemic elimination The rate at which circulating drugs are metabolized as they traverse the liver; first pass elimination kinetics assume the amount of parent drug arriving to the liver is proportional to its concentration in the circulation, and further assumes there is optimal blood flow, uncompromised hepatic function, free access of the drug to the liver's metabolic 'machinery', appropriate transportation by carrier molecules

First use syndrome An anaphylactoid reaction described in patients undergoing hemodialysis, which occurs with the first use of a dialyzer, attributed to various dialyzer substances or to residual ethylene oxide, which is used for sterilization (MMWR 1991; 40:147)

Fisch-Renwick syndrome A variant of Klein-Waardenberg syndrome characterized by congenital deafness, hypertelorism, high palatal arch, ocular heterochromia and a white forelock

Fish A 'high quality' source of protein and essential oil HAZARDS OF EATING FISH (DAMNED IF YOU DO...) a) Fish oil Despite its cardioprotective effects, high levels of fish oil may cause nosebleeds due to impaired platelet function (J Pediatr 1990; 116:139) b) Envenonation, see Ciguatera poisoning, Scombroid poisoning c) Heavy metal poisoning, eg mercury, which concentrates up the food chain, especially in certain fish, eg tuna d) Parasitosis, see Sushi BENEFITS OF EATING FISH (...DAMNED IF YOU DON'T) The beneficial effects of fish consumption are attributed to fish oil's omega-3 or n-3 fatty acids, including eicosapentanoic and docosahexanoic acids Note: Deep water trout has three-fold more n-3 oil than other fish; effects of fish oil on disease, see review, J Am Med Assoc 1989:261:698rv; fish oil's benefits may be a function of the length of the fatty acid acyl chain (C20 and C22) rather than polyunsaturation (N Engl J Med 1990; 322:403c) a) Atherosclerosis Omega-3 oil inhibits production of platelet-derived growth factor (PDGF) in endothelial cell cultures; PDGF causes smooth muscle proliferation, a factor in atherogenesis, possibly related to free radical production b) Cardiovascular effects The incidence of myocardial infarcts in Danes and Americans is ten-fold greater than that of Greenland Eskimos, despite similar levels of dietary fat; Danes consumed twice the saturated fat and more n-6 polyunsaturated fat than Eskimos, who consumed 5-10 g/d of long-chain n-3 polyunsaturated eicosapentanoic acid (C20:5n-3) and docosahexaenoic acid (C22:6n-3), essential fatty acids are concentrated up the food chain from phytoplankton to fish to marine mammals c) Diabetes mellitus n-3 lipids prevent the insulin resistance induced in rats by non-'aquatic' fat (n-6 fat derived from vegetables and meats rather than fish), replacement of 6% of the vegetable oil with n-3 fish oil circumvents the insulin-resistance otherwise seen in the rats d) Hypertension Marine oils are high in n-3 polyunsaturated fatty acids (PFA); salad oils are high in n-6 fatty acids; vegetable PFAs are reported to decrease platelet aggregation, vaso-occlusive events and blood pressure, evoking low-level decreases in both diastolic and systolic pressures, as well as decreasing the levels of thromboxane A_2 metabolites (N Engl J Med 1989; 320:1037; ibid, 1990; 322:795) e) Longevity When n-3 fish oil replaces corn oil or lard in the laboratory rodent diet, they live longer, have less atherosclerosis, arterionephrosclerosis and produce fewer autoantibodies

FISH Fluorescent in situ hybridization An experimental technique for determining the ploidy by evaluation of interphase (non-dividing) nuclei in samples used for cytological analysis and cytogenetic studies

Fisher syndrome Ophthalmoplegia-ataxia-areflexia syndrome A variant of Guillain-Barré syndrome seen in middle-aged males after a viral infection of the upper respiratory tract **Clinical** Headache, fever, dyspnea, facial paralysis and cerebellar ataxia; most resolve spontaneously within 3 months or progress to coma (N Engl J Med 1956; 255:57)

Fisher syndrome CM Fisher, J Neurol Neurosurg Psychiatry 1967; 30:383; see One and a half syndrome

Fisher-Volavsek syndrome An autosomal dominant condition characterized by syringomyelia, sparseness of facial and scalp hair and thickening of the terminal digits

Fish-eye disease A rare autosomal dominant condition with intense corneal opacification and vague non-specific atherosclerosis-related cardiac disease **Laboratory**

Reduced high-density lipoprotein (HDL), increased triglycerides (2.8-4.0 mmol/L US: 250-350 mg/dl) and cholesterol (8.7-13.8 mmol/L US: 340-540 mg/dl) Pathogenesis Defective esterification of free cholesterol into HDL Note: Similar corneal opacities occur in Tangier's disease and in combined apolipoprotein A-I and C-III deficiency (N Engl J Med 1982; 306:1513); Cf LCAT deficiency

Fish facies A physiognomy characterized by antimongolic palpebral fissures, colobomata, fishmouth, total deafness and malformation of ears, fancifully likened to that of aquatic poikilothermic vertebrates, seen in mandibulo-facial dysostosis, Treacher-Collins syndrome and Franceschetti syndrome

Fish flesh A descriptor denoting both the tactile sensation and gross appearance of mesenchymal tumors, seen in sarcomas, but also lymphomas and florid reactive lymphoid hyperplasia

Fishhook sign Radiology An upwardly curved or J-shaped distal ureter, seen by cystography, characteristic of prostatic hypertrophy

Fish-mouth deformity A facial deformity characterized by cleft lip or palate and accompanied by patellar dimples, supernumerary ribs, arachnodactyly, talipes equinovarus, cardiac malformations, hypoplastic external genitalia, hypotonia and seizures, findings typical of the Prader-Willi syndrome (Curr Prob Ped 1984; 14:1), as well as in the 18q- syndrome

Fishmouth incision A wide horizontal incision made on the tip of the finger to provide drainage for a subungual abscess

Fishmouthing' Critical care medicine Lower jaw depression with inspiration, an ominous sign of increasing medullary damage with apneic potential in the face of autonomic respiratory failure

Fishmouth stenosis Buttonhole deformity Cardiology A flattened and stenosed mitral valve caused by fibrous bridging across valvular commissures, commonly associated with rheumatic heart disease

'Fish smell see Fishy odor

Fishtail lesions Ophthalmology Scattered pisciform yellow spots, seen in the optic fundus of young subjects with the autosomally inherited fundus flavimaculatus Clinical Bilateral, slowly progressive posterior pole degeneration, which overlaps with Stargardt's macular atrophy, and with time, causes a loss of visual acuity

Fish tank granuloma An opportunistic infection by an 'atypical' mycobacteria, ***M marinum,*** after inoculation in contaminated fresh or salt water, that may occur in occupational exposure, and in ***M avium-intercellulare-scrofulaceum*** (N Engl J Med 1982; 307:1456) Clinical A solitary nodule develops at sites of abrasion (fingers and hands), later becoming indurated and ulcerated, resembling 'garden variety' cutaneous tuberculosis; occasionally developing satellite lesions, thus being clinically identical to the Swimming pool granuloma

Fish tapeworm ***Diphyllobothrium latum*** A tapeworm that parasitizes freshwater fish of temperate zones in the Northern hemisphere (***D pacificum*** has been described in marine fish off Peru); the definitive hosts are humans, domestic pets and other mammals *D latum* is the largest known vertebrate tapeworm, measuring 10 meters in length with 4000 proglottids, the most distal of which disintegrate, releasing eggs into the feces that mature and hatch into ciliated coracium; the coracium are ingested by the first intermediate host, an aquatic arthropod, the copepod, which is then ingested by a second intermediate host, a freshwater fish, eg salmon, trout and whitefish; the eggs develop into procercoid larvae in the fish muscle and viscera and are eaten by man as raw fish and the cycle continues Clinical In general, infection is limited to one worm, causing nervous and gastrointestinal symptoms, abdominal discomfort, weakness, loss of weight, malnutrition and megaloblastic anemia Treatment Niclosamide

Fish vertebrae Radiology A descriptor for biconcave, fish-like vertebrae, resulting from infarction and central bone collapse secondary to thrombosis of the vertebral arteries, a finding typical of sickle cell anemia, which often occurs before the second decade; the periphe-ral perforating metaphyseal arteries are relatively spared, explaining the lesser involvement of the anterior and posterior faces of the vertebrum; fish vertebrae may also be seen in hereditary spherocytosis, homocystinuria, Gaucher's disease, osteoporosis and osteopenia, renal osteodystrophy or hyperparathyroidism, osteomalacia and thalassemia major

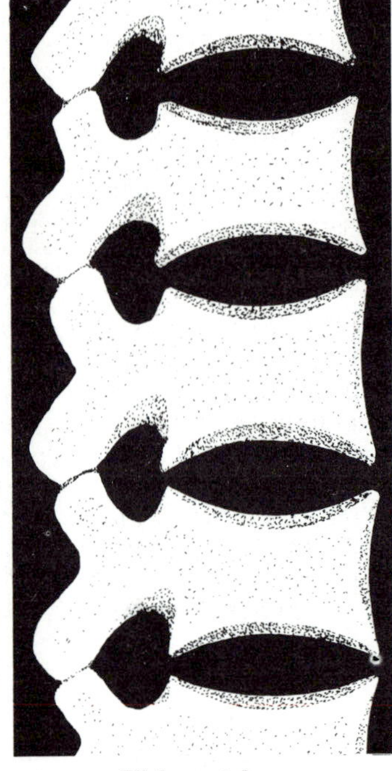

Fish vertebra

Fishy odor A piscine odor described in wide variety of clinical conditions, eg vaginosis, caused by a newly-described ***Mobiluncus*** genus, ***Gardnerella vaginalis,*** excretion of trimethylaminuriae (due to large ora doses of L carnitine, 'rotting' fish), di-N-butylamine, diethylamine, stools infected by ***Vibrio cholera***, which have a 'rice-water' appearance, a rancid fish odor is described in tyrosinemia, which may occur in hereditary tyrosinosis (tyrosinemia type I) or in severe hepatic failure; see Odors

FITC Fluorescein-isothiocyanate A stable 'label' that binds both basic and acidic protein side chains at pH 8.0, which fluoresces at 490 and 520 nm; FITC is a 'workhorse reagent' in immunology and is used to 'tag' proteins of interest and follow their movement in the cell or site(s) of deposition; it may be used clinically to evaluate complement and immunoglobulin deposits in a)

The skin in patients with vesiculobullous lesions and b) The kidneys to detect immune complex deposition, both by direct immune fluorescence; see Flow cytometry, Immunofluorescence

Five day fever see Trench fever

5p- syndrome see Cri-du-Chat syndrome

Five Fs Food, fingers, fomites, flies, feces; a mnemonic for the most common mode of transmission of ***Salmonella typhi***

Fixed drug reaction A skin eruption of unknown pathogenesis that more commonly afflicts blacks, characteristically recurring at the same site each time a particular drug or a related congener is administered; the fixed reaction may also occur with chemically unrelated drugs or disappear with repeated administration of the same drug **Clinical** The fixed reaction lesion is a sharply circumscribed edematous red-brown or purplish plaque that may be surmounted by a bulla, most often located on the extremities, the hands and glans peniswhich with time, becomes lichenified, scaly, and occasionally accompanied by hypermelanosis; common drugs and chemicals evoking the reaction include phenazone, barbiturates, sulfonamides, quinine, tetracycline, oxyphenbutazone, chlordiazepoxide, food dyes, toothpaste and mothballs **Histopathology** Erythema multiforme-like changes, including hydropic degeneration of the basal cell layer, pigmentary incontinence and scattered dyskeratotic keratinocytes

'Fixover' SURGICAL PATHOLOGY A specimen that is not processed on the day of surgery because it requires fixation in formalin prior to cutting, eg large resections of the gastrointestinal tract, which if sectioned prematurely are associated with 'rolling' of the mucosa away from the muscularis propria, making staging, ie evaluation of the depth of tumor invasion difficult; in contrast, some tissues, eg uterine leiomyomas become 'hardened' by prolonged fixation and brittle to cutting by a microtome

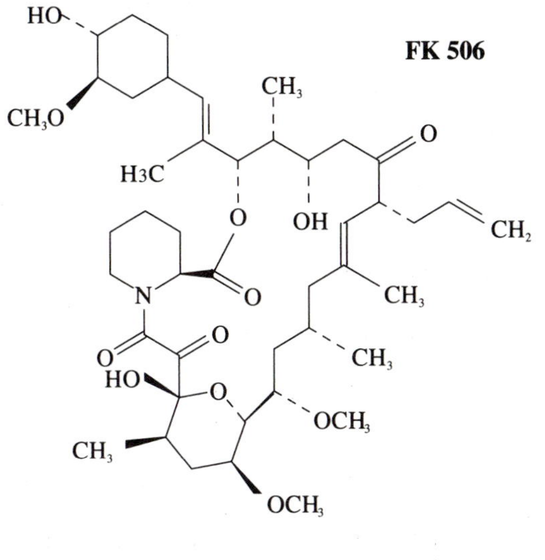

FK 506

FK 506 An immunosuppressive agent (figure) produced by ***Streptomyces tsukubaensis*** (Fujisawa, Osaka), developed to counteract transplant rejection; FK506 inhibits interleukin-2 (IL-2) synthesis and binding and is both similar to, and synergistic with cyclosporine, but is reported to be 50-fold more immunosuppressive than cyclosporine; FK 506 is used in kidney (J Am Med Assoc 1990; 264:63) and liver transplantation and is of potential use in lung transplantation **Side effects** Nephrotoxicity (not dose limiting), neurotoxicity, possible induction of diabetes (effects similar to cyclosporine), as well as headache, nausea, paresthesiae of hands and feet and insomnia

FKBP FK 506 binding protein A rotamase enzyme and receptor for FK 506 and rapamycin (Science 1991; 252:836); FKBP's amino acid sequence is similar or identical to that of protein kinase C (Nature 1991; 351:195c)

Flabby heart An atonic, dilated and fat-laden heart characteristic of ***Corynebacterium diphtheriae***-induced myocarditis; the flabbiness of the heart is attributed to a diphtheria exotoxin that interferes with a translocating enzyme responsible for elongation of polypeptide chains; the same exotoxin inhibits carnitine metabolism, thereby interfering with the oxidation of long-chain fatty acids, with the consequent accumulation of triglycerides in the cardiac muscle

'Flag' LABORATORY MEDICINE A determined value on a diagnostic test at or above which a certain action is taken; eg fasting glucose > 7.8 mmol/L (US: > 140 mg/dl), is a flag for notifying the attending physician; see Decision level, Panic value, Red flag

Flagella The organelle responsible for bacterial locomotion; average bacterial flagella measures 10-30 µg in diameter, best appreciated by a modified Leifson stain; flagella are classified according to location on the bacterium: Peritrichous, polar and mixed; like eukaryotic cilia, prokaryotic flagella have the characteristic 9 + 2 arrangement of fibrils; see Cilia

Flagellin MOLECULAR BIOLOGY A fibrous bacterial protein, which is the major component of flagella and which has structural homology with keratin, myosin and fibrinogen

Flag sign CLINICAL NUTRITION The finding of sharply demarcated alternating bands of pigmented and depigmented hair, evidence of intermittent malnutrition, seen in kwashiorkor and marasmus type of malnutrition, or rarely, associated with chemotherapy, eg methotrexate (Cancer 1983; 51:1356)

Flail chest TRAUMATOLOGY The result of multiple anterior rib fractures; for 'flailing' to occur, there must be a two-point fracture involving at least two adjacent ribs, although these fractures are usually symptomatic if four or more ribs are involved in one hemithorax; this causes instability of a large area of the anterior chest wall, paradoxic movement during inspiration, ie the free-floating 'flailed' part moves inward as the chest expands, in response to the negative intrathoracic pressure; the extent and location of the fractures determines the adequacy of ventilation, ranging from asymptomatic to severe dyspneic; hypoxemia is common, but not hypercapnia or alveolar hypoventilation; when conscious, the patient may 'splint' the segment, causing the examiner to pass over the lesion; the inability to maintain adequate ventilation in concert with the paradoxic (and ineffective) respiratory effort and atelectasis, hypoxia and hypercapnia develop; posterior flail segments are less of a concern as the muscles and scapula provide 'scaffolding', and patients lie on their backs, supported by the mattress; flail chest most often secondary to motor vehicle accidents or aggressive cardiopulmonary resuscitation

Flake maneuver EMERGENCY MEDICINE A variant of the Heimlich maneuver, in which the victim lies with his head down, eg stairs and pumps his own diaphragm; the Heimlich maneuver has the considerable disadvantage of a) Requiring two people to perform and b) May worsen the situation by causing the food to pop up, then sink even further down the trachea as the patient gasps for air; Cf Cough CPR, Heimlich maneuver

'Flaky paint' dermatitis A dermatopathy characterized by irregular, dry, hyperkeratotic, hyperpigmented psoriasiform lesions located on the face, extremities and perineum that may become excoriated and infected, seen in Kwashiorkor

Flame cells Thesaurocytes Plasma cells with intensely eosinophilic (flaming) cytoplasm containing glycoprotein globules; although these cells were initially considered specific for IgA myelomas, flame cells also occur in Waldenström's disease and the leptomeningitis of African trypanosomiasis adjacent to clusters of neutrophils; Cf Mulberry cells, which are cytologically similar, although the material appears to be membrane-bound

Flame figure DERMATOPATHOLOGY Aggregates of smudged necrobiotic material from decomposed eosinophilic granules and nuclear debris and collagen, seen in eosinophilic cellulitis or Wells syndrome (Acta Derm Venereol (Stockh) 1986; 66:213) **Clinical** Episodic waves of pruritic cutaneous tumefactions (and eosinophilia) spreading over the body for 2-3 days, resolving within 1-2 months

Flame photometry A laboratory technique used to identify elements in a solution, eg calcium and potassium, where a fluid of interest is atomized and sprayed into a flame produced from a mixture of gases including oxygen, hydrogen, natural gas and acetylene; the emission spectrum is analyzed as the electrons excited by the flame fall to a lower energy level

Flame-shaped lesion Splinter lesion A hemorrhage in the nerve fiber layer of the optic fundus, seen in grade III hypertensive retinopathy, whichresolves 4-6 weeks after acute hypertensive crisis, and may occur in anemia, leukemia, arteriolosclerotic retinopathy and diabetes mellitus Note: Dot and blot hemorrhages, cotton-wool spots and waxy exudates are fundoscopic findings also seen in grade III hypertension

Flanking DNA Any fragment of DNA that is immediately adjacent, either upstream or downstream of a DNA segment of interest

Flap PLASTIC SURGERY A pedicle of tissue, used to cover a defect, usually of the skin; flaps are cut in such a way as to leave a well-vascularized base of the 'peninsula', and sewn at the site of the defect, allowing time for free end to become vascularized before separating the tissue from the 'donor' site

Flapping Flapping tremor Asterixis Icarus sign HEPATOLOGY An abnormal, involuntary jerking tremor of wide amplitude elicited upon dorsiflexion of the pronated wrist and spreading of extended fingers; in full-blown flapping, there is abrupt flexion of the fingers at the metacarpophalangeal joint and flexion of the wrist, occurring asynchronously with each other every few seconds, due to exaggerated reflexes; bilateral flapping is quasi-pathognomonic for metabolic, often alcohol-related, hepatic encephalopathy seen in end-stage (post fibrotic) cirrhosis due to increased blood ammonia NEONATOLOGY Coarse bilateral tremors, accompanied by limb rigidity, hyperreflexia, resistance to flexion and extension, described in infants born to heroin-addicted mothers who undergo 'withdrawal' at birth

Flare OPHTHALMOLOGY A 'spume' of translucent proteins in the aqueous humor, appearing as a whitish shadow as a beam of light traverses the anterior chamber, the intensity of the flare is a function of the amount of protein in the anterior chamber, being faintly visible in the normal eye and prominent in anterior uveitis, accompanied by conjunctival hyperemia, inflammation and posterior corneal keratinization, congestion of the iris, neovascularization and band formation; see Band keratopathy RHEUMATOLOGY An acute exacerbation of the symptoms of lupus erythematosus and disease activity **Laboratory** Increased levels of anti-double-stranded DNA antibodies, plasma C3a, serum complex of complement 5b-9 and plasma Bb and decreased levels in the serum of complement C3 and C4 UROLOGY A worsening of clinical disease seen in the early stages of hormonal manipulation for metastatic prostate carcinoma; therapeutic gonadotropin-releasing hormone analog, eg buserelin, down-regulates the pituitary-gonadal axis and within one week of therapy, plasma levels of gonadotropin and later testosterone and dihydrotestosterone fall to castration levels; 'flare' affects 10% of patients in the first week of therapy, and is attributed to a surge in plasma gonadotropin and androgen levels, manifested by increased levels of prostatic acid phosphatase, worsening of clinical symptoms and potentially, death; an anti-androgenic agent nilutamide (RU 23908) may prevent this complication (N Engl J Med 1989; 321:413)

Flare phenomenon NUCLEAR MEDICINE Pseudo-enlargement of tumor masses, in which a temporary increase in the radioisotope uptake by radionuclide scanning in advanced prostatic carcinoma may accompany the early stages of successful treatment; the flare phenomenon invalidates bone scans as follow-up vehicles in tumors with osteoblastic metastases

Flashback SUBSTANCE ABUSE An adverse effect of psychedelic drugs, eg LSD and PCP, which is characterized by a brief reappearance of distortions and hallucinations; flashbacks occur days to weeks after the last dose, are most common in heavy users and disappear with time; the term also refers to non-drug-related repetition of frightening experiences or images, as may affect ex-soldiers, as is well-described in veterans of the Vietnam conflict

Flask-shaped heart A heart with an enlarged, water-bottle shaped cardiac silhouette, with loss of the usual 'signature' of the chambers when seen on a plain chest film, a finding characteristic of marked pericardial effusion

Flask-shaped lesions see Erlenmeyer flask deformity

Flat chest syndrome see Straight back (and flat chest) syndrome

Flat face A non-specific group of facial dysmorphias of variable intensity characterized by attenuation of the malar prominences and a broadening of the facies, which may be due to achondroplasia, Apert, arterio-hepatic dysplasia, camptomelic dysplasia, chondrodysplasia punctata (Conradi-Hünermann type), Down syndrome, Escobar syndrome, Kniest dysplasia, Larsen syndrome, lethal multiple pterygium syndrome, Marshall syndrome, partial 10q syndrome, rhizomelic chondrodysplasia, Stickler syndrome, trisomy 20p syndrome, XXXXX syndrome, XXXXY syndrome, Zellweger syndrome

Flat feet Pes planus A common orthopedic complaint affecting many age groups; true flat feet are uncommon; often the parent will perceive flattening of the foot when a child first ambulates; laxity of the ligaments may result in collapse of the foot with valgus on the hindfoot and eversion or pronation of the forefoot; a valgus deformity of > 10% requires therapy; often a shoe will suffice as therapy; acquired flat feet may be a) Ligamentous, due to tendino-ligamentous trauma b) Muscle-related, due to poor control or incoordination, as in poliomyelitis or cerebral palsy c) Osseous, due to trauma or degeneration and d) Postural, due to internal tibial torsion as occurs in obesity, muscle fatigue, faultyfootwear and footwork and arthritis; flat feet are divided into four grades of disability, ranging from mere strain or tenderness to osseous rigidity: the peroneal spastic flatfoot variant is commonly due to abnormal coalescence between two or more tarsal bones, often at the calcaneocuboid, calcaneonavicular and talocalcaneal bars

'Flat line' A colloquial term for complete lack of cerebral activity as measured by electroencephalography, a finding that is equated with 'brain death'; see Harvard criteria

Flatulence Physicians rarely regard excess flatus rationally; one 'xylophonist' with numerous, noisy and noisome events (N Engl J Med 1976; 295:261) meticulously recorded a production of 35 events/day (control population, 13 events/day); despite use of antibiotics, simethicone, charcoal and ***Lactobacillus acidophilus***, the flatteur's fecal floral fanfare continued unabated; gas chromatography revealed: CO_2 44%, H_2 38%, N_2 17%, O_2 1.3% and CH_4 0.3%, a production that partially responded to lactose elimination; borborygmi are associated with legumes (chick-peas, lentils, navy, string and soy beans, which contain indigestible polysaccharides with raffinose, stachyose and verbascose side chains, rendered digestible by soaking in water), nonabsorbable carbohydrates, eg fruits, vegetables, lactose, wheat, cryptococcal infection and iron and vitamin E deficiencies; in most subjects, methane production is low, but increases dramatically in colon carcinoma, reflecting a change in the colonic flora (flatulographic screening assays have a lower yield than occult blood testing) Note: H_2 and CH_4 are explosive gases, and detonation may occur during electrocauterization or colonoscopic polypectomies, disasters prevented by using bowel 'preps' containing nonfermentable agents (Am J Surg 1952; 84:514); see 'Downwind of matters gaseous' (Western J Med 1986; 145:502) **Treatment** A fabis abstinetis; gastric gas may respond to simethicone, intestinal gas to activated charcoal

Flat waist sign The loss of concavity of the left cardiac border, seen on a plain antero-posterior chest film corresponding to a slight rotation of the heart anteriorly, to the right and obliquely, that accompanies the left lower lobe collapse of the lung

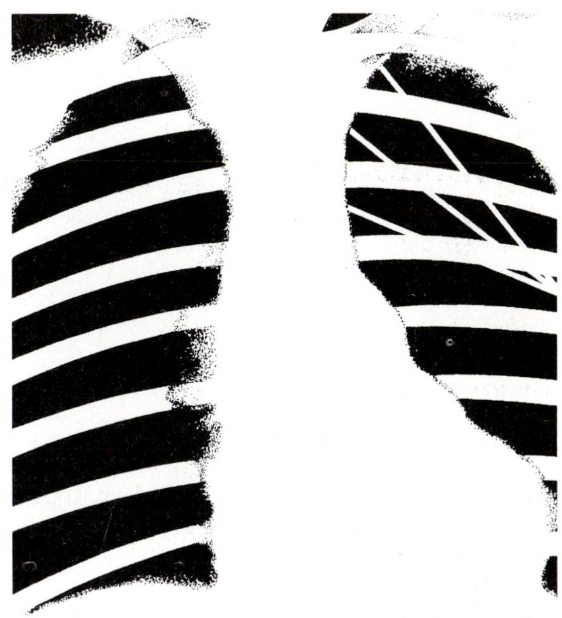

Flat waist appearance

Flaviviridae A large group of viruses with a single-stranded 10-11 kilobase RNA genome housed within a central nucleocapsid surrounded by a lipid envelope; the entire flaviviral life cycle occurs in the cytoplasm, without an intermediate DNA form; human flaviviral infections include dengue and possibly hepatitis C (J Am Med Assoc 1990; 263:3065)

Flea A wingless blood-sucking member of the order Siphonaptera, measuring 1-4 mm, vectors of the Bubonic plague and rickettsial disease;fleas of medical import: Human flea (***Pulex irritans***), oriental rat flea (***Xenopsylla cheopis***) and water flea (Cocepod)

Flea bite appearance A descriptor for multiple punctate hemorrhages of various sites, eg gastrointestinal tract, a descriptor for the endoscopic findings of multiple lesions of Kaposi sarcoma within the lumen

'Flea-bite' dermatitis Erythema toxicum A papulo-vesicular, slightly erythematous waxing and waning rash

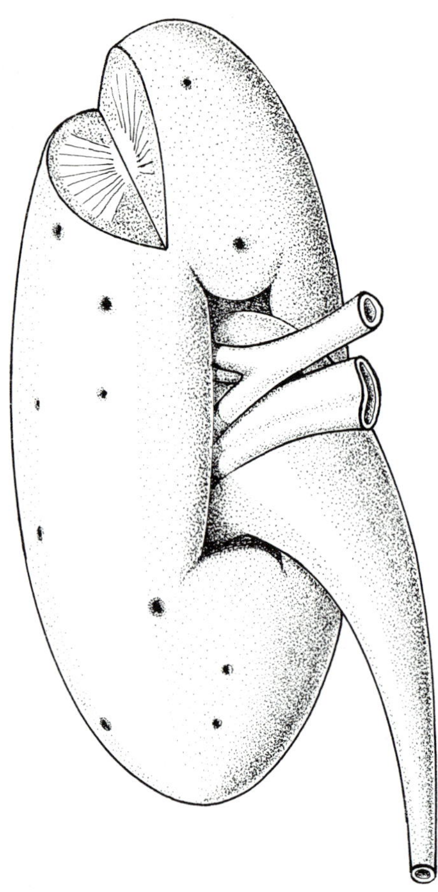

'Flea-bitten' kidney

seen on the trunk and extremities of neonates, disappearing by the end of the first week of life, possibly induced by histamine

'Flea-bite' encephalitis A circumscribed influenza-induced hemorrhagic leukoencephalitis, with macroscopic cortical petechiae likened to flea bites

Flea-bitten kidney A descriptor for the petechial hemorrhages and microinfarctions seen on the renal cortical surface (figure), which are characteristic of malignant hypertension, arising secondary to thrombosis in the arcuate and interlobular arteries; the flea-bitten appearance has also been described in lupus erythematosus, polyarteritis nodosa, leukemia and lymphoma

Flecainide CARDIOLOGY An antiarrhythmia agent that has fallen into disfavor after the CAST trials demonstrated a 3.5-fold greater incidence of death due to arrhythmia in the treated subjects than those 'treated' with placebo (N Engl J Med 1991; 324:781); Cf CAST, Encainide

Fleck dystrophy OPHTHALMOLOGY An autosomal dominant condition characterized by bilateral variably-sized, white-gray, wreath-like and non-progressive transcorneal opacities that do not interfere with vision Note: Family members may have other corneal abnormalities, atopy and pseudoxanthoma elasticum Histopathology Swollen vacuolated keratinocytes filled with complex lipids and acid mucopolysaccharides

Fleckmilz German, Spotted spleen A spleen with a mosaic or 'shower' of scattered 1-5 mm in diameter yellow-white lesions, caused by septic infarcts, secondary to acute infections, which induce acute vasculitis and splenic vessel thrombosis and uremia Histopathology Infarcted areas are bound by palisaded histiocytes and the vessels are 'cuffed' with lymphocytes

Fleck phenomenon Focal aggregation of cytologically similar leukocytes in fever, pregnancy, inflammation, epilepsy, anaphylactic shock, cerebral edema, cerebrovascular accidents; this condition has no known significance but is important as it may simulate a lymphoproliferative process

Fleur-de-lis A stylized iris, used in heraldry to denote French royalty, and in medicine in reference to a trefoil pattern ORTHOPEDICS A stenotic pattern due to impingement of lumbar spinal canal by laminar fibrosis accompanied by anterior and posterior bony overgrowth PULMONARY PATHOLOGY A pattern of involvement of the pulmonary parenchyma seen in *Pseudomonas* pneumonia, which affects the terminal airways with a striking alternation between whitish necrotic and dark red hemorrhagic zones

FLEX exam Federal licensing exam An examination required of physicians who are licensed to practice medicine in the USA, consisting of a three day, written multiple-choice examination, which assesses a physician's knowlege in 'basic' and 'clinical' sciences

Flexner report A study of US medical schools conducted by A Flexner in the early 1900s and commissioned by the Carnegie Foundation, which was largely responsible for the reform of medical education, in which an orientation towards research and education led to appointment of full-time faculty dedicated to the furtherance of medical science (J Am Med Assoc 1991; 265:1555)

Flip-flap PLASTIC SURGERY A popular single-stage procedure for the repair of hypospadias; an incision is made in the glans and penile shaft; another incision releases the prepuce and a flip-flap of skin and soft tissue is molded to the distal urethra

Flip-flop COMPUTERS A simple electronic logic circuit; a simple flip-flop is known as a toggle, where the input flips the toggle to 0 or 1; flip-flop devices may be connected to each other to yield complex circuitry MEMBRANE BIOLOGY The rotation of a transmembrane molecule through the lipid bilayer (membrane) at a 180° angle, such that the exterior portion of the molecule faces the cytoplasm or vice versa

Flippase MOLECULAR BIOLOGY A protein integral to certain biological membranes, eg endoplasmic reticulum that catalyzes the movement of small phospholipids through the lipid bilayer

'Flipped' LDH CARDIOLOGY An inversion (figure, page 227) of the ratio of lactate dehydrogenase (LD) isoenzymes LD_1 and LD_2; LD is an enzyme composed of H and/or M subunits; LD_1 is a tetramer of four H (heart) subunits, is the predominant cardiac LD isoenzyme and migrates more rapidly at pH of 8.6 than LD_5, a tetramer of M subunits that is present in high concentrations in

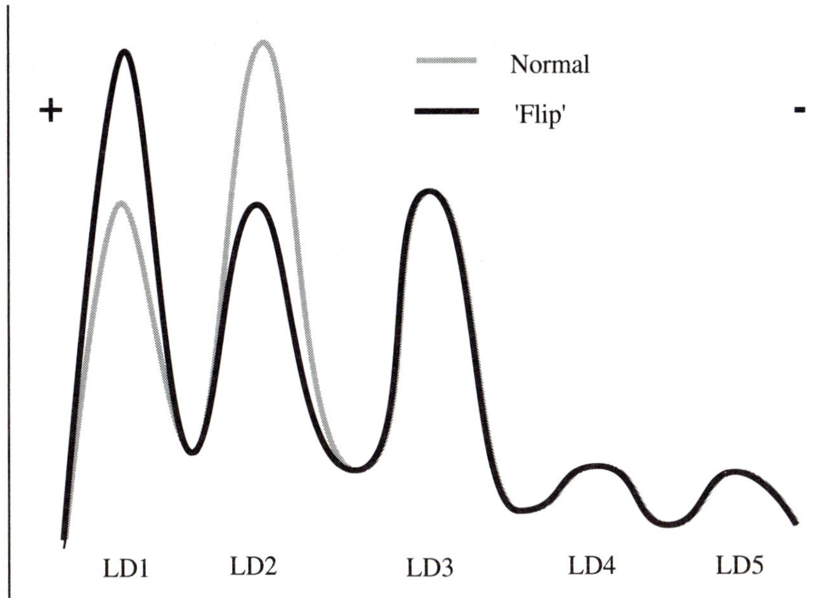

'Flipped' LDH

liver and skeletal muscle (tissues with predominantly anaerobic metabolism) Note: LD_2, LD_3 and LD_4 are present in differing amounts in other non-muscle tissues; normally the LD_1 peak is less than that of the LD_2, a ratio that is inverted (flipped) in 80% of myocardial infarcts within the first 48 hours; less common causes of LD flipping are: Renal infarcts, hemolysis, hypothyroidism and gastric carcinoma

'FLK' Funny-looking kid PEDIATRICS A colloquial descriptor for non-specific facial dysmorphias that may be accompanied by growth and/or mental retardation; the term arose in the US in the 1950s and has been used in reference to children with facial features that are not typical of any particular condition Note: The term is strictly confined to clinical parlance as there are no citations in the English language literature referring to 'Funny looking kids', presumably because of its derogatory nature

'Float' A skilled and responsible person, eg house staff officer, resident physician or supervisory nurse, who 'floats' about an institution addressing various concerns, assuring continuity of care, allowing for breaks and relief of personnel

'Floater' FORENSIC PATHOLOGY Assuming there is no air trapped in the clothing, dead bodies sink; a 'floater' is a body that rises as a result of bacterial putrefaction and gas production, often accompanied by a malodorous nauseating stench; putrefaction is more rapid in fresh, stagnant water, slower in salt water and may not occur in very cold water HISTOLOGY Extraneous tissue fragments inadvertently introduced onto a histological glass slide of material from person B, which is derived from paraffin-embedded material floating on a water bath from patient A; although an uncommon problem in surgical pathology, 'floaters' may potentially result in incorrect interpretation of the tissue and benign tissue being diagnosed as malignant and vice versa

'Floaters' Muscae volitantes Proteinaceous aggregates within the vitreous humor of the eye, corresponding to degenerative changes

Floating β-lipoprotein An abnormal very low density lipoprotein (VLDL) that contains an excess of triglycerides seen in the ultracentrifuge serum fraction (density $<$ 1.006 g/ml), which contains the pre-β VLDL-migrating band; floating β-lipoprotein bands are associated with familial dyslipoproteinemia (hyperlipo- proteinemia, type III), have a β mobility by serum protein electrophoresis, are smaller and heavier than VLDL and have a cholesterol:triglyceride ratio of $>$ 0.3 (a criterion for diagnosing type III hyperlipoproteinemia) Clinical Flat xanthomas on the palmar creases, nodular xanthomas of the elbows, knees, tendons and trunk, coronary artery disease and peripheral vasculopathy, due to a mutation in the apolipoprotein E gene, causing defective binding of apo-E to its hepatic membrane receptor, retarding the uptake and clearance of chylomicrons and VLDL Treatment Diet, weight loss

Floating gall bladder An abnormally positioned gall bladder with increased peritoneal covering, a finding of no known pathological significance

Floating teeth Marked osteolysis surrounding the mandibular teeth, imparting a radiographic appearance of teeth levitating atop cystic loculations; floating teeth are classically described in circumscribed histiocytoses X, ie Hand-Schüller-Christian disease and eosinophilic-granuloma, but may appear in Burkitt's lymphoma and neuroblastomas

Float nurse see 'Float'

Flocculation IMMUNOLOGY An immune reaction between antigen and certain antisera (antibody in solution) in which precipitation occurs over a narrow range of antigen-antibody ratios; the term was originally used to describe the 'H' precipitation test; the term flocculation has also been applied to aggregation of lipids, eg cardiolipin and others in the serological tests for syphilis, although the term 'agglutination' is preferred

Flocculent densities 'Fluffy' dense patches within mitochondria, seen by electron microscopy in infarction and mercuric chloride intoxication, considered a sign of early cell death

Floor plate EMBRYOLOGY A specialized group of midline neuroepithelial cells that regulates cell differentiation and axonal growth in the vertebrate nervous system, which is induced by local signals from the notocord (Science 1990; 250:985)

Floppy baby syndrome A condition thought to be the

most common manifestation of botulism in the USA, causing 100 cases/year, resulting from intestinal colonization and production of neurotoxin by ***Clostridium botulinum***, a bacterium that may be found in commercial honey, which may account for one-third of cases Clinical Lethargy, weakness, feeble cry, failure to thrive, loss of head control and later flaccid paralysis Treatment Supportive; antibiotics, antitoxin and guanidine have little effect Prognosis 2% mortality

Floppy head syndrome A non-specific condition characterized by isolated weakness of the neck musculature, affecting the oropharynx and/or shoulder girdle and upper trunk, which may be idiopathic or seen in myasthenia gravis, motor neuron disease and polymyositis

FLOPPY INFANT TYPES

Bone disease Osteogenesis imperfecta, rickets

Central nervous system Atonic diplegia, cerebellar ataxia, cerebral lipidosis, kernicterus, chromosomal defects, Lowe's oculocerebrorenal syndrome, Prader-Willi syndrome, Zellweger's cerebrohepatorenal syndrome, cerebral lipidosis

Muscle disease Central core disease, glycogen storage disease type IIa or Pompe's disease, mitochondrial myopathies, muscular dystrophy, myotonic dystrophy, nemaline myopathy

Neuromuscular junction disease Botulism, myasthenia gravis

Peripheral nerve disease Familial dysautonomia, Guillain-Barre syndrome, Oppenheimer's amyotonia congenita, anterior horn cell diseases, polyneuritis, congenital sensory neuropathy

Spinal cord disease Poliomyelitis, spinal cord trauma and tumors, transverse myelopathy, Werdnig-Hoffmann disease

Non-neuromuscular disease Endocrinopathies, metabolic disease, vitamin deficiencies

Floppy infant PEDIATRICS A generic term for any newborn with poor muscular tone and/or response to stimulation of extremities caused by a heterogeneous group of neuromuscular and musculoskeletal disorders (table)

Floppy valve syndrome see Mitral valve prolapse syndrome

Florette giant cells Multinucleated giant cells, with marginally placed, often overlapping nuclei and an eosinophilic center, characteristic of the pleomorphic lipoma, a benign tumor of the upper back, most common in older men

Flotation method PARASITOLOGY A simple method for isolating parasite eggs, devised in 1906; when shaken with water, feces sink, hookworm and other parasitic eggs float

Flow cytometry A procedure based on laser-induced excitation and fluorescence of cells that have been 'tagged' with monoclonal antibodies raised against cell surface and intracellular antigens; the cells can be sorted by size, intensity and type of fluorescence and the DNA ploidy can be analyzed; see Backscatter, FACS, FALS; the flow cytometer is used clinically to a) Diagnose clonal expansion Marked increase of cells displaying only one set of surface or cytoplasmic markers confirms the presence of a monoclonal lymphoproliferation; Cf Gene amplification b) Surveillance of immune status The helper:suppressor ratio (a measure of the ratio of the helper subset of T lymphocytes (CD4) to suppressor T lymphocytes (CD8), is a commonly used parameter in AIDS patients for titrating the dose of zidovudine c) DNA ploidy analysis In general, more anaplastic tumors are more aggressive and display greater aneuploidy; a benchmark for aggression is the percentage of cells in the S1 growth phase; see Ploidy analysis

Flowerette appearance see Pilot's wheel appearance

Flower-petal pattern A fanciful descriptor for the pattern of fluorescein leakage out of the vessels in cystoid macula, seen shortly after injection in a retinal angiogram in endogenous uveitis (Mayo Clin Proc 1990; 65:671)

Fluconazole INFECTIOUS DISEASE A antimicrobial agent that is considered by some workers to be the antifungal agent of choice for treating cryptococcal meningitis and local or systemic candidiasis in AIDS patients, which has a long serum half-life and good penetration of the cerebrospinal fluid (N Engl J Med 1991; 324:580); see *Candida krusei*

Fluffy infiltrate Patchy perihilar parenchymal infiltrates on a plain chest film, which corresponds to alveolar lesions of well-advanced pulmonary sarcoidosis

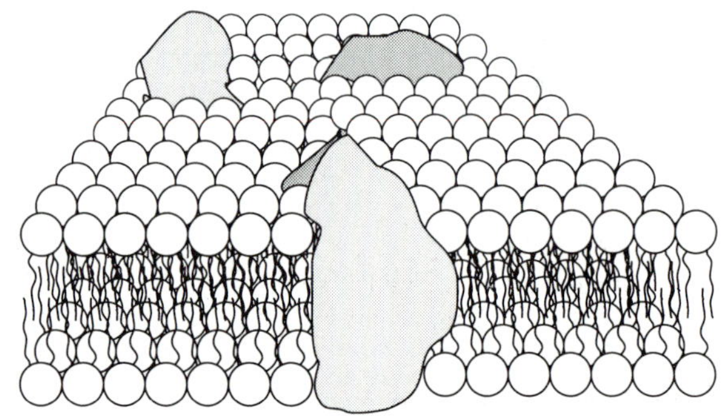

Fluid mosaic model

Fluid mosaic model The Singer-Nicholson 'fluid mosaic' (figure) is the accepted model for cell membranes, which consists of a bilayer of phospholipids and glycolipids, with the hydrophilic portions of the molecules oriented either toward the exterior or interior of the cell, while the hydophobic lipid tails face the interior of the membrane; both amphipathic lipids and globular proteins are 'scattered' throughout the membrane, and its fluidity allows the relatively unrestricted lateral movement of the proteins, glycoproteins, receptors and other molecules embedded therein

Fluke A widely distributed family of Trematodes that infect man as either the definitive or accidental host; trematodes include the genuses ***Heterophyes, Metagonimus, Fasciola, Opisthorchis, Paragonimus, Schistosoma, Clonorchis***

Fluorescence microscopy A type of microscopy in which a tissue or cell of interest is stained with a fluorochrome and illuminated by ultraviolet or short-wave visible light, eg by use of a laser, which contrasts with conventional microscopy as the tissue emits (fluorescent) light upon returning from an excited to a ground state; see Microscopy

Fluorescence recovery after photobleaching (FRAP) Fluorescence microphotolysis A method used to study the lateral movement of membrane-bound proteins and lipids in which a small area of a cell membrane is 'bleached' by light and the amount of time necessary for fluorescent marker-tagged proteins to reappear in the bleached site is a measurement of the cell membrane's fluidity

Fluoridation The addition of small amounts of fluoride to drinking water to reduce the incidence of cavities; although most data suggest that fluoridation reduces the incidence of caries, it remains unclear whether fluoride actually has this effect and soft data suggest possible carcinogenesis (Science 1990; 247:276); more than one-half of the US water supply has more than 0.7 ppm of fluoride, a level that is considered adequate to reduce the incidence of caries (J Am Med Assoc 1991; 265:2934/FDA)

Fluoride intoxication Excess fluoride may be fatal, given its affinity for calcium, notably causing one of the lowest serum calcium levels ever recorded, 0.85 mmol/L (US: 3.4 mg/dl, Pediatrics 1976; 58:90); fluoride-associated death may be either accidental or suicidal; acute fluoride intoxication (contained in some rodenticides, insecticides, fertilizers, industrial and anesthetic gases) may occur by inhalation (coughing, choking chills and fever), ingestion (nausea, vomiting, salivation, diarrhea and abdominal pain) or contact (hydrogen fluoride is similar to hydrogen chloride, causing severe, intense burns of the skin); chronic intoxication results in weight loss, brittle bones, anemia, weakness, general ill health and stiffness of joints; low level fluoride intoxication causes fluorosis

Fluoroquinolones see Quinolones

Fluorosis A chronic low-level intoxication that occurs where drinking water has fluoride is excess of 2 ppm **Clinical** Mottled enamel and chalky white discolored teeth that have a normal resistance to caries; fluorosis is common, given its availability in mouth rinses, toothpastes, the injudicious use of fluoride treatments and an extant philosophy that '...**more of a good thing must be better**'

Fluorocarbons see CFCs

Fluorouracil 5-FU ONCOLOGY A pyrimidine antagonistic antimetabolite, derived from uracil that blocks demethylation of dUMP to dTMP, interfering with DNA synthesis, depriving DNA of functional thymidine; 5-FU is used in a wide range of malignancy, including carcinoma of the bladder and in terminal epithelial malignancies **Side effects** Bone marrow toxicity and mucosal inflammation

Fluoxetine A drug that blocks the re-uptake and increases the availability of serotonin (5-hydroxy-tryptamine) and may cause regional inhibition of dopamine synthesis; fluoxetine is used to treat depression, anxiety, obsessive-compulsive disease and bulimia; co-administration with inhibitors of monoamine oxidase may be fatal; it has been suggested that the recommended dose of 20 mg may be excessive (Medical Letter 1990; 32:83)

Flush method PEDIATRICS A method for obtaining the blood pressure in a restless infant; an appropriately-sized cuff is placed on the infant's upper arm or thigh and inflated until the skin blanches; the pressure is slowly released until a flush is seen; the pressure at the flush stage is slightly below that found by the direct auscultation method

Flutter CARDIOLOGY A family of cardiac tachyarrhythmias **Atrial flutter** occurs at 200-350 beats/min (with a 2:1 block, so that the ventricle fires at circa 150 beats/min); atrial flutter results from a circus pathway, occurs in atrial dilatation, primary myocardial disease or rheumatic heart disease and responds poorly to antiarrhythmic agents **Ventricular flutter** is characterized by a continuous and regular firing rate of greater than 200 beats/min and demonstrates high-amplitude zigzag pattern on the EKG, without clear definition of the QRS and T waves, a pattern that may revert spontaneously to a normal sinus rhythm or progress to ventricular fibrillation

FLV 23/A An AIDS drug derived from cyclohexane-based hexylene oxides, that was claimed in clinical trials to assist in a patient's recovery from AIDS (Nature 1990; 347:606n); FLV 23-A was used to treat children infected with HIV-1 in Romania; the trials were halted when the manufacturer failed to provide data regarding the drug's chemical formula, mechanism of action and efficacy

Fly-catcher tongue A fanciful descriptor for the intermittent in-and-out darting of the tongue characteristic of tardive dyskinesia, a complication of chronic antipsychotic drug therapy; see Tardive dyskinesia

FMF see Familial mediterranean fever

FMG see Foreign medical graduate

Foamy appearance A descriptor for the granular appearance of lymph nodes affected by lymphoma (a pattern described as more characteristic of T cell lymphomas), as seen by lymphography

Foamy histiocyte Foam cell A generic term for a histiocyte filled with a wide variety of materials, including iron, ceroid and lipid; in adults, lipid-laden foam cells in the vascular intima accompanied by injury of the microvasculature occur in 8% of patients dying of atherosclerotic heart disease; morphologically identical cells are commonly seen in congenital lipid storage diseases, including cholesteryl ester storage disease, Farber's, Gaucher's, Niemann-Pick and Wolmann's diseases, histiocytosis X, sea-blue histiocytosis, malignant histiocytosis, infectious mononucleosis, type I hyperlipoproteinemia, hyperlipemia, mineral lipidosis, diabetes mellitus, metachromatic leukodystrophy, thalassemia, sickle cell anemia, hypoplastic anemia, idiopathic thrombocytopenic purpura, rheumatoid arthritis, corticosteroid therapy, acute leukemia, chronic granulocytic leukemia and infections with ***Mycobacterium leprae*** and ***Cryptococcus neoformans***

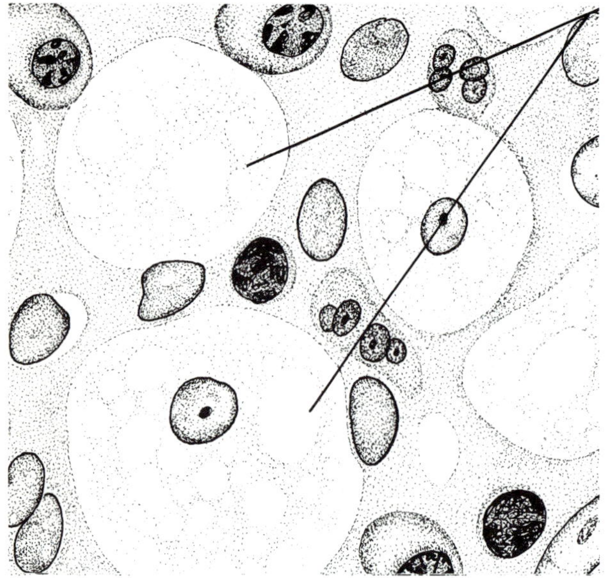

Foam cells

Foam stability index Bubble stability test OBSTETRICS A semiquantitative bedside test for determining fetal lung maturity, based on the stability of bubbles when amniotic fluid is shaken in test tubes with increasing concentrations of ethanol (which reduces the foaming or bubbling action of phosphatidyl choline, using 42% to 58% alcohol) in a series of amniotic fluid-filled test tubes; each is shaken vigorously; the higher the concentration of alcohol in which the bubbles are maintained, the more mature the lungs; see Surfactant

FOBT Fecal occult blood testing; see Occult bleeding

Fodrin Non-erythrocyte spectrin A fibrous actin-binding protein that is structurally and functionally similar to spectrin, which cross-links adjacent actin bundles in the 'terminal web' subjacent to the intestinal brush border and has been identified in leukocytes, sensory nerve cells and keratinocytes

Fogging RADIOLOGY Haziness or clouding of diagnostic X-ray films due to aging of unexposed film, or leakage of radiation or light prior to developing the films

Foldase see Chaparonin

Foldback DNA Any single strand of DNA folds upon itself and forms a hydrogen-bonded segment that is either a simple inverted repeat, ie a palindrome, known as hairpin DNA or an interrrupted series of inverted repeats resulting in a structure known as stem and loop DNA, together forming cruciform DNA

'Fold-lock-cut' A synthetic pathway for the production of the high-affinity conotoxins, a diverse family of venom peptides produced by the cone snail (***Conus geographicus*** and others), which act on voltage-sensitive calcium channels, sodium channels, NMDA receptors, acetylcholine receptors and vasopressin receptors (Science 1990; 249:257; EMBO 1990; 9:1015)

Folded lung syndrome Shrinking pleuritis with rounded atelectasis A condition that may be associated with asbestosis and pleural plaques **Radiology** see Comet tail sign **Histopathology** Chronic fibrosing pleuritis, varying degrees of inflammation; asbestos fibers are conspicuously absent from the pleural plaque and effusions but may be seen in the subpleural lymphatic plexus (Br J Dis Chest 1966; 60:19, N Engl J Med 1983; 308:1466cpc)

Folie 'a deux' PSYCHIATRY An exotic form of paranoid schizophrenia in which two closely related people share a delusional system, eg a mother who believes her son to be a prophet of God, a belief shared by the son

Folk medicine Any system of health care practiced among the aborigines, see Ethnomedicine

'Folk' medicines Self-prescribed 'natural' drugs and products that are consumed in the USA, and to a lesser degree in developed countries, by a segment of the population that has a categoric distrust of physicians and medical science and when sick, seek alternate therapeutic modalities, treating themselves with 'folk' or natural medicines, potentially causing significant comorbidity, eg heavy metal poisoning with lead, mercury, arsenic and cadmium (J Am Med Assoc 1990; 264:2212c); see Dolomite, Herbal medicine, Holistic medicine

'Follicle lysis' A finding by light microscopy consisting of invagination of small, mantle zone lymphocytes into and disruption of the germinal centers, which may be associated with hemorrhage; follicle lysis is a 'soft' histopathological criterion thus far unique to AIDS-related complex lymph nodes (Am J Surg Path 1987; 11:94); see AIDS, Benign lymphadenopathy

Follicular phase see Proliferative phase

Follistatin A 30-35 kD glycosylated protein, structurally distinct from inhibin, with similar action, as both inhibit FSH release; follistatin is the binding site on the ovary for Activin, see there

Food see Chinese restaurant, Ciguatera poisoning, Diet, Fats, Fish, Scombroid poisoning, Spicy food, Succotash, Sushi

Food irradiation A method of food preservation, using 1000 Gray to prevent sprouting in potatoes, onions and garlic and higher doses to kill bacteria in cereals, poultry and frog's legs; although irradiation is considered safe, mass hysteria prevents its broader use

Food preservatives A group of chemical preservatives that the US Food and Drug Administration classified under a GRAS (generally regarded as safe) definition of food additive, first conceptualized in the 1958 Amendment to the FFD&C Act; GRAS preservatives include the antioxidants butylated hydroxyanisole (BHA) and butylated hydroxytoluene (BHT), propylparaben, sodium nitrate, sodium nitrite, benzoic acid, stannous chloride and others; see GRAS

Foot and mouth disease An infection of cloven-hoofed barnyard beasts, including cattle, goats, pigs and sheep by a picornavirus, genus Aphthovirus, or by a rhabdovirus, vesicular stomatitis virus, which has an RNA clothed in a naked icosahedral nucleocapsid **Clinical** After a 24 hour incubation, human infections are self-limited with fever, oropharyngeal and palmo-plantar vesicle formation; Cf Hand, foot and mouth disease

Football sign PEDIATRICS A radiologic finding in massive pneumoperitoneum described in children with perforated hollow organs, due to free air accumulation in the supine upper abdomen, which gives rise to an ovoid increase in the radiolucent abdominal cavity

Foot-drop NEUROLOGY A manifestation of peripheral neuropathy seen in diabetic mononeuropathy, Charcot-Marie-Tooth syndrome and severe vitamin B_{12} deficiency, which causes subacute combined degeneration of the spinal cord with symmetrical loss of myelin sheaths and (to a lesser degree), axons; the pathology is most prominent in the posterior and lateral columns and results in paresthesias of the feet, loss of vibratory and position sensation, spasticity and exaggeration of the tendon reflexes in the legs; see Wrist drop

Footprinting MOLECULAR BIOLOGY A method for detecting sites of interaction between regulatory or promoter proteins and DNA (DNA footprinting), DNA and RNA (RNA footprinting) DNA footprinting A DNA molecule is 'incubated' with a binding protein, which binds to a specific site along the double helix, and then subjected to restriction endonuclease digestion, which reduces the entire DNA to mono- and oligonucleotide fragments except for the portion of the DNA molecule that was 'protected' from digestion by the binding protein; removal of the protein by simple chemical means, eg by gel electrophoresis, allows the study of DNA and binding protein interaction RNA footprinting A purified fragment of double-stranded DNA is labeled with an isotope at the 5' end of one strand and allowed to interact with RNA polymerase or histones; this same strand (with the attached RNA proteinase) is then subjected to scission by either DNAse I or by the synthetic reagent MPE (methidiumpropyl-EDTA) causing DNA to be cleaved at every base pair, except at those sites where 'protecting' proteins, ie promoter or regulatory proteins or histones prevent base pair cutting; the sites where DNA remains intact are the sites that are bound by the regulatory proteins and thus these experiments are known as 'DNA protection experiments'

Footprints INFECTIOUS DISEASE A descriptor for the appearance of ***Mycobacterium lepra***-laden macrophages seen in the absence of caseation necrosis, which may also occur in patients with AIDS and anergic Hodgkin's disease, infected by ***M avium-intercellulare*** (J Am Med Assoc 1986; 255:1192)

Foot process fusion RENAL PATHOLOGY The foot process or podocyte is a cytoplasmic extension from the epithelial cell of the glomerulus that attaches to the basement membrane and it is diffusely effaced or fused in minimal change glomerulopathy or 'nil disease'; foot process fusion is seen by electron microscopy, is reversible and may be the only morphological change seen in this condition

FOP Fibrodysplasia ossificans progressiva An autosomal dominant condition of irregular penetration with a prepubertal onset, characterized by microdactyly, focal, transient and occasionally painful ossifying tumors in the neck, back and extremities, with bony replacement of fasciae, ligaments and fibrotendinous tissue, associated with baldness, deafness, mental retardation, fever **Differential diagnosis** Osseous metaplasia, myositis ossificans, extraskeletal osteosarcoma

Forbidden clone theory A hypothesis that explains autoimmunity as a re-appearance (through mutation) of clones of lymphocytes that had been functionally deleted in the thymus during ontogeny; forbidden clones of cells are those with self antigens, against which an organism should not react

Foreign bodies Objects introduced into the human economy can be microscopic or macroscopic, by intent, by accident or as the inevitable accompaniment of an invasive procedure; foreign bodies may be categorized as a) Iatrogenic, eg sutures, sponges, instruments left during surgery, metals and plastics that replace or enhance failing or non-functioning body parts, eg artificial joints, limbs and pacemakers b) Accidental or unintentional, as in abrasions and open wounds in various accidents, or in gun shot wounds, which may elicit foreign body-type granuloma formation; foreign bodies may be introduced in the context of sexual deviancy, for inflicting pleasure or pain, commonly, in the anorectum or vagina, including an array of 'jeux d'amour', eg vibrators, bottles, light bulbs, eggs and others; see Sexual deviancy

Foreign medical graduate (FMG) International medical graduate A physician who graduated from a medical school outside of the United States, Canada or Puerto Rico; FMGs may suffer discrimination resulting from poor linguistic skills or because of the perception of inferior education and skills (Am Med News 28/Dec/90); FMGs are divided into alien FMGs (natives of non-North American countries) and USFMGs (North Americans who studied medicine outside of the USA, Canada and Puerto Rico); see USFMG

Forequarter amputation A major surgical procedure in which the upper extremity and a variable portion of the supporting shoulder 'girdle' is amputated, almost invariably for either advanced malignancy, eg malignant melanoma or for a primary malignancy of the soft or bony tissues, eg chondrosarcoma or osteosarcoma; an alternative to forequarter amputation of an upper extremity with a sarcoma is the Tikhoff-Lindberg procedure, in which the distal clavicle, proximal humerus and the majority of the scapula is resected (Surg Gyn Obstet 1989; 169:1, Yonsei Med J 1990; 31:110); forequarter amputations of the leg and pelvis are generally considered more 'heroic' than those of the upper extremity and are not commonly performed, although they were once considered the treatment of choice for certain bone tumors, eg Ewing sarcoma; see Heroic surgery, Mutilating surgery

Forensic anthropology The scientific study of human remains, usually with the express purpose of identifying the remains of the deceased and the cause of death if unknown

Formaldehyde $H_2C=O$ Methanal A highly toxic, flammable gas that is highly irritating to the respiratory and conjunctival mucosa at concentrations above 2 ppm; formaldehyde is soluble in water and forms methylene bridges between denatured proteins; see Formalin

Formalin A 37% solution of formaldehyde gas in water that reacts with the amine groups of proteins and DNA, serving as a disinfectant and when buffered, to denature ('fix') tissues for histological examination

Formamide The amide of formic acid that reacts with adenine in DNA, disrupting the adenine-thymine base pairs and denaturation of DNA

Forme fruste The aborted, attenuated or atypical expression of a clinical entity or pathological condition

Forskolin A molecule used experimentally to study modulation of a) voltage-gated potassium ion channels, and b) acetylcholine receptor that acts directly instead of via a second messenger (Science 1988; 240:1655)

Fort Bragg fever Anicteric leptospirosis A condition first described in an outbreak of pretibial rashes in military recruits in Fort Bragg, Texas during World War II, caused by ***Leptospiralis autumnalis***; in peacetime, leptospirosis is more common in children with an abrupt onset of a 'toxic' state, fever, shaking chills, headache, nausea, vomiting and severe myalgias (especially of the legs), lethargy, dehydration, photophobia, orbital pain, generalized lymphadenopathy and hepatosplenomegaly; because the distinct serotypes of ***Leptospira*** species do not produce clinically distinct syndromes (eg canicola fever, Fort Bragg fever, Weil's disease and others), it has been suggested that these diseases be referred to simply as leptospirosis

Fortification phenomenon see 'Maginot line' phenomenon

Fortified food Any food, eg cereals that has been supplemented with essential nutrients, eg iron and vitamins, either in quantities that are greater than those present normally, or which are not present in the fortified food (this latter is considered the more correct usage of 'fortification'); Cf Enriched food, Refined food

FORTRAN A high-level language used to program mainframe computers, ideally suited for complicated mathematical computations; see BASIC, Computers

Forward angle light scatter see FALS

Forward failure CARDIOLOGY A concept of dubious value referring to decreased cardiac output and inadequate perfusion of organs implying either a) Symptoms of congestive heart failure, ie low cardiac output with easy fatigability, weakness and even shock or b) A pathogenic mechanism of cardiac failure, in which decreased cardiac output produces tissue edema and increased capillary permeability, secondary to tissue hypoxia, a mechanism that has proven conceptually incorrect; forward failure is best understood as decreased cardiac output due to decreased renal blood flow and altered glomerular filtration with retention of salt and water, causing a secondary increase in the blood volume; Cf Backward failure

fos The *fos* oncogenes include the cellular *fos* oncogene, c-*fos*, which is the normal cellular counterpart or proto-oncogene of the viral oncogene, v-*fos*; c-*fos* encodes a 380 amino acid nuclear phosphoprotein that modulates the expression of other genes, requiring phosphorylation for efficient activity (Nature 1990; 348:80); c-*fos* is rapidly and transiently expressed in response to various stimuli, including epidermal, neural and platelet-derived growth factors (PDGF, EGF and NGF), as well as by neurotransmitters, neuronal stimulation and the cancer promoter-phorbol ester; *fos* encodes a nuclear phosphoprotein with DNA-binding properties and is thought to function as a 'third messenger' molecule in signal transduction systems, coupling short-term intracellular signals elicited by a variety of extracellular stimuli, serving as a 'master switch', turning on other genes; see Serum response element Note: The *fos* oncogene is named after the FBJ and FBR osteogenic sarcomas

Foscarnet AIDS An experimental drug used in AIDS patients with cytomegalovirus-induced inflammatory conditions, including colitis, hepatitis, pneumonia and retinitis who don't respond to or cannot tolerate gancyclovir, the usual drug of choice for cytomegalovirus infections; Cf ddC, ddI, Zidovudine

Fossil fuel ENVIRONMENT A fuel derived from decomposing fossilized organic material of fossilized plant or animal origin, including oil, coal and natural gas, the burning of which is widely regarded as the single greatest contributor to the Greenhouse effect, and a major contributer to Acid rain

Founder cell A cell that has undergone minimal differentiation, passing the primitive 'stem' cell stage, while retaining the ability to colonize an entire tissue, eg primitive hepatocytes or chondrocytes that could give rise to the liver or cartilage

Founder effect CLINICAL GENETICS The result of a small subgroup of a species establishing itself as a separate and isolated entity in an ecosystem or location; the founder colony carries with it only a fraction of the gene pool of the parent population, which tends to result in an increased frequency of certain diseases, in particular those diseases known to be autosomal recessive; the founder effect is described in CETP deficiency in the Japanese, Tay-Sachs disease in the Jews, yellow mutant albinism in the Amish

Four cell diagnostic matrix

	Disease Present	Disease not present
Test positive	True positive (TP)	False positive (FP)
Test negative	False negative (FN)	True negative (TN)

Sensitivity TP / TP + FN (Total patients with disease)
Specificity TN / TN + FP (Total patients without disease)
False positive rate FP / TP + FN (Total patients with disease)
False negative rate FN / TN + FP (Total patients without disease)

Four cell diagnostic matrix LABORATORY MEDICINE A simple decision-making model (figure) for the evaluatng the relative merits of a diagnostic test, which allows comparison of the ability of various methodologies to diagnose the presence of a disease, defining such terms as false negativity and positivity, sensitivity and specificity (Ann Int Med 1981; 94:553); see ROC curve

Four Fs The four Fs (Fat, female, flatulent and forty) is a mnemonic which has clinical currency as the factors associated with cholelithiasis and acute cholecystitis

Four food groups NUTRITION A grouping of comestibles by the US Department of Agriculture that delineates in a simplefied form, its recommendations for eating priorities, graphically presented as a pyramid, at the base of which are carbohydrates with 6-11 portions recommended daily (group one), on top of which are fruits and vegetables with 5-9 portions, followed by dairy products, fish and meat 4-6; at the pyramid's peak are the 'discouraged' foods to be eaten sparingly, including fats, oils and sweets (Science 1991; 252:917n)

4p- syndrome see Deletion syndromes

Fourier transform A mathematical function that describes the amplitude (height of a sinusoid) and the phase (starting point) of a sinusoidal pattern of any fluctuating phenomenon in the physical universe (light, tidal and solar waves, molecular vibration); the transform states that any distribution (Fourier analyzed temperature) can be described mathematically in an equation and its higher frequency harmonics; the Fourier transform has had broad applications in biology and medicine; analysis of the X-ray crystallography data was pivotal in identifying the double helical nature of DNA , and has assisted in analysis of other molecules including viruses (Sci Am 1990; 260/6:86); the modified back-projection algorithm, universally used in CT-imaging is based on the Fourier transform; Jean-Baptiste-Joseph Fourier was a French mathematician of post-revolutionary vintage who formulated the transform in 1807 Noter: The merging of mathematics with biology may occur when DNA folding patterns are analyzed in the contexts of chaos, fractal analysis, Fourier transforms and knot and wavelet theories; Cf Fractals, Wavelet theory

Fourth disease Parascarlatina, Filatov-Duke disease

'Fourth therapy' Background Cancer is traditionally treated with one or more of the three tumor-ablative modalities, ie surgery, radiotherapy and chemotherapy; the use of biological response modifiers (interferons, interleukins, monoclonal antibodies, colony-stimulating factors and tumor necrosis factor), is known as the 'fourth therapy', which attempts to take advantage of certain aspects of the immune system, including immunomodulatory, antiproliferative and tumorilytic activities; see Biological response modifiers

Fourth ventricle 'syndrome' Symptoms that arise from expansile lesions (neoplastic or inflammatory) or infarction in the floor of the fourth ventricle, involving cranial nerves V-VII

'Fourth World' SOCIAL MEDICINE A colloquialism coined for the phenomenon of 'Third World' poverty within the borders of a developed, ie 'First World' country, as occurs among the homeless in the USA; see Homeless

Fowler's solution A potassium arsenite solution, formerly used to treat leukemia and various dermatological conditions; after a latency period of up to 43 years, malignancy may appear in those treated with or occupationally exposed to arsenicals, in the form of hepatic angiosarcoma, small cell, squamous cell and bronchoalveolar carcinomas of the lungs, esophageal and genitourinary carcinoma (J Am Med Assoc 1984; 252:3407)

F protein see Atypical measles

Fractal THEORETICAL MEDICINE An invention of IBM mathematician Benoit Mandelbrot, which are a) Self-symmetrical, ie an enlargement of a small part is similar to the whole and b) Have fractional dimension; man has traditionally related nature to artificial and invalid geometric shapes (circles, squares, triangles); with fractals, a true representation of the natural universe can be reduced to a mathematical model (figure); in the human economy, the ever-increasing number of branches in the blood vessels as they become capillaries, as well as the branching of the bronchi are each considered to be recapitulations of fractal geometry; see Chaos

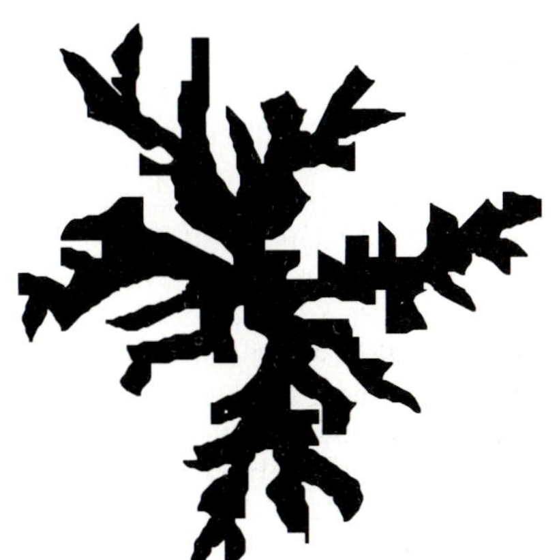

Fractal pattern

Fractional kill hypothesis Background Dosing of cancer chemotherapeutic agents is based on experimental studies where the tumor's size, kinetics and percentage of cells killed can be determined within reasonable limits; the hypothesis assumes a homogeneity of the tumor cell population and a constant percent decrease in tumor bulk with each course of therapy; in treating cancer, tumor populations are actually heterogeneous; although chemotherapy does kill a certain large percentage of actively dividing cells; cells not in a susceptible period of the growth cycle are not killed, while other cells are resistant, expressing the MDR (multidrug resistance) gene; one way to reduce the tumor load is to debulk by surgery or radiotherapy, then 'consolidate' the treatment with chemotherapy or subject the patient to a 'second look' procedure

Fragile data Data that has been generated in a well-designed study and achieves or nearly achieves statistical significance, but which reaches unexpected conclusions, causing the authors to present the data with caveats on the 'fragility' of the findings; see Data

Fragile sites MOLECULAR BIOLOGY Specific chromosomal loci (of the 320 bands per haploid set) of a routine human metaphase chromosome preparation that may be expressed as gaps or breaks, which are co-dominantly inherited, including those found on chromosomes 3p14.2, 6q25.3 and 16q23.2; cells grown in folic acid- and thymidine-deficient culture media have an increased expression of 13 of the 16 common heritable (constitutive) fragile sites and increased spontaneous chromosomal breakage; extended haploid sets with 850 bands, when incubated in caffeine, an inhibitor of DNA repair in replicating cells, reveal that 20 of the 51 fragile sites in the human genome correlate with known chromosomal defects in leukemias, lymphomas and solid tumors

Fragile X syndrome A condition related to mutation in a highly unstable 550-base pair locus on chromosome Xq27.3, which is susceptible to insertions, methylations, amplifications and varies in length across generations; insertions of less than 400 base pairs are not associated with phenotypic expression of a gene that requires the abnormal cytosine methylation of a single CpG island (Science 1991; 252:1097, 1070) Note: Fragile X is the most common (1:1500) cause of inherited mental deficiency in males (30% of female carriers are also mentally deficient); the defect appears in 10-50% of chromosomes tested and is diagnosed by growth in a folic acid-poor growth medium, which enhances chromosomal breakage Molecular biology The gene's methylation may explain both the pattern of inheritance and the lack of expression of an as-yet-unknown structural gene, as methylation of a gene functionally stops its activity (Science 1991; 251:1236) Clinical Moderate mental retardation, neuropsychiatric disorders (hypotonic or hyperactive state, autism), large forehead, macroorchidism, enlarged chin, jaw and ears

Frame shift mutation MOLECULAR BIOLOGY The loss or gain of one or more nucleotide base pairs in a gene, which results in the 'misreading' of all codons downstream from the mutation, and the encoding of different amino acids or stop codons in the elongating polypeptide chain; see Point mutation

Framework regions (FR) The regions of an immunoglobulin where the amino acid residues are relatively constant and are β-pleated, forming the folding portion of the immunoglobulin molecule; FRs in the light chain are located at amino acid residues 1-28, 38-50, 56-89 and 97-107; FRs in the heavy chain are located at amino acid residues 1-31, 35-49, 66-101 and 110-117; Cf 'Hot spots'

Frankenstein The central character of Mary Shelley's novel by the same name; 'Frankenstein' is used as an adjective in a variety of biomedical contexts, eg **Frankenstein complex** The fear that machines via artificial intelligence may replace physicians **FRANKENSTEIN FACTOR** Any unforeseen consequence of genetic engineering **FRANKENSTEIN 'SYNDROME'** The potential result of experimentation on humans; used as a noun, a Frankenstein is any enterprise that circumvents or expands beyond the mechanisms designed to control them, eg the health-care reimbursement system (Am Rev Respir Dis 1975; 111:689)

FRAP see Fluorescence recovery after photobleaching

Fraud in science The intentional misrepresentation or manipulation of data; scientific fraud ranges from 'innocent correction' of data by the investigator, see Cooking, Trimming, to complete fabrication of data; in the USA, misinterpretation of complex data in difficult niches of research has been scrutinized by non-scientists and 'whistle-blowers', see Qui tam lawsuit, engendering a label of fraud, despite commonly held opinions that such inquiries are best left to peer review; retraction of fraudulent data reduces subsequent citation by 35%

'Freak out' SUBSTANCE ABUSE A highly colloquial verb, first used in North America in the 1960s, during which time the chief proponents of social changes were known as hippies or 'freaks', who used psychedelic drugs for 'mind expansion', which in excess, would cause hyperexcitation or 'freaking out' (N Engl J Med 1991; 324:926); see 'Bad trip', 'Flash back'

Freckles Ephilides Brown macules, often exacerbated on sun-exposed zones of the skin surface, disappearing during the winter; most commonly affecting the fair-skinned, especially those of Celtic stock; freckles are not associated with atypical melanocytic hyperplasia, nor with malignancy Histopathology Increased melanin and fewer but enlarged melanocytes

Free base (cocaine) SUBSTANCE ABUSE An aqueous form of cocaine that allows it to be injected intravenously or smoked, producing a more intense 'high' (and more intense addiction) that is prepared through the chemical conversion of cocaine-HCl by alkalinizing and extracting through heated ether and organic solvents Note: The danger of explosion at the ether extraction phase forced clandestine chemists to create a newer formulation of cocaine, Crack, see there

Freeman surgery see Psychosurgery

Freemartin Stable chimera Dizygotic bovine twins that are of the opposite sex, the female of which often has reproductive abnormalities, that shared in utero circulation and are immune tolerant to each other's red cell antigens; the system of shared in utero circulation was reduced in size by Billingham, Brent and Medawar (Nobel prize) to a mouse model

Free radical One of a highly reactive family of molecules containing an unpaired electron in the outer orbital, eg the excited variants of oxygen; free radicals cause random damage to structural proteins, enzymes, macromolecules and DNA and play major roles in inflammation, hyperoxidation, post-ischemic tissue damage, infarcs, and possibly also in carcinogenesis and tissue damage induced by organ transplantation; superoxide dismutase is the major 'scavenger' enzyme, catalyzing reduction of reactive oxygen species to O_2 and H_2O; the havoc wreaked by radicals includes polyunsaturated fatty acid peroxidation of organelles and plasma membranes, oxidation and inactivation of sulfhydryl group-bearing enzymes, polysaccharide depolymerization and

DNA damage; the action of free radicals on DNA in the form of hydroxylation of bases, cross-linking, nicking may block transcription and by extension, synthetic activities Note: Free radical production by endothelial cells during coronary artery ischemia and inculpated in myocytolysis may be reduced in experimental systems by pre-treatment with superoxide dismutase

Free radical inactivator Any molecule that reduces free radical-induced damage, including ceruloplasmin, cysteine, glutathione, superoxide dismutase, transferrin, vitamin E and D-penicillamine (Mayo Clin Proc 1988; 63:381, 390rv)

Free radical scavenger Any compound that reacts with free radicals in a biological system and provides protection against the indirect effects, ie free radicals, of ionizing radiation

Free radical theory GERONTOLOGY A biological theory that assumes that the changes seen in aging cells and organisms result from the accumulation of molecules damaged by free radicals; the host cell's defenses against free radical damage include glutathione peroxidase, α-tocopherol (vitamin E) and superoxide dismutase; intracellular superoxide levels correlate well with lifespan; Cf Cross-linkage, Error catastrophe, 'Garbage can' hypothesis, Pacemaker theory

Free-standing HEALTH CARE INDUSTRY An adjective for any physically and often financially discrete entity, eg a surgicenter, that is separated from, but which may be affiliated with a hospital; free-standing facilities may provide ambulatory surgery, emergency or primary care; see Walk-in clinic

Free thyroxine index (FTI), FT_4I, T7 assay, T12 assay LABORATORY MEDICINE A clinical parameter measured by radioimmunoassay, used to evaluate thyroid function, calculated by $T_4 \times T_3RU$ (resin uptake); the FTI is not susceptible to fluctuations of T_3/T_4 binding globulin and is more reliable than thyroxine when the binding proteins are altered; the FTI is increased in hyperthyroidism and factitious hyperthyroidism and decreased in hypothyroidism; it is falsely elevated in heparin therapy and falsely decreased in phenytoin and valproic acid therapy and in the euthyroid sick syndrome

Freeze-clamp technique A method used in experimental biology to analyze metabolic processes in quasiphysiological conditions, by immersing the tissue of interest in liquid nitrogen, abruptly stopping any in vivo reaction, allowing the study of concentrations of the metabolites in various intracellular compartments; Cf Patch-clamp method

Freeze-fracture 'imaging' CELL BIOLOGY A technique that allows ultrastructural examination of membrane-bound proteins and subcellular particles as they appear within cells Method A cell or tissue of interest is frozen in nitrogen and 'fractured' with a blow from a sharp knife removing membranes interfering with visualization of organelle topography; the surface is then overlaid with carbon to form a continuous layer and then 'shadowed' with platinum, imparting a three-dimensional image of the organelles

'Freezing' NEUROLOGY Hesitation on gait initiation, ie start-hesitation, upon stopping, ie terminal hesitation or when walking in crowded places, a manifestation of well-developed Parkinson's disease

French-American-British classification see FAB classification

French congenital nephrotic syndrome An often fatal autosomal recessive proliferative mesangial glomerulosclerosis of onset in early infancy Histopathology Atrophy of the tubules with interstitial fibrosis and increased mesangial matrix; Cf Finnish congenital nephrotic syndrome

French sizes EMERGENCY MEDICINE The system for sizes of tubes used in endotracheal intubation, the use of which varies according to the age of the patient; at one month, size 4; at age 2, size 5.0; at age 6, size 6; at age 12, size 7.0

Fresh frozen plasma see FFP

Friction rub CARDIOLOGY A scratchy triphasic (occasionally, biphasic or monophasic) sound extending over the entire precordium, best heard along the left midsternum with the patient leaning forward, which changes in quality with inspiration and positional changes; the rub is considered pathognomonic for pericarditis and must be differentiated from to-and-fro or machinery-like murmurs and 'crunching' sounds heard in emphysema; the 3 phases of the triphasic rub are due to pericardial-epicardial contact during ventricular systole, diastole and atrial systole

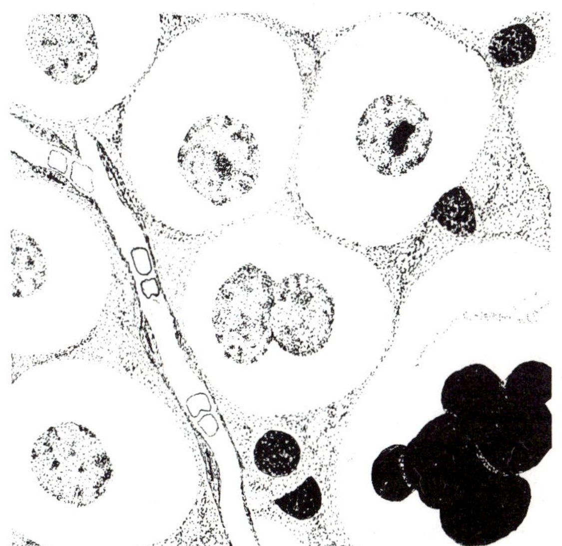

Fried egg appearance, oligodendrogliocytes

'Fried egg' appearance A descriptor for a pattern likened to eggs fried with an intact yolk Note: Fried eggs may be either 'scrambled' or 'sunny side-up' (with the yolk intact), although the adjective usually refers to the latter NEUROPATHOLOGY The appearance by light microscopy of oligodendrogliocytes, in which a large central nucleus is surrounded by cleared cytoplasm, a finding thought to be an artefact due to slow fixation of tissue; a similar finding may rarely occur in astrocytomas MICROBIOLOGY A descriptor for the gross colony morphology that is characteristic of ***Mycoplasma hominis*** and ***M pneumonia*** on Shepherd's differential growth medium, where the growth occurs in two planes, both deep to and on the surface of the agar; ***M hominis*** is further characterized by its ability to utilize arginine

'Friendly' fire MILITARY MEDICINE The misdirection of the firepower, eg gunfire, dropping of bombs and shelling by long-range weapons, in an armed confllict towards combattants of the same side; it has been estimate that as many as 10% of combat casualties are the result of such faux pas, despite technical advances as 'surgical' bombing

Fringe medicine see Holistic medicine

Frivolous lawsuit see Malpractice

Frogbelly PEDIATRICS A fanciful term for the pendulous abdominal fat of children with congenital hypothyroidism (cretins)

Frogface The end-result of long-standing angiofibromas (large, pedunculated gray-pink spongy fibrous 'tumors' with superficial ulceration) of the intranasal cavities which may ultimately protrude into the orbits, causing bilateral exophthalmos, associated with nasal congestion and a flat, croaking voice

Frog leg position A descriptor for a position that may occur a) As an incorrect sleeping position in infants with an 'out-toeing' deformity of the leg, which may evolve into a Charlie Chaplin gait, prevented by sewing together the legs of the pajamas b) In infants with fulminant scurvy, where tenderness and irritability cause the children to assume the least painful position, resulting in a pseudoparalysis with the hips and knees semiflexed and the feet rotated externally, often accompanied by edematous swelling of the femoral shafts and occasionally, palpable subperiosteal hemorrhage and c) In children with congestive heart failure

Frog neck appearance A deep-set neck and hairline, described as characteristic of Klippel-Feil disease

Front typing TRANSFUSION MEDICINE Use of known antibodies (from commercially available 'panels') to detect ABO antigens on the red blood cells; a discrepancy between front and back typing can be due to acquired group B or group B antigenic subtypes, cold or saline agglutinins, decreased immunoglobulins, polyagglutination of anti-B and anti-A_1 antibodies, rouleaux formation, the presence of Wharton's jelly, mosaicism or two different cell populations, as seen after transfusion

Frontal bossing see Bossing

Frost see Uremic frost

'Frosting' Finely granular salt deposits on the skin overlying sweat glands in children with cystic fibrosis

'Frozen' see Frozen section

Frozen blood TRANSFUSION MEDICINE A blood product that was a 'spin-off' of the Cold War, in anticipation of the need for transfusions in a world without donors, assuming that the only survivors of a total 'exchange' would be those living in nuclear submarines; in order to extend the shelf life of packed red cells, most of the plasma is replaced with glycerol; frozen red cells are licensed by the FDA for routine transfusion for up to 10 years after collection, when stored at -80°C in certain agents, eg 40% glycerol plus 15% DMSO-dimethylsulfoxide, allowing survival of viable red cells (80% recovery) for up to 40 years; upon rethawing, hemoglobin (due to rethawing lysis) is 100 mg/dl; inadequate removal of cryopreservatives may induce hemolysis; frozen erythrocytes may be used in a) Rare blood types, eg Bombay phenotype b) Paroxysmal nocturnal hemoglobinuria c) IgA deficiency, with production of anti-IgA antibodies d) Those with graft-versus-host transfusion reactions

Frozen pelvis ONCOLOGICAL SURGERY A term for massive involvement of the pelvic floor by malignancy, usually carcinoma, often of the female genital tract, in which there is contiguous extension of the tumor from the bladder, female genital tract and sigmoid colon; adequate surgical resection of a frozen pelvis is virtually impossible, although surgery, chemotherapy and radiotherapy are palliative at best Clinical The symptoms are related to compression and stenosis of pelvic floor organs, formation of fistulous tracts (which may unchain one of the common terminal events, sepsis), difficulty in defecation and dyspareunia; see All-American operation

Frozen section SURGICAL PATHOLOGY A rapid diagnostic procedure performed on tissue obtained intra-operatively, where the tissue is frozen in a synthetic material, eg OCT (Miles Laboratories), sectioned with a cryostat, stained with hematoxylin and eosin and viewed with a light microscope, allowing a rapid diagnosis of a pathologic tissue; the technique provides the surgeon with information necesary to guide therapy and to determine the extent of further surgery at the time of surgical procedure; the information obtained from a 'frozen' includes 1) Differentiating between benign and malignant 2) Determining the type of malignancy, eg lymphoma versus carcinoma 3) Evaluating tissue margins for involvement by malignancy, eg basal cell carcinomas 4) Determining the adequacy of tissue for further studies after the patient is closed and 5) Determining the type of tissue, eg differentiating lymphoid tissue from parathyroid gland; 'quick sections' shorten the turn-around time for a diagnosis from 1-3 days to 15 minutes, with the disadvantage that the tissue is suboptimal, as it contains freezing artefact and is thus more difficult to interpret than paraffin-embedded tissue

Frozen shoulder A generic term for a shoulder afflicted with incapacitating pain secondary to bursitis and marked inflammation, which may be due to primary or secondary osteoarthritis, rheumatoid arthritis, cuff tear arthropathy and the clinically similar 'Milwaukee shoulder', avascular necrosis and calcific tendonitis and tearing of the rotator cuff muscles

Fructose-3-phosphate A monosaccharide phosphate not present in normal lenses but found in the lens of diabetic rats, F-3-P glycosylates proteins and inactivates enzymes; its metabolic product, 3-deoxyglucosone is implicated in the visual defects of diabetes mellitus (Science 1990; 247:451)

Fructose intolerance 'syndrome' The autosomal recessive deficiency of fructose-1-phosphate aldolase; the subject is asymptomatic until exposed to fructose (or sucrose) Clinical Hepatomegaly, jaundice, edema; with time, the patients may develop cirrhosis Treatment Dietary, avoidance of fructose-containing foods

Fruit-laden tree appearance see Cherry blossom appearance

FSH Follicle-stimulating hormone A 30 kD glycoprotein that binds membrane receptors, activating adenyl cyclase and increasing intracellular AMP; FSH stimulates ovulation and spermatogenesis and is increased in primary gonadal failure, testicular or ovarian agenesis, Klinefelter syndrome, FSH-secreting tumors and decreased in anorexia nervosa, hypogonadotropic hypogonadism, panhypopituitarism, malignancy of the ovaries, testes and adrenal glands

FSI see Foam stability index

FSV Fujinami sarcoma virus A transforming virus that acts on rat fibroblasts, forming a fusion product from viral GAG and cell-derived FPS, encoding a chimeric protein with tyrosine kinase activity and oncogenic transforming capacity

FTA-ABS Fluorescent treponemal antibody-absorption A highly sensitive (circa 100%) and sensitive (96 to 97%) serological test for the diagnosis of congenital, secondary, tertiary and neurosyphilis; see VDRL

FTE see Full-time equivalent

F Test A statistical test that allows comparison of the standard deviations of two different sets of data or populations, defined as F = s^2 new data/s^2 old data; the smaller the standard deviation, the more precise or reliable the test or data being studied

FTI see Free thyroxine index

FTT see Failure to thrive

ftz Fushi tarazu, Japanese, Insufficient segments A 2 kilobase gene of ***Drosophila melanogaster*** that controls the number of body segments during embryogenesis and cell fate during neurogenesis; *ftz* is transiently expressed in neuronal precursors (Science 1988; 239:170), and when mutated, allows production of one half the normal body segments, resulting in death before birth, in the neurons, absence of *ftz* caused the cells to change identity

Fugu Puffer fish A raw fish delicacy eaten in Japan that contains tetrodotoxin, a highly selective sodium channel blocker that is concentrated in the ovaries, liver, skin and intestines and is fatal when improperly prepared, causing about 100 deaths annually in Japan

Fugue state NEUROLOGY A state in which the patient denies any memory of his activities for a period of time ranging from hours to weeks; to external appearances these activities were either completely normal or the patient disappeared and traveled extensively; most are of a functional nature although rare cases of short-lived fugues occur with temporal lobe epilepsy; Cf Jamais vu

Fullerenes Hollow cage-like all-carbon molecules that are generated when carbon burns, including C60, C76, C84, C90, C94 and C70; fullerene variants include **Buckyball** C60 or Soccer ball structure **Hairyball** A C60 structure festooned with a dozen or more ethylene diamine molecules whose nitrogen groups have spare electrons **Dopeyball** C60 with boron inside, so named as it is a fullerene that has been 'doped' with another molecule; it is unclear what applications in biology and medicine this new class of compounds will have (Science 1991; 252:547, 548)

'Full House' syndrome FFFDD Familial focal facial dermal dysplasia An autosomal dominant condition characterized by lesions devoid of hair with fingerprint-like puckering of the skin, especially at the temples, due to alternating bands of dermal and epidermal atrophy, one family described was cancer-prone and had gastric and familial polyposis (Birth Defects 1971; 7:96) Note: The name is inspired by poker, a card game in which a 'full house' is three cards of one value and two of another

Full-time equivalent (FTE) Health care management The amount of time worked by the combined full and part-time staff, divided by the time worked (in the USA, 40 hours) by a full-time employee; in hospitals, FTEs are calculated for services which provide 24 hour/day service, including the nursing staff and laboratory

Fumagillin A natural antibiotic from ***Aspergillus fumigatus*** that inhibits endothelial cell proliferation and tumor-induced angiogenesis; fumagillin also inhibits tumor growth but because it causes severe weight loss, fumigillin analogues ('angioinhibins') are designed to inhibit tumor growth without the side effects (Nature 1990; 348:555); see Neovascularization

Functional illiteracy SOCIAL MEDICINE The inability to read and write with enough proficiency to effectively function in an office or business; in contrast, complete illiteracy is a major cause of 'disenfranchisement', where patients cannot use the health benefits available to them

Fungible An adjective for any product that is readily exchanged for another, eg plasma, generic drugs, sterile gloves, without compromise of function or inconvenience

Fungoides Bacteria that mimic true fungi, eg ***Actinomadura, Actinomyces, Nocardia*** and ***Streptomyces*** species, both morphologically and clinically

Fungus ball Aspergilloma, mycetoma A tumor-like mass of fungi, classically the saprobic form of ***Aspergillus*** species that colonizes a preexisting pulmonary cavity Radiology Solid rounded mass within a cavity, rimmed by an 'air density' crescent; surgical excision of large lesions carries a 5-10% intraoperative mortality rate and a 25-35% complication rate, but without surgery, potentially fatal hemoptysis occurs in 50-83%; radiologically similar lesions occur in abcesses, ankylosing spondylitis, congenital lung cysts, cystic bronchiectasis, emphysematous bullae, cavitary histoplasmosis, neoplasia, radiation fibrosis, sarcoidosis and AIDS (N Engl J Med 1991; 324:654)

Funnel chest Pectus excavatum A congenital, often isolated, skeletal anomaly associated with upper airway obstruction or segmental bronchomalacia; surgical correction is not clearly beneficial and some cases may resolve spontaneously

Funny looking kid see FLK

FUO see Fever of unknown origin

Furry tongue see Black hairy tongue, Hairy tongue

Fused protein see Hybrid protein

Fushi tarazu see ftz

Fusion peptide A strongly hydrophobic, highly conserved amino acid sequence contained in influenza viruses; at pH 7.0 the sequence is virtuously tucked away in a crevice of the hemagglutinin spike, at pH 5.0 (presumably intracellularly), the fusion peptide swings outward and pierces the cell membrane

Futility Futile resuscitation BIOMEDICAL ETHICS A subjective term that encompasses a range of probabilities that a patient will benefit from efforts designed to improve his life and will survive to discharge from a health care facility; the definition for futility has proven to be a stumbling block on whether a person should be subjected to cardiopulmonary resuscitation if the likelihood for a 'meaningful existence' is minimal (J Am Med Assoc 1991; 265:1868); see DNR orders; Cf Euthanasia

Fuzzy space An intracellular, submembranous region in excitable tissue, eg heart muscle that acts as a calcium ion 'purgatory'; on one side, there is sodium-calcium exchanger located on the cell membrane and on the other side is sarcoplasmic reticulum that responds to the influx of calcium by contracting (Science 1990; 248:372, 283)

F waves CARDIOLOGY The waves of atrial flutter on the EKG, which appear as a 'sawtooth' pattern in leads II, III and aVF; less commonly, F waves are undulating, firing at a rate of 280-320/min; this rate is often associated with a 2:1 block and alternating F waves merge with the QRS or T wave NEUROLOGY F wave F response An undulation of the electromyogram that corresponds to time between the application of the stimulus to the axon of the α motor neuron as it propagates andromically to the anterior horn of the spinal cord, and then returns orthodromically along the same axon

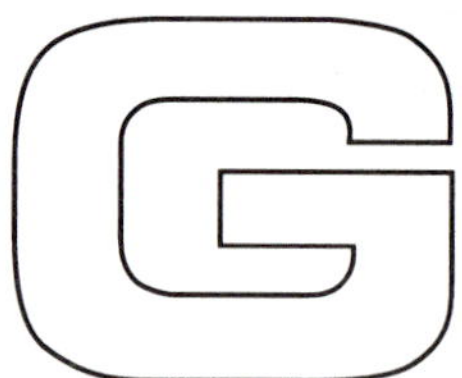

G Symbol for: Gauss; giga-; glycine; guanine

g Symbol for: gram; gravity/centrifugal force

G6PD Glucose-6-phosphate dehydrogenase

G7 The seven wealthiest and industrially advanced nations: Canada, France, Germany, Italy, Japan, United Kingdom, United States

GABA Γ-aminobutyric acid An amino acid that is the major inhibitory neurotransmitter in the vertebrate gray matter; GABA-ergic neurons are classified according to the direction of the cell processes and the signal transmitted and received **Type I GABA-ergic neurons** send and receive signals **Type II GABA-ergic neurons** send messages to other neurons within adjacent gray matter **Type III ('projection') GABA-ergic neurons** have axons that project from the gray matter to the white matter; benzodiazepines potentiate GABA's action by lowering the concentrations of GABA necessary to increase chloride permeability, but therapeutic stimulation or inhibition of GABA release is difficult to achieve, given the ubiquity of GABA's actions; see Stiff man syndrome; GABA is increased in the gastrointestinal tract in hepatic failure and may have a role in hepatic encephalopathy

GABA receptors Membrane receptors which are composed of one or more α/β subunits, each capable of forming receptor-type ion channels (Science 1988; 242:577); once the ligands bind to the receptor, chloride channels are activated

Gadolinium A rare element, atomic weight, 157.25 used as a contrast medium for magnetic resonance imaging of the central nervous system to enhance visualization of neoplasms, parenchymal and congenital lesions, infections and post-operative 'failed back' syndromes (Mayo Clin Proc 1989; 64:986)

gag A retroviral gene that encodes a structural protein within the virus core, which in HIV-1 corresponds to the heterogeneous p24 protein; see HIV-1, Retrovirus

'Gag rule' A US Supreme Court decision in Rust *v.* Sullivan that prohibits physicians employed by the Title X projects, the federal family planning grant program initiated during the Reagan Administration, from fully-counseling women who are unintentionally pregnant, preventing them from offering nondirective advice on prenatal, infant, foster care, adoption and pregnancy termination; see Title X projects

Gaia hypothesis ENVIRONMENT Background: According to Darwin, evolution of the species, ie life, is driven by a static environment or nonlife; Gaia is the theoretical opposite of Darwinism, postulating that living organisms control and modify the relative compositions of the sea, air and environment, thus viewing all life (flora and fauna) on the planet as an interacting homeostatic macrocosm or organism driving mutual coordinated evolution of both the geophysical sphere and the diverse multitude of living organisms (Science 1988; 240:393); Gaia is viewed by its chief architect, J Lovelock as not being endowed with the foresight to regulate the planet's temperature and composition, but rather to optimize it; Gaia-ists are often scientifically 'innocent', while non-Gaia-ists are often mainstream biologists; '....*WE SHOULD BE CAREFUL, HOWEVER, NOT TO PRETEND* (that) *GAIA IS A TESTABLE HYPOTHESIS, MUCH LESS A BASIS FOR MANAGING THE BIOSPHERE. THE RISK IS THIS: A METAPHOR LIKE GAIA, FLEXIBLE ENOUGH TO WRAP AROUND ANY DATA SET, IS ALSO VERSATILE ENOUGH TO BE INVOKED, AD HOC, TO LEND A SPURIOUS AIR OF SCIENTIFIC LEGITIMACY TO ALMOST ANY RECKLESS CONJECTURE.'* JW Kirchner, Cal Tech (Nature 1990; 345:470c); Gaia, the Greek Goddess of the Earth, is an 'organism' from J Lovelock's book on a magical kingdom, Gaia, A New Look at Life on Earth, Oxford University Press, 1979; see Autopoietic Gaia, Creationism; Cf Darwinism, Neo-Darwinism

Galanin A 29-residue peptide neurotransmitter produced in the gastrointestinal tract that induces both contraction and inhibition of the circular and longitudinal smooth muscle and is thus involved in peristalsis

Gale filarienne INFECTIOUS DISEASE Nodules located on the flanks tht correspond to subcutaneous lymphatic vessels plugged with ***Ochocerca volvulus*** microfilaria

Gallium scan NUCLEAR MEDICINE Radioscintillation imaging method that uses ^{67}Gallium citrate ($T_{1/2}$, 25 days); once injected, the gallium binds primarily to transferrin and any tissue that concentrates lactoferrin also concentrates gallium; the gallium scan was formerly used to localize abscesses and osteomyelitis and is used for staging of lymphomas, lung carcinoma, hepatoma, melanoma, metastases (to bone, brain, lung), head and neck, gastrointestinal and genitourinary neoplasia

Gallo probe Robert C Gallo and Luc Montagnier head the AIDS research teams at the National Institute of Health in Bethesda and the Pasteur Institute in Paris respectively; in 1984; Gallo et al, announced the discovery of the retrovirus held responsible for AIDS, which his group called HTLV-III (human T cell lymphotropic virus, now known as human immunodeficiency virus-1 or HIV-1); it was alleged that HTLV-III had been isolated from a cell line designated H9 (or HUT78) that was inadvertently infected with LAV (lymphadenopathy-associated virus, now known as HIV-1) from Montagnier's laboratory, an event with commercial and academic ramifications in the primacy of HTLV-III's discovery; the 'Gallo probe' by the interested parties concluded that the event was the result of unintentional contamination of the tissue culture medium (Science 1990; 248:1494, Nature 1990; 347:603n); see HUT78

Gallop(s) Cardiac auscultatory phenomena in which the tripling or quadrupling of heart sounds have been likened to the canter of a horse; although gallops are often the first sign of cardiac disease, they are often unrecognized, misinterpreted or ignored; gallops occur in diastole (the term 'systolic' gallop is considered incorrect and the appropriate descriptive terminology, eg ejection sound or systolic click is preferred); diastolic sounds are separated by the phase in which they occur; the ventricular (S3 or protodiastolic) gallop follows the normal first and second heart sounds, occurs in early diastole, coinciding with rapid ventricular filling, causing high-pitched vibrations of the ventricular wall as the blood is abruptly stopped; the S3 gallop connotes serious heart disease or decompensation and is associated with coronary, hypertensive, rheumatic and congenital cardiac disease, but may be normal in young adults; once diagnosed, the average ventricular 'galloper' survives 4-5 years; the atrial (S4) gallop occurs during presystole or atrial systole and is characteristic of left ventricular hypertrophy or ischemia; if ventricular failure accompanies ventricular hypertrophy, an S3 gallop may also be heard; the S4 gallop may occur in absence of cardiac decompensation or in primary myocardial disease, coronary artery disease, hypertension and severe valvular stenosis, accompanied by an increased P-Q interval; if the P-R interval is prolonged or the heart rate sufficiently rapid S3 and S4 merge resulting in a 'summation' gallop Note: Traditionally both the three- and four-beat sounds are called gallops, after the footfall of horses; however, while a four-beat heart sound is properly known as a gallop, a three-beat heart sound is equivalent to the equestrian's canter, which in French translates as 'le galop' (J Am Med Assoc 1989; 262:352c)

Galloping consumption Diffuse tuberculous bronchopneumonia

GALT Gut-associated lymphoid tissue The gastrointestinal immune system which is present in the mucosa and submucosa of the gastrointestinal tract, but especially prominent in the oropharynx (tonsils), subjacent to the mucosa (Peyer's patches) and appendix; GALT's components include a) M cells which overlie Peyer's patches, considered 'gatekeepers' for molecular traffic, b) Intraepithelial lymphocytes including CD8 T cells and IgA-producing B-cells, which mediate T-cell cytotoxicity and immune recognition and c) Lamina propria lymphocytes including CD4 T cells, null cells and IgA-producing B-cells

Gamblegram A diagram that represents the cationic and anionic composition of the body, dividing each into rectangles

Gamekeeper's thumb An avulsion fracture at the ulnar aspect of the base of the proximal phalanx, characterized by valgus instability, treated by a cast in adduction; if point instability is marked, open repair of the ligament is indicated; while now more common in 'week-end warriors', ie football or skiing injuries, the original gamekeeper's thumb resulted from repetitive low-grade force, described in gamekeepers who used their thumbs to dislocate the necks of rabbits

Gamma (γ) Symbol for: The heavy chain of immunoglobulin G (IgG); hemoglobin monomeric chain; photon; the third carbon in an aliphatic organic molecule

gamma 'hemolysis' Streptococci hemolyze blood by one of two hemolysins a) The antigenic O_2-labile streptolysin O, which produces α or partial hemolysis and b) The nonantigenic O_2-stable streptolysin S, which produces β or complete hemolysis; streptococci that are non-hemolytic, are said to be gamma-hemolytic, despite the misnomer

gamma-hydroxy-butyrate (GHB) An agent that is in research protocol as a possible therapy for narcolepsy; in Europe, GHB has been used as an anesthetic adjunct and experimentally to treat post-hypoxic cerebral edema and ethanol withdrawal; GHB has been marketed illicitly to body builders since mid-1990 as a sleeping aid, for weight control, as a replacement for L-tryptophan and for allegedly producing a 'high', acting on the endogenous opioid system Toxic effects Potentially severe respiratory depression, seizure-like activity, nausea, vomiting, amnesia, vertigo, hypnagogic effect and coma; the US Food and Drug Administration has issued a warning against the complications when the GHB is used outside of protocol (J Am Med Assoc 1991; 265:1802)

γ-Interferon see Interferon-γ

Gamma knife NEUROSURGERY A stereotactic radiotherapy device that destroys intracranial targets by three-dimensionally focused beams of γ (^{60}Cobalt) radiation with stereotactic precision; thousands of patients have been treated worldwide with minimal intraoperative mortality for such diverse conditions as arteriovenous malformations, meningiomas, acoustic neuromas, pituitary adenomas, craniopharyngiomas and malignancy; the reported delayed morbidity is 3% versus 15% for helium beam therapy; the obliteration rate of arteriovenous malformations by standard helium beam is 30%, while the γ knife has an 80-90% rate of obliteration with negligible recurrent hemorrhage

Gammopathy An abnormal increase in immunoglobulin production; Monoclonal gammopathies are usually malignant and include multiple myelomas, Waldenström's disease, chronic lymphocytic leukemia, heavy-chain disease, but may also be benign, appearing in amyloidosis and monoclonal gammopathy of undetermined significance; polyclonal gammopathies are usually benign and appear in inflammatory conditions, including rheumatoid arthritis, lupus erythematosus, cirrhosis, tuberculosis, leishmaniasis, angioimmunoblastic lymphadenopathy Note: Polyclonal gammopathies may occur as epiphenomena in lymphomas, Hodgkin's disease, metastatic adenocarcinoma

Gancyclovir (9-[2-hydroxy-1-(hydroxymethyl) ethoxymethyl] guanine An anti-viral agent used to treat cytomegalic inclusion viral (CMV) infections in the immunocompromised; gancyclovir is effective in treating CMV-induced retinitis, gastroenteritis and hepatitis and eliminates CMV from the blood, urine and respiratory secretions within 5 days of therapy; CMV progression despite adequate therapy may indicate drug resistance by CMV (N Engl J Med 1989; 320:289) Side effects Changes in mental status, neutropenia, thrombocytopenia Note: AIDS patients and bone marrow recipients respond poorly to gancyclovir; Cf Acyclovir

Ganglion A mass of organized neural tissue

Ganglion cyst A common soft tissue 'tumor' of the hand that is a) Not a ganglion, ie neural in origin and b) Not a cyst, but rather represents mucoid degeneration of tendinous tissues; ganglion cysts are often located on the wrist in middle-aged women and may cause the carpal tunnel syndrome

Gangrene Tissue death most common in the distal lower extremities or internal organs, usually the large intestine; the type of gangrene is a function of the environment or host **DRY GANGRENE** A condition caused by chronic occlusion that slowly progresses to severe tissue atrophy and mummification, often associated with peripheral vascular disease, eg diabetes mellitus, atherosclerosis **GAS GANGRENE** A condition most often appearing in open or poorly cleaned wounds infected by gas-producing gram-positive anaerobes, including ***Clostridium perfringens, C histolytica, C septicum, C novyi*** and ***C fallax*** that release histolytic enzymes, including collagenase, fibrinolysin, hyaluronidase and lecithinase **WET GANGRENE** A condition caused by relatively acute vascular occlusion, eg burns, freezing, crush injuries and thromboembolism, resulting in liquefactive necrosis, causing bleb and bullae formation with violaceous discoloration

GAP GTPase-activating protein A 110 kD cytoplasmic protein that has a role in human cancer, acting as a growth signal, enhancing the GTPase activity of the N-ras p21 protein by interacting with the ras effector binding domain (Science 1988; 240:518); GAP has a 25% homology with the catalytic region of the neurofibromatosis gene

Gap-43 Growth-associated protein A neuron-specific protein associated with the membrane of the nerve growth cone, having a role in cytoskeleton and intermediate filament regulation

Gap filling MOLECULAR BIOLOGY An activity that occurs on the discontinuous strand of DNA during replication, which entails joining of the gaps between the Okazaki fragments; see Okazaki fragments

Gap junction A cluster of transmembrane channels or connexons, separated by a 2-4 nm space that allow communication between cells and the free passage of small (< 1.2 kD) molecules, including ions, water, amino acids and nucleoside phosphates; each connexon is composed of a six subunits, each containing 12 molecules of 28-32 kD connexin, arranged in a hexamer that opens as cellular calium ions fall; Cf Tight junction

GAPO syndrome A condition characterized by growth retardation, alopecia, pseudo-anodontia (the teeth are present but unerupted) and optic atrophy; the few cases described have also had hydrocephalus, high palate, low-set ears

'Garbage' Computers A colloquial term for a) Scattered storage space, usually due to deleted files, that is not available for use, the sum aggregate of which is large enough to store extra files, either on the hard drive or on floppy disks, despite 'insufficient memory' messages and requires a 'garbage collecting' program to utilize the dead space created by the deleted files and b) 'Nonsense' produced by a printer, eg incorrect ASCII characters versus text, often due to loose cables to the printer or due to use of an incorrect printer driver

'Garbage can' hypothesis Accumulation theory A theory regarding the pathogenesis of senescence, which holds that as a cell line ages, it converts to a multigenerational wastebasket, where the older cells accumulate metabolic products capable of damaging the cell's macromolecules, eg proteins and nucleic acids and are less efficient in repairing damage; the most critical intracellular 'garbage' accumulated are the oxygen free radicals; mechanisms designed to remove the free radicals, including antioxidants and superoxide dismutase; another contributor to senescent 'garbage' is glucose, which attaches to proteins by non-enzymatic glycosylation, forming advanced glycosylation end products causing a loss of collagen elasticity (Science 1990; 250:622) Note: Enzyme systems have been shown to be less efficient in aging cells lines, lending credence to this theory; Cf Pacemaker theory

Garden hose appearance The appearance of tubular lumens with extensive transmural fibrosis and stenosis, seen in a) The small intestine,usually affecting the terminal ileum in advanced Crohn's disease and b) Esophagus in well-developed progressive systemic sclerosis

'Garden variety' An adjective for lesions or diseases that are both common and/or have relatively routine clinical, radiologic or pathological findings, and which constitute the bulk of disease seen in medical practice, thus there is 'garden variety' appendicitis, 'garden variety' myocardial infarction, 'garden variety' colonic adenocarcinoma and so on

Gardner effect see Sellafield studies

Gargoyle cells Cells that are engorged with mucopolysaccharide-laden lysosomes, abundantly present in those afflicted with Hurler syndrome or mucopolysaccharidosis type I-H, due to α-L-iduronidase deficiency, in which there is an accumulation of dermatan and heparan sulfates

Gargoyle face The characteristic facies seen in gargoylism, an obsolete term for mucopolysaccharidoses (MPS); the classic gargoyle face is seen in MPS type I-H (Hurler) and MPS type IV (Morquio) and characterized by thickening and coarsening of the facial features due to subcutaneous deposit of MPSs, most commonly appearing after the first year of age; the head is large and dolichocephalic, with frontal bossing and prominent sagittal and metopic sutures, with mid-face hypoplasia, depressed nasal bridge, flared nares and increased prominence of the lower third of the face, thickened facies, widely spaced teeth and attenuated dental enamel and gingival hyperplasia; similar facies may be seen in the cherry red spot myoclonus syndrome, Coffin-Siris syndrome, GM1 gangliosidosis, Goldberg syndrome, hyperimmunoglobulin E syndrome, hypothyroidism, Kniest syndrome, mannosidosis, type II, mucolipidosis (I-cell disease), MPS types I-S (Scheie syndrome), II (Hunter syndrome) and III (Sanfilippo syndrome), multiple neuroma syndrome, multiple sulfatase deficiency, Robinow syndrome, Rolland-Desbuquios syndrome, sialic acid storage disease with sialuria, sialidosis, type II, Sotos' syndrome and Williams syndrome Note: Gargoyles are grotesque spouts in the form of mythical animals, fantastic beasts or grotesque human that project from the gutters of Gothic buildings; the term arrived to Middle English in 1412, via Spanish, gargola, throat

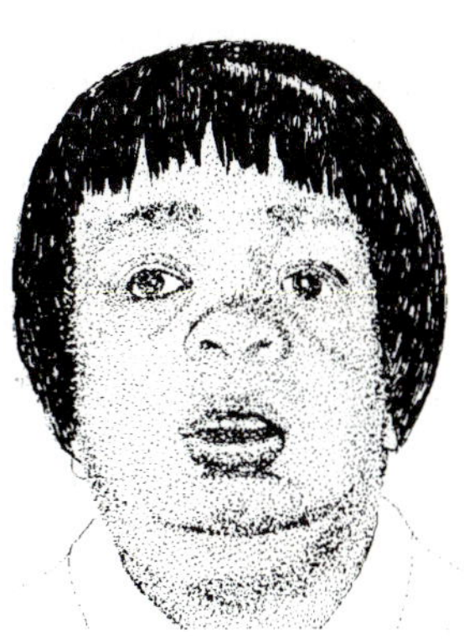

Gargoyle-like face

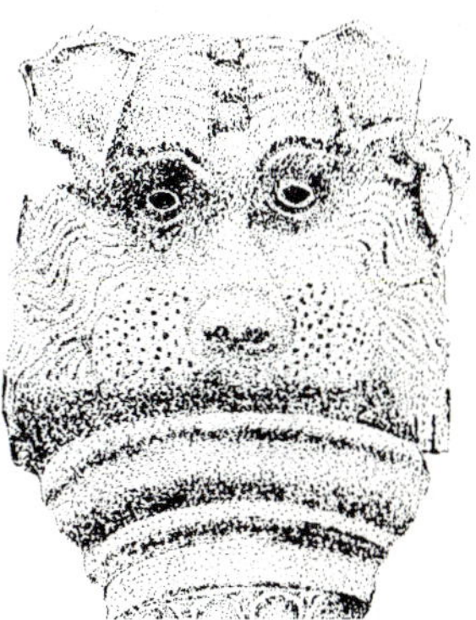

Gargoyle

Garlic *Allium sativum* A pungent herb used in cooking that is attracting research interest given its positive systemic effects on metabolism, the immune and other systems; in experimental systems allicin, the active ingredient of garlic oil extract, a) Inhibits tumor growth and activity of tumor promoters and has chemopreventive activity against methylcholanthrene-induced carcinogenesis b) Enhances defenses against systemic toxins, acting in antihepatotoxin, stabilizing liver microsomal membranes from lipid peroxidation and ameliorates cyclophosphamide toxicity in mice c) Has non-specific anti-infectious activity, inhibiting growth of ***Entamoeba histolytica***, lipid synthesis by ***Candida albicans*** and attachment of ***Candida*** species to buccal mucosa and d) Inhibits platelet aggregation, inhibiting platelet release reaction (J Natl Med Assoc 1988; 80:439); garlic owes its aroma to the high content of selenium, which is eliminated through the lungs and skin as volatile dimethyl selenide Note: Garlic's protective effect against upper respiratory tract infection may be an epiphenomenon as those with 'hypergarlicosis' may be given a wider berth by peers and are thus less exposed to infected aerosols; Cf Spicy foods

Garlic clove fibroma A fanciful term for a benign, pedunculated tumor arising in the fingernail bed Histopathology Either a fibroepithelial polyp or irritation fibroma

Garment nevus see Bathing trunk nevus

GASA Growth adjusted sonographic age Obstetrics A sonographic estimation of fetal age based on two determinations of biparietal diameter, one at 26 weeks and one at 30-33 weeks; Cf Biophysical profile

Gas-bloat syndrome GASTROENTEROLOGY The inability to vomit after gastric fundoplication for reflux esophagitis, a complication of the Nissen repair of a hiatal hernia, a procedure that corrects 96% of cases of esophageal reflux; the bloating is thought to be due to vagal injury and is characterized by post-operative dysphagia and a build-up of gas

Gas-liquid chromatography (GLC) INSTRUMENTATION A type of column partition chromatography in which the stationary phase is an inert vehicle covered by a non-volatile gas and the mobile phase is volatile; GLC is a highly sensitive and specific analytic technique for quantifying volatile substances (and substances that can be transformed into volatiles) that is used in toxicology and in research, eg in microbiology to identify short-chain fatty acids, non-volatile organic acids and alcohols produced by bacterial metabolism

Gasoline pump appearance A descriptor for the apically-oriented eosinophilic secretory 'snouts' seen by light microscopy in apocrine metaplasia of the breast, the presence of which suggests benign behavior in breast lesions, although 'snouting' may occur in the rare cases of apocrine carcinoma Note: The term derives from the bulbous tops of gasoline (petrol) pumps of pre-1950s vintage

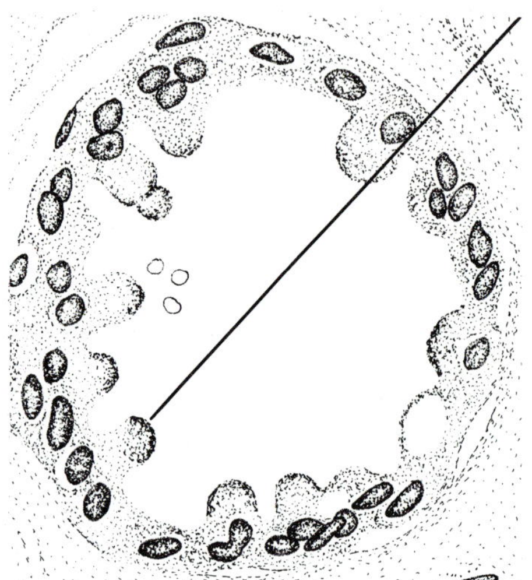

Gasoline pump appearance

Gasping syndrome NEONATOLOGY A condition due to toxic systemic accumulation of benzyl alcohol (used to clean neonatal skin), which because of the immaturity of their metabolic systems and relative fragility of their skin, is most severe in preterm infants **Clinical** Gradual neurological deterioration, severe metabolic acidosis, sudden onset of gasping respiration, hematological abnormalities including pancytopenia, hyperbilirubinemia and hyperammonemia, skin sloughing, hepatic failure, renal failure, hypotension, cardiovascular collapse and a 'negative' autopsy (N Engl J Med 1982; 307:1384)

Gas(-producing) 'syndromes' Excess gas in the gastrointestinal tract is due to aerophagia or increased production by intestinal bacteria which may be facilitated by a deficiency of pancreatic enzymes; gastric gas is accompanied by bloating, pain, eruction and flatulence; intestinal gas is often accompanied by abdominal distension, flatulence and hypomotility or hypermotility; see Flatulence

Gastric bubble of Garren A doughnut-shaped inflatable polyurethane cylinder designed to decrease the available stomach volume, a therapeutic modality for morbid obesity, reducing the gnawing hunger pangs by inflating a balloon in their stomachs; when the gastric bubble is placed for prolonged periods, it may induce hyperplasia of the G or gastrin-producing cells or rarely, pressure ulcers (J Am Med Assoc 1986; 256:3284); see Diet, Ileal bypass operation, Morbid obesity

Gastric 'cannonball(s)' Radiology A descriptor for smoothly contoured, large and non-ulcerated filling defects in the stomach, seen in radiocontrast studies, most often due to metastasizing hepatoma, but also seen with hematomas, multiple submucosal leiomyomas, lymphomas, neurofibromas, metastatic intraperitoneal malignancy and other lesions that deform the gastric mucosa; Cf 'Golfball' metastases

Gastric inhibitory polypeptide see GIP

Gastric outlet obstruction (GOO) A manifestation of gastric dysmotility; the rate of gastric emptying is controlled by duodenal receptors for fat or acid; GOO is diagnosed when there is a) More than 50% retention of a barium 'meal' more than 4 hours after ingestion b) An overnight fasting gastric residue volume of more than 200 ml or c) Fractional emptying of a ^{99m}Tc-labelled liquid of less than 10%/min; GOO is due to ulcers, benign or malignant tumors, inflammation (cholecystitis, acute pancreatitis or Crohn's disease), caustic strictures, pyloric stenosis **Clinical** Vomiting (often daily), intermittent epigastric pain

Gastrin G34 (34 amino acid residues, 'big' gastrin) is the circulating form in both patients with Zollinger-Ellison syndrome and in normal subjects; G17 (17 residues, 'little' gastrin) is the tissue-based form produced in gastrinomas, the normal gastric antrum, duodenum and jejunum; G13 or G14 (14 residues, 'minigastrin', formed from the carboxyl-terminal); a non-functional 13 residue amino-terminal fragment is also produced; gastrin is released by local (partially digested proteins and calcium salts) and neural (bombesin) stimulation and inhibited by secretin, somatostatin and vasoacitive intestinal polypeptide; gastrin stimulates acid secretion, mitotic activity of the gastric mucosa and increases blood flow through gastric mucosa; excess gastrin causes the release of calcitonin and insulin, spasm of the lower esophageal sphincter, hyperacidity with formation of multiple peptic ulcers, hypertrophy of the gastric mucosa, steatorrhea and secretion of water and electrolytes and enzymes; normal levels 100 pg/ml, occur while in the Zollinger-Ellison syndrome, levels of up to 60 000 pg/ml occur; gastrin is increased in antral or G-cell hyperplasia, atrophy of mucosa achlorhydria, gastric carcinoma, gastric outlet syndrome, pernicious anemia, pheochromocytoma, 'retained antrum' syndrome, short bowel syndrome and uremia

Gastrinoma An often multicentric tumor of the pancreatic islet delta cells that arises spontaneously or may be associated with MEN-1 (multiple endocrine neoplasm, type 1); rarely the tumors may be very small, eg 2-6 mm and located in the duodenum (N Engl J Med

1990; 322: 723) and/or are associated with the Zollinger-Ellison syndrome

Gastrinoma triangle The anatomic region defined by the junction of the cystic and common bile ducts superiorly, the junction of the second and third segments of the duodenum infero-laterally and the neck and body of the pancreas medially (Am J Surg 1984; 147:584, Am J Med 1987; 82:supp 5B:17); this triangle defines the region where most gastrinomas are located

Gas washout technique PHYSIOLOGY A method that uses inert gases (N_2, He, Ne, Xe) to measure the functional, freely-communicating airway and lung volumes; Fowler's 'single nitrogen wash-out test' measures the uniformity of ventilation throughout the lungs; the patient first expires to maximum residual volume, then fills the lungs maximally with 100% O_2; during the next breath, the concentration of nitrogen at the mouth is continuously recorded and plotted against the volume of expired gas; while Fowler's initial measurements in 1949 concentrated on changing N_2 concentrations, addition of xenon to the mixture increases the test's utility as it provides information on functional size of the small airways or the closing volume, which in normal healthy young adults is about 10% of the vital capacity, a volume that increases with age and in smokers

GATA-1 A zinc-finger transcription factor that binds to the GATA consensus elements in regulatory regions of the α- and β-globin gene clusters and other erythrocyte-specific genes and which is critical in differentiation of erythrocytes (Nature 1991; 349:257)

Gate COMPUTERS An electronic circuit that performs an operation when the criteria for a logical relation, eg AND, or OR are fulfilled; see Computers

Gate control theory NEUROPHYSIOLOGY The theory that holds that the amount and quality of nociception is determined by multiple physiologic and psychologic variables, modulated at the dorsal horns and at other levels of the ascending afferent pathway (Science 1965; 150:971); this theory attempts to explain why neural impulses generated by painful stimuli and transported by small A-delta and C fibers can be blocked at the synapse in the dorsal horn by simultaneous firing of large diameter, low-threshold myelinated A fibers, inhibiting nociception; it is also evoked to explain the effects of acupuncture and transcutaneous electrical nerve stimulation on recalcitrant pain; the gate control theory contrasts to the more widely accepted 'specificity' theory in which individual branches of peripheral nerves are thought to be devoted to carrying only one type of sensation, eg pain, touch or temperature

Gated blood pool scanning A radionuclide technique used in cardiology to calculate various hemodynamic parameters including cardiac output, right and left ventricular ejection fractions; one parameter, stroke volume ratio, allowing quantification of valvular regurgitation at rest and during exercise; finally the technique detects abnormalities of regional wall movement

'Gatekeeper' Any person, organization or legislation that selectively limits access to a service; in health care, primary-care physicians, peer-review organizations and utilization review committees function as direct or indirect gatekeepers

'Gateway' drug Any drug or addictive subtance, eg nicotine and alcohol that may be abused prior to a person initiating abuse of illicit 'soft' drugs, eg marijuana and/or 'hard' drugs, eg cocaine and heroin; see Glue sniffing, 'White-out'

Gating PHYSIOLOGY The opening and closing of voltage-activated channels, an activity that is regulated by transmembrane voltage and neurotransmitters

Gating INSTRUMENTATION A process of electronic selection, in which the observer selects a level of an electronic signal above which a certain action is allowed, as in flow cytometry, where only those lymphocytes that fall within a 'gated' region are counted as such on the histogram, while those outside of this region are not PHYSIOLOGY The opening and closing of an ion channel in a cell membrane, caused by conformational change in one or more transmembrane proteins; see Ball and chain model, Voltage-dependent calcium channel

Gavage Nasogastric feeding of patients, eg premature infants with weak sucking reflexes or nasogastric hyperalimentation

Gay bowel syndrome An array of infectious and non-infectious gastrointestinal symptoms first described in homosexual males prior to the early reports of AIDS (Am J Gastroenterol 1977; 67:478) Clinical Proctalgia 80%, change in bowel habits 50%, condyloma acuminata 52%, cramping diarrhea, bloating, flatulence, nausea and vomiting, adenomatous polyps, fissures, fistulas, hemorrhoids, perirectal abscess, shigellosis, proctitis, rectal ulcers, giardiasis and sexually-transmitted disease, including Herpes simplex, syphilis, gonococcus and *Chlamydia trachomatis*; other 'gay bowel' organisms, include 'gay CLOs', ie *Campylobacter*-like organisms, eg *C fennelliae* and *C cinaedi*, human papilloma virus (associated with anal carcinoma and dysplasia), cytomegalovirus, hepatitis A and B, parasites, eg ***Entamoeba histolytica, Entamoeba coli, Endolimax nana, Enterobius vermicularis, Strongyloides stercoraliz, Iodamoeba beutschlii*** and bacteria (***N meningitis, Haemophilus ducreyi*** and ***Salmonella*** species); other findings include rectal dyspareunia, pruritis ani, anal incontinence, trauma, eg secondary to 'fisting' that, like insertion of variably-sized and shaped foreign objects, may cause colorectal perforation and abscess formation Treatment Acute proctitis may require penicillin, probenicid and doxycycline, changing to specific agents if an organism is identified (J Am Med Assoc 1988; 260:348); anal cancer is more common in the male gay population and has been related to receptive anal intercourse; the relative risk for squamous cell anal cancer is 1.8; genital warts are often positive for human papillomavirus and may precede squamous cell carcinoma, but not transitional cell carcinoma

GC 1) see Gas-liquid chromatography 2) Neisseriae gonorrheae see Penicillinase-resistant Gonococcus neisseriae

GC box see GGGCGG box

G cells Flask-shaped gastrin-secreting cells thought to be of neural crest origin, which have features of APUD system; G cells are located in the gastric mucosa, especially in the pyloric antrum

G:C ratio Guanine:Cytosine ratio MOLECULAR BIOLOGY The DNA nucleotide base pairs guanine and cytosine in the double helix share three hydrogen bonds and denature at higher temperatures than adenine and thymine, which share two hydrogen bonds, therefore the higher the G:C base pair content of the double helix, the higher the temperature required for thermal denaturation of DNA; this occurs at 70°C when the double helix is composed entirely of adenine and thymine base pairs and at 110°C when the entire DNA molecule is composed of cytosine and guanine base pairs; the G:C ratio has been used to compare relatedness between various organisms, eg in microbiology for classifying bacteria

G-CSF Granulocyte colony-stimulating factor A biological response modifier, the recombinant DNA-produced form of which, Filgastim (Neupogen, Amgen Inc) was licensed in 1991; G-CSF stimulates granulocyte production in bone marrow suppressed by chemotherapy and/or radiation, serving to reduce infections in patients with malignancy; G-CSF is encoded on chromosome 17, produced by endothelial cells, fibroblasts and macrophages, and stimulates granulocyte production in the bone marrow, acting synergistically with IL-3 to stimulate proliferation of other marrow cells (N Engl J Med 1990; 323:871; J Am Med Assoc 1991; 265:2315); see Biological response modifiers, Colony-stimulating factors; Cf GM-CSF

G deletion syndrome CLINICAL GENETICS A complex resulting from various anomalies of the G chromosome, eg partial deletion and ring formation Clinical Ptosis, epicanthal folds, flattened nasal bridge, growth and mental retardation

'Geezer' A derogatory term for elderly, cantankerous, often poorly-educated male patients (J Am Med Assoc 1988; 259:1228)

Gefilte fish A traditional Jewish dish eaten on Friday nights, made from various fishes that are chopped, ground, mixed with eggs, salt, onions and peppers, often garnished with chrayn (horseradish), and then cooked; gefilte fish may be a vector for the fish tapeworm, *Diphyllobothrium latum*, which may ingested while the chef is preparing the garnee prior to cooking and is well-described in Jewish mothers; the parasite destroyed by cooking for 10 minutes at 56°C, or blast-freezing to -35°C for 15 hours or -23°C for 7 days; freezing for 24 hours, salting, smoking and pickling does not kill parasites; see Fish, Sushi

Gegenhalten German, to hold against Paratonia Resistance to passive movement that increases with the velocity of movement and continues through the full arc of motion, thought to be due to diffuse forebrain dysfunction as occurs in anterior cerebral artery occlusion ('arteriosclerotic parkinsonism or pseudoparkinsonism); Gegenhalten may be accompanied by grasp reflex; Cf Clasp-knife phenomenon, Cogwheel rigidity

Gel Agar gel A semisolid medium made from the seaweed agar that is used as a support in CLINICAL CHEMISTRY for serum protein electrophoresis for separating proteins into albumin and α, β and γ bands, see SPEP HEMATOLOGY for separating hemoglobins IMMUNOLOGY for antigen-antibody reactions MICROBIOLOGY where various nutrients are added to the agar to enhance or select for the growth of certain bacteria and fungi MOLECULAR BIOLOGY for separating DNA, RNA and proteins by electrophoresis

Gelastic epilepsy A form of complex partial seizure due to epileptic discharges in the temporal lobe characterized by inappropriate laughter as a manifestation of automatism

Gel filtration chromatography Molecular sieve chromatography A column chromatographic technique in which gel particles of a certain size and porosity comprise the stationary phase, allowing the fractionation of a solution of molecules according to size, shape and rate of diffusion into the gel, where larger molecules pass through the column and are eluted before smaller molecules

'Gelling' Stiffness following rest, characteristic of rheumatic diseases, eg in juvenile rheumatoid arthritis (Still's disease) variably accompanied by polyarthritis and guarding of the joints against activity

Gelsolin A protein produced by macrophages that caps, severs and nucleates actin filaments, participating in actin's assembly and dissembly and increasing the motility of some cells, eg fibroblasts in a concentration-dependent fashion (Science 1991; 251:1233); gelsolin is activated by calcium ions and inhibited by membrane polyphosphoinositides; precise regulation of actin assembly may result from an interplay between gelsolin and the related, structurally homologous gCap39 protein (Science 1990; 250:1413)

Gemfibrozil A drug that inhibits very low density lipoprotein synthesis, used to lower serum cholesterol, triglycerides and lipoproteins; in healthy volunteers, gemfibrozil causes a 30-40% reduction in VLDL and IDL and 10% increase in the HDL (J Am Med Assoc 1989; 262:3148); in type V hyperlipoproteinemia, gemfibrozil is an agent of first choice in lowering both cholesterol and triglyceride (ibid, 262:3154); see Cholesterol-lowering drugs, Lovastatin

Gene The classic mendelian definition of a gene as a unit of heredity carrying a single trait and recognized by its ability to mutate and undergo recombination is primitive; as currently defined, a gene is a segment of DNA nucleotides, comprised of 70 to 30 000 base pairs including introns, that encodes a sequence of messenger RNA, capable of giving rise to a functional (enzyme, hormone, receptor) polypeptide; genes may be structural, forming cell components or functional, having a regulatory role

Gene amplification The increase in copy numbers of a gene, an event associated with cellular oncogenes in malignancy, where the copy number is a crude benchmark of tumor aggression; chromosomal abnormalities typical of amplified genes include double minutes, C-bandless (fragments of DNA without centromers) chromosomes and homogenously-staining chromosomal regions; the precise mechanism of amplification is unknown, but may be due to multiple repeated unequal sister chromatid exchanges; an example of gene amplification au natural is that of the multi-drug resistance gene in tumors treated with methotrexate Note: The polymerase chain reaction (PCR) is a form of 'gene amplification', but given the potential for confusion, 'gene amplification' is best used for a phenomenon occurring in vivo in aberrant, often malignant cells that appear to be mounting a defense against a hostile environment; 'DNA amplification' is best reserved for an in vitro process in which the double helix of DNA is manipulated as per the desires of the researcher; see PCR (polymerase chain reaction)

GenBank A repository for nucleic acid sequence data created in 1982 from the Los Alamos (USA) DNA sequence library, which currently accumulates 20 million nucleotide of DNA sequences per year in its database, providing a format for electronic publishing so that a sequence of nucleotides is published within 2 weeks of submission of the information rather than the one year required in usual (paper) publishing (Science 1991; 252:1273)

Gene diversity The breadth of immune response that an antigen is capable of evoking, based on a simple principle of mixing and matching of exons from gene segments designated as variable, diversity, joining and constant regions (table); elucidation of this mechanism of gene diversity (Proc Natl Acad Sci 1976; 73:3628) garnered its author, Susumu Tonegawa, the 1987 Nobel Prize

Gene diversity How immunoglobulin responds to many antigens (Proc Nat Acad Sci 1976; 73:3628)
- Multiple germ-line V genes
- VJ and VDJ recombinations (Nature 1983; 302:575)
- Recombinational inaccuracies
- Somatic point mutation
- Heavy and light chain combinations
- Signal sequence replacement (Science 1988; 242:261)

Gene expression The multistep (transcription of a segment of DNA to mRNA and translation into a protein) process by which a functioning protein product is produced

Gene knockout technique An experimental technique used in yeast genetics in which a normal gene is replaced by a defective gene at the exact same chromosomal site (hence, the normal gene is 'knocked out' by the defective gene); in contrast, insertion of DNA in mammalian cells occurs in random sites

Gene library see Library

Gene machine A semi-automatic or automatic device that is capable of synthesizing high-quality chains of nucleic acids of up to 100 bases in length; Cf Sequenator

Gene mapping see Mapping

Gene pool 'The sum total of the genes present in a sexually-reproducing population', Stenesh, 1989; see Consanguinity, Founder effect

Gene product A polypeptide or protein encoded by a gene

Gene promotion Induction or activation of genes, which is facilitated by breaks in the ordered arrays of nucleosomes, these sites being sensitive to DNase I

General adaption 'syndrome' see Fight-or-flight response

General health screen A battery of serum assays that are considered to be the most cost-effective in determining a person's basic state of health, including albumin, alkaline phosphatase, AST (GOT), BUN/creatinine, calcium, total bilirubin, cholesterol, glucose, lactate dehydrogenase, potassium, total protein, sodium, triglycerides, uric acid; see Executive profile, Organ panel

Generally regarded as safe list (GRAS) CLINICAL PHARMACOLOGY An extensive list of compounds compiled by the US Food and Drug Administration that are often used in foods, cosmetics and drugs and widely regarded as having little or no adverse effects on humans, first legally defined under the 1958 Amendment of the Federal Food, Drug and Cosmetics Act; GRAS compounds include food preservatives, coatings and films that may be used on fruits and vegetables, special dietary and nutritive additives, anticaking agents, eg sodium ferrocyanide, flavoring agents, gum bases and other multipurpose agents; see Food preservatives

Gene rearrangement The shuffling of genetic material, where introns (intervening sequences) are removed and exons are spliced together to form mRNA; gene rearrangement indicates a lymphocyte's commitment to production of one specific cell type, either immunoglobulin production by B-cells or a β-chain receptor in T-cells; malignancy, then, may be viewed as an irreversible clonal expansion detectable by changes in a cell's genotype; in lymphocytes, if the cell population is heterogeneous, as it is under normal circumstances, there will be no predominance of any one cell type and by extension, no 'signal' as detected by Southern blot hybridization; however if one clone of cells is expanding, ie malignant, a 1-5% increase in the number of those cells is detectable by Southern blotting; for lymphoproliferative disorders, a) T-cell malignancies, somatic rearrangement and clonal expansion of the T-cell receptor β-chain is diagnostic for T-cell lymphoma/leukemia (Proc Nat Acad Sci 1985; 82:1224) and b) B-cell malignancies, somatic rearrangement and clonal expansion of immunoglobulin genes (V, D, J and C regions) is virtually diagnostic for a B-cell lymphoproliferative disease

Gene recombination see Recombinant DNA

Generic Nonproprietary

GENESIS A computer program (Loomis and Gilpin, University of California, San Diego) that has rules for DNA sequence duplications, deletions, exons and mutations

Gene splicing see Recombinant DNA technology, Splicing

Gene therapy A family of therapeutic modalities and products derived from recombinant DNA technology; these products include tissue plasminogen activator and

Recombivax Note: The diseases targeted for gene therapy include inborn diseases of metabolism, where a defective gene cannot encode a crucial protein, usually an enzyme; the first disease in the protocol stage for gene therapy is adenosine deaminase (ADA) deficiency; strategies for gene therapy include a) Introduction of a recombinant retrovirus bearing the missing gene, the promoter and the gene regulator sequence in the package or b) Implant the colonies of cells producing the missing factor(s), eg α_1-antitrypsin deficiency with the missing enzyme introduced into 'carrier' fibroblasts

Genetic disease A generic term for any (inherited) condition caused by a defective gene, most of which are known as an 'inborn error of metabolism'

Genetic engineering The manipulation of the genome of a living organism, resulting in the modification of both 'domesticated' and wild-type bacteria by insertion of genes or by genetic selection; genetic engineering has broad potential applicability a) Agriculture, as natural enemies to crop parasites or by increasing nitrogen-fixing b) Industry, for production of fuels, eg ethanol, chemicals, eg amino acids and for mineral processing, eg bioleaching c) ENVIRONMENT for the production of biodegradable plastics and treatment of municipal and industrial wastewater and d) Medicine (Science 1989; 244:1305)

Genetic heterogeneity The presence of a variety of genetic defects which cause the same clinical disease, often due to mutations at different loci on the same gene, a finding common to many human diseases including Alzheimer's disease, cystic fibrosis, lipoprotein lipase and polycystic kidney disease

Genetic marker A visible mutable site on a chromosome which when mutated, leads to gross changes to the host organism and on the chromosome itself

Genetic polymorphism see RFLP

Genetic recombination The process by which blocks of homologous chromosomes exchange material by crossing over, an event that occurs during meiosis in sexually-reproducing organisms and forms the basis of genetic maps

Geneva Conventions A protocol established in 1864 and revised and expanded in 1949 regarding the conduct of the military towards medical personnel and the obligations of medical personnel during acts of war; the initial Geneva Conference of 1864, simply recognized the neutrality of medical personnel, acknowledged the need for common protection in time of battle, and agreed upon rules for the protection and exchange of wounded personnel; in the 1949, 60 nations agreed upon conventions that bound all nations to the laws of humanity and to the dictates of public conscience; under the revision, medical personnel and treatment facilities are designated as immune from attack and captured medical personnel are to be promptly repatriated; medical personnel likewise have a series of specific obligations 1) As 'noncombatants', medical personnel are forbidden to engage in or be parties to acts of war 2) The wounded and sick, both soldier and civilian, both friend and foe, shall be respected, treated humanely and cared for by the belligerants 3) The wounded and sick may not be left without medical assistance, and only urgent medical reasons authorize any priority in the order of their treatment 4) Medical aid must be dispensed solely on medical grounds, without distinctions founded on sex, race, nationality, religion, opinion or any other similar criteria 5) No physical or moral coercion shall be exercised against protected personnel (civilians), in particular to obtain information from them or from third parties; see Helsinki Declaration, Nuremburg Code of Ethics, Unethical medical research

Genome project see Human genome project

Genomic imprinting see Imprinting

Genote MOLECULAR EVOLUTION A cytological term for an organism with modern translation machinery, based on the 'evolutionary clock', where organisms are phylogenically classified according to the evolving complexity of ribosomal RNA; Cf Progenote, Universal ancestor (Science 1990; 250:1070c)

Gentleman scientist A term arising in post-renaissance Europe, referring to a financially independent gentleman who had the luxury of studying scientific phenomena as a hobby; during most of the 20th century, science became more egalitarian and any person who could do 'good science' was be able to support himself and his 'significant others' on his salary; in the 1980s and 1990s, budget deficits in developed nations have burgeoned, and monies to support new grants have receded (in the US and in part in Europe), with the result that many excellent grants are awarded the hollow accolade of *'APPROVED BUT NOT FUNDED'* (approximately 20% of grant proposals are ultimately funded), or suffer the lesser indignation of 'downward negotiation' and 'dunning fees' from their own institution in the form of bills for overhead costs Note: Given the current economic environment for scientists, independent wealth may become necessary in order to 'do science' and the gentleman scientist may once again become a fixture in academia; see 'New scientist', Cf 'Lab rat'

Genu genuflectum Infrapatellar bursitis in clergy, which can be so intense (as with Saint Tekla Haymanot, 12th century) as to cause gangrene of the foot Note: According to legend, St Tekla was compensated for the lost legs by being given a pair of wings, ie alae neoplasticae post-gangrenosa eremeticum (N Engl J Med 1983; 309:561c)

Geode Giant subchondral pseudocysts often of weight-bearing joints, with articular destruction, characteristic of rheumatoid arthritis, but also seen in osteoarthritis and hemophilia (Mayo Clin Proc 1987; 62:407)

Geographic exclusion A ban on the collection or use of blood donated by subjects native to certain countries, which currently includes all of Africa with the exception of Algeria, Egypt, Libya, Mauritania, Morocco, Sudan, Somalia, Tunisia and Western Sahara (Arab nations with a low incidence of AIDS) Note: Since the beginning of the AIDS epidemic, there has been a well-publicized, higher-than-normal incidence of HIV seropositivity in Haitians, leading the US FDA to ban blood donation from this population group, a ban that was lifted in 1990 (Am Med News 28/Dec/90)

Geographic pattern A descriptor for lesions in which large areas of one color, histological pattern or radiological density with variably scalloped borders are superimposed on another color, pattern or density, likened to national boundaries and coastlines DERMATOLOGY A pattern of skin involvement in psoriasis FORENSIC PATHOLOGY A descriptor for the variegated pattern of skin ulceration seen in drug addicts who inject heroin subcutaneously (skin popping), which may be surrounded by 'ameboid' rim of hyperkeratotic and inflammed skin PATHOLOGY Sharply defined 'fjord-like' histologic separation of one tissue morphology from another, seen at low-power (40 X) in a) Lymph nodes affected by lymphogranuloma venereum, less commonly described in cat-scratch disease b) Lungs of Wegener's granulomatosus where irregular necrotic patches are interspersed with scattered islands of preserved pulmonary parenchyma, also described in rare fulminant pulmonary infections c) Soft tissue in epithelioid sarcoma, in which geographic lesions may result from fusion of several necrotizing nodules, often accompanied by hemorrhage and cystic degeneration in epithelioid sarcomas; the geographic islands have central necrosis and are rimmed by chronic inflammation; epithelioid sarcomas are slow-growing tumors of young adults, often of the upper extremities **Prognosis** Poor if necrotic RADIOLOGY Broad areas of patchy destruction, seen in such diverse conditions as Gaucher's disease, histiocytosis X, osteolytic tumors, eg metastatic bronchogenic carcinoma and osteosarcoma

Geographic tongue Erythema migrans, glossitis areata exfoliativa, lingua geographica, migratory glossitis ORAL DISEASE **Clinical** Idiopathic tender or irritated lesions, possibly related to emotional stress, more common in children and adolescents or asymptomatic inflammation with denudation of the filiform papillae (smooth bright red patches) in an irregular circinate pattern, surrounded by yellow, gray or white membranous frontiers which slowly extend, resolving spontaneously only to later recur **Histopathology** Focal absence of granular and horny layers, mimicking psoriasis (hyperkeratosis and Kogoj's microabscesses) **Treatment** Empirical, eg vitamins, psychotherapy, not often successful **Differential diagnosis** Lingual syphilis with dense white patches Note: In the pre-antibiotic era, 21% of oral cancer occurred in a background of syphilis

Geographic ulcer OPHTHALMOLOGY A sharply demarcated corneal ulcer with scalloped margins caused by Herpes simplex, which arises in dendritic herpetic keratitis, approximately one-half of which respond to idoxuridine therapy

Geophagy Clay-eating A formerly common custom practiced in many cultures, still extant in some regions of the Southern US Note: Although clay may be beneficial during pregnancy, providing trace minerals, mainstream medical thinking considers geophagy a form of pica (ingestion of indigestibles as comestibles, itself is commonly associated with iron-deficiency anemia)

Geotrichum A candida-like arthroconidia-producing imperfect fungus of the Cryptococcaceae family, which has a 'hockey stick'-like morphology, as it buds from the corners; *Geotrichum* grows well in corn meal agar and when isolated, is clinically significant as it often affects immunocompromised patients with lymphoreticular neoplasia; the arthroconidia have a 'box car'-like appearance

'Gerbiling' see Sexual deviancy

GERD Gastroesophageal reflux disease

Geriatric abuse The physical or psychological mistreatment of elderly subjects, which like child abuse, most often occurs at the hands of family members and is difficult to diagnose, as it rarely suspected; between 0.5 and 2.5 million events are estimated to occur annually (Ann Emerg Med 1988; 17:1006)

Geriatrics The medicine specialty involved in the care and management of the elderly; the life expectancy in the USA in 1900 was 45 years; the life expectancy in the USA in 1983 was 71 years in males and 78 years in females; Cf Gerontology, Todeserwartung

'Geritol' fix see Iron hypothesis

GERL Golgi-endoplasmic reticulum lysosome Transtubular network A hydrolase-rich region of the endoplasmic reticulum, which is the last compartment of the Golgi apparatus, representing the sorting site for proteins, where they are separated into membrane proteins, secretory proteins and lysosomal enzymes

German measles Rubella An acute, benign, but potentially teratogenic viral infection, most commonly affecting children **Virology** The rubella virus is a single-stranded RNA virus (genus, Rubivirus) of the Togavirus family, which unlike other Togaviridae, doesn't require an arthropod vector **Clinical** (acquired form) After a 2-3 week incubation, an evanescent rash begins on the face and neck and spreads caudally, accompanied by mild fever, malaise, sore throat, cervical lymphadenopathy and palatal enanthema (rose spots) coalescing into a reddish blush in the fauces and an evanescent, rapidly extending maculopapular rash with innumerable variably sized lesions resolving by day 3 **Management** If a mother is pregnant while acutely infected, abortion is often advised, given the frequency of the congenital rubella syndrome; see Congenital rubella syndrome, Expanded rubella syndrome, TORCH

German syndrome see Fetal trimethadione syndrome

Germ cell tumors (GCTs) A group of tumors arising from malignant degeneration of the germ cell epithelium, with an annual incidence rate of $3/10^5$; GCT mortality has doubled since the 1940s; 10% occur in cryptorchid testes and cryptorchid testes have a 33-fold increased incidence of these tumors; GCTs are common in males, comprising 90-95% of all testicular tumors and are the most common malignancy of men ages 25-35, but relatively less common in blacks; GCTs are classified by the Dixon and Moore ('American') scheme as either a) Seminoma, the most common GCTs, which have a good prognosis (90-95% five-year survival) or b) Non-seminomatous GCTs, which have a less favorable prognosis, and include embryonal carcinoma, mature and immature teratoma, teratocarcinoma and choriocarcinoma, the last of which has a 0% five-year survival; yolk sac tumor and mixtures thereof; GCTs are less common in females, comprising 20% of ovarian tumors, the majority of which are benign cystic teratomas; other female GCTs include immature (ie, malignant) teratoma, dysgerminoma (the female counterpart of the seminoma), the highly malignant endodermal sinus (yolk sac) tumor and others, including choriocarcinoma, embryonal carcinoma and polyembryoma; see Sex cord-stromal tumors

Germinal centers Follicular centers The site in lymph nodes and lymphoid aggregates where normal B lymphocyte transformation occurs; the germinal center is composed of a mixed cell population composed of cleaved and noncleaved or transformed lymphocytes; when the lymphoid follicles are hyperplastic, the germinal centers are replete with tingible body macrophages; several terms are used by pathologists **'Burned-out' germinal centers** are characteristic of angioimmunoblastic lymphadenopathy, are composed of loose aggregates of pale histiocytes, thus resembling granulomas and scattered immunoblasts or epithelioid cells mixed with amorphous eosinophilic and PAS-positive intercellular material **'Progressively transformed' germinal centers** (PTGC) are morphologically distinct, enlarged and reactive, often centrally located within the lymph node, with loss of the usually distinct frontiers seen between different cell types, accompanied by a 'starry sky' pattern, scattered epithelioid histiocytes, increased dendritic reticulum cells, mantle zone lymphocytes and increased T cells; PTGC is of particular interest as it may be associated with nodular lymphocyte predominant Hodgkin's disease, but is not itself considered neoplastic **'Regressively transformed' germinal centers** are small, virtually devoid of lymphocytes and have an onion-skin layering of dentritic reticulum cells, fibroblasts, vascular endothelial cells and eosinophilic, hyalinized, PAS-positive intercellular material

Germinoma Any neoplasm with the morphologic features of a germ cell tumor, eg seminoma; the term is reserved for midline tumors of germinal origin, including those of the central nervous system and pineal galnd, mediastinum, retroperitoneum and thymus; see Germ cell tumor; Cf Teratoma

Germ-line configuration A 'primitive' arrangement of genes that have not yet undergone the rearrangement required for cell maturation; the term is usually applied to genes of the immunoglobulin superfamily that are in a pristine state; these genes include those encoding the immunoglobulin heavy and light chains in B cells and the genes encoding the T cell receptor in T lymphocytes; see Gene rearrangement

Germ tube test MICROBIOLOGY The germ tube is a short projection on a germinating spore of either *Candida albicans* or *C stellatoidea* (figure, right) that appears after three hours of incubation at 37°C on an appropriate culture medium; the germ tube test is a rapid bench test that allows a rapid presumptive diagnosis of *C albicans* as *C stelloidea* is a rare clinical isolate

Gerontology The systematic study of the aging phenomenon as it affects cells and organisms; gerontologists have found that rodents are less 'instructive' than other 'unusual' animals, including lizards, bats, turtles and fish; senescence is thought to be the result of 1) Accumulation of degradation products, coupled with a cell's increasing inability to metabolize the products, see Garbage can hypothesis and/or 2) Activation of longevity-determining or aging genes which may be intimately linked to certain oncogenes, eg c-fos, which evokes uncontrolled cell proliferation (Science 1990; 250:622); current data indicates that the agony of the human condition may be prolonged by a) Eating less A 30% reduction in caloric intake decreases the incidence of cancer, autoimmunity, cross-linking of collagen, post-absorptive cholesterol levels, loss of striatal dopamine receptors and loss of lens γ crystallins; increased lipolysis in response to glucagon and epinephrine and the age-related changes in lipid levels and insulin are seen in rodents on low-calorie diets b) Reduction of protein intake, especially tryptophan-rich products c) Exercise When begun early in life and performed regularly, exercise retards or reverses age-related changes in lipid deposits, insulin levels, bone mineral loss, cardiovascular deterioration d) Ingestion of antioxidants 'Soft' data implies that increased antioxidant ingestion, eg vitamin E, vitamin C, glutathione may increase longevity

Gerovital A formulation of procaine-HCl that is used as an analgesic in dentistry; gerovital has been given the fanciful synonym of vitamin H_3, gerovital is alleged to have anti-aging and antineoplastic properties by some alternative (holistic) health advocates and some self-proclaimed cancer specialists

Geschlechtsverkehr Sexual traffic, Sexual activity

Gestalt therapy German, Configuration A form of psychotherapy that focuses on the whole person, thus representing a 'holistic approach' to a patient's psyche, taking into account his perceptions and the effects of his environment and related stresses on his behavior; see 'Holistic' medicine

Gestational diabetes mellitus A usually transient con-

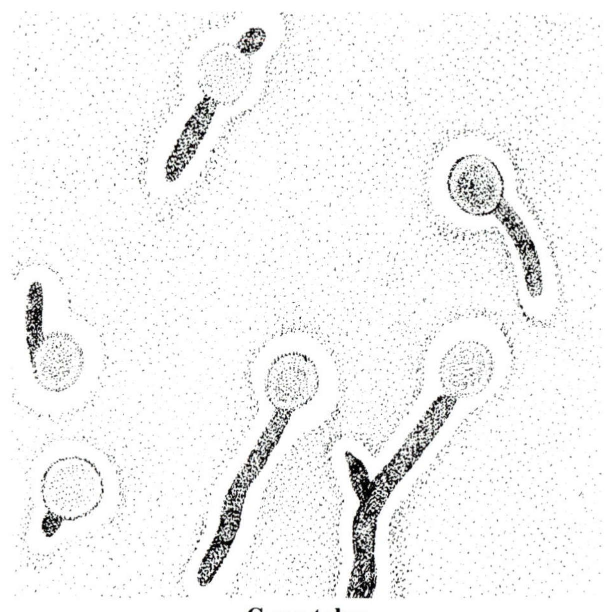

Germ tubes

dition characterized by glucose intolerance that coincides with the onset of pregnancy, which is associated with a) Increased perinatal complications for the mother, as well as the infant, see Fetal diabetes 'syndrome' and b) Tendency to develop glucose intolerance in absence of pregnancy 5-10 years after gestational diabetes Note: Early diagnosis of pregnancy in insulin-dependent diabetes mellitus allows optimal metabolic control, reducing the risk for spontaneous abortion, a common event in diabetic gestation (N Engl J Med 1988; 319:1617); see Glucose tolerance curve

Gestational thrombocytopenia Immune thrombocytopenic purpura (ITP) that first appears in pregnancy and carries the risk of neonatal thrombocytopenia and intracranial hemorrhage; conservative management is appropriate when idiopathic thrombocytopenic purpura (ITP, a not uncommon event in women of child-bearing years) first appears in pregnancy and no circulating antiplatelet antibodies are detected (N Engl J Med 1990; 323:229, 264ed)

GFAP Glial fibrillary acidic protein An intermediate filament characteristic of glial cells that may rarely be co-expressed with S-100 protein in peripheral nerve tumors; see intermediate filament

GGGCG box MOLECULAR BIOLOGY A highly conserved sequence of DNA, which like the CCAAT and TATA 'boxes', is located between 60 and 120 nucleotides upstream from the start site for gene transcription;these boxes are known as promoter-proximal sequences, which when mutated, result in lower rates of transcription, implying that they are DNA-binding sites

GGM see Glucose/galactose malabsorption

GGT γ-glutamyl transferase see Glutamyl transferase

GHB see GABA, γ-hydroxy-butyrate

Ghost HEMATOLOGY The pale white membrane of a hemoglobin-depleted red cell, which is virtually identical to all other mammalian cell membranes (52% protein, 40% lipid, 8% carbohydrate), and is thus useful in studying cell membranes; erythrocyte membranes differ in that most of the membrane is attached to the proteins glycophorin and band 3, identified by gel electrophoresis; see Band

Ghost cell A shadowy, light pink (by the hematoxylin and eosin stain) cell wraith with a well-demarcated cytoplasmic border that may appear in the presence of coagulation, ie anoxic necrosis, accompanied by abolition of cell detail CYTOLOGY An anuclear yellow-orange squame seeni n well-differentiated squamous cell carcinoma DERMATOPATHOLOGY see Shadow cells ORAL PATHOLOGY A pale, eosinophilic and swollen keratinocyte that lacks a nucleus but retains the cellular and nuclear contour, a finding characteristic of the calcifying odontogenic cyst PARASITOLOGY Hemoglobin-depleted erythrocyte 'husks' that are infected with the schizonts of ***Plasmodium ovale***; Cf Ghost

Ghost surgery LEGAL MEDICINE A surgical procedure that Dr 'A' has the patient's permission to perform, which is performed by Dr 'B'; without the proper provisos for a substitute (as in university hospitals where much of the surgery is performed by the residents) in the patient consent form, the patient may initiate a lawsuit for assault and battery, as he was operated on by someone other than the physician to whom he gave permission

Ghost teeth Regional odontodysplasia An uncommon dental anomaly affecting predominantly the maxillary teeth, both deciduous and permanent, especially the central and lateral incisors and cuspids; the teeth while normally mineralized, are delayed or fail to erupt; the resulting deformity causes cosmetic defects necessitating tooth extraction

Ghost villi OBSTETRICS Rounded pale eosinophilic masses seen by light microscopy that are surrounded by inflammatory cells and correspond to chorionic villi in a placental infarct; ghost villi may also be seen with retained products of conception (missed abortion)

GHRH Growth hormone regulatory hormone

Giant axonal neuropathy An autosomal recessive disease of early onset characterized by symmetric distal polyneuropathy, mental retardation and tightly coiled kinky hair and segmental axonal dilatations packed with neurofilaments; a histologically identical neuropathy may be seen in n-hexane intoxication; Cf Kinky hair disease

Giant cell Giant cells may occur in benign or malignant lesions and come in many forms; although they are highly nonspecific, their presence in the proper setting may support the diagnosis of certain lesions Epithelioid giant cells of Langerhans and Touton are associated with infections and other 'benign' processes, eg sarcoidosis, have abundant cytoplasm and a rim or clutch of enlarged histiocyte-like nuclei; giant cells in tumors are less inhibited by the rules of cytologic etiquette and are anointed with adjectival modifiers, eg bizarre, monster, osteoclastoma-like and Reed-Sternberg; in tumors, the nucleus and/or cytoplasm may be markedly enlarged and the cell mitotically active; a general rule is that the larger and 'uglier' the cell, the worse the clinical outcome

Giant cell arteritis Temporal arteritis A self-limited disease of middle-aged women that evolves to systemic arteritis in 10-15% of cases, with blindness as a potential late complication Histopathology Nodular transmural swelling of arteries, infiltration by neutrophils, eosinophils, mononuclear cells and giant cell granulomas

Giant cell carcinoma A highly malignant epithelial tumor with fulminant clinical course, bizarre histologic appearance and poor prognosis that is most common in a) Lung An aggressive, poorly differentiated carcinoma that arises peripherally, grows rapidly and is often too large for adequate therapy by the time of clinical presentation Histopathology Bizarre pleomorphic multinucleated giant cells, large mononuclear cells in a background of neutrophils and b) Thyroid An anaplastic carcinoma arising in a pre-existing well differentiated thyroid carcinoma Clinical Aggressive infiltration and compromise of vital neck structures with 100% mortality, most dying within six months Histopathology Storiform infiltration, neutrophilic inflammation, vascularization and osteoclast-like giant cells; most tumors produce cytokeratin; the giant cell tumor of the pancreas does not behave as an anaplastic tumor, but rather like a 'garden variety' ductal carcinoma

Giant cell fibroblastoma A benign mesenchymal tumor exclusive to children under the age of 10, often located in the superficial soft tissues of the back and thigh

Giant cell glioblastoma A firm, well-circumscribed variant of grade III-IV astrocytoma or glioblastoma multiforme Histopathology Highly cellular with abundant bizarre, multinucleated giant cells, hemorrhage and necrosis

Giant cell granuloma see Central giant cell granuloma, Peripheral giant cell granuloma

Giant hemangioma of Kasabach-Merritt A condition characterized by thrombocytopenia and 'giant' (circa 5 cm in diameter) hemangiomas associated with disseminated intravascular coagulation Treatment Mild cases may respond to steroids, or spontaneously regress in five years

Giant cell hepatitis Giant cell transformation of the liver NEONATOLOGY A nonspecific reaction of the newborn liver to increased conjugated hyperbilirubinemia of any etiology, that is most common in infants with intra- or extrahepatic biliary atresia, erythroblastosis fetalis, TORCH (toxoplasmosis, rubella, cytomegalovirus, herpes) and other in utero and neonatal infections, eg coxsackie, hepatitis, ***Escherichia coli***, syphilis, metabolic defects, eg α1-antitrypsin deficiency, cystic fibrosis, hereditary fructose intolerance, galactosemia, parenteral nutrition and tyrosinosis, choledocal cysts, idiopathic, congenital hepatic fibrosis, Byler's disease, Lucy-Driscoll disease, Niemann-Pick disease, trisomy 18, Zellweger's disease Pathogenesis Theories abound, but no simple mechanism exists Pathology The liver is enlarged with dense bodies, lobular disarray, multinucleated hepatocytes, mononuclear cell infiltration and marked biliary stasis; the presence of bile-duct proliferation indicates exhepatic biliary atresia, a lesion that may be amenable to surgery Cf Syncytial giant cell hepatitis

Giant cell myocarditis An idiopathic condition that may represent a virally-induced immune reaction associated with underlying diseases including encephalitis, hepatitis, infection, intoxication, nutritional defects, thymoma, thyroiditis and Wegener's disease Clinical Rapid deterioration and high mortality Histopathology Focal granulomatous necrosis, multi-nucleated giant cells, epithelioid histiocytes, eosinophils, lymphocytes

Giant cell (interstitial) pneumonia An idiopathic, interstitial pneumonia with lymphoid infiltrates, bizarre, actively phagocytic giant cells, associated with respiratory syncytial virus, influenza and other viral infections, easily confused with measles, or associated with bacterial or mycoplasmal infections, drugs (nitrofurantoin, chemotherapy, methysergide) and collagen vascular disease

Giant cell pneumonia of Hecht A fulminant respiratory disease with tachycardia, dyspnea, which is most commonly due to fulminant measles infection that compromises the cellular and humoral immune response Prognosis Poor with high mortality, especially in those with underlying leukemia, cystic fibrosis, immuno-deficiency and persistent measles viremia; Cf Atypical pneumonia

Giant cell reaction A nonspecific term for a reparative tissue reaction with multinucleated epithelioid histiocytes that may be due to exogenous material, eg sutures or due to endogenous material, eg the sebaceous contents of a ruptured epidermal inclusion cyst, chalazion or fat

Giant cell reparative granuloma see Central giant cell granuloma, Peripheral giant cell granuloma

Giant cell thyroiditis Synonym for de Quervain's subacute or granulomatous thyroiditis

Giant cell tumor (GCT) of bone A lesion comprising 5% of all osseous tumors, which is most common in the weight-bearing epiphysis of females over age 20, affecting the distal femur, proximal tibia and distal radius PATHOLOGY GCTs are red-brown with pale necrotic areas, with stromal mesenchymal cells and tumor giant cells that have nuclei identical to those of the mesenchymal cells and a high acid phosphatase content; 60% recur with curettage and 10% metastasize, an event that is far more common in deep (to the fascial planes) tumors Differential diagnosis A GCT-like histopathology may be seen in the brown tumor of hyperparathyroidism, chondroblastoma, giant cell reparative granuloma, benign and malignant fibrous histiocytoma, non-ossifying and chondromyxoid fibroma, unicameral bone cyst, aneurysmal bone cyst, fibrous dysplasia, osteoblastoma, osteosarcoma, osteoid osteoma and eosinophilic granuloma

Giant cell tumor of tendon sheath A potentially recurring lesion of the acral flexor tendon sheath that is a variant of fibrous histiocytoma, which reaches a maximum of 3 mm in size and may erode into the bone Histopathology Osteoclast-like giant cells with hyalinization, pseudoglandular formation, lipid and hemosiderin accumulation (simulating malignancy)

Giant condyloma acuminata of Büscke-Loewenstein A verrucous carcinoma (squamous cell carcinoma of low histological aggressiveness), affecting the male anogenital region, demonstrating human papillomavirus (HPV) types 6 and 11 Treatment Early lesions, require radical local excision, while recurrent or metastasizing lesions require abdominoperineal resection (Dis Colon Rectum 1989; 32:481)

'Giant' hairs Fusion of sensory hairs in the cochlea and vestibule, described in aminoglycoside-induced ototoxicity (guinea pigs, Adv Otorhinolaryngol 1973; 20:14), presumed to occur in humans but not searched for in post-mortem examinations

Giant (pigmented) hairy nevus A large congenital melanocytic nevus measuring more than 5 cm in greatest dimension that has a 'garment-like' distribution (bathing trunk, cap, coat sleeve, stocking), often with scattered satellite lesions and is considered premalignant, as up to 12% develop melanoma; leptomeningeal involvement may be accompanied by epilepsy and mental retardation; the three histological patterns are compound and intradermal nevus, neural nevus and blue nevus

Giant hypertrophic gastritis A condition characterized by rugal folds of the stomach and late development of parietal cell autoantibodies and gastric atrophy; giant hypertrophic gastritis is associated with Menetrier's disease (Gastric mucosal hypertrophy, decreased acid secretion, protein loss in the stomach, edema, weight loss, abdominal pain, nausea) and hypertrophic hypersecretory gastropathy, morphologically similar to Menetrier's disease but with increased acid secretion, more common in men, age 30-50 Treatment Varying success is achieved with anticholinergics, cimetidine, vagotomy and pyloroplasty

Giant metamyelocyte An atypical myeloid cell with clumped chromatin in a large, often bizarre, immature nucleus and relatively mature cytoplasm, typically seen in megaloblastic anemia, as the nucleus cannot properly mature without the single-carbon transport provided by the deficient vitamin B12 and folic acid

Giant mitochondria Massively enlarged mitochondria that appear as pale rounded eosinophilic masses by light microscopy that mimic both red cells and Mallory's hyaline; the finding of giant mitochondria in hepatocytes is non-specific but characteristic of all phases of alcoholic liver disease ranging from fatty liver to cirrhosis

Giant platelet syndrome of Bernard-Soulier An autosomal recessive condition with mucocutaneous and visceral hemorrhage due to deficiency of glycoprotein Ib, the receptor for von Willebrand factor Laboratory Prolonged bleeding time (due to poor platelet adhesion to subendothelium), no platelet aggregation with ristocetin Note: Up to 10% of a normal platelet population is comprised of giant, often 'squashed' platelets; abnormalities in this syndrome include increased size, basophilia of membrane, aggregation (or absence) of cytoplasmic granules, pseudopod formation and cytoplasmic vacuolization; when more than 20% of the platelets are giant, certain other conditions must be considered, eg idiopathic thrombocytopenic purpura, lympho- and myeloproliferations, reticulocytosis, disseminated intravascular coagulation, lupus erythematosus, Bernard-Soulier syndrome, gray platelet syndrome, May-Hegglin anomaly and Montreal platelet syndrome

Giant reparative granuloma see Central giant cell granuloma, Peripheral giant cell granuloma

Giant T wave inversion CARDIOLOGY An electrocardiographic finding characterized as an inversion of the normal T wave, seen in the mid- to left precordial leads and suggestive of apical hypertrophic cardiomyopathy

Gibbus An anterior angular deformity of the lower back due to hypoplasia or 'wedging' of one or more lower thoracic or upper lumbar vertebrae, resulting in beaked projections on the infero-anterior aspects and hypoplasia of the upper portions of vertebral bodies, seen in mucopolysaccharidosis, type I-H Hurler syndrome, tuberculosis (Pott's disease) or trauma; the gibbus or 'buffalo hump' seen in Cushing's disease and syndrome is due to accumulation of soft tissue secondary to prolonged endogenous or exogenous corticosteroid and is located in the cervicothoracic region

Gigantism Sotos syndrome An inherited condition with rapid somaticgrowth of neonatal onset without endocrinopathy Clinical Macrosomia, where growth is accelerated for the first 4-5 years of life, followed by a normal growth pattern, enlarged acral parts, macrocephaly, mild mental retardation and perceptual defects; patients are at increased risk for various neoplasms

GIGO Garbage in, garbage out COMPUTERS An acronym referring to incorrect entry of data in a database, which cannot be coherently retrieved; GIGO has been colloquially borrowed by various fields, in particular, laboratory medicine for improperly obtained materials, eg stool cultures, urine and cytologic specimens for which a diagnosis cannot be rendered Note: This colloquialism is equally applicable to other fields of medicine and been used by cytotechnologists in reference to poor quality specimens that preclude diagnosis

Ginkgolide B A chemical extracted from the ginkgo tree (Gingko biloba) of potential use for treating asthma and circulatory deficiency in the elderly

Ginseng Any one of 22 different deciduous plants, usually of the Panax family, commonly Panax ginseng that are native to Southeast Asia, used in Chinese folk medicine as a tonic and restorative, consumed for its purported antifatigue, immunologic and hormonal effects, claimed to cure respiratory infections, gastrointestinal disease, impotence, fatigue and stress; the active chemicals include panaxin, panax acid, panaquilen, panacen, sapogenin and ginsenin; the physiologic effects include increased testosterone, corticosteroid levels in experimental animals and increased gluconeogenesis, central nervous system activity, blood pressure, pulse, gastrointestinal motility and hematopoiesis and decreased cholesterol levels; because of ginseng's androgenic activity, ginseng may be passed through maternal milk, causing transient androgenization in infants (J Am Med Assoc 1979; 241:1614); Cf Garlic

Ginseng abuse 'syndrome' A clinical complex secondary to daily ingestion of 3 or more g/day of ginseng Clinical Diarrhea, nervousness, insomnia, eruptive dermatosis, increased cognitive and motor activity

GIP 1) see Giant cell (interstitial) pneumonia 2) Gastric inhibitory polypeptide A 43-residue insulinotropic polypeptide hormone of the incretin family produced by the pancreas, that is secreted in response to oral (but not parenteral) administration of nutrients, eg glucose and lipids; see Incretin

GIPP Gonadotropin-independent (ie nonpulsatile) precocious puberty A possibly familial condition due to a lack of suppression in response to LHRHa with noncyclic steroidogenesis, Clinical Ranges from complete testicular immaturity to maturity (N Engl J Med 1985; 312:65); see Precocious puberty

Gitterzellen German, lattice cells Cells seen in early central nervous system necrosis, where the normal microglia is converted from small round cells with fine branching processes to rounded plump macrophages filled with variably sized fat globules and disintegrating myelin

Glairy material Greasy, clear yellow, fat-laden semi-fluid material, characteristically seen in mature cystic teratomas, which is often admixed with hair

Gland A secretory 'organ' that may be a simple, single cell unit that discharges its production directly into the circulation or more complex, consisting of an organized cluster of cells that discharge their production into a duct, which may be classified according to a) Complexity Simple A gland with a single unbranched duct or Complex A gland with multiple and/or branched ducts, which when multiple and large are termed organs, eg the pancreas b) Shape, ie tubular, acinous or alveolar c) Type of secretion, ie mucinous glands, which produce viscous and sticky material, serous glands, which produce clear watery fluid and mixed glands; each of which is invested with a basket-weave pattern of myoepithelial cells d) Postulated manner of production, which is no longer entirely valid Apocrine A gland that was thought to secrete part of its cytoplasm at the same time as the secretion itself, a concept that is somewhat incorrect Holocrine A gland in which the cells themselves detach as part of the secretion Merocrine A gland that produces secretions without altering its own morphology, ie through the delivery transmembrane vesicles Paracrine A gland that secretes hormones acting on cells in the immediate vicinity

Glanders An infection by ***Pseudomonas mallei***, a gram-negative strict aerobic bacillus, which affects large domestic animals, most common in horses and is an entity distinctly uncommon in the US; human disease occurs in the form of acute septicemia, chronic mucocutaneous disease (see Farcy) or pulmonary infection Clinical Ranges from cellulitis to necrosis and granuloma formation with draining mucosal ulcers, pleurisy, necrotizing lobar or bronchopneumonia, nasal septal necrosis, fever, chills, malaise, headaches, pustular rash, lymphadenopathy, splenomegaly; chronic disease is associated with hepatosplenomegaly, pulmonary abscess formation and granuloma formation Treatment Sulfadiazine, tetracycline, chloramphenicol, aminoglycoside

Glasgow coma scale CRITICAL CARE MEDICINE A method for evaluating the severity of central nervous system involvement in head injury that measures three parameters for a maximum score of 15 for normal cerebral function and zero for brain death; the PARAMETERS ARE A) BEST MOTOR RESPONSE, ie the subject obeys commands 6, if none 0 B) BEST VERBAL RESPONSE, ie oriented 5, if no response 0 and C) EYE OPENING, if spontaneous 4, if none 0; the system is of lesser use in children (Am J Dis Child 1990; 144:1088); Cf Pittsburgh score

Glassy appearance An adjectival descriptor for a smooth or vitrioid grayish radiolucency or pale eosinophilic hyalinized cytoplasm or stromal tissue

'Glass ceiling' phenomenon ACADEMIA The constellation of barriers to career advancement that confront women who strive for leadership positions (Am Med News 3/Mar/91)

'Glass pusher' A highly colloquial, somewhat derogatory synonym for a 'service' surgical pathologist, whose primary function is to 'push glass', ie interpret the histology of biopsies and tissues removed during surgery, which have been embedded in paraffin, mounted on a glass slide and stained

Glassy cell carcinoma (GCC) A female genital tract malignancy a) GCC of the uterine cervix, comprises 1.2% of primary cervical cancers and is an aggressive, poorly differentiated adenosquamous carcinoma, originating from the subcylindric reserve cell with a 5-year survival of 25% Histopathology Large, mitotically active polygonal cells with abundant, finely granular amphophilic 'glassy' cytoplasm, distinct cell borders, large nuclei with one or more prominent nucleoli and b) GCC of the endometrium is also very rare and histologically similar to that of the cervix with an equally poor prognosis

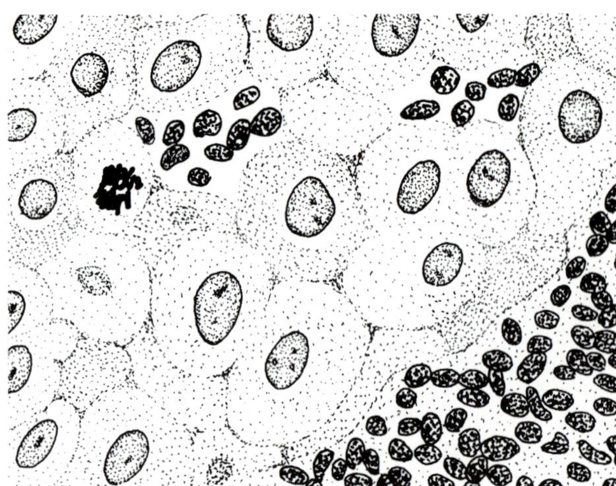

Glassy cell carcinoma

GLC see Gas-liquid chromatography

Gliding motility A pattern of movement typical of *Capnocytophaga* species, in which the yellowish colonies display finger-like projections that appear to glide on the primary isolation media; these gram-negative fusiform bacilli are indigenous to the oral cavity, are implicated in periodontal and oral infections and lack flagella, and thus are intrinsically motile; Cf Swarming

Glioblastoma Astrocytoma, grade III-IV A highly aggressive tumor comprising 30% of the 5000 primary brain malignancies diagnosed annually in the US; those at possible occupational risk include anatomists, pathologists, dentists and ophthalmologists (N Engl J Med 1991; 324:1441) Treatment Glioblastoma is unaffected by surgery, chemotherapy and radiotherapy, but may respond to genetically-engineered viruses (Science 1991;252:854)

Glitter cells Neutrophils that are swollen in hypotonic (dilute) urine and contain granules in Brownian motion that 'glitter' when seen by low-power light microscopy, a finding described as typical of pyelonephritis

Globalization The dissolution of national borders in all aspects of human endeavor; in science, this translates into international collaboration efforts, eg Human Frontier Science Project with funds being provided by funding agencies and/or private companies from different countries; the term represents a recognition that a) Changes in one part of the world have a broader impact, both regionally, eg the burning oil wells of

Kuwait, or over the entire planet, eg CFC use by developed nations and ozone layer depletion and b) Resolution of issues of international concern, eg environment, population, research, loss of human rights, requires participation of all members of the 'global village'; see G7

Globi Masses of acid-fast staining ***Mycobacterium leprae*** present within histiocytes ('lepra cells') in advanced lepromatous leprosy lymphadenitis; globi are usually located in the subcapsular region of the lymph node; when stained by haematoxylin & eosin, the histiocytes are foamy with gray cytoplasm and similar globi-like masses occur in ***M avium-intercellulare*** infections in patients with AIDS

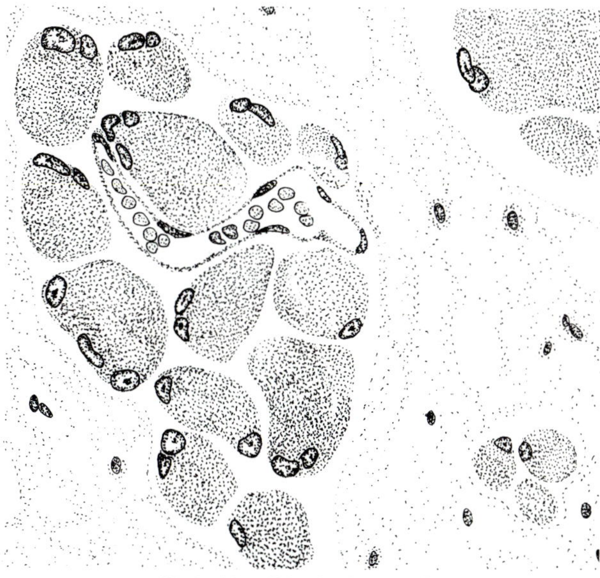

Globoid cell leukodystrophy

Globoid cell leukodystrophy Krabbe's disease An autosomal recessive sphingolipid metabolism defect due to galatocerebroside β-galactosidase deficiency, causing in utero demyelinization, and death in early infancy Clinical Spastic paralysis, seizures and pyrexia, vomiting, cortical blindness, deafness, dysphagia, pseudobulbar palsy, quadriplegia, mental deterioration Neuropathology The lesions are confined to the central nervous system with a loss of myelin, fibrous gliosis and abundant, perivascular clusters of 20-25 μm rounded or globoid macrophages and multinucleated cells with faintly granular cytoplasm filled with galactosyl ceramide Ultrastructure Hollow crystalline tubes or twisted tubular arrays similar to inclusions found in Gaucher's disease; autosomal recessive; Cf Leukodystrophy

Globoside(s) Ceramide-(glucose)m-(galactose)n-(N-acetyl-hexosamine) A family of ceramide-based molecules, designated as GL-1, GL-2 and so on, according to the number of sugar residues added to the ceramide; globosides represent the predominant glycolipid in the red cell membrane and other plasma membranes

Globoside dysfunction syndrome A group of enzymopathies characterized by defective addition of sugar residues to ceramide, eg Fabry's disease and Lactosyl ceramidosis

Globular protein In the early days of clinical chemistry, proteins were separated into either albumin or 'globulins' (immunoglobulins, enzymes and other proteins) the latter calculated as 'total protein', determined by the Biuret method, minus albumin, separated by using a salt solution; the term is obsolete as electrophoresis is used to separate proteins into more clinically relevant groups

Globus hystericus A subjective sensation of compression or a lump (bolus) in the throat, considered a psychoneurotic symptom; Note: A bolus sensation is characteristic of carcinomas or strictures in the oropharynx or pharyngeal pouch, or may occur in pharyngeal paralysis, hypochromic anemia or cervical spinal disease, eg osteoarthritis; see Factitial syndromes

Glomerular polyanion A negatively charged glycoprotein lining the glomerular foot processes of the epithelial cells of Bowman's capsule, responsible for the selective permeability of the glomeruli; loss of negative charges in the foot process region is responsible for increased filtration, ie loss of albumin and proteinuria, as occurs in minimum change nephrotic syndrome

Glomeruloid bodies Glomerular bodies A loosely used term that refers to an organized cluster of often primitive cells that simulate primitive glomeruli (figure); the classic glomeruloid body is a key histological feature of Wilms' tumor, a tumor accompanied by nests of primitive cells and a fibroblast-like stroma), and consists of a Bowman-like space, epithelial cell tufts and PAS-positive basement membrane material without a capillary lumen and lining endothelial cells; the Schiller-Duval bodies, characteristic of endodermal sinus tumor and yolk sac tumors and clear cell carcinoma are sometimes also called glomeruloid bodies and contain a central capillary surrounded by loose connective tissue, rimmed by a layer of epithelial cells with scattered intracytoplasmic hyaline globules (Cancer 1978; 41:1395); Cf Embryoid bodies

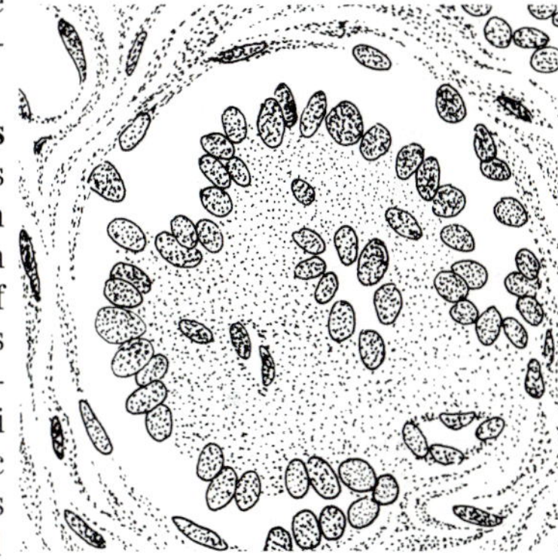

Glomeruloid body

Glomerulonephritis see Capsular 'drops', Casts, Crescents, Deciduous tree in winter appearance, Dense deposits, Fingerprints, Fusion of foot processes, Humps, 'Shunt' nephritis, Spike, Tramtrack pattern

Glomus tumor A neoplasm arising in the neuromyoarterial glomus, an arteriovenous shunt Clinical When located in the 'usual' subungual site, the abundant innervation makes the tumor exquisitely painful; when located elsewhere, eg middle ear, stomach, the glomus tumor is painless

'Glove(s)' FORENSIC PATHOLOGY Broad sheets of epidermis, especially of the hands and feet that may include the fingernails that slough from bodies that have been submersed for long periods of time, a phenomenon that occurs more rapidly in warm water; Cf 'Floater'

Glove box A sealed glass or plastic chamber that has two or more pairs of rubber gloves for the manipulation of cells, microorganisms or mammals without physically violating the environment within the box; the box is designed to either maintain an atmosphere that a 'fastidious' organism requires for optimal growth, eg an anaerobe, or to protect an immune defenseless organism from all pathogens, see 'Bubble boy; alternately, a glove box is used to protect the manipulators from chemical toxins or from dangerous pathogens

Gloved finger shadow of Simon A descriptor for retained plugs of mucopurulent secretion within ectatic bronchi in patients with chronic obstructive pulmonary disease (COPD), best seen by an air bronchogram; the thickened bronchial walls may be accompanied by atelectasis and pneumonitis

Glucagon A 29-residue polypeptide hormone produced by the pancreatic islet α cells that activates hepatic phosphorylase, decreases gastric motility, secretion and muscle mass, increases ketogenesis and hepatic incorporation of amino acids and urinary excretion of sodium and potassium

Glucagonoma A pancreatic α cell tumor with two distinct clinical and histological patterns, presenting either as a benign tumor, not associated with the glucagonoma syndrome, which has a bland gyriform histologic pattern or a potentially malignant tumor associated with the glucagonoma syndrome

Glucagonoma syndrome A symptom complex associated with glucagonoma, a tumor of postmenopausal women who often have diabetes mellitus, blistering dermatitis (necrolytic migratory erythema), weight loss, normochromic anemia, ileus, constipation or diarrhea, glossitis, angular cheilitis, venous thrombosis, hypoproteinemia, neuropsychiatric disease PATHOLOGY Glucagonomas are small, solitary tumors with atypical neuroendocrine granules Note: One-half of glucagonomas are malignant; many produce more than one hormone

Glucose tolerance test (GTT) A standardized test that measures the body's response to an oral (challenge) dose of glucose, used to diagnose diabetes mellitus; in the most commonly used GTT, 100 g of glucose is ingested per os in a fasting individual, which stimulates insulin secretion; the peak glucose levels in normal subjects are reached within an one hour; in diabetics, the peak is reached after two to three hours and the peak glucose level is much higher; in the accompanying figure, Siperstein's (Adv Int Med 1975; 20:297) 'liberal' criteria are used, which recognize that the GTT differs with age, while other workers feel that the GTT should be abandoned completely

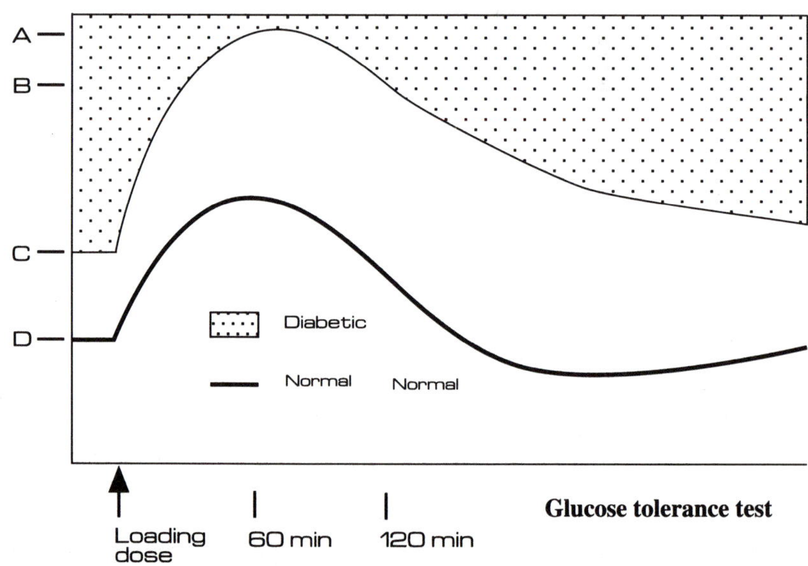

Glucose tolerance test

A Level at 1 hour ≥ 14.4 mmol/L (US: 260 mg/dl)
B Level at two hours ≥ 12.2 mmol/L (US: 220 mg/dl)
C Fasting glucose level ≥ 7.8 mmol/L (US: 140 mg/dl)
D Baseline glucose level, normal subject

Glucosuria see Glycosuria

Glucocorticoid regulatory element see GRE

Glue ear Chronic otitis media with effusion, a common cause of conduction-type deafness in school-age children **Clinical** Variable pain, accompanied by upper respiratory infection and tonsillitis **Treatment** Adenoidectomy plus bilateral myringotomy with grommet insertion for young children (Brit Med J 1990; 300:1551)

Glue-sniffing SUBSTANCE ABUSE A potentially fatal form of substance abuse practiced by young male adolescents, in which model airplane glue is placed in a paper or plastic bag and deeply sniffed in order to obtain the maximum desired effect, which consists of a combination of euphoria and central nervous system depression caused by toluene, an organic solvent; exposure to toluene vapors causes irritation of mucosae, lacrimation, arrythmias, nausea, vomiting, mental confusion, hallucinations, chemical pneumonitis, respiratory arrest and sudden death; direct contact may cause erythema, defatting dermatitis, skin paresthesiae, conjunctivitis and keratitis; the NIOSH recommendations for toluene exposure is 200 ppm at an 8-hour time-weighted average; abusers may be exposed to 1000 ppm for prolonged periods; toluene is also present in adhesives, explosives and dyes; see Gateway drugs; Cf 'White-out'

Glucose/galactose malabsorption (GGM) An autosomal

recessive condition of neonatal onset characterized by malabsorption of glucose and galactose, resulting in severe, potentially fatal diarrhea and dehydration if these sugars are not eliminated from the diet Pathogenesis Normal glucose absorption is mediated by the Na^+/glucose cotransporter, which is encoded by the SGLT1 gene on the distal q arm of chromosome 22; in GGM, there is a single missense mutation in the SGLT1 gene, resulting in a complete loss of Na^+/glucose transport (Nature 1991; 350:354)

GLUT A family of cell membrane-bound glucose transporting proteins, of which five isoforms have been identified; on the basis of hydropathy plots, all forms have 12 membrane-spanning domains, six exoplasmic loops and five endoplasmic loops; GLUT-1, GLUT-3, GLUT-4 and GLUT-5 all have low Km, which allows their facile transportation throughout the corporal economy and into various tissues; GLUT-2 regulates glucose homeostasis (Science 1991; 251:1200)

GLUT-2 A protein with a high Km (Michaelis constant) that transports glucose into the β cells of the pancreatic islets, providing an essential signal for the normal insulin secretory response; GLUT-2 is elevated in those cells, eg pancreatic β cells, liver, basolateral aspect of the epithelial cells of the small intestine and renal tubules that participate in the regulation of blood glucose homeostasis; GLUT-2 is reduced in both insulin-dependent (autoimmune) and non-insulin-dependent diabetes mellitus due to a down-regulation that is defective in non-insulin-dependent diabetes mellitus (Science 1991; 251:1200)

Glutamate cascade NEUROLOGY A sequence of events postulated to be a major cause of ischemia-induced neuronal death in cerebrovascular insults (strokes) that can be topographically divided into a core region immediately adjacent to an occluded vessel, which is almost invariably doomed to infarction unless the thrombus is removed immediately (which is usually impossible) and a penumbral region, which receives some blood from non-occluded collateral vessels, the region in which the glutamate cascade is thought to occur in a three step process 1) Induction The cascade begins when the terminals of ischemic neurons oversecrete the excitatory neurotransmitter glutamate into the intercellular spaces, in response to which NMDA receptors open and allow the free passage of sodium and calcium ions, AMPA/kainate receptors allow passage of sodium ions and metabotropic receptors trigger the generation of intracellular messengers diacylglycerol (DAG) and inositol 1,4,5-triphosphate (IP3) 2) Amplification The excess intracellular sodium activates a sodium-for-calcium transporter, which activates voltage-gated calcium channels; the excess IP3 releases calcium from intracellular stores, which may combine with DAG, activating enzymes and triggering the release of more glutamate 3) Expression Excess calcium activates enzymes that degrade DNA, proteins and phospholipids, the last of which is catabolized to arachidonic acid generating highly-destructive oxygen free radicals and eicosanoid molecules, which combine with activated platelet-activating factor, recruiting previously uninvolved vessels and widening the extent of the ischemia (Sci Am 1991; 265:1/56rv)

Glutamic acid decarboxylase autoantibody An autoantibody against a 64 kD antigen associated with insulin-dependent diabetes mellitus and with the 'stiff man' syndrome

γ-glutamyl transferase (GGT) A hepatic enzyme that is the best single screening assay for detecting latent or chronic liver disease, including malignancy; elevated GGT often indicates continued imbibition in chronic alcoholics as it increases in response to microsomal enzyme induction

Glutathione γ-Glutamyl-cysteinyl-glycine A ubiquitous tripeptide that is involved in central nervous system metabolism, serving as a coenzyme for some enzymes of oxidation-reduction systems, transmembrane amino acid transport, maintenance of erythrocyte integrity and prevention of H_2O_2 accumulation in red cells

Gluten A wheat endosperm protein composed of gliadin and glutelin, which is inculpated in the pathogenesis of celiac disease

Glycated hemoglobin see Glycosylated hemoglobin

Glycerol 1,2,3 propanetriol, a sweet oily liquid used as an industrial solvent, plasticizer and emollient; it is hygroscopic, ie soluble in both alcohol and water; it is a component of neutral fats, phosphatides and cardiolipin and is used in transfusion medicine for long-term storage of frozen red cells

Glycine An inhibitory neurotransmitter that acts primarily at the level of the spinal cord, the receptors for which are distributed in a heterogeneous pattern (Science 1988; 242:270)

Glycocalicin A 135 kD hydrophilic glycoprotein split from the α-chain of platelet glycoprotein Ib that is markedly reduced (5-20% normal levels) in aplastic anemia or amegakaryocytosis; patients with peripheral-destruction type thrombocytopenia (and normal marrow precursors) have less than 50% normal levels

Glycocalyx HISTOLOGY The 'fuzzy coat' formed by oligosaccharide side chains and the negatively-charged sialic acid that is attached to membrane-bound proteins and lipids and located on the surface of secretory epithelial cells, eg of the gastrointestinal tract **Ultrastructure** Granular extracellular 'fuzz'

Glycogen granules Glycogen-filled 'organelles' that appear as granular dots by electron microscopy that may be seen in benign tumors, eg hepatic adenomas, parathyroid adenomas and 'sugar' tumor and malignant tumors, eg sarcomas, classically Ewing sarcoma as well as extraskeletal chondrosarcoma, clear cell sarcoma, leiomyosarcoma and rhabdomyosarcoma, clear cell carcinoma of the urogenital tract, endometrial carcinoma and choriocarcinoma

Glycogen rosettes Garland-like clusters of granular 'specks' seen by electron microscopy in the cytoplasm of malignant cells, classically seen in Ewing sarcoma

Glycogenosis Glycogen storage disease (GSD) A group of 12 inherited defects in the ability to store glucose and/or retrieve glucose from intracellular storage depots, all of which have an autosomal recessive pattern of heredity, resulting in the accumulation of glycogen in the liver,

Glycogen storage disease

Type	Deficient enzyme
0	Hepatic glycogen synthetase
I	Glucose-6-phosphatase or intracellular transportation
II	Lysosomal acid maltase alpha-1,4 glucosidase
III	Amylo-1,6 glucosidase see 'Debrancher' disease
IV	Amylo-1,4->1,6-trans-glucosidase see 'Brancher' disease
V	Myophosphorylase
VI	Hepatic phosphorylase
VII	Phosphofructokinase
VIII	Inactive hepatic phosphorylase is implicated
IX	Hepatic phosphorylase kinase
X	Cyclic 3'5'-AMP-dependent kinase
XI	No deficiency identified

muscle, heart, kidney and other tissues enzyme defects, resulting in an array of symptoms, including hepatosplenomegaly, cardiomegaly, mental retardation, eg Dancing eyes syndrome (GSD VIII) or Doll face syndrome (GSD Ia); see Brancher, Debrancher diseases

Glycogen storage disease see Glycogenosis

'Glycogen tumor' A colloquialism for the glycogen-rich rhabdomyoma; see Spider cells

Glycophorin A sialoglycoprotein (60% carbohydrate, 40% protein) that spans and comprises a major component of the red cell membrane

Glycosaminoglycan (GAG) Formerly, mucopolysaccharide Any of a number of disaccharide polymers, one of which is either a D-acetylglucosamine or a D-galactosamine, linked by ester or amide bonds; GAGs are the carbohydrate component of proteoglycans and include hyaluronic acid and chondroitin sulfate, dermatan sulfate, heparan sulfate, heparin sulfate and keratan sulfate; see Basement membrane

Glycoside CLINICAL PHARMACOLOGY A molecule formed from the condensation of either a furanose or a pyranose with another molecule as an acetal, nitrogen glycoside or phosphate ester glycoside; cardiac glycosides include digitoxin, digoxin and ouabain

Glycosuria Glucosuria The spillage of excess glucose into the urine, an event common in uncontrolled diabetes mellitus and in 'renal' glycosuria, which may be divided into Type A T_m mutation or V_{max} type, result of a lowering of the renal threshhold for glucose Type B K_m or degree of splay mutation; as with the T_m mutation type, K_m may be inherited as an autosomal recessive

Glycosylated hemoglobin hemoglobin A1c see Advanced glycosylation endproducts, Fast hemoglobins

Glycosyl-phosphatidylinositol(s) A group of glycosylated Phosphatidylinositol (GPI) glycophospholipids, responsible for a) Anchoring particulate cell-surface proteins to the membrane, eg alkaline phosphatase, 5'-nucleotidase, acetyl-cholinesterase, Thy-1, carcinoembryonic antigen, TAP, N-CAM, Decay accelerating factor and b) Signal transduction for insulin, nerve growth factor and IL-2 (Science 1991; 251:78), where they act as 'second messengers'

Glypiation MOLECULAR BIOLOGY A convoluted coinage referring to the anchoring of glycosyl-phosphatidylinositol residue to a protein or substrate, which serves as a signal for sorting glycoproteins

Gm An allotype of an immunoglobulin IgG heavy chain, resulting from an inherited variation in the amino acid sequence Note: allotypes exist for IgA heavy chain and kappa light chains, but not for IgM, IgD and IgE heavy chain or the lambda light chain

GM-CSF Granulocyte macrophage-colony stimulating factor A hematopoietic growth factor, which in the native form is produced by monocytes, lymphocytes, fibroblasts and endothelial cells; recombinant GM-CSF (sargramostim) may be of use in increasing leukocytes in AIDS patients, or stimulating hematopoiesis after high dose chemotherapy in autologous bone marrow transplantation; it may also be useful as an immune 'tonic' in cancer and AIDS patients, anemia, increasing the survival of bone marrow grafts and reducing infections in congenital neutropenia (J Am Med Assoc 1989; 262:1295); see Biological response modifiers, Sargramostim; Cf G-CSF

GME Graduate medical education The formal hospital-sponsored training period that follows graduation from medical school, which includes internship, residency and fellowship (J Am Med Assoc 1990; 263:2927); Cf CME, Fifth pathway

GM-1 ganglioside A complex acidic glycolipid that may be of use in reducing the morbidity and hastening the functional recovery in patients with spinal cord injury (N Engl J Med 1991; 324:1829)

GM-1 gangliosidoses Lysosomal disorders caused by β-galactosidase deficiency with accumulation of GM1 ganglioside, a monosialoganglioside of the gray and white matter, divided into Type I (infantile form), characterized by severe mental retardation and neurological, somatic and osseous defects, accumulation of β-galactoside and death by age two Type II (juvenile and adult form) is milder than type I, with death occurring by age ten

GM-2 gangliosidoses Type I Tay-Sachs disease, infantile amaurotic idiocy An autosomal recessive (carrier frequency, Ashkenazi Jews, 1:25) condition due to hexosaminidase A deficiency, resulting in a 100-fold increase in GM-2 ganglioside in the brain **Clinical** Onset in early infancy with generalized hypotonia, apathy and poor head control, 'cherry-red spots' in the optic macula Note: Genetic screening has virtually eliminated the disease **Type II** Sandhoff's disease An autosomal recessive condition caused by a complete deficiency of hexosaminidase isoenzymes A and B, with the central nervous system changes of Tay-Sachs disease as well as visceral involvement; 100 to 200-fold increase in GM-2 gangliosides and a 50-100-fold in GA2, the asialo-derivative of GM-2 in the brain, liver, spleen and kidney;

type II is not more common in eastern European Jews **Type III** Juvenile GM-2 gangliosidosis An autosomal recessive condition of later onset (between ages 2 and 6), with ataxia and psychomotor retardation and death by age 5-15; it is not associated with organomegaly and, like type I, is more common in Ashkenazi Jews

GMP-140 see CD62

GMS stain Gomori-Grocott methenamine silver stain A chromic acid, sodium bisulfite stain used in histology and cytopathology for identifying fungi; the glass slide with the tissue or cytologic smear is then placed in a hot bath (58°C) for the penetration of tissue, staining fungi a distinct black with sharp margins and a cleared center, an appearance that may be mimicked by erythrocytes that also absorb silver and stain black, but are rounder and have a dark center; see Sealed envelope appearance

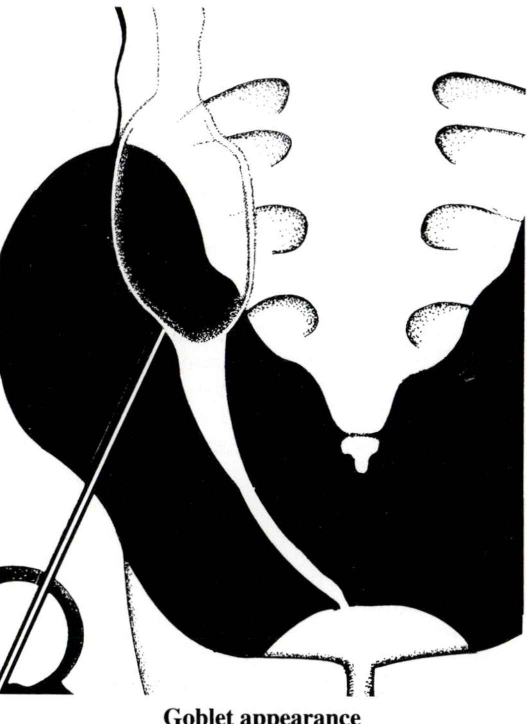

Goblet appearance

Gnotobiotic Germ-free; gnotobiotic organisms are either experimental models, eg mice with naive immune systems or 'experiments of nature', in which the natural immune defense mechanisms are grossly defective, eg severe combined immune deficiency and continued survival of the host requires complete avoidance of exposure to pathogens; see 'Bubble boy'

GnRH see Gonadotropin-releasing hormone

GnRH analogs Polypeptide analogs of gonadotropin-releasing hormone (GnRH) that are 15 to 200-fold more potent than GnRH in stimulating the release of gonadotropins; these analogs include leuprolide and histrelin, which can be administered in a pulsatile fashion, with the purpose of restoring lost GnRH, normalizing pituitary-gonadal function, as in congenital GnRH deficiencies, eg hypogonadotropic hypogonadism with anosmia (Kallmann syndrome) or without anosmia or in acquired GnRH deficiency secondary to irradiation of the central nervous system, pituitary tumors or panhypopituitarism; GnRH may be administered continuously in order to induce biochemical 'castration', by 1) suppressing a pituitary-gonadal axis that at normal levels of activity is exacerbating an undenying medical condition, eg endometriosis or prostatic carcinoma or 2) suppressing a pituitary-gonadal axis acting in pathological excess, eg polycystic ovarian disease or hyperthecosis (N Engl J Med 1991; 324:93rv); see Gonadotropin-releasing hormone

GNR Gram-negative rods MICROBIOLOGY An abbreviation for bacilli that do not absorb the gram stain, ie, pink in color; the most common GNRs of clinical importance are of the coliform family ***Enterobacteriaceae***, eg *Escherichia, Proteus, Pseudomonas, Salmonella, Shigella*, growth of GNRs usually implies fecal contamination, as in peritonitis induced by appendicitis, a ruptured diverticulum or gunshot wound

Goblet appearance RADIOLOGY A radiolucent filling defect seen in tumors of the ureters, where the superior meniscus 'front' of the contrast outlines a goblet-shaped lower or upper margin of the tumor, best visualized by retrograde pyelography, an appearance fancifully likened to that of a wine goblet

Goblet cells Caliceal mucin-laden cells, located in the lateral wall of the intestinal crypts and elsewhere in the gastrointestinal tract

Goiania A city near Brazilia that was the scene of a civilian radiation accident second only in severity to that of Chernobyl; in 1987, some unemployed men entered a partially demolished radiotherapy unit and extracted the core canister containing 1400 curies of cesium-137, which was sold to a junk dealer who opened it and distributed the glowing cesium as 'carnival glitter'; 10 people died, 54 were hospitalized, 244 received 'major league' exposure and a large region of the city required decontamination; the treatment administered was Prussian blue (to chelate the radioactive cesium and induce excretion, bone marrow transplantation and stimulation of marrow recovery by GM-CSF (Science 1987; 238:1028)

Go 'bare' Bare, Old High German, without clothing LEGAL MEDICINE To practice medicine without malpractice insurance; the cost of malpractice insurance in the USA is a function of a) Specialty, ranging from a low of $1-2000 per year in rehabilitation medicine, to $100 000 in neurosurgery, orthopedic surgery, plastic surgery and obstetrics and b) Location Long Island (New York), Florida and California are most expensive; because of these costs, some physicians transfer all their assets to third parties, incorporate themselves and practice their specialty without insurance, ie 'go bare' Note: This practice may prevent 'frivolous' lawsuits initiated through avarice, but also prevents truly damaged parties from recuperating compensation; see Malpractice, Cf Surplus line companies

'God committee' see Seattle committee

Goiter Latin, Guttur, throat Non-neoplastic thyroid enlargement of any etiology; a goiter may be euthyroid, hypothyroid or hyperthyroid, endemic or sporadic and simple (colloid) or multinodular; goiters are most often due to increased pituitary secretion of thyroid-stimulating hormone (TSH), stimulated by decreased levels of circulating thyroid hormone; congenital goiter occurs in the rare Pendred syndrome (accompanied by deafness) or with in utero exposure to antithyroid drugs or iodides; acquired goiter is idiopathic or may be due to goitrogens, eg lithium carbonate, amiodarone Endemic goiter is subdivided into a) A nervous system syndrome, consisting of ataxia, spasticity, deaf-mutism and mental retardation and b) A myxedematous syndrome characterized by poor growth, mental and sexual development and myxedema; in nodular goiters the lack of available iodine induces hyperplasia with excess colloid being stored in nodular, enlarged follicles; goiters are common in Graves-Basedow disease, occur in hyperactive middle-aged females and are multinodular and 'hot', displaying hyperactivity on a ^{67}Gallium scan

Gold RHEUMATOLOGY Gold compounds are used to treat arthritic conditions, acting to protect membrane proteins and lipids from oxidative degradation and quench singlet oxygen generated as free radicals **Side effects** Gastrointestinal tract, eg diarrhea, abdominal pain, nausea and vomiting, partially relieved by cromolyn sodium, renal, eg nephrotic syndrome and proteinuria, skin rashes, blood dyscrasias, hepatitis **Histopathology** IgG and C3 deposits in a 'moth-eaten' glomerular basement membrane and feathery crystals in the renal tubules

Gold curve see below, Gold-sol curve

(Goldberg-Maxwell-)Morris syndrome Testicular feminization An X-linked condition occurring in genotypic XY males who have a female phenotype, characterized by feminine habitus, sexual behavior and secondary sex characteristics, associated with a blind vaginal pouch, scanty pubic and axillary hair and internal undescended testicles **Laboratory** Testosterone levels are normal in the face of defective end-organ response; see Pseudohermaphroditism, male

Goldberg syndrome An autosomal recessive condition due to a defective gene on chromosome 10, resulting in neuroaminidase and β-galactosidase deficiencies **Clinical** Neonatal onset with mental and physical retardation, seizures, visual defects, deafness, gargoyle facies, corneal clouding, a cherry red spot of the macula; see Cherry red spots

Goldblatt kidney A classic model for studying renovascular hypertension, where the renal artery from kidney 'A' is partially obstructed by an atheromatous plaque (or less commonly, an occlusion external to the vessel, eg a tumor); the juxtaglomerular apparatus of kidney 'A' perceives decreased circulating blood volume and secretes renin, increasing the blood pressure (systemic hypertension) and, over time, the morphologic changes of malignant hypertension, ie arterionephrosclerosis in kidney 'B' due to increased activity of the renin-angiotensin-aldosterone system, while kidney 'A' is 'protected' by first pass inactivation of renin and aldosterone; the 'Goldblatt kidney' effect allows one to distinguish between benign and malignant hypertension, as in the malignant form, the affected side has 1.5-fold more renin than the unaffected side

'Goldbricking' Benign self-mutilation A condition in which a benign skin disorder, eg an occupational dermatosis, is exacerbated by self-induced excoriation prior to workman's compensation review in order to ensure that pension benefits will continue, rather than return to work

Goldenhar syndrome Oculoauriculovertebral dysplasia An autosomal condition characterized by multiple developmental defects **Clinical** Malar hypoplasia and dysplasia, macrostomia, micrognathia, cleft palate, vertebral body anomalies, eg spina bifida, scoliosis, epibulbar dermoids, external ear defects, antimongoloid slant, and less commonly, mental retardation, clubfoot and congenital heart defects

Golden hour CRITICAL CARE MEDICINE An uncommonly used term for a timespan after a trauma victim's arrival to a health care facility, during which the physician has an opportunity to make the right decisions, ie order appropriate diagnostic tests and initiate patient management, either surgical or continued observation; Cf Golden period

Golden-Kantor syndrome Steatorrhea with the radiologic 'moulage' sign, small intestinal segmentation, colonic dilation, redundancy, osteoporosis and dwarfism

Golden period CRITICAL CARE MEDICINE A term referring to a period of time during which an injury or other potentially urgent condition may go untreated without harmful effects; the 'golden period' differs according to the organ system or body site, eg revascularizaton of an extremity may be delayed up to six hours without compromising a limb's potential for functional recuperation; thrombolytic therapy with urokinase or streptokinase may be delayed up to 24 hours

Golden pneumonia see Lipoid pneumonia

'Golden shower' see Sexual deviancy

Golden tongue A bright yellow lingual lesion, seen in an immunocompromised patient with acute lymphocytic leukemia who was treated with chemotherapy and became infected with the otherwise saprobic fungus, ***Ramichloridium schulzeri*** (Arch Dermatol 1985; 121:892) Note: A general rule in mycology is that the brighter the colony of fungus, the less likely is the organism to be pathogenic

Golden triangle SUBSTANCE ABUSE A region of Southeast Asia that produces high-grade heroin; see Body-packing syndrome

Goldflam-Erb disease Obsolete for myasthenia gravis

Goldmann-Favre syndrome A rare autosomal recessive condition characterized by ocular hyaloid-retinal degeneration

'Goldrush effect' A term coined in a report about a mathematical proof of Johannes Keplers' sphere-packing problem, expounded in 1611; the proof is so complex that it is anticipated that other mathematicians would become involved in proving side theorems and other related geometric complexities; the term is applicable to any area of science in which a large conceptual leap forward is followed by those rushing to find 'gold', where none had been previously known to exist (Science 1991; 251:1028)

Goldscheider syndrome An autosomal recessive dystrophic variant of Fox's disease with hemorrhagic, scarring, pigmented or depigmented bullous lesions due to loose anchoring of the epidermis to the upper dermis; the lesions are acral and accompanied by onychodystrophy, leukoplakia, claw-hand, bony deformities and dwarfism

Gold-sol curve Lange's colloidal gold test An empiric, obsolete and nonspecific method for measuring protein in cerebrospinal fluid, where progressive dilutions of fluid are added to 10 test tubes containing colloidal gold solutions; precipitation within the tubes indicates the presence of gammaglobulin, causing a bright red colloidal gold color 0, to change to red-blue 1+, purple 2+, deep blue 3+, pale blue 4+ or colorless 5+; the highest concentration of protein in the fluid is on the left; a 'mid-peak' curve is normal 0001210000, a 'first zone' curve, eg 44332000000 is classically associated with neurosyphilis, but is now more common in multiple sclerosis (50% are positive), and may be seen in subacute sclerosing panencephalitis, central nervous system hemorrhage, meningitis and polyneuritis

'Gold standard' The best or most successful diagnostic or therapeutic modality for a clinical condition, against which any new tests or therapeutic results and protocols are compared; a gold standard is loosely equivalent to a 'standard of practice' and may be delineated in textbooks, having withstood the test of time; deviation from such standards without reason may be considered malpractice, thus potentially forcing a physician to adhere 'to the book', even though he might believe that a newer therapy is appropriate, eg the X-ray venography for diagnosing deep vein thrombosis is considered to be a 'gold standard', although the diagnosis of deep vein thrombosis may be established using radionuclide venography, liquid crystal thermography, ultrasonography and impedance plethysmography

Goldstein's disease A cerebellar disease with defects of equilibrium, perception of time, space and weight (ergo, unsteady gait), adiadochokinesia, megalographia, hyperreflexia of joints and intention tremor Note: The disease was described in 1915 and it is difficult to determine whether this entity was not a form of another disease, eg neurosyphilis or meningoencephalitis

Goldstein syndrome Hereditary hemorrhagic telangiectasis

G_{olf} A G protein involved in olfaction, a neural activity that is similar to vision in that it requires that external signals be converted to electrical signals recognizable by the brain; one model of olfaction proposes that the olfactory signal is transduced as follows: An odorant is received at the membrane receptor of the sensory dendrite, after which GTP is degraded to GDP by the inner membrane-bound G_{olf} protein, which activates adenyl ate cyclase, generating a cAMP from ATP, activating a Na^+/K^+ cation-conducting channel, generating a neural signal (Nature 1991; 350:16n&v)

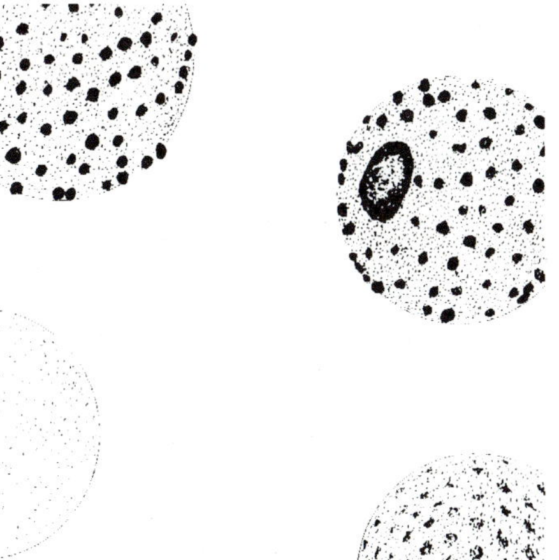

Golf ball bodies

Golf ball bodies A fanciful descriptor for erythrocytes of severe α thalassemia that are filled with large rounded inclusions or Heinz bodies, composed of precipitated hemoglobin H, resulting from oxidative denaturation of unstable hemoglobin H (four β chains); these structures are more prominent after splenectomy, best seen in peripheral blood smears stained with brilliant cresyl blue and comprise more than half of the erythrocytes in these patients

'Golf ball' metastases A pattern of pulmonary metastases, seen on a plain chest film, where the nodules are between the size of the 'cannonball' metastases of renal cell carcinoma and the 'miliary' or millet-seed sized metastases of thyroid, lung and breast carcinomas, typically seen in sarcomas, clear cell carcinomas and seminomas and melanomas

Golf 'elbow' Medial epicondylitis SPORTS MEDICINE A sports injury characterized by pain and tenderness of the medial humeral epicondyle at the origin of the flexor tendons, caused by excessive golfing Treatment Rest, steroid injection if severe; Cf Tennis elbow

Golgi-derived coated vesicle A vesicle involved in nonspecific intracellular transport of biosynthetic molecules, mediated by non-selective 'bulk flow' carrier molecules, designated as COPs (coat proteins), one of which, β-COP has sequence similarity to adaptin proteins of clathrin-coated vesicles (Nature 1991; 349:215); see COPs; Cf Clathrin

Gompertzian growth ONCOLOGY A growth curve expressed as an exponentially decreasing function, ie as the size increases (to a theoretical limit), the relative speed of the increase falls exponentially; the curve is named after an 18th century mathematician, and describes the growth of cell masses, eg a fetus or the growth dynamics of most malignancies; Cf Farr's law of epidemics

Gonadal dysgenesis see Intersex syndromes

Gonadotropin-releasing hormone (GnRH) A decapeptide synthesized in the hypothalamus, secreted into the anterior hypophysis via the hypophysioportal circuit, where it stimulates the release of the gonadotropins, FSH and LH; GnRH is secreted in a) A pulsatile fashion (when the pituitary gland is under constant stimulation by GnRH or its analogs, the anterior pituitary becomes desensitized, with subsequent gonadal suppression) and b) With peaks of secretion during the neonatal period followed by a quiescent phase, later reaching adult levels in puberty Mechanism of action GnRH binds to a cell receptor that mobilizes calcium ions, with the subsequent release of gonadotropins; because of GnRH's short half-life (2-4 minutes) and its vital physiological role, GnRH analogs have been developed (N Engl J Med 1991; 324:93rv); see GnRH analogs

Goodness of fit STATISTICS The degree to

which statistical data supports a specified theoretical model; a 'good fit' assumes that the probability model is valid

'Good' patient A patient who provides reliable information to the physician, who follows the prescribed regimen, drug therapy or recommended change in lifestyle, if appropriate for the patient's condition, and who can be counted on to return for 'check-up' visits at appropriate intervals; Cf Difficult patient

Good Samaritan laws FORENSIC MEDICINE Legislation tailored to the needs of individual jurisdictions that applies to health care professionals and citizens providing emergency medical care in 'good faith'; these laws are designed to protect 'good samaritans' from civil liability while attempting resuscitation Note: If the statutory requirements of 'acting in good faith' at the 'scene of an accident or emergency' are met, a plaintiff's lawsuit against a physician or other 'good samaritan', for allegedly causing damage to the plaintiff, is often dismissed as 'frivolous'

Goose-flesh Cutis anserina Diffuse 1-3 mm bosselations or papules, fancifully likened to a goose's skin after the feathers have been plucked FORENSIC PATHOLOGY 'Goose-flesh' is an early postmortem finding caused by rigor mortis of the erector pili, especially common in drowning victims INFECTIOUS DISEASE Diffuse, finely papular rash of scarlet fever overlying an erythematous base SUBSTANCE ABUSE Horripilation, one of the early symptoms of heroin withdrawal or 'cold turkey', a reflection of marked sympathetic discharge, occurring about 8 hours after the last dose, accompanied by yawning, lacrimation, mydriasis, insomnia, hyperactivity of the gastrointestinal tract, diarrhea, tachycardia and systolic hypertension

Goose neck deformity The convoluted twisting of a short tubular structure, likened to a goose's neck has been used in two cardiovascular contexts, a) 'Goose neck' describes the distorted left ventricular outflow tract seen by selective left ventriculography in patients with partial atrioventricular (AV) canal defects (ostium primum and common AV valve), where the failure of the endocardial cushions to fuse produces an abnormally low AV valve with an abnormally high anterior position of the aortic valve and b) The goose neck lamp deformity is a nodularity palpated externally in Mönckeburg's arteriosclerosis, caused by dystrophic calcified rings within the media of the medium to small blood vessels, likened to the flexible 'goose neck' lamps Histopathology No inflammation, no involvement of the adventitia and intima

Gordon Research conferences A series of meetings held annually in New England (USA) for research scientists with common interests in chemistry and related sciences to meet and interact for discussion and free exchange of ideas, stimulating advanced thinking at universities,research foundations and industrial laboratories; initially organized and chaired by Dr Neil Gordon of Johns Hopkins University, the 'Gordons' began with one meeting in 1931 and have grown to 130 annual meetings; the camaraderie of these conferences is such that critics at one session may become collaborators by the next and are felt by some to represent the spirit of science practised in its purest and most selfless form; current director A Cruickshank, U Rhode Is (Emeritus); see Rs (the three Rs of research)

Gore-tex A proprietary form of expanded polytetrafluoroethylene that is a versatile synthetic material, which is biologically similar to fascia and used for abdominal and thoracic wall, pediatric and diaphragmatic reconstructions, rectal, vaginal and urethral suspension and hernia repair

'Gork' God only really knows A transiently popular colloquialism used by medical students and interns on the wards of some US teaching hospitals that referred to patients with a difficult diagnosis; the term acquired a derogatory flavor and came to refer to terminally comatose patients'

Goserelin A gonadotropin releasing hormone analog that may be used to suppress testosterone activity in advanced prostate carcinoma Note: The prognosis of prostatic adenocarcinoma is poor in the presence of bone pain, elevated testosterone and alkaline phosphatase levels (J Am Med Assoc 1991; 265:618)

'Go sour' A generic American colloquialism for unanticipated deterioration of a patient's clinical status that is used in a broad range of situations, eg an uncomplicated myocardial infarction that 'goes sour' with the development of intractable arrhythmia or a routine hip replacement on an elderly patient who undergoes an abrupt and unanticipated intraoperative deterioration

Gossypol An aromatic triterpene derived from cotton (*Gossypum hirsutum*) seed oil that is 90% effective in reducing sperm counts to the level of infertility, thus having potential as a male contraceptive DISADVANTAGE Nephrotoxicity, hypokalemia, 25% suffer irreversible sterility (Med Clin North Am 1990; 74:1205)

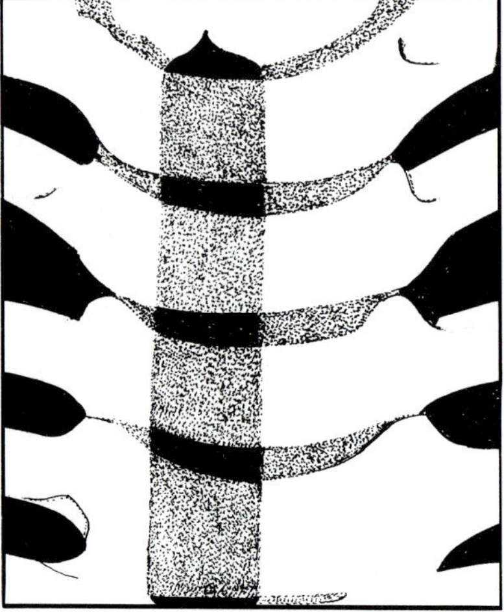

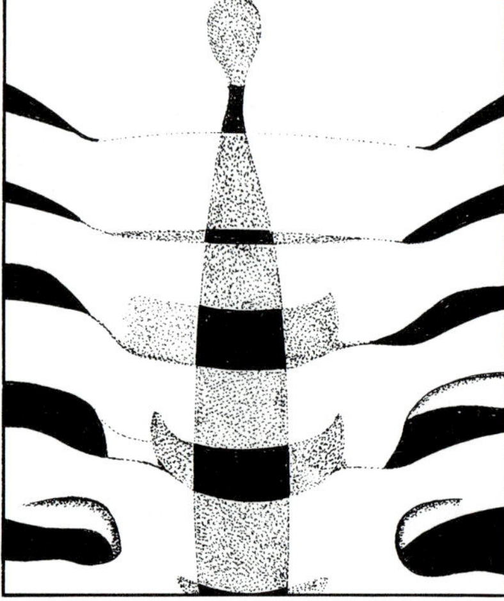

Normal **Gothic arch sign** **Epiglottis**

GOT Glutamic oxaloacetic transaminase see AST (aspartate amino transferase)

Gothic arch appearance Steeple sign OTORHINOLARYNGOLOGY Narrowing of the glottis and subglottis due to edema and acute and chronic inflammatory cells in the soft tissue, seen in a lateral neck film of young children with croup infections, eg due to parainfluenza, other viruses and bacteria (J Can Assoc Radiol 1961; 12:86, Ped Clin North America 1974;21:707), an appearance fancifully likened to that of a gothic arch, see figure, facing page

Gout, congenital Latin, gutta, droplet A usually acquired condition that the ancients considered to occur 'droplet by droplet'; congenital gout is associated with two X-linked enzymes a) Hypoxanthine-guanine phosphoribosyl transferase (HGPRT), which is defective in Lesch-Nyhan disease and b) 5-phosphoribosyl-1-pyrophosphate (PRPP); gout is intimately linked to increased serum levels of uric acid that is often above 410 µmol/L (US: 7.0 mg/ml), a level that occurs in a significant minority of men (90% of gout occurs in men); the indigestible monosodium urates in the synovium stimulate the release of lysosomal enzymes from neutrophils, the crystals of which remain undigested, causing a vicious cycle, in which crystals are ingested but not digested, although lytic enzyme is released, the end-result of which is joint destruction; family history can be evoked in about one-half of cases, one-half of cases present with the classic 'podagra' (first metatarsophalangeal joint) and up to 90% will suffer podagra at some time during their disease **Acute treatment** Colchicine, non-steroid anti-inflammatory drugs, Corticosteroids **Interval treatment** Dietary **Chronic treatment** Allopurinol, sulfinpyrazone, salicylates

'Gowns' ACADEMIA The academic faculty of a medical school; many US teaching hospitals are university-based and the teaching faculty may spend more time writing papers and in research than seeing patients; Note: 'Gowns' are the ceremonial robes of education and learned professions; according to Sir William Osler '...*TO PRACTICE MEDICINE WITHOUT PATIENTS IS TO NOT SAIL AT ALL*'; Cf 'Towns'

gp90mel see Selectins

gp120 A 120 kD glycoprotein on the surface of human immunodeficiency virus type 1 that binds to cells (T cells, macrophages) with the CD4 receptor; blockage of the gp120 antigens by soluble synthetic CD4 peptides (sCD4) results in reduced infection of CD4 cells in a 'dose-dependent' fashion, implying that sCD4 may have a role in blocking HIV-1 infection (Nature 1990; 346:277); gp120 is divided into a 'loop region', which although readily accessible to the immune system, is the product of the highly mutable env gene, frustrating the host's attempts to produce effective antibodies; in vitro antibodies to this region block HIV's fusion to CD4-bearing cells and infection and a 'pit region'

gp160 vaccine A vaccine prepared from a cloned fragment of HIV-1's envelope protein, which increases the cellular and humoral immunity to HIV products in patients with early HIV infection, slowing the rate of reduction of CD4 T cells, a major predictor of AIDS progression (N Engl JMed 1991; 324:1677)

G protein(s) Guanosine phosphate GDP, GTP-binding proteins A family of more than 20 different membrane-bound proteins that regulate ten or more different ion channels and as many enzymes; G proteins function as heterotrimers (α, β and γ subunits), transducing biological signals, including light, hormones and neural neural signals (table, page 262); according to the accepted model, a transmembrane receptor undergoes a conformational change, interacts with a G protein, which, depending on the ligand, either activates (as do ACTH, glucagon or epinephrine, left side of below

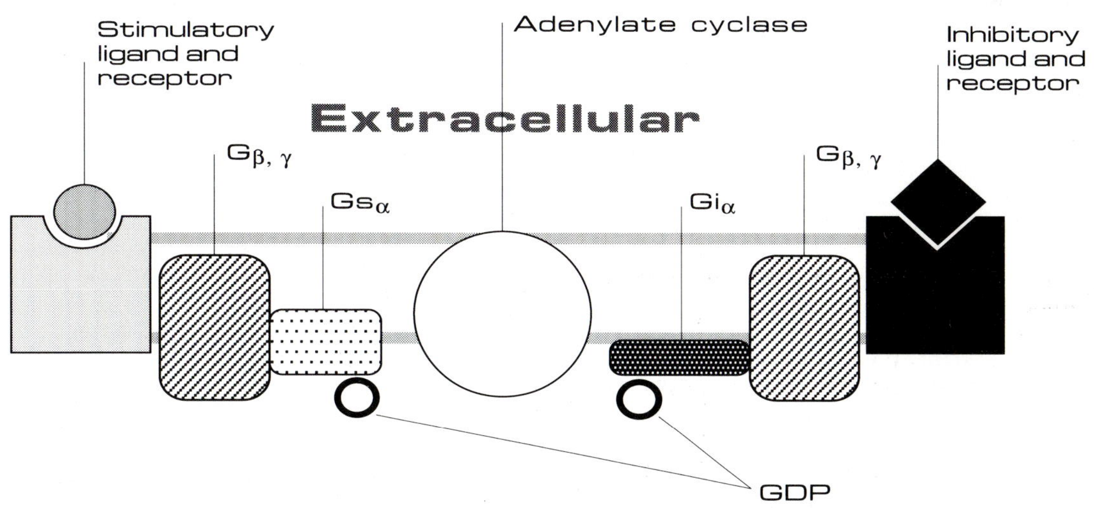

figure) or inhibits (eg, prostaglandine E_1 or adenosine) adenylate cyclase, which is mediated by GTP and GDP; the α G protein subunit is thought to be the most central component of the complex and is linked to critical intracellular effectors including receptors via adenyl cyclase, effector enzymes, phosphoinositide cycle proteins, calcium and sodium ion channel proteins and transportation of proteins and sugars; subtypes of G-proteins include G_s, stimulatory for adenylate cyclase; G_i, inhibitory for adenylate cyclase; G_o, otherwise, function unknown and G_t, a transducin or photoreceptor; G proteins '...*HAVE SEVEN TRANSMEMBRANE DOMAINS WITH MARKED SEQUENCE SIMILARITY, AN EXTRACELLULAR N TERMINUS WITH CONSENSUS SEQUENCES FOR N-LINKED GLYCOSYLATION, SEQUENCE DIVERGENCE IN THE CONNECTING HYDROPHILIC LOOPS, A CYTOPLASMIC CARBOXYL TAIL AND/OR A LARGE INTRACELLULAR LOOP RICH IN SERINE AND THREONINE RESIDUES, WHICH ARE SITES FOR PHOSPHORYLATION AND CONSERVED SITES FOR POST-TRANSLATIONAL MODIFICATIONS, INCLUDING FATTY ACYLATION AND DISULFIDE BOND FORMATION; THE DIVERSE LIGANDS APPEAR TO INTERACT WITHIN A POCKET CREATED BY SOME OF THE A-HELICAL MEMBRANE-SPANNING REGIONS, WHILE OTHER REGIONS ON THE INNER SURFACE OF THE RECEPTOR INTERACT WITH AND ACTIVATE SPECIFIC G PROTEINS, DETERMINING THE NATURE OF THE BIOLOGICAL RESPONSE...*' (Nature 1991; 351:353); G-protein diseases are processes that block G-protein activity at the membrane, eg pertussis and cholera, preventing signal transduction

G protein receptors A family of membrane receptors including D_1, D_2, D_3 (dopamine) receptors, β, α_1 and α_2-adrenergic and muscarinic and serotonergic receptors that evoke intracellular responses by degrading GTP to GDP; see G proteins

Graafian follicle GYNECOLOGY A fluid-filled cystic 'unit' containing the ovum, partially covered by a cap of granulosa cells (cumulus oophorus, discus proligerus) that measures 5-10 mm, is lined by an inner layer of granulosa cells and outer layer of theca cells (theca interna) and surrounded by an avascular capsule (theca externa), a structure that is partially recapitulated in the endodermal sinus tumor

Graft versus host disease (GVHD) A condition that is a major cause of morbidity and mortality in bone marrow transplantation, although it is less problematic in transplantation of kidneys, heart, liver and skin; viable donor T lymphocytes react immunologically against the host, rejecting the hand that feeds Clinical Fever, skin rash (central erythematous maculopapular eruption that may spread to the extremities with bulla formation), anorexia, nausea and vomiting, watery or bloody diarrhea, lymphadenopathy, infections, hepatosplenomegaly, elevated liver function tests and hemolytic anemia; for GVHD to exist, the graft must contain immunocompetent cells, the recipient must express antigens that are not present in the transplant donor and the recipient must be incapable of mounting an effective response to destroy the transplanted immunocompetent cells (Billingham, 1966) Prophylaxis Combination of cyclosporin and methotrexate Treatment One-half of the 40% of patients who develop post-bone marrow transplantation GVHD respond to high-dose steroids (N Engl J Med 1991; 324:667); other agents in development include FK506, rapamycin and anti-T-cell ricin (ricin conjugated to a monoclonal antibody against CD5, a pan-T-cell marker seen on the cell surface of 95% of all T-cells); see Bone marrow transplantation, FK506, rapamycin Note: An HLA mismatch is more compatible with graft survival than a blood group ABO mismatch; GVHD occurs in 1) Immature immune systems, eg runt disease of mice or 2) Immunodeficiency states, either a) Congenital, eg thymic alymphoplasia, severe combined immunodeficiency disease, Wiskott-Aldrich and T-cell defects and b) Acquired, due to cytotoxic drug therapy, bone marrow transplantation, lymphoproliferative disease, eg acute lymphocytic or myelocytic leukemias, non-Hogdkin lymphoma and Hodgkin's disease as well as in neuroblastoma and glioblastoma Gradation of skin changes in GVHD 1) Vacuolization of the basal cell layer 2) Dyskeratosis 3) Subepidermal cleft formation and 4) Complete epidermal separation (N Engl J Med 1985; 313:645), which serves as a method for predicting GVH in bone marrow transplant victims Prevention Irradiation of the donated blood may prevent the functionally active leukocytes from rejecting recipient cells and tissues **Acute GVHD** is associated with rashes, elevated 'liver function' tests, diarrhea, dermatitis, hepatitis, response to immunosuppressive therapy occurs in 35-60% Clinical **Chronic GVHD** Occurs in 20-40% of those who survive transplantation > 180 days Note: GVH may also occur when maternal lymphocytes are transferred into a fetus with a congenital deficiency in the immune systems, ie intrauterine transfusion; see Transfusion-associated graft-versus-host disease

G PROTEIN-COUPLED LIGANDS (or stimuli)

ARACHIDONIC ACID DERIVATIVES Thromboxane A2
BIOGENIC AMINES Acetylcholine, adenosine, dopamine, epinephrine, histamine, 5-hydroxytryptamine, norepinephrine
BRAIN/GUT PEPTIDE HORMONES Angiotensin, arginine, vasopressin, bombesin/gastrin releasing hormone, thyrotropin-releasing hormone, vasoactive intestinal polypeptide
HORMONES Choriogonadotropin (lutropin), follicle-stimulating hormone, parathyroid hormone, thyrotropin
Miscellaneous: cAMP, cannabinoids, complement 5a, endothelins, platelet-activating factor, thrombin (see G protein receptors)
SENSORY STIMULI Light (retinal), odorant s
TACHYKININS Substance K, substance P, neuromedin K

Gramicidin(s) A family of linear antibiotics produced by Bacillus brevis that carry an N-terminal formyl group and a C-terminal ethanolamine group and are active against gram-positive bacteria, acting by increasingion permeability of the cells **Gramicidin A** is composed of a dimer of hydrophobic amino acids with alternating L- and D-forms, used in membrane research as it is the simplest protein capable of forming transmembrane ion channels, which is selective for monovalent cations (NH_4^+, H^+ and others) (Science 1990; 250:1256) **Gramicidin S** is a cyclic polypeptide, more properly named tyrocidin as it uncouples oxidative phosphorylation of tyrosine

Gram stain A stain formulated by the great Dane, HCJ Gram, used to identify bacteria; gram-positive bacteria (purple) have cell wall peptidoglycan and an inner cell membrane and are digested by lysosomal enzymes from macrophages; gram-negative bacteria are red, have a membrane similar to the above and in addition, an outer lipid bilayer with lipopolysaccharide which is destroyed by cationic proteins and complement (the 'fluid-phase'); once an organism is identified by its 'gram-ness' and morphology, laboratory algorithms may be followed to identify and speciate the organism

'Grandfather' clause A colloquialism for any policy or rule that exempts a group of individuals, organizations or drugs from meeting new standards or regulations; eg when a new subspecialty board in internal medicine is created, the physicians practicing in that area are 'grandfathered' into the subspecialty and not required to meet residency requirements

Grand mal seizure A form of epilepsy with an onset between infancy and early adulthood, with attacks triggered by fever or unidentified environmental cues, eg psychological and emotional stress **Clinical** Prolonged tonic-clonic seizures with the risk of intra-ictal cerebral hypoxia; sequelae include intellectual impairment, behavioral changes or more rarely ataxia and spasticity **Encephalogram** Tonic-clonic seizures demonstrate low-voltage fast (10 Hz or faster) activity during the tonic phase evolving to slower, larger sharp waves associated throughout both hemispheres; during the clonic phase, the bursts of sharp waves are associated with rhythmic muscular contractions while the slow waves coincide with the pauses; between seizures, the EEG is usually abnormal demonstrating polyspike, spike or rarely, sharp and slow-wave discharges; Cf Petit mal epilepsy

Grand rounds ACADEMICS Formal presentation of an aspect of clinical medicine, with discussion of pathogenesis, symptomatology and therapy Note: Although the term was first used for the formal presentation of a patient's clinical, radiological and laboratory data in an academic setting, for review by colleagues, this latter is regionally known 'professorial rounds', while in grand rounds, the patient is a peripheral player to the topic being discussed; see Rounds; Cf Clinicopathologic conference

Granular cell tumor Abrikossof's giant cell myoblastoma A small (< 3 cm) painless subepithelial tumor of the tongue, skin, breast and other epithelia and muscle, affecting older blacks with a male:female ratio of 2:1 **Histopathology** Small round nests of large, polyhedral cells with pale pink granular cytoplasm (figure, top), thought to be of Schwann cell origin, which are separated by bundles of mature collage, and which may be covered by pseudoepitheliomatous hyperplasia of the superficial dermis (figure, bottom right) **Ultrastructure** Autophagocytic lysosomal vacuoles filled with cellular debris (figure, bottom left); the cells are positive by the periodic acid Schiff/diastase resistant (PAS/dr) and neuron-specific enolase (NSE) stains **Differential diagnosis** Any mass composed of enlarged cells with granular cytoplasm, eg oncocytoma, metastatic Hürthle cell tumor, rhabdomyosarcoma, hybernoma, xanthogranuloma; less than 2% become malignant (Virch Arch Path Anat 1926; 260:215)

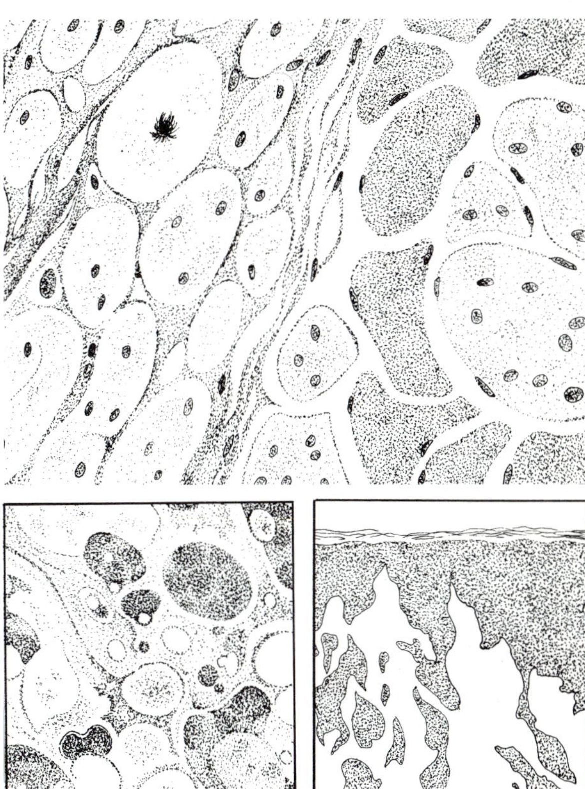

Granular cell tumor

Granular dystrophy An autosomal dominant variant of early-onset corneal stroma dystrophy with central 'bread-crumb'-like opacities, episodic irritation and photophobia

Granulation tissue A post-inflammatory reaction characterized by edema, chronic (lymphocytes, macrophages, scattered plasma cells, neutrophils) inflammation and numerous proliferating endothelial cells and blood vessels

Granules HEMATOLOGY Intracytoplasmic inclusions typical by light microscopy of myeloid cells, divided into 1) Primary azurophilic or immature granules in promyelocytes contain membrane-bound lysosomes filled with acid phosphatase, α-mannosidase, aryl-sulfatase, β-glucuronidase, cathepsin, elastase, esterase, lactoferrin, myeloperoxidase, 5'-nucleosidase, N-acetyl-β-glucosaminidase, sulfated mucosubstance, lysozymes and other basic proteins 2) Secondary (specific) granules contain lactoferrin and alkaline (but lack acid phosphatase and peroxidase and 3) Tertiary granules contain amino peptidase, lysozyme, collagenase and basic protein

Granulocyte A mature cell of the myeloid series that comprises 25-40% of the circulating leukocytes or white cells; neutrophils, both the immature 'band' form and the mature polymorphonuclear neutrophil, have a multilobed mature nucleus, and comprise the majority of circulating granulocytes; eosinophils and basophils each comprise 1-3% of the circulating leukocytes

Granulocytic sarcoma see Chloroma

Granuloma A nodular aggregate of epithelioid macrophages with abundant endoplasmic reticulum, giant multinucleated epithelioid cells and scattered CD4 T cells in the center, which function in antigen recognition, surrounded by a rim of collagen, rare CD8 T lymphocytes and proliferating fibroblasts; granulomas are common in chronic infection, especially if the organism remains viable, has metabolic machinery allowing circumvention of the macrophage's phagocytic defense and is capable of residing in histiocytes; granulomas (with Langhans' giant cells) are characteristic of tuberculosis but occur in a) Other infections, eg brucellosis, cat-scratch disease, glanders, fungal infections, leishmaniasis, lepra, listeriosis, mesenteric lymphadenitis, schistosomiasis, tularemia and b) Noninfectious conditions, eg berylliosis, Crohn's disease, rheumatoid arthritis, sarcoidosis, silicosis, sprue; Cf Giant cells

Granuloma gravidarum see Pregnancy 'tumor'

Granulosa cell tumor (GCT) GYNECOLOGY A sex cord tumor of older women comprising 1-2% of ovarian neoplasms, which is 'driven' by unopposed estrogen stimulation; the endometria of patients with GCTs often has cystic hyperplasia and 5-25% of cases have a concomitant well-differentiated endometrial carcinoma Pathology GCTs measure up to 4-5 cm, 5% are bilateral and have cystic and solid areas, with a gross appearance fancifully likened to watered silk; 10% rupture, causing hemoperitoneum; 10% of GCTs are malignant, and these are histologically characterized by more prominent nucleoli; a) Adult GCTs are more common with an onset after age 30, characterized by Call-Exner bodies and pale cells with grooved nuclei and b) Juvenile GCTs occur in younger patients, and are characterized by irregular follicles, large, dark cells with ungrooved nuclei and common luteinization

Granulovacuolar degeneration NEUROPATHOLOGY Lucent 3-5 μm in diameter vacuoles with a dense central granule, which comprise one of three cardinal neuropathological features seen in 10-50% of pyramidal neurons of the hippocampus in Alzheimer's dementia, and are possibly of lysosomal origin; granulovacuolar degeneration (figure, right) may also occur in Down syndrome, Pick's disease, amyotrophic lateral sclerosis, Guam-type Parkinson's dementia complex, in the red and pontine nuclei in progressive supranuclear palsy and in cerebral nodules of tuberous sclerosis

Grape-like appearance A morphologic descriptor for massively enlarged, hydropically degenerated chorionic villi seen in hydatidiform mole (molar pregnancy); a similar morphology may be seen in benign cystic mesothelioma and in embryonal rhabdomyosarcoma

Grape cell HEMATOLOGY A large (30-80 μm) variant 'reticulum cell' with a small nucleus, condensed chromatin and regular, rounded spaces filled with immunoglobulins separated by wisps of bluish cytoplasm, occasionally seen in multiple myeloma and other clinical states causing increased immunoglobulin production, occasionally seen in bone marrow

GRAS see Generally recognized as safe

GRATEFUL MED INFORMATION SCIENCE A low-priced and 'user-friendly' software package that facilitates literature searches and accession of the data at the National Library of Medicine's database, MEDLARS; MEDLARS' most popular database is MEDLINE

Gravewax Adipocere A waxy induration of adipose tissue that occurs when an unembalmed body resides one or more months in cold wet ground, see Bog bodies

Gray Gy The International system (SI) unit for radiation as it is presumed to affect life forms, based on the actual absorption measured by a thermoluminescent dosimeter placed within a patient or a phantom; 1 Gray is equal to 1 joule/kg of the absorber (100 rads) Note: The formerly used unit for radiation exposure, the rad, is an 'indirect measurement' based on dosage measured in the air or on the skin surface and equated to a dose of radiation resulting in absorption of 100 ergs of energy/gram in the medium of interest, usually tissue Note: Because of the potential for confusion in the conversion of units, it is customary in some circles to use the unit centiGray (cGy), which is quantitatively equivalent to the rad

Graybiel's criteria A set of criteria used to diagnose seasickness delineated by Graybiel in Aerospace Med 1968; 39:453

Gray 'hepatization' A phase in lobar pneumonia, typically occurring at the first week of infection, at which time the lobe is covered with fibrin, the cut surface is gray, dry and granular, the alveoli are filled with fibrinous exudate composed of degenerating polymorphonuclear leukocytes and the inflammation is interconnected through the pores of Kohn

'Graying of America' see Oldest old

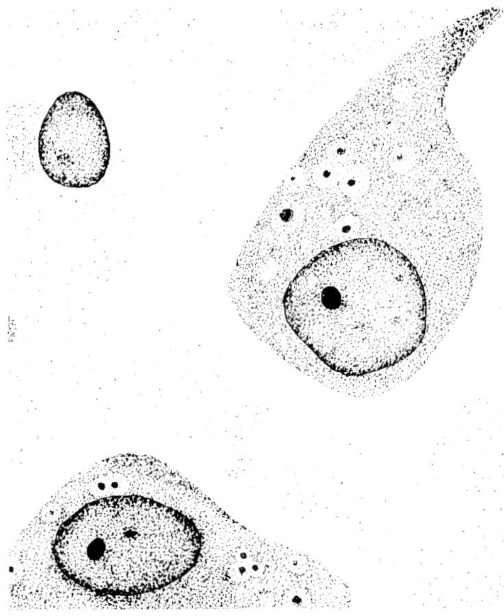

Granulovacuolar degeneration

'Graying-out' Slow visual impairment accompanying papilledema caused by slow-growing intracranial masses, eg brain tumors and abscesses; Cf 'Gray-out'

Gray journal A colloquialism of little utility used in the US for certain journals that may be requested in a medical library by color; the classic 'gray journal' is the gray-green Annals of Internal Medicine, although there are many other widely circulated 'gray' journals, including the American Journal of Obstetrics and Gynecology, the Journal of Pediatrics and RADIOLOGY; Cf Green journal

Gray lethal mouse The murine model for osteopetrosis, which has normal appositional bone growth without physiological resorption of bone; osteoclasts are present but afunctional

Gray matter The component cells and circuitry that comprises the 'central processing unit' of the central nervous system, composed of the nerve bodies, initial axon segments, dendritic arborizations, glial and vascular support; in the brain, the gray matter is peripheral, in the spinal cord it is central

Gray-out A descriptor for faintness due to vasodepressor illness/vasovagal syncope that may be seen in cardiac disease, eg in idiopathic hypertrophic subaortic stenosis; 'grayout' also refers to visual 'misting' seen in acceleration or deceleration injuries in high speed vehicles; Cf Graying out

Gray patch ringworm Fungal folliculitis in children, caused by ***Microsporum canis*** and ***M audouinii***, which progresses from an erythematous papule at the hair follicles, extends peripherally and forms annular lesions

Gray platelet syndrome of Raccuglia A condition in which the platelets lack α and dense platelet granules and by extension, lack certain platelet proteins, eg von Willebrand factor, fibrinogen, fibrin, fibronectin, platelet factor 4 (PF4), β-thromboglobulin, platelet-derived growth factor, thrombospondin and contact-promoting proteins Clinical Lifelong bleeding diatheses with epistaxis, bruisability, petechiae Laboratory Thrombocytopenia, enlarged platelets with a grayish hue on Wright-Giemsa stained peripheral blood smears, increased bleeding time Treatment DDAVP (desmopressin acetate)

Gray scale see Ultrasonography

Grayson-Wilbrandt syndrome An autosomal dominant anterior membrane dystrophy of the cornea Treatment Corneal transplant

Gray syndrome A condition that may occur when chloramphenicol levels exceed 70 µg/ml; premature infants are most susceptible, given their limited capacity to glucuronidate and excrete chloramphenicol (the functional deficiency in glucuronyl transferase activity corrects itself within the first 3-4 weeks of life); high levels of chloramphenicol inhibit mitochondrial electron transport, disrupting energy metabolism Clinical Vomiting, tachypnea, dyspnea, abdominal distension, cyanosis, diarrhea (pseudomembranous colitis), flaccidity, hypothermia, ashen gray skin and potentially death due to circulatory collapse; in children under one month of age, doses should be under 25 mg/kg Laboratory Chloramphenicol may be quantified by colorimetry, gas-liquid chromatography, high-performance liquid chromatography, microbiological and radioenzymatic methods

Gray top tube LABORATORY MEDICINE A blood collection tube containing powdered sodium fluoride and/or potassium oxalate, which inhibits glycolysis; 'gray tops' are used for glucose tolerance testing, as erythrocytic glycolysis would cause falsely-low glucose levels, as well as for measuring lactate (transported on ice) and lactate tolerance

GRE Glucocorticoid regulatory element(s) A group of steroid hormone-responsive DNA sequences that bind to the glucocorticoid receptor, enhancing DNA transcription from linked promoters in both mammals and yeasts (Science 1988; 241:9650), implying high conservation of biological mechanisms among species

Great imitator A non-specific term for any nosology that is difficult to diagnose, given the polymorphous nature of its presentation; the classic 'great imitator' is syphilis, which has a broad palette of clinical manifestations, affecting in particular the skin and central nervous system; of more recent vintage are a host of lesser 'great imitators', including neuroborreliosis (tertiary Lyme disease), hypothyroidism, given the non-specificity of signs and symptoms and pheochromocytoma, due to the nonspecificity of hypertension, migraines, tachyarrhythmias, endocrine dysfunction and central nervous system symptoms that mimic both benign and malignant conditions

Great pox Syphilis The first clinical descriptions of 'the mother of venereal disease' appeared when Charles VIII's mercenaries invaded Naples in the late 1400s; while the origin of the disease is uncertain, historical evidence vaguely implicates Haiti as the place where Columbus' sailors first contracted syphilis, anointed the 'great pox' to contrast to smallpox

Greek cancer cure An unproven cancer therapy involving blood tests of an undisclosed type that allegedly serve to diagnose the presence, stage and progression of malignancy; the treatment consists of injecting an unknown substance, possibly pure nicotinic acid that is purported to cure the cancer; the principal proponent of this therapy is a physician whose license to practice medicine has been twice suspended in Greece, who treats foreign tourists in various hotels in Athens; according to the evidence available to the American Cancer Society, this modality has no known effect in treating malignancy (CA 1990; 40:368, Am Cancer Society); see Unproven methods of cancer management

Greenberg's method An obsolete method for semiquantifying serum proteins, where proteins are separated with $NaSO_4$, treated with phenols and the resulting colors are compared

Green bottle fly A fly that is an opportunistic pathogen, causing a form of myasis, ie maggot infestation, pupating in open sores or purulent discharges

Green book Directory of Graduate Medical Education Programs A book published annually by the American Medical Association that catalogs the accredited internships and residency training programs sponsored by university and teaching hospitals in the USA and Canada; 'Green book' is also a schedule of adult immunizations published by the American College of Physicians, Cf Red book

'Green' card A white and salmon-colored document that identifies an alien as a permanent resident of the US, and in the case of physicians in specialty training, allows them the option of staying in the USA after finishing their training, thereby contributing to the Brain drain, see there

Greenfield syndrome Infantile metachromatic leukodystrophy NEUROLOGY An autosomal recessive condition characterized by marked sulfated sphingolipid accumulation and loss of myelin in neural tissue **Clinical** Onset by age 2, death by age 5 with upper and lower motor neuron disease, reduced nerve conduction, spasms, ataxia, oculomotor paralysis, bulbar palsy, blindness, deafness and dementia; see Leukodystrophy

'Green foot' Verdous discoloration of the soles and toenails of those wearing sweat-dampened rubber-soled basketball shoes that are actively colonized by a pigmented strain of Pseudomonas aeruginosa; see Green nail syndrome

Greenhouse effect ENVIRONMENT The ability of increased environmental gases to trap solar radiation, which is likened to a greenhouse, and attributed to an imbalance of the O_2:CO_2 ratio; production of O_2 is decreased by deforestation (rain forest destruction occurs at the rate of 100 000 km^2/year!) and production of CO_2 and other 'greenhouse' gases (CH_4, NO_2, CFCs); CO_2 concentration has increased from 315 ppm in 1958 to 352 ppm in 1988; the global temperature has risen 0.6°C within the past 100 years (1990 was the hottest year on record, Science 1991; 251:274; 1991 appears to have surpassed 1990 (author's note); a global rise of another 2-5°C would partially melt the polar caps, causing a one meter rise in the sea level, endangering coastlines, creating from 50 to 500 million 'environmental' refugees, leaving arable land inundated and much of the low-lying remainder susceptible to the elevated (salt) water table that would further deteriorate both the potable water supplies and croplands (in a worst-case scenario, there may be a rise of 5-10°C by the year 2100, with an inland migration of the oceans in a densely crowded, polluted and contaminated environment (Science 1989; 243:1544); sea level has risen 2.4 mm/year since 1920 (Sci 1989; 244:751); while increased CO_2 may stimulate photosynthesis, the positive effect on plant growth is offset by the acid rain pollutants (SO_2 and NO_2), vegetation toxins (H_2S, NH_3, dimethyl sulfide), industrial NO_2, natural and industrial hydrocarbons and increased atmospheric ozone, explaining the dying forests of Europe; in addition to the direct effects of greenhouse gases, minor contributing gases eg NO_2 and CFCs (chlorofluorocarbons) are major actors in depletion of the ozone layer in the stratosphere that blankets the earth at 20-50 km, filtering out the 'hard' ultraviolet-B; the ozone holes at the polar caps may increase the UV-B to levels toxic to the phytoplankton that initiates the marine food chain (N Engl J Med 1989; 321:1577rv, Scien Amer 1989; 261/3); see CFCs, Iron hypothesis, Montreal protocol

Greenhouse gases Those gases that are held responsible for causing the planet's warming, including CO_2, CH_4, NO_2, SO_4 and others; per capita emission of CO_2 Italy 2.01 tons per person, France 2.04 tons, Japan 2.45 tons, UK 2.97 tons, West Germany 3.45 tons and USA 6.14 tons; anthropogenic gas production in 1987 was estimated to be: 7.9×10^9 metric tons of CO_2 (due to changes in land use/deforestation, fossil fuel combustion and cement manufacture, resulting in a net addition of 47% to the atmospheric gases), 270×10^6 metric tons of CH_4 (from livestock, wet rice cultivation, solid waste and coal mining, caused a net addition of 18% to the atmospheric gases)

Greenhouse index A method proposed by the Intergovernmental Panel on Climate Change (IPCC) for measuring a nation's contribution to the Greenhouse effect by comparing the infrared heating effectiveness of a greenhouse gas with CO_2 and multiplying the relative productions by the population (Nature 1990; 347:705) Note: This index has potential for allowing an equitable reduction in global anthropogenic gases by fining the nations with high values

Greenhow's disease Skin excoriation and discoloration due to pediculosis-induced scratching

Green journal An Americanism of little utility, referring to commonly requested journals in medical libraries; the classic 'Green journal' is the British green American Journal of Medicine; other green-colored journals, include the kelly green Obstetrics and Gynecology, the sherbet green Pediatrics and the forest green American Journal of Psychiatry

Green monkey disease see Marburg virus disease

Green nail syndrome Verdous discoloration of the fingernails, most often associated with ***Pseudomonas paronychia***, seen in persons who regularly submerge their hands; the greenish discoloration is merely the result of diffusion of pyocyanin produced by Pseudomonas in the adjacent paronychia; Cf Green foot

'Green paper' Parliamentary policy When the British government has plans for or is considering reform in any field, eg Health policy or consolidation of funds allocated to basic sciences, a 'green paper' (a discussion document) is published, which then becomes a matter for comment or open debate; this is followed by a 'White paper', see there

Green sickness see Chlorosis

Greenstick fracture An incomplete angulated fracture that causes bone bowing with rupture of the periosteum on the convex side of the bone, ie the opposite cortex is intact, without the fracture line traversing the bone, which is more common in vitamin D-deficiency rickets Note: The small tender 'green' branches of trees when bent, buckle but don't break, leaving the internal wood intact

Green stool syndrome Transient neonatal passage of thickened, bile-stained stools, thought to be caused by an unknown bacterium that alters urobilin metabolism, responding within 24 hours to penicillin

Green technology Environment The modification of energy consumption, manufacturing processes and products being and waste disposal to minimize or eliminate its impact on the environment; among the 'green tech' targets are substitutes for CFCs, bioremediation of soil and water contaminated by pollutants and biodegradable plastics; the most concerted effort in this vital arena is being spearheaded by the Japanese (Nature 1991; 350:266n)

Green top tube Laboratory medicine A blood collection (test) tube with a green stopper containing sodium or lithium heparin that is used to obtain blood for ammonia (collected on ice), carboxyhemoglobin and oxygen saturation, cholinesterase, hemoglobin, methemoglobin, pH, as well as histocompatibility testing, including HLA-A, B, HLA-D (mixed lymphocyte culture), NBT (nitrotetrazolium blue) assay, phagocytosis, T- and B-cell studies surface markers

Green urine disease Massive increase of verdohemoglobin in the urine which fluoresces with ultraviolet light, a sign of fulminant *Pseudomonas aeruginosa* infection; the finding of green urine in such patients may be accompanied by poor response to aminoglycosides

Greenwood-Yule method Epidemiology A method that attempts to resolve whether a disease process is related to the order of birth within a sibship

Grenz radiation Radiation oncology Low-dose superficial radiation (10 kV range) that has been used to treat psoriasis, in which the positive effect is transient and the carcinogenic effect real (J Am Acad Dermatol 1989; 21:475); Cf Bremstrahlung

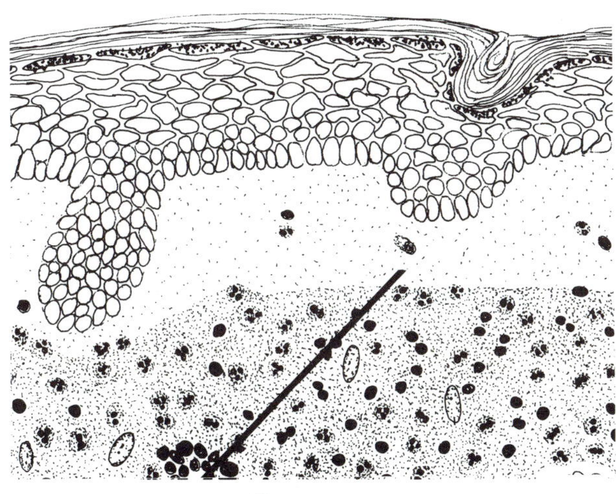

Grenz zone

Grenz zone German Border, frontier Dermatopathology A well-demarcated zone of separation in the upper dermis (figuree), delineated by the collagen of the flattened basal epidermis from the upper dermis, the latter of which often has a dense, usually lymphocytic infiltrate; a grenz zone is seen in granuloma faciale, lepromatous leprosy and lymphocytoma cutis and may separate a pilar tumor or leiomyoma from the atrophic overlying skin

GRID Gay-related immune deficiency A transiently-used acronym for the AIDS (acquired immunodeficiency syndrome), the first cases of which occurred in homosexual (gay) men; see AIDS

Griseofulvin An oral antifungal agent isolated from *Penicillium griseofulvum dierckx* and *P janczewski* with an affinity for skin, used for dermatophytic infections (Epidermophyton, Microsporum and Trichophyton) **Mechanism** Griseofulvin disrupts the mitotic spindle by interacting with polymerized microtubules **Side effects** Headache, nausea, diarrhea, vomiting, photosensitivity, fever, rashes, dysfunction of hepatic, nervous, hematopoietic systems; it is teratogenic and carcinogenic in rodents

Grommets see Tympanostomy tubes

Groomed whisker appearance Sun ray pattern Hairlike periosteal projections perpendicular to bony trabeculae seen by radiology most commonly associated with Ewing sarcoma, as well as osteosarcoma, neuroblastoma and renal cell carcinoma metastatic to bone

Groove Molecular biology see Major groove, Minor groove

Groove sign Rheumatology Branched zone linear loss of dermal fibrosis overlying the veins in eosinophilic fasciitis; when the affected extremity is raised, the reticulated pattern of the intersecting veins seen has been likened to dry, merging river beds Sexually-transmitted disease A finding characterized as linear fibrotic depressions parallel to the inguinal ligament, bordered above and below by enlarged and matted lymph nodes and covered by adherent, erythematous skin, seen in 10-20% of cases of lymphogranuloma venereum (*Chlamydia trachomatis,* serotypes L1, L2, L3)

Gross negligence Medical malpractice The reckless provision of health care that is clearly below the standards of accepted medical practice, either without regard for the potential consequences or with wilful and wanton disregard for the rights and/or well-being of those for whom the duty is being performed; see Malpractice

Gross dictation Surgical pathology A formal 'script' generated by a pathologist that describes surgically-excised tissues, providing details on size, shape, morphology, color and consistency; 'grossing' serves to document the nature of surgery-removed tissues, from which representative sections are made and processed through aqueous and non-aqueous solutions, embedded in paraffin, sectioned with a microtome, placed on a glass slide, stained, usually with hematoxylin and eosin and interpreted by light microscopy; the pathologist may elect, in certain tissues, eg uncomplicated hernia sac or a fractured femoral head in an older person, not to submit tissue, which may be designated as 'gross only'; see Glass pusher

Ground glass A adjectival descriptor commonly used in medicine, which is equivalent to the German, Milchglassartig Hematology Ground-glass histiocytes have 'washed-out' cytoplasm and are typical of reticulocytic granuloma Bacteriology A shadowy ground glass-like appearance on culture plates that is midway

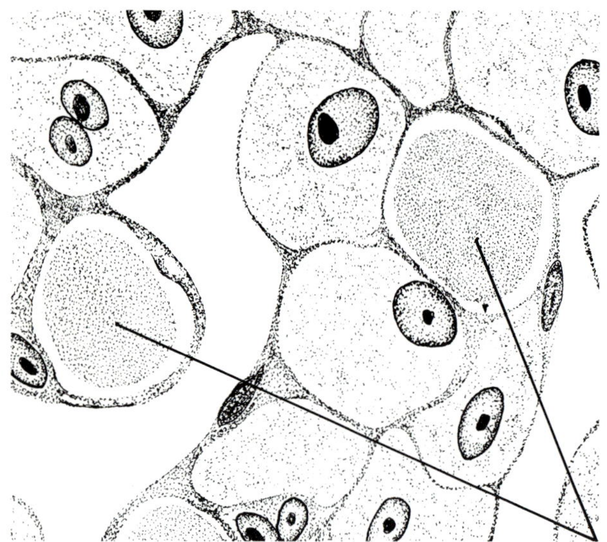

Ground glass hepatocytes

between the greenish hue of α hemolysis and the ochre-brown of β-hemolysis, incorrectly termed γ-hemolysis HEPATOLOGY Ground glass cytoplasm is classically associated with hepatitis B virus and results from swelling of the smooth endoplasmic reticulum, see figure, above HISTOPATHOLOGY Uniform, finely granular eosinophilic (orcein and aldehyde fuchsin positive) cytoplasm with a peripheral clear halo; a similar morphology may be seen in dilated lysosomes in Gaucher's disease or in the lung with viral inclusions, which by electron microscopy, reveal spherules of HBsAg or Dane particles; similar PAS inclusions may be seen in alcoholics treated with alcohol aversion-inducing disulfiram (Antabuse), an acetaldehyde dehydrogenase inhibitor (Arch Pathol Lab Med 1986; 110:906); see Pseudo-ground glass inclusion NEUROPATHOLOGY Ground glass cytoplasm is characteristic of gemistocytic cells in astrocytomas PANCREAS A ground glass appearance is typical of the abolished architectural details seen by low-power light microscopy in enzymatic fat necrosis or in postmortem autolysis OPHTHALMOLOGY Ground glass opacification of the cornea occurs in children in mucopolysaccharidosis (MPS) type I-H (Hurler) with global MPS deposition in the ocular structures, photophobia, retinal degeneration, attenuation of vessels, optic atrophy, loss of vision and hydrocephalus RADIOLOGY, ABDOMEN A ground glass appearance with haziness and erasure of organ silhouettes, which is typical of massive ascites, and related to an increased water density and peritonitis RADIOLOGY, BONE The ground glass appearance corresponds to a relatively uniform loss of osseous density which may be accompanied by intravascular calcification and subcutaneous ossification, seen in bones affected by fibrous dysplasia, scurvy (located at the epiphyses), osteomalacia, agnogenic myeloid metaplasia, osteoporosis RADIOLOGY, CHEST The ground glass appearance corresponds to an alveolar, acinar or amorphous pattern seen in bronchiolitis obliterans and obstructive pneumonia RADIOLOGY, PEDIATRIC Ground glass is a descriptor for poorly circumscribed radiopacifications of the right lower quadrant, mixed with fine trapped bubbles within the meconium 'plug', seen on a plain film in meconium ileus; Cf Applesauce VIROLOGY Ground glass-like appearance is seen in the nuclei of epithelia infected with Herpes simplex

Ground itch A hypersensitivity reaction to hookworms, occurring in previously sensitized individuals **Clinical** Inflammation, erythema, blistering and intense pruritus at the larval penetration site (feet) Agents ***Necator americanus, Ancylostoma duodenale***

Group atrophy A light microscopic pattern seen in denervation, where the normal 'checkerboard' pattern of type I mixed with type II skeletal muscle fibers is lost and there is a histochemical 'regrouping', so that there are large bundles of each type, a change typical of reinnervation

Group C drugs Investigational drugs that have reproducible efficacy in one or more specific tumor types; these drugs alter or are likely to alter the pattern of treatment of a disease and can be safely administered by properly trained physicians without specific supportive care

Growing fork MOLECULAR BIOLOGY Replication on double-stranded DNA is bidirectional, starting at one origin (replicons), giving rise to two de novo synthesized DNA chains; the rate of replication is a function of the organism's complexity, the growing forks of ***Escherichia coli*** duplicates at a rate of 1000 base pairs/second (bp/s), while human cells duplicate at 100 bp/s; the human genome of 3 X 10^9 base pairs requires 8 hours to complete duplication and involves 10 to 100 thousand replicons; of the growing forks, the 'leading' strand is reproduced as an unbroken strand of new DNA growing continuously in the 5' to 3' direction, while the 'lagging' strand forms short discontinuous segments also in the 5' to 3' direction, which are primed by short segments of RNA; these short DNA-RNA primer sequences are known as Okazaki fragments

Growing pains Benign leg pains occurring in young children; experts disagree on whether this condition actually exists; if it does exist, it is a diagnosis of exclusion, requiring that trauma, infection, avascular necrosis of bone, tumors, collagen vascular disease, Lyme disease, psychosomatic nosologies, congenital and developmental abnormalities be ruled out **Clinical** Growing pain complaints are bilateral, intermittent, most often occurring after going to bed, thought to be due to edema of muscles encased within 'tight' fascia, often following a day of strenuous exercise, although a temporal or activity-relatable pattern may not be detected; the pain may be accompanied by restlessness and disappears with the cessation of growth (Ped Clin N Amer 1986; 33:1365) **Treatment** Local heat, massage and if severe, quinine sulfate

Growth see Mitosis

Growth factors A broad family of cytokines that facilitate cell growth and proliferation, including epidermal growth factor (S Cohen, 1986 Nobel prize), erythropoietin, fibroblast growth factor, insulin-like GF I, IGF II, nerve growth factor (R Montalcini-Levi, 1986 Nobel prize), platelet-derived growth factor, relaxin, somatomedin A and B, transforming growth factors

(TGF-α and TGF-β)

Growth hormone Somatotropin A 21.5 kD protein hormone that is under the hypothalamic control via growth hormone-releasing hormone (GHRH), acting via insulin growth factor-1 (IGF-I or somatomedin-C), increasing protein and glycogen synthesis, lipolysis, opposing the effect of insulin on muscle and 'priming' macrophages for superoxide production Note: Short children may respond to growth hormone therapy and are identified with stimulation (arginine-insulin) tests rather than baseline measurements; the use of human-derived growth hormone to treat these children was stopped when Creutzfeldt-Jakob disease developed in some recipients; recombinant growth hormone (rGH) is being used to treat reduced height; early data has linked the use of rGH to a two-fold increase in childhood leukemia and slippage of the femoral head epiphysis (J Pediatr 1990; 116:397) Normal 5-10 μg/L (US: < 5 ng/ml, male; < 10 ng/ml female); growth hormone levels decrease with age, reflected in the decreased levels of IGF-I (< 350 U/L, normal for age: 500-1500 U/L), a decrease that may result in decreased bone density and lean body mass and increased adipose tissue mass typical of older subjects (N Engl J Med 1990; 323:1) Circadian rhythm A daily growth hormone peak occurs in the first 2 hours of sleep, increases with stress, exercise, hypoglycemia, amino acid (arginine) and protein infusions, and may be 4-to-12-fold normal in acromegaly

Growth hormone insensitivity syndrome Laron dwarfism Severe growth retardation and physical manifestations typical of one who is deficient in growth hormone, with low serum insulin-like growth factor-I (IGF-I), which responds to IGF-I infusion with increase in calcium excretion and decrease of serum and urea nitrogen, suggesting therapeutic potential for this agent (N Engl J Med 1991; 324:1483cr)

Grübelsucht German PSYCHIATRY A colloquial translation for hair-splitting, a feature of obsessive-compulsive neuroses Note: The literal translation of the root verb, grüben, refers to brooding, and thus imparts a melancholic Gef'ühl to this variant of neurosis

GSD see Glycogen storage disease

GSH see Glutathione

G syndrome of Opitz-Frias An autosomal dominant condition of neonatal onset, characterized by pulmonary aspiration at birth due to a laryngotracheoesophageal cleft, stridor, cleft lip, cardiac defects, hypospadias, imperforate anus, a broad nasal bridge and ocular hypertelorism

GTPase superfamily A family of conserved 'molecular switch' enzymes that bind and hydrolyze GTP, acting as 'on-off' switches for various intracellular activities; the switch is turned on when GTP is bound and off when GTP is hydrolyzed to GDP; GTPases sort and amplify transmembrane signals, direct the synthesis and translocation of proteins, guide vesicular traffic through the cytoplasm, control cell proliferation and differentiation and have a pivotal role in pathogenesis of malignancy and infectious diseases since they are targets of mutations and microbial toxins; GTPases are divided into three classes, a) The 21K family, which includes the products of *ras* oncogenes and protooncogenes b) The GTPases involved in ribosomal protein synthesis and c) The α subunits of the signal-transducing G proteins (Nature 1991; 349:117rv); the high conservation of structural motifs across diverse species, suggests that the family originates from a single primordial protein (Nature 1990; 348:125)

GTT Gastrostomy tube; see Glucose tolerance test

GU-AG rule MOLECULAR BIOLOGY The finding that an intron begins at the guanine and uracil nucleotides at the 5'-end of the 'donor' junction and closes when the spliceosome reads an adenine and uracil at the 3'-end of the recipient junction

Guam An island in the Marianas (Oceania), the native inhabitants (the Chamorros) of which have had their brains poked and prodded by Japanese and American neuropathologists, who wonder why this population is so susceptible to the amyotrophic lateral sclerosis-Parkinson's-Alzheimer's dementia complex (ALS-P-A); a proposed explanation for the disease's decline since insidious 'Americanization' began 35 years ago is that the use of the plant *Cycas circinalis*, containing BMAA, an unusual amino acid (related to BOAA, a grass pea neurotoxin causing lathyrism in animals), a native medicine and food is being used with decreasing frequency; Cycas-fed macaques develop corticomedullary dysfunction, the parkinsonian shuffle, behavioral and neuropathological manifestations that mimic ALS-P-A complex

Guaiac-positive stool see Occult blood

Guarding Involuntary muscle spasm elicited by fulminant acute peritonitis, leaving the anterior abdominal muscles in a state of tonic contraction, imparting a board-like consistency to the rectus abdominis muscles, to be distinguished from voluntary guarding, seen in 'ticklish' patients

Guillotine amputation A sharply defined loss of a portion or entire segments of extremities, ranging from digits to major amputations, seen in the congenital aglossia-adactylia syndrome

Guinea pig A rodent occasionally used in research Note: The idiom in English 'to be a guinea pig', which implies that one is being used as an experimental animal, is largely incorrect; the guinea pig, ***Cavia cobaya***, is cuddly and resembles the human hormonally, immunologically and in reproductive physiology, but is a poor experimental model, comprising but 2% of the rodents in the research rat race; they are stupid, ie rather incapable of learning, have less complex immune systems than mice, have a long gestation period, produce small litters, are picky eaters, are susceptible to infections and are more costly to maintain than smaller rodents (Handbook of Inbred and Genetically defined Strains of Laboratory Animals, Altman and Katz, 1979), and thus, most research is performed on rats or mice, the choice differing based on the needs of the researcher; eg mice are of interest as their immune system (major histocompatibility complex is on chromosome 17 in mice and very similar to the human system located on chromosome 6; although guinea pigs, eg ***C porcellus***, are traditionally classified as a New World hystricomorph rodent, phylogenetic analysis of the amino acid sequence data implies that the guinea pig diverged before the separation of the primates and artiodactyls from the myomorph rodents (Nature 1991; 351:649); see Rat

Gull syndrome Obsolete for adult-onset hypothyroidism

Gull wing pattern Seagull appearance A descriptor for a gull wing-like pattern with a broad, flattened and gently curved V-shape IMMUNOLOGY The presence of two distinct and connected, relatively flat precipitin arcs in the serum protein electrophoresis, typically seen in lambda light chain myeloma or IgD or IgE myelomas MICROBIOLOGY The classic high-power light microscopic morphology of the gently undulated gram-negative ***Helicobacter*** and ***Campylobacter*** species RADIOLOGY A double curved shadow seen on a plain lateral film of the entire pelvis in either fracture-dislocation of the posterior acetabular rim or dislocation of the femoral head; the 2 wings are contributed by the intact and fractured acetabulum (Radiol 1965; 84:937)

Gumboil Parulis A dental abscess, converted into a cyst with chronic drainage through a fistulous tract, seen by a plain film of the jaw

Gumma Lentil-to-cherry-sized masses characteristic of tertiary syphilis, which represent a hypersensitivity response to treponemal products (the organism itself is rarely found) Histopathology Central caseating necrosis surrounded by epithelioid histiocytes and multinucleated giant cells and vessels 'cuffed' with inflammatory cells; gumma also occur in the skin, liver, bones, testes, mucosal membranes and stomach

'Gun barrel' vision see Tunnel vision

Gun control FORENSIC MEDICINE The USA is unique in the access its citizens have to firearms, an anachronistic right guaranteed by the US Constitution, the consequence of which is that a) Suicide rate by handguns is 5.7-fold greater in the US than Canada (adjusting for other methods, the USA suicide rate ages 15-24 is 1.38-fold greater N Engl J Med 1990; 322:369) Homicide rate (per 100 000 population) Philippines 38.7, Lesotho 36.40, Jamaica 18, US 8.6, France 4.05, Italy 1.52, Germany 1.5, UK 1.33, Ireland 0.54 (Vital World Statistics, The Economist Books, London, 1990)

Gunn rat Animal model for the study of jaundice due to this rodent's inherited deficiency of glucuronyl transferase (J Heredity 1938; 29:137)

Gunstock deformity ORTHOPEDICS A reversal of the arm's carrying angle, resulting from a) Inadequate correction of the medial angulation of the distal fragment of a supracondylar fracture of the humerus or b) stimulation of the lateral condylar epiphysis from the fracture itself (even when the fracture has not been displaced)

GVH disease see Graft versus host disease

Gynandroblastoma 'Yin-yang' tumor A rare ovarian sex-cord tumor with masculinizing (hirsutism, clitoral hypertrophy and deepening of the voice) and/or feminizing (vaginal bleeding due to endometrial hyperplasia) hormonal effects; Gynandroblastoma is an over-diagnosed term that should be reserved for when well-differentiated testicular and ovarian tissue is present within the neoplasm, requiring that at least 10% of the minor component be present Histopathology Functionally-active and mature masculinizing elements, granulosa-(Call-Exner body formation) thecal cells and Sertoli-Leydig (Reinicke crystalloids) cells Clinical The tumor presents in the second to the sixth decade as a unilateral cystic and solid pink-to-yellow 0.6-18.0 cm pelvic mass Treatment Excision (Pathology 1986; 18:348)

Gynecomastia A breast lesion that most commonly affects boys and adolescents, often regresses at puberty; gynecomastia is caused by various conditions (table, below), often related to an increased estradiol:testosterone ratio, which occurs in the obese, due to peripheral aromatization of androgens, which converts them into estrogens; gynecomastia of the elderly male is due to testicular failure

GYNECOMASTIA ETIOLOGY

Endocrinopathy Orchitis, hypogonadism (androgen deficiency), androgen resistance syndromes, tumors or hyperplasia of the adrenal gland, testes, eg Leydig cell tumors (increased hCG production), lung cancer, Klinefelter syndrome (increased risk of breast carcinoma) and thyroid hyperplasia

Drugs alpha-methyldopa, amphetamine, androgens, benzodiazepines, cimetidine, chemotherapeutic agents, digitalis, INH, marijuana, penicillamine, phenothiazine, reserpine, spironolactone, tricyclic antidepressants

Other conditions Starvation diet (mechanism: testicular and hepatic hypofunction) or on resuming normal diet, hemodialysis, hepatopathies (cirrhosis, hepatomas, hemochromatosis, due to decreased hepatic metabolism of estrogens), mycosis fungoides, myotonic dystrophy and spastic paraplegia and leprosy

Gyrase Topoisomerase II An enzyme first isolated from *Escherichia coli*,cutting double-stranded DNA, passing a portion of double helix through the uncut double helix, resealing it on the other side, a maneuver that transforms a 'positive' supercoil into a 'negative' supercoil; in mammalian cells, the density of supercoiling is a function of histone binding; see Supercoiling

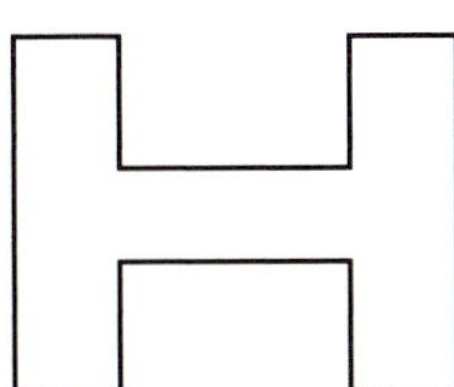

H Symbol for: Histidine; Hounsfield unit; hydrogen; magnetic field strength

h Symbol for: hecto-; hour

H1, H2A, H2B, H3, H4 see Histones

H-2 complex The major histocompatibility complex (MHC) in mice, which is located on chromosome 17 and is highly correlated with the MHC that is located on chromosome 6 of humans

HA-1a A human monoclonal IgM antibody that binds to the lipid A domain of endotoxin and prevents death in laboratory animals with gram-negative bacteremia and endotoxemia; its use in humans with septicemia (frequency USA, 400 000 cases annually, 30% caused by gram-negative bacteria, mortality 20-60%) is less spectacular, but the use of HA-1A may be associated with a slightly improved clinical course (N Engl J Med 1991; 324:429)

Habenula NEUROANATOMY A dorsomedial thalamic prominence that receives afferents from the amygdala via the medullothalamic striae and from the hippocampus via the fornix, forming a central point where olfactory, visceral and somatic afferent pathways are integrated, mediating gastrointestinal secretion and deglutition and possibly also thermoregulation

Haber-Weiss reaction A devastating intracellular event occurring when superoxide dismutase and catalase in tissue are insufficient to decompose superoxides and peroxides and other toxic free radicals in the tissues: $H_2O_2 + O_2^- = OH^\cdot + OH^- + O_2$; see Free radical, 'Garbage can' hypothesis, Superoxide dismutase

Habituation An adaptive response characterized by a decreased reactivity to a repeated stimulus, eg a substance of abuse or repeated electrical stimuli of a nerve

Habitus The general corporal type of the adult body; an asthenic habitus is seen in tall thin subjects whose organs are said to hang low in the body; the hyperthenic subject is plethoric and his organs are higher in the body and the hyposthenic habitus lies between the two

HACEK group An acronym for a group of bacteria that may cause infective endocarditis: ***Haemophilus, Actinobacillus, Cardiobacterium, Eikenella*** and ***Kingella*** species

HADD see Hydroxyapatite deposition disease

Haff disease German, Bay, Harbor A disease of historic interest that occurred in Königsberg Bay in Lithuania Clinical Myalgia, dyspnea, dysuria and myoglobulinuria; death due to renal failure occurred in about 1% of the cases and was due either to eating fish tainted with cellulose-derived toxic resins from paper-processing plants or ingestion of an unidentified toxin in certain eels and fish

Hafnia A motile, gram-negative, facultative anaerobic fecal saprobe of the Klebsiella tribe; formerly an Enterobacter, ***Hafnia*** is separated therefrom by DNA homology studies and has but one species, ***H alvei***, which is rarely pathogenic and responds to Enterobacter-type antibiotics

Hair Types of hair **ANAGEN HAIR** Actively growing hair **LANUGO HAIR** Fine hair of the fetus, usually shed at birth **TELOGEN HAIR** Non-growing hair that is easily removed **TERMINAL HAIR** Coarse, deeply pigmented, stiff and thick, seen in the scalp and eyebrow, chest, facial and pubic hair; androgens typically induce transition of vellous to terminal hair, although there is marked variation in the response of different body regions to androgens **VELLOUS HAIR** Fine, soft and downy hair of children and women Note: Except for the knuckles, elbows, knees, lips and palmoplantar regions, the body is covered with hair; see Hirsutism, Minoxidil

HAIR-AN Hyperandrogenic insulin-resistant acanthosis nigricans A subtype of hyperthecosis affecting 5% of hirsute females, often associated with polycystic ovaries, characterized by a) Hyperandrogenesis (increased testosterone, increased androstenedione; early, premenarcheal hyperandrogenism) b) Insulin-resistance, where the patients are either normal or have clinical diabetes and c) Acanthosis nigricans, possibly an epiphenomenon Treatment Bilateral oophorectomy, contraceptives, corrects the hyperandrogenism, but often not the excess insulin

Hair analysis The only legitimate diagnostic use of hair is for detection of chronic heavy metal intoxication, eg arsenic, lead and mercury; it may be possible to use hair as a source for drug testing, as hair analysis is nonintrusive, clean and difficult to cheat on, providing a long-term 'record' of drug ingestion Note: Hair analysis has been claimed by charlatans ('quacks') to reveal information regarding a person's health and nutritional status, claims that remain unsubstantiated

Hair-brain syndrome see BIDS syndrome

Hairbrush appearance A fanciful descriptor for the elongated periosteal bony spicules projecting from the femoral metaphyses in achondrogenesis, seen radiologically and equivalent to a focal Hair-on-end reaction

Hair-on-end appearance Crewcut appearance A radiologic pattern seen as calcified spicules perpendicular to the bone surface, corresponding to a periosteal reaction to disturbed bone repair with neoosteogenesis of the outer cranial table, marked calvarial thickening, external displacement and thinning of the inner table, seen in congenital hemolytic anemias (pyruvate kinase deficiency, sickle cell anemia, thalassemia, hereditary elliptocytosis and spherocytosis), iron-deficiency anemia, cyanotic (right-to-left shunt) congenital heart disease, osteomyelitis, early onset polycythemia vera, thyroid acropachy, hemangiomas, metastatic neuroblastoma; bone spiculation in malignant tumors of bone has three broad patterns a) Hair-on-end Parallel spiculations, eg Ewing sarcoma b) Sunburst Radiation from a central point, eg osteosarcoma and c) Velvet-like Low, slanting spicules, eg chondrosarcoma (Semin Roentgenol 1966; 1:293)

Hairpin loop MOLECULAR BIOLOGY DNA hairpin A short segment of inverted repeat DNA that forms under low-stringency denaturing conditions (low stringency conditions allow 'sloppy' binding between complementary DNA strands), when the complementary segments are adjacent to each other on the DNA; if the regions of complementarity are distant to each other, they form heteroduplexes RNA hairpin A short segment of RNA transcribed from a DNA palindrome, which folds upon itself, forming a double strand; RNA hairpins are found within the nucleus and are an integral component of the 'cloverleaf' configuration of tRNA

Hairpin vessels Minute blood vessels that are doubled upon themselves, seen at the metaphyseal-diaphyseal junction of normal bone

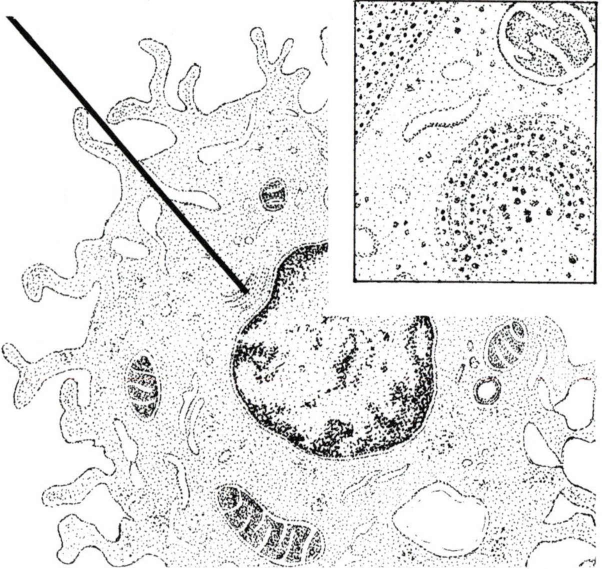

Hairy cell leukemia Leukemic reticuloendotheliosis A low-grade B-cell leukemia that comprises 2% of adult leukemia, commonly affecting men (Male:female ratio, 4:1) age 50-55 and leading to progressive pancytopenia **Clinical** Insidious onset with weight loss, bruising, abdominal fullness due to splenomegaly, pancytopenia with normocytic, normochromic anemia, rarely aplastic anemia; 10% have platelet counts of $< 20 \times 10^9$/L (US: < 20 000/mm^3), 20% have thrombocytosis; 1-80% of nucleated blood smear cells are hairy Cause of death Infections, gram-negative bacteria, atypical mycobacteria and fungal **Laboratory** Increased acid phosphatase, especially isoenzyme 5 (which is also increased in bone metastases and in children with Gaucher's disease), 'dry tap' from a bone marrow biopsy and the cells are positive for tartrate-resistant acid phosphatase (TRAP) an enzyme that may be weakly expressed in infectious mononucleosis, macroglobulinemia, prolymphocytic leukemia and Sézary syndrome; hairy cells measure 10-20 μm and are in late stages of B-cell ontogeny, have undergone immunoglobulin gene rearrangement and are positive for mature pan-B cell markers (CD19, CD20) and may express monocytic and T-cell markers Note: The hairy cell gene may be X-linked and close to the glucose-6-phos D gene (N Engl J Med 1990; 322:1159c) Ultrastructure Villous processes and intracytoplasmic lamellar ribosomal complexes, zipper-junctions (figure) **Treatment** A-IFN; pentostatin (deoxycoformycin); 2-chlorodeoxyadenosine, a purine nucleoside used in low-grade lymphoproliferative processes, eg chronic lymphocytic leukemia and non-Hodgkin's lymphoma is more effective than interferon-α (N Engl J Med 1990; 322:1117)

Hairy leukoplakia ORAL PATHOLOGY An Epstein-Barr virus (EBV)-associated infection seen in HIV-infected subjects (Oral Surg Oral Med Oral Pathol 1989; 67:404), characterized by a condyloma-like tongue mass (75% of patients have papilloma virus, 95% have EBV in epithelial cell nuclei) preceding the onset of clinical AIDS **Histopathology** Koilocytosis with ballooned prickle cells, perinuclear halos, pyknotic, hyperchromatic and occasionally atypical nuclei, basal cell disorganization and increased mitotic activity; the hyper- and parakeratotic 'hairy' projections appear as a corrugated surface

Hairy penis Hirsutoid papillomata of the penis Pearly papules possibly representing an anatomic variant of the penile corona that is first seen at ages 20-50 as a verrucous lesion **Histopathology** Well-vascularized connective tissue covered by epidermis with central thinning and peripheral acanthosis Note: Whether there is human papilloma virus in these lesions is unknown **Treatment** None required

Hairy polyp Teratoid tumor A benign congenital malformation of young, often female children arising from ecto- and mesodermal totipotent cells, located in the nasopharynx, oropharynx and tonsils **Differential diagnosis** Intranasal glioma, rhabdomyosarcoma, meningoencephalocele, Rathke's pouch cyst, pharyngeal hypophysis and craniopharyngioma

Hairy tongue A benign elongation of the tongue's filiform papillae and failure of the superficial layer to desquamate, serving as a nidus for microorganisms, potentially resulting in halitosis; although idiopathic, hairy tongues may be associated with heavy smoking, alcohol abuse, radiotherapy to the head and neck, dehydration, systemic illness and antibiotic therapy, resulting in decreased flow of saliva, occasionally allowing unrestrained fungal growth Note: When the papillae are stained brown or other colors by extrinsic substances, including tobacco and chromagens, the condition may be designated as 'Black hairy tongue'

Haiti see Geographic exclusion

Halberd bone Battle ax bone PEDIATRIC RADIOLOGY Marked flaring of the iliac crests, typical of metatropic dwarfism, a rare metaphysealdysplasia with bulbous joints and multiple, markedly deformed and shortened bones

Half and half nails An idiopathic onychopathy occasionally seen in chronic renal insufficiency (uremia), characterized by a transverse distal red-brown band occupying most of the nail with a dull, white proximal band

Half-life ($T_{1/2}$) The amount of time required for a substance to be reduced to one-half of its previous level by degradation and/or decay (radioactive half-life), by catabolism (biological half-life) or by elimination in a system, eg half-life in serum HEMATOLOGY $T_{1/2}$ is the time that cells stay in the circulation, eg erythrocytes 120 days, which increases after splenectomy, platelets 4-6 days, eosinophils 3-7 hours and neutrophils 7 hours IMMUNOLOGY $T_{1/2}$ is the time an immunoglobulin stays in the circulation: 20-25 days for IgG, 6 days for IgA, 5 days for IgM, 2-8 days for IgD and 1-5 days for IgE PHYSICS $T_{1/2}$ is the time required for a radioisotope to decay to one-half of the original amount having the same radioactivity; a radioisotope's effective $T_{1/2}$ is either the time required to decay (physical $T_{1/2}$) or the time required for elimination from the biological system

Half moon sign BONE RADIOLOGY A semilunar shadow that may disappear in posterior dislocation of the humerus with the glenoid capsule, as under normal circumstances, the medial humeral head overlaps the glenoid fossa

'Halfway house' A semi-sheltered environment for subjects who are in rehabilitation for mental illness or addiction disorders including drug and alcohol abuse, who do not require in-patient hospitalization; halfway houses are often staffed by their own 'graduates' or professionals who provide guidance and if necessary, treatment

'Halfway technology' A coinage by Lewis Thomas for a therapeutic approach to diseases that are incompletely understood or for which appropriate therapy is beyond technological reach; halfway therapeutic modalities ameliorate or modify illness without curing, as incomplete understanding of the pathogenesis precludes prevention

Halitosis see Odors

Halo appearance A descriptive adjective for a doughnut-shaped light density within and surrounded by a rounded darker dense zones DERMATOLOGY see Target lesions BONE PATHOLOGY The 'halo' is a rimming of osteocytic lacunae, seen by light microscopy in X-linked hypophosphatemia, caused by delayed maturation BREAST PATHOLOGY The halo is an annular rim of stromal edema seen in gynecomastia (figure), due to acidmucopolysaccharides, eg hyaluronic acid, which surrounds ducts with epithelial hyperplasia; a similar effect is seen in fibroadenomas of the female breast CARDIAC RADIOLOGY A halo of radiolucency seen on a plain antero-posterior chest film in pneumopericardium GASTROINTESTINAL RADIOLOGY The 'halo' may be seen either in duodenal ulcers, where the radiocontrast settles in a fixed location, typically occurring in an acute ulcer within a mound of radiolucent edema surrounding the crater; alternately, 'halo' refers to a saccular collection of radiocontrast surrounded by radiolucency, seen in the rare intraluminal duodenal diverticulum, which causes a windsock deformity GYNECOLOGIC RADIOLOGY The 'halo' or wall sign is a smooth-contoured delineation of one tissue density from another, seen in a mature cystic teratoma or dermoid on a plain abdominal film, that is enhanced by the firm fibrous capsule investing these usually benign tumors HEPATIC RADIOLOGY An avascular radiolucency surrounded by radiodensity, which corresponds to increased vascularity, seen by hepatic angiography in hemangiomas Note: Computed tomography and magnetic resonance imaging techniques have reduced the utility of hepatic angiography to very specific applications; a 'paradoxical' halo may appear as an extrahepatic density, simulating an intrahepatic mass OBSTETRIC RADIOLOGY Spaulding's halo sign is a semispherical shadow seen on a plain film of the maternal abdomen, corresponding to the skull of a dead infant that is covered by edematous skin and soft tissue overlying the skull RENAL RADIOLOGY The hypernephroma halo is a radiolucent rim surrounding perinephric fat caused by a diffuse renal mass, first described in renal cell carcinoma (hypernephroma) that may be seen in abscesses, hematomas, disseminated malignancy and, if left-sided, pancreatitis

Halo device An orthopedic device used to manage cervical spine injuries to minimize neurological damage, requiring long-term immobilization; in the halo device, pins are inserted on the outer skull for skeletal traction, using a 2-3 kg weight for upper cervical injuries and 10-15 kg for lower cervical injuries

'Halo effect' The beneficial effect of a physician or other health care provider on a patient during a medical encounter, regardless of the therapy or procedure provided Note: A halo is a shimmering ring of light floating above the heads of angels of Judeo-Christian dogma, endowed with mystical healing powers, as in the 'healing hands' of the physician; see Hawthorne effect, Placebo effect

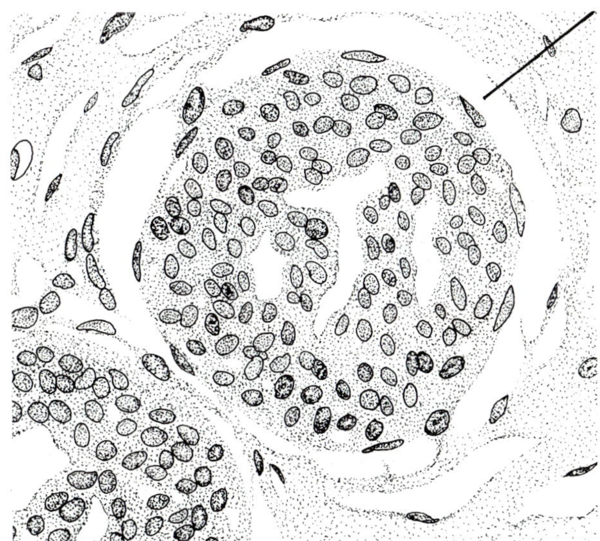

Halo appearance

Halo nevus Leukoderma acquisitum centrifugum A pigmented melanocytic nevus surrounded by a peripheral zone of depigmentation (melanocytes absent with a lymphohistiocytic infiltrate), measuring ± 5 mm in diameter surrounding a common nevus, most often affecting adolescents on the back; when inflamed, it is called an inflammatory halo nevus; the halo may also occur in congenital, blue and Spitz nevi, neurofibromas, primary and metastatic melanomas

Haloperidol A butyrophenone, dopamine-blocking antipsychotic agent, used for schizophrenia and Giles de la Tourette; haloperidol's well-known extrapyramidal side effects may be immediate (parkinsonism, akathisia and acute dystonia), or late with long-term therapy: Tardive dyskinesia, 'rabbit' syndrome (see there) and orthostatic hypotension

Halophyte see *Salicornia bigelovii*, subspecies Torr

Halothane hepatitis A carbon tetrachloride-related halocarbon, used as a maintenance-type anesthetic (thiopental is usually used for induction), preferred for the ease of awakening, relatively low toxicity and low blood:gas partition coefficient; although classically, halothane causes hepatotoxicity (post-operative jaundice and hepatic necrosis), the incidence of this reaction is low (1/35 000 halothane administrations); hepatotoxicity occurs in 7-14% of hypoxic animals pretreated with phenobarbital

HALV Human AIDS/lymphotrophic virus Prior to settling on the acronym of HIV for human immunodeficiency virus, Montagnier favored LAV and Gallo preferred HTLV-III, in the spirit of collaboration, Wong-Staal suggested (Nature 1985; 314:574c) a non-partisan acronym, as a '...perfect solution for the two groups to meet HALV (sic)-way'

Halzoun TROPICAL MEDICINE An upper respiratory tract infestation by the sheep liver fluke, ***Fasciola hepatica***, occurring in Lebanon and Syria, through ingestion of raw goat and sheep liver, containing third stage larvae, which inhabit the oropharyngeal mucosa causing deafness by blocking the eustachian tube, causing dysphagia and dyspnea, the last potentially fatal by closure of the nasopharynx

HAM syndrome Hypoparathyroidism, Addison's disease and mucocutaneous candidiasis see MEDAC syndrome

HAM HTLV-I-associated myelopathy see Tropical spastic paraparesis

HAM-1 and **HAM-2** Histocompatibility antign modifier Two genes in mice that encode permeases that transport antigen (oligopeptides) from the cytoplasm into a membrane-bound compartment in which the antigen interacts with major histocompatibility complex (MHC) class I and II molecules (Science 1990; 250:1723); the human equivalent of HAM-1 and -2 are designated ATP-binding cassette transporters, see ABC superfamily

HAMA Human anti-mouse antibody A family of antibodies that that may be used in research protocols in which patients with advanced malignancy are treated with monoclonal antibodies directed against an epitope on the tumor cells; host production of HAMAs limits the amount of monoclonal antibodies that can be administered, causing adverse immune reactions including anaphylaxis, sub-acute allergic and delayed hypersensitivity reactions, flu-like syndrome, gastrointestinal symptoms, rash and urticaria, hypotension, dyspnea and renal failure; see also Biological response modifiers, 'Humanized' antibody

Haman Tashen-induced opium intoxication Haman Tashen are cookies filled with poppy seeds traditionally consumed during the Jewish holiday of Purim; when consumed in excess, trace amounts of opium alkaloids may accumulate, resulting in clinical intoxication with vomiting, abdominal pain, pallor, hallucinations, sweating and pinpoint pupils (J Am Med Assoc 1983; 250:2469c), see Jewish traditions

Hamartoma Tumor-like, non-neoplastic disordered proliferation of mature tissues that are native to a site of origin, eg exostoses, nevi and soft tissue hamartomas; although most hamartomas are benign, some histological subtypes, eg the neuromuscular hamartoma may proliferate aggressively

Hamartoses Congenital disease complexes with hamartomas often associated with benign or malignant neoplasms, including dyskeratosis congenita, incontinenti pigmenti, linear nevus sebaceous syndrome, von Recklinghausen's neurofibromatosis, tuberous sclerosis, xeroderma pigmentosa and the Gardner, Goltz, Klippel-Trenaunay-Weber, Mafucci, neurocutaneous (McCune-Albright), melanosis, multiple lentigines (LEOPARD), multiple neuroma, Sturge-Weber and von Hippel-Lindau syndromes

Hammerhead motif MOLECULAR BIOLOGY A molecular configuration seen in ribozymes that has a unique secondary (possibly also tertiary) structure crucial for cleavage; this motif may have therapeutic potential for reducing HIV-1 tat gene's transcript (Science 1990; 247:1222)

Hammer toe Hallux valgus The lateral deviation of the great toe, common in middle-aged to elderly females in whom life-long use of high heeled shoes is suspect; with time, the deformity elicits callosities on the plantar surfaces of the second and third metatarsal heads Treatment Keller arthroplasty, consisting of removal of exostosis and proximal phalangectomy

Hamstring muscles The muscles of the posterior thigh, consisting of biceps, semitendinosus and the semimembranosus muscles

H&D Curve Hurter and Driffield curve RADIOLOGY An exposure response graph, supplied with X-ray film for plotting absorbance (optical density) vs. log of relative exposure, used for quality control of the film

Hand-arm vibration syndrome White finger syndrome A Raynaud phenomenon-like complex due to cold-induced vasospasm resulting from a prolonged use of vibrating hand-held tools, which may be seen in assembly line workers, grinders, mechanics, jack-hammer operators and others; plethysmographic studies demonstrate changes in digital blood flow (N Engl J Med 1990; 322:675)

Handedness see Chirality

Hand-foot syndrome Sickle cell dactylitis A 'crisis' in sickle cell anemia caused by sludging of red cells in vessels and characterized by symmetric infarction of the small bones of the hand and foot, periosteal neoosteogenesis, pain and swelling that may occur as early as 18 months of age, often resolving spontaneously within 1-4 weeks

Hand-foot-flat face syndrome of Emery Nelson An autosomal dominant condition characterized by a flattened physiognomy, flexion and extension deformities of the hands and feet, mental and growth retardation

Hand, foot and mouth syndrome A clinical complex appearing in infants due to Coxsackievirus A16, A5, A9, A10, B2, B7 and enterovirus, resulting in vesicular stomatitis and exanthema with a summer-fall cycle Clinical After a 4-6 day incubation, most infected toddlers suffer a low-grade fever, 0.5 cm intraoral vesicular ulcers (sore throat and refusal to eat), vesicular lesions of the hands, buttocks and feet, resolving in a week Note: Hand, foot and mouth disease due to enterovirus 71 is more commonly associated with meningoencephalitis and paralysis

Hand-foot-uterus syndrome An autosomal dominant condition characterized by minor digital anomalies of the hands and feet and uterine duplication extending into the cervix and vagina, causing increased stillbirth and perinatal death in the gestational products of afflicted mothers

H & H Hemoglobin and hematocrit; see 10/30 rule

Handicap SOCIAL MEDICINE According to the US legal system, a handicap is construed to include a broad range of physical and mental disabilities which substantially limit a person's major life abilities (1974 Amendment, 29 USC S706(7)(B)) Note: AIDS patients are legally considered to be handicapped and thus are protected from discrimination in the workplace, in housing and education

'Handicapped' health care provider A physician or health care worker who is impaired by physical limitations, usually of long enough duration that he has learned to compensate for the defects; Cf 'Impaired health care provider, Incapacitated' health care provider

Hand mirror cell A lymphocyte with the nucleus at the 'mirror end' and an elongated cytoplasmic appendage or uropod mimicking a mirror's handle; hand mirror cells are seen in benign or malignant hematopoietic conditions and may correspond to immature T lymphocytes, large granular lymphocytes, including natural killer cells and atypical lymphocytes of infectious mononucleosis; hand mirror cells are most often seen in acute lymphocytic leukemias, FAB L1 or L2 subtypes, although similar cells are seen in lymphosarcoma, multiple myeloma, Hodgkin's disease, acute and chronic lymphocytic leukemias and acute myelogenous leukemia, FAB M5a subtype; the 'hand mirror' cells seen in acute myelogenous leukemia may reflect locomotive disturbances while those of acute lymphocytic leukemia may be related to immune defects; the hand-mirror morphology per se has no prognostic value (Am J Clin Path 1977;68:551, ibid, 82:131)

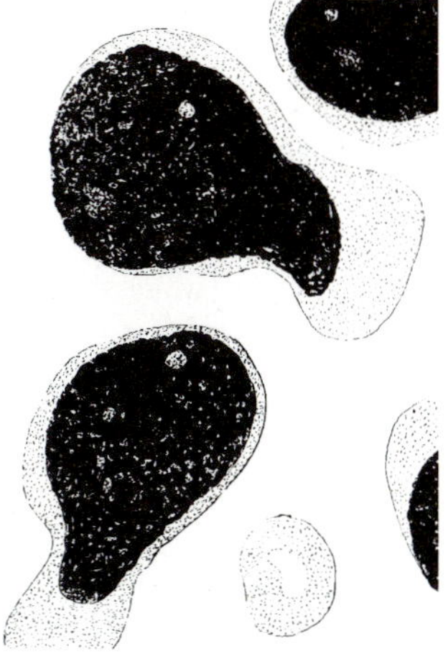

Hand mirror cells

Hand mirror cell leukemia A morphologic descriptor that has been used for two biologically distinct tumors a) A variant of acute monoblastic leukemia (FAB M5a), which is thought to have a better prognosis (than the 'garden variety' leukemia), a diagnosis that requires that 40% or more of the blasts have the hand-mirror morphology, average age of onset, 12, female:male, 2:1 b) An acute lymphoblastic leukemia seen as a blast crisis in chronic myelogenous leukemia (Arch Pathol Lab Med 1990; 114:676)

HANE Hereditary angioneurotic edema An immune complex-induced condition caused by a deficiency of C1q esterase inhibitor (C1q-INH) characterized by episodic consumption of activated C1, C4 and C2, triggered by physical stimuli (trauma, cold, vibration), histamine release, menstruation, with fewer attacks occurring in the last two trimesters of pregnancy Clinical HANE causes transient non-pitting, non-pruritic, non-urticarial swelling that peaks at 12-18 hours, affecting extremities, lips, face, fingers, toes, knees, elbows, buttocks, gastrointestinal mucosa and oropharynx, causing potentially fatal epiglottic edema (33% mortality), often accompanied by abdominal pain with nausea and vomiting; HANE has been divided into four types, two of which are congenital; HANE Type I Common (85%) with C1q-INH decreased to 30% of normal levels; HANE Type II Variant form The gene product is present but dysfunctional; type II may be a) Acquired, associated with lymphoproliferative disorders, eg IgA myeloma, Waldenstrom's macroglobulinemia, chronic lymphocytic leukemia and other B-cell proliferations or b) Autoimmune associated with IgG1 autoantibodies, due to uncontrolled activation of C1s Treatment Androgens Note: Osler described the first case in a young woman over 100 years ago (Am J Med Sci 1888; 95:362); see C1-INH

HANES Health and nutrition examination survey A series of dietary surveys first carried out in 1971 by the National Institute of Health (USA); HANES I determined that Americans consumed suboptimal levels of iron, calcium and vitamins A and C; HANES III is in progress and under the auspices of the National Center for Health Statistics and will determine the weights of the average American

'Hang a shingle' A colloquial Americanphrase for the opening of a private office by a professional, eg physician, lawyer Note: The phrase derives from the name plate used, which is symbolically a roofing shingle, as the person is traditionally so impoverished when opening his own practice that he can't afford anything more luxurious

Hanging drop technique MICROBIOLOGY A method for evaluating bacterial motility, where a flagellated bacterium is placed in a drop of clear physiologic or nutrient solution on a cover glass ('upside-down', therefore, 'hanging') and examined by light microscopy

Hangman's fracture A bilateral avulsion fracture through the neural arch (lamina or pedicles) of the axis (C2, without injuring the odontoid process), causing acute central cervical spinal cord damage with axial dislocation in the C3 vertebral body; major injury to the upper cervical vertebrae is a relative contraindication for surgical correction, unless the vertebral column is unstable or requires neural decompression; formerly, such fractures were seen when hangings used a submental knot; the classic hangman's fracture is now only seen in high speed trauma, eg automobile accidents Note: Hanging as a form of capital punishment was introduced in England in the 5th century; early hanging caused death by strangulation; later technical refinements included a long drop of the body and a submental knot to ensure the desired avulsion or 'Hangman's' fracture, avoiding the unesthetic writhing of a slowly strangulating criminal

Hangover headache Intense cephalgia and malaise upon awakening (often prematurely) after a night of binge drinking or with prolonged use of benzodiazepines, often accompanied by mental dulling, hyperacusia, mild incoordination, tremor and nausea, due to the toxic effects of alcohol and its metabolites, dehydration and decreasing blood levels of alcohol

Hantaan virus see Korean hemorrhagic fever

H antigen IMMUNOLOGY Histocompatibility antigen MICROBIOLOGY A protein present in bacterial flagella TRANSFUSION MEDICINE The trisaccharide stem molecule chain of the ABO blood group, which islocated on red cell membrane surfaces; the enzyme, α-L-fucosyl-transferase is encoded by the H gene and produces the oligosaccharide structure

H antigen
Gal(β1-3)N-acetyl-D-glucosamine-R (Lacto-N-tetraose)
[(α,1-2)
Fucose

HAPC see Hospital-acquired penetration contact

HAPE see High-altitude pulmonary edema

Haplotype A cluster of alleles that are located at the same locus on a chromosome and which are usually inherited together; ; assuming simple mendelian genetics, ie, without unexpected translocations, one in four siblings will share both haplotypes; see MHC

Happy puppet syndrome Angelman syndrome A rare form of infantile epilepsy characterized by severe mental retardation, microcephaly, occasionally, unilateral cerebral atrophy, flattened occiput, protruding jaw and tongue, a smiling vacuous facial expression, ataxia and spastic 'bouncing' movements likened to those of a marionette

Hapten X see CD15

Haptotaxis A type of chemotaxis in which the cells respond to a concentration gradient of an insoluble ligand (eg developing cells responding to various tissue concentrations of fibronectin)

Hard clot An insoluble, usually intravascular thrombus in which the fibrin monomers have been terminally cross-linked by coagulation factor XIII in the presence of calcium ions

Hard copy A term derived from 'computerspeak' that has been modified in various fields and come to be equated to any paper printout of a file in magnetic storage, eg hard or floppy disks or printout from devices as diverse as electrocardiographs, laboratory instruments or medical records retrieved from microfiche storage; see Smart card

Hard disk COMPUTERS A permanent or non-removable data storage device, which for microcomputers ranges from 10 to 600 megabytes or more; hard disk memory can be either a) Magnetic, which has a faster access time and a practical ceiling of up to one gigabytes of memory and b) Optical, which is currently slower than magnetic devices but may practically store 1 or more gigabytes of information and is less expensive

'Hard' drug Any intensely addictive substance of abuse that may compel its user to commit crimes in order to obtain the drug, due to its high cost, eg heroin or through loss of societal inhibitions, eg cocaine Note: 'Soft drug' is an uncommonly used term for less addictive agents that may be legal, viewed as less addicting and/or more socially acceptable, eg tobacco, alcohol and marijuana

Hardening Hydrogenation of the unsaturated fatty acids in triglycerides into saturated fatty acids; see Browning reaction, Tropical oils

'Hard' liquor A colloquial term for beverages with a high, often greater than 30% alcohol by volume (60 proof), eg gin, rum, vodka, whiskey; hard liquors are preferred by alcoholics as a steady state of low-level inebriation is easier to maintain

Hard spin see Heavy spin

'Hard' tubercle see Naked granuloma

Hardware COMPUTERS The electronic and mechanical, non-software components of a computer, which include the central processing unit, monitor, disk drives, printer, modem, scanning devices

Hard water 'syndrome' A clinical complex seen when 'hard' water (which contains high levels of iron, calcium and magnesium) is used during hemodialysis, resulting in post-dialysis nausea, vomiting, asthenia, hypertension

Hardwiring NEUROPHYSIOLOGY Permanent neural connections between the sensory input and motor output that are present in the brain of infants after a critical period of perinatal rewiring; the hardwiring concept is part of neuroscience dogma, which holds that reorganization in an adult organism is minimal, although recent data from the Silver Spring monkeys indicates that reorganization occurs in the cerebral cortex, extending 10 to 14 mm into the somatosensory region formerly dedicated to the region of limbs that had been denervated (Science 1991; 252:1789n&v)

Hard X-rays RADIATION ONCOLOGY Short wavelength, high-frequency and highly penetrating X-rays that may be used in radiotherapy or which may be generated by nuclear 'incidents'

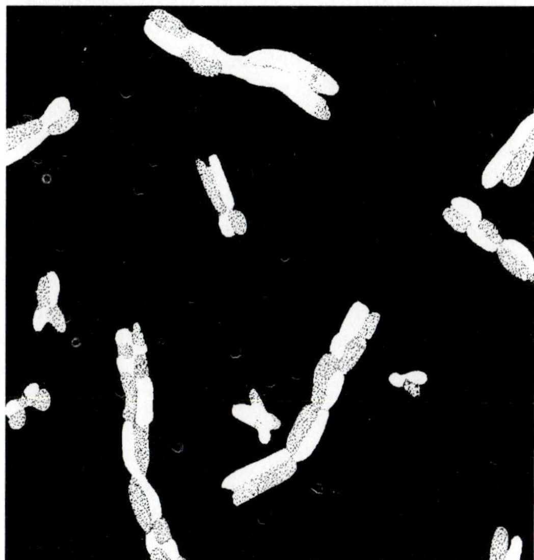

Harlequin chromosomes

Harlequin chromosome technique GENETICS An experimental method used to demonstrate 'sister chromatid exchange' in chromosomes, where one of the 'sisters' is chemically altered and made to fluoresce more brightly than its twisted sister (figure); here there is no gain or loss of genes, only axial rotation of alleles

Harlequin color changes PEDIATRICS A benign erythema that longitudinally 'sections' the prone infant into a pale upper and a vividly flushed lower half (most prominent from the forehead to the pubis), related to autonomic vascular lability; this color change is rare, occurring most commonly in premature or low birth weight neonates, and like erythema neonatorum, is a transient vasomotor phenomenon with no clinical significance

Harlequin fetus Ichthyosis congenita A rare autosomal recessive disease of infants in which the baby is encased in a thickened keratinaceous 'coccoon' with deep fissures, accompanied by ectropion; once thought a variant of lamellar ichthyosis, this is a severe dyskeratosis, the defect of which lies in lipid metabolism; there is massive hyperkeratosis; the stratum corneum is up to 30-fold thicker than the stratum malpighii; the stratum granulosa is reduced to a one-cell layer or absent (Arch Dermatol 1985; 118:952)

Harlequin nail A fingernail in a subject who has abruptly stopped smoking; the proximal zone of new growth is pink while the outgrowing nail formed during nicotine exposure (the 'nicotine sign') is a dirty yellow-brown (Chest 1990; 97:236)

Harrison Narcotic Act, 1914 The first legislation in the USA that regulated importation, manufacture, sale and use of opium, cocaine and all related derivatives; the act stood with many amendments, later encompassing marijuana, LSD and other hallucinogens until its replacement by the Controlled Drug Substances Act of 1970, see there

Hartmanella see Primary aseptic meningitis

Harvard criteria see Table

Harvard criteria for brain death

The Harvard medical school ad hoc committe established four criteria for irreversible coma

- ✻ Unreceptivity and unresponsiveness
- ✻ No movement or breathing
- ✻ No reflexes
- ✻ Flat electroencephalogram (confirmatory)

IN ADDITION, THE FOLLOWING MUST BE PRESENT

- ❍ Body temperature greater than or equal to 32° C
- ❍ Absence of central nervous system depressants

Harvard fraud case J Am Med Assoc 1983; 249:1797

Harvard guidelines A series of guideline issued by Harvard University in 1988 intended to prevent scientific fraud, rather than act in response to it; in addition to guidelines on supervision of research trainees, care in gathering, record-keeping and analysis of data and establishment of criteria for authorship credits, see Relman's criteria, there is an objective limit on the number of publications reviewed for faculty appointment or promotion; five publications are reviewed for assistant professor, seven for associate professor and ten for full professor (N Engl J Med 1988; 318:1462ed)

Harvard law '...under optimal laboratory conditions of constant temperature, light, humidity and substrate availability, an organism will do as it damned well pleases...' Note: This colloquialism is well-known in some circles in the natural sciences, although the author was unable to find it in written form

Harvest TRANSPLANTATION Procurement of an organ from a cadaveric or live donor; because the word harvest connotes gathering of a mature crop, alternate terms, eg donation, 'procurement' or 'recovery' appear to be less degrading to the donor

Harvest Moon phenomenon A decrease in mortality in certain subjects prior to the occurrence of a symbolically meaningful event or occasion; epidemiologists usually examine the impact of external factors in establishing cause-and-effect relations to disease; cultural factors are rarely examined and usually viewed as having a negative impact on disease; one study (J Am Med Assoc 1990; 263:1947) revealed a positive impact of culturally significant events on mortality to two populations, older Chinese women (event: Harvest Moon festival) and older Jewish men (event: Passover); each group proved itself capable of staving off death, especially of cardiovascular disease and cancer with mortality dipping 35% before the event and increasing by 34.6% thereafter

Hashimoto's disease A condition most common in women over age forty, often presenting as a diffuse firm thyroid enlargement which, when extreme, cause esophageal or tracheal compression **Pathogenesis** Probably autoimmune, given the presence of antibodies against thyroid peroxidase (microsomal antibodies), thyroglobulin and colloid **Histopathology** Lymphocytic infiltration, oxyphilic changes of thyroid follicular epithelium, lymphoid follicles with prominent germinal centers, often accompanied by atrophy of the thyroid epithelium **Treatment** Hormonal replacement **Prognosis** Excellent **Complications** Rarely, lymphoma

Hashitoxicosis Hashimoto's thyroiditis (chronic autoimmune thyroiditis) presenting as hyperthyroidism

HAT medium Hypoxanthine, aminopterin and thymidine A culture medium optimal for hybridoma (monoclonal antibody) production; aminopterin blocks de novo synthesis of GMP by the myeloma cells, while hypoxanthine and thymidine are nutrients required by both myeloma cells and the monoclonal antibody-producing cells; the cells producing the monoclonal antibodies have hypoxanthine guanine phosphoribosyl transferase, bypassing the aminopterin-induced blockage of GMP production that would otherwise kill the non-fused myeloma cell line; see Hybridoma

Hatband sign A unilateral sweat stain on a hat, seen in Horner syndrome, associated with pulmonary carcinoma

Hatchet face The characteristic physiognomy of advanced myotonic dystrophy; the face is drawn and lugubrious, with hollowing of the muscles around the temples and jaws; the eyes are 'hooded', the lower lip droop ; the global weakness of the facial muscles causes sagging of the lower face, accompanied by marked wasting of the neck muscles, especially the flexors imparting a 'swan-necked' appearance; a similar facies may rarely occur in amyotrophic lateral sclerosis and Curschmann-Batten-Steiner syndrome

HAV Hepatitis A virussee Hepatitis

Haverhill fever Erythema arthriticum epidermicum First described in Massachusetts in an epidemic in 1925 (Bost Med Surg J 1926, 194:285) caused by *Haverhillia multiformis*, currently known as *Streptobacillus moniliformis* (a non-motile, gram-negative rod of varible length, growing in liquid culture medium as 'puff-ball'-like colonies, transmitted in crowded urban slums by ingesting milk contaminated by rat excreta; *S moniliformis* is present in the nasopharynx of up to 50% of laboratory and healthy wild rodents **Clinical** 2-10 day incubation, then abrupt onset of an acute prostrating disease with shaking chills, spiking fever, upper respiratory symptoms, pharyngitis, vomiting, headache, myalgias, generalized, predominantly palmoplantar blotchy, maculopapular, morbilliform petechial rashes, nonspecific migratory polyarthritis **Mortality** 10% **Late complications** Endocarditis, pericarditis, pneumonia, abscesses, anemia, biological false positive tests for syphilis, urticaria **Treatment** Penicillin, tetracycline; see Rat-bite fever, Sodoku

Hawkinsuria An autosomal dominant form of tyrosyluria, named after the index family, presenting in infancy with severe metabolic acidosis, ketosis, failure to thrive, transient tyrosinemia, excess excretion of *p*-hydroxyphenylpyruvic and p-hydroxyphenylacetic acids as well as unusual tyrosine metabolites, one of which is hawkinsin; the disease responds to dietary restriction of phenylalanine and tyrosine and resolves spontaneously with age without mental retardation or hepatopathy

Hawthorne effect A beneficial effect that health care providers have on the workers in virtually any environment when an interest is shown in the workers' well-being; the 'Hawthorne studies' were conducted in the 1930s at the Hawthorne plant of the Western Electric company and attempted to delineate the effects of improving the social environment and laborer-management relations in the workplace Note: This phenomenon differs from both a) The 'Halo' effect, in which the contact with health care personnel is personal and occurs in a legitimate medical context and b) The placebo effect, in which the subject may believe a therapeutic effect is present, where none exists, ie *cogito ergo sum*; Cf 'Nocebo'

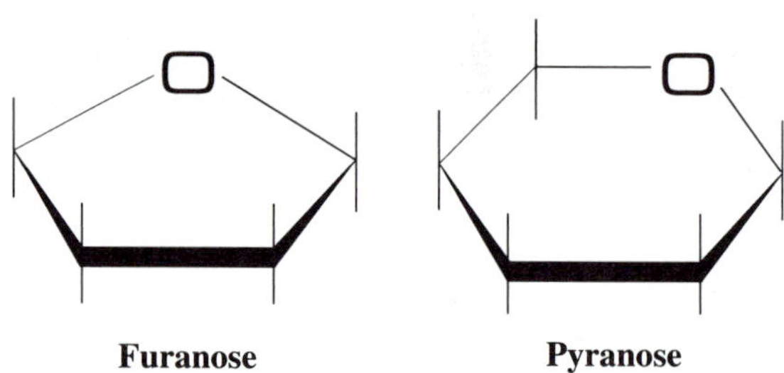

Furanose **Pyranose**

Haworth projections

Haworth projection Biochemistry A convention used in chemistry to partially represent the three dimensional configuration of cyclic sugars, in particular furanoses (cyclical five-carbon sugars, eg ribose and fructose) and pyranoses (cyclical six-carbon sugars, eg glucose and galactose); Haworth projections are shown as planar molecule with the oxygen bridge in the rear and the three carbon bonds in the front (figure, above)

Hazardous waste Environment Any unwanted product that poses a hazard or potential hazard to human health, which may be generated by a manufacturing process, eg radioactive gas cylinders, chemicals, pesticides, acids and liquid or by a health care facility, including regulated biohazardous waste; this contrasts with municipal solid waste, eg paper, plastics and metals; see Regulated waste, Toxic dump

HBGF Heparin-binding growth factor(s) A family of seven structurally-related polypeptide cytokines that are activated after binding heparin

HBGF-8 Heparin-binding growth factor-8 see Pleitrophin

HBIG Hepatitis B immunoglobulin A 3-5 ml preparation of antibodies to hepatitis B virus (HBV), derived from donor pools and administered at the time of and one month after presumed exposure to HBV; HBIG is heat-treated and negative for human immunodeficiency virus;

HBIG is available in low- (anti-HBs > 1:128 — $5/dose) or high titer (anti-HBs > 1:100 000 — $150/dose) forms; there is little evidence that the high-titer immune globulin is more effective

'H blocker' see Histamine receptor blocking agents

H bodies Heinz bodies (Clumps of denatured hemoglobin); see Golf ball bodies

H-bomb sign RADIOLOGY A finding in a radiocontrast study of a stomach with atrophic gastritis, where the fundus appears as a 'bald' dome with thinned rugae and an attenuated gastric wall; the speckled background is due to poor mixing of gastric secretions with the barium; when erect and distended with air, the 'mushroom' appearance has been fancifully likened to the appearance of a hydrogen bomb explosion figure

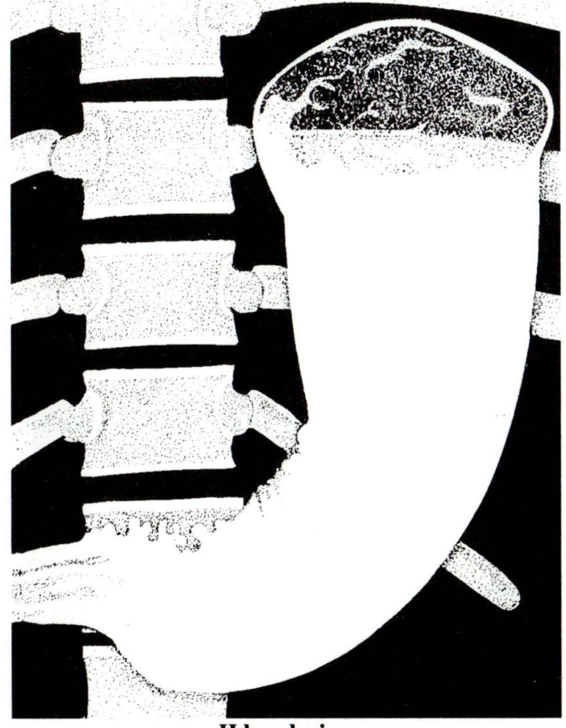

H bomb sign

HBLV Human B-lymphotropic virus see Herpesvirus-6

HBV Hepatitis B virus

HBx A hepatitis B regulatory gene that encodes an HBx protein that acts as a transcriptional transactivator of viral genes, altering the host gene expression and inducing the development of hepatocellular carcinoma in transgenic mouse induced hepatomas (Nature 1991; 351:317); see Hepatitis

HCA see Hypothalamic chronic anovulation

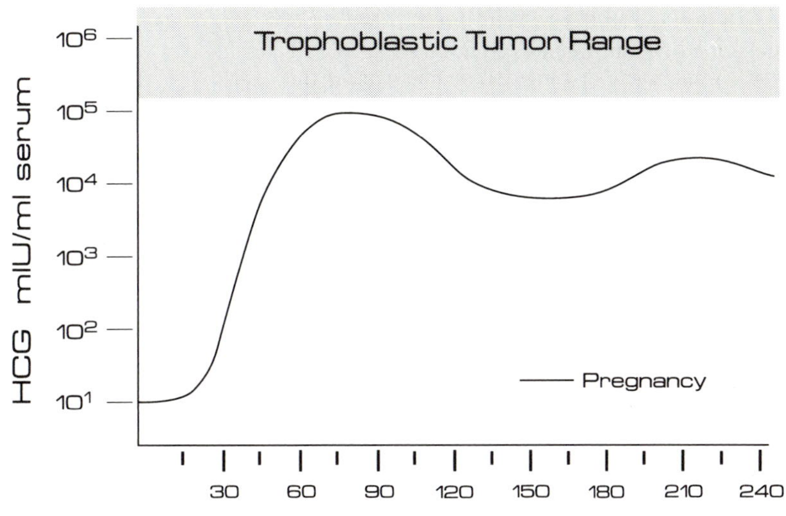

HCFA Health Care Financing Administration A bureaucracy created by the US government 1977 from Medicare, Medicaid and the Office of Long-Term Care, which administers these programs at the federal level; see JCAHO, Medicaid, Medicare

HCFC Hydrochlorofluorocarbons see CFCs, Ozone layer

hCG Human choriogonadotropic hormone A glycoprotein hormone containing lactose and hexosamine that is produced by the syncytiotrophoblast, the fetal liver and kidney and certain tumors; hCG is released in a pulsatile fashion in normal pregnancy, peaking at the tenth gestational week with serum levels of 50-140 000 IU/L, thereafter falling to 10-50 000 IU/L Note; hCG levels during pregnancy are below 100 000; higher levels are seen in trophoblastic tumors and in moles of pregnancy; hCG may be low to undetectable in ectopic pregnancy or markedly elevated in multiple gestation, polyhydramnios, eclampsia, erythroblastosis fetalis or trophoblastic disease, including hydatidiform moles, choriocarcinoma and placental site trophoblastic tumor; hCG levels may be extremely elevated in tumors producing either the β subunit or both α and β subunits, measured by radioimmunoassay or enzyme-linked immunosorbent assay (ELISA); ectopic elevation of hCG may occur with carcinomas of the stomach, liver, pancreas, breast, kidney, lungs and adrenal cortex, as well as seminoma, leukemia, lymphoma and melanoma

hCG-like activity Cross-reactivity of the α subunit of thyroid-stimulating hormone, luteinizing hormone and follicle-stimulating hormones with the detector molecule of the α subunit of hCG, such that elevation of these hormones mimics an elevation of hCG when measured by radioimmunoassay Note: The 18 kD α subunit of hCG has an 80% amino acid homology with these cross-reactors, which explains why the β subunit is used for analysis

HCHWA-D Hereditary cerebral hemorrhage with amyloidosis, Dutch type An autosomal dominant form of cerebral amyloid angiopathy in which the patients develop recurrent intracerebral hemorrhages leading to death by the sixth decade of life; HCHWA-D has been described in four families from two coastal villages in the Netherlands; cloning and sequencing of the exons reveals a mutation causing an amino acid substitution in the amyloid protein (Science 1990; 248:1124); see also Cerebral amyloid angiopathy

H-2 Complex The major histocompatibility complex (MHC) in the mouse, which is located on chromosome 17 and analogous to the human HLA system on chromosome 6; the H-2 complex is 2-4000 kilobase pairs in length and contains the thousands of genes involved in immune recognition, each 600 base pairs in length; the H-2 subregions of K, D and L correspond to HLA's subregions A, B and C3, and the I-A and I-E regions correspond to the HLA-D region in humans Note: The MHC was discovered in the 1930s in inbred mice by Gorer who was studying the effects of graft rejection on erythrocytes; the gene for histocompatibility that rejected the red cell antigen was designated as number 2 (ergo H-2)

HCT Hematocrit

HCV see Hepatitis C

HDC-ABMT High-dose chemotherapy with autologous bone marrow transplantation An experimental therapeutic modality used in patients with terminal malignancy, of currently unknown efficacy

HDL High-density lipoprotein A plasma lipoprotein that has a density of 1.063-1.210 kg/L (US: 1.063-1.210 g/dl); HDL is 33% protein (predominantly apolipoprotein A-I and A-II), 29% phospholipid, 30% cholesterol and 8% triglycerides and transports cholesterol from the intestine to the liver; the larger the HDL molecule, the more efficient the lipid transport and by extension, lipolysis; HDL levels are the single most important predictor of coronary heart disease (CHD), given that a) Several risk factors for CHD, eg smoking, obesity and lack of exercise may actually lower HDL b) HDL has an inverse relation with VLDL and LDL, lipoproteins known to be atherogenic and c) HDL may interfere with atherogenesis by promoting reverse cholesterol transport or prevent aggregation of LDL particles in the arterial wall (J Am Med Assoc 1990; 264:3053); small HDL molecules (HDL_3) are metabolically 'early' forms and more prominent in alcoholics; increases in the larger HDL_2 molecule are associated with a reduced risk of coronary heart disease and in sedentary older adults, HDL_2 is inversely related to truncal (waist-to-hip) fat, insulin levels and glucose intolerance (N Engl J Med 1990; 322:229); apolipoprotein E may prove a better measure of atherosclerotic risk than HDL_2, as it correlates well with exercise Note: Anabolic steroids eg stanozolol, testosterone reduce HDL_3, HDL-cholesterol and apo-A-I, an effect partially ameliorated by oral rather than parenteral administration (J Am Med Assoc 1989; 261:1165)

HDL/LDL ratio The ratio of cholesterol carried by high-density lipoprotein to that carried by low-density lipoprotein, which allows a rapid risk stratification for atherosclerosis-related cardiac disease; the HDL/LDL ratio is decreased by saturated fatty acid

HDN Hemolytic disease of the newborn

Headbanger's tumor A lesion that may develop in children who bang their heads as part of a 'routine' for falling asleep, which consists of a mass of organizing fibrous tissue covered by hyperpigmented skin, identical in pathogenesis to the lump described on the foreheads of devout Moslems; headbanging occurs transiently in 3.5% of infants of normal intelligence and is 3.5-fold more common in boys, in 5% of whom it may be of longer duration, especially in the mentally-retarded or psychiatrically disturbed (Br J Plastic Surg 1982; 35:72)

Head drop sign NEUROLOGY A finding evoked by raising an infant's trunk at the shoulders; a head that drops backward suggests nuchal limpness typical of both paralytic and non-paralytic poliomyelitis

'Headhunter' An employment agency or person who actively recruits physicians, upper echelon executives or other professionals, matching potential employees with employers

Head shaping External cranioplasty The intentional employment of external forces or devices to conform the head (of children) to a desired shape, producing permanent modifications of the craniofacial bony architecture; head molding was formerly widely practiced in various cultures as a sign of aristocracy and continues to be practiced in certain aboriginal tribes and cultures of North and South America; although head shaping may cause proptosis, epilepsy, mental retardation and even death when performed with excess diligence by the medically inept, the procedure is generally regarded as safe (J Am Med Assoc 1991; 265:1179)

Head space analysis LABORATORY MEDICINE Gas chromatographic analysis of the air (head space) from a stoppered specimen tube warmed to 40-60°C, which detects the presence of volatile organic substances

Health advocacy see Health promotion

Health care access SOCIAL MEDICINE The ability of an individual to receive health care services, which is a function of a) Availability, which in the US is in chronic short supply in rural regions due to logistics and in the inner cities, due to financing and the ability to pay for those services; health care access ranges from universal access in socialized medicine to the 'free market' system prevalent in the USA; each of these 'extremes' has considerable disadvantages, with the free market model becoming increasingly problematic as the cost of health care continues to spiral upward, such that it constitutes between 11 and 13% of the US gross national product, while more than 20% of the population has no access to health care, thus creating a two-tiered system of inequity, between the 'haves' and the 'have-nots' (see May 15, 1991, Journal of the American Medical Association; summary: pp 2564-5)

Health care rationing The limitation of access to or the equitable distribution of medical services, through various 'gatekeeper' controls Note: The limitless expansion of technology, the aging population and the upward spiralling costs of health care (the health care industry expenditure was estimated at $\$5.5 \times 10^{11}$ in 1990, representing 11.3% of the US gross national product) in the developed nations has brought to the fore the ethical issue of '*WHO IS ALLOWED TO GET HOW*

MUCH OF WHAT', and deciding, for example, between financing five liver transplantations or prenatal care for one thousand pregnancies, becomes a morally unsolvable conundrum, as the five will die without treatment, while the benefits of prenatal care are difficult to translate into concrete and immediate benefits; Cf Coby Howard, Oregon plan, Rule of Rescue, 'Squeaky wheel'

Health food A non-medical term defined by the lay public as a food that has little or no preservatives, which has not undergone major processing, enrichment or refinement and which may be grown without pesticides; health foods have been mystically endowed by certain segments of the population with the ability to prevent the development of most diseases, including atherosclerosis, aging phenomena, rheumatic disease and cancer, as well as to treat malignancy and prolong life; see Food preservatives, Organic food; Cf Diet, Junk food

Health fraud Deceit for profit, including false representation of efficacy and concealment of adverse effects of medications or 'natural curatives; see Pseudovitamins, Unproven methods of cancer therapy

Health maintenance organization see HMO

Health promotion Any activity that seeks to improve a person's or population's health by providing information about and increasing awareness of 'at risk' behaviors associated with certain diseases, with the intent of reducing those behaviors; in the USA, health promotion has met with success in reducing the incidence of cardiovascular and tobacco-related diseases

'HEALTHY PEOPLE PLAN'

Confining HIV infection to < 800/100 000 and new cases to less than 98 000/year

Alcohol abuse Reduce alcohol-related motor vehicle accidents to < 8.5/100 000; reduce alcohol abuse to 13% in those under age 17

Chronic disease 15% reduction in chronic disease-related disability

Drug abuse Reduce drug-related deaths to 3/100 000, marijuana abuse to less than 8% in those aged 18-25 and cocaine abuse in this same group to 3%

Immunizations Eliminate measles; reduce pneumonia and influenza-related death to 7.3/100 000; increase number of children immunized to 80%

Obstetric care Reduce infant mortality to 7/1000; reduce low birth weight to less than 5%; extend first-trimester care to 90% of all pregnancies; reduce teen pregnancies to less than 50/1000 teen-aged girls

Sexually-transmitted disease Reduce gonorrhea to 225/100 000 and syphilis to 10/100 000 Tuberculosis Reduce tuberculosis from its 1988 high of 9.1/100 000 to 3.5/100 000

'Healthy people 2000' PUBLIC HEALTH A series of health goals (table) promulgated by the US Public Health Services that provides insight into the state of American health (J Am Med Assoc 1990; 264:2057); the priorities include health promotion, ie targeting risk behaviors and health protection, which includes environmental or regulatory measures that confer broad-based protection, as well as preventative services and surveillance systems, addressing numerous specific issues; see Mortality, YPLL

Healthy worker effect The finding that death from disease is markedly reduced in certain occupations; the mortality in young men enlisted in the US Army is one-fourth that of civilian men of similar age, a fact attributed to self-selection, pre-enlistment screening (eliminating the less physically or psychologically fit), exercise, health care and health promotion (J Am Med Assoc 1990; 264:2241; Br J Ind Med 1987; 44:289)

Health 'yuppie' A 'yuppie' (young, upwardly-mobile professional) who is a physician, dentist or other highly paid health care worker (NY State J Med 1991; 91:43), whose inferred goals pivot around material gains and egocentricity, rather than the altruistic principles that traditionally guide physicians and others in the health care field

'Heaped-up' appearance GASTROENTEROLOGY The endoscopic morphology seen in malignant gastric ulcers where the margins of the lesion are irregular, with overhanging borders, and a 'dirty', necrotic base; Cf Punched-out appearance; see Meniscus sign of Carmen

'Heartburn' Burning retrosternal, often postprandial discomfort due to reflux of gastric contents into the esophagus, associated with dysfunction of the lower esophageal sphincter; heartburn may be idiopathic or associated with Barrett's esophagus, duodenal ulcers, reflux, scleroderma and Zollinger-Ellison syndrome

Heartcutting INSTRUMENTATION A method for improving the resolution of gas chromatography by switching a portion of the analyzed specimen into a second separation column with a different polarity, measuring a second parameter; thus is also known as multidimensional gas chromatography (Science 1984; 227:1570)

Heart failure cells Intra-alveolar hemosiderin-laden macrophages seen in the lungs (figure) of patients with compromised cardiac function that results in low-grade pulmonary hemorrhage, as in congestive heart failure; the cell content is confirmed by an appropriate iron stain, eg Prussian blue

'Heart laws' Legislature that attempts to distinguish cardiac injuries and consequences due to work-related physical exertion and/or psychologic stress from those due to the natural progression of underlying cardiac disease; these laws do not provide for workman's compensation if the disability is related to coronary artery disease or hypertension, ie naturally-progressing disease, except for certain 'favored' occupational groups, including uniformed police and firefighters whose death or disability is presumed to have been suffered in the line of duty

Heart-lung machine Extracorporal circulation A device used during cardiothoracic surgery in which the blood is pushed by a roller pump and gently separated into tubing, where the blood is then bubble-oxygenated, reheated, filtered and pumped back into the body

Heart-lung transplantation A procedure being successfully performed at specialized centers, eg Stanford University and the University of Pittsburgh; post-transplant patients have adequate ventilation, despite a loss of innervation and increased tidal volume; heart-lung transplantation may be effective for a) Primary respiratory disease with chronic disturbance in gas exchange and alveolar mechanics and a secondary increase in pulmonary vascular resistance (those with primary vascular resistance fare poorly with heart-lung transplants) and b) Pulmonary vascular disease with primary high-resistance circulatory disorder, for whom the procedure is beneficial as tracheo-bronchial and alveolar abnormalities are not present; Cf Domino donor transplantation, Lung transplantation, UNOS

Heart-shaped face A descriptor for a physiognomy described in Turner syndrome (45,XO), characterized by prominent ears, broad malar bones and a small chin

Heart tumors Cardiac neoplasms are rare; most primary lesions are benign (myxoma > rhabdomyoma > osteoclastoma) although malignant tumors occur (angiosarcoma, rhabdomyosarcoma); secondary neoplasms are usually malignant and hone in on the pericardium, arising in the lung, or extend from a hilar-based lymphoma or melanoma

Heart valve A prosthetic device used to replace a stenosed or 'insufficient' cardiac valve, which may be mechanical, eg Bjork-Shiley tilting disk valve, bioprosthetic, or porcine; when compared, survival with an intact valve is slightly better with certain mechanical devices, but these carry the risk of morbidity due to the need for long-term anticoagulant therapy (N Engl J Med 1991; 324:573); in 1988, 51 000 valves were transplanted in the US; the mechanical valves include tilting disks, the Starr-Edwards caged ball and St Jude's pivoting bileaflet; in addition to the porcine bioprosthesis, there is a commercially available cryopreserved human aortic valve (ibid, 324:624)

Heat shock MOLECULAR BIOLOGY The inhibitory effect that high ambient temperatures have on the transcription and translation machinery; severe heat shock blocks gene splicing, blocking translation of intervening sequences (introns) of mRNA precursors; since the mRNA in the cytoplasm doesn't have the usual cuts at the 5' and 3' splice junctions and translation of the mRNA proceeds into the exons (which are usually spliced out), resulting in the production of abnormal proteins, therefore repression of normal transcription during heat shock is beneficial to the host cell or organism, as defective proteins are not produced (Science 1988; 242:1544)

Heat shock proteins (hsp) A small group of highly-conserved proteins, containing a 'heat shock consensus' region, the production of which increases when a cell is subjected to various metabolic stresses, especially heat; hsp activities include assembly of proteins into protein complexes, correct protein folding, uptake of protein into organelles and protein sorting (Nature 1991; 349:627); the largest group of hsps has a molecular mass of about 70 kD; when cells are treated with antibodies to hsp 70, they accumulate heat shock proteins and die by thermal stress; when the HSP104 gene of ***Saccharomyces cerevisiae*** is eliminated by deletion mutation, thermotolerance is lost, implying that the gene is required for thermotolerance (Science 1990; 248:1112); hsp70s stimulate translocation and folding of precursor proteins into the mitochondrial matrix and endoplasmic reticulum, and are thus thought to facilitate transport competence to precursors (Nature 1990; 348:137); hsp60 proteins have 'foldase' activities, see Chaperonins; hsp90 proteins are thought to act in the signal transduction pathway for steroid, eg glucocorticoid and estrogen receptors, facilitating response of the aporeceptor to the hormonal signal (Nature 1990; 348:166); hsp 70 proteins that help cells recover after exposure to high temperatures are Ss1p and Ss2p, which increase the rates of translocation of proteins into microsomes and possibly salvage precursor proteins that prematurely fold into translocation-incompetent conformations during translation, allowing passage, possibly by binding and unfolding hydrophobic receptor sites of certain proteins produced outside of the cells where needed; two groups of hsps respond to different stressants, a) Group I Ethanol which induces translational errors and amino acid analogs, eg puromycin causing production of abnormal proteins and b) Group II Heat shock (protein unfolding), heavy metals and inorganic toxins (copper-chelaters, arsenite, iodoacetamide, p-chloromercuribenzoate, which causes conformational changes in the proteins by binding to sulfhydryl groups, recovery from anoxia, H_2O_2, superoxide ions and other free radicals (oxygen toxicity, free radical fragmentation of proteins), ammonium chloride (inhibition of proteolysis), others (inhibition of oxidative phosphorylation, changes in redox state, protein modification)

Heat shock response A constellation of responses that occur when an organism is exposed to high temperatures, including repression of synthesis of some proteins, increased synthesis of other proteins andtranscription and translation of genes to form 'new' proteins that are not produced at lower temperatures

Heat stress disease CRITICAL CARE MEDICINE A group of conditions due to overexposure to or overexertion in excess environmental temperatures, of increasing severity, from a) Heat cramps, which are non-emergent and treated by salt replacement b) Heat exhaustion, which is more serious, treated with fluid and salt replacement and c) Heat stroke, a condition most commonly affecting extremes of ages, especially the elderly, accompanied by convulsions, delusions, coma and treated with cooling the body and replacement of fluids and salts Note: The body's reaction to heat is a function of controllable (use of anticholinergics, phenothiazines, alcohol, heavy exercise, clothing, obesity, direct exposure and acclimatization) and uncontrollable factors (high ambient temperatures or humidity, lack of air circulation, underlying fever, old age or infancy, ectodermal dysplasia

Heavy chain diseases A family of monoclonal gammopathies or paraproteinemias that are characterized by excess production of an immunoglobulin Fc fragment that may be detected in the serum and/or urine, and accompanied by lymphoproliferative disease **Alpha heavy chain disease** Seligmann's disease The most common heavy chain disease or paraproteinemia, in which there is an excess production of an incomplete IgA1 molecule (partial heavy chain and no light chain), affecting Sephardic Jews, Arabs and those living in the Mediterranean rim, South America and Asia Clinical Onset in childhood or adolescence as either alympho-proliferative disorder confined to the respiratory tract or an enteric form (see IPSID) with severe diarrhea, malabsorption, steatorrhea, weight loss, hepatic dysfunction, hypocalcemia, lymphadenopathy, marked mononuclear infiltration which may eventuate into lymphoma (see Mediterranean lymphoma); α chain disease may remit spontaneously, respond to antibiotic therapy or if clearly monoclonal, may require combination chemotherapy, potentially causing death by ages 20-30 Laboratory Increased alkaline phosphatase, hypocalcemia Treatment Antibiotics, or if advanced, chemotherapy **Delta heavy chain disease** A single case has been reported in an elderly man with osteolytic lesions, marrow infiltration by abnormal plasma cells, who died in renal failure **Gamma heavy chain disease** of Franklin A disorder of older males, ranging from fulminant, ie death in weeks to prolonged, lasting 20 years, although usually death occurs in the first year, often due to infection Clinical Presents as a lymphoproliferation with fever, fatigue, anemia, angioimmunoblastic lymphadenopathy, hepatosplenomegaly, uvular and palatal edema, eosinophilic infiltrates, leukopenia, associated with autoimmune disease, tuberculosis and lymphoma Laboratory Increased IgG1; most cases excrete less than 1 g/day of paraprotein, rarely up to 20g/day Treatment Cyclophosphamide, vincristine, prednisone **Mu chain disease** A rare paraproteinemia that affects the middle-aged to elderly, most of whom have or slowly progress to chronic lymphocytic leukemia Clinical Lymphadenopathy, hepato-splenomegaly and bone marrow infiltration by vacuolated plasma cells, often accompanied by increased kappa chain production Treatment As with chronic lymphocytic leukemia

'Heavy guns' A highly colloquial term, most commonly used in the context of highly aggressive therapy, as in chemotherapy of an advanced malignancy that the oncologist 'hits with heavy guns', using multiple agents and several therapeutic modalities; see Induction

Heavy metals Antimony, arsenic, bismuth, lead, mercury When exposed to heavy metals, cells respond by increasing transcription of a variety of genes, including the eukaryotic heat shock system, metallothioneins, prokaryotic mercury resistance gene and iron uptake systems Clinical General, fine tremor, speech slurring, stomatitis, drooling, cataracts and neurasthenia Treatment Chelation with EDTA; see Mad Hatter, Minamata Bay disease, Queen of Poisons, Pink disease

Heavy spin TRANSFUSION MEDICINE A term referring to the intensity of centrifugation (5000 g) used in a blood bank for separating various blood components from a donated unit of erythrocytes; a heavy spin of 5-7 minutes is required for separation of red cells, platelets, plasma, cryoprecipitate and leukocyte-poor red cells

'Hectic-septic' fever An erratic fever pattern that, while uncommon and non-specific, may be seen in abscesses, as well as malaria, kala-azar and endocarditis

Heel-pad sign A characteristic clinical finding in acromegaly, where soft tissue under the heel is thickened to greater than 30 mm (normal < 23 mm)

Hegsted's score A formula for determining a diet's relative lipid composition, where a high value indicates increased saturated fatty acids and cholesterol and low polyunsaturated fatty acids (N Engl J Med 1985; 312:811)

Hegsted's score

2.16 X S (% kcal, saturated fatty acids)
 - 1.65 X P (% kcal, polyunsaturated fatty acids)
 + 0.0677 X C (mg cholesterol/1000 kcal) X (K/1000)

Heimlich maneuver A technique for removing a bolus of food stuck in the oropharynx potentially causing acute asphyxia; the Hiemlich-*er* stands behind the victim and clasps his hands around the Heimlich-*ee*, slightly above the umbilicus and abruptly pulls backwards, forcing residual air in the lungs out the trachea (J Am Med Assoc 1975; 234:398) Note: While the maneuver is often successful, the victim may have developed an air hunger so intense that the benefit of the expulsive rush of air dislodging the bolus is immediately offset by a gasp by the victim, that jams the food further down the traheo-bronchial tree, exacerbating the situation Complications Fatal aortic regurgitation (N Engl J Med 1986; 315:1613cr); see Cafe coronary, Flake maneuver

HeLa cells TISSUE CULTURE **An aneuploid epithelial cell line isolated by GO Gey (John Hopkins) from Henrietta Lack, a young Baltimore woman who died in 1951 of an anaplastic carcinoma of the** uterine cervix; the Hela cell line has been in continuous culture in numerous laboratories around the world and is a 'gold standard' cell line widely used in experimental oncology, which has contributed much to the understanding of cancer

Helical scanning see Spiral computed tomography

Helical structure BIOCHEMISTRY The α helix is a major structural motif present in many proteins, eg myoglobin that is most stable in a right-handed conformation, which usually has 3.6 amino acid residues per 360° turn; the peptide bonds are parallel and side chains perpendicular to the helical axis of the α helix; each amino acid forms a hydrogen bond to the fourth amino acid above and to the fourth amino acid below at a distance of 0.29 nm; Cf β-pleated sheets

Helicase An enzyme that binds DNA downstream of the replicating fork, catalyzing the unwinding of the DNA duplex; Cf Gyrase

Helicobacter pylori A gram-negative microaerophilic curved bacillus that was first classified as a *Campylobacter*, but later separated therefrom (Int J

Syst Bacteriol 1989; 39:397), due to major differences in ultrastructure, fatty acid content, respiratory quinines, growth properties, RNA sequence and enzymes, eg urease production; ***H pylori*** is held responsible for most cases of gastritis and is present in 10% of healthy young persons and up to 60% of those 60 years or older (N Engl J Med 1991; 324:1043rv) Note: 90% of patients with intestinal-type gastric carcinoma have been infected by ***H pylori***, which may be a co-factor for gastric cancer, acting either by stimulating the production of cellular mutagens or by inducing a high rate of proliferation following damage to the cells (J Nat Can Instit 1991; 83:640, N Engl J Med 1991; 325:1127, 1132, 1170ed); H pylori may be spread by intrafamilial contacts (N Engl J Med 1990; 322:359) and is increasingly implicated in duodenal ulcers which may respond to antibiotics

Heliotrope rash The classic rash seen on the face of patients with dermatomyositis, so named for its purplish hue, likened to that of the fragrant herb, ***Heliotropium peruvianum***

Helix-turn-helix motif Helix-loop-helix motif MOLECULAR BIOLOGY A group of 20-residue peptides characterized by two α helices separated by a non-helical segment, of nearly invariant geometry but with considerable amino acid sequence variation, which have conserved amino acid residues at the points of contact with the repressor-operator complexes (Science 1990; 247:1210); like other DNA-binding motifs, eg the Leucine zipper and Zinc finger, the helix-turn-helix configuration regulates gene expression by binding in the major and minor grooves of the DNA (Science 1988; 242:899); the motif occurs in the MyoD protein and myogenin (Cell 1990; 60:733)

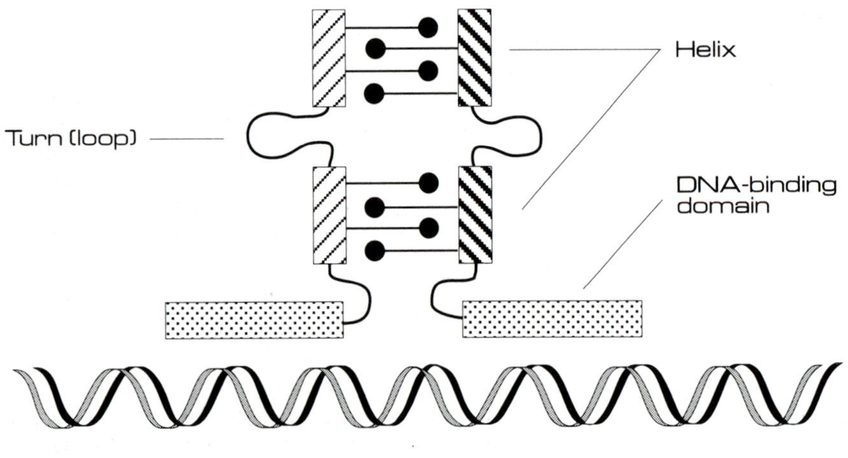

HELLP syndrome OBSTETRICS A clinical entity associated with eclampsia or severe pre-eclampsia, characterized by the acronym of Hemolysis, Elevated Liver function tests, Low Platelets, which may transiently worsen following delivery; other HELLP symptoms include blood pressure greater than 160 systolic and/or 110 diastolic, urinary volume less than 400 mL/24 hours, nonspecific cerebral abnormalities, pulmonary edema and/or cyanosis **Laboratory** Proteinuria greater than 5 g/24 hours, schistocytes (red cells that have been sheared and fragmented by intravascular fibrin deposition), increased liver function tests (ALA, AST, ALT, bilirubin), increased prothrombin time, partial thromboplastin time and fibrinogen levels are normal (Am J Obstet Gynecol 1982; 142:159

Helmet bodies Large compact, dense homogeneous, perinuclear inclusions in epithelial cells, surrounded by a mononuclear cell infiltrate (lymphocytes, plasma cells and macrophages), seen in mucocutaneous infections by ***Chlamydia*** species that may be identified by conjunctival scrapings stained with Romanovsky stain

Helmet cells see Schizocytes

Helmet field A radiotherapeutic field that covers parallel opposing lateral whole brain fields, reaching as low as C2 to include the meninges, of use in treating lymphoma of the central nervous system (CNS), either prophylactically (2400 cGy) or if the CNS is known to be involved (4000 cGy)

Helmet skull A fanciful descriptor for the cranial deformity seen in craniocarpotarsal dysplasia, characterized by brachycephaly, prominent forehead, hypertelorism and microstomia; other anomalies include bilateral hip dislocations and muscle wasting

Helmet vertebrae A descriptor for spondylosclerosis, which has a hemispherical 'dome' above the body proper, end-plate erosions, neo-osteogenesis and narrowing of the disk space caudad to the affected vertebra

Helper T cells Helper T lymphocytes A subset of T lymphocytes bearing the antigenic determinant CD4, which are presented with a foreign antigen in the context of both a self MHC class II antigen and IL-1; once immune recognition or response occurs, helper cells produce various cytokines, eg interferon-γ, IL-2 and osteoclast activating factor, which are critical in hematopoietic differentiation, collagen synthesis and antibody formation; see CD4, Flow cytometry, Suppressor cells, T cells

Helper:suppressor ratio IMMUNOLOGY The ratio of CD4 helper T-lymphocytes to CD8 suppressor T-lymphocytes, normally 1.5-2.0; in AIDS; this ratio is the single best monitor for clinical deterioration, where less than 0.5 is commonly seen and values of 0.1 or less presage fulminant clinical deterioration; the helper:suppressor ratio is also decreased in other conditions, including viral infections (cytomegalovirus, herpes, Epstein-Barr virus, measles), graft-versus-host disease, recuperation from bone marrow transplant, lupus erythematosus with renal involvement, exercise, severe sunburn, burns, myelodysplasia, acute lymphocytic leukemia in remission, sleep deprivation; the ratio is increased in atopic dermatitis, psoriasis, Sézary syndrome, chronic autoimmune hepatitis, primary biliary cirrhosis, rheumatoid arthritis, lupus erythematosus without renal involvement and insulin-dependent diabetes mellitus

Helsinki Declaration A document based on the Nuremburg Code of Ethics that offers recommendations for conducting experiments using human subjects that was adopted in 1962, revised by the 18th World Medical Assembly (WMA) in Helsinki in 1964, and subsequently re-revised in the 29th WMA in Tokyo in 1975; see Geneva Convention, Nuremburg Code of Ethics, Unethical research

Hemagglutination LABORATORY MEDICINE A serological test used to screen for the presence of various antigens Principle: A latex bead is coated with an antigen 'X' and coincubated with an antibody having a weak affinity for antigen 'X', but having a stronger affinity for the antigen X of interest; if X antigen is also present in the test serum, the linking antibody will preferably bind to X rather than 'X', thereby causing a non-agglutinating reaction, ie a positive reaction; a negative result appears as 'clumping' of the latex particles; hemagglutination is of use in a) Transfusion medicine for detecting antigens on the red cell's surface and b) Microbiology to identify hepatitis B virus, leptospirosis, rubella and others

Hemagglutination inhibition reaction LABORATORY MEDICINE An immune reaction in which antigen-bearing red cells are prevented fromagglutinating; this reaction is used to diagnose a) viral infections, including i) Exanthematous viruses (Rubella, rubeola, variola-vaccinia) ii) Herpesvirus (Herpes simplex, types 1 and 2, H zoster, cytomegalovirus and Epstein-Barr virus) iii) Respiratory viridiae (Adenovirus, coronavirus, influenza, mumps, parainfluenza) and iv) Togaviridiae (Eastern, St Louis, Venezuelan and Western equine encephalitides), b) Bacteria (***Neisseria gonorrhea, Streptococcus pneumoniae, Vibrio cholera, Rickettsiae***) and c) parasites

Hemagglutinin A protein that agglutinates erythrocytes VIROLOGY A glycoprotein located on the surface of a virus that has an intrinsic affinity for red cells, or other cells, eg respiratory epithelium at the receptors Hematology A hemagglutinin is an antibody that agglutinates erythrocytes, acting either at body temperature as 'warm hemagglutinins' or at subcorporal temperatures as 'cold hemagglutinins'

Hemangioblastoma An uncommon vascular tumor of the cerebellum, representing 2% of all central nervous system neoplasms, appearing in the third and fourth decades and seen alone or in association with von-Hippel-Lindau syndrome, pheochromocytoma, syringomyelia and erythrocythemia **Pathology** Grossly, the tumor is well-circumscribed, yellow-brown and hemorrhagic **Histopathology** Anastomosing network of capillaries and abundant plump stromal cells that are thought to represent the neoplastic component of the lesion **Treatment** Surgical **Prognosis** Good

Hemangiopericytoma A tumor of perivascular cells or pericytes appearing in the legs and retroperitoneum of adults; recurrence is common, one-half develop metastases **Histopathology** Jagged endothelial channels with 'staghorn'-like blood vessels, best seen when the tissue is stained for reticulin or by the periodic acid Schiff technique, which are variably surrounded by increased basement membrane **Differential diagnosis** Synovial sarcoma, mesenchymal chondrosarcoma, fibrous histiocytoma, rarely thymoma

Hemapheresis Apheresis The removal of whole blood from a donor or patient, followed by its separation into components, retention of certain components and return of the recombined remaining elements to the patient; Hemapheresis is a therapeutic modality for removing a) Leukocytes in hyperleukemic leukostasis with > 100 x 10^9/L blasts b) Platelets in thrombocytosis with > 1000 x 10^9/L platelets, if symptomatic c) Defective red cells and replacement by normal red cells as in sickle cell anemia with sickle cell crisis d) Immunoglobulins causing a hyperviscosity syndrome in macroglobulinemia or multiple myeloma e)autoantibody production in myasthenia gravis, Goodpasture syndrome, lupus erythematosus, factor VIII antibodies and f) Lipoproteins in patients with homozygous familial hypercholesterolemia (Am J Med 1990; 88:94); other conditions may occasionally benefit from hemapheresis, including allograft rejection, Guillain-Barre syndrome, hemolytic disease of the newborn, autoimmune hemolytic anemia, idiopathic thrombocytopenic purpura, post-transfusional purpura, glomerulonephritis (crescentic or rapidly progressive), Goodpasture's disease, HUS-TTP complex, intoxication from various agents and thyroid storm; the devices used in apheresis include those with intermittent flow and continuous flow; see Cytapheresis, Hemodialysis, Leukapheresis, Plasmapheresis

Hematin Brown granular crystals seen by light microscopy in tissue fixed by formalin that is too acidic or seen in fixed parasites that have ingested blood in vivo, thus also being known as malarial or schistosomal pigment; Cf Hematoidin

Hematochezia Passage of bright red or maroon stool, usually equal to blood; upper gastrointestinal tract hemorrhage resulting in hematochezia implies a blood loss of 1000 ml or more, often accompanied by hypovolemia, hypotension and tachycardia, while lower gastrointestinal or rectal hemorrhage may be guaiac-positive with as little as 25 ml, ie the blood is a brighter red when it is more caudal

Hematoidin A golden-yellow pigment chemically identical to bilirubin formed in tissues from hemoglobin under conditions of reduced oxygen

Hematopoietin see Interleukin-3

Hematoxylin HISTOLOGY A natural dye derived from logwood (***Hematoxylin campechianum***), that was the first major stain used to examine tissues by light microscopy, which continues to be the major 'workhorse' stain in histopathology, staining nuclei and calcium-bearing material a blue-purple color; hematoxylin is usually used in conjunction with eosin, the so-called counterstain, which stains other tissues and cell components varying shades of pink

Hematoxylin bodies RHEUMATOLOGY A pathognomonic finding of lupus erythematosus characterized as homogeneous globular masses of nucleic material containing nucleoproteins, DNA and anti-DNA; these structures are blue-purple when stained with hematoxylin and may be seen in the atrial endocardium, kidneys, lungs, spleen, lymph nodes, serous membranes and synovium; hematoxylin bodies are less common in fulminant cases of lupus erythematosus and represent the tissue equivalent of the LE cell Note: LE cells have also been described in chronic active hepatitis, rheumatoid arthritis and in Sjögren syndrome

Hemiballism NEUROLOGY A form of secondary chorea characterized by violent flinging movements of the limbs of one body half, often due to hemorrhage or infarction, rarely tumors of the contralateral subthalamic nucleus, developing after recovery from a stroke-induced hemiparesis and hemisensory defect; hemiballism (like other abnormal involuntary movements) disappears during sleep; in the usual scenario, hemiballism fades to hemichorea and finally extinction as the weeks pass Treatment Persistent hemiballism may respond to reserpin or antipsychotics

Hemi '3' syndrome A form of hemihypertrophy occurring in females, possibly related to neural tube defects characterized by unilateral musculoskeletal hypertrophy, hyperesthesia, areflexia and progressive scoliosis

Hemihypertrophy Hemimacrosomia A unilateral increase in some or all paired organs or tissues of the body; hemihypertrophy may be idiopathic, possibly related to neural, vascular, lymphatic, endocrine or chromosomal abnormalities and may occur in the Curtius syndrome, Klippel-Trenaunay syndrome and Silver-Russel syndrome and in hepatoblastoma

Hemivertebra A congenital vertebral body deformity arising from a simple, ie nondysplastic, nonmetabolic embryonal defect, in which the anterior half of a vertebral body is absent and adjacent vertebrae expand attempting to fill the vacated space, accompanied by preservation of the interspaces; Cf Butterfly vertebra

Hemlock Any of a family of poisonous herbs of the carrot family; in particular, ***Conium maculatum***, contains the alkaloid conine that first produces central nervous system hyperactivity, followed by medullary depression and respiratory failure Treatment Activated charcoal Note: Socrates died from hemlock in 399 BC when he was tried and convicted for corrupting Athenian youth, two of whom, Alcibiades and Critias, betrayed Athens

Hemlock society see Euthanasia

Hemochromatosis An autosomal recessive (homozygous frequency 0.0045 gene frequency of 0.067, N Engl J Med 1988; 318:1355) excess of gastrointestinal iron absorption with progressive iron loading in parenchymal organs, the gene for which is linked to the HLA locus on the short arm of chromosome 6 Clinical Cardiomegaly, 300-fold more common, cirrhosis is 13-fold more common (once cirrhosis occurs, there is a 200-fold increase in hepatocellular carcinoma), gray-bronze skin pigmentation and diabetes mellitus with a 7-fold increase, 'bronze diabetes', arthropathy and hypogonadism (impotence, testicular atrophy) Laboratory Transferrin saturation of greater than 62% warrants a 'workup' Note: Other metals may accumulate in hemochromatosis, eg copper, lead, molybdenum (Am J Med 1991; 90:445rv, Am J Med Sci 1991; 301:47)

Hemochromatosis triad Troisier-Hanot-Chauffard 'syndrome' Hepatomegaly, diabetes mellitus and skin pigmentation that occurs in hemochromatosis, due to deposition of iron pigment that may also deposit in pancreas, heart, pituitary, glands (adrenal, parathyroid and thyroid), joints and skin

Hemodialysis A therapeutic procedure for removing small molecular weight toxins by allowing the blood to flow adjacent to a semipermeable membrane where the toxins diffuse away from the blood down a concentration gradient; hemodialysis is used in renal failure to reduce BUN, creatinine, hyperkalemia and correct metabolic acidosis; prolonged dialysis is associated with poor quality of life with anemia, frequent infections, myalgia, peripheral neuropathy, cerebral edema, myocardial infarcts, aluminum toxicity (see Dialysis dementia); therefore, renal transplantation is always the preferred long-term therapeutic modality Note: The attempt to reduce the dialysis time to less than 3.5 hours is associated with increased mortality (relative risk 1.17 to 2.18, J Am Med Assoc 1991; 265:871) Complications Pyogenic reactions due to gram-negative bacterial endotoxemia, with chills, fever, hypotension, nausea and myalgia, depressed natural killer cell activity, decreased serum calcitriol; Cf Hemapheresis

Hemoflagellates PARASITOLOGY Flagellated parasites of the Kinetoplastidea family, characterized by kinetoplasts which are composed of mitochondrial DNA; hemoflagellates of human importance include ***Leishmania, Trypanosoma, Leptomonas*** and ***Crithidia*** species

Hemoglobin A tetrameric protein composed of two α chains, each 141 amino acids in length, encoded from the zeta chain gene on chromosome 16 and two β chains, each 144 amino acids in length, encoded from the contiguous eta, Gγ, Aγ and delta chain genes on chromosome 11; while the more common hemoglobin defects, eg HbS, HbC and the thalassemias, cause a characteristic clinical picture, 'rare hemoglobin variants are variously ignored, misunderstood, misdiagnosed, feared, shunned or rejected...' (Mayo Clin Proc 1990; 65:889ed) Hemoglobin (Hb) nomenclature The first Hb described was HbA (normal Hb); HbB was proposed for sickle cell hemoglobin (but never assigned, as HbS was considered more euphonic); abnormal Hbs subsequently recognized in the 1950s were designated HbC, HbD, HbE, HbF (fetal Hb), HbG, HbH, HbI and HbJ, based on migrations on zone (paper) electrophoresis, a practice that stopped when more specific methods became available (Nature 1956; 178:792); hemoglobin variants subsequently received geographic names or names of cities, a practice that continues, with the disadvantage that some cities have up to four different Hbs and identical Hbs may be discovered in two different cities (Mayo Clin Proc 1990; 65:889ed); most hemoglobinopathies are due to a single base substitution, eg a point mutation; as of early 1990, there were 119 α, 225 β, 32 γ and 14δ chain variants that are divided into a) Fusion hemoglobinopathies, eg Hb Constant Spring and Lepore b) Chain with longer than normal hemoglobin chains as translation continues beyond the termination codon or

c) Shorter than normal hemoglobin chains as translation stops prior to the termination codon, all three of which may be due to point mutations, frame shifts and insertions **Clinical** a) Sickling phenotypes, eg HbS, HbSC, HbS-Thalassemia b) Thalassemic phenotypes, eg Constant Spring, HbE, Lepore, Kenya, Vicksburg, Indianapolis c) Low oxygen affinity hemoglobins, eg Bristol, Bucuresti/Louisville, Caribbean, Etobicoke, Hammersmith, Moscva, Okaloosa, Peterborough, Seattle, Torino d) High oxygen affinity hemoglobins, eg Altdorf, Istanbul, Baylor, Belfast, Boras, Buenos Aires, Cranston, Duarte, Djelfa, Freiburg, Geneva, Hopkins II, Koln, Lyon, Niteroi, Nottingham, Pasadena, Sabine, Santa Ana, St Louis, Shepherds Bush, Tak, Tours, Toyoake, Tübingen, Zürich and e) Unstable hemoglobins

Hemoglobin A_{1c} see Advanced glycosylated endproducts, Glycosylated hemoglobin

HEMOLYSIS

Intracorpuscular hemolysis

a) Membrane defects, eg hereditary elliptocytosis, spherocytosis, stomatocytosis and paroxysmal nocturnal hemoglobinuria

b) Metabolic defects, eg G6PD, pyruvate kinase deficiency

c) Abnormal hemoglobins see Hemoglobin

Extracorpuscular hemolysis

a) Immune reactions, primary, eg autoimmune hemolytic anemia

b) Immune reactions, secondary, due to

i) Infections, eg Bartonella, Clostridia, malaria, sepsis

ii) Neoplasia, eg lymphoma, leukemias

iii) Drug reactions due to the 'innocent bystander' phenomenon (drug-antibody complex activates complement, causing intravascular hemolysis, eg quinidine), hapten-mediated (a protein-bound drug attaches to the red cell membrane, eliciting an immune response when the 'signature' of the hapten-protein complex is recognized as foreign, as occurs when penicillin acts as a hapten

iv) Induction of autoimmunity by red cells antigen alterations, eg Rh antigen

c) Physical, eg Thermal, high concentrations of glycerol (inadequate washing of frozen blood), bladder irrigation, cardiac valves

Hemolysis Lysis of erythrocytes (table) may be immune-mediated or non-immune-mediated, due to defects intrinsic or extrinsic to the erythrocyte Clinical types of hemolysis: Immune hemolysis may be a) Intravascular and is often more severe, IgM-mediated and requires complement activation, eg ABO blood groups **Laboratory** Increased free hemoglobin or b) Extravascular hemolysis is less severe, IgG-mediated and does not activate complement, eg Rh, Kell, Duffy Note: Clinically significant hemolysis is usually detected by hemagglutination, less commonly by hemolysis, which detects anti-P, -P_1, -PP_1P^k, -Jk^a, -Le^a, occasionally also anti-Le^b and -Vel **Laboratory** Decreased haptoglobin, decreased half-life of circulating red cells, increased indirect bilirubin as the hepatic capacity to conjugate bilirubin (forming direct bilirubin) may be overwhelmed if the hemolysis is massive, increased lactate dehydrogenase, hemoglobin in blood and urine, hemosiderinuria, methemoglobin and metalbumin, increased urobilinogen in urine and feces MICROBIOLOGY Hemolysis is characteristic of certain strains of streptococci and is divided into α- and β-hemolysis; γ 'hemolysis' is a complete misnomer

Hemolytic disease of the newborn (HDN) A hemolytic condition due to the incompatibility of fetal red cells with the maternal immune system, caused by the production of maternal IgG antibodies in response to the fetal erythrocytes that innocently enter the maternal circulation; if the IgG response and the sharing of circulations (as in low-grade feto-maternal hemorrhage) is intense, erythroblastosis fetalis occurs; the most intense HDN occurs in incompatabilities of the RhD blood group antigen, which is responsible for 70% of all HDN; within the Rh group, anti-D causes 93% of anti-Rh reactions and anti-DC, -E, -Ce cause the remainder; Rh-induced HDN is reported in 11/10 000 births, but this figure is thought to be an underestimate of the actual incidence (J Am Med Assoc 1991; 265:3270); routine screening for only anti-RhD and -D^u, causes a proportionate increase in anti-C, -c, E and -e related Rh disease, see RhIG; two other red cell antibodies potentially requiring exchange transfusions are anti-Fy^a and Kell Frequencies of HDN: ABO (mild, transient) > Rh-D > Rh-c > Rh-E > K (Kell); rarely incriminated in HDN are anti-PP_1, -Be^a, -K, -k, -Kp^a, -M, -S, -s, -U, -FAR, Mt^a, Js^a, Js^b, Jk^a, -Jk^b, -Fy^b, -Fy_3, Mv, -Lu^a, Di^a, -Di^{bm}, Yt^a, -Do^a, -Wr^a, -Jr^a, Cs^a; HDN has not been described due to anti-Le^a, -Le^b and anti-P_1 antibodies, as these are IgM and do not pass to the placenta; the serum half-life of IgG is 20-25 days and significant amounts of maternal immunoglobulin remain in the infant's circulation for up to 3 months after birth **Clinical** see Hydrops fetalis **Pathology** Placenta Large, edematous with immature red cells, lipid-laden pink Hofbauer cells in the stroma of the villi Basal ganglia kernicterus **Laboratory** 'Panic' values of bilirubin are 16-20 mg/dl of indirect bilirubin; the immaturity of the blood-brain barrier allows penetration of bilirubin and deposition on the basal ganglia; in utero antibody titers above 1/32 may presage a difficult recovery period

Hemolytic-uremic syndrome A clinical complex that affects children under the age of two, often accompanied by a prodrome of bloody diarrhea, most commonly occurring in the summer and microangiopathic hemolytic anemia, thrombocytopenia and platelet abnormalities **Laboratory** Impaired aggregation, depletion of platelet serotonin, ADP and β-thromboglobulin **Histopathology** Renal arteries occluded by fibrin thrombi in the interlobular arteries, afferent arterioles and capillaries, widespread cortical necrosis, that may also involve the liver, brain, heart, islet cells and muscle **Pathogenesis** Uncertain, *Escherichia coli* O157:H7, which produces a 'verotoxin' has been implicated and in one enteric nursing home outbreak, 50% died Note Hemolytic-uremic syndrome (HUS) has been re-interpreted as a polar form of a clinical spectrum, at the other end of which is thrombotic thrombocytopenic purpura, see TTP-HUS

Etiology, hemolytic-uremic syndrome

1) Prototypic or 'classic' form
2) Post-infectious, eg *Shigella dysenteriae*-1, *Streptococcus pneumoniae*, *Salmonella typhi*, occasionally viruses
3) Hereditary forms: Autosomal dominant, or autosomal recessive associated with hypertension
4) Immune-mediated forms
5) Associated with other diseases, eg hypertension, connective tissue disease, immunosuppression or radiotherapy to kidneys
6) Related to pregnancy and oral contraceptives

Hemophilus influenza vaccine see Hib

Hemorrhagic disease of the newborn A neonatal condition caused by vitamin K deficiency, the combined result of a lack of unbound maternal vitamin K, immaturity of the fetal liver and lack of vitamin K-producing bacteria in the infant colon **Clinical** Abrupt early post-partum onset with spontaneous nasogastric or intracranial hemorrhage, affecting up to 1/1000 neonates and carrying a 5-30% mortality, if untreated; the condition is thought to be more common in breast-fed infants and is more severe and of earlier onset in infants of mothers receiving anticonvulsives (antagonistic to warfarin) during pregnancy **Laboratory** Increased prothrombin time due to extrinsic factor depletion, inceased clotting time, decreased liver-dependent coagulation factors

Hemorrhagic fever with renal syndrome see Korean hemorrhagic fever

Hemosiderosis An iron overload syndrome that is arbitrarily differentiated from hemochromatosis by the reversible nature of this accumulation in the reticuloendothelial system

Hemostatic plug After tissue trauma and rupture of vessels, the platelets fill the gap, forming a plug; formation of a 'hemostatic plug' is an orderly process divided into stages, a) Adhesion After tissue injury, collagen and basement membrane are exposed and serve as signals for platelets to 'huddle' about the open vessel, b) Release Platelets come in contact with collagen and are stimulated to release thrombin, epinephrine and ADP, releasing their granular contact, c) Aggregation ADP is released, promoting platelet aggregation that becomes irreversible as local ADP concentrations rise above 2 X 10^{-6}M, d) Fusion Fibrin, thrombin, ADP and Thromboxane A_2 cause coalescence of the plug, e) Clot retraction Fibrin threads contract, squeezing out the liquid caught in the meshwork

HEMPAS Hereditary erythrocytic multinuclearity with positive acidified serum lysis Congenital dyserythropoietic anemia, type II An autosomal recessive condition characterized by an IgM autoantibody directed against the red cell membrane i antigen ('anti-HEMPAS'), present in 1/3 of normal sera **Clinical** Mild or subclinical congenital dyserythropoietic anemia Laboratory Normocytic aniso-poikilocytosis and multinucleated erythroblasts; increased agglutinability of serum with anti-i antibodies Note: A positive acidified serum lysis test may be seen in paroxysmal nocturnal hemoglobinuria **Treatment** None; splenectomy partially beneficial; see CDA

Hepadnaviridiae A recently formed family of small DNA viruses with a circular genome that includes hepatitis B and hepatitis D (delta agent); Cf HHV

Heparin A 4-30 kD, heavily-sulfated glycosaminoglycan anticoagulant that inhibits activated factors IXa, Xa, XIa, XIIa and thrombin, decreasing local anti-thrombin-III, promoting its inactivation by neutrophil elastase; the interaction of heparin with endothelial cells results in the displacement of platelet factor 4, which in turn inactivates heparin; heparin therapy is indicated for venous thromboembolism, coronary artery disease, after myocardial infarction (12 500 U bid) and pulmonary thromboembolism (10-15 000 U sid); heparinization is monitored by measuring activated partial thromboplastin time (aPTT), titrating heparin levels so that the aPTT is 1.5-2.0 X normal **Side effects** Hemorrhage, thrombocytopenia, osteoporosis, skin necrosis, alopecia, hypersensitivity, hypoaldosteronism (N Engl J Med 1991; 324:1565rv)

Heparin-associated thrombocytopenia (HAT) Heparin-induced thrombocytopenia and/or thrombosis (HITT) An acquired thrombocytopenia affecting 1% of heparin-treated patients, induced by heparin-dependent antibodies to endothelial-bound heparin; HAT-like phenomena may occur in heroin addicts, in whom an IgG antibody induces thromboxane synthesis and platelet aggregation

Heparin-binding fibroblast growth factor(s) A family of seven related gene products with a broad range of biological activities including stimulation and inhibition of proliferative and secretory functions in hepatocytes (Science 1991; 251:665); see Pleitrophin

Heparin cofactor II (HC II) A 66 kD protein produced in the liver which, like antithrombin III (heparin cofactor I), neutralizes thrombin and chymotrypsin but not factor Xa or other coagulation factors and its activity is accelerated by dermatan sulfate and heparin; HC-II deficiency is associated with thromboembolic disease and reduced in cirrhosis and disseminated intravascular coagulation

Hepar lobatum A deformed lobated liver described in the currently rare end-stage tertiary syphilis **Histopathology** Broad bands of fibrotic scar tissue coalesce and bridge poorly-healed small and large gummata, alternating with nodules and masses of well-normal preserved parenchyma, mimicking macronodular cirrhosis Note: Arsenic, the preantibiotic therapy for syphilis caused massive hepatic necrosis and obstructive cholangitis

Hepatic panel see Liver panel

Hepatic rickets Vitamin D-deficient rickets due to reduced bile salt secretion, resulting from inadequate absorption of fat-soluble vitamins, seen in extrahepatic biliary atresia, neonatal hepatitis and injury induced by parenteral nutrition, see Total parenteral nutrition Laboratory Reduced vitamin 25(OH)D, reduced calcium, increased alkaline phosphatase

Hepatitis A generic term for any hepatic inflammatory process, most often by viral hepatitis A and B; hepatitis A is usually acquired through the oral-fecal route, has a shorter incubation period and is rarely associated with long-term morbidity; hepatitis B is usually acquired through parenteral contact, has a longer incubation period and is linked pathogenically to hepatocellular carcinoma; other viral hepatitides include hepatitis non-A, non-B (many of which are considered hepatitis C, hepatitis D (delta agent), hepatitis E, infectious mononucleosis, Epstein-Barr virus, cytomegalovirus, herpesvirus, measles, mumps, Coxsackievirus, rubella, rubeola, bacteria, parasites and fungi Non-infectious hepatitides may be induced by hyperthermia, radiation, alcohol, toxins Clinical Anorexia, nausea, vomiting, malaise, jaundice, myalgia, arthralgia, photophobia and bleeding diathesis Laboratory Increased transaminases (ALA, AST, GGT), bilirubin and immunoglobulins (specific if hepatitis is infectious) and decreased vitamin K-dependent coagulation factors, ergo prolonged prothrombin time

Hepatitis B MOLECULAR BIOLOGY Hepatitis B is a small DNA virus with four open reading frames: S gene encodes HbsAg, P gene encodes a DNA polymerase, an X gene and the core gene that encodes HBcAg and the pre-core region which encodes HBeAg; patients with fulminant hepatitis B have a point mutation that results in a stop codon in the pre-core region, implicating a mutant virus in non-self-limited hepatitis B (N Engl J Med 1991; 324:1699, 1705) SEROLOGY see Hepatitis immunopathology panel

Hepatitis B vaccine(s) Of the hepatitis B vaccines that became available during the 1980s, the human plasma-derived hepatitis B vaccine (Heptavax-B) proved unpopular, attributed in part to 'AIDS-phobia' and is no longer used; the yeast (***Saccharomyces cervesiae***)-derived recombinant DNA vaccine, (RecombivaxTM) has reported protective levels of close to 100% and those who do not respond initially may respond with intradermal vaccination

Hepatitis B virus protein X see HBx

Hepatitis C The agent(s) responsible for most transfusion-induced hepatitides, which may play a role in the pathogenesis of hepatocellular carcinoma (J Am Med Assoc 1991; 265:1974); the complementary DNA for hepatitis C was used to develop an RIA-based immunoassay for HCV antibodies, which detects one-half of cases, despite the prolonged HBC 'window' period; patients receiving HBC-positive blood products have a 20-fold greater incidence of non-A, non-B hepatitis (NANBH) (Lancet 1990; 335:558); during the early or window period of primary HCV infection, the only evidence of disease may be HCV RNA in the serum; disappearance of HCV RNA from the serum correlates with the resolution of NANBH (N Engl J Med 1991; 325:98) Note: Not all patients with NANBH have antibodies to C100-3, a commercial marker for hepatitis C, therefore the incidence of hepatitis C is underestimated (Lancet 1990; 335:1) Treatment Interferon α appears to suppress the fibrosis induced by transforming growth factor (TGF-β1) that is typical of hepatitis C which could eventuate in cirrhosis in these patients (N Engl J Med 1991; 324:933) Note: Many cases of NANBH hepatitis are due to hepatitis C and there is considerable overlap between the two conditions, although they are not synonymous; see Hepatitis non-A, non-B

Hepatitis D virus see Delta hepatitis

Hepatitis E virus HEV Enteric non-A, non-B hepatitis A virus with a highly conserved single-stranded RNA transmitted by the oral-fecal route and implicated in major epidemics where sanitation is poor, the drinking water contaminated and the population malnourished (Science 1990; 247:1271)

'Hepatitis', giant cell neonatal see Giant cell hepatitis

Hepatitis, non-A, non-B (NANBH) The major cause of transfusion-related hepatitis; incidence, 7/10^5/year, USA NANBH risk factors: 42% intravenous drug abuse, 40% no known risk factors, 6% sexual contact, 6% blood transfusion, 3% household contact, 2% health professional (J Am Med Assoc 1990; 264:2231); of the estimated 150 000 annual cases in the US, 30-50% become chronic carriers and 20% of these develop cirrhosis; NANBH may also rarely be epidemically transmitted (J Am Med Assoc 1990; 263:3281); NANBH comprises a group of not fully characterized hepatitides; in general, parenteral NANBH is most commonly hepatitis C and enteric NANBH is hepatitis E; testing blood for antibodies to HCV is part of the battery of tests used in screening of blood to reduce NANBH, since about one-half of transfusion-related NANBH is associated with antibodies to hepatitis C virus (J Am Med Assoc 1990; 263:77), many of the remainder are in 'window' period for hepatitis C; this screen reduces the false positivity due to non-specific ALT elevation (ibid, 263:49)

Hepatitis (immunopathology) panel A battery of tests that are the most efficient, ie cost-effective, in the evaluation of the clinical and immune status of a person thought to have hepatitis; the acute hepatitis panel includes hepatitis B surface antigen (HBsAg), anti-hepatitis B surface antigen (anti-HBs), antibody to hepatitis B core antigen (anti-HBc), anti-HBe, anti-hepatitis A (IgM) and anti-hepatitis C; the chronic hepatitis (carrier) panel includes the above but not the anti-hepatitis A assay; Cf Organ panels

Hepatitis serology Hepatitis B serological markers LABORATORY MEDICINE A generic term that refers to the hepatitis B antigens and antibodies to these antigens Core antigen (HBc) The HBc particle contains double-stranded DNA and DNA polymerase, is associated with the HBe antigen, but is not directly detected by currently-used assays; the presence of core antigen indicates persistently replicating hepatitis B virus, and antibody to Hbc is a long-term serologic marker for hepatitis B, rising early and detectable as an IgM antibody, remaining detectable up to 20 years after infection, especially in those with active liver disease; partially protective anti-HBc antibody levels can be induced by recombinant vaccination (Heptavax), but are short-lived; the IgM anti-HBc is the single best serological marker for acute hepatitis B; HB e antigen(HBe) rises and falls parallel to HBsAg, derives from the proteolytic cleavage of the nucleocapsid, and its presence implies a carrier state; anti-HBe rises as HBe falls, appearing in convalescent patients, persisting for up to several years after resolution of hepatitis; surface antigen (HBs) is the first marker to appear after hepatitis B infection, preceding clinical disease by weeks, peaking with the onset of symptoms and disappearing six months post-infection; anti-HBs (antibody to surface antigen) begins to rise as the HBsAg falls and may persist for life

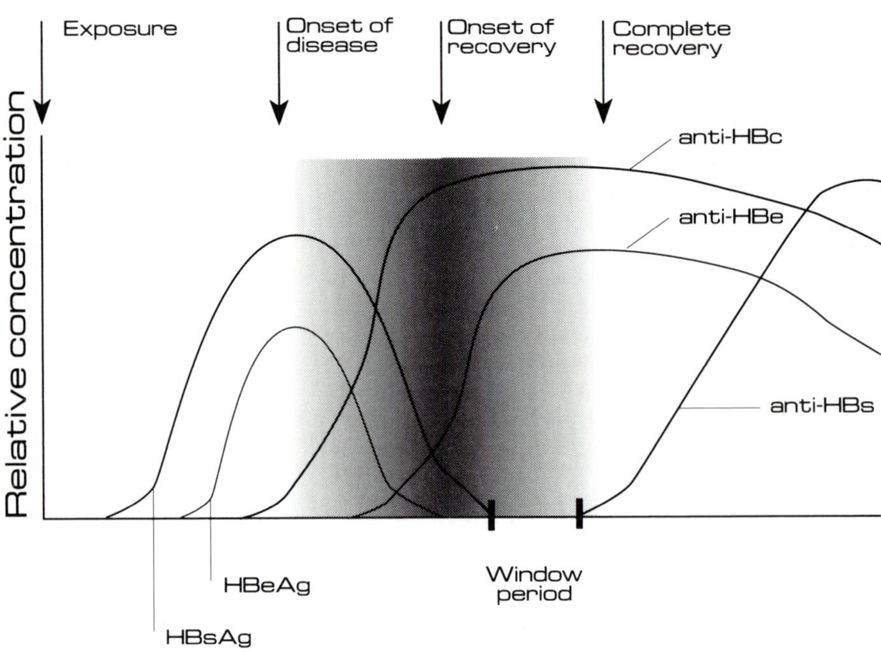

Hepatitis B serology

'Hepatization' An acquired firmness of the lungs, commonly seen in lobar pneumonia, especially that caused by ***Streptococcus pneumoniae*** types 1, 3, 7 and 2, as well as other streptococci, ***Klebsiella*** species, staphylococci and gram-negative rods, occurring in the elderly and infants; in healthy adults lobar pneumonia is largely of historic interest that has been classically divided into Stage 1 Congestion Stage 2 Red hepatization occurs in early lobar pneumonia and is characterized by hemorrhage, fibrin accumulation and neutrophils within alveoli and fibrinopurulent pleural exudate Stage 3 Gray hepatization occurs before the first week, representing early resolution with leukocytes, indurated fibrinopurulent exudate and rare erythrocytes; the pleural surface is gray, dull and granular Stage 4 Resolution occurs after the first week

Hepatoblastoma A malignant hepatic tumor almost exclusively found in infants that may be associated with hemihypertrophy, Wilm's tumor and glycogen storage disease Diagnosis Hepatic angiography, computed tomography, elevated α-fetoprotein and ectopic hormone production Pathology The tumors are single, solid, well-circumscribed Histopathology Immature hepatocytic, fetal, embryonal, macrotrabecular or mixed patterns Prognosis Better than hepatocellular carcinoma Treatment Surgery and adjunctive chemotherapy

Hepatoma Hepatocellular carcinoma

Hepatocyte growth factor (HGF) A plasminogen-like protein that is thought to act as a humoral mediator of hepatic regeneration; the HGF receptor is the protein product of the c-met proto-oncogene (Science 1991; 251:802)

Hepatorenal syndrome A condition characterized by renal dysfunction without renal pathology, caused by a combination of decreased renal perfusion, hypovolemia and hyperaldosteronism, secondary to liver disease including acute liver failure due to cirrhosis, acute fatty liver, hepatic failure, obstructive jaundice, sepsis and infectious hepatitides Note: Kidneys from these patients may be used for transplantation; membranous nephropathy occurs in hepatitis B; one-third relentlessly deteriorate (N Engl J Med 1991; 324:1457); Cf Cirrhotic glomerulonephritis

HEPES N-2-Hydroxyethylpiperazine-N'-ethanesulfonic acid An agent used to prepare biological buffers between pH 6.8 and 8.2

HER-2/*neu* An oncogene of the ***erb*B** oncogene family, which is related to epidermal growth factor; HER-2 is amplified 2-20 fold in one-third of breast carcinomas and is associated with decreased survival and shortened time to relapse Note: The prognosis of breast carcinomas is best predicted based on tumor size, number of lymph nodes involved and estrogen and progesterone receptor status

Herald bleed An episode of hemorrhage, often accompanied by abdominal pain, preceding by hours to weeks a catastrophic hemorrhage; herald bleeds are characteristic of arterial-enteric fistulas with false aneurysms, often at the site of the proximal anastomosis of a prosthetic graft of the abdominal aorta

Herald patch DERMATOLOGY A typical early lesion of pityriasis rosea that appears as a solitary oval, 1-10 cm annular macule with raised border and fine, adherent scales, preceding by 7-10 days the other lesions, which are multiple, smaller, a dull red color and distributed along the lines of cleavage of the trunk in a Christmas tree or chevron fashion Differential diagnosis Contact dermatitis, impetigo, secondary syphilis, psoriasis and tinea corporis

Herald state of leukemia A term referring to the nonspecific manifestations of dyshematopoiesis that precede the onset of acute myelogenous leukemia, including anemia, which may be accompanied by weakness and pallor, malaise, exertional dyspnea and fever unrelated to infections

Herald wave phenomenon EPIDEMIOLOGY The finding that the strains of influenza virus present in a population at the end of one season's epidemic are the same strains responsible for the next season's influenza syndromes

Herbal medicine see Holistic medicine, Homeopathy, Unproven cancer therapy

Herbal tea An infusion made from a plant not containing caffeine may be purported to have beneficial effect(s) on one or more organ systems for various conditions; some plants have toxic as well as tonic effects, affecting the cardiovascular, gastrointestinal, hematologic and nervous systems CHAMOMILE Anaphylactic shock, contact dermatitis COMFREY Veno-occlusive disease, hepatic failure, possible hepatic carcinogen FOXGLOVE (***Digitalis purpurea***) Malignant arrhythmia, cardiac arrest JIMSONWEED Atropinic and hallucinogenic effects, central nervous system intoxication, ataxia, blurred vision MANDRAKE Scopolaminic effect with anticholinergic blockade MATE Veno-occlusive disease with possibe hepatic failure POKE ROOT High saponin content causes gastroenteritis, bloody diarrhea POKEWEED Respiratory depression, mitogenic effects SASSAFRAS Hepatic carcinogen SNAKEROOT Reserpinic effect, causing central nervous system intoxication (Arch Environ Health 1987; 42:133); see Holistic medicine, Natural food, Organic food

Hereditary cancer syndrome(s) A group of often autosomal dominant entities characterized by tumors that are often site-specific, of early onset and multiple and/or bilateral; these conditions include nevoid basal cell carcinoma syndrome, dysplastic nevus (B-K mole) syndrome, Cowden syndrome, familial polyposis, Gardner syndrome, Gorlin syndrome, Li-Fraumeni syndrome, multiple endocrine neoplasia, type I and II (MEN I & II); see Hereditary neoplasms, Hereditary preneoplasia

Hereditary motor and sensory neuropathy (HMSN) A group of conditions dignified by eponym and subdivided into TYPE I CHARCOT-MARIE-TOOTH DISEASE, hypertrophic form An autosomal dominant condition that is the most common form of HMSN, characterized by a slowly progressive disease of childhood onset with predominantly motor symptoms, pes cavus, calf atrophy, very slow motor impulse conduction with segmental demyelination and remyelination with 'onion-bulb' formation TYPE II CHARCOT-MARIE-TOOTH DISEASE, neuronal form or Roussy-Levy syndrome An autosomal dominant condition characterized by slowly progressive disease of adolescent onset with predominantly motor symptoms, clubfoot deformity, calf atrophy, mild reduction in impulse transmission and 'onion-bulb' formation TYPE III DEJERINE-SOTTAS DISEASE A rare relentlessly progressive autosomal recessive condition of infant onset with short stature, scoliosis, pes cavus, calf atrophy, very slow conduction of motor impulses with segmental demyelination and remyelination 'onion-bulb' formation; see Hereditary sensory neuropathy

Hereditary neoplasms Chemodectomas, medullary carcinoma of the thyroid, neurofibroma, pheochromocytoma, polyposis coli, retinoblastoma, trichoepithelioma; other tumors may occur more frequently in certain families, including leukemia and melanoma

Hereditary neutrophilia A rare benign autosomal dominant condition characterized by lifelong neutrophilia, hepatosplenomegaly, pseudo-Gaucher cells, thickened calvaria, increased leukocyte alkaline phosphatase (LAP score), increased vitamin B_{12} (Am J Med 1974; 56:729)

Hereditary persistence of fetal hemoglobin see HPFH

Hereditary pyropoikilocytosis (HP) HEMATOLOGY A rare congenital hemolytic condition that is most common in blacks caused by impaired self-assembly of the spectrin tetramer in the red cell membrane, withmore ; there are more dimers and defective forms and fewer multimers, resulting in increased membrane instability and susceptibility to thermolysis, occurring at circa 45°C, which in normal red cells occurs at 49°C; HP may represent a variant of hereditary elliptocytosis **Laboratory** Anisocytes, elliptocytes, poikilocytes, schistocytes, microspherocytes and polychromasia, findings that resemble the peripheral blood smears in burn patients (Br J Haematol 1975; 29:537)

Hereditary preneoplasia Neoplasms that arise in the context of an underlying syndrome, including phakomatoses, eg Cowden's disease, multiple exostoses, Peutz-Jegher syndrome, von Hippel-Lindau syndrome, neurofibromatosis, tuberous sclerosis, genodermatoses, eg albinism, dyskeratosis congenita, epidermodysplasia verruciformis, polydysplastic epidermolysis bullosa, Werner syndrome, xeroderma pigmentosa, chromosome instability syndromes and immune deficiencies, eg ataxia-telangiectasia, common variable immunodeficiency, Wiskott-Aldrich syndrome, X-linked aγglobulinemia and X-linked lymphoproliferative syndrome; see Cancer families; Cf One-hit, two-hit model

Hereditary sensory neuropathies (HSM) A group of diseases with chronic pain, skin ulcers due to hypoesthesia, dyskinesia, autonomic dysregulation, loss of pain, touch-pressure and temperature sensations, affecting the small nerves with degeneration of large myelinated nerves HSM type I Autosomal dominant and characterized by perforating foot ulcers HSM type II is autosomal recessive, early onset of mutilating ulcers, sensory loss and loss of tendon reflexes HSM type III (Riley-Day disease) is autosomal recessive, affecting Jewish children, causing autonomic dysfunction, xerophthalmia, loss of temperature control, skin blotching, diaphoresis, hypertension, postural hypotension, pain insensitivity, poor feeding, vomiting, lung infections and early death, possibly related to defective nerve growth factor; see Hereditary motor and sensory neuropathy

Hereditary transmission EPIDEMIOLOGY The maintenance

of an infection, usually viral, within the insect vector population through transovarial transmission; Cf Horizontal transmission, Vertical transmission

Heritability The likelihood of suffering from a hereditary disease when the defective gene is in the patient's gene pool

Hermaphroditic flukes Sexually self-contained worms that in humans may migrate and flourish in the a) Hepatobiliary tract, eg *Clonorchis sinensis, Dicrocoelium dentriticum, Fasciola hepatica, Metorchis conjunctus, Opisthorchis* species b) Intestine, eg *Echinostoma ilocanum, Fasciolopsis buski, Gastrodiscoides hominis, Heterophyes heterophyes, Metagonimus yokogawai* c) Lung, eg *Paragonimus westermani, P skrjabani* and d) Systemically, eg *Alaria americana*

Hermaphroditism A clinicopathological nosology with both testicular tissue, ie seminiferous tubules and ovarian tissue, ie follicular structures within the same organ yielding an 'ovotestis', in which the tissues are arranged end-to-end and may be accompanied by a left-sided ovary and a right-sided testis; 60% of patients are 46 XX, 12% 46 XY, the remainder are mozaics **Clinical** Most true hermaphrodites have asymmetrical external genitalia, eg labioscrotal folds; phenotypic males may have gynecomastia, phenotypic females may be amenorrheic or have successful gestation; 2.6% develop germ cell tumors; Cf Pseudohermaphroditism

Herniated disk 'syndrome' An acquired condition most commonly affecting active middle-aged adults, classically occurring after a minor trauma or tortion stress of the vertebral column, punctuated by the sensation of a 'snap', which corresponds to a prolapse of the nucleus pulposus into the nerve roots or spinal cord, causing progressive and distal radiation of pain; the backache subsides as the sciatica 'syndrome' develops with its sensorimotor consequences

'Heroic' therapy Aggressive treatment of an often malignant disease that is regarded by a patient's care-givers as incurable with standard treatment at usual and prudent doses of toxic drugs; heroic surgery infers wider than normal resective margins, as a malignancy has spread beyond a resectable size, eg radical mastectomy; these therapies are performed in order to alleviate pain or improve the quality of life of the terminally ill; see All-American operation, Commando operation, Forequarter amputation

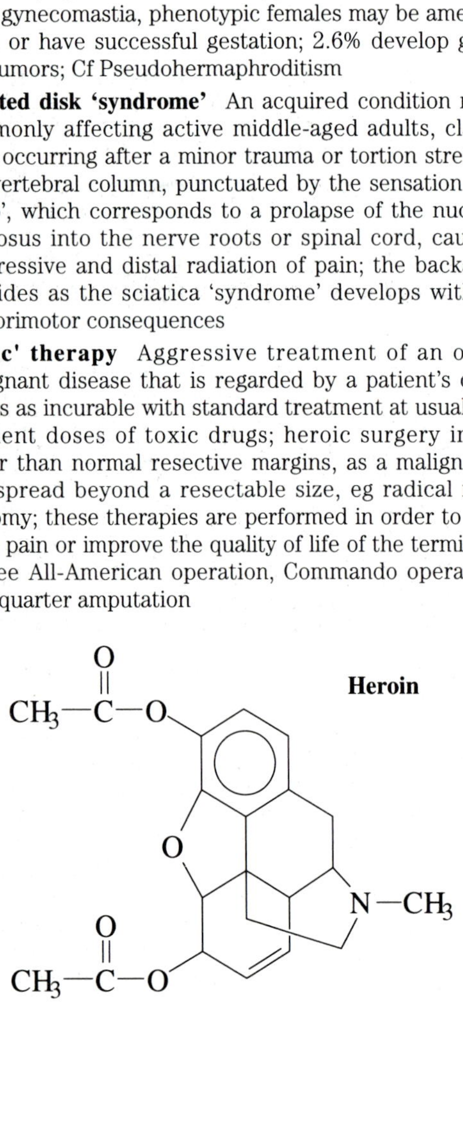

Heroin

Heroin Diacetyl morphine A semisynthetic narcotic drug that was formulated and marketed in 1898, one year before aspirin was introduced; the adverse effects of heroin abuse include sepsis, shock and systemic pathology affecting all organ systems CARDIOVASCULAR *Staphylococcus aureus* endocarditis, especially of the right side and tricuspid valve LIVER Viral hepatitis (HAV, HBV, HCV or non-A, non-B hepatitis and delta hepatitis) LUNGS Pulmonary edema, due to direct heroin toxicity to capillaries or myocardium, hypoxic endothelial damage, congestive heart failure, central vasomotor effect (increased protein in edema fluid) MUSCULOSKELETAL Acute rhabdomyolysis, septic arthritis, chronic osteomyelitis RETICULOENDOTHELIAL SYSTEM Regional lymphadenopathy with chronic non-specific hyperplasia due to injected contaminants SKIN Track marks and circular scars with necrotic ulcers **Histopathology** Hypoxic endothelial damage and asteroid body formation (heart), non-specific anoxic changes (brain), focal membrano-proliferative glomerulonephritis and glomerulosclerosis, periglomerular fibrosis, basement membrane thickening, nephrotic syndrome, IgM and C3 deposition within vessels (kidney), chronic nonspecific portal 'triaditis', chronic active hepatitis with septal fibrosis, piecemeal necrosis, lobular inflammation, chronic persistent hepatitis and non-specific hepatitis (liver), hypoxia, edema and talc granulomas (lung), rhabdomyolysis and chronic osteomyelitis (musculoskeletal system) and regional lymphadenopathy with chronic non-specific hyperplasia; see Brown heroin, Opium

HERP index Human exposure/rodent potency index RISK ASSESSMENT A formula that extrapolates the data obtained from toxicologic studies of potential carcinogens in food or other ingested substances in the rodent and attempts to determine the daily amount that must be ingested by humans to induce a similar carcinogenic effect; Cf Ames test

Herpesvirus A family of DNA viruses with a central icosahedral (containing 162 capsomeres) core of double-stranded DNA, a trilaminar 100 nm in diameter lipoprotein envelope, a 30-43 nm in diameter nucleus and prolonged dormancy, lasting up to years; the Human herpes viruses (HHV) have been classified as **HHV-1** H simplex-1, which typically affects the body above the waist, is responsible for most cases of oral herpes and fever blisters, and is often accompanied by stomatitis, conjunctivitis, necrotizing meningoencephalitis, encephalitis Portal of entry Fibroblast growth factor receptor (Science 1990; 248:1410, Nature 1990; 348:344) **HHV-2** H simplex-2 is sexually transmitted—only 5% of venereal herpes is caused by HHV-1, and is uncommon under age 15, predominantly affecting the body below the waist, causing venereal, vulvovaginal and penile herpetic ulcers; HHV-2 is more often prevalent in multiply married, female, black city dwellers with lesser educations (N Engl J Med 1989; 321:7); HHV-1 and HHV-2 have a 50% homology and may bind to different membrane receptors, generally transmitted by contact; one form, Kaposi's varicelliform eczema herpeticum is potentially fatal and seen in atopic individuals Herpes in pregnancy Early gestational infection may cause spontaneous abortion, while the products of late gestational infection suffer microcephaly, mental retardation, retinal dysplasia and hepatosplenomegaly; recurrence rate in subsequent pregnancies approaches 70%; HS-2 causes most neonatal herpes, infecting via the birth canal; the infants are healthy at birth and become symptomatic 1-4 weeks post-partum Early neonatal herpes causes vesiculo-bullous lesions (absent in 20%), lethargy, irritability, hypotonia and loss of gag and sucking reflexes; late neonatal herpes may cause generalized seizures, jaundice, hypotension, disseminated intravascular coagulation, acidosis,apnea, thrombocytopenia and shock Diagnosis Enzyme-linked immunosorbent assay (ELISA) linked to an amplification culture system, complement fixation, radioimmunoassay, culture in fetal fibroblasts, fluorescent antibody against membrane antigen; RFLP (restriction fragment length polymorphism) analysis allows epidemiologic tracking of sources of infection Cytopathology STAGE 1 Granular chromatin STAGE 2 Multinucleated giant cells with 'ground glass' chromatin, where the 'grains' correspond to viral particles, 50-200 000 viruses per infected cell STAGE 3 Inclusion bodies surrounded by a halo, cf HBLV **Molecular biology** The double-stranded DNA viral genome is 108 kD, with many guanine and cytosine nucleotides, having therefore a high GC:AT ratio; the herpes genome encodes 60-70 gene products divided into α, β and γ genes, based on timing of expression after infecting the host cell: the γ genes are 'late expressors', require previous production of the 'early' α and β proteins and encode structural proteins; HS-1 and HS-2 remain latent for years once the viral DNA is integrated into the host DNA, usually confined to the sensory nerves; the latency may be due to the presence of a mirror image of the viral protein ICPO (Infected-cell protein number zero) that 'commandeers' host cell replicative machinery, producing virions **Treatment** Antiviral agents, eg cytosine arabinoside (5-iodo-2'-deoxyuridine), adenine arabinoside (Acyclovir) and trifluorothymidine (Trifluidin) shorten the duration of an attack **HHV-3** Herpes varicella-zoster has two clinical forms: Acute HHV-3 infection or chickenpox and Chronic HHV-3 infection or shingles **HHV-4** see Epstein-Barr virus **HHV-5** see Cytomegalovirus **HHV-6** Human B cell lymphotropic virus measures 200 nm and transforms infected B-cells into enlarged refractile mono- or binucleated cells, generating abundant extracellular virus from infected cells, seen as cytoplasmic and nuclear inclusion bodies; the initial report of HBLV (Science 1986; 234:596) described six cases with co-morbid conditions including HIV-positivity, cutaneous T-cell and immunoblastic lymphomas, acute lymphocytic leukemia lymphoma, dermatopathic lymphadenitis, angioimmunoblastic lymphadenopathy; most HHV-6 isolates have been from AIDS patients and HHV-6 is synergistic with HIV-1 as both have affinity for CD4 T cells and activate HIV-1's long terminal repeat sequence (Nature 1989, 337:370); HHV-6 may be a co-factor in the pathogenesis of AIDS, as it both upregulates expression of the CD4 receptor in neoplastic T cell lines and induces de novo expression of the CD4 receptor in CD8 cells, rendering them susceptible to HIV (Nature 1991; 349:533); although usually benign, HHV-6 may cause malignant fulminant hepatitis (N Engl J Med 1991;324:1290c) and roseola (exanthema subitum), causing acute infectious mononucleosis-like symptoms

Herpes gestationalis Duhring-Brocq disease A rare vesiculo-bullous, often severely pruritic eruption occurring in pregnancy and the puerperium, associated with vesiculo-bullous lesions and an increased infant mortality **Pathogenesis** Uncertain, although it is probably immune-mediated **Histopatho-logy** Edema, hyperemia and eosinophils in dermis Immunofluorescence Linear C3 (C1q, C4 and properdin) and IgG ocur in 50% of cases **Treatment** Corticosteroids

Herpes gladiatorum Herpes simplex-1-induced lesions of the eyes and skin of the head, neck, trunk or extremities, accompanied by lymphadenopathy, sore throat, fever, chills and headache, described in modern 'gladiators', eg wrestlers and rugby players (N Engl J Med 1991; 325:906)

Herringbone pattern A fanciful descriptor for the arrangement of malignant fibroblasts when viewed by low power light microscopy, where the elongated nuclei are positioned at sharp angles to each other in linear arrays, a pattern characteristic of fibrosarcoma that has been observed in malignant schwannomas and in benign nodular fasciitis; a herringbone pattern is composed of rows of parallel lines with adjacent rows slanting in reverse direction

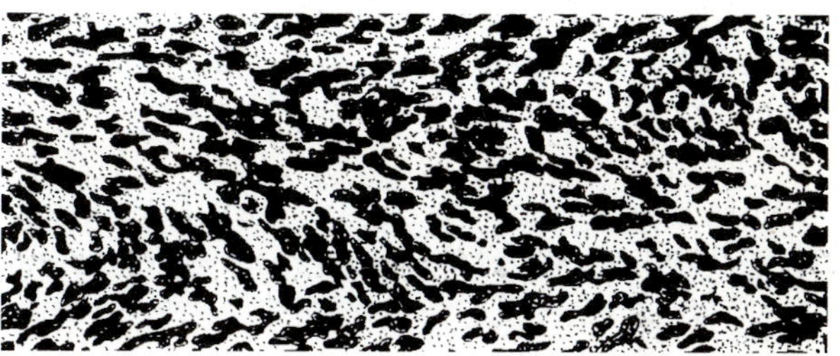

↑ Tissue Herring bone pattern Cloth ↓

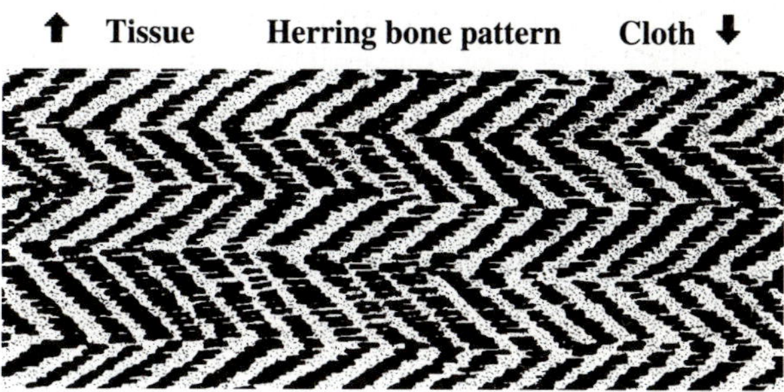

Her's disease Glycogen storage disease, type VI; Cf His disease

HES Hydroxyethyl starch TRANSFUSION MEDICINE A synthetic starch that is added to the input line during leukapheresis to promote red cell rouleaux formation, which facilitates their separation from leukocytes Side effects Minimal and limited to occasional urticarial and anaphylactoid reactions due to slow elimination, patients requiring granulocyte transfusions should be monitored with erythrocyte sedimentation rates; HES has been used as a cryopreservative for frozen packed red cells, but glycerol is preferred; see Colloid solutions; Cf DMSO

(dimethylsulfoxide)

HETE 8, 15-dihydroxyeicosatetraenoic acid PHYSIOLOGY A leukotriene precursor formed in the 15-lipoxygenase pathway of arachidonic acid metabolism within eosinophils that is similar in potency to leukotriene B_4 for neutrophil chemotaxis

Heterochromatin GENETICS Chromatin that remains tightly coiled during interphase, seen by light microscopy; heterochromatin can be a) Facultative, arising from inactivation or 'lyonization' of one of the X chromosomes, the Barr body that corresponds to a 'clump' of heterochromatin and b) Constitutive, where the heterochromatin is integral to each chromosome, located adjacent to the centromeres,telomeres, in the long arm of the Y chromosome and contains highly repeated DNA sequences

Heterogeneous nuclear RNA (hnRNA) A 5-15 kilobase segment of RNA that is confined to the nucleus and is the presumed precursor of messenger RNA; hnRNA and mRNA are similar in structure and both may be transcribed by RNA polymerase II; hnRNA is associated with proteins (hnRNP) and like snRNPs (small nuclear ribonucleic proteins) may have a role in splicing, an activity that results in mRNA maturation

Heterophile antibody An antibody, usually an IgM 'agglutinin' that is produced in one species of animals and capable of reacting against the red cells of another, phylogenically unrelated species; heterophile antibodies are classically observed in humans with infectious mononucleosis (IM) where the antibodies react against sheep erythrocytes; high titers of heterophile antibodies also occur in serum sickness; the two conditions are differentiated by adsorbing the serum with beef red cells (bearing the so-called Forsemann antigen) and retesting; the sera of infectious mononucleosis no longer react

Heterophyes A genus of minute (1-3 mm) intestinal trematodes (flukes) that may parasitize humans ingesting poorly or uncooked fish, eg sushi, occurring in Southeast Asia, Egypt and India; the worms adhere to the small intestinal mucosa by a ventral sucker, causing diarrhea and abdominal pain **Treatment** Praziquantel

Heterosis Hybrid vigor The greater fertility and strength of progeny obtained when highly inbred strains are crossed; the vigor is partially attributed to the elimination of homozygous traits that are deleterious to survival of each parent cell; Cf Bottlenecks, Consanguinity, Inbreeding

Heuristic method A form of problem solving based not on scientific proof but rather on plausible, possible or creative conclusions to questions that cannot be answered in the context of, or the 'logic' of which lies outside of, a currently-accepted scientific paradigm; the heuristic process is of use as it may stimulate further research; Cf Aunt Millie approach, Stochastic method

HEXA gene A gene that encodes the α unit of hexosaminidase A, the enzyme deficient in Tay-Sachs disease; three different mutations account for 98% of Tay-Sachs disease (GM-2 gangliosidosis, type 1), two of which cause infantile Tay-Sachs, the third causing adult Tay-Sachs (79% have exon 11 insertion, 18% have intron 12 splice-junction mutation and 3% have the less severe disease characterized by an exon 7 mutation); DNA-based analysis of the HEXA gene is more specific and has a higher predictive value than the currently used enzyme test for hexosaminidase A(N Engl J Med 1990; 323:6)

HEXB gene A gene that encodes the β chain of hexosaminidase A and both β chains of hexosaminidase B

Hexachlorophene An antibacterial agent used as a preoperative scrubbing solution and as a detergent; its use is contraindicated in premature infants, as it is associated with neurotoxicity; Cf Gasping syndrome

Heymann glomerulonephritis A membranous glomerulonephritis model induced by immunizing rodents with proximal tubule brush border homogenates containing subepithelial antigen or the 330 kD Heymann factor in Freund's adjuvant; granular subepithelial (lamina rara interna) immune complex deposits may be detected on the glomerular basement membrane by immunofluorescence

Hfr High frequency of recombination Molecular Biology A conjugating organism, eg ***Escherichia coli*** with its DNA-exchanging equipment in 'overdrive' because the episomal fertility factor is integrated into the bacteria's chromosome

H gene A gene that encodes the enzyme, α-L-fucosyltransferase, which produces an oligosaccharide known as the H antigen; homozygous deficiency of H gene results in an hh or Bombay phenotype individual who, lacking the above transferase, cannot attach the fucose to the galactose on the precursor H substance; when the H gene is present, ABO precursor molecule is encoded; when the A gene is also present, the 'A-transferase' is encoded, which adds N-acetyl-**D**-galactosamine to the H antigen, resulting in group A red cells; when the B gene is present, 'B-transferase' adds **D**-galactose to the H antigen, resulting in group B red cells; the amount of H substance on red cells differs according to the blood type, where group $O > A_2B > B > A_1 > A_1B >$ Bombay; see Bombay phenotype, H-antigen, Secretor, Ulex europa

HGBF see Heparin-binding fibroblast growth factor family

HGP-30 An experimental AIDS vaccine (CEL-SCI Corp, Alexandria, Virgina), based on a synthetic HIV core protein, p17

HGPRT see Hypoxanthine guanine phosphoribosyl transferase

HHH syndrome Hyperornithinemia, hyperammonemia and homocitrullinemia An autosomal recessive condition characterized by a defect in ornithine transport from the cytoplasm into the mitochondria (where the urea cycle occurs) **Clinical** Mental retardation, seizures, failure to thrive, chronic vomiting, acute episodic hyperammonemia and coma **Treatment** Protein restriction, ornithine supplementation

HHHO syndrome Hypomentia, hypogonadotrophic hypogonadism, muscular hypotonicity and obesity A clinical complex seen in Prader-Willi syndrome often accompanied by short stature, adult-onset diabetes mellitus, acromicria (small hands and feet), micrognathia, strabismus, fish-like or Cupid's bow mouth, clinodactyly, absence of auricular cartilage and hypoventilation with pulmonary hypertension

HHT Hereditary hemorrhagic telangiectasia Osler-Weber-Rendu syndrome A clinical complex characterized by episodic epistaxis in childhood, chronic gastrointestinal hemorrhage, palmo-plantar, muco-cutaneous and hepatic telangiectasias and pulmonary arteriovenous malformations

HHV Human herpes virus see Herpes virus

Hiatal hernia Herniation of the esophagogastric junction affects up to 1% of the population, 5% of whom are symptomatic and is divided into a) Sliding hiatal hernia, comprising 90% of cases, characterized by axial displacement of the esophagogastric (EG) junction in the cranial direction, where it slides in and out of the chest depending on changes in the intrathoracic and intraabdominal pressures; the sliding hernia is ensheathed in its own peritoneal sac Treatment Symptomatic cases are repaired by surgically returning the distal esophagus back to the peritoneal cavity with a valvoplasty and b) Para-esophageal hiatal hernias are less common and often accompanied by a sliding component; pure hiatal hernias are rare and associated with chronic hemorrhage and gastric volvulus, both indications for surgical repair

Hib *Hemophilus influenzae*, type b A bacteria causing 20 000 annual infections in the USA, commonly affecting those under age 5, resulting in 1000 deaths/year; prevalence in infants, $275/10^5$; the polysaccharide vaccine (HibVac) licensed in 1985 had a low efficacy attributed to its limited immunogenicity (J Am Med Assoc 1988; 260:1423, 1413, 1419); anti-Hib vaccine composed of Hib's capsular polysaccharide covalently linked to a carrier protein (polyribosylribitol-diphtheria toxoid or PRP-D) provided 94% protection to a cohort of Finnish infants (N Engl J Med 1990; 323:1381) and 35% protection to Eskimo infants (ibid, 323:1393); the lower immunogenicity of the PRP-D has been surpassed by PRP-tetanus toxoid which provides up to 75% protection; the PRP-diphtheria toxoid vaccine is reported to be 88% effective (ibid, 1991; 265:987)

Hibernating myocardium Regional dysfunction of myocardial tissue due to prolonged local hypoperfusion, which is completely reversible upon restoration of adequate blood flow; hibernation occurs in patients with coronary artery disease and impairment of left ventricular function at rest (J Am Med Assoc 1990; 264:455c); Cf 'Stunned' myocardium, Thallium imaging

Hibernoma A benign, well-circumscribed and asymptomatic tumor measuring 5-10 cm, consisting of brown fat and affecting young adults Prognosis No recurrence, Treatment excision

Hiccup/hiccough Singultation An abrupt inspiratory muscle contraction, followed within 35 msec by closure of the glottis; the hiccup center is located in the spinal cord between C3 and C5; the afferent impulse is carried by the vagus and phrenic nerves and the thoracic sympathetic chain; the efferent impulse is carried by the phrenic nerve with branches to the glottis and accessory respiratory muscles; many conditions elicit hiccups, including gastric distension, gastrointestinal hemorrhage or inflammation, abrupt temperature change, alcohol, inferior wall myocardial infarct, irritation of the tympanic membrane, diaphragmatic irritants, excess smoking, excitement or stress, toxins, metabolic defects, eg azotemia, hyponatremia, uremia, pharmacologics, eg general anesthesia, barbiturates, diazepam, α-methyldopa, tumors, pneumonia, herpes zoster, central and peripheral nervous system disease (encephalitis, brainstem infarcts, phrenic nerve compression), intractable hiccupping may result in inability to eat or sleep, may cause arrhythmia or reflux esophagitis, or may be compatible with a normal life; no hiccup therapy gives consistent results, but chlorpromazine (a dopaminergic blocker) and diphenhydramine may be as effective as (and more dignified than) standing on one's head; other dopaminergic blockers include haloperidol, metoclopramide and apomorphine, rare cases may respond to amantidine (N Engl J Med 1988; 318:711) or amitriptyline; the most recalcitrant known case of hypersingultation occurred in an American pig farmer, starting in 1922, continuing to 1987

'Hide-bound' skin A descriptor for the smooth shiny indurated skin associated with adherent fibrosis and sclerosis that 'glues' the subcutaneous tissue to underlying structures, classically described in scleroderma

HIE see Hyperimmunoglobulin E syndrome

HIG see Human immune globulin

'High' SUBSTANCE ABUSE A generic term for any state of pleasant and/or manic euphoria that is often a desired end-point for users of narcotics, hallucinogens or other potentially addicting substances of abuse; while a subject is high, he may experience megalomania and commit acts that may be in wanton disregard for the safety of himself and others; a 'high' may be evoked by alcohol, amphetamines, cocaine, heroin, LSD, marijuana and others; see Bad trip, 'Stoned'

High altitude acclimatization see Höhendiurese, Mountain sickness

High altitude pulmonary edema A clinical complex caused by rapid ascent of unacclimatized individuals to altitudes above 2000-2500 meters that is accompanied by headache, insomnia, dyspnea and tachycardia; see also Höhendiurese, Mountain sickness

High amplitude swelling HISTOPATHOLOGY An intracellular finding seen by electron microscopy indicative of irreversible hypoxia-induced cell death, which causes a shut-down of the calcium pump and consists of vacuolization of mitochondrial cristae, accompanied by aggregates of amorphous densities, disruption of the outer limiting membrane and nuclear pyknosis

'High-ceiling' diuretics see Loop diuretics

High disseminator EPIDEMIOLOGY A subject who is the carrier of a highly virulent and easily transmissible infectious agent, eg *Salmonella typhi*, transmitted by a cook infelicitously known as Typhoid Mary who was responsible for more than ten epidemics of typhoid fever; in the current AIDS epidemic, high dissemination is thought to be more common among heterosexuals and related to the virulence of the strain of human immunodeficiency virus (N Engl J Med 1989; 321:1460); see Typhoid Mary; Cf Fabian Bridges

'High dry' field A colloquiallism used by histopathologists for 400X (of less commonly, to 600X) magnification, the combined result of a 10X ocular and 40X objective; 'high dry' fields are generally used to study nuclear details and to count mitotic figures; the maximum obtainable resolution by light microscopy without resorting to immersion oil is 1200X, using a 15X ocular and a 60X 'dry' objective; Note: 25-40X magnification is referred to as 'scanning power'; 100X is known as 'low power' and 970X is termed 'oil power'

High endothelial venules (HEV) Postcapillary venules that are located in the paracortical region of lymph nodes and in the GALT (gut-associated lymphoid tissue, eg Peyer's patches) that contain specialized columnar cells with receptors for antigen-sensitized lymphocytes, providing the main signal for the egress of lymphocytes from the circulation; lymph nodes have a 'homing' receptor for circulating lymphocytes involving ubiquitin; synovial HEV receptors are distinct from lymphoid HEV receptors, implying 'specialization' within the lymphoid tissue

High-energy bond BIOCHEMISTRY A covalent bond that serves as a ubiquitous intracellular 'storage battery', as hydrolysis of these bonds provides the energy necessary to activate various enzymatic reactions; high-energy bonds are most efficiently formed during aerobic glycolysis and are oftenattached to phosphate groups, eg ATP, ADP, NADP and NADPH and designated by a 'squiggle' (~) shape

High energy phosphate Any phosphate (PO_4)-containing compound which has one or more energy-rich (21 to 54,400 J/mol) phosphate bonds, eg ATP, ADP, cyclic AMP, ITP, GTP, NADP, phospho-creatinine and acetyl phosphate; high energy phosphate bonds form during energy-releasing reactions eg glycolysis and serve as intracellular stores of energy required for synthetic reactions

Higher multiple OBSTETRICS A term for multiple or higher order gestations greater than triplets, lumping together quadruplets and quintuplets; although traditionally, the frequency of triplets was considered the square of the 1:85 ($1:85^2$) frequency of twins, ie, circa 1:7000 and that of quadruplets, the cube ($1:85^3$) ie, circa 1:600 000, the use of fertility drugs, in vitro fertilization and other modalities has made higher multiples more frequent; differences in multiple gestations includes in-hospital stay for mothers: 1.4 days for mothers of singletons, 9.5 days for twins, 29.5 days for triplets and 54.5 days for quadruplets; in higher multiples, the incidence of lower birth weight is increasingly higher, and by extension the incidence of cerebral palsy; the more 'products', the greater the health care costs and the greater the puerperal complications for the mother including hemorrhage, anemia, infections and high blood pressure

High frequency antigen Public antigen TRANSFUSION MEDICINE An erythrocyte antigen present on the surface of red cells, in such a high percentage of the population that antibodies to these antigens are rare, thereby presenting difficulties in identification; high frequency antigens include AT^a, Co^a, Dib, Ge, Gy^a, Hy, K and Kell group antigens including Js^b, Kp^b, Kelly, Lan, Sc_1 (Sc_2 or Bu^a is a low frequency, probably allelic), SD^a, Vel, Yk^a, Yt^a and Yus

High-grade lymphoma A group of aggressive lymphomas that respond poorly to chemotherapy and comprise 20% of all lymphomas classified by the Working Formulation (Cancer 1982; 49:2112); high-grade lymphomas include the diffuse large cell immunoblastic lymphoma, lymphoblastic lymphoma and the diffuse small, non-cleaved cell lymphoma, which includes the Burkitt's lymphoma and non-Burkitt's lymphomas Note: High-grade lymphomas have a mean survival of less than one year without therapy, but may respond well to therapy; see Lymphoma, Working Formulation

High mortality outlier A hospital that has been identified by the US Health Care Financing Administration (HCFA) as having a mortality rate far in excess of what is considered 'normal' for the remaining nearly 5500 health care facilities in the US; because these 'outliers' may be due to characteristics of the patient population, eg elderly (older than 85), 'high-risk' diagnoses or skewing of data by those who require nursing care upon discharge (J Am Med Assoc 1991; 265:1843); it is thought that mortality rates are of little utility as a determinant of patient quality of care; see Hospital mortality rate

High output cardiac failure (HOF) Congestive heart failure due to a marked increase in circulating blood volume without functional myocardial abnormalities, where the demand outstrips the capacity, resulting in a hyperkinetic state; the cardiac pump activity is a function of preload (ventricular end-diastolic fiber tension), myocardial contractility, afterload and the heart cardiac rate; HOF may be a physiologic response to such 'insults' as anemia, cor pulmonale, exercise, fever, high humidity, systemic hypertension, obesity, pregnancy, emotional stress and temperature extremes, or non-physiological in Albright's disease (polyostotic fibrous dysplasia), carcinoid syndrome (serotonin-producing usually hepatic metastases), arteriovenous fistulas (trauma, Paget's disease of bone, hemangiomatosis, glomerulonephritis, hemodialysis, hepatic disease (alcohol-related thiamine deficiency decreases peripheral arterial resistance), hyperkinetic heart syndrome, polycythemia vera and thyrotoxicosis (T_3 increases heart rate, cardiac sensitivity to epinephrine and causes peripheral vasodilation)

High output gastrointestinal fistula Background Gastrointestinal fistulas are defined as abnormal communications between the gastrointestinal tract and another segment of intestine or other intraabdominal organ, an internal fistula, or the skin, an external fistula, caused by trauma, gastrointestinal pathology or surgery; high output fistulas produce more than 200 ml of fluid, most often arising in the stomach, proximal small intestine and pancreas; the pancreas may produce up to 1500 ml of electrolyte-rich fluid/day; see Low output gastrointestinal fistula

High performance liquid chromatography see HPLC

High power field (HPF) A unit of measurement, usually understood to be a 'high dry' field (400x magnification); used by histopathologists to assess a tissue's growth, which by extension is an indicator of tumor aggression; the number of mitotic figures per HPF serves to prognosticate certain tumors, in particular, *A) HODGKIN'S DISEASE* The number of classic Reed-Sternberg cells (RS) per single HPF allows subclassification of Hodgkin's lymphoma into lymphocyte predominance less than or equal to 5 RS/HPF (often far fewer), mixed cellularity 5-15 RS/HPF and lymphocyte-depleted, which is greater than or equal to 15 RS/HPF *AND B) SMOOTH MUSCLE TUMORS* of i) Stomach These tumors are considered malignant if there are greater than five mitotic figures/10 HPF, although 40% of gastric leiomyosarcomas have less and ii) Uterus These tumors are regarded as frankly malignant if there are more than 10 mitotic figures/10 HPF; the diagnosis of 'smooth muscle tumor of uncertain malignant potential' (STUMP) or low-grade leiomyosarcoma (which has a low mortality, but often recurs) is rendered in smooth muscle tumors with less than 10 mitotic figures/10 HPF (in absence of cellular atypia), or 5 to 9 mitotic figures/HPF in the present of atypia

'High power institution' ACADEMIA A colloquial Americanism used in academic circles for highly competitive hospitals, eg Massachusetts General Hospital, the Mayo Clinic, National Institutes of Health, reseach institutions, eg Massachusetts Institute of Technology, the Whitehead Institute and universities, eg U of Chicago, Harvard U, Stanford U and U of Utah that perform 'cutting edge' ('world class') science, are highly selective in who they train

High pressure liquid chromatography see HPLC

High-resolution computed tomography (HRCT) A computer tomography (CT) study at slice (collimation scan interval), widths of 4mm or less, which is narrower than the usual 1-3 cm interval 'slices' obtained in conventional CT imaging; HRCT is the optimal technique for evaluating interstitial lung disease and emphysema and is preferred to conventional CT in detecting subpleural nodules, small linear densities, 'honeycombing' and bronchiectasis (Mayo Clin Proc 1989; 64:1284, Diag Imaging 1991; 13:102), and is of use in any body region where greater detail is desired; Cf Spiral computed tomography

High risk infant NEONATOLOGY An infant at increased risk of suffering co-morbid conditions and potentially fatal complications, resulting from fetal, maternal or placental anomalies FETAL HIGH RISK FACTORS APGAR score of less than 4 at one minute, birth weights of less than 2500g or greater than 4500g, gestational age less than 37 or more than 42 weeks, fetal malformation, fetal-maternal blood group incompatibility and twinning MATERNAL HIGH RISK FACTORS Previous in utero or neonatal death, infection, true diabetes mellitus (gestational diabetes is less risky to the infant), premature rupture of membranes, maternal age less than 16 and greater than 40, alcohol, drug or tobacco use, gestation beginning within six months of previous delivery, poor prenatal care, severe emotional stress, accidents or general anesthesia, ingestion of teratogenic medication PLACENTAL AND INTRAUTERINE HIGH RISK FACTORS Placenta previa, short umbilical cord, single umbilical artery, abruptio placentae, oligohydramnios

High-risk sex see Safe sex practices

High-stringency hybridization MOLECULAR BIOLOGY A hybridization between two molecules capable of forming nucleotide base pair dimers, eg DNA with DNA or DNA with RNA under conditions that require virtually exact alignment of bases; the stringency of a hybridization can be controlled by titrating the temperature and salts; Cf Low stringency hybridization

High-titer, low-avidity antibodies (HTLA) Transfusion medicine A group of antibodies that cause red cell agglutination at high dilutions in the antiglobulin test (Coomb's) phase, but which evoke weak aggregation and are rarely associated with clinically significant hemolysis; HTLA antibodies include anti--Bg^{a}, -Ch, -Cs, -JMH, -Kna, -McC^{a}, -Rg, -Yk; occasionally, anti-Hy, Lutheran group and the leukocyte antibody

High touch SOCIAL MEDICINE Patient contact on a individual basis, in which there is physical and or direct emotional interaction, distinct from modern medicine's trend toward technological and innovative aspects of healing; 'high-touch' fields of health care include nursing and psychiatry; see Doctor-patient interaction

Hill-Burton Act A program that arose from US Public Law 79-725 (the Hospital Survey and Construction Act of 1946), which provided financial assistance for modernizing health care facilities in areas that had undergone a rapid post-World War II population growth; the Hill-Burton Act was superceded by US Public Law 93-641 of 1974, which attempted to reverse the migration of health providers and services to large population centers by supporting rural facilities or areas deficient in health services, eg inner-city

Hilus cell An interstitial (Leydig) cell located in the ovarian hilum, associated with the rete ovarii, containing Reincke crystalloids (eosinophilic rods measuring 1-4 μm in length X 0.5 μm in diameter), without which the cells are indistinguishable from lutein cells or adrenocortical cells; hilar cells are present as unencapsulated aggregates in the embryonal ovary that disappear in childhood and reappear in puberty, increasing in number with pregnancy and aging and are abundant in postmenopausal women; hilar cells produce androstenedione, estrogen and progesterone; when 'driven' by human choriogonadotropin, hilar cells undergo mitosis and hypertrophy, and are an integral histologic feature of gonadoblastoma and androblastoma

Hilus cell tumor SURGICAL PATHOLOGY A subtype of ovarian Leydig cell tumor (the other is the non-hilar Leydig cell tumor) Clinical Benign, autumn colored (red, yellow and brown) tumor, causing hirsutism or virilization in most cases, average age, 58 years Treatment Excision Prognosis Excellent Note: The other form of Leydig cell tumor is the ultrarare, non-hilar cell tumor, which behaves clinically like the hilus cell tumor

***Hind*II, *Hind*III** MOLECULAR BIOLOGY Two commonly used bacterial restriction endonucleases (figure) derived

*Hin*dII	*Hin*dIII
GTPyr*PurAC	A*AGCTT
CAPur*PyrTG	TTCGA*A

from *Hemophilus influenzae* that selectively hydrolyze or cut double-stranded DNA at the appropriate mirror-image or 'palindromic' sites (*); Cf *Eco*RI, RII, pBR 322

Hinge region IMMUNOLOGY A region of an immunoglobulin heavy chain that is often located between the first and second constant domains (CH1 and CH2) of the immunoglobulin chain and highly flexible due to the high content of proline residues

Hippocratic facies A physiognomy characteristic of advanced, untreated, preterminal peritonitis, who Hippocrates described as having '...hollow eyes, collapsed temples; the ears, cold, contracted and their lobes turned out; the skin about the forehead being rough, distended and parched; the color of the whole face being brown, black, livid or lead-colored...'; these facial features are also described in celiac sprue; Cf Triangular facies

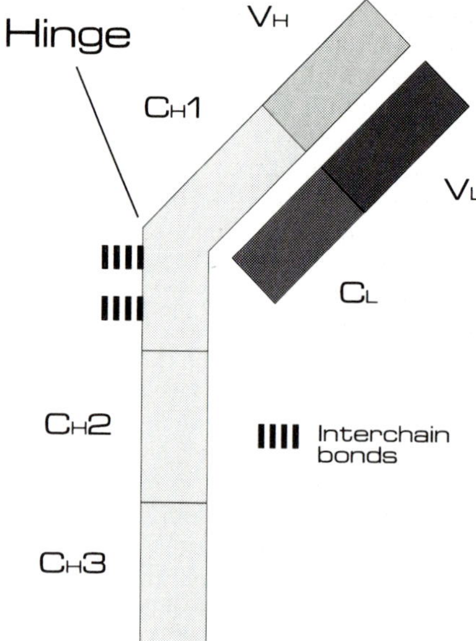

Hippocratic nails see Clubbing of fingers

Hippocratic oath The ethical guide for physicians, as timely today as in the 5th century BC; althoughit has been attributed to Hippocrates, the father of medicine and his school, the 'Oath' is of uncertain origin; see Code of Hamma-rubi

Hip-pointer contusion SPORTS MEDICINE A bruise of the iliac crest which occurs in contact sports due to a blow delivered by the knee, elbow, football helmet or other blunt object causing a subperiosteal hematoma and either avulsion of abdominal muscle or a fracture of the iliac crest

Hippus A spasm of the iris, resulting in exaggerated rhythmic contractions and dilatations of the pupil that are not consonant with accommodation and light; see Hiccup

'Hired gun' LEGAL MEDICINE A highly colloquial term for a physician whose major souce of income derives from his role as the plaintiff's 'expert witness' at court trials for medical malpractice; mercenary 'experts' may have little knowledge of the medical field in which the tort occurred and may have their own fees tied to the monies 'won' in a successful lawsuit Note: Most physicians truly welcome the opinion of well-respected peers in their specialty, as they may temper the jury's view of the events in medically-related torts with their experience and offer reasons why many acts of alleged negligence are inevitable risks of a diagnostic or therapeutic procedure; see Malpractice, Cf Physician expert witness

Hirsutism Excessive growth of body hair, a common complaint in

HIPPOCRATIC OATH

'I swear by Apollo the physician, by Aesculapius, Hygeia and Panacea, and I take to witness all the gods, and all the goddesses, to keep according to my ability and judgement the following Oath: To consider dear to as my parents him who taught me this art; to live in common with him and if necessary to share my goods with him; to look upon his children as my own brothers, to teach them this art if they so desire without fee or written promise; to impart to my sons and the sons of the master who taught me and the disciples who have enrolled themselves and have agreed to the rules of the profession, but to these alone, the precepts and instructions. I will prescribe regimen for the good of my patients according to my ability and judgment and abstain from whatever is deleterious and mischievous. I will give no deadly medicine to anyone if asked nor give advise which may cause his death. Nor will I give a woman a pessary to procure abortion. I will preserve the purity of my life and practice my art. I will not cut for stone, even for patients in whom the disease is manifest, but will leave this operation to be done by practitioners of this art. Into whatever house where I come, I will enter only for the benefit of the sick, keeping myself far from all intentional mischief and corruption, and especially from the pleasures of love with women or with men, be they free or slaves. All that come to my knowledge in the exercise of my profession or outside of my practice or in daily commerce with men, which ought not to be spoken abroad, I will keep secret and not divulge. If I keep this oath unviolated may I enjoy my life and practice my art, respected by all men and in all times, but should I trespass this oath, may the reverse be my lot'

women, divided into a) Androgen-independent hirsutism in which the entire body is covered with vellous hair evenly distributed over both androgen-dependent and androgen-independent regions Etiology Congenital disease, eg Cornelia de Lange and Seckel syndromes, drugs, eg androgen analogs, anti-convulsants, corticosteroids, cyclosporine, minoxidil, phenytoin and progesterone analogs, metabolic disorders, eg anorexia nervosa, porphyria cutanea tarda and b) Androgen-dependent hirsutism where there is increased terminal hair over the 'androgenic' regions of the face and upper chest, which may be **I) NONENDOCRINE HIRSUTISM OF ETHNIC OR RACIAL ORIGIN**, with excess hair growth on the face, upper body, chest nipples, or lower abdomen; the intensity and distribution is a function of a person's sensitivity to circulating androgens; a male pattern of hirsutism is more common in southern Europe and distinctly less common in aborigines and Orientals Treatment Rule out hormonal dysfunction, then bleach, pluck and shave; spironolactone or combined spironolactone-progestagen combination therapy (Presse Med 1990; 19:1529) or **II) HIRSUTISM OF ENDOCRINE (OVARIAN) ORIGIN**, either non-neoplastic, eg polycystic ovaries syndrome of Stein-Leventhal (accompanied by hyperthecosis, increased testosterone and variably increased 17-ketosteroids), hyperthecosis, idiopathic, Achard-Thier syndrome or hormonally active neoplasms, eg granulosa cell tumor, gynandroblastoma, gonadoblastoma, Sertoli-Leydig cell tumors (arrhenoblastoma), stromal/pregnancy luteoma, teratoma, hilar cell tumors, lipoid cell tumors **III) HIRSUTISM OF ENDOCRINE (ADRENAL) ORIGIN**, either non-neoplastic, eg adrenogenital syndrome (congenital adrenal hyperplasia, deficiency of 11- or 21-hydroxylase), normal testosterone, increased 17-ketosteroids, normal or increased pregnanetriol, Cushing's disease or neoplastic, eg adrenal tumor (carcinoma or virilizing adenoma, with increased 17-ketosteroids) **IV) DRUG-INDUCED HIRSUTISM** due to excess of androgens, corticosteroids, contraceptives, menopausal 'cocktails', '19-nor' progestins, cyclosporine, diazoxide, minoxidil, 'stress'; (hyperthecosis and insulin resistance) phenothiazines, phenytoin **V) METABOLIC** (AND OTHER CAUSES OF) **HIRSUTISM** Acromegaly, hypothyroidism, porphyria cutanea tarda

Hirudin The most potent known inhibitor of thrombin, produced by the medicinal leech, ***Hirudo medicinalis***; crystallographic analysis of the hirudin-thrombin complex reveals that 27 of the 65 residues have contacts of less than 4 A, forming 10 ion pairs and 23 hydrogen bonds, explaining hirudin's potency as an anticoagulant, as the affinity is much stronger than that for thrombin's natural inhibitor, anti-thrombin III(Science 1990; 249:277)

Hirudinea A class of segmented annelids, ie leeches, the most well-known of which is ***Hirudo medicinalis*** that evolved from earthworms and is found in fresh water and soil in the subtropics and tropics; the genera include ***Haemadipsa***, the medicinal leech as well as ***Dinobdella, Haementeria, Helobdella, Hirudinaria, Hëmopis, Limnatis, Macrobdella, Poecilobdella, Pontobdella***; the leech is flat, has two suckers, the cranial sucker houses a mouth (the impression left by a leech bite has been fancifully likened to the Mercedes-Benz insignia); the caudal sucker is involved in crawling; the leech has a highly branched digestive system and a simple nervous system with one neurotransmitter, serotonin, which has made the leech a good model system in neurobiology; leech phlebotomy first began with the Greeks, and is undergoing a limited renaissance for various indications, including removal of excess blood from an operative site, stimulating capillary regrowth into reimplanted, traumatically amputated extremities, in plastic surgery for harvesting hirudin, a potent anticoagulant and in cancer research, as leech saliva inhibits tumor extension; not all leeches are so happily symbiotic; ***Limnatis nilotica*** (***Hirudo aegyptica***), an aquatic leech of North America, Europe and the Middle East may be ingested with drinking water and attach to the oropharynx and urogenital region, causing blood loss and anemia and, if excessive, asphyxia

HIS see Hospital information system

His bundle electrocardiography A relatively recent and sophisticated use of the bipolar cardiac catheter electrode system for recording His bundle activity, studying the cardiac physiology of a patient with recurrent arrhythmias, optimizing pacemaker implantation and for differentiating true atrioventricular blocks from pseudo-atrioventricular block

His disease His-Werner disease A louse-borne, rickettsial (*R quintana*) infection Clinical Intermittent fever, generalized myalgia, shin pain, vertigo, malaise and relapses; Cf Her's disease

Histamine A bioactive amine that is stored in mast cells and basophils that may be secreted by monocytes, neural and endocrine cells; histamine causes smooth muscle contraction, including bronchiolar and small vessel constriction, increased vascular permeability and secretion by nasal and bronchial mucous glands and is held responsible for the symptoms of hay fever, urticaria, angioedema and the bronchospasm of anaphylactic reactions

'Histamine' headache see Cluster headache

Histamine (H_1 and H_2) receptors Cell membrane receptors that are located on the basolateral membrane of the acid-secreting gastric parietal cell; when histamine is bound to H_2 receptors, adenylate cyclase is activated, increasing the intracellular concentration of cyclic AMP, activating the parietal cells' proton pump, an H^+K^+-ATPase which secretes H^+ ion against a large concentration gradient; H_1 and H_2 receptors are expressed on a variety of cells (lymphocytes, monocytes, basophils, eosinophils, smooth muscle cells and gastric parietal cells **H_1 receptor** A histamine receptor present on the surface of some smooth muscle cells that responds to histamine by dilation of arterioles and constriction of veins and bronchioles **H_2 receptor** A histamine receptor present on gastric parietal cells that increases the rate of HCl secretion in response to histamine **H_3 receptor** A histamine receptor present in the lungs, spleen, skin, brain and on nerve endings surrounding blood vessels (Nature 1987; 327:117)

Histamine (H_1 and H_2) receptor antagonists A family of therapeutic agents that counter histamine's activity; H1 receptor mediation of 'mal de mer' can be attenuated by H_1 blockage with diphenhydramine; H_2 receptor-mediated gastritis and benign gastric ulceration usually respond to H_2 blockage by cimetidine and ranitidine, which inhibit gastric acid secretion by blocking the histamine H_2 receptors on the gastric parietal cells; H_2 blocking agents are used to treat recurring duodenal ulcers, gastric ulcers, gastroesophageal reflux and other conditions associated with increased release of histamine, eg mast cell disease and basophilic leukemia **Side effects** Antiandrogenic, eg gynecomastia and impotence Note: H_2 receptor antagonists are used to treat Zollinger-Ellison syndrome, but require high doses, making a new agent, omeprazole, see there

Histidine An amino acid that is not essential for adults, which is required for optimal growth in infants (cross-linking of collagen); histidine is also responsible for the Bohr effect (conformational changes required for optimal O_2 binding by hemoglobin)

Histidemia A common (1:10 000), often asymptomatic autosomal recessive condition characterized by a deficiency in histidase, the enzyme that converts histidine to urocanic acid in the liver and skin **Clinical** Variable, which when symptomatic, is of neonatal onset with impaired speech, growth and mental retardation **Laboratory** Some of the accumulated excess histidine is transaminated to imidazole, the urinary metabolite of which, imidazolepyruvic acid is detectable by the ferric chloride test or by Phenistix, otherwise used to diagnose phenylketonuria Note: 99% of cases are clinically normal despite having biochemical disease; in the symptomatic 1%, treatment (histidine-free formula) is of little benefit

Histiocytic lesions Lesions composed of histiocytes may be benign, indeterminant and malignant in proliferative potential; in order to reduce the confusion related to these lesions, it has been suggested that histiocytoses be subdivided into Class I or Langerhans-cell histiocytoses, encompassing histiocytosis X and non-Langerhans histiocytoses, separated into class II, including infection-associated hemophagic disease and familial erythrophagic lymphohistiocytosis **Clinical** Coagulopathy, pancytopenia, fever and hepatomegaly, and class III, including the rare malignant histiocytic proliferations, eg acute monocytic leukemia (FAB M3), malignant histiocytosis and histiocytic sarcoma **Clinical** Fever, wasting, lymphadenopathy and hepatosplenomegaly (N Engl J Med 1990; 322:683cpc); histiocytic lesions may be grouped according to potential behavior

1) Benign histiocytic lesions a) FAMILIAL HISTIOCYTOSIS WITH EOSINOPHILIA A chronic disease of infants with recurring bacterial infections, diarrhea, eczema, alopecia, associated with immunodeficiency b) SINUS HISTIOCYTOSIS WITH MASSIVE LYMPHADENOPATHY (SHML) Rosai-Dorfman disease A disease most common in adolescent blacks with massive cervical lymphadenopathy as well as enlargement of extranodal (orbit, skin, bone, salivary gland, testis) lymphoid tissues and c) VIRUS-ASSOCIATED HEMOPHAGOCYTIC SYNDROME (VAHS) A condition induced by viral infections, often accompanied by abnormal liver function tests, coagulation assays and pancytopenia **Histopathology** Histiocytic hyperplasia, hemophagocytosis and replacement of native bone marrow elements

2) INTERMEDIATE HISTIOCYTIC LESIONS see Histiocytosis X

3) MALIGNANT HISTIOCYTIC LESIONS a) HISTIOCYTIC MEDULLARY RETICULOSIS (HMR) A systemic proliferation of mature histiocytes with hemophagocytosis, bone marrow necrosis, pancytopenia, hepatitis and coagulopathy; HMR has proven confusing, the combined result of differing criteria used to establish a diagnosis, its relative rarity, regional preferences for different terms for the same condition and misapplication of criteria used to establish the diagnosis; HMR is subdivided into i) MALIGNANT HISTIOCYTOSIS OF ROBB-SMITH A premalignant neoplasm composed of large atypical circulating histiocytes that actively phagocytose red cells, white cells and platelets **Clinical** Aggressive with generalized lymphadenopathy, hepatosplenomegaly, pulmonary involvement and pancytopenia, often fatal **Differential diagnosis** Virus-associated hemophagocytic syndrome and reactive histiocytosis of T-cell proliferations ii) 'REGRESSING ATYPICAL HISTIOCYTOSIS' An indolent pre-histiocytic lymphoma accompanied by chromosome defects **Clinical** Vaguely-defined heterogenous clinical picture with a peak onset in the third decade of life, commonly with extranodal disease of the gastrointestinal tract, skin and bone marrow disease **Prognosis** Relatively good, b) REACTIVE HEMOPHAGOCYTIC SYNDROME (RHS) A condition with a potentially pernicious clinical course, associated with infections, often viral, eg adenovirus, cytomegalo-virus, Epstein-Barr virus, Herpes zoster and parainfluenza, gram-negative bacteremia, tuberculosis, fungal infection, leishmaniasis, as well as drugs and malignancy, eg acute lymphocytic leukemia, Hodgkin's and Lennert's lymphoma and carcinoma of stomach **Histopathology** Dilated subcapsular sinusoids, lined by cells with abundant cytoplasm and a bland nucleus, erythrophagocytosis and increased angiotensin converting enzyme, more specific than lysozyme **Clinical** Patients are severely ill with high mortality, fever, lymphadenopathy, hepatosplenomegaly

Histiocytic lymphoma see Lymphoma

Histiocytoid angioma of Rosai A variant of pyogenic granuloma consisting of a heterogeneous group of non-regressing large vascular tumors which have increased vascular spaces lined by cuboidal histiocyte-like epithelial cells containing large, pale cleaved nuclei

Histiocytosis X Langerhans' cell granulomatosis An autonomous proliferation of a specific cell of the lymphoreticular system, the Langerhans cell, which is a multinucleated giant cell that stains positively with antibodies to ATPase, S-100 and CD1a; the aggregates of Langerhans' cells are accompanied by eosinophils, foamy cells, neutrophils, fibrosis; histiocytosis X is commonly divided into three clinical forms (table)

'Histiocytosis Y' Verruciform Xanthoma A solitary lesion of the oral cavity (occasionally extraoral), described in 1971 by WG Shafer as a red, asymptomatic lesion occurring at age 40 **Histopathology** Verrucous, hyperkeratotic lesion with parakeratin plugging, shaggy with superimposed bacterial colonies, elongated rete pegs with lipid-laden macrophages confined to papillae, no clinical significance **Treatment** Complete excision (Oral Surg 1971; 31:784)

Histocompatibility The desirable prerequisite for tissue allograft transplantation is perfect immune compatibility of tissues; in absence of a perfect HLA (Human leukocyte antigen) match, recipient lymphocytes are stimulated to reject donor tissue by recognizing its 'non-selfness'; these identification characteristics are encoded by a cluster of genes known as the major histocompatibility complex (located on chromosome 6 in humans and 17 in mice), see HLA

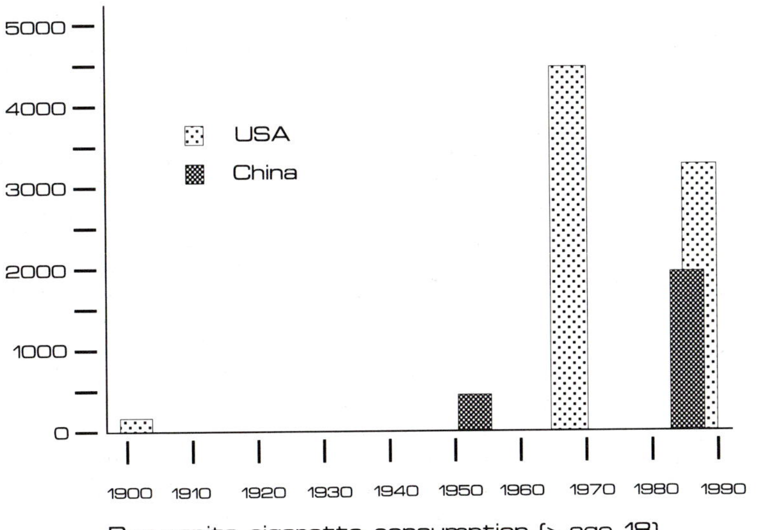

Histiocytosis X

Solitary bone involvement Eosinophilic granuloma A lesion of younger patients that may affect any bone (sparing the hands and feet), most commonly those of the cranial vault, jaw, humerus, rib and femur Radiolog Mimics Ewing sarcoma Treatment Simple curettage Prognosis Excellent

Multiple bone involvement Polyostotic eosinophilic granuloma A lesion that variably affects the skin, eponymically dignified as Hand-Schueller-Christian disease, accompanied by proptosis, diabetes insipidus, or chronic otitis media or combination thereof, marked by a prolonged course with waxing and waning symptoms and a relatively good prognosis

Multiple organ involvement Letter-Siwe disease A lesion that affects the bone, lung and skin, which while histologically indistinct from the other forms, behaves far more aggressively than the other forms Indicators of a poor prognosis include Age under 18 months at time of diagnosis, hemorrhagic skin lesions, hepatomegaly, anemia, thrombocytopenia, bone marrow involvement

Histogram A bar graph representing the frequency of sample distribution found between each of many determined values, as in a chronologic histogram, or as shown below, the per capita consumption of cigarettes

Histologist Anyone who prepares tissues for light and/or electron microscopic examination who is not certified by examination(s) sponsored by the American Society for Clinical Pathologists (ASCP)

Histological technician A person who prepares tissue for microscopic examination with one or more years of formal training, designated by the American Society of Clinical Pathologists as HT(ASCP)

Histopathologist A physician who has undergone a formal training period (in the USA, three or more years) in histopathology, who is eligible or certified by the American Board of Pathology and who interprets histologic slides prepared from diseased tissue

Histotechnologist A histologic technician HT(ASCP) with far more extensive training than a histologic technician, designated as HTL(ASCP)

Histone(s) MOLECULAR BIOLOGY A group of five 11-21 kD basic globular proteins of unknown function that interact in a periodic fashion with eukaryotic DNA; every 150-180 base pairs of DNA are bound to one molecule of H1 and two molecules of H2A, H2B, H3, H4; the evolutionary conservation of the histone 'motif' is considerable, as, for example, there is considerable sequence homology between bovine H3 histone and the garden pea; see Spliceosomes

HITT see Heparin-induced thrombocytopenia/thrombosis

Hitch-hiker thumb A condition characterized by bilateral abduction of the thumbs (proximally placed and hypermobile) associated with deformed and dense carpal and metacarpal bones, seen in diastrophic dwarfism, occasionally Fanconi's anemia and acrocephalosyndactyly

HIV-1 Human immunodeficiency virus The retrovirus intimately linked to AIDS, formerly, AIDS-related virus (ARV), human T-cell lymphotrophic virus, type III (HTLV-III, R Gallo, National Institutes of Health, USA) and lymphadenopathy-associated virus (LAV, L Montagnier, Pasteur Institute, Paris) **Acute HIV infection** Primary symptomatic HIV infection Early HIV infection may be asymptomatic or accompanied by a 'viral syndrome' **Clinical** Fever, severe fatigue, sore throat, myalgia, arthralgia, nausea, vomiting, diarrhea, anorexia, weight loss, headache, photophobia, lymphadenopathy, pruritic maculopapular or urticarial rash, lymphocytic meningoencephalitis and peripheral neuropathy, all of which remit, reappearing as AIDS after a variable latency period of up to several years Pathogenesis High titers of cytopathic virus, which form syncytia in the H9 cell line (N Engl J Med 1991; 324:954,

Clinical classification, HIV-1 infection

Group I Acute HIV-1 infection
Group II Asymptomatic HIV-1 infection
Group III Persistent generalized lymphadenopathy with HIV-1 infection
Group IV HIV-1 infection and either clinical AIDS or other AIDS-related symptoms, eg involuntary weight loss, fever or diarrhea for > one month, dementia, peripheral neuropathy, hairy leukoplakia and oral candidiasis that fall short of the CDC's definition of AIDS
Subgroup A Constitutional symptoms
Subgroup B Neurological symptoms
Subgroup C Infectious disease
(MMWR 1987; 36:3S-15S)

961) **Clinical classification of AIDS** (table, above) **Diagnosis** Enzyme-linked immunosorbent assay (ELISA) is a screening tool that detects the presence of IgM antibodies to HIV Note: Antibodies cross-reactive to HIV-1 core antigen are rare, but occur in normal subjects or those with autoimmune disease, cutaneous T-cell lymphoma and multiple sclerosis; low-level false positive ELISA occurs in alcoholic hepatopathy, pregnancy, non-HIV infected IV drug abusers and hemodialysis patients; ELISA-positive sera are then subjected to Western immunoblot hybridization (see below), which detects specific antibodies to HIV antigens, including p24 (often the first antibody to appear), p41 and p17 antigens Note: ELISA followed by Western blotting (if the serum is positive by the ELISA test) is the standard 'work-up' of blood donors for HIV status; other HIV-1 antigens, eg gp160, gp120, gp50-65 and p31 may evoke antibody production, but are only variably present or less specific; Western blot's rate of false positivity is 1/135,187 (N Engl J Med 1988; 319:961); in terminal AIDS, sero-reversion may occur with loss of antibodies to p24 and p17 (Mayo Clin Proc 1988; 63:373); HIV-1 antigen titers in the blood may be quantified, levels of 30, 3200 and 3500 tissue culture infective doses are observed in subjects with asymptomatic HIV infection, AIDS-related complex and AIDS, respectively, suggesting a direct effect of HIV-1 in the progression of AIDS (N Engl J Med 1989; 321:1621); HIV viremia is more indicative of AIDS than p24 antigenemia which is present in only 45% of those with detectable viremia (ibid, 321:1626); other AIDS tests include a) Agglutination reaction between HIV peptides conjugated to red cells or latex particles, an inexpensive test allowing HIV antibody detection in 10 μl of blood in 2 minutes (false negative rate, 2%) b) HIV culture in cell lines and chloramphenicol acetyltransferase-signal bioassay (low sensitivity, expensive) c) HIV-Antigen assay (slow, expensive) **Disinfection** HIV is inactivated by bleach (750 ppm, or 1:10 dilution for 40 minutes) and formaldehyde (2% for 10 hours); high laundry temperatures (90% reduction in viable HIV), eg 25 minutes at 71°C or 10 minutes at 80°C may be effective; low temperature washing without bleach does not remove HIV (Lab Med 1988; 19:88) **Infections in HIV** Second disease model HIV-positivity tends to worsen the response to other infections, and T-cell response to infections in HIV-positive subjects may trigger multiplication of dormant HIV; AIDS patients have an increased susceptibility to disseminated vaccinia after immunization, neurosyphilis, tuberculosis, herpes and other infections that respond to standard therapy (N Engl J Med 1991; 324:289); several viruses may co-infect with HIV-1, transactivating HIV-1's long terminal repeat (LTR) sequence, eg Herpesvirus, HHV-6, papovavirus, adenovirus and HTLV-I (Nature 1989; 337:370) **Mycoplasma** Simultaneous HIV-1 and Mycoplasma fermentans (incognitus strain) infection results in increased cytocidal effects on CD4+ lymphocytes (Science 1991; 251:1074) **Pathogenesis** HIV-1 infects cells by attaching to susceptible host cells at the extracellular amino acid residues 37-53 of the CD4 receptor, a glycoprotein receptor found on the surface of the helper subset of T cells, most monocytes and macrophages; HIV may also invade cells by IgG's Fc receptor (Science 1988; 242:580); once inside the cell, HIV uses reverse transcriptase to transcribe its RNA into a DNA provirus, which then integrates itself into the host DNA, either remaining dormant or entering into a 'lytic' cycle forcing host cells to produce retrovirus; see Reverse transcriptase **Precautions** Universal blood and body and fluid precautions (MMWR 1985; 34:681, 691; ibid,

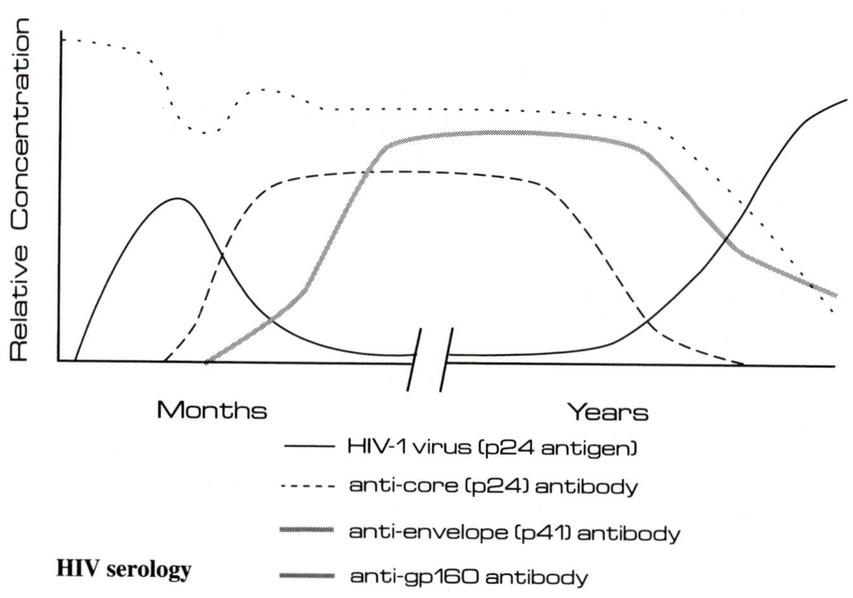

HIV serology

35:221) **Serology** The figure on the facing pag demonstrates the relation between the antigens and the clinical response and the patient's ultimate demise **Seroprevalence Africa** Sub-Saharan Africa Male 1:40; female 1:40, focally up to 1:5; North America Male 1:75; Female 1:700 (Science 1991; 252:372) **Seroprevalence USA** 650 000-1 400 000 (0.2-0.5% of the population) are infected with HIV-1 (MMWR 1990 39:110), ranging from 0.1% in rural regions with low 'risk' activities to 7.8% in urban populations; in low prevalence regions, HIV-1 positivity is more common in men; in high prevalence regions, the male:female ratio is 2.9:1; 20% of men in high prevalence regions are HIV-positive (N Eng J Med 1990; 323:213); seropositivity is up to 9-fold greater in those refusing to be tested **Army (US) personnel** Seroconversion rate among soldiers is 0.29 per thousand person-years (J Am Med Assoc 1991; 265:1709) **Child-bearing women** (USA) Inner-city 8.0/1000, urban (not inner-city) and suburban 2.5/1000 Suburban and rural 0.9/1000; 4.5-5.8/1000 in New York, New Jersey, Washington DC and Florida and 1.5/1000 in the entire US; rate of HIV transmission to the child is 30% (J Am Med Assoc 1991; 265:1704) **Emergency room patients** (USA, 1987) 3% of all and 16% of 25-34 year-old emergency room patients are HIV positive, 80% of whom were unsuspected **Health care workers** (HCW) HIV positivity in HCW reflects HIV positivity in the general population; in the USA, less than 100 HCW without other known risk behaviors have seroconverted; seroconversion after needle or mucosal exposure to HIV-infected patients is approximately 0.3% (Ann Intern Med 1990; 113:740); one dentist in the US infected at least three low-risk persons (J Am Med Assoc 1991; 265:563) **Newborns** Rural New York 0.16% positivity, New York City 1.25% positivity (J Am Med Assoc 1989; 261:1745) **Prison population** Prevalence 2.1-7.6% in men; 2.5-14.7% in women (J Am Med Assoc 1991; 265:1129) **Sexually active adults** 5% of those with sexually-transmitted disease are HIV-1 positive, especially those who also had syphilis or a history of genital herpes **Transmissible fluids and tissues** Blood, tissues, breast milk are recognized HIV 'vectors'; casual household contacts, feces, skin, tears and urine are not known to transmit HIV; saliva inhibits the ability of HIV to infect lymphocytes, see Bergalis case **Treatment** All therapy directed against HIV is experimental, and includes soluble CD4 injected into the circulation, of potential use in binding HIV before it invades cells via the CD4 receptor; CD4 linked to an Fc immunoglobulin fragment, forms an 'immunoadhesin' that has the theoretical advantage of both combining with HIV and stimulating the immune system by activating cytotoxic T-cells Note: HIV-1 survives despite brisk humoral and cellular immune responses by the host **HIV-vaccine** Three facets of the human immunodeficiency virus (HIV) make it a difficult candidate for vaccine production a) It can hide within normal(but infected) cells, protected from the immune system, cloaked within vesicles made from host membrane (the 'Trojan horse' effect) b) The gene encoding the envelope glycoprotein, gp120, is highly mutable and the change of but one or two of gp120's amino acids alters the immune response, forcing the immune system into a constant (and losing) battle to produce antibodies against HIV-1's ever-changing proteins in gp120's 'loop' region; in particular, gp120's env region contains many such hypervariable regions ('hot spots'); any antibody to such 'hot spots' would be useless, although an antibody 'cocktail' to portions of gp120 is of potential use Note: Recombinant gp120 provides protection against HIV-1 in monkeys, but gp160 does not (Nature 1990; 345:622), which is possibly related to the constancy of gp120's 'pit' region c) Has marked affinity for the CD4 molecule; for a vaccine to skirt that affinity, it would need a molecular motif similar to the CD4 molecule Disadvantage: When a non-mutating CD4 'look-alike' is introduced, the immune system may recognize the CD4 antigen as foreign, destroying self CD4 T cells and macrophages d) HIV inserts its genome into the host's genome; development of an anti-HIV vaccine is further hampered by factors extrinsic to the virus, i) in vitro testing of anti-HIV activity cannot prove whether there is adequate in vivo defense ii) Dangers and/or uncertainties of clinical trials with an HIV vaccine, eg paucity of altruistic volunteers for a live attenuated vaccine and iii) Lack of a suitable animal model, although chimpanzees appear to be suitable for testing, given the similarity of HIV to SIV/STLV-III; an effective vaccine must elicit antibodies capable of recognizing HIV before it binds to the CD4 receptor on CD4-bearing T cells and macrophages, which must be very rapid given the high affinity that HIV has for CD4 Recombinant virus expressing a limited number of epitopes ('epitope' vaccines) may result in immune-mediated damage clinical disease by T cells; this family of vaccines, to prevent HIV infection in the early exposure period may elicit unwanted immune destruction (Science 1991; 251:195); potential types of HIV vaccines a) Live attenuated HIV; the possible danger of this approach is exemplified by the finding that live attenuated polioviruses in vaccines may rarely reactivate and themselves cause polio b) Whole inactivated (killed) HIV c) Live recombinant viruses, ie ones containing HIV fragments of sufficient immunogenicity to evoke a protective immune response d) Synthetic peptides or antigenic subunits, eg gp120 or its C21E subfragment Note: Peptides might combine with an inappropriate adjuvant and the tandem molecule may elicit an anomalous and exhuberant immune reaction and e) Others, eg natural products, recombinant DNA products, anti-idiotype molecules and passive immunization; as of year's end of 1991, no effective vaccine was available and none anticipated for at least five years; see gp160 vaccine **Western blot** An immune assay that confirms HIV infec-tion, used

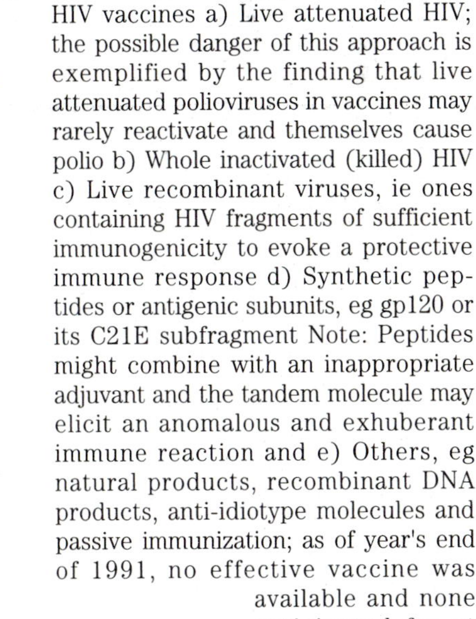

Western blot

when an ELISA screening assay is positive (see figure, above) TECHNIQUE Crude HIV is 'sieved' by gel electrophoresis, separating the HIV molecule into distinctive molecular weight protein bands that are then blotted onto a nitrocellulose strip, some bands are considered diagnostic by the CDC: Definitely positive p24 or p31 and gp41 or gp 120/gp 160 Possibly positive gp41 and gp 120/gp 160 or any combination, one from each gene product Indeterminant One HIV-related band; with time, HIV-1 products may disappear from the serum, especially p24, with a concomitant decrease in anti-core antibody **Window period** A time span of three or more months (see above, HIV serology) during which an HIV-1-infected person is capable of transmitting the virus, but cannot be undetected by currently available tests Note: All blood is screened by the enzyme-linked immunosorbent assay (ELISA), which detects the antibody and not HIV-1 antigen; HIV-antibody-negative but HIV-1 positive donors in the 'window' period may still transmit HIV; see AIDS, Mosquito connection, Monkey connection, Zagury, Zidovudine

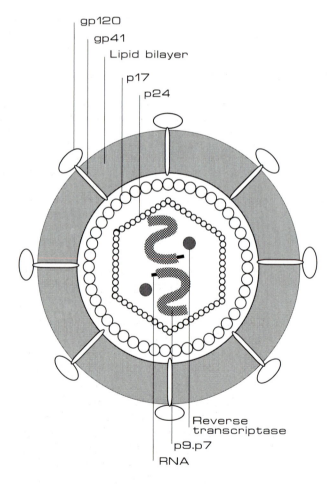

HIV-1 genes ***art/trs*** **gene** see rev gene ***env*** **gene** Encodes viral coat proteins gp 120 and gp 41, which mediate CD4 binding and membrane fusion, controlled by tat and rev ***gag**** **gene** Encodes nucleocapsid core proteins including p24 **LTR** Long terminal repeat Provides the binding sites for host transcription factors, which regulate HIV replication ***nef**** **gene** 3` orf, B gene, ORF-2 gene Encodes a protein of unknown function found in infected patients that may down-regulate viral expression (nef deletion results in a five-fold increase in viral DNA synthesis and replication) ***pol**** **gene** Encodes reverse transcriptase, protease, integrase and ribonuclease **R# gene** Encodes the TAR (transcription activating response) element, which has a nonspecific immunodeficiency effect ***rev#*** **gene** art/trs gene Encodes a 19 kD post-transcriptional protein regulator required for HIV replication, up-regulating HIV synthesis by transactivating anti-repression, increasing the levels of envelope RNA byregulating the env gene; inactivation of the rev gene prevents viral replication (as measured by the successful production of the p24 glycoprotein) by infected monocytes can be massively increased by addition of cytokines to the culture medium ***tat#*** **gene** Encodes a potent 14 kD transcription activator that amplifies HIV replication, the inactivation prevents viral replication ***vif#*** **gene** A gene that facilitates infectivity of free HIV ***vpr#*** **gene** Encodes a weak transcription activator ***vpu#*** **gene** A gene unique to HIV-1 that encodes a 16 kD product, which when mutated, has a 5-10-fold reduction in replicative capacity and is critical for efficient bedding of virions (N Engl J Med 1991; 324:308rv)

*Gene encoding structural protein(s)
#Gene encoding regulatory proteins

HIV virion, structure HIV has a 100 nm in diameter lipid envelope surrounding a dense cylindrical nucleoid containing core proteins, reverse transcriptase (figure) and a genome that has sequence similarity to non-cell-transforming lentiviridae, eg visna and caprine encephalitis viruses; envelope proteins gp41, gp120; nucelocapsid proteins p24, p17, p9, p7

HIV-2 Formerly LAV-2, HTLV-IV, SIV/AGM An immunodeficiency virus first identified in West Africans with abnormal reactions to HIV-1 and simian immunodeficiency virus (SIV), HIV-2 is genetically closer to SIV/MAC (70% sequence 'homology') than to HIV-1 (40% sequence 'homology'), with 50% conservation for gag and pol and even less for other genes; HIV-2 has structural antigens p24, gp36 and gp140 Clinical Similar to AIDS Epidemiology HIV-2 is largely confined to West Africa and has an AIDS pattern II (heterosexual promiscuity) epidemiology; HIV-2 contains X-ORF (as does SIV/Mne) and vpx, which are unique to HIV-2

HIV-3 A 'third' human immunodeficiency virus has been described by various workers, who are peripheral to major HIV research efforts; if an HIV-3 exists, it is poorly studied

HLA Human leukocyte antigen complex A system of

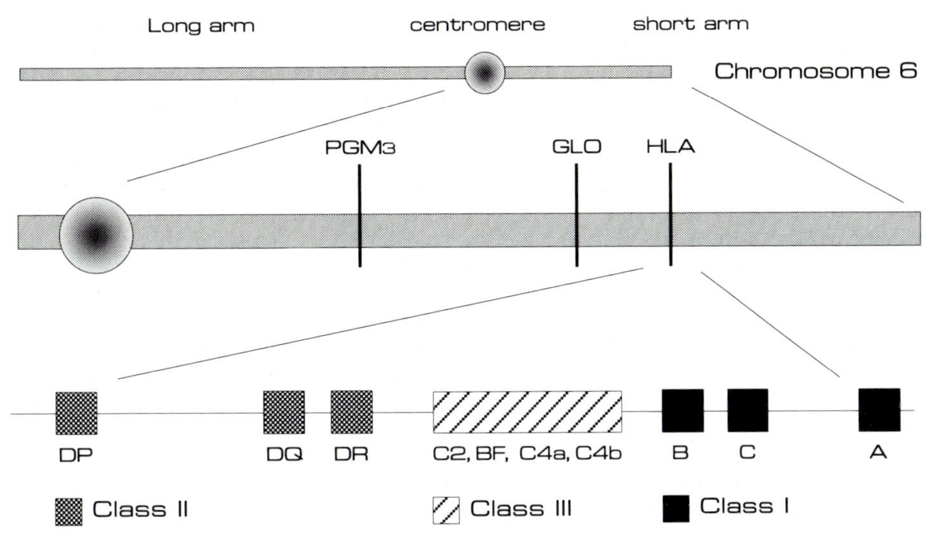

HLA specificities

genes unique to each individual human that are statistically shared with one in four of his/her siblings; the HLA regions are found within the major histocompatibility complex (MHC) and were first recognized when the serum from multiply transfused subjects and multiparous females were found to agglutinate leukocytes; multiparous women continue to be the best source for HLA typing antisera, which is harvested from placentas; the MHC is located on the short arm of chromosome 6, 32 centimorgans from the centromere and divided into three classes Class I proteins include HLA-A, HLA-B and HLA-C, have a transmembrane hydrophilic region with two disulfide-linked and one non-disulfide linked extracellular domain bound to β_2-microglobulin, encoded on chromosome 15 and expressed on all nucleated cells; class I antigens are defined serologically by the microcytotoxicity assay, are recognized during graft rejection, are responsible for refractoriness to platelet transfusions and serve as homing targets for HLA-specific cytolysis (efferent limb of virally-infected cells) and may be lysed by killer cells; the class I region also encodes a group of non-polymorphic proteins, HLA-E, F and G; some structural motifs in class I antigens appear in insulin receptors, epidermal growth factors and γ-endorphin Class II proteins, HLA-DR, HLA-DQ and HLA-QP, consist of two similar (α and β) chains with transmembrane hydrophilic regions and two extracellular, disulfide bond-linked domains, are expressed on sperm, B-cells, myeloid cell precursors, activated T-cells and antigen-presenting cells (monocytes, macrophages, Langerhans and dendritic cells), endothelial cells; class II antigens act in the sensitization phase (afferent limb) of cell-mediated cytotoxicity, coordinating the presentation of antigen to T-cells, facilitating T-helper function, suppression and cooperation, and mediating graft-versus-host disease; class II antigens (HLA-DR and HLA-DQ) are identified by mixed leukocyte reaction Lymphocytes (responder cells) from a potential organ recipient are incubated with irradiated lymphocytes from a donor that are antigenic, but immunoparalyzed, thus being capable of eliciting proliferation of immune competent cells, measuring the increase in H_3 uptake in recipient cells b) HLA-DP specificity is determined by primed lymphocyte typing, which identifies differences in antigens among members of a species; primed lymphocyte typing is essentially in vitro immunization, using lymphocytes from any two subjects to prepare reagents that detect antigenic differences in the HLA class II Note: HLA-DQ and HLA-DR are heterodimers composed of a 34 kD α chain and a 29 kD β chain MHC Class III encodes 21-hydroxylase, complement proteins C2, C4 and factor B of the alternate complement pathway

HLA and disease The association of HLA haplotypes with specific diseases is determined by calculating a) Relative risk Patients with a particular HLA antigen 'X' Number of control subjects without the antigen, divided by Patients without the antigen 'X' Control subjects with the antigen (but not the disease) and b) Absolute risk Patients with the HLA antigen divided by the control subjects with the antigen X Prevalence of the disease in the population; in certain conditions, virtually all

Diseases associated with HLA specificities

Addison's disease (B8, DR3, Dw3), ankylosing spondylitis (B27), Behcet's disease (B5), Buerger's disease (B12), celiac disease or gluten-sensitive enteropathy (B8, Dw3), chronic active hepatitis (DR3), deQuervain thyroiditis (Bw35), dermatitis herpetiformis (Dw3), Goodpasture syndrome (DR2), mesangioproliferative glomerulonephritis (DR4), Grave's disease (B8 in caucasians, Bw35 and Dw12 in Japanese, Bw46 in Chinese), hemochromatosis (A3, B7, B14), insulin-dependent diabetes mellitus (B8. B15, DRw3, DRw4), juvenile rheumatoid arthritis (B27, DR5, DR8), late onset adrenal hyperplasia with hirsutism (Aw33/B14), myasthenia gravis (A1, A3, B8, Dw3, DR3), psoriasis (Cw6), psoriatic arthritis (B27), Reiter syndrome (B27), rheumatoid arthritis (DR4), Salmonella arthritis (B27), Sjogren syndrome (DR3, B8), lupus erythematosus (DR2, DR3), Takayasu's disease (B52), Yersinia arthritis (B27) patients have the same HLA antigens, eg HLA-B27 associated with ankylosing spondylitis, HLA-DR4 with pemphigus vulgaris and HLA-DRw52a with primary sclerosing cholangitis (N Engl J Med 1990; 322:1842); other HLA associations include HLA-B8 Chronic active hepatitis, sicca syndrome, dermatitis herpetiformis, coeliac disease, idiopathic Addison's disease, Graves' disease, multiple sclerosis HLA-B27 see below HLA-DR3 insulin-dependent diabetes mellitus, Graves disease, Addison's disease, celiac disease (table, above)

HLA-B27-related arthropathies A group of joint diseases that more commonly occur in subjects with the HLA-B27 antigen, including ankylosing spondylitis, juvenile rheumatoid arthritis, psoriatic arthritis, Reiter syndrome, ***Salmonella***-related arthritis, ***Yersinia*** arthritis

HLA-G An HLA class I antigen expressed on trophoblast, ie placental cells, and tumors of trophoblastic origin; this unique antigen is not polymorphic and is found only on cells that don't express HLA-A, B and C, eg extravillous cytotrophoblast from the placenta and choriocarcinoma; HLA-G is most prominently expressed in the first trimester of pregnancy; since it is thought that the trophoblast cells at the maternal-fetal interface play a role in the survival of the semiallogenic fetus, HLA-G-positive cells may form a barrier, preventing 'rejection' of the fetus; the high expression of HLA-G implies a global immune tolerance by the mother (Science 1990; 248:220)

HLH see Helix-loop-helix motif

HLHS Hypoplastic left heart syndrome see Baby Faye heart

HMG CoA reductase inhibitors A family of drugs that inhibits the activity of 3-hydroxy-3-methylglutaryl coenzyme A, an enzyme involved in an early step of cholesterol synthesis; the first approved agent with this activity permits enough mevalonate to be synthesized so that there is adequate cholesterol for cell membrane function and steroidogenesis; HMG CoA reductase evokes a significant reduction in LDL-cholesterol, the main atherogenic factor in the atherosclerotic process; these agents are indicated in younger men with total cholesterol levels above 6.47 mmol/L (US: 250 mg/dl), at a dose of 20 mg/d lovastatin (J Am Med Assoc 1991; 265:1145)

HMwK High molecular weight kininogen A 150 kD plasma glycoprotein involved in initiating the intrinsic coagulation pathway

HMO Health maintenance organization An organized system that provides comprehensive prepaid health care; an HMO provides or ensures delivery of a set of basic and supplementary health maintenance and treatment services in a defined geographic region to a voluntarily-enrolled group of persons, requires that its enrollees use the services of designated physicians, hospitals and other providers of medical care and receives reimbursement through a predetermined, fixed periodic prepayment by or on behalf of each individual or family unit regardless of the amount of services provided; HMOs are large multi-specialty groups that homogenize medical care by utilizing physicians as interchangeable parts; in 1987, 650 HMOs provided medical services to 30 million US citizens; there is an trend for younger physicians to work for HMOs as the burden of patient billing is eliminated, on-call schedules at night are shared with a larger group of colleagues and the average medical school debt ($42 000, 1989) may be paid (N Engl J Med 1985; 312:590)

HMR see Histiocytic medullary reticulosis

hnRNA see Heterogeneous nuclear RNA

Hobnail A fanciful adjectival desciptor for a two- or three-dimensional jutting of mutiple large rounded masses above a flattened surface

Hobnail cells A non-specific term for cells that jut above an adjacent epithelial or endothelial surface or lining; the hobnail pattern's significance differs according to the organ, and it can be neoplastic as in mesonephroid-type ovarian cystadenocarcinoma, clear cell carcinoma, endometrial carcinoma, mesotheliomas or reactive, as the jutting of type II pneumocytes above the alveolar lining in lungs with diffuse alveolar damage or the bulging of succulent, secretion-filled, vacuolated, enlarged and pleomorphic cells in the lobules of a lactating breast

Hobnail metaplasia A benign transition of endometrial glands into hobnail-like cells that prolapse into the lumen and which may be associated with endometrial hyperplasias or endometrial carcinoma, but alone has no prognostic significance

Hobnail pattern Liver pathology Bumpy nodularity separated by broad trabecular scars seen macroscopically on the liver surface in posthepatitis cirrhosis Note: A hobnail has a massive head and short tang and is used to protect soles of heavy boots

Hockey stick appearance A descriptive term for an elongated cylindrical mass ending in a gentle curve, fancifully likened to a hockey stick

Hockey stick cells Hematopathology Unicellular Reed-Sternberg cells with a large vesicular nucleus and peripheral nucleolus Hooked cells Neuropathology Neuro-fibroblasts in von Recklin-ghausen's disease

Hockey stick deformity Orthopedics A descriptor for the femoral deformity that may be seen (figure)in Jaffe-Lichtenstein syndrome (monostotic and polyostotic fibrous dysplasia), and if severe, simulates a shepherd's crook

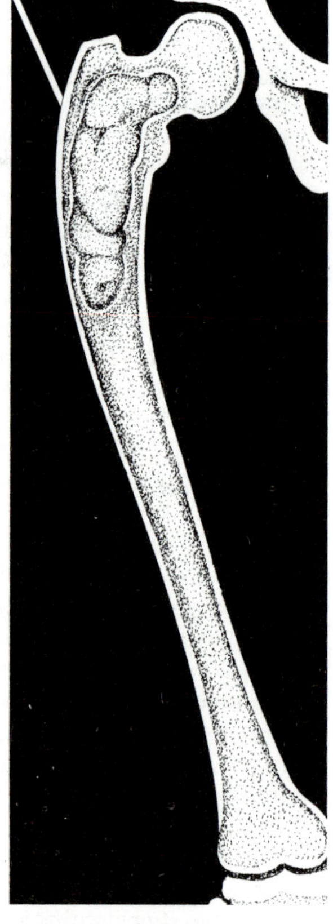

Hockey stick deformity

Hof German, courtyard The focal perinuclear clearing seen at the nuclear concavity in plasma cells; a hof may also be seen in lymphoblasts, Reed-Sternberg cells or in the inclusions in chlamydia-infected epithelial cells in trachoma inclusion conjunctivitis, where the 'hof' is created by the nucleus

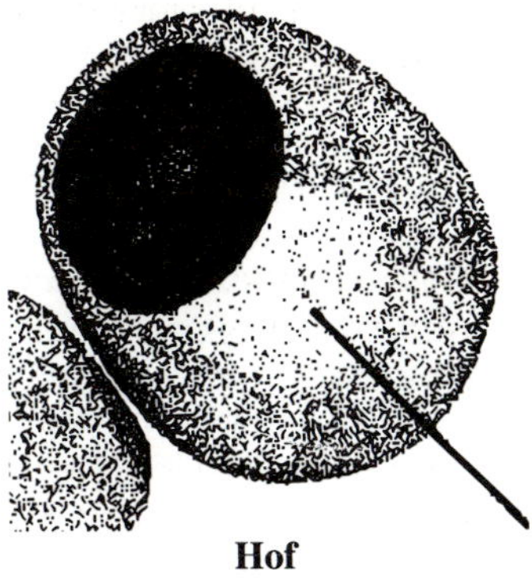

Hof

Hogness box see TATA box

HOHD syndrome Hair-onychodysplasia, hypohydrosis-deafness syndrome An autosomal recessive condition characterized by life-long baldness, microdontia, dysplastic toenails, hypohidrosis, palmo-plantar as well as knee-elbow hyperkeratosis that may be accompanied by sensorineural defects

Höhendiurese A physiological reaction to high altitudes, in which there is increased excretion of fluids; in acute mountain sickness, there is increased weight, infrequent urination, peripheral edema and rales on chest examination, ie fluid accumulation possibly related to the loss of this physiological response

Holandric GENETICS Passing of chromosomal material exclusively from father-to-son, as in the passage of the Y chromosome

'Hole-in-the-stomach' man PHYSIOLOGY Alexis St Martin, a French-Canadian fur trapper whose accidental shotgun blast to the stomach in 1822 never properly healed; Wm Beaumont, a US Army surgeon, took the opportunity to study gastric physiology and for the next eight years popped things in and out of Alexis' stomach including Limberger cheese, tripe, inebriants and other comestibles; these crude studies served to identify pepsin and hydrochloric acid

Holiday heart 1) Atrial fibrillation or flutter after binge alcohol abuse (Am J Heart 1978; 95:555) 2) Atrial fibrillation or flutter as a startle response to loud noises, eg firecrackers on July 4th, the US day of Independence (N Engl J Med 1989; 320:402c)

Holistic medicine Fringe medicine A group of alternate health care systems in which there is a 'whole body' approach to healing, and health maintenance, requiring integration of the body, mind and spirit, based on the holistic doctrine, which holds that the entire organism cannot be understood merely by studying and understanding the lower levels of organization; holistic medicine 'disciplines' include aural analysis, biofeedback, clairvoyant diagnosis, homeopathy, hypnosis, iridology, naturopathy, psychic healing, rolfing, tai chi and zone therapy Note: Acupuncture and chiropractic medicine are also 'holistic', but are generally regarded with less suspicion by mainstream medicine as some data suggests they may be effective in certain types of diseases; holistic medicine is criticized as being more 'mystical' or magical than scientific in its approach to understanding disease; see Unproven methods of cancer therapy

Holliday model MOLECULAR BIOLOGY A model that seeks to explain the mechanism of gene conversion during a recombination event, in which there is reciprocal exchange of distinct markers; according to the model delineated by R Holliday, homologous chromosomes I and II are aligned, adjacent chains are nicked at homologous sites, the strands are allowed to cross, then rejoin and the newly exchanged branches migrate back

Hollingshead index SOCIAL MEDICINE A simple scoring system for determining socioeconomic status based on two objective criteria a) Occupation The occupation of the head of household, allowing a score of 1 for major professionals (physicians, lawyers, certified public accountants), higher executives, major military or political officials, proprietors of large businesses, to a score of 7 for unskilled laborers and b) Education The amount of formal education, with a score of 1 for those who had completed graduate/professional schooling to 7 for those who had not completed six years of formal education

Hollyleaf appearance 1) A descriptor for the scalloped regenerative nodules separated by broad bands of fibrosis, typical of the macronodular cirrhosis of well-advanced hemochromatosis 2) A descriptor (fingure, below) for the irregularly spiculated erythrocytes (drepanocytes) due to polymerization of 'sickling' hemoglobins Hbs when red cells are exposed to low-oxygen environments; sickling Hbs, eg hemoglobins C, D and S, sickle-trait (Hb AS), S-thalassemia, Hb C-Harlem, hemoglobin S-Memphis

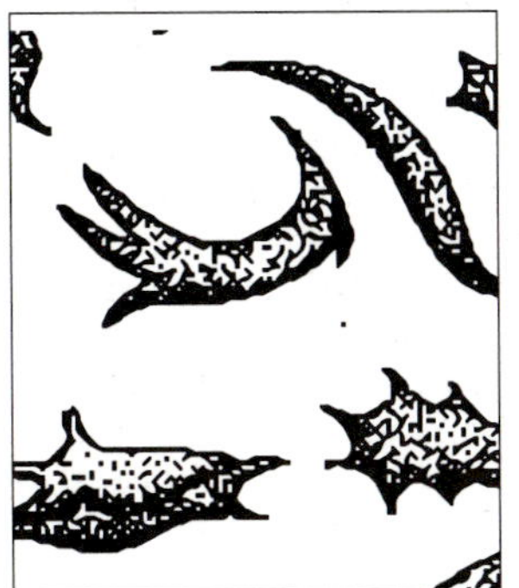
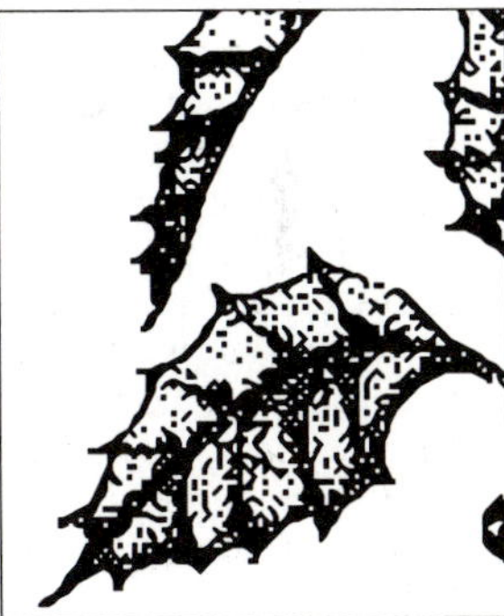

Hollyleaf appearance

'Holstein cow pattern' A descriptor for the gross appearance of the patchy midbrain demyelinization typical of multiple sclerosis, seen with myelin stain

Home-bound syndrome see House-bound syndrome

Home health care A segment of the health care industry that provides equipment, eg miniature intensive care units with ventilators, central venous pressure lines, telemetry, health care providers, eg licensed practical nurses, registered nurses and other services including socialization and communication, with the intent of maintaining a person in an environment, eg the patient's home, that is comfortable and cost-effective (J Am Med Assoc 1990; 263:1241rv; ibid 1991; 265:769rv)

Homeless(ness) SOCIAL MEDICINE A tragedy of developed

nations where person(s) lack a permanent residence, often living on the streets without protection from the environment and/or ready access to sanitation facilities; up to 3 milion people are estimated to be homeless in the USA, and they are often victims of violence, 'disaffiliation', suffer multiple infections, sexually-transmitted disease, especially AIDS and high levels of substance abuse (J Am Med Assoc 1989; 262:1352, 1358); 40% are considered mentally disturbed; most deaths in the homeless occur in males under age 60 and are alcohol-related; the US vagrancy laws are often abused in dealing with those who are guilty of no other crime than lack of money or a job and/or a place to go; see 'Fourth World', Shelterization

Homeobox A lineage-restricted 183 base pair segment of DNA that contains homeotic genes, which control identity, polarity and segmentation of body parts, ie spatial organization and which plays a role in embryogenesis and spermatogenesis; the homeobox is highly conserved, with 75% amino acid homology between frogs, fruitflies and more 'advanced' species; the homeobox is a fairly 'ancient' DNA sequence, which has been found in yeasts, estimated to be 100 milion years old; the homeobox encodes a 61- residue homeo domain, a DNA-binding protein that controls the homeobox by transactivation, binding by a 'helix-loop-helix' motif (Science 1988; 242:925) to the DNA near the gene's start codon; human homeoboxes are similar to the *Drosophila* boxes, discovered in the 1980s in the *Antennapedia*, fushi tarazu and engrailed genes; Cf Oct-1, Oct-2 genes

Homeopathy A form of 'holistic' medicine, formulated by SF Hahnemann (1755-1843) that was heretical at the time for its opposition to blood-letting, emetics and cathartics; homeopathy is based on the principle of '*SIMILIA SIMILIBUS CURANTUR*', Like cures like, ie a disease caused by a substance, eg arsenic, could be cured by that same substance in infinitely diluted doses; homeopathy has lost support for the lack of reproducibility of reported results and in the current environment, some of its practitioners have been severely criticized (J Am Med Assoc 1987: 257:1635); in one report (Nature 1988; 333:816) ultra-low (homeopathic) concentrations of immunoglobulin E evoked basophil degranulation; there was no plausible explanation of the phenomenon, the results were poorly reproducible (Nature 1988; 335:200); homeopathy thus remains unsubstantiated; see Holistic medicine, Naturopathy

Homeotic genes Those genes that establish primitive embryonic structural pathways giving rise to adult structures, the mutation of which causes a transformation of body parts into structures that are appropriate for other positions in the organism; see Homeobox

Homeric laughter Uncontrolled spasmodic laughter induced by mirthless stimuli, a symptom of organic brain disease that indicates a poor prognosis; mirthless laughter may be seen in multiple sclerosis,pseudobulbar palsy, epilepsy, intracranial hemorrhage, frontal lobotomy and is especially characteristic of Kuru, a disease that causes 'laughing death'

Homicide A rare event in civilized nations that reaches epidemic proportions in the US; in males aged 15-24, homicide rate ranges from 0.3-0.5/10^5 in Austria and Japan to 5.0/10^5 in Scotland, in the USA, 22/10^5, 86/10^5 in blacks and 231/10^5 in the state of Michigan (J Am Med Assoc 1990; 263:3292); 12-40% of homicides in the US are drug-related and the victims often have cocaine metabolites (benzoylecgonine), in their body fluids at the time of death (J Am Med Assoc 1991; 265:760); see Manslaughter, Murder; Cf Suicide

Homing receptor selectin see Selectins

Homologous recombination GENETICS A recombination event that occurs at regions of chromosome homology, through the breakage and union of DNA, an event that has been used in transgenic models, where existing genes are knocked out and replaced with a modified gene; see Recombinant DNA technology

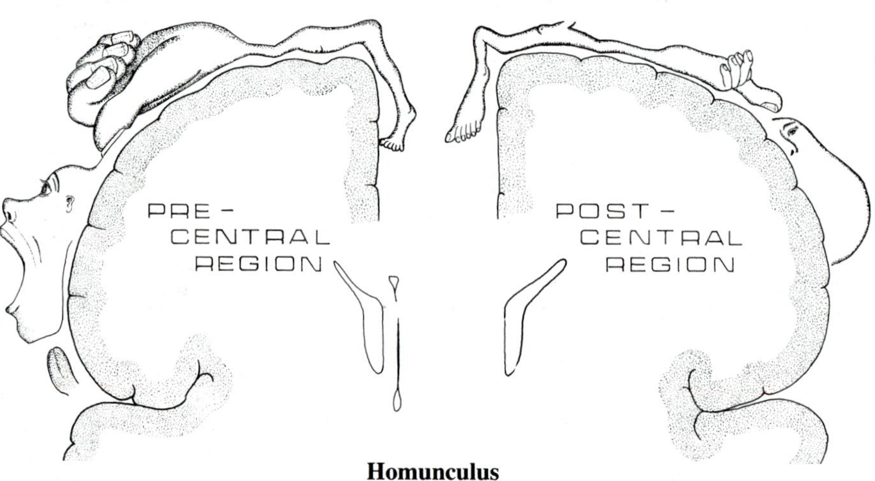

Homunculus

Homology EVOLUTIONARY BIOLOGY A term that implies common ancestral origin of DNA and proteins, which has been incorrectly used by molecular biologists for the degree (in percentage) of sequence relatedness either for DNA (nucleotide or DNA 'homology') or proteins (amino acid or protein 'homology'); evolutionary biologists decry this misuse of 'homology' and suggest 'sequence similarity' as a viable substitute (Cell 1987; 50:667; Science 1987; 237:1570) Note: Given the firm entrenchment of the incorrect use of homology in the biological literature, and that evolutionary biologists are a more exotic species in the research food chain, the 'wrong' definition may ultimately prevail

Homosexuality The latent or manifest sexual attraction of one to another of the same sex, referring in common parlance to male homosexuality; Kinsey's seminal studies in the 1940s on sexual behavior in the US were based on data from white middle-class men; at the time, 4% of US males were exclusively homosexual; data from 1970 and 1988 indicate that 20.3% of adult males had had homosexual contact prior to age 19, 6.7% after the age of 19 and 1.6-2.0% within the last year; never-married men are more likely to be homosexual, but also one-half of the current homosexual group was married Note: Minimum estimates are assumed as under-reporting of homosexual activity is probable (Science 1989; 243:338); an organic component to homosexual orientation has been proposed, as the male homosexual brain may have both an enlarged suprachiasmatic nucleus and a region of the anterior hypothalamus' interstitial nucleus that is similar in size to that of women (Science 1991; 253:1034, 956ed); see AIDS, Gay bowel disease, Circumstantial homosexuality, HIV; Cf Sexual deviancy

Homosexual panic A form of schizophrenic anxiety where a patient is greatly agitated, fearing that he/she is homosexual, will inadvertently commit an act viewed as being homosexual in nature or will be accused of being homosexual; these anxiety attacks are transient and are often accompanied by delusions, hallucinations, irrational behavior or thought and shallow or inappropriate affect; see Circumstantial homosexuality; Cf 'Don Juan' syndrome

Homunculus 'Little man' NEUROANATOMY A diagrammatic representation of the volume of the cerebral cortex dedicated to either motor (precentral or Brodman's areas 4 and 6) or sensory (postcentral or Brodman's area 3) zones with respect to each corporal region; the grotesque little man (facing page) has hands and tongue that are far more prominent han the trunk and extremities, indicating their relative importance

Honeybee syndrome A model for experimental teratogenesis, created by adding D-mannose to rat-embryo culture, causing growth retardation and faulty neural tube closure, attributed to low-level inhibition of glycolysis (hypoxic glycolysis is a major source of ATP during early rodent development and presumed to be so in humans); the defects are thought to result from aberrant 'fuel mixtures' during critical stages of embryogenesis, explaining some of the defects seen in children of diabetic mothers, in whom increased glucose causes defective glycolysis (N Engl J Med 1981; 310:223); the term 'honeybee' was chosen as the deleterious effects of D-mannose were initially seen only in apidae (honeybees); other hexoses (fructose, sorbitol, galactose) cause low-level growth retardation; the D-mannose effect can be overcome by increasing the O_2 or glucose in the system, suggesting that mannose and glucose compete with each other for available hexokinase

Honeycomb atropy A rare autosomal recessive symmetrical skin lesion characterized by cutaneous atrophy with sharply demarcated 'pits', variably accompanied by cardiac defects, mental retardation and neurofibromas

Honeycomb pattern A reticulated or net-like pattern with relative periodicity in a two-dimensional plane BONE RADIOLOGY A honeycomb pattern may be seen in a plain skull film as patchy new bone fills in the underlying osteoporosis circumscripta characteristic of Paget's disease of the bone GYNECOLOGIC CYTOLOGY 'Honeycombs' are monotonous clusters of benign endometrial cells seen on papanicolaou-stained cervical smears, seen as monolayers of small epithelial cells with uniform, oval nuclei,bland or slightly granular chromatin PULMONARY DISEASE 'Honeycombing' (figure, below) is a localized or diffuse coarsening of pulmonary parenchyma with partial alveolar wall destruction and incomplete replacement, and alveolar wall thickening by interstial fibrosis (in contrast, emphysema demonstrates alveolar wall attenuation), a pattern typical of advanced interstitial pneumonia; the radiologic honeycomb pattern is more vague, and may be seen in a plain chest film in interstitial fibrosis, as well as lupus erythematosus, progressive systemic sclerosis, lymphangiomatosis syndrome, end-stage sarcoidosis and adenocarcinoma; Cf Chicken wire pattern

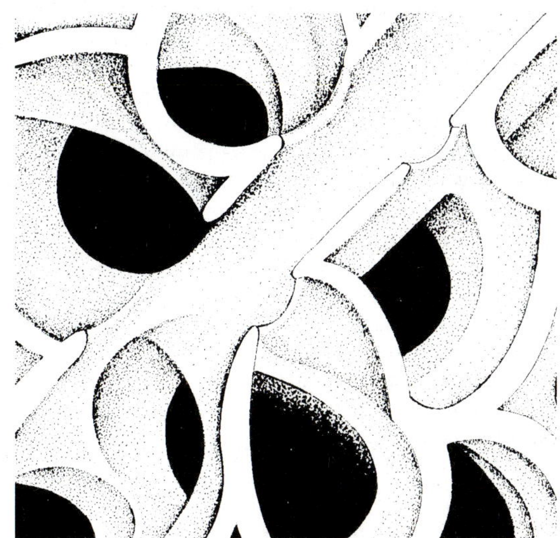

Honeycomb pattern, lung

Honey intoxication Infant botulism may be due to ingestion of *Clostridium botulinum* spores, which germinate in the gastrointestinal tract, producing toxin, causing constipation, feeding difficulties, floppy baby symptoms, facial grimacing, dysphagia, decreased sphincter control, reflexes and sudden apnea; at least one-third of cases of infant botulism worldwide directly inculpate honey, as the same serotype of *C botulinum* is isolated from both the honey and the infant Mortality Less than 3%

Honeymoon cystitis A non-specific urethritis caused by local irritation due to prolonged, frequent or first-time sexual activity in women with a low baseline of sexual traffic; damage to the vesicovaginal wall may evoke cystitis, hematuria, dysuria, increased frequency and urgency; although cultures are often negative, the condition may respond to antibiotics; resolution may be hastened by a rest period

Honeymoon period A phrase used in various fields of medicine referring to a time period following the diagnosis of a disease, but preceding its full effect or impact, fancifully likened to the period of early marriage when the husband and wife are most cordial and passionate with each other DIABETOLOGY A period of residual β cell function and insulin secretion in early-onset insulin-dependent diabetes mellitus that follows stabilization of the patient's hyperglycemic presentation; in the honeymoon period, most children require one-half of the calculated insulin dose, ie 0.5 U/kg or may even go into temporary 'remission', signalled by recurring hypoglycemia at the initial dose, a time period that is short-lived, usually less than one year in duration NEPHROLOGY A period of optimism and euphoria accompanying the early stage of chronic dialysis affecting patients in renal failure; the honeymoon period lasts from 6 weeks to 6 months and is followed by a Mourning period, see there PEDIATRIC SURGERY A postoperative time period in an infant with congenital diaphragmatic hernia characterized by stable vascular resistance, relative ease of ventilation and normalization of blood gases; this deteriorates within hours to days and the infant develops pulmonary hypertension and resultant right-to-left shunting through the ductus arteriosus and foramen ovale (J Pediatr Surg 1977; 12:149); see Extracorporeal membrane oxygenation

Honk PEDIATRICS A widely-transmitted precordial whoop, described as a high-pitched, musical, late systolic murmur in some patients with mitral valve prolapse, a sound attributed to resonation of the valve leaflets and chordae; non-honking patients with mitral valve prolapse may be made to honk by having them stand or lean (Br Heart J 1971; 33:707) Note: 'Honk' is the sound produced by geese or automobile horns

H2O syndrome Hypogonadotrophic hypogonadism, muscular hypotonicity and obesity; see HHHO syndrome

Honorary co-authorship ACADEMIA The practice in which the name of senior researchers are added to research reports that are the work of others, eg undergraduates and postdoctoral fellows working in their laboratories, regardless of whether they have participated in the research itself (Nature 1987; 325:207); this practice may prove embarassing to the co-author if the research proves to be fraudulent; see Authorship, CV-weighing, Darsee affair

HOOD syndrome Hereditary onycho-osteodysplasia see Nail-patella syndrome

Hoogsten base pairing MOLECULAR BIOLOGY A variant DNA conformation that occurs in a region where proteins interact with the double helix; Hoogsten pairing requires higher energy to maintain the physicochemical conformation by protonation of the cytosine ring; most double helices of DNA are in the classic Watson and Crick conformation

Hook effect IMMUNOPATHOLOGY An artefact occasionally seen in the immunoradiometric assay (IRMA) that appears when the hormone being measured is present in very high concentrations; the detector system will not measure that excess, as it will have reached a theoretical limit; the decreased counts bound with the labeled antibody at high hormone levels results in a spuriously low result being reported; IRMA should not be used for measuring hormones which may be in high concentrations (hCG, prolactin or gastrin) in clinical samples; the hook effect requires that two different concentrations be measured to establish linearity

Hookworms Nematodes, eg Old World hookworm (***Ancylostoma duodenale***) and New World hookworm (***Necator americanus***), which target the small intestine, causing sensitization of the penetration site, eg skin, causing 'ground itch, or lungs, eg Loeffler syndrome as they wiggle therethrough, causing eosinophilia and anemia **Laboratory** Rhabditidiform larvae may be confused with ***Strongyloides stercoralis*** and the eggs may be confused with those of ***Trichostrongylus*** and ***Meloidogyne*** species

HOPG Highly-ordered pyrolytic graphite The most common substrate used in scanning tunneling microscope studies (SEMs) for analysis of the surface morphology or 'signature' of biomolecules, eg DNA Note: Because HOPG, which is attached electrophoretically to the molecules being studied, has its own 'signature' with features including periodicity and meandering of molecules over steps that were previously attributed to biomolecules, it is unclear whether SEM studies using HOPG are completely valid (Science 1991; 251:641)

Horizontal ray RADIOLOGY A central projection ray that remains horizontal regardless of the patient's position; horizontal rays are of use in determining fluid levels, as these appear as sharply-demarcated lines, delineating two different densities and in films of joints to assess rugosity of an articular surface

Horizontal transmission EPIDEMIOLOGY The transmission of an infection in individuals of the same generation; Cf Hereditary transmission, Vertical transmission

Hormonal therapy ONCOLOGY A therapeutic modality for certain malignancies, some of which partially respond to manipulation of hormonal receptors on the surface of the tumor cells BREAST CARCINOMA Hormonal manipulation intends to block membrane receptors for estrogens and, to a lesser extent, progesterone, reducing cancer aggressiveness LYMPHOPROLIFERATIVE DISORDERS Adjuvant therapy uses corticosteroids in both induction of remissions and maintenance doses PROSTATIC ADENOCARCINOMA Hormonal therapy attempts to either inhibit gonadotropin at the pituitary by using potent analogs, eg buserelin, leuprolide acetate, blocking gonadotropin-releasing hormone, or block the peripheral action of androgens at the cellular level, eg flutamide, nilutamide (N Engl J Med 1989; 321:419); other therapeutic uses of hormones include treatment of deficiency states and use of pharmacologic doses of steroids as an anti-inflammatory agent or an immune suppressant; see Ectopic hormones, Estrogen receptors

Hormone family A group of hormones that share considerable sequence similarity ('homology') in terms of peptide motifs, including gastrointestinal tract hormones and neuropeptides; hormone families are thought to have arisen through gene duplication during evolution and have been divided into a) Gastrin, cholecystokinin b) Secretin, glucagon and VIP, as well as gastric inhibitory polypeptide (GIP), growth hormone releasing factor (GRF), Glicentin and oxyntomodulin c) Pancreatic polypeptide, peptide YY, neuropeptide Y d) Tachykinin, bombesin, substances K and P, neuromedins B and K e) Opioid peptides f) Proenkephalins, eg met- and leu-enkephalins g) Pro-opiomelanocortins, including ACTH, α- and β-MSH, β-endorphin g) Predynorphin group, including β-endorphin, dynorphin, leu-enkephalin, leumorphin h) Calcitonin, epidermal growth factor (EGF), insulin and somatostatin

Hormone response element (HRE) Short, circa 20 base pairs in length cis-acting sequences of DNA that are required 'receptor' sites for hormonal activation and transcription; insertion of HREs to otherwise hormone-nonresponsive sites causes a gene to become responsive to a hormone; HREs function in a position- and orientation-independent fashion, thus acting like transcription enhancers, although differing therefrom as HRE activity requires a protein ligand

Horn cell Keratocyte Normocytic, normochromic erythrocytes with lateral notches and two pointed ends, corresponding to ruptured vacuoles; the cells have a semilunar or spindled shape; associated with intravascular protuberances, eg cardiac valve protheses, synthetic intravascular grafts and fibrin in disseminated intravascular coagulation

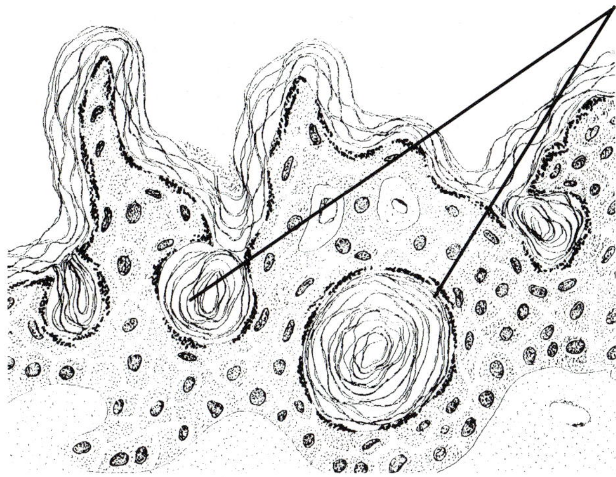

Horn pseudocysts

Horn pseudocyst DERMATOPATHOLOGY Laminated, whorls of 'basket-weave' cornified keratin that dip below the epithelial surface, forming pseudocystic spaces, a characteristic histologic finding seen in irritated seborrheic keratosis; Cf Squamous eddies, Squamous pearls

Horror autotoxicus Fear of self-poisoning IMMUNOLOGY Paul Ehrlich's explanation for why an individual does not (usually) produce autoantibodies, despite the proven immunogenicity of his antigens, because of the horror or fear of self-destruction; loss of this horror results in autoimmune diseases

Horse riding stance see 'Plucked chicken' appearance

Horseshoe kidney A relatively common (1/700 live births) lesion (male:female ratio, 2:1), seen alone or associated with trisomy 18, characterized by fusion of the renal poles; this developmental anomaly occurs after the metanephric ducts have joined the metanephric blastema, but before the kidney's cephalic ascent, which occurs in the second gestational month; in most cases, the fusion is at the lower pole, the isthmus consists of

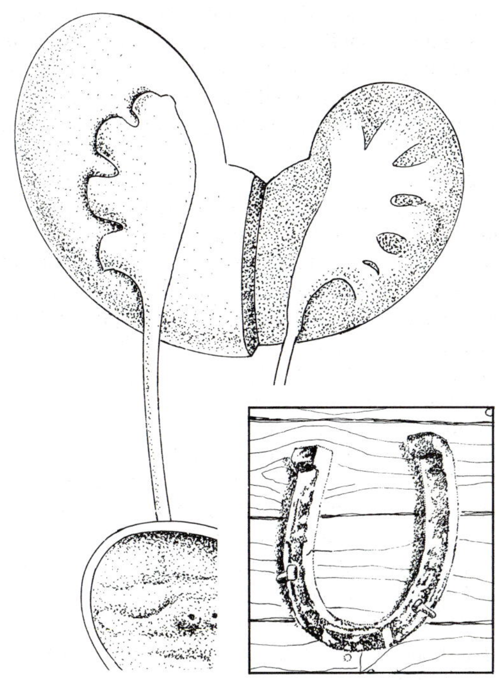

Horseshoe kidney

renal parenchyma, lies anterior to the aorta and often is located in the lower pelvis as ascent is prevented by the inferior mesenteric artery; associated anomalies include urogenital anomalies, eg polycystic kidneys, ureter reduplication, as well as gastrointestinal, cardiac and skeletal anomalies and a slight increase in transitional cell carcinoma of the renal pelvis **Clinical** The clinical spectrum is broad, from asymptomatic to advanced renal disease, eg hydronephrosis, infection and concrement formation, which may be accompanied by chronic gastrointestinal symptoms and pain; the 'classic' Rovsing sign, ie abdominal pain localizing to the kidneys accompanied by nausea upon spinal retroflexion is rarely of help, but when present is due to the pressure of the isthmus of the kidney on the nerves and vessels and may occur in S-shaped or L-shaped kidneys

Horseshoe lung Partial fusion of lungs behind the pericardial sac; one lung is smaller than the other but both have their own bronchial supply; the horseshoe lung is a morphologic anomaly seen in the scimitar lung that may be accompanied by pulmonary dysplasia

Hospice An institution expressly intended to provide care and comfort for those who are dying of cancer and, more recently, AIDS; hospice care recognizes that death is inevitable and rather than attempt to cure a disease, alleviates the patient's and family's physical, mental, social and spiritual suffering in the final moments of life, by providing nursing care and relief of pain; an estimated 1700 hospices in the US (J Am Med Assoc 1990; 264:369) provide care for an estimated 200 000 people, one-third of whom receive Medicare benefits Note: Hospices were created in the Middle Ages as places where the Christian crusaders could receive care and replenishment

Hospital-acquired penetration contact (HAPC) A break

of skin or mucosal barriers by needle sticks, paper cuts, broken glass, resulting in contact infection by highly infectious, blood-transmitted, usually viral infections, eg HIV-1, hepatitis B or Jakob-Creutzfeldt agent; the frequency of acquiring AIDS through this route is low, generally regarded as being much less than 1 per 100 infected penetrations; a cardiology resident in Baltimore was the first physician to be infected by HIV-1 through an HAPC

Hospital-based physician One who provides 'clinical support', performing his medical services within a hospital or medical facility; hospital-based physicians include radiologists (interventional and diagnostic), anesthesiologists, pathologists and emergency room physicians ('RAPERs'), as well as physicians specialized in nuclear medicine, physical medicine and rehabilitation, occupational medicine, radiation oncology, public health and forensic pathology; see RAPERs; Cf House physician, Medical specialties, Primary care, Surgical specialties

Hospital chart A specific type of medical record, which is a legal document open to public examination; hospital charts should be complete (see S.O.A.P.), dated often and the prose should be terse Note: Changing of dates and details in the chart at a later date is unethical and puts the defendant at risk for punitive damages, or loss of the license to practice medicine; a good hospital record should '*...CONTAIN SUFFICIENT INFORMATION TO IDENTIFY THE PATIENT, SUPPORT THE DIAGNOSIS, JUSTIFY THE TREATMENT AND DOCUMENT THE RESULTS ACCURATELY*' (Standard II of the JCAHO Accreditation Manual)

Hospital information system (HIS) The computer hardware and software that processes a hospital's information, including financial, patient and 'strategic' management, including patient accounts, tracking of patients, payroll, reimbursements, taxes and statistics; a complete hospital computer integrates monitoring of medication usage, laboratory results, patient and nurse scheduling, on-line library information, inventory control and food management; budget costs for an HIS average $550 000 in hospitals of less than 250 beds to $4.1 million in hospitals of greater than 500 beds; Cf Laboratory information system

Hospitalization The period of confinement in a health care facility that begins with a patient's admission and ends with his discharge; hospitalization also refers to a group health insurance program that pays employees all the expenses incurred during a period of hospitalization, including both the hospital costs per se, the so-called part 'A', as well as a portion or the entirety of the physicians' costs (part 'B'); see Bed, Per diem

Hospitalization hazards Medication prescribing errors and others References J Am Med Assoc 1990; 263:2329; Ann Int Med 1988; 109:582; N Engl J Med 1981:304:638); see July phenomenon

Hospital mortality rate A parameter used by some agencies in the US to measure the quality of medical care; hospital mortality rates: osteopathic facility 129/1000, for-profit facility 121/1000, public facility 120/1000, private non-teaching facility 116/1000, private not for-profit facility 114/1000, private teaching facility 108/1000 (N Engl J Med 1989; 321:1720); see High mortality outlier

Hospital utilization A group of statistics referring to a population's use of hospital services; in the US (1985), hospital utilization was 148 days/1000 persons in a population; average length of stay: 6.5 days and was due to cardiovascular disease (5.5 million admissions), childbirth (4.3 million admissions) and gastrointestinal disease (3.9 million admissions)

Host defense The protection an organism is afforded against infections may be a) Nonimmunologic, including mucocutaneous (integumental) barriers, cilia, microvilli and mechanical, eg urinary outflow, vascular perfusion of tissues and native flora that are capable of 'outcompeting' and b) Immunologic, including chemotaxis, phagocytosis, immunoglobulins, complement, cell-mediated (T cell) defense

Hostility see 'Toxic core'

Hot air balloon sign RADIOLOGY A fanciful descriptor for the radiological appearance of a massively dilated diverticulum of the sigmoid colon, where the point of attachment is the 'gondola'; that occurs in association with a slowly expanding abscess (Am J Gastroenterol 1981; 76:59)

'Hot and heavy' MOLECULAR BIOLOGY A method for examining DNA-protein (histone) interactions, by using two different radioactive labels, one is detected by radioimmunoassay and labeled with ^{3}H ('hot'); the other radioisotope is detected by density separation, and labeled with ^{13}C and ^{15}N which are 'heavy' isotopes (Proc Nat Acad Sci 1982; 79:3143)

Hot antigen suicide IMMUNOLOGY A technique devised to determine whether antibody-producing cells descend exclusively from the antigen-binding cells; the antigen in the experimental system is labelled with a highly radioactive isotope, eg ^{131}I and if the antigen-binding cell is the ancestor of the antibody-producing cell then no antibody will be produced, since binding of the 'hot' antigen would be tantamount to cellular suicide; the hot antigen suicide theory is considered proof of the clonal selection theory

Hot-cold disease system A therapeutic philosophy rooted in classical Greco-Roman/Persian-Arabic medicine that arrived with 'los Conquistadores' and merged with the local Mayan medicine; the system is practiced in its waning years by 'curanderos' in Central America; all illness is viewed as either 'hot' and treated with their opposite, ie 'cold' remedies, eg limes, cauliflower and roses or viewed as 'cold', treated with 'hot remedies', eg rue (***Ruta graveolens***), garlic and crude brown sugar (Soc Sci Med 1985; 21:807)

Hot comb alopecia A rare condition affecting women who straighten their hair with a 'hot comb', which may cause centrifugal scarring of the scalp

Hot cross bun skull Towerhead, Türmschädel Thickened and prominent frontal bones caused by periostitis of the superciliary arches, hence also known as the Olympian 'brow'; this skull deformity is often accompanied by mild hydrocephalus and although classically described in late congenital syphilis, may be seen in homozygous β-thalassemia and craniosynostosis

Hotdog headache Pulsating cephalgia with facial flushing, caused by sodium nitrite-preserved meat, especially hotdog meat; in addition to preserving meat, nitrites impart a red tinge that imparts a desirable ('marketable') appearance for displaying meats to shoppers

Hot flashes/flushes GYNECOLOGY A symptom afflicting 80-85% of middle-aged women, first occurring during the perimenopause, continuing with decreasing intensity for years, manifesting itself as transient waves of erythema and uncomfortable warmth beginning in the upper chest, face and neck, followed by fine sweating and chills; hot flashes are precipitated by emotional stress, meals and environmental cues, and are more intense when the ovaries are surgically removed than when the decline of ovarian function occurs more gracefully Etiology Idiopathic, due to the response of the autonomic nervous system to decreased estrogens, a decrease that is also held responsible for osteoporosis, atrophy of vaginal epithelium, leukorrhea and pruritus; the relation of decreased estrogen to coronary artery disease is unclear; although estrogen replacement skirts the complications of menopause, it also 'drives' atypical endometrial proliferation in the form of adenomatous hyperplasia and even endometrial carcinoma Note: Hot flashes occur in eunuchs and in most men who have been acutely deprived of testosterone as in castration, a therapeutic modality for advanced prostatic carcinoma (Lancet 1985; 1:1201); diethylstilbestrol may stop the flashes, but exacerbate cardiovascular disease, which in Europe is treated with cyproterone acetate (J Am Med Assoc 1989; 261:1799)

'Hot' food see Spicy foods

'Hotline' A telephone system often manned by volunteers and dedicated to answering questions about a particular disease or group of diseases, eg AIDS 'hotline'

Hot nodule NUCLEAR MEDICINE A focal increase in radioisotope uptake on a ^{123}I scintillation scan; in the thyroid, hot nodule(s) often correspond to toxic nodular or multinodular goiter, in which functional thyroid lesions suppress TSH (thyroid-stimulating hormone) synthesis; Cf Cold nodule, Warm nodule

'Hot paper' SCIENTIFIC JOURNALISM A paper or article published in a peer-reviewed journal that receives an increased number of citations (see Citation impact) by other authors, implying that it has presented unique or important data; see 'Fast track' paper, Landmark article; Cf Uncitedness index

'Hot seat' SURGICAL PATHOLOGY A location in some academic departments of pathology that provides tentative diagnoses for all tissues received from the previous days' surgery and endoscopic procedures; the 'hot seat' allows a patient's attending physician to treat the patient without delaying clinical decisions, waiting for the paper copy of a histologic diagnosis, and is a legacy from Lauren Ackerman, the recognized father of Surgical pathology

Hot spot IMMUNOLOGY A hypervariable region present in the DNA segments that encode the variable region of the heavy (V_H) and light (V_L) chains of an immunoglobulin molecule, also known as complementarity-determining regions (CDR);these points provide the necessary specificity for binding antigens and determine an immunoglobulin's idiotype, while the background support regions of the heavy and light chains are known as framework regions FR; the hot spots on the kappa and lambda light chains are located near amino acid residues 30, 50 and 95 MOLECULAR BIOLOGY A region of DNA where mutation and recombination occurs at a much higher than normal rate; HIV has an entire hypermutable region of 'hot spots', the env of the gp120 protein; thus HIV is constantly 'ahead' of the host immune system (Science 1988; 240:719); see Designer antibodies THERMOGRAPHY A circumscribed increase in skin temperature of the breast, which may be seen in both carcinoma and mastitis; the unacceptable high false positive and and false negative rates of thermography caused it to be abandoned

Hottentot apron Excessive elongation of the labia minora seen in the Hottentot tribe of southern Africa, which when seen elsewhere has been attributed to masturbation

Hot tub dermatitis A generalized pruritic infection caused by ***Pseudomonas aeruginosa*** acquired in communal hot tubs and whirlpools Clinical Hot tub folliculitis begins hours to days post-ablution with vesiculopustular eruptions over the trunk, buttocks, arms and legs, and may resolve without therapy in a week

Hounsfield units CT number A unit of tissue density used in computed tomography; Hounsfield units measure the amount of attenuation by a biological material: bone is +1000 H units, water is 0 H units, air is -1000 H units; the units were named in honor of Hounsfield, the British physicist who fathered computed tomographic imaging analysis, while working at EMI, the British recording and engineering firm; the first person 'imaged' was his secretary who had a glioma of the brain

Hourglass A popular adjectival descriptor for any cylindrical mass with a central constriction

Hourglass deformity CARDIOLOGY A focal stenotic ring within large arteries, typical of supravalvular aortic stenosis Treatment Insert a Dacron or pericardial patch RADIOLOGY A finding by 'barium swallow' in patients with combined sliding and para-esophageal hernia of the esophagogastric junction, where the 'waist' of the hourglass corresponds to constriction from the hiatal ring UROLOGY A congenital malformation of the urinary bladder in which there is incomplete transverse reduplication of the vesical; most cases occur in men and have no clinical significance

Hourglass gallbladder Dumbbell gallbladder A deformity without clinical significance, consisting of transverse septation between the body and fundus; Cf Phyrigian cap

Hourglass mark An identifying red spot on the ventral aspect of the female black widow, ***Lactrodectus mactans***; see Black widow

Hourglass nucleolus An elongated nucleolus with a central constriction that may be seen in the lymphocytes of Burkitt's lymphoma accompanied by coarse chromatin

House-bound syndrome PSYCHIATRY A type of panic disorder that most commonly occurs in women (ratio, 2-4:1), affecting 2-6% of women between ages 18 and 64; house-boundness is characterized by agarophobia, difficulty in functioning in public and generalized anxiety, which evokes cardiovascular symptoms, eg chest pains, tachycardia, arrhythmia, as well as gastrointestinal distress, headache, vertigo, syncope and paresthesiae; see Panic disorder

Housekeeping genes MOLECULAR BIOLOGY Those genes that are expressed (or have the potential for being expressed) in all cells, theoretically at all times; constitutive genes encode proteins involved in basic cellular functions, eg glycolysis and electrolyte balance and are thus required by all cells

Housemaid's knee Occupation-related traumatic bursitis see 'Beat knee', Genu genuflectum

House physician A loosely-defined term referring to physician who 'covers' the medical needs of patients in a hospital; most commonly, a house physician is not board-certified, but has had a number of years of formal training in clinical medicine in a teaching hospital and works in a secondary care facility, usually carrying out the wishes of the patient's 'private' physician

House staff The body of physicians and other health care providers who participate in patient management within the confines of a hospital; in teaching hospitals, the house staff includes interns, residents and fellows who act with an increasing degree of autonomy under the tutilage of licensed, board-certified physicians in an officially accredited graduate medical education program; in non-teaching hospitals, the house staff is comprised of physicians a) Whose practice is confined to the hospital but who are not hospital-based specialists, eg anesthesiologists, pathologists or radiologists, see RAPERs b) Who do not have private patients, but rather provide service to the patients of other, 'attending' physicians, see House physician and c) Who are may not be eligible for certification in a specialty of medicine board or received prolonged specialty training; house staff may include dentists, osteopaths and podiatrists; see Hospital-based physician, RAPERs

Howard Hughes Medical Institute HHMI A philanthropic institution created in 1953 by American aviator-industrialist-billionaire, Howard Hughes; unlike other research institutes, the HHMI is largely 'de-centralized' and is based in 30 university-hospital complexes throughout the USA; HHMI's stated areas of interest include genetics, immunology, metabolic regulation, neuroscience and structural biology and in 1990 had a budget of $230 million for 180 investigators and 1350 ancillary staff (HHMI, Bethesda, MM, USA 20817); Cf Imperial Cancer Research Fund

Hox A family of vertebrate genes which, like the homeobox genes first discovered in Drosophila with which they share significant homology, are important regulators of vertebrate development, by an as-yet unknown mechanism (Nature 1991; 350:473, 458); see Homeobox

Hoxsey method An unproven method of cancer therapy in which a 'brown tonic' containing potassium iodide, licorice and herbs is administered for internal malignancies or one of three topical escharotic formulations is administered for external malignancy, in conjunction with a 'positive attitude' and special elimination diet; there is no data to support its efficacy; see Unproven method of cancer therapy

HPETE Hydroperoxyeicosatetranoic acid The parent molecule for the leukotrienes arising from the 5-lipoxygenase pathway of arachidonic acid metabolism, where HPETE is converted to leukotriene A_4, B_4 and the slow-recting substances of anaphylaxis (leukotrienes C_4, D_4 and E_4); see Arachidonic acid

HPF see High power field

HPFH Hereditary persistence of fetal hemoglobin ($Hb\alpha_2\gamma_2$) A condition possibly due to a defect in the hemoglobin 'switch' mechanism, where the usual transition from γ to β chain production does not occur; four types of HPFH have been described, Greek HPFH, Swiss HPFH. British HPFH, as well as the most common form, HPFH in blacks, in which heterozygotes represent 0.1% of the population; the hemoglobin F (HbF) level in heterozygotes ranges from 15-30% and is evenly distributed in all erythrocytes; see Class switching

HPLC High-pressure (500-1500 pounds/square inch, psi) or performance liquid chromatography INSTRUMENTATION A highly sensitive analytic method used in pharmacology, toxicology, and hormonal analysis (steroids, catecholamines and small peptides), as well as in industrial and clinical laboratories **Method** A microliter volume liquid sample is injected into a moving stream of solvent flowing through a 'column', separating the sample molecules by adsorption, partition, ion exchange or size exclusion; the molecules are eluted or 'pulled off' the column and detected by an ultraviolet light detector, fluorometer or electrochemical analyzer; HPLC may be used in tandem with various forms of liquid chromatography, eg gel filtration, adsorption, partition and ion exchange

HPRT see Hypoxanthine-guanine phosphoribosyl transferase

HPSF Hepatocyte proliferation stimulatory factor A heat-labile trypsin-sensitive protein, the production of which is increased in rodent livers that have suffered toxic insults (Biochem & Biophys Res Comm 1988; 150:133); a similar factor is presumed to exist in humans

HPV Human papilloma virus A virus that is potentially oncogenic to humans, which is most prevalent in those with the greatest number of sexual partners (Pediatr Res 1990; 28:507); 46 genotypes of HPV (a genotype is considered distinct if it has less than 50% DNA sequence similarity or 'homology' with its closest relative) have been described; HPV has been identified by in situ hybridization in epithelial proliferations that are benign, eg condyloma acuminatum, malignant, eg squamous cell carcinoma of the anus, penis and uterine cervix or of uncertain clinical behavior, eg inverted papillomas of the nasopharynx; uterine cervical carcinomas that are negative for HPV sequences have a 2.6-fold increased risk of relapse, a 4.5-fold higher risk for distal metastases and have a greater incidence of positive regional lymph nodes; anal HPV infection is associated with anal intraepithelial neoplasia for anal carcinoma (JAMA 1990; 263:2911); HPV types 6 and 11 are not considered premalignant (although these types have been, while HPV types 16, 18, 31, 33 and 35 are associated with cervical dysplasia, cervical intraepithelial neoplasia (CIN) and anogenital cancer; the mechanism by which cancerous degeneration occurs is unclear, but HPV encodes a viral protein E6 produced by clinically aggressive HPV that binds to the tumor suppressor protein p53 (Science 1990; 248:76) implying that HPV evokes de-repression phenomena

H_1 receptor see Histamine receptor

H reflex NEUROLOGY An electrically-induced spinal reflex thought to be monosynaptic that is used to diagnose S-1 radiculopathy and for studying nerve conduction, as in Guillain-Barré syndrome

HRE see Hormone response element

HSE Heat-shock consensus element CTNGAANNTTCNAG A 14, or possibly 10 (Science 1988; 239:1139) base pair segment of DNA that is present in multiple copies and located upstream from all heat-shock genes; single base pair substitutions of the HSE (and of immediately flanking regions) cause considerable variation in the production of heat shock proteins; see Heat shock, Heat shock proteins

H-shaped esophagus see H type fistula

H- or U-shaped vertebra PEDIATRIC RADIOLOGY Flattening of the central vertebral body with mineralization of the posterior aspects of vertebral body, which may be seen in sickle cell anemia and in thanatophoric dwarfism

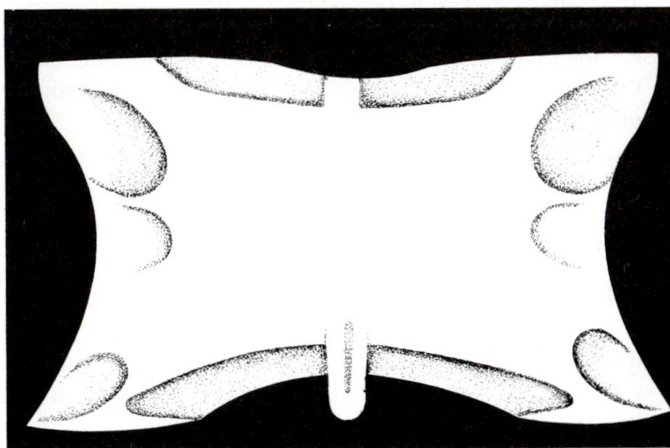

H-shaped vertebra

hsp see Heat shock proteins

HSR Homogeneously staining region(s) MOLECULAR BIOLOGY Duplicated chromosomal regions present in up to 100 copies that often correspond to oncogenes, eg N-myc; HSRs may span a several hundred kilobase segment of DNA and are most prominent in malignant cells; duplicated regions confined to the chromosome, are HSRs; when the same fragments split off as independent particles, they are termed 'double minutes'; Cf Tandem repeats

HSV Herpes simplex virus see Herpes virus

HTLA antibody see High-titer, low-avidity antibody

HTLV Human T cell leukemia/lymphoma virus A family of enveloped, single-stranded retroviruses, subfamily Oncoviridae that produce a DNA copy from viral RNA by using reverse transcriptase; the HTLV as a group are capable of immortalizing and transforming T cells Epidemiology The HTLV family all appear to be transmitted by blood and mucosal contacts and thus concomitant infections may occur, eg HTLV-I and HIV-1 (formerly HTLV-III, N Engl J Med 1986; 315:1073) and HTLV-I may be a cofactor facilitating production of large quantities of HIV-1 by infected leukocytes (Science 1988; 240:1026) **HTLV-I** A retrovirus that immortalizes T cells, which is associated with a) Adult T cell lymphoma/leukemia in endemic regions of southern Japan (where up to 40% of leukemic patients are HTLV-I-positive) and the Caribbean b) Chronic progressive myelopathy (tropical spastic paralysis), a condition endemic to the Caribbean, tropical Africa and South America (N Engl J Med 1988; 318:1141) and c) HTLV-I-associated neuropathy; HTLV-I, like HIV-1 (formerly HTLV-III), is a blood-borne infection; the carrier incidence of HTLV-I in the US and Europe ranges from 0.03% to 0.10%; 1% of HTLV-I-infected subjects develop clinical disease, which may reflect host susceptibility and variant strains of the virus; neurological disease is attributed to the presence of high circulating levels of HTLV-I-specific cytotoxic T lymphocytes that are CD8+, HLA class I-restricted and which recognize products encoded in the regulatory pX region (Nature 1990; 348:245) **HTLV-II** A retrovirus that may transform CD4 T cells, that may rarely be linked to disease, eg hairy cell leukemia (J Am Med Assoc 1990; 263:60); HTLV-I and HTLV-II have a 60% homology with each other, both use the same cell membrane receptor (encoded on chromosome 17cen-qter) to penetrate T cells, evidenced by interference with syncytium formation, have a tax gene encoding the transactivating protein, p37xII required for replication, immortalize T cells, causing malignant transformation by trans-activation, and increase the expression of genes attached to appropriate viral control sequences (these proteins are probably encoded near the 3' end of the viral genome) **HTLV-III** see HIV-1 **HTLV-IV** see HIV-2 **HTLV-V** A retrovirus described in a case of CD4+/Tac- mycosis fungoides associated with cutaneous T cell lymphoma

H-type fistula PEDIATRICS A congenital variant of esophageal atresia and tracheoesophageal fistula (EATF) that corresponds to Gross-Vogt's type E fistula, where the esophagus communicates with the stomach in the usual fashion and has a small fistulous tract to the trachea, causing recurrent aspiration pneumonia Note: The most common EATF is type C, in which the upper esophagus ends in a blind pouch and the lower portion of the esophagus communicates with trachea **Treatment** Surgical closure, nutritional support

Huckleberry Finn 'syndrome' Truancy syndrome A psychodynamic complex in which the obligations and responsibilities avoided as a child, eventuate into frequent job changes and absenteeism as an adult, a response that may represent a defense mechanism arising from parental rejection, a deeply-ingrained feeling of inferiority and depression in a relatively intelligent person Note: Huckleberry Finn is the key character in Mark Twain's book by the same name, who shirked responsibilities

HUGO Human Genome Organization

Human catastrophe see Disaster

Human chorionic (hC) hormones hC hormones A family of glycoprotein hormones produced by trophoblastic (placental) tissue, specifically the syncytiotrophoblastic cell **hC corticotropin** Immunologically similar to ACTH **hC gonadotropin** A 36-40 kD dimeric protein, composed of an α subunit that is similar to pituitary hormones (TSH, FSH and LH) and a unique β subunit that is used as an early diagnostic test for pregnancy **hC somatomammotropin** formerly, placental lactogen A single-chain 21 kD polypeptide hormone produced by the syncytiotrophoblast that is lactogenic, somatotrophic, luteotropic and mammotropic **hC thyrotropin** Immunologically similar to TSH

Human Frontier Science Project A foundation created by Japan's Ministry of International Trade and Industry (MITI), based in Strasbourg, France that has a primary goal of promoting research on the brain and molecular biology, through multinational collaboration and sharing of the incurred financial burden (Nature 1991; 350:97n)

Human Genome project A multinational collaborative effort that will sequence (map) all 3×10^9 nucleotides of a haploid set of the human genome, an effort begun in 1987 and projected to be completed circa the year 2000 at a total cost of US \$3 $\times 10^9$; if the sequencing were to be carried out by hand it would require 30 000 person-years of labor, at an error rate of approximately 1 base per 1000; the recently-developed sequencers substantially reduce the error rate and time required for sequencing; the actual database created from the Genome project is less useful than the technological advancements engendered by the project itself; in the early stages, the map intends to 'blanket' each of the 23 chromosomes with evenly spaced genetic 'signposts', the more markers (a minimum of 500 to several thousand), the finer the resolution; one group (Cell 1987; 51:319) published an early list with 404 markers, each about 10 centimorgans apart; the strategy proposed by M Olsen is to use short, tagged segments of DNA sequence as landmarks, 'creating an STS map' and relying on the language and techniques of the polymerase chain reaction (see PCR) as a standard; the STS (sequence tagged site) approach allows facile integration and cooperation (Science 1989; 245: 1434) among 'big' and 'little' science laboratories; it is hoped by the year 2000, a map and the function of 6000 genes will be developed (Science 1990; 250:210n&v); another approach is that of creating a complementary DNA (cDNA) map of only those genes that are expressed in cells, thereby by-passing all of the information-poor ('junk') DNA, which comprises circa 95% of the human genome; the advantage to the cDNA map approach is that the genetic infromation obtained from the genome in terms of enzymes and various proteins could be used immediately Note: An argument against such 'big science' projects is that they divert funds and manpower away from researcher-driven ('little science') projects; see Sequencers

Human immune globulin (HIG) A therapeutic agent prepared from a donor pool screened for the presence of human immunodeficiency virus, both at the time of 'harvesting' and once the plasma is pooled; one form of HIG, Sandoglobulin is produced by the Kistler Nitschmann method of cold ethanol fractionation at acid pH, a process that completely inactivates viruses (Vox Sang 1988; 54:78); 7.5 million grams of human immune globulin have been infused and no case of HIV, HAV, HBV or non-A, non-B hepatitis has been reported (personal communication, Sandoz Pharmaceuticals) Note: Prior to 1987, several lots had been contaminated with HIV antibody Indications, HIG Primary immunodeficiencies, eg X-linked aγglobulinemia, severe combined immune deficiency and combined variable immune deficiency, as well as in acute or chronic idiopathic thrombocytopenic purpura

Human immunodeficiency virus see HIV

Humanized antibody A product created by recombinant DNA technology in order to reduce the immunogenicity of non-human monoclonal antibodies, transferring the hypervariable genes of a rat antibody (which encodes peptide segments capable of recognizing the desired epitope), into the normal human gene; the resulting immunoglobulin is largely human, thereby reducing the 'xenophobic' response or allograft rejection when the hybrid molecule is administered to a human, confining the nonhuman portion to the necessary recognition site (N Engl J Med 1990; 323:250cr); the constant region may be selected for desired effector functions including complement fixation, antibody-dependent cell-mediated cytotoxicity and maximum serum half-life; Cf Designer antibody

'Humanized' milk NEONATOLOGY A modified formulation of cow milk, the fat ratio of which closely mimics human milk (40% casein, 60% whey), indicated in infants below 2000 g; see Milk; Cf White beverages

Human placental lactogen see Human chorionic somatomammotropin

Humidifier lung A transient condition related to mechanical ventilation of buildings related to the heating and cooling systems, possibly caused by a water-born amoeba occurring 1-3 days after exposure Clinical Malaise, cough, chest tightness, shortness of breath and with time, weight loss; the symptoms appear 4-6 hours after re-exposure to a workplace, often after the weekend, thus the common synonym of 'Monday sickness'; the symptoms resolve spontaneously, regardless of continued exposure Radiology Negative Laboratory Antibodies to ***Negleria gruberi*** and ***Acanthamoeba*** spp; other humidifier lung organisms include ***Aspergillus fumigatus, Aureobasium pullulans*** (J Am Med Assoc 259:1965), ***Micropolyspora faeni, Thermoactinomyces vulgaris*** and other water-born organisms; see Sick building syndrome

Humor A fluid or gel-like substance

Humoral immunity B cell immunity An arm of the immune system that develops within vascular compartments or in extracellular fluid spaces, which is mediated by specific, eg immunoglobulins and nonspecific, eg complement molecules, contrasting with cellular or T cell immunity Note: Subdivision of immune labors into the neat 'B' and 'T' boxes is not completely correct as the two systems are intimately related; Cf Cell-mediated immunity

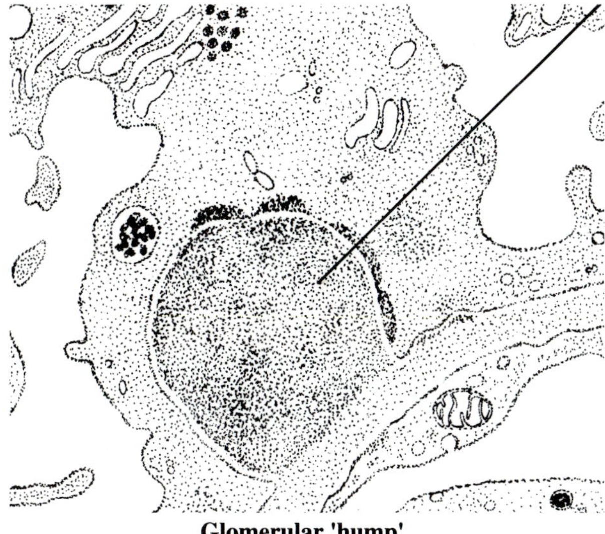

Glomerular 'hump'

Hump NEPHROPATHOLOGY A finding in poststreptococcal glomerulonephritis, characterized by deposits of subepithelial immune complexes on Bowman's capsule **Histopathology** Masses attached to the glomerular epithelium that are red by Masson's trichrome stain or blue by toluidine blue stain **Ultrastructure** Discrete electron-dense, 'domed' deposits, projecting outward from the epithelial aspect of the glomerular basement membrane at the site of slit pores, separated by an electrolucent zone, often demarcated from the overlying epithelial cell by cytoplasmic condensation **Immunofluorescence** Variably present deposits of complement C3 and IgG as well as alternate pathway proteins, eg properdin and factor B, implying that complement is being activated; humps may disappear four-to-eight weeks after infection and when humps are persistent and confluent, may be associated with incomplete clinical resolution Note: Humps also occur in nonstreptococcal infectious glomerulonephritis (with infective endocarditis), Henoch-Schönlein purpura and membranoproliferative glomerulonephritis

Hump sign RADIOLOGY A distortion of the gas-fluid levels in a plain abdominal film caused by an intraluminal bolus of *Ascaris lumbricoides* within the intestine, an uncommon finding in massive intestinal involvement by roundworms (Am J Radiol 1980; 135:37)

Humpty-Dumpty etymology The redefinition of terminology that already has widely accepted definition(s), according to the whims of the lector or writer, a term arising from Humpty-Dumpty's statement, '*WHEN I USE A WORD, IT MEANS JUST WHAT I CHOOSE IT TO MEAN, NEITHER MORE NOR LESS*'; the Humpty-Dumpty conundrum is typified by the problem facing evolutionary biologists, for whom 'homology' refers to common evolutionary origin, while molecular biologists later applied the term to the degree of sequence relatedness, see Homology

Humpty-Dumpty 'syndrome(s)' A group of allegorical terms derived from the children's nursery rhyme Humpty-Dumpty, who '*...ALL THE KING'S HORSES AND ALL THE KING'S MEN COULDN'T PUT HIM TOGETHER AGAIN*'; the term has been applied to a) A form of disability neurosis in which there is physical recovery from an injury, but the 'scars' of childhood psychological trauma intervene, preventing mental recuperation b) Borderline psychiatric personalities that cannot be salvaged c) Polytraumatized patients who require multiple, not fully corrective procedures and d) Specialty 'fragmentation' see Frankenstein, Twigging

Hunchback An obsolete (trivial) term for angular kyphosis that has retained its popularity in non-medical parlance; angular kyphosis in children is either congenital, due to a lack of segmentation or lack of formation of one or more vertebral bodies **Treatment** Surgical fusion of vertebrae Acquired angular kyphosis in children is idiopathic and often accompanied by a compensatory increase in lumbar lordosis; in adults, the hunchback deformity may be due to infections, eg midthoracic tuberculosis or neoplastic, eg myeloma or infiltration by an osteophilic carcinoma, eg breast or kidney

'Hungry bones' syndrome Post-parathyroid surgery recalcification tetany Transient hypoparathyroidism secondary to resection of significant portions of a hyperactive parathyroid gland; 'hungry' bones occur in the face of high pre-operative PTH (due to excess PTH secretion as occurs in parathyroid hyperplasia and adenoma), high alkaline phosphatase and extensive bone demineralization, which results in a rapid 'rebound' recalcification of bones after prolonged hypocalcemia; bone hunger is exacerbated by a pre-existing compromise in renal function **Radiology** Mottled zones of hypodensity in bones **Laboratory** Increased calcitriol, marked hypocalcemia, eg 1.5 mmol/L (US: 6 mg/dl) or lower, decreased phosphorus and magnesium and a reactive increase in PTH (if there is residual secretion); the danger lies in attributing the symptoms to acidosis, which may accompany and exacerbate the complex **Treatment** Vitamin 1,25(OH)D_2

Hunting phenomenon PATHOPHYSIOLOGY An auto-thermoregulatory 'maneuver' on the part of a hypothermic body attempting to conserve a cold extremity, where with prolonged corporal exposure to temperatures below 15°C, blood flow increases intermittently to the extremities; if the hypothermia persists, the limb will lose its blood flow entirely in order to maintain the core temperature

HUS see Hemolytic uremic syndrome

HUT78 A cell line established in 1978 from a patient with mycosis fungoides by J Minna's research group; the cell's name was changed to H9 by workers at the US National Institutes of Health, and was successfully infected with HIV-1 and has become the 'workhorse' cell line in HIV-1 research (Science 1990; 248:1499)

hut operon Histidine utilization operon An example of autogenous regulation, where a regulatory protein controls its own synthesis; bacterial (***Klebsiella aerogenes*** and ***Salmonella typhimurium***) degradation of histidine into NH_3, glutamic acid and formamide is dependent upon two (hut) enzymes, which are the gene products encoded by two separate hut operons, each with its own operator and promoter; without histidine in the medium, a single repressor protein binds to both hut operons, preventing transcription; when present, histidine combines with the repressor and transcription is allowed to continue

Hyaline arteriosclerosis A degenerative change of aging that most affects the spleen and kidneys, commonly seen in accelerated ('malignant') hypertension and diabetes mellitus; hyaline changes may occur in the pancreas, adrenal glands, liver, gastrointestinal tract, brain, choroid and retina Histopathology Glassy eosinophilic hyalinoid material corresponding to iC3b is deposited in the arteriolar walls by slowspontaneous activation of the alternate complement activation pathway and random deposition of the metastable C3b to hyaluronic acid in the arteriolar wall, inactivated by alternate complement pathway factors I and H

Hyaline cell Plasmacytoid cell ORAL PATHOLOGY A myoepithelial cell seen in pleomorphic adenoma that is small, dark, polygonal with an eccentric nucleus and 'glassy' pink cytoplasm, some of which have squamous differentiation

Hyaline globules Variably sized, rounded periodic acid Schiff (PAS)-positive, diastase resistant 1-7 mm masses seen intra- and extracellularly in Kaposi sarcoma, possibly representing effete red erythrocytes

Hyaline membranes PULMONARY PATHOLOGY Layered, eosinophilic, pink, glassy membranous material on the alveoli that corresponds to degenerated cells and exudate, constituting a major feature of hyaline membrane disease and diffuse alveolar damage Etiology Any condition or 'insult' that can cause diffuse alveolar damage may also evoke hyaline membrane production, eg viral infection, uremia, toxic gas, eg phosgene inhalation, and connective tissue disease, eg rheumatoid arthritis

Hyaline membrane disease (HMD) A morbid process occurring in up to 50% of neonatal deaths in the US, ie 40 000 annually Clinical Atelectasis, hypoventilation (increased pCO_2, decreased pH and O2), hypotensive shock, pulmonary vasoconstriction, alveolar hypoperfusion, shut-down of cellular metabolism; 60% of HMD occurs in infants, most are under 28 weeks of age; 5% occur in infants older than 37 weeks Pathogenesis Surfactant deficiency, due to the combined effects of prematurity (insufficient phosphatidyl glycerol), intrapartum hypoxia, 'subacute' fetal distress, acidosis, hypoxia familial predisposition; α_1-antitrypsin deficiency, thyroxine, prolactin, cortisol, estrogen; HMD is more frequent in the second twin delivered, twin-to-twin transfusion recipient infant, male infants, children of diabetic mothers and in cesarian sections; a vicious cycle begins where decreased surfactant results in atelectasis and therefore decreased ventilation (increased CO_2, decreased O_2, hypoxia exacerbating the lack of surfactant), causing shock and more hypoxia Clinical Early onset of tachypnea, prominent grunting, intercostal retractions (air hunger), cyanosis; the infants may not respond to oxygen; blood pressure and corporal temperature fall, asphyxia intervenes and causes death or the symptoms peak at 3 days and the infant recovers Differential diagnosis Neonatal pneumonia, birth-related asphyxia, group B streptococcal sepsis, cyanotic heart disease Treatment Supportive with O_2, correction of acidosis and administration of surfactants

Hyalinosis cutis A rare skin disorder causing subcutaneous deposits of amorphous PAS-positive material that corresponds to a mixture of monoclonal kappa light chains, an adhesive 90 kD glycoprotein and type I collagen and high serum levels of IgM antibodies to cytokeratin

H-Y antigen Histocompatibility-Y antigen A male-specific histocompatibility antigen which was postulated to exist and encode a testis-inducer, a hypothesis (Nature 1975; 257:235) that has been abandoned; see Testis-determining factor

Hybrid-arrested translation see Hybrid-selected translation

Hybridization MOLECULAR BIOLOGY A group of techniques for determining the relatedness or sequence 'homology' between two strands of nucleic acids, allowing precise identification of relatively short (up to 20 kilobases) segments or sequences of DNA (Southern blot) or RNA (Northern blot) Technique, DNA hybridization A sample of DNA is denatured by a salt, eg NaOH, which causes the double helix to separate into single strands that are subsequently 'chopped' at specific sites by restriction endonucleases into short (up to 20 kilobases) segments of single-stranded DNA and electrophoresed on a slab of agarose, separating the DNA fragments by size; the gel is then bathed in a solution containing a probe (an exact base pair 'mirror image' of the single-stranded DNA that now lies at a certain point on the slab of agarose; the probe is labelled by a radioactive isotope, eg ^{32}P or ^{35}S, or a fluoresceinated or a biotinylated 'tag', each of which is coupled to a detection system); if the probe finds its complementary strand, it 'hybridizes', reforming a double strand; after hybridization, the material on the gel is transferred to a nitrocellulose or nylon membrane (Southern transfer) and either autoradiographed or further manipulated; DNA hybridization under low-stringency conditions, ie not requiring exact complementarity of base pairs may be used to isolate related gene segments, eg identification of the mineralocorticoid receptor gene from the known structure of the glucocorticoid receptor gene; see Dot hybridization, Immunoblotting, in situ hybridization, RNA hybridization

Hybridoma A 'tumor' cell line (figure, facing page) originating from two cells that are interdependent upon one another's metabolic machinery, created by fusing a mouse cell line producing copious amounts of antibody against an antigen of interest, with an immortal mouse

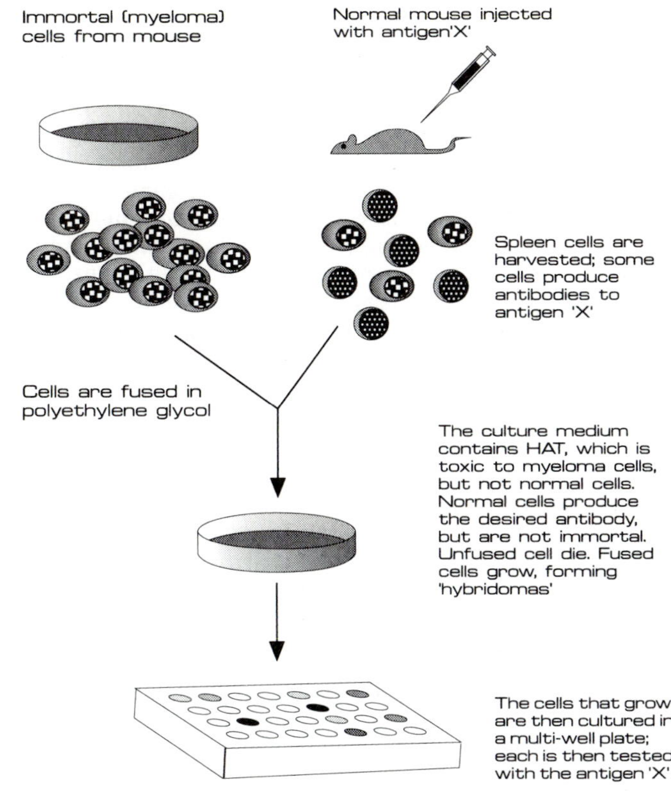
Immortal (myeloma) cells from mouse
Normal mouse injected with antigen'X'
Spleen cells are harvested; some cells produce antibodies to antigen 'X'
Cells are fused in polyethylene glycol
The culture medium contains HAT, which is toxic to myeloma cells, but not normal cells. Normal cells produce the desired antibody, but are not immortal. Unfused cell die. Fused cells grow, forming 'hybridomas'
The cells that grow are then cultured in a multi-well plate; each is then tested with the antigen 'X'

Hybridoma

myeloma cell line; the broadly applicable hybridoma technique and its authors, Köhler and Milstein were accorded the 1984 Nobel Prize together with Jerne (who provided the theoretical groundwork on idiotypic networks) Method Antibody-producing cells that lack the ability to secrete hypoxanthine guanine phosphoribosyl transferase (HGPRT, an enzyme required for DNA nucleotide synthesis) are fused with an immortal myeloma cell line; if the pathway of nucleotide synthesis is blocked, the myeloma cells become HGPRT-dependent and the mutual survival is a symbiotic relation, where the antibody-producing cell line provides the HGPRT and the myeloma cell line provides immortality (Science 1986; 233:1281); the advantages of hybridomas is that one highly-specific antibody is produced in unlimited supplies that may be stored permanently

Hybrid production see Hybridoma

Hybrid protein see Fusion protein

Hybrid-selected translation Molecular biology A method for screening the clones from a cDNA (complementary DNA) library, where a sequence of DNA of interest is hybridized to a complementary mRNA strand under 'R-looping' conditions; the two hybrid strands are then separated and the mRNA is allowed to translate the sequence into a polypeptide; hybrid-arrested translation is a permutation of this theme in which the same selection process occurs, but the DNA-mRNA hybrid is deleted from the system and the polypeptide is not translated

Hydantoin syndrome see Fetal hydantoin syndrome

Hydatid cyst disease Hydatid, Latin, Drop of water A condition characterized by cysts of tapeworm larvae, ***Echinococcus granulosa, E multilocularis*** Epidemiology Most common in cattle, especially sheep of the Southern hemisphere Definitive hosts Canine carnivores, eg coyote, wolves Intermediate hosts Sheep, cattle, pigs, and is an accidental 'tourist' in man; once the tainted meat is ingested, the ova hatch, penetrate the intestinal wall, migrate to the liver, proliferate there or pass to the lung, kidney, heart, skeletal muscle and central nervous system before beginning reproduction; the unilocular hydatid cyst is most often located in the liver, but may also develop in the lungs Treatment Caution; violation of the thick fibrous capsule liberates protoscoleces, causing disseminated disease with significant morbidity; alveolar hydatid disease is caused by the larval stage of the sylvatic, or more rarely, the domestic small animals; the lesions are similar but are often multilocular as the larvae proliferate and spread by budding off from the mother or 'brood' capsule; identification of hydatid cyst is often a fortuitous radiologic finding of a cystic hepatic mass, confirmed by immune assays

Hydatid 'sand' Granular mixture of echinococcal scolices and necrotic debris which results in a radiological 'fluid' level

Hydatidiform mole A benign neoplasm or 'allograft' of trophoblastic tissue, characterized by edematous chorionic villi with a varying amount of proliferative trophoblast Moles are divided into 1) Complete mole The chorionic villi are swollen, often accompanied by trophoblastic proliferation but not fetal tissue; most complete moles have a 46 XX genotype, of which both X chromosomes are of paternal origin, and in 10-15% of the complete moles that are 46 XY, both the X and Y chromosome are of paternal origin; it is thought that complete moles are due to abnormal gametogenesis and fertilization, where in the 46 XX moles, there is fertilization of an empty ovum with no effective genome by a haploid sperm that duplicates without cytokinesis; in the 46 XY complete moles, there may be fertilization of an empty ovum by two haploid sperms with subsequent fusion and replication 2) Partial mole A mass characterized by a mixture of fetal tissue with normal edematous villi and/or hydropic degeneration; most partial moles are triploid (47 XXY > 47 XXX, > 47 XYY, rarely also trisomy 16), and are thought to be the result of unsuccessful dual fertilization of a single ovum; the conceptus does not die, but remains as a proliferating 'tumor' Note: Hydropic degeneration of chorionic villi is relatively common, occurs in 20-40% of spontaneous abortions and is associated with chromosome defects and ovarian disease; 20% of moles have theca lutein cysts

Hydergine The only approved drug for treating Alzheimer's disease, a combination of ergoloid mesylates, described as a 'metabolic enhancer', hydergine's efficacy has not been well established (N Engl J Med 1990; 323:445); there is no effective drug for Alzheimer's dementia (AD), a common diagnosis at the time of death in the US, estimated to cost the US health care system \$24-48 x 10^9 per year

Hydramnios The presence or two of more liters of amniotic fluid; Note: At the 38th week, 500 ml/hour is produced by a combination of fetal kidneys, amnion and transudate of maternal serum; the mechanism of hydramnios is unexplained; 20% of fetal malformations are accompanied by hydramnios, 20% are associated with anencephaly, 10% with multiparity, 5-10% with diabetes mellitus; other conditions associated with hydramnios include esophageal and duodenal atresia, hydrops fetalis, hydrocephalus, spina bifida, achondroplasia and toxemia; about 50% have no fetal or maternal abnormalities

Hydrocephalus Distension of the cerebral ventricles by increased cerebrospinal fluid, due to a) Decreased absorption, eg blockage by congenital malformations, obliteration of the aqueduct, hemorrhage, infection, neoplasms and trauma or b) Increased production, which is distinctly uncommon; as the ventricle enlarges, the ependymal lining separates from the ventricles, permeability increases, the brain becomes edematous and the gyri flatten; incomplete resolution results in chronic hydrocephalus; in the infant whose cranial sutures have yet to close, the cranial circumference increases, cerebral parenchyma is destroyed, gyri flatten, sulci are obliterated and the 'setting sun' sign appears, which is usually associated with a poor prognosis; treatment by ventriculo-peritoneal shunting is palliative; hydrocephalus in adults may be a) ex vacuo, seen in severe cerebral atrophy, with loss of noble tissue, as in Pick's or Alzheimer's diseases, thus being hydrocephalus by default, as the production and absorption of cerebrospinal fluid are normal or b) normal pressure, occurring secondary to trauma or infection with reflux into the ventricles

Hydrolethalus Hereditary hydrocephalus A condition that is fatal in the early neonatal period, characterized by polydactyly, cardiac malformations, airway stenosis and abnormal pulmonary lobation

Hydrops fetalis A 'puffy', plethoric or hydropic state occurring in newborns that may be a) Immune-induced response The mother produces IgG antibodies against infant antigen(s), often a red cell antigen, most specifically anti-RhD, which then passes into the fetal circulation, causing hemolysis; hydrops may also be a b) Non-immune response Hydrops may result from various etiologies that may be of i) Fetal origin, including congenital heart disease (premature foramen ovale closure, large atrio-ventricular septal defect), hematological (erythroblastosis fetalis, α-thalassemia, due to hemoglobin Barts, chronic fetomaternal or twin-twin transfusion), infection (cytomegalovirus, herpesvirus, rubella, sepsis, toxoplasma), pulmonary (cystic adenomatoid malformation, diaphragmatic hernia, with pulmonary hypoplasia, lymphangiectasia), renal (vein thrombosis, congenital nephrosis) and teratomas, skeletal malformations (achondroplasia, osteogenesis imperfecta, fetal neuroblastomatosis, storage disease, meconium peritonitis, idiopathic) ii) Placental Chorangioma, umbilical or chorionic vein thrombosis and iii) Maternal Diabetes mellitus, toxemia **Clinical** Ascites and edema, due to heart failure, decreased protein or chronic intrauterine anemia, hepatosplenomegaly, cardiomegaly, extramedullary hematopoiesis, jaundice, pallor Cause of death Heart failure; see Hemolytic disease of the newborn

Hydroxyapatite deposition disease (HADD) RHEUMATOLOGY A crystal-induced arthropathy **Clinical** Mono- or polyarticular periarthritis accompanied by joint erosions and destruction; HADD may be secondary to collagen vascular disease, renal failure and osteoarthritis

17-Hydroxycorticosteroids (17-OHCS) Steroid hormones formed in the adrenal gland by action of 17-hydroxylase, including cortisol, cortisone, 11-deoxycortisol and tetrahydro derivatives thereof; urinary excretion of 17-OHCSs is a rough guideline of both the functional status of the adrenal gland and rates of catabolism 17-OHCs are increased in pregnancy, Cushing's disease, obesity and pancreatitis and decreased in Addison's disease and hypopituitarism Normal, under age 1, 1.4-2.8 µmol/day (US: < 1 mg/day); Adult 8.2-27.6 µmol/day (US: 3-10 mg/day)

5-Hydroxy-indol-acetic acid (5-HIAA) An oxidative deaminated metabolite of serotonin that is excreted in the urine and accounts for 1% of degraded tryptophan Normal 10.5-42 µmol/d (US: 2-8 mg/day); 5-HIAA may be markedly (25-50-fold normal) elevated in carcinoid tumors, Hartnup's disease, nontropical sprue and reserpine therapy and decreased in massive gastrointestinal tract resections, renal insufficiency and phenylketonuria

Hydroxyproline A hydroxylated proline that is present in high concentrations in collagen and has a major role in cross-linking collagen

Hydroxyprolinemia A clinical condition caused by a deficiency of hydroxyproline oxidase, resulting in increased hydroxyproline in serum and urine and mental retardation

Hydroxyurea A non-alkylating, relatively non-toxic chemotherapeutic agent that inhibits ribonucleotide reductase, the enzyme responsible for the conversion of ribonucleotide diphosphates to deoxyribonucleotides, which is commonly used as a single agent to control blast transformation in chronic myeloid leukemia, to manage polycythemia vera, essential thrombocythemia and, in conjunction with prednisone, to treat idiopathic hypereosinophilic syndrome; hydroxyurea may be used to increase hemoglobin F production and red cell survival and decrease bilirubin and lactic dehydrogenases in patients with sickle cell anemia (N Engl J Med 1990; 323:366)

Hymenolepis A genus of human tapeworms infecting humans, including ***H diminuta*** and ***H nana***, both of which are global in distribution Intermediate host

Rodents, infection occurs by ingesting grains with rodent feces containing eggs; the worms measure up to 60 cm in length; the eggs measure 30-50 µm in diameter by 60-85 µm in length **Clinical** When massive, the tapeworms cause nausea, vomiting, diarrhea and convulsions, otherwise asymptomatic **Treatment** Niclosamide

Hymenopterans Insects of the venom-carrying family, including honey bee, yellow jacket, yellow hornet, white-faced hornet, polistes wasp and ants; see Immunotherapy, Killer bees

Hyperactivity syndrome see Attention deficit-hyperactivity disorder

Hyperadrenalism Cushing syndrome

Hyperaldosteronism Conn syndrome

Hyperalimentation see TPN (Total parenteral nutrition)

Hyperammonemia(s), congenital A heterogeneous group of five autosomal recessive (except ornithine transcarbamylase deficiency, which is X-linked) inborn errors of metabolism, each of which is deficient in one of the urea cycle enzymes (arginase, argininosuccinase, argininosuccinic acid sythetase, carbamyl phosphate synthetase, ornithine transcarbamylase); all have a late infancy or childhood onset (except arginase deficiency, which is neonatal) **Clinical** The accumulation of urea precursors, eg ammonia, glutamine causes progressive lethargy, hyperthermia, apnea and marked hyperammonemia Neuropathology Cerebral edema, swollen astrocytes Diagnosis may be established in utero by restriction fragment (RFLP) analysis **Treatment** Restrict dietary protein; activate alternate pathways of waste nitrogen excretion, eg sodium benzoate or dietary supplementation with arginine

Hyperbaric oxygen Therapeutic modality; intermittent administration of O_2 in a chamber at greater than sea-level atmospheric pressures (three atmospheres), increasing the dissolved O_2/dl of blood to 6 ml (normally 1.5 g/dl); hyperbaric oxygen is considered effective therapy for treating air (or gas) embolism, smoke, cyanide intoxication, acute carbon monoxide poisoning (J Am Med Assoc 1989; 261:1039); traumatic ischemia, as in compartment syndrome(s) and crush injury, decompression, see Caisson's disease, to enhance healing of recalcitrant or necrotic wounds, clostridial gangrene (acute tissue hypoxia and myonecrosis), chronic osteomyelitis, extreme blood loss, osteoradionecrosis, compromised skin flaps **Complications** Barotrauma (Air embolism, pneumothorax, tympanic membrane damage), O_2 toxicity (central nervous system, pulmonary, reversible visual changes), fire or explosion and claustrophobia (J Am Med Assoc 1990; 263:2216)

Hypercalcemia Normal levels of (total) calcium 2.10-2.55 mmol/L (US: 8.4-10.2 mg/dl) levels of ionized calcium 1.12-1.23 mmol/L (US: 4.48-4.92 mg/dl) **Etiology** Hypercalcemia may be due to excess parathyroid hormone, calcitriol, thyrotoxicosis, drugs, eg corticosteroids, thiazides and may be associated with granulomas, eg berylliosis, sarcoidosis, silicon injection, tuberculosis, thyrotoxicosis **Clinical** Nausea, anorexia, vomiting, central nervous system depression, fatigability, muscular weakness, corneal calcification, peptic ulcers, pancreatitis; a calcium level above 2.95 mmol/L (US: 12 mg/dl) is a medical emergency and when prolonged, causes bony lesions (cystic degeneration of bone or 'brown tumors', osteopenia and 'punched-out' lesions), joint pain, finger clubbing,dystrophic calcification in various tissues, the kidneys may react to these deposits with polyuria EKG Long Q-T intervals **Laboratory** Increased alkaline phosphatase, cAMP in urine; Cf Long Q-T syndrome

Differential diagnosis, hypercalcemia

Ca^{++}	PO_4	
▲	▲	Parathyroid carcinoma, adenoma or hyperfunction, tertiary hyperparathyroidism
▲	▼	Multiple myeloma, hypervitaminosis D, bone metastases, sarcoidosis, milk-alkali syndrome
▼	▲	Malabsorption, chronic diarrhea
▼	▼	Post parathyroidectomy
Normal	Normal	Hypervitaminosis A, healing of fractures, adolescence

Hypercalcemia of malignancy (HCM) A clinical complex, 50% of which results from hypersecretion of parathyroid hormone-related protein (PTHRP, also known as parathyroid hormone-related peptide, Mayo Clin Proc 1990; 65:1399); normal subjects have low (<2.0 pmol/L) levels of PTHRP, while those with HCM may have plasma levels above 20.9 pmol/L (N Engl J Med 1990; 322:1106); Note: PTHRP is assumed to have a normal function, given its high levels in human breast milk; in HCM, lymphokines stimulate activated macrophages to produce 1,25-dihydroxyvitamin D_3; PTHRP increases cAMP and phosphorus, decreases calcium and may be produced by carcinomas of the lungs, breast, kidney, ovary, leukemia, lymphoma and sarcoma; less common causes of HCM include direct resorption (common in breast carcinoma), increased prostaglandin E_2 production, which stimulates osteoclast resorption, increased cytokine production, eg osteoclast-activating factor, interleukin-1, tumor necrosis factor and lymphotoxin (TNF-β) **Diagnosis** Radioimmunoassay **Treatment** HCM may respond to bleomycin

Hypercalcemia syndrome see Elfin face syndrome of Williams

Hypercholesterolemia, primary see Familial hypercholesterolemia

Hypercholesterolemia, secondary see Hyperlipidemia

Hypercoagulability see Disseminated intravascular coagulation

Hyperdipsia see Polydipsia

Hyperemesis gravidarum A potentially pernicious condition of early pregnancy that respects no race, parity status or social class, characterized by vomiting in the first trimester (3.5/1000 pregnancies), of a severity that may induce renal failure and require hospitalization; if the patient stabilizes, there is no risk of toxemia during the latter part of gestation, nor is there an increased risk of spontaneous abortion or deformities

Hyperendemicity A state of prevalence of active disease, often infectious in nature in a population that surpasses that considered to be endemic for the region, but which falls short of being considered an epidemic

Hypereosinophilia syndrome(s) (HES) An idiopathic and heterogeneous group of conditions that may represent a form of myeloproliferative disorder, as a) 25% have chromosomal abnormalities, eg aneuploidy and decreased vitamin B_{12} with persistent eosinophilia (> 1500 x 10^9/L) for longer than six months b) Absence of secondary causes of eosinophilia,despite aggressive workup and c) Symptoms due to organ involvement or dysfunction Pathogenesis The microvasculature stimulated by an increase in eosinophilic stem cells or the colony-stimulating factor Clinical Age of onset is between 20 and 50 with generalized weakness, dyspnea, cough, malaise, myalgia, angioedema, rash, low-grade fever, night sweats and rhinitis; eosinophils cause organ dysfunction, affecting the heart, bone marrow, liver and spleen, central nervous dysfunction, which is either focal, due to emboli or diffuse, causing altered behavior and cognition, psychosis, ataxia, spasticity, peripheral symmetrical polyneuropathy, coma, as well as gastrointestinal tract symptoms (diarrhea, abdominal pain and malabsorption), lungs (interstitial inflammation with eosinophils) and nonspecific rashes; once the heart is involved, eg endocardial fibrosis, thrombosis and restrictive cardiomyopathy; death occurs within 9 months Treatment Some cases respond to corticosteroids

Hyperglycinemia Nonketotic hyperglycemia An autosomal recessive condition with glycine accumulation due to a catabolic pathway defect, possibly a glycine decarboxylase deficiency Clinical Presents shortly after birth with marked central nervous system depression, seizures and convulsions, later developing atonia and areflexia

Hyperglycinuria Glycine wastage as either Iminoglycinuria, an autosomal recessive renal tube defect that 'spills' imino acids (proline and hydroxyproline) and glycine or Glucoglycinuria, an autosomal dominant increase of the glycine in both the urine and serum

Hypergonadotropic hypogonadism Primary hypogonadism A condition that results from the lack of target organ response to the pituitary hormones, eg follicle-stimulating hormone and/or luteinizing hormone; see Hypogonadism

Hyperhidrosis Increased sweating may be a primary symptom in asymmetric hyperhidrosis, due to a local neural or visceral lesion, gustatory hyperhidrosis, due to surgery to the parotid glands, elicited by spicy foods and 'mental' hyperhidrosis, due to emotional stress or anxiety; in thermoregulatory hyperhidrosis, sweating is merely a symptom occurring in chronic disease including central nervous system disease (psychiatric stress, lesions of the cortex, hypothalamus, medulla and spinal cord), dermatopathies (dyskeratosis congenita, pachydermoperiostosis), drugs (anticholinesterase, overdose, eg aspirin, pilocarpine or withdrawal from narcotics), dumping syndrome, endocrinopathy (acromegaly, hypoglycemia, reactive hyperadrenalism, Graves' disease, pheochromocytoma, menopause), familial dysautonomia (Riley-Day syndrome), infections (brucellosis, tuberculosis), lymphomas(classically, the Pel-Epstein fever of Hodgkin's lymphoma) and others

Hyperimmunoglobulin E syndrome (HIE) Job syndrome A condition characterized by an early onset of eczema, frequent abscesses of the skin, lungs, sinuses, eyes and ears by ***Staphylococcus aureus, Haemophilus influenzae, Streptococci pneumonia***, group A streptococci and ***Candida*** species Laboratory Increased eosinophils, IgE > 5000 IU/mL, decreased antibody response to vaccines and major histocompatibility antigens, decreased T cell helper:suppressor ratio Prognosis HIE is compatible with long-term survival

Hyperimmunoglobulin-M syndrome An immunodeficiency characterized by normal to elevated serum IgM with markedly decreased/absent IgG and IgA, associated with frequent infections and neoplasia at an early age; heredity: X-linked, autosomal dominant or related to congenital rubella; the defect lies in the inability of the T-lymphocytes to provide the 'switch' signal for IgM-secreting cells to become IgG- and IgA-secreting cells

Hyperinfection syndrome Disseminated parasitosis in immunosuppressed, malignant or malnourished hosts, caused by autoinfection with ***Strongyloides stercoralis*** Clinical Abrupt onset of high fever, abdominal pain and distension, intestinal ulcerations, gram-negative sepsis and shock; intense transpulmonary nematodal migration is characterized by dyspnea, cough and hemoptysis Treatment Thiabendazole Prevention Shoes

Hyperkalemic periodic paralysis see Periodic paralysis

Hyperkinetic heart see Athletic heart syndrome

Hyperlipidemia/hyperlipoproteinemia Increased circulating fatty acids, triglycerides and cholesterol (hyperlipidemia) is related to increased carrier lipoproteins (hyperlipoproteinemia) and the presence of degradative enzymes, including lipoprotein lipase; increased circulating lipids are responsible for cardiovascular disease, the major cause of morbidity and mortality in older adults in developed nations; secondary hyperlipidemias may be a symptom of an otherwise unrelated condition Note: Only 30-40% of the population is sensitive to dietrary cholesterol and thus increasing dietary cholesterol increases that in the circulation; increased lipids occur in I) SECONDARY HYPERCHOLESTEROLEMIA, seen in acute intermittent porphyria, cholestasis, hypothyroidism and pregnancy, II) SECONDARY HYPERTRIGLYCERIDEMIA, seen in diabetes mellitus, acute alcohol intoxication, acute pancreatitis, gout, gram-negative sepsis, glycogen storage disease I, oral contraceptives and III) COMBINED HYPERCHOLESTEROLEMIA AND HYPERTRIGLYCERIDEMIA, seen in nephrotic syndrome, chronic renal failure, steroid therapy and immunosuppression

CLASSIFICATION OF HYPERLIPOPROTEINEMIA

I FAMILIAL LIPOPROTEIN LIPASE DEFICIENCY An autosomal recessive inability to release triglycerides from chylomicrons, causing marked hypertriglycerides (> 20 g/L) Clinical Childhood onset, diarrhea, pancreatitis (potentially fulminant), xanthomata, lipemia retinalis, hepatosplenomegaly, but no increased risk of atherosclerosis; this condition is similar to apolipoprotein C-II deficiency Laboratory Triglycerides > 4.0 g/L (US: 400 mg/dl), cholesterol normal, increased chylomicrons, decreased post heparin lipolytic activity; this lipoprotein pattern may be mimicked by lupus erythematosus

II Familial hypercholesterolemia An autosomal dominant condition characterized by tuberous xanthomata of tendons, accelerated coronary atherosclerosis, early myocardial infarcts and ischemic events, onset between ages 20 and 50, due to an absence or defect in low-density lipoprotein (LDL) receptors due to mutant alleles Rbo, Rb- and Rtio, resulting in the inability to absorb cholesterol from LDL, which is complicated by increased hepatic production of LDL, a response to the loss of the negative feedback loop Laboratory Cholesterol 5 to 6 g/L in homozygotes, 3 to 4 g/L in heterozygous; type IIa Increased cholesterol, normal VLDL (normal triglycerides); this lipoprotein pattern may be mimicked by hepatic tumors; type IIb Increased cholesterol, increased VLDL (increased triglycerides)

III Remnant removal disease Dys-β–lipoproteinemia Broad or fused β band disease An autosomal dominant condition characterized by decreased intermediate-density lipoprotein catabolism Clinical Obesity, accelerated atherosclerosis, thromboembolism and strokes, palmo-plantar xanthomas, measuring up to 10 cm, associated with diabetes mellitus, obesity and hypothyroidism Laboratory Increased triglycerides, cholesterol and abnormal (diabetic) glucose tolerance test; this lipoprotein pattern may be mimicked by myeloma

IV Hypertriglyceridemia An autosomal dominant condition that is the most common form of hyperlipoproteinemia Clinical Most patients are asymptomatic, rarely suffering peripheral and coronary vascular disease Laboratory Nonspecific elevations of triglycerides and very-low density lipoprotein Treatment Clofibrate, gemfibrozil Acquired causes of hypertriglyceridemia include diabetes mellitus, chronic uremia, dialysis, obesity, estrogen use and alcohol, use of diuretics, glucocorticoids and β-adrenergic agents

V Mixed hyperlipoproteinemia A heterogeneous group of conditions characterized by eruptive xanthomata, pancreatitis, lipemia retinalis, increased VLDL and chylomicrons

Hyperlysinemia An autosomal recessive condition of childhood onset characterized by increased lysine or metabolites Type I hyperlysinemia is due to a lysine α-ketoglutarate reductase deficiency with increased lysine, homoarginine and NH_3, causing mental retardation, hypotonicity and coma; high-protein diets result in attacks which begin with vomiting Treatment Decrease dietary lysine Type II hyperlysinemia is thought to be due to an as yet undiscovered enzymopathy, with milder symptoms; see Lysinemia

Hypernatremia, congenital Idiopathic neonatal hypernatremia of Ballard A potentially life-threatening clinical complex of perinatal onset with markely elevated serum sodium, usually greater than 134-146 mmol/L (US: 310-340 mg/dl) Clinical Central nervous system dysfunction, seizures, neuromuscular spasms, production of low volumes of concentrated urine, weight loss, hypotension, increased BUN; the symptoms are exacerbated by concomitant sepsis, asphyxia or central nervous system hemorrhage Etiology Increased loss of sodium, as occurs in diabetes insipidus, either decreased ADH secretion or decreased sensitivity to ADH, osmotic diuresis, diaphoresis, diarrhea; decreased intake, due to disordered thirst sensation, increased salt ingestion without adequate fluid, electrolytic imbalance, increased calcium and potassium

Hypernephroma Obsolete for renal cell carcinoma

Hyperornithinemia see Ornithinemia

Hyperostosis A proliferation of bony matrix

Hyperostosis corticalis deformans juvenilis An early-onset osteopetrosis syndrome with multiple fractures, enlarged head, broadened diaphyses, bowed legs, decreased height, increased alkaline phosphatase, histologically divided into Bakin-Enger syndrome and juvenile Paget's disease

Hyperostosis corticalis generalisata of van Buchem An autosomal recessive osteoporosis complex of early onset with bony overgrowth of a) bone marrow, resulting in chronic cytopenias and b) cranial foramina, causing stenosis and paresthesia of the facial nerve, loss of vision and deafness Laboratory Increased alkaline phosphatase

Hyperostosis corticalis infantalis of Caffey-Silverman An autosomal dominant complex characterized by early onset of hyperostosis and neoosteogenesis, affecting the facial and, less commonly the long bones, accompanied by soft tissue swelling, hyperirritability, dysphagia, fever,pleuritis Laboratory Increased erythrocyte sedimentation rate and alkaline phosphatase

Hyperostosis frontalis interna of Morgagni-Stewart-Morell A osteopetrosis syndrome that is confined to the cranial bones, structurally compromising the hypophysis (dysmenorrhea, virilism, hirsutism, diabetes insipidus, glucose intolerance), cranial nerve foramina (vertigo, tinnitus, anosmia, visual disorders) associated with fatigue, hemiplegia and hemiparesis

Hyperparathyroidism Parathyroid gland hypersecretion causes several relatively specific clinical complexes, including a myopathic 'syndrome', a skeletal 'syndrome', a urologic 'syndrome' and a central nervous system 'syndrome', in addition to the classic findings of peptic ulcer, hypercalcemia and acute pancreatitis Primary hyperparathyroidism is most commonly due to parathyroid hormone (PTH) hypersecretion secondary to parathyroid adenomas or hyperplasia (parathyroid carcinomas are extremely uncommon), PTH may also be ectopic and occur with MEN I and II syndromes, see there Clinical Hypercalcemia symptoms, including nausea, anorexia, vomiting, central nervous system depression, fatigability, cornea calcification, muscular weakness, peptic ulcers, pancreatitis; levels above 2.9 mmol/L (US: 12 mg/dl) require immediate therapy and when prolonged, cause bone abnormalities, eg osteitis fibrosa cystica or 'brown' tumors, significant osteopenia with 'punched-out' lesions of the bone, joint pain and finger clubbing as well as ectopic calcium deposits in various tissues, in particular, the kidney, resulting in polyuria and eventually renal failure EKG Decreased Q-T intervals Secondary hyperparathyroidism is usually due to end-organ defects (renal failure and hemodialysis) or the rare malabsorption syndrome Note: The histopathological criteria separating parathyroid adenomas from parathyroid hyperplasia differ widely among pathologists; Cf Hypercalcemia

Hyperphenylalaninemia(s) A group of eight different congenital enzymopathies characterized by an accumulation of phenylalanine and related metabolites, eg phenylpyruvate, phenyllactate, phenylacetate, phenylacetylglutamine, in addition to a deficiency of tyrosine, an amino acid that forms catecholamines, thyroxine (T_4) and triiodothyronine (T_3), melanin and other proteins; the most common or 'classic' phenylketonuria (PKU or hyperphenylalaninemia, type 1) is an autosomal recessive condition characterized by a deficiency in phenylalanine hydroxylase, which if not recognized early (urine has a 'mousy' odor) and treated by restricting dietary phenylalanine, results in a child with tremors, seizures, eczema, hyperactivity and hypopigmentation and an IQ of less than 50; other hyperphenylalaninemia types, eg types 2, 3 and 7, are relatively benign

Hyperphosphatasia Hyperostosis corticalis deformans juvenilis

Hyperphosphatasemia Benign familial hyperphosphatasemia A rare condition described in a small cohort (J Am Med Assoc 1989; 261:1310) with a benign increase in the intestinal isoenzyme of alkaline phosphatase, which causes no clinical disease unless the altered enzyme levels evoke an aggressive work-up for bone or liver disease, malignancy, pregnancy, resulting in a 'Ulysses syndrome'

Hyperphosphatemia The elevation of phosphate(s) above 1.5 mmol/L (US: 4.5 mg/dl) Etiology Increased growth hormone, either physiologic with growth spurts or pathological in gigantism and acromegaly, decreased parathyroid hormone and pseudohypoparathyroidism or in renal failure

Hyperprolinemia A condition characterized by a defect in imino acid metabolism **HYPERPROLINEMIA, TYPE I** A condition characterized by a defect of proline oxidase, which produces pyrroline carboxylate from proline and is associated with renal tube defects, without mental retardation; **HYPERPROLINEMIA, TYPE II** A condition characterized by a defect of delta'-pyrroline-5-carboxylic acid dehydrogenase with variable mental retardation, seizures and renal tube defects

Hypersensitive sites MOLECULAR BIOLOGY Regions of a eukaryotic genome that have an increased sensitivity to DNase cleavage and which often correspond to regulatory sequences

Hypersensitivity pneumonitis A group of disorders caused by an exuberant pulmonary reaction to aerosolized immunogens (table), that with time may develop interstitial lung disease; the prototypic hypersensitivity pneumonitis is Farmer's lung, which is accompanied by fever, malaise, cough, chest tightness and myalgias; see Farmer's lung, Humidifier lung

Hypersensitivity pneumonitis

Syndrome	Suspected antigen
Bagassosis	*Thermoactinomyces vulgaris*
Bird fancier's lung	Bird droppings
Pigeon handler's lung	*Histoplasma capsulatum*
Cheese worker's lung	*Penicillium*
Detergent worker's lung	*Bacillus subtilis* enzyme
Fish meal lung	Fish proteins
Farmer's lung*	*Micropolyspora faeni, Thermoactinomyces vulgaris*
Humidifier lung*	*Thermophilic actinomycetes*
Malt worker's lung	*Aspergillus clavatus*
Maple bark disease	*Cryptostroma corticale*
Mushroom picker's lung	*Micropolyspora faeni*
Sequoiosis	*Graphium, Auerobasidium*
Suberosis (oak bark)	*Micropolyspora faeni*
Vineyard sprayer's lung	Copper
Wood dust pneumonitis	Oak and mahogany dust
Wood pulp worker's lung	*Alternaria* species

*See separate heading

Hypersexuality A phenomenon inducible in experimental mammals by bilateral lesions in the limbic region, localized in the piriform cortex overlying the amygdala, causing the animals to mount females that are not in estrus, other males, animals of other species and inanimate objects; non-psychogenic hypersexuality has been reported in some patients with bilateral lesions adjacent to the amygdaloid nucleus; see Temporal lobe syndrome; Cf 'Don Juan' syndrome

Hypersomnia(s) a) Primary hypersomnia-bulimia syndrome of Klein-Levine A condition characterized by semiannual bouts of hyperphagia followed by a 2-5 day 'sleep-off' described in young males b) Hypersomnia-sleep apnea syndrome A condition described in obese and hypertensive middle-aged males characterized by daytime grogginess and loud snoring; these patients are at an increased risk for myocardial infarcts and cerebrovascular accidents; see Sleep apnea syndrome c) Secondary hypersomnia is a symptom caused by focal central nervous system disease, eg brain tumors, especially those affecting the posterior hypophysis or diencephalon, encephalopathia lethargica and meningitis or systemic disease, eg hypothyroidism, trypanosomiasis; see Narcolepsy, Sleep disorders; Cf REM sleep

Hypersplenism An enlargement of the spleen by any etiology, characterized by splenomegaly, pancytopenia and hyperplasia of the marrow precursor cells, with clinical improvement upon splenectomy Congestive hypersplenism is due to stasis of blood flow and most often secondary to cirrhosis of the liver, as well as thrombosis and other vascular abnormalities; less common causes of hypersplenism include lymphoproliferative disorders, eg lymphoma, leukemia, especially chronic myeloid leukemia, infections, eg infectious mononucleosis, kala azar, tuberculosis and infiltrations, eg Gaucher and Niemann-Pick diseases **Clinical** Isolated hypersplenism is asymptomatic, but the primary diseases may be accompanied by general malaise, fever, fullness, purpura or may present with hematemesis or gastrointestinal bleeding **Laboratory** Decreased red cell survival, reticulocytosis and 'left shift' of the myeloid series; Cf Splenosis

Hypertelorism Any excess separation of paired organs, eg the eyes or breast Ocular hypertelorism A common cranio-facial defect seen in many congenital anomalies, many of which have been eponymically dignified, eg Apert syndrome (acrocephalosyndactyly), Crouzon's disease (craniofacial dysostosis), Opitz' syndrome (Hypertelorism-hypospadia or BBB syndrome) and Taybi syndrome (otopalatodigital syndrome) Mammary hypertelorism is relatively uncommon, and is typical of the Turner syndrome

Hypertension A condition affecting a reported 60 million persons in the US, defined as a systolic blood pressure of greater than 160 mm Hg and/or diastolic blood pressure of 95 mm Hg and graded according to the intensity of increased diastolic blood pressure Class I (mild) Diastolic pressure 90-104 mm Hg Class II (moderate) Diastolic pressure 105-119 mm Hg Class III (severe) Diastolic pressure greater than 120 mm Hg Evaluation of hypertension requires clinical history for patient and family history, two blood pressure determinations, fundoscopic examination, identification of bruits in the neck and abdominal aorta, evaluation of peripheral edema, peripheral pulses and residual neurologic defects in stroke victims, chest films to determine cardiac size and laboratory parameters to rule out causes of secondary hypertension (table) Pathogenesis The mechanism by which hypertension causes morbidity is not understood; one-third of cases have an increased cardiac load, the remainder have increased peripheral arterial pressure and generalizedvasoconstriction due to autonomic nervous system dysfunction and end defective organ response in the vessels, related to increased renal cytochrome P-450 and P-450-induced arachidonic acid metabolites (Biochem Pharmacol 1988; 37:521), activation of the renin-angiotensin (see table, renin levels) and kallikrein-kinin systems, with contributions from arginine vasopressin and atrial natriuretic peptides Risk factors Race (blacks more common), males, family history of hypertension, obesity, metabolic defects of lipid metabolism, diabetes mellitus, sedentary lifestyle, cigarette smoking, electrolyte imbalance, including increased sodium, phosphorus, decreased potassium and tin (Mayo Clin Proc 1988; 63:700); sodium's link to hypertension is unclear (in one report, administration of sodium chloride, but not sodium citrate, to patients with essential hypertension increased systolic and diastolic blood pressure by 16 mm and 8 mm Hg, respectively) **Treatment** Hypertension may respond to diet, eg sodium restriction (see previous caveat), reduced calories, alcohol and cigarettes (although the weight gain accompanying smoking cessation tends to offset the minimal reduction in blood pressure), calcium supplementation, or lifestyle manipulation, eg biofeedback, increased exercise; antihypertensive medications, eg diuretics (benzothiadiazines, loop diuretics, potassium-sparing diuretics), sympatholytic agents (central and peripheral-acting α-adrenergics, β-adrenergics, mixed α- and β-blocking agents), direct vasodilators, converting enzyme inhibitors, calcium channel blockers; Cf Pseudohypertension, 'White coat' hypertension **Essential hypertension** Idiopathic hypertension The major form comprising 90% of all hypertenion, see above **Malignant hypertension** A sustained blood pressure of greater than 200/140 mm Hg, resulting in arteriolar necrosis, most marked in the brain, eg cerebral hemorrhage, infarcts and hypertensive encephalopathy, eyes, eg papilledema and hypertensive retinopathy and kidneys, eg acute renal failure and hypertensive nephropathy; if malignant hypertension is uncorrected or recalcitrant to therapy, the patient may enter into a hypertensive crisis in which prolonged high pressure causes left ventricular hypertrophy and congestive heart failure **Paroxysmal hypertension** Transient or episodic waves of increased blood pressure of any etiology, punctuated by periods of normotension, classically described in pheochromocytoma **Portal hypertension** A condition caused by a back-flow of blood through the splenic arteries and collateral circulation, usually associated with hepatic cirrhosis, or rarely portal vein disease, venous thrombosis, tumors or abscesses **Pulmonary hypertension** A condition defined as a 'wedge' systolic/diastolic pressure of reater than 30/20 mm Hg (Normal: 18-25/12-16 mm Hg), often secondary to stasis of blood in the peripheral circulation, divided into passive, hyperkinetic, vaso-occlusive, vasoconstrictive and secondary forms, see Pulmonary hypertension **Renovascular hypertension** see there **Secondary hypertension** (see table, page 326)

Hypertension & Renin levels

Low	High
Mineralocorticoid hypersecretion decreased K^+, decreased Ca^{++} alkalosis	Unilateral renal artery stenosis Malignant hypertension Chronic renal failure, volume (secondary hyperaldosteronism, increased glucocorticoids, estrogens)

Hypertension panel A battery of 'cost efficient' serum tests used to evaluate a person with hypertension, which include the most common causes of secondary hypertension, measuring BUN/creatinine, chloride, CO_2 content, free urinary cortisol, potassium, sodium, thyroxine, vanillylmandelic acid, urinalysis/bacterial colony count; Cf Organ panel

Hypertensive crisis A rare clinical event characterized by a severe and/or acutely increased diastolic blood pressure above 120-130 mm Hg; it constitutes a medical emergency if there is evidence of rapid or progressive central nervous system (encephalopathy, infarction or hemorrhage), cardiovascular (myocardial ischemia,

SECONDARY HYPERTENSION (after S Oparil, in JB Wyngaarden, LH Smith, 1988)

Aging

Cardiovascular Open heart surgery, coarctation of the aorta

Cerebral Increased intracranial pressure

Combined systolic and diastolic hypertension

Decreased vascular resistance Arteriovenous shunts, Paget's disease of the bone, beri-beri

Endocrine Mineralocorticoid excess, congenital adrenal hyperplasia, glucocorticoid excess, eg Cushing syndrome, hyperparathyroidism, acromegaly

Gynecological Pregnancy, oral contraceptives

Increased cardiac output Anemia, thyrotoxicosis aortic valve insufficiency

Neoplasia Renin-secreting tumors, pheochromocytoma

Renal disease Vascular, parenchymal

Systolic hypertension

infarction, aortic dissection, pulmonary edema) and renal deterioration, eclampsia or microangiopathic hemolytic anemia; hypertensive crises most commonly occur in pre-existing chronic hypertension, but may be due to renovascular hypertension, parenchymal renal disease, scleroderma and collagen vascular disease, ingestion of sympathomimetic and tricyclic antidepressant drugs or after withdrawal from antihypertensive drugs, use of recreational drugs, eg crack, spinal cord syndromes and pheochromocytoma Histopathology Intravascular fibrin deposition and fibrinoid necrosis of vessels walls Treatment Therapy must target the organ most affected by the crisis, using calcium channel antagonists, laβlol, loop diuretics, nitroglycerine and sodium nitroprusside (N Engl J Med 1990; 323:1177rv) Prevention Stannous chloride has an antihypertensive effect in rats, reducing cytochrome P-450-derived metabolites of arachidonic acid (Science 1989; 243:388) Prognosis Untreated, five-year mortality is 100%

Hypertensive retinopathy The constellation of retinal changes induced by hypertension, which includes 'copper wire' and 'silver wire' changes of long-standing hypertension or retinal and disc edema following an abrupt increase in systemic blood pressure, ie malignant hypertension; hypertensive retinopathy is divided into GRADE I Generalized narrowing of arterioles, vasoconstriction, 'hyaline' deposition in walls GRADE II As above with hyaline thickening of vessels, arteriovenous 'nicking', ie thin-walled veins compressed by engorged arterioles, imparting a 'silver wire' or if the blood column is no longer visible, a 'copper wire' appearance GRADE III As above with flame-shaped, 'splinter' hemorrhages in the nerve and around the optic nerve head and macula, retinal edema with exudates, pools of fluid rich in lipid, protein and fibrin, hemorrhages and scattered gray-white grayish macular spots with fluffy borders, known as macular stars; arteriovenous 'nicking' is prominent, with 'cotton-wool' patches, tiny, white, disk-shaped and superficial retinal infarcts, corresponding to foci of nerve fiber-layer necrosis containing cytoid bodies GRADE IV As in III with edema of optic disk, both of which may be accompanied by retinal detachment

Hyperthecosis A condition characterized by hyperplasia of the theca interna of a maturing ovarian follicle that may be associated with hirsutism and amenorrhea; see Hirsutism

Hyperthermia A clinical condition defined as a corporal temperature of greater than 42°C; as a defense, there is peripheral vasodilation (decreased effective volume), resulting in an increased pulse rate, a response to perceived blood loss, decreased cardiac efficiency, hypoxia, increased permeability of cell membranes with increased potassium and cardiac failure; see Malignant hyperthermia

Hypertrichosis see Hirsutism

Hypertrophic cardiomyopathy Formerly, idiopathic hypertrophic subaortic stenosis A group of diseases characterized by either symmetric (concentric) or asymmetric (eccentric) hypertrophy, the latter with disproportionate thickening beneath the mitral valve, which occurs in the absence of any other cardiac disease; one-half of cases are congenital, with an autosomal dominant pattern Clinical Younger patients, ranging from asymptomatic to diastolic dysfunction, dyspnea, fatigue, chest pain and syncope, an increased incidence of severe obstruction, congestive heart failure and sudden death, simulating myocardial infarction EKG Increased QRS complexes, T-wave inversion and Q waves in the inferior and left precordial leads Histopathology Asymmetric septal hypertrophic ventricle, myofiber disarray, thick-walled intramural coronary arteries Treatment Symptomatic, ie relief of dyspnea or chest pain Drugs β-adrenergic agents are effective short-term; calcium channel blockers, which increase diastolic filling of the ventricles Surgery Recalcitrant cases may require a transaortic ventricular septal myotomy-myectomy

Hypertrophic (pulmonary) osteoarthropathy A clinical complex characterized by clubbing of the fingers and toes, periostitis of the ends of the long bones, arthritis, pain and occasionally, autonomic dysfunction including pallor, flushing and profuse diaphoresis; although it may rarely occur as an idiopathic condition (pachydermoperiostosis), it is classically associated with pulmonary disease, including cancer, abscesses, emphysema, chronic interstitial pneumonitis; Cf Clubbing

Hypertyrosinemia see Tyrosine

Hypervalinemia see Valinemia

Hypervariable region see Hot spot

Hyperventilation syndrome Tachy-dyspnea 'syndrome' A clinical complex affecting neurotics with anxiety attacks; the hyperventilation, in addition to the characteristic EEG changes (bilateral synchronous theta wave followed by delta activity with spike and slow-wave discharges) causes respiratory alkalosis, tightness in the chest, dizziness without syncope, numbness of the hands and feet and tetany Treatment Rebreathe air in a paper bag, as the increased CO_2 facilitates physiologic compensation

Hyperviscosity syndrome A clinical complex evoked by a marked increase in plasma viscosity, which is 18 to 33-fold greater than blood (Normal plasma viscosity is about 1.8 X more viscous than water); hyperviscosity is most commonly seen in Waldenström syndrome due to a massive increase in circulating IgM, less commonly in IgG or IgA plasma cell dyscrasias Clinical The findings reflect sluggish blood flow, seen in the retina (engorged 'sausage-link' veins), ear (tinnitus and vertigo), and petechial hemorrhage (due to microcirculatory sluggishness, hypoxia and capillary damage) Treatment Plasmapheresis, with removal and washing of 2-3 units of plasma/day until the viscosity normalizes, then maintaining as needed Note: Viscosity is the measurement of a fluid's resistance to flow, a function in biological systems of protein concentration and the intrinsic 'stickiness' of each constituent protein

Hypervitaminosis see Vitamin

Hyphae see Dimorphic fungi

Hypnosis A modality that has theoretical currency in behavior modification and biofeedback; its success is difficult to evaluate, as valid double-blind studies cannot be performed, given that all studies must evaluate the success (or failure) to achieve the intended effect(s) on a per-case basis; hypnosis is claimed to be useful in speech therapy, smoking cessation, ameliorating panic disorders and in lower back pain

Hypnotics Therapeutic central nervous system depressants Benzodiazepines are the drug of choice for 'primary' insomnia; short-acting hypnotics, eg triazolam and oxazolam are used to induce sleep; to maintain sleep throughout the night, longer-acting hypnotics, eg flurazepam are required Note: When insomnia is secondary, treatment of the underlying condition, eg Parkinson's disease, causes resolution of insomnia

Hypo-β–lipoproteinemia see Hypolipoproteinemia

Hypochlorite Bleach

Hypochondroplasia An autosomal dominant condition characterized by short limbs, decreased height, caudal syringomyelia

Hypogammaglobulinemia Reduced production of proteins, usually immunoglobulins migrating in the 'γ' region of a protein electrophoretic gel, which may be congenital, as in Bruton's disease, other B cell defects or acquired, as in chronic lymphocytic leukemia, which may be accompanied by monoclonal gammopathies (table) Treatment Human immune globulins; see Immunodefi-ciency, B cell

Hypoglycemia A decrease in circulating glucose that often is a symptom of systemic disease; fasting hypoglycemia occurs in endocrinopathies, including hypopituitarism, Addison's disease, adrenogenital syndrome, islet cell tumors, factitious insulin ingestion, non-pancreatic neoplasms, eg retroperitoneal sarcoma, producing ectopic insulin, hepatic disease, glycogen storage disease; postprandial hypoglycemia may be functional and idiopathic, associated with preclinical diabetes, status post-gastrectomy or drug-related, by for example sulfonylureas, oral hypoglycemic agents, including chlorpropamide, tolbutamide, tolazamide, acetohexamide, as well as alcohol, aspirin, phenformin and insulin

Hypoglycin A toxic derivative of propionic acid that evokes Jamaican vomiting sickness, see there

Hypogonadism A clinical condition with decreased or absent phenotypic expression of a person's sexual genotype, which may be primary, due to a lack of end organ response to FSH or LH produced normally by an intact pituitary gland (hypergonadotropic hypogonadism), or secondary to defective hypothalamic or pituitary hormonal activity (hypogonadotropic hypogonadism, see table, next page

Hypogonadotropic eunuchoidism Kallmann syndrome Secondary hypogonadism with testicular failure, due to inadequate gonadotropin secretion by hypothalamic or pituitary dysfunction; in most, decreased FSH and LH impairs both sperm and androgen production Clinical Delayed puberty, micropenis, eunuchoid features, cryptorchism, anosmia, midline defects, including cleft lip and palate, renal agenesis, nerve deafness and color blindness, skeletal abnormalities; highly variable hereditary pattern Treatment Androgens may be used to induce anatomic maturation and gonadotropins or luteinizing hormone releasing

HYPOGAMMAGLOBULINEMIA CONGENITAL

X-linked agammaglobulinemia of Bruton An autosomal recessive condition in which the B cells are arrested at the pre-B cell stage of development anddisease becomes manifest as the passively transfered maternal immunoglobulin falls below 200 mg/dl, which occurs at about 6 months of age, given IgG's serum half-life of 20-25 days Clinical Recurrent pyogenic organisms with intact T cell and NK cell-mediated immunity; malabsorption associated with Giardia infections Complications Polyarthritis collagen vascular disease and fatal dermatomyositis Treatment Immunoglobulins

Transient hypogammaglobulinemia A quasi-physiological state which is similar to Bruton's disease in presentation, but merely represent a normal delay in immunoglobulin production by the infant rather than rather than the inability to produce them

Swiss-type lymphopenic agammaglobulinemia A condition in which there are both B and T cell defects see Severe combined immunodeficiency

Other congenital hypo-globulinemias Selective deficiencies in the production of IgA, IgM, subclasses of IgG, associated with 5'-nucleotidase deficiency or X-linked with lymphoproliferative disorders, eg Duncan syndrome,

Combined variable immunodeficiency (CVID) B cell precursors are present but don't differentiate into plasma cells and is associated with T cell defects; acquired hypogammaglobulinemia may be associated with drug and protein-losing states

HYPOGONADISM

FEMALE HYPERGONADOTROPIC (PRIMARY) HYPOGONADISM Turner syndrome, XX Turner sydrome, XX pure gonadal dysgenesis, mixed gonadal dysgenesis, autoimmune ovarian disease

FEMALE HYPOGONADOTROPIC (SECONDARY) HYPOGONADISM Carpenter syndrome, hypopituitarism, Lawrence-Moon-Biedl, multiple lentigines syndrome, polycystic ovaries (Stein-Leventhal syndrome)

MALE HYPERGONADOTROPIC (PRIMARY) HYPOGONADISM Congenital anorchia, rudimentary testes, germ cell hypoplasia (del Castillo syndrome), XY Turner phenotype (Noonan syndrome), Klinefelter syndrome and variants, XX males, XYY males

MALE HYPOGONADOTROPIC (SECONDARY) HYPOGONADISM Amyloidosis, Carpenter syndome, fertile eunuch syndrome, Froehlich syndrome, Sheehan syndrome, Kallmann's disease, Laurence-Moon-Biedl disease, Lowe syndrome, Prader-Willi syndrome

factor for spermatogenesis

Hypohidrosis Reduced sweat production (table)

Hypohidrotic dysplasia An uncommon familial condition characterized by peg-shaped teeth, focal anodontia, facial dysplasia, hyperthermia, decreased sweat glands

Hypolipoproteinemia A group of conditions characterized by decreased lipoproteins, either acquired, eg secondary to malabsorption, anemia(s), hyperthyroidism or congenital, eg Tangier's disease, a-β-lipoproteinemia (Bassen-Kornzweig syndrome) and lecithin-cholesterol acyl transferase (LCAT) deficiency **Hypo-β–lipoproteinemia** An autosomal dominant condition due to decreased low-density lipoprotein Laboratory Decreased serum cholesterol 1.81-3.11 mmol/L (US: 70-120 mg/dl) and acanthocytosis **a-β-lipoproteinemia** Bassen-Kornzweig syndrome Absence of apolipoprotein B (apo-B) and low-density lipoprotein (LDL) cholesterol (when homozygous) Clinical Fat malabsorption, ataxia, retinitis pigmentosa, neuropathy, acantholysis; in one kindred with the disease, a truncated apo-B results from a four nucleotide deletion, a frameshift mutation and production of a premature stop codon **Tangier disease** a-α-lipoproteinemia Absent HDL and very low levels of apoA-I and apoA-II, with generalized deposits of cholesteryl esters in the tonsils, other lymphoid tissues and corneal opacifications

Hypoperfusion syndrome A 'prerenal' circulatory disorder that is secondary to a) Occlusive renal arterial disease with stenosis and ischemia, resulting in increased renin, hypertension and azotemia, affecting one or both kidneys b) Reduced effective circulatory volume, due to increased vascular capacitance, eg induced by sepsis, sequestration of fluids in compartments, eg in the hepatorenal syndrome or ascites, or the inability to effectively transfer fluids from the venous 'compartment' to the arterial 'compartment' due to congestive heart disease or pericardial limitations due to constrictive pericarditis or effusions; the reduced volume form of hypoperfusion is associated with oliguria, azotemia, reduced sodium excretion and increased renin, but not hypertension

Hypophosphatasia A congenital rickets-like metabolic disease, defined by low serum alkaline phosphatase and disease manifestations of variable intensity; clinical forms A) CONGENITAL (IN UTERO) ONSET 50% neonatal mortality, often due to respiratory insufficiency due to inadequate thoracic ossification Clinical Bone deformities, softened skull and delayed closure of the fontanelles, bowing of legs, irregularity of metaphyseal mineralization, short extremities, blue sclera, failure to thrive, irritability Differential diagnosis Osteogenesis imperfecta, achondroplasia, cleidocranial dysplasia, campomicromelic dwarfism, skeletal dysplasias B) INFANT ONSET, PRESENTING BETWEEN AGES 6-24 MONTHS, Clinical Less severe bony changes than those seen in the congenital onset form, with premature loss of deciduous teeth, metaphyseal defects, growth retardation, craniosynostosis, periostitis, increased fractures and infections, anorexia, polyuria Differential diagnosis Rickets, renal osteodystrophy, metaphyseal dysostosis, cystic fibrosis, phosphate depletion and C) ADULT ONSET Clinical Mild disease, early loss of permanent teeth, radiolucencies, osteoporosis, fractures and pseudofractures

Hypohidrosis

Inherited conditions Hereditary anhydrotic ectodermal dysplasia, ichthyosis, or angiokeratoma corporis diffusum universale

Adquired conditions

Collagen vascular diseases Sjögren syndrome, progressive systemic sclerosis

Dermatopathies Anhidrotic asthenia, miliaria profunda, pemphigus vulgaris, psoriasis

Drugs Anticholinergics, eg atropine, scopolamine and ganglionic blockers

Endocrinopathies Diabetes insipidus, hypothyroidism, hypothalamic lesions

Environmental stress Heat stroke and dehydration

Peripheral neuropathies Alcohol, amyloid, diabetes mellitus, Horner syndrome, leprosy

Hypophysis The pea-sized powerhouse orchestrating the endocrine symphony, saddled in the sella turcica and separated into an a) Anterior lobe, containing cells producing ACTH, FSH, growth hormone (GH or somatotropin), LH and TSH Note: The formerly used division of cells into chromophobes or chromophils (subdividing these into acido- or basophils) is obsolete as some cells produce more than one hormone; monoclonal antibodies may be used to identify the hormone produced by each cell type b) Intermediate lobe, which produces MSH and c) Posterior lobe Neurohypophysis, which, under the hypothalamic baton, produces antidiuretic hormone (vasopressin) and oxytocin

Hypoplastic left heart syndrome see Baby Fae heart

Hypoplastic right heart syndrome(s) A group of congenital cardiac defects that have right ventricular hypoplasia, left ventricular hyperplasia and an atrial right-to-left shunt; right-sided cardiac hypoplasia occurs in tricuspid or pulmonary valve atresias, pulmonary stenosis or in the rare right ventricular hypoplasia

'Hypothalamic fever' Elevated temperature due to an alteration in the hypothalamic thermostat, caused by hemorrhage, trauma or tumor Note: Most patients with hypothalamic damage are hypothermic

Hypothalamic-pituitary 'axis' A group of feedback systems that co-ordinate the activity of the major peptide hormones, where the hypothalamus synthesizes releasing hormones that act on the pituitary, which in turn evokes end-organ responses; the five axes include the hypothalamic-pituitary (HP) adrenocortical-ACTH-adrenal gland axis, HP-FSH/LH-gonadal axis, HP-TSH-thyroid gland axis, HP-growth hormone-somatotroph axis and the hypothalamic-lactotroph-breast axis

Hypothermia A clinical condition defined as a core temperature of 35°C or less that causes 750 annual deaths in the US; those most at risk for hypothermia are the exposed extremes of age, the homeless, alcoholics, those with hypothyroidism and young adults involved in winter sports

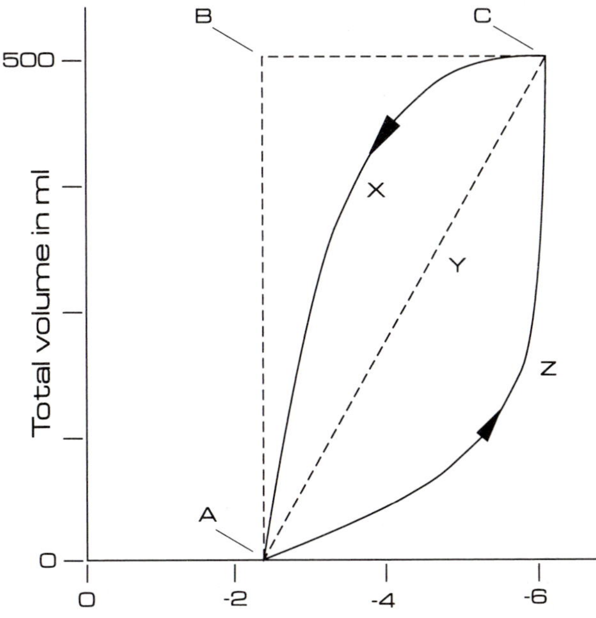

Hysteresis curve

Hypoxanthine-guanine phosphoribosyltransferase (HGPRT) An enzyme encoded on the X chromosome and found in high concentrations in the brain, responsible for transfer of phosphoribosyl groups; deficiency of the HGPRT enzyme results in two syndromes a) Lesch-Nyhan disease, with hyperproduction of uric acid and central nervous system abnormalities, including mental retardation, spasticity, choreoathetosis and compulsive self-mutilation and b) gout without the neurologic disease; variant forms of the enzyme: HGPRT Toronto, London, Ann Arbor, Munich; HGPRT-deficiency has been established in a mouse embryonal stem cell (transgenic mouse), allowing experimental dissection

HYPP Hyperkalemic periodic paralysis see Periodic paralysis

Hysteresis A phenomenon in which the values or data points in a cyclical or periodic process occur along a different route in one direction as the other, described by a hysteric response curve

I Symbol for: Electric current; hypoxanthine; inosine; intensity; ionic strength; isoleucine; luminous intensity

i Symbol for: Isochromosome

IADL Instrumental activities of daily living A series of life functions necessary for maintaining a person's immediate environment, including obtaining food, cooking, laundering, housecleaning, managing one's own medications, use of the telephone; IADL is a measure of a person's (elderly, mentally handicapped or terminally ill) ability to live independently

Ia antigen Immune-associated antigen Cell surface antigens encoded by the I region genes of the major histocompatibility complex (located on chromosome 17) of the mouse which corresponds to the human HLA-DR (chromosome 6), Class II MHC; Ia antigens are expressed on B cells, monocytes and some subsets of T cells, acting as gene-specific mediators of the immune response

IAT see Intra-operative autologous transfusion

Iatrogenic illness Any complication related to diagnosis and treatment of disease, regardless whether the condition occurs as a known risk of a procedure or through errors of omission or commission; iatrogenic disease is a major source of morbidity and mortality for hospitalized patients, the most common of which is cardiac arrest, comprising 14% of the in-hospital cardiac arrests, most often related to errors in medication, especially of digoxin (J Am Med Assoc 1991; 265:2815)

IBD see Inflammatory bowel disease

IBM Ideal body mass

IBS see Irritable bowel syndrome

IBT see Ivy bleeding time

IBW Ideal body weight

ICAM-1 Intercellular adhesion molecule-1 A protein ligand the production of which is induced by γ-interferon and required for neutrophils to migrate into inflamed tissues; in Sézary syndrome, clinical aggression is associated with decreased ICAM-1 expression, possibly due to decreased interferon-γ production by the malignant T cells (J Am Med Assoc 1989; 261:2217)

Icarus complex PSYCHIATRY A constellation of mental conflicts, the degree of which is a function of the disproportion between a person's desire for success, achievement or material goods and his ability to achieve those goals; the greater the gap between the idealized goal and reality, the greater the likelihood of failure; the Icarus analogy has been applied to a 'driven' or aggressive 'type A' person who cannot recognize his own limitations; alternately this conflict has been considered an internalization of father-son rivalry; Daedalus and Icarus were a father and son in Greek mythology who had been imprisoned by King Minos on Crete to prevent their return home; they fashioned wings of feathers and attached them with wax; Icarus, despite his father's ministrations, flew too close to the sun, melted his wings and fell to his death; see Type A, 'Toxic core'

ICD-9-CM International Classification of Disease, 9th edition, Clinical Modification A systematic and standardized classification of disease that allows clinicians, statisticians, politicians, health planners and others to speak a common language, both in the USA and internationally; infectious diseases are 001-139, neoplasia 140-239, endocrine 140-279, blood-related 280-289, mental disease 290-319, nervous 320-389, circulatory system 390-459, respiratory system 460-519, gastrointestinal tract 520-579, genitourinary tract 580-629, pregnancy-related 630-676, skin 680-709, connective tissue disease 710-739, congenital anomalies 740-759, conditions of perinatal origin 760-779, vaguely defined conditions 780-799, injury and poisoning 800-999; other details may be added to the classification, including a V prefix for a virulent or communicable disease and E for external causes of injury

$$C_6H_5{-}CH_2{-}CH(CH_3){-}NH{-}CH_3$$

'Ice'

'Ice' The 'street' name for the smokable, crystal form of the psychostimulant, (+)- or D-methamphetamine HCl; oral abuse of methamphetamine has occurred in epidemic waves in Japan, Sweden and the US since the 1950s; an inhaled smokable form of the crystalline form, which has an ice-like appearance (hence, 'ice') represents a new form of abuse; ice induces an effect similar to intravenous injection of methamphetamine, ie far more intense than that achieved by oral ingestion; the mechanism of action differs from cocaine, but has a stimulant effect similar and of longer duration (hours versus minutes for cocaine); because methamphetamine is synthetic, an unlimited supply may be manufactured in illicit laboratories as a 'designer drug'; ice is being touted as the 'drug of the 1990s' and in Hawaii has become the most common drug of abuse (Science 1990; 249:631); the low cost of the raw material (phenylacetic acid, $1300/kg) and the high street value of the finished product, Ice ($500 000), make it likely that ice addiction will increase; 1.2% of US high school students have used it, 3% in the Western states; ice, like 'crack' has a prolonged 'high' and is more socially acceptable to upper class; Ice's neurotoxicity is prolonged with severe depression of the caudate dopamine levels, lasting six months or more after last use in animal models (J Am Med Assoc 1990; 263:2717) Complications Pulmonary edema, dilated cardiomyopathy, acute myocardial infarction, cardiogenic shock and death (J Am Med Assoc 1991; 265:1152); see 'Designer' drug

Ice ball method GYNECOLOGY A method for treating benign lesions of the uterine cervix, in which special probes previously frozen with either liquid nitrogen or freon are placed on the cervix for 2-3 minutes, freezing and then excising a lesion Advantage Reduced postoperative pain, infection, discharge and better hemostasis Disadvantage Freezing introduces considerable histological artifact that makes the ice-ball technique controversial in treating dysplasia and carcinoma

Iceberg (thoraco-abdominal) sign A sharply-demarcated radiopacity seen in plain films of the chest or abdomen that may be either sub- or supradiaphragmatic and corresponds to a paravertebral tuberculous abscess, aneurysm, esophagogastric lesion or the azygous continuation of the inferior vena cava

Iceberg lesion see Dumbbell tumor

Ice cream headache A migraine headache triggered by oropharyngeal irritation due to cold foods, the ingestion of which causes bifrontal headaches in most patients with migraines

Ice hockey see Silo-filler's disease

Iceland disease Epidemic neuromyasthenia, benign myalgic encephalomyelitis An epidemic disease, described as common in the summer among student nurses, that resembles poliomyelitis **Etiology** Unknown, psychosocial dysfunction has been implicated **Clinical** Severe headache, myalgia, fatigue, myasthenia, variable cranial and peripheral nerve dysfunction and depression; recuperation requires up to a year

I-cell disease Leroy's disease Type II mucolipidosis A condition caused by a defective protein traffic and sorting factor (N-acetylglucosamine-1-phosphotransferase)

which directs correct compartmentalization of catabolic enzymes, by phosphorylating mannose, without which, the lysosomal enzymes are present but 'forget' their final destination in the lysosomes, resulting in massive accumulation of intracellular and extracellular waste products, especially glycolipids **Clinical** Hurler-like disease (type I-H mucopolysaccharidosis) with a gargoyle face, early onset of psychomotor retardation, joint contracture, hepatosplenomegaly and cardiac decompensation which causes death in childhood Note: 'I-cell' derives from the microscopic finding of numerous dark cytoplasmic inclusions in fibroblasts grown from biopsies

'Ice man' FORENSIC PATHOLOGY A free-lance 'con' artist who dealt in contraband guns and stolen cars, and who was alleged to have been responsible for an unknown number of murders in the New York metropolitan area in the early 1980s, whose business associates often 'disappeared'; the sobriquet stems from his modus operandi--after incapacitating his victims with cyanide and/or strangling them, he stored the bodies for a year or two in a freezer, as the ice crystals destroyed the evidence for a time of death

Ichthyosis A group of hereditary diseases characterized by dyskeratosis and non-inflammatory scaling of the skin, subdivided into four major primary forms, including ichthyosis vulgaris, X-linked ichthyosis, epidermolytic hyperkeratosis and lamellar ichthyosis and three minor primary forms, including harlequin ichthyosis, erythrokeratodermia variabilis and ichthyosis linearis circumflexa; the secondary ichthyoses occur in conjunction with neuroectodermal or mesodermal defects, eg Conradi-Hünermann, Netherton, Refsum, Rud, Sjögren-Larsson syndromes, rhizomelic chondrodysplasia punctata, as well as acquired conditions including Hodgkin's disease, lymphoma, leprosy, hypothyroidism

Ichthyosis hystrix Systematized epidermal nevus A bilateral symmetrical epidermal nevus arranged in a geometrical pattern

Icon-driven COMPUTERS A system design in microcomputers that enables the user to transfer, copy, open, close and otherwise manipulate files and software programs while in the computer's 'root directory', by pointing and clicking on an icon (a small schematic, often trademarked representation of a software program, file, directory, or subdirectory); the icon-driven environment may be combined with pull down menus, both of which may be controlled by 'user-friendly' devices, most commonly, a 'mouse', allowing a non-computer-literate person to use a microcomputer and circumvent the need to memorize arcane disk-operating system commands; see Computers; Cf Menu-driven

ICRF see Imperial Cancer Research Fund

ICRP International Commission on Radiological Protection; see BEIR studies, Chernobyl, Sellafield studies

ICSH Interstitial cell-stimulating hormone Obsolete for luteinizing hormone

ICU Intensive care unit A ward of a secondary or tertiary health care facility, in which 20% of all patients spend some time during their hospitalization; Criteria for admission and continued stay in the ICU include chest pain and suspected myocardial infarct, pulmonary edema and syncope (J Am Med Assoc 1990; 264:992)

id PSYCHIATRY The source of mental energies and libido, the id corresponds to the first (selfish and supremely egocentric) mind of the neonate; the id is later modified by the ego (the conscious being) and the superego (the parental and social conscience), which impose a sense of reality and control on the id's egocentric drives; Freud created the id concept and felt that repression of the id led to neurosis, inhibition of the id led to sexual deviation and sublimation of the id led to artistic creativity; Cf id reaction

IDDM Insulin-dependent diabetes mellitus Juvenile, type I or 'brittle' diabetes mellitus is due to a deficit in endogenous insulin production and comprises about 10% of diabetes mellitus **Genetics** IDDM is more common in HLA-DR3, DR4-positive subjects; concordance between identical twins is 55% **Clinical** Extreme hyperglycemia, lability of glucose control and ketosis; IDDM of recent onset may have IgG autoantibodies directed against glucose transport proteins (N Engl J Med 1990; 322:635); see Honeymoon period; Cf NIDDM

Ideational apraxia NEUROLOGY The inability to execute a sequence of movements in an orderly fashion; although individual components of the movement are executed, the entire act remains uncompleted, eg a match may be removed from its cover but not struck

Identifier sequence see ID sequence

Ideokinetic apraxia NEUROLOGY The dissociation of an idea and the motor act, eg a patient cannot whistle when commanded to do so, but may do so spontaneously

Idiogenic osmoles FLUID PHYSIOLOGY Amino acids and unidentified solutes that accumulate in neurons during chronic hypernatremia, minimizing the shrinkage that occurs in these cells, since the oncotic pressure exerted by these molecules prevents fluid loss by neurons

Idiopathic cyclical edema see Cyclical edema syndrome

Idiopathic hypertrophic subaortic stenosis see Hypertrophic cardiomyopathy

Idiopathic midline destructive disease

a) Local destruction of the upper respiratory tract
b) Lack of progression to system disease (average follow-up, seven years)
c) Acute/chronic inflammation with variable necrosis, without vasculitis, atypia or malignancy
d) No evidence of infection or malignancy

Idiopathic midline destructive disease (IMDD) Lethal midline granuloma of Stewart A primary nosology that is a diagnosis of exclusion (criteria, table), representing a midline granuloma for which no etiology can be elucidated; most midline granulomas are secondary manifestations of a primary process, including vasculitis, eg Wegener's disease, malignancy, eg lymphoma, nasal carcinoma and infections, eg destructive fungal infections in immunocompromised patients Treatment Radiotherapy; see Lethal midline granuloma, Midline granuloma

Idiopathic panarteritis Takayasu's disease

Idiopathic interstitial fibrosis of lung A disease more common in middle-aged men, possibly related to collagen vascular disease, with positive 'rheumatoid' serology Clinical Aggressive with a rapid onset of dyspnea, orthopnea, hemoptysis, cyanosis, clubbing of the fingers and toes, pulmonary hypertension, bibasilar rales, non-productive cough and death in 3-6 years Radiology Diffuse reticulonodular infiltrates Histopathology, early Fibrinous edema, erythrocytes and desquamated macrophages and hyaline membrane disease Histopathology, late Bronchial cells undergo columnar or mucinous metaplasia, muscular hyperplasia, later collagenous replacement of the alveolar wall causes compression, collapse and alveolar 'honeycombing' and has a bossellated or 'hobnailed' pleural surface; pulmonary fibrosis is subdivided into usual, desquamative, lymphocytic and giant cell interstitial pneumonitides

Idiot savant see Savant syndrome

Idiotype The specific type of an immunoglobulin, defined by the myriad of possible combinations of the V (variability), D (diversity) and J (joining) exons as elucidated by Tonegawa; idiotypic specificity resides in the variable region of the heavy and light chains and is specific for an epitope, see Immunoglobulin; Cf Mimotope

Idiotype suppression IMMUNOLOGY The suppression of idiotype antibody synthesis by suppressor T lymphocytes that have been activated by anti-idiotype antibodies

IDL Intermediate-density lipoprotein A plasma lipoprotein that has a density of 1.006-1.019 kg/L (US: 1.006-1.019 g/dl), which is formed by VLDL hydrolysis with lipoprotein lipase that is partially depleted of triglycerides; IDL is composed of 15% protein (predominantly apolipoproteins B and E), 25% phospholipid, 30% cholesterol and 30% triglycerides and transports cholesterol from the intestine to the liver, and once in the liver, is delipidated by hepatic lipoprotein lipase to form low-density protein

Idling reaction MOLECULAR BIOLOGY The transient binding to a ribosome's 'A' site, of a tRNA lacking an attached amino acid, resulting in the temporary halting of the growth of the polypeptide chain and breaking ATP's high-energy phosphate bonds converting GDP to pppGpp; this phenomenon has been fancifully likened to the idling of an automobile motor that makes no progress but expends energy

id reaction Dermatophytid reaction A rash of sudden onset associated with, but located at a distance from, a cutaneous inflammation in a sensitized patient with similar lesions elsewhere; id reactions occur on the hands and arms, as sterile papulovesicular pustules, classically associated with dermatophytosis, eg tinea pedis, tinea capitis and may be associated with stasis dermatitis, eczema and contact dermatitis, which disappear after successful therapy; Cf Isomorphic phenomenon

ID sequence Identifier sequence MOLECULAR BIOLOGY Any of circa 80 base pair in length segments of DNA that are transcribed in the brain and thought to control tissue-specific gene expression

IEF see Isoelectric focusing

IF see Intrinsic factor

IFE Immuno-fixation electrophoresis

IFN see Interferon

Ifosfamide An antineoplastic agent approved under a treatment investigational new drug (IND) protocol as a third-line chemotherapeutic for treating germ-cell testicular malignancy

IGCN see Intratubular germ cell neoplasm

IGF-I Insulin-like growth factor I, Somatomedin-C A 7.6 kD single-chain polypeptide hormone structurally similar to proinsulin, which is synthesized in the liver and fibroblasts, giving fibroblasts a paracrine function; IGF-I is considered to be the sole effector of growth hormone (GH) action, ie GH acts indirectly; IGF-I is an age-dependent primary growth regulator; serum levels correlate with the development of secondary sex characteristics in puberty; IGF-I is bound to a carrier-protein and therefore has relatively constant serum levels; because GH fluctuates widely during the day, IGF-I reflects GH activity Normal levels < age 5 < 100 µg/L, peaks during puberty < 225 µg/L, over age 50 < 100 µg/L); IGF-I is decreased in starvation, anorexia nervosa and African pygmies and increased with decreased somatomedins in Laron dwarfs, kwashiorkor and hepatic disease in children Note: Somatomedins include somatomedins A and B and IGF-I and -II

IGF-II Insulin-like growth factor II A protein structurally homologous to IGF-I that may be produced by tumors, eg leiomyosarcoma, mesotheliomas and others and may cause reactive hypoglycemia; IGF-II receptor is similar, if not identical to the receptor for mannose-6-phosphate

IgG index LABORATORY MEDICINE A value determined by the ratio of production of IgG and albumin in the brain and in the peripheral tissues, which is elevated in a wide range of infectious, inflammatory and neoplastic disorders of the central nervous system; Cf Oligoclonal bands

IgM index A measure of the total IgM synthesis in the blood-brain barrier (BBB), which is characteristically increased in infectious meningoencephalitis by bacteria or *Borrelia burgdorferi*; the IgM may also be elevated in multiple sclerosis and lupus erythematosus of the central nervous system

IHSS see Idiopathic hypertrophic subaortic stenosis

Ii antigens A pair of non-allelic antigens present on the surface of hematopoietic, typically red cells and non-hematopoietic cells; the i antigen is immature and present on fetal red cells and red cell precursors; I antigen results from the enzymatic conversion of aliphatic galactose-N-acetyl-glucosamine to a complex branched form; therefore two 'alleles' don't exist, merely immature (i) and mature (I) forms; expression of the I antigen indicates red cell maturation, occurring by age 2; in the absence of the I antigen, only i antigen is expressed; anti-i antibodies cause hemolysis in infectious mononucleosis; anti-I antibodies are uncommon, but when seen are of high titer and have a wide thermal amplitude

IIFL see Idiopathic interstitial fibrosis of the lung

IL see Interleukins

Ileal bypass operation A surgical procedure that may be indicated for extreme obesity or high serum cholesterol Method The distal one-third of the small intestine (circa 2 m) is bypassed and bowel continuity is restored by an end-to-side ileocecostomy; ileal bypass surgery improves the lipid profile of those with a previous myocardial infarction (reduction of total and LDL-cholesterol by 23% and 38%, with 5% increase in HDL-cholesterol; post-operative coronary artery disease is reduced but not significant (N Engl J Med 1990; 323:946) Side effects The jejuno-ileal bypass procedure is a more extensive variation on the 'morbid obesity surgery' theme, resulting in significant weight loss, although fraught with complications, eg steatorrhea, diarrhea, hepatic failure, cirrhosis, oxalate deposition and concrement formation, bile stone formation, electrolyte imbalance: decreased calcium, potassium, magnesium, hypovitaminosis, psychogenic problems, polyarthropathy, hair loss, pancreatitis, colonic pseudoobstruction, intussusception, pneumatosis cystoides intestinalis and blind loop syndrome Note: Many of these same symptoms occur to a lesser degree with less extensive surgery; see Gastric bubble, Jaw wiring, Morbid obesity

Ileal loop test see Rabbit ileal loop test

Ileocecal valve lipohyperplasia Excessive adipose tissue at the submucosa of the ileocecal valve with thickening and protrusion into the cecum and obstructive potential

Ileus Impairment of the caudad flow of the intestinal contents, which is either a) Adynamic or paralytic, secondary to electrolyte derangements, mesenteric arterial vascular accidents, peritoneal irritation, surgery, trauma or as a paraneoplastic phenomenon or b) Obstructive, due to adhesive bands, foreign bodies, hematomas, intussusception or tumors Clinical Symptoms are a function of the level of obstruction and the type of ileus; paralytic ileus causes little pain and is first evident through abdominal distension and vomiting; a post-operative paralytic ileus may manifest itself through increased naso-gastric secretions or oliguria; mechanical ileus is associated with vomiting, abdominal colic, distension and constipation, that may be episodic with intermittent relief through production of voluminous, watery stools Treatment Stabilize, decompress, repair

Iliac horn PEDIATRIC RADIOLOGY A clinical feature of the nail-patella (HOOD or hereditary onychoosteodysplasia) syndrome, seen in early infancy as bilateral chondro-osseous extensions from the iliac wings; iliac horns may also be seen in thanatophoric dwarfism and achondroplasia; bilateral horns without other clinical findings, are known as Fong's disease; unilateral horns have no significance

Illness The state of being unwell, a term used by regulatory agencies, eg the US Food and Drug Administration, which modifies 'illness' with certain adjectives, in order to allow patients to receive experimental drugs that do not have FDA approval; see Life-threatening illness, Severely debilitating illness

ILO International Labor Organization

ILGF Insulin-like growth factor see IGF-I

Imaginary pregnancy see Pseudocyesis

Imaging Production of non-invasive images of body regions through use of ionizing radiation, eg computed tomography or mammography or electromagnetic radiation, eg magnetic resonance imaging or ultrasonography, with or without radiocontrast medium; the information obtained may then be analyzed by a computer to produce a two-dimensional display; the information provided may be anatomic (computed tomography, magnetic resonance imaging, mammography, ultrasonography), metabolic (positron emission tomography, SPECT) or data on electrical activity (SQUID)

Imaging center A facility that has the equipment necessary to produce various types of radiologic and electromagnetic images and the professional staff to interpret the images obtained; in the US, imaging centers may be free-standing and independent financially from, but affiliated with a health care facility, operated on a fee-for-service basis and owned by a group of investors, some or all of whom may be radiologists Note: Because of the wide profit margin and potential for proliferation of imaging centers as vehicles for profit, some states require that an imaging center obtain a 'Certificate of Need' prior to reimbursing the services provided

Imanishi-Kari affair see Baltimore affair

IMAOs Inhibitors of monoamine oxidase A family of therapeutics, eg phenelzine, that are used to treat atypical depression or when tricyclic agents fail; IMAOs have traditionally been relegated to a secondary role treating depression, given the tendency towards inducing hypertensive crises when IMAO-treated patients ingest tyramine-containing products; IMAOs' appear to be most effective when depression is accompanied by anxiety

IMDD see Idiopathic midline destructive disease

IMG International medical graduate

Iminoglycinuria A benign autosomal recessive condition characterized by defective tubular resorption and urinary spillage of proline, hydroxyproline and glycine

Immediate-spin crossmatch TRANSFUSION MEDICINE A test that is used as a final serologic check for incompatibility between the donor red cells and the intended recipient's serum, which detects ABO incompatibility in close to 100% of cases, but fails to detect IgG red cell alloantibodies; the efficiency of this test in detecting ABO incompatibility may be improved by delaying the 'reading' time and resuspending the red cells in a saline-EDTA solution (Transfusion 1991; 31:197)

Immersion foot An affliction of sailors who wear cold and damp rubber sea boots for extended periods, resulting in peripheral vasoconstriction and ischemia, which when severe may require amputation; Cf Trench foot

Immersion oil An oil with a refractive index of 1.52 that allows highpower (from 600x to 1800x) magnification for light microscopy, of particular use in cytopathology, hematology and microbiology Note: Examination of tissues 'under oil' is of limited use in histopathology, as most diagnoses are rendered between 40x and 400x magnifications

Immobilized enzyme An enzyme that has been fixed by physical or chemical means to a solid support, eg a bead or gel to confine a reaction of interest to a particular site

Immotile cilia syndrome Kartagener syndrome An uncommon (1:20 000) autosomal recessive disease of childhood onset due to defective or afunctional cilia in the respiratory tract, resulting in chronic sinusitis, defective mucociliary transport and bronchial clearance, bronchiectasia, chronic otitis media and chronic, potentially incapacitating headaches, related to immotility of ependymal cilia in the walls of cerebral ventricles **Reproduction** Men are infertile, one-half of females are impregnatable, the other half sterile; one-half of cases have Kartagener's triad, ie chronic sinusitis, bronchiectasis and situs inversus totalis, the last of which is possibly due to an in utero defect with the cilia beating in the contrary direction **Ultrastructure** Cilia lack dynein arms; the related Young syndrome is characterized by sinusitis, bronchiectasis and azoospermia, that may follow a fertile phase; other defects associated with immotile cilia include cardiovascular, renal and ocular defects, and absence of frontal sinuses (J Am Med Assoc 1987; 258:1329c; see Cilia

Immune complex-mediated conditions

Arthus reaction Acute hemorrhagic necrosis that follows re-exposure to an antigen, which attracts neutrophils, activates complement, binds ICs by the Fc receptor, causing phagocytosis and increased production of chemotactic factors, especially C5b67 and increasing anaphylotoxins C3a and C5a, resulting in vasodilation

Serum sickness A reaction that is milder than the Arthus reaction, occurring 8-12 days after exposure to the antigen, at the time of 'equivalence' (antigen and antibody are in a 1:1 ratio), after injection of a foreign protein mixture, eg horse serum for antitoxin to tetanus

Immune complex disease (ICD) A morbid state caused by circulating antigen-antibody complexes, which in the face of mild antigen excess, lodge in the small vessels and filtering organs of the circulation and activate complement, chemotactically attracting neutrophils; immune complexes (IC) are involved in complement activation, phagocytosis, neutrophil, basophil and mast cell degranulation, platelet aggregation, increasing humoral responses and activation of CD8 suppressor T-cells; immune complex 'disease' occurs if the immune system has had time to develop antibodies against an antigen and is then re-exposed to the antigen; 'immunocytes' with C3 or Fc receptors are attracted to the site of the immune response and attempt to resolve the immune complexes (ICs); in ICD, size is critical: large ICs are insoluble and are rapidly cleared, small ICs circulate without eliciting a reaction, while intermediately-sized ICs activate the complement cascade; immune complex-mediated conditions (table, above) **Clinical** Fever, enlarged and tender joints, splenic congestion, proteinuria due to glomerular IC deposition, eosinophilia, hypocomplementemia, lymphadenopathy, glomerulonephritis (hypertension, oliguria, hematuria, edema), skin (purpura, urticaria, ulcers), carditis, inflammation of the liver and muscles and necrotizing vasculitis **Methods for detecting ICs** C1q binding assay, solid phase C1q assay, Raji cell assay, conglutinin assay, Staphylococcal protein assay, polyethylene precipitin assay Immune complexes appear in connective tissue disease and inflammation (lupus erythematosus, periarteritis nodosa, mixed connective tissue disease, scleroderma, rheumatoid and juvenile rheumatoid arthritis, temporal arteritis, Behcet's, Reiter's and Wegener's diseases, Sjögren syndrome, ankylosing spondylitis, eosinophilic fasciitis), bacterial infections (***Neisseria meningococcus***, ***N gonorrhoeae***, streptococcus, leprosy, syphilis, salmonellosis), viral infections (hepatitis B virus, infectious mononucleosis, cytomegalovirus, subacute sclerosing panencephalitis, dengue), neoplasia (carcinoma, melanoma, neuroblastoma, lymphocytic leukemia, lymphoma), inflammation (inflammatory bowel disease, optic neuritis, idiopathic glomerulonephritis, interstitial pneumonitis), neurological conditions (multiple sclerosis, myasthenia gravis, Guillain-Barre disease) and others (bullous pemphigoid, diabetes mellitus, intestinal bypass, pemphigus, primary biliary cirrhosis, Schönlein-Henoch syndrome, sickle cell anemia, thrombotic thrombocytopenic purpura)

Immune tolerance see Immunologic tolerance

Immunoadsorbent Any material, eg a gel or inert solid used to adsorb or purify antibodies from a solution

Immunoassay Any assay that measures an antigen-antibody response, the sensitivity of which varies according to the method; the least sensitive is immunoelectrophoresis which can detect antigen levels of 5-10 000 ng/ml, agglutination 1-10 000 ng/ml, single agar diffusion 1-10 000 ng/ml, double agar diffusion and nephelometry < 1000 ng/ml, enzyme immunoassay 1-10 ng/ml, complement fixation 5 ng/ml, immunofluorescence, enzyme-linked immunosorbent assay (ELISA) and radioimmunoassay (RIA), which are sensitive to < .001 ng/ml

Immunoaugmentive therapy (IAT) An unproven method of cancer therapy being administered in clinics in the Bahamas, Mexico and Germany (Science 1990; 249:1369); there is little scientific evidence of efficacy nor safety of IAT, an expensive ($50 000) therapy that entails parenteral administration of tumor cell lysates and serum from both cancer patients and normal subjects; the putative active agents include 'blocking' and 'deblocking proteins', tumor antibody and 'complement' (which is not complement as understood by immunologists); independent analysis of some of the sera used in IAT were found to be contaminated with various organisms (Science 1988; 241:1285; J Am Med Assoc 1988; 260:3435); see Unproven methods of cancer treatment

Immunoblast Lymphoblast

Immunoblastic lymphadenopathy see Angioimmunoblastic lymphadenopathy

Immunoblastic sarcoma A lymphoma composed of cells with features of immunoblasts (transformed lymphocytes) that is subdivided into **B-CELL IMMUNOBLASTIC SARCOMA** Malignant lymphoma, large cell, immunoblastic plasmacytoid type The predominant cell is immunoblast-like, mixed with Reed-Sternberg-like and plasmacytoid cells; this is the most common lymphoma arising in a background of natural immunodeficiency, immunosuppression and immunoproliferative states, eg angioimmunoblastic lymphadenopathy and other diseases of the immune system, including Hashimoto's disease, Sjögren syndrome, α-chain disease and lupus erythematosus Prognosis Poor; 14 month median survival **T-CELL IMMUNOBLASTIC SARCOMA** Malignant lymphoma, large cell, immunoblastic clear cell type Less common than the B-cell immunoblastic lymphoma, characterized by cells with a 'water-clear' cytoplasm, round-to-oval nuclei, fine chromatin, 1-3 nucleoli, nuclear folding, lobulation and occasional multinucleation, interspersed with benign histiocytes, plasma cells, delicate fibrous bands; this lymphoma may arise in a background of mycosis fungoides, with generalized lymphadenopathy and polyclonal hypergammaglobulinemia

Immunoblot see Western blot

Immunochemistry The field that studies the complex properties of immune molecules, attempting to resolve the sites that are active in immune responses, formulate the rules that limit antigen and antibody reactions and ultimately, to design newer structures, including catalytic antibodies and other biological catalysts (Science 1991; 252:659)

Immunocyte adherence see Rosetting

Immunodeficiency, acquired A generalized diminution of the immune response to antigenic stimuli due to a wide variety of conditions including aging, AIDS, Alzheimer's disease, amyotrophic lateral sclerosis, burns, chemotherapy, coeliac disease, corticosteroids, depression and psychologic stress, inflammatory bowel disease, leprosy, nonsteroid antiinflammatory drugs, radiation, sarcoidosis, sepsis, hematological and lymphoproliferative disease (Hodgkin's and non-Hodgkin's lymphomas, leukemia, myeloma, Waldenström's disease, aplastic and agranulocytic anemias, sickle cell disease), systemic disease (malnutrition, chronic diarrhea, fulminant mycosis, sepsis, terminal cancer, diabetes mellitus, uremia and nephrotic syndrome), splenectomy, surgery and trauma

Immunodeficiency, congenital A heterogeneous group of relatively uncommon diseases (table), that are often accompanied by autoimmune disease, allergy, increased incidence of malignancy, gastrointestinal abnormalities Incidence IgA deficiency 1:500, agammagobulinemia

CONGENITAL IMMUNE DEFICIENCIES

I DEFECTIVE CELL TYPE

Stem cell Reticular dysgenesis, severe combined immunodeficiency with thymic dysplasia or adenosine deaminiase deficiency, Swiss type, common variable immunodeficiency (CVID) associated with ectodermal dysplasia and dwarfism, X-linked agammaglobulinemia

B cell defects comprise 50% of congenital immunodeficiencies, including Bruton's disease or other forms of congenital hypogammaglobulinemia variably associated with thymoma, CVID, X-linked hyper-IgM syndrome

T cell defects comprise 10% of congenital immunodeficiencies, including Nezeloff's disease (thymic hypoplasia), DiGeorge syndrome, nucleoside phosphorylase deficiency, chronic mucocutaneous candidiasis

Complex immunodeficiencies with combined B and T cell defects, comprising 30% of congenital immunodeficiencies, including Wiskott-Aldrich syndrome, cartilage-hair hypoplasia syndrome, ataxia-telangiectasia, hyper-IgE syndrome

II DISORDERS OF MOLECULAR SYSTEMS AND NON-SPECIFIC IMMUNE CELLS

Phagocytic defects, comprise 6% of total

i) Leukocyte disorders, eg neutropenia, Chediak-Higashi, lazy leukocyte syndrome, hyper-IgE syndrome

ii) Defective bactericidal activity, eg chronic granulomatous disease (combined neutrophil and macrophage defect), myeloperoxidase deficiency, Chediak-Higashi disease (neutrophils and macrophages with defective lysosomes, chemotactic defects, defective bactericidal activity) and glucose 6-phosphate dehydrogenase deficiency

Complement defects comprise 4% of total Defects of the 'early' complement proteins are associated with autoimmune disease, especially lupus erythematosus; 'late' complement proteins are associated with recurrent infections, especially by *Neisseria* species; complement protein defects may be combined with other immune defects, including

i) Chemotactic defects

ii) Complement defects, eg C1r, C2, C3, C5 combined with B and T cell disorders, including Wiskott-Aldrich disease, chronic mucocutaneous candidiasis, opsonization defects, sickle cell disease, defects in purine metabolism, see adenosine deaminase, combined variable immunodeficiency, purine nucleoside phosphorylase deficiency, severe combined immune deficie

1:50 000, severe combined immunodeficiency 1:100 000, see Adenosine deaminase, Combined variable immunodeficiency, Purine nucleoside phosphorylase deficiency, Severe combined immune deficiency

Immunodiffusion assay A technique for detecting either an antigen or antibody; a serum or fluid presumed to contain the molecule of interest is placed in well A cut in a slab of agar gel; a standardized antigen or antibody is placed in well B; if there is an affinity between the antigen and antibody, precipitation occurs as the two diffuse toward each other; see Radial immune diffusion, Rocket electrophoresis

Immune electron microscopy A technique that uses ferritin-labeled antibodies to study the ultrastructure of various intracellular organelles

Immunofixation electrophoresis (IFE) A type of electrophoresis that follows gel electrophoresis, in which the gel is overlaid with monospecific antisera and the precipitation reaction appears at a characteristic site, producing a sharper image than that obtained by simple immunoelectrophoresis; IFE is used for detecting monoclonal light chains or small monoclonal peaks in the face of a polyclonal expansion, which may be otherwise undetectable due to an 'umbrella' effect, detection of immune complexes, borderline Bence-Jones proteinuria, transferrin bands, specific immunoglobulins (measles, rubella, mumps, herpes simplex), separating very close biclonal populations, phenotyping α-1-antitrypsin

Immunofluorescence Immunofluorescent microscopy A technique in which tissues and cells are examined by a fluorescent light microscope for deposition of immunoglobulins, complement and other immune mediators; in direct immunofluorescence, an anti-human antibody, with a fluorescent tag, eg fluoresceinated isothiocyanate (FITC) is incubated directly with an antigen of interest; in the more sensitive indirect method, unlabelled anti-human antibody is first incubated with the antigen, then incubated with an antibody that has a fluorescent tag allowing 'amplification' of the signal; immunofluorescence microscopy is used to study immune deposits in Berger's and Goodpasture's diseases and hemolytic uremic syndrome and to study the epidermal-dermal junction in bullous pemphigoid, pemphigus vulgaris and dermatitis herpetiformis; standardized tissues may be overlaid with the serum of patients suspected of having circulating autoantibodies, allowing classification of connective tissue diseases; see Antinuclear antibodies; Cf Microscopy

Immunogenicity The degree to which a molecule (usually a protein) is capable of evoking an immune response and production of a specific antibody; immunogenicity is influenced by certain characteristics of the antigen itself (table, below); other factors that impact on immunogenicity include the host's capability for producing antibodies and the manner of antigen presentation, eg a high-dose may overload the system and prevent an immune response; see Immune tolerance

Immunoglobulin A highly-specific molecule of the immune system produced by mature B cells in response to an antigen; the production of an immunoglobulin requires previous rearrangement of the variable, diversity and joining gene segments that form part of the enormous potential repertoire of 10^{10}-10^{12} antibody molecules that may be encoded in response to a molecule's surface binding site or epitope; immunoglobulins are defined as idiotypes, which are imunoglobulins that have been evoked by a particular epitope, isotypes, which are immunoglobulin subtypes (IgG, IgA, IgM, IgD, IgE) that all normal individuals have, and allotypes, which are subtypes that are shared by population groups, eg with racial differences

Immunoglobulin A deficiency The most common (1:600, USA) primary disease of the immune system, characterized by a decrease of IgA to less than 50 mg/L (normal 760-3900 mg/L; US 76-390 mg/dl); 40% of patients produce subclass specific anti-IgA antibodies, (anti-A1, -A2, -A2m(1), -A2m(2)) and may also have IgG2 and IgG4 deficiencies or an HLA-A1/B8 haplotype Clinical Potentially fatal hemolysis occurs if these patients receive blood transfusions due to the production of natural anti-IgA antibodies; other clinical features include myotonic dystrophy, intestinal lymphangiectasia, gluten-sensitive enteropathy, allergies, arthritis, 7S IgM antibodies to food, especially to milk, cirrhosis, autoimmune disease and sinopulmonary infections Treatment Intravenous immune globulin, eg Gammagard (Baxter), has minimal IgA and thus may be well-suited for boosting the humoral immune system (N Engl J Med 1991; 325:110rv)

IgM deficiency syndrome A rare clinical condition usually without clinical consequences that may have decreased complement activation and an increased susceptibility to respiratory infections, fulminant septicemia and various tumors, which may be associated with deficiency in 5-ecto nucleotidase on the B-cell surface

Immunoglobulin-like domain MOLECULAR BIOLOGY A structural motif in certain β-sheet-rich proteins that is 100 amino acid residues long, has intrachain disulfide bonds, associates in pairs by noncovalent bonds, which is present in immunoglobulins, interleukin-1, interleukin-6, platelet-derived growth factor and T cell receptor

Immunohematology see Transfusion medicine

Immuno-isolation The encapsulation of potentially antigenic tissues or cells within a semipermeable, nonimmunogenic membrane as a means of

IMMUNOGEN, REQUIREMENTS: It must be

Foreign Non-self

Large Minimum size 1 kD; most immunogens are greater 10 kD

Chemically complex The more twisted and complex the surface of the molecule, the more immunogenic, eg amino acid homopolymers elicit no antibody, in contrast to heteropolymers of three or more amino acids do

Chemistry of the amino acid Aromatic side chains increase immunogenicity, where the degree of immunogenicity is proportional to the protein's tyrosine

introducing allogenic (non-self) tissues, eg insulin-producing pancreatic islet cells, which are capable of responding to small molecular weight stimuli but which remain isolated from the host immune system; see Biohybrid artificial pancreas, Islet cell transplantation; Cf Liposome

Immunologic (self) tolerance Immune paralysis An active process by which limits are placed on the responsiveness of lymphocytes to self antigens, through multiple complementary pathways and feedback loops; since autoantibody formation is a common event, the loss of self-tolerance is best considered quantitative (Science 1989; 245:147rv); T cell tolerance is more rapid (inducible in 1 day vs. 10 days for B cells), occurs at lower doses of immunogen (1/100th as much as for B cells) and lasts longer (150 days vs. 50-60 days for B cells); natural tolerance to self antigens is related to suppression of T helper cell activity that may be mediated by T suppressor cells and it is thought that the continued presence of these antigens is necessary for maintaining the tolerant state; B cell tolerance occurs by several mechanisms, where a) Immature B cells at very low doses of antigen are very susceptible to tolerization, with subsequent clonal 'abortion' (in contrast, T cell tolerance is not maturation-dependent) b) Clonal exhaustion All B cells capable of responding to an immunogen are stimulated into cell maturation and short-lived antibody production, 'exhausting' or functionally deleting that portion of the B cell repertoire, seen in T-independent antigens c) Antibody-forming cell blockade A short-lived form of B cell intolerance in which antibody-bearing cells are profusely covered with antigens, such that the cell is incapable of response

Immunomodulation Immunotherapy Manipulation of the immune system with either a) Non-specific biological response modifiers, includingnatural molecules, eg lymphokines or synthesized hybrid molecules ('magic bullets'), eg anti-CD5-ricin or b) Specific molecules that have been generated against a patient's self cells

Immunonephelometry LABORATORY MEDICINE A diagnostic modality that detects relatively small antigen-antibody aggregates in a solution by measuring the light scattered at a 90° angle to the light source (a laser, although optional, increases sensitivity), measured by a spectrophotometer at 340-360 nm; in contrast, turbidimetry detects large clumps and particles in a system based on a drop in light from a direct beam of light, ie by 'forward angle light scatter'

Immunoperoxidase method A technique that detects antigens in tissue sections by a) Bathing a histologic section in a monoclonal antibody solution, followed by a wash step to remove unbound monoclonal antibody b) Bathing the tissue with anti-mouse antibody (monoclonal antibodies are of murine origin) which has an attached peroxidase enzyme, followed by another wash step and finally c) Bathing the tissue with an uncolored substrate; if the monoclonal antibody is bound in the first step, the substrate is digested by the peroxidase and a red-brown color develops that may be viewed by light microscopy; see Avidin-biotinylated complex, PAP, Sandwich method

Immunophilins Cytoplasmic receptor proteins that bind with high affinity to immunosuppressants, including cyclosporin A, FK 506 and rapamycin and inhibit rotamase activity, inhibiting the interconversion between the cis- and trans-rotamers of the peptidyl-prolylamide bond of peptide and protein substrates; immunosuppressants are thought to act by inhibiting the T cell receptor-mediated signal transduction pathway, preventing the activation of the nuclear factor of activated T cells; immunophilins thus far identified include cyclophilin and FK 506-binding protein (Science 1991; 251:283, Nature 1991; 351:248); see Cyclophilin, FKBP

Immunoradiometric assay see IRMA

Immunotherapy ALLERGY MEDICINE Hyposensitization therapy A treatment modality in which an allergen, eg hymenopteran venom, is administered in increasing doses to subjects with potentially fatal hypersensitivity reactions to the allergen; immunotherapy attempts to elicit production of blocking IgG antibodies, interfering with antigen-Fab (a portion of an immunoglobulin) combination, preventing fixation of IgE, l'enfant terrible of anaphylaxis, thereby attenuating or eliminating anaphylactic reactions; immunotherapy is of little use if the insect-sting reactions are confined to the skin (N Engl J Med 1990; 323:1601) ONCOLOGY A therapeutic modality that attempts to non-specifically stimulate the immune system to destroy malignant cells; immunotherapies with anecdotal success in treating malignancies include BCG immunotherapy which has had occasional success in treating melanomas, acute myeloblastic leukemia and solid tumors, Coley's toxin and heat-killed formalin-treated *Corynebacterium parvum*, an immunopotentiator and immunomodulator in animals that evokes reticuloendothelial hyperplasia, stimulation of macrophages and B cells and which may enhance T cell function by increasing its blastogenic response to T cell mitogens (concanavalin A, PHA and pokeweed mitogen) Note: BCG is of use in urology for controlling superfical transitional cell carcinomas by instillation in the bladder; see bCG, Coley's toxin, Malariotherapy

Immunotoxin One of the 'magic bullets' envisioned by Paul Ehrlich, which may be designed to be tumor-specific, where a monoclonal antibody or portion thereof is attached to various toxic molecules, including radioactive isotopes, chemotherapeutic agents, bacterial or plant toxins, produced with the hope that these 'bullets' will concentrate in the malignant tumor, destroying it; recombinant DNA techniques allow creation of highly specific hybrid molecules with therapeutic potential, although the immunotoxins thus far created in the laboratory have encountered in vivo difficulties, including accessibility of the immunotoxin to the tumor, instability of the cross-linking protein, rapid metabolism and development of anti-immunotoxin antibodies

Immunotyping Immunophenotyping HEMATOPATHOLOGY A method for qualifying cell surface or cytoplasmic antigens; the information derived allows determination of clonality and classification of B or T cell lineage; immunotyping of chronic lymphocytosis (145 cases,

Mayo Clin Proc 1988; 63:801) revealed that the majority are malignant and of B cell origin, lymphocytosis (121 B-CLL, 11 lymphosarcoma), T cell lymphocytosis (5 cases, 4 indolent), hairy cell leukemia (2), reactive lymphocytosis (6); see CD (cluster of differentiation)

Impaired health care provider A physician or health care worker whose ability to function in his usual role has been reduced or otherwise compromised by various internal and external forces Note: Although 'impairment' implies any physical or mental reduction in capacity to provide medical care, the term has acquired a distinctly unsavory connotation and in some circles, is a euphemism for substance (addictive drugs, alcohol) abuse or acute psychiatric decompensation, both of which potentially place patients at increased risk of poor judgement by the care-giver; Cf 'Handicapped' health care provider, 'Incapacitated' health care provider

Imperial Cancer Research Fund (ICRF) A London-based charity that is Europe's largest independent cancer research organization, which employs 1500 staff including researchers, physicians and technicians, funding one-third of all cancer research in the United Kingdom, often working in conjunction with the British Medical Research Council; the income is generated by charity shops, stocks, assets and legacies (estates); ICRF supports basic research (two-thirds of budget) and clinical research (one-third of budget); Cf Howard Hughes Medical Institute

Impingement syndrome A clinical complex caused by the limitation of a space between bones and fascia, compromising the flow of blood and irritating the nerves passing through the space; common impingement syndromes include the carpal tunnel syndrome which affects middle-aged women and that of the shoulders in which the space beneath the coraco-acromial arch for the supraspinatus and biceps tendons is reduced, resulting in a painful arc of movement and paresthesias, common in competitive swimmers Mechanism Ischemia or osteophyte rubbing the acromium

Implantation recurrence SURGICAL ONCOLOGY A rare phenomenon occurring at the site of a surgical resection for malignancy, where tumor cells, often of epithelial origin, 'spill' from an operative field or are carried by needles or stapling devices, 'seeding' malignancy into previously uninvolved sites; these lesions often appear anecdotally, as recently reported in a patient who had a laparoscopic cholecystectomy and, apparently, implantation seeding in the skin through which the gall bladder (subequently shown to have adenocarcinoma) was removed (N Engl J Med 1991; 325:1316c)

Import CELL PHYSIOLOGY *Noun* A product that has been transported into a cell *Verb* To transport a (required) substance into a cell

Impotence The inability to achieve or maintain a penile erection adequate for the successful completion of intercourse, terminating in ejaculation; for an erection to achieve a successful outcome, it requires a) An intact central nervous system, ie without underlying medical or psychological disease, or central-acting drugs, intact sympathetic and parasympathetic circuitry, ie without spinal trauma or degenerative disease b) An intact vascular supply to the penis and c) An intact, anatomically correct penis; 25% of impotence may be psychological or 'partner-specific', 25% has an organic component and 50% of impotence is organic in nature; in organic impotence, nocturnal penile tumescence is not present Treatment Microvascular surgery to bypass occluded vessels (most effective in younger men), penile prosthesis and combined therapy with phentolamine and papaverine (self injected by the patient, wielding an erection of one hour's duration Side effects Priapism, penile plaques or Peyronie's disease) Note: Drugs associated with impotence include antihypertensives, eg methyldopa, guanethidine, reserpine, clonidine, due to decreased blood pressure, antidepressants, eg phenelzine, isocarboxazide, amitriptyline, causing altered moods and decreased libido), tranquilizers, eg chlordiazepoxide and lorazepam and the muscle-relaxing diazepam, cimetidine, which increases prolactin levels, and is associated with impotence and loss of libido

Imprinting Genomic imprinting MOLECULAR BIOLOGY The variable phenotypic expression of a gene depending on whether it is of paternal or maternal origin, which is a function of the methylation pattern; imprinted regions are more methylated and less transcriptionally active; the 'imprints' are erased and generated in early embryonic development of mammals; imprinted genes include those for insulin-like growth factor-2 and its receptor, fragile X syndrome, Prader-Willi syndrome, Angelman syndrome and Wilms tumors (Science 1991; 252:1250n&v) PSYCHOLOGY Imprinting A form of learning restricted to certain critical or sensitive time periods of life, and which stops when definitive learning occurs or when a critical phase has passed; imprinting may occur before the organism is capable of an appropriate response, is irreversible and is characteristic of the species of organisms being imprinted

IMViC Reaction	I	M	V	C
Arizona	-	+	-	+
Edwardsiella	+	+	-	-
Enterobacter	-	-	+	+
Escherichia coli	+	+	-	-
Klebsiella	-	(+)	+	+
Proteus spp	-	+	-	(v)
Providentia spp	+	+	-	+
Salmonella	-	+	-	(+)
Shigella	(-)	+	-	-
Yersinia	(-)	+	(-)	-

IMViC reactions MICROBIOLOGY A mnemonic for the classic 'bench' tests (table), including indole produc-tion (I), methyl red production (M), Voges-Proskauer (V) and citrate utilization (C) that are used to differentiate among the major genuses of ***Enterobacteriaceae***

IN see Intraepi-thelial neoplasia

Inactivated vaccine see Killed vaccine

Inactive ingredient Additive, Excipient CLINICAL PHARMA-

COLOGY Any substance that is regarded by the US Food and Drug Administration as having no effect on a drug's absorption or metabolism, which is added for the manufacturer's expediency; these 'inert' ingredients are added to either a) Impart satisfactory processing and compression characteristics to the drug formulation, including binders, diluents, glidents or lubricants or b) Confer desirable physical characteristics to the finished product, including disintegrants, colorants, flavors and sweetening agents; Cf GRAS substances

INAD Investigational new animal drug A therapeutic modality with potential for use in food animals that is under an FDA protocol prior to being approved; see Bovine growth hormone; Cf IND

Inborn error of metabolism A term coined in 1908 by A Garrod based on his studies of alkaptonuria, in which he anticipated the one-gene, one-enzyme concept; inborn errors of metabolism are an ever-expanding group of inherited metabolic and biochemical disorders, numbering in the hundreds that may be loosely divided into those affecting a) Small molecules, including simple sugars, amino or organic acids that often have an acute onset in infancy and early childhood and b) Large molecules, most commonly increased in 'storage diseases', eg mucopolysaccharidoses and glycogen storage diseases that usually affect older children;

Inborn errors of metabolism (consequences)

Loss of certain molecules, eg albinism (defect of tyrosinase) or Ehlers-Danlos disease (defect of lysyl-hydroxylase) or others of a vast array of enzymes

Accumulation of normal metabolites, eg alkaptonuria (defect of homogentisic acid oxidase) or galactosemia (defect of Galactose-1-phosphate uridyl transferase)

Transport defects, eg cystinuria (dibasic amino acids) or intestinal disaccharidase deficiency

Defects in erythrocyte metabolism, eg glucose-6-phosphate dehydrogenase deficiency e) Pigment defects, eg acute intermittent porphyria

Defects in mineral metabolism, eg Wilson's disease

Vitamin defects, eg vitamin D-dependent rickets

Defects in intestinal absorption, eg cystic fibrosis

Other defects of unknown origin, eg achondroplasia

Inbreeding GENETICS A process in which littermates or siblings are mated to each other over multiple generations, resulting in a strain of animals that is virtually identical genotypically; highly inbred animal lines allow the study of certain traits in a relatively pure form; see Bottlenecks, Consanguinity; Cf Hybrid vigor

'Incapacitated' health care provider A physician or health care worker who is acutely impaired in his ability to provide care either for physical or mental reasons; Cf 'Handicapped' health care provider, 'Impaired' health care provider

Incarcerated hernia The herniation of a tissue, classically a loop of intestine, into a mesothelial sac, that cannot return to its original position without surgery; Cf Strangulated hernia

Incidence PUBLIC HEALTH The number of new cases of a disease that occur in a population divided by a unit of time, usually a year; Cf Prevalence

Incident HOSPITAL CARE ADMINISTRATION An event that represents a marked negative deviation from the 'standard of care' that occurs in a health care facility; if the incident is regarded as serious and has potential for harming a patient, an 'incident report' is generated and put in the responsible party's employment record for possible disciplinary action or dismissal; incidents include major substitution of medications or leaving a patient without attendance for a prolonged period of time; Cf Misadventure

'Incidentaloma' An incidentally-discovered tumor mass, detected by computed tomography, magnetic resonance imaging or other modality performed for an unrelated reason; the 'classic' incidentaloma is a sellar mass that may be accompanied by visual disturbances and altered pituitary hormone secretion; most subjects with incidentalomas remain asymptomatic, some may have a pituitary adenoma or chemodectoma (J Am Med Assoc 1990; 263:2772); see Pathologist's tumor; Cf Ulysses syndrome

Incident report see Incident

Inclusion body HISTOPATHOLOGY A generic term for any circumscribed mass of foreign (eg lead or viruses) or metabolically inactive materials (eg ceroid or Mallory bodies), within a cell's cytoplasm or nucleus

Inclusion body myositis A type of idiopathic myositis that is not autoimmune and does not respond to immunosuppressive therapy, which is a clinical diagnosis of exclusion, confirmed by characteristic histological features **Clinical** Slowly progressive disease of middle-aged males, beginning in the legs, causing atrophy and weakness of the quadriceps, while sparing the facial and oropharyngeal muscles **EMG** Abnormal electrical 'irritation', slowing of nerve conduction and increased wave amplitude **Histopathology** Rimmed vacuoles within fibers, occasional eosinophilic intranuclear and intracytoplasmic inclusions, scattered atrophic fibers, endomysial inflammation composed of cytotoxic T lymphocytes **Ultrastructure** Myelinoid inclusions and virus-like particles (N Engl J Med 1991; 325:1487rv)

Incretins A family of gastrointestinal hormones that are secreted in response to oral but not parenteral administration of nutrients (taking their signals directly from the gastrointestinal lumen) and accompanied by insulinotropic activity: gastrin-inhibiting polypeptide (GIP) is the most potent of the incretins; others include gastrin, peptide histidine methionine (PHM), YY peptide and neurotensin, each of which have lesser incretin activity (Mayo Clin Proc 1988; 63:794)

IND Investigational new drug CLINICAL PHARMACOLOGY A status assigned to a drug by the US Food and Drug Administration (FDA) prior to its study in humans; the first step in this long (up to ten years in duration) process of bringing a drug to the marketplace is sponsored submission of an **IND APPLICATION**, which allows only the 'sponsor' and investigators named in the application to study the drug; without a sponsor, clinical investigation cannot be carried out, since the FDA does not investigate new drugs (FDA Guidelines for IND, J Am Med Assoc 1988; 259:2267) **COMMERCIAL IND** status allows a drug's sponsor to collect data on its clinical safety and effectiveness, which is required for a New drug application (NDA), permitting a drug to be marketed for specific uses **NONCOMMERCIAL IND** status allows a sponsor to use a drug in research or in early clinical investigation; the **IND REWRITE** (1987) clearly delineated the phases of clinical trials for an IND and addressed the study's design prior to performing the clinical phases required for an NDA; see Phase 1, 2, 3 studies

Indeterminant syndrome see Overlap syndrome

Index medicus INFORMATION SCIENCE A database maintained by the US National Library of Medicine that is available in printed form on a monthly and annual basis; the Index catalogs the articles that appear in 3200 biomedical journals, over one-half of which are written in English; an expanded form of the Index Medicus can be retrieved electronically from the Medline database, allowing searches of the biomedical literature and relevant abstracts to its inception in 1966; see GRATEFUL MED, MEDLARS, MEDLINE

Index of suspicion A catch-phrase broadly used in various medical fields to indicate how seriously a particular nosology is being entertained as a diagnosis; as an example, there would be a high index of suspicion that rapid and unexplained weight loss in an elderly patient would be due to a carcinoma of the pancreas and a low index of suspicion that it would be due to AIDS

India ink cells Densely hyperchromatic, loosely cohesive cells seen in small (undifferentiated non-keratinizing) cell carcinoma of the lung; see Small ('oat') cell carcinoma

India ink spot nuclei Nuclei that have dark, homogeneous chromatin and a smooth contour, which may be seen in occasional cytological preparations of keratinizing epidermoid carcinoma from endobronchial washings; the nuclei may be surrounded by 'dirty' blue-gray or orange cytoplasm, the latter indicating the cells' partially consummated desire to produce keratin Note: Similar hyperchromatic nuclei may be seen in mesothelial cells as well in lentigo maligna (Hutchinson's melanotic freckle)

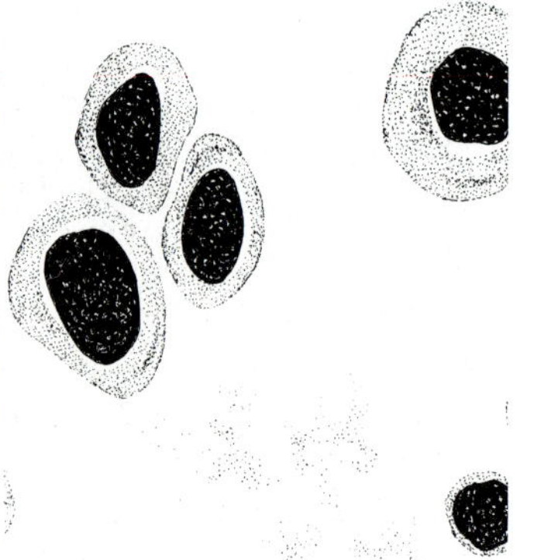

India ink nuclei

Indian childhood cirrhosis A fatal disease of early childhood onset with familial tendencies that was first described in the middle classes of rural India and occurs elsewhere in the tropics and subtropics **Clinical** Irritability, fever, anorexia, hepatomegaly, jaundice, fulminant cirrhosis, hepatic failure, coma and death **Laboratory** Hyperimmunoglobulinemia, increased serum and hepatic copper levels **Pathogenesis** Idiopathic, copper cookware has been incriminated **Histopathology** Massive hepatocyte degeneration, global inflammation, Mallory body formation, diffuse fibrosis and 'micro-micronodular' cirrhosis

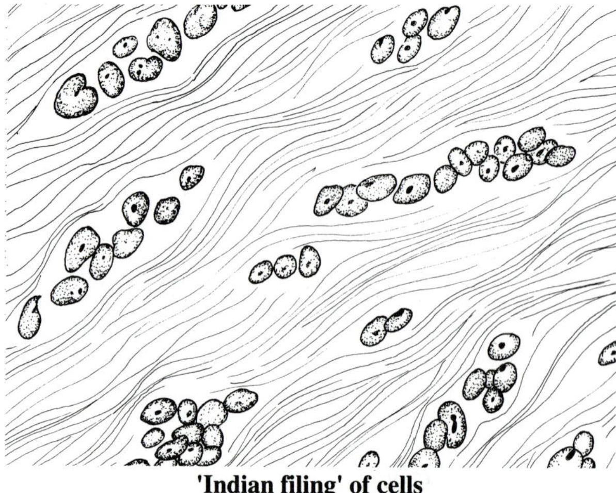

'Indian filing' of cells

Indian filing Indians in a file SURGICAL PATHOLOGY Single cell 'cords' that are compressed within a densely hyalinized or desmoplastic stroma, a finding typical of infiltrating lobular (21%) or ductal (36%) breast carcinomas (Cancer 1967; 20:363); single cell 'Indian file' arrangement may also occur without the dense stromal reaction in bronchoalveolar carcinoma, meningioma, medulloblastoma, Spiegler-Fendt's pseudolymphoma of the skin, well-differentiated lymphocytic leukemia of the skin, at the periphery of terminal duct carcinoma of the salivary gland and at the normal mantle zone of lymphocytes in lymph nodes

'India rubber man' A fanciful descriptor for the hyperlaxity of joints and hyperextensible, fragile and bruisable skin accompanied by cutaneous and vascular friability characteristic of patients with Ehlers-Danlos disease

Indirect Coombs' test see Coombs' test

Indirect costs Overhead costs ACADEMIA The monies required to construct and maintain buildings, including the costs for heating, water and electricity, as well as administrative costs and salaries, eg lawyers, bureaucrats, financial office personnel that are levered by a university against the budgets of investigators receiving government grant support; as an example, an indirect cost of 50% for a $100 000 grant requires that an extra $50 000 be included in the grant proposal (Science 1990; 248:293, ibid 1991; 252:636n&v); see Circular A-21; Cf Direct costs Note: Indirect costs are a normal financial consideration in preparation of hospital budgets and differ somewhat from the term as used by grant-giving bodies and grant recipients; in a health care facility, indirect costs include depreciation of equipment or the cost of construction or renovation; direct costs include overhead, employee salaries, disposibles, drugs, laboratory reagents and waste disposal

Indirect immunofluorescence IMMUNOLOGY A technique that is a modification of the indirect Coomb's (antiglobulin) test, in which the antigen reacts with a primary antibody; the primary complex then reacts with an antibody that has been labeled with a fluorescent tag; because the indirect method eliminates the need to purify and conjugate antibodies to a particular antigen, it is widely preferred to 'direct' methods; Cf Direct immunofluorescence

Indolent malignancy A lesion that is malignant by cytological, genetic, histopathological or other criteria, but which rarely displays the classic sine qua non criterion that defines a malignant lesion, which is metastasis; indolent malignancies include lymphomatoid papulosis and pagetoid reticulosis (Woringer-Kolopp disease)

Indolent myeloma A slowly progressive myeloma with an average survival of 10 years, which contrast to untreated multiple myeloma, 6 month survival and treated myeloma which has a 3 to 5 year survival; stable myeloma comprises 5% of multiple myelomas and is often detected by routine laboratory test for unrelated reasons; most patients have stage I disease and the mitotic activity, as measured by 3H-thymidine labelling index, is low at less than 0.8%

Indoor air pollutants CLINICAL TOXICOLOGY Any of a number of usually low-level toxins that may become relatively concentrated in the air of commercial or residential buildings; these pollutants include cigarette smoke, cooking and combustion products, eg natural gas, oil, wood and kerosene, volatilized chemicals, eg solvents, cleaning fluids, paint strippers including methylene chloride, asbestos in old buildings and formaldehyde in new furniture; see Passive smoking, Radon, Sick building syndrome

Induced fit model Sequential model BIOCHEMISTRY A model for the interaction of an allosteric enzyme with its substrate, proposed by Koshland, Nemethy and Filmer (KNF), which holds that an enzyme's active site undergoes a series of sequential changes in conformation that affect the rate of binding of substrate, positive and negative effectors; the 'KNF model' is a modification of Fisher's 'lock-and-key' hypothesis for enzyme action, where instead of a rigid site for the interaction between an enzyme and its substrate, both enzyme and substrate are distorted on binding and the substrate molecule is forced by the enzyme into a 'stressful' conformation that approximates the transition state; see Lock-and-key model

Induction Induction of remission ONCOLOGY The initial phase of a three-step therapeutic chemotherapeutic regimen used in treating acute leukemia; in acute lymphoblastic leukemia, prednisone and vincristine induce complete remission in 90% of children and 50% of adults, which may be increased up to 80% by the addition of a third drug, eg L-asparginase, daunorubicin or doxorubicin; in acute myelogenous leukemia, the dosage levels of chemotherapeutic agents are close to levels that are also toxic to the bone marrow, thus by extension, successful induction of remission may be a pyrrhic victory associated with aplastic anemia; cytosine arabinoside followed by an anthracycline (daunorubicin or doxorubicin) induces remission in 50-85% of patients under age 60 and 30-40% of those above age 60; see Consolidation chemotherapy, Maintenance chemotherapy

Induction chemotherapy Drug therapy given as a primary treatment for patients who present with an advanced cancer for which no alternative treatment exists; selection of agents is based on the effectiveness of the drugs in rodent models; combinations of agents are usually empirical and based on effectiveness, limiting toxicity and cross-resistance; induction chemotherapy is most successfully used in lymphoproliferative disease, where it comprises a component of standardized protocols, see above; induction chemotherapy with cisplatinum and 5-fluorouracil (5-FU) in combination with radiotherapy is of use in lymph node negative patients with advanced (stage III or IV) squamous cell carcinoma of the larynx, allowing preservation of the vocal cords, improving the quality of life, while reducing the co-morbidity associated with surgery (N Engl J Med 1991;

INFANTICIDE

'SOFT' CRITERIA (for determining if an infant's death was intentional)

Denial of pregnancy If the woman is obese or a dullard, she may not know she was pregnant

Rigor mortis A finding that is poorly appreciated in neonates

Impression of the body in soil, blood or fomites (ie bed clothing), requiring diligent and timely scene investigation

Maceration of skin A finding typical of stillbirth

Putrefaction Stillborns do not putrefy as they have sterile bowels

Umbilical cord A cut cord indicates active intervention-time undetermined; an intact cord is consistent with stillbirth

Determination of age Viability, most fetuses born before 18 weeks gestation die despite resuscitative efforts, age is determined by skeletal dating, antenatal studies corroborating fetal death, eg,Spaulding sign of *in utero* death characterized by overlapping cranial bones

'HARD' CRITERIA (for determining if an infant's death was intentional)

Comparison of the composition of gastric fluids with those of a toilet bowel Active drowning

Peural surfaces with petechiae Seen in induced suffocation, most significant when coupled with hematomas and petechiae on the mouth and epiglottis; the lingual frenulum may be torn and the lips bruised, indicating active attempts at suffocation

Lungs Stillbirth lungs are not aerated and do not float

Edematous foam on nostrils An indicator of active breathing

Meconium Resuscitation of a true stillborn may push meconium into the perianal region, but extensive staining of the placenta and umbilical cord is due to antenatal stress

324:1685); see Salvage treatment

Infanticide FORENSIC MEDICINE The active or semi-passive killing of a viable conceptus that is older than 20 gestational weeks and breathes spontaneously; in differentiating stillbirth from live birth and subsequent death, ie suspected infanticide, 'soft'and 'hard' criteria are examined (table, page 341); see Battered child syndrome, Child abuse

'Infectious mononucleosis syndrome(s)' A group of often viral agents that acutely induce a marked monocytosis in the peripheral blood and cause symptoms typical of classic Epstein-Barr virus-induced infectious mononucleosis, eg cytomegalovirus, herpes virus HHV-6, HIV-1 and Toxoplasma gondii

Infertility The involuntary inability to conceive, which contrasts to sterility, the total inability to reproduce; 10% of married couples in the US seek medical assistance because they are inconceivable; successful impregnation requires the production of an adequate number of normal motile spermatozoa that are ejaculated through patent ducts into an unobstructed reproductive tract of an accomodating female who contributes by ovulating at the appropriate time and releasing an ovum that the incoming sperm is capable of fertilizing, which then develops and implants in a well-prepared endometrium; one half of infertility is due to female factors, eg fallopian tube defects (20-30%), uterine and cervical pathology (10%), vaginal disease (< 5%), amenorrhea and anovulation (15%), nutritional and metabolic defects (5%), immunologic defects (< 5%) and ovulatory defects < 5%); 40% of infertility stems from male factors including decreased production of spermatozoa, abnormal sperm, ductal obstruction, ejaculatory defects (psychogenic or anatomic) or immunologic defects; 10% of cases are idiopathic

Inflammatory bowel disease (IBD) A generic term applied to several including Crohn's disease (CD), ulcerative colitis (UC) and idiopathic inflammatory bowel disease, the last of which is a diagnosis of exclusion that mimics and/or overlaps with CD and UC both clinically and pathologically **Heredity** First-degree relatives of those with CD and UC have an 8- to 10-fold increased risk of developing the same form of colitis; the risk of first-degree relatives of UC patients of developing CD or the risk of first-degree relatives of patients with CD of developing UC is 1.7 and 3.8 respectively (N Engl J Med 1991; 324:84; see ibid, 325:928rv, 325:1008rv); intestinal inflammation may also be induced by ischemia, irradiation, uremia, cytotoxic drugs, heavy metal intoxication; IBD patients often have two or more of the following: Visible abdominal distension, relief of pain upon defecation, looser and more frequent bowel movements when the pain occurs; male:female ratio is 2:1 and is more common among Jews; IBD is associated with mucocutaneous disease (pyoderma gangrenosa, erythema nodosum, oral ulcers, annular erythema, vascular thromboses, epidermolysis bullosa acquisita), ocular disease (uveitis, iridocyclitis), hepatopathy (chronic active hepatitis, cirrhosis, sclerosing cholangitis), arthropathy (ankylosing spondylitis); Cf Irritable bowel syndrome

Inflammatory bowel disease

	ULCERATIVE COLITIS	CROHN'S DISEASE
Clinical		
Rectal bleeding	Common	Rare
Abdominal mass	Rare	10-15%
Abdominal pain	Left-sided	Right-sided
Abnormal sigmoidoscopy	95%	< 50%
Perforation	12%	4%
Colon carcinoma	5-10%	Rare
Response to steroids	75%	25%
Surgical outcome	Excellent	Fair
Rectal involvement	> 95%	!0%
Radiology		
Ileal involvement	Rare	Usual
Cross-hatched ulcers	Rare	Occasional
Thumbprinting	Absent	Common
Fissuring	Absent	Common
Skip areas	Absent	Common
Strictures	Absent	Common
Pathology		
Distribution	Diffuse	Focal
	'Superficial'	Transmural
Mucosal atrophy	Regeneration	Marked Minimal
Hyperemia	Often marked	Minimal
Crypt abscess	Common	Rare
Cytoplasmic mucin	Decreased	Intact
Lymphoid aggregates	Rare	Common
Lymph nodes	Reactive hyperplasia	May have granulomas
Edema	Minimal	Marked
Granulomas	Absent	60%

Inflammatory carcinoma Erysipeloides A carcinoma characterized by invasion of the dermal lymphatics with malignant cells, most often of breast origin, less common in malignancies of the lung, gastrointestinal tract and uterus **Clinical** Diffuse swelling, erythema, pain and edema, simulating acute mastitis or cellulitis, and potentially delaying the diagnosis and therapy **Prognosis** Poor

Inflammatory fibroid polyp A benign presumed reactive gastric, usually antral 'tumor', associated with hypo- or achlorhydria **Histopathology** Polymorphic inflammatory cell population, predominantly eosinophils with submucosal edema **Differential diagnosis** Eosinophilic gastroenteritis

Inflammatory oncotaxis The attraction of malignant tumor cells to sites of tissue trauma, inflammation and capillary disruption, as seen after radiation and surgery; cutaneous metastases from colon, kidney and uterine cervix may settle on surgical incisions; Cf

Implantation recurrence

Inflammatory polyp 'Allergic polyp' A non-neoplastic, reactive, recurrent often bilateral 'tumor' that forms in response to infection, allergy and mucoviscidosis Histopathology Mucous glands covered by respiratory epithelium, a loose myxoid stroma, and when associated with allergy, a marked eosinophilic inflammatory infiltrate

Inflammatory pseudotumor A solitary, expansile but resectable tumor, composed of mature lymphocytes, which clinically and pathologically mimics malignancy, located in lungs, ocular orbit, abdominal cavity Etiology Trauma, surgery, local infection, myocardial infarct, aortic aneurysm, connective tissue disease Histopathology Edema, plasma cells, bizarre fibroblast-like cells and lipid-laden histiocytes; Cf Pseudo-lymphoma, Pseudosarcoma

Influenza A An avian virus, especially of ducks (which in China live in close proximity to the pig reservoir and 'vector'); periodic mutations of the virus (13 hemagglutination and 9 neuraminidase subtypes) are responsible for 'flu' epidemics and pandemics, the most memorable of which was the 1918 global pandemic which killed 20-30 million; each year, minor random mutations in the virus occur (genetic or antigenic drift); about every 20 years a major mutation occurs resulting in an alteration of the surface hemagglutinin (genetic or antigenic shift); Influenza type A (H3N2 immunotype) was the most prevalent cause in the 1989-90 season; see Antigenic drift, Antigenic shift

'Influenza syndrome' A clinical complex characterized by fever,headache, malaise, dizziness, ataxia, leukopenia, thrombocytopenia, muscular weakness, gastrointestinal symptoms (nausea, vomiting and diarrhea) and potentially renal failure, a potential side effect of intermittent therapy with rifampin Note: Influenza-like syndromes may occur with virtually any infection, especially of viral origin and are highly non-specific

'Informed' An adjective for an employer, co-worker or family member of a person with an infectious disease that is not spread by casual contact, who is (theoretically) completely at ease with the infected person in the workplace or in a social setting; 'informed' is a euphemism that first appeared in the AIDS epidemic for persons in contact with HIV-positive citizens, which contrasts to an 'uninformed' person, who responds in a hysterical and irrational fashion to the knowledge that a colleague or acquaintance is infected with the human immunodeficiency virus (Science 1991; 252:1798)

Informed consent A voluntarily-obtained and legally documented agreement by the patient to allow performance of a specific diagnostic or therapeutic procedure or procedures; the doctrine of informed consent has had enormous impact on the provision of health care in the US and has been cited as a major factor in erosion of the 'doctor-patient relation', which was formerly paternalistic in nature); a procedure performed without valid informed consent makes the physician liable for a lawsuit with a formal charge of assault and battery; for exceptions to the requisite for informed consent, see Emergency doctrine, Therapeutic privilege doctrine

INFORMED CONSENT

Requires patient understanding of:

- The nature of his illness/injury
- The nature and purpose of the treatment
- The risks and potential for death or injury during the procedure and the consequences of the proposed treatment
- The probability of success
- Other treatment options and their associated risks and benefits and
- The risks, benefits and prognosis when treatment does not occur

Note: Obtention of informed consent from minors (< 18 years of age) is potentially problematic as, under the US legal system, an 'emancipated' or 'mature' minor may give permission for a procedure, if he understands its nature and outcome, although it may be against the wishes of his parents, who could sue the physician for assault and battery; alternately, the parent may give permission to perform a procedure which the minor obviously understands and does not want, who could then sue the medical team for assault and battery; see Malpractice

Infusion pump A device designed to deliver various drugs and/or 'biologicals', at low doses and at a constant or controllable rate; increased rates of delivery in such devices may be associated with local hemolysis, compromising the potential benefits of a calibrated delivery system; Cf Pancreatic transplantation

Ingelfinger rule SCIENTIFIC JOUNALSIM A set of guidelines delineated by Franz J Ingelfinger, MD, the late editor of the New England Journal of Medicine, who felt that two criteria were imperative in accepting papers for publication in a scientific journal of high quality: 1) A news embargo on articles scheduled for appearance in the journal and 2) Strict application of the Ingelfinger rule: '*THE JOURNAL UNDERTAKES REVIEW WITH THE UNDERSTANDING THAT NEITHER THE SUBSTANCE OF THE ARTICLE NOR THE FIGURES OR TABLES HAVE BEEN PUBLISHED OR WILL BE SUBMITTED FOR PUBLICATION DURING THE PERIOD OF REVIEW. THIS RESTRICTION DOES NOT APPLY TO ABSTRACTS PUBLISHED IN CONNECTION WITH SCIENTIFIC MEETINGS OR TO NEWS REPORTS BASED ON PUBLIC PRESENTATIONS AT SUCH MEETINGS*'; the Ingelfinger Rule has become the standard of high-quality medical and scientific journalism (N Engl J Med 1991; 325:1371); see Authorship, Clinical alert, Vancouver group; Cf Embargo arrangement

'Inheritance powder' Arsenic A metal available in a powdered form that has enjoyed intermittent popularity as an unsuspected poison that induces slow mental deterioration and vague gastrointestinal symptoms in its victims, who may have been poisoned by next-of-kin eager to inherit (hence the macabre sobriquet) the victim's worldly possessions

Inhibin REPRODUCTIVE PHYSIOLOGY A heterodimeric peptide hormone released by the testicular Sertoli cells that inhibits FSH that is also produced by the ovarian granulosa cells in response to FSH; inhibin peaks at 800 U/L in the follicular phase of the menstrual cycle and forms a negative feedback loop that prevents the maturation of cohort follicles; inhibin is a tumor transforming factor with a reciprocal relation with activin (Cell 1988; 34:233) and may be increased in granulosa cell tumors; see Follistatin

Inhibitory transmitter NEUROPHYSIOLOGY A substance, eg GABA (γ-amino butyric acid), produced by one neuron that attenuates or inhibits the firing of another neuron

Iniencephaly sequence A primary neural tube malformation that occurs at the level of the thoracic and cervical vertebrae, which results in a 'sequence' of secondary features including retroflexion of the upper spine, shortened neck and trunk, cervical anomalies, defects of thoracic cage, anterior spina bifida, diaphragmatic defects, with or without hernia, hypoplasia of the lung and/or heart; see Sequence

INIT Initial device see Computers

Initial body see Reticulate body

Initiation MOLECULAR BIOLOGY The first step in the synthesis of a polypeptide chain, requiring the formation of a ribosome-mRNA-initiator tRNA complex ONCOLOGY The first 'hit' in a two- or multi-'hit' carcinogenic cascade, which theoretically is due to a short intense exposure of the DNA to a carcinogen, resulting in mutation; for a tumor to develop, subsequent steps are required, and the cell(s) must be acted on by a promoter; see Tumor promoter

Initiation codon see Start codon

Initiation complex see Initiation factor(s)

Initiation factor(s) A family of proteins that help the ribosome find an initiation site, which is necessary to induce protein synthesis, without which the 'initiation complex' of mRNA, Met-tRNA, GTP, and the small ribosomal subunits does not form

Initiative 119 A 'landmark' legislation proposed in the state of Washington, and voted upon in late 1991 (it did not pass), which would have allowed physicians to legally perform active euthanasia without criminal sanction, on a 'conscious and mentally competent, qualified patient'; under Initiative 119, a candidate for euthanasia would be terminally ill or have an irreversible condition that, in the opinion of two physicians would result in death within six months; under the proposal, the patient would be required to be fully conscious, mentally competent and voluntarily request the service in writing at the time of its being rendered (Am Med News 7/Jan/1991) Note: Although euthanasia is practiced in the Netherlands, it is technically illegal; see Dr Death, Euthanasia and 'Slippery slope'

Ink blot test see Rorschach test

'Inkwell' GASTROINTESTINAL SURGERY A surgically constructed vagination ('intussusception') of a short sleeve of esophagus sewn into the stomach, which as intragastric pressure increases, is compressed, forms a functional valve, for example, the Nissen fundoplication Note: Inkwells are reservoirs for ink pens, designed in such a way as to prevent the glass container from tipping on its side and were replaced by the self-contained (fountain) pen

Inlet patch An island of heterotopic but normal gastric mucosa occurring in 4-20% of normal subjects in the lower esophagus above the Z-line; since this finding (early embryonic esophagus having been lined by columnar epithelium with secondary ingrowth by squamous epithelium) may be confused with Barrett's esophagus, esophageal biopsies should be well above the Z-line; see Barrett's esophagus

Innocent bystander hemolysis A non-immune phenomenon caused by adsorption of carrier protein-bound drugs to the red cell surface; drugs causing innocent bystander hemolysis include sulfonamides, phenothiazines and quinidine, which act as haptens, eliciting drug-specific complement-fixing immune hemolysis of 'innocent' erythrocytes (activated by the alternate complement pathway); the direct antiglobulin test (Coomb's test) reveals only membrane-associated cleavage products, eg C3dg; the indirect antiglobulin test (indirect Coomb's test) is negative

Innocent murmur Any cardiac murmur that occurs in a normal person; these are divided into six systolic murmurs, eg vibratory systolic murmur (Still's murmur) and the mammary souffle and two diastolic murmurs, eg the venous hum; innocent murmers occur in all normal people at some time in their lives, most commonly occurring during mid-systole; the greatest danger in innocent murmurs lies in their mis-interpretation as representing serious cardiac pathology, resulting in recommendation of restriction of life-style, thereby becominga cardiac cripple

Inosine prabonex (IP) Isoprinosine AIDS A para-acetamidobenzoic salt of N,N-dimethylamino-2-propanolo:inosine in a 3:1 molar ratio that enhances various immune functions in vivo and in vitro (possibly increasing interleukin-1 and/or interleukin-2 production, resulting in T-cell proliferation and increased natural killer cell activity); in a trial of HIV-positive subjects, $<$ 0.5% of those treated with IP developed AIDS vs. 4% in the placebo group (N Engl J Med 1990; 322:1757, 322:1807ed)

Inositol 1,4,5-triphosphate (IP_3) MEMBRANE PHYSIOLOGY A major and ubiquitous intracellular second messenger involved in signal transduction, divided into two forms: chiro-inositol and myo-inositol that act in part by liberating calcium ions stored in cells; after an extracellular signal (hormone, neurotransmitter, inflammation, immune modulator) is received at the appropriate receptor and interacts with protein G, membrane phosphatidylinositol 4,5 biphosphate is targeted for signal-dependent hydrolysis, producing a) IP_3, which mediates calcium release in an all-or-nothing fashion (Science 1990; 250:977) from the cytoplasmic membrane and mitochondria and b) 1-2 Diacylglycerol (DAG), which activates protein kinase C, playing a key role in cell growth; IP_3 has high affinity binding sites and directly opens calcium channels in nanomolar concentrations, allowing amplification of signals by minute amounts of calcium Note: Non-insulin-dependent diabetes mellitus (NIDDM) has decreased excretion of chiro-inositol and decreased myo-inositol in the muscle, which may be related to insulin resistance (N Engl J Med 1990; 323:373); see 1,2-Diacylglycerol, Protein kinase C, Second messenger

Inoue balloon CARDIOLOGY A device for performing percutaneous mitral valve commisurotomy that is becoming the preferred modality for treating mitral valve stenosis, since it is non-invasive and allows resumption of full-time employment within 1 week in contrast to the 6-8 weeks of recuperation required after an open-heart surgical procedure (Mayo Clin Proc 1991; 66:276, 332); see Balloon valvoplasty, percutaneous; Cf Percutaneous transluminal coronary angioplasty

Insanity FORENSIC PSYCHIATRY A legal and social term for a condition that renders the affected person unfit to enjoy liberty of action because of the unreliability of his behavior with concomitant danger to himself and others, denoting, by extension, a degree of mental illness that negates an individual's legal responsibility or capacity Note: The term insanity is not sanctioned by the psychiatry community; the closest equivalent is 'psychosis'

Insanity defense FORENSIC PSYCHIATRY An argument advanced by the defense in a trial of law that seeks to explain the defendant's criminal actions with the claim that at the alleged time that the alleged act was alleged to have been perpetrated, the defendant was insane; the insanity plea is made in less than 1% of criminal trials in the US, rarely results in acquittal, and may be evoked as an act of desperation by the defense attorneys; after its successful use in the 1982 acquittal of the defendant in the assassination attempt on US President Reagan, the insanity defense has fallen into disfavor in the US legal system; Cf Television intoxication, 'Twinkie' defense

INSERM Institut National de la Santé et de la Recherche Medicale Founded in 1941 as the Institut Nationale d'Hygiene and renamed in 1964; INSERM has nine scientific commissions and is France's major medically-oriented research organization; INSERM laboratories may be free-standing, often closely proximous to affiliated hospitals; many INSERM projects overlap with CNRS, see there; Budget 1990: FF 1830 million employing 1900 researchers in 260 French research units; Cf NIH, Max Planck Institute(s), SERC

Insertin An actin-capping protein that allows the barbed end of actin to maintain an equilibrium with the monomer pool, with growth still being allowed

Inserting sequence BIOTECHNOLOGY A 500 base-pair segment of DNA that has an inverted repeat sequence at each plus end of the DNA; inserting sequences are used in molecular biology for manipulating DNA and under natural conditions, are responsible for antibiotic resistance transfer and thus act as information 'shuttles', but are themselves incapable of autonomous existence; see Transposons

Insertion The interposition of one or more nucleotides or base pairs in a chain of DNA or RNA, resulting in a 'frame shift' mutation

Insertion sequence A 'jumping gene', or extra piece of DNA which, when inserted in the middle of a gene, causes inactivation of that gene; insertion sequences have been identified in bacteria (six in *Escherichia coli*), the inserted molecule contains at one end, an inverted repeat (of the other end) of several hundred to a few thousand nucleotides; ISs have no known raison d'etre and have thus been called selfish genes; Cf Transposons

***in situ* hybridization** A method for detecting the presence of a sequence of DNA, mRNA or proteins; cells or tissues are heat- or acid-fixed on a glass slide, denatured with 70% formamide, bathed in a hybridization solution containing a label, eg 2-acetyl-aminofluorene-tagged, biotinylated or radiolabelled DNA or RNA that is complementary to the mRNA in the tissue; if present, the complementary strands hybridize in the cells or tissue, linking to their complementary strand, which may then be detected by autoradiography, then counterstained with a standard histological stain to delineate cellular, tissue or other architectural landmarks

***in situ* transcription** MOLECULAR BIOLOGY A technique for reverse transcription in fixed tissue where the mRNA serves as a template for the complementary DNA (cDNA, Science 1988; 240:1661)

Insomnia The inability, either perceived or actual, to sleep for the accustomed amount of time Note: 2-3% of the population either takes hypnotics or seeks consultation for sleeping disorders **CHRONOLOGIC CLASSIFICATION** a) TRANSIENT INSOMNIA, eg 'jet lag', which does not require treatment b) SHORT TERM INSOMNIA, of less than three weeks in duration, related to travel to high altitudes, grieving the loss of a loved one, hospitalization, pain c) LONG TERM INSOMNIA, of more than three weeks in duration, eg related to medical, neurologic or psychiatric disorders or addiction **ETIOLOGIC CLASSIFICATION** a) PHARMACOLOGIC INSOMNIA, due to ingestion of coffee, nicotine, alcohol b) REBOUND (WITHDRAWAL) *INSOMNIA*, related to abrupt discontinuation of hypnotic drugs c) DELAYED SLEEP PHASE INSOMNIA, due to shift work, chronic pain, sleep apnea and restless leg syndrome; see Circadian rhythm, Jet lag, REM sleep, Sleep disorders

$InsP_3$ see Inositol 1,4,5-triphosphate

Inspissated milk syndrome Intestinal obstruction in infants fed either powdered or concentrated milk Radiology Dense, amorphous intraluminal masses surrounded by halos of gas Treatment Hydration, increasing the water in milk products

Institute of Medicine A Washington, DC-based organization founded in 1970 under the auspices of the US National Academy of Science that identifies, studies and reports on the (US) nation's major problems in medicine and the health sciences and recognizes outstanding achievements in the field of medicine

'Institutional effect' A colloquial term for bias(es) in therapeutic decisions, diagnoses or interpretation of data that are related to guidelines or 'cut-off' values for laboratory parameters promulgated within a health care facility or hospital (J Am Med Assoc 1991; 265:97); see Referral bias

Institutionalization 'syndrome' SOCIAL MEDICINE The constellation of psychological changes that occurs in individuals who have been maintained in segregated communities, eg mental institutions, state-run nursing homes **Clinical** Apathy, dependence, depersonalization and retreat from reality Note: This complex is similar, if not identical, to 'shelterization', described in homeless persons; see Homeless(ness), Shelterization

Institutional review board (IRB) BIOMEDICAL ETHICS A committee in a university hospital or academic health care facility that is specifically charged with ensuring the safety and well-being of human subjects involved in research projects at the institution; the existence of an IRB is required by US Federal regulations operating under the Department of Health and Human Services; research proposals require that a) The risks to individuals are minimized b) The risks are reasonable in relation to the anticipated benefits c) The selection of individuals is equitable d) Informed consent is obtained and documented from the subject or his legal representative e) There are provisions for maintaining the individual's privacy and f) There are safeguards that prevent undue influence on vulnerable subjects by nature of educational or economic disadvantage or by dint of severe illness; see Ethics committee, Helsinki Declaration, Nuremburg code

Insulin A disulfide-linked polypeptide hormone produced by the pancreatic islet β cells that stimulates the expression of genes encoding glyceraldehyde-3-phosphate dehydrogenase, c-Fos, glucokinase and α-amylase and inhibits expression of phosphoenolpyruvate carboxykinase, see PEPCK Mechanism of action Unknown; it appears to act via serine protein kinases, eg insulin receptor serine kinase, acetyl CoA carboxylase kinase, microtubule associated protein-2 (MAP-2) kinase, protein kinase C, Raf-1, myelin basic protein kinase; insulin activates type 1 protein phosphatases that control glycogen metabolism, by phosphorylating (or dephosphorylating) specific serine residues (Nature 1990; 348:302)

Insulin-like growth factor-I see IGF-I

Insulin-like growth factor-II see IGF-II

Insulin pump An implantable device that delivers insulin at low levels at a regulated rate, designed as an artificial 'pancreas' to provide optimal delivery of insulin; two early devices, the external pump with continuous peritoneal infusion of insulin and the closed loop insulin infusion delivery systems have not proven useful; variable-rate open-loop devices are in clinical trials and although the MiniMed (Sylmar, Cal) pump, used in the PIMS study was reported to achieve reasonable control of glucose levels (J Am Med Assoc 1989; 262:3195), a wait-and-see policy prevails; Cf Biohybrid artificial pancreas, Islet cell transplantation

Insulin receptor A heterodimeric membrane receptor composed of α and β chains that has tyrosine kinase activity after binding insulin; receptor deficiency is an uncommon cause of diabetes mellitus and may be due to a gene rearrangement, causing a deletion in the tyrosine kinase domain (Science 1989; 245:63), a point mutation with a loss of the ATP binding site (ibid; 245:66) or other genetic defect

Insulin-regulatable glucose transporter (IRGT) A protein expressed in muscle and fat that migrates from the cytoplasm to plasma membrane in response to insulin, resulting in increased intracellular transport of glucose

Insulin resistance (IR)

Type A 'Pre-receptor' phase IR, related to defects in synthesis and secretion of insulin, seen in the HAIR-IN syndrome, with hyperandrogenism (to a degree suggesting hyperthecosis, ovarian neoplasia or polycystic ovaries), which is of pubertal onset, with high levels of endogenous insulin, overt diabetes mellitus and resistance to exogenous insulin, related to anti-insulin antibodies

Type B 'Receptor' phase IR, related to decreased insulin binding to receptors, number of receptors, or marked insulin resistance, which may be associated with acanthosis nigricans, autoimmune disease and overt diabetes mellitus due to circulating anti-receptor antibodies

Type C 'Post-receptor' phase IR, related to defects arising after the insulin-receptor complex has formed, eg a defect in the insulin action cascade

Insulin resistance A condition characterized by suboptimal response to physiological levels of insulin that may be due to increased circulating glucagon or a relative insulin receptor deficiency, where plasma insulin is high relative to glucose; in uremia, insulin resistance may be due to non-specific receptor antagonism, as the insulin binds poorly to receptors and hypocalcemia increased secretion of proinsulin (table); defects in glycogen synthesis are pivotal in the insulin-resistance of non-insulin-dependent diabetes mellitus (NIDDM), as muscle glycogen synthesis is the main pathway of glucose disposal in normal and diabetic subjects (N Engl J Med 1990; 322:223); see Subcutaneous insulin-resistance syndrome; Cf Syndrome X

Insulin shock A rarely observed clinical event in which excess insulin is administered, causing profound hypoglycemia to levels below that required for normal brain function, causing anxiety, delirium, convulsions, coma and death

Insult CLINICAL MEDICINE A generic term for any stressful stimulus, which under normal circumstances does not affect the host organism, but which may result in morbidity when it occurs in a background of preexisting compromising conditions; the term most commonly refers to an acute hypoxic episode in a patient with underlying atherosclerosis, who may suffer such 'insults' as a transient ischemic attack of the brain (a 'stroke'), angina or an acute myocardial infarction

***int*-1** A recently reclassified proto-oncogene, see *wnt*-1

Integral (membrane) proteins Any transmembrane protein that is so intimately linked to a biological membrane that it cannot be removed without disruption of the phospholipid bilayer membrane itself, eg the Rh antigens of red cells

Integrase A bacteriophage enzyme that creates and resolves Holliday junctions, which are present in a form of genetic recombination

Integrated circuit see Computer, Chip

Integrins 'RGD superfamily' A family of more than 15 cell surface adhesion receptors composed of heterodimeric (α and β subunits) membrane-spanning glycoproteins that recognize the tripeptide, arginine-glycine-aspartic acid (occasionally serine), known as the RGD sequence on the β subunit, which acts as a receptor recognition signal; integrins mediate cell binding to major components of the extracellular matrix; integrins are subdivided based on differences in the β subunit, which confers specificity, acting as receptors for collagens, fibronectin, fibrinogen, platelet glycoprotein IIb-IIIa, laminin, LFA-1, Mac-1, osteospondin, p150,95, thrombospondin, VLA1-6 (very late antigens 1 to 6), vitronectin and von Willebrand factor; this group and their receptors, constitute a recognition system critical in cell anchorage, traction for migration, signals for polarity, position, differentiation, growth, phagocytosis, platelet aggregation and complement binding; the receptors are intracellular and anchored to cytoplasmic proteins (actin, talin, ankyrin, vincullin, fibroconnexin) Note: Absence of the β subunit (LFA-1, and Mac-1) results in Leukocyte adhesion deficiency syndrome; the β1 subfamily (VLA proteins) mediates cell binding to collagen (VLA-1, -2, -3), fibronectin (VLA-3, -4 and -5) and laminin (VLA-1, -2, -6) (Science 1991; 251:1600); Cf RGD family

Integrin family of leukocyte adhesive proteins see CD11/CD18 family

Intelligent terminal see 'Smart' terminal

Intercalation The interposition of a flat molecule between two adjacent nucleotides in the DNA double helix, eg ethidium bromide, which generates positive superhelical turns in closed circular DNA molecules, or acridine orange, which results in frameshift mutations; see Acridine Orange, Ethidium bromide

'Interesting' disease A generic term for any clinical or pathologic nosology that is rare, difficult to diagnose, challenging to treat, poorly understood pathogenically or any combination of the above; it has been observed that when a condition is characterized by pathologists as 'interesting', it often implies a poor prognosis

Interface A boundary, eg between two phases, as in a solid-liquid interface in chemistry or between two electronic devices as in a computer interface

Interference Cross-over effect GENETICS The effect that the crossing over of a chromosome at one locus has on the frequency of cross-over at another locus, termed positive interference if the frequency is decreased and negative interference if the frequency is increased

Interferons (IFN) A family of at least 15 immune-regulatory proteins produced by T-cells, fibroblasts and other cells in response to double-stranded DNA, viruses, mitogens, antigens or lectins; interferons are designated as α-, β- or γ-interferons and act as immunomodulators, increasing the bactericidal, viricidal and tumoricidal activities of macrophages (J Am Med Assoc 1991; 266:1375rv); IFN-α and IFN-β have alternately been termed type I interferons as both are growth inhibitory cytokines whose biological activities depend on induced changes in gene expression; see MAF and MIF

Interferon(s)-alpha (IFN-α) A family of leukocyte-derived immunomodulating glycoproteins, numbering 13 at last count, which have antiproliferative and antiviral activity, the gene for which is located on the short arm of chromosome 9 and the receptor on the long arm of chromosome 21 Therapeutic indications Recombinant IFN-α has been used to treat hairy cell and chronic myeloid leukemias, Kaposi sarcoma, human papillomavirus-related epithelial proliferations, eg condyloma acuminatum, respiratory papillomatosis and pulmonary hemangioendotheliosis (N Engl J Med 1989; 320:1197); IFN-α induces prolonged clinical and histologic remission in one-third of patients with chronic hepatitis (N Engl J Med 1990; 323:295), and may be used to treat renal cell carcinoma, either alone or in combination with vinblastine, yielding a 21% response rate and the osteoclastic lesions may regress (N Engl J Med 1991; 324:633c) Side effects Flu-like symptoms, malaise, fatigue, headache, anxiety, vertigo and depression, increased aminotransferase, bone marrow suppression, supraventricular tachyarrhythmia with hypotension or hypertension and potentially fatal congestive heart failure, exacerbation of multiple sclerosis (J Am Med Assoc 1989; 261:2065); one-half of cases, especially those with cirrhosis and hypersplenism don't tolerate therapy as it causes fatigue, profound thrombocytopenia and neutropenia (Mayo Clin Proc 1990; 65:1330)

Interferon-beta (IFN-β) A 20-kD protein with anti-viral activity that has 30% 'homology' with interferon-α, is encoded on chromosome 9 and produced by fibroblasts in response to viruses or polyribonucleotides

Interferon-gamma (IFN-γ) A 21-25 kD glycoprotein lymphokine encoded on chromosome 12q, consisting of a heterodimeric protein with six α helices in each chain (Science 1991; 252:698) that is produced by activated T and natural killer (NK) cells; IFN-γ is antiviral, regulating the expression of class II MHC antigens, Fc receptors and immunoglobulin production and class switching, activates monocyte cytotoxicity and enhances NK cell activity; IFN-γ is decreased in IgA deficiency, lymphoma, chronic lymphocytic leukemia, infections, eg Epstein-Barr and cytomegalovirus, rubella, lepromatous leprosy and tuberculosis, lupus erythematosus, rheumatoid arthritis, sickle cell anemia, post-transplantation Therapeutic indications Recombinant IFN-γ is used to treat giant condylomata acuminata, chronic lymphocytic leukemia, Hodgkin's disease, mycosis fungoides, rheumatoid arthritis and may be of use in treating leprosy, tuberculosis, toxoplasmosis and chronic granulomatous disease (to prevent infections); IFN-γ suppresses collagen synthesis by fibroblasts, reduces the size of keloids, causing a local increase in inflammatory cells and mucin production, and may be of use in controlling abnormal fibrosing conditions (Arch Dermatol 1990; 126:1295) Side effects Acute renal failure (N Engl J Med 1988; 319:1397), rash, headache, chills; IFN-γ receptor is encoded on chromosome 6q

Interferon-stimulated response element A *cis*-acting DNA element encoded by genes transcribed when interferon-α interacts with its membrane receptor, a signal thought to be mediated through arachidonic acid metabolism (Science 1991; 251:204)

'Interim' methadone treatment A form of administration of methadone for heroin addicts, in which the drug is provided with minimal service to the ex-addict; this became necessary given the lack of funds and manpower combined with the finding that effective methadone-maintenance is associated with a reduced incidence of HIV infection

Interleukin(s) (IL) A family of cytokines produced by lymphocytes, monocytes and other cells that induce growth and differentiation of lymphoid cells and primitive hematopoietic stem cells; see Biological response modifiers, Tumor necrosis factor

IL-1 Leukocyte-activating factor An 11 kD cytokine produced by monocytes, B, natural killer, endothelial, epithelial, microglial, mesangial and antigen-presenting cells, fibroblasts and large granular lymphocytes, as well as by malignancies, eg acute myeloid leukemias (FAB M3, FAB M4), squamous cell carcinoma, Hodgkin's disease and melanoma; IL-1 elicits the acute phase response, acts on the central nervous system as a pyrogen, stimulates fibroblast, B cell and T cell proliferation and differentiation and increases lymphokine, collagenase and prostaglandin production; IL-1 enhances the activity of natural killer cells against tumor targets, stimulates myocytolysis (via prostaglandins), elicits hormone release from the pituitary gland (including ACTH, LH, GH and TSH release and prolactin inhibition, via corticotropin releasing factor), evokes the release of neutrophils from the bone marrow, and neutrophil degranulation, increases oxidase activity and hexose monophosphate shunt activity; in synovial cells, IL-1 stimulates proliferation and production of collagen, prostaglandin and plasminogen activator; IL-1 production is stimulated by various agents, eg calcium ionophores, IFN-α, IFN-γ, lipopolysaccharides, muramyl dipeptide, aluminum hydroxide,phorbol myristate acetate, staphylococci, silica and others and inhibited by corticosteroids, prostaglandin E_2 (acting via the cyclooxygenase pathway), suppressor T cells, cyclosporin (which specifically inhibits T cell-induced IL-1 production) IL-1 and disease IL-1 may have a role in a) Insulin-dependent diabetes mellitus (IDDM, increased IL-1 production by macrophages occurs in the early β-cell destructive lesions of IDDM) b) Atherosclerosis (n-3 fish oils reduce circulating IL-1) and c) Rheumatoid arthritis, where IL-1 acts in conjunction with substance P **IL-1 receptor** IL-1 mediates its action on target cells by high-affinity receptors on fibroblast and T cell membranes; receptor expression may be increased by prostaglandins and glucocorticoids; it binds both IL-1α and IL-1β and has 319 extracellular amino acid residues with 3 immunoglobulin-like domains, a transmembrane region and a 217 residue cytoplasmic 'tail'; other interleukin receptors (IL-2 β chain, IL-3, IL-4, IL-6 and erythropoietin) share a common structural motif (Science 1990; 247:324)

IL-2 T cell growth factor A 15 kD glycoprotein that is produced at low baseline levels by the CD4 T (helper) cells; after presentation of antigen by antigen-presenting cells, accompanied by IL-1, T cell production of IL-2 and IL-2 receptor (IL-2Rβ) on the membrane increases, peaks at 6 hours and falls to baseline levels; IL-2 is also produced by medullary thymocytes and a subset of large granular lymphocytes, the NK cell activators; IL-2 up-regulates the immune system, causing lymphokine-activated killer (LAK) cells to lyse tumor cells, see IL-2/LAK cells **Side effects** IL-2 requires weeks of intensive care due to toxic effects, including a 'capillary leakage syndrome', malaise, gastritis, gastrointestinal symptoms, anemia, thrombocytopenia, rigors, fever, hypotension, azotemia, jaundice, hyperbilirubinemia, rash (erythroderma globalis), confusion, ascites, fluid retention, pruritus, agitation, respiratory insufficiency, cardiac failure and irreversible demyelinization (N Engl J Med 1990; 323:1146c) and hypothyroidism Note: Cytotoxic T lymphocytes (CTLs), when incubated with certain MHC Class II molecules, eg HLA-DR may down-regulate their lytic activity; IL-2 causes antigen-activated B cells to progress through the cell cycle and differentiate into antibody secreting cells, actions carried out by a receptor and a transduction 'complex'; see IL-2/LAK cells **IL-2 receptor** A heterodimer of 75 kD β and 55 kD α (also known as CD25, or Tac antigen) proteins that is transiently expressed on T cells, induced by IL-2, tumor necrosis factor, IL-1, IL-4 and IL-6; IL-2 receptor enhances lymphokine production and transmits protein kinase-C activation; IL-2 receptor is increased up to six-fold normal in Kawasaki's disease, a condition causing mucocutaneous erythema, fever and cardiac damage; the critical signal for IL-2R activity is phosphoryation of the IL-2Rβ chain by the *src*-family protein tyrosine kinase $p56^{lck}$, the activity of which is initiated by IL-2 stimulation of T cells (Science 1991; 252:1523)

IL-2/LAK cells Interleukin-2/Lymphokine-activated killer cells Natural killer (NK) cells that have been activated by co-incubating in interleukin-2 and injected into cancer patients in a therapeutic modality known as adoptive immunotherapy, which may evoke temporary tumor regression in non-Hodgkin's lymphoma, melanoma, colorectal carcinoma and renal cell carcinoma, as well as cause regression of hepatic and pulmonary metastases; IL-2/LAK cells are in experimental protocol for treating advanced renal cell carcinoma (partial remission 15%, complete remission 4%) and malignant melanoma **Complication** The typical transient defect in neutrophil chemotaxis may explain the high morbidity typical of IL-2/LAK therapy (N Engl J Med 1990; 322:959, Science 1990; 250:20n&v) **Adverse effects** Pulmonary edema, congestive heart failure

IL-3 Multi-CSF, Hematopoietin, P-cell stimulating factor, Burst-forming unit A lymphokine produced by activated CD4 T (helper) cells and others that bind to high- and low-affinity receptors, inducing tyrosine phosphorylation, promoting colony formation of multiple (erythroid, megakaryocytic, myeloid and lymphoid) hematopoietic lineages, mast cell proliferation and histamine release; IL-3 induces 20-α-hydroxysteroid dehydrogenase, assisting T cell maturation; the IL-3 gene is on the long arm of chromosome 5 **IL-3 receptor(s)** see Blood 1991; 77:989

IL-4 B-cell growth factor A 20 kD cytokine produced by T helper cells and mast cells that is co-mitogenic for B cells and thymocytes, activates macrophages and stimulates hematopoiesis; IL-4 competes with IL-2 at its receptor in the transduction pathway, possibly altering the signal of whether a lymphocyte will mature to synthesize pentameric IgM or monomeric IgG1 or IgE (Science 1989; 243:781)

IL-5 Eosinophil differentiating factor An 18 kD cytokine produced by CD4+ T lymphocytes that co-stimulates B cell proliferation and differentiation and IgA class switching; IL-3 and IL-5 may function in concert to potentiate production of eosinophils (Science 1989; 245:308) via eosinophil-CSF

IL-6 IFN-β-2 A 26 kD cytokine mediating host response to injury and infection that plays a role in growth and differentiation of B cells, T cells, myeloma-plasmacytomas, hepatocytes, hematopoietic stem cells and nerve cells; the presence of IL-6 in psoriatic plaques, suggests a pathogenic role in that condition (Proc Natl Acad Sci 1989; 86:6367) **IL-6 receptor** A membrane receptor that measures 468 amino acid residues and is homologous to an immunoglobulin domain (constant 2) Note: IL-6, nerve growth factor and growth hormone have no tyrosine kinase domains, and thus process extracellular signals by a less well understood mechanism

IL-7 A predominantly T cell growth factor that is produced by the stromal cells of the bone marrow, acting as a lymphopoietic factor, converting stem cells into early pre-T, as well as B cells and which is active in primitive lymphocytic leukemias **IL-7 receptor** see Cell 1990; 60:941

IL-8 Neutrophil activating protein-1 A 72 residue protein produced by most cells that targets T cells, as well as neutrophils, up-regulating the binding activity of leukocyte adhesion receptor CD11b/CD18; IL-8 also dynamically regulates its own receptor (CR1) expression on neutrophils (J Biol Chem 1990; 265:183); IL-8 is antiviral, antiproliferative and immunomodulatory, inhibiting neutrophil adhesion to cytokine-activated endothelial cells, preventing neutrophil-mediated damage (Science 1989; 246:1601)

IL-9 Murine growth factor P40, T cell growth factor III A hematopoietic growth factor glycoprotein isolated from a megakaryoblastic leukemia, expressed in several human T cell lines and in mitogen-stimulated peripheral lymphocytes that is structurally and functionally related to mast cell growth-enhancing activity (Eur J Immunol 1990; 20:1413), the gene for which maps to both chromosome 5 and 13 **IL-9 receptor** see J Immunol 1990; 145:2494

IL-10 Cytokine synthesis inhibitory factor A protein produced by TH1 helper T cells that inhibits the synthesis of interferon γ by other activated helper T cells and stimulates mast cell precursors (J Exp Med 1991; 173:507); in mice, IL-10 is produced by B cell lymphomas and normal B cells; first identified in mice, the predicted IL-10 structure has extensive homology with an open reading frame (BCRFI) in the Epstein-Barr virus genome and with the EBV virus protein BCRF1 (Science 1990; 250:830)

IL-11 A lymphopoietic and hematopoietic cytokine derived from tissue stroma (Proc Nat Acad Sci (USA) 1991; 88:765)

Interlocking OBSTETRICS A rare (estimated to occur in 1 in 817 twin gestations) complication of vaginal delivery of twins, where the first twin presents in breech and descends 'locking' his head above the head of the second twin; if the second baby is already in the pelvis, loss of the first baby is almost inevitable and interventional decapitation of the first infant may be necessary to salvage the second infant, an event that virtually never occurs as the vast majority of twin gestations are delivered by cesarian section prior to the spontaneous onset of labor Note: there are rare cases of salvage of both twins by either epidural anesthesia and cesarian section or use of β-sympathomimetic drugs (Br J Obstet Gynaecol 1981; 88:76); Cf Selective termination

Intermediate body The final stage of the development of *Chlamydia trachomatis* infection, comprised of reticulate bodies that have molded themselves in a perinuclear fashion and become septated; see Elementary bodies

Intermediate care facility An institution providing the minimal health care and services required for mental or physically handicapped individuals; Cf Hospice, Nursing home, Shelter, Tertiary care center

Intermediate cells Primitive cells described in neonatal and infant intestines, in and adjacent to colonic inflammation and seen in adult small intestinal neoplasia, which stain positively for Paneth cell granules within goblet cells

Intermediate density lipoprotein see IDL

Intermediate filaments A diverse group of abundant, cell lineage-specific intracellular filaments that are seen by electron microscopy, which measure 7-11 nm in diameter, a size intermediate between the 6 nm actin microfilaments and the 25 nm microtubules; intermediate filaments have considerable (40-70%) sequence similarity ('homology') with each other and differ according to embryologic origin, which can be determined by the cells with monoclonal antibodies raised against each filament; epithelial cells produce 40-68 kD cytokeratin intermediate filaments (IF), muscle cells produce 53 kD desmin IF, mesenchymal cells produce 55 kD vimentin IF, glial cells produce 55 kD glial fibrillary acidic (astrocytic) protein IF and neurons produce 68-100 kD neurofilament Note: Primitive cells may be negative for all IFs or may express more than one IF, as malignant cells dedifferentiate and 'forget' their cell lineage; such co-expression of IFs is not uncommon in sarcomas, which may co-express vimentin and desmin, eg mesothelioma, synovial and epithelioid sarcomas; malignant tumors, eg renal cell, ovarian, lung, endometrial, anaplastic, thyroid carcinomas, as well as benign tumors, eg pleomorphic adenomas may co-express vimentin and cytokeratin

Intermediate-grade lymphoma A group of lymphomas of intermediate aggression that are classified according to the Working Formulation (Cancer 1982; 49:2112), which have survival periods between the indolent low-grade lymphomas (survival 5 to 7.5 years) and the aggressive high-grade lymphomas (survival less than one year); intermediate lymphomas include the follicular predominantly large cell lymphoma, diffuse small cleaved lymphoma, diffuse mixed large and small cell lymphoma with epithelioid cells (Lennert lymphoma) and diffuse large cell cleaved and non-cleaved cell lymphoma; see Lymphoma, Working Formulation

Intermediate syndrome CLINICAL TOXICOLOGY A clinical complex due to organophosphorus insecticide poisoning, so-called as it is neither acute, which is associated with neurotoxic symptoms nor delayed, ie occurring 2-3 weeks after exposure, which is associated with chronic distal motor polyneuropathy; since the symptoms occur in a 'window period', they are thus relatively unexpected **Clinical** 10% of those exposed develop paralysis of the cranial motor nerves, proximal limb, cervical flexor and respiratory muscles; onset, 1-4 days after a cholinergic phase **Prognosis** Less than 5%, possibly due to a neuromuscular junction defect (N Engl J Med 1987; 316:761)

Intern A term essentially equivalent in context to 'apprentice', used in North America for a graduate of a medical, osteopathic or dental school who is serving his first year (an 'internship') of graduate clinical training, usually in a teaching hospital; following internship, the physician may then enter private practice (a route chosen by few physicians in 1991) or enter a period of post-graduate education, ie residency training Note: The term has been widely used in other fields and may refer to virtually any period of training that follows the closure of a period of formal education; see GME; Cf CME, Extern, Fellowship, Internist

Internal standard INSTRUMENTATION A standardized, stable and constant substance added to a chromatographic (gas chromatography or high-performance liquid chromatography) sample that neither interferes with nor has a molecule 'signature' overlapping that of the molecular species being analyzed, serving as a positive 'control'; see Blanks, Control, Quality control

Internal version OBSTETRICS A procedure that attempts to convert a difficult fetal presentation to a vaginally deliverable situation, hand-rotating the fetus while in utero; in the US, given the high potential for litigation should an internal version 'go sour' and compromise the fetus, most obstetricians prefer to perform an elective cesarian section rather than risk a potentially complicated delivery

International medical graduate see Foreign medical graduate

International Red Cross and Red Crescent Movement see Red Cross

International unit Any arbitrarily defined and internationally-sanctioned unit of measurement for a naturally-occurring substance, eg hormone, enzyme or vitamin; see SI (Systeme International)

International Workshop classification, chronic lymphocytic leukemia (CLL) A clinical staging system that blends features of the Rai and Binet classification of CLL STAGE A No anemia or thrombocytopenia and less than three involved lymphoid regions STAGE B patients No anemia or thrombocytopenia and more than three involved lymphoid regions and STAGE C Anemia and/or thrombocytopenia, regardless of the amount of involved lymphoid tissue

INTERNIST see Expert systems

Internist A practitioner of general medicine who is certified by the American Board of Internal Medicine (ABIM) and who has had three years of training in internal medicine; in the US, board eligibility or certification by the ABIM is an implied prerequisite for further training in the form of one or more years of fellowship for various specialties of internal medicine, eg gastroenterology, hematology/oncology, infectious diseases; Cf Family practitioner, Intern

Intersex syndromes A group of clinical complexes that occur in subjects with ambiguous genitalia Note: Testis-determining factor (TDF) is present by the sixth embryologic week and stimulates wolffian duct (male) development; without TDF, the embryo 'defaults' to müllerian duct (female) differentiation despite genotypic maleness; intersex syndromes include **TRUE HERMAPHRODITISM** Gonads contain both ovarian and testicular tissue, genotypically either 46, XX or 46, XY; 75% are raised as boys; the testicular tissue is dysgenic, doesn't produce sperm and may undergo malignant degeneration (requiring prophylactic removal); ovarian function in those raised as girls may be adequate to produce term pregnancy **MALE PSEUDOHERMAPHRODITISM** Testicles are present and cryptorchid, but testosterone production is inadequate (due to decreased LH or hCG receptors on the Leydig cells); patients are raised as females (Morris syndrome) and may have defects of the central nervous system, eg defective gonadotropin response, primary gonadal defects, eg idiopathic, defective pregnanediol (3-β 17-α, 17,20 des and 17 β) synthesis, regression of müllerian tubes, Leydig cell agenesis, androgen insensitivity, increased susceptibility to breast cancer, Sertoli adenoma, germinoma in situ, seminoma, Leydig cell tumor **FEMALE PSEUDOHERMAPHRODITISM** Ovaries are present, but the infant is masculinized by in utero androgen exposure during fetal development (maternal ingestion or the result of congenital adrenal hyperplasia with virilization) **GONADAL DYSGENESIS** Underdeveloped or imperfectly formed gonads; the prototypic gonadal dysgenesis is Turner syndrome 45, X0, seen in 1/2-7000 female births **Clinical** Short stature, webbed neck, cubitus valgus, micrognathia with high arched palate, epicanthal folds, lymphedema of the hands and feet, aortic coarctation, renal malformation, osteoporosis, diabetes, widely-spaced nipples, sexual infantilism **Histopathology** Ovaries are small and thin ('streak' ovaries); a variant, mixed gonadal dysgenesis is characterized by a mosaic phenotype 45,X/46,XY, and a streak ovary on one side and a testis or germ cell tumor on the other side, accompanied by intense virilization

Interstitial lung disease (ILD) A generic term for an increase in the volume of pulmonary interstitial tissue, conceptually divided into **A) Distortion ILD** A reversible condition in which the alveolar walls are distended by inflammatory cells without damaging normal structures or the cells lining the alveolar spaces, seen in sarcoidosis and early hypersensitivity pneumonitis and **B) Fibrosis ILD** A condition that is either idiopathic or induced by inorganic dusts, eg silica, asbestos, diatomaceous earths, coal dust, metals and rare earths, with fibroblast proliferation in the alveolar walls and deposition of connective tissue; the normally flattened type I pneumocytes are partially replaced by type II pneumocytes; FILD is often progressive and ultimately fatal

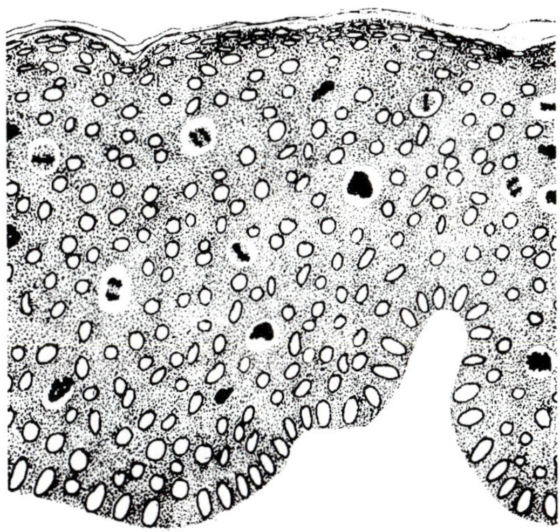

Intraepithelial neoplasm

Interventional radiology A subspecialty of general radiology that provides either a) Diagnostic information, eg computed tomography-guided 'skinny' needle biopsies and dye injection for analysis of various lumina and tracts, eg arteriography, cholangiography, antegrade pyelography and b) Therapeutic options, eg percutaneous nephrostomy or biliary drainage (N Engl J Med 1990; 322:1364)

Intestinal 'angina' Chronic intermittent occlusion of intestinal arteries, analogous to angina pectoris, causing sporadic claudication of the vascular supply to the intestine; ingestion of food results in angina as digestion increases the blood flow through the gut, which is supplied by the celiac axis, superior and inferior mesenteric arteries; postprandial abdominal pain implies major atherosclerotic narrowing of more than one vessel given the rich anastomoses among these vessels

Intestinal knot syndrome Compound volvulus A clinical condition characterized by torsion of the terminal ileum around the sigmoid colon, which itself is rotated on its own axis Clinical Intense abdominal pain, distention-type ileus with rapid progression Radiology Barium studies demonstrate dilated small intestine, right-sided distended sigmoid

'Intracellular immunization' A coinage of recent vintage to describe a potential use of a dominant negative mutant viral gene to interfere with the replication of wild-type virus; the most attractive potential application of this concept would be to protect cells against HIV-1, since the target, CD4-bearing peripheral cells is easily accessible; that goal has been achieved with ***gag, tat*** and ***rev*** mutant genes (Nature 1990; 345:573n&v) and with a CD4 mutant containing the KDEL sequence (see there), allowing its retention within the endoplasmic reticulum preventing transport of HIV envelope proteins to the cell surface (Nature 1990; 345:625)

Intracellular pathogens Microorganisms that are adept at eluding the host's immune system, residing most often with histiocytes, in particular, ***Mycobacterium tuberculosum, M lepra, Listeria monocytogenes, Salmonella typhi, Trypanosoma cruzi, Toxoplasma gondii*** and ***Chlamydia*** species

Intraepithelial neoplasia An in situ carcinoma (figure, left) that is confined to an epithelium that may superficially penetrate adnexal glands, measuring less than either 3 mm or 5 mm depending on the criteria used; intraepithelial neoplasia (IN) is adjectivally modified according to the site of origin (table, below); see CIN

INTRAEPITHELIAL NEOPLASIA

AIN	Anal intraepithelial neoplasia
CIN	Cervical intraepithelial neoplasia
OIN	Oral intraepithelial neoplasia
PAIN	Perianal intraepithelial neoplasia
PIN	Penile intraepithelial neoplasia
VAIN	Vaginal intraepithelial neoplasia
VIN	Vulvar intraepithelial neoplasia

Intramural esophageal diverticulosis Pseudodiverticulosis A complex characterized by multiple small diverticuli lined by squamous epithelium present in the superior esophagus or occupying its entire length; apparently arising from the mucous gland ducts; Cf Inlet patches

Intraoperative autologous transfusion (IAT) Transfusion medicine Intraoperative blood salvage A procedure in which the blood shed or otherwise lost into a surgical operative field is collected under sterile conditions, filtered and reinfused as a packed unit of red cells; IAT may be used in 'bloody' procedures, including cardiovascular surgery, eg for aortic aneurysms or coronary artery bypasses or orthopedic surgery, eg hip arthrodesis, reducing a patient's exposure to multiple donors and may be used in conjunction with pre-deposit autologous donation, in which packed red cell units are collected from the patient before surgery; Cf Autologous transfusion

Intraperitoneal loose bodies Peritoneal 'mice' Asymptomatic often indurated intraperitoneal structures in the peritoneal cavity formed by torsion or infarction, detached appendices epiploicae or small detached uterine leiomyomas; Cf Joint mice

Intratubular germ cell neoplasm An in situ carcinoma affecting up to 80% of the residual seminiferous tubules in testicles with germ cell tumors; 1% of infertile men have IGCN and many evolve to invasion within five years **Diagnosis** Biopsy of contralateral testis, clinical follow-up and serial serum levels of α-fetoprotein, human chorionic gonadotropin and human placental lactogen

Intravenous immune globulin (IVIG) A formulation of immune globulins, predominantly IgG, prepared by pooling plasma from approximately 1000 donors, which has a broad spectrum of activity against cytomegalic inclusion virus, hepatitis A and B, measles, rubella, tetanus and varicella zoster; IVIG is not regarded as appropriate therapy for replacing plasma proteins in adults with AIDS (as the defect is predominantly cellular) or with chronic lymphocytic leukemia, in whom its use costs an estimated $6 million for every year gained of quality adjusted life (N Engl J Med 1991; 325:81); IVIG is indicated in low-birth weight children with repeated infections or in children with major defects in the humoral immune system, eg AIDS, X-linked agammaglobulinemia, common variable immunodeficiency syndrome(s) (ibid, 1991; 325:110rv, 123ed); in children with AIDS and low CD4+ T cells, IVIG increases the duration of bacteria-free periods (ibid, 1991; 325:73); IVIG is also of use in idiopathic thrombocytopenic purpura, autoimmune phenomena (hemolysis, neutropenia and thrombocytopenia), Kawasaki's disease and pediatric AIDS **Side effects** Pyrogenic, hypersensitivity and anaphylactic reactions and minor systemic reactions, including headache, myalgia, fever, vasomotor disease and cardiovascular abnormalities, lability of blood pressure and tachycardia (J Am Med Assoc 1990; 264:3189); Cf Human immune globulin

Intravesicular therapy ONCOLOGY The irrigation of urinary bladder with topical agents, eg thiotepa, mitomycin C and BCG, to halt the progression of superficial transitional cell carcinoma; the most widely studied agent is thiotepa; it has little effect on normal bladder epithelium, but destroys established cancers, inhibits tumor reimplantation and retards the development of new lesions; patients receive 30-60 mg/30 to 60 ml intravesically, once weekly for four weeks, thereafter once monthly; 30% achieve complete and 30% achieve partial remission; other agents include adriamycin, epodyl and 5-FU

Intrinsic factor (IF) A 45 kD low-affinity vitamin B_{12}-binding glycoprotein secreted by the gastric parietal cell, which closely parallels the secretion of HCl; IF secretion is stimulated by histamine, gastrin and methionine, and usually greatly exceeds that required for B_{12} absorption; IF is re-absorbed by specific receptors in the ileum (the absence of which causes Imerslund syndrome, an autosomal recessive, familial vitamin B_{12}-IF complex malabsorption syndrome); the high-affinity B_{12} binder, R protein, attaches to vitamin B_{12} in the acidic environment of the stomach, later releasing B_{12} to IF after cleavage by pancreatic enzymes; IF is decreased in patients with low gastric acid production or by agents which reduce gastric acid secretion by blocking parietal cell receptors, eg H_2-blockers, but is unaffected by agents that block H^+/K^+-ATPase-induced gastric acid secretion; see H_2-blockers

Intrinsic factor antibodies A family of antibodies directed against either the binding site (known as type I or 'blocking' antibodies) or any other epitope site (type II antibodies) on intrinsic factor, which are present in 75% of patients with pernicious anemia

Intrinsic pathway An arm of the coagulation cascade, initiated by negatively charged surfaces (contact factors eg sulfatide micelles, kaolin) which bind factor XII and high molecular weight kininogen (HMWK); HMWK binds prekallikrein and factor XI activating the latter; XIa then activates IX which in turn activates factor X, initiating the common pathway of coagulation: see Common pathway, Extrinsic pathway

Intron MOLECULAR BIOLOGY An 'intervening sequence' or segment of mRNA that is spliced out and not part of the primary transcript from which mRNA reads the DNA-derived message, the exon that is ultimately transcribed to become a protein; because introns do not serve a known function, they are considered less interesting biologically, to the point of being considered to have derived from 'junk DNA'; introns have been free to evolve without selective pressure, but are nevertheless felt to have an as yet unknown function as the intron-exon junction is at least 1.7 X 10^9 years old Note: Introns themselves are capable of generating split genes, which encode proteins (Science 1989; 246:1106); Cf Exon

Inulin A plant-derived homopolysaccharide of D-fructose used to measure renal clearance

inv IMMUNOLOGY A group of allotype antigenic sites in the constant region of the kappa light chain of an immunoglobulin

Invariant chain An intracellular protein that associates with a class II major histocompatibility complex (MHC) in the endoplasmic reticulum, preventing the binding of endogenous peptides to the class II molecule, shepherding it to the relevant intracellular compartments; truncation of the invariant chain generates a second targeting signal that may be operative in the trans-Golgi network, preceding the transport of class II molecules to the cell surface (Nature 1990; 348:600)

Invasion The penetration of a basement membrane by a neoplastic process usually, but not invariably implies a malignancy with metastatic potential; an exception to this rule is the identification of 'foreign' tissues within lymph nodes, eg clusters of melanocytes or thyroid tissue, see Lymph node inclusions or in the perineurium with breast glands, as may occur in sclerosing adenosis; see Metastasis

Inverted comma sign A radiologic finding seen by a plain chest film in a not uncommon (1/200 subjects) variation of the azygous lobe, which is invested with its own pleural membrane in the medial aspect of the right upper lobe

Inverted mushroom and stem sign GASTROINTESTINAL RADIOLOGY A cap-like radiopacity surrounded by a 'coiled spring'-like appearance, seen by barium enema in intestinal intussusception

Inverted papilloma SURGICAL PATHOLOGY A proliferation characterized by a thin investment of epithelium overlying papillary fronds of epithelium; inverted papillomas may occur in either transitional epithelium (renal pelvis, ureters, bladder and urethra) or in stratified cuboidal epithelium (paranasal region, 3/4 of patients had concomitant HPV infection, types 6b and 11 and lesions of the upper respiratory tract); inverted papillomas tend to recur in the nasopharynx, but not in the urinary tract; the bladder papillomas have been subdivided histologically into glandular and trabecular patterns, a distinction of no clinical utility

Inverted repeat see Palindrome

Inverted '3' sign of Frostberg RADIOLOGY An acquired deformity of the duodenum and adjacent ampulla of Vater with fixation of the pancreatic and common bile ducts at the ampulla of Vater and associated edema of the medial duodenal wall; first described as characteristic of carcinoma of the head of the pancreas, it occurs in only 10% of these patients and may be seen in acute pancreatitis or duodenal ulcers Note: The adjective 'reversed' is more semantically correct

Inverted 'U' sign RADIOLOGY A massively dilated (possibly extending to the diaphragm), redundant loop of sigmoid colon that twists on its mesenteric axis and may be seen in a volvulus of the sigmoid colon; see Hot air balloon sign

Inverted umbrella sign of Fleischner A gaping ileocecal valve with immediately proximal stenosis, simulating an umbrella turned inside-out by a gust of wind, seen in barium contrast studies; this sign was first described in tuberculous ileitis, but may also be seen in Crohn's disease

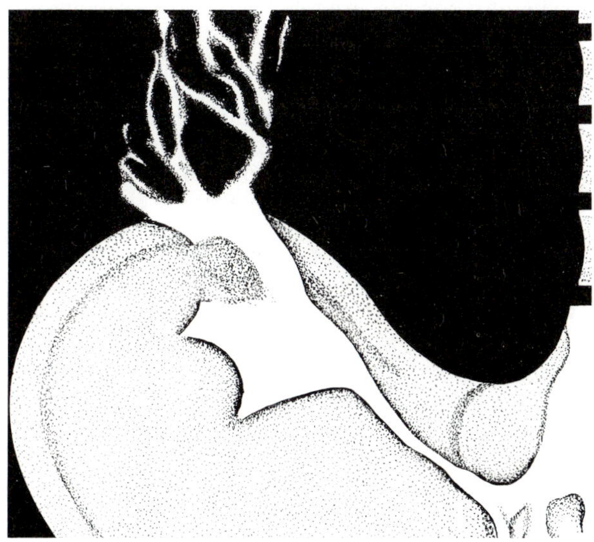

Inverted umbrella sign

Inverted 'V' sign RADIOLOGY Lateral umbilical ligaments made prominent by gas percolated on either side of the ligaments, characteristic in a plain supine film of pneumoperitoneum, when the patients are too sick for erect studies; see also Double wall sign

Inverted 'Y' field NUCLEAR MEDICINE A large radiotherapy field for treating contiguous lymph nodes involved in Hodgkin's disease or other lymphomas, which covers the para-aortic, splenic hilar, iliac, inguinal and femoral lymph nodes Note: Less than 3600 cGy (rads) is a prophylactic dose, used when lymphoid tissue is not involved by tumor, 3600-4400 cGy constitutes a tumoricidal dose; see Abdominal bath, Mantle port

Investigational new drug see IND

'Invisible' profession Nursing (J Am Med Assoc 1990; 264:2851)

***in vitro* fertilization** (IVF) A form of artificial fertilization in which an inseminated egg in early embryogenesis is implanted into the uterus; the success rate (in experienced centers) is 20-25% overall (7.7% success when cryopreserved pre-embryos are used and 24% when fresh embryos are used, N Engl J Med 1990; 323:1153); IVF bypasses certain causes of infertility Ethics and human IVF The experimental use of human embryos created by IVF has engendered heated debate, resulting in a ban on its use in federally-funded research in the US; in the United Kingdom, Parliament allows regulated research on human embryos up to 14 days post-conception Legal issues, IVF When gametes are joined in vitro and frozen for future transfer into a mother, 'product' ownership is unclear and may be decided in a court of law, should the couple then get divorced after creation of the pre-embryos, the couple got divorced (J Am Med Assoc 1990; 263:2484) Note: An estimated 20 000 babies have been born by various forms of IVF since its first implementation; see Artificial reproduction, Surrogate motherhood, Test tube baby

Involuntary smoking see Passive smoking

'Iodine mumps' Bilateral swelling of the parotid glands that may accompany administration of organic or inorganic iodine, eg triiodothyronine for treating hypothyroidism

IOM see Institute of Medicine

Ion channels PHYSIOLOGY A large heterogeneous family of voltage-activated proteins that control the permeability of cells to specific ions (Na^+, K^+, Ca^{++}, Cl^-) by opening or closing in response to differences in potentials across the plasma membrane, an action which in sodium, potassium and calcium channels appears to be controlled by the S4 sequence of polypeptides; ion channels participate in the generation and transmission of electrical activity in the nervous system and in the hormonal regulation of cellular physiology; all are composed of four or five homologous domains or subunits, each of which contains numerous membrane-spanning α-helices; the polar faces of the α-helices from neighboring subunits aggregate to form a pore or alternately, are less polar and composed of serine, threonine and cysteine residues; ion channel control of intracellular concentrations of ions, eg calcium, in turn controls such diverse cell functions as secretion and cell division (Mayo Clin Proc 1990; 65:1127); ion channels are embedded in the cell membrane and are either a) Ligand-gated, eg nicotinic acetylcholine receptor, GABA receptor and glycine receptors all of which mediate local increase in ion conductance at chemical synapses, thereby either depolarizing or hyperpolarizing the (pre)synaptic region or b) Voltage-sensitive ion channels which mediate rapid changes in ion permeability during action potentials in excitable cells and modulate membrane potentials and ion permeability in inexcitable cells; see Ball-and-chain model, Na^+/H^+ antiporter, Na^+/K^+ ATPase, Potassium channel, Voltage-dependent anion-selective channel, Voltage-dependent calcium channel

Ionization chamber A sealed, usually cylindrical chamber for measuring the electric currents produced when a gas is bombarded by ionizing radiation (electrons, protons and X-rays); such chambers comprise the detection unit in a Geiger-Müller counter

IP Interstitial pneumonia; see Interstitial lung disease

IP_3 see Inositol 1,4,5-Triphosphate

IPA Independent practice association; see IPO

IPCC Intergovernmental Panel on Climate Control ENVIRONMENT A formal forum of scientists from different countries that are currently assembling data on the potential effect of greenhouse gases (Nature 1991; 350:219); see CFCs, Greenhouse effect, Montreal protocol

IPO Independent practice organization A legally defined entity in the US, in which physicians and/or dentists enter an arrangement to provide services through an entity, eg a prepaid health plan, while at the same time maintaining their own private practices; see HMO, PPO

IPPNW International Physicians for the Prevention of Nuclear War An organization that won the 1985 Nobel Prize for Peace; Cf Amnesty international, Red Cross, Medicine sans Frontieres

IPPV Intermittent positive pressure ventilation see PEEP

IPSID Immunoproliferative small intestinal disease Mediterranean lymphoma α heavy chain disease A heterogeneous group of conditions characterized by monoclonal increases in production of immunoglobulin (usually α) heavy chain, without accompanying light chains, ie 'truncated' immunoglobulins; all or part of the variable region is lost as well as one (usually C_H1) or two constant domains; the mRNA is very short and has mutations, deletions or insertions; IPSID is usually a 'secretory' or α chain proliferation, but may also be a γ or mu chain (N Engl J Med 1989; 320:1534) Clinical Malabsorption, diarrhea, weight loss, abdominal pain, due to marked expansion of the proximal small intestine and mesenteric lymphoid tissue, clubbing of fingers and toes Treatment Without antibiotic therapy, eg tetracycline, IPSID may evolve to malignant lymphoma (B cell immunoblastic sarcoma)

IRAP Interleukin-1 receptor antagonist protein A natural inhibitor of IL-1 bioactivity on T lymphocytes and endothelial cells (Nature 1990; 344:633)

IRB see Institutional review board

IRGT see Insulin-regulatable glucose transporter

Irish's node Left anterior axillary lymph node, which is a site of predilection for involvement by metastatic gastric carcinoma; see Sentinel node, Sister Mary Joseph node

Iris lesion Target lesion, Bull's-eye lesion DERMATOLOGY An erythematous annular macular or papular lesion that develops an inner red-purple ring, papule or macule, a finding characteristic of erythema multiforme

Iris pearls A fanciful term for the multiple whitish, opalescent, miliary lepromata seen in the optic fundus in ocular leprosy

IRMA Immunoradiometric assay LABORATORY MEDICINE A quantitative 'sandwich' assay using radioiodinated label to measure certain plasma proteins; IRMA differs from RIA in that the antibody in the detector system is radioactive and not the competing hormone derived from the patient; see Hook effect

Iron hypothesis ENVIRONMENT A proposal that CO_2, the primary major gas responsible for the greenhouse effect could be markedly reduced by stimulating the growth of algae in the Antarctic with iron (fancifully termed the 'Geritol fix' after a proprietary iron supplement, Science 1991; 253:1490), the limiting nutrient for algal growth; according to the initial estimate (Paleoceanography 1990; 5:1), the reduction would be 150 ppm of CO_2; another model (Nature 1991; 349:228, 198) estimates a mere 30 ppm reduction after 100 years of successful iron 'fertilization' and potentially nefarious side effects of algal overgrowth; 1990 CO_2 level: 345 ppm; 2100 (estimated) CO_2 level: 1200 ppm

Iron lung A tank ventilator that encases a patient up to his neck, enabling artificial respiration by intermittent applied negative pressure around his body, externally expanding the thoracic cavity Note: IPPV has a similar effect internally with positive internal pressure; see Mechanical ventilation, PEEP

Iron-responsive element see CAGUGX

Iron stores Hematology The amount of bone marrow iron is a crude indicator of a disease state and is graded on a scale of 0 (no discernable iron) to 4+ (ponderous clumps of hemosiderin); a marked decrease or absence of marrow iron occurs in chronic disease, hemorrhage, decreased iron intake, hypochromic anemia and polycythemia vera; a marked increase in marrow iron may be due to conditions affecting erythrocyte production, eg β-thalassemia, hemolytic anemia and sideroblastic anemia, the liver, eg hemochromatosis, alcoholic cirrhosis, viral hepatitis, and other diseases, eg porphyria cutanea tarda, Gaucher's disease Note: The decalcification step that is required in the preparation of bone marrow for light microscopy dissolves some of this iron

Irritable bowel syndrome IBS, Spastic colon An intestinal dysmotility complex, thought to be related to psychophysiologic stress with maladaptive reinforcement of autonomic visceral responses Clinical Most often seen in anxious 20-40 year-old females with colicky abdominal pain and altered bowel habits Pathophysiology Altered secretory patterns, increased sensitivity to cholinergic agents, hyperalgesia with intestinal distension and increased secretion of prostaglandin E_2 (altered bowel habits, increased transit time, decreased slow wave activity of the intestinal smooth muscle, increased segmenting contractions, delaying gastrocolic response) Histopathology Although there are no consistent findings, edema, varying degrees of inflammation, hyperemia and subepithelial collagen deposits may be seen Treatment None consistently effective; attempted modalities include high-fiber diet, laxatives (with caution), psychotherapy, emotional support, biofeedback, sedatives, tranquilizers and antidepressants, and anticholinergics to relieve pain; Cf Inflammatory bowel disease, 'Unhappy gut'

IS see Insertion sequence

Iscador see Unproven methods of cancer treatment

Ischemic colitis A condition characterized by transient and recurring colicky abdominal pain accompanied by nausea, tenesmus, fever and bloody diarrhea, resulting from atherosclerosis of the mesenteric arteries supplying the intestine, that most intensely affects the descending colon

ISCOM CLINICAL PHARMACOLOGY A lipid bilayer that has a rosette conformation, which has been manipulated to integrate proteins; ISCOMs have potential as drug delivery vehicles or as 'vectors' for viral products in vaccinations

Islet cell transplantation A technique that as of 1991 has had limited success in treating diabetes mellitus; successful transplantation requires 1) An adequate number (800 000+) of functioning islets from at least two cadaveric donors, verified by purification, culturing and assays for insulin production and 2) Adequate immune suppression, the most successful agent is FK 506 **Method** Islet cells are injected into the portal vein and the liver acts as the 'host organ'; Cf Biohybrid artificial pancreas, Insulin pump, Pancreatic transplantation

Isoelectric focusing (IEF) LABORATORY MEDICINE A technique that separates amphoteric compounds, eg proteins, by charge along a stable pH gradient, allowing them to migrate to an isoelectric point where their overall charge is zero or neutral; IEF is used to detect abnormal hemoglobins, myoglobin and glycohemoglobin and to separate amylase isoenzymes; Cf Two-dimensional gel electrophoresis

Isolation INFECTIOUS DISEASE The segregation or 'quarantining' of a patient, his body fluids or fomites to prevent transmission of an infection to other patients or hospital personnel; various terms are used by the CDC for the levels of required: Blood/body fluid isolation or precautions (Creutzfeldt-Jakob disease, hepatitis B, HIV); see Biosafety levels, Disinfection, 1Precautions, Sterilization; Cf Reverse 'precautions'

Isomorphic phenomenon of Köbner Induction of skin changes at site 'B', following minimal non-specific trauma (heat or light), when identical lesions are already present elsewhere at site A; the isomorphic phenomenon is characteristic of psoriasis and may be seen in lichen planus, active eczema and in verruca; Cf Id reaction

Isoprenoids Terpenes A large and diverse group of lipids, eg steroids and bile acids, lipid-soluble vitamins, coenzyme Q and others that derive from five-carbon isoprene units and which may help anchor proteins to cell membranes (Science 1990; 247:318, 320)

Isoretinoin A proprietary agent that has been used to treat severe recalcitrant acne; isotetinoin is considered a category X drug (ie teratogenic, and not to be used in pregnant women), as it has ben associated with cardiovascular defects (ventricular septal, aortic arch and conotruncal defects), external ear deformity, cleft palate, micrognathia and central nervous system malformations; see Vitamin A analogs

Isosbestic points LABORATORY MEDICINE The wavelength at which the spectral curve for two substances,eg barbiturates, intersects or has the same absorption

Isospora belli PARASITOLOGY An enteropathogenic sporozoite parasite of unkown prevalence that is more common in the tropics and subtropics of the Western Hemisphere and in Southeast Asia; ***I belli*** infection is probably underreported, as in uncompromised hosts, it mimics viral gastroenteritis, although when associated with AIDS may cause fulminant disease **Clinical** Watery diarrhea with variable hemorrhage, colicky pain, weight loss, steatorrhea and eosinophilia **Histopathology** Mucosal atrophy, attenuated villi, crypt hypertrophy and inflammation of the lamina propria **Treatment** Trimethoprim-sulfamethoxazole

Isothiocyanate see FITC, Spicy food

Isotope A nuclide of an element, which has the same number of protons and atomic number, while differs in the number of neutrons and the atomic mass; isotopes of medical importance include Positron emitters

Isotype IMMUNOLOGY A numerical subtype of an immunoglobulin that is present in all normal individuals, regardless of race, which are differentiated based on the size and number of domains and the number of intra- and interchain disulfide bonds in the constant region; IgG has four isotypes: IgG1, IgG2, IgG3 and IgG4; IgA has two isotypes: IgA1 and IgA2; the remaining heavy chains as well as light chains have only one isotype; Cf Allotype, which differs according to the gene pool and Idiotype, which differs according to epitope

ISS Injury severity score EMERGENCY MEDICINE A group of indices that are used to 'triage' severely injured patients, calculated as the sum of the squares of the highest abbreviational injury scores in each of the 3 most severely injured body parts, resulting in scores from 1-75, which correlate well with length of hospitalization, time to death, disability and need for surgery (J Trauma 1974; 14:187); an ISS of greater than 20 implies a poor prognosis; Cf Trauma score

Itai-itai byo Japanese, 'Ouch-ouch' disease CLINICAL TOXICOLOGY A form of renal osteodystrophy with marked bone pain, described in multiparous Japanese women due to accumulation of cadmium in bone, related to eating fish contaminated by industrial pollutants **Pathogenesis** Its occurrence in multiparous women suggests that the iron, calcium and other divalent cations lost in multiple pregnancies may be replaced by cadmium

ITP Idiopathic thrombocytopenic purpura Werlhof's disease Acute ITP is more common in children, causing a self-limited wave of ecchymotic hemorrhage secondary to viral infection or vaccination; chronic ITP is more common in adults and often is autoimmune with mucocutaneous, central nervous system, cardiac and renal hemorrhage (and potentially infarction), bruisability and transient thrombocytopenia (with normal or increased megakaryocytes in bone marrow); 2/3 of cases have IgG antiplatelet antibodies and hemolysis within the splenic sinusoids **Clinical** Female:male, 3:1, microangiopathic hemolytic anemia, fever, transient neurologic defects, renal failure, microthrombolic 'showers' to the brain, heart, lungs, kidneys, adrenal glands, spleen and live Note: ITP should be differentiated from the microthrombi of thrombotic thrombocytopenic purpura of young females, microangiopathic hemolytic anemia, neurologic defects and renal failure **Treatment** 75% markedly improve with splenectomy

'It's Over, Debbie' BIOMEDICAL ETHICS The title of an anonymous, personal account of the mercy killing of a young woman dying of terminal ovarian cancer, by the author, a young resident in gynecology, written in the 'Piece of my Mind' column of the Journal of the American Medical Association (1988; 259:272); 'it's over, Debbie' has become a battle cry of the euthanasia movement; for those who would defend the physician's action, the 'victim' was emaciated, racked with pain and according to the author, wanted to get it (presumably the dying process) over with; the ensuing controversy was enormous and physicians were 4:1 against the act; see DNR, 'Doctor Death', Euthanasia

IUD Intrauterine device A contraceptive that is being used with decreasing frequency in the US, given that the wave of litigation initiated by the doomed, deemed defective device, the Dalkon shield, engendered secondary waves of lawsuits that forced the manufacturers of similar contraceptive devices to withdraw from the market in the USA, see Copper-Seven, Dalkon shield, although these IUDs are widely used elsewhere; IUDs are associated with actinomycosis, a fungal infection affecting 85% of women with an IUD in place for more than three years; approximately 20% of ectopic pregnancies occur in wearers of IUDs; pelvic infections are three to seven-fold more frequent in IUD users, often of a polymicrobial nature, including aerobic and anaerobic bacteria, mycoplasma and *Chlamydia* species **Histopathology** Focal acute and chronic inflammation in 25-40% of IUD users, also, squamous metaplasia, premature predecidual reaction, focal fibrosis and pressure atrophy **Electron microscopy** Giant mitochondria are seen in proliferative phase endometrium, premature predecidual changes in secretory phase endometrium; copper IUDs induce increased mitochondria (with vacuolated matrix) and lysosomes; 75% epithelial cells reveal the myelin figures that correspond to the 'wear-and-tear' pigment, lipofuscin Note: Although no IUD-related neoplasia has been reported in humans, stainless steel or polyethylene loops implanted in virgin Wistar rats induce sarcomas and carcinomas; see Pearl index

IUGR Intrauterine growth retardation A phenomenon afflicting high risk infants, associated with perinatal asphyxia, hypoglycemia, hypothermia, pulmonary hemorrhage, meconium aspiration, necrotizing enterocolitis, polycythemia and multiple complications of infections, malformations and syndromes seen in the children;see Low birth weight

IUPAC International Union of Pure and Applied Chemistry

IVBAT Intravascular bronchiolar and alveolar tumor An uncommon tumor of women presenting as multifocal slowly-growing intrapulmonary nodules that mimic pulmonary metastases; first described as a variant of bronchoalveolar cell carcinoma, IVBAT is a neoplasm a sui generis caused by proliferation of blood vessels **Clinical** Often asymptomatic or minimal shortness of breath, 40% of patients are < 30 years old; 50% of patients die of disease, 25% within the first year; it may be related to endotheliomatosis or identical to epithelioid hemangioendothelioma **Radiology** Multiple bilateral pulmonary nodules < 2 cm in diameter **Histopathology** Tumor nodules with peripheral growth and central coagulative necrosis, dystrophic calcification or ossification; cells have rounded nuclei with overlapping contours, fibrillar, ground-glass, hyalinized, myxomatous or vacuolated cytoplasm **Immunoperoxidase** Vacuoles stain for factor VIII-r’ iated antigen, suggesting primitive endothelial differentiation

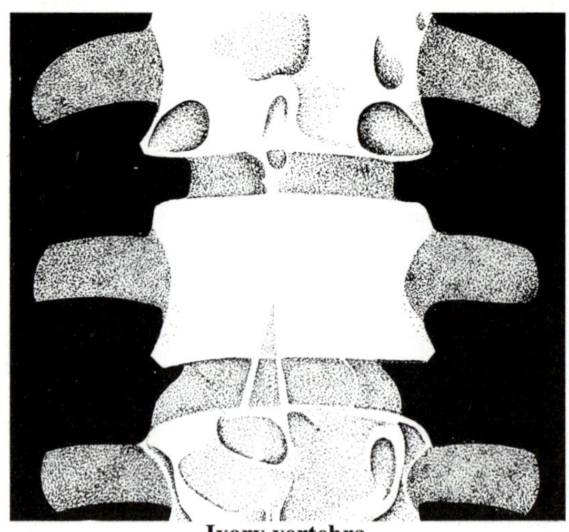
Ivory vertebra

Ivermectin TROPICAL MEDICINE A single dose antifilarial drug, that is now preferred by many workers to the previous standard, diethylcarbazine, which requires a 12-day course and patient compliance; ivermectin is effective against *Onchocerca volvulus, Wuchereria bancrofti, Brugia malayi*, requires a lower dose and has fewer side effects (N Engl J Med 1990; 322:1113); treatment of an entire community markedly reduces the prevalence of infection and may form the basis of effective eradication of *O volvulus*, the agent of river blindness (Science 1990; 250:116)

IVF see In vitro fertilization

IVH Intraventricular hemorrhage

IVIC syndrome An autosomal dominant condition characterized by multiple congenital defects including a defect in the radial 'ray' (an embryologic structure from which the radial bone and related musculoskeletal structure arises), strabismus, deafness, thrombocytopenia Note: The complex was first described in the IVIC (Instituto Venezolano Investigationes Cientificas)

IVIG see Intravenous immunoglobulin

IVLEN Inflammatory verrucous linear epidermal nevus DERMATOLOGY Persistent and pruritic linear lesions composed of erythematous slightly verrucous scaling papules, that may be associated with immune compromise **Differential diagnosis** Lichen striatus

Ivory vertebrae Osteosclerosis of vertebrae(figure, facing page) most common in osteoblastic metastases, classically seen in adenocarcinoma of the prostate, rarely also in colonic carcinoma, in particular those treated with hormonal or chemotherapy, Hodgkin's disease, sclerotic Paget's disease of the bone and multiple myeloma

Ivy bleeding time HEMATOLOGY A quantitative coagulation assay based on a standardized skin wound that measures the platelet and vascular response to injury Method A sphygmomanometer is placed around the upper arm and inflated to 40 mm Hg pressure, a 5 mm incision is made on the flexor surface of the forearm; the time required to stop bleeding is then measured Normal 1-6 minutes Increased in patients with Bernard-Soulier disease, Glanzmann's thrombasthenia, platelet defects, eg thrombocytopenia, storage pool disease, vascular defects, eg Ehlers-Danlos disease and von Willebrand's disease

Izumi fever Scarlatina-like water-born disease endemic to rural Japan, first described in 1929 that may have sporadic epidemic foci; the long form is characterized by a diphasic fever, while the short form has a single febrile peak; increase in atypical lymphocytes, appears to be similar or identical to infectious mononucleosis, with EBV antibody titers exceeding those seen in Burkitt's lymphoma

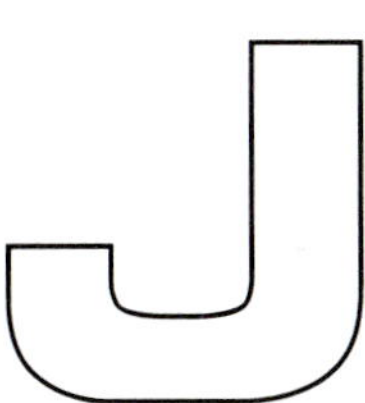

J Symbol for: Joule

Jaagziekte Afrikaans, Hunted sickness Pulmonary adenomatosis A disease first described in sheep in the Republic of South Africa; the name derives from the manner in which the animals become dyspneic, perceive themselves pursued and run until they die Etiology Unclear; pleuropneumonia-like organisms (PPLO) have been isolated from the animals Histopathology The lungs have microscopic features that are analogous to bronchoalveolar cell carcinoma of humans

Jack-knife phenomenon see Clasp knife phenomenon

'Jackpot' experiment RESEARCH An experiment designed in the hope (or with the assumption) that the results of the experimental sequence will corroborate an unusual scientific phenomenon; such goal-oriented research is rarely rewarded with the desired result, ie the 'Jackpot'; most research proceeds with a slow deliberate pace likened to the plodding of the Tortoise in Aesop's fable of '*The Tortoise and the Hare*'

Jackson Laboratory The world-renowned resource of live genetic material that maintains over 1000 colonies of inbred strains and stocks of mutant mice for sale and distribution to scientists; located in Bar Harbor, Maine, Jackson Laboratory is also a genetic information resource and maintains banks of frozen mouse embryos and a mouse DNA bank; Cf ATCC

'Jack-straw' crystals ANATOMIC PATHOLOGY A descriptor for haphazardly arranged, intracytoplasmic crystals, seen by the phosphotungstic acid-hematoxylin (PTAH) stain and thought to represent Z-band material, which in addition to increased mitochondria and glycogen is characteristic of the rhabdomyomas; see Spiderweb cells

Jail bars sign RADIOLOGY Dense osteosclerosis of the ribs, seen on a plain antero-posterior chest film, resulting in horizontal bands fancifully likened to the bars of a prison window, first described as characteristic of agnogenic myeloid metaplasia, it may also be seen in sickle cell anemia and osteopetrosis

Jail fever Epidemic louse-born Typhus fever

Jamaican neuropathy A condition characterized by spasticity and other signs of corticospinal tract disease, which has been divided into an a) Ataxic form, thought to be more common in Nigeria, accompanied by sensory ataxia, numbing and burning of the feet, deafness, visual defects with optic atrophy and a central scotoma, spasticity, leg atrophy and footdrop, findings that may be due to subclinical malnutrition and b) Tropical spastic paraparesis, a subacute neuropathy with predominantly pyramidal tract disease affecting the posterior column, causing paresthesia, loss of sensation, bladder dysfunction and girdling lumbar pain; 80% of patients have antibodies to HTLV-I

Jamaican vomiting sickness An intoxication by 'bush tea' made from unripe fruit of the Jamaican ackee tree (*Blighia sapida*), caused by hypoglycin, a propionic acid derivative that inhibits isovaleryl CoA dehydrogenase, provoking violent vomiting, prostration, drowsiness, convulsions and hypoglycemia as low as 0.56 mmol/L (US: 10 mg/dl) Mortality High, often within 24 hours of ingestion, caused by the metabolites of hypoglycin A, an amino acid that is converted to coenzyme A thioesters and carnitine derivatives, which sequester intracellular carnitine, inhibiting fatty acid oxidation, causing accumulation of isovaleric acid with continued fatty acid esterification, resulting in a fine-droplet fatty liver (N Engl J Med 1976; 295:461)

Jamais vu French, never seen PSYCHIATRY A group of

paramnesias in which there is a complete absence of memory for events known to have been experienced by the subject, each of which has been associated with neurotic depersonalization and temporal lobe epilepsy; **Jamais entendu** Intense feeling of never having previously heard something **Jamais eprouvé** Intense feeling of never having previously experienced something **Jamais fait** Intense feeling of never having previously done something **Jamais pensée** Intense feeling of never having previously thought something **Jamais racontée** Intense feeling of never having previously related something (as in having told someone) **Jamais vécu** Intense feeling of never having previously lived through something **Jamais voulu** Intense feeling of never having previously wished something **Jamais vu** Intense feeling of never having previously seen something; Cf Deja

Japanese cerebrovascular disease see Moya-Moya disease

Japanese encephalitis (JE) The single most common epidemic form of viral encephalitis, reaching an incidence of $50/10^5$ (in contrast, the peak of the poliomyelitis epidemic did not surpass $10/10^5$); JE is often fatal or crippling, especially in Thailand, where an annual summer peak may affect 2000 people, carrying a 20% mortality; vaccination in Thailand has caused a ten-fold reduction in JE, as well as a reduction in the incidence and severity of dengue fever (both are flaviviruses, a family that includes yellow fever and St. Louis encephalitis virus) Clinical Abrupt onset with fever, headache, meningeal irritation, convulsions, muscular rigidity, mask-like facies, coarse tremor, paresis, hyperactive deep tendon reflexes Histopathology Cortical neuronolysis, chronic perivascular inflammation of the brain, especially affecting the sustantia nigra, thalamus, hypothalamus, cortices and basal ganglia (N Engl J Med 1988; 319:608) Vector ***Culex*** mosquito

Japanese illusion Neurology A clinical test used to elicit right-left confusion in unilateral anesthesia; the patient crosses arms, opposes the palms and clasps fingers; the clasped hands are then rotated inward and the arms extended, making it difficult for the subject to tell the right from the left fingers

Jarvik-7 An artificial heart that was first transplanted into a dentist who survived 620 days; the second patient was transplanted in 1982 and died four months later; other subsequent deaths contributed to the US Food and Drug Administration's decision to revoke approval for the Jarvik-7 as a permanent replacement organ, although it had been considered an adequate temporary 'hold-over' or bridge device and 6 of 8 of those for whom it was used for this purpose lived to hospital discharge (J Heart Transplant 1988; 7:12); see Penn State heart

Jaw winking Marcus-Gunn phenomenon Neurology Elevation of a ptotic eye by jaw movement, as seen in autosomal dominant congenital ptosis, due to faulty innervation of levator palpebrae; inhibition of the levator muscle of the jaw accompanied by 'winking' is known as the inverse Marcus-Gunn phenomenon

Jaw wiring An extreme treatment of morbid obesity that utilizes the same methods and devices as those used for jaw fractures, allowing only the intake of liquids; although this technique is effective while the patient is 'wired', the patients usually regain the weight unless it is combined with another modality, eg ileal bypass surgery; see Gastric bubble, Ileal bypass surgery, Morbid obesity

JCAHO see Joint Commission on Accreditation of Healthcare Organizations

J-chain A 15 kD polypeptide that allows polymerization of immunoglobulins by disulfide bonds between polymeric serum IgA and all secretory IgA, as well as IgM and IgG-secreting glandular tissue; the J-chain has a high content of arginine, aspartic acid and glutamic acid and has 77% 'homology' to the mouse J-chain, formed in the mouse by splicing 4 exons; its synthesis is increased by interleukin-2

J-curve phenomenon Cardiology A relation (figure) that is postulated to exist between blood pressure and both cardiac morbidity and mortality, where the lowering of blood pressure below a critical point may be associated with an increased risk of morbidity and death of uncertain origin (J Am Med Assoc 1991; 265:489)

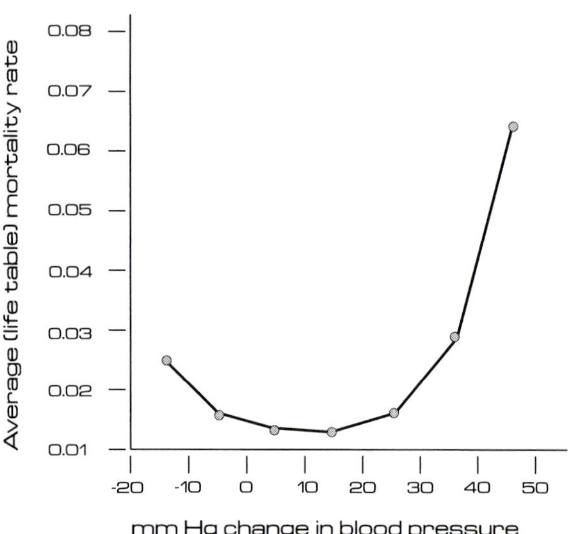

JC virus A polyoma virus, named after the index patient that causes progressive multifocal leukoencephalopathy (a subacute demyelinating infection of oligodendroglia, affecting immunocompromised hosts); during its long latency, the virus is maintained within monocytes and eventually penetrating the glial cells by the Virchow-Robin space; when the virus is injected into rodents and primates, many develop central nervous system tumors (astrocytomas, ganglioblastomas and retinoneuroblastomas (J Virol 1989; 63:863)

Jeep seat An inflammation of a pilonidal cyst and sinus that arises in a congenital malformation of the sacrococcygeal region with focal persistence of the neuroendocrine canal and ingrowth of hair into the cyst/sinus; 'Jeep driver's seat' is often first seen after repeated trauma as may occur in young military recruits who bounce over the countryside in shock absorber-less military vehicles or 'jeeps'

'Jekyll-and-Hyde' syndrome A symptom complex described in the elderly who cyclically improve with hospitalization (general stabilization, rehydration, appropriate administration of drugs) and undergo mental and physical deterioration while at home Note: This reference to the hero/villain of RL Stevenson's short story of Dr Jekyll and Mr Hyde, is inappropriate, as the elderly are not so Janus-faced

Jeffries probe see DNA fingerprinting

Jejuno-ileal bypass see Ileal bypass surgery

Jello sign OBSTETRICS A characteristic undulation of the scrotum that occurs with fetal limb movement, a 'soft' but relatively reliable criterion for determining an infant's sex by ultrasonography, seen after the 22nd gestational week; the movement has been fancifully likened to that of a proprietary brand of gelatin

Jentigo DERMATOLOGY A histological finding that consists of a combined junctional nevus and simple lentigo, coined by the Ackerman group of dermatopathology; in the natural history of a simple lentigo, increased melanocytes, originally distributed singly in the basal layer, tend to aggregate into nests at the epidermal-dermal junction; differentiating this lesion from a melanoma in situ rests on finding single and nests of melanocytes scattered along a broad front, poor circumscription and larger size in the malignant melanoma

Jerne network theory IMMUNOLOGY A hypothesis born from experimental data suggesting that after production of an antibody, 'Ab-1' to an antigen, 'X', the Ab-1 antibody-producing cells would be down-regulated by a second group of antibodies, 'Ab-2' that are formed against Ab-1, which recognize an epitope near the binding region of Ab-1; this network of interrelated and down-regulating antibodies allows immunologic 'homeostasis', so that endless antibody production to differing 'self' antigens does not occur, preventing uncontrolled antibody production

'Jet lag' An acute shift in the circadian rhythm, caused by travelling across multiple (usually three or more) time zones Clinical Alterations in mood, performance efficiency, temperature rhythms, rapid eye movement and slow-wave sleep; the patterns revert to normal either in a linear or monotonic fashion after several days 'acclimatization' in the new time zone; see Circadian rhythm, Insomnia, Shift work, Sleep disorders

Jet lesions Zahn-Schmincke pockets CARDIAC PATHOLOGY Vegetations that develop where a regurgitant 'jet' of turbulent blood flow strikes the endocardium, causing fibrosis and roughening of the endocardial wall, typical of anomalies of blood flow from a high-to-low pressure region, eg aortic stenosis or coarctation, mitral stenosis, ventricular septal defect and patent ductus arteriosus, as occurs in rheumatic fever or congenital heart disease; the roughened lesions may give rise to small emboli and produce cerebral thromboembolism

Jet phenomenon RADIOLOGY A narrow-shouldered column of barium seen as it gushes past the stenosis caused by an esophageal web, or a dysfunctional cricopharynx

Jet sign UROLOGIC RADIOLOGY A thin, obliquely-oriented high-pressure stream of radiocontrast seen in excretory urograms of a normal bladder, the result of peristaltic emptying of the ureters

Jet ventilation A technique used during tracheal reconstructive surgery where a catheter tube is passed through the endotracheal tube into the distal main stem bronchus; a small tidal volume is delivered at a high (60-150 'breaths'/min) frequency which serves to maintain lung expansion, alveolar ventilation and oxygenation

JGA Juxtaglomerular apparatus

Jigsaw puzzle cells Poikilocytes Bizarre, variably sized and shaped erythrocytes, fancifully likened to the jagged pieces of a jigsaw puzzle that may be due to mechanical damage, as in severe hereditary spherocytosis or elliptocytosis, denaturation of spectrin, as in in vitro thermal injury to red cells in hereditary pyropoikilocytosis or in Woronet's trait, an asymptomatic genetic curiosity (Blood Cells 1980; 6:281)

Jigsaw-puzzle contours OPHTHALMOLOGY A variegated, mosaic pattern of hyperpigmentation seen in angioid streaks of the retinal fundus, located posterior to the retina itself

Jigsaw-puzzle model MOLECULAR BIOLOGY A hypothesis that proteins undergo a random set of folding intermediates before assuming their native or in vivo configuration (Proc Natl Acad Sci 1985; 82:4028); the protein folding process in barnase (and presumably others, if not all proteins) appears to follow a defined pathway in which there is one or more distinct intermediate transition states (Nature 1990; 346:440, 488, 409)

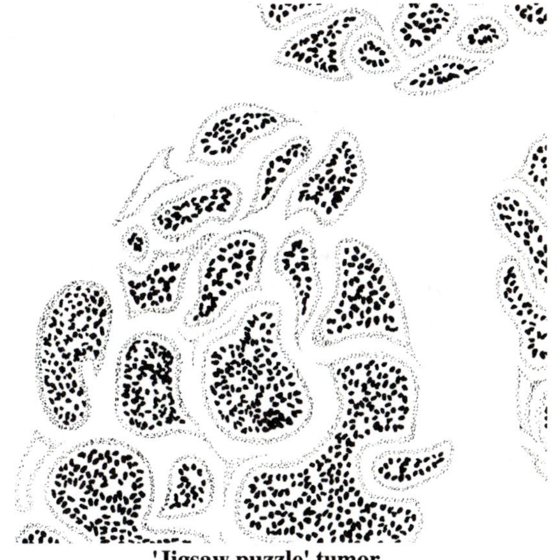

'Jigsaw puzzle' tumor

'Jigsaw puzzle' tumor DERMATOPATHOLOGY A fanciful descriptor for cylindroma, a skin adnexal tumor, referring to the histological pattern of cell islands composed of a) undifferentiated, palisaded and peripherally-oriented cells with small dark nuclei and b) central lighter staining cells with larger nuclei differentiating towards glands that may focally demonstrate secretion; cylindromas are usually solitary, smooth, variably shaped nodules on the face, trunk and extremities, corresponding to skin appendage proliferations; when extensive and on the scalp, known as Turban tumors, see there; apocrine, rarely merocrine differentiation;

some cylindromas are autosomal dominant, they may be associated with trichoepitheliomas and may undergo malignant degeneration

Jitter NEUROLOGY A finding in motor neuron disease characterized as instability in subcomponents of motor unit action potentials when measured by single-fiber electromyography and thought to be due to inefficient transmission of impulses in recent neural collaterals or due to abnormal neuromuscular transmission (Mayo Clin Proc 1991; 66:54)

Jitter phenomenon NEUROPHYSIOLOGY A normally variable interval in the firing of the muscle impulse, attributed to 'chaos' that exists among action potentials of the muscle fibers in the same motor unit, as recorded in single-fiber electromyography; in myasthenia gravis, the jitter time is increased and the impulses may not appear at the appropriate interval ('blockings')

Jo-1 syndrome A clinical complex related to the production of antibodies against the Jo-1 antigen (histidyl-tRNA synthetase), which is associated with myosotis, arthritis and interstitial lung disease Note: Anti-Jo-1 antibodies are present in 25% of adult patients with various forms of myositis, including polymyositis, dermatomyositis and the 'overlap' syndrome

Job stress The work-related combination of high psychological demands and low decision latitude; intuitively, hypertension has been related to job strain, objectively determined to have a relative risk of 3.1 (J Am Med Assoc 1990; 263:1929); see 'Toxic core', Type A personality

Job syndrome Hyperimmunoglobulin E syndrome An immunodeficiency syndrome characterized by multiple recurring 'cold' abscesses **Clinical** Multiple episodes of otitis media, sinusitis, severe, life-threatening staphylococcal infections, chronic eczemoid lesions and recurring abscesses of the lungs, skin and joints **Laboratory** Defects in neutrophil and monocyte chemotaxis, hyperimmunoglobulin E; although the first cases described (Lancet 1966; 1:1013) occurred in two red-headed girls, it also occurs in males and in those with other hair colors Note: The biblical Job was cursed and covered with boils (abscesses) from head to toe (one of the calamities he suffered to test his faith in God); hyperimmunoglobulin E syndrome is the accepted synonym for Job syndrome because of the characteristic multiple recurring abscesses; however, since the description of his affliction was vague, historians have postulated that Job syndrome was due to syphilis, yaws, leprosy, smallpox, pemphigus, dermatitis herpetiformis, pellagra or scurvy

Jocasta complex PSYCHIATRY 1) The sexual love or desire, usually latent that a mother has for a son or 2) The domineering non-incestuous, quasi-adulatory love that an affect-hungry mother has for an intelligent son, often in the face of an absent or weak father figure; Jocasta of Greek mythology was the mother of Oedipus; while Oedipus' desire for his mother was completely innocent, Jocasta's incestuous act was conscious; see Oedipus complex; Cf Phaedra complex

Jodbasedow disease Hyperthyroidism in iodine- (German, Jod) deficient patients that occurs after iodine replacement, resulting in a hypermetabolic goitrous state with exophthalmos, causing an autoimmune disease with antibodies directed against the TSH receptor Note: von Basedow described the condition in 1840, Graves in 1835

Jogger's foot see Tarsal tunnel syndrome

Johnson Controls decision see Maternal-fetal conflict(s)

'Joint' SUBSTANCE ABUSE A cigarette made from dried marijuana (*Cannibas sativa*) leaves, which is 'toked' in order to produce a 'high', and if smoked in excess, 'get stoned'; see Hallucinogen, Marijuana, Substance abuse, THC receptor

Joint Commission on Accreditation of Healthcare Organizations (JCAHO) A private, nonprofit organization sponsored by a number of medical associations (American Hospital Association, American Medical Association, American Dental Association and by the American College of Physicians and American College of Surgeons), the purpose of which is to maintain a high standard of institutional care, by both establishing guidelines for the operation of hospitals and other (psychiatric, ambulatory and long-term) health care facilities and by 'policing' those facilities through surveys and periodic inspections; 'accreditation' of a facility is a requirement adopted by health insurers, funding agencies and public programs History, see J Am Med Assoc 1987; 258:951

Joint mice ORTHOPEDICS A fanciful term for free bodies within the synovial cavity, especially of the knee, which are composed of fibrous tissue covered by cartilage and measure 0.5 to 1.5 cm in diameter, classically described in degenerative joint disease; joint mice are a relatively non-specific finding, since they may also be seen in synovial osteochondromatosis, chondrometaplasia, neuropathic arthro-pathy, osteoarthritis dissecans, pigmented villonodular synovitis and gout

Jones criteria RHEUMATOLOGY Those criteria used to establish the diagnosis of rheumatic fever, requiring that a patient have 1) Two (or more) major criteria, eg carditis, erythema marginatum, polyarthritis, Sydenham's chorea and subcutaneous nodules, or one major criterion and 2) Two (or more) minor criteria, either a) **Clinical** Previous rheumatic fever or known rheumatic heart disease, arthralgia or fever b) **Laboratory** Acute phase reactants, erythrocyte sedimentation rate, antistreptolysin O, C-reactive protein, increased P-R interval on the electrocardiogram

Joseph complex PSYCHOLOGY An allegorical descriptor for intense sibling rivalry, derived from the favorite and youngest of the twelve sons of Jacob, the Israelite, Joseph, who was cast out by his brothers

Journal club A form of graduate (and less commonly, continuing) medical education used by physicians during the residency training period, in which a small group convenes and discusses, analyzes and reviews a limited number of articles from major medical journals, often on a weekly or monthly basis; while there are no rules, the journal club attempts to increase a professional's reading of timely information, presenting it from different vantage points, improving the resident's knowledge of epidemiology and biostatistics with the hope that he will be critical in his assimilation of new information (J Am Med Assoc 1988; 260:2537); the first journal club was organized by Sir William Osler at McGill University in 1875

J pouch A reservoir formed from a J-shaped loop of the terminal ileum where the loops are sectioned, forming a pouch and then anastomosed to a continent anorectum, preserving anal sphincter function; the procedure is used following total proctocolectomy for familial polyposis coli or ulcerative colitis totalis; see S pouch

J-shaped sella A shallow, elongated or 'boot-shaped' sella turcica with an elongated anterior recess, extending below the anterior clinoid process, classically seen in Hurler's mucopolysaccharidosis (due to the accumulation of dermatan and keratan sulfates or glycosaminoglycans); the change may also occur in the orodigitofacial syndrome and mannosidosis

J syndrome Jamaican syndrome A form of diabetes mellitus thought to be identical to the 'Third diabetic syndrome', see there

Judaism, practice of see Haman-Tashen intoxication, Seder syncope, Shmita salmonellosis, Shofar-blowing emphysema, Yom Kippur effect (J Am Med Assoc 1983, 250:2469, ibid, 1984; 251:2348c); Cf Harvest Moon phenomenon

Jughandle view RADIOLOGY A modified basal view of the skull used to visualize the zygomatic arches, of particular interest in evaluating midfacial fractures

'Juicy baby' NEONATOLOGY A fanciful term for an infant who produces excess mucus in the early post-partum period; 'juiciness' is a soft criterion for esophageal atresia, which when accompanied by respiratory distress (cyanosis and tachypnea), implies concomitant tracheoesophageal fistula

'July phenomenon' A popular myth in North America holds that the quality of medical care deteriorates and mortality rate increases in teaching hospitals during the month of July (the time when interns, fresh from medical school begin their training period); one study indicated that the length of hospital stay and costs may actually be reduced during July (J Am Med Assoc 1990; 263:953) Note: Given the financial pressures in the US to discharge patients as soon as possible, reduced hospital length of stay has become an indirect measurement of quality of patient care; see Libby Zion; Cf 'Quicker and sicker'; Cf DRGs

Jumper syndrome Vertical deceleration injury A distinct form of blunt trauma from jumping or falling from heights, usually greater than five stories; the injury severity score is 41 (predicted survival, 50%; actual survival is less); all had multiple fractures, eg 'ring fracture' of the skull base, separating the rim of the foramen magnum from the remainder of the base and compression fractures of the vertebrae, both of which occur when the victim lands on his feet or buttocks; many jumpers may also have coup and/or contrecoup injuries of the brain; over one-half arrive to the emergency ward in shock and most have angiographic evidence of retroperitoneal hemorrhage; see Lover's heels

Jumping see Chromosome jumping

'Jumping Frenchmen of Maine' syndrome A culture-specific complex that is evoked in the members of a religious sect paradoxically originating from Wales and residing in North America, the rites of which includes jumping, rolling on the ground, barking like dogs and so on until a state of ecstasy is achieved, which subsides after the ceremonies, or which may be re-evoked on command; the reflex may be considered an exaggeration of the normal startle reflex (hyperexplexia) seen in 'startle diseases' that may be elicited by any, often auditory stimulus, causing a stiffening of the body, arm flexion, a jump, involuntary shout or fall to the ground; such complexes may be inherited in an autosomal dominant fashion and must be differentiated from Gilles de la Tourette and startle epilepsy (Brain 1986; 109:561)

Jumping genes Mobile DNA elements, which were first recognized by B McClintock in maize (*Zea mays*) in 1931, which she viewed as agents capable of moving into and out of (ie, 'jumping') genes, concomitantly alternating the genetic activity of those genes; jumping genes include insertion sequences, transposons, viral and non-viral retroposons

Jumping library A cloned 'library' of transposible DNA elements, produced by cloning a locus by reverse genetics, crossing over hundreds of kilobases; here reverse genetics with chromosomal map positions and genetically-linked DNA markers are used to identify and clone DNA sequences 100 or more kilobases away from starting point Method Pulsed field electrophoresis

'Jump position' Posture of a spastic child who stands with his knees and hips flexed and the ankles in equinus position, a characteristic stance in spastic paraplegia of cerebral palsy

jun An oncogene that induces avian sarcoma and transforms certain avian cell lines in vitro; the viral oncogene, v-*jun* and the related cellular genes c-*jun*, *jun* B and *jun* D encode transactivating or repressing DNA-binding proteins, forming homodimeric (Jun-Jun) or heterodimeric (Jun-Fos) protein complexes that recognize the AP-1 consensus sequence, a response element that makes cells susceptible to the tumor-promoter, phorbol ester TPA, as well as cell growth factors; v-*jun* lacks a nucleotide sequence for 27 amino acids encoded by c-*jun*, has mutations causing amino acid substitutions not seen in c-*jun* and its protein product is highly expressed in v-*jun*-infected cells; the c-*jun* protein product is structurally similar to GCN4, a protein that activates yeast genes by binding to a DNA binding site similar to that of AP-1 a human transcription factor; *jun* binds to *fos* by a leucine zipper, together effecting greater control over gene transcription than either can alone; the jun protein is structurally and functionally similar to the *fos* protein; c-Jun-mediated transactivation may be augmented independently of c-Fos by Ha-Ras, which stimulates phosphorylation of c-Jun's activation domain and possibly explains how oncoproteins participate in the transformation of cells in culture (Nature 1991; 351:122) Note: *jun* was named by a post-doctoral fellow, as an abbreviation of ju-nana, Japanese for 17, as it was the 17th in a group of 30 avian sarcoma viruses recovered from the tumors encountered in a poultry house by Vogt et al, which causes a fibrosarcoma in chickens; see *fos*, Oncogene, One-hit/two-hit model

Junk DNA Long stretches of non-protein-coding DNA that comprise 95% of the human genome (Science 1990; 250:1337), are mobile, capable of self-replication, but serve no known function, thus also being known as selfish DNA; these quasi-autonomous segments include spacer DNA, satellite and exons that are spliced out when the primary transcript of the RNA becomes mRNA; see Human Genome Project, LINES, SINES

Junk food A popular term for any food that is low in essential nutrients and high in carbohydrates; junk foods may be highly salted, eg potato chips/crisps, pretzels, high in refined sugar (empty calories), eg cake, candy, soft drinks and high in saturated fats and cholesterol, eg cake and chocolates; see Cafeteria model, 'Couch potato', 'Fast' food

Junkie A US colloquialism for a person, usually an intravenous narcotic abusing addict, whose life is disorganized in terms of family and societal structure and whose existence revolves around obtention (often through theft, prostitution or other illicit means) of another 'fix' of narcotics, known in some circles as 'junk'; see Cold turkey, Shooting galleries Note: Junkie has been further colloquialized to imply anyone with an 'addiction' for a particular food or habit, eg a Junk food 'junkie'

Juvenile aponeurotic fibroma Calcifying fibroma, Keasbey's tumor A benign tumor of fibrous tissue of the hand or wrist in children or adolescents HISTOPATHOLOGY Fibrous tissue, calcification and cartilage; although one-half recur locally, local surgical incision is curative

Juvenile carcinoma Secretory carcinoma A rare breast carcinoma seen in children, average age 9 PATHOLOGY Small, well-circumscribed, fibroadenoma-like tumor with tubuloalveolar and focal papillary formations lined by vacuolated cells producing eosinophilic, PAS-positive secretions Treatment 'Lumpectomy' is usually adequate

Juvenile hyalin fibromatosis A rare autosomal recessive condition, characterized by generalized subcutaneous and gingival nodules, which vaguely resembles myofibromatosis, but lacks mature collagen; other soft tissue proliferations are not uncommon in childhood and adolescence, most of which are benign, including calcifying aponeurotic fibroma, congenital fibromatoses (solitary or multiple), digital fibromatosis (see Kissing tumor), fibromatosis coli, fibrous hamartoma, infantile (desmoid-type) fibromatosis, infantile myofibromatosis, juvenile angiofibroma, hyaline fibromatosis and giant cell fibroblastoma

Juvenile laryngeal papillomatosis A neoplasm in children caused by human papillomavirus types 6 and 11 that may also occur in adults in the upper respiratory tract (known as recurrent respiratory papillomatosis); the lesion is analagous to condyloma acuminatum of the genital tract; the tumor rarely undergoes malignant degeneration, although it may be accompanied by severe airway compromise, the major complication of this lesion, a lesion of such recalcitrance that hundreds of surgical resections may be required; although leukocyte interferon significantly reduces the growth rate of the tumors during the first six months of therapy, the effect is not sustained (N Engl J Med 1988; 319:401)

Juvenile 'melanoma' An obsolete misnomer for the spindle and epithelioid cell nevus or Spitz nevus, a benign pigmented nevus that occurs before puberty, commonly presenting as a raised pink or red nodule on the facial skin

Juvenile myoclonic epilepsy Impulsiv petit mal de Janz A seizure disorder comprising 4% of epilepsies Clinical Normal IQ, onset in adolescence, affecting the flexor muscles of the head, neck and shoulders; the attacks tend to occur as clonic-tonic-clonic seizures upon awakening EEG 4-6 Hz multispike and wave pattern; 40% of relatives, especially female, have myoclonus Treatment Valproate

Juvenile pemphigoid A pruritic variant of bullous pemphigoid that affects the genitalia and face of children

Juvenile periodontitis Early onset periodontitis, affecting adolescents, male:female, 3:1, characterized by an early loss of alveolar bone surrounding permanent teeth; 84% have underlying endocrinopathies and 12% had systemic disease, eg diabetes mellitus, neutropenia, Down and Ehlers-Danlos syndromes, hyperkeratosis palmaris et plantaris, histiocytosis X and hypophosphatasia Etiology *Actinobacillus actinomycecomitans* and others; when accompanied by palmo-plantar hyperkeratosis, the disease is called Papillon-Lefèvre syndrome, characterized by loss of alveolar bone, premature dental exfoliation, clinical features of hereditary ectodermal dysplasia and calcifications of the falx and dura

Juvenile xanthogranuloma A yellowish tumor of early childhood involving the face, head, neck and extremities Histopathology Abundant dermal histocytes apposing adnexal structures, extending into the subcutis Prognosis Spontaneous involution

Juxtaovarian adnexal tumor An adnexal tumor of probable wolffian origin, which is located in the leaves of the broad ligament and often asymptomatic, affecting patients between ages 30 and 60 Pathology The tumors measure up to 12 cm, from rubbery to friable in consistency, appearing by light microscopy as clusters of epithelial-like mesothelial cells Prognosis Often benign, rarely, these tumors may recur or metastasize

J wave of Osbourne A quasi-pathognomonic electrocardiographic (EKG) change seen in one-third of patients with hypothermia, appearing as a positive 'hump' at the end of a QRS complex that disappears on rewarming the patient; other cardiovascular changes include brady-arrhythmia, atrial flutter and fibrillation EKG Prolongation of the P-R and S-T intervals and T-wave inversion

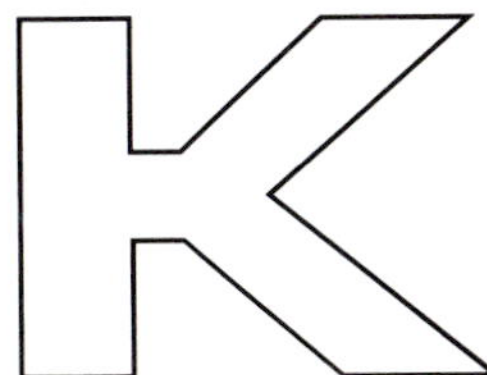

K Symbol for: Equilibrium constant; degrees, Kelvin; Kilobyte, which is actually 1024; Lysine; potassium

k Symbol for: kilo

K562 An immortalized cell line, originally obtained from a patient with chronic myelogenous leukemia inblast crisis, which is a 'standard' target for measuring natural killer cell activity, see NK cells

Ka The symbol for the ionization constant of an acid in an equilibrium reaction

Kabuki mask facies A congenital complex of unknown etiology with a characteristic facial dysmorphia (long palpebral fissures, eversion of the lateral lower eyelids, broad depressed nose, fancifully likened to a mask worn in a Kabuki theater), large ears, a high arched or cleft palate, mental and growth retardation, scoliosis and recurrent otitis (Clin Genet 1982; 21:315)

Kabure An urticarial skin reaction that occurs 4-8 weeks after penetration of the skin by the burrowing cercariae of *Schistosoma japonicum*, which may be accompanied by fever, purpura, malaise, arthralgia, abdominal cramps, diarrhea and hepatosplenomegaly

Kala-azar Hindi, Black fever Dumdum disease Visceral leishmaniasis (*L donovani*), seen in Asia, Mediterranean rim countries, Africa and South America Life cycle, Stage 1 Amastigote (leishmanial) stage Maturation in vertebrates Stage 2 Promastigote (leptomonad) stage Transmitted by insects After a 2-week to 1-year incubation, the parasites invade the spleen, causing massive splenomegaly, liver, bone marrow and lymph nodes **Clinical** Chills, fever, vomiting **Diagnosis** Spleen biopsy (potentially fatal) and Montenegro test (positive in treated cases) **Treatment** Parenteral pentavalent organic antimonials, eg sodium antimony gluconate, aromatic diaminidines, eg pentamidine, amphotericin B **Mortality** 75% without therapy

Kallikrein A hydrolytic enzyme that cleaves kininogen to produce bradykinin, a nonapeptide that acts on vessels, evoking vasodilation, increasing capillary permeability; kallikrein also acts on smooth muscle, pain receptors and is chemotactic for neutrophils

Kallikrein-kinin system An interconnected family of endogenous vasopressive peptides that maintain blood pressure by controlling regional blood flow and electrolyte and water excretion; kallikrein stimulates renin release and kinin production (kinins are potent vasodilators and natriuretics, inhibiting sodium transport in the distal nephrons, altering the osmotic gradient of the renal medulla; in addition kinins interface with the immune system; the kallikrein-kinin and renin-aldosterone-angiotensin (RAA) systems interact to control blood pressure and are closely linked, as evidenced by kininase II that inactivates kinin and converts A-I to A-II; see RAA system

Kanagawa phenomenon MICROBIOLOGY A laboratory finding in *Vibrio parahemolyticus*, which becomes hemolytic on a Wagasumi agar, first described in Kanagawa, a prefecture of Japan and is of diagnostic use during epidemics (N Engl J Med 1985; 312:345)

Kanemi oil intoxication see Yusho

Kane surgery Any surgical procedure performed by the surgeon on himself; Dr E O'Neill Kane operated upon himself for an inguinal hernia, appendicitis and amputated his own finger; Dr Rennie, commentator on this form of surgery, noted that an autosurgeon who represents himself for negligence has a fool for a surgeon, a patient, a prosecutor and a defender (J Am Med Assoc 1987; 257:825)

Kangri cancer Neve syndrome Heat-induced squamous cell carcinoma seen in natives of Kashmir, occurring on the skin of the inner thighs and umbilicus, caused by the heat and volatile products produced by the kangri, a-n earthenware charcoal 'hibachi' worn for warmth by Kashmiris (Brit Med J 1923; 2:1255)

Kanteserin A serotonin antagonist that acts at the cognate receptors in the arterial wall but not in the endothelium; see Serotonin

K antigens German, Kapsul MICROBIOLOGY A group of antigens present on the surface of gram-negative bacteria, which are of two types a) Protein (fimbriae) and b) acid polysaccharides, expressed on the surface of *Klebsiella* species and *Escherichia coli*; K antigens are located external to the somatic 'O' antigen and are heat-labile and cross-react with other encapsulated bacteria (*Haemophilus influenzae, Streptococcus pneumoniae* and *Neisseria meningitidis*); certain K antigens are associated with more virulent urinary tract infections; anti-K antibodies, while protective against the strain of bacteria, are often weak

Kaposi sarcoma (KS) A once rare, indolent malignancy that predominantly affected older Italian or Jewish men or those immunocompromised through the vicissitudes of transplantation, immunosuppression of lymphoproliferation; KS has become extremely common, occurring in 46% of male homosexuals with AIDS, 12% of female intravenous drug-abusers (IVDA) with AIDS and 4% of male IVDA with AIDS; KS is characterized by a proliferation of lymphatic or vascular channels, driven by growth and regulatory factors, including IL-1-β, IL-6 and tat protein **Histopathology** Jagged blood vessels filled with red cells that percolate into the adjacent tissue, subdivided into inflammatory and polymorphous types;

see Promontory sign Note: Kaposi also described lupus erythematosus profundus (Kaposi-Irving syndrome), a variant of xeroderma pigmentosum (Kaposi syndrome, type II) and eczema herpeticum (Kaposi syndrome, type III)

Kappa chain One of the two light immunoglobulin chains; present in a 2:1 ratio with lambda

Kappa rhythm NEUROLOGY An electroencephalographic pattern with α or theta frequency, recorded over the temporal regions during normal mental activity

Karnovsky scale A scale of objective criteria for the quality of life, which is used for patients with incapacitating diseases; the scale was developed for patients with cancer and of use in AIDS; a Karnovsky score of 100 indicates that there is no clinical evidence of disease; those with scores above 80 are able to maintain normal activities; a score between 50-70 precludes work and is accompanied by decreasing levels of autonomy; a person with a score between 10-40 is severely ill and requires hospitalization; a person with a score of 0 requires interment

Karyotype An organism's chromosome complement, best studied by high-resolution photography in the metaphase of mitosis (nonsexual, somatic or body-cell division), the stage of maximum condensation and point when the chromosomes' morphology is most distinct; a haploid number (n) bears one half of a full set of the organism's chromosomes, 23 in humans; a full or euploid set of chromosomes in most mammals is 2n, one n being contributed during meiosis by the male and one n by the female to form a 2n complement of chromosoms; polyploidy refers to full multiples of n, eg 3n, 4n, 5n...; aneuploidy is a lopsided number of chromosomes (n X Y) + Z, where Z is not = n and Y is a whole number

Karyotype analysis is indicated for children born with congenital anomalies, mental retardation without due cause, intersex, primary amenorrhea, male or female infertility, habitual abortion without anatomic abnormalities, previous spontaneous abortions, advanced maternal age or family history of chromosome abnormalities; see also Banding, Chromosomes

Katal The International System (SI) unit for measuring enzymatic activity, which is equal to 1 mol/ml of substrate consumed per second under specified conditions; depite the SI's 'blessing' of the katal, the International Unit (U) continues to be the preferred unit of measurement

Katayama disease Acute schistosomiasis caused by *S japonicum* and *S mansoni*, and rarely *S hematobium* after a 2-10 week incubation, corresponding to oviposition of juvenile worms; the disease severity is a function of worm load and evokes a serum sickness-like disease due to immune complex deposition *INTERMEDIATE HOST* The oncomelania snail *DEFINITIVE HOST* Water buffalo, domestic animals, human **Clinical** Acute onset of fever, chills, sweating, headache, cough, lymphadenopathy, hepatosplenomegaly, eosinophilia, potentially fatal if the tumor load is heavy

Katzenellenbogen German, Cat's elbow sign Lichen planus actinicus DERMATOLOGY A variant of lichen planus, seen in the Middle East, on sun-exposed parts, especially the face, characterized by annular lesions with pigmented centers, central thinning of epidermis and well-demarcated pale, raised margins

Kawasaki disease Mucocutaneous lymph node syndrome An endemic and epidemic disease of children under age 5 that often follows a 1-2 week incubation, presenting with fever, cervical lymphadenopathy, palmo-plantar and mucosal erythema and edema, aneurysms of small and medium-sized coronary arteries with arteritis (occasionally causing sudden death; mortality, 1-5%), and may affect peripheral arteries; CDC definition requires four or more of the following a) Fever of greater than 5 days b) Bilateral ocular conjunctival injection c) One or more changes of the oral mucosa including erythema, fissuring and xerostomia, conjunctival edema, mucosal edema of the upper respiratory tract, eg pharyngeal injection, dry, fissured lips and 'strawberry tongue', and d) One or more changes of the extremities, including acral erythema or edema, periungual and/or generalized desquamation, polymorphous exanthematous rash, truncal and cervical lymphadenopathy Note: Any of the above may occur as isolated findings in toxic shock, fever that is refractory to antibiotics, vasculitis of large and medium vessels, death due to acute myocarditis with congestive heart failure, arrhythmia, pericarditis, cardiac tamponade, thrombosis, infarction, development of coronary arterial aneurysm **Etiology** Various microorganisms have been implicated, eg ***Proprionobacterium acnes*** or retroviruses, but none definitively **Laboratory** Increased erythrocyte sedimentation rate, C-reactive protein, complement, globulin levels **Treatment** Early γ-globulin in a single intravenous bolus (N Engl J Med 1991; 324:1633) or aspirin 80 000 cases have been reported in Japan with three epidemics in 1979, 1982 and 1986; fatality rate 0.4% especially in children under age 2 (J Am Med Assoc 1991; 265:2699rv)

Kb The symbol for: Ionization constant of a base in equilibrium reactions; Kilobase

KB cell A cell line in permanent culture that was derived from a carcinoma in 1954; Cf HeLa cell

K cell IMMUNOLOGY see Killer cell PULMONARY MEDICINE see Kulchitsky cell

K complex NEUROLOGY A burst of high-voltage diphasic slow waves over the cranial vertex seen by electroencephalography that are either spontaneous or due to sensory stimuli during stage 2 and 3 of the sleep cycle; asymmetric K complexes may indicate organic cerebral lesion or may rarely occur in patients with cortical atrophy, eg Alzheimer's disease

KCT Kaolin clotting time

Kd The symbol for dissociation constant in an equilibrium reaction

kD see Kilodalton

KDEL sequence A tetramer of amino acids (Lys-Asp-Glu-Leu, abbreviated as KDEL in the one letter system) that is present at the carboxy-terminus of proteins, eg heavy chain-binding protein, protein disulfide isomerase, calreticulin and glucose-regulating protein 94, which serves as a retention signal for proteins residing in the endoplasmic reticulum, bound by a KDEL receptor (Nature 1990; 345:495, 480n&v); Cf RGD family

k-DNA see DNA

Kedani disease see Scrub typhus

Kelley index of malignancy ALTERNATIVE MEDICINE A questionnaire developed by a researcher in the late 1960s who believed that cancer resulted from a deficiency of pancreatic enzyme(s); the questionnaire was used to allegedly locate and determine the growth rate of tumors, that were then treated with laetrile; see Laetrile, Metabolic therapy, Tijuana, Unproven cancer therapy

Keloid Greek, Crab's claw An exuberant skin scar most common in adults aged 15-45 that is six-fold more common in dark-skinned individuals and in women; keloids may occur in other conditions, eg Rubinstein-Taybi syndrome and be associated with infection, burns, trauma, insect bites **Pathology** Rubbery, sharply demarcated, elevated scarred mass with pincer-like extensions, composed of whorled collagen fibers, often located on the seborrheic areas (shoulders and upper chest) and extremities; caused by excessive synthesis of collagen and increased proline hydroxylase activity; unlike hypertrophic scars that flatten with time, keloids are stable **Treatment** Local steroid injection to relieve pruritus or reduce the size in early lesions; post-excisional recurrence is common

Kemron A low-dose formulation of interferon-α, touted by researchers in Kenya as treating and occasionally curing AIDS, a claim that has not been substantiated

Keratin pearl see Squamous pearl

Keratoacanthoma A benign proliferation of squamous epithelium due to infundibular hyperplasia and squamous metaplasia of sebaceous glands which may histologically mimic well-differentiated squamous cell carcinoma Note: 10-15% of keratoacanthomas cannot be distinguished from squamous cell carcinoma; findings favoring keratoacanthoma are the rapid development of the lesion (over several weeks), keratin-filled 'craters' surrounded by buttresses with eosinophilic and 'glassy' keratinocytes; findings favoring squamous carcinoma are the histological findings of perineural invasion, nuclear atypia, abnormal mitoses, single cell necrosis, inflammation and horn cysts

Keratocyte Kerato-, Greek, horn An erythrocyte with one or two notches or horns that result from the red cells being squeezed through strands of intravascular fibrin, as seen in disseminated intravascular coagulation, microangiopathic hemolytic anemia, immune complex nephritis or foreign materials within vessels; as a result of this trauma, pseudovacuoles are formed which burst, leaving a horny erythrocyte

Keratohyalin granules Dense osmiophilic aggregates of cytokeratin seen within horn cells of the granular cell layer of normal epidermis, eccrine duct cells, rarely also in clear cell type sweat gland tumors

Keratosis A condition characterized by an increased production of keratin **ACTINIC (SOLAR) KERATOSIS** Seen in sun-exposed parts of light-skinned subjects, characterized by hyperkeratosis, parakeratosis, upper dermal atrophy and squamous cell atypia which may be a precursor of squamous cell carcinoma **ARSENIC-INDUCED KERATOSIS** A lesion of historic interest seen at a time when arsenic was used to treat arthritis, asthma, psoriasis and syphilis, characterized as warty palmo-plantar excrescences, occasionally evolving to squamous or basal cell carcinomas **KERATOSIS PILARIS** A lesion associated with ichthyosis vulgaris and atopic dermatitis, often on the extremities (in lichen spinulosus, similar lesions are located on the trunk and buttocks) with pinpoint indurations likened to a nutmeg grater **SEBORRHEIC KERATOSIS** A lesion common in the face and upper trunk of the middle-aged and elderly, histologically demonstrating hyperkeratosis, acanthosis and papillomatosis

Kerion A severe form of tinea capitis in which well-circumscribed portions of the scalp are transformed into a painful, boggy inflamed and confluent mass with loosening of the hair, purulent folliculitis, crusting, often accompanied by lymphadenopathy, due to a zoophilic superficial mycotic species, *Trichophyton verrucosum* or *T mentagrophytes*; geophilic or anthropophilic fungal infections may abruptly become kerions

Keshan disease A disease of children and young women, first described in the Keshan province of the People's Republic of China, due to selenium deficiency in that region's water supply, resulting in dilated cardiomyopathy and increased platelet aggregation due to impaired free radical salvage by glutathione peroxidase **Histopathology** Focal myocardial necrosis, fibrosis and contraction band formation **Treatment** Selenium

Ketoacidosis A syndrome seen in poorly controlled diabetes mellitus, with 'starvation amidst plenty'; despite hyperglycemia, insulin deficiency makes the excess glucose unavailable to the cells and they must rely upon lipid metabolites (ketone bodies) resulting from incomplete lipid metabolism for energy **Clinical** Systemic acidosis, depressed cardiac contractility and vascular response to catecholamines with thready pulse, hypotension, poor organ perfusion and diabetic ketoacidosis may be the presenting sign in previously undiagnosed diabetes mellitus, accompanied by an acute abdomen and a marked leukocytosis **Laboratory** Ketonuria and ketonemia, hyperglycemia, glycosuria, decreased pH and plasma bicarbonate, increased anion gap; hyperlipidemia

Ketone body, ketone One of three organic molecules (acetone, acetoacetate, β-hydroxybutyrate) with a carbonyl group, C=O, designated 'oxo-' in formal nomenclature; formation of ketone bodies is a physiological defense in starvation, in diabetes mellitus and in defective carbohydrate metabolism; in diabetes mellitus, the fatty acid levels are very high, as the lack of insulin prevents glucose utilization, metabolic needs are met by fatty acids; glucagon induces ketogenesis by lowering malonyl CoA, markedly increasing carnitine acyl transferase I activity, translocating fatty acids from the hepatic cytosol into the mitochondria converting them into ketone bodies by β-oxidation, providing energy to the nervous system while sparing proteins **Quantification** Sodium nitroferrico-cyanide reaction; see

Ketoacidosis

Ketorolac tromethamine A non-opioid anti-inflammatory drug with the analgesic equivalence of morphine that does not depress ventilation at analgesic concentrations (Br J Anaesth 1990; 65:445)

17-ketosteroids 'Male' hormones (androsterone, epiandrosterone, dehydroepiandrosterone, etiocholanolone, 11-keto- and 11-β-hydroxyandrosterone, 11-keto- and 11-β-hydroxyetiocholanolone; male urine levels 28-70 μmol/day (US: 8-20 mg/day) reflect adrenocortical and testicular function; female urine levels 21-52 μmol/day (US: 6-15 mg/day) reflect adrenocortical function; 17-ketosteroids are increased in adrenal or testicular tumors or hyperplasias, pregnancy, stress, polycystic ovarian disease and are decreased in primary or secondary adrenal hypofunction, Klinefelter syndrome, castration, hypothyroidism and anorexia nervosa Quantification Colorimetry (Zimmerman reaction), gas-liquid chromatography

Keyhole limpet hemocyanin see KLH

Keyhole sign RADIOLOGY A pseudolesion of the duodenal bulb in which the radiocontrast in an upper gastrointestinal 'series' is trapped within contiguous parallel folds of the duodenal mucosa, a sign that disappears with peristalsis

Key sign TROPICAL MEDICINE Hyperesthesia due to *Trypanosoma brucei gambiense* infection, where the patients are so sensitive to touch that familiar activities, eg locking of doors (which requires the use of keys) are avoided

Khaini cancer A squamous cell carcinoma of the oral cavity seen in men of the Indian states of Uttar Pradesh and Bihar, caused by a non-smoking tobacco habit, where a mixture of slaked lime and tobacco is habitually left in the lower gingivolabial fornix, the site of the malignancy's appearance; see Betel nut chewing

Ki-1 lymphoma see Lymphoma

KIA Kligler iron agar; see Triple iron agar

Kickback HEALTH CARE INDUSTRY A practice in which a person or business pays a person who finds new clients (known as referrals) a percentage of the increased transactions resulting from those referrals; in medicine, this is considered an unethical form of fee-splitting and, when performed in an organized fashion with hospitals and multiple health care providers may result in litigation through the US government's 'anti-kickback' law of 1986, which was written with the intent of stopping this practice in the defense industry (Am Med News 28/Jan/91); Cf Fee-splitting, Finder's fee

Kidney panel A battery of tests that, according to the US form of health care reimbursement (the 'DRGs'), is the most cost-effective in evaluating the kidney's functional status, including albumin, BUN/creatinine, chloride, CO_2 content, creatinine clearance, glucose, potassium, total protein, sodium, 24-hour urinary creatinine and protein; see Organ panel

KID syndrome PEDIATRICS A non-specific term for a trilogy of symptoms (keratitis, ichthyosis and deafness), which when one is identified, should evoke a search for the remaining two

Killed vaccine A vaccine consisting of dead, but antigenically 'active' viruses or bacteria, which are capable of evoking production of protective antibodies without causing disease; killed viruses may consist of whole inactivated organisms, eg pertussis, exotoxins, either alone or linked to a carrier protein, eg tetanus and diphtheria toxoids, soluble capsular components, eg pneumococcal polysaccharide, extracted material, eg hepatitis B (which is no longer used) or various subunits of the organism; Cf Live attenuated vaccine

Killer bee see Africanized bee

Killer cell K cell IMMUNOLOGY A large granular lymphocyte that mediates antibody-dependent cell cytotoxicity and non-complement-mediated cytolysis of IgG-coated target cells, including virus- or tumor- laden self cells **Cytolytic mechanism** Insertion of a transmembrane protein polymer perforin, perforating the target cell's membrane, similar to the insertion of C9 polymers in complement-mediated cytolysis; perforin is stored in 'small dark organelles' and released under appropriate local conditions, but the K cell's own perforin is prevented from polymerization and autoperforation by the proposed protein protectin **Surface markers** Fc receptors; K cell activity is tested by measuring lytic activity against chicken erythrocytes; Cf Cytotoxic T cells, Natural killer cells

'Killer' urine A popular term for the incompletely understood bactericidal effect of urine on bacteria, a function of acid pH, urea and other factors

Kilobase MOLECULAR BIOLOGY A reference unit of 1000 nucleotides on a single RNA or DNA strand, which has a molecular mass of approximately 3300 kD on RNA and for a double DNA strand (kilobase pair) of approximately 6 600 kD; Cf Centimorgan

Kilobyte (Kb) A unit of computer memory equal to 1024 bytes (circa one-half page of written text) that is evolving towards obsolescence; in the microcomputers available in the mid-1970s, random access memory (RAM) began at 16 Kb, floppy diskettes stored 64 Kb of data and hard disks stored 5-10 megabytes (Mb) of data; current microcomputers have 1-128 Mb of RAM, floppy diskettes store 1.2 or more Mb of data and hard drives begin at a modest 40 Mb and reach into gigabyte ranges

Kilodalton (kD) A unit of protein mass, where one dalton or atomic mass unit is equal to one-twelfth the mass of an atom of ^{12}C, weighing 1.661×10^{-24}; a 100 kD protein would have approximately 850 amino acids; Cf Kilobase

Kinase The trivial name for the phosphorylase subclass of transferase enzymes that transfer high-energy phosphates from a donor molecule, eg ATP or GTP to an acceptor molecule (alcohol, carboxyl/acyl, nitrogenous or other phosphate group)

Kinase cascade The intracellular signalling pathway that occurs via protein phosphorylations and dephosphorylations, initiated by a hormonal signal at the cell membrane and amplified by adenylate cyclase, cAMP and kinases

Kindling NEUROLOGY A relatively prolonged reduction in the threshold for depolarization for a given impulse or impulses, that can be evoked by repeated administration of an initally subconvulsive electrical stimulus, leading to progressive intensification of seizure activity, culminating in a generalized seizure; kindling can be induced in most regions of the brain; chemical kindling is relatively selective, GABA antagonists kindle the cortex but not the amygdala; muscarinic agonists kindle the amygdala but not the cortex; kindling may be suppressed with phenobarbital and benzodiazepines and variably reduced with other agents; kindling is linked to drugs of abuse (alcohol, cocaine and to a lesser degree, amphetamines and the phenomenon may explain some of the links between partial seizure complexes, eg temporal lobe epilepsy and their psychiatric symptoms; kindling may cause fatal tonic-clonic seizures in chronic cocaine abusers, induced in the limbic system, especially the amygdala by euphoria and an intermittent stimulus eg procaine or cocaine; see Cocaine

Kinesin PHYSIOLOGY A 'motor' molecule that is a microtubule-activated ATPase composed of two heavy and two light chains, converting the chemical energy from ATP hydrolysis into mechanical force to drive vesicle transport and other forms of microtubule-based motility in endoplasmic reticulum and for mitosis (Science 1990; 249:42), by a 'stroke-release' mechanism (Nature 1990; 348:346, 348, 284)

Kinetochore A specialized region of the chromosome that overlies the centromere, which is critical in mitosis and has two 'motors', one located at a dividing mitotic pole, the other at the chromosome that is regulated by factors that influence phosphorylation (Nature 1991; 351:206, 187)

Kinetoplastida An order of unicellular flagellated protozoa, eg Trematosomatidae (genera ***Trypanosoma, Leishmania, Crithidia***), many of which are people parasites and characterized by the presence of kinetoplasts, which are perinuclear accessory bodies consisting of an enlarged specialized mitochondrial subunit composed of DNA; the high concentration of DNA in the kinetoplast of ***Crithidiae luciliae*** is used as a substrate for the indirect immunofluorescence test for detecting the presence of anti-DNA antibodies in patients with lupus erythematosus

Kingella A genus of non-motile gram-negative, facultative anaerobic rods, normally oropharyngeal saprobes; ***K kingae*** is β-hemolytic and occasionally pathogenic; ***K dinitrificans*** is non-pathogenic but shares many features with ***Neisseria gonorrhoeae***, with which it may be confused

King Kong gel A three foot in length DNA sequencing gel (which by today's standards is very big; currently used gels are 20-30 centimeters) based on the Sanger sequencing method

King Kong peptide A 27 amino acid toxin produced by the cloth of gold cone snail (***Conus textile***), which was so named (Hillyard et al, 1988) as, when it is injected into lobsters, it causes an otherwise subordinate lobster to assume an exaggerated dominant position with bizarre aggressive behavior, a stance fancifully likened to that of King Kong, the venerated Hollywood behemoth; when the King Kong peptide is injected into snails (the cone snail's prey), the victim snail suffers periodic convulsive undulations instead of the normal reaction of retreating within its shell (EMBO J 1990; 9:1015); the peptide's structure or mechanism of action is as yet poorly characterized

King Lear complex PSYCHIATRY Incestuous libido of a father for his daughter Note: The term is a misapplication of the persona of Shakespeare's King Lear, as his was truly paternal love for his daughter, Cordelia ; Cf Electra complex

King's evil Scrofula The lymphadenopathic form of tuberculosis (lymph nodes are the most common extrapulmonary site of tuberculous lesion and are often confined to the cervical region); the appellation derives from the popular belief in the Middle Ages that scrofula was curable by the royal touch

King syndrome An autosomal dominant form of malignant hyperthermia characterized by facial dysmorphia (malar hypoplasia, micrognathia, ptosis, antimongolic slant of palpebral fissures), pectus carinatum, delayed motor development and cryporchidism Note: Malignant hyperthermia may be evoked in these patients by halothane or succinylcholine

Kinin system see Kallikrein-Kinin system

Kinky hair disease of Menke Trichopoliodystrophy An X-linked recessive condition due to defective copper metabolism with excess copper accumulation in certain tissues, eg fibroblasts, kidneys and intestinal mucosa and a relative deficiency of copper in other tissues, eg brain and liver, accompanied by defective copper enzymes, eg lysyl oxidase, tyrosinase; the defects result in arteriopathy (fragmentation of the elastica, intimal thickening), neuropathology (cerebral degeneration with loss of cortical neurons, gliosis and cystic changes), loss of the amorphous elastin of the skin (hypopigmented brittle skin), a relative increase of aortic and cutaneous myofibrils with tortuous blood vessels and occasional vascular occlusion, decrease in collagen and elastin cross-linking (osteoporosis), mitochondria from the brain and muscle have decreased cytochrome oxidase a and a_3 activity; the hair is morphologically similar to the wool of copper-deficient sheep Clinical Failure to thrive, seizures, hypothermia, increased infections, kinky hair (pili torti due to defective disulfide bond formation), seborrheic dermatitis, mental and growth retardation, myoclonic seizures, scurvy-like radiological changes of the long bones, death often occurs in early infancy with progressive neurologic and vascular degeneration; kinky hair also occurs in autosomal dominant trichodento osseous syndrome; Cf Giant axonal neuropathy, Uncombable hair syndrome, Woolly hair disease

'Kissing balloon' coronary angioplasty CARDIOLOGY A technique used in interventional cardiology to treat stenoses of the coronary arteries at bifurcations (which normally have a difficult access); the kissing balloon technique is difficult and unwieldy as it requires two guiding catheters or a single catheter with two long exchange guidewires; the alternate dual probe method allows two balloons to be passed through the same catheter and may improve angioplastic results at bifurcations (Mayo Clin Proc 1989; 64:277,360)

Kissing bug Reduviid bug A cone-nosed hematophagous insect with various hosts in the tropics and subtropics that measures 1-4 cm, 'autumn-colored', the bite of which elicits papules, painful urticaria, hemorrhagic, bullous lesions, occasionally angioedema, anaphylactoid reaction and shock; the bug is also the vector for trypanosoma (Chaga's disease), causing inflammation, atrophy and fibrosis of Auerbach's plexus ganglion cells, resulting in acquired megacolon

Kissing chancre A mirror-image lesion seen in syphilis, caused by autoinoculation due to prolonged apposition ('kissing') of a primarychancre; Cf Kissing ulcer

'Kissing' disease A trivial synonym for infectious mononucleosis, which refers to a common mode of transmission of Epstein-Barr virus (EBV), ie through osculation and salivary exchange; the first contact with EBV occurs in childhood in lower socioeconomic strata and in adolescence whilst osculating in the upper strata; see Epstein-Barr virus, Infectious mononucleosis

Kissing sequestra An articular lesion characterized by extensive denudation of cartilage and joint fusion seen in the resolving phase of tuberculous osteoarthritis, classically located in the knee, accompanied by extensive cortical destruction, in the middle of which are two preserved islands of apposed ('kissing') sclerotic bone, seen on a plain film

Kissing spine A descriptor for the enlarged facets, arches and spinous processes of vertebral bodies in generalized hypertrophic osteoarthritis, seen on a plain spine film

Kissing tumor Infantile digital fibromatosis A tumor of infants affecting the fingers and toes measuring less than 2 cm **Histopathology** Proliferation of poorly-circumscribed fibroblasts with the pathognomonic hyalinoid eosinophilic inclusions seen by PTAH (phosphotungstic acid hematoxylin) or Masson's trichrome stains **Prognosis** Benign, although 60% recur locally

Kissing ulcer Kissing lesion An ulcer seen on an apposing side of the vulva, due to autoinoculation by *Haemophilus ducreyi*, which may be associated with occasionally suppurative (chancroid) lymphadenopathy; see Groove sign; Cf Kissing chancre

'Kiss of death' tests CRITICAL CARE MEDICINE A sobriquet for any laboratory test which, when positive, infers a poor prognosis and may presage a patient's demise, eg a) Lactate levels > 10 mEq/L b) 'LDH6' An abnormal lactic dehydrogenase band that migrates cathodic to the usual LDH isomers (85% mortality) c) Delta osmolality, which when greater than 40 mosm/ml indicates a poor prognosis d) Multifocal atrial tachycardia (43% mortality)

'Kiss of death' surgery A surgical procedure, which under certain clinical conditions, is relatively contraindicated and associated with an increased mortality, eg abdominal surgery during acute pancreatitis has been considered a kiss of death procedure

c-*kit* A proto-oncogene of the tyrosine kinase receptor family that binds to the hematopoietic growth factor SCF, see there

'Kiting' A form of health care fraud in which zeros are added to a physician's prescription for a drug, increasing the quantity of drug or reimbursement; 'kiting' may be performed by a pharmacist who provides the patient with the prescribed quantity of medicine, then 'kites' the bill in order to receive a larger reimbursement from a third party payer, eg Medicaid; 'kiting' by a patient is usually for the purpose of obtaining more of a dependency-type of drug

Kittniere German, putty or cement kidney Calcified, contracted scarred and afunctional kidneys filled with encapsulated, mortar-like or stony masses, surrounded by fibrosed renal pelvis, seen as a 'healed' phase of tuberculosis of the kidneys

Klenow fragment The proteolytic fragment of *Escherichia coli* DNA polymerase I, which has DNA polymerizing and 3'→5' exonuclease activities; it is a well-studied DNA-synthesizing enzyme in terms of high-resolution structural information and a good experimental enzyme for analyzing template-directed DNA synthesis; 2 domains are inferred from the crystal structure, corresponding to the larger -COOH terminal domain with polymerase function and the smaller $-NH_2$ terminal domain with 3',5'-exonuclease function (Science 1988; 240:199)

KLH Keyhole limpet hemocyanin An agent used experimentally to test primary sensitization in delayed cutaneous hypersensitivity

'K Mart model' A state in which the loss of relatively low-paid personnel, eg 'floor' nurses in a hospital is compensated for by increasing the salary of those who remain (J Am Med Assoc 1990; 264:3117)

KNF model see Induced fit model

Knife-and-fork model Kornberg mechanism A fanciful term for an in vitro system used to study DNA replication, which contains DNA ligase, DNA polymerase and endonuclease

Knife-blade atrophy Walnut brain Extreme and global thinning of the gyri of the cerebral cortex seen in the frontal and temporal lobes in Pick's disease; Cf Windswept cortex

Knob Parasitology A specialized red cell membrane modification that allows red cells infected with ***Plasmodium falciparum*** to adhere to the vascular epithelium, resulting in relative blood stasis through less-well oxygenated tissues

Knob sign RADIOLOGY Decreased or lost visualization of the aortic 'knob' on a plain antero-posterior chest film, typical of secondary atelectasis of the left lower lobe of the lung

Knock Pericardial knock A cardiac sound resembling a premature third sound, heard in constrictive pericarditis, accompanied by increased systemic venous pressure, exertional dyspnea, orthopnea, fatigue, ascites and hepatosplenomegaly; Cf Gallop

Knock knees Genu valgum Internal deviation of the knee joint; some degree of 'knock-knee' is present in all children from 2-6 years of age and most autocorrect with time; when marked, the work in walking may fatigue the child, causing pronation, shoe top bulging and medial collapse over the medial longitudinal arch; to compensate for the shift in gravity, the child deviates the foot medially (toe-in) or laterally (toe-out); the degree of knock knee is best determined by measuring the distance between the medial malleoli (ankles); knock-knee may be a congenital component of Ellis-van Creveld syndrome, due to rickets or may occur as a complication of epiphysiodesis

Knock-out drop effect see Mickey Finn

Knots Umbilical cord knots OBSTETRICS False knots of the umbilical cord result from twisting and meandering of the umbilical vein and are of no clinical significance; the umbilical arteries are relatively linear; true knots require that the umbilical cord be sufficiently long to permit the infant to pass through a loop of cord; since the cord is composed of erectile tissue, irreversible cord knotting is rare

Knudsen's theory see One-hit, two-hit model

'Koala bear' syndrome A fanciful synonym for the physiognomy of the autosomal dominant Conradi-Hünermann syndrome in which there is a flat face and nasal bridge, a hypoplastic nose and a mild mongoloid slant that may be accompanied by pulmonary calcifications, mental retardation and right ventricular hypertrophy (Eur J Pediatr 1986; 145:116)

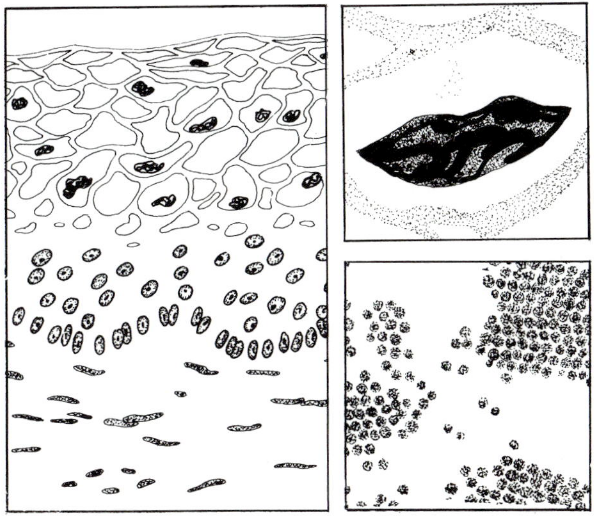

Koilocytosis

Koilocytosis Koilo-, Greek, Hollow A cytological abnormality of the superficial epithelial cells of the uterine cervix, less commonly, of the oropharynx and elsewhere, which is characterized by large cells (koilocytes) with cleared cytoplasmic, pyknotic, rugose nuclear membranes with inconspicuous nucleoli; koilocytosis is induced by human papilloma virus (HPV) infection, ie condyloma acuminata, and while not per se a premalignant lesion, it is typically seen in HPV infection and some serotypes of HPV (types 16 and 18), which are premalignant, its presence should put the clinician on the alert about the possibility of future malignancy; figure demonstrates low-power histology, left, high-power histopathology, upper right and ultrastructure of HPV particles, bottom right; koilocytotic changes may occur in atrophy-related vacuolar degeneration of the cervix, as seen in menopause, or occur in non-HPV infections, including trichomoniasis, *Gardnerella vaginalis* and candidiasis

Konzo A distinct upper motor neuron spastic paraparesis described in Africa due to cyanide poisoning, related to consumption of high-carbohydrate cassava, which a) In droughts produces more cyanogenic glycosides and b) Due to the food shortage, causes the food manufacturers to take short-cuts in the steps designed to remove the cyanide (Brain 1990; 113:223)

Korean hemorrhagic fever Hemorrhagic fever with renal syndrome A condition seen in Central and Far Eastern Asia, caused by a Bunyavirus, the Hantavirus, isolated in the Hantaan river, acquired through aerosolized rodent feces and urine (*Rattus rattus, Apodemus agrarius, Clethrionomys glariolus, Microtiae*); in China, 100 000 cases are reported/year and are thought to be increasing in number Clinical Fever, flushing, edema, petechiae, conjunctivitis, headache, aches/pains, thrombocytopenia and renal tubular dysfunction, ranging from mild proteinuria to transient anuria; the mortality rate may be determined by the rodent vector itself, *Apodemus*-associated infections (3-7% mortality) appear worse than the so-called nephropathia epidemica, which has a vole (*Clethrionomys*) vector Diagnosis IgM is measured by ELISA, indirect immunofluorescence assay and plaque reduction neutralization assay (J Am Med Assoc 1988; 259:1622)

Koro A sociocultural desomatization complex, described in Malaysia, in which the subject attempts to counteract a fear that his penis is shrinking and disappearing within his body by tying the penis to the outside of his body with various devices; ; Cf Piblokto

Korotkov sounds CARDIOLOGY Low frequency vibrations (< 200 mHz) originating in vascular walls and heard distal to cuff compression of a peripheral artery, subdivided into: An initial or transient murmur (opening tap) and a compression murmur (rumble); evaluation of Korotkov sounds was a crude and subjective method for determining the severity of occlusive peripheral arterial disease, having had its heyday in the pre-Doppler era

kpn family A family of intermediate-sized repeated fragments of DNA, measuring less than 6 kilobases in length, so called as they result from kpn I restriction enzyme digestion

Kraurosis vulvae Lichen sclerosis (et atrophicans) GYNECOLOGY A lesion of older, often post-menopausal women, more common in whites, that may have a vague genetic component in a background of autoimmunity; this lesion in men is known as balanitis xerotica obliterans Histopathology Blunting or loss of the rete ridges with homogenization of the upper dermis with loss of melanocytes, occasionally hyperkeratosis and mild epithelial atypia; it is not considered a premalignant lesion

Krazy glue™ Ethyl-2-cyanoacrylate A commercial 'superadhesive' that is also used as a surgical adhesive; compared to longer chain cyanoacrylate derivatives, eg butyl-2-cyanoacrylate, Histoacryl, Krazy glue is thought to evoke greater histotoxicity in the form of seromas, acute inflammation, necrosis and foreign-body giant cell reaction (Arch Otolaryngol Head Neck Surg 1990; 116:546)

Krebs' carcinoma A transplantable anaplastic carcinoma of mice, probably arising in the mammary gland

Bay region

Benzo(a)pyrene **K region**

K region MOLECULAR BIOLOGY A region of benzo(a)pyrene, an aromatic hydrocarbon with potent carcinogenic effects; the metabolic system, cytochrome P-450 can 'choose' two routes of metabolism for this molecule—one that results in a highly electrophilic (ie carcinogenic) diol-epoxide, a reaction centering around the opposite face of the molecule, the 'Bay' region, and the other which acts at the K region, leading to the non-carcinogenic 4,5-dihydrodiol, lending support to the model of carcinogenesis as defective DNA repair

'Krimsky index' An informal system delineated by a Dr Krimsky of Tufts University as a measure of an academic department's non-academic ties and potential for 'conflict of interest', calculated as the number of faculty members with commercial ties divided by the total number of faculty members (Science 1990; 248:152); see CRADA

Kringle MOLECULAR BIOLOGY A triple-looped, disulfide-linked protein domain (figure) that is involved in binding membranes, proteins and phospholipids and in regulating proteolysis; the kringle is a common structural motif, so-named for its resemblance to the kringler, a Danish pastry and is present in coagulation-related and fibrinolytic proteins and other plasma proteinases, eg tissue plasminogen activator (t-PA, N Engl J Med 1988; 319:926), urokinase and apolipoprotein A (possibly explaining the increased coagulation seen in atherosclerosis) and may be present in multiple copy numbers, eg apolipoprotein-A has up to 37 kringle domains, while t-PA has five

KUB Kidneys ureters bladder UROLOGY A colloquialism for a plain, ie without radiocontrast, antero-posterior film of the abdomen, used as a crude method for detecting nephroliths (kidney stones); the KUB film may be used as a 'scout' examination prior to performing the more definitive intravenous pyelogram

Kulchitsky cell An enterochromaffin, ie one containing neurosecretory granules that is native to the respiratory tract, produces bombesin, vasoactive intestinal polypeptide and leu-enkephalin, and gives rise to bronchial adenoma, pulmonary carcinoid (tumorlet), oat cell carcinoma (of the lung and elsewhere), APUDomas, sugar tumor; Kulchitsky cell tumors may be subdivided into typical, atypical and small-cell carcinoids (Cancer 1985; 55:1301); see Carcinoid, Dense core granules

Kurtosis STATISTICS A measurement of the degree to which a one-dimension probability curve with a gaussian distribution of data is concentrated in a single peak; if the peak is flat, it is 'platykurtic', if sharp, 'leptokurtic'

Kuru New Guinea dialect, Trembling with fear A subacute spongiform encephalopathy, recently recognized as being induced by a prion, see there; kuru was responsible for the deaths of 90% of females in the once cannibalistic Fore tribe of New Guinea (females were most affected as they prepared and ate the infected brains) **Clinical** Cerebellar ataxia, shivering tremors, dysarthria, progressing to complete motor paralysis and death in 3-9 months due to infection or malnutrition; the disease may terminate with uncontrollable, compulsive laughter (known as a 'laughing death') **Histopathology** Spongiform encephalopathy, cytoplasmic vacuolization of neurons, especially of the striatum and cerebellum; the kuru plaques are positive with a periodic acid Schiff/diastase staining reaction Note: Kuru symptoms have been induced in primates after a 20 year latency

Kuskokwim syndrome An autosomal recessive form of arthrogryposis described in Alaskan Eskimos, who due to the early onset of impaired movement and joint contractures, waddle like ducks

Kwashiorkor Protein malnutrition often associated with marginally adequate caloric intake, occurring in African children weaned from the 'high-octane' protein-rich maternal milk and fed protein-poor cereals, cassava and

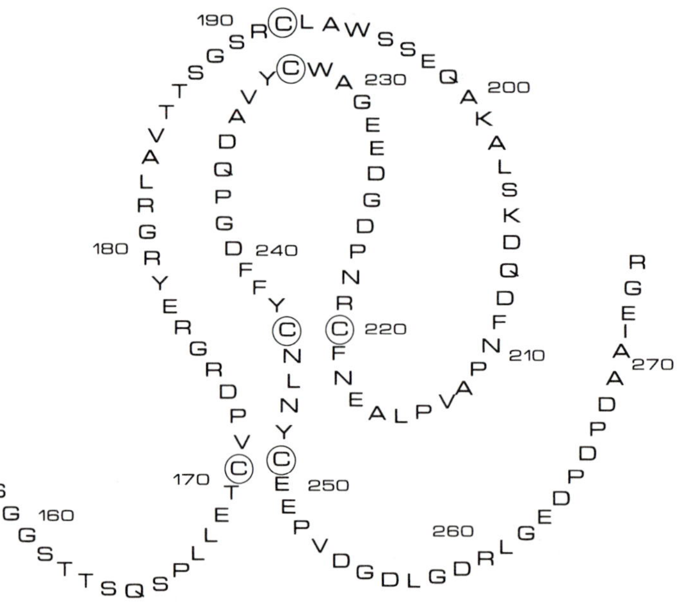

Kringle domain

sweet potatoes **Clinical** Pitting edema, massive ascites, retarded growth, apathy, skin rashes, dry skin with desquamation and ulcers, hepatomegaly, anorexia, diarrhea, decreased size of the heart and kidneys **Histopathology** Severely flattened, small intestinal villi may be due to coincident infection and not Kwashiorkor per se **Laboratory** Anemia, decreased hematocrit, blood volume, decreased albumin Note: In the Gia dialect of Ghana, kwashiorkor translates as 'deposed child' or *'THE SICKNESS OLDER CHILD GETS WHEN NEXT CHILD IS DUE'* (as the child's weaning results in the deterioration in the quality of nutrition; in another dialect, kwashiorkor translates as 'red-boy' since the afflicted children often have reddish hair **Treatment** Succotash, dietary mixture that provides all the deficient amino acids Note: Marasmus, kwashiorkor's cousin, is a global decrease of proteins and carbohydrates

Kyasanur forest disease A tick-born flaviviral disease of the Mysore and Karnataka states of India, maintained by infected monkeys and rodents; those living in wooded farmlands are at the highest risk **Clinical** High fever, myalgia, prostration, enteric, uterine or pulmonary hemorrhage, meningismus, leukopenia, thrombocytopenia, albuminuria **Diagnosis** Isolation of virus from blood, complement fixation **Prognosis** 5-10% mortality

L Symbol for: Liter (USA); Lambert, a unit of luminance or photometric brightness; Leucine; levorotatory

L- A descriptive prefix to indicate one of two entantiomeric forms of optically active organic compounds (sugars and amino acids), the mirror image is the D-entantiomer

l Symbol for: Length; Liter (International System)

'Ls of dermatology, the 5' A group of skin lesions associated with dense patchy infiltrates of upper dermal lymphocytes, including lupus erythematosus, lymphoma, pseudolymphoma of Spiegler-Fendt, polymorphous light eruption of plaque type, Jessner's lymphocytic infiltration; other dermal lymphocytic infiltrates include actinic reticulosis, angioimmunoblastic lymphadenopathy, arthropod bites, lymphomatoid papulosis, phenytoin-induced drug eruption

Label A marker, eg an enzyme or a radioactive isotope of a normal molecule, eg ^{35}P that replaces a non-radioactive ^{32}P, which is used to mark or indicate the presence of a protein or molecule of interest, by one of a variety of identification systems, eg immunoperoxidase staining or radioimmunoassay

Labeling index A measurement of the mitotic activity of a cell population, defined as the number of cells in the S phase of the growth cycle divided by the total cells in the population

Labor Parturition Expulsion of a conceptus from the uterus via the cervix and vagina, the onset of which is triggered by oxytocin, released from the posterior hypophysis **PRECIPITATE LABOR** Parturition of less than three hours in duration in a primigravida **PROLONGED LABOR** Parturition of greater than 24 hours in duration in a primigravida **FALSE LABOR** Parturition that results from disordered uterine action where regular painful contractions are not accompanied by effacement or dilation of the cervix that may either cease or be followed by the onset of true labor

Laboratory information system (LIS) A 'dedicated' computer, often a minicomputer that controls the flow of various data through the laboratory; the capacity required of an LIS is a function of a) The type of instruments the system supports, noting that the computer must convert an instrument's analog data to digital data b) The type of communication the computer must provide with the rest of the hospital in the form of direct communication with the 'floor', patient billing, admitting and discharge and elsewhere c) The need for long-term information storage and retrieval d) The needs for statistical analysis in terms of quality control and quality assurance and, perhaps most importantly, e) The number of laboratory sections, eg chemistry, hematology, microbiology and blood bank, and the number of instruments being served Note: Most LISs do not integrate blood bank modules given the potential danger to a patient of lost data regarding, for example, the presence of life-threatening antibodies or rare blood types, or the potential liability to the hospital if a unit of autologous blood donated pre-operatively, is 'lost' and a random packed red cell unit is transfused to the patient during surgery; the anatomic (cytology and surgical) pathology section is also less commonly integrated in the LIS, as pathology deals with a limited number of the patients admitted to the hospital, requires relative self-containment of information and is 'text-intensive', rather than data intensive; see Computers; Cf Hospital information system

'Lab rat' A highly colloquial term referring to a graduate student or 'post-doc' dedicated to bench research to the virtual exclusion of a personal and family life, who may be acting out an idealized fantasy or image of a dedicated scientist; because 'lab rats' may be ostracized for their social ineptness and lack of 'political savvy', they are often ill-equipped to address the realities of practicing science in the 1990s, which requires organization, social graces and political skills; see Gentleman scientist, 'New scientist'

Labrea hepatitis A form of hepatitis seen in South America characterized by massive hepatic necrosis and steatosis, thought to be caused by either hepatitis delta or by intoxication with rotenone, a toxic plant (*Deris negrensis* and others) found along the Amazonian river banks (J Am Med Assoc 1988; 259:3559c)

Labyrinth The internal ear, the essential organ of hearing and the final destination of the vestibulocochlear nerve, is composed of the membranous labyrinth, a series of communicating membranous sacs and ducts, separated from the bony labyrinth by the perilymph (fluid), both of which lie within the petrous portion of the temporal bone

Lace-like appearance see Lacy appearance

LACI see Lipoprotein-associated coagulation inhibitor

***lac* operon** A complex of three *Escherichia coli* genes that encode the enzymes involved in lactose metabolism: β-galactosidase, β-galactosidase transport protein and β-galactosidase transacetylase; the *lac* operon has proven to be a useful experimental system for deciphering the mechanisms of gene regulation

Lacquer crack appearance OPHTHALMOLOGY A pattern in the optic fundus characterized by branching clefts in the lamina vitrea (figure) with choroidal atrophy seen in progressive myopia

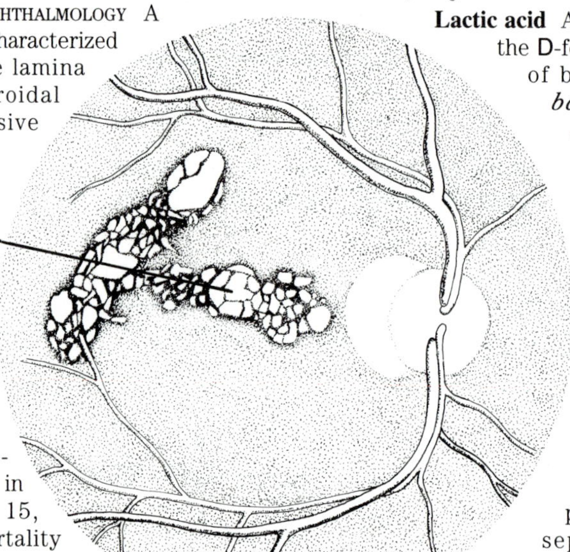

Lacquer crack appearance

La Crosse encephalitis The most common form of the mosquito-born California encephalitis Vector *Aedes triseriatus*, which breeds in old tires and small puddles Agent Bunyavirus Clinical Summer-fall epileptiform meningoencephalitis in children under age 15, male:female ratio, 2:1, mortality less than 1%

α-Lactalbumin A protein found only in milk; the amino acid composition of lactalbumin is considered ideal for humans and thus is a standard used in evaluating all protein substitutes in the diet

Lactase deficiency β-D-galactosidase deficiency Lactose intolerance syndrome A condition that is either congenital and common in non-Caucasians or acquired, due to a deficiency of lactase on the intestinal brush borders Clinical Cramps, bloating, flatulence, inability to metabolize disaccharides (resulting in osmotic diuresis, diarrhea and acidic stools) Diagnosis Lactose tolerance test, in conjunction with a glucose tolerance test Treatment Symptomatic, lactose restriction

Lactate dehydrogenase (LD) CARDIOLOGY A hydrogen transferase present in the cytoplasm of all cells, consisting of an enzyme tetramer composed of two different 34 kD subunits, H (heart) and M (muscle), which are separable by electrophoresis; the HHHH tetramer (LD_1) is the most rapidly migrating or anodic fraction and has a mobility similar to α_1 globulin; the slowest migrating or cathodic fraction is composed of the MMMM tetramer (LD_5) and migrates to the gamma (γ) region in a serum protein electrophoretic gel; there are thus five LD isoenzymes; after the total LD is measured as a screen for the presence of non-specific enzyme abnormalities, the serum is then separated by electrophoresis into isoenzyme fractions, localizing the abnormality to a particular tissue; total LD is markedly increased in myocardial infarction, megaloblastic anemia and severe hypoxia, moderately increased in myelocytic leukemia, hemolytic anemia and minimally increased in liver disease (hepatitis, obstructive jaundice, cirrhosis, delirium tremens); LD_1 is classically increased in myocardial infarcts, peaking by the fourth post-infarct day; abnormal LD bands occur when serum proteins complex with isoenzymes, seen in 25% of tested patients with cirrhosis and these LD-IgG complexes may be associated with shock (cardiogenic, septic or hemorrhagic) and a concomitant increase of LD_5; see Flipped LD, LD_6

Lactic acid A glycolytic product from lactose; the D-form is produced by some genera of bacteria, eg *Listeria, Lactobacillus, Erysipelothrix* and *Streptococcus*, the DL racemic mix is produced in sour milk and stomach and the L-form is an end-product of anaerobic glucose metabolism that is increased in congenital, eg glycogen storage disease and acquired conditions, either in physiologic, eg strenuous exercise or pathologic conditions, eg hypoxia with decreased clearance in hepatic failure, cardiac decompensation, respiratory failure, septicemia, glycogen storage disease, oral hypoglycemic agents, eg phenformin, infarction and neoplasia Laboratory Decreased bicarbonate and pH, increased anion gap and PO_4

Lactoferrin A non-specific immunoprotective protein found in milk and neutrophil granules that binds iron molecules, making them unavailable to bacteria that may be lurking about

Lacto-ovo vegetarian A vegetarian who eats non-flesh animal protein including eggs and dairy products; Cf Vegan vegetarian

Lactose Milk sugar A reducing disaccharide composed of D-galactose and D-glucose, synthesized by the mammary glands

Lactulose A synthetic disaccharide, used to treat hepatic encephalopathy, administered per os, acting as a laxative, reducing intraluminal NH_3, which via the extracellular fluid, reduces NH_3 in the blood

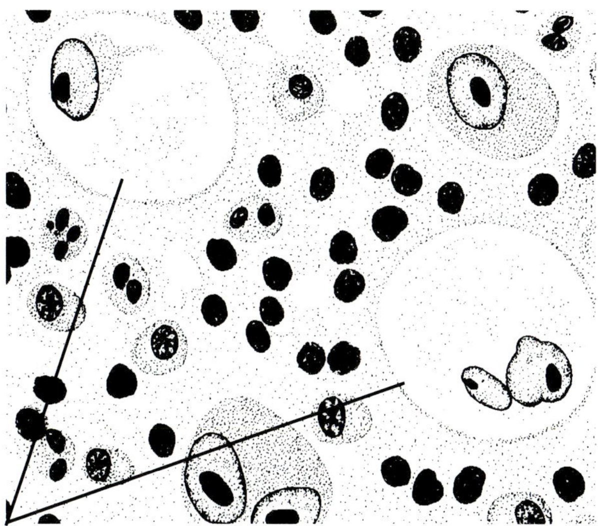

Lacunar cells

Lacunar cell An enlarged, 40-50 µm in diameter Reed-Sternberg cell variant, which has a polylobated nucleus, lacy chromatin and one or more variably sized nucleoli, is surrounded by a rim of clear to eosinophilic cytoplasm and is located in clear lacunae that are thought to be an artefact of formalin fixation; lacunar cells were first described in nodular sclerosing Hodgkin's disease, but may occur in aggregates in the other types of Hodgkin's disease; similar cells are seen in undifferentiated nasopharyngeal carcinoma; in the accompanying figure, a classic Reed-Sternberg cell (RS) is seen at 6 o'clock and a mononuclear RS cell is present at 1 o'clock; Cf Popcorn cell

Lacunar infarcts NEUROPATHOLOGY Multiple small cerebral infarcts in the corona radiata, internal capsule, striatum, thalamus, basis pontis, cerebellum, occasionally preceded by transient symptoms, see Lacunar state; the infarcts are due to involvement of the penetrating branches of the middle and posterior cerebral and median branches of the basilar arteries; resolution of infarcts is characterized by residual 1-3 mm cavities or lacunae, characteristic of long-standing hypertension; see Multi-infarct dementia

Lacunar skull A skull, the diploë of which is characterized by irregular rarefactions or shadowy depressions and a smooth outer contour, seenradiologically over the fronto-parietal region in 50% of those with meningocele or meningomyelocele, which may be complicated by hydrocephalus; the area is lined by dura and bordered by osseous tissue; the entire bony skull becomes attenuated and the lacunae disappear upon separation of the cranial sutures Note: This is identical to that of the 'beaten brass' appearance and separation between the two is of dubious utility; Cf 'Punched-out' lesions

Lacunar state État lacunaire NEUROLOGY A clinicopathological nosology characterized by multiple minute infarcts (lacunes) in the basal ganglia, often seen in severe hypertension; when numerous, the lacunar state causes dementia or a lacunar 'syndrome' **Clinical** Loss of recent memory, altered time-space orientation, paranoia, headache, vertigo, giddiness, convulsions; the focal nature of the infarcts explains various neurological defects including homolateral cerebellar ataxia, isolated hemiplegia, pure segmental sensory stroke and dysarthria-clumsy hand syndrome **Neuropathology** Multiple small infarcts associated with fibrinoid degeneration and lipohyalinosis of small penetrating vessels of the basal ganglia, internal capsule, thalamus and pons

Lacy appearance MICROBIOLOGY A descriptor for the delicate, filigreed pattern that contaminating fungi impart on a Thayer-Martin (***Neisseria***) agar plate BONE RADIOLOGY A descriptor for the coarsely trabeculated shadows seen in the long bones in secondary syphilis, corresponding to gumma and syphilitic periostitis, a term also used for subperiosteal bone resorption and loss of the cortical definition, seen in early hyperparathyroidism or chronic osteomyelitis; when marked, the bony resorption is said to have a 'scooped-out' appearance with trabeculation and radiolucency of the medullary cavity; Cf Ground-glass appearance, Veiled appearance

Laddergram CARDIOLOGY A schematic method used to analyze complex arrhythmias in which a simple rhythm strip from a standard electrocardiogram is subdivided into an A (atrial) line, an A-V (atrio-ventricular junction) line and a V (ventricular) line; the lines representing conduction are diagrammed under the actual tracing and accurately drawn so that the 'A' line begins at the P wave and the 'V' line at the beginning of the QRS; ladder diagrams were first described in 1896 by Engelmann to explain cardiac tracings inscribed by the electrocardiograph

Ladder pattern CLINICAL TOXICOLOGY A characteristic linear serrated wheal produced by the adherent tentacles of the box jellyfish (***Chironex fleckeri*** and ***Chiropsolmus quadrigatus***), coelenterates native to the Pacific basin PEDIATRICS A clinical sign seen on the abdominal wall in children with obstruction of the lower gastrointestinal tract, seen as parallel loops of distended small intestine, causing a 'stepped' pattern

Ladder sequencing MOLECULAR BIOLOGY Any method, eg those delineated by Sanger or Maxam and Gilbert, where the sequence of the nucleotides in a nucleic acid is read from the step-like bands in an electrophoretic gel, fancifully likened to a ladder

LADS see Leukocyte adhesion deficiency syndrome

'Lady Godiva syndrome' A fanciful, albeit incorrect synonym for exhibitionism, which unlike Lady Godiva's threadless equestrian peregrination through Coventry, decrying her husband's excess taxes of the citizens, is considered a lascivious act; see Sexual deviancy

Laennec's cirrhosis Nutritional cirrhosis Portal cirrhosis A clinicopathologic entity which (usually) evolves from the early lesion of alcoholic fatty liver, in which the liver is 'greasy' and weighs up to three kg, with intact lobules and veins, portal infiltration by neutrophils and prominent Mallory body formation to the end-stage alcoholic cirrhosis, characterized by collapse, bile duct proliferation, hemosiderin deposition, in which the liver is fibrotic and shrunken, weighing less than one kilogram; 'classic' cirrhosis is defined by the histopathologic triad of 1) Diffuse fibrosis with lobular collapse 2) Regenerative nodules of hepatocytes and bile duct proliferation and 3) Hepatocellular necrosis (and mild hemosiderin deposition); Cf Micro-micronodular cirrhosis

Laetrile 1-Mandelonitrile-β-glucuronic acid Amygdalin 'Vitamin B-17' A preparation from apricot pits that is high in cyanide and claimed to be effective in treating cancer; the use of laetrile arises from a modernization of the 'Trophoblastic theory of cancer' espoused by the Scottish zoologist and embryologist, James Beard (1857-1924); laetrile has no proven effect in cancer treatment, and is alleged to have been associated with a number of cancer-related deaths; the agent was named by its discover, ET Krebs, as it is levo-rotatory (left-handed) and amygdalin is chemically a mandelonitrile; see Manner cocktail, Tijuana

Lager syndrome see Concentration camp syndrome

Lagging strand see Replication

Lag phase BURN PHYSIOLOGY The earliest phase (first 12 hours) of wound healing, preceding histopathological changes, a period during which chemical mediators of inflammation, eg arachidonic acid metabolites, cytokines, kinins and edema accumulate in the burn site(s) EMERGENCY MEDICINE The period between the time a person is exposed to a toxic inhalant, eg cadmium fumes, dimethyl sulfate, methyl bromide, ozone, nitrogen oxides, phosgene, phosphorus compounds and others and development of pulmonary edema, a period lasting up to 12 hours MICROBIOLOGY The period prior to the logarithmic growth phase where the bacteria are too busy gearing up their enzymatic machinery (producing macromolecules, eg proteins and ribosomes) to proliferate

Lai tai see Sudden unexplained nocturnal death

LAK cells Lymphokine-activated killer cells; see IL-2/LAK cells

Lake Nyos ENVIRONMENT A crater lake in the Northwest Province of Cameroon, which in 1986, was the site of a massive natural release of CO_2 gas, causing an estimated 1700 deaths; the lake contains 300 million cubic meters of CO_2 gas that is increasing at a rate of 5 million annually, another disaster may occur at any time (Nature 1990; 348:201c)

Lake Tahoe mystery disease see Chronic fatigue syndrome

LAM-1 Leukocyte adhesion molecule A membrane protein with a 'homing' function, related to its lectin-like domain that binds specific glycoconjugates on target cells, regulating leukocyte migration by mediating the binding of lymphocytes to high endothelial venules and binding of neutrophils to endothelium in sites of inflammation (Nature 1991; 349:691); see Selectins

Lamarckism A philosophy advanced by French naturalist JP Lamarck in 1809, which holds that phenotypic adaption, eg hypertrophy or atrophy, made during an organism's lifetime could be imprinted on the genome, a posit that is diametrically opposed to mendelian genetics, which may be supported by the phenomenon of DNA methylation; see Imprinting, Lysenkoism, Methylation

Lamaze technique OBSTETRICS A program of instruction and orientation towards an uncomplicated vaginal delivery with participation of the father or 'significant other', teaching the mother how to breathe and relax during parturition, thereby reducing the anxiety associated therewith and the amount of anesthesia required for women delivering their first child; see Doula, Midwifes, Natural childbirth

Lambda (λ) Symbol for: Wavelength; Decay constant; Immunoglobulin light chain

Lambda bacteriophage Lambda vector MOLECULAR BIOLOGY A DNA virus with affinity for ***Escherichia coli*** which, once inside the host, either directs the production of phage particles, causing bacteriolysis or integrates itself into the genome, with the phage dividing in tandem with the host ***E coli*** genome; the lambda phage has proven a good model forstudying protein-DNA interactions; see Bacteriophages

Lambda chain One of two immunoglobulin light chains, the normal lambda to kappa light chain ratio is 2:1

Lambda waves Sharp, low amplitude EEG waves in the occipital region in non-REM sleep and in newborn children; of no known significance

LAMB syndrome Carney's complex A clinical triad of young adults, consisting of spotty mucocutaneous lentigenes, cutaneous and cardiac myxomas, endocrine hyperactivity, as well as multifocal myxoidfibroadenomas of the breast, adrenocortical hyperplasia and calcifying Sertoli cell tumors of the testes

Lamellar body Myelinoid body Myelin figure A non-specific descriptive term for concentrically layered, fingerprint-like, osmiophilic material derived from membranes and organelles, eg the endoplasmic reticulum, seen by electron microscopy DERMATOPATHOLOGY Lamellar or Odland bodies or keratinosomes are seen by electron microscopy in the stratum spinosum and in the intercellular spaces; although their function is not known, they may play a role in keratinization and are increased in lamellar ichthyosis HEMATOPATHOLOGY see Ribosomal

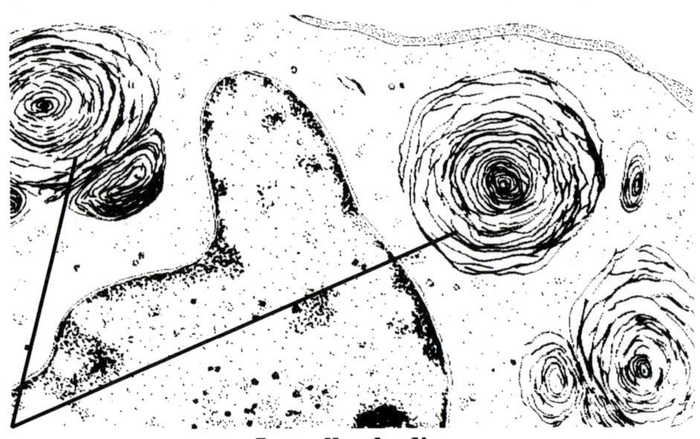

Lamellar bodies

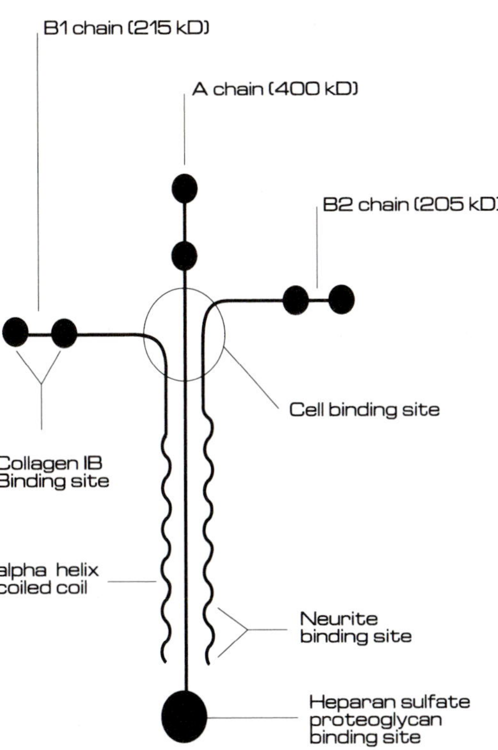

Laminin

lamellar complexes PULMONARY PATHOLOGY Lamellar bodies are membrane-bound layered material seen by electron microscopy (figure, facing page), corresponding to surfactant, a normal product of type II pneumocytes that is increased in interstitial lung diseases (desquamative interstitial pneumonitis, usual interstitial pneumonitis and diffuse alveolar damage), primary pulmonary proteinosis, pulmonary toxicity (methotrexate, bleomycin, cytoxan, busulfan), type II glycogen storage disease, cystic fibrosis, bronchoalveolar cell carcinoma and diffuse pleural mesothelioma Note: Lamellated structures have been seen by electron microscopy in the adrenal cortex related to spironolactone therapy, in the liver secondary to phenobarbital therapy, in the proximal renal tubules in gentamicin- and aminoglycoside-induced nephropathy, in uteri with intrauterine devices and in normal oocytes and neurons; by light microscopy, lamellar bodies correspond to concentrically laminated lipoprotein-phosphatide complexes with increased uptake of H_2O, ceroid, seen in the autophagic vacuoles of Fabry's disease, granular cell tumors, malignant fibrous histiocytoma and spermatocytic seminoma

Lamin(s) A fibrous protein of the intermediate filament family, divided into lamins A, B and C, which form a two-dimensional network on the inner face of the nuclear membrane, binding DNA in the nucleoplasm; lamin phosphorylation by a kinase triggers disassembly of the nucleus and condensation of chromatin at the time of mitosis; see Intermediate filaments

Laminectomy ORTHOPEDIC SURGERY A procedure for treating herniation of an intervertebral disk; the 'classic' laminectomy entails removal of the entire lamina of a vertebral body; the permutations of the procedure depend on the case and the field of exposure desired by operator **LAMINOTOMY** (FENESTRATION) Removal of a portion of the superior and inferior aspects of the lamina adjacent to the diseased disk **HEMILAMINECTOMY** Unilateral excision of the lamina with removal of variable parts of the adjacent facet **LAMINECTOMY** Bilateral removal of the lamina as well as varying portions of both facets **MICROSURGICAL LAMINECTOMY** (DISKECTOMY) A technique that avoids vertebral exploration prior to disk surgery, reducing the risk of the feared 'Failed disk syndrome' as there is minimal excision of bone and epidural fat and minimal nerve root adhesion (J Am Med Assoc 1990; 264:1469DATTA)

Laminin CELL BIOLOGY An 820 kD basement membrane glycoprotein of the integrin receptor family that has a cruciform structure (deduced by 'rotary shadowing'), and has binding sites for Type IV collagen, heparin sulfate proteoglycan and surface receptors of normal and malignant cells; laminin promotes cell attachment and migration, and plays a role in differentiation and metastasis; it is produced by macrophages, endothelial, epithelial and Schwann cells, and appears as early as the morular stage of the embryo, serving as the 'glue' for the primitive endothe-lium, epithelium and meso-thelium; soluble laminin fragments have theoretic currency in preventing the attachment of malignant cells

Laminin receptor A heterodimeric membrane-bound protein composed of a large subunit joined by a disulfide bond to a small subunit; laminin receptor functions include cell attachment and neurite outgrowth; structural motifs of the laminin receptor are shared by other integrins, eg fibronectin and vitronectin

Lampbrush chromosome A large amphibian chromosome with expanded, mitotically paired chromosomes that are transiently expressed in the early prophase (diplotene stage) of meiosis of spermatocytes and oocytes; lampbrushes are very active in RNA synthesis, with 'innumerable' very long loops of chromatin covered by newly transcribed RNA packed in dense RNA-protein complexes; these loops, like polytene puffs, correspond to fixed units of folded chromatin that are opened up and transcriptionally active, a transition that requires topoisomerase II, without which the cell cannot replicate; the lampbrush and supercoiled DNA chromosomal conformations are seen by Dapey stain; Cf Feather pattern

LAN see Local area network

'L&D' Labor and Delivery A commonly used colloquialism for the obstetric unit of North American hospitals

Landmark article An article or abstract in a scientific journal that is considered by the workers in a field to have been a seminal study or to have had substantial impact on that area of knowledge, eg Banting and Best's *THE INTERNAL SECRETIONS OF THE PANCREAS* (J Lab Clin Med 1922; 7:251), JW Conn's *PRIMARY ALDOSTERONISM, A NEW CLINICAL SYNDROME* (J Lab Clin Med 1955; 45:3) and RF Schilling's *INTRINSIC FACTOR STUDIES II. THE EFFECT OF GASTRIC JUICE ON THE URINARY EXCRETION OF RADIOACTIVITY*

AFTER THE ORAL ADMINISTRATION OF RADIOACTIVE VITAMIN B_{12} (J Lab Clin Med 1953; 42:860); like citation classics, landmark articles are benchmarks of original work with potential for a Nobel prize; see Citation classic, 'Hot paper'; Cf Uncitedness index

Lane LABORATORY TECHNOLOGY A 'corridor' in an electrophoretic support medium, eg agar gel or paper, at the beginning of which is a well or point on which a fluid containing a molecule of interest is 'spotted', after which the support is subjected to a unidirectional electric current, causing the molecular migration within the lane and separation into 'bands' according to size

Langerhans' cell Dendritic reticulum cell A specialized macrophage that presents antigen to lymphocytes in the upper dermis at the suprabasilar layer, which sends dendritic processes both to the granular layer and to the basal lamina Note: Paul Langerhan (1847-1888) described the cell while a medical student under Virchow in Berlin

Langerhans' granules see Tennis racquet granule

Langerhans, islets of Nests of pancreatic endocrine cells, more numerous in the tail, invested with a well-developed capillary network, composed of a) α cells, comprising 20% of islet cells, which produce glucagon, b) β cells, 70% of total, which produce insulin and c) delta cells, 10% of thecells, which produce somatostatin

Langhans' giant cell A giant cell composed of fused epithelioid histiocytes, whose multiple (up to 50) nuclei are arranged in a garland-like fashion, surrounding glassy cytoplasm; when accompanied by caseating necrosis, the Langhans' giant cell is virtually diagnostic for tuberculosis, but may be seen in other contexts in secondary syphilis (T Langhans, Swiss pathologist 1839-1915)

LAP 1) Leukocyte alkaline phosphatase, Neutrophil alkaline phosphatase A phosphomonoesterase with optimal activity at pH 10.0 that is concentrated in granules of normal neutrophils; LAP is decreased in chronic myeloid leukemia, paroxysmal nocturnal hemoglobinuria, idiopathic thrombocytopenic purpura, infectious mononucleosis and aplastic anemia; LAP is increased in chronic myeloid leukemia in remission, polycythemia vera, Hodgkin's disease, myeloid metaplasia, corticosteroid therapy and pregnancy 2) see Leucine aminopeptidase

Laparoscopic cholecystectomy A minimally invasive technique for removing the gallbladder, in which the entire procedure is performed through the laparascope, with an average in-hospital stay of 1.2 days, in contrast to the usual 5.6 days; 5% of cases in one series needed conversion to an open cholecystectomy due to anatomic variations Complications 5%, versus 6-21% in conventional cholecystectomy (N Engl J Med 1991; 324:1073)

Lap traveler PUBLIC HEALTH A child travelling in an automobile seated on an adult's lap and who is not restrained in an infant or car-seat; often the person holding the child will survive as they are cushioned from the dashboard injuries by the child who dies; in older statistics, up to 40% of infants who died in automobile accidents were lap-travellers; see MVA

Lardaceous spleen A spleen with diffuse amyloidosis, where there is prominent red pulp involvement of a firm enlarged spleen, the cut surface of which is waxy and translucent; Cf Sago spleen

Large cell undifferentiated carcinoma of lung A pleomorphic aggressive carcinoma that is considered a poorly differentiated squamous cell carcinoma, adenocarcinoma or small cell carcinoma; the lesions may be associated with marked peripheral eosinophilia or leukocytosis Clinical Similar to pulmonary adenocarcinoma in that 50% metastasize to the brain; if more than 40% of the cells are 'giant', it is designated giant cell carcinoma and has a very poor prognosis, with an average survivial of less than one year

Lariat MOLECULAR BIOLOGY An intermediate structural motif arising in the pre-mRNA splicing reaction, consisting of a novel 2"-5' phosphodiester bond that enables one adenosine nucleotide to formphosphodiester links with three other nucleotides rather than the ususal two, resulting in a branched intermediate, which is followed by 3' splice-site cleavage (intron excision), ligation of the exons and freeing of the lariat structure

Larva currens An infestation by female larva of ***Strongyloides stercoralis*** that penetrate the skin, causing intense, transient pruritus and urticaria; see Hyperinfection syndrome

Larva migrans Human infestation by non-human nematodes that penetrate but cannot complete their life cycle in man CUTANEOUS LARVA MIGRANS results from the dog and cat hookworm, ***Ancylostoma braziliense***, the larvae of which migrate a few millimeters/day, producing pruritic serpiginous tracks in the stratum germinatum that are visible below the skin VISCERAL LARVA MIGRANS is due to the dog (***Toxocara canis***) or cat parasites (***T cati***), the life cycles of which in their usual hosts resemble that of ***Ascaris lumbricoides*** in humans; in this form, the embryonated eggs are accidentally ingested and hatch in the intestine, penetrating the mucosa, aimlessly wander through the circulation, passing to the hepatic and/or pulmonary vasculature and are potentially fatal if they involve the myocardium or central nervous system; in the eye, the resulting retinal granuloma mimics retinoblastoma

Laryngeal nerve transplant A surgical attempt to repair surgical severance of the recurrent laryngeal nerve (RLN); damage to this nerve may be uni- or bilateral, temporary or permanent and occurs in 0.2% of cases of thyroid surgery for non-malignant conditions and 5% of cases treated for thyroid malignancy; asymptomatic unilateral paralysis requires no treatment; bilateral RLN injury may result in defects of the respiratory toilet and if extreme, airway obstruction; the surgeon usually attempts a direct repair if severance is recognized at the time of surgery or performs a tracheostomy and awaits spontaneous return of nerve function; repair of the recurrent nerve is better than the nerve transplant procedures, eg splitting of the vagus nerve and end-to-end anastomosis to the distal end of the RLN or the Tucker procedure, in which the omohyoid muscle is implanted into the cricothyroid muscle

Laryngeal nodule see Singer's node

Laryngeal web An uncommon congenital laryngeal anomaly resulting from incomplete separation of the fetal mesenchyme between both sides of the larynx, consisting of a fibrovascular lamina at the anterior aspect of the vocal cords, causing respiratory obstruction that may present as a neonatal emergency

Laryngismus stridulus Pseudocroup PEDIATRICS A childhood cough with a whooping character that is due to spasmodic laryngeal closure with crowing inspiration, cyanosis accompanied by apnea, paresthesia, tingling of hands and feet, due to a marked decrease in serum calcium with normal magnesium levels; see Latent tetany syndrome, Whooping cough

Lasers Light amplification by stimulated emission of radiation PHYSICS The principle on which lasers are based was postulated by Einstein in 1917; the first working model was built in 1961 at Princeton University **Principle** Atoms of a suitable material are excited to a higher energy level by energy 'pumping'; if during the excitation phase, an additional photon with an appropriate frequency impinges on the excited system, it is forced into resonance and releases identical photons as the system reverts to a lower energy state; the photons 'bounce' back and forth between a highly reflecting and a semitransparent mirror, stimulating the release of more resonant photons, causing an 'avalanche' effect; the beam of laser energy differs from thermal light as the beam is highly coherent, collimated, ie 'focused', and monochromatic; in addition to the thermal effects, lasers may evoke photodissociation of molecules, and generate shock waves by creating an ionized plasma capable of disintegrating mineral deposits, causing a target tissue to fluoresce and to interact with a dye, destroying a target cell or tissue; lasers have been used since the early 1960s in ophthalmology for the destructive effects of the intense heat, and its selective nature; an argon laser that generates a green beam that is selectively absorbed by the retina's melanin pigment, causing damage without destroying adjacent structures, and is of use for 'riveting' detached retina and for treating both opened and closed angle glaucomas; lasers are being increasingly used in other areas of health care, eg dentistry to treat cavities, dermatology for coagulation-bleaching of tattoos and port-wine nevi (see Selective photothermolysis), endoscopy for coagulating vascular malformations (see Nd-YAG laser), gynecology (see Roller ball technique) and in the laboratory, where they form part of the instrument itself, serving as the light source in flow cytometry and spectrophotometry; short wavelength lasers include argon, krypton, neodymium and ruby; long wavelength lasers include CO_2, erbium-yttrium-aluminum-garnet (YAG) laser (Prog Pediatr Surg 1990; 25:5; Sci Am 1991; 264:6/84rv)

Lassa fever An acute arenavirus infection, first described in northeastern Nigeria, endemic in western Africa(10% of fever in Sierra Leone is Lassa-related), causing 250 000 annual cases in small epidemic clusters RESERVOIR & VECTOR House rat (***Mastomys natalensis***), transmitted by the oral-fecal route, rarely human-to-human **Clinical** Many cases are mild, subclinical or have an insidious onset of fever, weakness and malaise followed by headache, dry cough, pharyngitis, back pain, myalgia, vomiting, lymphadenopathy, sensorineural deafness (J Am Med Assoc 1990; 264:2093) and, if severe, shock (N Engl J Med 1990; 323:1120) Mortality 5-30%

Latah A psychiatric reaction occurring in Malaysians after a sudden stressful stimulus, resulting in either automatisms and passive obedience to commands or uncontrollable motor and verbal responses (J Ment Sci 1952; 98:515); see Cultural psychosis, Zombies

'Latchkey' children SOCIAL MEDICINE Children who come home from school and are unattended until the parents' arrival several hours later; whether this transient lack of supervision has a negative influence on the child's behavior, socialization or on performance in standardized test scores is controversial, as well-designed studies have not been performed (J Am Med Assoc 1988; 260:3247, 3399); the major concern is for the safety of the younger and lack of supervision of the older children; studies do not reveal significant differences in school performance, although the younger age group of non-parentally-supervised (day-care) children have lower grades and test scores (Child Development 1988;59:868); Cf 'Supermom'

Late gene VIROLOGY A gene produced by the cell long after the integration of a virus into the host genome, which encodes structural proteins of interest to the virus; see Early gene

Latency NEUROPHYSIOLOGY The time between application of a stimulus and reaction thereto is divided into a) Sensory latency The time required to process the message of irritation and b) Motor latency The time between a message's arrival and the corresponding muscle response

Latent tetany syndrome A physiological state of neuromuscular hyperexcitability, delineated by physical examination and electromyography **Clinical** Trousseau and Chvostek signs of hypocalcemia, bowel irritability, laryngismus stridulus, anxiety, asthenia, migraines and mitral valve prolapse

Late phase reaction (LPR) A delayed or secondary response in asthmatics after an antigenic challenge, in which neutrophils release histamine, stimulating secondary mast cell and basophil degranulation, in turn evoking bronchial hyperreactivity; LPR differs from the primary response in that prostaglandin PGD2 is not produced; LPRs may also be evoked by irritants, eg cold air, ozone, viruses **Treatment** β-adrenergic aerosols

Latex Lactescent gels of molecular homogeneity, obtained from plants and composed of microglobules of natural rubber LABORATORY MEDICINE The term 'latex' has been broadened in scope to include neoprene, polystyrene, polyvinylchloride and synthetic 'rubbers'; latexes are the inert vehicles that may be used to carry antibodies or antigens in latex agglutination immunoassays

Lathyrism A disease of livestock that grazes on *Lathyrus* species of sweet peas, which induces spastic paralysis, skeletal and cardiovascular abnormalities due to accumulation of β-aminopropionitrile and due to collagen defects, the latter making lathyrism an excellent experimental model for studying collagen disease; lathyrism in humans is due to excessive consumption of fava beans, which contain β-aminopropionitrile, an irreversible inhibitor of the copper-bearing amino oxidase (in blood) and lysyl oxidase (in bone and connective tissue), which prevents hydroxylation of proline and lysine, in turn preventing the cross-linking of tropocollagen **Clinical** Spastic paraplegia, pain, paresthesia, marked increase in the urinary excretion of hydroxyproline, skeletal deformities, eg marfanoid habitus, kyphoscoliosis and aortic aneurysms **Laboratory** Increased hydroxyproline excretion

Latrodectus A genus of highly venomous spiders (Family Theridae, which includes the black widow spider, *Latrodectus mactans*), endemic to the USA, with a characteristic orange-red hourglass-shaped marking on the abdomen; the venom is a non-hemolytic neurotoxin **Clinical** Latency of hours, followed by severe myalgia, myospasm, truncal rigidity, nausea, vomiting, diaphoresis and shock; most resolve spontaneously, small children are at higher risk **Treatment** Establish airway, supportive care

LATS Long-acting thyroid stimulator A 7S IgG anti-thyroglobulin autoantibody that mimics thyrotropin, which is produced by most patients with Grave's hyperthyroidism, often associated with exophthalmos; the original LATS assay was developed in the mouse; in humans, levels of LATS-related thyroid-stimulating autoantibodies are measured

LATS protector An antibody present in 90% of patients with Grave's disease which in vitro prevents the inactivation of LATS; the LATS-P assay is a sensitive marker for Grave's disease, but is too cumbersome to utilize as a diagnostic tool

Lattice BIOCHEMISTRY An organized three-dimensional scaffold of usually similar molecules; Cf Domain, Motif

Lattice dystrophy OPHTHALMOLOGY Localized deposition of amyloid between an irregular epithelium and Bowman's membrane of the cornea

Laughing death see Kuru

Laughing disease see Pseudobulbar palsy

'Laundry list' A fanciful colloquialism for a long and relatively complete list of symptoms, diseases or differential diagnoses that share something in common, eg etiology of acute abdomen

LAV Lymphadenopathy-associated virus; see HIV-1

Lavage The washing out of a body cavity or hollow organ to obtain fluids for diagnostic cytology from the pleura and pericardial cavity, to detect hemorrhage in blunt trauma or to remove toxins, eg gastric lavage in overdose; see BAL (bronchoalveolar lavage)

Lavender top tube LABORATORY MEDICINE A phlebotomy tube with EDTA anticoagulant, used in a) Chemistry Measure carcinoembryonic antigen, lead, renin, b) Hematology Measure parameters that require separated cells, including counts of white and red cells, hemoglobin, hematocrit, mean corpuscular volume (MCV), mean corpuscular hemoglobin (MCH), mean corpuscular hemoglobin concentration (MCHC), differential counts, sedimentation rate, glucose-6-phosphate dehydrogenase, sickle cell preparation, hemoglobin electrophoresis, platelet and reticulocyte counts

Lawn plate MICROBIOLOGY A bacterial culture plate in which the organisms are inoculated with a McFarland turbidity standard of 1.0 (approximately 10^8 organisms/ml of a clear fluid) that were previously incubated in a Müller-Hinton broth and are then grown to confluence (a 'lawn') on a nutrient medium, eg blood agar; lawn plates are used to detect minimum bactericidal concentration of antibiotics (MIC); see MIC

Law of mass action A universal physicochemical law that states, 'At equilibrium in a reversible chemical reacting system, the rates of forward and reverse reactions, substrate utilization and product formation are constant'; this law applies to any equilibrium that does not require the input of energy

Layer cake education The technique for teaching science in the USA, where in the final years of secondary education, biology, chemistry and physics are taught in separate academic years, likened to the 'layers on a cake', as opposed to integrating the disciplines over a period of years, a methodologic philosophy that has been highly criticized as a cause of the deterioration of the quality of secondary education in the US in the 1980s

Lazarus complex see Near-death experience

Lazy bladder That which occurs in children with a history of infrequent voiding, as infrequently as one-two times per day and overflow incontinence; because of the bladder decompensation from chronic overdistension, the bladder does not properly empty and the children are prone to urinary tract infection

Lazy eye Amblyopia Subnormal visual acuity in one or more eyes despite appropriate correction of refractive errors, subdivided into **ORGANIC AMBLYOPIA**, in which there is pathologic change affecting the visual pathways including macular scarring seen in chorioretinitis, retrolental fibroplasia, retinoblastoma, optic atrophy, meningoencephalitis and other organic lesions and **FUNCTIONAL AMBLYOPIA**, in which there is no underlying pathology and visual impairment is either sensory deprivation amblyopia, which may be the long term result of anisometropia (mismatch of the refractive state of the eyes) or due to inhibition of visual sensation, ie misuse

Lazy leukocyte syndrome An idiopathic disease due to defective neutrophil chemotaxis after appropriate stimuli, eg endotoxin or epinephrine and inefficient egress of neutrophils from the bone marrow **Clinical** Increased pyogenic infections, including gingivitis, abscess formation and pneumonia, mild neutropenia **Prognosis** Uncertain

LBW see Low birthweight

L-CA see Leukocyte common antigen

LCAM see Leukocyte cell adhesion molecule

LCAT see Lecithin cholesterol acyl transferase

L cells 'Null' or non-T, non-B cells; variant lymphocytes with labile cell surface IgG and high affinity Fc receptors, which unlike B cells, are resistant to trypsin digestion

LCM see Lymphocytic choriomeningitis

LCR amplification Ligase chain reaction A proprietary DNA amplification technique from Biotechnica, Inc, similar to the more popular polymerase chain reaction; see PCR

'LD_6' An extra lactate dehydrogenase (LD) band seen by electrophoresis in myocardial infarcts and in cardiogenic shock that migrates cathodally to LD_5; the LD_6 band is associated with a very poor prognosis, in one review 95 of 108 patients died shortly after the appearance of LD_6; see 'Kiss of death' tests, Lactate dehydrogenase

LDH isoenzymes see Lactate dehydrogenase

LDL Low-density lipoprotein A plasma lipoprotein with a density of 1.019-1.063 kg/L (US: 1.019-1.063 g/dl); LDL is 23% protein (predominantly apolipoprotein B-100), 27% phospholipid, 62% cholesterol and cholesterol esters and 11% triglycerides, and transports cholesterol from the intestine to the liver, and is a major transporter of cholesterol that binds to the LDL receptor at apolipoprotein-B100, inhibiting cellular 3-hydroxy-3-methyl-glutamyl coenzyme A reductase (HMG CoA, which synthesizes cholesterol) and regulating LDL-receptor expression on membranes; defective LDL-receptor is implicated in certain forms of hypercholesterolemia and may be responsible for accelerated atherosclerosis **Pathogenesis** In early atherosclerotic lesions, fatty streaks and foam cells accumulate in the arterial wall, in a sequence that is mediated by a variant LDL-receptor, the acetyl (or 'scavenger') LDL-receptor, which has a high affinity for oxidized and abnormal LDL, possibly induced by macrophages through lipo-oxygenase and/or generation of oxygen free radicals, changes that can be abolished with antioxidants, eg vitamin E Note: Acetyl LDL-receptor does not recognize normal LDL, but does recognize oxidized LDL, a molecule with other biochemical modifications including conversion of LDL lecithin to lysolecithin, oxidation of cholesterol, increasing negative charge and LDL density, while decreasing polyunsaturated fats (due to oxidation), LDL receptor-mediated uptake, degradation of apo-B100 (histidine, lysine and proline); oxidated LDL chemotactically attracts monocytes; this model of atherogenesis may be valid in vivo as probucol (an antioxidant) slows the atherogenic process in rabbits (N Engl J Med 1989; 320:915) Note: The LDL-receptor that netted the 1984 Nobel prize in medicine and physiology may not play a major role in the early stages of atherosclerosis, a condition occurring in the animal model for atherosclerosis, the Watanabe rabbit, which lacks LDL receptors; LDL receptors regulate the amount of circulating ligands (apoB-100 and apoE) by internalizing them **Biochemistry** LDL is subdivided by ultracentrifugation into an LDL_A profile composed of large, light LDL molecules, present in 70% of humans and an LDL_B profile composed of small, dense and heavy LDL molecules, a pattern associated with a higher risk for heart disease in a small cohort; studies in a Mormon cohort suggest that a single gene regulates a subject's LDL 'A-ness' or 'B-ness'

LDRG Laboratory diagnosis-related groups; see Organ panels

Lead CARDIOLOGY Specific sites for the placement of electrodes in electrocardiography (EKG); the standard 12-lead EKG includes three bipolar limb leads (I, II, III), three augmented unipolar limb leads (aV_R, aV_L and aV_F) and six precordial leads (V_1-V_6); the EKG is calibrated so that a 1 mV potential results in a 1 cm deflection and the paper moves at 25 mm/sec CLINICAL TOXICOLOGY A heavy metal that paints a broad clinical palette EPIDEMIOLOGY Inorganic lead sources include burning car batteries, 'Moonshine' liquor distilled in tubing soldered with lead, foods and beverages served on Mexican ceramic or leaded crystal; lead in canned and packaged foods in the USA derives from fossil fuels with lead additives (which were banned from motor vehicles but continue to be used in agriculture and thus find their way to crops, lead-bearing water and equipment in processing the foods and lead in the solder on canned products); lead levels in canned vegetables are 15 to 30-fold greater than levels in fresh-frozen vegetables (N Engl J Med 1991; 324:416c); serum levels above 25 mg/dl are considered excessive (MMWR 1991; 40193cr); the peripheral blood reveals red cells with coarse basophilic stippling, anemia, reticulocytosis, erythroid hyperplasia, autofluorescence of erythrocytes and erythroid precursors **Clinical** Chronic disease is characterized by neuromuscular disease with wrist drop and encephalopathy (convulsions, mania, delirium), abdominal pain, Fanconi syndrome (aminoaciduria, glycosuria, fructosuria, phosphaturia) and occasionally protoporphyria-like symptoms **Pathology** Lead deposits may be seen in various tissue, eg renal tubules (figure, Lead inclusions) and in erythrocytes, see Basophilic stippling **Treatment** Chelation, including dimercaprol, calcium EDTA, D-penicillamine and succimer; see Saturnine gout, Succimer

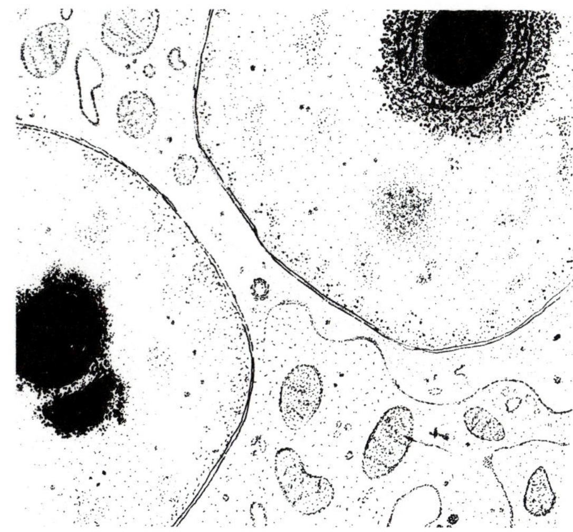

Lead inclusions

Leader sequence MOLECULAR BIOLOGY An untranslated segment of RNA nucleotides located at the 5' end of mRNA preceding the AUG start codon that contains the 'Shine-Delgarno sequence', which pairs with 16S ribosomal RNA, assuring the proper alignment of the mRNA transcript to the ribosome prior to initiation of translation into a protein and may also contain regulatory elements

Leading front technique IMMUNOLOGY A technique used to evaluate cell migration (chemotaxis), detecting the differences in the migration of stimulated and nonstimulated cells; the disadvantage is that it assumes that the fastest cells represent the majority of cells capable of migrating

Leading strand see Replication

Lead line A horizontal hyperpigmented line on the gingiva, caused by chronic intoxication with lead, mercury or other heavy metal, often accompanied by intranuclear inclusions in renal tubular epithelium and radiodense 'lead lines' in the epiphysis of growing children

Lead pipe rigidity A 'smooth' rigidity in flexion and extension that continues through the entire range of the stretching muscle, seen in atherosclerotic parkinsonism; virtually identical to Gegenhalten; Cf Garden hose

Leaf appearance see Ash leaf appearance

Leafless tree appearance RADIOLOGY The finding of multiple abrupt cutoffs of terminal bronchioles in an air bronchogram, fancifully likened to a leafless deciduous tree in winter (figure); this sign was first described in bronchoalveolar carcinoma, but is relatively non-specific, as it has been seen in chronic bronchitis and bronchiectasis, and in the era of computed tomography is a rarely evoked finding

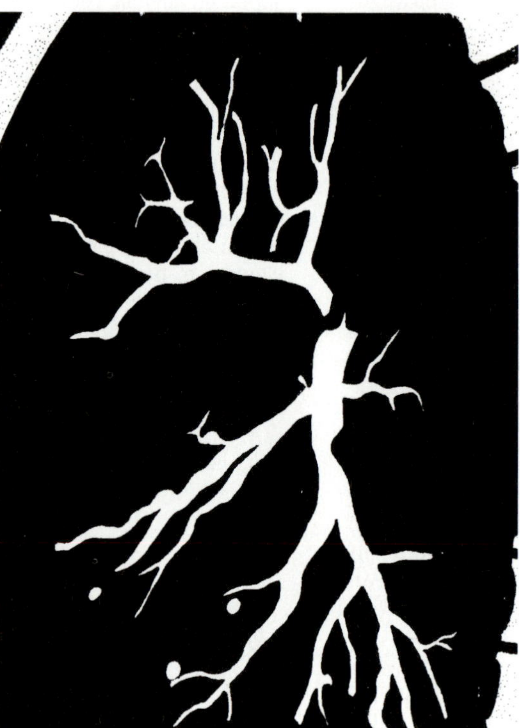

Leafless tree appearance

Leaflet PHYSIOLOGY One of the two layers of the phospholipid bilayer of the cell membrane; each sheet is characterized by a hydrophilic head that is oriented either to the exterior or interior of the cell and has hydrophobic residues that are 'buried' within the membrane itself; see Fluid mosaic model

Leaky patch A focal increase in the permeability of the cell membrane produced by the transmembrane assembly of complement in the phospholipid bilayer, which allows free passage of water and ions; Cf Doughnut model

'Leap-frog method' TRANSFUSION MEDICINE A technique for maximizing the amount of autologous blood available for elective surgery (table); because of the shelf life of red cells (circa 42 days), a practical maximum available by this method is four units

Leap-frog method

Week 1 a unit 'A' of red cells is drawn
Week 2 'A' unit is re-infused and two 'B' units are drawn
Week 3 'B' units are re-infused and three 'C' units are drawn
Week 4 'C' units are re-infused and three 'D' units are drawn

'Lear complex' see King Lear complex

'Learned profession' BIOMEDICAL ETHICS A calling or vocation requiring specialized knowledge and often long and intense academic preparation; as such, a learned profession entails individual and group self-governance, service to the poor without expectation of compensation, deliverance of quality; high level of learning, autonomy of activity, self-sacrifice, altruism with threadbare nobility, heroism as needed and ethical practice with public accountability (J Am Med Assoc 1990; 263:86); learned professionals are historically distinguished from tradesmen and businessmen and include doctors, lawyers and clergy; according to E Pelligrino (Kennedy Institute of Ethics), a fundamental difference between a business and a profession is that '*AT SOME POINT IN A PROFESSIONAL RELATIONSHIP, WHEN A DIFFICULT DECISION MUST BE MADE, THE TRUE PROFESSIONAL CAN BE RELIED UPON TO EFFACE HIS OWN SELF-INTEREST*'; the relationship of the professional with the poor is considered unique; service to the indigent is known as stewardship for the clergy and *pro bono publico* for lawyers (J Am Med Assoc 1988; 260:3178)

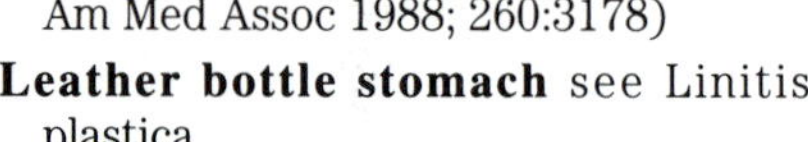

Leather bottle stomach see Linitis plastica

LEC-CAMs see Selectins

LE cell RHEUMATOLOGY A neutrophil characteristically seen in the synovium or peripheral blood in patients with lupus erythematosus; the cytoplasm is distended by a red-purple homogeneous or 'glassy' inclusion ('hematoxylin' body) with an eccentric nucleus, corresponding to phagocytosed deoxyribonucleoprotein (DNA-histone complex); LE cells are also seen in scleroderma, drug-induced lupus erythematosus and in lupoid hepatitis

LE cell 'prep' RHEUMATOLOGY A test in which heparinized blood is gently agitated with glass beads, releasing neutrophil nuclei which are then incubated with antinuclear protein in the serum; the 'glassy' appearance of LE bodies results from homogenization of the chromatin; these bodies are then phagocytosed by the remaining neutrophils

Lecithin-cholesterol acyl transferase (LCAT) An enzyme,

the gene for which resides in chromosome 16 that catalyzes phosphatidyl choline and cholesterol, yielding lysolecithin and cholesteryl ester Note: LCAT and lipoprotein lipase are markedly decreased in a-β–lipoproteinemia (Tangier's disease), resulting in a decreased rate of cholesterol esterification due to relative lack of cholesterol, causing a pseudo-lecithin cholesterol acyl transferase deficiency

Lecithin-cholesterol acyl transferase deficiency syndrome An autosomal recessive condition of adult onset characterized by corneal opacifications, proteinuria, renal insufficiency with hypertension, premature atherosclerosis, hemolytic anemia, obstructive jaundice and hepatic failure Laboratory Increased ratio of free cholesterol to cholesteryl ester, variably increased phospholipids and triglycerides and presence of lipoprotein X; Cf Fish eye disease

Lecithin:sphingomyelin ratio see L:S ratio

Lectin A family of simple, ie non-immunogenic carbohydrate-binding proteins and glycoproteins derived from plant seeds, mollusks and other animals that contain two or more binding sites for animal proteins; lectins are mitogenic and stimulate lymphocyte transformation, cell-cell recognition and agglutination of certain red cell antigens; in the blood bank, lectin specificity may be used to identify blood types (eg ***Dolichus bifloris*** binds anti-A_1, ***Ulex europeus*** binds anti-H and ***Arachis hypogea*** binds anti-T) Note: Some cytokines, eg tumor necrosis factor, interleukin-1 and interleukin-2 have lectin- and/or carbohydrate-binding sites

Lecturer An individual who is primarily (if not entirely) involved in the teaching activities of an academic center, who is not expected to perform research or patient management; in general, lectureships are non-tenured positions

Leech Segmented annelids that evolved from earthworms and are found in either fresh water or soil in the tropics and subtropics; leeches have two suckers, a cranial sucker housing a mouth, the bite mark of which has been likened to the Mercedes-Benz emblem and a caudal sucker involved in crawling; the classic medicinal leech is ***Hirudo medicinalis***, other leeches include ***Poecilobdella, Dinobdella, Limnatis, Haemadipsa*** and ***Macrobdella***; the leech has recently acquired some respect in the biomedical sciences; the simplicity of the its nervous system, it has only one neurotransmitter, serotonin, has made it a useful model for neurobiologist, and leech phlebotomy is undergoing a renaissance for a) Removing excess blood from an operative field b) Stimulating capillary ingrowth in reimplanted, traumatically amputated extremities and in plastic surgery c) To obtain hirudin, a potent anticoagulant, and as yet poorly delineated substances in leech saliva that inhibit tumor spread Note: Not all leeches are so happily symbiotic; ***Limnatis nilotica***, an aquatic leech of the Northern Hemisphere may be ingested with drinking water and attach to the oropharynx, nasal passage, larynx and esophagus, causing anemia that may be fatal in children, asphyxia, local wounds, pruritus, hoarseness, dyspnea, hemoptysis, dysphagia and hematemesis Note: The leech has had an honored place in medicine and was used by Greek and Moor physicians; its use extended into the late 1700s, when bleeding was the standard of proper medical care; in one session, a leech can ingest up to 17 grams of blood and was a practice that was instrumental in hastening the deaths of George Washington and Louis XIII; see Hirudin

Left axis deviation CARDIOLOGY Any shift in the pattern of the electrocardiographic leads; when seen in conjunction with a counterclockwise loop abnormality in the frontal plane of the vector cardiogram, a left axis deviation is characteristic of the ostium primum type of partial atrioventricular canal defect

Left-handed DNA An alternate secondary structure of DNA, which is the reverse of more common right-handed helical form (B-DNA); conformational microheterogeneity or 'left-handedness' is thought to play a role in regulation of major cell processes, including replication andrecombination, mutagenesis and carcinogenesis (and repair thereof), transcription, chromosomal organization and viral packaging; the sites where the right-handed DNA twists to become left handed DNA are mutagenic 'hot-spots' (Science 1987; 238:773) Note: Z-DNA is a type of left-handed DNA, which has been the most extensively studied and is a term often used interchangeably with left-handed DNA; see DNA forms

'Left shift' CLINICAL CHEMISTRY see Neuroblastoma HEMATOLOGY An increase in the peripheral blood smear consisting of immature granulocytes with decreased nuclear segmentation, ie 'band' forms, due to increased production of the myeloid series in the marrow, caused by acute infection Note: 'right' shifts are not described, although hyper-lobation of neutrophils seen in megaloblastic anemia might warrant this designation RESPIRATORY PHYSIOLOGY An increase in hemoglobin's affinity for oxygen (as represented by the oxygen dissociation curve), where the P_{50} is decreased and shifted to the left, as occurs with increased pH (Bohr effect) or decreased temperature; Cf Right shift

Left-sided 'appendicitis' A descriptor of acute diverticulitis with impending rupture, which clinically is a mirror image mimic of (left-sided) appendicitis

Left-sided colon see Malrotation

'Legend' drug Obsolete for 'Prescription' drug

Legionella A genus of small, fastidious, facultative intracytoplasmic gram-negative bacilli, comprised of more than 20 species, 14 of which have been implicated in human disease, including ***L micdadii*** (Pittsburgh pneumonia agent), ***L anisa, L bozemanii, L dumoffi, L gormanii, L jordanis, L longbeachae, L oakridgensis, L rubrilucens*** and others; 12 of the 39 serotypes correspond to ***L pneumophila*** (Legionnaire's disease agent); ***Legionella*** species are aerobic, motile nonsaccharolytic bacilli, cultured with techniques usually reserved for ***Rickettsia*** species, ie within embryonal eggs or injection into guinea pigs; ***Legionella*** also grow on CYE (charcoal yeast extract) agar, supplemented with branched-chain fatty acids; chief energy source is amino acids; although they are gram negative, ***Legionella*** are best seen with other stains, eg Gimenez, silver stains and direct-fluorescent techniques; liposaccharide wall components function as endotoxin, hemolysin and protease

Legionnaire's disease A dramatic epidemic that occurred in an American Foreign Legion convention in Philadelphia in 1976; legionnaire's disease is either sporadic or epidemic with a mortality of up to 15%; depending upon the population, ***Legionella*** species are thought to cause 1 to 27% of community acquired pneumonias; male:female ratio, 3:1 **Clinical** 2-10 day incubation, followed by an abrupt onset of malaise, headache, myalgia, a dry initially non-productive, later productive cough; hemoptysis is relatively common; fever to 40°C, rigors are seen in most, associated with bradycardia; less commonly: nausea, diarrhea and confusion, delirium, septicemia, abscess formation, acute myocarditis and pericarditis and rhabdomyolysis **Radiology** Patchy interstitial infiltrate, often progressing to nodular condensations **Laboratory** Decreased sodium, and phosphorus, increased liver enzymes, proteinuria, microscopic hematuria, relative leukocytosis (leukopenia is often associated with a poor prognosis) **Complications** Empyema, shock, disseminated intravascular coagulation, renal failure, neurological sequelae, peripheral neuropathy **Histopathology** Acute fibrinopurulent, necrotizing pneumonia with macrophages and neutrophils, diffuse alveolar damage and possibly permanent pulmonary fibrosis **Treatment** Erythromycin, trimethoprim-sulfamethoxazole **Prevention** Chlorination and ultraviolet irradiation of water supplies; Cf Pontiac disease

Legless mutation see Transgenic mice

LEM Leukocyte endogenous mediator A polypeptide implicated in anemia of chronic disease, released by neutrophils and macrophages after stimulation by bacterial toxins

Lemon sign OBSTETRICS An ultrasonographic finding seen when a major neural tube defect accompanies the Arnold-Chiari malformation, with herniation of the cerebellar tonsils and midbrain structures into the foramen magnum, causing ventriculomegaly due to compression of the outflow from the third and fourth ventricles; downward traction of the brain causes a reduction in the anterior calvarium, in turn resulting in a triangular-shaped head in the biparietal diameter, fancifully likened to a lemon

Lennert's lymphoma Malignant lymphoma with high content of epithelioid cells A diffuse mixed cell non-Hodgkin's lymphoma with a large number of benign epithelioid histiocytes (Virch Arch Path Anat 1968; 344:1) that affects older patients **Clinical** Generalized lymphadenopathy, hepatosplenomegaly and 'B' symptoms (fever, night sweats and weight loss), which is often first seen in stage III or IV; for a time, the very existence of Lennert's lymphoma's was controversial (Cancer 1980; 45:1379), as many of the original cases were later reclassified as Hodgkin's, non-Hodgkin's and immunoblastic lymphomas, as well as histiocytosis X; see Lymphoma, Working classification; Cf Progressive transformation of germinal centers

Lentigo Freckle A pigmented, flat or slightly elevated macule, with increased melanin, melanocytic hyperplasia, epidermal pigmentation and elongation of the rete ridges **LENTIGO MALIGNA** (Hutchinson's freckle) A pre-melanoma located on sun-exposed aging skin that begins life as an unevenly pigmented macule with an irregular border, which slowly extends peripherally, one-third of which progress to melanoma, the transition may require 10-15 years **LENTIGO SENILIS** A pigmented red-brown macular lesion, often multiple, affecting sun-exposed skin, often seen in caucasians, closely mimicking seborrheic keratosis, both of which have been referred to as 'liver spots' and are of merely cosmetic concern **LENTIGO SIMPLEX** A clinical mimic of junctional nevus that has three forms: lentiginosis profusa, mutiple lentigines syndrome (see Leopard syndrome) and speckled lentiginous nevus

Lentiviridae A subfamily of retroviruses first recognized 50 years ago in epidemic lung (maedi) and central nervous system (visna) infections of sheep in Iceland; lentiviruses are 'slow infections' with prolonged incubation periods, remaining within the host macrophages, disseminating by a 'Trojan horse mechanism' (see there), often persisting in the central nervous system, where one of the most common manifestations of lentivirus infection is neurologic deterioration; other RNA lentiviruses include HIV, bovine immunodeficiency virus, feline lymphotropic virus (FTLV), simian lymphotropic virus (STLV) and others; see HIV, Retroviruses, STLV; Cf Prions

Leonine facies A deeply furrowed 'lumpy' face with prominent superciliary arches, classically seen in lepromatous lepra; a similar facial deformity may occur in Job syndrome, chronic granulomatous disease, van Buchem's disease, leontiasis ossium (idiopathic leonine facies); the features may be due to overgrowth of bones, as in Paget's disease or McCune-Albright syndrome, polyostotic fibrous dysplasia or soft tissue, as in hypothyroidism with myxedema of periorbital tissues, epidermoid carcinoma, Sézary syndrome, which is characterized by generalized exfoliative dermatitis, edema, erythema, pachydermia and palmoplantar keratoderma

Leopard skin Focal macular hyperpigmentation of the skin in a hypopigmented background, accompanied by scaling, seen in infection by *Onchocerca volvulus*

'Leopard spotting' A fanciful descriptor for the postmortem, non-inflammatory and geographic brown-black mottling seen in esophagomalacia due to superficial mucosal autolysis, the result of acid digestion of hemoglobin, seen when the gastric juices flow onto the esophageal mucosa

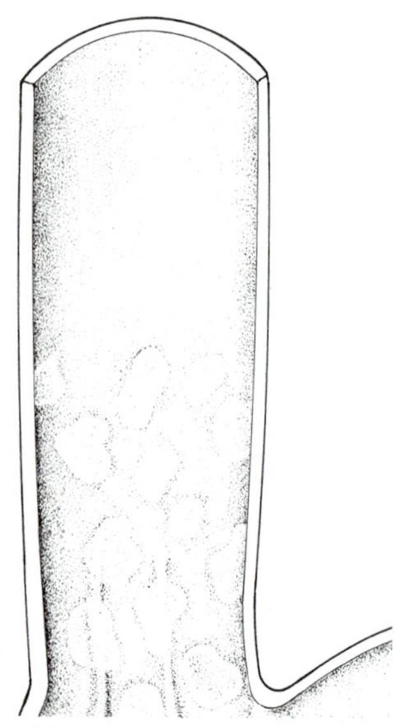

Leopard spot appearance

Leopard syndrome Multiple lentigines syndrome An autosomal dominant condition with thousands of 1-5 mm darkly pigmented macules on the skin but on the mucosal surfaces **Clinical** characterized by the mnemonic acronym **LEOPARD**, for **L**entigines, **E**lectrocardiographic (EKG) disturbances, **O**cular hypertelorism, **P**ulmonary sten-osis, **A**bnormalities of genitalia (gonadal or ovarian hypoplasia), **R**etarded growth and neural **D**eafness

Lepra cells Foamy macrophages replete with clumps (known as 'globi') of ***Mycobacterium lepra***; the macrophages are unable to digest the bacteria due to the loss of cell-mediated immunity, typical of lepromatous leprosy; lepra cells are distinctly less common in borderline leprosy and never seen in the tuberculous leprosy; see Intracellular pathogens

Leprechaunism Donohue syndrome An autosomal recessive polydysmorphic complex with parental consanguinity that is more common in females (increased male fetal wastage in utero) and characterized by a coarse gnome-like face with a saddle nose, broad mouth, large, low-set ears, hirsutism, cutis laxa, atrophy of subcutaneous adipose tissue, dwarfism, extreme wasting, mental retardation, dysphagia, enlarged nipples, breasts, kidneys, pancreatic islets and ovaries (with premature follicular maturation), hepatic nodules, insulin receptor dysfunction and early death

Lepromin A heat-killed extract of ***Mycobacterium lepra*** skin nodules that is injected intradermally ('lepra test') and evokes granuloma formation within three to four weeks in normal subjects and those with borderline and tuberculous leprosy, but not in subjects with anergy and lepromatous lepra

Leprosy A disease common in the Middle Ages that migrated with 'los Conquistadores', spread during slavery and transmitted by contact with skin ulcers, maternal-fetal or maternal-infant contact or rarely by droplets; ethnic or genetic susceptibility to the variant forms of leprosy is postulated; GHA Hansen described the bacterium in 1873; sylvatic leprosy occurs in armadillos and chimpanzees; 15 million cases worldwide, 4 million in Africa, 3.6 million in India, 6 000 in US (national leprosarium, Carville, Louisiana); see Dapsone

Leptocyte Greek, Leptos, thin Wafer-thin erythrocyte with peripheral marginated hemoglobin, seen in thalassemia and obstructive liver disease

Leptophaeria Genus of fungi causing maduromycosis

Leptopsylla Genus of flea, vector of the plague

Leptospira Member of the Spirochaetaceae family; diagnosed with difficulty (darkfield microscopy and Giemsa stains are unreliable), cultured on Fletcher and Stuart medium, intraperitoneal inoculation of blood or urine into guinea pigs or hamsters, serologically rising titers, most commonly due to ***L interrogans*** (formerly ***L icterohemorrhagiae***), following ingestion of water contaminated with infected livestock or rat urine

LES Lower esophageal sphincter A 3-5 cm in length zone of increased pressure at the junction of the distal esophagus with the gastric cardia, located at the hiatus, which forms a physical barrier in preventing gastric reflux

Lesbianism Sapphism Tribadism Female homosexuality is far less studied from a medical standpoint than male homosexuality; the scanty data available indicates that there is no increased incidence of enteric or other sexually-transmitted disease, possibly due to a combination of relative monogamy and sexual practices; Cf Homosexuality, Sexual reassignment, Transexuality

Lesch-Nyhan disease A condition due to a deficiency of the 24 kD hypoxanthine-guanine phosphoribosyl transferase, resulting in an accumulation of uric acid crystals in the renal pelvises, pseudo-gouty arthritis, erosive changes of fingertips, compulsive self-mutilation, choreoathetosis, mental retardation **Laboratory** Increased oxypurines, hypoxanthine and xanthine in the cerebrospinal fluid due to purine overload Note: The first transgenic mouse was 'engineered' to be deficient in HGPRT; recently embryonal stem cells without the enzyme were introduced into mouse fibroblast females to produce germline chimeras

'Lesionectomy' NEUROSURGERY A neologism referring to stereotactic resection of poorly-circumscribed intra-axial (a region often considered inoperable) brain masses including vascular malformations and glial neoplasms, identified by magnetic resonance imaging that may be associated with epileptiform seizure activity (Mayo Clin Proc 1990; 65:1053); Cf Lumpectomy

Let-down reflex NEONATOLOGY A physiological response occurring in the puerperium, which is evoked by sucking (or negative mechanical pressure) on the female nipple or by psychological stimuli, causing the release ('let-down') of breast milk in a nursing mother; the reflex is due to myoepithelial cell contraction of the alveolar glands elicited by oxytocin and may be lost if the mother is under stress or fatigue, resulting in milk retention

Lethal agranulocytosis IMMUNOLOGY An autosomal recessive condition of early infant onset, characterized by profound neutropenia ($< 0.3 \times 10^9$/L) (US:$<$ 300/mm^3), absolute monocytosis and eosinophilia, recurring pyogenic infections of skin and lungs **Histopathology** Vacuolation of myeloid precursors with normal colony-stimulating factor and colony-forming units **Treatment** None, universally fatal in childhood

Lethal dose A dose of a toxin, virus or any substance that is lethal to all the members of a species within a specified or well-defined time period'; see Poisons

Lethal equivalent The sum of 'semilethal' genes (lethal genes present in the heterozygous state, and therefore clinically silent); three to five lethal equivalents are thought to be present in all individuals

Lethal gene A mutant gene that when autosomal dominant, is invariably lethal; when an gene is lethal only when in the homozygous state, the heterozygous state is 'semilethal'

Lethal hit A critical event caused by an ionizing particle that inactivates a virus or impacts on a genome, resulting in death; Cf 'One-hit, two-hit' model

Lethal midline granuloma (LMD) Rhinitis gangrenosa progressiva A condition that is confusing to those who read about it and (seemingly) to those who write about it; LMD is best considered a clinical syndrome rather than a specific histological entity, consisting of a destructive lesion of the upper respiratory tract (nose, nasopharynx, palate and midface); LMD is either idiopathic or secondary to a) Wegener's granulomatosis, an ulcerating, necrotizing and osteolytic lesion of the upper respiratory tract and lungs, defined as having systemic necrotizing vasculitis, a male:female ratio of 2:1, hemoptysis, fever, rash, prostration, arthritis, neuropathy, splenomegaly and progressive glomerulonephritis ending in terminal renal failure b) Any lymphoma occurring in this region, including large cell lymphomas, eg T cell lymphoma or c) Malignant histiocytosis, see there; see Idiopathic midline destructive disease, Midline granuloma

Lethal mutation Any mutation of a genome, including frameshift mutation, deletion, insertion and others that leads to the premature death of the host

Letter E sign see Figure E sign

Leu-CAM Leukocyte-cell adhesion molecules; see CD11/CD18 family

Leucine aminopeptidase (LAP) A hydrolase that catalyzes N-terminal peptide hydrolysis, especially aliphatic amino acids, that is increased in bile duct obstruction, pancreatitis, pancreatic carcinoma, hepatopathies and infectious mononucleosis

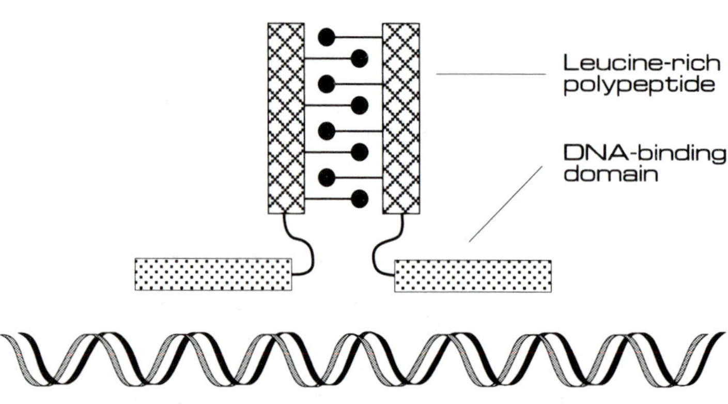

Leucine zipper motif

Leucine zipper MOLECULAR BIOLOGY A structural motif (figure) found in oncogenic proteins and in some DNA-binding proteins consisting of a segment of approximately 40 amino acids that form an α-helix containing a periodic array of 4 or 5 leucine residues at every seventh amino acid position ('heptad spacing') along the enhancer regulator protein, over a distance of 8 helical turns (of the DNA); the zipper promotes homo- or heterodimerization through hydrophobic interaction between arrays of leucine residues on participating zippers, intertwined as coiled coils; dimerization through a zipper interaction is a prerequisite for sequence-specific DNA-binding of oncogenic transforming proteins (Fos, Jun, Myc) and enhancing or regulating transcription factors (C/ERP, CREB, GCN4) and the zipper is required for cell transformation and regulation (Oncogene 1990; 5:683); Cf DNA-binding motifs

Leucovorin 'rescue' ONCOLOGY A therapeutic modality used to prevent excess 'collateral damage' to normal cells when treating patients with methotrexate (Mtx), an antimetabolic chemotherapeutic agent used to treat lymphoproliferative disorders and other malignancies, causing potentially severe myelosuppression and gastrointestinal symptoms; leukovorin (reduced folate) is a direct Mtx antagonist, and is administered immediately after chemotherapy, 'rescuing' the normal cells; up to 1500 mg/m^2 of methotrexate may be given in one session, if it is followed by leucovorin 15-50 mg/m^2 qid x 48 hours, a classic leucovorin 'rescue' protocol, a dose that must be increased in the presence of renal dysfunction, due to delayed elimination of methotrexate

Leukapheresis TRANSFUSION MEDICINE A technique that removes circulating white cells from either a) Healthy subjects to pool and transfuse the cells to immunocompromised and leukopenic patients, which may be effective in short-term therapy of acute infections; long-term, patients become either immunized against the donor antigens or infected with virulent organisms; 10^{10} granulocytes are needed for adequate 'coverage' against infections; to maximize the harvest, the donor receives corticosteroids, or b) Patients with leukemia in whom excess cells compromise normal circulation and is indicated to temporarily relieve the symptoms of hyperleukemia in excess of 100 x 10^9/L; Cf Cytapheresis, Hemapheresis

Leukemia An relatively uncommon (incidence, US 3.5/10^5/year) malignant clonal expansion of myeloid or lymphoid cells characterized by an increase in circulating leukocytes, often first diagnosed either as an incidental finding when evaluating an unrelated clinical problem, or when the expansion compromises marrow production of one or more cell lines causing anemia, thrombocytopenia or granulocytopenia; leukemias are divided by chronology (acute or chronic), by cell lineage (lymphoid, myeloid, monocytic or megakaryocytic) and subdivided by stage of maturation or cell size; see FAB classification **Clinical** Bone marrow infiltration by leukemic cells, causing anemia, thrombocytopenia, granulocytopenia, immune paralysis, decreased B cells and helper T cells, increased suppressor T cells, infiltration and leukostasis, cranial nerve palsies, meningitis, lymphadenopathy, hepatosplenomegaly, testicular and cutaneous involvement, metabolic derangements, eg increased calcium, potassium, lactate dehydrogenase, ammonia, weight loss, less commonly autoimmune hemolytic anemia, pallor and arthralgia **ACUTE LEUKEMIA** is more common in children, 80% of which are acute lymphocytic leukemia, often occurring before age 10, with a peak between ages 3 to 7 in caucasians, male:female ratio, 1.3:1 Cell types Early pre-B cell 67%; pre-B cell 18%; B cell 1%; T cell 14%; 50-85% are cALLA positive (common acute lymphocytic leukemia antigen, CD10); 5% have the Philadelphia chromosome

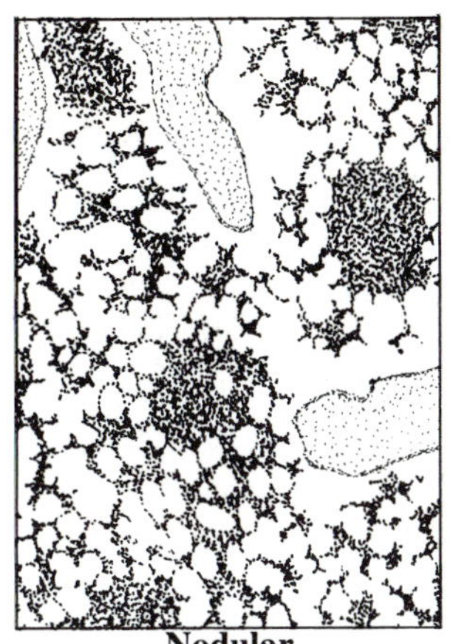
Nodular

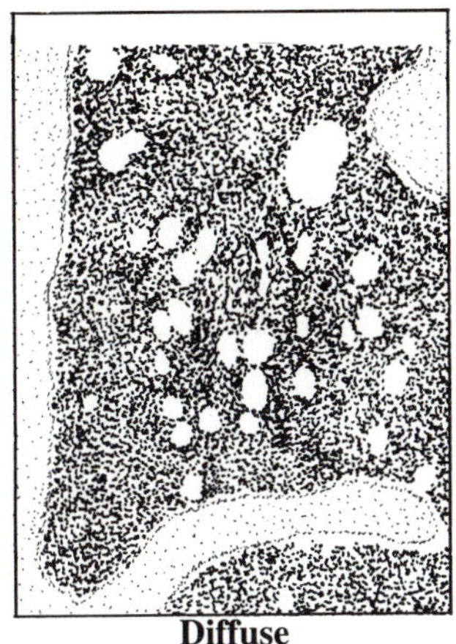
Diffuse

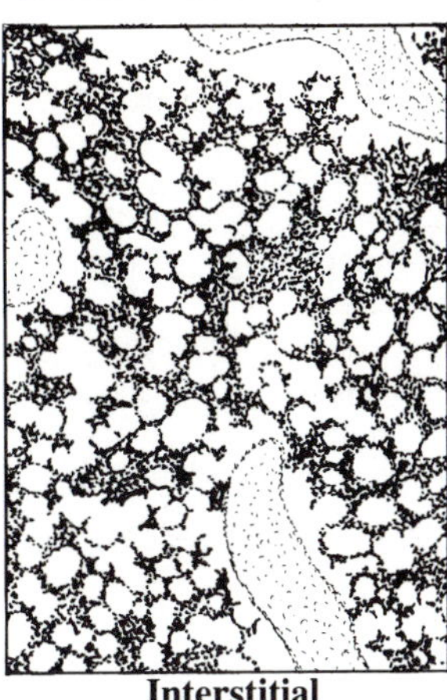
Interstitial

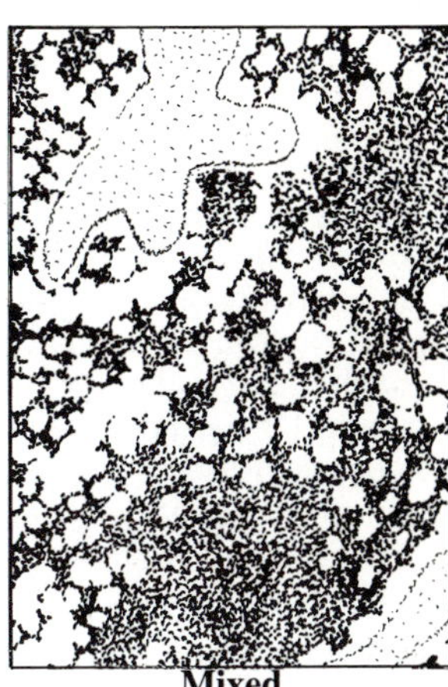
Mixed

Patterns of leukemic infiltrations of the bone marrow

Clinical More abrupt than acute myelogenous leukemia, with petechial hemorrhage, bone and abdominal pain, headache and vomiting due to intracranial pressure, lymphadenopathy, splenomegaly and hepatomegaly Laboratory 70% have decreased lymphocytosis (less than 20 x 10^9) at the time of diagnosis Treatment

PROGNOSTIC FEATURES, ACUTE LEUKEMIA

ACUTE LYMPHOCYTIC LEUKEMIA

Good prognostic features Ages 2-10, CD10 positivity, hyperdiploid karyotype

Poor prognostic features Ages less than 2 or greater than 10, B-cell phenotype, especially the L2 phenotype by the FAB classification, presence of chromosomal translocations, central nervous system involvement, mediastinal masses and a high initial white cell count

ACUTE MYELOID LEUKEMIA

Good prognostic features Young age, presence of Auer rods, short time required to objective therapeutic response

Poor prognosis features Older age, prior malignancy, prior therapy and many chromosomal defects

Protocols vary according to standard- or high-risk clinical features, and may include bone marrow transplantation Prognosis Table **CHRONIC LEUKEMIA** usually affects adults and older children and is often myelogenous; chronic myeloid leukemia (CML) is Philadelphia chromosome positive and may occur before age 5 with myelomonocytosis, anemia, thrombocytopenia and lymphadenopathy; white cell count is < 50 x 10^9, hemoglobin F and muraminidase are increased; adult CML comprises 20% of all leukemias Clinical Gradual onset of fatigability, anorexia, splenomegaly, lymphadenopathy is not common Laboratory > 25 x 10^9/L leukemic cells in blood (often with an absolute lymphocytosis of > 15 x 10^{10}/L, < 10% blasts in bone marrow, myeloid:erythroid ratio is 10-30:1, 90% of cases have low-to-absent leukocyte alkaline phosphatase and rarely also, increased vitamin B_{12} and B_{12}-binding capacity Treatment see Chemotherapy, Induction Prognosis see Remission

RISK GROUPS, LEUKEMIA

LYMPHOCYTIC LEUKEMIA

Hematologic disease Idiopathic thrombocytopenia, paroxysmal nocturnal hemoglobinuria, refractory sideroblastic anemia, polycythemia vera

Malignancy, eg carcinoma of the breast or ovary, Hodgkin's disease, multiple myeloma

Congenital disposition Twin of leukemic patient, underlying congenital genetic predisposing condition, eg ataxia-telangiectasia, Bloom syndrome, Down syndrome, Fanconi's anemia, fragile X syndrome, Klinefelter syndrome, osteogenesis imperfecta, von Recklinghausen's disease, Wiskott-Aldrich syndrome

Radiation exposure Radiologists, children of nuclear power plant workers, see Sellafield or other radiation exposure, see Chernobyl and Goiana

Immunosuppressive therapy Alkylating agents in chemotherapy for malignancy

Toxic exposure Chronic benzene exposure and chloramphenicol, see Secondary malignancy

MYELOID LEUKEMIA

Exposure to ionizing radiation and in those with HLA-Cw3 and HLA-Cw4; unlike ALL, other genetic factors and exposure to chemotherapeutics or chemicals do not play a major role

Congenital leukemia is extremely rare (usually myeloid)

Leukemia, chemotherapy-induced A leukemia that is linked to the previous use of chemotherapeutic agents to treat a malignancy; most commonly inculpated are the alkylating agents, which induce acute nonlymphocytic leukemia (ANLL), often accompanied by mutations of chromosomes 5 and 7; 15 years after chemotherapy-treated Hodgkin's disease, the risk of leukemia is from 5-11% (versus 0.9% when radiotherapy alone is used), see table 385, leukemia risk groups; ANLL may follow chemotherapy for non-Hodgkin's lymphoma, polycythemia vera, multiple myeloma, breast and ovarian carcinoma, or use of these agents for certain recalcitrant non-neoplastic diseases eg multiple sclerosis, rheumatoid arthritis and Wegener's granulomatosis; see Secondary malignancy

Leukemic coagulopathy Leukemic coagulopathic 'syndrome' A variant presentation of leukemia, which is accompanied by hemorrhagic diathesis resulting from 1) Abnormalities related to the leukemia per se, eg bone marrow infiltration, dysmorphic megakaryocytes, decreased platelet lifespan, qualitative platelet defects (decreased platelet aggregation with ATP and collagen stimulation or defects in ADP release) and disseminated intravascular coagulation due to sepsis or transfusion reactions and coagulopathy due to leukemic therapy 2) Bone marrow toxicity due to combination chemotherapy that may deplete fibrinogen, factors IX, XI, plasminogen, antithrombin III, increased factor V, uric acid nephropathy (due to massive cytolysis of malignant cells), vitamin K deficiency (treatment of infections due to granulopenia, reduces the vitamin K-producing intestinal bacteria)and heparin anticoagulation

LEUKOCYTE STAINS		ESTERASES				
	PX/SBB	α-NA	α-NB	N-ASD	PAS	Acid phos
Promyelocyte	+	(-)	-	+	(+)	+
Neutrophil	++	(-)	-	+	+++	+
Monocyte	(-)	+++	+++	(-)	(-)	++
Lymphocyte	-	(-)	(-)	-	(-)	(++)
Erythroblast	-	(-)	-	-	-	(-)
Megakaryocyte	-	+++	(-)	-	++	++
ALL	-	(+)	-	-	+	(+)
AML(M1)	+	-	-	+	+	-
AML(M2)	++	(+)	(+)	+	+	+
APL(M3)	+++	(++)	-	+++	(++)	++
AMML(M4)	++	+++	++	++	(++)	++
AMoL(M5)	(-)	+++	+++	(-)	++	+
EL(M6)	-	++	+	-	++	-
MegL(M7)	-	+	(-)	-	++	+
AUL	-	-	-	-	-	-

Leukemoid reaction An abnormal polyclonal proliferation of leukocytes, defined as greater than 25 x 10^9/L; leukemoid reactions reflect a normal marrow response to trauma, stress, metabolic disease, drugs, inflammation, connective tissue disease or malignancy, resulting from secretion of colony-stimulating factor and they are often associated with immaturity of other cell lines; in contradistinction to leukemia, leukemoid reactions almost invariably have leukocyte counts of less than 50 x 10^9/L; often only the granulocytes are increased without marked basophilia or eosinophilia Laboratory Increased leukocyte alkaline phosphatase (LAP), which is decreased or absent in leukemia, 'left shift' of myeloid cells (increased bands, metamyelocytes, myelocytes), plasma cells and plasmacytoid lymphocytes, toxic granulation, Döhle inclusion bodies, vacuolization (implies intracellular bacterial phagocytosis) PHYSIOLOGICAL LEUKOCYTOSIS may be idiopathic or hereditary, neonatal, induced by heat or solar irradiation, diurnal, increased in the afternoon, related to stress, eg pain, nausea, vomiting, anxiety, womanhood (increased during ovulation and near term, very high during labor), ether anesthesia, increased adrenalin, convulsions, paroxysmal tachycardia, pain, nausea, vomiting, anoxia, exercise and convulsions PATHOLOGICAL NEUTROPHILIA Infections, often bacterial, inflammation, severe burns, post-operative, myocardial infarct, strangulated hernias, intestinal obstruction, gouty attacks, acute glomerulonephritis, serum sickness, rheumatic fever, immune disorders and connective tissue diseases, metabolism (ketoacidosis, uremia, eclampsia), heavy metals (lead, mercury), petrochemicals (benzene, turpentine), drugs (phenacetin, digitalis), black widow spider venom, endotoxin or toxoid injection, Jarisch-Herxheimer reaction, hemorrhage (often into cranial cavity), serosal surfaces (pleural pericardium and peritoneum) or acute hemolysis, malignancy (gastrointestinal tract or hematopoietic) and Cushing syndrome

Leukocidin An exotoxin produced by pathogenic staphylococci and streptococci, which induces a profound, albeit transient neutrophilia; leukocidin destroys neutrophils by inserting pores in the membranes of the enzyme-filled lysosomes

Leukocyte adhesion deficiency syndrome (LADS) An autosomal recessive, often consanguineous condition presenting in infancy with delayed separation of the umbilical cord, recurring staphylococcal or *Pseudomonas* bacteremia related to defects in the 'integrin family of leukocyte adhesive proteins', alternately known as the CD11/CD18 family, specifically in the gene encoding the CD18 protein; a genetically engineered retrovirus with this gene has been successfully inserted into a LADS patient cells and may eventually be inserted into patient stem cells (Science 1990; 247:1413); see CD11, CD18, Leu-CAM, LFA-1 deficiency syndrome

Leukocyte alkaline phosphatase see LAP

Leukocyte common antigen (LCA) T-200 CD45 A single

chain glycoprotein with five different 180-220 kD forms arising from alternative mRNA splicing; because LCA is present on the membranes of all leukocytes (B and T cells, monocytes, macrophages and granulocytes), it has been used as an immunoperoxidase marker for differentiating between poorly differentiated carcinoma, which is often positive with antibodies to cytokeratin and/or epithelial membrane antigen and the LCA-positive lymphomas; see CD45

Leukocyte inhibitory factor (LIF) A heat-stable 68 kD protein produced by sensitized lymphocytes that immobilizes neutrophils during early inflammation

Leukocyte stains A battery of histochemical stains that are used in hematology to identify leukocytes and to classify leukemias, table, facing page, a requirement for optimal therapy Key to stains Acid phos Acid phosphatase α-NA α-naphthyl acetate α-NB α-naphthyl butyrate N-ASD Naphthol ASD chloroacetate PAS Periodic acid Schiff PX/SBB Peroxidase/Sudan Black B Key, leukemias ALL Acute lymphoblastic leukemia AML(M1)Acute myeloblastic leukemia AML(M2) Acute myeloblastic leukemia with maturation AML(M3) Acute promyelocytic leukemia AMML(M4) Acute myelo- monocytic leukemia AMoL(M5) Acute monocytic leukemia EL(M6) Acute erythroleukemia MegL(M7) Acute mega-karyocytic leukemia AUL Acute undifferentiated leukemia; see FAB classification, Leukemia, T cell leukemia

Leukocytoclastic vasculitis Allergic cutaneous arteriolitis, necrotizing angiitis and urticarial vasculitis A form of vasculitis with fragmentation of neutrophil nuclei, immune complex deposition (direct immunofluorescence demonstrates IgG, IgM and complement deposition), that elicits neutrophilic 'suicide' and deposition of abundant nuclear 'dust', necrotic debris and fibrin, most common in small post-capillary venules; the condition may be local, eg cutaneous or systemic Etiology Henoch-Schönlein disease, lupus erythematosus, rheumatoid arthritis, erythema elevatum diutinum, periarteritis nodosa (often within large arteries), allergies, Wegener's disease, cryoglobulinemia, Waldenström syndrome, drug therapy (penicillin, sulfonamides, phenylbutazone), acute febrile neutrophilic dermatosis (Sweet syndrome), leprosy (Lucio's phenomenon), granuloma faciale, granuloma annulare, necrobiosis lipidica, Herpes simplex and H zoster

Leukocytosis Any leukocyte count > 11 x 10^9/L (US: 11 000/mm^3), benign or malignant; see Leukemoid reaction, Leukemia

Leukodystrophy NEUROPATHOLOGY A heterogeneous group of disorders of myelin or myelin metabolism, including 'sphingolipidoses', which share certain pathological features, including global distribution, bilateral and symmetrical myelin degeneration, relative sparing of arcuate fibers, and eventually, segmental peripheral nerve degeneration Clinical 'White matter disease', ie predominantly motor, dominated by progressive paralysis and ataxia rather than dementia Note: The leukodystrophy concept was introduced in 1887 by Heubner, expounded upon in 1912 by Schilder, and confused by everyone since then, including Schilder himself, who included under the rubric of leukodystrophy (which he called 'encephalitis periaxialis diffusa'), such diverse conditions as multiple sclerosis, inflammation-induced demyelinization, and hereditary defects of myelin metabolism, the group that comprises the current leukodystrophies, which are separated based on differences in clinical presentation, histopathology and defective enzymes Note: Leukodystrophies that cannot be further classified are 'lumped' together as 'unclassified leukodystrophy', or sudanophilic leukodystrophy

LEUKODYSTROPHIES

I Globoid cell leukodystrophy of Krabbe A condition of infant to adult onset due to galactocerebrosidase deficiency, characterized by abundant globoid cells in the demyelinated areas; see Globoid cells

II Metachromatic leukodystrophy A condition of infant to adult onset due to sulfatase deficiency characterized by metachromasia of the demyelinated tissue Clinical If the involvement is mild, it may be completely symptomatic

III X-linked leukodystrophy a) With adrenal involvement (adrenoleukodystrophy) due to a defect in the peroxisomal fatty acid oxidation system and accumulation of very long chain fatty acids or b) Without adrenal involvement (Pelizaeus Merzbacher disease) due to a unknown defect with accumulation of proteolipid

Leukoedema Edema of the oral mucosa of undetermined significance that may clinically mimic early leukoplakia, an often premalignant, characterized by acanthosis, intracellular edema and superficial parakeratosis

Leukoencephalopathy see Progressive multifocal leukoencephalopathy

Leukoerythroblastic reaction Vaughan's leukoerythroblastosis The increased presence in the peripheral blood of immature red cells, ie normoblasts, and immature leukocytes, metamyelocytes and band forms, which may be associated with metastatic cancers, hematopoietic malignancy, hemolytic anemia, Gaucher's disease, polytraumatized patients, marrow infiltration by a variety of processes, infection, eg fungal, viral, tuberculosis, sarcoidosis, histiocytosis, hypoxia; one-third of patients with this reaction have no known underlying disease; Cf Leukemoid reaction

Leukokinin see Tuftsin

Leukoplakia A white patch or plaque seen by gross examination of the oral cavity and upper respiratory tract, vulva and uterine cervix and renal pelvis and urinary bladder; in each site the significance is different ORAL CAVITY Leukoplakia is often tobacco-induced (either smoked or chewed) and is regarded as a premalignant lesion, especially in pipe smokers, 15-20% of which are dysplastic, carcinoma-in-situ or frankly invasive carcinomas at initial evaluation and 15-20% of remainder develop cancer within 10 years of follow-up; other 'white patch' lesions of the oral cavity include lichen planus, syphilis, candidiasis, lupus erythematosus, chemical burns, alcohol, endocrine dysfunction, vitamin A and B complex deficiencies EXTERNAL FEMALE GENITAL Leukoplakia is not per se premalignant, although intraepithelial neoplasia (Bowen's disease, carcinoma-in-situ) and invasive squamous cell carcinoma may produce 'white patches', as do lichen sclerosis et atrophicus and kraurosis vulvae UTERINE CERVIX Leukoplakia usually corresponds to hyper-or parakeratosis and may be seen with in-situ or invasive cervical carcinoma as a coincidental finding

Leukorrhea GYNECOLOGY A non-specfic whitish malodorous vaginal discharge accompanied by dyspareunia and intense pruritus, which may be induced by infection, eg ***Candida albicans, Gardnerella vaginalis, Trichomonas vaginalis, Neisseria gonorrhoeae***, foreign body-related infections, estrogen depletion, neoplasms and as a postpartum phenomenon

Leukotomy see Psychosurgery

Leukotrienes (LT) A family of low-weight, biologically-active molecules produced by leukocytes, macrophages, mast and other cells in response to immunologic and non-immunological stimuli; LTs are synthesized by 5-lipoxygenase-induced oxidation of arachidonic acid at C-5, which is subsequently transformed into an unstable epoxide intermediate LTA_4, followed by either hydration to LTB_4 or addition of glutathione to form LTC_4 (elimination of a γ-glutamyl residue yields LTD_4; further removal of a glycine yields LTE_4); LTA_4 is produced in the asthmatic lung, in neutrophils and mast cells, causing smooth muscle contraction and bronchoconstriction; LTB_4 is produced by neutrophils, causing adhesion and chemotaxis, stimulating neutrophil aggregation, enzyme release and superoxide generation within neutrophils; LTC_4, LTD_4, LTE_4 and platelet activating factor comprise the 'Slow-reacting substances of anaphylaxis' or SRS-A; LTC_4 may have a central neuroendocrine function; 5-lipoxygenase pathway products are linked to adult respiratory distress syndrome, allergic rhinitis, asthma, gout, inflammatory bowel disease, neonatal pulmonary hypertension, rheumatoid arthritis (N Engl J Med 1990; 323:645rv); see Eicosanoid, Lipoxin

Levan DENTISTRY A fructose homopolymer linked by β-2,6 bonds, formed by the partial digestion of sucrose by ***Bacillus*** and ***Streptococcus*** species, which is a component of dental plaque representing the first biochemical event in cariogenesis; see Caries, Plaque; Cf Periodontal disease

Level of care The intensity of medical care being provided by the physician or facility PRIMARY CARE Coordinated, comprehensive and personal care, available on both a first-contact and continuous basis; it incorporates the tasks of medical diagnosis and treatment, psychological assessment and management, personal support, communication of information about illness, prevention and health maintenance; primary care is generally equated to that provided by the family physician, general practitioner and by physicians in the emergency room SECONDARY CARE That medical care that is available in the community hospital, comprising the bulk of in-patient medical care provided in the US; secondary care centers are equipped to provide all but the most specialized of care, surgery and diagnostic modalities TERTIARY CARE Highly specialized medical care for patients who are usually referred from secondary care centers, which consists in subspecialty expertise in a) Surgery Organ transplantation, pediatric cardiovascular surgery, stereotactic neurosurgery and others b) Internal medicine Genetics, hepatology, adolescent psychiatry and others c) Diagnostic modalities PET (positron emission tomography) and SQUID (superconducting quantum interface device) scanning, color Doppler electrocardiography, electron microscopy, gene rearrangement and molecular analysis and d) Therapeutic modalities Experimental protocols for treating advanced and/or potentially fatal disease, including AIDS, cancer and inborn errors of metabolism

'Leveno method' A design for a clinical study in which the patient's permission is not obtained for entry in either of the two blinded arms of a protocol, since both arms represent widely accepted 'standards of care' (N Engl J Med 1987; 315:615, ibid; 316:480); Cf Zelen design

Levonorgestrol see Norplant

Lewis system A group of erythrocyte antigens that differs from other red cell antigen groups as a) The antigen is present in the soluble form in saliva and blood, and red cells acquire their phenotype by adsorbing the antigen from the plasma onto the red cell membrane (table, below) b) The Lewis phenotype expressed depends on whether the subject is a 'secretor' or 'non-secretor' of the Lewis gene product and c) Lewis phenotype expression depends on another blood group, the ABO phenotype; Lewis antigens are carbohydrates and those with the Lewis blood 'secretor' status are at increased risk of urinary tract infections by ***Escherichia coli*** and other bacteria which attach to carbohydrate residues of glycolipids and glycoproteins on the urothelial cell (N Engl J Med 1989; 320:773)

Lewis blood group

Genotype	Secretor status	Phenotype
Le, H, se	Non-secretor	Le^{a+b-}
Le, H, Se	Secretor	Le^{a-b+}
le, H, Se	Secretor	Le^{a-b-}
le, H, se	Non-secretor	Le^{a-b-}

LFA-1 deficiency A co-dominant or recessive immune deficiency due to a defect in the lymphocyte function-associated antigen, a 95 kD β chain that is normally linked by covalent bonds to the CD11a molecule that facilitates NK binding, cytolytic T-cell mediated killing and the helper T cell response Clinical Inflammation and delayed separation of the umbilical cord, pyogenic mucocutaneous infections, pneumonia and poor wound healing due to abnormal cell adherence, chemotaxis and a reduced respiratory burst

L-form MICROBIOLOGY A special slow-growing (transitional phase) variant bacterium, eg streptococci, that has lost its rigid walls, replicating as small filterable elements in hypertonic media; L-forms arise spontaneously or may be induced, eg using gradients of penicillin in the agar, which inhibits bacterial wall formation and may be recovered in pyelonephritis and endocarditis; may revert to normal either spontaneously or with magnesium; the 'L' designation honors the Lister Institute of London

LFT Liver function tests Clinical parlance for a battery of biochemical determinants, that are measured in the serum and reflect the liver's metabolic reserve capacity; thus defined, LFTs include those that a) Measure hepatic ability to i) Excrete endogenous (bilirubin, bile acids, ammonia) or exogenous (drugs, dyes, galactose) substances and ii) Perform metabolic functions including conjugation and synthesis of proteins b) Measure substances elevated in i) Hepatic disease, inflammation or necrosis (elevation of transferases and other enzymes, vitamin B_{12}, iron and ferritin) or ii) Biliary tract obstruction (bilirubin, cholesterol, enzymes and lipoprotein-X) Note: Other non-LFT biochemical and immunologic determinants for specific hepatic disease include serological markers for hepatitides (HAV, HBV, HCV, HDV, HEV) and HIV, autoimmune diseases (anti-mitochondrial antibodies, primary biliary cirrhosis), malignancy (α-fetoprotein, relatively specific hepatocellular carcinoma) and metabolic diseases (ceruloplasmin in Wilson's disease and transferrin levels in hemochromatosis)

LGC see Lymphoid glandular complex

LGL Large granular lymphocyte, Null cell, Third population cell Lymphocytes that lack the usual B- or T-cell markers, but have IgG Fc fragment receptors; LGLs comprise 3.5% of lymphocytes and are thought to be of marrow origin and are further divided into *NATURAL KILLER CELLS*, comprising 70% of LGLs and defined by the monoclonal antibodies, B73.1, anti-Leu 11 and N 901,. which bind to corresponding antigens on the cell surfaces and *KILLER CELLS* which mediate antibody-dependent cell-mediated cytotoxicity; see ADCC, Killer cells, Natural killer cells

LGV see Lymphogranuloma venereum

LH see Luteinizing hormone

LHRH Luteinizing hormone-releasing hormone A decapeptide synthesized by hypothalamic neurons that stimulates the release of FSH and LH in response to central nervous system stimulation; LHRH may be used to stimulate normal testicular function and to suppress testosterone production in prostatic carcinoma, thus functioning in a similar fashion as estrogen, eg diethylstilbestrol therapy or orchiectomy

LI see Labeling index; see Locomotion index

LIA Lysine iron agar MICROBIOLOGY A growth medium for gram-negative rods that overlaps the characteristics of Kligler iron agar and Triple sugar iron agar, see TSI

Libby Zion A young woman who died shortly after admission to the emergency room in a New York hospital in 1984, related to inadequate care provided by overworked and undersupervised medical house officers; based on her medical history, she was diagnosed as having a viral syndrome with hysterical symptoms, but at autopsy had fulminant bilateral bronchopneumonia; the 'Libby Zion case' became a cause célèbre and the catalyst for increasing the supervision of physicians-in-training (residents), especially those who are working in emergency rooms (N Engl J Med 1988; 318:771) and reducing their work-load to 80 hours/week; the cost of increasing the 'coverage' of a hospital's physician staff to full-time (in order to compensate for the mandated reduction in hours), would add an estimated hundreds to thousands of millions of dollars annually to the cost of health care in the US, if the precedent set in New York State becomes a norm (J Am Med Assoc 1990; 263:3177)

'Liberated' CR1 A truncated complement receptor CR1 that lacks the transmembane and intracytoplasmic domains, which may have a role in limiting the size of myocardial infarcts by reducing complement activation; 'liberated' CR1 may have a therapeutic role in other forms of ischemia, burns, autoimmunity and inflammation, since it is a natural inhibitor of complement activation

Library DNA library MOLECULAR BIOLOGY A complete set of genomic clones from an organism or of complementary DNA clones from one cell type; a DNA library is prepared by extracting all of an organism's DNA, derived from cells presumed to have a full set of sequences, eg sperm or embryonal cells; the DNA is then digested using a restriction endonuclease of bacterial origin, eg ***Eco***RI, which cleaves the double-stranded DNA into 2 to 20 kilobase pair fragments, each end of which has a short, single-stranded four nucleotide (AATT) segment known as a 'sticky' end; the DNA fragments are then mixed with an equal amount of lambda bacteriophages that have also been subjected to ***Eco***RI digestion; ***Eco***RI digestion of the lambda phage yields three fragments, a disposible middle segment and two flanking segments; the flanking segments attach to the 'sticky' ends of the previously digested 2-20 kilobase pair fragments of DNA; DNA ligase is then added to the mixture to rejoin the recombinant DNA molecules; the recombinant molecules are then coated with bacteriophage proteins; only the molecules of an appropriate size will be 'packaged' into a coherent and viable recombinant bacteriophage Note: 'Library' also refers to the full complement of sequence elements that encode the two variable regions on the immunoglobulin light chain or the three variable regions on the immunoglobulin heavy chain

Library search see Literature search

Lichen Greek, Tree moss A generic term that may be applied to any skin condition characterized by thickened papular eruptions

Lichen sclerosis et atrophicus (LS et A) Hallopeau's disease A pruritic lesion of the mucosa that is more common in women, which when confined to the genitalia is termed kraurosis vulvae in women and balanitis xerotica obliterans in men; the cutaneous lesions consist of flat-topped white macules that coalesce, forming white patches **Histopathology** Hyperkeratosis with follicular plugging, atrophy with hydropic degeneration of basal cells, edema and homogenization of the upper dermal collagen and mid-dermal inflammation; LS et A evolves towards malignancy in 5% of men, but rarely, if at all in women

Licorice A preparation from the root of the European legume ***Glycyrrhiza glabra***, which has a high content of glycyrrhizic acid (glucuronic acid + glycyrrhetinic acid), which is structurally similar to steroids; excessive ingestion of licorice may cause a syndrome of mineralocorticoid excess, with sodium and water retention, hypokalemia and myopathy with myoglobulinuria, acting not by molecular mimicry, as had been previously postulated, but rather by suppressing both 11 β-hydroxysteroid dehydrogenase and the renin-angiotensin-aldosterone axis (N Engl J Med 1991; 325:1223)

LID Late-onset immune deficiency An idiopathic condition associated with gastric carcinoma, atrophic gastritis, pernicious anemia, autoimmunity, malabsorption variably accompanied by lactose intolerance, small intestinal atrophy, thymoma and agnostic myeloid metaplasia with immunoglobulin defects and the Prasad syndrome

Life extension see Gerontology

Life support measures The care provided to a person in profoundly obtunded or nearly moribund state that is usually administered in an intensive care unit to maintain the patient in a stable and/or 'compensated' clinical state, requiring 24-hour monitoring and extraordinary therapeutic measures; see Advance directive, DNR orders

Life table Actuarial life table, Kaplan-Meier survival estimate PUBLIC HEALTH A table that presents the results of a clinical study in which the subjects enter and leave the trial at different times; each subject has a well-defined point of entry (onset of treatment) and end point (relapse, death or other) and all subjects may be evaluated at determined intervals with respect to the expected survival of an idealized person, based on actuarial analysis of census data and mortality rates

Life-threatening illness A morbid condition in which the likelihood of death is high unless the course of disease is interrupted, eg AIDS, high-grade or preterminal cancer, or conditions in which the end-point is mere survival, eg severe cerebrovascular accidents with significant residua; this term is of use for regulatory agencies that may choose to allow a patient to enter a therapeutic protocol based on the severity of his disease, eg under a 'Compassion treatment' IND protocol; see Illness; Cf Severely debilitating illness

Li-Fraumeni syndrome SBLA syndrome An autosomal dominant condition with a marked predisposition towards multiple malignancies (Ann Med 1969; 71:747), including sarcomas, carcinomas of the adrenal cortex, breast, larynx and lung, brain tumors, leukemia and lymphomas occurring at any time from infancy to adulthood **Molecular biology** Skin fibroblasts from these patients are resistant to killing by ionizing radiation and have 3-8 times greater than normal expression of the c-myc gene product and activation of the c-***raf***-1 gene; the gene defect lies in the tumor suppressor gene, p53 (Science 1990; 250:1233) and the early onset of malignancy may be a confirmation of Knudsen's one-hit/two-hit model of carcinogenesis, initially enumerated in retinoblastomas (Medical Hypothesis 1979; 5:15); see One-hit/two-hit model

Ligandin Glutathione S-transferase Y protein A hepatic protein that binds unconjugated bilirubin in the hepatic cytosol; increased ligandin retards bilirubin efflux into the plasma and has a role in hepatic excretion of other anionic substances

Ligase A generic term for the class of enzymes (EC 6) that joins two different substrate molecules, coupled to the hydrolysis of a high-energy pyrophosphate bond, eg the carboxylation reaction in which CO_2 is joined to pyruvate forming oxalacetate, accompanied by the degradation of ATP to ADP

Light chain disease Bence-Jones myeloma ONCOLOGY A paraproteinemia, comprising 20% of all myelomas, in which monoclonal light chains are produced in excess and associated with renal amyloidosis and failure due to tubular blockage by certain Bence-Jones proteins (N Engl J Med 1991; 324:1845)); 80% have monoclonal light chains in the circulation; 60% demonstrate decreased γ-globulin and lytic bone lesions; those with light chain disease fare less well than those with IgG or IgA myelomas, and the lambda type generally is more aggressive than kappa light chain disease, with marked proteinuria, poor renal function and shorter survival

Lightening OBSTETRICS An abrupt sensation of 'lightness' or relief from the weightiness felt by the mother that occurs about two weeks before delivery, corresponding to the drop of the baby's head into the pelvis

Lightning foot Burning feet, Barashek or Gopalan syndrome Intense burning pain of the feet with hyperesthesiae, increased skin temperature and vasomotor changes, occasionally accompanied by scotoma and amblyopia; the lightning foot is of uncertain etiology, but may be due to a combination of vitamin B and protein deficiency and/or a toxin present in polished rice, a condition reported in late Colonial India

Lightning mark FORENSIC PATHOLOGY An arborescent charring of skin, secondary to high voltage electricity (lightning and hydroelectric generators), which may be seen in subjects dying of electrocution

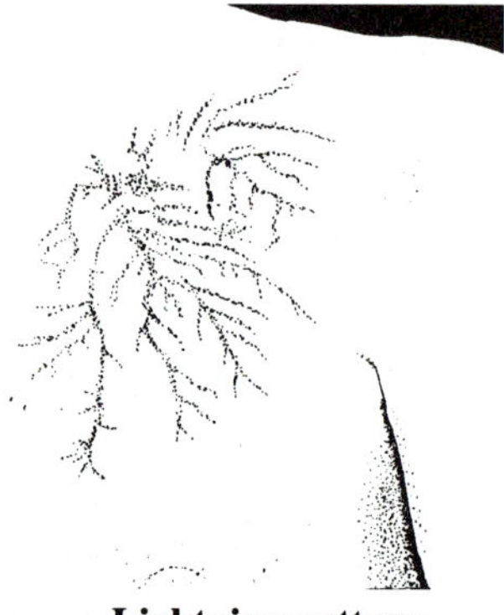
Lightning pattern

Lightning movement Myoclonus Shock-like muscle contraction (or inhibition, 'negative myoclonus', eg asterixis), involving one or multiple muscle groups ranging from a muscle flicker to a synchronous jerk of an entire body segment **Types** **ESSENTIAL MYOCLONUS** Idiopathic and non-progressive, eg restless legs syndrome **PHYSIOLOGIC MYOCLONUS** Associated with sleep jerks and hiccough **EPILEPTIC MYOCLONUS** Associated with epilepsy and **SYMPTOMATIC MYOCLONUS** Associated with encephalopathy, spinocerebellar degeneration, metabolic, toxic or viral encephalopathy or trauma

Lightning pains Sudden, sharp painful crises that are either idiopathic or elicited by cold and stressants, potentially requiring opiates for relief, a classic symptom of tabes dorsalis, which is usually accompanied by progressive degeneration of the posterior and lateral columns of the spinal cord Clinical Loss of reflexes, vibration and position sense, ataxia, urinary incontinence, impotence; lightning pains also occur in post-herpetic neuralgia, glossopharyngeal and trigeminal neuralgia (tic douloureux, triggered by peri- or intraoral stimulation, occurring as clusters of stabbing pain followed by refractory pauses, exacerbated in the spring and fall)

Light scatter The dispersion of light in any direction, which may be used to determine the size of a particle in a clear solution; when an instrument's 'detector' is directly in front of the incident light, dispersion of light is minimal and such so-called 'forward angle light scatter' is a measurement of the particle's diameter; a 'backscatter' detector is located at a 90° angle and measures the light reflecting from a particle's surface, which may be enhanced by adding a fluorescent label and used to detect the presence of specific molecules (antigens), when linked to a monoclonal antibody, serves to quantify the amount of antigen present in a cell sample

Lilac ring pattern A round-to-oval violaceous cutaneous induration that surrounds the ivory-white shiny lesions of early scleroderma ('morphea'); Cf Heliotrope rash

Lilliputian syndrome Micropsia A hallucination in which all persons viewed by the subject appear very small, likened to the Lilliputians in Swift's 'Gulliver's Travels'; the finding is non-specific and has been described in febrile dementia, chorea, prolonged fasting, dementia and various drug intoxications; separation of this psychovisual phenomenon from the 'Alice in Wonderland' syndrome is arbitrary and of questionable usefulness

Limb-girdle disease/syndrome(s) A group of often autosomal recessive muscular dystrophies that initially involve either the shoulder (Erb type) or the pelvic (Leyden-Möbius type) 'girdle' Clinical Limb-girdle 'syndromes' are of later onset than Duchenne's disease, with marked muscular atrophy of the affected region accompanied by relentless deterioration, eventually involving the extremities Diagnosis EMG, muscle biopsy; 'Limb-girdle' disease also occurs in acid maltase deficiency, Becker, Duchenne and Emery-Dreifuss dystrophies, endocrine myopathies, lipid storage disease, late onset (nemaline, central-core) myopathies, polymyositis and sarcoidosis Note: The subtypes of childhood muscular dystrophy, scapulohumeral muscular dystrophy, adult-onset limb girdle dystrophy are uncommon

Limbic system NEUROLOGY The 'peripheral' component of the central nervous system, which is linked to the autonomic nervous system and carries out the non-motor and non-sensory aspects of cerebral function, including emotion, feeding, sexual and other behavior and olfaction; the limbic system is comprised of the olfactory system, hippocampus, dentate nucleus, cingulate gyri, amygdalus, septum and parts of the thalamus and hypothalamus; the limbic system has autonomic effects, including changes in blood pressure and respiration

Limit dextrinosis see Debrancher disease

Lindane The gamma-isomer of benzene hexachloride; a carcinogenic, lipid-soluble insecticide used topically to control lice and scabies and occasionally by the suicidally inclined, requiring circa 20-30 g to produce serious toxicity or death Clinical Onset is similar to DDT poisoning with tremors, ataxia, violent tonic-clonic convulsions, pulmonary edema and vascular collapse of neurogenic origin; with time, massive hepatic necrosis ensues, accompanied by hyaline degeneration of the renal tubules and aplastic anemia

Line HEALTH CARE ADMINISTRATION A funded or paid employee position, regardless of whether the person is full- or part-time SUBSTANCE ABUSE A 'unit' of cocaine consisting in an elongated trail of relatively pure powdered cocaine that is snorted through a tube or drinking straw

LINE Long interspersed repeated elements MOLECULAR BIOLOGY 1-5 kilobase pair repeated sequences of DNA; there are an estimated 20-40 000 LINES in the human genome, constituting the 'LINE 1 family' of retroposons, most of which do not encode protein, thus forming a type of junk DNA; see Junk DNA, SINE

Linear accelerator RADIATION ONCOLOGY A device for accelerating charged particles, which employs electrodes and gaps arranged in a straight line, so proportioned that when the potentials are varied in the proper amplitude and frequency, particles passing through the waveguide receive successive increments of energy, and are therefore accelerated; the device is designed to deliver therapeutic radiation in the range of 4 to 25 million volts, as either radiation or high-energy electron beams (most commonly, cobalt-60), delivering 2-10 grays/min (200-1000 rads/min) at the center of an internal malignancy; linear accelerators are used to treat Hodgkin's disease and other lymphoproliferative malignancies, seminomas and localized carcinoma of the breast, in combination with a 'lumpectomy'

Linearity STATISTICS A straight line relation between two quantities, where when a value 'X' is increased or decreased, 'Y' is proportionately increased or decreased; linearity assumes that the relation between X and Y (abscissa and ordinate) can be summarized in a straight line, known as a least-squares regression method; linearity is a requirement for quality control in laboratory medicine and is applicable to most 'chemistries' where the coefficient of variation is less than 10.0

Linear regression A generic term for statistical methods that are used to 'fit' a straight line to scattered data points of paired values Xi, Yi, where the values of Y (the ordinate or vertical line) are observations of a variable, eg systolic blood pressure and the values of X (the abscissa or horizontal line) increase in a relatively non-random fashion, eg age; the crude technique of 'eyeballing' a scattergram of data points is rapid but subjective, inelegant, imprecise and not amenable to statistical analysis; linear regression is a simple way of evaluating the validity of data by determining the trueness of its 'fit' to a straight line and can be used to summarize data or calculate the change between the outcome, response or dependent variable and the main variable known as the predictor variable

Formula for linear regression
Predicted outcome
= Intercept + Slope X Predicted value

Linear staining IMMUNOLOGY A pattern of immune deposition described as continuous, smooth, thin, delicate and ribbon-like; linear deposits of IgG and C3 are seen in patients with either anti-glomerular basement membrane disease or Goodpasture syndrome, when viewed by immunofluorescent microscopy; weakly staining linear deposits of IgG may occur in diabetes mellitus, celiac disease, human allografts and minimal change nephrotic syndrome; linear staining in the skin corresponds to IgA deposition at the dermal-epidermal junction in bullous dermatosis, which is seen by indirect immunofluorescence; Cf Band test, Lumpy-bumpy pattern

Linear transformation The mathematical conversion of an equation into one providing data that can be plotted in a straight line, eg transformation of the Michaelis-Menten equation into Lineweaver-Burk plot

Lingua geographica see Geographic tongue

Linguatula A genus of tongueworm, a primitive parasite lacking circulatory and respiratory tracts that invades the respiratory tracts of carnivores; linguatuliasis is the direct human infection by the third-stage larvae, which most commonly affects those of the Middle East who ingest undercooked liver or lymph nodes from sheep or goats, migrating from the stomach to the nasopharynx, resulting in pain, itching and irritation in the throat with dyspnea, dysphagia and vomiting, or with intense infestation cause asphyxia; alternatively, the worms may emerge in the intestine and encyst in the liver, spleen, lymph nodes and lungs

Linitis plastica Greek Linen cloth A descriptor for the appearance of certain hollow viscus organs, consisting of a rigidly thickened wall, classically described in a common variant of gastric carcinoma **Radiology** Upper gastrointestinal series demonstrates neither ulcer nor mass but a fixed, non-distensible stomach, absent folds and narrowed lumen, fancifully likened to the Spanish leather wineskin, la bota **Histopathology** Extensive desmoplastic reaction with numerous scattered signet ring cells and clusters of moderately-differentiated adenocarcinoma; linitis plastica may rarely occur in other hollow epithelial cell-lined organs, eg colon or bladder

Linkage disequilibrium (LD) GENETICS The tendency for certain alleles at different loci to occur far more (or less) frequently in the same haplotype than expected based on statistics alone, the result of proximityof those alleles, as occurs on the major histocompatibility complex, located on chromosome 6; in a random population breeding under ideal conditions, the occurrence of individual genes is a product of the frequencies, ie random; thus the relation of one gene to another should be purely statistical; as an example, if HLA-A1 occurs in 16% of a population and HLA-B8 in 10%, an expected 1.6% of the population should have the allelic combination, although the combination actually occurs in 9%; other examples include a) MNSs blood group, where an association of group N with s is five times more common than the N with S, b) The extended haplotype HLA A1, Cw7, B8, DR3, Dw3, MB2, MT2 occurs four times more frequently than expected based on chance Mechanisms of linkage disequilibrium a) Selection Linkage may occur via immune response genes, by interaction of HLA gene products with environmental agents or b) Crossover suppression Crossing-over during meiosis occurs at a significantly lower rate

Linkage map A genetic map based on the coinheritance of allele combinations across multiple polymorphic loci; parental combinations usually delineate the locations of chromosomal 'landmarks', measured in centimorgans (the number of cross-overs/100 meioses) from the chromosomes centromere; see Human Genome Project, Lod score

Linkage number see Winding number

Linkage study GENETICS A study that identifies the chromosome responsible for a disease, requiring a large family with multiple living relatives who have the disease, high diagnostic reliability and sufficient genetic markers to ensure that at least one is close to the gene; see Lod score

Linker DNA A segment of DNA that links adjacent nucleosomes in a chromosome to each other, which is held in place at the H1 histone molecule

Linking number see Winding number

Link sausage appearance MICROBIOLOGY A descriptor for the light microscopic appearance of the elongated blastospores with focal constrictions typical of *Candida* species; Cf Box-car appearance OPHTHALMOLOGY see Sausage link appearance

Linoleic acid An essential 18-carbon fatty acid with 2 unsaturated bonds, derived from plant oils; see Essential fatty acids

Linolenic acid An essential 18-carbon fatty acid with 3 unsaturated bonds, derived from either plants (α-linolenic acid) or animals (γ-linolenic acid); see Essential fatty acids

LIP see Lymphocytic interstitial pneumonia

Lipase A pancreatic esterase that hydrolyses glycerol esters of long chain fatty acids; pancreatic lipase cleaves the outer 1, 3 ester linkages of long chain fatty acids; lipase is elevated only in pancreatitis (markedly so in acute pancreatitis) and pancreatic duct obstruction; see Lipoprotein lipase

Lipid bilayer see Fluid mosaic model

Lipid cell tumor Lipoid tumor A group of steroid hormone-producing tumors **Clinical** Most cases are associated with virilization, less commonly with Cushing's syndrome, 20% are malignant and those which are malignant are often greater than 8 cm in diameter **Pathology** The tumors are yellow-brown, unilateral, composed of cells with theca-lutein, Leydig or hilar cell and/or adrenal cortical cell features including pale pink cytoplasm in polyhedral rounded cell clusters, positive fat stains and well-developed smooth endoplasmic reticulum and mitochondria with tubulo-vesicular cristae, features typical of cells that produce steroid hormones; the true cell of origin is obscure and it is proposed (Int J Gynecol Pathol 1987; 6:40) that steroid cell tumor is a more appropriate term; see Steroid cell tumor

Lipid hypothesis CARDIOLOGY A widely accepted postulate that hyperlipidemia in the form of increased cholesterol, and to a lesser degree, other lipids in the circulation responsible for atherosclerosis, the major cause of death in the US, levels which, when altered by dietary or pharmacologic manipulation, result in a decreased risk of atherosclerosis-related morbidity; the hypothesis appears to be valid, as a) Atherosclerotic plaques contain lipids, most of which are derived directly from plasma lipoproteins b) Atherosclerotic lesions may be produced in hyper-cholesterolemic experimental animals c) Hyperlipidemia is more prevalent in groups with documented atherosclerosis d) Atherosclerosis is more prevalent in subjects with certain familial hyperlipidemias and e) Epidemiologic studies demonstrate a graded increased risk in atherosclerosis-related morbidity and mortality with increasing levels of LDL-cholesterol and decreasing levels of HDL-cholesterol

Lipid 'profile' LABORATORY MEDICINE An abbreviated battery of tests performed on an automated multichannel chemical analyzer, including total cholesterol, LDL-cholesterol, HDL-cholesterol and triglycerides, which helps stratify patients according to risk of atherosclerosis-related mortality and morbidity

Lipid storage diseases A group of rare conditions, including Fabry's disease, Niemann-Pick disease and the sea-blue histiocytosis syndrome, which are often fatal in early childhood, usually due to a catabolic defect of lipid metabolism and characterized by the accumulation of lipids in one or more organs, some of which, eg Gaucher disease, GM-1 gangliosidosis type I and fucosidosis demonstrate foamy histiocytes in the bone marrow, while others, eg Tay-Sachs disease, Krabbe and metachromatic leukodystrophy do not; the diagnosis can be established in utero by performing enzymatic studies on cultured amniotic fluid cells, which can be completed by the 20th week of gestation; see Pseudo-Gaucher's disease, Sphingolipidosis

Lipochrome A generic term for any natural, fat-soluble pigment including lipofuscin, carotenes and lycopene s

Lipofuscin A pigmented lipid degradation product thought to derive from peroxidative destruction of the mitochondrial polyunsaturated lipid membrane or the mitochondria itself; the malonaldehyde produced by mitochondrial peroxide damage may block DNA template activity contributing to heart failure; lipofuscin accumulates with age in the heart, muscle, liver, nerve and in lysosomes

Lipoid adrenal hyperplasia (LAH) A subtype of congenital adrenal hyperplasia, most common in the Japanese, due to a defective cholesterol side-chain cleavage enzyme $P450_{SCC}$, formerly 20, 22 desmolase; LAH is associated with decreased peripheral conversion of cholesterol to pregnenolone, accumulation of cholesterol and lipids in the adrenal cortex and, given the lack of testicular hormone production, all infants are phenotypic females **Prognosis** Death in early infancy in adrenal 'crisis' due to insufficient mineralocorticoid and glucocorticoid production

Lipoid pneumonia Golden pneumonia A pneumonitis caused by exogenous oils that percolate into the lungs through intranasal instillation of mineral oil, forced administration of cod liver, castor or other oils or due to a congenital defect in the oropharyngeal diaphragm, eg cleft palate or an intense gag reflex; the intensity of the response is a function of the oils' irritability, ranging from the least irritating vegetable oils to liquid petrolatum, which may act as a foreign body and animal oils and milk, which may evoke a pneumonitis **Histopathology** Accumulation of abundant foamy lipid-laden macrophages in the alveolar spaces, and lesions that progress from interstitial proliferation to exudation, with proliferative fibrosis and eventually, miliary paraffinoma-like nodules; see Mineral oil

Lipoid proteinosis An autosomal recessive condition of childhood onset characterized by coalescent aggregates of lipid and mucopolysaccharides, resulting in numerous yellowish plaques, papules, nodules and induration of the skin (pachydermia), eyelids, oropharynx and larynx with hoarseness, hyperkeratosis of the knees and elbows, hyalinization of the blood vessels; calcification of the hippocampal gyri, while uncommon, is pathognomonic and held responsible for the associated convulsions

Lipoleiomyoma A uterine leiomyoma-like lesion of obese, post-menopausal women with cholecystitis, which may cause vague abdominal pain, backache, vaginal discharge or hemorrhage

Lipomatosis dolorosa Dercum's disease A disease of perimenopausal women with multiple localized masses of adipose tissue accompanied by local pain at the sites of accumulation **Clinical** Neuroasthenia, headache, depression, ecchymoses and cardiovascular decompensation due to cardiac overload **Treatment** Weight reduction

Lipomatosis multicentrica A heterogeneous clinical condition in which there are multiple aggressively proliferating masses of non-encapsulated adipose tissue

Lipooxygenase pathway An arachidonic acid metabolic pathway leading to 5-HPETE (5-hydroperoxyeicosatetraenoic acid), that is further metabolized to 5-HETE, lipoxins or leukotrienes (LTC_4, LTD_4 and LTE_4), see SRS-A (slow-reacting substances of anaphylaxis)

Lipophilin A proteolipid that comprises a major component of myelin

Lipopolysaccharide-binding protein A trace plasma protein that binds to the lipid A moiety of bacterial lipopolysaccharide (LPS) or to endotoxin (a glycolipid present in the outer membrane of all gram-negative bacteria); the complexes formed between LPS and its binding protein may stimulate monocyte release of tumor-necrosis factor (Science 1990; 249:1429)

Lipoprotein(a) Lp(a) A lipoprotein that has a wide range of serum levels 0.05-1.90 mmol/L (US: 20-760 mg/L), which has a lipid content similar to LDL, and binds to the LDL receptor with lesser affinity than LDL; Lp(a) has considerable sequence similarity ('homology') to plasminogen, a finding of unknown significance; although its metabolism and relation to atherosclerosis is unclear, it is increased in those at risk for coronary heart disease (N Engl J Med 1990; 322:1494, Science 1989; 246:904)

Lipoprotein-associated coagulation inhibitor HEMATOLOGY A protease inhibitor of the extrinsic coagulation pathway that inhibits factor Xa and factor VIIa/tissue factor (J Biol Chem 1989; 264:18832)

Lipoproteins A family of lipid-carrying, water-soluble proteins including chylomicrons, high-, intermediate-, low- and very low-density lipoproteins that are responsible for the transport of cholesterol and cholesterol esters, phospholipids and triglycerides throughout the circulation; lipoprotein composition (table, below); lipoproteins are classified based on the density by ultracentrifugation; some are subdivided by gel electrophoresis **HDL** High density (1.063-1.21 kg/L) lipoprotein is synthesized in the liver and intestine and is responsible for cholesterol metabolism; HDL migrates-electrophoretically as an α globulin, major protein components are apoA-I and apoA-II; HDL is further subdivided into HDL_1 (1.050-1.063 kg/L, which has a density overlapping LDL as well as HDL_2 (1.063-1.120 kg/L) and HDL_3 (1.120-1.210 kg/L); the higher the HDL-cholesterol level, the lower the risk of myocardial infarct and HDL is used to screen for atherosclerosis (J Am Med Assoc 1989; 261:497), see HDL **IDL** Intermediate density (1.006-1.019 kg/L) lipoprotein is a β-globulin-migrating metabolic intermediate formed by the action of lipoprotein lipase on chylomicrons and VLDL **LDL** Low density (1.019-1.063 kg/L) lipoprotein migrates as a β-globulin with apolipoprotein-B being the major protein component and cholesteryl linoleate the major lipid component; increased LDL is a major risk factor for atherosclerosis and coronary artery disease, when LDL is subdivided by gel-electrophoresis, patients with increased small dense LDL subclass are at highest risk for myocardial infarcts **VLDL** Very low density (< 1.006 kg/L) lipoprotein migrates in the pre-β region of the electrophoretic gel; the main lipid component is triglyceride and the major proteins are apolipoprotein-B, apolipoprotein-C and apolipoprotein-E

Composition of Lipoproteins

	Chol	TGs	Prot	PPLs	
HDL	20	5	50	25	α migration
VLDL	25	50	7	18	α_2 migration
LDL	55	5	20	20	β migration
IDL	30	40	10	20	
Chylo	5	90	1	5	

Chol Cholesterol — PPL Phospholipids
Prot Protein — TGs Triglycerides

Lipoprotein lipase A hydrolytic enzyme that breaks ester bonds of di- and triglycerides from chylomicrons and low-density lipoprotein to form free fatty acids and glycerol, acting in the capillary endothelium of adipose tissue, skeletal and cardiac muscle

Lipoprotein lipase deficiency An autosomal recessive condition characterized by absence of lipoprotein lipase (LPL), resulting in massive hypertriglyceridemia of neonatal onset and recurrent episodes of pancreatitis; in 73% of the French-Canadian cohort of patients with lipoprotein lipase deficiency, the defect lies in a missense mutation on residue 207 of exon 5 (N Engl J Med 1991; 324:1761), detectable in homozygous and heterozygous subjects by dot-blot analysis Clinical Fatty food intolerance, eruptive xanthomas and hepatosplenomegaly that regresses with dietary control; because hydrolysis of triglycerides from chylomicrons and endogenous VLDL requires both LPL and its activator apoC-II, apoC-II deficiency has a similar clinical picture

Lipoprotein X An abnormal lipoprotein composed of 65% lecithin, 30% cholesterol and 5% protein (apolipoprotein-C and albumin) that is seen in lecithin-cholesterol acyl-transferase deficiency and in obstructive biliary disease, which is associated with cholestatic jaundice

Liposome THERAPEUTICS A synthetic, relatively uniform bilayer lipid membrane-bound vesicle formed by emulsification of cell membranes in dilute salt solutions; liposomes are being developed as an approach for drug delivery in which relatively toxic drugs, eg amphotericin B, doxorubicin and pentavalent antimony are 'wrapped' inside a liposome and tagged with an organ-specific antibody

Liposuction Suction-assisted lipectomy A plastic surgical technique used to remove focal fat deposits; a metal cannula with side holes is connected to a high-pressure vacuum, removing fat from the face, neck, breasts, abdomen, thighs

β-Lipotropin A 91-residue protein of unknown function produced by the anterior pituitary and co-secreted with ACTH, which has sequence homology to endorphins and enkephalins

Lipoxins A group of arachidonic acid-derived products formed by 5- and 15-lipoxygenase and peroxidase that contain a conjugated tetraene structure and three alcohols; lipoxin A (LXA) and lipoxin B (LXB) inhibit natural killer cell-induced cytotoxicity; alone, LXA dilates arterioles, induces glomerular hyperperfusion and hypertension and contracts pulmonary muscle, and when added to neutrophils, stimulates superoxide generation

Lip stripping DERMATOLOGY Excision and advancement of the buccal mucosa, a technique used in plastic surgery when the vermilion border becomes indistinct, due to squamous metaplasia or labial hyperkeratosis, a potentially preneoplastic lesion of light-skinned sun-exposed elderly subjects

Liquefactive degeneration Immune-induced liquefaction at the dermal-epidermal interface, which 'loosens' the basal cells, resulting in coalescing subepidermal vesicles in dermatitis herpetiformis, dermatomyositis, dyskeratosis congenita, erythema multiforme, fixed drug reaction, incontinentia pigmenti, lichen nitidus, lichen planus, lichen sclerosis et atrophicans, lichenoid drug reaction, lupus erythematosus, pinta, poikiloderma atrophicans vasculare, poikiloderma congenita of Rothman-Thompson and Riehl's melanosis

Liquefaction necrosis A pathological state characterized by fulminant enzymatic hydrolysis of tissue, due to ischemia, resulting in myocardial and cerebral infarction or due to bacterial, often pyogenic, infections which, when associated with gas production, yield cystic spaces; liquefaction is a necrotizing process evoked by hydrolytic enzymes that may be produced by coagulase-positive staphylococci, β-hemolytic streptococci and *Escherichia coli*

Liquid-protein diet A very low calorie weight reduction diet that provided 800 calories and protein in the form of hydrolyzed collagen; the quality of protein in collagen is so poor that it is immediately converted to glucose, resulting in a negative nitrogen balance; liquid-protein diets were inculpated in a number of sudden cardiac arrests in dieters on this regimen and have been abandoned; see Diet

Liquid scintillation counter An instrument that detects low-energy β-particle emissions from ^{14}C and ^{3}H, for immunoassays of substances, eg proteins, of biological interest **Principle** Radioactive samples are dissolved in toluene, a substance that absorbs low-energy β-emissions; the energy is then transferred to a fluor, which emits a photon detectable by a photomultiplier; see POP, POPOP, Quenching, Radioimmunoassay

LIS see Laboratory information system

LISS Low-ionic strength saline TRANSFUSION MEDICINE A low-concentration saline solution used in the blood bank to reduce the zeta potential (the electron cloud separating erythrocytes) allowing weak antibodies to agglutinate and be detected by the usual agglutination tests; see Zetacrit

Listeria A genus of small gram-positive motile bacilli with a palisading growth pattern, similar to the chinese letter appearance of *Corynebacteria* species; *L monocytogenes* is named for its marked affinity for and residence within monocytes and macrophages **Epidemiology** Outbreaks may be associated with contaminated milk products and cheese (N Engl J Med 1988; 319:823) **Clinical** One-third of reported cases of listeriosis occur in pregnant women, causing transplacental infection with abortion, stillbirth and premature delivery Perinatal infection Infants may present with septicemia, diarrhea, vomiting, cardiorespiratory distress and meningoencephalitis Immunocompromised adults may suffer meningoencephalitis, endocarditis, disseminated granulomatosis, lymphadenitis, peritonitis and cholecystitis **Treatment** Ampicillin, gentamicin, erythromycin, chloramphenicol

Literature search A review of the literature that is relevant to a particular subject for the purpose of writing a report, preparing for a conference or guiding patient management; most medicine-related literature searches in the US begin with the venerated Index Medicus and are then carried out by 1200, 2400 or 9600 baud modem, accessioning the US National Library of Medicine; the average cost per search is 2-4$ and requires the GRATEFUL MED software, a user identification number and a password

Lithium carbonate CLINICAL PHARMACOLOGY An alkali used to treat manic-depression that blocks neurotransmission at the 'second messenger' phosphoinositide-mediated cholinergic neurons in the hippocampus (Science 1988;239:1428), inhibiting the release and uptake of norepinephrine at nerve endings by inhibiting receptor-mediated synthesis of cAMP **Clinical** Hyperirritability, hyperpyrexia, stupor, coma, gastroenteritis, cardiovascular disease, eg arrhythmia, hypotension, decreased ST wave, T inversion, osteoporosis **Analysis** Flame photometry, atomic absorption spectrophotometry **Teratogenesis** Relatively severe cardiac malformations occur in 10% of infants born to lithium-treated manic-depressive women **Toxicity** Overdose causes death in one-fourth of patients **Treatment** Potassium-sparing drugs

Lithotripsy Shock-wave lithotripsy A non-surgical, non-invasive method for dissolving renal, and more recently biliary tract calculi; the patients lie prone and partially immersed in a large bathtub-like vat; shock waves are generated extracorporally by high-energy underwater spark discharge focused on the patient's ventral aspect by a reflector (N Engl J Med 1988; 318:393, Ann Int Med 1990; 112:126)

Litogen LEGAL MEDICINE A drug used during pregnancy that is not teratogenic, but which nevertheless results in lawsuits (N Engl J Med 1986; 315:1234); the term was coined by the editor of Teratology, in response to the Wells *v* Ortho case, in which the plaintiff was awarded $5 million for alleged teratogenesis by spermicides, which have not been inculpated in congenital malformation; thus any Litigation-generating agent, might be viewed as a litogen, regardless of its teratogenic, carcinogenic or toxic potential

Little Boy RADIATION MEDICINE The bomb that flattened Hiroshima Note: The biggest bomb in the US arsenal, the B-53 (deployable on the B-52 bomber), was built in the 1960s and is currently 'moth-balled' as safer bombs are available; the B-53 is equivalent to 9 megatons of TNT, ie 750-fold more destructive than Little Boy and 30 times more destructive than the current MX family of nuclear warheads; see IPPNW, Nuclear war

Little gastrin see Gastrin

Little League elbow PEDIATRIC ORTHOPEDICS A form of medial epicondylitis manifesting as apophyseal tenderness with ulnar nerve irritation, which may require surgery if severe, with potential for lifelong arthralgia due to injury of the physeal cells under the articular cartilage; permanent damage results from repeated and excessive axial loading, which compresses the cells against the osseous matrix; later sequelae include osteochondritis dissecans

Little League shoulder PEDIATRIC ORTHOPEDICS Fracture of the proximal humerus through the epiphyseal growth plate (the weakest point of growing long bones), the result of a growing shoulder articulation chronically insulted by throwing a baseball Note: Little League is an international organization dedicated to the sportsmanlike practice of baseball for children under the age of 12

'Little science' A phrase used by US government science policy-makers, for investigator-initiated research, which contrasts with 'big science' that is applied in scope and goal-oriented; see 'Big science'

Little's disease Bilateral congenital spastic diplegia A variant of cerebral palsy with agenesis of the lower motor neurons in the inferior extremities, which affects about 300 000 in the USA **Clinical** Spasticity, muscle weakness, mental retardation and ocular defects, due to neonatal hypoxia, mechanical trauma and prematurity; congenital cerebrovascular malformations and immune-related kernicterus account for a low percentage of cases **Histopathology** Focal cerebral atrophy, microcystic and spongiotic changes of the white matter, potentially associated with basal ganglia atrophy **Differential diagnosis** Brain tumors, 'Floppy infant' syndromes, leukodystrophy and muscular dystrophy

'Little women' syndrome A Laron-type dwarfism variant seen in a highly inbred population of Spanish descent living in the province of Loja in southern Equador that predominantly affects females as the gene mutation may be linked to a trait lethal in males; features unique to this variant include blue sclera, limited elbow extensibility, shortened extremities, high-pitched voices and hip dysplasia in adults (N Engl J Med 1990; 323:1367) Note: Laron dwarfism is an autosomal recessive condition with a high incidence of consanguinity, small facies, micrognathia, prominent forehead, saddle nose, sparse slow-growing hair, poor dentition, small hands and feet, high-pitched voice in children and hypoglycemia **Pathogenesis** Both forms result from a marked reduction in growth hormone-binding protein with reduced insulin-like growth factor I (IGF-1)

Littoral cells Normal fixed macrophages of the spleen that are involved with sequestration and destruction of effete and/or abnormal erythrocytes

Live attenuated vaccine A vaccine that induces an immunologic response more closely resembling that of a natural infection than that elicited by killed vaccines, as the organisms contained therein actively reproduce until held in check by the recipient's own antibodies, thus often conferring life-long immunity; live attenuated vaccines include measles, mumps, polio and rubella; see Killed vaccine

Live birth the '...*COMPLETE EXPULSION OR EXTRACTION FROM ITS MOTHER OF A PRODUCT OF CONCEPTION...WHICH, AFTER SUCH SEPARATION, BREATHES OR SHOWS ANY OTHER EVIDENCE OF LIFE SUCH AS THE BEATING OF THE HEART, PULSATION OF THE UMBILICAL CORD, OR DEFINITE MOVEMENT OF VOLUNTARY MUSCLES, WHETHER OR NOT THE UMBILICAL CORD HAS BEEN CUT OR THE PLACENTA IS ATTACHED*'—American Public Health Association

'Liver eater' TRANSPLANTATION A highly colloquial term of little clinical utility for a patient who has rejected two or more transplanted livers

Liver panel A battery of tests that is considered to be the most cost-effective in evaluation of the liver's functional status, ie produce proteins and metabolize toxic substances, and detect inflammation, measuring the transferases (AST/GOT, AST/GPT and γ-glutamyl transferase), alkaline phosphatase, total bilirubin, conjugated bilirubin, total protein, albumin, prothrombin time; Liver function tests, Organ panel

Liver-spleen scan A radionuclide imaging technique that uses a scintillation camera to detect metabolically-active potentially malignant masses of 2 cm or greater in diameter Note: For detection of mass lesions, the images provided by CT and MRI are far superior; radioisotopes used include ^{99m}Tc and ^{198}Au

'Liver spots' A relatively non-specific lay term for red-brown skin lesions associated with aging, including pigmented seborrheic keratosis and lentigo senilis; see Lentigines

Liver tongue A rarely observed blue-red tongue with engorged capillaries seen in advanced cirrhosis, equated to palmar erythema or spider hemangiomas, which may be accompanied by papillary atrophy or hypertrophy

Liver transplantation A procedure that replaces a metabolically defeated liver which is being performed with increasing frequency and impunity; patients with acute liver disease respond better to liver transplantation as the manifestations of chronic liver disease have not yet developed; transplantations have been performed for chronic active hepatitis, primary sclerosing cholangitis, primary biliary cirrhosis, hepatitis B, hepatitis D, α_1-antitrypsin deficiency (Mayo Clin Proc 1989; 64:84) and LDL-receptor deficiency; in poor operative candidates for orthotopic liver transplantation, auxiliary heterotopic liver transplantation, leaving the patient's own liver in place, may be compatible with up to 12 years survival Transport medium University of Wisconsin solution (J Am Med Assoc 1989; 261:711) **Operating time** 6.5 hours; average blood use during transplantation, 13 units of packed red cells Rejection phenomena occur in 60%, which usually respond to various 'cocktails' including corticosteroids, OKT3 antibody, cyclosporin, FK 506, rapamycin and experimental agents **Early complications** Hypothermia, hyperglycemia **Late complications** Infection, eg cytomegalovirus, gram-positive bacteremia, renal insufficiency, due in part to cyclosporine nephrotoxicity, hypertension, hypokalemia, metabolic alkalosis and fever (Mayo Clin Proc 1989; 64:433); 1 year survival, 83%; 2 year survival 70%; despite ample indication that alcoholics can survive well with liver transplantation, there is an ethical dilemma of whether a person who is solely responsible for his terminal illness has a 'right' to the procedure (J Am Med Assoc 1991; 265:1295, 1299); 90% of rehabilitated alcoholics who survived transplantation returned to a productive life; 20% were retransplanted

Living will A term coined in 1969 to describe an 'advance directive' document in which a mentally-competent adult formally expresses his preferences regarding medical treatment in the event of future incapacitation or should he become incompetent to make medical decisions; a living will is essentially a statement of a person's right to die without what might be considered senseless resuscitation efforts or artificial life support; such a document is 'living' since it is prepared prior to the time of incapacitation and a 'will' as it delineates the person's directions ante incapacitatum (N Engl J Med 1991; 324:1210ed); it is statutorily binding in most US states and goes into effect once competence is lost (J Am Med Assoc 1990; 263:2365); the language recommended by the National Conference of Commissioners on Uniform State Laws is, *'IF I SHOULD HAVE AN INCURABLE OR IRREVERSIBLE CONDITION THAT WILL CAUSE MY DEATH WITHIN A RELATIVELY SHORT TIME, AND I AM UNABLE TO MAKE DECISIONS REGARDING MY MEDICAL TREATMENT, I DIRECT MY ATTENDING PHYSICIAN TO WITHHOLD OR WITHDRAW PROCEDURES THAT MERELY PROLONG THE DYING PROCESS AND ARE NOT NECESSARY TO MY COMFORT OR TO ALLEVIATE PAIN'*; see Advance directive, DNR, Cf Durable powers of attorney, Euthanasia

Lizard skin appearance A fanciful descriptor for the lichenoid changes of the skin, eg drying, scaling, cutaneous atrophy and depigmentation seen in the chronic dermatitis of ***Onchocerca volvulus***, which is characterized by layers of keratin that are loosely separated from the epidermis, accompanied by scarring and loss of dermal elastin fibers

Load LABORATORY SCIENCE To place the specimen(s) of interest, the positive and negative controls at the starting point of a support medium for chromatographic or electrophoretic procedure; alternatively, to position multiple samples in carosel or tray for automated feeding into a a multichannel analyser

Lobster claw deformity A deep cleft between the third and fourth digits of the hands or feet, due to an absence of the central embryologic 'ray'; this deformity is more common in the foot, and is often accompanied by syndactyly of varying severity; the deformity classically occurs in ectodermal dysplasia, eg in the EEC syndrome (ectrodactyly, ectodermal dysplasia and cleft palate), which may be associated with a variety of organ defects

Local area network (LAN) A series of computers that are linked over limited distances by telephone lines or direct cabling, allowing them to share hardware, eg a printer, data, software and software applications; each member in a LAN has its own independent central processing unit, in contrast to mini- and mainframe computers which often communicate in unidirectional fashions, where peripheral 'dummy' terminals largely function as input and query devices

Lochkern German, hole-ridden nucleus A vacuolated nucleus that is a commonly seen in both mature fat and lipomas, which may simulate lipoblasts; see Brown fat

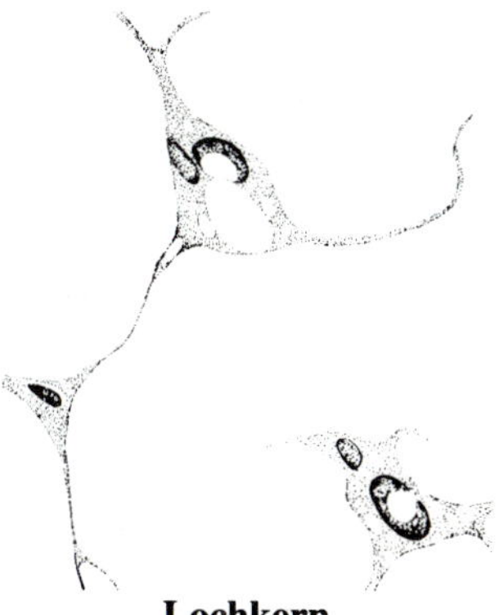

Lochkern

Lock-and-key model BIOCHEMISTRY A model that assumes an enzyme and substrate have a rigid interaction with each other, where a substrate fits in a key-like fashion to its lock, the enzyme, turning on the reaction; while this concept, formulated by Emil Fisher in the 1890s is essentially correct, the 'induced fit model' is more accurate, as the enzyme molds to the substrate before binding and fully activating an enzyme; see Induced fit model

'Locked-in' syndrome REHABILITATION MEDICINE Flaccid tetraplegia with facial paresis and complete incapacity to express voluntary response (anarthric and aphonic), the result of damage or dysfunction of descending motor pathways or peripheral nerves, due to bilateral destruction of the basis pontis or medulla and sparing of tegmentum, caused by infarcts or central pontine myelinolysis; the patients are conscious and alert and only capable of communicating by moving their eyes and eyelids

'Locked lung' Paradoxic bronchospasm, Refractory status asthmaticus A clinical state due to excess use of nebulized isoproterenol, resulting in complete loss of response to epinephrine, aminophyllin, corticosteroids and intermittent positive pressure, which requires weaning from isoproterenol

Lockjaw Spasm of the masseter muscles with stiffness of the jaw caused by tetanospasmin, a neurotoxin produced by ***Clostridium tetani***, resulting in unrestrained muscle firing and sustained muscular contraction, which when severe, causes dysphagia or acute respiratory insufficiency by causing prolonged diaphragm contraction

LOCM see Low-osmolality contrast medium

Locomotion index Leukotactic index A measurement of the ability of leukocytes to migrate in response to chemotactic stimuli; neutrophils are used for in vitro assays of chemotaxis, by either the micropore filter technique or the 'under agarose' method; the leukotactin is obtained from the supernatant of ***Escherichia coli*** in culture, which measures the white cell's ability to move along a chemoattractive gradient, complement C5 is used to test monocyte chemotaxis; locomotion or chemotaxis is decreased in the congenital lazy leukocyte syndrome or in the face of circulating chemotactic factor inactivator, which is increased in cirrhosis, lepromatous leprosy, sarcoidosis, lupus erythematosus, Hodgkin's disease and hairy cell leukemia

Lod score GENETICS A value representing the logarithm (log_{10}) of the odds (probability) of a gene being linked or associated with a disease; linkage analysis calculates the odds for or against the association of a DNA 'marker', ie a segment of DNA, expressed as a 'lod score'; a lod score of +3 or more indicates a significant probability that the DNA marker is linked to a disease, while a lod score of -2 or less indicates a significant probability that there is no linkage

Log Logbook A journal or ledger containing data and dates when the data was collected; logs are used to record scheduling information, document patient-physician encounters, to record quality control data in the laboratory and may be used as a legal document; Cf Notebook

Log-cell kill (hypothesis) ONCOLOGY A malignant tumor

mass exposed one time to a chemotherapeutic drug will undergo under the best of circumstances a maximum of a 2 log-cell kill, ie reduction to 1% of the original 100% or 10^2 tumor volume; since often a tumor mass may be 10^{12} cells in volume, adequate tumor shrinkage depends on multiple log-cell kills by various effective agents Note: In contrast to bulk tumor destruction, which is the intended goal of chemotherapy, immunotherapy is effective against small tumor masses but useless when a tumor is > 0.1 cm, and thus theoretically of use in the lower 'log kill' range

Logic CLINICAL DECISION-MAKING The sum total of education and experience that is integrated into a physician's medical decision-making processes; see Aunt Millie approach, Heuristic logic, Markov process, ROC analysis, Stochastic process

Logic board COMPUTERS The electronic circuitry designed to perform logical functions by a series of logical operations, using logical variables following logical instructions, operating on a two-valued (true or false) system

'Logs in a stream' pattern MICROBIOLOGY A fanciful descriptor for the elongated blastoconidia that readily dissociate from the pseudohyphae, seen by light microscopy in *Candida pseudotropicalis*

Loin pain-hematuria syndrome A benign condition in young women taking oral contraceptives, characterized by episodic gross hematuria, pelvic pain and mild hypertension that resolves upon discontinuation of contraceptives

'Lollipop' appearance MICROBIOLOGY A fanciful descriptor for the microscopic appearance of stalks of varying lengths of *Blastomyces dermatitidis* conidia when cultured at room temperature

Lollipop culture A synonym for an experimental technique for isolating mutant forms of the outer dynein arms in *Chlamydomonas reinhardtii*, a biflagellate unicellular alga used to study the functional, genetic and structural aspects of flagella and their assembly; by shearing a population of cells ('lollipops'), relatively pure amounts of flagella may be obtained for study

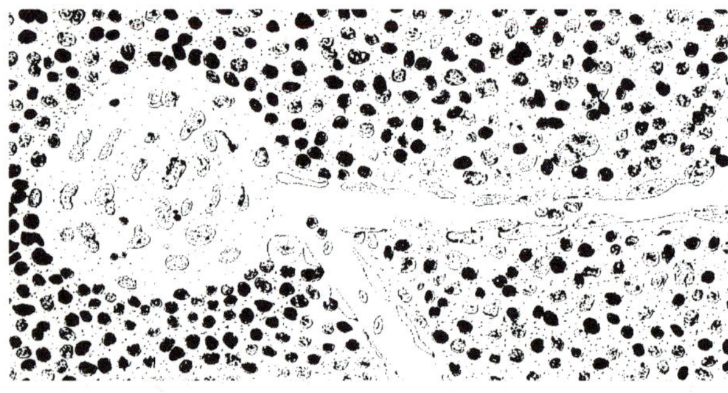

Lollipop follicle

Lollipop follicles HEMATOPATHOLOGY A fanciful descriptor for the histologic appearance of capillaries ensheathed by collagen extending into a germinal center in the hyaline-vascular form of Castleman's disease or angiofollicular lymphoid hyperplasia, figure

Lollipop tree appearance A cholangiographic pattern consisting of multiple, variably-sized cystic spaces that freely communicate in and along the intrahepatic biliary ducts in Caroli's disease and congenital hepatic fibrosis (RADIOLOGY 1973; 109:565)

'Loner' Solitary hunter Lone wolf syndrome A single young man who is estranged from society, suffers from psychogenic pain, tending to live 'on the edge', vacillating between aggression and depression; loners often have unrealistic goals, but are unable to work towards those goals **Prognosis** Guarded; progressive depression, poor functionality, suicidal tendencies

Lone star tick *Amblyomma americanum* A tick occasionally implicated in the transmission of Lyme disease, see there

Long-acting thyroid stimulator see LATS

Long interspersed repeated elements see LINES

Long leg syndrome Short leg syndrome A condition caused by inequity of leg length resulting in mechanical disturbances of gait and posture **Clinical** The first manifestations are back and knee pain, where a persistent deformity causes a compensatory pelvic tilt, lumbar scoliosis, backache and rheumatologic symptoms; the longer leg is held in flexion with excess lateral strain, causing premature degenerative changes and valgus deformity due to a collapse of the lateral compartment

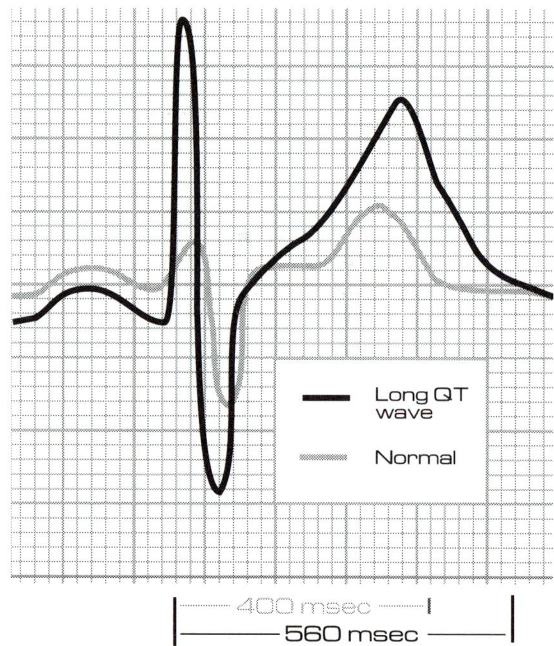

Long Q-T (interval) syndrome (LQTS) CARDIOLOGY An often underdiagnosed clinical complex that is most common in otherwise healthy young females evoked by fright or physical exertion, resulting in episodic syncope, or if the stimulus is extreme, sudden death related to increased autonomic tone that occurs during periods of exercise and excitement, eg sudden death while exercising on a hot day due to sudden onset of ventricular arrhythmia; once diagnosed, all related family members should have an EKG (figure), as a prolonged Q-T interval is associated with an increased incidence of malignant ventricular arrhythmia, eg 'torsades de pointes' **Molecular biology** LQTS is tightly linked (Lod score: 16.4) to the Harvey ras (H-*ras*-1) oncogene (a gene linked to many different signal transduction pathways) on the short arm of chromosome 11 (Science 1991; 252:704); LQTS may also be induced by drugs, eg antiarrhythmics, phenothiazine, tricyclic antidepressants and lithium, metabolic and electrolyte imbalances, low-energy diets, central nervous system and autonomic nervous system disease, coronary artery disease and mitral valve prolapse; the complex also occurs as a symptom in congenital disease, in a) Jervell-Lange-Nielsen syndrome, an autosomal recessive condition accompanied by deafness and b) Romano-Ward syndrome, which is autosomal dominant, but not accompanied by deafness

Long terminal repeat see LTR

Long-term potentiation (LTP) NEUROPHYSIOLOGY A type of synaptic plasticity that is thought to form the molecular and cellular basis of learning and memory, in which neural connections (synapses) corresponding to new information are strengthened; the LTP model supported by quantal analysis, a technique that determines the physical signal passing across a synapse from one neuron to another, implies that synaptic strengthening is presynaptic and relatively permanent (Nature 1990; 346:177, 724); induction of LTP requires transient activation of the NMDA receptor system; during low-frequency transmission, NMDA activation is prevented by GABA-mediated synaptic inhibition; during high-frequency transmission, the GABA block is reduced by a GABA autoregulatory mechanism, permitting induction of LTP (Nature 1991; 349:609); see Synaptic plasticity

'Look-back' program PUBLIC HEALTH An organized study of subjects exposed to a disease, usually infectious, from whom specimens, eg sera, epidemiologic, demographic or other data is examined retrospectively to determine whether the subjects are currently infected; look-back programs have been developed during the AIDS epidemic to evaluate HIV antibody seroconversion in subjects exposed to potentially contaminated blood products (prior to the availability of serum screening assays) or who were treated by HIV-positive health care providers, from whom the possibility of HIV antibody seroconversion, is considered minimal, but which will have a major impact on the liability industry (Am Med News 10/June/91)

Loop ENDOCRINOLOGY The loop 'classification' was established at a time when the pituitary gland and target organs were thought to control the secretion of releasing and stimulating hormones from the hypothalamus and hypophysis, respectively, a posit that has proven largely correct *LONG FEEDBACK LOOP* Target organs produce hormones that act on the hypothalamus and the pituitary, modifying pituitary secretion, eg thyroid hormone inhibits the synthesis and secretion of thyrotropin-releasing hormone (TRH) from the hypothalamus and thyroid-stimulating hormone (TSH) from the pituitary *SHORT FEEDBACK LOOP* There is negative inhibition of pituitary hormones at the hypothalamus, eg increased growth hormone results in decreased somatostatin secretion *ULTRASHORT FEEDBACK LOOP* A term occasionally used referring to hypothalamic hormones that regulate their own secretion

Loop diuretics NEPHROLOGY A family of therapeutic agents that are the most potent diuretics in clinical use, which act on Henle's loop, causing excretion of 20-25% of the filtered sodium; these 'high-ceiling' diuretics are most indicated in pulmonary edema, congestive heart failure and renal impairment and include furosemide and ethacrinic acid, which increase levels of renin, angiotensin II and prostaglandins and increase natriuresis by inhibiting the sodium-potassium-chloride cotransport system, which is responsible for solute resorption in the thick ascending loop of Henle; since both agents are secreted in the tubular lumen by the organic acid pathway, they are less effective in the presence of endogenous or exogenous organic acids; because loop agents cause marked hypokalemia, they are often used in tandem with other potassium-sparing diuretics

Loop-to-loop pattern A fanciful descriptor for the arrangement of clusters of endometrial cells seen in endometrial cytology specimens from patients with intrauterine devices

Lop ear A prominent deformity of the external ear resulting from the lack of bending of the cartilage forming the antihelix **Treatment** Cosmetic surgery before age 5, when auricle is more fully developed; Cf Cauliflower ear

'Loss leader' A business term for an item sold to the public at or below the original cost in order to entice the customer to purchase other, more expensive items; in the health care industry, a 'loss leader' is a service provided below cost, in order to attract (well-insured) patients to return and refer other patients in need of services that produce income above the cost of the 'loss leader'; in hospitals, the emergency room was considered a 'loss leader' that would increase the hospital's census, filling beds and increasing hospital revenues; with the Medicare reforms under TEFRA in 1982, it became apparent that emergency rooms often attracted financially 'undesirable' patients with inadequate insurance coverage; consequently some private hospitals have closed their emergency rooms; see Dumping, Skimming, TEFRA

Lot syndrome Lot's wife syndrome Hypercalcinosis A rare condition characterized by florid 'metastatic' calcification of soft tissues due to a) Hyperparathyroidism and/or hypervitaminosis D with massive bone resorption or b) Chronic hypodipsic hypernatremia A condition with normal blood volume and renal function (Bristol Med Chir J 1984; 99:88); N Engl J Med 1986; 315:433); the two causes of massive soft tissue mineralization are named after the biblical Lot and his wife, who turned for one last look at the sinful city of Sodom and turned into a 'pillar of salt'

Lou Gehrig disease The popular (trivial) name used in the USA for amyotrophic lateral sclerosis, named after Lou Gehrig, the 'Iron Horse', a first baseman for the New York Yankees (1925-39), who played 2130 consecutive major league games (a record still unbeaten); he died of the disease in 1941, thereby immortalizing the disease Note: Stephen Hawking, cosmologist also suffers from the condition

Louse Flat wingless parasitic insects, which include a) Biting lice, Order Mallophaga, which rarely afflict humans and b) Sucking lice (Order Anoplua, family Pediculidae) that are global in distribution, acting as vectors for *Borrelia recurrentis* (*Bhermisi turcatae, B parkeri*); *Pediculus humanis capitis* head lice, *Pediculus humanis corporis* body lice, *Phthirus pubis* crab or pubic louse

Louse-borne fever see Relapsing fever

Lovastatin A lipid-lowering drug of the 3-hydroxy-3-methyl-glutaryl coenzyme A (HMG-CoA) reductase inhibitor family; lovastatin is a partial inhibitor of HMG-CoA reductase activity in early cholesterol synthesis, allowing sufficient mevalonate production to provide adequate cholesterol for cell membrane function and steroidogenesis; it is well tolerated, lowering LDL-cholesterol an average of 41%, while raising HDL-cholesterol 10% (Am J Cardiol 1990; 66:Symposium) and is of use in treating other dyslipidemias including primary mixed and primary moderate hyperlipidemias, diabetic dyslipidemia and hyperlipidemia of the nephrotic syndrome; in healthy volunteers, it decreases LDL-cholesterol by 35%, apolipoprotein-B by 25%, VLDL-cholesterol and IDL-cholesterol by 30-40% and raises the HDL-cholesterol by 10% (J Am Med Assoc 1989; 262:3148), Cf Cholesterol-lowering drugs, Gemfibrozil; Cf HMG CoA reductase inhibitors

Love canal ENVIRONMENT A major site of toxic contamination of soil and water, which became one of the first targets for the US Environmental Protection Agency's 'Superfund'; the canal was dug in 1892 by William Love for an industrial complex near Niagara Falls, New York and was used from 1947-53 as an industrial dump by a chemical and plastic manufacturer; after a heavy rainfall in 1976, the canal began to leak 82 different chemicals, 11 of which were carcinogens; the local residents whose drinking water was contaminated from the canal had an increased rate of spontaneous abortions, birth defects, cancer, urinary tract and hepatic disease; see Bhopal, Bitterfeld, Haff disease, Minamata disease, Times Beach

'Love handles' Bilateral overhangs of adipose and soft tissues on the antero-lateral flank that are refractory to dieting and of little importance, except as occasional barriers to medical communication, causing accidental detonation of beepers (N Engl J Med 1991; 324:1517c)

Love-hate relationship Ambivalence PSYCHIATRY A clinical complex characterized by essential changes in freudian impulses; love-hate is normal for children passing through the 'anal-sadistic' phase of development, in which there is both love and 'murderous' hatred toward the same object, often occurring simultaneously; in the normal course of personality development, most of this aggression is neutralized and what remains becomes a desire to win out over (rather than destroy) the other person; in obsessive-compulsive disorders, the person consciously expresses both the love and hate components and thus is stuck in repeating cycles of doing and undoing behaviorisms; Cf Passive-aggression

Lovejoy's classification A classification (table) for the severity of neurological disease in Reye syndrome

Lovejoy's classification
(Coma stages in Reye' syndrome
1) Vomiting, lethargy and sleepiness
2) Combativeness, hyperventilation, hyperreflexia, responsive to noxious stimuli
3) Obtunded, comatose with decorticate activity; intact cranial nerves
4) Deepening coma, decerebrate activity, no cranial nerve response
5) No deep tendon reflexes, respiratory arrest

'Love' surgery Vulvovaginoplasty A rarely-used vaginal operation for treatment of '*COITALLY CONNECTED INFLAMMATION OF THE BLADDER AND INTERNAL PAIN WITH INTERCOURSE, IE DYSPAREUNIA*'; the operation entails '*ROTATION OF THE VAGINAL AXIS AWAY FROM ALIGNMENT WITH THE INTERNAL GENITALIA AND BLADDER*'; one physician claimed that it increased penile-clitoral contact during intercourse, although in some cases, allegedly left the patient with painful sequelae (Am Med News 27/Jan/89); Cf Female circumcision

Lover's heels FORENSIC MEDICINE A comminuted intraarticular fracture of the os calcis with severe crush injury to the bones of the foot with major anatomic distortion, described in 'jilted' lovers who jump from major heights, see Jumper syndrome INFECTIOUS DISEASE A fanciful synonym for gonococcal tenosynovitis of the Achilles tendon Note: Migratory gonococcal arthritis is usually pauciarticular, affecting the knees, ankles, elbows and wrists and resolves spontaneously

'Low back syndrome' A generic term for any complaint referable to the lower back, attributable to degenerative, infectious, neoplastic or traumatic origin; the low back syndrome may be acute or chronic, temporary or permanent, congenital or acquired and is quite common in the older, especially female population

Low birth weight (LBW) NEONATOLOGY A 'condition' in a newborn infant that is often a risk factor *a sui generis* for morbidity in early infancy; LBW is defined as an infant who at birth weighs less than 2500g; moderate LBW is 1500-2500g; very low LBW infants weigh less than 1500g, a group accounting for 50% of neonatal mortality (85-95% survival if more than 1250g, 65-75% survival if more than 800g, 2% survival if less than 600g) World Records The lowest birthweight recorded for a child with normal mental and psychomotor development is 380 g (N Engl J Med 1990; 322:1753c), a delivery necessitated by hypertension and coagulopathy; the lowest birthweight recorded for a long-term surviving infant, albeit with a low IQ is 280 g (ibid, 1991; 324:1599c); central to neonatal survival is control of fluid balances and modern neonatal 'hardware', including radiant warmers, phototherapy, ventilators, arterial catheters, cardiorespiratory monitors; 6-7% of

of white infants, an incidence that declined until 1985, followed by reversal (MMWR 1990; 39:137, 148) Relevant definitions **APPROPRIATE FOR GESTATIONAL AGE** (AGA) An adjective applied to an infant whose gestational age and weight are synchronous according to standardized age and growth curves **INTRAUTERINE GROWTH RETARDATION** (IUGR) A generic term for any delay in achieving intrauterine developmental milestones, most commonly related to maternal drug, tobacco and alcohol abuse **SMALL FOR GESTATIONAL AGE** (SGA) An adjective applied to an infant whose gestational age and weight gain are below that expected for age, most common in infants exposed in utero to drugs of abuse (cocaine 93g decrease, marijuana 79g, tobacco 200-400g, N Engl J Med 1989; 320:762); 26% of SGA infants have severe mental impairment, which can be reduced to 4% if they are given daily activities in intensive care unit, massages, and audiotaped conversation from their parents and classical music (Pediatrics 1987; 80:68); weight gain is faster and neurological development improved with increased levels of dopamine, norepinephrine and epinephrine in the urine of premature infants treated with massage, which reduces incubator time and shortens the length of intensive hospital-based care; prophylactic ligation of the patent ductus arteriosus at the time of birth may reduce the incidence of necrotizing enterocolitis (N Engl J Med 1989; 320:1511), but has no effect on bronchopulmonary dysplasia, retinopathy or intraventricularhemorrhage; SGA infants are at risk for future developmental disability, which can be reduced by early intervention (including neonatal nursery, home visits, child development centers and parent groups), increasing the average IQ and is associated with fewer behavioral problems in the future (J Am Med Assoc 1990; 263:3035)

Low cardiac output syndrome Forward failure 'syndrome' A clinical condition in which the cardiac output falls below the tissue needs for oxygen **Laboratory** Increased vascular resistance and oxygen consumption, lactic acidosis, decreased cardiac index and oxygen saturation **Treatment** Digitalis, vasopressors, dopamine, dobutamine, vasodilatation **Prognosis** Poor if unresponsive to drugs

Low density lipoprotein see LDL

Low frequency antigen Private antigen TRANSFUSION MEDICINE A red cell antigen that is uncommon in the general population, and thus rarely associated with antibody production, eg C^x, C^w, He, Lu^{a+b-}, Sw^a, Wr^a

Low-grade lymphoma A group of relatively indolent lymphomas classified according to the Working Formulation (Cancer 1982; 49:2112) that have a prolonged survival of 5 to 7.5 years, often with minimal therapy; low-grade lymphomas include the small lymphocytic (plasmacytoid) lymphoma, follicular small cleaved cell lymphoma, follicular mixed small cleaved and large cell lymphoma; see Lymphoma, Working Formulation

Low-osmolality contrast medium RADIOLOGY Any of a group of radiologic contrast media first used in Europe which are said to have fewer side effects after intravenous injections, but which are more expensive and may cause hypercoagulability

Low-output gastrointestinal fistula An external (ie communicates with the skin) gastrointestinal fistula that produces less than 200 ml of fluid, originating from the distal small intestine and large intestine; Cf High-output fistula

Low quality protein CLINICAL NUTRITION A protein usually of plant origin that lacks one or more essential amino acid, eg corn, which is low in lysine, or beans, which are low in tryptophan; the poor quality of protein is a major impediment to progress in developing nations, which responds to a simple expediency of succotash, a gruel containing both foods; low quality protein in the form of the 'liquid diet' had transient currency in the US 'weight loss industry' and resulted in a number of deaths prior to its abandonment; see Liquid diet; Cf Succotash

Low-stringency hybridization MOLECULAR BIOLOGY A hybridization between two molecules capable of forming nucleotide base pair dimers, eg DNA with DNA or DNA with RNA under conditions that allow 'sloppy' alignment of bases; the stringency of a hybridization can be controlled by titrating the temperature and salt concentrations

Low T_3 syndrome see Euthyroid sick syndrome

Low T_4 syndrome A 'laboratory disease' in patients undergoing regular hemodialysis or continuous ambulatory peritoneal dialysis, in which 40% have serum T_4 (thyroxine) less than 5 μg/dl but who have normal free T_4 levels (Nephron 1987; 46:225)

Low-tar cigarettes Cigarettes that are lower than average in nicotines and tars; a 50% reduction in tar is thought to result in a 20% reduction in lung cancer mortality; smokers of 'low-yield' cigarettes do not have a lower incidence of myocardial infarction (N Engl J Med 1989; 320:1569), possibly due to deeper inhalation of pollutants by these smokers; see Non-smoking tobacco, 'Pack-year', Passive smoking, Smoking

L-phase bacteria see L-form

LPR see Late phase reaction

LPSTGE A highly conserved six-residue (Leu-Pro-Ser-Thr-Gly-Glu) oligopeptide that is adjacent to the hydrophobic region of all known surface proteins of gram-positive bacteria and required for their attachment; see M protein

LQTS see Long Q-T interval syndrome

L/S ratio OBSTETRICS The ratio of lecithin to sphingomyelin, a parameter used to determine infant lung maturity and predict the infant's ability to survive without developing respiratory distress; surface-active lecithin appears in the amniotic fluid at 24-26 gestational weeks; sphingomyelin is similarly produced but remains relatively constant; before the 32nd week, the L/S ratio is less than 1.5, after the 34th week, the L/S ratio is greater than 2.0, which corresponds to an adequate level of surfactant for adequate extra-uterine pulmonary function **Laboratory** The L/S ratio may be determined by thin-layer chromatography and two-dimensional chromatography, the latter of which has fewer false negatives; see Biophysical profile, Lung profile, Respiratory distress syndrome

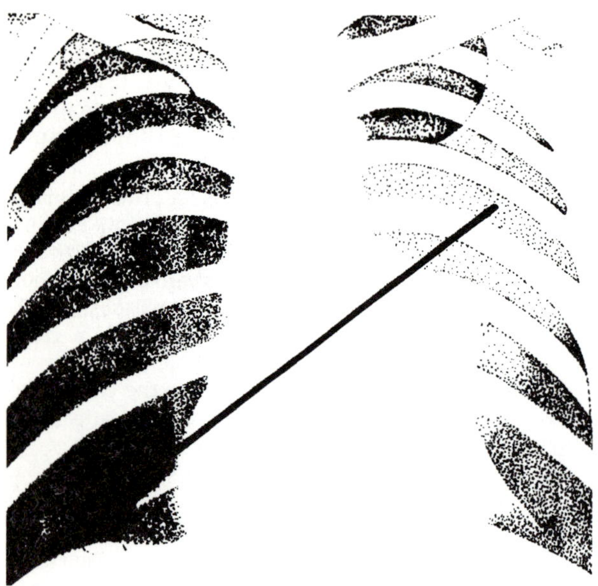

Luftsichel sign

LS and A see Lichen sclerosis et atrophicus

LTP see Long-term potentiation

LTR Long terminal repeats MOLECULAR BIOLOGY The two end segments of 250-1200 base pairs in length double-stranded retroviral DNA that are synthesized by reverse transcriptase of retroviral origin; LTRs contain many of the signals required for retroviral function, including promoter and enhancer sequences, polyadenylation sites, and encode peptides integral to integrating the virus into the host genome; see HIV, HTLV, Retrovirus

LTS see Latent tetany syndrome

Lucid interval NEUROLOGY A period of time preceding the loss of consciousness and coma that occurs in subdural and epidural hematomas, intracranial edema; Cf Window period

Luciferase The enzyme responsible for the bioluminescent reaction of the firefly, which catalyzes the oxidation of luciferin, releasing a photon of light; this reaction can be modified to allow detection of molecules present in low levels in both the clinical and research laboratories; see Chemiluminescence

Lucilia Genus of flies causing myasis

Lucke tumor A transplantable renal cell carcinoma of frogs

Lucy AL 288-1 ANTHROPOLOGY The trivial name given to a female hominid (***Australopithecus afarensis***) skeleton that was discovered in the Afar Triangle of Ethiopia in 1974, the pelvis of which indicates that modern man probably walked erect about 3 million years ago; in contrast to the relatively vertical chimpanzee pelvis, in which babies are delivered without rotation, Lucy's children needed a one-quarter turn for delivery, while the relatively flat modern human pelvis, adapted for bipedalism, requires the fetus to make a full turn in order to successfully pass out of the birth canal; see Anthropology, Eve

LUF syndrome Luteinized unruptured follicle syndrome A condition characterized by the development of a dominant follicle without disruption and release of the ovum, an abnormality diagnosed by ultrasonography or laparoscopy; LUD is thought to be an extremely rare and sporadic cause of infertility

Luftsichel sign German, Air crescent RADIOLOGY A curved often left-sided perihilar opacification seen on a plain antero-posterior chest film (figure, left) that is characteristic of upper lobe atelectasis, due to interposition of the lower lobe apex over the atelectatic upper lobe

Lugol solution GYNECOLOGY An iodine solution that colors the normal uterine cervix a homogeneous brown color when seen by colposcopy; any alterations in the color may indicate an underlying defect in the glycogen content of the cervical epithelium that may be associated with cervical carcinoma and appear as a whitish discoloration

Lumone A hormone of the gastrointestinal lumen; see Incretins

'Lumpectomy' Segmental mastectomy SURGICAL ONCOLOGY A cosmetically acceptable, but variably complete excision of breast carcinoma; lumpectomy of early (< 4.0 cm) breast carcinoma combined with radiotherapy offers a 90% five-year survival (N Engl J Med 1985; 312:655; J Am Med Assoc 1991; 265:391) Note: Recurrence of breast carcinoma is often a late event, thus 10- and 15-year survival statistics are more relevant than five-year survival statistics; the American College of Surgeons has taken no official position regarding the definition or applicability of 'lumpectomy'; some data suggest that a lumpectomy with axillary lymph node dissection may be as effective as a mastectomy in treating carcinoma of the breast; Cf Lesionectomy

'Lumping' Reductionism CLINICAL DECISION-MAKING The practice of aggregating diseases or pathologic nosologies with variably distinct features under a common term; 'lumpers' take a pragmatic approach to the diagnosis and treatment of various diseases, rather than attempt to differentiate among subtle subclassifications, recognizing that these distinctions may be arbitrary and/or artificial; Cf 'Splitting'

Lumpy-bumpy pattern RENAL PATHOLOGY A pattern seen by immunofluorescent microscopy (figure, opposite), which consists in granular deposits of IgG and C3 along the glomerular basement membrane, caused by a wide variety of conditions, including serum sickness nephritis (exogenous foreign proteins), exogenous antigens (bacterial endocarditis, leprosy, syphilis, hepatitis B, malaria), endogenous antigens (DNA, thyroglobulin, tumor-associated antigens)

Lumpy deposits see Humps

Lumpy jaw INFECTIOUS DISEASE A jaw characterized by painful, 'wood-hard' fibrotic induration of the parotid and submandibular regions, arising in a background of dental disease (caries, periodontitis or extractions), characteristic of cervicofacial actinomyces, the most common form of actinomyces infection; lumpy jaw in humans is caused by ***A israeli, A meueri, A naeslundi, A odontolyticus*** and ***Arachnia propionica***; lumpy jaw in cows is caused by ***A bovis***; other manifestations of cervicofacial actinomycosis include trismus, multiple draining sinus tracts bearing the classic yellow-white sulfur granules, fever, leukocytosis, extension to the facial soft tissue, bone and if untreated, the central nervous system **Treatment** Penicillin

Lung carcinoma Lung cancer is the most common cause of cancer death accounting for 30% of the cancer deaths in the USA, the vast majority of which is directly attributed to tobacco abuse; once diagnosed, the average patient survives one to two years, with 5-10% surviving five years after diagnosis; the prognosis of small cell (undifferentiated) carcinoma is slightly better than the more differentiated squamous cell and bronchoalveolar carcinomas, assuming they respond to chemotherapy

Lung profile NEONATOLOGY A two-dimensional chromatograph prepared on a thin layer plate of silica gel containing 5% ammonium sulfate from an acetone-precipitated lipid extract of bloody amniotic fluid; the lung profile allows determination of relative amounts of lecithin, sphingomyelin, phosphatidyl glycerol, phosphatidyl inositol and phosphatidyl serine (measured by densitometry after charring) and in experienced hands allows determination of fetal lung maturity; in the presence of phosphatidyl glycerol, respiratory distress syndrome does not occur; see L/S ratio; Cf Organ panels

Lung stones Broncholiths Calcification of necrotic and/or infected tissue within bronchioles, secondary to tuberculosis, histoplasmosis, sarcoidosis and papillary carcinoma

Lung transplantation Approximately 200 patients per year (USA) receive lung transplants for various indications, one lung is transplanted in pulmonary fibrosis, both lungs in diffuse pulmonary disease, eg cystic fibrosis, bronchiectasis, emphysema and both the heart and lungs in cases where there is combined pulmonary disease and end-stage heart disease (N Engl J Med 1990; 322:727, 772); cost $240 000, $47 000 annual maintenance; Survival 70% at one year, 55% overall; some cases have survived more than five years; see Cyclosporin, Domino-donor transplantation, FK506, UNOS

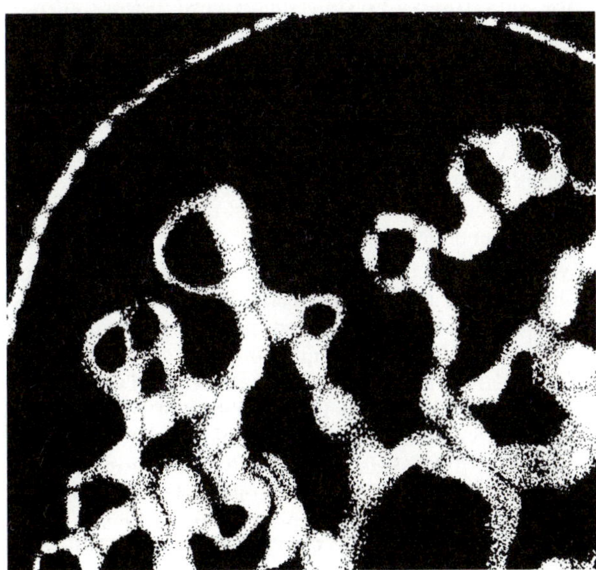

Lumpy-bumpy pattern

Lung carcinoma, classification

% Total	Type	5-year survival, I	II	III
38%	Squamous cell (epidermoid)	38%	16%	9%
23%	Adenocarcinoma	32%	7%	3%
	a) Papillary adenocarcinoma			
	b) Alveolar cell			
	c) Bronchiolar carcinoma			
	d) Mucinous adenocarcinoma			
	e) Adenosquamous carcinoma			
29%	Undifferentiated Small ce	0%	0%	0%
	a) Oat cell carcinoma			
	b) Intermediate cell type			
	c) Combined oat cell type			
9%	Undifferentiated Large cell	30%	6%	5%
Rare	Giant cell carcinoma	Highly lethal		

Lung volumes PHYSIOLOGY A group of air 'compartments' into which the lung may be functionally divided (figure, below) **EXPIRATORY RESERVE CAPACITY** (ERV) The maximum volume of air that can be voluntarily exhaled **FUNCTIONAL RESIDUAL CAPACITY** (FRV) Volume left in the lungs at the end of a normal breath which is not normally part of the subdivisions **INSPIRATORY CAPACITY** (IC) The maximum volume that can be inhaled **INSPIRATORY RESERVE CAPACITY** (IRC) The maximum

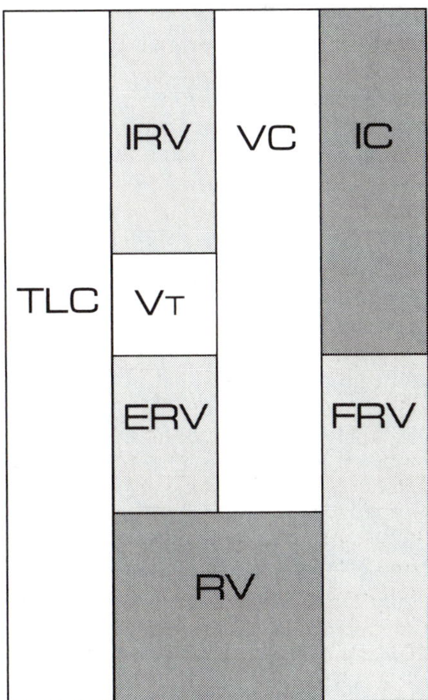

volume that can be inhaled above the tidal volume **Tidal volume** (V_T) The normal to-and-fro respiratory exchange of 500 cc **Total lung capacity** (TLC) The entire volume of the lung, which is approximately 5 liters **Vital capacity** (VC) The maximum volume of air that can be inhaled and exhaled or the maximum amount of exhalable air after a full inspiration, which added to the residual volume, is the total lung capacity

'Lupoid' hepatitis An autoimmune hepatitis most common in young women, many of whom produce antinuclear, anti-smooth muscle and antimitochondrial antibodies, termed 'lupoid' for the presence of the LE cell phenomenon, which occurs in 15% of cases; the lesion is histologically characterized by chronic active hepatitis, a low incidence of carcinoma and good response to corticosteroids

Lupus anticoagulant Lupus inhibitor A generic term for IgG or IgM class antibodies that arise spontaneously in patients with lupus erythematosus ('lupus' is retained for convention, as these antibodies also occur in neoplasia, drug reactions or in normal subjects); directed against phospholipoproteins or phospholipid components of coagulation factors; although these antibodies produce in vitro interference with phospholipid-dependent coagulation, eg activated partial thromboplastin time (aPTT) and kaolin clotting time assays in specimens from patients with lupus erythematosus, they don't produce in vivo coagulopathy in absence of other platelet defects or coagulation defects or the presence of drug-induced antibodies Laboratory A lupus anticoagulant is often present if patient:control clotting time is 1.5 x normal at a dilution of 1:1000 and the altered aPTT is corrected by 1:1 mix with normal plasma; lupus anticoagulants include anticardiolipin and other anti-phospholipid antibodies (J Am Med Assoc 1988; 259:550); Cf Anticardiolipin antibodies

Lupus eythematosus and pregnancy Patients with lupus erythematosus have an increased risk of fetal wastage due to thromboses; in particular, two previous spontaneous abortions and anti-cardiolipin antibody or anti-Ro antibodies is associated with future fertility failure and frequent fetal fatality (Q J Med 1988; 250:125); see Anticardiolipin antibody

Lupus erythematosus, drug-induced A lupus erythematosus-like syndrome that may develop in patients taking certain drugs, including procainamide, hydralazine, isoniazid, phenytoin, mesantoin, D-penicillamine and ergot compounds; nearly 50 different agents have been implicated, either idiosyncratically or in a dose-dependent fashion; 80% of drug-induced lupus have antinuclear, as well as anti-histone antibodies; only one-third have clinical changes of lupus, eg arthralgia, fever, serositis; the renal and central nervous system changes of classic lupus are distinctly uncommon; many of these patients are 'slow acetylators', resulting in accumulation of non-acetylated metabolites that bind to macromolecules, acting as haptens; by extension, this condition is a situation in which a metabolic abnormality induces autoimmunity

Lupus psychosis A clinical complex seen in lupus erythematosus, attributed to an antibody to P protein, a polypeptide present in ribosomal phosphoproteins; lupus patients may have a transient increase in anti-P antibodies during periods of psychotic exacerbation; cerebral lupus may also cause acute vasculitis and immune complex deposits in choroid plexus

Luteinizing hormone-releasing hormone see LH-RH

Luteoma A non-neoplastic yellow-gray mass measuring up to 20 cm in diameter due to hyperplasia of luteinized cells that involutes spontaneously after parturition; this 'luteoma of pregnancy' is most common in young multiparous black women, multiple in one-half and accompanied by virilization or exacerbation of hirsutism in one-fourth; testosterone levels may be 70-fold greater than normal with transient virilization of the female infants

Luxury genes Genes that are not universally expressed, ie those that encode proteins only in specialized cells, eg gastrin production in parietal cells, immunoglobulin production in plasma cells and melanin production in melanocytes; Cf Housekeeping genes

Luxury perfusion syndrome A cerebrovascular state in which there is increased blood flow to the brain but decreased oxygen uptake by cerebral tissue, resulting from acute lactic (metabolic) acidosis accompanied by cerebral edema; luxury perfusion is non-specific and may occur in strokes, trauma, tumors, alcoholism, sickle cell anemia, diabetic ketoacidosis and meningoencephalitis; Cf Carotid steal syndrome, Robin Hood syndrome

LW antibody An antibody that was thought to be directed against the Rhesus factor (anti-Rh), later recognized as a distinct erythrocyte antigen, which although closely linked to the Rh gene family, is inherited separately; the antigen was designated 'LW' to honor Landsteiner and Wiener's work in the rhesus monkey; anti-LW antibody is very rare and can react with Rh+ or Rh-, but not with Rh_{null} cells

Lyase A class of enzymes responsible for non-hydrolytic or oxidation-reduction cleavage of carbon-carbon, carbon-oxygen and carbon-nitrogen bonds, resulting in two products, one or both of which have double bonds; lyases include aldolase, deaminase, decarboxylase, dehydratase, hydrase, nucleotide cyclase, synthase

LYDMA A membrane antigen expressed by Epstein-Barr virus-infected B-cells that is a target for activated T cells and thought to play a role in host defense against infectious mononucleosis

Lye injury Toxicology A condition often secondary to the ingestion of bleach, of suicidal intent in adults and of accidental nature in children; periodic follow-up is obligatory as 5% develop squamous cell carcinoma 20-40 years after the insult Clinical, acute Tachycardia, intense retrosternal pain, production of copious frothy mucus, vomiting of blood, sloughing of esophageal mucosa, dysphagia, followed by fibrosing stricture Barium 'swallow' studies demonstrate a pencil-thin esophageal lumen Treatment Bougienage is a therapeutic mainstay; given the potential for perforation, it is best begun five or more days post-insult; large-bore nasogastric tubes appear preferable to bougienage, as the strictures formed are of a large and useful diameter; pharmacologic doses of corticosteroids appear to minimize fibrosis

Lyme disease Afzelius' disease A condition caused by *Borrelia burgdorferi*, and possibly mediated by interleukin-1, that was first seen in Lyme, Connecticut where it presented as an 'epidemic' of juvenile rheumatoid arthritis (Still's disease); one astute mother alerted Yale epidemiologists who then 'discovered' the disease; DNA sequences of *B burgdorferi* were identified by polymerase chain reaction in archival specimens of *Ixodes dammini* that had been stored since the 1940s, making Lyme disease older by two decades than previously thought (Science 1990; 249:1420); 6000 cases occur annually, making it the most common zoonosis in the US, especially along the Eastern 'seaboard'; *B burgdorferi* has also been identified in Northern Europe and Australia Vectors Deer tick (*Ixodes dammini*, Eastern USA, up to 60% of which carry the spirochete), white-footed mouse tick (*I pacificus*, Western USA, about 1% of which carry the organism), wood tick (I *ricinus*, Europe), lone star tick (*Amblyomma americanum*) and rarely deerflies and horseflies (N Engl J Med 1990; 322:1752c) Host Deer, field mice **Clinical** Lyme disease is divided into Stage I Erythema chronicum migrans Rash stage, a condition first described in 1910 by Afzelius, associated with wood tick bites and confined to Northern Europe until 1970 when the first US cases were described, presenting as a solitary reddish papule and plaque with centrifugal expansion (up to 20 cm), peripheral induration and central clearing, persisting for months to years; potentially pruritic with IgM and C3 deposition in vessels Stage II Cardiovascular (myocarditis, pericarditis, transient atrioventricular block, ventricular dysfunction); neurological (Bell's palsy, meningoencephalitis, optic atrophy, polyneuritis) symptoms; HLA-DR4 and HLA-DR2 may be more common in chronic Lyme arthritis and resistance to antibiotics (N Engl J Med 1990; 323:219) Stage III Migratory polyarthritis **Laboratory** Non-specific findings include increased erythrocyte sedimentation rate, IgM and cryoglobulins, decreased C3 and C4, increased IgG and IgM antibody titers to *B burgdorferi*, agreement among laboratories as to whether a subject has Lyme antibodies, when tested by indirect fluorescent antibody (IFA) or enzyme-linked immunosorbent assay (ELISA) is low (J Am Med Assoc 1989; 262:3431) and lacks standardization; histologic stains of involved tissue (Warthin-Starry and Dieterle) have a low diagnostic yield; definitive diagnosis requires identification of IgG antibodies to *B recurrentis* by the 'Western' immunoblot **Treatment** Tetracycline, penicillin, erythromycin

Lyme disease, chronic A predominantly neurological condition ranging from mild, eg fatigue, paresthesia, arthralgia, memory loss, mood swings and dysomnia to severe, eg spastic paraparesis, tetraparesis, ataxia, chorea, cognitive impairment, bladder dysfunction, cranial nerve deficits, myelitis, brainstem encephalitis and demyelination Lyme disease triad: Lymphocytic meningitis, cranial neuritis (especially of the 7th and 8th cranial nerve) and radiculitis **Diagnosis** Specific IgG antibody ('Western' immunoblotting) to *B burgdorferi* that may disappear with time; persistent, ie treatable infection should be ruled out by a specific T-cell lymphoblastic response assay Note: Chronic neurological abnormalities of encephalopathy, leukoencephalopathy and polyneuritis may improve with antibiotics (N Engl J Med 1990; 323:1438)

'Lyme embryopathy' A complex of congenital malformations described in infants born to women suffering from Lyme disease while pregnant, including syndactyly, cortical blindness, intrauterine fetal death, prematurity and neonatal rash

Lymphadenopathy Enlargement of the lymph nodes of virtually any etiology; the differential diagnostic considerations are enormous and have been divided for convenience into reactive patterns (see Human Pathol 1974; 5:519; a 'classic' paper recommended for its clarity); benign lymphadenopathy is characterized by a) Variability of the follicle (germinal center) size b) Lack of capsular or fat invasion c) Mitotic activity that is confined to the germinal center and d) Cortical localization and inhomogeneous distribution of the follicles; see Benign lymphadenopathy

Lymphangiomatosis Diffuse or multifocal lymphangioma A rare lesion confined to children, characterized by well-demarcated osteolytic lesions variably accompanied by sclerosis, often misdiagnosed as fibrous dysplasia; while the condition is histologically benign, the prognosis is poor if the lesions affect the liver, spleen or thoracic duct as these sites are not amenable to adequate resection; the bone lesions may be stable unless they are in the vertebral body in which case the patients may develop cord compression

Lymphangiomyomatosis syndrome A rare thoracic duct defect causing chylothorax in women of child-bearing years related to estrogen production or occurring in tuberous sclerosis **Clinical** Exertional dyspnea, hemoptysis, cough, chest pain, pneumothorax, chylothorax and progressive respiratory insufficiency RADIOLOGY Reticulonodular changes, cysts or bullae, effusion and hyperinflation **Pathology** Diffuse smooth muscle proliferation within small blood vessels and lymphatics, lymphangiectasia, 'honeycombed' pulmonary parenchyma, lipid pneumonia **Prognosis** Although this condition was initially thought to have a poor prognosis, most patients survive 8+ years (N Engl J Med 1990; 323:1254) **Treatment** Possible response to hormonal manipulation, eg tamoxifen, medroxyprogesterone acetate

Lymphedema A condition characterized by the accumulation of lymph, due to interference with lymphatic drainage, resulting in expansion of the interstitial fluid compartment; lymphedema may be a) Congenital, eg Milroy's disease, related to poor development of the lymphatic channels b) Idiopathic, affecting young females with unremitting swelling in one or more extremities or c) Acquired through microfilarial infection or involvement by malignancy or by modalities for treating malignancy, eg lymphadenectomy or regional lymphoid irradiation **Complication** Chronic lymphedema may on occasion be associated with the highly malignant lymphangiosarcoma

Lymph node inclusions The presence of benign tissues within lymph nodes, a phenomenon that may lure the unwary or inexperienced into misdiagnosing malignancy; benign 'metastases' include salivary gland tissue, thyroid follicles, müllerian epithelium, endometriosis, nevus cell aggregates and breast tissue; other non-neoplastic inclusions with lymph nodes include adipose tissue, ectopic thymus, hyaline and proteinaceous material; Cf Benign lymphadenopathy

Lymph node necrosis A non-specific finding that can be divided into a) Focal necrosis, usually benign, seen in infection by bacteria, cat-scratch disease, Epstein-Barr virus, fungemia, lymphogranuloma venereum, toxoplasmosis, tuberculosis and tularemia, trauma, vascular compromise, post-vaccination lymphadenitis or autoimmunity, eg lupus erythematosus, muco-cutaneous lymph node syndrome (Kawasaki's disease), necrotizing lymphadenitis (Kikuchi's disease) and b) Global necrosis, 80% of which is associated with lymphoma

Lymphocyte The leukocyte responsible for specific immune responses in the form of antibody production, 'self' (MHC) restriction and other specific and non-specific immune interactions; lymphocytes comprise 30% of the circulating white cells (neutrophils comprise 60%), of which 65% are T cells (35-50% CD4 T cells with a 'helper' phenotype, 15-30% CD8 T cells with a 'suppressor' phenotype), 25% are B-cells and the rest, natural killer and killer cells; see B cell, K cell, NK cell, T cell

Lymphocytic choriomeningitis An aseptic meningitis of low morbidity caused by an arenavirus (single-stranded RNA virus containing two glyco- and nucleoproteins) that is transmitted through rodent excretia, affecting adults in winter, when rodents move indoors **Clinical** Biphasic presentation with flu symptoms followed by meningitis with fever, headache, lymphocytosis in the cerebrospinal fluid, often associated with leukopenia and thrombocytopenia, this latter may be a hyperimmune response **Differential diagnosis** Infectious mononucleosis, enterovirus, Herpes zoster

Lymphocytic interstitial pneumonia (LIP) A diffuse pulmonary disease of insidious onset that is most common in middle-aged women and which may be accompanied by Sjögren's disease, hypergammaglobulinemia or hypoγglobulinemia **Clinical** Progressive shortness of breath, cough RADIOLOGY Reticulonodular infiltrates on a plain chest film, which may be accompanied by Kerley 'B' lines **Histopathology** Nodular interstitial process of the alveolar and interlobular septae in a perivascular pattern characterized by mature lymphocytes admixed with plasma and other 'round' cells Note: LIP may mimic lymphoma, as it is characterized by cellular monotony with aggregates of small lymphocytes, bronchial mucosal ulceration, parenchymal infiltration and is considered by some to be a premalignant lesion; with time, the patients progress to end-stage lung disease or develop lymphoma

Lymphocytotoxicity assay A complement-mediated assay commonly used in HLA (human leukocyte antigen) typing laboratories, which tests for the presence of cytotoxic antibodies in the serum of the potential recipient that are capable of reacting with the lymphocytes of the potential donor; see Mixed lymphocyte culture

Lymphoepithelioma Undifferentiated nasopharyngeal carcinoma A malignancy with a marked lymphocytic component, subdivided into a) SCHMINCKE TYPE Diffuse mixing of epithelial and lymphoid elements, making the lesion difficult to distinguish from lymphoma, since the epithelial cells may mimic lymphoblasts or the lacunar cell variants of Reed-Sternberg cells and b) REGAUD TYPE Cohesive carcinoma cell aggregates that are large enough to make the epithelial nature of the tumor obvious **Diagnosis** Immunoperoxidase positive for cytokeratin **Treatment** Prognosis; Cf Eskimoma

Lymphogranuloma venereum (LGV) A sexually transmitted disease caused by one of three immunotypes (L_1, L_2 and L_3) of ***Chlamydia trachomatis***; LGV is uncommon in USA, regionally endemic in Asia, Africa and South America **Clinical** Papulo-ulcer that forms and spontaneously heals at the inoculation site, followed by matted and painful loco-regional (inguinal and perirectal), lymphadenopathy, described as 'kissing' lesions with a 'groove' sign, sloughing of skin, purulent drainage, hemorrhagic proctocolitis, malaise, fever, headache, aseptic meningitis, anorexia, myalgia, arthralgia, hepatitis, conjunctivitis and erythema nodosum **Laboratory** Antibody assays, eg immunofluorescence, counterimmunoelectrophoresis, complement fixation titers of greater than 1:32, Frei test (intradermal injection of crude antigen into the forearm, read at 72 hours, where greater than 6 mm induration is positive **Histopathology** Inclusion bodies in Giemsa-stained histiocytes, 'stellate abscesses' in lymph nodes **Treatment** Tetracycline, excision

Lymphoid granular complex A large intestinal microbursa that was initially described as a morphological marker for inflammatory bowel disease, but which is recognized as the local recipient site for antigens destined for future immune recognition, forming an integral component of the gastrointestinal-associated lymphoid tissue; see GALT

Lymphokines A heterogeneous group of nonspecific hormone-like polypeptides that are secreted by various cells of the immune system during anantigen response 'cascade', enhancing or suppressing the immune system, having either paracrine (locally cytostimulatory) or autocrine (self-stimulatory) activities; lymphokines are produced by activated T cells and natural killer cells, promote cell proliferation, growth and/or differentiation, regulate cell function by acting on gene transcription and in inflammation; lymphokines include γ-interferon, interleukins IL-2 to IL-6, granulocyte-macrophage colony-stimulating factor and lymphotoxin Note: Cytokine is the preferred term as certain 'lymphokines' are also produced by monocytes and macrophages and thus may also be termed 'monokines'; see Biological response modifiers, Colony-stimulating factors, Interferons, Interleukins, Tumor necrosis factor

Lymphokine-activated killer cells see LAK cells

Lymphoma A malignant neoplasm of B or T lymphocytes, arising from a monoclonal, ie derived from a single progenitor cell, proliferation of lymphocytes; the proliferative process is considered lymphomatous in the appropriate clinical setting, given that not all monoclonal expansions have a malignant behavior Note: The process of producing and secreting immunoglobulin (B cells) or membrane receptor (T cells) is preceded by a DNA rearrangement, in which the introns are spliced out, ie eliminated and the exons linked together (V/J or V/D/J rearrangement), forming a mature messenger RNA molecule that is unique to one individual cell; when a cell produces abundant daughter cells, the monoclonal 'expansion' is detectable by Southern blot hybridization; B and T cell malignancies are driven by the common mechanism of translocation and oncogene regulation; the prognosis is favorable in follicular lymphomas, especially those with cleaved, mixed and large non-cleaved cell types, and may also be favorable in certain diffuse lymphomas, eg small lymphocytic, cleaved cell, Burkitt's, non-cleaved cell and convoluted cell types; a distinctly unfavorable prognosis is characteristic of diffuse plasmacytoid lymphocye, mixed cell, mixed small noncleaved cell and large noncleaved cell types; Advanced age, anemia and high mitotic activity are associated with a poor prognosis **Angiotropic lymphoma** see there **B cell lymphoma** A lymphoma composed of follicular center cells Note: It is unclear whether there is a difference in clinical behavior between B or T cell lymphomas that have a similar morphology by simple light microscopy; this is supported by the Working Formulation classification, which is clinically valid but does not require identification of B or T cell lineage; the overall survival and survival by stage are similar in cutaneous T cell lymphomas and in histologically favorable B cell lymphomas **Biclonal lymphoma** see there **Burkitt's lymphoma** A lymphoma of children that is 'driven' by the Epstein-Barr virus endemic to certain regions of Africa (see Lymphoma belt), which presents in the young African jaw or in young American abdomen, affects the bone marrow and usually responds well (initially) to chemotherapy; Burkitt's lymphoma is characterized by sheets of monotonous small round cells punctuated by a 'starry sky' pattern, see there **Centrocytic lymphoma** see below, Diffuse small cleaved cell lymphoma **Composite lymphoma** A rare lymphoma composed of two or more malignant cell lines in the same lymph node **Diffuse lymphoma** A lymphoma composed of sheets of cells and lacking all attempts to recapitulate germinal centers, which often spill into the adjacent adipose and other tissues; in general, diffuse lymphomas are more aggressive than follicular lymphomas **Diffuse large cell lymphoma** A complex and heterogeneous group of non-Hodgkin's lymphoma that corresponds to the 'histiocytic' lymphoma and reticulum cell sarcoma of older classifications affecting those circa age 60, which is composed of small round cells with little cytoplasm that may present in advanced stages, 20% of which may be accompanied by monoclonal gammopathy Prognosis 60% five year survival **Diffuse mixed (small and large cell) lymphoma** A clinico-pathologically heterogeneous group of lymphomas, most of which are the diffuse counterparts of follicular lymphoma or peripheral T cell lymphoma **Diffuse small cleaved cell lymphoma** A usually B cell lymphoma composed of follicular center cells with one-half the survival rate of follicular small cleaved cell lymphoma **Discordant lymphoma** A rare lymphoma composed of two or more histiological subtypes in separate anatomic locations; therapy is directed at the lineage with the worst prognosis **Extranodal lymphoma** A lymphoma that is often histologically diffuse, appears in the stomach, tonsils, skin, small intestine and salivary glands and which is usually slightly more aggressive than nodal lymphomas **Follicular lymphoma** A heterogeneous group of lymphomas arising in follicular center cells, which comprises 50% of all non-Hodgkin's lymphomas in adults in the US, more common in the elderly and distinctly uncommon in those under age 20 and in the black population; follicular lymphomas are usually confined to lymph nodes, have a 8:14 chromosomal translocation and when accompanied by del 13q32, are more aggressive and may enter a leukemic phase; follicular lymphomas are histologically divided into those with predominantly small cleaved cells (large cells comprise less than 20% of the cells), those with more than 50% large cells, and those with mixed, small cleaved and large cells **Gastric lymphoma** A diffuse low-grade lymphoma with 5- and 10-year survivals of 57% and 46%, respectively, in which the histologic subtype, clinical stage and mode of therapy are of little prognostic value, composed of monotonous mature or atypical lymphocytes **Histiocytic lymphoma** A very rare lymphoma consisting of discrete mass(es) in lymphoid tissues, skin and bone of histiocytes, which may also have T cell or B cell markers; many of the lesions first described by Rappaport, now known as 'Rappaport's histiocytic lymphoma', ultimately proved to be comprised of transformed lymphocytes mimicking histiocytes **Intermediate lymphocytic lymphoma** An indolent B cell lymphoma of the middle-aged and elderly, related to small cell follicular lymphoma, composed of cells similar to those of well-differentiated lymphocytic lymphoma **Ki-1 lymphoma** Pleomorphic histiocytic lymphoma(s) A heterogeneous group of childhood lymphomas, the cells of which are reactive against the monoclonal antibody Ki-1, (an antibody that also reacts with Reed-Sternberg cells), leukocyte common antigen and epithelial membrane antigen; despite the anaplastic 'ugly' histology, the tumor may respond to chemotherapy with prolonged remission or complete cure **Large cell lymphoma with filopodia** A rare type of large cell lymphoma, characterized by abundant filiform projections on the cell surfaces, a functional variant of dubious distinction **Lennert's lymphoma** Lymphoepithelioid lymphoma A lymphoma of large cells that are more pleomorphic than those of large cell lymphoma (with which it was confused in the early reports), which have immunocytochemical evidence of monocyte-histiocytic differentiation; these lymphomas are nodally based and tend to involve the skin and bone, carrying a relatively good prognosis **Lymphoblastic lymphoma** A lymphoma most common in children and adolescents, arising in the mediastinum, which without therapy, is highly aggressive, causing rapid multisystem dissemination and death within a year of presentation composed of diffuse monomorphous sheets of large cells, punctuated by a focal starry sky pattern

MEDITERRANEAN LYMPHOMA see IPSID (Immunoproliferative small intestinal disease) **MONOCYTOID B CELL LYMPHOMA** A distinct B cell lymphoma that represents the malignant counterpart, ie a clonal expansion of the monocytoid cells seen in reactive lymphoid hyperplasias that arise in a background of toxoplasmosis and other benign lesions **NODULAR LYMPHOMA** see Follicular lymphoma **NON-HODGKIN'S LYMPHOMA** 60% of all lymphomas are non-Hodgkin's lymphomas, of which 55% are diffuse lymphomas and 45% are nodular lymphomas; 27 000 new cases of non-Hodgkin's lymphomas are diagnosed annually in the US **PEDIATRIC LYMPHOMA** An uncommon lymphoma that is often extranodal, diffuse and responds well to chemotherapy **PLEOMORPHIC (NON-BURKITT'S) LYMPHOMA** A lymphoma composed of pleomorphic cells, midway in size between small cleaved and large cells, which tends to involve the gastrointestinal tract and the bone marrow and may be more aggressive clinically **PULMONARY LYMPHOMA** see Lymphocytic interstitial pneumonia **RAPPAPORT'S HISTIOCYTIC LYMPHOMA** see above, Histiocytic lymphoma **SIGNET RING CELL LYMPHOMA(S)** A group of lymphomas that share nothing in common beyond having scattered-to-abundant 'signet ring' lymphocytes; the cleared vacuoles are derived from multivesicular bodies, a form of lysosomes, which in some cases, may be filled with immunoglobulins; these lymphomas are otherwise heterogeneous by histological (many are follicular center lymphomas), clinical and immunohistochemical criteria and thus the designation of signet ring-cell lymphoma represents a curiosity of questionable significance, comprising up to 1% of all B cell and T cell lymphomas **SMALL LYMPHOCYTIC (WELL DIFFERENTIATED) LYMPHOMA** A relatively indolent lymphoma that affects the middle-aged to elderly with a good prognosis, some cases of which represent the tissue equivalent of chronic lymphocytic leukemia; most are of B cell type and have monoclonal antibodies on the cell surface; in those cases with T cell markers, the cells are larger and more aggressive clinically **SMALL INTESTINAL LYMPHOMA** see IPSID **SMALL NON-CLEAVED CELL LYMPHOMA** A high grade B-cell lymphoma composed of B cell markers, which is arbitrarily subdivided into Burkitt's lymphoma and Pleomorphic (non-Burkitt's) lymphoma **T CELL LYMPHOMA** 90% of all patients with T cell lymphoma have extracutaneous involvement at the time of diagnosis Note: The overall survival and survival by stage is similar in cutaneous T cell lymphomas and in histologically favorable B cell lymphomas Pathology Vascular proliferation, TdT (Terminal deoxynucleotidyl transferase), T helper (CD4) or T suppressor (CD3) cell subsets; pleomorphic nucleus and cleared cytoplasm; see T cell lymphomas **UNDIFFEREN-TIATED LYMPHOMA** see Small non-cleaved cell lymphoma; see AIDS, Hodgkin's disease, Monoclonality, Pre-lymphoma, Working classification; Cf Leukemia

Lymphoma belt A region of Central Africa between 10 north and 10 south of the equator that has a high incidence of Epstein-Barr virus-induced Burkitt's lymphoma (BL); in Uganda, BL is the most common cause of childhood malignancy; similar environmental and climatic conditions are seen in Papua New Guinea, another focus of BL Note: Epstein-Barr virus is present in 90% of African BL, but in less than one-half of non-African BL (Br J Med 1962; 2:1019, Nature 1962; 194:232)

Lymphomatoid granulomatosis A condition initially thought to be a variant of pulmonary angiitis and granulomatosis, now considered a lymphoproliferative disorder, which presents in middle-aged subjects with well-circumscribed bilateral nodules seen on a plain film of the chest and some cases occur in immunosuppressed renal transplant recipients and in those with Sjögren syndrome Clinical 80% of cases have extrapulmonary involvement, eg skin, central nervous system, kidneys, liver, spleen, adrenal glands, heart, gastrointestinal tract and other organs Histopathology Vasocentric polymorphic infiltrate comprised of plasma cells, immunoblasts and large atypical lymphocytes Prognosis 64% mortality with a median survival of 14 months, the death being due to pulmonary destruction accompanied by sepsis; the malignant deterioration is associated with severe impairment of the T cell function possibly explaining the tendency for malignant degeneration; Cf Lymphoid interstitial pneumonia

Lymphomatoid papulosis A recurring papular eruption of the skin with a benign clinical course that histologically resembles malignant lymphoma; although most lesions behave in an indolent fashion, gene rearrangement studies demonstrate a clonal expansion of T cells; 10-20% are associated with or evolve toward T cell lymphoma

Lymphotoxin A heterodimeric glycoprotein cytokine with a 5 kD and a 15 kD protein fragment produced by T cells that evokes B cell proliferation, which also specifically inhibits tumor growth, in vivo and in vitro, inhibiting transformation of cells induced by chemical carcinogens and ultraviolet light

Lyonization A normal genetic event described by Mary Lyon, a British geneticist that consists of inactivation of all X chromosomes (although portions of the 'inactivated' chromosome may remain functional) that are in excess of one; lyonization occurs during embryogenesis and results in the formation of 'Barr bodies', present in all nucleated somatic cells, but best visualized in polymorphonuclear granulocytes and scraped squamous cells of the buccal mucosa

Lyophilization Freeze drying A method for preserving foods or biologicals, where a substance, eg coagulation factor VIII, is 'snap-frozen' in liquid nitrogen (-70°C) and placed in a high vacuum to remove the water vapor as it sublimes; once the water is removed, the substance is brought to room temperature and stored; Cf Quick-freeze technique

Lysenkoism A pseudoscientific doctrine based on Lamarckism that was espoused by the Russian geneticist TD Lysenko, which formed the basis of Soviet genetics from 1932 to 1965; see Lamarckism

Lysergic acid diethylamide (LSD) SUBSTANCE ABUSE A synthetic hallucinogen derived from ergot alkaloids that produces mood elevations, sensory distortion, depersonalization, which may provoke panic attacksand flashbacks; LSD was most popular during the 1960s among the 'hippies', as it was touted as having a 'mind-the 'hippies', as it was touted as having a 'mind-expanding' potential, and as a euphorogenic drug of abuse is less popular than certain other agents; see Designer drugs, 'Ice' Note: It is unclear how teratogenic LSD is, as most of the data is anecdotal

Lysinemia A heterogeneous group of diseases with increased lysine or its metabolites in the blood, including hyperlysinemia, types I and II, saccharopurinuria, hydroxylysinuria, pipecolic acidemia and α-ketoadipic aciduria

Lysogeny The inherited ability of certain strains of bacteria to act as viral vectors, integrating themselves into the bacterial genome itself; lysogenic bacteria may differ from their non-infected comrades, eg ***Corynebacterium diphtheriae*** only produce toxin in the presence of lysogenic phages; lysogeny can be stimulated by suboptimal growth conditions or through inhibition of bacterial protein production, eg adding chloramphenicol to a culture

Lysosomal storage diseases A generic term for a heterogeneous group of diseases with specific defects in lysosomal enzymes; these diseases including a) Sphingolipidoses, in which there are defects in sulfated mucopolysaccharide catabolism eg Niemann-Pick, Gaucher's, Krabbe's, Fabry's diseases and others b) Mucopolysaccharidoses, in which there are defects in the glycosaminoglycans, which can be identified by culturing skin fibroblasts, eg Hurler, Scheie, Hunter, Sanfilippo and other syndromes and c) Disorders involving multiple storage products, including various mucolipidoses; Cf Inborn errors of metabolism

Lysosome A membrane-bound cytoplasmic organelle that contains a vast array of digestive enzymes, including ribonuclease, deoxyribonuclease, phosphatase, glycosidase, arylsulfatase, collagenase and cathepsins; once a 'virgin' lysosome or primary granule encounters a substrate for digestion, it becomes known as a secondary lysosome or granule

Lysozyme A class of hydrolytic enzymes responsible for hydrolysis of mucopolysaccharides and mucoproteins, found in tears, milk, saliva and serum as well as neutrophils and cells of the monocyte phagocytic system

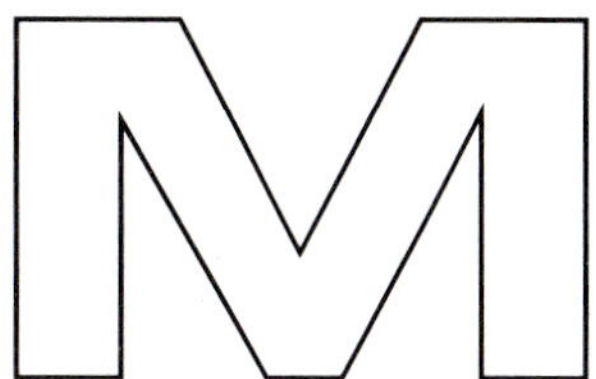

M symbol for: Mega (10^6); methionine; molar concentration; M (mitosis) phase of the cell cycle

m symbol for: Mass; median (statistics); mean of a sample, meta- (organic chemistry, benzene ring position); messenger (RNA); meter; milli-; molal concentration

MAAC Maximum allowable actual charge HEALTH CARE FINANCING The practical limit on the amount of money that physicians who don't accept Medicare 'assignment' may collect from Medicare patients

MAB Monoclonal antibody, Monoclonal antibodies

Mabiki Japanese, thinning out SOCIOLOGY The killing of unwanted offspring, usually female, practiced by rural peasants in old Japan, by suffocation or a blow to the head, where the ideal ratio of progeny was two male children to one female; female infanticide has also been practiced among the Aborigines, Arabs, Chinese, in India and Oceania; women have been historically weaned earlier, underfed and overworked throughout the world, a practice that continues today in Africa, the Middle and Far East

MAC ***Mycobacterium avium*** complex A common cause of systemic infection of AIDS patients, affecting as many as two-thirds of AIDS patients with CD4-positive T cells in the circulation; MAC responds poorly to combination anti-tuberculous drug 'cocktails', but responds well to clarithromycin (Am Med News 22-29/Apr/91)

Machine error COMPUTERS A hardware error versus a software 'bug'

Machine language COMPUTERS A set of instructions written in symbols and graphic representations in the logical language for and understood by a computer Advantage Flexibility Disadvantage It is error-prone and considerable skill is required to write the programs

Machinery murmur of Gibson A harsh, rasping, continuous cardiac murmur characteristic of patent ductus arteriosus that begins shortly after the first sound, reaches a maximum at the end of systole and wanes in late diastole; it is best heard in the second left intercostal space, transmits to the chest and neck and may be felt by the patients as a palpable thrill or 'buzz'; it may also be heard in ventricular septal defect,rarely in pulmonary hypertension and in penetrating soft-tissue injury with formation of an arteriovenous fistula

MAC program Maximum Allowable Cost program A US federal program that purchases drugs from several commercial sources in order to obtain the lowest possible price and limit reimbursement for prescription drugs under the Medicare and Medicaid programs

Macroamylase A 200 kD plasma amylase, usually of salivary type that circulates complexed to various high molecular-weight plasma proteins, eg IgG, IgA, polysaccharides, glycoproteins and α_1-antitrypsin; persistent six-to-eightfold elevation of macroamylase occurs in 1% of older subjects, often accompanied by abdominal pain, associated with alcoholism, pancreatitis, malignancy, diabetes mellitus, cholelithiasis, autoimmune disease

Macrobdella A genus of fresh water leech; see Leech

Macrobiotics ALTERNATIVE MEDICINE A diet and philosophy taught by G Ohsawa and M Kushi and popularized in the 1960s in the US, based on an idiosyncratic version of the ancient concept of yin and yang, arbitrarily assigning foods as having a 'male' or 'female' quality; the diet consists predominantly of whole grains, vegetables and enough food of animal origin to prevent malnutrition; nonmacrobiotic diets have been linked to the development of cancer by the followers of the macrobiotic philosophy, who mistakenly believe that any diet that can prevent cancer is also appropriate in its treatment Note: Kushi himself recognizes that the diet is to be used in conjunction with cancer treatment regimens; see Unproven methods of cancer treatment

Macrocephaly Macrencephaly An enlarged head; in the pediatric age group, macrocephaly is defined dynamically and in vivo as an occipitofrontal circumference of greater than three standard deviations above the mean; in the adult, macrocephaly may be static and is defined in vitro as any brain weighing more than 1800 g, due to the expansion of any subdural component, including cerebral tissue, liquid, blood, tumor or storage disease; the largest brain reported weighed 2.1 Kg (4 lbs, 8.29 oz), recognizing that size is no indicator of intellectual prowess **Differential diagnosis**, non-hydrocephalic macrocephaly A benign familial form in which the sibs also have large heads, achondroplasia, Banayan syndrome, cerebral gigantism (with macrosomia or Sotos syndrome), cutis marmorata telangiectatica congenita, fragile X syndrome, Klippel-Trenauny-Weber syndrome, mucopolysaccharidosis, neurofibromatosis and Weaver syndrome

Macro-creatine kinase An atypical electrophoretic creatine kinase(CK) band that migrates between CK-MM and CK-MB and consists of either CK-BB or CK-MM complexed to another serum protein, often IgG, rarely IgA or lipoprotein

Macrocyte An enlarged (> 100 μm^3 volume) red cell with increased hemoglobin and decreased lifespan, which may be secondary to various stresses, eg hemolytic anemia, hyperthyroidism, massive bleeding, erythroblastosis fetalis, which is accompanied by increased erythropoietin production

Macroenzyme Obsolete for aspartate aminotransferase (AST)

Macrogamete PARASITOLOGY The female gamete of ***Plasmodium*** species, which conjugates with the microgamete (male), forming a zygote that develops into an oocyst, a part of the ***Plasmodium*** life cycle that occurs in the human; the asexual phase occurs in the mosquito

Macroglia An obsolete generic term for all the central nervous system cells that are not neurons and not microglia (tissue-based macrophages), eg astrocytes, oligodendroglia and glioblasts; 'macroglia' provide nutrition, support and synthesize myelin

Macroglobulin Any large serum protein, eg IgM (900 kD), α_2-macroglobulin (820 kD); macroglobulins are detected by sharp peaks on a simple zone electrophoresis, usually in the γ-region Note: Because of the differing charges on the radicals, the electrophoretic mobility, pI, on the agar may shift and monoclonal spikes may occur in the β or, less commonly, the α regions

Macroglossia Enlargement of the tongue due to accumulation of various substances, edema, presence of ectopic tissues, tumors and others; macroglossia occurs in amyloidosis, Beckwith-Wiedemann syndrome, congenital hypothyroidism, cystic hygroma, Down syndrome, ectopic thyroid, glycogen storage disease, type II (Pompe), hemangioma (of the tongue), Hurler syndrome, intestinal duplication, lymphangioma, mannosidosis, neurofibromatosis, rhabdomyoma and Sandhoff's disease

Macrolide antibiotic Any of a group of broad-spectrum antibiotics, eg erythromycin that are produced by Streptomyces species, which contain a lactone ring and inhibit protein synthesis in target bacteria

Macronucleoli GYNECOLOGIC CYTOLOGY Enlarged nucleoli seen in tissue repair and in invasive carcinoma on a papanicolaou smear, but not generally seen in 'intermediate' (dysplasia, carcinoma in situ) lesions SURGICAL PATHOLOGY Macronucleoli are highly characteristic of certain malignancies, eg carcinoma of the kidney, breast and thyroid, malignant melanoma, Hodgkin's disease and immunoblastic lymphoma

Macrophages IMMUNOLOGY Non-specific immune defense cells that interact with proteins and polysaccharide antigens, internalizing and partially degrading them, and/or presenting the antigens to T cells in a major histocompatibility complex (MHC) context, secretion, immune interaction with T and B cells, provide lymphokine receptors (once activated, macrophages are highly microbicidal and tumoricidal), often closely associated with the blood vessels, epithelial and mesothelium, appropriate sites for non-specific immunocytes; macrophages can be divided into a) Monocytes, comprising 3-5% of circulating leukocytes, b) Tissue-bound macrophages, located in the alveoli, central nervous system (designated as microglial cells), liver (Kupffer cells), lymph nodes, peritoneum and skin (Langerhans cells) and c) Histiocytes Substances secreted by macrophages include binding proteins (transferrin, transcobalamin II, fibronectin), chemotactic factors (for neutrophils), complement components (C1-C5, factors B and D, properdin, C3b inactivator, β1H), endogenous pyrogens, enzymes (neutral proteases, plasminogen activator, collagenase, elastase, angiotensin-convertase, acid hydrolase, proteases, lipases, ribonuclease, phosphatase, glycosidase, sulfatase, arginase, lysozyme), enzyme inhibitors (plasmin inhibitor, α_2-macroglobulin, oxygen radicals: H_2O_2, superoxide, hydroxyl radical, singlet oxygen), bioactive lipids (arachidonic acid metabolites, eg prostaglandin E_2 and F_1, thromboxane A_2, leukotriene, HETE, SRS-A and platelet activating factors), mitogens (colony-stimulating factors, lymphocyte activating factors, growth factors for fibroblasts, endothelium, granulocytes, IL-1), nucleosides and metabolites (thymidine, uracil, uric acid), regulatory proteins (haptoglobin, collagenase, elastase)

Macrophage activation The array of processes that form part of the up-regulation of macrophage activity, which has multiple structural components, including increased size and cytoplasmic granules, spreading, membrane ruffling, as well as functional changes, including increased amino acid and glucose metabolism and transport, increased enzymatic activity, eg adenylate cyclase, collagenase and lactate dehydrogenase production and increases in plasminogen activator, prostaglandins, cGMP, intracellular calcium ions, pinocytosis, phagocytosis, bacteriolysis and tumorlysis

Macrophage activating factor(s) (MAF) A heterogeneous group of lymphokines secreted by sensitized lymphocytes; the most potent MAF is interferon γ but other interferons and molecules have this activity; interferon-activated macrophages have increased bactericidal and tumoricidal activity and demonstrate morphological evidence of 'maturation', including enlargement, increased spreading, pseudopod formation and vacuolization

Macrophage chemotactic factor(s) Any cytokine that functions in tandem with the macrophages, mediating migration; mutiple factors are involved and include interleukins and interferons, appearing in the supernatant of graft-versus-host disease

Macrophage function assays Tests that determine the functional activity of macrophages, testing a) Chemotaxis A chemoattractant is placed at one end of a Boyden chamber and macrophages at the other, and the ability of the cells to migrate towards the test substance is evaluated b) Lysis A chemoattractant is placed in a chamber and the radioactivity of the supernatant is measured after a target (bacteria, tumor cell) has been destroyed and c) Phagocytosis Active ingestion by macrophages of a radiolabelled target, yields a radioactive macrophage

Macrophage inflammatory protein-1-α (MIP-1) An endogenous heparin-binding pyrogen (other pyrogens include interleukin-1 and tumor necrosis factor) that is not affected by cyclooxygenase inhibition, which is secreted in response to endotoxin (Science 1989; 243:1066) MIP-1 is identical to SCI (stem cell inhibitor), an inhibitor of hematopoietic stem cells and may be a key actor in the growth regulatory network for hematopoietic cell production (Nature 1990; 344:380, 442)

Macrophage mannose receptor see *Pneumocystis carinii*

Macula densa RENAL HISTOLOGY A specialized region in the distal renal tubule at which point specialized cells converge; the macula densa is part of the juxtaglomerular apparatus, the components of which include the afferent and efferent glomerular arterioles, Lacis cells and non-granular cells

'Mad cow' disease see Bovine spongiform encephalopathy

Mad Hatter syndrome A descriptor for the neurologic component of chronic mercuric nitrate poisoning, which is clinically similar to prolonged exposure to mercury vapor, erethism; exposed persons undergo psychological changes including anxiety, depression, eccentricity, reclusiveness, emotional instability, irritability, as well as circumoral, glossal and limb tremors, gingivitis, arthralgias, headaches and extrapyramidal signs; a major labor-related mercury intoxication occurred in a felt hat factory (hence the fanciful trivial name) during World War II in Italy; of 100 affected, 30 had permanent sequelae (Med Lav 1949; 40:65) Note: Despite the popularized version, it is uncertain whether the Mad Hatter described by Lewis Carroll in Through the Looking Glass was a victim of mercury poisoning (Br Med J 1984; 288:324); see Minamata Bay disease

Mad honey Nectar derived from pollens of certain plants, including rhododendron, western azalea, California rosebay, mountain laurel and sheep laurel containing toxic diterpenes (grayanotoxins); ingestion of 'mad honey' causes an abrupt attack that may simulate acute myocardial infarction **Clinical** Vertigo, weakness, diaphoresis, nausea, vomiting, profound hypotension, bradyarrhythmia, heart block and potentially, convulsions; all victims recover within 24 hours (J Am Med Assoc 1988; 259:1943c)

Madura foot see Mycetoma

MAF see Macrophage activating factor

MAFH see Multicentric angiofollicular lymphoid hyperplasia

Magenstraße German, Gastric 'street' The pliable, linear rugal folds of the gastric mucosa that follow the lesser curvature and are bound externally by the gastrohepatic ligament, which is the site of most spontaneous gastric rupture, due in part to the lesser distensibility of the lesser curvature

Magenta bodies CYTOLOGY A characteristic, variably-sized red-to-purple perinuclear inclusion seen by the Romanovsky stain in breast carcinomas, both primary or metastatic

Magenta tongue A deeply red-to-purple, smooth tongue seen in riboflavin deficiency

Maggot The larval stage of the green (*Phaenicia sericata*) and black (*Phormia regina*) bottle flies, which were once used to treat osteomyelitis and chronic suppurative infections, since the larva only thrive in necrotic tissue, secreting allantoin, thought to be a stimulant for epithelial growth; pernicious maggots that thrive on live tissues include ***Auchmeromyia luteola*** (Congo floor maggot) nocturnal blood suckers, ***Eristalis*** and ***Helophilus*** (Rat-tail, hover-fly maggots) which frequent stagnant water and have a predilection for the nasopharynx and intestine; Cf Leeches, Roaches

Magical thinking A form of deretic thought, similar to a normal phase of childhood development (Piaget's preoperational phase), in which thoughts, words or actions assume power, ie they can prevent or cause events to happen without a physical action occurring, ie 'by magic'; magical thinking may be unnerving to those with obsessive-compulsive disorders who fear aggressive thoughts; dereism is thought that is not concordant with logic or experience

Magic bullet IMMUNOLOGY A term coined by Paul Ehrlich, circa 1900, for what he considered would be an ideal therapeutic agent, arriving only to a designated cell or target; the higher the organism is phylogenetically, the more difficult it is to achieve this goal, as the metabolism of the target and host cells are similar; antibiotics are a form of 'Magic bullet'; the term is modified by modern immunologists to signify any agent that would act with the specificity of an antibody and have the lethal potential of a toxin; monoclonal antibodies linked to a toxin were crude first-generation magic bullets that have fallen short of their intended aim, as the constant region of the monoclonal antibody doesn't support cytocidal activity; later magic bullet candidates linked cytokines or monoclonal antibodies to toxins (diphtheria toxin, pseudomonas toxin A or ricin); one apparently successful 'magic bullet' therapeutic approach uses monoclonal anti-B cell antibodies, 'raised' against the CD21 and CD24 antigens to suppress the B cell lymphoproliferative syndrome (N Engl J Med 1991; 324:1451); see Orthozyme CD5plus

Magic mushrooms see Peyote

'Magic number' BIOCHEMISTRY The number (20) of different amino acids present in proteins of all plants and animals Note: Although other amino acids are present in proteins, these represent minor biochemical modifications of the 'magic 20'; see Degenerate code

Magic spot nucleotides A pair of spots (which when first described were of unknown nature, therefore 'magic') seen on thin-layer chromatograms that were later identified as guanosine 5'-diphosphate 3'-diphosphate (ppGpp) and guanosine 5'-triphosphate 3'-diphosphate (pppGpp), two nucleotides that accumulate during the stringent response reaction in bacteria, in which multiple metabolic pathways shut down when one or more amino acids are present in limited quantities

Maginot line pattern Fortification phenomenon A fanciful descriptor for teichotic scotomata, which are jagged, slightly off-center scintillating lines characteristic of the visual aura that often precedes visual migraines Note: The Maginot line is a 20 mile stretch of tooth-like concrete 'barriers' built after World War I, by the worried, war-wearied French with the intent of preventing a third German invasion

Magnet Magnesia, the ancient city in Asia minor that had stones with magnetic properties; see Electromagnetic fields, Magnetic resonance imaging, Mesmerism

Magnetic core memory see Computers

Magnetic flux Theta A measurement of the strength of a magnetic field, expressed by the International System (SI) unit, weber, which is equal to one volt-second

Magnetic resonance The absorption or emission of electromagnetic energy by nuclei in a static magnetic field after excitation by a suitable resonance frequency magnetic field; the peak resonance frequency is proportional to the magnetic field and is given by the Larmor equation Note: Only nuclei with a non-zero spin exhibit magnetic resonance

Magnetic resonance imaging The creation of images by the phenomenon of magnetic resonance (MR), which is a function of the distribution of hydrogen nuclei (protons) in the body; the MR image is a computerized interpretation of the physical interaction of unpaired protons with electromagnetic radiation in the presence of a magnetic field; the image brightness in a given region depends on 1) Spin density and 2) Relaxation times, the relative importance of which is determined by the imaging technique employed as well as 3) Motion such as blood flow; it was postulated in 1971 that MR might be clinically useful for analysing the whole body; the early work was performed by EMI Ltd of England before the MR imaging became a reality; the images derive from analysis of the amplitudes and frequencies of the weak signals produced by MR, allowing deduction of the sample's chemical composition, with protons providing the best images; the strength of a signal reflects the amount of hydrogen modified by the tissue relaxation parameters, T1 (the spin lattice parameter, which depends on the interaction of hydrogen with other molecules) and T2 (the spin-spin parameter, a function of the interaction of the protons with each other); MR signal intensity is influenced by the proton bulk motion effect, which is a function of the 50 msec lag time between signal production and its registering on the detector **Principle** When tissue is placed in an intense magnetic field, the hydrogen nuclei behave like weak magnets, orienting themselves along the lines of flux; if the tissue is then 'zapped' with a pulse of a specific wavelength of radiofrequency (RF) electromagnetic energy (measured in tesla, high field strengths being 1-2 tesla, low energy < 0.5 tesla), which changes the alignment of hydrogen nuclei by absorption of that energy; as the nuclei return to their previous state of alignment, they emit a characteristic RF length signal which, when compared to other signal 'densities' within the sample, allows construction of an image; the magnetic signal is strongest immediately after the tissue has received the RF impulse and the time to achieve 'relaxation' depends upon differing hydrogen concentration in various tissues, resulting in different decay times T1 and T2; the longitudinal (T1, spin-lattice) relaxation time is that required for the nuclei to return to the pre-RF pulse ground state; the transverse (T2, spin-spin) relaxation time refers to the signal decay, which is a function of the interaction of the nuclei in tissues; signal decay is rapid for rigid molecules (proteins and nucleic acids) and these molecules are not major contributors to the image quality; the MR signal is largely a function of the tissue's water content, with lesser signals contributed by lipids and muscle, allowing excellent soft-tissue differentiation; MR has multiplanar capabilities without the ionizing radiation of computed tomography **Clinical applications** Because conventional MR imaging requires a few minutes to obtain the image, mobile organs, eg heart, gastrointestinal tract are relatively 'fuzzy' although the image obtention time can be 'gated' to reduce this problem MRI according to sites *ABDOMEN* see J Am Med Assoc 1989; 261:420 *BREAST* MRI is not likely to replace mammography, despite promising early reports *CENTRAL NERVOUS SYSTEM* MRI is preferred to CT in imaging posterior fossa lesions, eg tumors, multiple sclerosis, inflammatory lesions, eg lupus erythematosus, spinal cord and canal lesions, head trauma, hemorrhage and other cerebrovascular disease *CHEST* MRI may have some currency in the evaluation of pulmonary edema, hemorrhage and changes of cystic fibrosis *HEAD & NECK* MRI resolves soft tissue densities (fat, muscle, vessels and lymph nodes) in various fossae quite well and the quality of the sagittal, coronal and transaxial images is excellent, but MRI is relatively insensitive to calcification and bone *HEART* If properly 'gated', MRI is useful in detecting anatomic defects of the heart, including septal defects, chamber size and wall thickness *JOINTS* MRI may prove useful in identifying soft tissue disruption in articulations, eg the shoulder and knee *LIVER, PANCREAS* The relatively long 'acquisition' time required to produce an image results in uncontrolled movement, in addition to intrinsic background 'noise' of heartbeats and peristalsis; the motion artifacts can be controlled by using short time to recovery/time to echo (TR/TE) and multiple data collections; detection of hepatic metastases may be more sensitive than computed tomography *PELVIS* MRI is of use in the evaluation of pelvic wall invasion by carcinoma of the urinary bladder, cervix and endometrium as well as the presence of leiomyomas and trophoblastic disease *PROSTATE* MRI is of little use in staging early prostate carcinoma (N Engl J Med 1990; 323:621) *VASCULAR* MRI has potential for imaging 'water' flow, measuring vacular flow and capillary flow, diffusion and exchange (Science 1990; 250:53) Potential hazards Patients undergoing MRI are exposed to static magnetic, pulsed, radiofrequency, electromagnetic and gradient (time-varying) fields; gradient fields allow ultrafast imaging, reducing the scan time of 10 minutes in a conventional MR imager to milliseconds, with the disadvantage of potentially triggering cardiac arrhythmias and unwanted electrical activity (Science 1991; 252:1244n&v) ***GLOSSARY FOR MRI*** (modified from J Am Med Assoc 1987; 258:3422) **ANGULAR MOMENTUM** A vector quantity given by the vector product of the momentum of a particleand its position vector; in absence of external forces, the angular momentum remains constant, therefore a rotating body tends to maintain the same axis of rotation; when a torque is applied to a rotating body, the resulting change in angular momentum results in precession; atomic nuclei possess an intrinsic angular momentum referred to as spin, measured in multiples of Planck's constant **CARR-PURCELL SEQUENCE** A sequence of 90° radiofrequency (RF) pulses followed by repeated 180° RF pulses, producing a train of spin echoes that is used to measure T2 **CARR-PURCELL-MEIBOON-GILL SEQUENCE** A modification of the Carr-Purcell RF pulse sequence with 90° phase shift in the rotating frames of reference between the 90° pulse and subsequent 180° pulses, reducing the accumulating effects of imperfections in the 180° pulses; suppression of effects of pulse error accumulation can alternatively achieved by alternating phases of the 180° pulses by 180° **CHEMICAL SHIFT (DELTA)** The change in the Larmor frequency of a given nucleus, when bound in different sites in a molecule, due to magnetic shielding effects of the electron orbitals; chemical shifts make possible the differences between various molecules and different sites within the molecules in high-resolution magnetic resonance (MR) spectra; the amount of shift is proportional to strength of the magnetic field strength and is usually specified in parts per million of the resonance frequency relative to a standard **ECHO PLANAR IMAGING** A technique of planar imaging in which a complete planar image is obtained from one selective excitation pulse **FREE INDUCTION DECAY** (FID) is observed while periodically switching the **y**-gradient field in the presence of a static **x**-gradient field; the Fourier transform of the resulting spin-echo train can be used to produce an image of the excited plane **FLIP ANGLE** The amount of rotation of the macroscopic magnetization vector produced by an RF pulse with respect to the direction of the static magnetic field **FOURIER TRANSFORM** A mathematical procedure that separates the frequency component of a signal from its amplitude as a function of time or vice versa; the Fourier transform is used to generate the spectrum from the FID in pulse MRI and is essential to most imaging techniques **FREE INDUCTION DECAY (FID)** A transient MR signal produced by transverse magnetization of the spins, eg by a 90° pulse, which decays toward zero with a characteristic time constant T2 (or T2*); in practice, the first part of the FID is not observable due to residual effects of the powerful exciting RF pulse on the electronics of the receiver **GRADIENT MAGNETIC FIELD** (GMR) A magnetic field that changes in strength in a given direction; such fields are used in MR imaging with excitation that 'selects' a region for imaging and encodes the location of MR signals received from the object being imaged; the GMR is measured in teslas/meter **HOMOGENEITY** Uniformity of the static magnetic field, a criterion of the magnet's quality; the requirements for homogeneity in MR imaging are less stringent than for MR spectroscopy, but must be maintained over a larger region **INTERPULSE TIME** The time period between successive RF pulses used in pulse sequences; of particular importance are the inversion time (TI) in inversion recovery, a time period between a 180° pulse and the subsequent 90° pulse; the period between repetitions of pulse sequences is known as the repetition time (TR) **INVERSION** A nonequilibrium state in which the macroscopic magnetization vector is oriented opposite to the magnetic field; usually produced by adiabatic fast passage or by 180° RF pulses **INVERSION RECOVERY** A pulse MR technique that can be incorporated into MR imaging, where the nuclear magnetization is inverted at a time on the order of T1 before the regular imaging pulse-gradient sequences; the resulting partial relaxation of the spins in the different structures being imaged can be used to produce an image that depends on T1, possibly enhancing the differences in the appearance of structures with different T1 relaxation times Note: Inversion recovery does not produce a direct image of T1, but rather one that is calculated from the change in the MR signal from the region due to the inversion pulse compared with the signal with no inversion pulse or an inversion pulse with a different T1 inversion time **Larmor equation** A formula stating that the frequency of precession of the nuclear magnetic moment is proportional to the magnetic field. Equation: $w_0 = \gamma B_0$ (radians/sec) or $f_0 = \gamma B_0/2\pi$ (hertz), where f_0 is frequency, γ is gyromagnetic ratio, and B_0 is the magnetic induction field Note: A negative sign (-) indicates the direction of rotation **Larmor frequency** (w_0 or f_0) The frequency at which magnetic resonance can be excited, given by the Larmor equation; by varying a magnetic field across the body with a gradient magnetic field, the corresponding variation of the Larmor frequency can be used to encode position (for protons, the Larmor frequency is 42.58 MHz/tesla **Longitudinal magnetization** (M_z) The component of the macroscopic magnetization vector along the static magnetic field; after excitation by a radiofrequency pulse, M_z will approach its equilibrium value designated M_0, with a characteristic time constant, T1 **Longitudinal relaxation** The return of longitudinal magnetization to its equilibrium value after excitation, which requires exchange of energy between the nuclear spins and lattice **Macroscopic magnetization vector** Net magnetic moment per unit volume (a vector quantity) of a sample in a given region,considered to be the integrated effect of all the individual microscopic nuclear magnetic moments **Magnetic field** (H) The region surrounding a magnet (or current carrying conductor); in a magnetic field, a small magnet experiences a torque that tends to align it in a certain direction; magnetic fields are vector quantities, the direction of which are defined as the direction to which the north pole points when in equilibrium; this field produces a magnetizing force on any object within that field, a cause for potential safety concerns given the large magnetic fields used in MRI; formally, the forces experienced by moving charged particles, current carrying wires and small magnets in the vicinity of a magnet are due to magnetic induction (B), including the effects of magnetization, while the magnetic field (H) is defined so as to not include magnetization (in practice, however, both B and H are often used to denote magnetic fields **Magnetic moment** A measure of the net magnetic properties of an object or particle; a nucleus with an intrinsic spin will have an associated dipole moment, so that it interacts with a magnetic field, acting as if it were a tiny bar magnet **Magnetic resonance signal** An electromagnetic signal in the radiofrequency (RF) range produced by the precession of the transverse magnetization of the spins; rotation of the magnetization induces a voltage that is amplified and demodulated by the receiver; the signal may refer only to this induced voltage **Magnetization** The magnetic polarization of a material produced by a magnetic field, ie the magnetic moment per unit volume; Cf Macroscopic magnetization vector **Magnetization dipole** North and south magnetic poles separated by a finite distance, corresponding to an electric current loop, including the effective current of a spinning nucleon or nucleus, which may create an equivalent magnetic dipole **Multiple plane imaging** A variation on the sequential plane imaging techniques that can be used with selective excitation techniques and does not affect adjacent planes; adjacent planes are imaged while waiting for relaxation of the first plane toward equilibrium, resulting in decreased imaging time **Nuclear spin** An intrinsic property of certain nuclei that gives them an associated characteristic angular momentum and magnetic moment; Cf Spin **Partial saturation** An 'excitation' technique consisting of administration of repeated RF pulses in time periods equal to or shorter than T1; in MRI, although partial saturation results in decreased signal amplitude, it is possible to generate images with increased contrast between regions with different relaxation times Cf Saturation recovery **Permanent magnet** A magnet composed of a permanently magnetized material **Precession** The comparatively slow gyration of the axis of a spinning body, allowing it to 'race out a cone'; precession is caused by the application of a torque that tends to change the direction of a rotation axis and continuously directs it at right angles to the plane of the torque; the magnetic moment of a nucleus with spin will experience such a torque when inclined at an angle to the magnetic field, resulting in precession at the Larmor frequency, eg effect of gravity on a gyroscope or spinning top **Pulse, 90° (π/2 Pulse)** A radiofrequency pulse that is designed to rotate the macroscopic magnetization vector 90° in space as referred to the rotating frame of reference, usually about an axis at right angles to the main magnetic field; if the spins are initially aligned with the magnetic field, the pulse produces transverse magnetization and an FID **Pulse, 180° (π Pulse)** A radiofrequency pulse that is designed to rotate the macroscopic magnetization vector 180° in space as referred to the rotating frame of reference, usually about an axis at right angles to the main magnetic field; if the spins are initially aligned with the magnetic field, the pi pulse produces inversion **Pulse length** (width) The duration (delta time) of a pulse; for an RF pulse near the Larmor frequency, the longer the pulse length, the greater is the angle of rotation of the macroscopic magnetization vector (> 180° brings the pulse length back to its original orientation) **Pulse sequences** A set of RF (and/or gradient) magnetic field pulses and time intervals between these pulses; used in conjunction with gradient magnetic fields and MR signal reception to produce MR images; Cf Interpulse time **Radiofrequency** (RF) The frequency on the electromagnetic spectrum that is intermediate between auditory and infrared, which in MRI is in the megaherz range; the principal effect of RF magnetic fields on the body is the deposition of power (heat), usually confined to the corporal surface, being the main safety concern **Radiofrequency coil** A component of the MRI hardware that transmits RF pulses and/or receives MR signals; commonly having a solenoid or saddle configuration **Radiofrequency pulse** A brief burst of RF magnetic field delivered to the object by the RF transmitter;

for an RF near the Larmor frequency, the RF pulse results in rotation of the macroscopic magnetization vector in the rotating frame of reference; the amount of rotation depends on the strength and duration of the RF pulse, most commonly 90° (π/2) and 180° (π) pulses **RECEIVER** The component of the MRI hardware that detects and amplifies RF signals picked up by the receiver coil, which is comprised of a preamplifier, amplifier and demodulator **RELAXATION TIME** The time period after excitation that is required for spins to return to a ground state or state of equilibrium distribution, in which there is no transverse magnetization and the longitudinal magnetization is at its maximum value and oriented in the direction of the static magnetic field; the transverse magnetization decays toward zero with a characteristic time constant T2; the longitudinal magnetization returns toward the equilibrium value M_0 with a characteristic time constant T1 **REPEATED FREE INDUCTION DECAY** A form of MRI in which repeated 90° pulses are applied, which results in partial saturation if the interpulse times are equal or less than T1 **RESOLUTION** Spatial resolution The ability of the imaging process to distinguish among adjacent structures within an object being imaged, which is a measure of image quality; the criterion for determining resolution depends on the type of test being used (bar pattern or contrast detail phantom); the ability to separate or discern objects depends on their contrast and different MRI object parameters affect different imaging techniques, thus for example, comparison of resolution phantom tests from different machines may be difficult as the images differ **ROTATING FRAME OF REFERENCE** A point and its corresponding coordinate system that is rotating about the axis of the static magnetic field B_0 (with respect to a stationary or 'laboratory' frame of reference) at a frequency equal to that of the applied RF magnetic field, B_1; although B_1 is a rotating vector, it appears stationary in the rotating frame, and allows simple calculations **SEQUENTIAL PLANE IMAGING** An MRI technique in which an image is built up from successive planes in the imaged object; these planes are selected by oscillating gradient magnetic fields or by selective excitation **SIGNAL-TO-NOISE RATIO** (SNR) The ratio obtained from the relative contributions of detected true signal to that of random superimposed signals ('noise'), which is a function of the electromagnetic properties of the sample or the patient being studied; the higher the SNR, the better the image's resolution; SNR may be improved by a) Averaging several measurements of a signal since random signals tend to cancel themselves, b) Sampling large volumes (with corresponding loss of spatial resolution) and c) Increasing the magnetic field's strength **SPECTRUM** An array of the components of the MR signal according to frequency; nuclei with different resonant frequencies appear as peaks ('lines') at different frequencies in the spectrum **SPIN** The intrinsic angular momentum of an elementary particle (or system of particles such as a nucleus) that is responsible for the magnetic moment; the spins of nuclei have characteristic fixed values and when pairs of neutrons and protons are aligned, they cancel out the values of their spins, so that nuclei with an odd number of neutrons and/or protons will have a net nonzero rotational component characterized by an integer or half-integer quantum 'nuclear spin number' **SPIN DENSITY** The density of resonating spins in a given region, which is a prime determinant of the strength of an MR signal from the region, measured in SI (International system) units (moles/m^3); for water, 0.11 moles of H_2O/m^3; spin density cannot be imaged directly, but is a complex series of calculations received from different pulse times **SPIN ECHO** The reappearance of an MR signal after the free induction decay (FID) is complete, due to effective reversal of the dephasing of the spins ('refocusing') by various techniques, eg reversal of a gradient magnetic field, which is a form of 'time reversal' or b) Specific RF pulse sequences such as the Carr-Purcell sequence (applied in a time shorter than or equal to T2); multiple spin echoes or a series of spin echoes at different times can be used to determine T2 without 'contamination' through the effects of the inhomogeneity of the magnetic field **SPIN-ECHO IMAGING** A type of MRI where the spin-echo signal is measured (in contrast to measuring the FID); spin-echo images are largely a function of T2 **SPIN-LATTICE RELAXATION TIME** see T1 **SPIN-SPIN RELAXATION TIME** see T2 **STATIONARY RECOVERY** A type of partial saturation pulse sequence in which preceding pulses leave the spins in a state of saturation, so that recovery at the time of the next pulse takes place from an initial condition of no magnetization **SUPERCONDUCTING MAGNET** A magnet whose magnetic field originates from current flowing through a superconductor, which is encased in a cryostat **SURFACE COIL MR** A small RF receiver coil placed over a region of interest on the object being imaged which has an effective selectivity for the area of interest, eg the shoulder, knee, brain, spine and elsewhere **T1** Spin-lattice or longitudinal relaxation time A time period after transverse magnetization, which is the characteristic time (a constant) for spins to align themselves back to the external magnetic field; starting from zero magnetization in the z direction, the z magnetization increases to 63% of its final maximum value in a time T1 **T2** Spin-spin or transverse relaxation time The time period (a constant) for the loss of phase coherence among spins oriented at a right angle to the static magnetic field, a result of interactions between the spins, with the resulting loss of transverse magnetization and MR signal; starting from a non-zero value of magnetization in the XY plane, the XY magnetization decays and loses 63% of its initial value in a time T2 **T2*** The time constant for the loss of phase coherence among the spins oriented at an angle to the static magnetic field due to a combination of magnetic field inhomogeneities, deltaB and spin-spin transverse relaxation, which results in a more rapid loss in transverse magnetization and MR signal **TE** Echo time The time between the middle of the 90° pulse and the middle of the production of the spin-echo, for multiple echoes, TE1, TE2 and others **TESLA** The International System (SI) unit for magnetic flux density, equivalent to 10 000 gauss, the formerly used unit **TI** Inversion time The time period between the middle of the inverting (180°) RF pulse and the middle of the 90° pulse, used to detect longitudinal magnetization **TR** Repetition time The period between the beginning of the pulse sequence and the beginning of the succeeding (virtually identical) pulse sequence **TRANSVERSE MAGNETIZATION** (Mxy) The component of the macroscopic magnetization vector at right angles to the static magnetic field (B_0); Precession of the transverse magnetization at the Larmor frequency is responsible for the detected MR signal; in absence of an externally applied RF energy, the transverse magnetization will decay to zero with a characteristic time constant (T2 or T2*) **VOLUME IMAGING** Simultaneous volume imaging An imaging technique in which the signals are gathered from the whole object at one time, with appropriate encoding of pulse/gradient sequences to encode the positions of the spins; in principle, many sequential plane images can be generalized to volume imaging Advantage of volume imaging Improvement of SNR by including the signal from the whole object at once and any plane may be subsequently generated including any oblique projection desired Disadvantage The image reconstruction takes longer and the computations are more complex **ZEUGMATOGRAPHY** A coinage from Greek that dignifies magnetic resonance imaging, translated as 'the spatial relation of the image to a gradient magnetic field'

Magnetic resonance spectroscopy (MRS) LABORATORY MEDICINE A technique for determining the structure of organic compounds, the first practical use of the principle of magnetic resonance; MRS has become an indispensable tool in pharmacokinetics, biochemistry and molecular biology (J Am Med Assoc 1987; 258:3283)

Magnification see Microscopy

'Magnificent Seven' A highly colloquial synonym for the G protein-coupled membrane receptors, which belong to the same gene family, so named as they all span the cell membrane seven times; the term is intended as a play-on-words after the Hollywood film by the same name, although the parochial nature of the sobriquet appears to make preferable the more widely-used (and scientific) term 'G protein receptor', see there (

MAIDS see Murine acquired immuodeficiency syndrome

Maillard reaction FOOD TECHNOLOGY A non-enzymatic heat-activated chemical reaction between sugars (especially ribose) and amino acids that occurs in food as it forms glycosylamines and Amadori compounds, which is responsible for 'browning' of baked or cooked foods, eg bread crusts and barbecued steak; browned foods are mutagenic by the Ames assay; it is possible that the age-related changes in collagen are partially mediated through the Maillard reaction; see Browning reaction; Cf Rancidity

'Mail order' medicine A derogatory phrase for the basing of therapeutic decisions solely on the results of tests, eg Radioallergosorbent test, sent to a referral laboratory; see RAST

Mainframe A large computer that can manipulate large blocks of data by 'multitasking' logical sequences; although one flow of logic can occur at one time (unless there are multiple sequential processors), the power and speed of a mainframe computer, eg an IBM 3060, is such that the transition from one task to another is virtually 'seamless'; 'dedicated' mainframes are used for processing the data in computed tomography, magnetic resonance imaging and for hospital information systems and have speeds measured in MIPS (million instructions per second), ranging up to hundreds of MIPS; speed Cf Computers, Microcomputer, Minicomputer

Main-en-lorgnette Lorgnette, French, opera glass RHEUMATOLOGY A classic descriptor for the hand afflicted by arthritis mutilans, with extensive compressive erosion, collapse of the proximal phalanges with 'telescoping' of the bones upon themselves and overriding of the fingers by metacarpophalangeal dislocation, resulting in destroyed contracted hands; although most characteristic of advanced rheumatoid arthritis, 'main-en-lorgnette' may also occur in psoriatic arthritis, erosive osteoarthritis, chronic infection, diabetes and leprosy

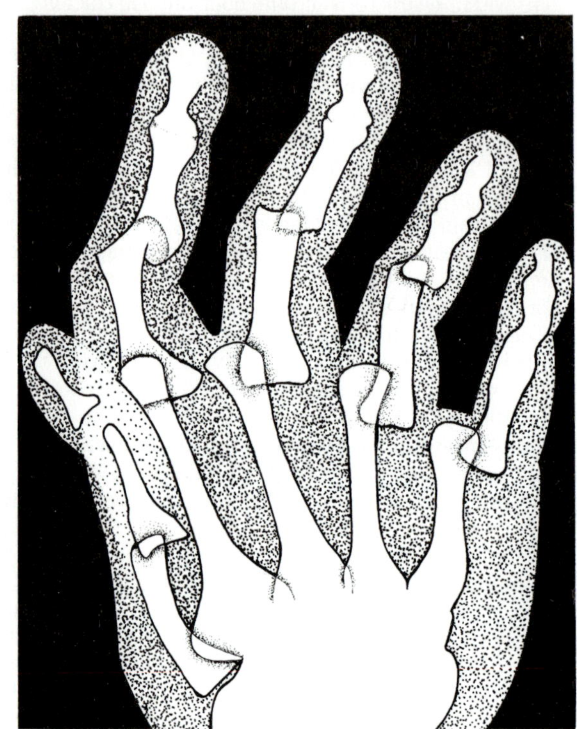

Main-en-lorgnette

Main-en-trident A short broad hand with a foreshortened middle finger, resulting in equal length of all digits; the characteristic shape of the index and ring finger results in an appearance fancifully likened to Neptune's trident, a finding classically seen in achondroplasia

'Mainstreaming' The placement of learning-impaired or otherwise handicapped children in the same classroom as other children, while supplementing their learning with various educational maneuvers, a process that is thought to improve socialization; by extension, mainstreaming refers to any effort to integrate a person with an affliction, eg mental health patients, into society

Maintenance see Remission

MAIS complex *Mycobacterium avium-intercellulare-scrofulaceum* Three mycobacterial species that are indistinguishable from each other in terms of surface lipids and antigens, pigment production, biochemical reactions, antibiotic susceptibilities, often in the same clinical company **Incidence** MAIS is relatively uncommon, but affects 5-8% of patients with AIDS, who are increasingly susceptible as the CD4+ T cells fall below 0.1 x 10^9 (US: 100/mm^3) **Clinical** Persistent fever possibly accompanied by night sweats, chronic diarrhea, abdominal pain, extrahepatic obstruction and potentially, severe anemia **Treatment** Ciproflozacin, clofazimine, ethambutol and rifampicin, to which amikacin is added if the initial therapy is unsuccessful by the fourth week; promising, not-yet-approved agents include rifabutin, clarithromycin and azithromycin (N Engl J Med 1991; 324:1332rv)

MAIS-intermediate A MAIS that differs from other MAISs as it is urease-negative, hydrolyzes Tween, has variable pigmentation and catalase activity (Lab Med 1985; 16:174)

Major basic protein (MBP) A 10-15 kD protein found in eosinophilic granules that forms a characteristic crystalloid; the adjectival 'basic' derives from MBP's isoelectric point of greater than pH 10; MBP causes bronchial epithelial damage and a wheal and flare response when injected subcutaneously and is related to asthma

Major crossmatch TRANSFUSION MEDICINE The testing of a patient's serum against a potential donor's red cells to detect the presence of ABO incompatibility and other major antibodies; see Immediate spin crossmatch, Minor cross-match; Cf Back typing, Front typing

Major diagnostic category see DRGs

Major groove MOLECULAR BIOLOGY A deep and wide furrow present in Watson-Crick DNA that extends over the entire length of DNA as long as the molecule remains in a normal or right-handed configuration; for the usual B-DNA, the major groove is 22nm wide; see Minor groove, Z-DNA

Major histocompatibility complex see MHC

Major life activities SOCIAL MEDICINE The constellation of human activities that constitutes economic, intellectual and functional self-sufficiency, including the ability to maintain a job, learning, mobility and self-direction; these activities or the inability to perform them are used by governing bodies to determine a person's eligibility for programs offering assistance to people with handicaps, mental retardation and developmental disabilities

'Major medical' Major medical expense insurance HEALTH CARE INDUSTRY A health insurance policy or 'rider' (extension) to an insurance policy that finances medical expenses incurred in injuries, catastrophic or prolonged illness, providing benefit payments above the base paid by the insurance company

Malakoplakia Malakos, Greek, soft plaque A lesion often seen in the urogenital tract (bladder, renal pelvis, ureter, uterus, broad ligament, endometrium, testes, epididymis and prostate, with female:male ratio of 4:1) and rarely also in the retroperitoneum, colon, stomach, appendix, lymph nodes, lungs, bone and skin, with a ratio of 1:1; malakoplakia is more common in the immunosuppressed transplant recipients **Pathogenesis**

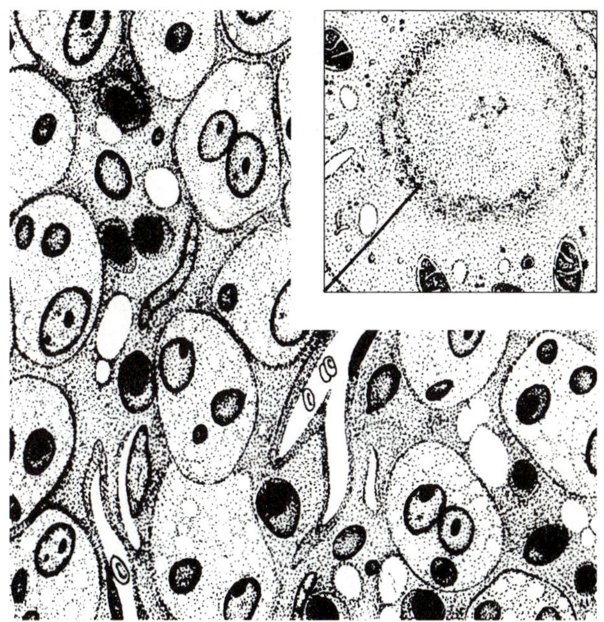

Malakoplakia

Defective macrophage response to coliform bacteria (often ***Escherichia coli***, but also ***Klebsiella*** spp and ***Mycobacterium intracellulare***); the condition was described in 1903 by von Hansemann and consists of soft, yellow, elevated and friable 3-4 cm in diameter mucosal plaques **Histopathology** Swollen submucosal histiocytes (von Hansemann cells) extending into con-

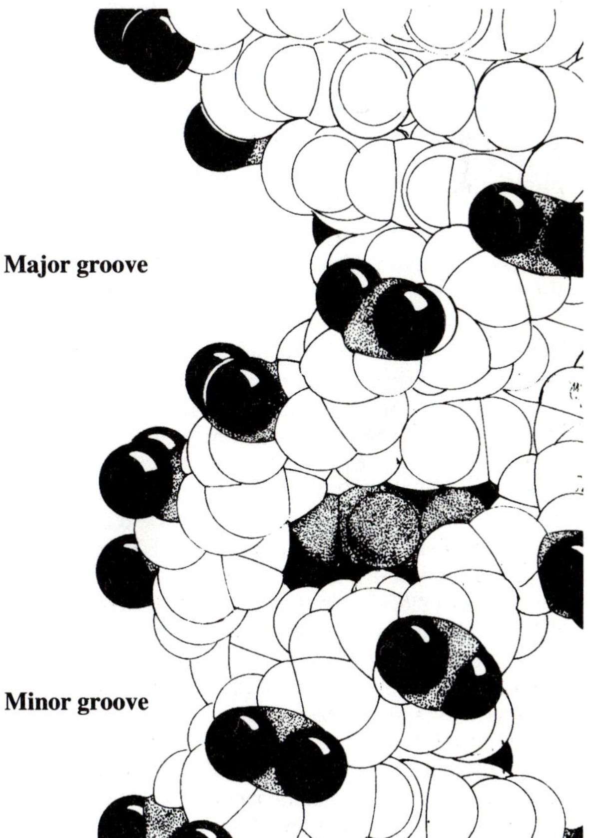

nective tissue replete with Michaelis-Gutmann bodies (spherical cytoplasmic structures layered by calcium/iron salts, contained within phagosomes, figure, page 417, upper right) Treatment Long-term antibiotics, ascorbic acid, cholinergic agents; if recalcitrant, surgical excision

Malaria Italian, bad air Roman fever A parasitemia afflicting 200-300 million people of the two billion exposed, which kills 2 million annually; malaria is caused by four genera of ***Plasmodium***; Vector ***Anopheles*** mosquito; ***P vivax*** is most common, ***P falciparum*** (malignant tertian malaria) has the greatest genetic plasticity, greatest morbidity and appears to be of avian origin (Scien Am 1991; 265/1:25); ***P malariae*** and ***P ovale*** are less common and carry a lower morbidity; the genetic diversity of the various plasmodia may cause differences in susceptibility to various drugs and host response to vaccines, as reflected in allelic variations of multiple genes on the merozoite surface antigen, mutation, variation in the expression of different genes and occasional absence of genes due to deletion (Nature 1991; 349;193n&v); eradication by massive DDT spraying to eliminate the vector is impossible and chemoprophylaxis of an entire population impractical; the high incidence of AIDS in Africa is problematic in that malaria-induced anemia commonly affects young children in this region, requiring transfusions of blood that has not been screened for HIV (10-20% of the population in Africa is HIV-positive)

Malarial pigment Black pigment in cerebral white matter composed of hematin and protein, a characteristic postmortem finding in ***P falciparum*** malaria; the malarial brain is congested and edematous with indurated, flattened gyri and petechiae

Malaria prophylaxis Prevention is preferable to treating malaria and prophylaxis is recommended by the Centers for Disease Control for travel to areas of ***Plasmodium falciparum*** endemicity Agents: Chloroquine, hydroxychloroquine, mefloquine, quinine sulfate, doxycycline (not recommended during pregnancy), proguanil, pyrimethamine-sulfadoxine, primaquine and more recently, mefloquine, currently the prophylactic agent of choice

Malaria vaccine A viable vaccine against malaria is not available; the current 'gold standard' for a ***Plasmodium*** that is immunogenic but not pathogenic is the radiation-attenuated sporozoite, although a combination of circumsporozoite protein and the 140 kD sporozoite surface protein 2(SSP-2) may be as effective (Science 1991; 252:715); another candidate is Pfs25, a 25 kD, cysteine-rich sexual stage surface protein of ***P falciparum*** that has been inserted into a vaccinia virus and elicits transmission-blocking antibodies in, but not restricted to mice (Science 1991; 252:1310); other approaches include eliciting natural antibodies against circumsporozoite (CS) protein, attempting to block the pre-hepatoinvasive stage; ***P falciparum*** is a highly mutable parasite for which there may never be a viable vaccine, given that a) the parasite reproduces sexually within the insect host, leading to maintenance and increase of heterozygosity and b) Natural immunity to the organism requires continued contact with the parasite for constant enrichment of genetic diversity, as opposed to a 'one-shot' exposure of a vaccine (Nature 1990; 348:494c)

Malariotherapy Iatrogenic malaria Therapeutic inoculation of benign tertian malaria (***Plasmodium vivax***), a modality used in the pre-antibiotic era for treating neurosyphilis; the data from these uncontrolled studies suggest that there was little, if any effect on the underlying syphilis, despite the non-specific immune reaction with fever and secretion of tumor necrosis factor and interleukin-1, as the reports of success were largely clinical without laboratory confirmation; although it was thought that patients with neuroborreliosis (advanced Lyme disease) might respond to malariotherapy, this appears to complicate or exacerbate an already poor clinical situation (MMWR 1990; 39:873); Cf BCG, Immunotherapy

Malate dehydrogenase (MDH) An oxidoreductase enzyme located in both the mitochondria and cytosol that catalyzes the reversible NAD^+/NADH reaction in the presence of L-malate; MDH is increased in myocardial infarction, hepatocellular necrosis, megaloblastic anemia and malignancy

Malathion An organophosphate insecticide; see Intermediate syndrome

Mal de Meleda An autosomal recessive condition causing symmetric palmoplantar hyperkeratosis and acanthosis accompanied by circumscribed hyperkeratosis of the wrists, knees, forearms and ankles, brachydactyly, koilonychia, growth and mental retardation, seen in the highly inbred population of the island of Meleda off the coast of Dalmatia in western Yugoslavia

Male see Anabolic steroids, Circumcision, H-Y chromosome, Testes

Male climacteric Male 'menopause' A psychogenic complex characterized by diminished libido, impotence, fatigue, hot flashes, irritability, depression, poor ability to concentrate and insomnia Laboratory Androgenic hormones are usually within normal limits Histopathology Testicle demonstrates variable decrease in spermatogenesis and tubular atrophy

Male 'uterus' Utricle

Malformation see Teratogenesis

Malfunction 54 RADIATION ONCOLOGY A software 'bug' that caused a 25 Megaelectron volt (MeV) linear accelerator, used in radiation oncology to accidently deliver 25 000 rads of 25 MeVs in one second, resulting in three known fatal radiation overdoses; the computer at fault used 'assembly' language and the software failed to access the appropriate calibration data

Malignancy see Cancer, Carcinogens, Congenital malignancy, Multiple primary malignancy syndrome, Metastasis, Oncogenes, Secondary malignancy

Malignant angioendotheliomatosis see Angiotropic lymphoma

Malignant cell A cell that has undergone 'transformation', is in a state of permanent proliferation and is capable of metastasizing; the malignant cell is defined by a series of phenotypic changes, including decreased intercellular adhesion and electrical repulsion (resulting in a loss of anchorage dependence), decreased intracellular potassium and calcium ions, aneuploidy, loss of response to (control by) the usual cytokines and mitogens, ectopic hormone production, the use of aberrant metabolic pathways, biochemical convergence (cells lose features of differentiation and organ-specific features, eg microvilli, desmosomes, intermediate filaments), cytopathological changes (nucleolar margination, a sign of rapid growth), cytologic atypia, nuclear irregularity, hyperchromasia and high nuclear:cytoplasmic ratio, swelling of mitochondria and flooding of the mitochondrial matrix; other features include alterations in growth parameters and cell behavior, cell-surface alterations, loss of actin myofilaments, increased transforming growth factor release, protease secretion, altered gene transcription and immortalization of cells

Malignant fibrous histiocytoma (MFH) Malignant fibrous xanthoma, fibroxanthosarcoma A pleomorphic mesenchymal malignancy of older adults, affecting the deep soft tissues (involving muscle 60% or fascia 20%) of the lower (50%) and upper (20%) extremities, retroperitoneum 15% and abdominal cavity **Metastasis** MFH metastasizes to the lung 80%, lymph nodes 30%, liver, bone **Histopathology** Storiform pattern with a pleomorphic mixture of primitive fibroblasts (collagen production), myofibroblasts, histiocytes (phagocytic capacity), xanthoma cells, siderophages, giant cells (bizarre, osteoclast-like), lymphocytes, plasma cells and eosinophils **Differential Diagnosis** Other sarcomas, pleomorphic or primitive carcinoma and bizarre melanoma **Prognosis** 40-65% ofresected tumors recur; 25-50% metastasize MFH variants **ANGIOMATOID MFH** A sarcoma of adolescent females, often subcutaneous in the lower extremity **Clinical** Systemic effects are common despite its small size, including fever, chills, weight loss, anemia **Pathology** Well-circumscribed mass with a fibrous pseudocapsule rimmed by lymphoid follicles and sheets of relatively monotonous fibroblast- or histiocyte-like cells with 0-3 mitotic figures/high-power field; the cytoplasm is filled with hemosiderin and lesser amounts of lipid, foam cells and rare multinucleated giant cells **Prognosis** Similar to usual MFH **OSSEOUS MFH** A rare primary MFH, affecting the lower extremity of young adults; male:female ratio, 2:1, which may arise in bone infarction **Radiology** Poorly-circumscribed radiolucency **Histopathology** Histiocytes with phagocytic capacity that may differentiate into fibroblasts, having a storiform pattern; 35% 5-year survival

Malignancy of unknown origin Cancers, the origin of which cannot be ascertained even by full autopsy examination; most such lesions are undifferentiated **Prognosis** Six month survival, 14%

Malignant hepatopathy Stauffer syndrome A paraneoplastic condition characterized by biochemical abnormalities (increased alkaline phosphatase, hypercholesterolemia and prolonged prothrombin time) and hepatosplenomegaly, which is associated with, and regresses following the successful treatment of, renal cell carcinoma and malignant schwannoma

Malignant histiocytoma see Histiocytic lymphoma

Malignant histiocytosis (MH) Histiocytic medullary reticulosis A rapidly fatal disease associated with aggressive proliferation of atypical histiocytes and precursors in lymph nodes, splenic red pulp, bone marrow, skin, gastrointestinal tract, kidneys, adrenal glands and lungs; although idiopathic, MH is associated with acute lymphocytic and myelocytic leukemias, post-renal transplantation immunosuppressive therapy and Epstein-Barr viremia **Clinical** Male:female ratio, 2-3:1; MH occurs at any age and presents with fever, weakness, weight loss, diaphoresis, chest and back pain, rashes, lymphadenopathy, hepatosplenomegaly, subcutaneous tumor nodules, pancytopenia, increased bilirubin followed by jaundice and may cause rapid deterioration **Histopathology** Large pleomorphic or anaplastic, erythrophagocytic cells with hyperchromatic and irregular nuclear membranes and enlarged nucleoli that more commonly infiltrate in a 'leukemic' or diffuse fashion in sinusoids of the reticuloendothelial system and vessels, in contrast to a 'lymphomatoid' or nodular fashion **Immunoperoxidase** Muraminidase positivity **Histochemistry** Acid phosphatase-positive, nonspecific (α-naphthylacetate or butyrate) esterase-positive (complete inhibition by sodium fluoride), PAS-positive **Ultrastructure** Langerhans granules are rare; more constant ultrastructural criteria include rudimentary junctional complexes and pseudopodia **Differential diagnosis** Acute myelogenous leukemia (FAB M5), hairy cell leukemia, 'histiocytic' and Hodgkin's lymphomas, melanoma, anaplastic or 'large cell' carcinoma, virus-associated hemophagocytic syndrome, infectious mononucleosis, sinus histiocytosis with massive lymphadenopathy, familial hemophagocytic reticulosis, histiocytosis X **Treatment** Multidrug regimens are used with protocols similar to those used in large cell lymphoma, including vincristine, cyclophosphamide, doxorubicin and prednisone achieving a high proportion of long-term remission; see further details under Histiocytosis

Malignant hyperthermia syndrome An autosomal dominant condition (of variable penetration) in which the subject when subjected to anesthetic (Halothane, diethyl-ether, cyclopropane, enflurane) and certain psychotropic agents develops a potentially fatal (70% mortality is described in acute episodes) clinical complex, occurring in 1/15 000 administrations of anesthesia in children, 1/50-100 000 adults; one-half of the cases had not been previously sensitive to anesthesia **Clinical** Tachycardia, tachypnea, cyanosis, labile blood pressure, muscle rigidity, becoming rapidly and markedly hyperpyretic, acidotic, hyperkalemic, potentially developing disseminated intravascular coagulation and renal failure; similar reactions may be evoked in these subjects by warm weather, exercise, emotional stress or without known environmental cue and are initiated by muscular hypermetabolism, due to idiopathic increase in sarcoplasmic calcium occurring under general anesthesia **Pathogenesis** Malignant hyperthermia (MH) may be related to a defective calcium channel in the sarcoplasmic reticulum; the genetic markers near the MH susceptibility locus are near the ryanodine receptor gene, which encodes a calcium channel (Nature 1990;

343:559); in MH, the total body O_2 consumption increases 2-3-fold normal, body temperature may spiral upward as rapidly as an increase of 1°C per five minutes peaking at 43°C (109°F) *Increases in*: Base excess to greater than -10, $PaCO_2$ to 70-110 mmHg, potassium ion to more than > 7 mEq/ml and enzymes, including CPK, LD, AST *Decreases in:* Serum pH to below 7.2 Diagnosis Muscle contraction test with halothane or caffeine challenge Treatment Hypothermia, hydration, sodium bicarbonate infusion, mechanical hyperventilation, diuretics to increase urine flow, dantrolene (an agent which blocks excitation-contraction coupling between the T tubules and the sarcoplasmic reticulum) Note: MH may also be a symptom in myotonic disorders, Duchenne dystrophy, brachial hypertrophic myopathy, central core disease and in congenital myopathy with dysmorphic features

Malignant lymphoepithelial lesion see 'Eskimoma'

Malignant melanoma see Melanoma

Malignant mimics Lesions that either grossly or microscopically mimic malignancy, which may be induced by inflammation, irradiation and chemotherapy, evoking cytologic features that are similar to malignant lesions Endoscopic lesions mimicking malignancy include 'ragged' well-circumscribed ulcers that histologically appear in an amorphous eosinophilic background, with sheets of closely packed variably-sized acini, cells with swollen granular cytoplasm, variably-sized, often hyperchromatic nuclei, mitotic activity and a lesion that fades into benign regenerative mucosa; other endoscopic malignant look-alikes seen in the esophagus, stomach and rectum consist of fibrinopurulent exudate, which covers aggregates of bizarre cells with variable amounts of granular cytoplasm, hyperchromatic pleomorphic nuclei Histopathology Various lesions mimic malignancy; classic 'dyads' include chondroma and chondrosarcoma, infarcted fibroadenoma and scirrhous carcinoma of the breast; necrotizing sialometaplasia and mucoepidermoid carcinoma of the oral cavity; nodal angiomatosis and Kaposi sarcoma; keratoacanthoma and squamous cell carcinoma; Spitz nevus and malignant melanoma; see Lymph node inclusions

Malignant narcissism Psychiatry A term that defines a range of psychopathic personality disorders characterized by the coexistance of marked narcissistic and antisocial traits; manifestations of this 'inhumanity and propensity toward evil' ranges from modest to extreme, the latter of which may affect notorious murderers, despots and dictators (Psychiatr Clin North Am 1989; 12:553rv, 643); Cf Serial killers

Malignant nephrosclerosis The form of renal disease associated with 'malignant' or accelerated phase hypertension; while the clinical condition may arise virtually de novo, it usually occurs in a background of benign essential hypertension; this condition comprises only 5% of hypertension and has a predilection for young black males Pathology Grossly, petechial hemorrhages on the renal capsule have been fancifully designated as 'flea-bitten' Histopathology a) Fibrinoid necrosis of arterioles and necrotizing arteriolitis, causing petechia on the renal cortex and b) 'Onion-skinning' of the interlobular arteries and arterioles with concentric layering of collagen (hyperplastic arteriolitis), variably accompanied by necrotizing glomerulitis

Malignant neuroleptic syndrome A complex which affects less than 1% of those exposed to neuroleptic agents (phenothiazine, butyrophenones) Clinical Onset 1-3 days after beginning antidepressant therapy causing hyperthermia, autonomic instability, muscle rigidity and myoglobinuria

Malignant osteopetrosis see Marble bone disease

Malignant osteoporosis Osteolysis secondary to infiltration by malignancy, which is often accompanied by pain; 80% of bone metastases arise from carcinoma of the breast, kidney, lung, prostate and thyroid, and most cause weakening of the bony trabeculae, with the exception of prostatic carcinoma, which classically is an osteoblastic lesion; 70% of bone metastases involve the axial skeleton, while the remainder affect the proximal appendicular skeleton Laboratory Elevated acid phosphatase, if extensive, hypercalcemia Treatment Remove primary carcinoma, radiotherapy (effective in most cases) and fixation of of unstable bone; see Hypercalcemia of malignancy

Malignant schwannomasee Peripheral nerve sheath tumor(s)

Malignant transformation Experimental oncology Changes in the growth properties of cells in culture evoked by various agents, eg radiation, toxins and viruses, which result in development of tumor-formation in cells; although this process is assumed to occur in vivo, direct correlation to tumor induction is difficult to confirm; transformation of cell lines by viruses, eg polyoma virus and cellular oncogenes, eg ras plus myc oncogenes, requires two proteins, a T protein that immortalizes the cells and another, the mid-T protein that changes the cells' properties; transformed cells have a characteristic phenotypic 'signature', including altered growth parameters and cell behavior, cell-surface alterations, loss of actin myofilaments, increased transforming growth factor release, protease secretion, altered gene transcription and immortalization of cells

Malignolipin A substance composed of fatty acids, phosphoric acid choline and spermine, described in the 1950s (Cancer 1966; 19:1149) as specific for malignancy and detectable early in the blood, inducing irreversible anemia, leukopoiesis and cachexia when injected into experimental models; malignolipin's diagnostic yield is less than 25% and the test has fallen out of favor

Malingering Fraudulant simulation of illness or exaggeration of the symptoms of a minor illness or injury, usually to avoid work or school; permutations of malingering include that which occurs in anticipation of collecting insurance benefits, known as 'goldbricking' and malingering with psychological underpinnings, of either endogenous origin, eg factitial dermatitis or exogenous origin, eg Munchausen syndrome; see Factitious disease(s)

Mallet finger Orthopedics A fracture often accompanied by avulsion of a bony fragment of the extensor insertion at the dorsal base of the distal phalanx, usually due to closed hyperflexion-type blunt trauma; in pre-adolescents, the injury is an open Salter-Harris type I or II injury where the extensor tendon insertion remains undisplaced and the remainder of the phalanx is acutely flexed by the unopposed flexor profundus tendon; in older subjects, hyperflexion injury causes a displaced type III dorsal physeal fracture, representing a 'true' mallet injury

Mallet toe A flexion deformity of the distal interphalangeal joint of the lesser toes, affecting one toe or two adjacent toes; the condition is less common than hammer toe (which is a flexion deformity of the proximal interphalangeal joint) and becomes symptomatic in adolescence or adulthood with the development of a painful 'corn' at the tip of the toe

Mallophaga An order of biting lice that may affect humans

Malnutrition see Kwashiorkor, Marasmus

Malocclusion ODONTOLOGY Misalignment of the maxillary and mandibular teeth, causing a 'poor bite', corresponding difficulties in mastication and, with time, periodontal disease

Malpractice Professional misconduct or unreasonable lack of skill in the performance of a professional act, a term that may be applied to physicians, lawyers and accountants; most cases of medical malpractice fall under the rubric of civil law, ie a legal action filed by one person against another, rather than criminal law, ie a legal action filed by a state or the federal government against an offending person(s); medical malpractice is based on the theory of negligence, which is conduct that falls below the 'standard of care' recognized by the law for protecting others against unreasonable risk of harm, ie deviation from accepted standards of care, resulting in harm to others *FOUR ELEMENTS MUST BE ALLEGED AND PROVEN IN A COURT OF LAW IN ORDER FOR THE COMPLAINING PARTY (THE PLAINTIFF) TO SUSTAIN (WIN) A LAWSUIT FOR NEGLIGENCE: 1) DUTY* The plaintiff must prove the existence of a legal relationship, ie duty between himself and the defendant *2) BREACH OF DUTY* Once duty is established, the plaintiff must prove that the physician breached that duty by failing to comply with accepted standards of care by malfeasance (an act not conforming to accepted standard of practice) or by non-malfeasance (failure to perform an act expected under the circumstances) *3) DAMAGES* The plaintiff must prove that he has sustained some injury as a result of the alleged negligent act, injury that is translated into a monetary value, either compensatory (tangible, either lost wages, lost earning capacity, medical expenses) or punitive (intangible, often in the form of 'pain and suffering', where multimillion-dollar awards are not uncommon) and *4) CAUSATION* The plaintiff must prove a reasonable connection between the alleged negligent act or omission of the defendant and suffered injury **Statistics, US** In one 5-year period, 48% of surgeons and surgical specialists, 34% of obstetricians-anesthesiologists and 15% of other physicians had had malpractice claims; 85% of the payments were made on behalf of 3% of the insurance policy holders, and those with previous claims had a greater risk for future claims (J Am Med Assoc 1989; 262:3291, 3320); in the USA, a physician may be sued for doing too much or too little or for ordering too few tests, potentially missing a relatively rare disease, see Ulysses syndrome, while the government penalizes those physicians who overorder tests; see Assault and battery, Blood shield laws, Consent, 'Defensive medicine', 'Difficult patient', DNR (do not resuscitate), Emergency doctrine law, Expert witness, 'Good Samaritan laws, Informed consent, Jehovah's witness, Medical record, Misdiagnosis, Negligence, Patient-physician relationship, Quinlan case, Respondeat superior, Standard of care, Therapeutic privilege doctrine, Wrongful birth **GLOSSARY ABANDONMENT** A physician's unilateral severance of a professional relation with a patient, without reasonable notice and at a time when the necessity for continuing medical attention remains; acts of abandonment include refusal, or more commonly, alleged refusal to treat after he has seen a person needing care, refusal to attend to a case in which the physician has already assumed responsibility, eg visit while the patient is in the hospital, failure to provide follow-up attention and failure to arrange for a competent substitute in times of absence **BORROWED SERVANT DOCTRINE** A principle under which the party usually liable for a person's actions, eg the hospital being responsible for a nurse, is absolved of that responsibility when that person is asked to do something, eg by a surgeon, which is outside of the bounds of hospital policy Note: A hospital is only liable if the plaintiff can prove that the hospital was negligent in removing a physician or employee known to be incompetent **BREACH OF CONTRACT** see Abandonment, above **CAUSATION** The establishment of a cause-and-effect relation between the allegedly negligent act and the purported injuries **CONFIDENTIALITY** An implied agreement between the physician and patient that all information related by a patient is to be held in the strictest of confidence unless it is illegal and dangerous to society **CONTRIBUTORY NEGLECT** Conduct on the part of the plaintiff, which occurred after he came under the physician's care that falls below that which a reasonable person would exercise for his own protection, thereby contributing to the alleged act of negligence **COUNTERSUIT** A lawsuit initiated by the defendant, who alleges that the original malpractice suit (see Frivolous lawsuit, below) was without reasonable or probable cause, was actuated by malice (improper motive) or the lawsuit ended in the physician's favor or the physician suffered damages (to reputation or otherwise) **DAMAGES, COMPENSATORY** An award that pretends to restore the victim to the state he would have been in had the 'wrong' not occurred, ie lost wages, pain and suffering, permanent disabilities, mental anguish and loss of consortium (conjugal fellowship, exchange of body fluids) **DAMAGES, PUNITIVE** An 'Insult-to-injury' award given by jury in order to castigate the defendant, designed to prevent him from repeating the offense; punitive damage awards are either a) Special (wages, lost profits, past and future medical fees) and other compensatory awards, the monetary value of which can be reasonably calculated and b) General (pain and suffering, humiliation, disfigurement) awards that elude standardized formulae **EMERGENCY PSYCHIATRIC COM-**

MITMENT The temporary admission of a person with an acute psychotic reaction to a mental institution for a period of observation, not to exceed seven working days; beyond this time, the patient must be formally committed or released; the patient must be dangerous, intoxicated or inebriated to justify commital **EMOTIONAL DISTRESS** *INTENTIONAL INFLICTION OF EMOTIONAL DISTRESS* The 'outrage' tort A legal action initiated against a defendant who allegedly said or did something so completely absurd (medically) or insulting to the plaintiff that he suffered emotional damage **FRIVOLOUS LAWSUIT** A groundless lawsuit in which injury did not occur or which was so negligible that it caused no damage, real or perceived to the plaintiff; such lawsuits have little prospect for success and are brought with the purpose of annoying or embarrassing a defendant; see de minimus rule **LIABILITY** A broad term referring to all character of obligation, amenability and responsibility for an act **REFERRAL AND CONSULTATION** A physician should always refer difficult cases to competent specialists Note: If the consultant proves to be incompetent, the referring physician may be sued for so advising the patient; consultation should be sought when the diagnosis is difficult, the illness is unfamiliar, complex or fraught with complications, the patient doesn't improve in a reasonable time and at the patient's request ***RES IPSA LOQUITOR*** *THE THING SPEAKS FOR ITSELF* A doctrine in which the plaintiff's burden to prove negligence is fairly light, not usually requiring expert witnesses, since the details of the incident are clear and understandable to a jury, eg foreign objects left behind in surgical procedures ***RESPONDEAT SUPERIOR*** *LET THE MASTER ANSWER FOR THE SERVANT* A doctrine in which the liability for a negligent act is passed to 'captain of the ship', eg the surgeon, despite the fact that the act is performed by another person, eg an operating room nurse; the hospital may under this doctrine claim that although the hospital is the nurse's employer, at the time of the negligent act, the nurse was under someone else's guidance **STATUTES OF LIMITATIONS** A doctrine that allows the plaintiff two years from the time of alleged malpractice to file a lawsuit, unless the plaintiff is 1) Minor, who has two years after reaching the adulthood to file a lawsuit or b) Later discovers the act of negligence **TORT** A civil wrong for which the wrongdoer (tortfeasor) may be held liable in damages; negligence is a type of tort equivalent to malpractice

Malrotation, intestinal The incorrect rotation of the intestines in utero, which may occur to a greater or lesser degree than normal; coincident with the growth in length, the primitive intestinal loop rotates 270° counterclockwise around an axis formed by the superior mesenteric artery; a counterclockwise rotation of only 90°, results in a left-sided colon; a reverse or clockwise rotation of 90° causes the transverse colon to lie behind the duodenum and superior mesenteric artery, causing a kinking of the arterial supply, potentially resulting in pseudoobstruction and malabsorption

MALT Mucosa-associated lymphoid tissue IMMUNOLOGY The umbrella term for extra-nodal aggregates of lymphoid tissue in the bronchus (BALT), gut (GALT) and skin (SALT) as well as breast and uterine cervix; MALT is the arm of the immune defense that is in closest contact with exogenous antigens, thus differing from the compartmentalized peripheral somatic lymphoid tissues which include lymph nodes, thymus and spleen; dimeric IgA or 'secretory' IgA appears to be under MALT's control and MALT may be the sites of origin of extranodal lymphomas

Malta fever Brucellosis caused by *B melitensis*

Maltese cross appearance A descriptor for a microscopic pattern likened to a maltese cross, which may correspond to granules of talc or cholesterol crystals JOINT Maltese crosses have been described in arthroscopic fluid, associated with traumatic arthritis MICROBIOLOGY The tetrad form of ***Babesia*** species, including ***B canis, B microti*** and ***B bovis*** has been termed 'Maltese cross' and is an uncommon but characteristic finding within infected red cells in a peripheral blood smear; Cf Rabbit ear appearance PULMONARY PATHOLOGY Maltese crosses measure 5-15 mm in diameter, appear as scintillating granules by polarized light microscopy and correspond to starch and talc granules, which are common in the lungs of intravenous drug abusers who 'cut' the heroin with various powders; the granules may be accompanied by foreign body-type giant cell reaction and appear in other tissues URINALYSIS 'Maltese crosses' are anisotropic or birefringent cholesterol-rich fat droplets, associated with finely granular renal casts, which have a cruciform appearance when seen by polarized light and are found both within and outside of the cells in the urinary sediment of patients with nephrotic syndrome, eclampsia, renal toxicity, fat embolism, after crush injury and in Fabry's disease (due to aggregates of glycosphingolipids)

Malt worker's lung An extrinsic allergic alveolitis due to hypersensitivity to spores from *Aspergillus clavatus* and *A fumigatus* in moldy barley and hay, which are ingredients for malt liquors; see Farmer's lung

MAMA see Mid-arm muscle area

Mammary dysplasia SURGICAL PATHOLOGY A non-specific term applied to various benign microscopic nosologies in the breast, including periductular fibrosis, ductal dilatation, apocrine metaplasia and others; since the term 'dysplasia' implies premalignancy, the term is invalid and should be deleted from the literature; see Fibrocystic disease

Mammary souffle CARDIOLOGY An innocent systolic or continuous cardiac murmur of presumed arterial origin heard during late pregnancy or in the early post-partum period that is differentiated from pathological lesions as it is unaffected by the Valsalva maneuver

Mammography The single best non-invasive screening procedure for breast cancer, which yields a false negative rate of 6% and a false positive of 11%; the most characteristic mammographic finding in malignancy is the presence of finely-stippled microcalcifications and suspicious, eg poorly-circumscribed, geographic densities in the mammogram; other findings (as classified by Wolf) are thought to be less reliable; the radiation dose during the usual mammographic study is 25-35 kV; the American Cancer Society and the National Cancer Institute (USA) both recommend self examination of the breast after age 20, a baseline mammogram between ages 35-45, and annual or biennial mammograms thereafter, the frequency of which is a function of the subject's relative risk factors for breast cancer (first-degree relative with breast cancer, caucasian, later pregnancy, etc); after the age of 50, annual screening mammography is recommended (Mayo Clin Proc 1990; 65:56); 24% of biopsies of non-palpable breast masses with calcification (more than 15 calcifications or calcifications in a linear or branching fashion) have ductal or lobular carcinoma (Arch Surg 1990; 125:170); see Cancer screening; Cf Lumpectomy

Mania PSYCHIATRY A hyperkinetic psychiatric reaction which may affect 1% of US citizens, either temporarily or on a permanent basis; the Diagnostic and Statistical Manual of Mental Diseases, 3rd ed separates two clinical types of mania **MANIC EPISODE** A persistently elevated, expansive or irritable mood, increased energy, decreased sleep, distractibility, impaired judgement, grandiosity, flights of ideas, leading to sexual indiscretions,buying sprees and unusual business transactions, most often affecting those under age 25; manic episodes are seen in those with primary (idiopathic) affective illness or bipolar disorder, in which patients vacillate between hypermania and abject depression **ORGANIC MOOD SYNDROME, MANIC TYPE** A persistently expansive or elevated mood, caused by nonpsychogenic conditions that may be evident by history, physical examination or laboratory tests, often affecting subjects older than age 35, due to infections of the central nervous system, eg viral and cryptococcal meningitides, neurosyphilis, trauma, eg thalamotomy, right hemispherectomy, tumors either primary or metastatic, vascular accidents, eponymic disorders, including Huntington and Klinefelter syndromes and Kleine-Levin, Parkinson's, Pick's and Wilson's diseases, carcinoid tumor, idiopathic cerebral calcification, hyperbaric oxygen therapy, systemic disease, endocrine, eg hyperthyroidism, hypothyroidism with starvation diet, puerperal and premenstrual psychoses, systemic infections, eg Q fever, infectious mononucleosis, renal failure, eg uremia, hemodialysis, drugs, eg bromide, bromocriptine, cocaine, corticosteroids, H_2-blocking agents, isoniazid, L-dopa, phencyclidine, procainamide, procarbazine, thyroid preparations, hypovitaminosis, including decreased vitamin B_{12} and niacin (Mayo Clin Proc 1988; 63:906)

Man-in-the-barrel 'syndrome' NEUROLOGY A form of reverse paraplegia with severe arm weakness without leg weakness, described in comatose patients who survive an episode of severe hypotension; the location of the lesion is uncertain but may be bilateral and prerolandic; the fanciful term derives from the fact that, like a man in a barrel, the patients have full use of their legs while their upper body is paralyzed

Manner cocktail A therapeutic modality used as alternate form of cancer therapy, consisting of a mixture containing vitamins A and C, laetrile and dimethylsulfoxide (see DMSO), administered on a daily basis as an unproven form of cancer therapy developed and practiced by a researcher who died in 1988; see DMSO, Tijuana, Mexico, Unproven cancer therapy

Manpower shortage A dearth of persons with a particular skill, which in a free market economy driven by 'supply-and-demand', increases their salary, while making it difficult to obtain their skills Note: A manpower shortage is said to be developing in pathology in the US, which may take effect in 1995; the manpower shortage of cytotechnologists has already arrived; Cf Physician 'glut'

Manslaughter The unjustifiable, inexcusable and intentional killing of a human being without deliberation, premeditation and malice, which is divided into a) Involuntary manslaughter That which occurs when a person is committing an unlawful act that is not felonious or tending to cause great bodily harm or when a person is committing a lawful act without due caution or requisite skill and inadvertently kills another and b) Voluntary manslaughter That which is committed voluntarily in a heat of passion; Cf Murder

Mantle port RADIATION ONCOLOGY A radiotherapy field that covers the axillary, mediastinal, hilar, cervical, supra- and infraclavicular lymph nodes, used to treat multiple contiguous lymphoid regions involved by Hodgkin's lymphoma Dosage 36-44 Gy are tumoricidal, while less than 36 Gy is considered to be prophylactic; see Abdominal bath, Inverted 'Y' field

Mantle zone lymphoma A variant of follicular lymphoma, which is an intermediate-grade lymphoma by the Working Formulation (Cancer 1982; 49:1429), and characterized by a proliferation of small lymphocytes in the mantle zone, surrounding benign germinal centers; these lymphomas often have a higher clinical stage but lower aggression, thus being exceptions to the Lukes and Collins (Br J Cancer, suppl II, 1975; 31:1) proposal that all nodular lymphomas are of follicular center origin **Clinical** Massive splenomegaly, generalized lymphadenopathy, one-third present with 'type B' symptoms, including fever, weight loss, night sweats **Histopathology** Cells are of B cell lineage and range from small to relatively large blasts with round-to-irregular contours, the chromatin is clumped; IgM is present in virtually all cases, with variable presence of IgG and IgD, Ia, BA1 and Leu-1 Median survival 31 months; 40% achieve complete remission with chemotherapy; see Lymphoma

MAO 1) Maximum acid output A measurement of the maximal secretory capacity of gastric hydrogen ions, defined as the sum of four 15-minute acid outputs (Normal: 5-60 mmol of titratable acid/hr), after either pentagastrin or histamine stimulation; MAO is markedly increased in the Zollinger-Ellison syndrome and conditions of increased gastrin production; see also BAO, PAO 2) Monoamine oxidase

Map A two-dimensional graphic representation of a topology or the location of multiple points in a 'universe' **cDNA MAP** MOLECULAR BIOLOGY complementary DNA map; see cDNA **'CONTIG' MAP** MOLECULAR BIOLOGY A map of a segment of a gene that is formed by arranging in order a number of contiguous and overlapping cloned segments of DNA **FATE MAP** EMBRYOLOGY A map that is drawn on the surface of a bisected blastoderm of an organism, consisting of physical landmarks of cell clusters that later give rise to mature adult structures;

the distance between these sites is measured in 'Sturts', after Alfred Sturtevant's studies in 1929 of ***Drosophila simulans*** **RESTRICTION MAP** MOLECULAR BIOLOGY A 'map' of achromosome that is delineated in terms of where a particular restriction endonuclease cleaves the oligomeric sites along the DNA; since there are numerous restriction endonucleases, there are potentially dozens of different restriction maps for a given chromosome **STS-MAP** see Sequence-tagged site map; see Human genome project

MAP Microtubule-associated protein(s) A family of proteins that promotes the assembly and polymerization of α- and β-tubulins and limits the growing and shrinking phases of dynamic microtubules, which are subdivided into 1) Large MAPS, greater than 200 kD, divided into a) MAP1, which has three subgroups (MAP1A, MAP1B and MAP1C) and b) MAP2 Two groups of unknown function confined to the axonal dendrites and 2) Small 'tau' 30-50 kD proteins; MAP2 and tau proteins share a binding motif and are present in the neurofibrillary tangles characteristic of Alzheimer's disease

Map-dot dystrophy Bilateral, symmetric intraepithelial, grayish cystic corneal opacities, thought to be aggregates of basement membrane material which wax and wane; the opacities have no pathological significance, but impart a foreign-body sensation

Maple bark stripper's lung An extrinsic allergic alveolitis due to hypersensitivity to spores from ***Cryptostroma corticale***; see Farmer's lung

Maple syrup urine disease (MSUD) Branched chain ketoaciduria A rare autosomal recessive inborn error of metabolism due to decreased branched-chain α-keto acid dehydrogenase complex activity Frequency in the general population 1:200 000; in the Pennsylvania Mennonite kindred of German descent 1:176; the defect in oxidative decarboxylation of branched chain amino acids (BCAA, valine, leucine and isoleucine) results in accumulation of BCAA **Clinical** Neonatal onset, decreased Moro reflex, dyspnea, spasticity, opisthotonos, mental and growth retardation, severe hypotonia, feeding difficulties, hypoglycemia, convulsions and decorticate rigidity **Laboratory** Increased BCAA in urine and serum and decreased threonine, serine, alanine in urine and serum, a positive dinitro-phenylhydrazine test for α keto amino acids, which form insoluble hydrazines **Neuropathology** Gliosis, defective myelinization **Treatment** Dietary reduction of BCAA, plus dietary overloading (twenty-fold excess) of thiamine **Prognosis** MSUD mortality was formerly 100%, often due to intercurrent infection; with BCAA-free infant formulas, the survival is virtually 100% and mental retardation completely preventable; since acute decompensation by BCAA and BCKA is due to a breakdown of endogenous proteins resulting in metabolic acidosis, ketosis, anorexia, emesis and potentially fatal encephalopathy, patients may respond to parenteral solutions of BCAA-free amino acids (N Engl J Med 1991; 324:175)

Map unit see Centimorgan

Marantic endocarditis A non-bacterial endocarditis with 1-5 mm sterile vegetations on both faces of the valve leaflets composed of fibrin and clots with possible rupture of the papillary muscles, a condition clinically indistinguishable from infectious endocarditis characterized by petechiae, fever, murmurs and emboli **Etiology** Debilitating diseases, eg terminal malignancy, protracted malnutrition, collagen vascular disease, chronic sepsis, renal failure

Marasmus A state of severe malnutrition, due to a decreased ingestion of protein and calories, resulting from an inadequate diet, improper feeding habits or parent-child relations or metabolic disturbances **Clinical** Failure to thrive, weight loss, emaciation, loss of skin turgor, subcutaneous atrophy; afflicted children appear wizened, with a distended abdomen and edema, develop 'starvation stools', become listless with muscular atrophy, hypotonia, hypothermia and reduced rate of metabolism; Cf Kwashiorkor

Marble bone disease Albers-Schönberg disease(s) Malignant osteopetrosis An autosomal recessive form of osteopetrosis of early onset with failure to thrive, bone fragility and multiple fractures, osteomyelitis and other infections, as well as proptosis, blindness, deafness and hydrocephalus due to bony overgrowth of cranial foramina; the osseous replacement of marrow spaces evokes extramedullary hematopoiesis, resulting in hepatosplenomegaly **Laboratory** Elevated acid and alkaline phosphatases, hypocalcemia, pancytopenia, defective T cell functions; see Osteopetrosis

Marble brain disease An autosomal recessive condition due to carbonic anhydrase II deficiency **Clinical** Mental and growth retardation, facial dysmorphia, dysodontogenesis, cerebral calcification with a 'veined' pattern, osteopetrosis, renal tubular acidosis, restrictive lung disease due to rib deformity **Laboratory** Metabolic acidosis, hyperchloremia, alkaline urine; Cf Etat marbre

'Marbling' FORENSIC PATHOLOGY A mosaic of discoloration due to prominent subdermal vessels, which is seen on the skin surface of a body in the early stages of decomposition, also termed 'venous patterning'

Marburg disease A rare viral hemorrhagic fever occurring in small clusters in Europe and Africa due to direct contact with infected monkey tissue, blood or human serum, first seen in Marburg Germany in 1967, when lab workers were exposed to African green monkey (***Cercopithecusa ethiops***) virus, a member of a newly designated family, Filoviridae, an elongated filamentotubular bacilliform rod **Clinical** Incubation 5-9 days; otherwise similar to Argentine or Bolivian hemorrhagic fever with insidious or abrupt onset of headaches, fever, diarrhea, myalgias, rash, pharyngitis, thrombocytopenia, leukopenia and hemorrhage; 7/31 of the Marburg cases died; Cf Ebola virus

March fracture A metatarsal stress fracture seen in military recruits who are unaccustomed to the repeated, otherwise trivial trauma to the feet associated with long marches when carrying heavy equipment

March hemoglobinuria Exertional rhabdomyolysis Hemolysis due to repeated trauma that impacts on red cells that travel through small vessels overlying the bones of the hands and feet in long-distance marching (soldiers), marathon running, calesthenics and karate **Laboratory** Myoglobinuria, proteinuria, increased BUN, elevation of enzymes (creatinine phosphokinase), local increase in lactic acid **Histopathology** Rhabdomyositis, rhabdomyolysis

'Marching' cavity The creeping expanding erosion of the contiguous thick-walled cavities of chronic pulmonary histoplasmosis

'Marching in place' NEUROLOGY Repetitive movements of the legs when standing, a clinical finding in tardive dyskinesia, a feared complication of chronic antipsychotic medication, which may be persistent or permanent; tardive dyskinesia may also manifest as body 'rocking', 'fly-catching' (darting movements of the tongue) and 'piano playing' (involvement of the digits)

MARCKS Myristoylated alanine-rich (protein) C kinase substrate

Marfanoid habitus A leptosomic body type that is tall and thin with long hands; marfanoid features may be familial in nature or pathological as occurs in homocystinuria and MEN type IIb, mimicking some of the changes of Marfan's disease, but not accompanied by luxation of the lens, funnel chest and dissecting aneurysm of the aorta

Marginal form see Applique form

CH_3, OH, H, H_3C, H_3C, O, C_5H_{11}

THC (Δ^9-tetrahydrocannibol)

Marijuana 'Pot', 'Weed' SUBSTANCE ABUSE A substance derived from the hemp plant ***Cannabis sativa***, the leaves of which are smoked, producing a hallucinogenic effect due to the neurochemical Δ^9-tetrahydrocannabinol (THC), which has a cognate THC receptor in the brain **Immune system** THC stops monocyte maturation NERVOUS SYSTEM Impaired motor skills, defective eye tracking and perception; THC receptors are most abundant in the hippocampus, where memory is consolidated, explaining marijuana's detrimental effect on memory and least abundant in the brainstem, explaining why death by overdose is unknown with chronic marijuana abuse PREGNANCY (Am J Perinatol 1990; 7:36) RESPIRATORY TRACT Marijuana is inhaled or 'toked' in a fashion that differs from that of tobacco; in order to maximize THC absorption and elicit the desired 'high', the subject prolongs inhalation, markedly increasing carbon monoxide and tar levels, and thus is comparable to tobacco smoke (N Engl J Med 1988; 318:347) THERAPEUTIC USES Although marijuana is an analgesic, it cannot be used as such, due to the inseparable hallucinogenic effect; it is of use for 1) Control of nausea and vomiting in terminal cancer patients; two antiemetic cannabinoids are commercially available, nabilone (Cesamet), a synthetic derivative of marijuana and dronabinol (Marinol) the principle psychoactive substance in marijuana; both are designated as second-line therapies, given their psychotomimetic effects and side effects (drowsiness, dizziness, vertigo, loss of ability to concentrate and mood swings) and 2) Control of intraocular pressure in open-angle glaucoma, administered orally, in topical drops or smoked in the crude form Note: The four-to-six marijuana cigarettes required to treat glaucoma, are sufficient to cause chronic marijuana intoxication, impacting on psychosocial development, motivation, memory, motor function and coordination; other possible therapeutic uses of marijuana include improved clinical response to neuroleptics in motor disorders, eg de la Tourette syndrome; marijuana's effects are equivalent to diazepam in torsion dystonia, and may relieve symptoms of Huntington's chorea, given its potent effect on the extrapyramidal motor system through a nicotinic cholinergic mechanism (Life Sciences 1989; 44:1521) **Toxicology** THC and metabolites are detectable in the urine one hour after smoking or later when used as a garnee for cooking, ie 'pot' in the pan; Sensitivity of method 100 ng/ml, urine in RIA and standard EMIT (homogeneous enzyme immunoassay); 50 ng/ml thin-layer chromatography; 5-20 ng/ml 'stepped up' EMIT; 5 ng/ml gas liquid chromatography and mass spectrometry; see Amotivational syndrome, Joint, Substance abuse, THC receptor, Toke*

Mariner's wheel appearance Mickey mouse appearance Pilot's wheel A descriptor for the yeast form of ***Paracoccidioides brasiliensis***, in which there is a large central yeast cell and multiple peripheral budding yeasts, with a double-contoured rim attached to the 'mother' by a base of varying thickness, yielding an morphology fancifully likened to a wheel of a sailing ship

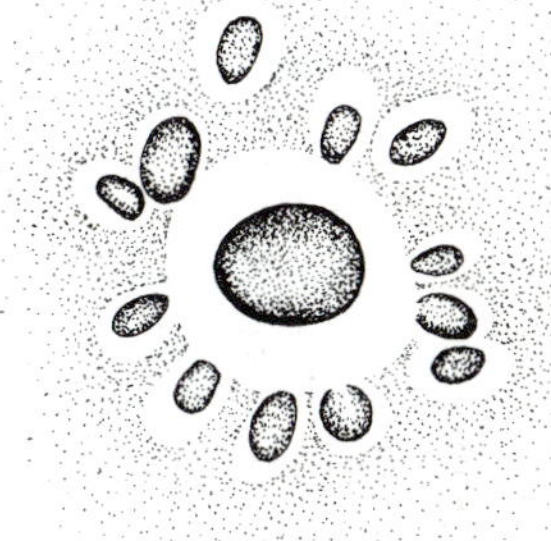

Mariner's wheel appearance

Marker gene MOLECULAR BIOLOGY A variant allele used to label a biological structure or process throughout an experiment; these genes are located in a constant genomic position in the studied organism

Marker rescue experiment MOLECULAR BIOLOGY Retrieval of a fragment of DNA which has been introduced and incorporated into a lambda phage DNA, by inducing lysis of the carrier bacterium; when different strains of bacteria are used, this technique allows analysis of the marker content of the DNA fractions

Marketing see Advertising, Detailing, Yellow professionalism

Markov process State-transition model A stochastic process in which the conditional probability distribution for a system's state at any given instant is unaffected by details on that system's previous state; the Markov process is a modeling technique that may be used in medical decision-making analysis for conditions in which the prognosis of a morbid condition is described by a 'natural history' or series of chance events (adverse outcomes) and the value of these outcomes depends on whether and when they occur; in Markov analysis, the patient's health is represented by a series of 'health states', which over time, move to other states (usually of lesser health, greater morbidity or death) according to the laws of probability; Markov models are of particular use in analyzing the effects of conditions involving multiple risks and time-dependent events, which are compared to an idealized 'illness-free life expectancy' (Statistics in Med 1988; 7:787) and are also useful in modeling diseases in which the same event recurs, eg osteoporotic fractures, thromboembolism, recurrence of malignancy in the same patient Note: Markov analysis may be used as part of an algorithm in decision-making by artificial intelligence; see Receiver operator characteristic

MARSA see Methicillin-aminoglycoside resistant *Staphylococcus aureus*

Masculinization see Virilization

Mask-like face A hypomimic, expressionless physiognomy or complete lack of facial affect, characteristic of Parkinson's disease, a finding that may be seen in depression, facioscapulohumeral-type muscular dystrophy, infantile botulism, Möbius' syndrome, myotonic dystrophy, Prader-Willi disease and Wilson's disease

Mask of pregnancy see Melasma

Mask phenomenon Post-emetic purpura that follows prolonged vomiting ('retching'), appearing as evanescent punctate macules on the face and upper neck, thought to be due to abruptly increased intrathoracic pressure; similar lesions occur in violent coughing, the Valsalva maneuver or in strangulation, and are accompanied by conjunctival petechiae

Masked depression A form of adolescent depression in which the young subject deals with despair by denial, somatization (headaches, abdominal or other pain) or 'acting out' (truancy, substance abuse, multiple accidents)

Masked mRNA Masked message sequence An mRNA sequence present in unfertilized eggs and other eukaryotic cells that is tightly bound by amacroprotein and floats about the nucleus as ribonucleoprotein complexes, which becomes activated and translated only after the egg is fertilized

Mass A cohesive aggregate of often similar components, composition, cells or molecules *ATOMIC MASS UNIT* Dalton 1.6604 x 10^{-27} kg *ELECTRONIC MASS* The mass of a negative electron (8.999 x 10^{-28}) when moving at a moderate velocity *ELECTRON MASS UNIT* 511 keV The energy required to annihilate an electron *MASS NUMBER* The number of protons and neutrons in a nuclide, eg 14 in ^{14}C

Massive transfusion TRANSFUSION MEDICINE The infusion, within a 24-hour period, of a blood volume that approaches or exceeds the recipient's own calculated blood volume; massive transfusions may be administered in medical or surgical emergencies or in the course of 'bloody' operations, and have a variety of effects on the recipient including depletion of coagulation factors, lowering of core temperature, due to the infusion of cool blood (uncommon in practice), and the inability to properly 'type' red cells, as the majority of the circulating erythrocytes are of donor origin

Mass spectroscopy Mass spectrometry An analytical method for measuring molecular mass and structure, in which a specimen is ionized and passed through either an electron beam (for liquid samples) or spark (for solids) **Principle** Ions are accelerated by a variable electrostatic field and deflected along a circular path by a constant magnetic field; the radius of the path is inversely proportional to the ion's velocity and its charge/mass ratio; the system may be coupled with gas chromatography (MS-GC) to measure a second parameter (dimension) of the specimen, thereby increasing its precision; the GC-MS hybrid is a 'gold-standard' device for confirming the results from screening techniques such as thin-layer chromatography and EMIT, and is used to quantify opiates, cannabinoids and narcotics; Cf EMIT, Gas-liquid chromatography

MAST 1) Military antishock trousers EMERGENCY MEDICINE A pressure device designed to provide life support in patients with external or internal subdiaphragmatic hemorrhage, which acts to stabilize movement of the lower extremities and pelvis as well as treat the hemorrhagic-traumatic shock by producing hemostasis and increasing systemic vascular pressure; Cf Pressure pants 2) Military Assistance to Safety and Traffic EMERGENCY MEDICINE A program in the US in which the military contributes helicopters and medical assistance to low-population density areas Note: The major MAST users are high-risk infants in rural settings

Mast cell A nonspecific immune cell that stains metachromatically due to its high proteoglycan content and abundant electron-dense granules; like basophils, mast cells are activated by cross-linking of IgE on the cell-surface and secrete neutrophil and eosinophil chemotactic factors, histamine, leukotrienes, neutral proteases, peroxidase, serotonin, superoxide dismutase, prostaglandins and platelet-activating factor; the release response may also be evoked in response to various substances including hormones, peptides, proteins, calcium ionophores, narcotics, muscle relaxants, dextran, complement C3a and C5a (anaphylotoxins); the mast cell is detected by measuring serum trypticase (a neutral protease in mast cell secretory granules); levels > 4 ng/ml indicate systemic mast cell activation; mast cell lesions see Mastocytosis

Master-servant doctrine see Respondeat superior

Master-slave hypothesis MOLECULAR BIOLOGY A theory that attempts to explain the lower than expected frequency of mutations in tandem arrays of repeated sequences of DNA; according to the master-slave hypothesis, sequence identity is maintained through either frequent unequal meiotic crossovers or gene conversion in which one gene (the master) corrects the other multiple copies (the slaves) that are arranged in an end-to-end fashion

Mastocytoma A focal aggregate of mast cells of undetermined significance, common in dogs, occasionally in cats and cows, rare in humans; see Mastocytosis

Mastocytosis Aggregation of mast cells is an uncommon, poorly understood event in humans that may be classified according to extent and behavior (table) **REACTIVE MASTOCYTOSIS** A focal increase in mast cells due to immediate or delayed hypersensitivity reactions, which may also occur in lymph nodes draining benign or malignant lesions, eg chronic liver or renal disease, leukemia, lymphoproliferative disorders or Hodgkin's disease Benign mast cell diseases include localized mastocytosis, which may be cutaneous or extracutaneous and urticaria pigmentosa **SYSTEMIC MASTOCYTOSIS** A potentially aggressive nosology, characterized by excess histamine production with flushing vertigo, palpitations, pruritus, colicky pain, dyspnea, nausea and vomiting, which may be asymptomatic, mild to moderate with intermittent symptoms or severe, disabling and progressive **'MALIGNANT' SYSTEMIC MASTOCYTOSIS** A form of mast cell disease that is fatal within two years of conversion to an aggressive form **MAST CELL LEUKEMIA** A neoplasm that develops in 15% of patients with malignant systemic mastocytosis Clinical Fever, anorexia, weight loss, fatigue, abdominal colic, diarrhea, pruritus, bone pain, duodenal ulcer, hepatosplenomegaly and lymphadenopathy; see Mastocytoma

Mastocytosis

I Localized mastocytosis
 a) Focal Single skin lesion: mast cell 'nevus'
 b) Generalized Urticaria pigmentosa
II Systemic mastocytosis:
 a) Indolent
 b) Progressive
 c) Malignant
III Mast cell leukemia
IV Mast cell sarcoma

Matagen Masking tape for gene expression Synthetic, chemically-modified sequence-specific analogs of gene segments composed of non-ionic oligonucleoside methylphosphonates, corresponding to enzyme-resistant RNA and DNA; modifications include methylation or adding sulfur at various points on the phosphate backbone of antisense DNA with the purpose of blocking viral expression

Match GRADUATE MEDICAL EDUCATION The 'Match' is a system used in North America by which both teaching hospitals rank their preferences for candidates to fill their first year post-graduate training positions, and graduating medical students rank their preferences for those (internship year) positions; some graduate programs allow certain graduate training positions to be filled 'outside of the match'

Matching grant ACADEMIA A form of usually non-peer-reviewed funding in which a foundation or philanthropy contributes a sum of money that 'matches' a financial contribution made by an institution, university or hospital; Cf 'Approved but not granted'

Mate A tea-like beverage obtained from an infusion of the leaves of a South American shrub (*Ilex paraguayensis*), habitually ingested at high temperatures in southeastern South America; high volume drinkers are 2.2-fold more likely to have esophagitis, and have a relative risk of 1.47 for esophageal cancer; ingestion of more than 2.5 liters/day is reported to be associated with a relative risk of 12.2 for esophageal cancer (Cancer Res 1990; 50:426)

Mater The trilaminar membrane enveloping the brain; the most external layer is the **DURA MATER** A tough fibrous membrane intimately attached to the inner aspect of the cranial bones that sheathes the brain, cranial nerves and spinal cord as it passes down the spinal canal **ARACHNOID MATER** A membrane that bridges the hemispheric sulci, and constitutes the connective tissue support for the blood vessels that communicate with the pia mater and contains the arachnoid granulations, a component of the blood-brain barrier **PIA MATER** The innermost layer that consists of loose connective tissue containing elastin, collagen and other basement membrane material; the pia mater is a continuation of the arachnoid sheathing the blood vessels and penetrates the gyri and cerebellar lamina and thus may be referred to as the pia-arachnoid mater

Maternal age Increased age is widely thought to adversely impact on pregnancy as a) The complication rate is greater in older pregnant women (see Elderly primigravida) and b) There is an increasing rate of fetal malformation in older women, possibly the result of an unknown effect of aging on the uterus and eggs (table); Cf Paternal age

MATERNAL AGE & CHROMOSOME DEFECTS

Age	Down syndrome	Others
<20	1/1900	1/526
25	1/1200	1/476
30	1/885	1/384
35	1/365	1/178
40	1/109	1/63
45	1/32	1/18
49	1/12	1/7

Maternal milk see Breast milk

'Maternal-fetal conflict' BIOMEDICAL ETHICS A dilemma with considerable medicolegal ramifications that arises when a mother wishes to carry out an activity, eg drinking alcohol or working at a job with an occupational exposure to high levels of lead, that is potentially harmful to the fetus; the current thinking in the US judicial system, as exemplified by the Supreme Court in the International Union *vs* Johnson Controls ruling, is that protection of the fetus over the mother's personal freedom is both paternalistic and inappropriate and that the ultimate decision-maker must be the woman herself (N Engl J Med 1991; 325:740); Cf Emancipated minor

Matt Dull MICROBIOLOGY A standard descriptor for a non-glistening surface seen on culture plates of bacteria that don't produce capsules, characteristic of many Enterobacteriaceae species; cultures of bacteria that produce capsules are described as glistening or 'mucoid'

Matthew effect Halo effect An allegorical term applied to the observation that an eminent scientist, eg Nobel laureate or other person of reknown will receive a disproportionate amount of credit for a discovery, despite a relatively small contribution to the ultimate success of a project; the name derives from Matthew, one of Christ's twelve disciples who said, *'For to every one who has, more shall be given and he shall have in abundance; but from him who has not, even what he has will be taken'*; the term has been borrowed by epidemiologists for tabulating the 'hard' and 'soft' risk factors of a disease, as those subjects with more risk factors will be more likely to suffer from the disease

Matting Enlargement and cohesion of lymph nodes, which is classically described in tuberculosis, which may occur in other infections, eg histoplasmosis or in metastatic carcinoma; see 'Shotty' lymphadenopathy

Maturational arrest Hematology The presence of relatively mature cytoplasm and an immature nucleus, seen in patients with megaloblastic anemia due to a deficiency of vitamin B_{12} and/or folic acid; the change affects all cells, is most prominent in the bone marrow and is characterized by enlarged cells with delicate, open chromatin and prominent parachromatin; this 'Nuclear:cytoplasmic asynchrony' is due to decreased DNA synthesis and a block in mitosis, attributed to the slowing of cobalamin-dependent pathway of methionine synthesis, which in turn sequesters folate as N^5-methyl FH_4 that cannot be used by thymidylate synthetase to generate dTMP from dUMP

Maturation index (MI) Squamous cell index Gynecologic cytology A crude evaluation of the female estrogenic status, using the papanicolaou ('pap') smear, using three values X, Y and Z that total 100, corresponding to the percentage of parabasal, intermediate and superficial squames respectively seen in the smear 1) *Parabasal cells* Immature round to oval squames with a large nucleus 2) *Intermediate squames* Mature, often polygonal squamous cells with a well- or partially lysed vesicular nucleus and 3) *Superficial squames* Mature squames with large polygonal borders and pyknotic nucleus; cells for the MI are taken from the lateral vaginal wall, 100 or more cells are counted; the MI is absolutely reliable in two situations: marked estrogen effect and total absence of estrogen; 'typical' MI patterns **0/60/40 Midcycle pattern** is seen on the middle day of a normal cycle or an elderly woman with estrogen supplementation **5/35/60 Ovulation pattern** is due to an estrogen effect, seen with endometrial hyperplasia or carcinoma, Stein-Leventhal syndrome, ovarian tumors, hepatic insufficiency **100/-/- Primary amenorrhea** the 'Pap smear' is composed of immature parabasal cells, due to complete lack of hormonal activity and **-/100/- Progesterone effect**; Parabasal cells predominate in early post-partum period, during lactation or in the prepubertal period; MI cannot be evaluated in cervical inflammation, due to excess cytolysis by Döderlein bacilli, drugs that alter squamous maturation, eg tetracycline, digitalis, thyroid, regional surgery and conization

Maxam-Gilbert sequencing Molecular biology A chemical method for determining the sequence of DNA, described by A Maxam and W Gilbert (Proc Nat Acad Sci, USA 1977; 74:560) Method The 5' end of a single strand of DNA (derived from a double-stranded segment) is labeled with ^{32}P; the DNA is then cleaved with a restriction endonuclease; one fragment of double helix DNA is isolated in a relatively pure form and one strand is separated from the other, yielding a population of identical strands that have been radioactively-labeled at one end; the sample is then divided into four samples, each of which is subjected to a chemical reaction that destroys one or two specific nucleotide bases, either cytosine, or guanine, or adenine and guanine or thymine and cytosine; the loss of the bases at this point facilitates the breaking of the deoxyribose-phosphate bond, thus being similar to restriction mapping; the broken pieces are then electrophoresed and arranged on a 'sequencing' gel in order of length; see King-Kong gel

Maximum acid output see MAO

Maximum allowable cost program see MAC

Maximum containment facility A 'level 3/4' research facility that is equipped to, and experienced in handling exotic, dangerous and potentially life-threatening infectious agents, eg HIV-1 and Lassa fever virus; all clothing changed prior to working with the organisms and at the day's end, appropirate decontamination procedures are carried out if warranted; see Biosafety

Maximum contaminant level (MCL) Environment The ceiling of an inorganic chemical that the US Environmental Protection Agency (EPA) will allow in drinking water, before declaring it unsafe for human consumption, eg 0.002 mg/L for mercury, 0.05 mg/L for arsenic, cadmium, chromium, lead and silver, 1 mg/L for barium and 10 mg/L for nitrates; in 1977, the EPA determined that 95% of US drinking water was affected by pollution

Maximum expiratory flow rate see Lung volumes

Maximum tolerated doses (MTDs) The highest dose of a substance that can be given without causing serious weight loss and other signs of toxicity

Max-Planck Institute(s) (MPI) Originally founded in 1911 as the Kaiser-Wilhelm Gesellschaft in Berlin, the MPI is comprised of 61 self-administering research institutes of social and natural sciences, including Institutes for Biochemistry, Biology, Biophysics, Biophysical chemistry, Brain research, Cell biology, Coagulation, Developmental biology, Endocrinology, Experimental medicine, Immunology, Molecular biology, Molecular genetics, Multiple sclerosis, Nutrition, Psychiatry and others Max-Planck Gesellschaft zur Forderung der Wissenschaften eV 8000 Munchen 1 Postfach 647, Rezidenzstr 1A

Maxwell An electromagnetic centimeter-gram-second unit of magnetic flux, equal to 10^{-8} weber

Mayo risk score A decision-making model for primary biliary cirrhosis based on five variables: bilirubin levels in the serum, age, albuminemia, prothrombin time, and the severity of edema, which allows determination of prognosis (Hepatology 1989; 10:1)

Mazoplasia An imprecise, rarely used term denoting a variant of mammary dysplasia with fibrosis and ductal desquamation

MB fraction see CPK-MB

M-BACOD A standard multiagent chemotherapeutic regimen used to treat lymphoma, consisting of methotrexate, bleomycin, doxorubicin (Adriamycin), cyclophosphamide, vincristine (Oncovorin) and dexamathasone, which is of use in treating AIDS-related lymphoma (J Am Med Assoc 1991; 266:84)

MBC see Minimum bactericidal concentration

MBEST A variant of magnetic resonance imaging (MRI) consisting of a heavily-weighted T2 sequence, which is based on the echo-planar technique of MRI, developed by P Mansfield (Nottingham), used for ultra-high-speed imaging of the brain; see BEST, MRI; the advantage of the ultra-high-speed image is to allow rapid screening, functional imaging and analysis of the CSF fluid and blood flow patterns and rapid 'shooting' of restless patients

MBP see Major basic protein, Myelin basic protein

MCAD see Medium-chain acyl-CoA dehydrogenase deficiency

MCAT Medical college admission test An examination administered by the Psychological Corporation, Inc, which is required in the US prior to entrance in the first year of medical school; the MCATs are an objectve evaluation of a candidate's verbal skills and scientific knowledge, which by extension, is assumed to be an adequate measure of the candidate's likelihood to succeed in medical school; see Graduate medical education, Medical student

McCollough effect A phenomenon observed in subjects who have worked for a prolonged period with a microcomputer monitor that displays green lettering on a darkened background, in which white paper acquires a pink hue, caused by adaption of cortical neurons to specific combinations of color and form; the effect may last for several weeks and is of no clinical significance (N Engl J Med 1983; 309:315c)

McCune-Albright disease An idiopathic disease possibly related to altered regulation of cAMP **Clinical** Precocious puberty, polyostotic (cystic) fibrous dysplasia (spontaneous fractures at an early age), cafe-au-lait spotting of skin, ovarian cysts and endocrinopathy including hyperthyroidism, hypophosphatemia and cyclical (4-6 week) fluctuations of plasma estrogen; afflicted young girls have decreased gonadotropins and reactivity to luteinizing hormone-releasing factor **Treatment** Aromatase inhibitor testolactone Note: Hormonal manipulation is logical use of the presence of estrogen and progesterone receptors on the osteogenic cells of McCune-Albright patients (N Engl J Med 1988; 319:421)

MCH

SI: $\frac{\text{Hemoglobin g/L of whole blood}}{\text{Red cell count } (10^{12})}$

OR

US: $\frac{\text{Hemoglobin g/L of whole blood X 10}}{\text{Red cell count } (10^{6}/\mu l)}$

MCH Mean corpuscular hemoglobin A measurement of the hemoglobin per individual erythrocyte Reference range 26-34 pg/red cell (SI: Internationsl System)

MCHC Mean corpuscular hemoglobin concentration A value that is derived on the Coulter cell counters from measured parameters Reference range: 31-36 g/dl

MCHC

$\frac{\text{Hemoglobin g/100 ml X 100}}{\text{Packed red cell volume (percent)}}$

OR

$\frac{\text{hemoglobin g/100 ml X 1000}}{\text{MCV X RBC (in millions)}}$

McKusick classification see MIM number Osler Professor of medicine at Johns Hopkins medical school and 'Linnaeus' of human genetics, who single-handedly organized the congenital diseases of man; his book, Mendelian Inheritancein Man forms the basis for international communication in genetic disease; each condition found in the work has been assigned an 'MIM number', subdivided into broad categories depending on whether the conditions are autosomal recessive, autosomal dominant or linked to the X chromosome, eg McKusick 23625 corresponds to 5,10-methylenetetrahydrofolate reductase deficiency; see Human Genome project, MIM number

MCL see Maximum contaminant levels

MCLN Mucocutaneous lymph node syndrome see Kawasaki's disease

M chain One of the two proteins required to form a tetramer of lactate dehydrogenase

M component A narrow peak or 'spike' seen on serum protein electrophoresis which is presumptive evidence of a monoclonal lymphoproliferation of mature B cells producing IgG, IgA or IgM; the M component may occur in multiple myeloma, Waldenström's disease, heavy chain disease and in lichen myxedematosus (a rare disease of proliferating fibroblasts)

M-current (I/M) NEUROPHYSIOLOGY A time and voltage-dependent potassium current that persists at slightly depolarized membrane potentials; IM is reduced by muscarinic cholinergic agonists and certain peptides and IM is partially responsible for the slow excitatory postsynaptic potentials in sympathetic neurons; IM in hippocampal neurons is increased by somatostatin, thus indicating that one ion channel has two different regulating receptors, the latter of which are mediated by arachidonic acid metabolites (Nature 1990; 346:464)

MCT 1) Medium-chain triglycerides, 2) Medullary carcinoma of the thyroid

MCTD see Mixed connective tissue disease

MCV

SI: $\frac{\text{Hematocrit (packed red cell)/L blood}}{\text{Red cell count } (10^{12})\text{/L}}$

OR

US: $\frac{\text{Hematocrit \%}}{\text{Red cell count } (\text{X } 10^{6})}$

MCV Mean corpuscular volume A calculated value for the average volume of peripheral red cells Reference range:

80-100 femtoliter/cell

MD Medical doctor, Mentally deficient, Muscular dystrophy, Manic-depressive

MDA or MDM 3,4-Methylenedioxymethamphetamine see Adam

MDD Major depressive disorder

MDF see Myocardial depressant factor

MDGC Multidimensional gas chromatography, see Gas chromatography

MD/PhD ACADEMIA An individual holding both a degree in medicine and a doctorate of philosophy; the two combined degrees may be obtained either by 1) Completing a four year medical school education (requiring four years in the US, since the prerequisite for entry to medical school is four years or more of university education), which is a relatively standardized experience, followed by the studies required for a doctorate of philosophy (Ph.D.), which can range from several years of a poorly-supervised and/or part-time educational experience in virtually any discipline to five or more years of intense post-graduate education and bench research or 2) Completion of a six-year combined program, in which the medical education is mixed with research activities extending over the entire six years of education, a philosophy that is thought to facilitate a physician's entry into research (J Am Med Assoc 1990; 264:1919)

MDR Multidrug resistance ONCOLOGY The simultaneous cross-resistance to multiple chemotherapeutic agents, including antitumor antibiotics, eg daunorubicinvinca alkaloids and epidophyllotoxins; mutants resistant to the effect of drug X occur with a frequency of 10^{-5}-10^{-8}; destruction of drug-sensitive cells 'selects' for resistant cells, explaining the increased efficacy (and necessity) of combination chemotherapy; in malignancy, cell membranes may 'bristle' with P-glycoprotein (P170), the protein encoded by the MDR gene, which zealously ushers toxins to the cell's exterior, related to increased expression of the mdr1 locus, causing gene amplification, with production of up to 60 copies in resistant cells; resistant drugs include colchicine, vincristine, actinomycin, daunorubicin **Mechanism** P170-mediated resistance is related to decreased drug accumulation (the P170 permeability glycoprotein pumps drug out of the tumor cells); MDR gene expression is amplified in methotrexate (MTX) resistance (MTX blocks formation of purine precursors), with the resistant cells producing more dihydrofolate reductase; non-P170 mediated resistance in MDR cells is related to an altered glutathione redox cycle Note: Increased expression of P170 may be ameliorated with verapamil, an antiarrhythmic that inactivates the P170 pump (J Clin Oncol 1989; 7:415) Note: An MDR-related gene is expressed in higher copy numbers in drug-resistant *Plasmodium falciparum* (Science 1989; 244:1184)

MDS see Myelodysplastic syndrome

MEA Multiple endocrine adenomatosis see Multiple endocrine neoplasia

'Meaningful existence' see Futility

Measles vaccine Measles is a condition that kills an estimated two million children annually in the 'global village'; in children hospitalized for treating complicated measles (with pneumonia, croup or diarrhea), treatment with large doses of vitamin A reduces the mortality by 50% and the hospital stay and co-morbid conditions by one-half (N Engl J Med 1990; 323:160)

Measurement The International System (SI) officially sanctions the use of certain prefixes for SI units (table); see SI

Measurement	
googa	100^{100}
exa	10^{18}
peta	10^{15}
tera	10^{12}
giga	10^{9}
mega	10^{6}
kilo	10^{3}
hecto	10^{2}
deka	10^{1}
deci	10^{-1}
centi	10^{-2}
milli	10^{-3}
micro	10^{-6}
nano	10^{-9}
pico	10^{-12}
femto	10^{-15}
atto	10^{-18}
zepto	10^{-21}

Note: 10^{12} corresponds to the British billion (USA, trillion); 10^{9} is the American billion (British millard)

Mechanical restraint A device applied to an individual to restrict free movement, including seatbelts and vests; US legal system requires documentation of 'medical' conditions justifying the use of restraints, which include unsteadiness, wandering and disruptive behavior, often secondary to psychiatric conditions and/or dementia, which may, in addition, require pharmacologic' restraints (J Am Med Assoc 1991; 265:469)

Mechanical theory of metastases see Seed-and-soil hypothesis

Mechanical ventilation Mechanically-assisted respiration in which inspiration is driven at a preset frequency or triggered by the patient; although expiration is passive, intraalveolar pressure may be purposely raised by positive end-expiratory pressure (PEEP) in those suffering from pulmonary edema or increased lung compliance; mechanical ventilation is indicated if the PO_2 is less than 60 mm Hg, despite best non-interventional efforts (mask, bronchodilators, diuretics and physical therapy); the Iron lung is a variation on this theme, where negative external pressure is applied to the thoracic wall in patients encased from the neck down in a negative pressure chamber Indications for mechanical ventilation Chest wall restriction (kyphoscoliosis, thoracoplasty), chronic obstructive pulmonary disease, central nervous and brainstem disease (central apnea, primary alveolar hypertension, tumors, vascular malformation), degenerative disease (Shy-Drager disease, spinocerebellar degeneration), neuromuscular disease (amyotrophic lateral sclerosis, multiple sclerosis, muscular dystrophy, myopathy, phrenic nerve damage, poliomyelitis), spinal cord disease (cervical trauma, quadriplegia, syringomyelia, Mayo Clin Proc 1988; 63:1209)

'Mechanism' A doctrine that holds that all the details of a process, eg evolution, the genetic code or pathogenesis of a disease, can be explained in terms of a limited number of physico-chemical cause-and-effect relations

Mechlorethamine An alkylating chemotherapeutic agent of the nitrogen mustard group, used to treat lymphomas and a component of the MOPP regimen **Side effects** Gastrointestinal symptoms, bone marrow suppression, skin vesiculation on contact

Meckel's diverticulum A pouch in the small intestine, which corresponds to the omphalomesenteric (vitelline) duct remnant, is located along the antimesenteric border and may contain gastric or pancreatic tissue; a popular mnemonic is the 'rule of twos', as the diverticulum is two feet (circa 0.65 m) from the ileocecal valve, two inches long (circa 5 cm), two cm in diameter, found in two percent of the population and two-fold more common in males; as Meckel's diverticulum is a favored site for carcinoids, it may be excised prophylactically when the surgeon is in the abdominal cavity for other reasons

Meconium Green viscid mucus-like material found in the intestine of all neonates; it is the first stool passed by the newborns and is passed in the first 24-48 hours of life

Meconium aspiration syndrome NEONATOLOGY A symptom complex caused by the aspiration of meconium at the time of delivery **Clinical** Low APGAR scores, tachypnea, dyspnea and cyanosis, which either resolves in the first three days of life, or if the amount of aspirated meconium was intense, progresses displaying patchy infiltrates on chest films accompanied by atelectasis, emphysema and rales; Cf APGAR

Meconium ileus Meconium plug syndrome A condition characterized by obstruction of the neonatal intestine by intensely viscid glue-like meconium that may be confined to the ileus, a finding highly characteristic of cystic fibrosis **Clinical** Non-passage of stool in the first two days of life, accompanied by nausea, vomiting and abdominal distension **Complications** Volvulus, intestinal infarction **Histopathology** Goblet cell hyperplasia Note: Meconium 'plugging' of the rectum may also signal the presence of Hirschsprung's disease, which is histologically characterized by segmental aganglionosis

MEDAC syndrome Multiple endocrine deficiency, Addison's disease and candidiasis A subtype of mucocutaneous candidiasis, which is characterized by increased gammagobulins and decreased IgA, accompanied by a progressive decline in parathyroid and adrenal function Note: the condition has also been termed HAM (Hypoparathyroidism, Addison's disease and mucocutaneous candidiasis)

Medea complex PSYCHIATRY Murderous hatred by a mother for her child(ren), arising from a desire for revenge on her husband; Medea of Greek mythology was a sorceress and the wife of Jason, who imprisoned her when she decided to marry Creusa; Medea responded by killing their children

'Media epidemic' A flurry of interest displayed by the news media (newspapers, television, radio), in an item of medical importance, eg a new therapeutic modality or 'breakthrough' or a new disease, which follows a report in a major medical journal; the 'media' are often less interested in reporting the facts than in exploiting the potential sensationalist impact of the news item in question, which may result in distortion of the details, as the reporters may not be scientifically sophisticated enough to balance the information they present in an appropriate context; see Embargo arrangement, Ingelfinger rule

Medial necrosis see Cystic medial necrosis

Median rhomboid glossitis A condition initially considered a developmental abnormality of the tongue, now considered a manifestation of chronic infection by ***Candida albicans***, facilitated by the high glucose levels as it is often seen in diabetics **Clinical** Rhomboid or diamond-shaped red plaque or patch on the dorsum of the tongue anterior to the circumvallate papillae **Histopathology** Loss of papillae, hyperparakeratosis, proliferation of the spinous layer, elongation of the rete ridges, lymphocyte and neutrophil infiltration of connective tissue, increased blood vessels and lymphatics, degeneration and hyaline formation of the underlying tongue **Treatment** Nystatin or amphotericin B may cause regression

Mediastinal 'crunch' SPORTS MEDICINE A substernal crepitant sound, often synchronous with the heartbeat, caused by percolation of air into the mediastinum (emphysema) as occurs in esophageal perforation or secondary to expansion of gas in rapid ascent in scuba divers (Caisson's disease)

Medicaid A federally-funded, state-operated and state-administered program of medical assistance in the US that is authorized by Title XIX of the Social Security Act of 1965 and provides medical assistance to certain low-income groups, including the elderly, blind, disabled, single-parent families and the unemployed, who are eligible for welfare cash programs, eg 'Aid to Families with Dependent Children' and 'Supplementary Security Income' programs, and to those with income sufficient for basic needs, but not for medical care; in 1987, Medicaid paid $45 x 10^9 to 23 million recipients Note: Some health care providers have found that the cost of processing the paperwork required to be reimbursed for services rendered to Medicaid patients is greater than the reimbursement obtained by the physician and thus Medicaid work may be viewed in a 'pro bono publico' context

'Medicaidization' A shift of financial liability for medical care of the financially disadvantaged to the public sector; in the USA, Medicaid bears the brunt of health care costs for the financially disenfranchised, paying a small fraction of the actual cost of the services provided; many AIDS patients are below poverty levels and there is an increasing tendency to shift the costs of providing care for these patients and indigents from private insurance companies to the agency (Medicaid) that pays the least for services (J Am Med Assoc 1990; 264:1261); Cf 'Dumping', 'Safety net' hospital, 'Skimming'

'Medicaid mill' A for-profit organization (in the USA) that provides health care, usually on an ambulatory basis in locations where few medical services are available, eg inner city ghettos and rural communities; these 'mills' are characterized by high productivity (as measured by the number of patients seen) and are frequently accused of a variety of abuses of the Medicaid reimbursement system; see also Family 'ganging', 'Ping-ponging'

Medical ethics, landmark cases A burgeoning field that attempts to formally address the moral dilemmas affecting broad medical decisions, which may be divided into a) The broad ethical principles that impact as a society on patients, physicians and health care institutions and b) The individual code of ethics of health care providers, delineated by the Hippocratic Oath; the expanding field of medical ethics is being delineated through 'lines in the sand' drawn by legal landmark cases in the US for patients' rights over control of their bodies, delineated in chronological order ROE *VS* WADE (1973, Texas) A woman's right to privacy includes abortion if the conceptus is incapable of reasonably functioning outside of the womb, defined as less than 27 weeks of gestation; see Roe *vs* Wade; Cf Webster decision QUINLAN (1976, New Jersey) A ruling to allowing removal of Karen Ann Quinlan's life support (possibly the most influential case in the euthanasia controversy, author's note), where a person's right to privacy was upheld through her father; see Persistent vegetative state, Quinlan BROTHER FOX (1981, New York) Removal of respirator in a comatose monk, ie active euthanasia; see Euthanasia JEFFERSON (1981, Georgia) Mother refused to allow her child to be delivered by cesarian section for religious reasons; the court held that the infant's right to life outweighed the mother's right to practice her religion; Cf Christian Science, Jehovah's witnesses BABY DOE (1982, Indiana) A child with Down syndrome and respiratory defects requiring surgery for survival; parents asked to relieve pain and suffering; county prosecutor asked to remove the child from parent's custody and authorize lifesaving procedures (the parental decision was upheld); see Baby Doe, Baby (Jane) Doe BARBER (1983, California) Physicians removed life support and feedings at the family's request; these same physicians were then charged with murder and later cleared by a higher court CONROY (1985, New Jersey) A feeding tube removed from a semi-comatose elderly male at nephew's request; the privacy right was upheld when the burden of continuing care outweighs the benefits BROUPHY (1986, Massachusetts) A ruptured berry aneurysm of the brain of a young public service worker caused permanent coma; the hospital and physicians refused the family's request for removal of life support, as the 'Barber case' was in the recent memory; life support was eventually withdrawn, but required that the comatose man be moved to another hospital before this would be performed BOUVIA (1986, California) A young quadriplegic woman in constant pain with cerebral palsy wished to have help in committing suicide, ie removal of the feeding tube; see Cruzan

Medical 'failure' A patient who does not respond to a non-interventional modality for treating a non-malignant, but potentially pernicious condition, and who, due to this failure, may benefit from surgery; the traditional philosophy is to attempt medical (drugs, change in lifestyle, diet and exercise) therapy when there is no clear benefit of performing surgery for a disease, as in the continuing controversy between coronary artery bypass surgery versus medical treatment to treat symptomatic atherosclerotic heart disease: if the patient does not respond to conservative ('medical') therapy, the patient's physician(s) then recommend bypass surgery or another semi-invasive modality, eg percutaneous transluminal angioplasty

Medical informatics The science that concerns itself with the cognitive processes of medical decision-making and the processing of medical information, which includes the technology and communication tasks of medical practice, education and research; see Artificial intelligence, Computers, Expert system, Electronic journal, Electronic publishing, MEDLINE, Online database

Medical record The written documentation of a person's medical history, the diagnostic and therapeutic procedures performed and the patient's clinical status at the time he was last seen by the medical team; the purpose of the medical record is to serve as the basis for planning and ensuring continuity of care, provide a means of communication among physicians and others contributing to patient management, provide documentation of the patient's course of disease and treatment, serve as a basis for review and evaluation, protect the legal interests of the patient, hospital and responsible physicians and provide data for use in billing, research and education; it is imperative that complete, accurate and timely records be kept, as lawsuits may be initiated years after the alleged occurrence of an event, at which time, independent recollection of the event is unlikely; the medical record should be accurate, timely, objective, specific, concise, consistent, comprehensive, logical, legible, clear, descriptive and reflective of rational thought process(es) Note: Although physicians tend to 'write like doctors', nothing erodes credibility in front of a jury more quickly than the inability of the defendant to read his own handwriting; see Hospital chart

Medical school debt The amount of monies owed (with interest) to various parties by a medical student; in the USA, higher education is costly and medical students are required to pay an annual university tuition fee (ranging from $10-25 000), in addition to living costs ($15-20 000/year), during the four years of medical school; the average graduating medical student owed $42 374 in 1989; less than 20% of graduates were debt-free at the time of graduation (J Am Med Assoc 1990; 263:2653)

'Medical' specialty A field of medical care that provides specialized patient care, treating patients in a non-interventional fashion, ie with drugs, or with minimum intervention, eg balloon catheterization; 'medical' specialties include internal medicine (allergy and immunology, cardiology, gastroenterology, hematology and oncology, neurology, infectious and pulmonary diseases), dermatology, pediatrics, psychiatry, preventive medicine, aerospace medicine; Cf Hospital-based physicians, 'Surgical' specialty

Medical staff The organized body of licensed physicians and health care providers who are permitted by law and by a hospital to provide medical care within that hospital or health care facility; the medical staff may be 'closed', ie allowing a defined number of specialists to practice, recruiting new members only when vacancies exist or it may be 'open', accepting new members on a continuing basis; see House staff, Staff courtesy, Staff privileges

Medical student abuse An widely extant practice of uncertain extent, in which medical students are psychologically 'abused' by superiors (interns, residents, fellows and attending physicians) in the form of badgering, belittling and being forced to perform menial, degrading tasks (J Am Med Assoc 1990; 263:527, 533) Note: The opinion has been privately voiced by some health care workers that abuse is part of the medical student experience, which helps 'harden' them for the realities of practicing medicine; see Pimping, Scut work

Medical team The group of physicians and health care workers who are responsible for a patient's medical needs while in the hospital and during a reasonable follow-up period; the 'team approach' has become the prevalent form of patient management in the US, which recognizes that no one person can be expected to diagnose and treat all aspects of a patient's condition

Medical technologist (MT) LABORATORY MEDICINE A laboratory worker who has received at least four years of formal college or university education and training in the performance of various techniques in clinical pathology, including hematology, microbiology, chemistry, blood banking, immunology and other areas of the clinical laboratory; MTs are eligible for certification by the American Society of Clinical Pathologists, and upon successful completion of the appropriate examination are entitled, MT(ASCP); technologists are empowered to perform and report the results of clinical tests; Cf Technician

Medicare A federal (US government-administered) program enacted as Title XVIII of the Social Security Act of 1965, providing hospital and medical insurance protection for those aged 65 and older, disabled persons under age 65 who receive cash benefits under Social Security and persons of all ages with chronic kidney disease; aliens and some federal civil service employees have been eligible since 1973; Medicare has 33 million enrollees (45% males, 55% females); $80 x 10^9 was paid by the US federal government to Medicare enrollees in 1987; Medicare consists of two parts a) Compulsory hospitalization insurance, known as 'Part A', which is financed by contributions from employers, employees and participants and b) Voluntary supplementary medical insurance, known as 'Part B', which is financed in part by monthly premiums paid by those enrolled and partly by the US federal government; insurance companies, Blue Cross and Blue Shield (see there) and several independent organizations act as fiscal intermediaries for the government; 6500 hospitals participate in the Medicare's 'Prospective payment system', the basis for which is the diagnosis-related groups, see DRGs; exceptions to Medicare coverage are health care facilities specialized in psychiatry, pediatrics, long-term care and rehabilitation; see Part A, Part B; Cf Medicaid, Socialized medicine

Medicins sans Frontieres (MSF) Doctors without borders The world's largest independent medical relief organization that provides short- and long-term medical aid to war zones, sites of natural disasters and refugee camps, in the form of emergency care, immunization services, food, hygiene, education and training; MSF was begun in 1971, has funded 4500 individual missions and often operates in volatile political environments, resulting in the deaths of some of its workers (Am Med News 18/Mar/91); one-fourth of MSF's funding is provided by the United Nations, the remainder from private donations; Cf Amnesty International, IPPNW, Red Cross

MedisGroups Medical illness severity grouping system (MediQual, Westborough, Mass) A system for classifying patients admitted to a hospital based on the severity of disease, formulated as an alternative to the diagnosis-related groups (DRGs) under which those hospitals admitting 'sicker' patients with the same DRGs were penalized since these patients had longer stays, thereby encouraging the practice of 'dumping'; under the MedisGroups, those patients admitted in group 0 to 1 (based on a list of key clinical findings) had a 1% mortality rate, while 60% of those in group 4 had imminent organ failure (J Am Med Assoc 1988; 260:3159) Note: MedisGroups admission severity does not adjust for interhospital case mix differences in outcome studies (ibid, 1991; 265:2965); see Kiss of death test; Cf DRGs, High mortality outlier

Mediterranean anemia Cooley's anemia Obsolete for β-thalassemia or thalassemia major

Mediterranean fever A term for either a) Generalized brucellosis or b) Familial mediterranean fever see there

Mediterranean lymphoma see IPSID Immunoproliferative small intestinal disease

Medium MICROBIOLOGY A liquid or solid matrix with nutrient designed to support the growth of microorganisms DIFFERENTIAL MEDIA are often solid and contain various chemical and other substances, eg colorants that may be produced by certain microorganisms, aiding in their identification ENRICHMENT MEDIA are often liquid and contain specific nutrients giving one or more of the microorganisms a growth advantage SELECTIVE MEDIA are those in which nutrients are added to either promote the growth of one or more group of bacteria, or inhibitors, eg nalidixic acid, malachite green and others to slow the growth of certain bacteria, giving the desired organisms a 'selective' growth advantage

Medium chain acyl-coenzyme A dehydrogenase deficiency An uncommon (1:6-10 000) disease of fatty acid oxidation that presents in the first two years of life as either sudden unexplained death at home, or when seen in the hospital, as Reye syndrome; the diagnosis is established by mutation analysis of postmortem tissue obtained from paraffin blocks (N Engl J Med 1991; 325:61c)

Medium chain triglyceride (MCT) CLINICAL NUTRITION A triacyl glycerol dietary substitute for long-chain triglycerides that is administered to very low-birth weight infants who cannot absorb longer chain fatty acids; MCT is derived from coconut oil and is theoretically useful in preventing steatorrhea, as 8-10 carbon triglycerides are more readily hydrolyzed by pancreatic enzymes, they don't require bile acids for absorption of the hydrolytic products and the metabolized products pass directly into the portal circulation; because MCTs provide less energy (8.3 kcal/g vs 9.0 for LCTs, no more than 400 calories of MCT may be used/day) Note: A small percentage of MCTs undergo omega oxidation, forming the metabolically useless dicarboxylic acid

MEDLARS Medical literature and analysis retrieval system MEDICAL INFORMATICS The computerized bibliographic retrieval system formed from the Index Medicus that provides access to the biomedical literature maintained by the National Library of Medicine in Washington, DC

MEDLINE MEDICAL INFORMATICS The most heavily-used of the more than 20 electronic (online) databases within MEDLARS, extending from 1966 to the present that is retrievable by a personal computer using a modem at data-throughput speeds of 300, 1200 or 2400 baud or more

Meds Colloquial for physician-prescribed medications

Medulloblastoma A brain tumor affecting adolescents, that presents with nausea, vomiting, headache, ataxia, papilledema, nystagmus, irritability, lethargy, cranial nerve palsy, dizziness, altered vision; two year-survival after relapse is 46% in those treated with salvage chemotherapy or irradiation and 0% in untreated patients (Mayo Clin Proc 1990; 65:1077)

Medullary carcinoma, breast A variant of ductal carcinoma affecting women under age 50, described as more common in Japanese women **Pathology** Often well-circumscribed, reaching a large size before metastasizing to the axillary lymph nodes **Histopathology** Prominent lymphohistiocytic inflammation peripheral to the 'pushing' tumor margins **Prognosis** 84% 10 year survival (ductal carcinoma, 63% 10-year survival)

Medullary carcinoma, thyroid (MCT) A tumor comprising 3-10% of thyroid malignancies, arising in the C (parafollicular) cells of ultimobranchial cleft (neural crest) origin; there are two clinical forms of MCT: **SPORADIC MCT** Comprises 80-90% of cases, mean age of onset 45, presenting as a solitary 'cold' (by thyroid scan) nodule variably accompanied by intractable diarrhea and Cushing's syndrome **FAMILIAL MCT** Comprises 10-20% of cases, mean age of onset 35, presenting as a multifocal and bilateral mass, accompanied by C-cell hyperplasia of the residual thyroid gland; familial MCT is often autosomal dominant and associated with multiple endocrine adenomatosis, usually type II (which has a germline abnormality on chromosome 10, with an earlier age of onset, often bilateral), or occasionally type III (less common, but more aggressive) and rarely a non-aggressive form of MCT that is not associated with other neural or endocrine lesions (J Am Med Assoc 1989; 261:3130) **Clinical** MCT presents as induration(s) that may metastasize to cervical lymph nodes, mediastinum, lungs, liver, bone and adrenal glands; the increased production of calcitonin by MCT is held responsible for the hypercalcemia, hypertension, paraneoplastic syndromes, eg Cushing syndrome and neuromas; MCTs may produce ACTH-like substance, biogenic amines, corticotropin-releasing factor, nerve growth factor, prolactin-releasing hormone, prostaglandins, carcinoembryonic antigen, melanin-stimulating hormone, histaminase, β-endorphin, 5-hydroxytryptamine, serotonin, somatostatin and thyroglobulin **Histopathology** Amyloid is a relatively constant feature, as the presence of neuron-specific enolase; microscopic patterns include carcinoid-like nests, trabecular, glandular and pseudopapillary (with psammoma body formation) patterns with variable inflammation **Ultrastructure** Abundant 80-400 nm dense-core neurosecretory granules, fibrillary material corresponding to amyloid, mitochondria and aggregates of polyribosomes **Treatment** Total thyroidectomy **Prognosis** 70-80% 5-year survival; sporadic MCT has a 50% 10-year mortality; in contrast, papillary thyroid carcinoma has 95% 5- and 10-year survival

Medullary cystic disease A group of autosomal dominant or recessive renal diseases characterized by renal cysts located at the corticomedullary junction in a background of scarring, which presents as functional tubular defects and Fanconi syndrome associated with azotemia, uremia and renal failure 3-5 years after presentation

Medullary sponge kidney see Polycystic kidneys

Medulloepithelioma An undifferentiated primitive neuroepithelial tumor of children that may contain bone, cartilage and skeletal muscle, which is highly malignant and tends to metastasize outside of the cranial cavity and when it occurs in the eye, arising from the ciliary epithelium, is known as a diktyoma

Medusa head appearance Medusa locks appearance A fanciful descriptor for anything with undulating or serpentine lines radiating from a central mass HEPATOLOGY Medusa head describes the appearance of the engorged veins that radiate from a recanalized falciparum ligament in portal hypertension most often seen in the context of advanced Laennec's or alcoholic cirrhosis MICROBIOLOGY Medusa head is a fanciful descriptor for the gross appearance of *Bacillus anthracis* (Anthrax agent) when grown on a 48-hour blood agar plate; 'medusa head' is also applied adjectivally to the light microscopic appearance of the serpentine clusters of the gram-positive *Clostridium sporogenes* PSYCHIATRY Freud viewed Medusa's decapitation as an allegory to

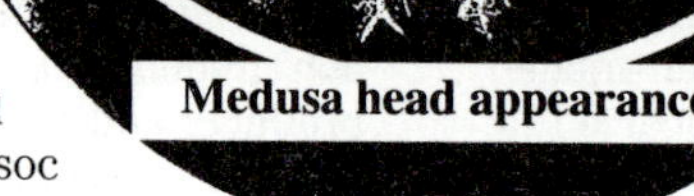

Medusa head appearance

the fear of castration, where Medusa's locks represent the female genitalia, especially those of the mother; the allegory is carried further, since Medusa's victims turned to stone, which Freud equated to an erect penis RADIOLOGY The medusa head or whirlpool sign describes a plain abdominal film finding of multiple aggregates of ***Ascaris lumbricoides*** worms in the intestinal lumen, admixed with gas, simulating the undulations of hair Note: In Greek mythology, Medusa was one of the three Gorgon sisters, who were so ugly that one look at them turned mortals into stone; Perseus found a loophole in the Mythical Law '...DON'T LOOK A GORGON IN THE EYE...', and beheaded Ms Medusa, taking aim through a mirror

Mefloquine The prophylactic agent of choice for prevention of malaria in those traveling to areas with drug-resistant ***Plasmodium falciparum***; see Malaria prophylaxis

MEFR Maximum expiratory flow rate

Megacolon A massively distended colon with decreased large intestinal activity, due to defective innervation, intraluminal overgrowth of microorganisms or of psychogenic origin **CONGENITAL MEGACOLON** Hirschsprung's disease Congenital aganglionosis A disease affecting 1:5000 live births, with a sibling risk of 1% for girls and 5% for boys; Hirschsprung's disease is ten-fold more common in Down syndrome; other anomalies in Hirschsprung's disease include hydrocephalus, ventricular septal defect, cryptorchism, diverticulosis of the urinary bladder, renal cysts and agenesis, polyposis coli and the Laurence-Moon-Biedl syndrome Treatment Resection of aganglionic colon **ACQUIRED MEGACOLON** A condition related to narcotics or disruption of ganglionic innervation, including idiopathic hypomotility, neuropathies (parkinsonism, multiple sclerosis, myotonic dystrophy, diabetic neuropathy and Chagas' disease), smooth muscle disorders (amyloidosis and progressive systemic sclerosis) and metabolic disease (hypokalemia, lead poisoning, porphyria, pheochromocytoma, hypothyroidism) and may be due to intraluminal overgrowth of microorganisms in Crohn's disease and ulcerative colitis (toxic megacolon), in the latter of which there is mucosal necrosis, transmural inflammation and systemic 'toxicity' associated with high fever, tachycardia, leukocytosis and diarrhea; in the psychogenic form of megacolon, no radiological or pathological abnormalities are present and the condition may be related to a 'fixation' in Freud's anal retentive stage of psychosexual development, with constipation of later onset than in Hirschsprung's disease, possibly secondary to abuse of the anthracine group of laxatives

Megaesophagus A condition classically occurring as a late complication of Chagas' disease, occurring 2-20 years after infection by ***Trypanosoma cruzi***, which evoke dysphagia when 50% of the ganglion cells in the esophagus are destroyed and megaesophagus when 90% are destroyed, possibly the combined result of toxic effects of the parasite and the chronic inflammatory and connective tissue response Clinical Dysphagia, aspiration pneumonia, pulmonary abscess and rarely esophageal carcinoma

Megakaryoblastic leukemia Megakaryocytic leukemia An uncommon clonal proliferation of platelet stem cells arising in severe myelofibrosis Clinical Pallor, weakness, excess bleeding, anemia and leukopenia Diagnosis Immunocytologic studies of von Willebrand factors and lineage-specific glycoproteins (GPIb, IIb/IIIa or IIIa); relatively mature, PAS-positive leukemic cells

Megaloblast An erythroid precursor with an enlarged nucleus related to vitamin B_{12} and/or folic acid deficiency, which causes an alteration in the nuclear:cytoplasm maturation, where cytoplasmic hemoglobinization proceeds normally, while nuclear maturation slows as the maturation-dependent methyl precursors (usually provided by B_{12} and folic acid) are not present; see Maturational arrest

Megaloblastic madness The neurologic manifestations of vitamin B_{12} deficiency, including alteration of personality and dementia, spastic weakness and ataxia, due to demyelination of the lateral and posterior columns of the spinal cord (subacute combined degeneration) Note: Folic acid deficiency, the other cause of megaloblastic anemia is less implicated in neurologic disease

Megamitochondria Massively enlarged mitochondria that are typically seen in the liver, classically associated with alcoholic liver disease, which also occur in malnutrition, in skeletal muscle in some myopathies and in tumor cells

Megarectum A feces-filled rectum in which electrical activity that would otherwise stimulate the external anal sphincter and puborectalis muscle has ceased, most common in the elderly, resulting in constipation; see Megacolon

Megaureter A large ureter of any etiology, divided by some urologists into reflux megaureter, obstructed ureter and the non-reflux or idiopathic megaureter

Megavitamin therapy The administration of excess or 'hyper-doses' of water soluble vitamins, either physician-guided or self-prescribed by health-food advocates; water-soluble vitamins include niacin (nicotinic acid) and niacinamide (nicotinamide), B_6 (pyridoxine, pyridoxal, pyridoxamine) and vitamin C are the most common components of megavitamin therapy, each of which may be ingested in toxic excess a) Excess niacin and niacinamide are hepatotoxic, evoking cholestasis, hepatocellular injury, portal fibrosis, causing gastrointestinal symptoms, eg nausea, vomiting, diarrhea, anorexia and increased uric acid levels b) Excess vitamin B_6 causes paresthesia, headaches, asthenia, irritability and c) Excess vitamin C increases iron absorption, possibly causing iron overload, evoking diarrhea, renal calculus formation and possibly inhibiting the bacteriolytic activity of neutrophils; Cf Decavitamin

Melancholia PSYCHIATRY Psychotic depression, which is similar or identical to the depression of bipolar disease; melancholia contrasts to the 'normal' melancholy of mourning, Freud views melancholia as an 'impoverishment' of the ego itself, as there is an internal loss (in mourning, the loss is external); because of the internal loss, the melancholic ego appears empty and has a shattered self-esteem, due to reproach and attack from the superego; melancholia is more common in women and is accompanied by helplessness, suicidal ideation or attempts

Melancholy This term, like the preceding term, melancholia, derive from Greek, melan (black) chole (bile), and, while both refer to states of depression, the former is of a degree sufficient to be considered a psychopathological state, while the latter, melancholy, is widely regarded as temporary condition, eg mourning the loss of a loved one; given the potential for confusion, health care workers may substitute 'transient depression' for melancholy, which the lay public might call 'the blues' or 'being down'--author's note

Melanin A complex polymer synthesized from DOPA and bound to a 'carrier' protein by melanocytes (skin, mucous membrane, pia arachnoid, retina, inner ear and mesentery); actinic stimulation drives production; detected in histological sections by the Fontana-Masson stain; see Albinism, DOPA, Melanoma

Melanocyte-stimulating hormone (MSH) A group of polypeptide hormones derived from the prepro-opiomelanocorticotropin (POMC) molecule and secreted in the middle lobe of the hypophysis; MSHs include a) α-MSH, which shares the 13 amino acids of the N-terminal end of ACTH and has some corticotropic activity b) β-MSH, which shares the 17 amino acids at the C-terminal end of γ-lipotropin and γ-MSH; MSH release is stimulated by MRH (an oxytocin-related releasing hormone) and inhibited by MRIH (a tripeptide release inhibitor), both of which are secreted by the hypothalamus; MSH's function in humans is unknown

Melanogen(s) A group of melanin-related compounds that are excreted in the urine of patients with well-advanced malignant melanoma

Melanoma Malignant melanoma A tumor first described by Hippocrates and identified in mummies from the pre-Colombian Peruvian Incas; melanoma comprises 1-3% of all newly diagnosed malignancies (18 000 annually) and causes 5500 deaths annually in the US, most of which in those age 30 to 50; the incidence of melanoma is increasing more rapidly than any other malignancy (Annual statistics, NCI, Wash DC, GPO, 1988; III.B.12-13, Pub # 88-2789); the incidence in Northern USA has increased from $3/10^5$ in 1950 to the current $9/10^5$, affecting the head and neck in men and rising from 4.4 to $11.7/10^5$ in females during the same period, predominantly affecting the legs (Mayo Clin Proc 1990; 65:1293);increasing at a rate of 7%/year and causing 6500 deaths/year Note: Ocular melanomas are not thought to increase the risk for cutaneous melanoma; melanoma metastasizes to liver, lung, intestine, pancreas, adrenal, heart, kidney, brain, spleen and thyroid **Molecular biology** Abnormalities of chromosomes 7 (site of the c-*erb*B oncogene) and 11 (site of H-*ras* and *ets*-1 oncogenes) have a less favorable prognosis (N Engl J Med 1990; 322:1508); loss of chromosome 6 (the responsible gene is as yet not known) is associated with melanoma (Science 1990; 247:568); an increased relative risk for melanoma is reported in those with persistent pigment changes in moles, especially in those patients older than age 15, in large or irregularly pigmented lesions or dysplastic moles, familial moles, lentigo maligna and congenital mole; caucasians are at a twelve-fold greater risk for melanoma than blacks; other risk factors include previous melanoma, melanoma in first-degree relative, immunosuppression and solar sensitivity or increased sun exposure **TYPES OF MELANOMA** (in order of aggressiveness) **PREMALIGNANT MELANOMA** One-third of lentigo malignum (also known as Hutchinson's freckle or melanosis circumscripta premelanoblasta of Dubreuilh) progress to malignant melanoma after 10-15 years **THIN MELANOMA** Stage I cutaneous melanoma A lesion measuring less than 1 cm in diameter, with virtually 100% survival Note: The prognosis is less favorable if the lesions is greater than 0.73 mm in thickness (73% five-year survival) or greater than 1.5 mm (63% five-year survival) **LENTIGO MALIGNA** comprises 10% of melanomas, and affects those older than age 60, appearing as flat, indolent lesions on the face, arising from a premalignant freckle with greater than 90% 5-year survival, etiologically linked to prolonged actinic exposure **SUPERFICIAL SPREADING MELANOMA** 70% of cases, affects those from age 30 to 60, especially female in lower legs or trunk, occurring as a flat lesion (radial growth phase) that may be present for months to years, average 5-year survival 75%, etiologically linked to recreational actinic exposure **NODULAR MELANOMA** 15% of cases, is similar clinically to the superficial spreading melanoma, boasting a 50% average 5-year survival **ACRAL LENTIGINOUS MELANOMA** is a rare, flat, palmoplantar or subungual lesion that is more common in non-whites, average 5-year survival less than 50%, unrelated to actinic exposure, but possibly related to ectopic pigmentation **AMELANOTIC MELANOMA** is rare, poorly differentiated and occurs in those with a previous pigmented melanoma; since the Fontana-Masson stain is rarely positive in amelanotic melanoma, special studies are necessary, including immunoperoxidase staining with antibodies to the S-100 antigen and ultrastructural examination for presence of premelanosomes (Mayo ClinProc 1988; 63:777) Note: Prolonged survival with metastatic melanoma may occur in rare patients, who have been reported to survive up to 20 years after histologically confirmed metastases (Cancer 1969; 24:574)

Melanoma-dysplastic nevus syndrome see Dysplastic nevus syndrome

Melanoma growth stimulatory activity see MGSA

Melanosis coli A benign condition characterized by segmental or global darkening of the colonic mucosa associated with chronic constipation, due to prolonged abuse of the cascara/sagrada family of laxatives, the anthraquinone content of which is converted to a melanin-like or lipofuscin-like pigment within histiocytic lysosomes

Melanosome see Premelanosome

Melanotic progonoma see Pigmented neuroectodermal tumor of infancy

Melarsoprol see O-11

MELAS NEUROLOGY An acronym for mitochondrial encephalomyopathy with lactic acidosis and stroke-like episodes, which first affects children and is associated with intermittent vomiting, proximal limb weakness and recurrent cerebral insults resulting in hemiparesis, hemianopia or cortical blindness; MELAS is due to an adenine-to-guanine substitution in a highly conserved portion of gene for tRNALeu(UUR), impairing the termination of mitochondrial transcription (Nature 1991; 351:236); Cf MERRF

Melasma Chloasma Mask of pregnancy A darkening of facial and neck skin with 'blotchy' coalescing hyperpigmented macules, seen in pregnancy, in oral contraceptive use, attributed to both estrogens and progesterones, due to oxidation of tyrosine to melanin, often regressing with delivery; a similar mask may appear in normal men without abnormal hormone levels, as well as those treated with phenytoin

Melatonin A hormone produced in a diurnal cycle by the pineal gland (a tissue with a verisimilitude to the 'third eye' or photosensory organ of lower vertebrates), in response to light; melatonin is synthesized from L-tryptophan → 5-hydroxytryptophan → serotonin → N-acetyl-serotonin-melatonin; its production peaks at night and controls reproductive cycling in mammals; its binding sites are concentrated in the suprachiasmatic nucleus of the hypothalamus (directly connected to the eyes and possibly also the biological clock (Science 1988; 242:78); see Circadian rhythm, Jet-lag, Shift work

Melbourne chromosome M1 chromosome A chromosome 17 or 18 with deleted short arms that had been in the past associated with an increased risk for Hodgkin's disease and follicular lymphoma

Melena see Black stool

Melioidosis An infection of the tropics by ***Pseudomonas pseudomallei***, an aerobic gram-negative bacillus found in wells and stagnant waters; epizootic infection occurs in sheep, goats and pigs; human infection is waterborne, ie not by direct animal contact Clinical Acute septicemia with disseminated abscesses in the liver, spleen and lungs (mortality without antibiotics, 90%, with antibiotics 50%), high fever, chills, tachypnea, myalgia; the chronic form has a lower (10%) mortality and is characterized by an intermittent, tuberculosis-like pneumonia, pulmonary cavitation and chronic drainage Treatment Tetracycline, chloramphenicol, aminoglycosides Note: The name melioidosis refers to the condition's similarity to ass distemper

Melittin A 26-residue polypeptide containing the toxic and hemolytic components of bee venom

Melituria A non-specific generic term for any sugar spilling into the urine, eg fructose, glucose, maltose and pentose

Meloidae see Spanish fly

Melorheostosis Lèri's disease An idiopathic condition characterized by cortical thickening of the long (tubular) bones, which when stripped of muscle, simulate a candle with wax dribbled down the side, which may be accompanied by pain, limitation of movement, contraction and/or fusion of joint spaces, generally affecting only one limb

Membrane attack complex (MAC) IMMUNOLOGY A complex of complement proteins that assembles at and later inserts into a cell membrane, causing (complement-mediated) lysis; the membranolytic sequence is initiated when complement C5b interacts with C6 and binds to C7, which becomes hydrophobic and inserts into the membrane; C8 binding causes slow cell lysis, although a fully active MAC, with accompanying rapid cell lysis requires the insertion of C9 polymers

Membrane potential Donnan potential NEUROPHYSIOLOGY That electrical potential due to the differences in the concentrations of ions on either side of a semipermeable membrane

Membrane protein A membrane-related protein that is either peripheral, ie easily stripped from the membrane and soluble in aqueous solutions or intrinsic, the removal of which requires membrane disruption by a detergent; intrinsic membrane proteins have a hydrophilic extracellular peptide segment with an end amine (NH_2) group, a hydrophobic transmembrane portion and an intracellular hydrophilic segment ending in a carboxyl (COOH) group; see Fluid mosaic model, Receptor; Cf Extracellular matrix

Membrane transport CELL PHYSIOLOGY The active translocation of a plethora of proteins from the site of production in the cell to the sites of storage or to the cell membrane for eventual release; such transport requires a) Translocation-competent membranes, eg endoplasmic reticulum, peroxisomal membrane and the mitochondrial inner membrane, b) Membrane-targeting signals to direct the molecules, often in the form of an NH_2-terminal oligopeptide with peroxisomal target proteins; the transported protein or presequence, has one of two basic structures: either a completely hydrophilic primary sequence or one which is hydrophilic at both the NH_2 and COOH ends, separated in the middle by an apolar hydrophobic core

Memory COMPUTERS The capacity of an electronic data storage device or component; memory is measured in a) **RANDOM ACCESS MEMORY** (RAM), ie that which is immediately available to the central processing unit, ranging to 128 Megabytes in the microcomputers of the early 1990s; RAM information is 'labile' and therefore lost when the device is turned off b) **READ-ONLY MEMORY** (ROM), which is information that is 'hard-wired' in the form of specifically designed circuitry, comprising a form of permanent software; see Computers EXPERIMENTAL BIOLOGY NEUROPHYSIOLOGY A process that is currently thought to be due to molecular transformation in the incoming neuronal branches (dendritic trees); each neuron may receive as many as 200 000 signals and since the sensory pattern probably stimulates relatively few sites on any 'tree', the numbers of patterns that may be stored are incalculable **SHORT-TERM MEMORY** Short-term potentiation is due to a modulation of synaptic strength by neurotransmitters, eg serotonin, acting by second messenger systems and protein kinases, to increase the duration of an action potential; protein phosphorylation decreases the number of potassium S channels causing a greater influx of calcium ions and increases the release of neurotransmitter **LONG-TERM MEMORY** Long-term potentiation is enhanced when mice are fed immediately after learning a task, a cholecystokinin-induced vagal nerve stimulation, possibly representing an evolutionary advantage by reinforcing actions that result in finding food and which should be retained in the memory; equally important to memory (for which long term potentiation—the repeated use of one of the neuron's synapses correlates with the activity of another—is becoming an accepted model) is the ability to forget, which may occur by long term depression, acting at a voltage-dependent threshold at the neuronal membrane (Nature 1990; 347:69)

Memory cell A B lymphocyte that has processed specific antigenic information, undergone a maturational sequence, ie the appropriate rearrangement of the V, D and J segments of the immunoglobulin repertoire, and which stands poised to defend the castle walls with its life if necessary, by mounting an immune reaction; see Antigen-presenting cells, Capping, V(D) J recombination; Cf T cells

MEN Multiple endocrine neoplasia Multiple endocrine adenomatosis A group of autosomal dominant, often overlapping diseases characterized by hyperplasia or neoplasia of more than one endocrine gland, many of which are members of the APUD (see there) system TYPE I Werner syndrome A complex characterized by pituitary adenoma or hyperplasia, adrenal adenoma or hyperplasia, parathyroid adenoma or hyperplasia, acromegaly, pancreatic islet cell tumors (insulinoma, carcinoid), Zollinger-Ellison syndrome, WDHA syndrome, increased gastrin secretion, peptic ulcer, Note: Non-hereditary factors may influence the expression of MEN I as the condition may be unequally expressed in identical twins; the defective gene is located on chromosome 11q13 (N Engl J Med 1989; 321:218) TYPE II/IIA Sipple syndrome A complex characterized by medullary carcinoma of the thyroid (bilateral and present in virtually 100% of cases) producing calcitonin, histaminase, prostaglandins, ACTH, potentially causing Cushing syndrome, pheochromocytoma and parathyroid adenoma or hyperplasia; the defective gene is located near the centromere of chromosome 10 (N Engl J Med 1989; 321:996) Prognosis Excellent TYPE III/IIB Mucosal neuroma syndrome A complex characterized by bilateral medullary carcinoma of the thyroid (producing calcitonin, histaminase, prostaglandins, ACTH and potentially, Cushing syndrome), pheochromocytoma, parathyroid adenoma or hyperplasia, mucosal (gut) neurofibromas, associated with thickened lips, submucosal oral nodules, intestinal ganglioneurofibromatosis, infantile intestinal dysfunction and cranial nerve hyperplasia) and connective tissue disease (Marfanoid habitus, scoliosis, kyphosis, pectus excavatum) Prognosis 20% mortality

Meningioma A tumor most common in middle-aged women, often presenting as an asymptomatic dural mass Histopathology Whorled fibroblastic tumor with psammoma body formation, divided into fibroblastic, syncytial or meningothelioma-like, psammomatous, transitional (between fibroblastic and syncytial types) and angioblastic (highly vascular); the subtyping of meningiomas is of no predictive value; aggressive meningiomas are characterized by bone destruction, florid mitotic activity and metastases; the hemangioblastic meningioma and hemangiopericytic meningioma variants are usually more aggressive

Meningismus A clinical nosology characterized by meningeal irritation without objective changes that is seen in young patients with systemic infections, eg the 'flu', pneumonia

Meningitis belt A region of sub-Saharan Africa in which cyclical epidemics of group A meningococcal infection occur about every 10 years

Meniscus sign Air crescent sign RADIOLOGY A semilunar radiolucency peripheral to a pulmonary mass lesion that was initially described as characteristic for echinococcal infection or hydatid cyst disease; the most common cause in the US for an air meniscus is a fungus 'ball', usually due to ***Aspergillus fumigatus***, although the meniscus may be seen in lung abscesses, benign and malignant tumors, hematomas, granulomatous infections and Rasmussen's aneurysm

Meniscus sign of Carmen RADIOLOGY A large semi-lunar hypodense zone that may be seen in ulcerated gastric adenocarcinomas, where there is a flattened, polypoid mass with a broad central ulceration; the gastric mucosa adjacent to the polyp is smooth, forming the smooth inner margin of the meniscus; see Whalebone in a corset; Cf Quarter moon sign

Menolipsis Menostasis GYNECOLOGY A non specific term for decreased menstruation at any time, at any age for any reason

Menopause Climacteric 'Time of life' The cessation of menstrual activity, an event that occurs between ages 45 and 50, characterized by menstrual irregularity, 'hot flashes', irritability or psychosis, increased weight, painful breasts, dyspareunia, increased or decreased libido, osteoporosis, atrophy of female tissues; see Hot flashes Note: Menopause under the age of 40 is considered premature; see Premature ovarian failure

Menstrual extraction ALTERNATIVE MEDICINE OBSTETRICS Suction extraction of an early (up to eight weeks of gestation) conceptus, performed by lay persons Equipment A sterile syringe, a rubber stopper, a one-way valve plastic tubing and jars; there are pros and cons to this unconventional, do-it-yourself-in-the-comfort-of-your-home procedure; while not wholly dissimilar to an abortion performed by a physician, the procedure is not without danger and women so treated may not seek timely medical intervention when needed; since the data is anecdotal, the claims for menstrual extraction's success may be bloated and the real or potential complications (uterine perforation, ectopic pregnancy, gram-negative sepsis and continued pregnancy) may be minimized by its advocates

Mental retardation (MR) A condition defined as two standard deviations below the mean intelligence quotient (IQ) as measured on a psychomimetic test, eg Stanford-Binet scale IQ less than 85, mild 57-67, moderate 36-56, severe 20-35 and profound < 20; formerly used terms indicating severity of mental retardation, eg 50-70 moron (Queen's English, dullard), 25-49 imbecile, less than 25 idiot, have fallen into disuse given their negative and derogatory nature; MR is classified based on ability to function or to be trained; 90% of MR is mild and 50% of those with IQs of 60-80 can function adequately in society CLASSIFICATION **IDIOPATHIC MENTAL RETARDATION** MR secondary to sociocultural, emotional and/or environmental deprivation **ORGANIC, STATIC MENTAL RETARDATION** MR that does not progress and which is largely attributable to intrauterine or antepartum events, eg hypoxia, infections, chromosomal defects, teratogens, especially alcohol, maternal malnutrition, neurotoxins and others **ORGANIC, PROGRESSIVE MENTAL RETARDATION** MR in which the infant may be normal at birth, but which undergoes inexhorable deterioration with time, eg metabolic as in the 'inborn errors of metabolism', hormonal imbalances, malnutrition, neuroectodermal dysplasia and slow viral infections Statistics 3% of any population is mildly retarded; in 15%, a genetic component is found; other causes include maternal substance abuse and exposure to environmental toxins, perinatal trauma and/or hypoxia (implicated in cerebral palsy), neonatal meningitides, metabolic diseases (eg phenylketonuria) and hyperbilirubinemia Quantification of MR: Stanford-Binet, Wechsler scales (WISC and WPPSI); Cf Psychological testing

Menu COMPUTERS A display on a computer monitor of the activities that the computer is currently capable of performing

Menu-driven COMPUTERS A feature of certain software programs that provides a simplified means ('user-friendly') of manipulating data, which for microcomputers is often used in conjunction with a 'mouse', a specialized input device; in the usual menu-driven program, a hand-held mouse is pointed to a location on the computer's monitor, a menu is 'pulled down' and a command is selected; menu-driven architectures contrast with more unwieldy and often arcane commands of non-menu driven programs, and are an integral part of all Macintosh (Apple Computer) microcomputer software and any IBM and 'IBM-clone' program that supports Microsoft Corporation's Windows 3.0; see Computers, Icon-driven

MEP Mucoid exopolysaccharide Alginate The outer polysaccharide coat of certain bacteria; the inability to produce an opsonizing anti-MEP antibody in patients with cystic fibrosis is inculpated in the increased morbidity in this disease (Science 1990; 249:537)

Meprobamate A potentially addictive sedative and muscle relaxant that blocks spinal interneurons Therapeutic levels 5-20 mg/ml Toxic levels > 50 µg/ml, which may cause hypotension, depressed brainstem functions, coma and death Quantification Thin-layer chromatography, gas-liquid chromatography and colorimetry

M:E ratio Myeloid:erythroid ratio HEMATOLOGY The ratio of maturing myeloid cells to erythroid cells within the bone marrow is normally 3-4:1; in certain conditions, the ratio may be decreased, eg hemolytic and megaloblastic anemias, increased, eg chronic myelogenous leukemia, leukemoid reactions or may be normal and not reflect any change in themarrow, since both the myeloid and erythroid series are equally affected, eg aplastic anemias, myelosclerosis, chloramphenicol toxicity

2-Mercaptoethanol (2-ME) A compound that breaks disulfide bonds, which is used to differentiate between IgM- and IgG-induced agglutination; IgM antibody agglutination doesn't occur after 2-ME treatment, while IgG agglutination remains intact

Mercaptopurine (6-MP) A chemotherapeutic agent that inhibits purine synthesis, which is a structural analog of hypoxanthine, converted in vivo to thioinosinic acid, a competitive inhibitor in purine synthesis, targeting rapidly dividing cells Toxicity Myelosuppression, anorexia, nausea, vomiting and jaundice Note: The wide variation in 6-MP bioavailability and suboptimal doses during maintenance regimens are attributable causes for the high incidence of relapse in children with ALL in remission (N Engl J Med 1990; 323:17)

Mercedes-Benz sign RADIOLOGY The finding of gallstones on plain films of the abdomen; gallstones contain intorgen gas which fills the spaces left by cholesterol crystals and appears as stellate (triradiate) translucent areas, fancifully likened to the emblem of a German motor vehicle (Am J Radiol 1973; 119:63)

Mercury ENVIRONMENT A highly toxic heavy metal widely used in household products, eg as a fungicide in latex paints (N Engl J Med 1990; 323:1096); see Mad hatter disease, Minamata disease, Pink disease

Mermaid syndrome see Sirenomelia

Merozoite A motile, pre- and extra-erythrocytic form of plasmodial parasites, resulting from the asexual division of *Plasmodium* species in the liver or red cells which either infect others erythrocytes or spontaneously develop into sexual forms: Microgametes (male) or macrogametes (female)

***mer*R gene** Mercury resistant gene The gene that encodes the MerR metalloregulatory DNA-binding protein, which mediates the induction of resistance by bacteria to mercury and other heavy metals

MERRF Myoclonus epilepsy with ragged red fibers A mitochondrial myopathy clinically characterized by myoclonus, epilepsy and ataxia, maternal inheritance; by light microscopy there are 'ragged red' muscle fibers when stained by the Gomori trichrome; electron microscopy demonstrates increased mitochondria (J Neuro Sci 1980;47:117); MERRF is attributed to a point mutation in the gene for tRNALys (Cell 1990; 61:931); see Ragged red fibers; Cf MELAS

Mesangial ring IMMUNOPATHOLOGY Annular deposition of C3, C4 and properdin in the glomerular mesangium, seen by immunofluorescence in membranoproliferative glomerulonephritis, type II Note: The mesangium is the renal stroma or matrix, in intimate contact with the filtration apparatus (foot processes and fenestrated epithelium) and is the site of immune contact, phagocytosis and immune complex deposition

MESC Ministry of Education, Science and Culture The agency of the Japanese government responsible for administering Japan's universities and funding university research; Cf SERC

Mescaline $C_{11}H_{17}NO_3$ A hallucinogen derived from the peyote cactus (genus *Lophophora*); see Hallucinogen

Meselson-Stahl experiment The definitive experiment that proved that DNA replication occurred in a conservative fashion; in the 1950s, it was not known how DNA replicated; three mechanisms had been postulated a) Conservative replication One daughter DNA double helix was an entirely new duplex and the other was entirely conserved b) Dispersive replication Both of daughter double helices had dispersed fragments from mother duplex DNA c) Semiconserved replication Each daughter DNA double helix had a conserved and a newly synthesized chain; Meselson and Stahl grew ***Escherichia coli*** in a medium containing radioactive and heavy ^{15}N (a 'hot and heavy' experiment) that was incorporated during bacterial growth; based on the flotation levels of the replicated DNA in a cesium chloride gradient, they concluded that DNA was replication in a semiconservative fashion in eukaryotic cells (Proc Nat Acad Sci 1958; 44:671)

Mesenchymal cystic hamartoma A rare lung lesion associated with hemoptysis, pneumothorax, hemothorax, pleuritic chest pain, dyspnea and combinations thereof **Histopathology** Primitive mesenchymal mass, associated with papillary excrescences in a subepithelial plexus of small airways lined by unremarkable respiratory epithelium; the masses are solid but undergo cystic degeneration above 1 cm in diameter; the mesenchymal cells are restricted to a subepithelial 'cambium' (see there) layer

Mesenchymoma A generic term for any benign or malignant tumor containing two or more mesenchymal elements in addition to fibroblasts that carries a relatively specific significance in each affected organ CARTILAGE 'Mesenchymoma' is a synonym for vascular or cartilaginous hamartoma, a benign chest wall tumor of infancy LIVER Hepatic mesenchymoma is a large, aggressive embryonal or 'primitive' sarcoma of the pediatric liver with a median survival of less than one year, characterized by necrosis, hemorrhage and cystic degeneration, histologically characterized by atypical fibroblasts and florid mitotic activity, entrapping hyperplastic bile duct-like structures MUSCLE Ectomesenchymoma A variant of embryonal rhabdomyosarcoma in which there is ganglionic differentiation; see Triton tumor

Mesenteric artery syndromes A group of clinical complexes pathogenically linked to occlusion of one or more mesenteric arteries, common in older subjects secondary to atherosclerosis, occasionally described in oral contraceptive users, possibly related to vasospasms **Clinical, early** Non-specific gastrointestinal complaints and abdominal pain **Clinical, late** Abdominal distension, shock and peritonitis **Clinical, too late** 45% mortality Note: the superior (midgut) mesenteric artery supplies the small intestine below the ligament of Treitz and the large intestine to the transverse colon; the inferior mesenteric artery supplies the remainder of the large intestine and rectum; based on the vascular supply, there is a superior mesenteric artery 'syndrome' and an inferior mesenteric artery 'syndrome'

Mesocestoides A genus of non-human tapeworms that may rarely afflict humans who eat poorly-cooked encysted muscle

Mesoderm The embryonal tissue layer that gives rise to muscle (myotome), cartilage and bone (sclerotome), subcutaneous tissue (dermatome), support tissue and matrix, cardiovascular system, urogenital system (excluding the urinary bladder), serous membranes or mesothelium (pleura, peritoneum and pericardium), spleen and adrenal glands

Mesoderm-inducing factor(s) (MIF) A group of proteins that are capable of changing the usual fate of an embryonal tissue from its 'programmed' epithelial end-stage to a mesodermal, eg muscle end-stage; MIFs are divided into the fibroblast growth factor family and the transforming growth factor β family which includes XTC-MIF, produced by ***Xenopus*** XTC cells and activin A, a ***Xenopus*** analog (Nature 1990; 345:729,732)

Mesogastropoda An order of snails, one of which, *Oncomelania hupensis*, hosts the parasite, *Schistosoma japonica*

Mesoblastic nephroma Fetal hamartoma A rare, usually benign congenital renal neoplasm first seen in early infancy, which consists of an indurated, well-circumscribed yellow-gray leiomyoma-like mass, composed of fascicles of spindled fibroblast-like cells **Treatment** Early and complete excision appears to prevent the rare cases of recurrence and metastasis

'Mesonephroma' GYNECOLOGIC PATHOLOGY An outdated term that referred to the mesonephros-like histologic appearance of two distinct ovarian tumors, clear cell (mesonephroid) adenocarcinoma and the endodermal sinus tumor

Mesonephros EMBRYOLOGY The second stage in renal development (pronephros, mesonephros, metanephros or adult kidney), which appears as an oblong mass that codevelops with the embryonal gonads and disappears with fetal maturation; residual mesonephric tissue or wolffian duct remnants are seen in adults, see Wolffian duct; Cf Muellerian duct

Mesothelioma A neoplasm of serosal surfaces, including the pleura,peritoneum, pericardium, tunica vaginalis and scrotum, occurring in 5-10% of those who were occupationally exposed to asbestos, with a latency period of 20-40 years; the incidence of mesothelioma increases exponentially if the subject is also a smoker; up to 10% of heavily asbestos-exposed workers die of mesothelioma Note: Mesotheliomas also follow radiation exposure and collapse (plombage) therapy for tuberculosis **Pathology** Fibrous encasement of organs **Histopathology** Papillary and tubular clusters of cells with hyperchromatic vesicular nuclei, prominent nucleoli, finely vacuolated cytoplasm, hyaluronic acid stain is positive, mucicarmine stain is negative; 50% of mesotheliomas are epithelial and given their tendency to exfoliate, may be diagnosed by a pleural 'wash'; 20% are fibrous with dense sarcoma-like pattern; the remaining 30% have mixed epithelial and fibrous patterns **Intermediate filaments** Epithelial mesotheliomas express both simple epithelial cytokeratins (7, 8, 18, 19), the cytokeratins expressed by pulmonary adenocarcinoma, as well as cytokeratins 4, 6, 14 and 17 and basic polypeptide 5; the fusiform cells of fibrous and biphasic mesotheliomas express vimentin (Am J Pathol 1985; 121:235) Ultrastructure Desmosomes, nuclear irregularity, free cell surfaces covered by microvilli, free glycogen bundles of tonofilaments, dense clusters of perinuclear filaments; see Asbestos

Messenger RNA (mRNA) The 'transcript' of a structural gene that has had the non-polypeptide-encoding intervening sequences of DNA (introns) spliced out, which comprises the template from which a protein is produced; see Exons, Introns, Pre-mRNA

met A gene first identified in murine osteosarcomas that belongs to the protein-tyrosine kinase class of oncogenes, which encodes a receptor for hepatocyte growth factor, transducing signals in a fashion similar to receptor kinases

met Metabolic equivalent The resting metabolic rate, which is equivalent to 3.5 ml of O_2 consumption/kg/min; the met unit is of use when planning the rehabilitation of patients who have had a myocardial infarction; Sleeping 1.0 met, desk work 1.5-2.5 met, coitus 2.0-5.0 met, walking 3 mph 3.0 met, medium housework 3.0-5.0 met, bicycling 3.5-15.0 met, shoveling snow 4.0-7.0 met, jogging 6 mph 10.0 met; see Exercise

Meta-analysis An analytical discipline ***a sui generis*** that critically reviews and combines the results of multiple studies, applying formal statistical methodology to sets of separate but similar experiments in the hope of reaching an unbiased conclusion, thus attempting to improve traditional methods of narrative review by aggregating information and quantifying impact, synthesizing large volumes of relatively recent literature; in being a retrospective discipline, meta-analysis is prone to the biases introduced by the authors of the original works; there is also up to 20% disagreement on what papers are suitable for inclusion (Science 1990; 249:455rv); R Peto and R Doll, champions of the meta-analytic process was recently awarded the Horten Research Award, an international prize, likened in scope by some to the Nobel prize (Science 1991; 254:373n)

Metabolic bone disease Any local or systemic defect in bone absorption or deposition, resulting in an alteration of the parathyroid hormone/calcium-phosphate/vitamin D axis, associated with increased bone fragility; metabolic bone disease occurs in fibrous dysplasia, histiocytosis X, acromegaly, corticosteroid therapy, heparin, hyperparathyroidism, hyperthyroidism, rickets, immobilization syndrome, bone metastases, metabolic disease, congenital (Ehlers-Danlos syndrome, homocystinuria, hypophosphatasia, Marfan syndrome, osteogenesis imperfecta), osteoporosis, Paget's disease of bone (osteitis deformans) Note: 'Workup' of these patients requires a measurement of calcium, phosphate, parathyroid hormone and other hormone levels, bone biopsy, tetracycline test

'Metabolic' therapy An unconventional and unproven form of cancer therapy that originated with Dr Max Gerson in the 1920s, which consists of bowel enemas to rid the body of unspecified toxins (putatively accumulated by an 'unhealthy' lifestyle, eating unnatural foods, preservatives, pesticides and industrial pollution), as well as dietary modifications, often supplemented with vitamins or minerals; metabolic therapies include the Gerson method, the Kelley treatment and the Manner method; see Tijuana, Unproven methods of cancer therapy

Metachromasia HISTOCHEMISTRY The property of a tissue that causes it to stain differently from the colors used in the dye; metachromatic dyes include methylene and toluidine blues and safranines; see Stains

Metachromatic leukodystrophy An autosomal recessive lysosomal storage disease caused by a deficiency of arylsulfatase A; this condition has been loosely subdivided into three clinical forms according to age of onset, where the infantile forms are the most severe, the adult form is least severe and the juvenile form is intermediate; the alleles designated I and A are defective in one-half of the cases with metachromatic leukodystrophy; early severe forms are homozygous for the I allele (N Engl J Med 1991; 324:18); see Leukodystrophy

Metagonimus yokogawai A 3 mm in length trematode or fluke found in the Mediterranean rim and in the Far East, which may be ingested with improperly cooked fish, as with sushi

Metal fume fever An influenza-like illness due to occupational exposure to copper dust or fumes, usually inhaled by miners as a sulfide ore (CuS, Cu_2S, $CuFeS_2$, Cu_3FS_3) Clinical Chills, myalgia, fever, nausea, dry throat and irritation of the upper respiratory tract, cough, weakness, lassitude and a low-grade leukocytosis; most workers develop a tolerance to the fumes that is quickly lost, thus a return to work is accompanied by a resumption of symptoms; Cf 'Monday death'

Metalloenzyme An enzyme that contains a metal ion, usually held by coordinate-covalent bonds on the amino acid side chains, or bound to a prosthetic group, eg heme; the metal ions have a function similar to coenzymes, imparting activity to the enzyme that is not present in its absence; metalloenzymes include alcohol dehydrogenase (zinc), ascorbic acid oxidase (copper), cytochrome oxidase (iron), glutamate mutase (cobalt), glutathione peroxidase (selenium), urease (nickel), xanthine oxidase (molybdenum)

Metallothionein A small, cysteine-rich, heavy metal-binding protein present in most species, the production of which is stimulated by heavy metals including cadmium and mercury, and is involved in the transportation, storage and regulation of copper and zinc

Metal shadowing Shadow casting RESEARCH A technique used to obtain information about the shape of purified viruses, fibers, enzymes and subcellular particles, where a thin layer of evaporated metal, eg platinum, is sprayed at an angle to the biological specimen; an acid bath then dissolves the biological material leaving the metal replica, which is then examined by transmission electron microscopy

Metamyelocyte The reniform M5 stage of a maturing granulocyte, morphologically between a myelocyte (M3 or M4) and a polymorphonuclear neutrophil (M6 or M7); metamyelocytes are usually confined to the bone marrow; the nucleus is kidney-shaped, with coarsely clumped chromatin; the cytoplasm is acidophilic and contains both primary and secondary granules

Metanephrine Methoxyepinephrine A metabolite of epinephrine that is normally excreted in the urine (normal, adults 0.03-0.69 mmol/mol creatinine), the excretion of which is increased in pheochromocytomas and neuroblastomas, as well as during stress, sepsis, shock or metastatic malignancy

Metanephros The embryonic precursor of the adult kidney that arises from the mesonephric ducts and nephrogenic cords

Metaplasia The conversion of one type of adult cells into another, usually occurring in epithelia Note: As it is unknown whether metaplasia has premalignant potential, there is a tendency among pathologists to consider the term metaplasia as a benign histological transformation of undetermined significance **INTESTINAL METAPLASIA** occurs in the stomach, and is more common in stomachs that ultimately develop adenocarcinoma **PANETH CELL METAPLASIA** and **ENTEROCHROMAFFIN CELL METAPLASIA** occur in the gall bladder, and are associated with adenocarcinoma of same **SQUAMOUS METAPLASIA** of the upper respiratory tract, with squamous epithelium replacing ciliated columnar epithelium; this event, which is particularly common in smokers, feeds the controversy regarding the possibility that this metaplasia may actually represent a dysplastic process with premalignant potential; squamous metaplasia of the endocervix is not associated with malignancy **TUBAL METAPLASIA** of the endometrium, ie replacement of the normal endometrial glands with ciliated (fallopian) tubal cells, may occur in endometrial polyps, mild adenomatous hyperplasia and in senile endometrium, but is rarely, and then only coincidentally, associated with malignancy

Metarubricyte Orthochromatic normoblast The last cell in erythrocytic development prior to extrusion of the nucleus; the metarubricyte is usually confined to the bone marrow, but may be seen in the peripheral blood in: Metastases to marrow, myelofibrosis, anemia of chronic disease; hemolytic anemia (increased erythropoiesis and 'spill-over' into the peripheral blood) should also be ruled out

Metastasis The distal spread of a malignant lesion, either by penetration of a blood or lymphatic vessel or by spread along a serosal membrane and eventual development into a secondary focus of malignancy; dissemination of lymphoproliferative malignancies is not regarded as metastatic, as they are by nature located within channels that facilitate widespread extension

Metastatic sequence A process that occurs in malignant cells, which consists of their extension into surrounding tissues, penetration and subsequent release into body cavities and vessels, with transportation, arrest/implantation and invasion into secondary sites, accompanied by evasion of local host defense which attempts to inhibit growth of the malignant cells at the new site; in the final step, the malignant cells create a suitable microenvironment; see Invasion

Metastatic disease panel LABORATORY MEDICINE A battery of cost-efficient tests that are used to detect, albeit in a crude fashion, the appearance of metastatic malignancy, usually of epithelial origin; the panel measures albumin, alkaline phosphatase, calcium, CEA (carcinoembryonic antigen), lactate dehydrogenase and transaminase (AST/GOT)

Metastatic tumor cell A cell that has undergone multiple changes allowing it to invade, disseminate, implant, survive and grow at sites distant from the site of origin *STEPS IN ENZYMATIC DEGRADATION OF BASEMENT MEMBRANE* collagen, type IV, progression from in situ to invasive carcinoma, include 1) *LOCAL DECREASE OF CALCIUM* causing a decrease of adherence of tissues 2) *AMEBOID MOVEMENT OF CELLS* 3) *INCREASED PRODUCTION OF VARIOUS FACTORS*; in addition the milieu surrounding the cells includes 'spreading' factors, eg hyaluronidase, type IV collagenase and autocrine motility factor and a TIMP (Tissue inhibitor of metalloproteinases) mutant which instead of inhibiting basement membrane-degrading enzymes, binds the receptors and leaves them in the 'on' position; *fos* oncogene turns on transin (an enzyme that lyses basement membrane) production (Science 1989; 244:147) 4) *CRABTREE EFFECT* Changes in metastatic cells include alterations of the cell surface carbohydrates (increased sialylation and β1-6-linked branching of complex-type asparginine-linked oligosaccharides; gp130 (a cell surface glycoprotein that is a major target of increased β-1-6 branching and the β1-6 expression) is directly related to metastatic potential; *TO METASTASIZE A CELL MUST* 1) *ADHERE TO THE BASEMENT MEMBRANE* via the laminin receptor 2) *LYSE THE BASEMENT MEMBRANE* through production of collagenase type IV and 3) *MIGRATE THROUGH THE DEFECT*; this sequence is thought to be mediated by cytokines and autocrine motility factors (J Am Med Assoc 1990; 263;1123)

Metastatic calcification Haphazard calcification occurring in sites other than bone, which may occur in the kidneys, blood vessels (vascular media), lungs, stomach, heart and eyes, usually not associated with malignancy Note: Given the considerable potential confusion that the adjective 'metastatic' (a term that the non-cognoscente often equate with the secondary spread of malignancy), might engender, the more non-committal, dystrophic calcification appears to be preferable

Meter The SI unit of length, defined as 1 650 763.73 wavelengths of the orange emission band of krypton (US 39.37 inches)

Methadone A synthetic, relatively long-acting oral opiate (figure, facing page) that was developed in Germany in World War II, which is used to detoxify heroin addicts; the L-isomeric form acts by occupying the opiate receptor, allowing methadone-maintained addicts to function in society; rehabilitation is rarely successful, and methadone maintenance is a lifetime proposition, implying a persistent opiate receptor disorder (J Am Med Assoc 1988; 260:3025); the clinical features of methadone overdose are similar to that of opiates, causing respiratory depression, stupor, and coma ANALYSIS Spectrophotometry, gas chromatography, enzyme-linked immunoassay or radioimmunoassay; Cf Heroin

Methamphetamine SUBSTANCE ABUSE A methyl derivative of amphetamine, which is more potent in its central nervous system stimulatory effect, and by extension more likely to be abused; methamphetamine has enjoyed intermittent popularity as a recreational drug and its abuse has increased exponentially in the past few years, rising to epidemic proportions **Abuser profile** Caucasian, age 20-35, high school education Form of abuse Intravenous 62%, 'snorting' 18%, oral 13% and smoking 7% **Fetal effects** Prematurity, low birth weight (J Am Med Assoc 1991; 265:1968); see Adam, Designer drugs, Eve, 'Ice'

Methanol A highly toxic polar alcohol used as an industrial solvent, in canned fuel and in antifreeze, where it may be abused as an inebrient by indigent alcoholics; methanol is metabolized to formaldehyde and formate causing significant metabolic acidosis and damage to the optical nerve and blindness; toxic range 60-250 ml, although as little as 15 ml has caused death **Treatment** Ethanol overload, as ethanol competes with methanol for sites on alcohol dehydrogenase, thereby reducing methanol metabolites and toxic effects

Methaqualone An addictive hypnotic-sedative of the quinazolone group, which is a 'schedule II' drug with similar effects to barbiturates that has enjoyed intermittent popularity as a drug of abuse **Clinical, overdose** Delirium, headache, nausea, pyramidal signs, convulsions, renal and cardiac failure and rarely, aplastic anemia **Treatment** Hemoperfusion for eliminating toxic overload **Diagnosis** Spectrophotometry, gas liquid chromatography

Methenamine A per os urinary tract antiseptic; in acid urine, methenamine decomposes, generating formaldehyde that is toxic to urinary tract bacteria

Methicillin-aminoglycoside resistant *Staphylococcus aureus* (MARSA) An organism with multiple antibiotic resistances, including aminoglycosides, chloramphenicol, clindamycin, erythromycin, rifampin, tetracycline, streptomycin, cephalosporin; in addition, some strains of MARSA have decreased sensitivity to certain antiseptics **Treatment** Vancomycin (N Engl J Med 1991; 324:601rv); see R factor

Methadone

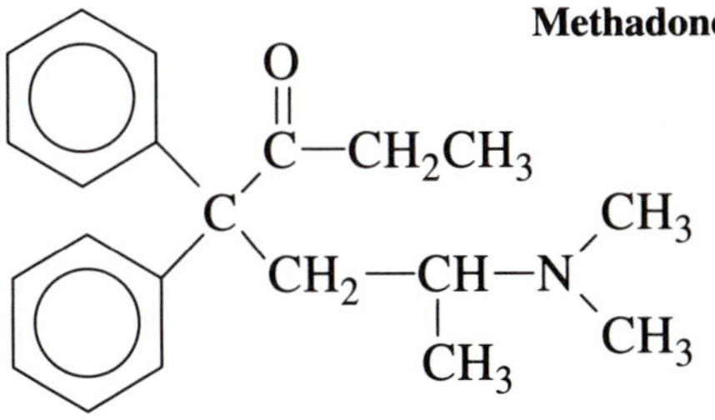

Methionine malabsorption syndrome An autosomal recessive disease characterized by albinism, hyperpnea, convulsions and mental retardation, the synonym 'oasthouse disease', derives from the hops or burnt sugar-like odor of the urine after methionine loading, which is accompanied by increased α-hydroxybutyric acid and causes the smell Note: An oasthouse is a building for drying hops, used for making beer

Method of least squares STATISTICS A method for drawing a straight line from a set of data points, such that the sum of the squares of the standard deviation from the mean of each point is minimized

Methotrexate ONCOLOGY The most widely used anti-metabolic chemotherapeutic agent, which may be used alone to cure choriocarcinoma and in combination with other agents for lymphoproliferative malignancy (acute lymphocytic and non-lymphocytic leukemias, as well as Hodgkin's, non-Hodgkin's, Burkitt's and histiocytic lymphomas, mycosis fungoides, myeloma), head and neck, ovarian and small-cell carcinomas, osteosarcoma, medulloblastoma Note: Nonmalignant conditions, eg recalcitrant psoriasis and rheumatoid arthritis often respond to methotrexate (J Am Med Assoc 1989; 261:2887); methotrexate is an anti-folate, competing with dihydrofolate (the natural substrate), for binding sites on dihydrofolate reductase (DHFR), blocking production of tetrahydrofolate (folate is the vitamin co-factor in methyl group transport for purine and thymidilic acid synthesis and DNA synthesis); see Leucovorin rescue and MDR gene Structure Pteridine ring, para-aminobenzoic acid and a glutamyl residue; MTX is metabolized to polyglutamate and derivatives Note: Tumor cells may become resistant to MTX by increasing DFHR synthesis and by decreasing the tumor cell affinity for DHR or for MTX or decreasing MTX transport into cells, polyglutamination and thymidylate synthetase activity; MTX may interfere with aspirin (by renal tubule competition), sulfonamides, phenytoin, ethanol, anticoagulants, Amphotericin B **Toxicity** Nausea, vomiting, anorexia, stomatitis, central nervous system, hypersensitivity, hepatocellular damage, ocular irritation, dose-limiting myelotoxicity may appear 4-7 days after beginning therapy, nephrotoxicity (crystallization within renal tubules) **Laboratory** Transient elevation of the 'liver function tests' **Analysis** MTX is measured by enzyme-linked immunoassay (EMIT), radioimmunoassay (RIA) and high-performance liquid chromatography (HPLC)

Methylation MOLECULAR BIOLOGY The addition of a methyl group to any molecule; this simple biochemical reaction has acquired a special significance in molecular biology, where it usually refers to the addition of a methyl group to a cytosine residue on double-stranded DNA; methylated genes are inactive and therefore the pattern of methylation is critical in gene expression, eg in the program of B cell maturation; these patterns may be passed from one generation to the next, in a process known as imprinting and genes may be demethylated or methylated de novo in accordance with the cell and/or tissue function or during normal development (Nature 1991; 351:239) Note: Phosphorylation is another form of semi-permanent gene control; see Imprinting, Phosphorylation

Methyl bromide CLINICAL TOXICOLOGY A highly toxic insecticide and rodenticide, delivered as a volatile fumigant that is three times more dense than air and absorbed through the skin, producing narcosis, pulmonary edema, renal tubule damage, jacksonian type of convulsions, central nervous system depression and peripheral neuropathy

Methylene blue A thiazine dye that is used as an indicator for theoxidation-reduction reaction, where an oxidized form is blue and the reduced form is in clinical medicine to reduce methemoglobin and used as a urinary tract antiseptic, in hematology for the 'Romanowsky' stains, eg Wright-Giemsa and in Histopathology for delineating connective tissue; Cf Toluidine blue, Trypan blue

3,4 Methylenedioxyamphetamine see Adam

Methyl green pyronine A variant of the Pappenheim stain that is used to identify RNA present in nucleoli, Nissl bodies and ribosomes

Methylmercury see Mercury

Methylphenidate CLINICAL PHARMACOLOGY An agent used to control the attention deficit/hyperactivity disorder (AD/HD) and hyperactive mentally retarded children Note: The use of this agent in mentally retarded adults is thought by some to be based on unreliable data (Science 1988; 242:27); the psychiatry community supports the data generated in pediatric use of methylphenidate for the attention deficit hyperactivity disorder

Methyl-tert-butyl ether see MTBE

'Me too' drug A colloquial term for a generic drug that has an identical formulation and stated indications for use as those agents that have passed the clinical testing phase, the appropriate regulatory hurdles and product safety standards; these drugs are usually approved 'automatically' based on their virtual identity with other previously approved therapeutic formulations

Metrizamide RADIOLOGY A water-soluble, iodinated radiopaque contrast medium used for myelography and for enhancing computed tomographic images

Metrizoate RADIOLOGY A water-soluble, triiodobenzene-based radiographic contrast medium used for angiography and urography

Metropolitan Life tables A correlative table generated from the Metropolitan Life Insurance Company that compares the weight of subjects to minimums of mortality in actuarial data, ie an obesity/mortality ratio (Sta Bull Metrop Life Insur Co 1983; 64:2-9); Cf Obesity

Metsovo lung Mesothelioma and/or pleural calcification affecting the lungs of inhabitants of a region of Northwest Greece, due to a tremolite type of asbestos contained in the whitewash used on the houses (J Am Med Assoc 1988; 260:339c)

Metyrapone 2-methyl-1,2,-di-3-pyridyl-1-propanone A diagnostic tool for evaluating the hypothalamus-pituitary-adrenal 'axis'; metyrapone inhibits 11-β-hydroxylase, the final enzyme in cortisol synthesis; the inhibition results in accumulation of 11-deoxycortisol (compound S) in the adrenal cortex, resulting in decreased negative feedback of ACTH synthesis by the pituitary, therefore increased ACTH and increased 11-deoxycortisol and its metabolite, tetrahydrocortisol, which can be measured in the urine as Porter-Silber compounds

Mevalonate 3-methyl-3,5-dihydroxy valerate A molecular precursor of many compounds, including cholesterol and coenzyme Q and carotenoids; mevalonic aciduria is a disease of infant onset characterized by failure to thrive, retarded development, hepato-splenomegaly, anemia, central cataracts, dysmorphias, marked increase in urinary cholesterol and nonsterol isoprene precursor molecules including mevalonic acid

Mexico City policy POPULATION CONTROL A 'white paper' that was released by the Reagan Administration in 1984 at the UN-sponsored International Conference on Population in Mexico City, which stated among other things, '...the relationship between population growth and economic development is not a negative one', a philosophy that is so contrary to conventional wisdom and logic that it has been termed 'voodoo demographics' (Science 1991; 252:1247n&v); see Amsterdam strategy, ZPG Note: The Mexico City policy typifies a current conservative trend in US (foreign and domestic) policy-making that holds that population growth need not be controlled, a position that explains the US Supreme Court's 'Webster' decision, see there

MFD Monostotic fibrous dysplasia

MFO see Mixed function oxidase

MG see Myasthenia Gravis

m7GpppX MOLECULAR BIOLOGY A 5' cap structure located on eukaryotic cellular RNA that facilitates binding to ribosomes and which is required for efficient translation; see eIF-4F

MGSA/gro Melanoma growth stimulatory activity/growth regulated gene A gene that encodes a protein produced in copious amounts in a melanoma as well as lung, kidney, prostate and skin cancer cell lines, which evokes autostimulation of its own production, inflammatory response, both inhibition and stimulation of cell division; MGSA/gro is a member of the larger family of growth regulators

MGUS see Monoclonal gammopathy of unknown significance

MHC Major histocompatibility complex The polymorphic gene complex that encodes the immune recognition unit located on the short arm of chromosome 6 in man and on chromosome 17 in the mouse, first identified in Japanese 'waltzing' mice; the products of the MHC gene complex are membrane-bound receptors for antigens and peptides, which when bound, are displayed to T lymphocytes; if the bound peptides are recognized by the T lymphocytes, an immune response is initiated against those peptides (Science 1989; 244:572) Class I MHC restricts the response of T lymphocytes to antigens by requiring that the foreign antigen be born by a self/native antigen-presenting cell; class I MHC includes the proteins encoded by HLA-A, -B, -C Note: chromosome 'walking' with overlapping cosmids has revealed a 435 kilobase segment of DNA that contains the genes for tumor necrosis factors (TNF-α and TNF-β) and HLA-B associated transcripts, abbreviated as BATs (Science 1989; 243:214) centromeric to the HLA-B region Class II MHC genes span an 1100 kilobase region of chromosome 6 and encode a group of membrane glycoproteins (HLA-DP, -DQ, -DR) that are

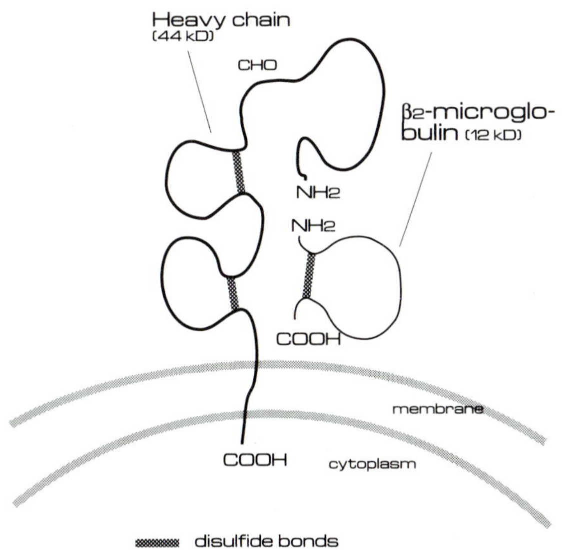

MHC I (Major histocompatibility complex I)

expressed on the surface of macrophages and B cells that bind antigenic fragments of foreign and self proteins, presenting the bound fragments to T cells; class II is a complex heterodimer with a 33 kD α and 27-30 kD β chain; polymorphism in these genes determines the specificity of an immune response and is related to development of autoimmunity; certain amino acid residues are associated with susceptibility to IDDM, rheumatoid arthritis and pemphigus vulgaris Class III MHC region is located between class I and II and the genes include those that encode complement proteins C2, C4 and factor B (alternate pathway of complement activation) as well as the gene encoding 21-hydrolase;

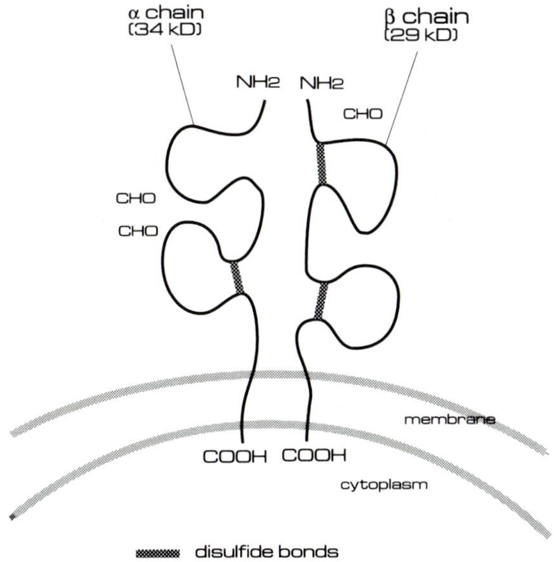

MHCII(Major histocompatibility complex II)

see HLA

MHC restriction The ability of T cells to recognize antigens when they are associated with the organism's own major histocompatibility complex (MHC) haplotype, providing a dual recognition system critical to T ell function; this selective process occurs in the thymus before a T lymphocyte becomes a functional antigen-specific cell in the peripheral immune system; the selection process operates on the α/β heterodimer of the T cell receptor assuring that the T cells will react with the product of the MHC and not with self antigens, ie the process is 'self-tolerant'; see Antigen-presenting cell

MHz COMPUTERS A measurement of clock speed for microcomputers, which is related to the efficiency of the circuit design and the microprocessor; the earliest microcomputers introduced in the 1970s, using the venerated Intel 8088 chip, had speeds of 4.77 MHz or less; the current generation of microcomputers from Apple and IBM have speeds up to 60 MHz and because of the increased 'width' of the information pathway and more advanced chips, carry far more information Note: MIPS (milion instructions per minute) and MHz do not translate well, as the systems' architecture and pathways of information flow differ substantially; the Quadra (Apple Computer, Cupertino, Cal) has a speed of 25 MHz and 20 MIPS; Cf MIPS

Microfold cell M cell An intestinal mucosal cell that overlies Peyer'spatches and has microfolds instead of microvilli, which allows the lymphocytes to approach the intestinal lumen without violating its integrity; M cells are thought to add the secretory piece to immunoglobulins, eg IgA; see MALT

MI see Myocardial infarction

MIC Minimum inhibitory concentration MICROBIOLOGY The minimal amount of antibiotic necessary to inhibit bacterial growth from a clinical isolate, extrapolated from the inhibition of bacterial growth on blood culture plate by an antibiotic-impregnated paper disk, which serves as a form of antimicrobial susceptibility testing **Method** A specimen is grown to confluence or a 'lawn' on a blood agar plate; standardized paper disks, each containing an antibiotic, are dropped on the plate and the amount of growth inhibition is measured in millimeters; antibiotic resistance and sensitivity of an organism obtained by the MIC allows modification of the antibiotic regimen; MIC can also be determined by broth or agar dilutions, but is more time consuming and labor-intensive Note: in vitro sensitivity does not ensure in vivo response to an antibiotic

Mice see Joint mice

Micelle An organized component of colloidal suspensions, consisting of spherical or laminar aggregates of polar surface-active molecules (soaps), in which the hydrophilic portion of the molecule interacts with the other members of the aqueous solution, ie are oriented 'outside' in water and the hydrophobic ends huddle together within the micelle; micelles of the small intestine are composed of bile salts with fatty acids and monoglycerides are released by pancreatic lipase; Cf ISCOMS

Michaelis-Menten equation An equation for evaluating the kinetics in an enzymatic system, which assumes that a rapid equilibrium is reached among the enzyme, its substrate and the enzyme-substrate complex, and that the initial velocity of the reaction is proportional to the concentration of the enzyme-substrate complex; the equation is defined as v = V[S]/Km + [S], or, as below, as an inverse relation, where v is the initial velocity of the reaction, V the maximum velocity, [S] is the substrate concentration and Km is Michaelis' constant

$$\frac{1}{V} = \frac{K_m}{V_{max}} \times \frac{1}{S} + \frac{1}{V_{max}}$$

Michelin tire baby An extremely rare cutaneous malformation, characterized by generalized folding of redundant skin, fancifully likened to the Michelin tire company's mascot; four cases of this condition have been reported; one had no histologic defects; another had hamartomatous smooth muscle; the two remaining cases had diffuse or focal lipomatous hypertrophy, one of whom had microcephaly, mental retardation, hemiparesis and a balanced translocation on chromosome 11

Mickey Finn A mixture of chloral hydrate in whiskey; chloral hydrate causes hypotension, pinpoint pupils, cardiac arrhythmia and in high doses, may evoke gastric irritability with perforation and hepatotoxicity and nephrotoxicity Note: Chlorals are the oldest class of hypnotics; trichlorethanol is the first metabolite of chloral and is responsible for its hypnotic effect; Mickey Finns were used in '*THE MALTESE FALCON*' to produce the alleged 'knock-out drop' effect on Humphrey Bogart, an effect not seen on volunteers (Clin Pharm and Therap 1972; 13:50)

Mickey Mouse appearance A descriptor for the facial appearance of sportsmen wearing combined intraoral and extraoral mouthguards designed to prevent dental trauma, especially in contact sports such as ice hockey and football; the extraoral guards were rejected by the players for esthetic reasons and thus never popularized as they made the players 'look like Mickey Mouse'

Mickey Mouse ears A fanciful descriptor for the appearance of the large and protruding external ears typical of Cockayne syndrome, an autosomal recessive progeria-like disease, which is accompanied by enlarged, cold and cyanotic hands and feet, dwarfism, microcephaly, mental retardation, photosensitivity, skin atrophy and scarring, retinitis pigmentosa and deafness

Mickey Mouse figures see Mariner's wheel

'Mickey Mouse' medicine A derogatory reference to non-patient-oriented duties that impact on physicians' time, eg paperwork, bureaucracies and committees, all of which are necessary to ensure quality of health care, but which do not utilize the skills for which physicians are trained; 'Mickey Mouse' physicians, an extension of the above, are those who dedicate themselves to 'Mickey Mouse medicine', ie 'medicrats' or practitioners of medical paperwork; 'Mickey mouse' in this context is an American colloquial synonym for *reductio ad absurdum*, ie anything that is not to be taken seriously, named after the Walt Disney cartoon character

Mickey Mouse sign RADIOLOGY Bilateral hydronephrosis in children seen on a plain film and made more evident by excretory urography, where the 'ears' correspond to the massively dilated ureters and the face to the bladder itself (JG Rabinowitz, Pediatric Radiology, JB Lippincott 1978) ULTRASOUND A normal landmark when evaluating the size of the common bile duct; in a transverse plane, the bile duct and hepatic artery correspond to the left and right ears, respectively and the portal vein to the head (Semin Ultrasound 1980; 1:102) Note: This landmark more closely simulates 'Mickey Mouse ears', a hat worn by members of the Mickey Mouse Club, a US television program in the 1950s

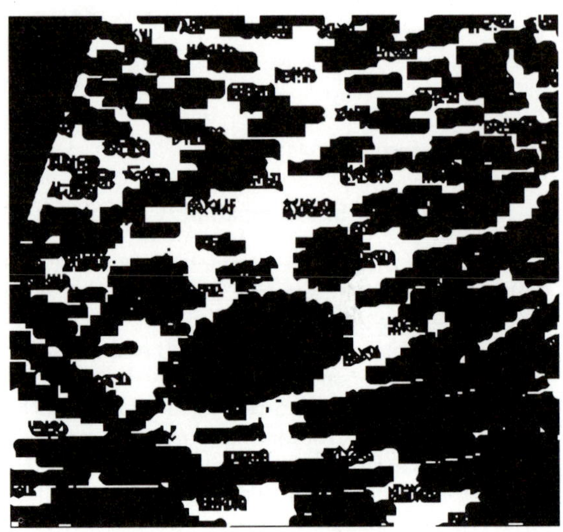

Mickey mouse sign

Miconazole A broad-spectrum antibiotic with anti-bacterial (for which it is rarely used) and antifungal activity; topical for cutaneous candidiasis, IV for systemic fungal disease (candida, coccidioides and paracoccidioides) or intrathecally for cryptococcal meningitis **Side effects** Local pruritus when topical, nausea, vomiting and fever when systemic

Microabscess A non-specific term for a focal aggregate of neutrophils that may appear in a variety of conditions, eg skin conditions, eg mycosis fungoides (Pautrier's microabscess), psoriasis (Munro's microabscess) and bullous pemphigoid (papillary microabscess) or may appear in other sites, eg in the perivascular tissues of the lung in Wegener's disease

Microaerophile MICROBIOLOGY A bacterium requiring oxygen only as a terminal electron acceptor; microaerophiles grow poorly at ambient (21%) oxygen levels and thus do not grow on the surface of culture plates and grow poorly in anaerobic conditions, eg *Campylobacter jejuni* that grows optimally at 5% O_2; see Anaerobes

Microaggregates TRANSFUSION MEDICINE Clumps of leukocytes, platelets and fibrin that may cause intravascular sludging and by extension, pulmonary insufficiency, most of which may be removed by 170 μm in diameter micropore filters

Microaneurysm An aneurysm, located in the retina of those with long-standing diabetes mellitus, which may be associated with edema and hemorrhage; see Cherry-red spot

Microangiopathy A generic term for any defect of very small blood vessels, usually capillaries, most common in diabetes mellitus; despite thickening of the vascular basement membranes, by a hyaline-like material which corresponds to advanced glycosylation end products (AGEs), the vessels are 'leaky' and allow transvascular passage of plasma proteins; AGEs or advanced diabetic microangiopathy-induced ischemia directly impacts on the retina, the kidney and the peripheral nerves

Microcell hybridization technique A method for introducing a limited number of chromosomes in a hybridization (Nature 1991; 349:340; Science 1990; 247:568, 707)

Microcephaly Any brain or head that is three or more standard deviations below the mean for the person's age, sex, height, weight and race; microcephaly is associated with many eponymic (Cockayne, Miller-Dieker, Smith-Lemli-Opitz, Rothmund-Thomson and Wolf-Hirschhorn) syndromes, chromosomal defects (cat-cry or 5p- and trisomy 13 syndromes), in utero infection (cytomegalovirus, rubella, toxoplasmosis),toxic exposure (fetal alcohol and fetal hydantoin syndromes), radiation or trauma

'Microcolon' PEDIATRIC RADIOLOGY The unused portion of the large intestine below a site of small or large intestinal atresia, which demonstrates a pencil-thin column of radiological contrast

Microcomputer A computer that uses a microprocessor (an integrated circuit chip) for its central processing unit and control circuitry; the two predominant microcomputer 'environments' in the 1990s are a) IBM-PC and IBM-PC 'clone' family of personal computers that operate in an MS/DOS (Microsoft disk operating system), using Intel's microprocessing chips 8088, 80286, 80386 and 80486, each with increasing power and speed (ranging from 4.77 Hz to 60 Hz) or b) the MacIntosh family of computers, based on Motorola's 68000 series of microchips that have clock speeds of 8 to 50 Hz; the first personal microcomputers introduced in the mid-1970s had 16 kilobytes of random access memory (RAM) with little permanent storage capacity, usually on floppy diskettes; the microcomputers available in the early 1990s have a 1.2 to 128 Megabytes of RAM, with larger RAM being required for three-dimensional manipulation of graphics, eg in space-filling models of molecules; the data is stored either on magnetic media where practical ceilings occur at around 600 Megabytes and optical storage devices which have capacities in the Gigabyte range Note: The term microcomputer is evolving toward obsolescence, as the memory and speeds of the silicon chips from Hitachi, Intel and Motorola have put minicomputer-sized computing mpower on a desktop machine; see Computers, Mainframe computer

Microconidia The reproductive form of certain fungi

Microfibrillar fibers (MFF) A group of discrete pleomorphic fibers, largely consisting of fibrillin, which is more widely distributed than elastin; by electron microscopy, MFF are linear bundles containing many microfibrils (10^{-12}m in diameter tubular threads) forming long rods, sheets and meshwork, serving as scaffolding for elastin and found in the mature tunica media of the aorta and other blood vessels, dermal-epidermal interface of the reticular dermis, ciliary zonules of the ocular lens, dura mater, cartilage, kidney, muscle, perichondrium, periosteum, pleura, skin and tendon

Microfilaments A group of elongated, 5-7 nm in diameter, cytoplasmic fibers composed predominantly of actin, which form a cytoskeletal latticework; Cf Intermediate filaments

Microfilaria Progeny of parasitic nematodes of the superfamily Filarioidea, which measure 200-300 μm in length, 5-7 μm in diameter and inhabit lymphatic channels **Clinical** Lymphatic filariasis may present as asymptomatic microfilaremia, tropical eosinophilia, filarial fever and lymphatic obstruction, which over time causes lymphatic dilatation, pitting edema and brawny edema with induration of subcutaneous tissue, hyperkeratosis, elephantiasis, fissuring of the skin and inflammation; human disease is caused by ***Brugia malayi*** Vector Mosquito ***Loa loa*** Vector Tabanid fly and ***Wuchereria bancrofti*** Vector Mosquito; ***Mansonella perstans*** (formerly ***Dipetalonema perstans***) and ***M ozzardi*** may both circulate in the blood, but being sheathless, are essentially asymptomatic; microfilaria circulate in the peripheral blood with circadian periodicity, *B malayi* and *W bancrofti* at night, *Loa loa* during the day Note: The microfilaria of ***Onchocerca volvulus*** Vector: blackfly and ***Dracunculiasis medinensis*** Vector: Copepod, a nematode, are usually confined to serous cavities and do not circulate **Diagnosis** Microfilaria are distinguished based on the pattern of the nematode's sheathing and arrangement of nuclei **Host defenses** Major basic protein and eosinophil peroxidase, stored in eosinophil granules, display in vivo toxicity against ***Brugia malayi*** microfilaria and are most effective when delivered with a peroxide-generating system and a halide, eg iodide (J IMMUNOLOGY 1990; 144:3166)

Microgamete The smaller (male), of the two motile conjugating gametes in the sexual cycle of ***Plasmodium*** species that fertilizes the macrogamete (female) during the insect phase of the plasmodial life cycle

Microglial cell A perivascular cell derived from the bone marrow, that is native to the central nervous system, belongs to the mononuclear phagocytic system, eg monocytes, macrophages, dendritic cells and granulocytes and presents antigen in a major histocompatibility antigen (MHC)-class II restricted context (Science 1988; 239:290)

Microglobulin see β_2-microglobulin

Microinvasive carcinoma A superficially invasive epithelial malignancy, which has a specific significance in gynecologic pathology UTERINE CERVIX Stage Ia A squamous cell carcinoma that penetrates less than 5 mm from the base of the epithelium or less than 7 mm in horizontal spread; anything larger is Stage Ib (Am J

Obstet Gynecol 1987; 156:263); cervical microinvasive carcinoma has a much greater than 95% 5-year survival; lymph nodes are involved in approximately 1% of microinvasive carcinomas VULVA A squamous cell carcinoma that measures less than 2 cm in diameter and with less than 5 mm of invasion into the stroma; 5% of cases have lymph node metastases Treatment Vulvectomy and lymph node resection, if involved; see Carcinoma in situ

Microlaminectomy see Laminectomy

Micromegakaryocyte A cell with a rounded, dense nucleus and 1-3 small nucleoli, seen in agnogenic myeloid metaplasia (AMM), rarely also in a blast crisis of chronic myeloid leukemia; the PAS-positive cytoplasm replete with miniplatelets or reduced to a narrow rim; also seen in AMM are megakaryoblasts with few α granules and a primitive nucleus with 1-2 nucleoli

Micromelia see Phocomelia

Micro method Micro methodology LABORATORY MEDICINE The use of smaller than usual samples (100 mg or 100 ul) for analyses, often for very sick patients or premature infants, in whom multiple specimens are required, potentially causing iatrogenic anemia; 'micro' samples may be obtain in early neonates by heel-sticks with capillary tubes

'Micro-micronodular' cirrhosis HEPATOLOGY A form of diffuse cirrhosis, which is characteristic of hepatic copper overload, or Indian childhood cirrhosis, in which oligocellular clusters of hepatocytes are surrounded by bands of fibrosis, accompanied by thickening of the hepatic vessels and diffuse ballooning degeneration of hepatocytes

Micromonosporaceae A family of fungi including *Micropolyspora faeni* and *Thermoactinomyces vulgaris*, which are responsible for Farmer's lung, see there

Micropenis A small penis; a normal infantile penis measures 3.9 cm ± 0.8 when stretched; micropenis may be idiopathic, a common finding in obese infants and boys or may be related to decreased activity of the hormonal axis, as in hypogonadotropic hypogonadism (Kallmann, Prader-Willi and Rud syndromes and septo-optic dysplasia), primary hypogonadism (Klinefelter's disease) and in partial androgen insufficiency; microphallus may be a component of a variety of congenital, eg Carpenter, Cornelia de Lange, Down, Fanconi, Hallermann-Streiff, 18q deletion, Noonan, Robinow, Williams syndromes, in hypopituitarism and in X-linked hypogammaglobulinemia

Microphthalmia A congenital decrease in ocular size, with the ocular bulb measuring as little as one-third of the normal volume in the most extreme cases, due to an abnormal development of the optic vesicle in the optic cup, which may be a) Congenital, as in encephalo-ophthalmic dysplasia, focal dermal hypoplasia, Hallermann-Streiff syndrome, incontinentia pigmenti, Lenz's microphthalmia syndrome, retinopathy of prematurity, trisomy 13-15 or b) Infectious, eg cytomegalovirus, rubella, toxoplasmosis

Microprocessor Computers The pivotal hardware component of a microcomputerthat contains the central arithmetic unit, a logic board and the associated circuitry which has been reduced in size so that it fits on one or several silicon chips; see Computer, Micro-computer, Silicon chip

Micro-protein sequencing A technique for sequencing proteins, based on Edman degradation, where amino acids are removed one at a time and analyzed by high-pressure liquid chromatography (HPLC), thereby providing a 'signature' of proteins in a cell

Microscopy van Leeuwenhoek, 1632-1723, is considered to be the father of microscopy, as he made the first practical microscope by placing a series of well-ground lenses in tandem; van Leewenhoek discovered sperm, erythrocytes and bacteria; today's laboratory light microscope is binocular and compound, having 10-15x ocular lenses and multiple objectives on a rotating 'nose-piece' ring; histopathologists often use the term 'scanning' power for 25 to 40x (ocular 10x multiplied by a 2.5x to 40x nose piece), 'low' power for 100x, 'high' power for 400x, 'high dry' power for 600x and 'oil' of 970x Types of microscopy **CONFOCAL MICROSCOPY** A variant of light microscopy, in which the light is focused in one plane allowing the organelles to be viewed in vivo below the cell membrane **DARKFIELD MICROSCOPY** A variant of light microscopy, in which the light is directed at an oblique angle and the specimen appears bright in a dark background, the method of choice for observing spirochetes (syphilis) **ELECTRON MICROSCOPY** A technique based on theories formulated by the French physicist, L de Broglie (Nobel prize, 1929), where electrons have shorter wavelengths than light and therefore a higher resolution; the first electron microscope was constructed in 1937 in Canada at 7000 magnifications; the three major types of electron microscopes include a) TRANSMISSION ELECTRON MICROSCOPE, the type with which most physicians are vaguely familiar, which has a resolution of up to 200 000 magnifications and is clinically useful for studying glomerulonephritidies and in classifying tumors, eg identifying cell junctions in poorly differentiated carcinoma, neurosecretory granules in tumors of neursl crest origin and for identifying premelanosomes in malignant melanoma Technique A beam of electrons passes through the specimen, providing a magnified image of an object on a fluorescent screen b) SCANNING ELECTRON MICROSCOPY see there c) SCANNING TUNNEL MICROSCOPY see there **FLUORESCENT MICROSCOPY** A variant of light microscopy, in which the light is projected onto the specimen by halogen-quartz, mercury or xenon lamps and re-emitted at another wavelength; although many objects naturally fluoresce; the technique is used to detect the presence of antigens or antibodies Principle A naturally fluorescing molecule, isothiocyanate (FITC) has a high affinity for the Fc fragment of immunoglobulins, which can be used to 'tag' a monoclonal antibody 'raised' against an antigen, 'X' of interest; if the antigen is present, the FITC tag allows detection in the tissue (the same principle is used in flow cytometry); fluorescent microscopy is of use in a) Detecting circulating autoantibodiesb) Differentiating vesiculo-bullous skin lesions, c) Delineating immune deposits in glomerulonephritides and d) Karyotype analysis (quinacrine staining or 'Q-banding') **INTER-**

FERENCE MICROSCOPY A variant of light microscopy, in which the light is affected by the meeting of wavelengths that enhance or attenuate interference; optical path differences in the object being viewed are converted into differences in the intensity of the image; the image produced is similar, but superior to that produced in a phase-contrast microscope **NOMARSKI INTERFERENCE MICROSCOPY** A form of light microscopy, in which the light from a reference beam is used to interfere with the light reflected from a surface, thereby producing a relief image of the reflecting surface that is not affected by variations in the refractive index of the surface **Operative microscopy** see Microsurgery **PHASE-CONTRAST MICROSCOPY** A permutation of light microscopy that is based on variations on the refractive index as light passes through an object, a technique widely-used in research to observe living cells; the phase contrast microscope separates the (normally) superimposed diffracted and undiffracted images that are about one-quarter wavelength out of phase with each other, allowing in situ observation of intracellular events **POLARIZATION MICROSCOPY** A technique that studies the anisotropic properties of objects, especially crystalline materials, see Polarization **POSITRON MICROSCOPY** A technique in the prototype phase, in which a beam of imaging particles passes through a specimen and the electromagnetic interactions with atoms in the target scatter the beam, producing a characteristic image **SCANNING ELECTRON MICROSCOPY** (SEM) A variant of electron microscopy in which the beam of electrons scans over the surface of an object, providing a three-dimensional image of the object of interest; SEM has had little use in medicine, given that the image is confined to cell surfaces, although SEM provides some information in renal pathology; SEM is of use in industry as a means of quality control of finely machined parts and in materials sciences, to detect fragmentaion **SCANNING TUNNEL MICROSCOPY** see there **SLIT-LAMP MICROSCOPY** A variant of low-power light microscopy, which has an attachment for examining the cornea **TRANSMISSION ELECTRON MICROSCOPE** see above, Electron microscopy

Microsomal enzymes A group of enzymes on the smooth endoplasmic reticulum, within cells; microsomal enzymes are abundant in the liver, are present in the kidneys and gastrointestinal tract, and are divided into a) Glucuronyl transferases and b) Mixed-function oxidases (MFO), which require NADPH and O_2; Microsomal MFOs catabolize endogenous substances, eg corticosteroids by hydroxylation and are the major pathway for catabolizing exogenous substances, eg for detoxification of various drugs, involving many reactions: N-, O-and S-dealkylation, aromatic or aliphatic hydroxylation, N- or S oxidation, deamination or desulfuration and epoxidation (epoxide: a cyclic ether composed of an O_2 molecule bound to 2 different carbons); usually, microsomal enzymes operate by first-order kinetics (catabolism at the first pass through the system) and only rarely by zero-order kinetics, which are reactions limited by substrate kinetics, as would be competition; many substances can induce hyperplasia of the microsomal enzyme system; MFO may be induced by at least two classes of compounds a) Phenobarbital and related molecules and b) Polycyclic hydrocarbons, eg 3,4 benzpyrene

Microsomes A heterogeneous group of variably-sized and variqbly-shaped lipoprotein-rich vesicles formed from ruptured endoplasmic reticulum andlarge polyribosomes, when a cell is subjected to ultracentrifugation at 100 000g for 60 minutes; at lower speeds (eg five minutes at 15 000g) mitochondria, lysosomes and peroxisomes settle to the bottom of the ultracentrifuge tube; at higher speeds (eg 2 hours at 300 000g) ribosomal subunits and small polyribosomes sediment to the bottom of the ultracentrifuge tube

Microspherocytes HEMATOPATHOLOGY Small, rounded erythrocytes observed in excess blood loss, burns, hemoglobin C, myelofibrosis and pernicious anemia

Microsporum A genus of fungi causing ringworm, see Tinea

Microsurgery Any surgical procedure that is performed with the aid of a low-power (circa 7x to 15X) microscope using special equipment, surgical thread, clamps, scalpels, to repair either severed blood vessels or nerves

Microtome HISTOLOGY An instrument used to cut histological sections; metal blades are used to cut paraffin-embedded tissues for light microscopy, at a thickness of 4 to 9 μm; glass or diamond blades are used in an ultramicrotome for cutting plastic-embedded tissues for electron microscopy at a thickness of 0.05 to 0.10 μm; see Thick sections, Thin sections

Microtubule A cylindrical, 24 nm in diameter tubule of variable length composed of α and β tubulin protein subunits that is a major component of the eukaryotic cytoskeleton and has key roles in cell division (the mitotic 'spindle' is a microtubule connecting centrioles with kinetochores during mitosis), motility, determination of cell shape, movement (microtubules are the key component of cilia and flagella), intracellular transport, eg in axons; microtubules facilitate two-way traffic of mitochondria and one-way traffic of other organelles; microtubules extend from the microtubule organizing center (MTOC) and are relatively dynamic, depending on the cell's whims and needs; microtubules may be transiently expressed, appearing as required for the mitotic spindle; others are permanent as are those associated with flagella and cilia; see also MAPs (microtubule-associated proteins); Cf Cilia, Intermediate filaments, MTOC

Microtubule organizing center see MTOC

Microvasculature The system of minute terminal capillaries, the endothelium of which secretes platelet anti-aggregates, prostaglandin I_2, procoagulant factor VIII, anticoagulant plasminogen activator, matrix proteins and fibronectin

Microvilli Finger-like projections from the surface of specialized epithelial cells, which are constructed of complex plasma membrane folds surrounding an actin microfilament core; microvilli greatly increase the cell surface and by extension, the capacity of absorptive cells; epithelial cells and their microvilli are known as the brush border, are located on the luminal aspect of the small intestine and are covered by glycocalyx, a fibrous network of glycoproteins containing glycosidases and peptidases

Microwave A wave on the electromagnetic spectrum 1-100 GigaHerz (10^9), which has a wavelength of 1-1000 mm; exposure to minimal amounts of microwaves is common with the advent of domestic microwave ovens; leakage of infrared waves ranges from 1 milliWatt/cm^2 at time of sale of a microwave oven to 5 mW/cm^2, measured at a distance of 2 inches; older pacemakers had a tendency to misfire when the wearer was exposed to the earliest microwave ovens available to the consumer Note: There is little substantive data to suggest that microwave exposure is associated with increased morbidity

MICU Mobile intensive care unit A vehicle, usually a specially-designed minivan or truck with the capacity for providing emergency care and life support to the severely injured or ill at the scene of an accident or natural disaster and which transports the patients to a medical facility where their treatment may continue; see Air ambulance

MID see Multi-infarct dementia

Mid-arm muscle area A derived value used to estimate the lean body mass as a function of skeletal muscle; 30% below a standardized value (52-55, males; 31-35, females) from the Health and Nutritional Examination Surveys (HANES) data indicates a depletion of lean body mass, ie malnutrition; Cf Triceps skin fold

Middle aged A nebulous adjective for a person between ages 40 and 65, commonly used in taking a patient's history; 'older' refers to someone between ages 60 and 80-85 and 'elderly' to those above 80 Note: To be accurate (given the average lifespan of 69 in males in developed nations); middle-aged should refer to ages 23 to 46

Middle lobe syndrome Chronic atelectasis and collapse of the right middle lobe of the lung due to extrinsic compression of the right middle bronchus by thymoma, hilar lymphadenopathy, eg tuberculosis, sarcoidosis or lymphoma, tumors or obstruction (due to intraluminal tumors or foreign bodies); the compression results in chronic pneumonitis, bronchial obstruction, bronchiectasis and decreased lung capacity; other findings, related to the primary pathology include calcified hilar lymph nodes, granuloma formation and erosion into the bronchopulmonary apparatus

'Middle molecule' toxins (MMT) A group of small, ie 3-3.5 kD molecules which include uric acid, guanidino compounds and metabolic end products, eg phenols, that are not removed during dialysis of patients with chronic renal failure and which are incriminated in the peripheral neuropathy and pericarditis commonly occurring in uremia; middle molecules may include 1-1.5 kD polypeptides; the 'MMT fraction' is also held responsible for inhibition of hemoglobin synthesis, deranged glucose metabolism, lymphoblast transformation, phagocytic activity and defective nerve conduction

Midge An insect of the Order Diptera, Family Ceratopogonidae, Genus *Culicoides*, blood-sucking intermediate host for filarial worms, eg *Mansonella perstans* and *M ozzardi*

Midgets see Dwarf

Midline granuloma Destruction and necrosis of tissues of the midline (north of the mediastinum, south of the cranial cavity, aftward of the nose and bowside to the vertebrae) of various etiologies, which may be due to 1) **IDIOPATHIC MIDLINE DESTRUCTIVE DISEASE**, see there 2) **WEGENER'S GRANULOMATOSIS**, a disease characterized histologically by vasculitis and 3) **MALIGNANT MIDLINE RETICULOSIS**, a pleomorphic lymphoma often of T cell lineage 4) **VARIOUS INFECTIONS**, see below, and other less common, less necrotizing, diseases including sarcoidosis, relapsing polychondritis and necrotizing sialometaplasia Clinical Progressive, ulcerating lesion of the nasopharynx and midline facial tissues; the pathogenesis is unclear and the disease may represent a poor immune response to various infections in an immune- or otherwise compromised patient, eg a diabetic Etiology Infection, bacterial (*Actinomyces, Brucella* spp, *Mycobacterium leprae, M tuberculosis, Klebsiella rhinoscleromatis, Treponema pallidum*), fungal (blastomycosis, candidiasis, coccidioidomycosis, histoplasmosis, phycomycosis, rhinosporidiosis), parasitic (leishmaniasis and myiasis) or malignant (squamous cell carcinoma, rhabdomyosarcoma, lymphomatoid granulomatosis and lymphoma); see Lethal midline granuloma

Mid-systolic click syndrome see Mitral valve prolapse syndrome

mid-T protein see Malignant transformation

Midwife OBSTETRICS A formally-trained person, usually a registered nurse, who assists in childbirth; midwifery is undergoing a renaissance, and provides obstetric services for lower income women, and is a delivery option chosen by some upper income women who desire a greater involvement in childbirth Note: There is an accelerating trend in litigation-oriented societies for obstetrician/gynecologists to shift their practice away from obstetrics, given the high cost of obstetric malpractice insurance and, regionally (eg inner cities, economically-depressed rural regions) increased numbers of financially-disadvantaged women, making obstetrics a 'loss leader' service; see 'Natural' childbirth; Cf Lamaze technique

MIF see Mesoderm-inducing factors

MIF Macrophage/monocyte inhibitory factor A 25 kD lymphokine produced by T-cells in response to antigenic stimulus that inhibits macrophage migration Mechanism Increased intracellular cAMP, polymerization of microtubules, halting macrophage progression; some interferons have MIF and MAF activity

Mifepristone see RU 486

Migraine A form of vascular headache of unknown etiology in which the pain is caused by dilatation of a branch of the carotid artery, stimulating the nerve endings supplying that artery; the release of vasomotor substances, eg bradykinin, histamine, prostaglandins, serotonin and substance P, which have a noxious effect on nerve endings; migraine headaches are subdivided into classic, common, complicated and variant forms of migraines **Clinical** 'Classic' migraines are most common in females, with the first migraine appearing before puberty and remitting at menopause **Treatment** Prevention by avoidance of precipitating factors; if conservative measures fail and the attacks are more common than once/week, pharmacologic prophylaxis is indicated, the safest agent is propranolol, while the most effective is methysergide, a serotonin antagonist with significant side effects, including vascular insufficiency, retroperitoneal and pleural fibrosis and fibrosis of the cardiac valves; treatment failures may respond to verapamil, amitriptyline or the recently available sumatriptan

Migrating testis Elevator testicle A testicle that is highly mobile within the inguinal canal, which may even migrate into the abdominal cavity; such cases require urological surveillance, as they have an increased risk for testicular torsion

Migratory thromboembolism Trousseau phenomenon Thrombophlebitis occurs in up to 10% of patients with malignancy, classically seen in mucin-secreting gastrointestinal adenocarcinomas, but may also occur in carcinoma of the breast, lung, ovary and prostate Note: Trousseau described this sign in himself, and it presaged his own death by pancreatic adenocarcinoma

Miliaria/miliary/milium Latin, millet seed

Miliaria Prickly heat DERMATOLOGY A skin lesion caused by the retention of sweat within keratin-plugged eccrine sweat glands and ducts; in the face of increased pressure, retained sweat leaks into the dermis causing erythema and inflammation, variably accompanied by pruritus, appearing as multiple papules on the skin surface, affecting overbundled children in winter, soldiers in the tropics and in fever **Clinical** Pruritus and hypohidrosis may cause irritability and insomnia Note: The clinical variant terms of miliaria crystallina (minute superficial, non-inflamed clear fluid-filled vesicles), miliaria profunda (deep lesions) and miliaria rubra (deeper lesion with papulovesicles and intense erythema, confined to flexures, accompanied by maceration, candidiasis and folliculitis in the diaper region) appear to reflect intensity and have no diagnostic utility; Cf Diaper dermatitis

Miliary An adjective for any disseminated process comprised of innumerable millet-seed sized lesions, classically seen in miliary tuberculosis in the pre-antibiotic period, where the 'millet seeds' correspond to granulomas; also refers to disseminated histoplasmosis and cytomegalovirus pneumonitis

Milium Whitehead DERMATOLOGY Multiple, small subepithelial keratin cysts, often located on the face, which may be present from infancy onwards, which may occur in young women after sunbathing, consisting of innocuous lesions arising in eccrine sweat ducts

Milk see Breast milk, Unpasteurized milk

Milk-alkali syndrome A condition characterized by hypercalcemia due to excess consumption of dairy products, overuse of calcium-containing (> 5g/day) antacids or alkalis (for treating peptic ulcer, eg Sippy antacid diet, of largely historical interest) **Laboratory** Hypercalcemia, severe compensated metabolic alkalosis, normo- to hyperphosphatemia; long-term metabolic derangement may cause renal failure through a combination of nephrocalcinosis, loss of ability to compensate for the alkalosis and dehydration

Milker's nodes Paravaccinia An infection by a bovine parapoxvirus that occurs through direct inoculation while manually milking cows, characterized by red-blue firm and tender nodules which may develop into a papulovesicular eruption of the arms and extremities and disappear in 1-2 weeks

'Milking' CARDIOVASCULAR SURGERY The gentle squeezing of any blood vessel, often a distal vein or the extremity itself, 'milking' it in the proximal direction in an attempt to extract a non-adherent thrombus

'Milk' leg OBSTETRICS Phlegmasia alba dolens Extensive deep vein or iliofemoral thrombosis due to stasis of uterine blood, accompanied by painful swelling and pallor of the entire extremity, a condition formerly common in parturition (hence, 'milk leg'), more often seen in recent abdominal or pelvic surgery; with progression, all the veins become thrombosed, blood cannot return to the heart and the leg becomes cool, painful and cyanotic, known as phlegmasia cerulea dolens or painful blue leg

Milk let-down see Let-down reflex

Milkmaid's grip NEUROLOGY A sign of generalized muscle weakness and the inability to maintain tetanic muscle contraction; the subjects, when asked to squeeze the examiner's fingers, do so by a 'milking' motion of contraction and relaxation, a finding typical of Sydenham's chorea, one of Jones' major criteria for diagnosing rheumatic fever

Milkman syndrome Generalized osteomalacia A radiologist's disease, characterized by alternating symmetrical radiolucent bands or pseudofractures, corresponding to resorption with mineralization adjacent to arteries, a condition that responds to vitamin D therapy

Milk-of-calcium appearance An appearance resulting from minute concrements composed of calcium carbonate, which have a 'sandy' or 'ground-glass' radiological appearance and seemingly float as a suspension, within pyelogenic cysts, simple cortical cysts of arterionephrosclerosis and in the cysts of polycystic kidney disease; the substance is best identified in plain films as a bilayer, with fluid on top and a granular layer on the bottom, separated by the whims of body position and gravity; a similar appearance may be seen in obstructed gall bladders

Milk-rejection sign An anecdotal clinical observation that breast-fed infants will not take milk from a breast affected by carcinoma (Cancer 1966; 19:1185); in a similar context, infants tend to suck less when the mother has ingested alcohol prior to breast feeding (N Engl J Med 1991; 325:981), related to objective changes in the quality of the milk

Milk spots Large lactescent patches on the left cardiac ventricular surface seen by gross examination in idiopathic dilated cardiomyopathy, corresponding to ischemia-induced fibrosis due to long-standing focal hypoxia

Milk stool PEDIATRICS The viscid dark green neonatal feces, ie meconium, gives rise to yellow-green and more liquid stools that later develop into the firm caramel-to-milk chocolate stool of the milk-fed infant Note: The stool of human milk-fed infants is looser and less malodorous than those fed cow's milk

Milk sugar Colloquial for lactose

Millwheel murmur CARDIOLOGY A descriptor for the precordial murmur heard in significant (ie greater than 200 ml) venous air embolism, which is accompanied by increased pressure, cyanosis, tachycardia, and syncope

Milwaukee shoulder A painful, destructive, bilateral upper girdle dysfunction of the elderly female consisting of capsular calcification, joint effusions (increased collagenase without inflammation), erosion of rotator cuff tendons and glenohumeral joint degeneration on the dominant side; the condition is worse at night or following heavy usage with accumulation of basic calcium phosphate crystals in inflamed joints

MIM number A numerical assignment given to any inherited disease that is listed in VA McCusick's comprehensive and monumental catalog Mendelian Inheritance in Man; each condition is given a five digit number, where 10005-19447 correspond to autosomal dominant conditions, 20010-27900 to autosomal recessive conditions and 30002-31500 to X-chromosome linked conditions

Mimotope A peptide sequence that immunologically mimics an antigen's epitope without having sequence homology to the antigenic site, an effect that is due to mimicry of the three-dimensional conformation of the epitope

Minamata disease ENVIRONMENT A disease that spanned 15 years, first recognized in 1953 in the city of Minamata, a coastal community in southwest Japan, caused by consumption of fish and shellfish contaminated with organic methylmercury (inorganic mercury is not considered to be a major teratogen) discharged into nearby rivers by industrial plants that produced acetaldehyde, which used mercury as a reactive catalyst; by 1972, 704 cases had been confirmed in all age groups in Minamata and 121 in Niigata City, 40 of whom were affected in utero (1200 more cases were unconfirmed) Clinical Severe mental and neurological impairment, degenerative changes of the cerebral and cerebellar cortex, paresthesias, blindness, deafness, inability to concentrate, dysarthria, tremors which may evolve to a persistent vegetative state; a similar epidemic occurred in Iraq when grain treated with a methylmercury fungicide, intended for planting was baked into bread, resulted in 6530 cases of poisoning and 459 deaths; Cf Bhopal, Haff disease, Mad hatter syndrome, Mercury, Toxic oil and Yusho oil syndromes

Mineralization An in vivo precipitation of mineral salts, usually calcium and phosphate due to a focal increase in concentration

Minerals, dietary Those metallic elements that are required for optimal functioning of the body; dietary requirements for minerals range from molar to trace amounts/day **MAJOR MINERALS, BONE** Calcium, phosphate, magnesium **MAJOR MINERALS, ELECTROLYTES** Sodium, potassium, chloride **MINOR MINERALS, METALLOPROTEINS** Iron, copper, manganese, iodine, cobalt, molybdenum, selenium, chromium, fluoride and zinc **TRACE MINERALS** Nickel, silicon, vanadium and tin

Mineral oil A mixture of liquid petroleum-derived hydrocarbons with a specific gravity of 0.818-0.96; mineral oil was formerly used with impunity as a vehicle for drugs applied to the nasal mucosa and internally as a laxative; when applied too liberally, mineral oil may evoke exogenous lipid pneumonia; although mineral oil may be used as a laxative without major adverse effect; excess use of mineral oil as a laxative may cause anorexia, malabsorption of fat-soluble vitamins and absorption of the oil itself; see Lipoid pneumonia

Minicomputer An increasingly obsolete term that was defined as a computer with a speed and memory capacity that fell between that of a microcomputer (speed measured in MegaHerz, the first of which had speeds of 4.77 MHz and 16 to 64 kilobytes of memory) and that of a mainframe computer (speed measured in MIPS or million instructions per second and a memory of hundreds to thousands of megabytes of data storage capacity); the current generation of personal (micro-) computers has surpassed some of the features, eg speed and memory capacity of minicomputers; the recently-released Apple Quadra has speeds measured in both MHz (25 MHz) and MIPS (20 MIPS); see Computers, Mainframe computer, Microcomputers

Minichromosome Artificial chromosomes that have been created by linking restriction endonuclease digested fragments of DNA

Minigene A segment of a gene that encodes a variable region of either the heavy or light chain of an immunoglobulin

'Minilap' An abbreviated laparotomy used to obtain cells, document intraperitoneal hemorrhage, obtain fluids for determining the presence of bile amylase, bacteria or fecal material by peritoneal lavage

Mini-mental test NEUROLOGY A brief clinical evaluation of mental status, where each correct answer in a series of questions is given one point for a total score of 30: Time orientation Year, season, month, date, day (total 5 points) Space orientation Country, state, county, town, place, hospital ward (5 points) Cognition Serial sevens (X 5) or spell world backwards (5 points) Short recall Name three objects (total 3 points) Memory Rename three above objects (3 points) Follow a three-part command Take a paper, fold it, put it on the floor (3 points) Common object recognition Name two familiar objects (2 points) Recognition of common phrase 'No ifs, ands, or buts' (1 point) Read and obey 'Close your eyes' (1 point) Write simple sentence (1 point) Copy drawing Intersecting pentagons (1 point); a person with a change in mental status and a score of greater than 27 points most often has affective depression; patients who are depressed and have cognitive impairment have scores of about 20 and those with true dementia often have scores of less than 10 (J Psych Res 1975; 12:189)

Minimum bactericidal concentration (MBC) MICRO-

BIOLOGY The lowest concentration of an antibiotic that is bactericidal to at least 99.9% of an original inoculum; MBC is a form of antibiotic susceptibility testing in which an antimicrobial agent in broth is serially diluted, or titrated in a standardized (McFarland) suspension of bacteria; tubes in which there is no growth are subcultured in an antibiotic-free growth medium; the MBC may vary as a function of certain intrinsic features of the bacterium, see Persistence phenomenon, Paradoxic effect and Tolerance Note: It is unclear whether determination of the MBC is indicated for streptococcal endocarditis, staphylococcal endocarditis or osteomyelitis and Enterobacteriaceae or *Pseudomonas* species from patients with meningitis, given the poor correlation between *in vitro* sensitivity and *in vivo* effectiveness

Minimum inhibitory concentration MICROBIOLOGY A laboratory test in which the lowest concentration of an antibiotic to be administered to a patient is extrapolated from a group of 'bench' tests, including serial dilution of an antibiotic in broth, the disk elution test and determination of the diameter of nongrowth surrounding a paper disk impregnated with antibiotics, known as the disk diffusion test

Minimum lethal dose The dose of any noxious substance or agent, eg bacterium, chemical, drug, ionizing radiation or virus that is lethal to 100% of a test population

'Minipill' An oral contraceptive that contains only the progestational agent, norethindrone in very low amounts (0.35 mg); the minipill reduces sperm penetration of the cervical mucus by interfering with luteinization, decreasing gonadotropin secretion and by interfering with implantation; the minipill may be slightly less effective than combined contraceptives and has been associated with dysmenorrhea; Cf Norplant, RU 486

Minisatellite MOLECULAR BIOLOGY A short (1-5 kilobase pair) region of simple sequence DNA comprised of 20-50 repeats of 15-100 nucleotide in length sequences, a size that distinguishes them from DNA satellites, which measure 10^5 to 10^6 bases in length; the small size of minisatellites allows facile Southern blotting and highly specific identification of individual subjects by determination of restriction fragment length polymorphisms (see RFLP), which are often associated with moderately repeated sequences; minisatellites are used for DNA 'fingerprinting', paternity testing, forensic medicine and human genome mapping; see Double minutes

'Minnesota experiment' A protocol which determined the physiological consequences of malnutrition; 32 male volunteers were semi-starved for six months, resulting in decreases in body weight (24%), cardiac stroke volume (18%), cardiac index (38%), vital capacity (8%) and tidal volume (19%); other changes of voluntary starvation include decreased enzymatic activity, decrease in organ size, slowing of metabolism, increased transit times, poor wound healing and immune dysfunction; see Kwashiorkor, Marasmus

Minnesota Multiphasic Personality Inventory see MMPI

Minor crossmatch TRANSFUSION MEDICINE The testing of a patient's cells against a potential donor's serum to detect the presence of ABO incompatibility and other major antibodies; see Immediate spin crossmatch, Major cross-match; Cf Back typing, Front typing

Minor groove MOLECULAR BIOLOGY A shallow 'furrow' in a DNA double helix measuring 1.2 nm across, which extends the entire length of DNA as long as the molecule remains in a normal or right-handed DNA conformation; see DNA forms, Major groove

Minor histocompatibility peptides H antigens Minor antigens identified include: That encoded by the H-3 gene, β_2-microglobulin and the male-specific H-Y antigen; nearly 50 other genes have been mapped but incompletely identified (Science 1990; 249:286)

Minor lymphocyte stimulating genes see Mls genes

Minoxidil A drug, which when administered per os, is a direct vasodilator, first used for severe refractory hypertension; side effects of oral minoxidil include sodium and water retention, pericardial effusion, hypertrichosis and hirsutism; as a 1-5% topical solution, minoxidil evokes terminal hair growth in 8-31% of men suffering early (less than five years duration) androgenic or male pattern baldness (J Am Med Assoc 1989; 261:2838); normal scalp hair density is 500/cm^2; minoxidil increases the thin areas by 83 hairs/cm^2, yielding satisfactory results for up to 48% of those treated **Mechanism** Unknown, although it may be related to local vasodilation

Minus-minus phenotype see Null phenotype

Minus strand A segment of DNA, produced by a single-stranded DNA virus infecting a eukaryotic host cell, which is complementary or antiparallel to the first strand; when such segments are derived from the virus, they are termed 'plus' strands and the complementary strand is designated the 'minus' strand

Minutes (pronounced min-uhhts) The record that summarizes the proceedings of a committee meeting and its important points

Minutes (pronounced mai-'n(y)üts) see Double minutes

MIP-1 Macrophage inflammatory protein A heparin-binding protein secreted by macrophages in response to endotoxin; MIP-1 differs from other endogenous pyrogens, eg tumor necrosis factor (TNF) and IL-1, as its effect is not mediated through prostaglandin synthesis (and therefore is not abrogated by cyclooxygenase inhibitors, eg ibuprofen) (Science 1989; 243:1066)

MIPS Million instructions per second A measurement of speed for mainframe computers, as used in computed tomography, which process information at speeds of 20 or greater MIPS; the speeds of the Cray and Hitachi supercomputers are giving press to a new acronym, GIPS for a billion (Brit: Milliard) instructions per second; Cf MHz

Mirror image biopsy A biopsy of the contralateral breast when lobular carcinoma-in-situ is found in one breast, a procedure that is necessary to rule out invasive carcinoma Note: Lobular carcinoma-in-situ is associated with a 1% annual risk of malignant degeneration and thus requires close follow-up; Cf Lumpectomy

Mirror syndrome The maternal mirror syndrome is a poorly understood clinical phenomenon in which the mother displays the same physiopathological conditions, eg hydrops, as her fetus, possibly causing high-output cardiac failure in the mother, which is postulated to be related to the release of hormones or vasoactive substances by the placenta

MIS Medical information system see Hospital information system, Laboratory information system

Misadventure An accident or unintentional act, as in an occupation-related 'homicide by misadventure'; in medicine, the term has become an elegant euphemism for a therapeutic 'boo-boo'*, as in a surgical misadventure, in which the wrong leg was amputated; see Mistake; Cf Miscall

Miscall A diagnostic 'boo-boo'*, as in a pathologist miscalling a benign tumor as malignant, see Misdiagnosis; Cf Misadventure

*'Boo-boo' is a widely used American contribution to low-brow lexicography, used for 1) Children who have small cuts, or bruise, as in '...baby has a boo-boo..' and 2) Adults who have commited a blunder, as above, a term of uncertain parentage

Misconduct see Fraud in science

Misdiagnosis The incorrect diagnosis of a morbid condition; misdiagnosis alone is insufficient to result in a successful lawsuit for malpractice if the physician can support the contention that he exercised reasonable and prudent medical judgement in arriving at a diagnosis in accordance with accepted medical standards; the plaintiff must then prove that the misdiagnosis caused injury; see Overcall, Undercall

Mismatch phenomenon NEUROPHYSIOLOGY A ratio of neurotransmitter to neuroreceptor that differs from the expected 1:1; high concentrations of neuroreceptors for substance P are found in the neocortex and hippocampus, although the neurotransmitters themselves are in low concentrations; such a mismatch implies the presence of another system(s) of cell communication, which may have a role in non-synaptic interaction among cells

Mismatch repair system (MRS) MOLECULAR BIOLOGY A set of proteins that detects errors in the nucleotide base sequences of newly synthesized strands of DNA; if the new strand does not complement the template strand on which it is being modeled, the MRS excises the defective segment with a portion of up- and downstream DNA; DNA polymerase then fills in the gaps; the MRS prevents incompatible DNA from existing, ie between even closely-related species from cross-breeding, thus erecting a reproductive barrier against 'erroneous' new strand formation; Cf Patch and cut repair

Misoprostol A prostaglandin E_1 analog used to reduce acute rejection of renal allografts, a phenomenon partially due to ischemic damage of kidneys that occurs between the time of 'harvesting' and re-establishment of the blood flow; misoprostol-treated group subjects suffered acute rejection one-half as often as the placebo group (N Engl J Med 1990; 322:1183); Misoprostol is also of value in preventing NSAID-induced gastric ulceration, in patients with a history of gastrointestinal bleeding (J Am Med Assoc 1990; 264:41)

Mispairing The mismatching of nucleotides or noncomplementary pairing of DNA strands that may occur in low-stringency hybridization studies; see Low stringency; Cf High stringency

MISS Modified Injury Severity Scale A method for quantifying pediatric multi-trauma injuries; MISS is the sum of the squares of the 3 most injured body regions, modified from the American Medical Association's abbreviated injury scale (AIS; burn victims are not included in the analyses), substituting the Glasgow coma scale for neurological evaluation

Missense codon Any altered codon (triplet of DNA nucleotides) that encodes an incorrect amino acid or stop signal, resulting in an altered or non-functioning protein product

Mistake Medical mistake An act, omission or error in judgement by a health care provider that has or may have serious consequences for a patient and that would be judged to be wrong by knowledgeable peers; for physicians in residency training, these errors include errors in diagnosis (33%), prescribing (29%), evaluation (21%), procedural complications (11%) and communication (5%); one-half discussed the mistake with superiors and one-fourth discussed it with non-medical peers or with the patients themselves (J Am Med Assoc 1991; 265:2089); Cf Misdiagnosis, 'Overcall', 'Undercall'

Mithridatism Tolerance developed against a toxin, which is induced by gradual incrementation of the toxin, a technique likened to tolerization therapy used in allergy medicine and named after Mithridates VI (131-63 BC), the king of ancient Pontus; Rasputin, the 'mad monk' was thought to have ingested increasing amounts of strychnine for this purpose

MITI Ministry of International Trade and Industry The central agency of the Japanese government encharged with coordinating research activities with industry; MITI recently opened up the rights to patenting R&D projects (Nature 1991; 350:102n)

Mitmachen German, to do with NEUROLOGY A finding in catatonic patients, who despite instructions to the contrary, allow an extremity to be placed in any position without resistance to light pressure, and then return the body part to the original resting position, once the extremity is released by the examiner

Mitochondria Intracellular organelles invested with their own DNA and energy-producing enzymatic machinery, including the electron transport chain complexes of oxidated phosphorylation, which are grouped as complex I, the NADH dehydrogenase system, complex II (Succinate dehydrogenase system), complex III (cytochrome b-c complex) and complex IV (cytochrome oxidase C); see mitochondrial DNA

Mitochondrial disease A group of multisystem disorders, defined as biochemical abnormalities of the mitochondria or muscle groups Group 1 Progressive external ophthalmoplegia a) Kearns-Sayre disease (due to multiple 1.3 to 7.6 kilobase deletions of mitochondrial DNA, N Engl J Med 1989; 320:1293) b) Ocular myopathy c) Leber's hereditary optic neuropathy (due to a point mutation, N Engl J Med 1989; 320:1300) Group 2

Mitochondrial encephalomyopathies a) Mitochondrial encephalomyopathy with lactic acidosis and stroke-like episodes, see MELAS b) Myoclonus epilepsy with ragged red fibers see MERRF c) Leigh syndrome Group 3 Undefined mitochondrial encephalomyopathies, eg congenital lactic acidosis Group 4 Mitochondrial myopathies a) Luft syndrome b) Enzyme defects, eg ATPase, cytochrome oxidase

Mitochondrial DNA (mtDNA) Mitochondria have their own DNA that is smaller and different from nuclear DNA; mtDNA measures 16.5 kilobases and is a circular double helix with 13 structural genes encoding respiratory chain elements, 22 tRNA genes and 2 genes that encode the 16S and 12S mitochondrial rRNAs that translate into the proteins responsible for the mitochondrial energy pathway, including NADH dehydrogenase, cytochrome c oxidase, ATP synthase and ubiquinol-cytochrome c oxidoreductase Note: Mitochondria are inherited in a non-mendelian fashion from the mother, evolves much more rapidly than nuclear DNA

Mitochondrial encephalopathies of Shapiro A clinically heterogeneous group of multisystem diseases that have in common, neuromuscular manifestations, due to abnormalities of the protein complexes of the electron transport chain of oxidative phosphorylation, including an array of syndromes, including Alper, Kearn-Sayres, Leigh, Lowe, Menke's kinky hair and Zellweger syndromes, lactic acidosis, Luft disease, MELAS, MERRF, rhizomelic chondrodysplasia punctata and stroke-like episodes

Mitochondrial Eve ANTHROPOLOGY A hypothetical 'mother of mankind', who is postulated to have lived in Africa circa 200 000 years ago (Science 1991; 253:1503); the ancestry of this first female ***Homo sapiens*** is inferred from phylogenetic trees constructed from restriction fragment length polymorphisms of mitochondrial DNA that are passed only by females; analysis of mitochondrial DNA may ultimately identify the female at, or close to the root of the phylogenetic tree; see Anthropology, Lucy; Cf Urkingdom

Mitogenesis theory A model for carcinogenesis that holds that the rate-limiting step in malignant transformation is the induction of increased cell division; the theory is supported by the fact that low-doses of environmental toxins, eg dioxins and others are not genotoxic and contrasts with the more 'mainstream' multistep process theory of carcinogenesis, in which low-level toxic exposures may be one of the 'steps' in malignant transformation

Mitotic activity The degree to which a cell population is proliferating, which is an indicator of tumor aggression, measured as the frequency of cell division; mitotic activity can be semiquantified by the relatively crude counting of mitotic figures per high-power field, or by flow cytometry; see Flow cytometry, High power fields

Mitotic spindle MOLECULAR BIOLOGY A transiently expressed structure that organizes the chromosomes and cytoplasm, which is composed predominantly of relatively labile microtubules, too thin to be studied by conventional light microscopy, requiring instead polarization microscopy; three types of microtubules or fibers are present in the spindle: 1) Polar fibers extending from one of the spindle poles to the equator, 2) Kinetochore fibers extending from the chromosome's centromere toward the pole and 3) Astral fibers extending from the mitotic pole to the periphery of the cell; see MTOC

Mitral facies CARDIOLOGY A physiognomy characterized by florid malar flushing associated with mitral valve stenosis; other physical findings in mitral valve stenosis include distended jugular veins with an 'a' wave, an accentuated first heart sound at the apex, an opening snap and a diastolic rumble

Mitral valve prolapse syndrome Barlow syndrome Floppy valve syndrome A condition most commonly affecting young females, in which the mitral valve prolapses into the left atrium, a condition that affects up to 5% of the general population, potentially causing sudden death by arrhythmia or rupture of cordae tendinae EKG Inverted T waves in II, III, aV_F leads, prolongation of Q- Histopathology Myxoid degeneration of valves with an increase of ground substance (Br Heart J 1968; 30:203)

Mittelschmerz German, Middle pain GYNECOLOGY Pain of the lower female abdomen at the time of ovulation, due to a ruptured graafian follicle

Mitten-hand deformity An end-stage lesion in the autosomal recessive dystrophic epidermolysis bullosa, with fusion of digits, loss of fingernails and dermal fibrosis Clinical Failure to thrive, growth retardation, repeated infections, subepidermal blistering and 'weeping' of lesions, involvement of the oro-genital mucosae, esophageal fibrosis with malnutrition and flexion contractions of joints

Mixed connective tissue disease (MCTD) Sharp syndrome Overlap syndrome A connective tissue disease that has features of systemic lupus erythematosus, dermatomyositis and rheumatoid arthritis; MCTD is considered unique as it has a speckled nucleolar pattern due to the presence of a specific circulating antibody, high titers of ribonucleoprotein and a relatively good clinical response to corticosteroid therapy; see Antinuclear antibodies, 'Chinese menu' diseases, Overlap syndrome

Mixed field agglutination TRANSFUSION MEDICINE An in vitro phenomenon, in which two or more different populations of red cells are present in the test tube, resulting in varying intensities of agglutinating reactions, eg one cell population may agglutinate strongly and another weakly or not at all; the most common cause of mixed field agglutination is a recent blood transfusion, other causes include hemolytic disease of the newborn, twin-to-twin in utero transfusion, weak subgroup of A (often A_3) or B, leukemia, Tn polyagglutination, true chimeras; pseudo-mixed field agglutination occurs with rare blood groups, eg Sd(a+) and Lu^a

Mixed function oxidase Monooxygenase PHYSIOLOGY An enzyme that oxidizes two substrates at once, in which usually one substrate accepts oxygen and the other furnishes two hydrogen ions, eg cytochrome P450, NADPH-cytochrome c reductase plus phosphatidyl choline; the p450 is the terminal electron acceptor of the system (absorbs at 450 nm); the activity of MFO may be induced by CCl_4 and bromobenzene

Mixed leukemia see Biphenotypic leukemia

Mixed lymphocyte culture (MLC) An in vitro assay of cell-mediated immunity that determines antigen specificity of HLA-A, B, C, DR loci in the major histocompatibility complex; the MLC is used in HLA typing in order to obtain the closest immune match between the recipient and host and to minimize organ rejection during transplantation, serving as a predictor of graft-versus-host disease **Method** The donor lymphocytes are 'paralyzed' by irradiation preventing them from dividing, so the only cell capable of proliferation is the recipient's CD4 (helper) T cell, which undergoes blast transformation, indicating immunologic disparity between the two cells, which is more intense as the antigenic disparity between the individuals increases; MLC is also used to diagnose T cell immunodeficiency; Cf Lymphocytotoxicity assay

Mixed mesodermal tumor (MMT) Malignant mixed müllerian tumor A rare carcinosarcoma of the elderly uterus **Clinical** Post-menopausal bleeding and uterine enlargement by a polypoid mass arising from the myometrium **Histopathology** The tumors are either 'homologous', ie containing stromal cells native to the uterus, eg smooth muscle cells and fibroblasts or 'heterologous', containing stromal tissue not native to the uterus, eg bone,cartilage, fat and striated muscle, the last of which is thought to have a slightly worse prognosis; MMT of the ovary has a 1 year survival with homologous elements and six month survival with heterologous elements; more important than the tissue of differentiation is staging; those tumors restricted to the inner half of the myometrium do relatively well; extrapelvic, lymphatic and hematogenous spread is relatively common and is associated with a 25% 5-year survival in uterine MMTs

Mixed tumor Pleomorphic adenoma A usually benign salivary gland tumor, that may also be seen in the breast and pancreas; mixed tumor comprises 60% of parotid gland tumors, where it is 10 times more common than in the submandibular gland, often affecting younger women **Histopathology** The tumors may have a 'frightening' appearance, characterized by dense clusters of epithelial and myoepithelial cells in a mucoid, myxoid, chondroid stroma; the recurrence rate reflects the adequacy of the initial excision; 2-10% are malignant; mixed tumors of the breast in humans are rare and usually benign Note: 20-25% of canine mammary lesions are mixed tumors; see Collision tumor; Cf Composite tumor

Mixed wound infection A skin infection containing many different organisms, including both aerobes, anaerobes and occasionally sabrobic fungi, most commonly associated with soil contamination; some of the organisms cultured by the laboratory are commensal flora and may be considered 'contaminants' by the laboratory personnel as they are uncommon causes of human disease, eg ***Corynebacterium*** spp, α-hemolytic streptococci, coagulase-negative staphylococci, ***Propionibacterium*** spp and ***Bacillus*** spp; other bacteria grown from wounds are best considered potential pathogens, eg ***Staphylococcus aureus***, β-hemolytic streptococci, ***Escherichia coli***, ***Pseudomonas aeruginosa***, other pseudomonads and enterococci; anaerobic culture must be carried out on all mixed wound infections, to rule out ***Bacteroides*** spp, ***Clostridium perfringens*** and other rare clostridia, eg ***C cava*** and ***C liniosa***, ***Actinomyces israeli***, ***Mycobacterium marinum*** and peptostreptococci

MJ The internationally-sanctioned unit for measuring energy, work or force, defined as the work produced by the force of one newton acting over a distance of one meter, where 4.2 MJ is equal to 100 kcal (N Engl J Med 1990; 322:1477)

MK-571 A potent synthetic leukotriene D_4-receptor antagonist that inhibits exercise-induced bronchoconstriction in subjects with asthma and causes a 20% decrease in the forced expiratory volume in one second or FEV1 (N Engl J Med 1990; 323:1736)

MK-801 A non-competitive NMDA antagonist that inhibits opiate tolerance and attenuates the development of morphine dependence (Science 1991; 251:85); MK-801 is of potential use for treating neurodegenerative disease as it interferes with excitatory and toxic action of certain amino acids; MK-801 binds to the PCP receptor in rats, eliciting a toxic reaction; see NMDA receptors

MLC 1) Minimal lethal concentration see Minimum bactericidal concentration 2) see Mixed lymphocyte culture

MLD see Metachromatic leukodystrophy, juvenile type

MLEL Malignant lymphoepithelial lesion, see 'Eskimoma'

MLNS Mucocutaneous lymph node syndrome see Kawasaki's disease

MLO Mycoplasma-like organism(s)

Mls antigens Minor lymphocyte stimulatory antigens A group of cell surface molecules first identified in mice that are immunogenic for unprimed T cells; Mls antigens have limited polymorphism and have two stimulatory forms (Mls_a and Mls_c); anti-Mls response correlates with expression of T cell receptor Vβ molecule, is a function of intrathymic contact of CD8 T cells and is pivotal in the development of immune tolerance; during maturation of the immune system, autoreactive T cells with the T cell receptor Vβ chain (encoded by the Mls genes) are clonally eliminated (Nature 1991; 350:207); see MMTV, Superantigens

***Mls* genes** Minor lymphocyte stimulatory genes A family of genes encoded by mouse mammary tumor (retro)-viruses (MMTV), the protein products of which, known as 'superantigens', are capable of markedly stimulating the proliferation of CD4 T cells in mixed lymphocyte cultures

MLT(ASCP) Medical laboratory technician A laboratory worker licensed in the US, equivalent to an LPN (licensed practical nurse), who is certified (through an examination) by the American Society of Clinical Pathologists to perform certain lab procedures and who must complete a formal two year-in-duration classroom and on-the-job training program; MLTs may report normal range values to physicians, but not panic values; Cf MT(ASCP)

MMM Myeloid metaplasia with myelofibrosis

MMPI Minnesota Multiphasic Personality Index A true-false test for evaluating a subject's psychological and personality 'profile'; the MMPI is used in 124 countries in 46 languages and consists of 550 questions (16 of which are repeated to ensure consistency); it is administered to those over age 15, yielding 14 ranks of personalities from 'social' to schizophrenic; it is imperative to update this fifty-year-old test, as at the time the MMPI was created, the average US citizen was 35 years old, married, lived in a small town, had had 8 years of general schooling and was employed in a skilled or semi-skilled trade; a revision (Mayo ClinProc 1989; 64:3) of the test divides it into a four-parameter Validity scale (measuring the subjects' willingness to complete the test, inability to read, psychological defensive behavior) and a 10-parameter clinical scale (measuring various abnormal psychological tendencies (Depression, sexual orientation, hypochondriasis, hypomania, hysteria, introversion, paranoia, psychasthenia or anxiety, psychopathy and schizophrenia); see Psychological testing

MMPS Medical mortality predictor scale A system used to predict the outcome of certain diseases (J Am Med Assoc 1988; 260:3617)

MMR vaccine Measles-mumps-rubella vaccine A vaccine prepared from live attenuated viruses and administered at 15 months of age or earlier in a measles epidemic, with a subsequent booster shot; the vaccine 'takes' in the vast majority; failure is due to poor timing of the dose, ie before 15 months of age, due to persistence of residual maternal antibodies or due to poor storage of the vaccine; MMR is contraindicated in pregnancy, immunodeficiency states, therapeutic immunosuppression or in acute febrile disease; see Killed vaccine, Live attenuated vaccine

MMTV Mouse mammary tumor virus A virus, the genome of which is integrated in the mouse genome, forming Vβ deletion ligands or minor lymphocyte stimulating genes, which are encoded in MMTV's open reading frame; in the MMTV experimental system, mice are congenitally infected with MMTV, and are immune tolerant to certain antigens common to the virus and to the characteristic tumor; the MMTV may produce suppressor T cells that blunt the T and B cell response to the tumor antigens, accelerating tumor growth; see Minor lymphocyte antigens, Superantigen

MMWR Morbidity and Mortality Weekly Report A 'journal' produced by the Centers for Disease Control in Atlanta, Georgia, which provides a vast array of epidemiological information, eg statistics on the incidence of AIDS, rabies, rubella, sexually-transmitted and other communicable diseases, causes of mortality, eg homicide and suicide, divided by region, sex, age and race

Mo1 A member of the adhesive glycoproteins found on neutrophils and monocytes, designated as Leu-CAM, which functions as the receptor for iC3b, a complement component that mediates complement-dependent monocyte functions, possibly by direct release of inflammatory mediator(s); see CD18/CD11 family

Mobiluncus A recently-identified genus of organisms that are gram-positive, curved, have spinning motility and have been implicated in bacterial vaginosis

Moccasin distribution A pattern of foot involvement in chronic tinea pedis due to ***Trichophyton rubrum***, most common in adult males, with Cushing's disease or lymphoproliferative disorders (implicating defective cell-mediated immunity) Clinical Asymptomatic, finely scaling diffuse erythematous lesion Note: Acute tinea pedis, caused by ***Trichophyton mentagrophytes***, is an intensely pruritic vesiculo-bullous and macerating lesion

Modeling PHYSIOLOGY The process of bone formation, which ends with bone maturation; re-modeling is a dynamic process of osseous turnover that maintains the structural integrity of bones, a function of the 'stress lines' and stresses that are perpendicular to the bone's long axis RESEARCH The simulation of an experiment based on hypothetical conditions, considered by some to be a 'third form of science' in addition to theory and experimentation; modeling allows the examination of a problem and the testing of highly complex hypothetical solutions thereto, performing only the experiments with a high probability of success based on predictions; modeling is used in neural networks, molecular dynamics, cell membrane interactions and in biosphere analysis

Modem Modulator/demodulator COMPUTERS An acoustic coupling device that converts a computer's digital signals to analog signals, allowing transmission of data through telephone lines, which are most commonly used in the health care setting for accessing electronic databases, the cost of which is a function of the time 'on-line'; the data is transmitted in bauds (equal to one bit/second); the standard speeds of transmission are 300 baud, 1200 baud, 2400 baud and 9600 baud

Modified radical mastectomy The standard surgical procedure for localized carcinoma of the breast, which includes the breast, an ellipse of skin, usually with the nipple and the axillary lymph nodes; the controversy continues to rage, as to whether the more cosmetically acceptable 'lumpectomy', or slightly larger 'quadrantectomy' procedures coupled with radiation represent adequate long-term therapy for breast cancer, see Lumpectomy Note: Radical mastectomies, which include the pectoral muscle are far less commonly performed, given the constant feature of extensive lymphedema of the arm on the side of the surgery, the compromise in quality of life and the possibility, albeit distant both chronologically and statistically, of developing a post-mastectomy angiosarcoma

Modigliani syndrome Pseudo-goiter Excessive cervical lordosis of the cervical spine in which there is a reversed 'C' or swan-like configuration or a somewhat elongated neck; the four cases in the original report were referred to the clinician for 'goiter' and the gracile neck seen in these patients was fancifully likened to the women drawn by Amedeo Modigliani, eg Lunia Czechowski, 1919 (Cleveland Clin Quart 1975; 42:319)

Modulation Regulation of the rate at which a specific gene is transcribed

MODY Maturity-onset diabetes of the young An autosomal dominant variant of non-insulin-dependent diabetes mellitus (NIDDM), the gene for which is located on the long arm of chromosome 20 (Proc Natl Acad Sci 1991; 88:1484); see NIDDM

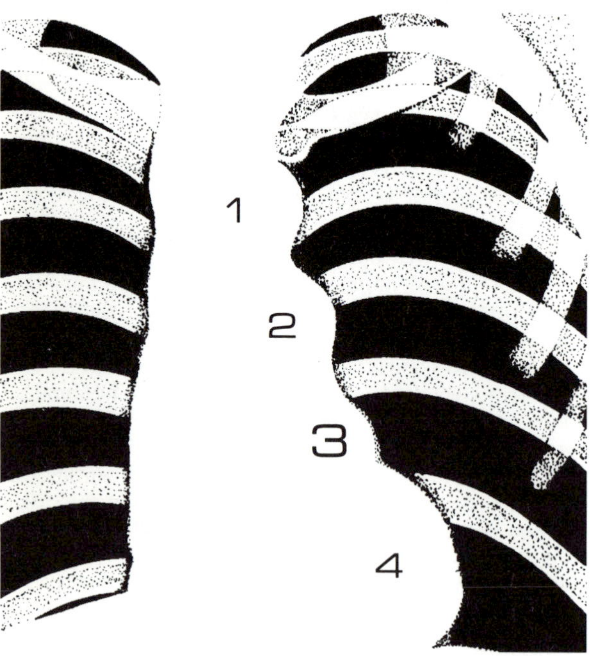

Third mogul sign

Mogul sign Third mogul sign A mogul is a mammillation of packed snow found on a ski slope; in radiology, moguls are sharply demarcated (suggestive of serosal covering, ie extrapulmonary) margins seen on a plain chest film; the left-sided moguls are of interest: the third mogul is an abnormal protuberance located below the left mainstem bronchus and pulmonary artery corresponding to an enlarged or herniated left atrial appendage seen in rheumatic heart disease, a pericardial defect, disease of the chordae tendineae or papillary muscle, papillary muscles, left atrial tumors, cardiomyopathy; alternatively, the left ventricle may be elevated in tetralogy of Fallot, Ebstein anomaly or in a left-sided ascending aorta in corrected transposition of the great vessels; the first mogul is paratracheal in location and corresponds to the aortic arch; the second mogul is left of the carina, located above the left mainstem bronchus and corresponds to the main pulmonary artery; the fourth mogul corresponds to the cardiac apex and lies on the left hemidiaphragm

Mohs surgery (Arch Surg 1941; 42:279) CANCER CHEMOSURGERY A therapeutic modality for treating broad-based, but shallow basal and squamous cell carcinomas, in particular lesions that are 1-2 cm, recurring or cancer recurring-prone sites (nose, eyes, ears) and aggressive histologic subtypes, eg morphea-like basal cell carcinoma Technique: The surface of the lesion plus 3-5 mm margin of normal tissue is coagulated with dichloracetic acid, overlaid with a 20% zinc chloride paste and covered with an occlusive dressing; the $ZnCl_2$ fixes the tissue similar to formaldehyde and after 24 to 48 hours, a 'saucer' of tissue is removed and submitted for frozen section diagnosis to determine sites, if any of deep tumor extension; although tedious in short-term, the Mohs' procedure reduces future recurrences while preserving non-involved tissue (Mayo Clin Proc 1988; 63:175)

Molality A fraction of a solution that is expressed in moles of solute per kilogram of solvent

Molarity The amount of substance of a solution that is expressed in moles of solute per liter of solution (mol/L)

Molar tooth appearance MICROBIOLOGY A descriptor for the appearance of colonies of ***Actinomyces israeli*** (figure, below), which are rounded, raised and have a glistening, white-yellow pearly bossellated surface, fancifully likened to molars

Molar tooth appearance

Molding OBSTETRICS Those changes that the fetal skull (composed of a relatively rigid face and base and the mobile cranial vault) undergoes to accommodate itself into the birth canal

Mole DERMATOLOGY A highly non-specific term used by lay persons for any pigmented lesion, benign or malignant OBSTETRICS A pathologic product of pregnancy or trophoblastic tumor, which occurs in 1:2000 pregnancies in the USA; moles are of two types: a) The hydatidiform mole (10-20 times more common in Southeast Asia), which grossly demonstrates innumerable grape-like avascular chorionic villi, the usual fate is passage of the product and b) The invasive mole which penetrates the myometrium; rarer still is malignant degeneration of a mole into a choriocarcinoma Laboratory In each of these tumors, human chorionic gonadotropin is markedly elevated; for the genetics of the mole, see Hydatidiform mole

Molecular biology The newest major discipline of science that marked its birth with the publication of Watson and Crick's seminal report, '*GENERAL IMPLICATIONS OF THE STRUCTURE OF DEOXYRIBONUCLEIC ACID*' in Nature (1953; 171:737), which elucidated the double helical nature of DNA; molecular biology seeks to understand the mechanisms controlling gene expression, in physiological and 'disease' states, and will ultimately provide the tools necessary for treating genetic diseases Note: A major new vantage point will be reached in this field when the entire human genome is sequenced, a project projected for completion by the year 2005; see Human Genome project

Molecular clock Evolutionary clock A term referring to the finding that mutations occur at a relatively constant rate in any gene; the more mutations there are in a given segment of DNA, eg that which encodes mitochondrial proteins, the older it is, and this would allow determination of the point of divergence of similar proteins in different species

Molecular disease A generic term for any condition that is traceable to a defect in the gene encoding one, or a limited number of molecules, eg sickle cell anemia or Gaucher's disease; see Inborn errors of metabolism

Molecular dynamics The science of simulating the motion of a system of particles, which provides biologists with the computational and theoretical framework necessary to explore molecular configurations; the complexity of biological macromolecules and their interactions caused the field to remain in its infancy until supercomputers became available, structural data based on NMR and X-ray analyses was refined, newer equations were integrated, which restricted the simulations to specific sites of interest, reducing the computation time by a factor of 10 to 100; the field of molecular dynamics promises to speed development of drugs through rational design, elucidate the role of flexibility in ligand binding, facilitate calculation of free energy changes, and identify causes of genemutations (Nature 1990; 347:631)

Molecular scissors see Ribozymes

Molecular sieve chromatography see Gel filtration chromatography

Molecular therapeutics see Recombinant pharmacology

Molluscum bodies Intracytoplasmic inclusion bodies (figure, top) seen within the epithelial cells of molluscum contagiosum, composed of aggregates of molluscum contagiosum virus (figure, bottom), a member of the pox viral family; the bodies first appear as minute ovoid eosinophilic structures in the lower stratum Malpighii immediately above the basal cell layer of the epidermis; as the cells mature, the molluscum bodies become larger than their host cell pushing the nucleus to the side; electron microscopy reveals a 230 nm in length nucleoid that is rectangular viewed en face, and dumbbell-shaped in profile

MOM Multiple of mean LABORATORY MEDICINE A statistic calculation of use for highly variable analytes, eg α-fetoprotein, which changes with fetal age; MOMs are used to establish a cut-off between normal and abnormal values, eg about 90% of anencephalics and about 80% of spina bifida infants have AFP-MOM values of greater than 2.5; Cf Cut-off values

MOMs Mitochondrial outer membrane proteins

'Monday death' OCCUPATIONAL MEDICINE An occupational hazard in the dynamite industry, attributed to exposure to nitroglycerin and ethylene glycol dinitrate; during the week, the workers developed 'tolerance' to these two substances which are known to cause throbbing headaches, tachycardia, palpitations, nausea, vomiting and alcohol intolerance; after a week-end of abstinence the affected workers suffered sudden death on Monday

Monday sickness see Humidifier lung

Monellin A carbohydrate-free, 94-residue heterodimeric protein with a high affinity for the sweet taste receptors, having a 100 000-fold greater molar potency than D-glucose; see Artificial sweeteners

Mongolian heart A complex of cardiac anomalies affecting 40-60% of those with trisomy 21, which includes ventricular septal defect and atrioventricular canal (endocardial cushion defects), less commonly, tetralogy of Fallot, secundum atrial septal defect and patent ductus arteriosus; in adults, aortic regurgitation and mitral valve prolapse may occur; cultured fibroblasts from trisomy 21 patients have an increased adhesiveness, implying an association with septal and cushion defects

Mongolian spots Dermatology Relatively large macules that are slate-gray in color due to the Tyndall effect, which have variably-defined margins, usually over the presacral regions, posterior thighs, legs, back and shoulders, most common in Blacks and Orientals, less in Caucasians, often fading with age (persisting in 4% of Japanese adolescents); mongolian spots are of no clinical significance; the lesion is thought to be due to arrested migration of melanocytes from the neural crest to the epidermis; the pigment changes are confined to

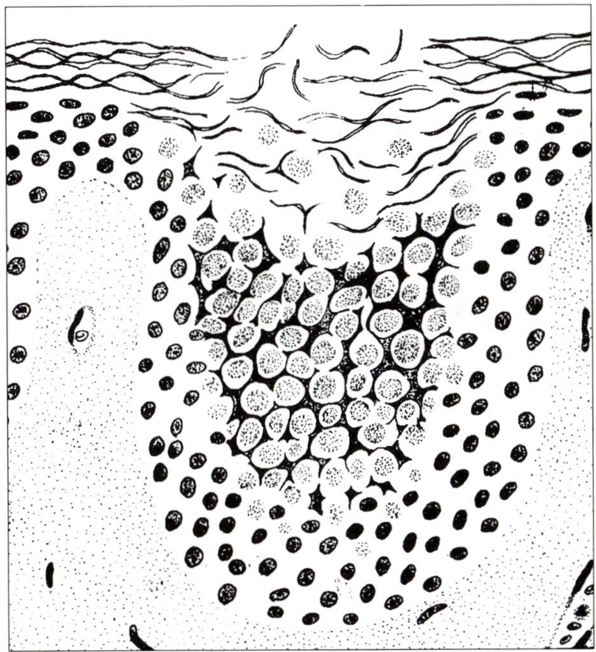

Molluscum contagiosum

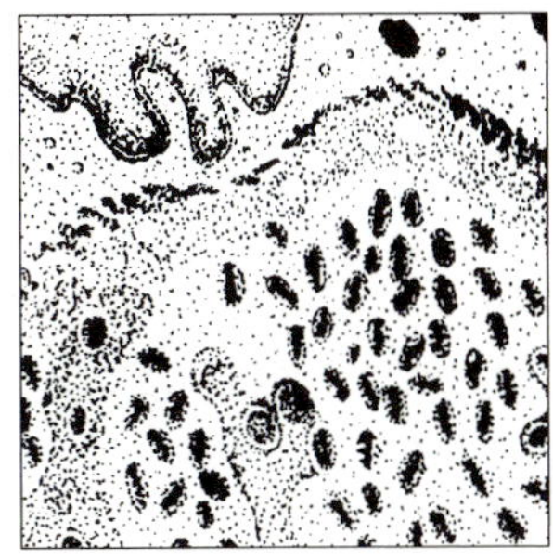

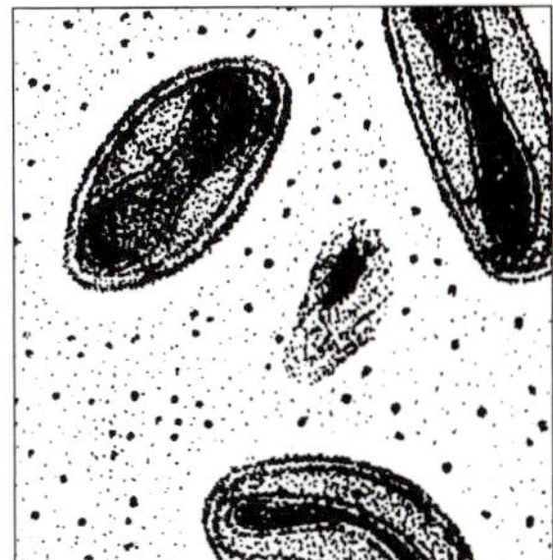

the dermis, and characterized by slender wavy dendritic cells admixed with melanin

Monilethrix see Beaded hair disease

Monitor COMPUTERS see Video display terminal HEALTH CARE INDUSTRY Any parameter that is regularly and consistently used to evaluate the quality of care LABORATORY MEDICINE A component of an instrument that detects physical or chemical fluctuations in electromagnetic radiation

Monkey see Executive monkey

(the) 'Monkey' connection The poorly understood relation between the simian immunodeficiency virus (SIV_{MAC}) and the human immunodeficiency viruses (HIV-1 and HIV-2), which cause similar clinical disease and share an R gene; Cf Africa connection, Mosquito connection

Monkey face A descriptor applied to the trophoblasts of *Giardia lamblia* which have a semi-piriform shape, bearing two nuclei at the broad end and flagella at the tapered end

Monoamine oxidase A catcholamine-metabolizing enzyme (other MAO substrates include MPTP, tryptamine and tyramine) that is located on the outer mitochodrial membrane; the two (or more) forms of MAO, MAO-A and MAO-B, differ in molecular weight and tissue distribution, and are present in varying amounts in the liver, basal ganglia, hippocampus, cerebral cortex and cerebellum (Brain 1988; 111:441) and are regulated by different genetic and hormonal factors

Monoclate-P A proprietary factor VIII:C produced by recombinant DNA technology (Armour, Kankakee, Illinois)

Monocle sign A morphological variation seen on a plain chest film of the central pulmonary artery, which when partially calcified and viewed 'on end' simulates a calcified lymph node

Monoclonal antibody (MAb) A highly specific antibody formed by fusing an immortal cell (mouse myeloma) to a cell producing an antibody against a desired antigen; the technique was pioneered by Köhler and Milstein (Nature 1975; 256:495), partially based on Jerne's network hypothesis (all workers shared the 1984 Nobel prize); certain immunogens elicit an inadequate response in mice; to this end, monoclonal antibodies have been produced in rabbits (Science 1988; 240:1788) MAbs are of use in diagnostics by radioactively-labelling MAbs to target malignant cells, detecting metastases, differentiating tumor subtypes with batteries of MAbs against intermediate filaments or membrane antigens, screening body fluids for microorganisms or measuring levels of circulating hormones; MAbs had been envisioned as having potential as 'magic bullets', which would destroy malignant cells; B72.3 is a MAb expressed in 50% of breast carcinomas and 90% of endometrial, gastrointestinal (colon, gastric), lung, ovary and pancreatic carcinomas; when radiolabelled with ^{131}I or ^{90}Yt, primary and metastatic malignancy is detectable in circa 70% of cases by gamma scans (J Am Med Assoc 1989; 261:744); see Hybridoma

Monoclonal gammopathy of undetermined significance (MGUS), benign monoclonal gammopathy Criteria Normal hemoglobin, serum albumin less than 20 g/L (US: < 2 g/dl), presence of an M-component, no Bence-Jones proteinuria, < 5% plasma cells in the bone marrow, no osteolytic lesions; with time, 20-40% of MGUS progress to malignant monoclonality Note: Monoclonal 'spikes' are usually malignant when the spike is greater than 20 g/L (US: 2 g/dl), the other immunoglobulins are decreased and Bence-Jones proteinuria is present Note: Non-secretory monoclonal gammopathies comprise 1-2% of all myelomas; long-term studies of IgM monoclonal elevations reveal that 56% continue as MGUS, 17% evolve to Waldenström's macroglobulinemia, 7% to lymphoma, 5% to chronic lymphocytic leukemia and 14% to other lymphoproliferative diseases (Mayo Clin Proc 1987; 62:719)

Monoclonal immunoglobulin A protein produced by clonally-expanded immunoglobulin-producing cells, as occurs in multiple myeloma, Waldenström's disease, chronic lymphocytic leukemia and other lymphoproliferative disorders; monoclonal immunoglobulin production may be evoked by other malignancies, eg adenocarcinoma and carcinomas of the bladder, cervix and liver, as well as angiosarcoma and Kaposi sarcoma; nonmalignant conditions associated with monoclonality, include infections, eg ***Acanthocheilonema perstans, Endolimax nana, Entameba hartmanni***, filariasis, schistosomiasis, septicemia, syphilis, trichuriasis, tuberculosis, viral hepatitis, hematologic disorders (anemia, autoimmune hemolytic anemia, hereditary spherocytosis, thalassemia), autoimmune disease (glomerulonephritis, pemphigus vulgaris, scleroderma) and others (chronic hepatopathies and nephropathies, amyloidosis, acute porphyria, chronic salpingitis, systemic capillary leak syndrome, Gaucher's disease, uterine fibromas, cerebrovascular disease, atherosclerosis Note: Although the terms monoclonal antibody and monoclonal immunoglobulin describe the same molecule, the former often refers to the product of an in vitro phenomenon, in which two disparate cells are fused, forming a 'hybridoma'; the term monoclonal immunoglobulin is of use to indicate a protein produced in vivo under natural conditions by a clonally expanded cell under malignant or benign circumstances; see Hybridoma

Monocyte The monocytic phagocyte is of marrow origin and derives from a common progenitor, CFU-GM (colony-forming unit, granulocyte-monocyte); the monocyte 'daughter' cells circulate in the blood, forming both resident and transient populations in various sites; resident monocytes (histiocytes) include Kupffer cells in the liver, Langerhans cells in the dermis, microglial cells in the brain, pleural, peritoneal, alveolar macrophages and osteoclasts; the circulating monocyte measures 15-25 μm, has a reniform nucleus with lacy chromatin and gray blue cytoplasm containing lysosomal enzymes, including acid phosphatase, arginase, cathepsins, collagenases, deoxyribonuclease, lipases, glycosidases, plasminogen activator and others and surface receptors, eg FcIgG and C3R; monocytes are less efficient in phagocytosis than neutrophils but have a critical role in antigen processing; monocytosis may be a benign reactive process, premalignant or frankly malignant (non-Hodgkin's or Hodgkin's lymphoma); reactive monocytosis may be due to infections, eg brucellosis, cat-scratch disease, HIV-1, infectious mononucleosis, malaria, Rocky mountain spotted fever, trypanosomiasis, tuberculosis; reactive monocytosis includes histiocytic lymphadenitis, non-specific lymphoid hyperplasia and Sjögren disease which may evolve toward lymphoma

Monocyte-derived neutrophil chemotactic factor see Interleukin-8

Monocyte-phagocytic system The most correct term for the non-specific branch of the immune system, which is carried out by the monocyte/macrophage cell line and based in the spleen; the term 'reticuloendothelial system' continues to be the more popular, albeit illogical and incorrect, synonym

Monokines see Cytokines

Monopsony HEALTH CARE INDUSTRY The power that a large paying segment of the users of a service, eg health care, have over controlling the price of that service without fear that the providers of the services, eg the physicians, will refuse to render the service for a fair market price (J Am Med Assoc 1990; 263:1981)

Monosodium glutamate see MSG

Monster, acardiac A variant form of twinning in which there is circulatory reversal through various interplacental anastomoses in a diamnionic-monochorionic placenta; malformations range from major malformations in the face of normal skeletal and cerebral structures to complete lack of limbs; usually the umbilical artery is single and the twins are of the same sex; four-legged monster, see J Bone & Joint Surg 1982; 64:88

'Monster' cells NEUROPATHOLOGY Large bizarre tumor giant cells, characterized by splayed nucleoplasm, a complex nuclear membrane, often with florid mitotic activity with tri- and quad-polar mitotic figures; the embryologic lineage is often indeterminant; monster cells are not necessarily malignant and rarely occur in normal epididymal cells, benign fibrous histiocytoma, but are rather more common in malignant fibrous histiocytoma, undifferentiated sarcomas and in grade III or IV astrocytoma (figure, right); despite their 'frightening' appearance, tissue cultures of monster cell tumors reveal that these cells have no growth advantage, and may actually represent effete end cells, in contrast to smaller tumor cells which grow aggressively (see tripolar figure, right) in culture; Cf Giant cells

Monstrocellular astrocytoma A morphologic, highly cellular variant of grade IV, less commonly of grade III astrocytoma, characterized by abundant pleomorphic and bizarre tumor giant cells with eosinophilic intra- and extranuclear inclusions, which has a very aggressive clinical course with a poor prognosis

Monte Carlo simulation A mathematical method that evaluates high-dimensional integrals by applying probabalistic sampling, a technique used in analyzing 'queuing' theory (see there) problems, which requires the construction of a model of a process in which the events are not completely predictable; the process is then simulated multiple times, each time assigning the values in a random fashion; each of these values is selected, usually by computer from a distribution of possible values, allowing estimation of the average values and distributions of the simulation; Monte Carlo simulations may be applied to a complex structure, eg a protein, allowing it to arrange in such a way that energy is minimized; in reverse Monte Carlo simulation, the structural model is adjusted so as to minimize the difference between the calculated diffraction pattern and that measured experimentally, so that good agreement is inevitable

Montevideo units OBSTETRICS A graphic portrayal of uterine activity, the product of the uterine contractions in 10 minutes multiplied by the intensity of the contractions (the average intrauterine pressure peaks of all contractions occurring in the same 10 minute span); coined by Caldeyro-Barcia and Alvarez of Uruguay

'Montezuma's revenge' see Traveller's diarrhea

Montreal platelet syndrome An autosomal dominant disease characterized by giant platelets, thrombocytopenia, a prolonged bleeding time, spontaneous platelet aggregation in vitro at pH 7.4 and normal platelet aggregation in response to ADP, collagen and ristocetin

Montreal protocol An international accord signed by 35 countries freezing chlorofluorocarbon (CFC) production at the 1986 level, with further reductions in their use by the end of the century; CFCs (and NO_2) are responsible for depleting the ozone layer that protects the earth from ultraviolet radiation; hydrochlorofluorocarbons (HCFCs) are an interim substitute for CFCs that also deplete the ozone layer but to a lesser extent; the Montreal protocol did not include dates for elimination of HCFC production; the most recent revision of the protocol cuts CFCs to 50% of its current use by 1995, to be phased out completely by 2000; halons will also be eliminated by 2000 except for their use in firefighting; carbon tetrachloride and methylchloroform will be phased out by the year 2000 and 2005 respectively; one 13-nation 'breakaway' group has announced an even

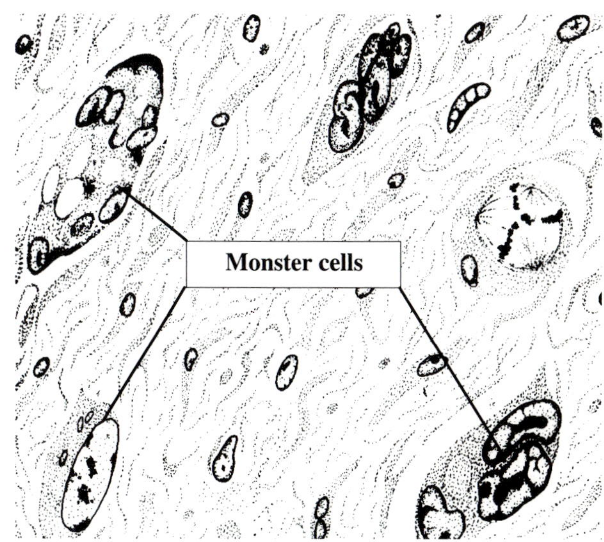

Monster cells

more rapid reduction in the use of these chemicals (see Nature 1991; 349:451), CFCs, Greenhouse effect, Ozone layer, Ultraviolet light

Moon crescent see Crescent

Moon face A rounded face with a double chin, prominent, flushed cheeks classically seen in both Cushing's disease and syndrome and in the cri-du-chat (5p-) syndrome; the name has also been applied to a broad, round face with bright-red cheeks in well-developed, broad chested children with pulmonic stenosis and a right-to-left shunt

Moonlighting An American colloquialism, meaning to take a second job after regular working hours, ie to work 'by moonlight'; a resident's salary at a typical US teaching hospital is sufficient to cover living expenses but not to repay medical school loans (circa $45 000 per person at the time of graduation from medical school); consequently, many young physicians 'moonlight' on a second job, working up to 110 or more hours per week, and are thus often overworked (performing secretarial, clerical and phlebotomy duties, colloquially known as 'scut-work', rather than providing patient care); while this 'sink or swim' method of training physicians has long been the standard in the USA and functions with surprisingly few errors, occasionally there are breakdowns that result in mismanagement of patients; see Libby Zion, Medical school debt

Moon's molars see Mulberry molars

'Moonshine' American colloquialism for illicitly distilled whiskey, intended to circumvent the high government taxes on alcoholic beverages; the equipment used for distillation may contain lead solder and be a source of chronic lead poisoning; moonshine is most commonly produced in the Southeastern USA; see Saturnine gout

MOPP nitrogen Mustard, vincristine (Oncovorin), Procarbazine and Prednisone A well-studied four-drug combination regimen used to treat stage III Hodgkin's disease; in stage IV, MOPP is given with alternating non-cross-reacting drugs, eg MOPP-ABVD (Adriamycin, bleomycin, vinblastine and DTIC); a slightly less toxic substitute for MOPP is the BCVPP regimen (BCNU, cyclophosphamide, vinblastine, procarbazine and prednisone); MOPP complications include myelosuppression, increased infections, nausea, vomiting and sterility

Morbid obesity Superobesity CLINICAL NUTRITION A condition defined as 45 kilograms over the ideal body weight, two times greater than the ideal or standard weight, or for children, a triceps skin fold that is greater than the 95th percentile of all children (National Health Examination Survey, Am J Dis Child 1987; 141:535) Physiopathology Superobese subjects react to the 'stress' of weight-loss by increasing lipoprotein lipase, which in the capillaries of adipose tissue, hydrolyzes triglycerides from circulating lipoproteins into free fatty acids that are taken up by adipocytes, enhancing lipid storage, making further weight loss more difficult (N Engl J Med 1990; 322:1053) non-surgical therapy is rarely successful and some previously used surgical procedures (jejunocolostomy, jejunoileostomy) have been abandoned; despite significant weight loss in the jejunoileal bypass, the procedure is fraught with complications (steatorrhea, hepatic failure, cirrhosis, oxalate deposition, bile stone formation, electrolyte imbalance: decreased calcium, potassium, magnesium, avitaminosis, psychogenic problems, polyarthropathy, hair loss, pancreatitis, colonic pseudoobstruction, intussusception, pneumatosis cystoides intestinalis and blind loop syndrome); see Gastric balloon, Obesity, Pickwick syndrome

Morbilliform rash Morbilliform Latin, measles-like An exanthema most commonly due to Echovirus 9 consisting of fine, discrete maculo-papules on the head and neck, rarely elsewhere, mimicking the rash of rubella, meningococcal petechiae (Waterhouse-Friderichsen syndrome) and Kawasaki's disease, which with the low-grade fever resolves in a week

'Morning-after pill' Interception pill A high-dose estrogen given in the early post-ovulatory period to prevent implantation of a potentially fertilized egg following unprotected intercourse Agents include: 1) Diethylstilbestrol (DES) 25-50 mg/day (now contraindicated given its teratogenic potential, see DES) 2) Ethinyl estradiol 1-5 mg/day and conjugated estrogens; the morning-after pill is taken within 72 hours after an isolated midcycle coitus and continued for 5 days; the pregnancy rate is 0.3-4% Side effects Nausea, vomiting, breast tenderness and menstrual irregularities Note: Non-expulsion of gestational products should be followed by interventional termination; see Contraception, Norplant, Pearl index, RU 486

Morning glory 'syndrome' A predominantly ocular disease complex characterized by mottled peripapillary pigment and an enlarged, funnel-shaped optic disc filled with pale tissue, surrounded by an elevated rim and tortuous radiating vessels (hence the name, morning glory, a flower); the lesion may be bilateral with impaired vision, strabismus and potentially, retinal detachment; other rare associations include cleft lip and palate, agenesis of the corpus callosum and omphalocele

Morning sickness Pregnancy-related nausea often accompanied by vomiting upon awakening, thought to be related to hunger; morning sickness occurs in one-half of pregnancies in the first 2-12 weeks of gestation, which if severe, may cause dehydration and acidosis; the only drug approved by the FDA for treating this problem was Bendectin (which withdrawn for this purpose due to mounting litigation for an alleged teratogenic effect); less effective control of morning sickness is by frequent small meals of low-fat, high-carbohydrate foods

Moroccan leather skin 1) see Pigskin 2) Thickening and grooving of the skin of the face, neck, axillary folds, antecubital fossa, inguinal and periumbilical regions, a characteristic finding in pseudoxanthoma elasticum

Moron see Mental retardation

Morphea A disease characterized by subcutaneous sclerosis, divided by some authors into 1) A generalized form: Scleroderma and 2) A localized form, subdivided into a) Circumscribed morphea Characterized by one or more round-to-oval firm reddish plaques measuring up to several centimeters in diameter with a yellow-white center and a lilac telangiectatic border, b) Linear morphea or linear scleroderma and c) Frontoparietal lesions (en coup de sabre) with or without hemiatrophy of the face

Morphine An opium alkaloid with potent analgesic properties that does not cloud the sensorium, which owes its narcotic properties to its particular aromatic ring structure; see Controlled drug substances, Designer drugs, Heroin, Substance abuse

Morphogen Any substance, eg retinoic acid, that triggers the growth, proliferation and differentiation of cells and tissues in a concentration-dependent fashion

Mortality Leading causes of mortality, USA: Cardiovascular (including arteriosclerosis and aneurysm) disease 39%, cancer 22%, cerebrovascular disease 7.6%, accidents 4.6%, pneumonia or influenza 3%, lung disease 3%, diabetes-related 1.8%, suicide 1.4%, cirrhosis 1.3%, nephritis 1.0%, homicide 1.0%, and others to 100% Mortality rate in viral infections: Rabies 99%, HIV 50+%, Ebola 20-80%, smallpox 1-30%, hepatitis B virus 3-5%, polio circa 0.1% Mortality, under age 19 Fatal injuries for 1986 (MMWR 1990; 39:442) Motor vehicle accidents 47% (33% occupants, 8% pedestrians), homicide 12.8% (usually firearms), suicide 9.6% (male:female ratio 4:1), drowning 9.2% (most common in those under age 4, 90% of which in residential pools), fire/burns 7.2% (most common under age 4, black:white ratio, 3:1)

Mort d'amour CARDIOLOGY Death due to coitally-induced cardiac overload; in one case, a robust but severely atherosclerotic man died while engaged (Am Heart J 1965; 69:287); while uncommonly reported, la mort d'amour may occur in anyone with underlying cardiac disease, especially in those with hypertension, arrhythmias and with cerebral aneurysms

Morular cells Spherical to ovoid variant plasma cells measuring 12-20 µm in diameter, containing an eccentric hyperchromatic nucleus and cytoplasm replete with 1-3 µm in diameter acidophilic globules (Russell bodies) filled with immunoglobulins and neurofibrillary material; when the cytoplasmic contour is smooth, the cells are 'morular', when the globules cause superficial bosselations, they are known as mulberry cells; morular cells classically occur in the brains of patients with Western African sleeping sickness (Agent *Trypanosoma gambiense* Vector Tsetse fly), but may also occur in *T brucei rhodesiense* infections

c-*mos* A proto-oncogene that encodes pp39mos, a tubulin-associated protein kinase, also known as cytostatic factor, which is responsible for the arrest of meiosis in metaphase II and contributes to the formation of the mitotic spindle (Science 1991; 251:671)

Mosaic GENETICS An individual with two or more genotypically (karyotypically) distinct cell lines, arising from a single zygote by somatic mutation, crossing-over or nondisjunction during mitotic division, an event more common in older mothers; 30-40% of Turner syndromes are mosaics: 45,XO/46,XX; 45,XO/47,XXX and 45,XO/46,XY; 5-10% of Klinefelter patients are mosaics: 46,XY/47,XXY; 46,XY/48,XXYY; 45,X/46,XY/47,XXY; 46,XX/47,XXY; see Chimera, Freemartin

Mosaic A patchwork of one sharply demarcated 'jig-saw'-shaped pattern imposed upon another of different color, tissue pattern or radiologic density Note: The mosaic is an art form in which a surface design is produced closely inlaying colored pieces of marble, glass, tile or semiprecious stone; in the Roman empire, floors were decorated with mosaics made of large marble slabs in contrasting colors or of small marble cubes (tesserae); mosaics reached their height as an art form inthe 6th century at Byzantium

Mosaic artifact DERMATOLOGY A mimic of fungal infection of mucocutaneous tissues when dystrophic epithelial tissue is stained with potassium hydroxide; the 'mosaic' consists of an irregular band surrounding epithelial cells which is less translucent than the squamous cells

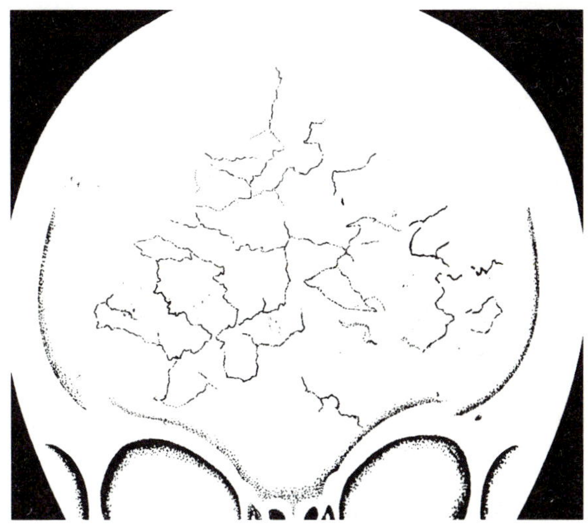

Mosaic bones, skull

Mosaic bone(s) Wormian bones (small irregular, intrasutural bones representing detached centers of embryological ossification in the skull, figure, above), seen in idiopathic osteolysis, hypothyroidism, progeria, cerebrohepatorenal (Zellweger) syndrome, pycnodysostosis, Prader-Willi syndrome, cleidocranial dysostosis, otopalatodigital syndrome

Mosaic pattern BONE A variegated pattern with hap-

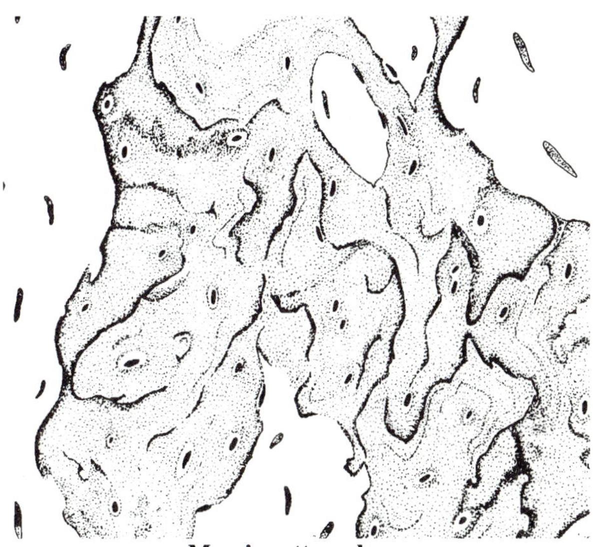

Mosaic pattern, bone

hazard cement lines (instead of the normal parallel arrangement in trabecular and cortical bone, figure, page 463)); the marrow space may be devoid of marrow elements or acellular and replaced by collagen, fibroblasts, fibroconnective and vascular tissue; these changes are due to a marked increase in bone turnover with increased osteoclastic and osteoblastic activity, calcification and accumulation of woven bone; this pattern is classically described in Paget's disease of bone and may occur in chronic osteomyelitis, irradiated bone, osteosarcoma and osteoblastoma CERVIX A colposcopic abnormality seen at an atypical transformation zone of the uterine cervix (atypical when the cervix is covered by 3% acetic acid); the fields of the sharply demarcated 'mosaic' are separated by reddish (vascularized) borders; this pattern may signify any epithelial proliferation ranging from mild dysplasia to carcinoma in situ MUSCLE A variegated pattern of distribution of dystrophin seen by immunostaining of muscle tissue from patients with Duchenne's muscular dystrophy (N Engl J Med 1989; 321:398c) MYCOLOGY An haphazard arrangement of the minute arthrospores seen ensheathing hairs in tinea capitis caused by ***Microsporum***, which differs from tinea capitis caused by ***Trichophyton***, where the arthrospores are larger and appear in parallel chains outside or within the hair shafts

Mosaic proteins A group of functionally diverse proteins which have evolved by duplication, insertion and deletion of a common pool of structural units or modules (defined as consensus sequences containing conserved disulfide bonds); mosaic proteins are involved in cell adhesion, migrations, embryogenesis and in the coagulation, fibrinolytic and complement pathways and include fibronectin, coagulation factor XII and tissue plasminogen activator (Nature 1990; 345:642)

Mosaic wart A verrucous lesion consisting of a large flat plaque composed of confluent contiguous plantar warts, thought to be caused by HPV-2 Note: 3-7% of the population has or has had plantar warts, most commonly during early adolescence

Moses 'syndrome' A poetic term of little utility referring to the difficulties that a health care system has in trying to maintain a balance between cost, quality and access to health care, likened to the tribulations of Moses who eventually led his people to the 'Promised Land'; Cf Franenstein 'syndrome'

Mosquito An arthropod that serves as a vector for various parasites including filariasis (***Brugia malayi, Wuchereria bancrofti***), *Plasmodium* spp, *Trypanosoma* spp and viruses, including αvirus, flavivirus and togaviruses, which cause California, eastern equine, Venezuelan and western equine encephalitides, o'nyong-nyong, dengue fever, Rift valley fever and yellow fever Note: ***Culex pipiens*** are resistant to organophosphorate pesticides arising from the overproduction of nonspecific esterases, mediated through amplification of the corresponding structural genes, designated B2 (Nature 1991; 350:151, 107)

Mosquito connection A postulated relationship between the high incidence of AIDS in a farm community in Florida and the number of mosquitoes, which were thought to act as vectors in blood-to-blood transmission of HIV, given that the 'no known risk' group was double the national average; intense epidemiological investigation revealed that all the infected patients were in a high risk group, eg homosexuals, intravenous drug abusers, Haitians or hemophiliacs (Science 1988; 239:193); Cf Africa connection, Monkey connection

Most significant other (MSO) SOCIAL MEDICINE The person in a patient's universe upon whom the patient most heavily depends, for moral and physical support during periods of crisis and stress; 'significant others' include parents, spouses, children, lovers, siblings or friends; the help of a patient's MSO may be enlisted by the medical team in patients with terminal disease

Moth ball syndrome An X-linked recessive disease caused by the congenital deficiency of glucose-6-phosphate dehydrogenase, resulting in hemolytic crises when exposed to naphthalene (moth balls), sulfonamides, primaquine, nalidixic acid and others; it affects American blacks 11%, Kurdish Jews 50%, others of Mediterranean rim bloodlines and in Orientals ClinicalAcute exposure by ingestion causes nausea, vomiting, diarrhea, hematuria, anemia, jaundice, oliguria and potentially renal shut-down Note: Moth balls are a commonly used household fumigant, composed of crystallized coal tar-derived naphthalene, effective against cloth moths and carpet beetles

Moth-eaten A commonly used descriptor for lesions or masses in whichone radiologic density, color or low-power histological pattern with 'ragged' margins is imposed upon a dark or light background

Moth-eaten alopecia Patchy hair-loss characteristic of secondary syphilis, where the hair falls out in small, scattered and irregular patches, commonly affecting the scalp but which may spread to the eyebrows to the beard; similar patchy loss may occur with trichomalacia and trichotillomania

Moth-eaten bone A non-specific descriptor for patchy osteolysis (figure, facing page) that is seen radiologically in Gaucher's disease, lethal hypophosphatasia (at the ends of the long bones with severe global defects in ossification and shortening of the long bones), leukemia, osteosarcoma, reticulum cell sarcoma and osteolytic metastases

Moth-eaten macrophage A non-specific descriptor for the histiocytes seen in amebiasis, where the ragged histiocytic contour differs from the smooth rounded margins of the ***Entamoeba histolytica*** trophozoites which are further distinguished from the histiocytes by the presence of ingested erythrocytes within the amoeba and their PAS positivity

Moth-eaten mouse A mutant from the inbred C57BL/6J strain of mice characterized by patchy hair loss, increased susceptibility to infection, polyclonal gammopathy, impaired cell-mediated immunity and autoimmunity with immune complex deposition in the glomeruli

Moth-eaten pattern RENAL PATHOLOGY A histological

descriptor for focal disintegration of the glomerular capillary basement membrane which follows spike deposition in membranous glomerulonephritis LYMPH NODES A histologic morphology characterized by partial architectural effacement, mottling, irregularity of follicles, follicular and paracortical hyperplasia, focal necrosis, capsular and pericapsular infiltration, seen in infectious mononucleosis **Differential diagnosis** Cytomegalovirus, Epstein-Barr virus, other viral lymphadenitides and poorly differentiated lymphocytic lymphoma SKIN An oozing and encrusted reddish skin erosion with a sharp cutaneous margin with raised borders, characteristic of Paget's disease of the breast; extramammary Paget's disease is similar but often accompanied by pruritus; moth-eaten skin also appears in Bowen's disease and in pagetoid spread of malignant melanoma

Moth-eaten skull Patchy variegated defects with a ground-glass center seen by a plain skull film in the diploe in hyperparathyroidism; this same descriptor is occasionally applied to the patchy, skull lesions seen in multiple myeloma, although the bony defects are usually more sharply-demarcated and may also be termed 'punched-out'

Motherhood The state of being a mother, which implies giving care to offspring that are perceived as belonging to the mother; this tenacious but difficult to study bond that is common to all mammals, and many vertebrates, although distinctly less common in aquatic animals, for obvious logistic reasons; in mammals, maternal touch stimulates the release of β-endorphin, without which the production of growth hormone is minimal; maternal contact also stimulates ornithine decarboxylase activity, directly affecting the synthesis of putrescine, spermadine and spermine, which regulate the synthesis of the nucleic acids in the brain, heart, lungs, spleen and other tissues; see Bonding

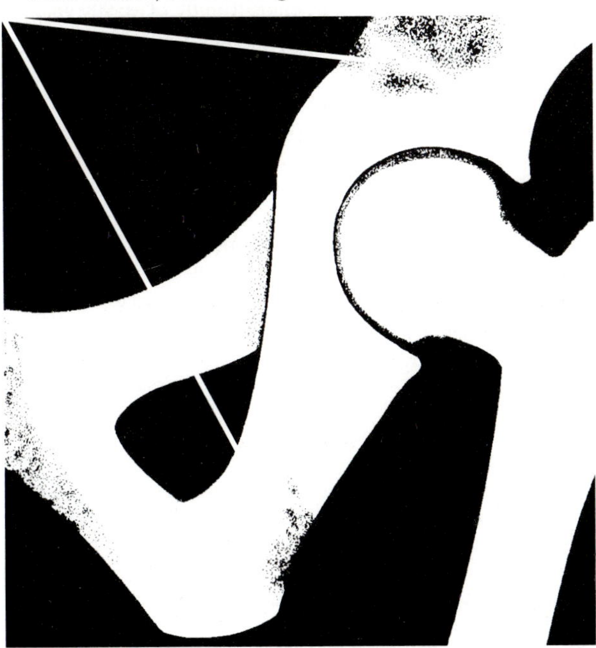

Moth-eaten osteolysis

Motif MOLECULAR BIOLOGY Any recurring design element present in a family of molecules that shares structural and usually functional similarity; eg in proteins, the 'leucine zipper' and the 'zinc finger' are DNA-binding and regulatory motifs; Cf Domain

Motilin A 22-residue gastrointestinal peptide that mediates gall bladder and smooth muscle contraction, stimulating intercibal, but not postprandial motility of the gastric antrum and the upper duodenum by stimulating specific smooth muscle receptors, a response that is lost in severe insulin-dependent diabetes mellitus; response to motilin may be restored by simple administration of macrolide compounds, eg erythromycin (N Engl J Med 1990; 322:1028)

Motion sickness A clinical complex that results from activation of the vestibular system, which may be related to the central triggering zone; the characteristic vomiting is often preceded by nausea, cold sweats, headache, hypersalivation and pallor; motion sickness may be studied by either placing the subjects in a slowly rotating drum, a linear accelerator or 'roller coasters'; electrogastrography is used to detect increased gastric slow wave activity **Treatment** H_1 family of antihistamines

Motor neuron disease (MND) A term for a group of conditions characterized by dysfunction of the motor neuron or anterior horn cell, the most common of which is amyotrophic lateral sclerosis (ALS); the terms are difficult to differentiate, and thus used interchangeably and subdivided into a) The Western Pacific form, seen in the Marianas and on Japan's Kii peninsula, which is associated with a high incidence of parkinsonism and dementia and b) Classic or sporadic form, with an incidence rate of 2/100 000, characterized by upper limb weakness, atrophy and focal neurological signs (Mayo Clin Proc 1991; 66:54rv)

Motor oil appearance A fanciful descriptor of the golden-brown greasy fluid present in the cystic spaces of craniopharyngioma, derived from Rathke's pouch, composed of a suspension of cholesterol

MOTT Mycobacteria other than ***M tuberculosis*** An acronym for non-tuberculous mycobacteria, which are being increasingly recognized due to an increased awareness and by extension, diagnosis of these organisms and decreasing incidence of ***M tuberculosis*** (The incidence of ***M tuberculosis*** reached its nadir in the US in 1986 and, given its relation with AIDS has begun to increase); the ratio of MOTT:***M tuberculosis*** is a function of the population and is lower in hospitals serving more indigent populations Note: ***M avium-intercellulare*** is often resistant to the usual antibiotics; see Runyon classification

Moulage French, a cast or mold A descriptor for the smooth contour of the small intestine, with loss of mucosal folds, a finding that is described as characteristic of radiocontrast studies in sprue-induced atrophy (see figure, top page 466)

Mountain sickness, acute A symptom complex of usually less than a week in duration associated with rapid ascent to greater than 2500 meters, occurring in 30% of subjects above 3000 meters and 75% of subjects above

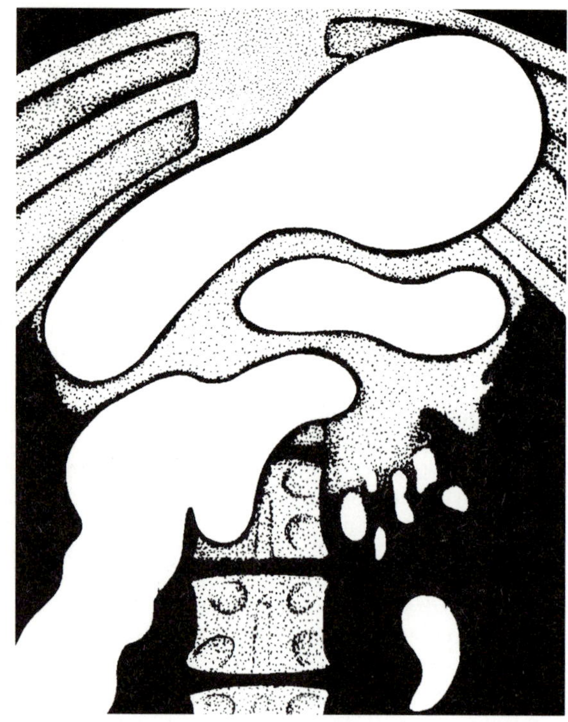

Moulage

4500; in the first 8-24 hours there is marked frontal throbbing headache, (worsened by exercise), nausea, vomiting and insomnia and in 4-40% of subjects, retinal hemorrhage; far less common is life-threatening high-altitude pulmonary, cerebral edema with convulsions and coma **Pathogenesis** The condition is attributed to the combined effect of hypoxia and hypercapnia; Cf Höhendiurese **Treatment** 4 mg dexamethasone, qid (Aviat Space Environ Med 1988; 59:950); while dexamethasone effectively treats the symptoms of central nervous system edema, physiological derangements are not corrected and the subject should descend immediately (N Engl J Med 1989; 321:1707); subjects who have ascended to ultrahigh (Himalayan) heights have mild, but significant residual deterioration of memory, long-term verbal memory, accompanied by aphasia (N Engl J Med 1989; 321:1714), perhaps the long-term effects of hypercapnia; the condition is diagnosed if a subject has three or more major symptoms including anorexia, dyspnea, fatigue, headache or insomnia; the symptoms may be ameliorated with dexamethasone (J Am Med Assoc 1989; 261:732, 734); see High-altitude pulmonary edema, Höhendiurese

Mountain sickness, chronic Monge's disease Andes' disease A clinical complex in which a previously-acclimatized person living for prolonged periods at 4000 or more meters loses his tolerance to hypoxia **Clinical** Drowsiness, dyspnea, asphyxia, cyanosis, cough, nausea, vomiting, palpitations, muscular weakness, pain in the extremities, headache, giddiness, intermittent stupor and loss of weight **Pulmonary function tests** Increased PCO_2, decreased pulmonary ventilation and arterial oxygen saturation and impairment of sensitivity of the respiratory center to hypoxia **Laboratory** Intense polycythemia, with hemoglobin to 25 g/dl and hematocrit to 80%

'Mount Everest experiment' RESEARCH An experiment that is 'ludicrously difficult', performed (as one might say in climbing Mount Everest) *'BECAUSE IT'S THERE'*; such experiments are reserved by the sane for those less so and justified by the investigator, who may perceive himself to be elucidating a greater truth, eg a disease mechanism (N Engl J Med 1987; 317:43)

Mourning reaction PSYCHIATRY A three to twelve month in duration period of depression, disillusionment and discouragement that follows an initial stage of euphoria in patients on chronic hemodialysis; the patients initially deny illness, then recognize that they have lost their health and independence and have an uncertain future, with difficulties in performing their usual employment and in meeting both familial and financial obligations; the mourning reaction is further characterized by role reversal, marital difficulties and changes in functions; the suicide rate among hemodialysis patients is said to be 300-fold greater than a similar, but healthy population; see Dialysis dementia, Honeymoon period; Cf Melancholia

Mouse COMPUTERS An input device ideally suited for menu-driven and icon-drived software programs, that consists of a weighted ball enclosed in a plastic shell allowing an arrow to be moved to various sites on the monitor's screen so that commands are given in a 'point and shoot' fashion

'Mouse incident' A case of apparent scientific misconduct that occurred at a cancer research center in New York City and pivoted around an experiment in which tissue immunogenicity was alleged to have been circumvented merely by incubating that tissue in culture medium for a few weeks; acting under pressure to produce results, the investigator allegedly used a felt-tipped marker and painted on a 'successful' engraftment of tissue from a black mouse onto a white one (J Am Med Assoc 1974; 229:1391); see Cooking, Fraud in science, Trimming

Mouse mammary tumor virus see MMTV

Movat pentachrome A five-dye connective tissue stain in which the nuclei are black, elastic fibers are purple, collagen is yellow, ground substance is blue-green and muscle is red

Moya-moya disease Moya-moya, Japanese, Hazy, smoky NEUROLOGY An idiopathic condition first described in 1961, the name of which derives from the cerebral angiographic appearance of prominent collateral vessels of the basal ganglia accompanying narrowed and distorted cerebral arteries with thin collateral vessels, appearing to arise in a wispy, net-like fashion from the circle of Willis, caused by slowly progressive occlusion **Clinical** Patients are in a 'fog', related to ischemia in younger patients or subarachnoid hemorrhage and altered mental status in older patients; most cases have occurred among the Japanese and appear as recurrent strokes in otherwise healthy female children and adolescents with a familial tendency, often following a febrile illness with abrupt onset of hemiparesis, transient aphasia, convulsions and spontaneous resolution **Histopathology** Intimal thickening and defects in the elastic lamina **Laboratory** Useless Note: The 'puff of smoke' pattern may also be seen in intracranial arteriosclerotic occlusive disease, radiation arteritis, intravascular tumor proliferation and tuberculous meningitis

Moxibustion A variant form of acupuncture that uses heat, in which the mugwort (***Artemisia vulgaris***) is rolled into a small cone, placed point up, burned almost to the skin, then removed

MNGC Multinucleated giant cell, see Giant cells

6-MP 6-Mercaptopurine A chemotherapeutic purine analog (thiol group replacing the 6-hydroxyl), which is activated by hypoxanthine phosphoribosyl transferase used in chemotherapy; the toxic effects of myelosuppression and epithelial damage appear after several cell cycles; 6-MP is used for

MPF M-phase promoting factor A protein kinase composed of $p34^{cdc2}$ and cyclin, which when activated, induces mitosis; the transition of the cell cycle from metaphase to anaphase occurs when cyclin is degraded by ubiquitin-mediated proteolysis, an event that marks the end of cell cycle (Nature 1991; 349:132); see PSTAIR

M-phase promoting factor see MPF

MPM Mortality prediction model INTENSIVE CARE A computer-based prognostic scoring system that stratifies patients receiving intensive care according to their risk of hospital death or need for emergency surgery; although MPM is attractive as it doesn't require disease classification and limits its questions to previous health states, it performs less well than APACHE II in statistical analysis of patient outcome; see Prognostic scoring systems

M protein 1) HEMATOLOGY Monoclonal IgM, Myeloma protein 2) MICROBIOLOGY An α-helical fibrillary molecule on the surface of group A streptococcus that confers resistance to phagocytosis; the 80 distinct serotypes of group A streptococci differ according antigenic variation in the M proteins, which share certain common structural motifs, having a coiled-coil rod in the center, flanked by a) A C-terminal anchor constructed of a highly conserved hexapeptide (Leu-Pro-Ser-Thr-Gly-GluA or LPSTGE), which may be the idoneous antigen to use for producing a vaccine and b) An N-terminal anchor, the antigens of which are highly variable; host antibodies against an N-terminal epitope would confer protection against only one of the 80 serotypes (Scientific American 1991: 264:58, Science 1989; 244:1487) 3) Physiology A structural protein present in the M band of striated muscle

M2 protocol ONCOLOGY A widely used chemotherapeutic protocol for treating multiple myeloma, which includes the alkylating agents vincristine, BCNU (carmustine), cyclophosphamide, melphalan and prednisone (VBCMP) Note: There is little evidence in well-conducted trials that any one multi-agent protocol improves survival more than another

MPTP 1-Methyl-4-Phenyl-1,2,3,6-TetrahydroPyridine A potent neurotoxin that acts on neuromelanin, producing the symptoms of Parkinson's disease; MPTP was first identified as a toxic byproduct in an amateur attempt to produce a meperidine analog, for use as a synthetic heroin and was responsible for a number of cases of permanent parkinsonism; pretreatment of monkeys with pargyline (a monoamine oxidase B inhibitor) prevents both the clinical and pathological evidence of neurotoxicity; see Designer drugs; the selective destruction of the dopamine neurons in the MPTP model is the direct result of its metabolite, MPP+ (1-methyl-4-phenylpyridium); the neurotoxic effect on the substantia nigra may be prevented by systemic treatment with N-methyl-D-aspartate (NMDA) antagonists, see MK-801 (Nature 1991; 349:414), or reversed by local treatment with brain-derived neurotrophic factor (BDNF, Nature 1991; 350:230, 195); see BDNF, Parkinson's disease

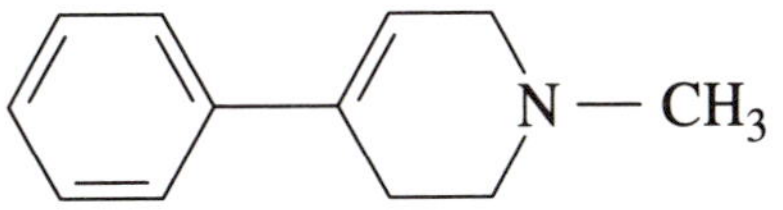

$N - CH_3$

MPTP

MRA Magnetic resonance angiography A non-invasive angiographic technique that provides information similar to that obtained by conventional cerebral angiography (CCA, a technique that uses iodinated contrast, causes paresthesia and carries a risk of ischemia, hemorrhage and idiosyncratic reactions) **Principle** MRA detects the movement of protons in the blood under a magnetic field; the signal is produced as the protons shift from a high-energy state (induced by radiofrequency pulses) to equilibrium, resulting in the production of an electrical signal in a receiver coil, which is transformed into diagnostic images by a computer using a variety of algorithms *ADVANTAGES* MRA is non-invasive, painless, has no known complications, is much more rapid than CCA and allows construction of images in any plane *DISADVANTAGES* The signal-to-noise ratio and spatial resolution at present are inferior to the 'gold standard' of conventional angiography and to digital subtraction angiography, as MRA tends to overestimate the degree of arterial stenosis in cerebral (carotid) vessels; due to the effect of turbulence on the magnetization vectors (the current algorithms are primitive, J Am Med Assoc 1990; 263:1890); MRA has been improved by using 'time of flight imaging', although the 'phase projection' techniques are slow; MRA is useful for imaging of atherosclerotic disease and dissecting aneurysms of the neck and intracranial aneurysms (J Am Med Assoc 1990; 263:2681); Cf Spiral computed tomography

MRA Medical records administrator

MRC Medical Research Council

MRD Mortality rate doubling The time required for an organism's mortality to double, which is a measure of senescence; MRD parallels the increased incidence of spontaneous degenerative disease; see Gerontology

mRNA messenger ribonucleic acid The reverse template 'message' from DNA that is required for protein synthesis; under most circumstances (and according to the 'Central dogma'), the 'message' flows from the DNA to the RNA, which is then translated into protein: DNA is wrapped around proteins (histones) in chromatin; the DNA unwinds, allowing transcription by one of the three RNA polymerases, forming a primary (nuclear) RNA transcript that is then processed by removing the intervening RNA sequences (introns), yielding a mature mRNA molecule that then passes through the nuclear pores into the cytoplasm where translation into proteins occurs; when a particular mRNA is no longer needed it is degraded by ribonucleases; see Central dogma, RNA

MRSA Methicillin-resistant ***Staphylococcus aureus*** see MARSA

MS Multiple sclerosis, Medical student

MSBOS Maximum surgical blood order schedule TRANSFUSION MEDICINE A list of commonly performed elective surgical procedures with the maximum number of units of blood to be cross-matched preoperatively; MSBOS's goal is to have a close correlation between the number of units ordered and number of units actually transfused (crossmatch to transfusion ratio), thereby minimizing the wasted labor in the laboratory, a goal best achieved by tying the MSBOS into the hospital computer system; see Cross-match/transfusion ratio

MSDS Material Safety and Data Survey

Mseleni disease A crippling form of idiopathic polyarticular osteoarthritis, endemic in Northern Zululand (now KwaZulu) which affects the appendicular joints of 20% of men and 40% of women; in the end-stage disease, most patients walk on their hands and knees Note: Pathological studies on the bones of Mseleni disease occur after the vultures have stripped the flesh since it is a local custom to leave the dead to be eaten by scavengers (Clin Orthop 1979; 141:223)

MSG Monosodium glutamate A flavor-enhancing amino acid that functions as an excitatory neurotransmitter and neurotoxin, which may cause convulsions when injected into the peritoneal cavity of experimental animals, stimulating neurons until they die, which has been implicated in brain damage in strokes, hypoglycemia, trauma, seizures as well as in Huntington's, Parkinson's and Alzheimer's diseases and in Guam-type amyotrophic lateral sclerosis Note: Domoic acid, a potent glutamate analog caused a toxic envenomation in mussel eaters, in some resulting in an Alzheimer-like disease, see Chinese restaurant syndrome, Domoic acid

MSOF see Multisystem organ failure

Mst II MOLECULAR HEMATOLOGY A restriction endonuclease used to detect sickle cell anemia, as the recognition site is abolished by a point mutation on the β globulin gene; Mst II-digested Southern blots of fetal DNA provide the most reliable currently available prenatal diagnosis of sickle cell anemia

MSUD see Maple sugar urine disease

MT see Medical technologist

MT A region of the brain where neurons specialize in detecting movement and in which the neurons are grouped in columns, each of which scans a part of visible space for objects moving in a certain direction

MTBE Methyl-tert-butyl-ether An aliphatic ether that rapidly dissolves cholesterol stones in vivo, which is introduced under local anesthesia via a percutaneous transhepatic cholecystectomy catheter, as a non-invasive method for treating gallstones; after injection, the dissolved 'slurry' is drained from the bladder Complications are rare and minor, including nausea, vomiting, bile leakage, drowsiness, transient elevation of liver enzymes, anorexia and hypotension (Br J Surgery 1990; 77:32); MTBE stone dissolution is effective when the patients are selected for cholesterol stones (N Engl J Med 1989; 320:633); dissolution of stones is improved and accelerated by adding transcutaneous ultrasound energy (Invest Radiol 1990; 25:146); see Lithotripsy

mtDNA see Mitochondrial DNA

MTHFR 5,10-Methylenetetrahydrofolate reductase An enzyme that catalyzes NADPH-linked reduction of methyenetetrahydrofolate to methyltetrahydrofolate, providing a methyl group for methylation of homocysteine; MTHFR deficiency is more common in females, characterized by developmental delay, motor, gait and typical EEG changes and early death **Laboratory** Increased serum homocysteine and homocystinuria with low plasma methionine

MTOC Microtubule organizing center CELL BIOLOGY A subcellular structure adjacent to the nucleus in resting cells, consisting of a centriole from which microtubules emanate, extending to the plasma membrane; see Microtubule

MTP-PE Muramyl tripeptide-phosphatidyl ethanolamine PHARMACOLOGY A synthetic lipophilic analog of a bacterial cell wall component, muramyl dipeptide that is 'bundled' in fat, in a liposomal vesicle and delivered into the pulmonary vasculature, theoretically turning on the tumorilytic machinery of the pulmonary macrophages; MTP-PE is in phase II trials for metastatic osteosarcoma (J Am Med Assoc 1990; 263:2289c)

MTS Mouse thyroid stimulator see LATS

MTX see Methotrexate

μ symbol for: linear attenuation coefficient (statistics); mean (statistics); micro- (10^{-6}); heavy chain of IgM

Mucicarmine HISTOLOGY A commonly used stain for SURGICAL PATHOLOGY that uses carmine in combination with aluminum hydroxide and aluminum chloride in 50% alcohol; the mucicarmine stain is most prominently positive with acid mucins secreted by the gastrointestinal tract and ***Cryptococcus neoformans***

Mucin(s) Mucosubstance A group of hydrated glycoproteins that may be 1) Stromal or dermal ('ground substance') composed of acid mucopolysaccharides, predominantly hyaluronic acid; it is hyaluronidase-labile, PAS-negative, stains with alcian blue at pH 2.5, but not at pH 0.4 and stains metachromatically with methylene and toluidine blues at pH of 3.0 but not at 1.5; with aging, this mucin undergoes basophilic degeneration and 2) Epithelial mucin, produced by glands, containing neutral and acid mucopolysaccharides; when stained, it is hyaluronidase-resistant, PAS-positive, stains with alcian blue at pH 2.5, but not at pH 0.4 and does not stain metachromatically with alcian, methylene and toluidine blues

Mucin clot see Rope's test

Mucin lake SURGICAL PATHOLOGY A non-specific term for

'pools' of mucin-staining material seen by light microscopy in various settings, eg in connective tissue as a component of aging or in degenerative diseases, in the peritoneum in a mucocele of the appendix or in protein-rich, lightly basophilic material admixed with adenocarcinoma cells seen in colloid type adenocarcinomas of the colon and breast

Mucocutaneous lymph node syndrome see Kawasaki's disease

Mucopolysaccharidoses (MPS) A heterogeneous group of diseases caused by an accumulation of mucopolysaccharides (glycosaminoglycans) due to an enzyme deficiency and accumulation of substrate molecules including dermatan sulfate, heparan sulfate and keratan sulfates **Clinical** Childhood onset of symptoms that include developmental delay, mental retardation, skeletal anomalies, coarse facial features, hepatosplenomegaly **Diagnosis** Urine screens, consisting of 'spot' tests in which basic dyes (alcian and toluidine blue) stain the acid mucopolysaccharides, modified turbidometric method may be false positive or false negative, modified Dische carbazole reaction, which measures uronic acid Note: Morquio syndrome doesn't excrete uronic acid and is not detected; see Gargoyle face

Mucormycosis Formerly, Phycomycosis, zygomycosis An opportunistic infection by fungi of the order Mucorales, which are found in decaying organic matter and grow in tissues as hyphae, thus being defined as molds; most grow within 2-5 days in the usual culture media; the most common pathogenic muycomycoses are ***Rhizopus*** species and ***Rhizomucor*** species; others include ***Absidia, Apophysomyces, Cunninghamella, Mucor*** and ***Saksenaea*** **Clinical** The fungi enter the respiratory tract and gain a foothold in the nasopharynx, usually in hosts who are immunocompromised by diabetes, corticosteroids, terminal cancer or AIDS Clinical forms Rhinocerebral, pulmonary, cutaneous, gastrointestinal, cerebral and miscellaneous forms; once the host defense has been circumvented, the hyphae are vasculocentric, explaining the commonly associated necrosis and thrombosis **Treatment** Amphotericin B, azoles (ketoconazole and others) and surgical debridement

Mucosa Mucous membrane An non-squamous cell epithelium, that usually corresponds to the glandular lining of the nasal and oral cavities, as well as the epithelium of the upper respiratory tract and external genitalia

Mucus A clear viscid fluid that is produced by the various mucosae; mucus consists of mucopolysaccharides, enzymes, IgA and other proteins, desquamated epithelial cells, inorganic salts in a fluid vehicle

Mucous An adjective that refers to either mucosa, eg mucous membrane or to mucus, eg mucous secretion

Mulberry stone

Muddy complexion A characteristic 'soiled' appearance of patchy hyperpigmentation seen on the face in older malnourished children, accompanied by pallor, lassitude, hypochromic anemia, delay in epiphyseal development, delayed puberty, irregularities in dentition, anorexia and increased susceptibility to infection; see 'Crazy pavement'

Muddy lung A descriptor for the lungs of those who have drowned or nearly drowned in stagnant water (and who subsequently die); muddy lungs are characterized by crystalline material, foreign body type giant cell and granulomatous reaction with carnification, massive fibrosis of the pulmonary parenchyma and abundant diatoms (Am J Clin Path 1985; 83:240)

Mud fever Weil's disease caused by ***Leptospira interrogans***

Müllerian ducts Paramesonephric ducts EMBRYOLOGY Structures that appear between the 6th and 7th weeks of embryologic development (during the sexually indifferent period as an invagination of coelomic epithelium, lateral to the cranial portion of the mesonephric duct); in the female the two müllerian ducts fuse during the 9th gestational week, forming the upper vagina, uterus and fallopian tubes, whilst the remaining degenerates; incomplete fusion of these ducts results in the didelphic uterus; in the male fetus, the müllerian ducts regress at 7-8th week, portions of which remain as müllerian duct remnants

Müllerian-inhibiting substance (MIS) A non-steroid compound secreted by the Sertoli cells of the fetal testes, which inhibits müllerian duct development, while potentiating wolffian duct development; when the fetal gonads are ovaries, no MIS is produced and the fetal external genitalia 'default' to female differentiation

Müllerian mixed tumor see Mixed mesodermal tumor

Mulberry appearance Any pathological mass or appearance characterized by a rounded mass with multiple superficial bossellations, likened to the appearance of a mulberry or cluster of grapes (unripe) OPHTHALMOLOGY A fanciful descriptor for the fundoscopic appearance of a retinal phakoma or glial hamartoma, consisting of a multinodular or multicystic yellow-white mass, classically seen in patients with tuberous sclerosis (Pringle-Bourneville syndrome)

Mulberry cell see Cluster of grapes cells appearance

Mulberry molars PEDIATRICS Abnormal lower deciduous molars characterized by a small biting surface and multiple cusps, seen in children with congenital syphilis (other dental anomalies of congenital syphilis include enamel defects causing increased caries and the peg teeth of Hutchinson)

Mulberry pattern GYNECOLOGIC PATHOLOGY A descriptor of the relatively characteristic pattern of calcifi-

cation seen in gonadoblastoma

Mulberry spots GYNECOLOGY see Powder burn appearance

Mulberry stones UROLOGY A descriptor for urinary bladder concrements (figure, page 469) composed of calcium oxalate that may be of dietary origin, due to intestinal malabsorption or seen in the rare primary hyperoxaluria; Cf Casts

Mulibrey nanism An acronym from the organs most commonly affected (muscle, liver, brain and eye) in an autosomal recessive disease first described in Finland, which is further characterized by constrictive pericarditis with pericardial effusions, yellow dots on the optic fundus, fibrous dysplasia of long bones and abnormalities in the shape of the skull and sella turcica

Muller's ratchet EVOLUTIONARY BIOLOGY A hypothesis that attempts to explain why sex exists; if most mutations are deleterious, a high rate of mutations could account for the evolution of sex; according to Muller, where the mutation rate is high, eventually mutation-free individuals become rare and lost in small populations, due to genetic drift; if the population is asexual, the loss is irreversible, ie occurs in a ratchet wrench-like fashion, and the load of deleterious mutations increases as the mutation-free individuals decrease in the population; according to Muller's ratchet, sexual differentiation increases the fitness of a population, as error-free individuals are created from mutated individuals, effectively stopping the ratchet effect; while the concept is theoretically attractive, it is unproven (Nature 1990; 348:454); see Hybrid vigor; Cf Bottleneck

Multicentric angiofollicular lymphoid hyperplasia Multicentric Castleman's disease

Multichannel analyzer LABORATORY MEDICINE An automated laboratory instrument, eg Beckman's 'CX' series, which simultaneously measures multiple analytes including calcium, glucose, phosphorus, lactate dehydrogenase, alkaline phosphatase and others by separating plasma into minute aliquots and passing each through a separate plastic tube (channel), within which a particular reaction occurs that is measured by a spectrophotometer that is pre-set to measure light at an optimal wavelength

Multi-copy prescription forms CLINICAL PHARMACOLOGY A triplicate form used in some states of the USA, eg California, Illinois, New York and Texas, to monitor prescriptions of controlled drug substances, where a copy of the prescription is retained by the pharmacist, by the physician and by the state government; see Controlled drug substances

Multicystic kidney see Polycystic kidney

Multicystic nephroma see Multilocular cyst of the kidney

Multifocal atrial tachycardia (MAT) A cardiac arrhythmia characterized by irregularity, variable 'P' waves and (in adults) a poor prognosis; MAT is seen in 0.05-0.32% of the EKGs interpreted in general hospitals and is more common in the acutely ill (burns, sepsis, respiratory failure) and elderly Treatment Magnesium and potassium, calcium-channel blockers, eg verapamil and β-adrenergic blockers, eg metoprolol Prognosis 43% of patients with MAT died during the hospital stay in which the arrhythmia was documented, but death was usually related to the underlying disease (N Engl J Med 1990; 322:1713)

Multi-infarct dementia (MID) A condition characterized by global cognitive impairment due to atherosclerosis-induced cerebrovascular disease, which is more common in women and associated with diabetes mellitus, hypertension, smoking and rarely, amyloidosis Clinical Gait and motor defects, abnormalities of language, mood, abstract thinking, apraxia, agnosia and urinary incontinence; the repeating 'mini-infarcts' of hypertension mimic the gradual deterioration typical of the more common Alzheimer's disease, which occurs without prominent motor changes and reflexes Histopathology Variably sized infarcts of sensorimotor areas and cortical zones involved with cognitive functions, especially in zones irrigated by the anterior and middle cerebral arteries, imparting a lacunated or 'Swiss cheese' appearance

Multi-lineage leukemia A leukemia that is clonally committed to myeloid differentiation and also demonstrates multiple clonal, eg megakaryocytic and/or erythrocytic, expansions, a finding more common when associated with monosomy 7; the finding of multi-lineage expansions, implies that the proliferative signal has occurred at the progenitor-cell stage of differentiation (N Engl J Med 1988; 318:1153); Cf Biclonality, Composite tumor

Multilocular cyst of the kidney Multicystic nephroma A unilateral idiopathic lesion that arises in infancy, producing symptoms by the presence of a mass or by ureteral obstruction, and consisting of multiple cysts ranging from 1 mm to 15 cm, which do not communicate with each other or with the remaining (unremarkable) renal parenchyma; it is unknown whether the cysts are neoplastic (as they may be associated with Wilm's tumor or renal cell carcinoma), segmental dysplasias (as they may occur in Potter type 2 renal dysplasia) or developmental defects (as they may be associated with hamartomas), although absence of other congenital malformations, favors an acquired etiology; see Polycystic kidneys

Multiorgan donation The best single source of multiple organs from a non-relative for allograft transplantation is a 'brain dead' donor, as the recipient is exposed to only one set of foreign antigens; 56-77% of such donations are from central nervous system catastrophes (subarachnoid bleeding or CNS tumors); the remaining donations are from cardiopulmonary arrest, anoxia, drug overdose, drowning or burn victims or those with prolonged ventilatory support Note: Donations from patients with prolonged brain death are less desirable given the potential for infectious complications; for management of multiorgan 'donors' and exclusionary criteria (J Am Med Assoc 1989; 261:2222)

Multiorgan failure see Multisystem organ failure

Multiple autoimmune disorders A pair of conditions, divided into MAD, type I Defined by at least two of the following Addison's disease, hypoparathyroidism, mucocutaneous candidiasis and MAD, type II Schmidt syndrome, characterized by two or more of the following, including Addison's disease, autoimmune thyroid disease, insulin-dependent diabetes mellitus with or without hypopituitarism and mucocutaneous candidiasis

Multiple basal cell nevus syndrome see Nevoid basal cell carcinoma syndrome

Multiple chemical sensitivity syndrome see Clinical ecology

Multiple comparisons method(s) STATISTICS A group of procedures for handling multiple inferences within the same data sets, including Bonferroni technique, Scheffe's contrasts, Duncan multi-range procedures, Newmann-Keuls procedure

Multiple hamartoma syndrome Cowden's disease An autosomal dominant condition characterized by an increased susceptibility to malignancy, oral papillomas, fibrocystic mastopathy and increased papillary or follicular thyroid carcinoma and breast cancer; Cf Chromosomal breakage syndromes, Li-Fraumani syndrome

Multiple lentigines syndrome see Leopard syndrome

Multiple malformation 'syndromes' (MMS) PEDIATRICS A group of disorders defined as having developmental anomalies of two or more systems possibly related to chromosomal damage, teratogens and other environmental influences, including the Cornelia de Lange, Prader-Willi, Rubinstein-Taybi and the Williams' syndromes; see Dysmorphology, Sequence

Multiple myeloma A well described clinical entity characterized by lineage 'infidelity', ie expression of multiple lineages, including megakaryocytic (88%), monocytic-myeloid (65%), lymphocytic (58%) and erythroid (39%) lines, both mature, eg surface immunoglobulins and immature, eg cALLA antigens, stages of development (N Engl J Med 1990; 322:664); see Myeloma kidney

Multiple primary malignancy syndrome ONCOLOGY The finding of two primary malignancies in the same patient is not uncommon, although more than two is distinctly unusual and becomes a 'syndrome', defined by Werthamer's criteria 1) The malignancies must be primary in different organs 2) Paired-organ (breast, kidney) malignancies (synchronous or metachronous) are considered to be a single primary 3) Multiple malignant tumors originating in the same organ are considered as a single primary 4) The lower intestine and uterus (with adnexae) are each considered single organs 5) The malignant nature of the lesions must be confirmed histologically 6) The lesion should be histologically proven to be non-metastatic (although this is sometimes impossible) Note: An additional criterion may prove valid 7) The malignancy should not have been induced by chemo- or radiotherapy (J Am Med Assoc 1961; 175:558); multiple primary malignancies occur in less than 1% of those with malignancy; the maximum recorded number of multiple primary malignancies is six (Am J Surg 1949; 78:894)

Multiple sclerosis (MS) An idiopathic, demyelinating disease in which the infiltrating lymphocytes (predominantly T-cells) and macrophages eat up the myelin, onset in younger, often female adults, affecting 1:2500 in the US, commonly associated with HLA-A3, B7, Dw2 haplotypes; MS is increased in a south-to-north gradient in the northern hemisphere **Clinical** Waxing and waning or slowly progressive paresthesias, gait and visual defects, muscular weakness, absent abdominal reflexes, hyperactive tendon reflexes and ataxia **Pathogenesis** Three major mechanisms have been evoked including autoimmunity, 'innocent bystander' demyelination and immune destruction of persistently infected (more than 20 viruses have been implicated in MS) oligodendrocytes (Mayo Clin Proc 1989; 64:570, 592) **Molecular biology** Antibodies are present in the cerebrospinal fluid that react with HTLV-I's GAG (p24) protein; gene amplification, cloning and DNA blotting analysis of peripheral monocytes from MS patients revealed HTLV-I sequences (Science 1989; 243:529); suggesting a retroviral relation to MS **Diagnosis** Oligoclonal elevation of IgG in the cerebrospinal fluid is present in 90% of patients, 'evoked potentials' seen by electroencephalography in the visual cortex and brainstem, multiple defects seen by computed tomography and magnetic resonance imaging Note: All of these tests are non-specific and must be correlated with the clinical findings **Neuropathology** Demyelinization, inflammation, and glial scarring, ie a 'dying-back gliopathy'; early lesions involve the paraventricular, frontal and temporal regions, later involving the optic tracts, brainstem, cortical white matter with patchy spinal cord lesions **Treatment** *...NO THERAPY IS TRULY WORTHLESS UNLESS IT HAS BEEN TRIED AND FAILED IN MULTIPLE SCLEROSIS...* **--anonymous**; some of the more recent agents that appear to be less than effective include cop-1, a mixture of 14-23 kD polypeptides containing alanine, lysine, glutamic acid and tyrosine in a ratio of 6:4.7:1.9:1, which is similar to that of myelin basic protein; cop-1 suppresses experimental allergic encephalitis, a murine model of MS, and hyperbaric oxygen (Arch Neurol 1991; 48:195); see Cop-1, Faroe Islands, Holstein cow, Oligoclonal bands, Shadow plaques

Multipotent reserve cell An undifferentiated cell of the adult breast capable of differentiating into myoepithelial, ductal and lobular cells (Cancer 1968: 22:125; ibid, 1954; 7:934)

Multiproblem family SOCIAL MEDICINE A family with a high potential for child abuse; these families are often urban and have an income level far below the poverty level; most of these families are headed by a single parent, half of whom have serious psychiatric disorders and a history of substance abuse and/or alcoholism; 81% had four or more episodes of child abuse in the previous three years, accompanied by severe child neglect in 30-80% of cases (N Engl J Med 1990; 323:1628); see Child abuse

Multirule procedure LABORATORY MEDICINE A set of rules for quality control (QC) of laboratory data which combines individual QC rules to increase the probability of error detection without increasing the rate of false rejections to unacceptably high levels; one commonly used procedure is Westgard's multirule procedure in which a 'run' of laboratory data is rejected if the control is 1) 3 standard deviations (SD) above or below the mean for that analyte 2) Two consecutive controls are greater than 2 SD in the same direction of the mean 3) Four consecutive controls are greater than 1 SD in the same direction of the mean 4) The range between 2 consecutive controls exceeds four SD 5) 10 consecutive controls are in the same direction of the mean

Multistage carcinogenesis The development of cancer through multiple steps; in contrast to the mechanistically correct, but simplistic model delineated by Knudson in the 'One hit, two hit' model of malignancy, malignant transformation of most tissues requires that multiple defects accumulate in the genome through various combinations of DNA defects including the loss of tumor suppressor genes, point mutations and juxtaposition of oncogenes with new sites, eg permanently turning on growth factors; recognizing of these early stages may ultimately allow for 'preneoplastic' therapy to be a viable option; see One-hit, two hit model, p53, Tumor

Multistix see Dipsticks

Multisystem organ failure (MSOF) A 'physiologic' shut-down of multiple body systems in the face of critical injury or uncontrolled sepsis; several factors are synergistic in producing organ dysfunction and death (average MSOF mortality 60%): shock, intestinal infarction, malnutrition, alcohol abuse and advanced age; MSOF may begin as cardiocirculatory failure and be followed by respiratory and renal shut-down, hepatic decompensation and metabolic derangements with thrombocytopenia occurring at any time; if the progression of MSOF can be stopped before a second organ fails, the mortality is 30%, otherwise death is virtually inevitable (J Am Med Assoc 1988; 260:530)

Multivesicular bodies (MVB) A form of lysosome appearing as a large,cleared, membrane-bound vacuole thought to result from defective membrane cycling and abnormal internalization of surface antigens in Golgi-derived vesicles; MVBs are characteristic of signet ring lymphoma

Multivitamin An over-the-counter and often self-prescribed combination tablet containing lipid-soluble vitamins (vitamin A, vitamin D, vitamin E and vitamin K) and water-soluble vitamins (vitamin B_1, vitamin B_2, vitamin B_6, vitamin B_{12}, vitamin C), folic acid, niacin, pantothenic acid and biotin; these dietary 'supplements' may also contain minerals, including calcium, phosphorus, iron, iodine, magnesium, copper and zinc; multivitamins may reduce the risk of anencephaly and spina bifida (N Engl J Med 1989; 321:430); see Decavitamin, Neural tube defects; Cf Megavitamin therapy

Mummified cell LIVER A degenerated eosinophilic hepatocyte described in acute hepatitis, preferably known as an apoptotic cell LYMPH NODE A large effete and degenerated cell (figure, right) that may represent an involuting Reed-Sternberg cell, which is most commonly seen in the diffuse subtype of lymphocyte predominance Hodgkin's disease; this form is characterized by diffuse effacement of the nodal architecture by a lympho-histiocytic proliferation, paucity of diagnostic Reed-Sternberg cells, presence of large abnormal polypoid cells without huge nucleoli (L/H cells, which are also seen in lymphocyte-predominant Hodgkin's disease) and abnormal, often ring-shaped mitotic figures

Mumps A condition described by Hippocrates, the English name of which refers to the mumbling speech characteristic in these patients; it is recommended that all children without immune compromise, anaphylactic reactions to eggs or other contraindications receive the live attenuated mumps virus vaccine which confers lifelong protection; adverse reactions, eg orchitis and parotitis are rare Note: Most of those born before 1957 have natural immunity

Munchausen syndrome A pseudo-disease complex seen in subjects who create bizarre lesions or fabricate symptoms in order to enjoy the perceived benefits from hospitalization; the chief complaints include those with vague symptoms, requiring numerous often complicated tests; once the charade is discovered, the 'patient' signs out of the hospital only to be admitted to another Statistics Female:male ratio, 2:1; 74% develop the condition by age 24, and on average are diagnosed as having the Munchausen complex by age 32; the patients often have a history of childhood neglect or abuse, linked to illness, where the hospital represents a place with a comforting and nurturing environment; to maintain their state of illness, some 'patients' may feign torsion dystonia, inject feces or perform surgery upon themselves; although less than 400 cases have been described since its initial recognition (Lancet 1951;1:339), these persons are very 'expensive', undergoing multiple hospitalizations and diagnostic procedures; their actual cost to the health care system cannot be estimated; The name derives from a fictional character, Baron Munchausen created by a German, RE Raspe (1737-1794) who wrote the original story in English as Baron Munchausen's Narrative of his Marvelous Travels and Campaigns in Russia, based on the true tales of a German soldier and raconteur, Freiherr von Münchhausen (1720-1797) of Hannover Note: The fictional character and the person who inspired the fiction should be distinguished, if only for the sake of accuracy (J Am Med Assoc 1983; 250: 1976)

Munchausen-by-proxy syndrome Polle syndrome A form of child abuse in which the children, often under the age

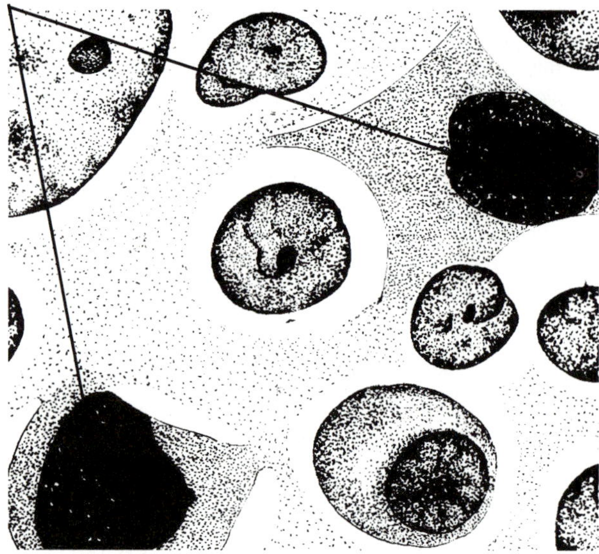

Mummified cells

of 5-6, are victims of factitious illnesses either fabricated by, eg reports of fever and seizure disorders or induced by the parents or guardians, eg administration of laxatives, withholding antibiotics, friction-induced 'rashes'; this condition may satisfy aberrant psychological needs on the part of the parents; the syndrome is misnamed after Polle, Freiherr von Munchhausen's daughter, who was said to have died at the age of one under suspicious circumstances, a 'fact' that is not supported historically (Lancet 1984; 1:166) as he did not have a daughter named Polle (Pediatrics 1984; 74:554)

Murder FORENSIC MEDICINE The unlawful killing of a human being by another with malice aforethought, either express or implied **MURDER OF THE FIRST DEGREE** 'Murder, one' Any homicide perpetrated by means of poison, lying in wait, or other kind of wilful, deliberate and premeditated act, or that which is committed while perpetrating a forcible felony, eg arson, rape, robbery or burglary **MURDER OF THE SECOND DEGREE** 'Murder, two' A homicide that falls short of criminal or premeditated intent; see Depraved heart murder, Manslaughter, Serial murder

Murine acquired immunodeficiency syndrome (MAIDS) A condition in mice caused by a defective retrovirus that has similarities to human AIDS, which include abnormal T and B cell function, polyclonal B cell proliferation, lymphadenopathy, splenomegaly, hyperγglobulinemia, increased susceptibility to infections and B cell lymphomas; MAIDS responds to cyclophosphamide (Science 1991; 251:305)

'Murky cell' carcinoma DERMATOPATHOLOGY A droll sobriquet for a pimary undifferentiated carcinoma of the skin, which is of undetermined origin, has a non-specific architectural pattern, indistinct cellular features, and vaguely resembles a Merkel cell tumor, a highly aggressive neuroendocrine neoplasm characterized by sheets of small-to-moderately-sized round 'blue' cells which have

Murphy's law of genetics 'Anything that may go wrong with a gene will go wrong'; Murphy's law is an American colloquialism attributed to a Colonel Murphy of the US Air Force, who observed that whenever something could go wrong, it (seemingly) would

Murray valley encephalitis A Japanese encephalitis-like disease occurring in small epidemic clusters in the Murray valley and elsewhere in Victoria and New South Wales, Australia, maintained by a wild-bird and mosquito cycle

Muscle A tissue of considerable research interest, given that it contains 'motor' proteins; when muscle is being examined for clinical disease, the biopsy should be obtained from a site moderately affected by disease, but not from the (inflamed) site of electromyography Type I muscle (slow-twitch or red muscle) is fatigue-resistant, has high mitochondrial oxidative (nicotinamide adenine dinucleotide-tetrazolium reductase or NADH-TR) activity and low glycolytic capacity, which stains lightly with ATPase at pH 9.4 (low myosin) and phosphorylase, and stains darkly with NADH-TR; type II muscle (fast twitch or white muscle) is fatigue-sensitive, has high glycolytic activity, displays light staining with NADH-TR and dark staining with ATPase at pH 9.4 (high myosin) and phosphorylase **Histology** Muscle is arranged in a mosaic of type I and type II fibers in a 1:1 ratio; Smooth muscle contraction is slower and more energy-efficient than that of skeletal muscle, which is related to the contractile apparatus, where muscle contraction occurs in a corkscrew-like fashion

Muscle antibodies see Smooth muscle antibodies

Muscle fiber type grouping see Type grouping

'Muscular cirrhosis' A term for the histopathology of end-stage interstitial pulmonary fibrosis, characterized by muscle cell proliferation with fibrosis, differentiating this from pulmonary leiomyomatosis in which the muscular proliferation is accompanied by minimal fibrosis

Muscular dystrophy, short classification

Name	Location	Heredity	Age, onset/‡
Becker	Pelvifemoral	X-Rec	16-20/50-60
Duchenne	Pelvifemoral	X-Rec	20-50/<20
Erb	Scapula	Auto Rec	20-30/
Landouzy-Dejerine	Facioscapulo-humeral	Auto Dom	15/Normal
Leyden-Mobius	Pelvic girdle	Auto Rec	20-50/<20

‡Age at death

Muscular dystrophy An X-linked, often recessive condition affecting 1:3500 male children, the most common form of which (clinical variants, see table, above), Duchenne's muscular dystrophy, often proves fatal by age 20; muscular dystroph(ies) are related to a defective muscle protein, dystrophin; in those with concomitant mental impairment (30%); which may be due to a defective dystrophin-like molecule is commonly found in the brain; functionally impaired smooth muscle of the gastrointestinal tract may cause impaired gastric emptying (N Engl J Med 1988; 319:15) **Histopathology** Muscle fibers demonstrate longitudinal splitting, ringed fibers, variability in size, juxtaposition of atrophic and hypertrophic cells, regeneration accompanied by endo- and perimysial connective tissue proliferation, fibrosis and fatty infiltration

Mushroom An adjectival descriptor for a thermonuclear explosion-like expansion of a cylindrical structure

Mushroom appearance PEDIATRIC ORTHOPEDICS The descriptor for a flattened femoral head that is contiguous with a broad neck, accompanied by a widened articular space, premature fusion of the ossification center and trochanteric overgrowth, seen in the re-ossification phase of Perthes disease, ie osteochondrosis of the femoral head, coxa plana; see Sagging rope sign

Mushrooming RADIOLOGY Burgeoning of bony excrescences in osteochondromata, often located adjacent to the epiphyseal plate in long bones

Mushroom lesion(s) Summit lesions GASTROENTEROLOGY 'Regurgitated' masses of acutely inflamed fibrinocellular exudate seen by low-power light microscopy in early pseudomembranous colitis, composed of fibrin, mucin, neutrophils, sloughed colonic epithelium and necrotic tips of the glands and abscessed crypts; see Pseudomembranous colitis

Mushroom of foam FORENSIC PATHOLOGY A frothy nasolabial 'spume' seen in drowning victims that may be inapparent when the body is first fished from the fjord, appearing as pressure is applied to the chest (in either resuscitative attempts or when removing the clothing); the foam is a mixture of air, mucus and water produced in the presence of respiratory movement and is considered proof that the victim was alive at the time of submersion; blood-stained foam is the result of increased intrathoracic pressure, a component of the drowning process; brown and malodorous foam indicates putrefaction; Cf 'Shaving cream' appearance

Mushrooms Fifty of the 2000 species of mushrooms are poisonous; the major toxin is the cyclic octapeptide-bearing amanitine, a selective RNA polymerase II inhibitor present in the ***Amanita*** and ***Galerina*** species; ***Amanita phalloides*** causes most mushroom deaths Mortality 40-90% Clinical Stage 1 Abrupt onset, ie within 6-24 hours after ingestion, accompanied by abdominal pain, nausea, vomiting, diarrhea, major fluid and electrolyte imbalances Stage 2 Apparent resolution, with asymptomatic renal and hepatic deterioration Stage 3 occurs by days 3-4 and is characterized by complete hepatorenal collapse, cardiomyopathy, disseminated intravascular coagulation, convulsions, coma and death

'Musician's wart' A heterogeneous group of calluses, hyperkeratoses and comedonic lesions appearing in regions where a musical instrument contacts or rests on the body, anointed with the highly descriptive terms, 'guitar nipple', 'cello scrotum' and 'fiddler's neck', which are variably accompanied by erythema and papule formation; see Performing arts medicine, Singer's nodule

Mutable gene An unstable gene that is both highly susceptible to mutation and which has a high rate of intrinsic mutation

Mutation A change in the base pair composition of DNA that differs from either of the parental haploid contributions to the progeny, most of which are not lethal **CONFORMATIONAL MUTATION** A single nucleotide substitution that alters the three-dimensional shape, ie conformation of the DNA's double helix, changing the mobility of restriction fragments in a polyacrylamide electrophoretic gel **MISSENSE MUTATION** A genomic mutation in which substitution of one (or more) base(s) encodes a different amino acid resulting in a dysfunctional protein **NONSENSE MUTATION** A point mutation in which a base pair substitution in transcription of the 'stop' codons UGA, UAA or UAG, which are signals for the mRNA to end translation into a protein **POINT MUTATION** A mutation that substitutes one base pair for another, but may not cause a restriction fragment length polymorphism; point mutations may be a) Silent, ie a 'synonymous mutation'; given DNA's 'degeneracy' is a base pair substitution which encodes the same amino acid; see Degenerate code, b) Yield a different new amino acid, a 'replacement mutation' which results in either a normally functioning protein (the substitution does not adversely impinge on the protein's active site) or a functionally defective protein, c) Result in the encoding of a missense codon, causing a premature termination of translation into a protein **SPONTANEOUS MUTATION** A de novo mutation that comprises 45% of major congenital malformations, which may be subsequently passed to future generations in an autosomal dominant and X-linked fashion (N Engl J Med 1989 320:19) **TRANSITION MUTATION** A type of substitution mutation involving an exchange between purines (adenine and guanine) or pyrimidines (cytidine and thymidine) **TRANSVERSION MUTATION** A specific base-pair mutation where a purine is substituted for a pyrimidine or vice versa

Mutations, detection of The 'gold standard' for detecting mutagenic activity is the Ames test, an in vitro assay designed to determine an agent's ability to induce mutations in bacteria; while the Ames test is expedient, its relevance to human environmental toxins is unclear; human gene assays are designed to detect mutations of the HGPRT (hypoxanthine guanine phosphoribosyl transferase) gene in T cells, as an indicator of an agent's mutagenic potential; toxins produce characteristic 'fingerprints' of the mutated gene that can be visualized by gradient denaturing gel electrophoresis (Science 1989; 243:737)

Mutation repair see SOS repair

Mutilating surgery '*...ANOTHER SUCH VICTORY AND WE ARE LOST...*'—Plutarch A form of 'heroic' surgery that consists of massive excision of tissue, usually from a broadly invasive malignancy, with the purpose of removing the tumor and/or metastases, regardless of the 'cost' in terms of deterioration of quality of life, potential infections and other co-morbid conditions; the availability of other modalities, eg chemotherapy, radiotherapy and various 'magic bullet' forms of immunotherapy, have made mutilating surgery a less preferred therapy for neoplasms

Muton A generic term of little practical use for a unit of a gene that is capable of undergoing mutation, ranging in size from a single nucleotide substitution, causing point mutations to deletions of large segments of DNA, causing frameshift mutations

Mutton fat lesion 'Greasy' rounded, yellow keratic precipitates of lymphocytes, plasma cells, epithelioid histiocytes and pigment adherent to the posterior aspect of the cornea seen in tuberculous iridocyclitis as well as in chronic granulomatous uveitis due to sarcoidosis

MVA Motor vehicular/vehicle accident A preventable morbid condition that claims 45 000 lives annually in the USA, 60% of whom are under age 35; MVAs account for 500 000 hospitalizations and most of the 20 000 spinal cord injuries in the US, at an annual cost of $75 billion; one-half of MVA fatalities in those ages 15-45 have excess blood alcohol levels and one-fourth have cocaine metabolites (J Am Med Assoc 1990; 263:250); The higher the population density in a given area, the lower the proportionate incidence of motor vehicular mortality ($2.5/10^5$ of Manhattan residents die annually of MVA, the adjusted rate for Nevada is $558/10^5$), due to a combination of poor road conditions, higher speeds, longer time in arriving to a hospital, less use of safety belts and higher use of vehicles with rolling tendencies, eg jeeps and trucks

M-VAC Methotrexate, vinblastine, doxorubicin (Adriamycin) and cis-platinum A chemotherapeutic regimen for bladder cancer

MVB see Multivesicular bodies

MVPS see Mitral valve prolapse syndrome

MVPS Medical volume performance standard

Myasthenic crises A clinical complex characterized by an acute exacerbation of myasthenia gravis symptoms, which is divided into 1) **MYASTHENIC CRISIS** An acute increase in requirement for anticholinesterase medication or refractoriness to same, which is diagnosed by a Tensilon test, with transient amelioration of symptoms and 2) **CHOLINERGIC CRISIS** An acute decrease in the need for anticholinesterase medication, resulting in 'overmedication' with the customary doses; the Tensilon test exacerbates this form of myasthenic crisis; cholinergic crises may be either a) **MUSCARINIC CRISIS**, causing abdominal pain, diarrhea, nausea, vomiting, lacrimation, blurred vision and bronchial hypersecretion due to over-response to the parasympathetic system or b) **NICOTINIC CRISIS**, characterized by muscle weakness, fasciculations, cramping and dysphagia, due to overdepolarization at the neuromuscular junction; see Tensilon test

c-*myb* MOLECULAR BIOLOGY A proto-oncogene that encodes a highly conserved 75-89 kD nuclear phosphoprotein (c-Myb) that is normally expressed in immature hematopoietic cell lines as these cells differentiate; c-Myb is down-regulated at the time of terminal differentiation; phosphorylation of Myb by casein kinase II at an N-terminal site prevents Myb from binding DNA and therefore from further activation; oncogenic transformation is associated with loss of this phosphorylation site, allowing Myb to bind to DNA (Nature 1990; 344:517)

myc MOLECULAR BIOLOGY An oncogene of cellular (c-myc) or viral (v-myc) origin that was first identified in the genome of a group of acutely transforming retroviruses capable of inducing neoplasia in birds possibly associated with RNA processing; c-*myc* is present in normal tissues and is dynamically expressed in the mid-gestation mouse embryo in various tissues undergoing expansion and folding of partially differentiated epithelial cells (Science 1989; 243:226); in humans, translocation of *myc*, designated as t(14;18)(q32;q21) results in the juxtaposition of bcl-2 to an activator of immunoglobulin heavy chains in follicular lymphoma; retroviruses with the *myc* gene inhibit terminal differentiation of myoblasts, locking the cells into continuous cycling (proliferation); c-myc in its normal site on chromosome 8 is transcriptionally silent; in Burkitt's lymphoma, c-*myc* is translocated, and becomes activated due to a) c-*myc*'s position to an immunoglobulin regulator b) truncation within the gene itself c) Mutation in the exon I and/or its flanking sequence or d) Due to a point mutation on the first intron of c-myc with a loss of a regulatory protein binding site; N-*myc* is amplified (3-300 copies) in stages II-IV of neuroblastomas (but not in stages I and IV-S), in lung cancer and in composite lymphoma, with simultaneous translocation of t(14;18) and t(8;14); c-*myc* proto-oncogene is amplified in early uterine cervix carcinoma (and may be a better prognosticator than lymph node status), lung cancer (more often in small cell carcinoma), promyelocytic leukemia, and is translocated in Burkitt's lymphoma Note: c-*myc* cooperates with H-*ras* in experimental transformation systems and the loss of c-Myc protein binding to DNA in vivo may explain its relation to malignant transformation (Science 1991; 251:186)

Mycetoma A condition first described by Gill in 1842 in the Madur district of India (hence the synonyms, Madura foot and maduromycosis); mycetoma is a generic term for a slow, relentless, ulcerating fungal (true fungi) infection, which when neglected, may result in osteomyelitis, occurring in a background of impaired host defense Agents ***Pseudallescheria boydii, Madurella mycetomatis, M grisea, Phialophora jeanselmei*** and others; Actinomycetoma is due to aerobic actinomycetes including ***Actinomadura madurae, A pelletieri, Streptomyces somaliensis, Nocardia brasiliensis, N asteroides*** and others, most common in the feet of young men (5:1) who work in the tropics and subtropics, which may aso be seen in the thigh and shoulders; clinical disease is uncommon unless accompanied by bacterial infection **Pathology** Indurated swelling, multiple draining sinus tracts and location in the foot **Histopathology** Suppurative granulomas surrounded by an amorphous rim of eosinophilic hyaline material produced as a host defense; the term mycetoma has also been applied to ***Acremonium*** and ***Fusarium*** species as well as the actinomycetes (***Actinomadura, Nocardia*** and ***Streptomyces*** species); the most common cause of mycetoma in the US is ***Pseudoallescheria boydii*** **Treatment** Trimethoprim-sulfamethoxazole

Mycobacterium All species of ***Mycobacterium*** are capable of producing the typical chronic inflammation, Langhans giant cells and varying amounts of caseating necrosis and are indistinguishable by the acid-fast stain; the most common portal of entry for non-tuberculous mycobacteria is the skin; see Acid-fast stain, Buruli ulcer, Langhans giant cells, MOTT, Prosector's wart, Runyon classification, Tuberculosis

Mycoplasma An incomplete intracellular and extracellular infectious particle that causes 'walking pneumonia' (which resolves in 4-6 weeks) and genitourinary infections; ***M pneumonia*** produces hydrogen peroxide, may be identified by hemadsorption and complement fixation and infects epithelial cells, without producing leukocytosis, ***M hominis*** may cause pelvic inflammatory disease, septicemia and urogenital infection MICROBIOLOGY ***Mycoplasma*** measure 0.25 µm, lack cell wall precursors (N-acetyl glucosamine and N-acetylmuramic acid), divide by binary fusion and fragmentation and have CO_2 and NH_3 as end products of ureaplasma enzymatic hydrolysis; the growth medium requires fresh yeast or fatty acids, sterols and nucleic acids; the 'spherule' seen on culture represents a microcolony and has a 'fried egg' appearance

***Mycoplasma*-AIDS link** A proposed pathogenic mechanism for the development of AIDS, proposed by L Montagnier, in which HIV-1 attaches to cells previously activated by infection with the cell-wall deficient mycoplasma, and associated infection first identified by SC Lo (Science 1991; 251:271n&v)

Mycosis cells T lymphocytes with scant cytoplasm, irregular hyperchromatic nuclei, a complex cerebriform nuclear membrane and increased mitotic activity, first described in mycosis fungoides and the related Sezary syndrome, which may also (rarely) be seen in lymphomatoid papulosis, psoriasis vulgaris, lichen planus, PLEVA, basal cell carcinoma, actinic keratosis, systemic and discoid lupus

Mycosis fungoides A rare ($0.3/10^5$/year), malignant neoplasm of paracortical T cells (usually of helper, less commonly, suppressor subtype) that is two-fold more common in older blacks Clinical Skin involvement precedes symptoms by up to 2 years; the leukemic phase (Sezary syndrome) occurs in 80% and is accompanied by fever, weight loss, lymphadenopathy, hepatosplenomegaly, eosinophilia and lymphocytosis, peripheral neuropathy and periarteritis nodosa; mycosis fungoides has been divided into four clinicopathologic stages of increasing aggression: Erythema stage, plaque stage, tumor stage, d'emblee stage Treatment Early aggressive radiotherapy and chemotherapy does not alter clinical disease (N Engl J Med 1989; 321:1784)

Mycotic aneurysm An intravascular inflammatory response seen in 3-15% of patients with infective endocarditis, which may arise from contiguous infected sites, but more commonly are of hematogenous spread, potentially resulting in thrombosis or rupture of arteries with walls weakened by an inflamed vasa vasorum or by an impaction-necrosis sequence; because the vessels are a poor culture medium for bacteria (commonly, ***Staphylococcus aureus***), smaller aneurysms may resolve spontaneously; those larger that 1-2 cm require excision, if surgically accessible; of greatest concern are the cerebral aneurysms; sites of symptomatic mycotic aneurysms include the sinus of Valsalva 25%, visceral arteries 24%, extremities 22% and brain 15%; Cf Berry aneurysm

Myelin basic protein (MBP) A 19 kD protein that is a major component of myelin, a lipoprotein that develops late in embryogenesis; MBP is elevated in multiple sclerosis and may evoke an altered T cell response to MBP in this condition (Science 1990; 247:718); many of the T cells responding to MBP have the Vβ17 variant of the T cell receptor (Science 1990; 248:1016)

Myelin figure Myelinoid body see Lamellar body

Myeloid antigen An antigen present on the surface of a leukocyte with myeloid differentiation, eg CD13, CD14 and CD33; the expression of myeloid antigens in acute lymphocytic leukemia carries a poor prognosis and represents the most powerful predictor of survival than any other parameters including initial white cell count, presence of extramedullary disease or T cell lineage (N Eng J Med 1991; 324:800); see CD antigens; Cf Pan-B cell markers, Pan-T cell markers

Myelodysplasia HEMATOLOGY see Myelodysplastic syndrome NEUROLOGY A generic term for a variety of developmental abnormalities of the spinal cord and nerve roots including myelomeningocele, sacral agenesis, spinal dysraphism and caudal regression syndrome; one-third of the infants with myelodysplasia develop external urethral sphincter dysfunction, often in the first three years of life, half of which are permanent (J Am Med Assoc 1987; 258:1630)

Myelodysplastic syndromes HEMATOLOGY A term that may be equated to preleukemia (which is only partially correct as pathologically, 'dysplasia' is neither clonal nor malignant, but may imply a premalignant condition); myelodysplasia is associated with monosomy 7 in granulocytes and monocytes which may cause defective granulocyte function (N Engl J Med 1987; 316:499); see Preleukemia

Myelofibrosis An increase in the reticulin fibers in the bone marrow, comprising up to 25% of the marrow volume, which may be idiopathic (see Agnogenic myeloid metaplasia) or secondary to chronic myelocytic leukemia, polycythemia vera, idiopathic thrombocytopenic purpura Laboratory Thrombocytosis (1-14 X 10^{12}/L) with giant and bizarre forms, hypochromic and microcytic anemia or erythrocytosis, elliptocytosis, Howell-Jolly bodies, target and teardrop cells; mild leukocytosis (15-40 X 10^{12}/L) with increased 'bands', ie left shift of granulocytes, juvenile metamyelocytes, occasionally eosinophilia, basophilia, splenic atrophy BONE MARROW Megakaryocytic hyperplasia, increased reticulin fibers, giant cells and immature forms, virus-like particles, granulocytic and erythrocytic hyperplasia, chromosomal abnormalities, eg of 21q which may correlate with reverse transcriptase activity Laboratory Increased leukocyte alkaline phosphatase, platelet acid phosphatase, uric acid, vitamin B_{12} and low grade disseminated intravascular coagulation

Myeloma see Multiple myeloma

Myeloma, IgD A condition that comprises 1-2% of all cases of myeloma, most commonly seen in older men Clinical Lymphadenopathy and hepatosplenomegaly, accompanied in 45% of cases by extra-osseous dissemination (which is present in 15% of IgA and IgG myelomas), hyperviscosity, severe anemia, azotemia, marked osteolysis, hypercalcemia and, commonly bizarre plasmacytes and plasmablasts; the M component is not markedly elevated

Myeloma kidney The combination of structural and functional renal defects that occurs in up to 40% of multiple myelomas and includes intraluminal eosinophilic 'blocked pipe' casts composed of PAS-positive homogeneous material and light chains (Bence-Jones proteins) within flattened distal tubules and collecting ducts (pressure atrophy), spilling over of proteinaceous material into the tubules, eliciting chronic interstitial nephritis, causing glomerulonephritis; the mesangial widening may mimic diabetic nephropathy; functional abnormalities cause renal failure in about 20%, due to hypercalcemia and renal calcinosis, heavy Bence-Jones proteinuria (causing tubular damage), hyperuricemia (increased tumor DNA turnover), proteinuria, amyloidosis and chronic pyelonephritis, acquired Fanconi syndrome, defects in acidification and concentration, acute and chronic renal failure Laboratory A peak may be seen in the γ-globulin region (usually) of urine electrophoresisor may appear between the α_2 and β regions

Myeloperoxidase deficiency syndrome A common (1:500 to 1:2000) autosomal recessive neutrophil dysfunction, resulting in a prolonged respiratory burst due to defective post-translational processing of an abnormal precursor protein Clinical Usually asymptomatic (several cases of *Candida* infections were reported in patients with concomitant diabetes mellitus) Treatment Unnecessary

Myelosclerosis with myeloid metaplasia see Agnogenic myeloid metaplasia

Myeloproliferative disorders (MPD) A generic term for hematopoietic stem cell disease(s) that are divided by chronicity ACUTE MPD Acute myelogenous leukemia (Myeloblastic, promyelocytic, myelomonocytic, monocytic, erythroid, megakaryocytic, eosinophilic, basophilic), acute biphenotypic (with myeloid and lymphoid markers) leukemia, and acute leukemia with lymphoid markers evolving from a prior clonal hemopathy SUBACUTE MPD Oligoblastic (smoldering) leukemia, refractory anemia with excess blasts (see RAEB), myelomonocytic leukemia CHRONIC MPD Polycythemia vera, agnogenic myeloid metaplasia, primary thrombocythemia, chronic myelogenous leukemia (Philadelphia chromosome positive or negative), chronic monocytic leukemia, chronic neutrophilic leukemia

Myocardial depressant factor(s) (MDF) As-yet unidentified molecule(s) that is/are thought to be present in the circulation of patients in shock; since MDF activity closely parallels the blood levels of lysosomal enzymes, MDF is thought to be a small peptide

Myocardial infarct Acute necrosis of myocardial tissue; in the early post-insult period, there may be a need to rely on 'soft' data, especially if the 'cardiac' enzymes have yet to increase, or there is a loss of sensation to the pain characteristic of : myocardial infarction, as occurs in circa 10% patients with diabetic mellitus; elderly older women may have normal levels of creatinine phosphokinase during recuperation from a myocardial infarct Risk factors for myocardial infarction Atherosclerosis, high cholesterol, hypertension, smoking, diabetes mellitus, low selenium and other factors (J Am Med Assoc 1989; 261:1161) Laboratory see Cardiac enzymes, 'Flipped' LD Pathology Chronicle of myocardial changes A) GROSS FINDINGS 6-12 hours Pallor by nitrotetrazolium blue test 18-24 hours Pallor by gross examination 2-4 days Yellow with hyperemic borders 4-10 days Yellow-gray to bright yellow with maximum softness 6 weeks Fibrosis and scar formation B) LIGHT MICROSCOPY 60 minutes Glycogen depletion 4-6 hours Myofibrillary degeneration 6-24 hours Coagulation necrosis 1-7 days Neutrophils, macrophages, fatty infiltration, nuclear pyknosis 1-6 weeks Scarring, granulation tissue formation C) ELECTRON MICROSCOPY 10-15 minutes Glycogen depletion 20-60 minutes Mitochondrial swelling with amorphous densities (tissue recovery is still possible) 3-4 hours Membranes rupture 5-6 hours Fragmentation of myofibrils Potentially fatal complications of myocardial infarction Shock, cardiac arrhythmias, rupture of ventricular aneurysms or papillary muscle, acute congestive heart failure, mural thromboembolism

Myocardial ischemia Hypoxia of the myocardium, characterized by an increase in tumor necrosis factor (TNF-β), local production of superoxide anions, loss of coronary vasodilation and myocardial necrosis; when given at the time of the ischemic event, recombinant TNF reduces circulating superoxide anions, maintains endothelial-dependent coronary relaxation and reduces the myocardial injury mediated by endogenous TNF (Science 1990; 247:61)

MyoD A sequence-specific DNA-binding protein that can activate muscle-specific gene expression in certain cells in vitro, which requires the interaction with other factors for complete and stable myogenesis (Nature 1990; 347:197)

***MyoD1* gene** A gene that regulates myogenesis, encoding the MyoD1 protein, a nuclear phosphoprotein with partial homology to the *myc* family of oncoproteins, which binds to the enhancer sequences of the muscle-specific creatine phosphokinase gene, inhibiting DNA synthesis and cell proliferation (Nature 1990; 345:813) Note: The 20 residue *myc*-like peptide segment converts fibroblasts to myoblasts; an action attributed to the presence of a helix-loop-helix domain in the encoded protein

Myoinositol (MI) One of the nine isomers of cyclohexane, synthesized from and structurally similar to glucose; these structures are present in most cells and in high concentration in the nervous system in patients with diabetes mellitus; diabetic neuropathy is attributed to a) Increased sorbitol in schwann cells, which through its osmotic effect, causes intracellular edema, slowing conduction and b) Decreased MI and its phospholipids within the Schwann cells, impairing Na^+-K^+-activated transport ATPase; MI is decreased in the nerves of diabetics during fasting (Mayo Clin Proc 1989; 64:905); Cf Advance glycosylation endproducts

Myopia An abnormality of refraction and accommodation in which parallel rays of light come to a focus anterior to the retina; myopic children are usually products of similarly afflicted adults and tend to as a group be more educated and have higher intelligent quotients (Arch Ophthalmol 1987; 105:1508); simple myopia increases through adolescence, and may be associated with degenerative phenomena in the retina; the use of cycloplegic agents and bifocals to retard the progression of myopia is controversial

Myositis ossificans Bone formed within muscle; the localized form of myositis ossificans is secondary to trauma resulting from a blow or muscle tearing; the generalized form is autosomal dominant, often accompanied by aplasia of the thumb, great toe, or rarely other digits, in which the first 'tumor' occurs in the paravertebral or cervical region, followed by multiple ossifying tumors, forming calcifying bridges across muscles and joints resulting in massive rigidity and the patient is turned into 'stone'; see Zoning phenomenon

Myotonic dystrophy An autosomal dominant condition with a gene defect , located on chromosome 19, which causes distal myopathy, preferentially affecting certain muscles, eg levator palpebrae, facial, masseter, sternocleidomastoid, forearm, hand and pretibial muscles, resulting in diffuse muscular weakness and atrophy beginning in early adulthood causing the characteristic 'hatchet face'; other changes include lenticular opacities, endocrinopathies (testicular atrophy with androgen insufficiency, ovarian dysfunction which rarely interferes with fertility, diabetes mellitus, hypothyroidism), mild cerebral cortical atrophy, frontoparietal baldness, cardiac and smooth muscle (gastrointestinal, especially esophageal motility) abnormalities, respiratory dysfunction and hyperostosis frontalis interna; death usually occurs by age 50 **Histopathology** Variable type I muscle fiber atrophy, with internal nuclei, ringed muscle fibers, increased intrafusal myofibers in the muscle spindles and hypertrophy of type II muscle fibers; internal (centralized) nuclei are characteristic, and occur early, as do sarcoplasmic masses ('pads') and annulets

Myotubular (centronuclear) myopathy A myopathy with various patterns of inheritance, which have a common feature of centrally-located nuclei within muscle fibers, which are surrounded by cytoplasmic material with features of maturing myotubules, accompanied by atrophy of type I and hypertrophy of type II muscle fibers; the X-linked form results in neonatal death due to respiratory muscle insufficiency; the autosomal dominant form is not pernicious

Myristate n-tetradecanoate acid The fatty acid component of glycosyl phosphatidylinositol, an integral membrane component of trypanosomes; see O-11

Myristoylated alanine-rich (protein) C kinase substrate see MARCK

Myxedema The hypothyroid state elicits several reactions ***a sui generis*** **Myxedema coma** A complication of severe hypothyroidism, in which an additional physiological stress is added to the clinical milieu, eg iatrogenic (sedatives in hypothyroidism are very slowly metabolized), infections, cold exposure or rarely, may occur spontaneously Mortality 20-50% **Myxedema madness** A condition that is most common in the elderly, characterized by impaired hearing and memory, acalculia, somnolence, psychological withdrawal and paranoia **Myxedema megacolon** Pseudoobstruction due to reduced gastrointestinal motility **Myxedema wit** Confabulation or use of humorous non-sequiturs by a patient with hypothyroidism in order to draw the interviewer's attention away from the patient's impaired memory

Myxoid A non-specific descriptor for any 'loose' pale-to-lightly basophilic by hematoxylin and eosinophilic stroma, the few cells present include fibroblasts and rarely chronic inflammatory cells; myxoid stroma occurs in nodular fasciitis, intramuscular myxoma, ganglion cyst, chordoma, neurofibroma, carcinomas, as well as spindle cell lipoma and lipoblastoma and in myxoid variants of sarcomas, where the distinction is of practical importance, as myxoid differentiation may have a better prognosis, including rhabdomyosarcoma, chondrosarcoma, malignant fibrous histiocytoma, liposarcoma; Cf Mucin lake

Myxoma A stromal proliferation that in the cardiac myxomas may demonstrate chromosomal abnormalities (telomere-to-telomere translocations, 45, XY) supporting a neoplastic origin

Myxopapillary ependymoma see Ependymoma

Myxovirus A large single-stranded RNA virus divisible into a) Orthomyxoviruses, eg influenza virus and b) Paramyxovirus, eg mumps virus

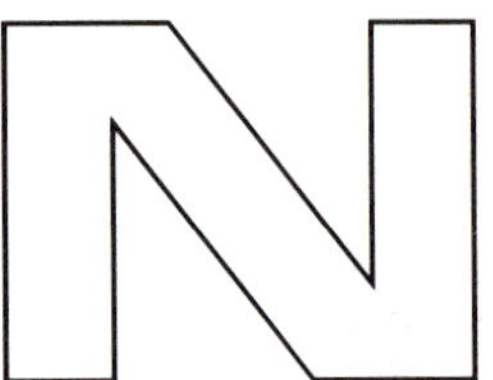

N Shorthand symbol for: Asparagine; neutron number; Avogadro's number (particles in 1 Mole = 6.023×10^{23}); nitrogen; population size; normal solution (equivalents/liter, a convention frowned upon by the International System)

n Shorthand symbol for: Haploid number; nano-; neutron, refractory index; sample size in data sets

ν (greek letter nu): Degrees of freedom; frequency; neutrino

NAD^+/NADH The oxidized/reduced forms of nicotinamide adenine dinucleotide, a redox coenzyme, crucial in intracellular storage (by high-energy phosphate bonds) and exchange of energy; a coenzyme used to transfer hydrogen (formerly, coenzyme I)

$NADP^+$/NADPH The oxidized/reduced forms of nicotinamide adenine dinucleotide phosphate; a coenzyme for transfer of hydrogen in the pentose phosphate reaction, which is also a coenzyme for glutathione reductase

Naegleria A genus of free-living flagellated soil-based amoebae of Class Rhizopoda that may cause primary amoebic meningitis, see there

Na^+/H^+ antiporter A 110 kD plasma membrane exchange glycoprotein transporter that regulates intracellular pH, important in signal transduction, which is modified in response to external mitogenic signals (phorbol esters, neurotransmitters, chemotactic peptides, lectins and growth factors) and by oncogenic transformation which induce persistent cytoplasmic alkalinization; antiporter activation is thought to be the result of phosphorylation (Science 1990; 247:723)

Na^+/K^+ ATPase PHYSIOLOGY A ubiquitous, integral membrane-bound enzyme that is present in all animal cells, and couples ATP hydrolysis to the countertransport of Na^+ and K^+ ions across the plasma membrane; in neurons, dopamine inhibits this pump, providing a mechanism by which neurotransmitters can regulate neuronal excitability (Nature 1990; 347:386); the responsible ATPase is an oligomer with two 90 kD (α) subunits and two 40 kD (β) subunits; cardiac glycosides are thought to act by blocking the receptor's β subunit

Nail-patella syndrome Österricher-Turner syndrome, Hereditary Osteo-Onychodysplasia HOOD syndrome An autosomal dominant disease affecting structures of both mesodermal and ectodermal origin with partial-to-complete absence of thumbnails and great toenails, flexion contractions of multiple joints, defective or absent patellae, lordosis, clinodactyly and campylodactyly, conical iliac horns, scapular thickening, radial head subluxation, renal abnormalities (mesangial proliferation, thickened glomerular basement membrane, collagen deposition with proteinuria, microscopic hematuria, glomerulonephritis, pyelonephritis and slowly progressive renal failure) and ocular disease (clover leaf pigmentation of iris, cataracts, microphakia, microcornea, keratoconus, ptosis)

Naked granuloma 'Hard' tubercle An epithelioid giant cell response consisting of Langhans' giant cell(s) and chronic, ie mononuclear cell inflammation without necrosis, therefore 'naked', a histologic finding typical of sarcoidosis and granuloma annulare

Naked nuclei CYTOLOGY A soft criterion for diagnosing ovarian endometriosis, seen in the slightly elongated, cytoplasm-poor cells with hyperchromatic nuclei Note: Definitive diagnosis of endometriosis requires endometrial glands, stroma and hemorrhage SURGICAL PATHOLOGY Naked cells are highly characteristic of undifferentiated or small cell carcinomas of any site, most commonly seen in small or 'oat' cell carcinoma of the lung and other sites which have friable ('taffy-pull') nuclei and scant or absent cytoplasm

Nalbuphine A narcotic agonist that is chemically related to naloxone with similar action to, but less addictive than morphine

NALC N-acetyl L-cysteine MICROBIOLOGY A mucolytic agent used for collecting sputa destined for tuberculosis culture that liquefies the mucus by breaking disulfide bonds

NAME syndrome see LAMB syndrome

NANB see Hepatitis, non-A, non-B type

Nancy Cruzan see Cruzan

Nantucket Disease A blood-borne infection by ***Babesia microti***, an intertriginous cyst-forming parasite, named after an island off Massachusetts in the US Northeast coast, occurring along the entire northeast seaboard of the USA Reservoir White-footed mouse **Vector** ***Ixodes dammini*** (the 'Lyme disease' tick) In Europe, babesiosis is most common in splenectomized subjects and is often fatal; in the US, it is rarely fatal and the splenectomized subjects comprise one-third of cases **Clinical** 1-3 week incubation, malaise, fatigue, anorexia, shaking chills, fever, headache, myalgias, depression and emotional lability **Diagnosis** Wright-Giemsa-stained smears of peripheral blood, where the ring form resembles that of ***Plasmodium falciparum***; indirect immunofluorescent antibody titers greater than 1:256 **Treatment** Clindamycin, quinacrine

NAP Neutrophil alkaline phosphatase see Leukocyte alkaline phosphatase

NAP-1 Neutrophil attractant or activation protein-1 see Interleukin-8

Naphtha Any petroleum distillation product; gasoline (British)

Naphthalene A crystal formed from 2 benzene rings, used for mothballs and insecticide **Toxicity** Headache, nausea, vomiting and hematuria, if severe or prolonged exposure, cataracts, convulsions, hepatocellular necrosis and marked hemolysis, especially in patients with glucose-6-phosphate dehydrogenase deficiency

Naphthol White crystalline phenol derivative intermediate in the synthesis of multiple compounds including pharmaceuticals **Toxicity** Abdominal pain, glomerulonephritis, convulsions, circulatory collapse and skin pigmentation

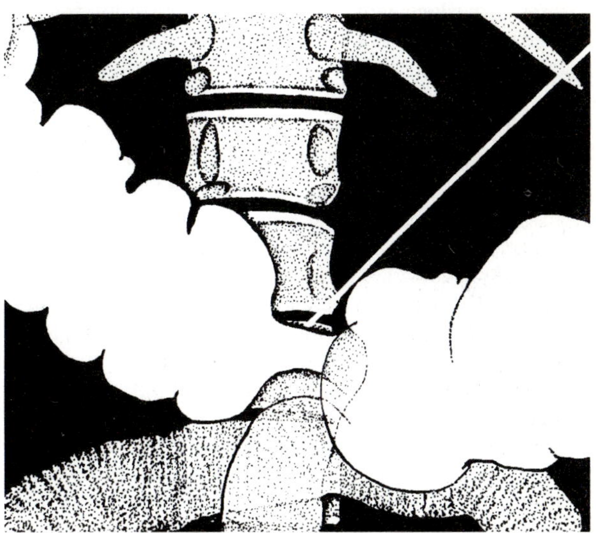

Napkin ring lesion

Napkin ring lesion Apple core lesion RADIOLOGY A pattern of intestinal constriction caused by mucosal erosion and stenosis with 'shouldering' of the margins, corresponding to an exophytic encircling mass within the large intestinal lumen, usually corresponding to an advanced invasive adenocarcinoma, more often present in the left colon; the mass may obstruct fecal flow, inducing pencil-thin stools and be partially mimicked by concentric amebomas in ***Entamoeba histolytica*** granulomas, by exuberant submucosal fibrosis in Crohn's disease, in the stenosing fibrotic stages of diverticulosis coli, and may occur in adenocarcinomas of the small intestine

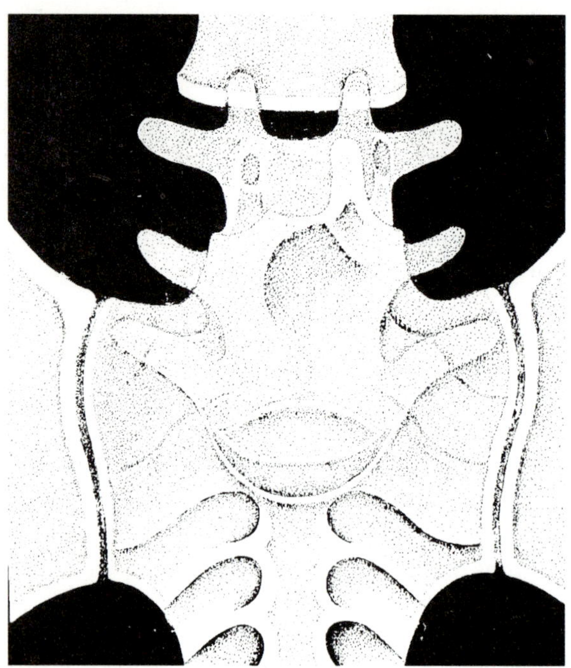

Napoleon's hat sign

Napoleon hat sign ORTHOPEDIC RADIOLOGY Marked antero-inferior displacement of the anterior edge of lumbar vertebrum L5, seen as a symmetrical navicular density in a frontal plain film of the lower vertebrae in congenital spondylolisthesis, fancifully likened to an inverted napoleonic hat

Naproxen see Non-steroid anti-inflammatory drugs

Narcolepsy A condition characterized by recurring attacks of irresistible desire for sleep and abnormalities of rapid-eye-movement (REM) sleep; narcolepsy affects 125 000 in the USA (prevalence 40/10^5) and is defined as a daytime mean sleep latency of less than 5 minutes, in conjunction with verification of REM in two of five daytime nap periods; 'classic narcolepsy' occurs in 70% of patients and is a combination of narcolepsy with cataplexy (abrupt loss of muscle tone, evoked by stong emotion, excitement, anger or laughter), causing them to collapse or fall to the ground, while completely conscious Note: Despite the common association, cataplexy differs from narcolepsy as it affects cell clusters in the medial medulla distinct from those affected in narcolepsy (Science 1991; 252:1315); narcoleptics may have amnesia for the 'absences', have fallen asleep while driving or while at work and prefer shift work as 'drowsiness' is more socially acceptable Prevalence From 1:600 (Japan) to 1:500 000 (Israel), affecting men and women equally, with an onset between the ages of 15 and 35, tightly linked to certain class II HLA antigens, eg 98-100% of narcoleptics have HLA-DR2 and/or HLA-DQw1 *NARCOLEPSY TETRAD* Narcolepsy, cataplexy, hypnagogic hallucinations and sudden paralysis; in cataplexy, which is often associated with narcolepsy, the patient feels a sense of absolute urgency for sleep in often inappropriate situations (while standing, eating, carrying on conversations) and is accompanied by blurring of vision, diplopia and ptosis **Treatment** Strategic pre-planned 'catnaps' throughout the day, analeptic drugs, ie long-term stimulants, eg methylphenidate, dextroamphetamine or tricyclic antidepressants that act by inhibiting re-uptake of norepinephrine and serotonin (N Engl J Med 1990; 323:389rv; Mayo Clin Proc 1990; 65:991); monoamine oxidase inhibiting agent may be useful in short term but can cause tardive dyskinesia; see Insomnia(s), Sleep apnea syndrome, Sleep disorders

Narcotic A substance causing euphoria and analgesia at the desired abuse levels and physical dependence and central nervous system depression, stupor, coma and death when administered in excess; narcotics may be a) Natural products extracted from the poppy plant, yielding morphine and heroin or the coca plant, yielding cocaine and crack b) Semi-synthetic products with opiate activity, eg meperidine and methadone or synthetics, see MPTP; under the umbrella term of narcotic, alkaloids, eg LSD, mescalin, barbiturates, alcohol, marijuana, cocaine, hallucinogens and stimulants, eg antidepressants and c) Completely synthetic narcotics, eg fentanyl

'Narcs' An American colloquialism for narcotics enforcement agents; Cf Narks

'Narks' A British colloquialism for nitrogen narcosis; see Rapture of the deep

Nasal cycle RESPIRATORY PHYSIOLOGY Alternating congestion and decongestion of the nasal airway that occurs in 70% of the adult population and is controlled by the autonomic nervous system; in the face of a unilateral fixed obstruction, the congestion phase of the side opposite the obstruction is interpreted as an abnormality of the normal side or 'paradoxical nasal obstruction' (Mayo Clin Proc 1990; 65:1095)

Nasal packing OTORHINOLARYNGOLOGY The filling of the nasal cavities with adaptic gauze impregnated with polysporin ointment, used in treating nasal fractures, reconstructive surgery, after septorhinoplasty and in posterior nosebleeds; with packing the airway improves in 96% of the packing group (versus 64% in the non-packed group); recurrent deviation occurred in 13% of the packed and 41% of the non-packed group (Plast Reconstruct Surgery1989; 84:41)

Nasopharyngeal carcinoma (NPC) A malignancy endemic to regions of southern China, where it is up to 100-fold more common than in Europe, often associated with HLA-A2, Bw46 and B17; NPC is associated with Epstein-Barr virus infection and 65% of NPCs express EBV's latent membrane protein (LMP); when keratinocytes in tissue culture are transfected with the LMP gene, the keratinocytes dedifferentiate, acquiring a 'malignant' morphology (Nature 1990; 245:447)

Natal teeth Teeth seen in 1:2000 neonates, often located in the position of the central mandibular incisors, with minimal gingival attachment, or less commonly, presage early eruption of remaining deciduous teeth **Clinical** If the teeth are loose, they are annoying to the nursing infant; if the teeth are well implanted, they are annoying to the nursing mother **Complication** Amputation of the tongue tip (Riga-Fede disease) by the natal teeth at the time of delivery

National boards examination A standardized examination that is administered in the US and Canada in lieu of state medical examinations to determine the level of competence of a candidate physician applying for a state's medical license Cf Stater

National Bureau of Standards A branch of the US government responsible for maintaining primary reference standards and developing reference methods and reference materials

National Cancer Institute (NCI) An organization with a focused interest in cancer research that has provided financial support of many experimental protocols in the US; see Cancer screening

National Formulary One of two (the other is the US Pharmacopeia) official compendia recognized by Federal Pure Food and Drug Act of 1906; in the National Formulary, the approved therapeutic agents used in medical practice in the USA are described and defined with respect to source, chemistry, physical properties, tests for identity and purity, dosage range and class of use

National Health Federation (NHF) An organization based in Washington DC with neither medical or scientific affiliations that represents the belief that organized medicine, the pharmaceutical industry and other 'special interest' groups have controlled legislation that does not serve the interests of the American public

National Institute for Occupational Safety and Health (NIOSH) The research arm and 'scientific conscience' of the US federal health and safety programs; NIOSH responsibilities include a) Development of 'criteria documents' that recommend exposure limits to hazardous substances b) Training and education of occupational health professionals c) Development of exposure measurement and sampling methods and d) Performance of industry-wide studies to evaluate the health effects of low level long-term exposure to potentially hazardous substances or processes; exposure to environmental toxins in the workplace is usually measured in parts (1 to 5000 or more, depending upon the substance) per million (ppm) of exposure/8 hours (Publications Division, NIOSH, 4676 Columbia Pkwy, Cincinnati, Ohio 45226)

National Institutes of Health see NIH

National Practitioner Data Bank A database established by the US Congress to facilitate professional peer review and restrict the ability of incompetent physicians and dentists to move from state to state, eluding discovery of previous substandard performance or unprofessional conduct; the Data Bank is accessible only to authorized persons and there are criminal penalties for misuse of the data or accession by unauthorized parties (J Am Med Assoc 1990; 264:945)

Native Unaltered or ground state of a molecular species, in which state in vivo biological systems are presumed to function

Natural antibody An antibody present in the circulation, without there being known previous exposure to the antigen, eg antibodies to the ABO blood group

Natural carcinogen A substance that is normally present in foods, which is carcinogenic when tested by standard mutagenic assays in rodents or in bacteria, eg Ames' test; it is unclear whether the 14 parts per million (ppm) of 5-8-methoxypsoralen, present in parsley and parsnips, and carcinogenic to rodents or the 50-200 ppm of caffeic acid, present in apples, carrots, cherries and others, actually present a carcinogenic potential in humans, or as Ames et al have implied (Proc Natl Acad Sci, USA 1990; 87:7777), there is a threshold at which critical mutation occurs (Science 1990; 250:743); see Ames' test, Toxicity testing

Natural childbirth A normal vaginal delivery in which the mother is more actively involved in the parturitional mechanics (than in the 'unnatural' birth); the 'natural' mother is awake during delivery often without general anesthesia, has actively 'trained' in the birthing process, and is 'attended' by the father at the time of delivery; see Bonding, Breast milk, Lamaze method

'Natural experiment' method EPIDEMIOLOGY A 'technique' in epidemiology that seeks to identify two or more naturally occurring cohorts with clear differences in sex, race, religion, occupation, geography and 'exposures', analyzing their risks for suffering certain diseases; 'natural experiment' populations include Mormons (non-smoking, non-drinking); Italians (low incidence of cardiovascular disease); Japanese and Icelanders (high incidence of gastric carcinoma); much of current knowledge about various morbid conditions, eg cancer and cardiovascular disease), their putative etiologies, early detection and prevention is initially recognized by statistical analysis of 'natural experiments'

Natural food movement see Health food movement

Natural gas An odorless (odorant is added to the gas as a safety precaution) combustible gas used for cooking and heating, the principal components of which are CH_4 (methane), ethane, propane, butane, CO_2, N_2 and H_2S **Toxicity** At high ambient levels, the volatile hydrocarbons induce hypoxia by replacing alveolar gas, crossing the alveolar-capillary barrier and causing central nervous system depression; Cf Flatulence

Natural killer cell (NK cell) A subset of 'null cells' or large granular lymphocytes (LGLs) that comprise 3-5% of peripheral leukocytes, 75% of which are NK cells with a high cytoplasmic:nuclear ratio and an intrinsic non-antibody-mediated ability to kill various cells, including virus-transformed fibroblasts, solid or hematopoietic tumor cells, microorganisms, embryologic, marrow and thymic cells; NK cells are stimulated by IL-2 to release eosinophilic granules (primary lysosomes) and interferon, increasing the number of target-binding NK cells, their cytotoxicity and speed of cytolysis Note: Cytolysis is normally slow (18 hours), triggered by protein kinase C, facilitated by lymphokines and mediated by perforins that insert transmembrane 'doughnuts' allowing free passage of ions into the cells; NK activity may also be stimulated by K-***ras*** oncogenic activation; NK activity decreases with age, malignancy (especially immunoproliferative) and immunodeficiency, eg severe combined immunodeficiency, X-linked and Chediak-Higashi syndromes NK cell surface markers IgG-FcR(2), low affinity T-cell markers (CD3), C3bi, Leu-7, HNK-1, OKM1, Mac

1, CD16 (Leu11) and B67.1 (T cell markers) **Quantification of NK cell activity** Measurement of lysis of the radioactive K-562 target cells

Natural selection see Darwinism

Nature-nurture debate PSYCHOLOGY An on-going controversy regarding the degree of influence the genome ('nature') has in determining behavior and shaping personality, and to what degree environmental factors('nurture') determine personality; this issue is unlikely to be resolved as it is not amenable to statistically valid experiments (Science 1990; 248:183)

Naturopathy 'Holistic medicine' An unorthodox approach to healing that espouses the philosophy that disease is the result of the violation of natural laws of living, ie drugs of any sort are harmful, while 'natural' products and activities are deemed therapeutic; 'naturopaths' are not licensed, but rather meet self-determined criteria; conventional drugs are proscribed and 'therapy' is prescribed, based on the use of natural forces and foods, herbs, teas and massage; see Holistic medicine; Homeopathy

Navicular cells Navicular, Latin, Boat-shaped CYTOLOGY Glycogen-rich variant of intermediate squamous cells seen in the papanicolaou-stained cytological preparations of the vagina and cervix (figure, below); navicular cells comprise the most abundant cells in pregnancy and are seen in early menopause, hormonal deficiencies and inflammation), see Maturation index

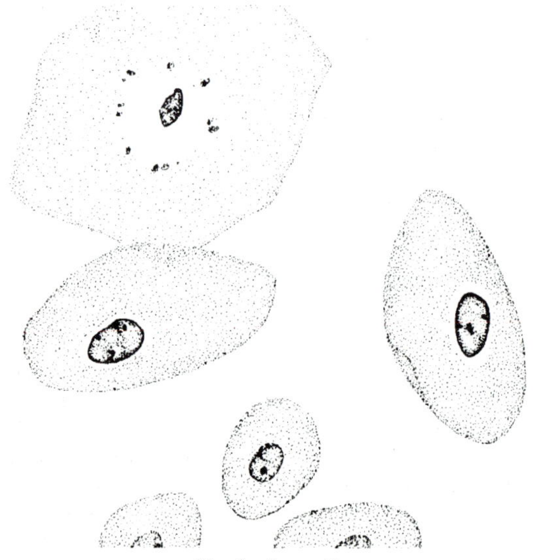

Navicular cells

NBE Non-bacterial endocarditis, see Mycotic aneurysm

NBS see National Bureau of Standards

NBT Nitroblue tetrazolium test A quantitative test that measures neutrophil peroxidase activity, indicating phagocytic capacity (the ability to reduce NBT which precipitates as deep blue granules if superoxide or O_2^- is produced in tested cell) which occurs via the hexose monophosphate shunt; NBT reduction is defective in Chronic granulomatous disease, see there

NBQX 2,3-Dihydroxy-6-nitro-7-sulfamoyl-benzo(F)-quinoxaline A non-NMDA (excitatory amino acid) receptor antagonist that has a protective effect against cerebral ischemia (Science 1990; 247:571); Cf NMDA

N-Cadherin see Cadherins

N-CAM Neural-cell adhesion molecule A glycoprotein present at the interfaces of cell clusters in early developing embryos; N-CAM's sequence, elucidated by cDNA (complementary DNA) analysis, reveals an extracellular region with 5 domains homologous to each other and to the immunoglobulin superfamily (immunoglobulins and T cell receptor); N-CAM modulates extracellular regions resulting in different extracellular signal 'messages' during embryogenesis and mediates post-translational changes in the oligosaccharides on the cell surface; N-CAM also mediates interneuronal and neuromuscular cell adhesions, influencing intercellular events, eg junctional communication and interaxonal associations with pathways, targets and signals altering neurotransmitter levels; low polysialic acid (PSA) levels in N-CAM triggers adhesion and contact-dependent events; high N-CAM PSA content inhibits cell-cell interactions; transition of the N-CAM isoform from 145 kD to 125 kD is associated with maturation from the myoblast to the multinucleated skeletal form (Nature 1990; 344:348)

N:C ratio see Nuclear:cytoplasmic ratio

NCI see National Cancer Institute

NDA New drug application PHARMACEUTICAL INDUSTRY A document generated usually from a pharmaceutical company that is the first step in developing a commercial drug; in the US, many years are required before a drug arrives to the 'marketplace'; after the chemist creates an 'interesting' compound, it is tested on the usual battery of beasts; if it is neither toxic nor teratogenic, the company may submit a commercial IND (investigational new drug) application, passing through phases 1 to 3 of clinical pharmacology; if both the FDA and drug's sponsor are satisfied that the drug has a desirable effect and an acceptable (low) level of toxic effects, an NDA is submitted; while this slow, tedious process is claimed to stifle creativity (as the cost of developing novel agents is financially burdensome), the US was spared the brunt of the thalidomide tragedy, which resulted in 10-15 000 cases of partial or complete phocomelia, largely in Germany; about 2/3 of the NDAs are returned to the sponsor for more information, often pertaining to issues regarding the drug's chemistry or manufacture; the average time from submission of an NDA until its approval is 32 months, during which time, labeling, indications, dosages, and methods of administration are delineated (N Engl J Med 1989; 320:281); see IND, Phase 1, 2, 3 studies

Nd-YAG laser Neodymium-yttrium aluminum garnet laser A photocoagulation unit used to control acute and chronic gastrointestinal hemorrhage, eg an endoscopically guided Nd-YAG laser may be used to control esophageal varices, vascular ectasias, angiodysplasia, radiation-induced telangiectasia, watermelon stomach, telangiectasia of Osler-Weber-Rendu, palliation of malignancy and management of benign and malignant obstructive biliary tract lesions (Mayo Clin Proc 1990; 65:509); see Lasers

Near-death experience A phenomenon of unclear nature that may occur in patients who have been clinically dead and then resuscitated; the patients report a continuity of subjective experience, remembering visitors and other hospital events despite virtually complete suppression of cortical activity; near-death experiences are considered curiosities with no valid explanation in the context of an acceptable biomedical paradigm; the trivial synonym, Lazarus complex refers to the biblical Lazarus who was raised from the dead by Jesus of Nazareth; see Harvard criteria

'Near miss' sudden infant death syndrome A prolonged, usually nocturnal apneic period in children, in whom the non-fatal outcome of apnea is attributed to continuous monitoring; 'near-miss' SIDS children may have enlarged adenoids or nasopharyngitis which responds to adenoidectomy; see SIDS

'Near poor' SOCIAL MEDICINE An increasingly large segment of the US population that has earnings sufficient only for daily needs, and therefore are not qualified for US government assistance programs; the near poor seldom have medical insurance and when ill, become a major burden for the health care system; Cf Engel's phenomenon, 'Fourth World', Homeless(ness)

Nebulin A 550 kD protein, located in the A and I bands that constitutes about 3% of skeletal muscle protein, forming long non-distensible filaments extending from the Z disks; nebulin is thought to regulate the number of actin monomers 'allowed' to polymerize into each thin filament during myogenesis and facilitate actin filament organization into its usual hexagonal geometry; nebulin is present in fetuses and infants with Duchenne-type muscular dystrophy, but disappears with disease progression (J Neurol Sci 1988; 87:315)

NEC see Necrotizing enterocolitis

Neck face syndrome A transient clinical complex characterized by oropharyngeal spasms, dysarthria, tachycardia and hypertension occurring after beginning chlorpromazine therapy

Neck hold(s) FORENSIC MEDICINE A form of constraint used to subdue overactive, unruly, violent or inebriated subjects with the intent of preventing them causing physical harm to themselves and others; neck holds are of two types: **CAROTID SLEEPER** Compression of the carotid baroreceptor causes asystole or marked slowing of the ventricular rate, a fall in the blood pressure and syncope; under controlled conditions, non-combative subjects lose consciousness within 6-10 seconds and **CHOKE HOLD** or bar arm control Occlusion of the upper airway by compressing the thyroid cartilage and displacing the tongue posteriorly, a hold that is considered more dangerous; neck holds are of medico-legal interest, as accidental death may be caused by police, orderlies or emergency medical technicians trying to restrain a subject undergoing acute psychotic attacks or other excited states (Am J Foren Med Pathol 1982; 3:253) Note: The carotid baroreceptor is located at the bifurcation of the internal carotid, the nerve endings of which join Hering's sinus nerve and the glossopharyngeal nerve, terminating in the cardio-inhibitory and vasomotor center in the medulla

Necklace pattern CLINICAL MEDICINE A descriptor for a distinct annular distribution of lesions seen in AIDS-related Kaposi sarcoma CYTOLOGY A descriptor for the perinuclear distribution of the PAS-positive granules in Lutzner's small cell variant of Sézary cells

Neck-tongue syndrome An acquired condition characterized by sharp pain and tingling of the upper neck and/or occiput upon sudden rotation of the neck, associated with numbness of the ipsilateral half of the tongue, thought to be the result of stretching of the C2 ventral ramus which contains proprioceptive fibers from the lingual nerve to the hypoglossal nerve and on to the second cervical root

Necrobiosis Physiologic cell death seen during normal turnover in the bone marrow, endometrium, gastrointestinal tract and skin; endometrial cells

Necropsy Autopsy

Necrosis Death of cells or tissue **ASEPTIC NECROSIS** Non-infected tissue death, usually related to ischemia **CASEOUS NECROSIS** Tissue death grossly appearing as dry-yellow-white, ricotta cheese-like in consistency material, due to a combination of coagulative and liquefactive necrosis, secondary to autolysis, ischemia and focal bacterial necrosis, forming a proteolipid 'paste', most often seen in the central portions of granulomatous lesions, classically in tuberculosis, but also seen in cat-scratch disease, deep fungal infections, lymphogranuloma venereum, plague, sporotrichosis, syphilis, tularemia; a similar material is seen in gouty lesions **COAGULATION NECROSIS** The most common type of tissue death, in which the cells are converted to pale eosinophilic 'ghosts' due to acute ischemia, affecting the heart, kidney and adrenal glands; the healing phase involves enzymatic liquefaction or neutrophilic phagocytosis of the debris **FAT NECROSIS** A process in which neutral fats of adipocytes are converted into fatty acids and glycerol, as in trauma-induced fat necrosis of the breast or acute pancreatitis attributed to the release of enzymes Histopathology 'Ghosted' fat cells surrounded by calcium, forming 'soaps', see Calcium soap **FIBRINOID NECROSIS** A misnomer that does not represent true necrosis but homogeneous, granular eosinophilic material, composed of fibrin, proteins, including complement and immunoglobulins and platelets that is seen in the various forms of necrotizing vasculitis **GANGRENOUS NECROSIS** see Gangrene **LIQUEFACTIVE NECROSIS** That which occurs during abscess formation, caused by enzymatic degradation **PATHERGIC NECROSIS** Pathergy Dissolution of tissue without apparent cause, which may be seen at the site of trauma, and accompanied by scattered histiocytes, eg Wegener's disease; pathergic necrosis must be differentiated from two similar processes: a) 'Garden variety' necrosis, mediated by neutrophils that actively pour histolytic enzymes into the milieu and b) Autolysis, due to enzymes released upon cell death, a common finding in the pancreas after death; see Acute tubular necrosis, Bridging necrosis, Cystic medial necrosis, Papillary necrosis, Piecemeal necrosis

Necrotizing enterocolitis (NEC) A disease of premature infants, affecting the terminal ileum 3-10 days after birth, representing 2% of neonatal ICU admissions and 10% of admissions of premature infant or low birth weight neonates and causing significant mortality and morbidity; NEC is usually prevented by either human breast milk or per os IgA-IgG immunoglobulin concentrate prepared from human serum (Cohn's fraction II by ion-exchange chromatography) Note: Hyperosmolar solutions used for these infants have been inculpated Mechanism, NEC Intestinal ischemia and breakdown of the mucosa with invasion by gas-forming bacteria causes the pneumatosis intestinalis **Clinical** From banal to fulminant with abdominal distension, vomiting, hematochezia, intestinal gangrene, perforation, sepsis and shock, survival 80%; NEC is less common in breast-fed children, who may be protected by secretory IgA in maternal milk; per os IgA-IgG solution in low birth weight infants may afford protection (N Engl J Med 1988; 319:1); prophylactic ligation of the patent ductus arteriosus at the time of birth may reduce the incidence of necrotizing enterocolitis (N Engl J Med 1989; 320:1511), but has no effect on other 'prematurity' lesions; Cf Pigbel

Needle aspiration cytology A diagnostic preparation of cells, eg smears and/or a 'cell block', see there, which is obtained from a clinically or radiologically identified mass, using a 'skinny' needle to spread the material on a glass; in well-trained hands, aspiration cytology specimens have a 90% sensitivity and 95% specificity for diagnosing thyroid and breast masses, using 21-25 gauge or 'skinny' needles; the procedure is helpful when positive, but when negative, requires further diagnostic procedures; a rare complication with larger bore needles is tumor implantation along the needle tract; the physical 'set-up' includes computerized tomographic guidance, a microscope and staining materials during the procedure in order to establish immediate diagnosis

Needle biopsy The principle is the same as that of aspiration cytology, but the larger bore (19 gauge) needle obtains architecturally intact tissue, yielding in some hands, a higher diagnostic success rate than with cytology alone Note: CT-guided transthoracic needles are better if the mass is less than 2.0 cm in diameter, while lesions larger than 2.0 cm are best diagnosed by fibroptic bronchoscopy if accessible (Mayo Clin Proc 1990; 65:173) Note: Despite the small size, needle biopsies may be analyzed by histochemistry and immunohistochemistry, cell culture and culture for organisms, electron and immunofluorescence microscopy, receptor analysis, in situ hybridization and polymerase chain reaction

Needle exchange programs INFECTIOUS DISEASE PUBLIC HEALTH A group of programs intended to slow the spread of AIDS among intravenous drug abusers (IVDAs), in which an agency, either governmental or charitable, exchanges sterile needles for 'dirty', potentially HIV-contaminated needles used by IVDAs when 'shooting' heroin (or less commonly cocaine); the controversy engendered by needle exchange programs is a) Whether it actually helps stop the spread of AIDS (soft data suggest that it does) and b) Whether government funds should be used to support an illicit activity

Needle-stick injuries An occupational injury that may affect any health care professionals; needles act as vehicles for at least 20 different microorganisms (N Engl J Med 1988; 319:284); most physicians have sustained at least one such injury during their training, one-third of which occurred during recapping; in urban US teaching hospitals, 20% or more of the population is HIV-positive; the risk of HIV transmission through a needle stick is currently estimated at 0.0035 (J Am Med Assoc 1990; 264:2111); see Hospital-acquired penetration contacts, Sharps

nef A human immunodeficiency virus gene that encodes the regulatory protein Nef, which had been thought to have a role in down-regulating viral reproduction, an effect now known to be an isolated phenomenon occurring in one cell line; mutations in the nef gene may be responsible for generating the different HIV-cell tropisms

NEFA Non-esterified fatty acids Fatty acids (straight or branched-chain monocarboxylic acid) that are not bound in the form of lipid esters, ie not esterified to a glycerol; NEFAs are absorbed in the ileum, represent about 5% of the total plasma lipids (0.3-0.95 mmol/L), primarily as straight-chain fatty acids (stearic and palmitic acids) are transported bound to albumin and represent an important source of energy

Negative-acting regulatory proteins Those proteins that bind to DNA at or near a promotion site, preventing access of RNA polymerase to the corresponding gene or operon, preventing transcription into mRNA

'Negative acute phase protein' see Transthyretin

Negative feedback see Feedback

Negative interference Gene mapping GENETICS A term referring to an overabundance of double cross-overs; without 'correction' for cross-overs, marker distances are not additive, ie they interfere in a negative fashion with evaluation of distance

Negative predictive value STATISTICS The number of true negatives divided by the sum of the number of true negatives (TN) and false negatives (FN), representing the proportion of subjects with a negative test result who do not have a disease; Cf Positive predictive value

Negative strand virus An RNA virus (class V virus) with a nucleotide base sequence complementary to that of the virus' mRNA, which requires that the genetic material be first copied by an RNA-dependent RNA polymerase before it is able to translate information into proteins; Cf Positive strand virus

Neglect see Child abuse

Negligence LEGAL MEDICINE *'THE FAILURE TO EXERCISE ORDINARY, REASONABLE, USUAL OR EXPECTED CARE, RESULTING IN HARM OR INJURY; NEGLIGENCE MAY BE AN ACT OF OMISSION OR COMMISSION, CHARACTERIZED BY INATTENTION, RECKLESSNESS, INADVERTENCE, THOUGHTLESSNESS OR WANTONNESS'* (JC Rhea et al, Dictionary of Health Care Management); in health care, negligence implies a substandard deviation from the 'standard of medical practice' that would be exercised by a similarly-trained professional under similar circumstances **CONTRIBUTORY NEGLIGENCE** An act or omission that constitutes the lack of reasonable care on the part of a plaintiff for his own preservation; in a malpractice lawsuit, a patient may have 'contributed' to a significant degree to his own condition by ignoring a physician's well documented advice or requests for the patient to return for follow-up visits **Gross negligence** Reckless provision of health care without regard for the consequences, an act that is more serious than an inadvertent error, but which does not imply intentional wrong, ie 'sloppy' **Wanton negligence** Provision of health care without regard for potential injury to the patient without an actual intent to cause injury, ie 'reckless' **Willful negligence** Provision of health care in an intentionally substandard fashion, the most serious form of negligence, which may carry with it criminal charges; the accusation of negligence comprises a major cause for malpractice litigation; see Adverse event, Malpractice

Nemaline myopathy Nemaline, Greek, rod-like A benign autosomal dominant muscular dystrophy affecting 'floppy infants' and characterized by non-progressive muscular weakness, reduced deep tendon reflexes and hypotonicity, causing skeletal abnormalities, a typical facies (oval face, micrognathia, malocclusion and a high arched palate), kyphoscoliosis, dislocation of hips and pes cavus; nemaline myopathy is compatible with a normal lifespan; 'Nemaline' refers to the ultrastructural finding of rod-like Z-band material in both type I and type II myocytes; Cf Central core myopathy, Floppy infant syndrome

N-end rule Protein catabolism The principle that the amino acid at a peptide's NH_2-terminus determines its metabolic stability and how rapidly it will be degraded; eg for β-galactosidase, methionine, alanine, serine, threonine, valine and glycine terminal amino acids are degraded within 20 hours; peptides with other N-end amino acids have shorter half lives; the half-life of an intracellular protein ranges from a few seconds to several days; most damaged or abnormal proteins are metabolically unstable and catabolically eliminated by various regulatory proteins, while other proteins are long-lived and maintained as components of macromolecule complexes such as ribosomes and multimeric proteins; when these proteins are dissociated from these macromolecular complexes, they too are metabolically unstable and catabolized; this selective degradation process is an ATP-dependent and nonlysosomal process in which ubiquitin covalently conjugates with the short-lived proteins 'tagging' them for catabolism; intracellular proteins are recognized as proteolytic substrates by the N-end rule, a phenomenon discovered in yeasts, where any 8 stabilizing amino acids at the N-terminal of the protein are associated with long (> 20 hours) intracellular half-lives while any of 12 destabilizing amino acids at the N-end have a short (3-30 minutes) half-life; in mammalian cells, the rule is more complex; there are three classes of N-end destabilizing residues and the types of proteins degraded as a function of the cell's physiology; the N-end rule requires that in addition to a destabilizing N-end amino acid, there is a lysine in position 15 or 17, the probable site of ubiquitination (J Biol Chem 1989; 264:16700; Nature 1990; 346:287); Cf PEST hypothesis

Neo-Darwinism A key paradigm of evolutionary biology that synthesizes the concepts of darwinian natural selection and mendelian genetics, and assumes that the environment is a static force that does not interact with organisms that survive based on their 'fitness' in an adverse environment; see Autopoietic Gaia

Neomembrane Neuropathology A thin sheet of reactive fibrous tissue overlying a chronic subdural hematoma

Neonatal 'hepatitis' A generic term for diseases that affect the newborn hepatic parenchyma, which are commonly associated with increased conjugated hyperbilirubinemia; diagnosis of this condition(s) requires three or more of the following: fatty changes, cholestasis, bile duct proliferation, fibrosis, pseudoacini and cirrhosis; neonatal 'hepatitis' is caused by infection (syphilis, listeriosis, hepatitis B virus, rubella, cytomegalovirus, echovirus, adenovirus, toxoplasmosis), metabolic disease (α1-antitrypsin deficiency, cystic fibrosis, Wilson's disease, galactosemia, fructosuria, tyrosinemia), mechanical (choledochal cysts,intrahepatic ductal atresia hypoplasia, familial intrahepatic cholestasis) and others (Bylers disease, hemolytic disease of the newborn) Histopathology Lobular disarray, focal hepatocellular necrosis, prominent giant cell 'transformation', mononuclear infiltration in the portal spaces, reactive hyperplasia in the Kupffer cells and cholestasis; Cf Giant cell hepatitis

Neonatal intensive care unit (NICU) A ward in a tertiary care center that provides intensive medical care; an NICU requires trained medical personnel at all levels, 24 hour availability of the appropriate specialists, monitoring devices, alarm systems for continuous assessment of vital functions, equipment for resuscitation and respiratory therapy, drugs and full laboratory coverage; the mortality of the very low birth weight (<1500 g) has fallen from 72% in 1960 to 27% in 1985; the mortality of those with moderate-to-severe residual handicaps (4-10%) was stable for that time period; the proportion of infants who survive in relatively good health has increased from 7.2% to 57% (J Am Med Assoc 1989; 261:1767); see Low birth weight

Neonatal withdrawal syndrome (NWS) A clinical condition affecting the infants of mothers who chronically abused central nervous system-active substances during pregnancy, for which the infant developed an in utero tolerance and who upon delivery, undergoes withdrawal; agents inculpated include opioids (heroin, methadone, meperidine, codeine, pentazocine, propoxyphene, cocaine and 'crack'), alcohol, clomipramine and sedative-hypnotics (barbiturates, meprobamate, benzodiazepines) Clinical Wakefulness, irritability, seizures, tremulousness, lability of temperature, tachypnea, hyperacusis, hyperreflexia, hypertonicity, diarrhea, sweating, respiratory distress and apnea, rhinorrhea, autonomic dysfunction, respiratory alkalosis, lacrimation, yawning and sneezing; the symptoms appear from twelve hours to one week after birth Treatment Swaddling (firmly wrapping in blankets), reduction of external stimuli and tincture of opium; see Crack babies

Neoplasm Any autonomous proliferation of cells, classified according to 1) Behavior (benign, borderline or malignant 2) Degree of differentiation Well-differentiated, ie the neoplastic cell simulates its parent or progenitor cell or poorly-differentiated, ie the neoplastic cell is bizarre and 'ugly' 3) Embryologic origin Epithelial, lymphoproliferative, mesenchymal, neural crest, etc and 4) Gross appearance Well-circumscribed or infiltrative; benign neoplasms are in general slow-growing, well-circumscribed, often invested with a fibrous capsule and are often only symptomatic if they compromise a confined space, eg massive meningioma of the cranial cavity, or encirclement of vital blood vessels; malignant neoplasms are often aggressive with increased mitotic activity, bizarre cells, necrosis and invasion of adjacent structures and have metastatic potential; see Cancer, Doubling time, Metastases

Neoplasm panel LABORATORY MEDICINE A battery of analytes that are considered to be the most cost-effective tests to perform when a person has a malignancy of unknown origin, including measurement of acid phosphatase (although prostate specific antigen appears to be of greater use), alkaline phosphatase, α-fetoprotein, carcinoembryonic antigen, chorionic gonadotrophic hormone and lactate dehydrogenase; because of the low yield of these assays, chemical 'cancer screens' have little active role in the early diagnosis of malignancy, and when 'negative', introduce a false sense of security that malignancy is not present

Neopterin A metabolite of guanosine triphosphate, produced by macrophages that have been stimulated by γ-IFN produced from activated T cells; levels of serum and urinary neopterin are elevated in progressing HIV-1 infection; the combination of decreasing CD4+ lymphocytes and increasing levels of either neopterin or β_2-microglobulin, which indicates lymphoid activation are relatively good predictors of progression of HIV-1 infection to clinical AIDS (N Engl J Med 1990; 322:166)

Neovascularization Capillary ingrowth and endothelial proliferation, typical of so-called 'angiogenic diseases', which include angiogenesis in tumor growth, diabetic retinopathy, hemangiomas, arthritis and psoriasis

Neper A unit of measurement expressing the ratio of two levels of electrical power, being the natural logarithm of the square root of that ratio, eg the ratio of the electricity in a comb charged with static electricity to a bolt of lightning

Nephelometry LABORATORY MEDICINE A technique that detects the amount of light scattered at 90 degrees to the incident light by particles dispersed in a clear solution, which is a function of the number and size of the particles; nephelometry is most commonly used to detect immune complexes when the participating antigen or antibody is unknown; Cf Turbidometry

Nephritic syndrome An obsolete and non-specific term that referred to a renal lesion histologically characterized by inflammation and necrosis of the glomeruli; Cf Nephrosis, Nephrotic syndrome

Nephroblastoma see Wilm's tumor

Nephroblastomatosis A congenital dysontogenic condition that may be bilateral and multifocal and both confused with *and* associated with Wilm's tumor, demonstrating a continuum between microscopic foci, termed nephrogenic rests or metanephric hamartomas and massive lesions or nephroblastomatosis, either of which may be surrounded by sclerosis, indicating regressive changes; focal lesions appear in 1% of normal fetal kidneys and 30% of kidneys affected by Wilm's tumor Treatment Conservative

Nephropathic cystinosis An autosomal recessive lysosomal storage disease characterized by early-onset renal tubular Fanconi's syndrome, progressive photophobia, renal failure severe enough to require either hemodialysis or transplantation by age 10, caused by defective trans-lysosomal membrane transport of cystine, resulting in tissue deposition of cystine causing corneal erosions, diabetes mellitus and neurologic deterioration Clinical Dehydration, acidosis, vomiting, electrolyte imbalances, hypophosphatemic rickets and failure to grow Treatment β-mercaptoethylamine (aminothiol cysteamine) to deplete intracellular stores and by extension dissolve tissue crystals, oral cysteamine therapy improves growth and delays renal deterioration; see Salla disease

Nephrosclerosis A generic term indicating global fibrosis and atrophy of the glomeruli, most commonly seen in arteriosclerotic kidneys, divided into 1) **BENIGN NEPHROSCLEROSIS**, a relatively common, symmetrical and indolent process causing 'benign' hypertension, average age of onset, 60, 5% of whom die of renal failure Histopathology Hyaline arteriolosclerosis, scarring of glomeruli and 2) **MALIGNANT NEPHROSCLEROSIS**, an uncommon process affecting 5% of hypertensives, often beginning under age 45 Histopathology Fibrinoid necrosis of small arteries (necrotizing arteriolitis), intimal hyperplasia of larger interlobular arteries (hyperplastic arteriolitis, 'onion-skinning'), collagen deposition and fibroblastic proliferation with luminal narrowing, thrombosis and necrosis of the glomeruli with atrophy and parenchymal scarring

Nephrosis A term used by clinicians as a synonym for nephrotic syndrome, which corresponds to a non-inflammatory derangement of glomerular function, characterized by increased glomerular leakage with loss of albumin and other macromolecules Note: The term is non-specific and uncommonly used by cognoscenti, appearing with adjectival modifiers, eg lipoid nephrosis, see Nil disease and myeloid nephrosis see Myeloma kidney; Cf Nephritis

Nephrotic syndrome A clinical disease characterized by the triad of edema, proteinuria (greater than 3.5g protein/1.73 m^2/24 hours) and hypoalbuminemia (less than 30 g/L) Laboratory Increased α_2 globulin and β globulin, decreased albumin; Increased cholesterol, triglycerides, phospholipids; the increases are confined to lipoproteins containing apoprotein B (chylomicrons and LDL cholesterol), due to increased production of apoprotein B (N Engl J Med 1990; 323:579); other findings in nephrotic syndrome include decreased HDL_2 and increased VLDL Urinalysis Maltese crosses (cholesterol), oval fat bodies, casts (fatty, waxy, cellular, granular) Etiology, children Minimum change 65-90%, membranoproliferative 7-10%, focal glomerulosclerosis, membranous, proliferative and other glomerulonephritides **Etiology, adult** Membranous 50%, minimum change 10-20%, focal glomerulosclerosis 10-20%, membranoproliferative proliferative, and other glomerulonephrites; other causes of nephrotic syndrome include amyloidosis, diabetes mellitus, infection, malignancy, lupus erythematosus and toxins, eg colloidal gold, 'street' heroin, penicillamine

Nerve conduction studies NEUROLOGY A noninvasive method for assessing a nerve's ability to carry an impulse, providing quantitative data on latency periods and conduction velocities; larger peripheral motor and sensory nerve s are electrically stimulated at various intervals along a motor nerve; the maximum (norma) velocity for peripheral nerves requires complete myelination, and is between 40 and 80 m/s; nerve conduction may be one-half or less than normal in segmental demyelination, as occurs in polyneuropathy, eg in Charcot-Marie-Tooth disease, diabetic neuropathy, Guillain-Barré syndrome, diphtheriae, metachromatic leukodystrophy; entrapment syndrome produce localized slowing of conduction; motor nerve conduction studies differentiate between peripheral nerve or muscle disease and anterior horn cells, measuring the resulting muscle twitch/action (M response) is measured; see F wave, H-reflex, Latency period

Nerve gas see Chemical warfare

Nerve growth factor (NGF) A 118-residue protein encoded on chromosome 1 and synthesized by neurons that regulates the proliferation and differentiation of the neuronal stem cells after the cells in the embryonic brain have been stimulated by fibroblast growth factor (Nature 1990; 347:762); NGF has a trophic role in embryogenesis, increasing mitotic activity, enhances differentiation, eg neurite outgrowth, is required for development and maintenance of sympathetic and sensory peripheral neurons, guides growing or regenerating neurites along a concentration gradient and may have antimitogenic activity; cholinergic neurons respond to NGF by increasing production of choline acyltransferase, and NGF's message may be mediated by signal transduction through trk, a tyrosine kinase receptor (Nature 1991; 350:158); NGF receptors are present on cells of neural crest origin, mast cells, cholinergic and adrenergic neurons Note: The original NGF work was done on chick embryos engrafted with fragments of mouse sarcoma by R Levi-Montalcini (Nobel Prize, 1986)

Nerve growth factor family A group of proteins that have various effects on neural tissues, currently under active study, including nerve growth factor, brain-derived neurotrophic factor, see BDNF, neurotropin-3 (NT-3) and ciliary neurotrophic factor, see CNTF; Cf Epidermal growth factor

Nerve growth factor receptor There are two receptors; a low molecular weight receptor of 80 kD and a high molecular weight receptor of 140 kD, may correspond to the trk protein product

Nerve regeneration NEUROPHYSIOLOGY Nerve transection was formerly considered an irreversible event; neuronal regeneration is increasingly evident, eg sensory cell regeneration after acoustic trauma in chickens (mitosis of support cells, Science 1988; 240:1772) and resynapsis of severed nerves; much of the groundwork has been by F Nottebohm in his seminal work with nerve regeneration and alteration of neural pathways in songbirds

Nesidioblastosis Islet cell hyperplasia (and neoformation of islets after birth) with variability of size and shape, vascular dilation, poor demarcation, clustering, abnormal interstitial location, arising from the exocrine ducts; nesiodioblastosis is associated with diabetes, affecting infants of diabetic mothers, diabetics with long-term oral hypoglycemic agents (sulfonylurea, tolbutamide) and in endocrinopathies, either congenital, as in the MEN (multiple endocrine neoplasia) syndrome or may be induced by glucagon and corticosteroids

Nesting COMPUTERS The inclusion of a block of data or programming subroutine within another subroutine, often in the form of a functional loop of logic, performing the routine a number of times before continuing with the program; see Computers OBSTETRICS Frenetic house cleaning by a woman in late pregnancy, which most often occurs with the first-born child, fancifully likened to birds building a nest

'Nettergram' A color medical illustration rendered by Frank H Netter, MD (1906-1991) which summarizes in a lucid and graphic form the clinical and pathological findings in a disease state; most of these illustrations are found within the 'CIBA collection', a 10-volume set, the first of which was released in 1953 and has helped educate more than three generations of medical students in the US and elsewhere

Network Any series of points in a system that is connected by numbered lines and arrows, indicating the flow of materials, personnel, energy, widgets

Network analysis A management tool designed to reduce a system's energy or labor expenditure to a minimum, attempting in addition to accurately estimate the amount of time that the growth of interrelated tasks or a 'network' will take by arranging the network in time-dependent routes, where the critical path is the one that requires the most time and which requires input from the previous steps; see Neural networks

Network hypothesis IMMUNOLOGY A theory proposed by Jerne (Nobel prize, 1984) that lymphocytes form a network of cells bearing idiotypes, each potentially capable of eliciting anti-idiotype antibodies; each 'new' antigen disrupts the balance of an immune network by stimulating an antibody response which then elicits an anti-idiotype-antibody response, which is followed by further anti-idiotypes, attenuating, and eventually quenching the response, bringing the system back into balance

neu A tyrosine kinase oncogene that is turned off by addition of tyrosine phosphatase, and which encodes the Neu protein

Neu protein HER-2, c-erbB-2, MAC 117 The gene product of the *neu* proto-oncogene, a membrane-bound receptor, which has extensive homology with epidermal growth factor; amplification of *neu* gene expression occurs in breast cancer, but not in ductal carcinoma in situ; tumors with neu amplification are larger but increased expression of neu has little bearing on the prognosis (N Engl J Med 1988; 319:1239)

Neural crest The dorsal region of the embryologic nervous system, appearing in the fifth week of development and giving rise to the sensory and autonomic nervous systems and melanocytes; as the embryo develops, neural crest cells migrate laterally, forming cells of the APUD system, melanoblasts, pia-arachnoid, odontoblast, Schwann cells and sensory neurons; tumors of neural crest origin include medullary thyroid carcinoma, derived from the ultimobranchial cleft, pheochromocytoma, medulloblastoma, neuroblastoma), undifferentiated neural crest tumors (Science 1989; 243:1608) and the pigmented neuroectodermal tumor of infancy

Neural network A computer design in which multiple microprocessors interact simultaneously, modifying each other's output; neural networks are inspired by the architecture of the nervous system and are designed to simulate how the brain is thought to function; neural networks are composed of units analogous to neurons in that they have multiple connections; the analogy to the brain is further enhanced by integration of the back-prop algorithm, which allows the network to auto-correct errors, avoiding future errors; neural-networks solve problems by generalizations and approximations, based on limited data (rather than requiring the exact answers dictated by the 'linear' algorithms of standard computing) and are thus best suited for pattern recognition and signal processing, as in noise filtration; newer algorithms have integrated self-correction or back-propagation Note: A true thinking machine based on independent ability to perform artificial intelligence algorithms may prove elusive (Science 1989; 243:481)

Neural tube defects A group of congenital central nervous system malformations, including anencephaly and spina bifida cystica that are attributed to multifactorial events and noxious environmental agents, which occur in 1:1000 to 1:5000 live births, male:female ratio 2-3:1, with regional differences, eg higher in Ireland and a 2-7% recurrence rate Laboratory Increased α-fetoprotein, which may be detected in antenatal screening of maternal serum or amniotic fluid Prevention The use of multivitamins during early pregnancy may decrease the risk of neural tube defects, although the effect of a 'healthier' lifestyle or demographics cannot be ruled out (J Am Med Assoc 1989; 262:2847, N Engl J Med 1989; 321:430)

Neuraminidase Acylneuraminyl hydrolase An enzyme that breaks the glucoside bonds between sialic acid and hexose and hexosamine, located on the extracellular portion of membrane-bound glycoproteins, glycolipids and proteoglycans; neuraminidase in addition to hemagglutinin is located on the 'spikes' of influenza virus; neuraminidase deficiency occurs in the autosomal recessive mucolipidosis, type I

Neurapraxia Partial or complete conduction block over a segment of a nerve fiber, producing temporary paralysis

Neurasthenia Effort syndrome Nervous prostration A chronic non-specific clinical finding, often associated with depression or anxiety neurosis, characterized by the subjective findings of fatigue and inability to function and accompanied by autonomic changes, including tachycardia, sighing, blushing, dysdiaphoresis; the patients are often convinced there is an organic and not a psychological underpinning to their condition

Neurilemmoma see Schwannoma

Neuroblastoma A neural crest-derived tumor that is the second most common neoplasm of children, after leukemia and other lymphproliferative disease Clinical Median age of onset is less than age 2; stage I survival is 80-90%, Stage IV, 15% Note: Stage IV-S is an exception, see below); higher stage neuroblastomas metastasize to bone, lymph nodes and liver Histopathology Two cell types are typical of neuroblastomas, either 'blue cell tumors', arranged in Homer-Wright rosettes or b) 'Small round cell tumors of infancy' Ultrastructure 100 nm 'dense core' granules, neurofilaments, microtubules, variably-sized glycogen granules Immunoperoxidase Neuron-specific enolase, S-100 Laboratory Catecholamines and metabolites are elevated by thin-layer chromatography, gas-liquid chromatography or high performance liquid chromatography, with a 5-fold increase in VMA (vanillylmandelic acid) and HVA (homovanillic acid); high HVA, the 'early end of catecholamine metabolism' relative to VMA, the 'late end of catecholamine metabolism' is known as a chemical 'shift to the left', and is thought to indicate a poor prognosis; also increased in neuroblastomas are epinephrine, norepinephrine, DOPA, dopamine, 3-methoxytyrosine, vanillactic acid, MHPG, metanephrine and LD Note: Tumors deficient in dopamine β-hydroxylase are more primitive and generally have a worse prognosis than tumors producing 'differentiated' hormones. eg epinephrine, norepinephrine and VMA; see 'One-hit, two-hit' model

Neuroblastoma, IV-S syndrome A type of neuroblastoma (IV-S for special (S) stage IV tumor) comprising 10-20% of all these tumors, where the primary tumor may be small, confined to the adrenal gland, but have widespread disease with massive involvement of the liver and skin; bone may be involved but osteolysis is not present; despite these 'metastases', the tumor regresses spontaneously through a maturation sequence from neuroblastoma, which is the most immature and composed of neuroblasts to ganglioneuroblastoma and finally ending in ganglioneuroma, which is the most mature of the sequence and is composed of ganglion cells; Knudsen postulated (N Engl J Med 1980; 302:1254) that the tumor represents a unique form of hyperplasia, as the cell clusters seen occur in sites to which cells of neural crest origin usually migrate, to later differentiate into Schwann cells or melanocytes

Neurocutaneous syndromes Phakomatoses A group of multisystem diseases characterized by involvement of the brain, skin, eyes and other organ systems, including neurofibromatosis (von Recklinghausen disease), tuberous sclerosis (Pringle-Bourneville disease), von Hippel-Lindau disease (all autosomal dominant), Sturge-Weber syndrome (not hereditary) and ataxia-telangiectasia

'Neurodermatitis' An eczematous dermatitis with a

hereditary component, accompanied by pruritus, which when disseminated, is known as atopic neurodermatitis and localized, known as lichen simplex chronicus

Neuroendocrine bodies (NEB) Intrabronchial structures that are thought to act as intrapulmonary hypoxia- and hypercapnia-sensitive chemoreceptors, which undergo physiologic hyperplasia in the lungs of those living at high altitudes; NEBs proliferate when exposed to certain nitroso compounds and contain neuron-specific enolase, serotonin, bombesin and calcitonin and may be the point of origin of microcarcinoids and bronchial tumorlets

Neuroendocrine cells Isolated neuroendocrine cells throughout the human economy that are thought to have a paracrine, regulatory function **Ultrastructure** Dense core neurosecretory granules **Immunoperoxidase** Variable amounts of ACTH, b; see ombesin, calcitonin, neuron-specific enolase, serotonin, leu-enkephalin and somatostatin, contained within the neurosecretory granules; each organ has a neuroendocrine component derived from the primitive neural crest; in the lungs, the neuroendocrine system is comprised of neuroendocrine cells and neuroepithelial bodies; see APUD system, Neural crest, Neurosecretory granules

Neuroendocrine tumors Neoplasms that share a characteristic morphology, often being composed of clusters and trabecular sheets of round 'blue cells', granular chromatin and an attenuated rim of poorly demarcated cytoplasm Neuroendocrine tumors include carcinoids, small ('oat') cell carcinomas, medullary carcinoma of the thyroid, Merkel cell tumor, cutaneous neuroendocrine carcinoma, pancreatic islet cell tumors, pheochromocytoma **Ultrastructure** Neurosecretory granules within the tumor cells **Immunoperoxidase** The cell tumor cells usually staining for pan-endocrine markers, eg neuron-specific enolase, chromogranins, synaptophysin and opioid receptors, as well as specific products of the tumor cells, eg calcitonin, bombesin, carcinoembryonic antigen and choriogonadotropic hormone; see neurosecretory granules

Neuroepithelium The embryonal ectoderm that gives rise to the cerebrospinal axis; in the mature mammal, neuroepithelium corresponds histologically to the simple columnar epithelial cell receptors for external stimuli (as well as the cochlea, olfaction and tongue); see Neural crest

Neurofibrillary tangles (NFTs) NEUROPATHOLOGY A characteristic histological finding seen in the perikaryon of large cortical neurons of patients with Alzheimer's disease, the number of which loosely correlates with the severity of dementia; NFTs consist of intensely argyrophilic aggregates of altered neurofilaments with an 800 A periodicity, forming 'twisted tubules' displacing cytoplasmic contents of the neurons; NFTs are also common in Down's syndrome (Arch Neurol 1989; 46:89) and post-encephalitic parkinsonism, or may be seen in normal adults (confined to the hippocampus); see Granulovacuolar degeneration, Paired helical filaments, Senile plaques

Neurofibromatosis, type 1 (NF1) von Recklinghausen disease, Peripheral neurofibromatosis An autosomal dominant condition affecting an estimated 100 000 in the USA, caused by a mutation of a large (circa two million base pair in length) gene on chromosome 17 t(1;17)(p34.3;q11), which has sequence similarity ('homology') to tumor suppressor genes, as well as genes encoding the catalytic region of GAP (GTPase-activating protein), this latter possibly explaining the aberrant proliferation of melanocytes and schwann cell typical of NF-1, as cAMP triggers division of these cells; NF1 is diagnosed in the presence of two or more of the following 1) Six or more 'Cafe-au-lait' macules measuring 5 mm in greatest diameter are identified in a pre-pubertal or > 15 mm in greatest diameter in post-pubertal patients 2) Two or more histologically-confirmed neurofibromas (or one plexiform neurofibroma) 3) Freckling in the axillary or inguinal regions 4) Optic glioma 5) Two or more Lisch nodules (iris hamartomas, the most common feature of NF1 in adults, N Engl J Med 1991; 324:1264) 6) Distinct bone lesions, eg sphenoid dysplasia, cortical thinning of long bones, pseudoarthrosis and 7) The subject has a first-degree relative with NF1

Neurofibromatosis, type 2 (NF2) Central neurofibromatosis Bilateral acoustic neurofibromatosis An autosomal dominant condition that is less common than NF1, which affects several thousand patients in the US, in 95% of whom the gene defect is located on chromosome 22q11.1→22q13.1, first seen in late adolescence; NF2 is diagnosed in the presence of either bilateral eighth nerve masses by computed tomography or magnetic resonance imaging or when a subject known to have a first-degree relative with NF2 presents with either a unilateral eighth nerve mass or two or more 'neural crest' tumors, eg neurofibroma, meningioma, glioma, spinal neurofibromatosis, schwannoma or juvenile posterior subcapsular lenticular opacity (Science 1987; 236:317)

Neurofibromatoses, types (3 and 4) Subtypes of neurofibromatosis of questionable validity, which have varying components of both NF1 and NF2

Neurofilaments see Intermediate filaments

Neurogenesis see Nerve regeneration

Neurogenic bladder A bladder with loss or impairment of voluntary control of micturition, which may be either 1) **SPASTIC NEUROGENIC BLADDER**, due to lesions of the spinal cord, accompanied by urgency, increased frequency, decreased functional capacity, spastic contractions and poor voluntary control and 2) **FLACCID NEUROGENIC BLADDER**, due to segmental lesions at S2 to S4, interfering with voluntary and reflex control, loss of the sensation of bladder fullness, causing 'overflow' incontinence, when the bladder contains two or more liters

Neuroleptic malignant syndrome ANESTHESIOLOGY A disorder seen in 1% of those treated with antipsychotic agents (especially haloperidol) and major tranquilizers, an effect attributed to antidopaminergic activity; the syndrome may also be associated with anesthesia, which affects an estimated 1:50 000 patients exposed to inhalation anesthesia, most common in young males, who have been transiently weakened by exhaustion or dehydration **Clinical** Fever in excess of 41°C, skeletal muscle hypertonicity, variable loss of consciousness, autonomic nervous system lability (pallor, sweating, tachycardia, arrhythmia, transient hypertension, which if severe may cause renal failure and dysfunction Mortality 20-30%, occurring between days 3-30, usually from renal failure **Treatment** Bromocriptine or dantrolene shorten the clinical disease from 6.8 days to less than 1.2 days (Arch Intern Med 1989; 149:1927)

Neuroleukin A 56 kD protein cytokine produced in the brain and in T cells, which has sequence similarity ('homology') to both phosphohexose isomerase and HIV-1's gp120; competitive inhibition by gp120 at the neuroleukin receptor may explain AIDS-related dementia

Neuromalacia An obsolete and non-specific term for the morbid softening of peripheral nerves, as may occur in ischemia

Neuromuscular junction Motor end plate The region of contact between a motor nerve and muscle effector PHYSIOLOGY A nerve impulse or wave of depolarization arrives via the axon to the junction, releases acetylcholine contained within synaptic vesicles into the synaptic cleft; acetylcholine binds to its receptors located on the post-synaptic membrane resulting in depolarization, the production of an end-plate potential on the muscle; neuromuscular blockade may be due to a) Reduction of post-synaptic receptors, eg myasthenia gravis, b) Defective acetylcholine release from storage vesicles, eg botulism, myasthenia or Eaton-Lambert syndrome and c) Competition for binding sites, either pharmacologic blockade, eg neostigmine, edrophonium or toxic blockade, eg organophosphate insecticides

Neuron A cell of the nervous system, which dogma has long held to be the smallest unit of the central nervous system; it has been shown that a single Purkinje cell may have six or more independently functioning dendritic units (Nature 1990; 346:108) Note: The subdivision of a single cell into multiple quasi-discrete units has broad implications, as it adds an extra 'layer' to the processing and storage capacity of the brain

Neuronal ceroid lipofuscinosis (NCL) A heterogenous group of progressive, idiopathic autosomal recessive degenerative encephalopathies, which are attributed to an accumulation of lipofuscin and/or ceroid, and accompanied by optic nerve atrophy **Clinical** Seizures, progressive mental retardation, macular degeneration of the retina, retinitis pigmentosa **Pathology** The affected brains are yellow-gray with a waxy consistency,demonstrating autofluorescent lipopigment in the brain, liver and muscle; NCL may be divided into 1) Major forms a) Chronic juvenile type of Batten b) Acute late infantile type of Bielschowsky c) Subacute-chronic adult type of Kufs and d) Acute infantile type of Santavuori-Haltia and 2) Minor forms, including congenital type, acute adult type, acute-subacute variant type, chronic childhood form with pervasiveness, chronic infantile form with autism and chronic juvenile form with ataxia and spasticity (J Child Neurology 1989; 4:165); NCL classified by chronology Acute a) Infantile or Finnish type Santavuori-Haltia disease Onset in early infancy with myoclonus, seizures, blindness, dementia, rapid deterioration, spasticity, rigidity, ataxia, seborrhea and peliosis **Histopathology** Multinucleated phagocytic histiocytes with granular autofluorescent lipofuscin-like material b) Late infantile form of Jansky-Bielschovsky Onset at age 2-3, characterized by minor seizures, myoclonic spasms, squirming ataxia, progressive loss of mental skills and optic atrophy, seborrhea, poliosis and hirsutism **Histopathology**, as above c) Adult onset form of Zeman-Dyken Onset in early adulthood (20-25 years), characterized by mental retardation **Histopathology** As above **Ultrastructure** Granular and curvilinear bodies Chronic a) Juvenile form of Spielmeyer-Sjögren Onset age 6, characterized by blindness, dementia, late seizures, motor defects **Ultrastructure** Granular and fingerprint bodies b) Adult form of Kufs-Böhme Characterized by seizures, ataxia, myoclonus, dementia and hypertension without blindness Atypical variants Subjects with amaurotic idiocy, sea-blue histiocytosis, cherry-red spot-myoclonus syndrome and others

Neuron-specific enolase (NSE) A homodimeric enolase isoenzyme composed of two γ chains that was first described as being specific for neurons and neuroendocrine cells and tumors as well as astrocytomas; NSE is also commonly present in medullary carcinoma of the thyroid, pituitary adenomas and endocrine neoplasms of the pancreas and gastrointestinal tract; NSE may also occur in many other benign and/or non-neuronal tissues and tumors (meningioma, fibroadenoma, carcinoma of the breast, kidney and ovary, occasionally lymphoma) and other non-malignant conditions; Cf S-100

Neuropathy A generic and highly non-specific term referring to virtually any disorder of peripheral nerves, which may be congenital (eg hereditary sensory radicular neuropathy or hypertrophic interstitial neuropathy), traumatic (entrapment, eg carpal tunnel syndrome), metabolic (eg, due to amyloid or diabetes mellitus), toxic (eg, ,tobacco or alcohol-related amblyopia, cis-platinum, vincristine)

Neuropeptides A family of low (less than 5 kD) molecular weight intracellular peptides that transmit information in the central nervous system, gastrointestinal tract and elsewhere, including ACTH, angiotensin II, bombesin, bradykinin, calcitonin gene-related products, carnosine, cholecystokinin, corticotropin-releasing factor, dynorphins, β-endorphin, leu-enkephalin, met-enkephalin, gastric inhibitory polypeptide, gastrin, glucagon, growth hormone, growth hormone releasing factor, insulin, luteinizing hormone-releasing factor, α-melanocyte-stimulating hormone, melanotropin-inhibiting factor, motilin, neurotensin, oxytocin, prolactin, secretin, somatostatin-14 and -28, substance P, thyroglobulin-releasing factor, thyrotropin, vasoactive intestinal peptide, vasopressin

Neuropeptide Y (NY) An abundant, widely distributed 36-residue tyrosine-rich neuropeptide, prominent in the hypothalamus and in limbic regions that co-exists with other neurotransmitters (epinephrine and norepinephrine, GABA, galanin, somatostatin) in discrete regions of the central, peripheral and enteric nervous systems; while the NY receptors are widely distributed in the brain, NY-like immune reactivity does not always overlap the presumed receptors, see Mismatch phenomenon; NY has considerable sequence homology with pancreatic polypeptide (PP) and peptide YY and is involved in a vast array of neuroendocrine activities, including autonomic functions (vasoconstriction and decreased absorption of electrolytes in the gastrointestinal tract), circadian rhythm, eating, drinking, sexual and motor activity and stress responses that may be altered by psychotropic drugs and excitatory neurotoxins and is being studied in Alzheimer's disease, Huntington's chorea, parkinsonism, eating disorders and depression (Prog Neuro-Psychopharmacol & Biol Psychiatr 1989; 13:31)

Neurophysin A carrier protein for oxytocin and vasopressin

Neuroregulator(s) see Neurotransmitters

Neurosarcoma see Triton tumor

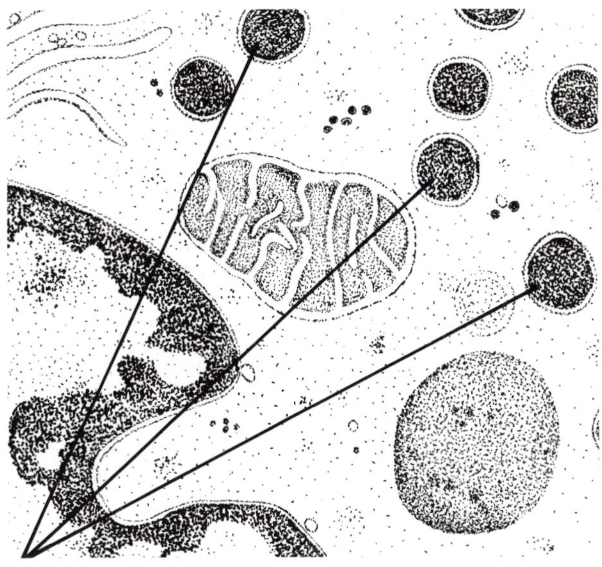

Neurosecretory granules

Neurosecretory granule Dense core granule A round, membrane-bound vesicle, which by electron microscopy appears as a dense black spot measuring 50 to 500 nm in diameter, surrounded by a cleared space, in turn surrounded by a dark thin rim (figure, above); neurosecretory granules contain various hormones, including calcitonin, gastrin, glucagon and vasoactive intestinal polypeptide (VIP) and are relatively specific for the neuroendocrine system, eg the neural crest and the APUD system; these structures have been divided into three sizes: a) 100-200 nm granules seen in the TSH-producing cells of the pituitary gland, PP cells of the pancreas and D_1 endocrine cells of the gastrointestinal tract b) 500-1500 nm granules seen in somatotrophic cells, prolactin-producing cells and carcinoid tumor cells and c) 200-600 nm granules that occur in all other cells; neurosecretory granule shape varies and may contain paracrystalline material with irregular sharp edges as in the α cells of the pancreatic islets; the dense core granule's limiting membrane may be tightly bound and indistinct, as in D cells of the pancreatic islets or have a gray halo, as in A cells of the pancreatic islets; in addition to the neuroendocrine system, dense core granules are seen in several types of neurons, adrenal neuroblastoma, pheochromocytoma, chemodectoma

Neurosis PSYCHOLOGY A disorder arising from an unresolvable conflict between the id (instinct) and the ego (conscious thought); subtypes include anxiety, manic-depression or pure depression, hysteria, obsessive-compulsive behavior and phobias

Neurosyphilis An uncommon manifestation of tertiary syphilis that may occur in secondary syphilis; neurosyphilis may be 1) Asymptomatic with only a positive VDRL in the cerebrospinal fluid, 2) Gummatous, 3) Meningovascular or thromboembolic form with cerebral infarction or cranial nerve defects, 4) Tabetic with degeneration of the posterior columns of the spinal cord and nerve roots, decreased peripheral reflexes and proprioceptive sensation, evoking Charcot's joints and e) General paresis or chronic meningoencephalitis **Clinical** Personality defects, aphasia, paralysis and seizures **Histopathology** Diffuse cortical atrophy (see Windswept cortex), neuronal depopulation and microglial proliferation; see STS-RPR, VDRL Cf Quaternary syphilis

Neurotensin A 13 residue neuropeptide secreted in the gastrointestinal tract that evokes vasodilation and inhibits gastric secretion and intestinal motility

Neurothekeoma Theke, Greek, sheath Nerve sheath myxoma A benign neural tumor of childhood, affecting the midline face, arms and shoulders at the dermal-epidermal interface **Histopathology** Large, mitotically active epithelioid cells with nuclear atypia and scattered spindled schwann cells in a mucinous matrix, divided into lobules by fibrous connective tissue **Immunoperoxidase** Tumor cells display variable amounts of S-100 antigen

Neurotoxin(s) Exotoxins that are present in many plants and animals, which block conduction of the nerve impulse or block synaptic transmission, by binding to the voltage-gated Na^+ channel protein; neurotoxins are produced by ***Corynebacterium diphtheriae, Clostridium tetani, C botulinum, Shigella dysenteriae***; other neurotoxins include conotoxin, saxitoxin and tetrodotoxin; see Conotoxin, Puffer fish and Red tide

Neurotransmitter PHYSIOLOGY Any of a number of small molecules present at synapses or neuromuscular junctions that are capable of transmitting an electrical impulse; to be defined as a neurotransmitter a) The synaptic vesicles in the presynaptic neuron must contain the substance and release it into the space at the time of an impulse b) Introduction of the substance into the synaptic space must elicit the same response as does stimulation of the presynaptic nerve and c) The substance must be rapidly degraded in the synaptic space with restoration of the membrane potential; virtually any intracerebral molecule capable of modifying neural signals may function as a neurotransmitter, including such diverse molecular species as amino acids (aspartic acid, GABA, glutamic acid, glycine), biogenic amines (acetylcholine, bradykinin, dopamine, epinephrine, norepinephrine, melatonin, serotonin or 5-HT), hypothalamic neuropeptides (luteinizing hormone, somatostatin, thyroid-releasing hormone), opioids (β-endorphin, neuroen- kephalin), neuropeptides (angiotensin, cholecystokinin, gastrin, nerve growth factor, neurotensin, substance P, vasoactive intestinal polypeptide) and others (ACTH, corticosteroids, estrogens, melanin-stimulating hormone, oxytocin, prolactin, prostaglandins, testosterone, vasopressin), epinephrine and norepinephrine; Cf Neuropeptides

Neurotrophic factor Neurotrophin One of a family of substances with roles in maintenance and survival of neurons, eg secretory proteins, nerve growth factor, brain-derived growth factor and neurotrophin-3 (Nature 1990; 344:339)

Neutral fats see NEFA

Neutral endopeptidase 24.11 see CD10

Neutralizing antibody An immunoglobulin produced by the host as a defense against bacteria, attenuating a microorganism's infectivity to the host; neutralization assays are used in the clinical laboratory as serologic tests to demonstrate a subject's previous exposure to the microorganism producing an exo- or endotoxin; alternately, the patient's serum or body fluid can be tested for the presence of an antigen, eg a virus by performing a neutralization assay with a standardized antibody or antitoxin

Neutron A non-charged elementary particle with a 1/2 spin and the approximate mass of a proton; alone it has a half-life of 12 minutes, but is stable when bound within an atom; in radiotherapy, neutrons have considerable advantages over γ radiation in that the oxygen enhancement ratio is lower for neutrons than for photons, there is little or no repair of DNA damage with neutrons and the variation in the cell sensitivity with the mitotic phases is less with neutrons than with other radiotherapeutic modalities; see Linear accelerator

Neutron activation analysis LABORATORY MEDICINE A highly sensitive reference method for quantifying elements in nanogram amounts, which is too complex for routine use Method The specimen is bombarded with neutrons that interact with the specimen's atoms, thus generating radioactive products that are identified based on the pattern of energy spectrum of the emitted γ rays

Neutron capture NUCLEAR MEDICINE A reaction that forms the basis on which radioisotopes of medical interest are produced in a reactor, where a neutron is temporarily absorbed by a nuclide (protons/neutrons comprising an atomic nucleus); once the neutron is absorbed, the radioactive nuclide emits γ rays (8 MeV), lower energy protons (β particles) and neutrons (α particles)

Neutropenic colitis with aplastic anemia Mulholland syndrome A clinical complex affecting young adults and consisting of right-sided colonic necrosis, profound agranulocytosis, aplastic anemia, fever, watery diarrhea, generalized abdominal pain without inflammation, accompanied by transmural bacterial infiltration often following antibiotic therapy Treatment Non-interventional (Ann Surg 1983; 197:84); see Pseudomembranous colitis

Neurotrophin-3 (NT-3) A member of the nerve growth factor family that stimulates the growth of a select number of nerves, at present incompletely studied; see BDGF (brain-derived growth factor), Nerve growth factor

Neurotrophic factor(s) see Nerve growth factor family

Neutrophil-activating factor-1 see Interleukin-8 (IL-8)

Neutrophil dysfunction syndromes A heterogenous group of diseases characterized by qualitative disorders of neutrophils, subdivided into defects of 1) Adhesion, eg cell adhesion deficiency, drug-induced adhesion defects 2) Locomotion, eg lazy leukocyte syndrome, abnormalities of actin polymerization 3) Phagocytosis 4) Microbial killing, eg chronic granulomatous disease, myeloperoxidase deficiency, hyperimmunoglobulin E syndrome, glucose-6-phosphate dehydrogenase deficiency 5) Structure of the nucleus or organelles, eg hereditary macropolycytes, hereditary hypersegmentation, specific granule deficiency, Alder-Reilly, May-Hegglin and Pelger-Huët anomalies, Chediak-Higashi disease and f) Multiple or mixed disorders (N Engl J Med 1987; 317:687rv)

Nevoid-basal cell carcinoma syndrome Gorlin-Goltz syndrome A rare autosomal dominant disease characterized by the childhood onset of multiple nevoid basal cell carcinomas associated with abnormalities of the skin ('pits' in the hands and feet in the form of 2-3 mm in diameter dells occasionally filled with carcinoma, milia, sebaceous cysts, lipomas, fibromas), lymphomesenteric cysts, central nervous system disease (mental retardation, electroencephalographic abnormalities, calcification of the dura, medulloblastoma and schizophrenia), endocrine system (ovarian cysts or fibroma, male hypogonadism, female escutcheon, scanty facial hair), eyes (canthal dystopia, hypertelorism, coloboma of nerve, congenital blindness), typical facies (hypertelorism, lateral displacement of the medial canthi, frontoparietal bossing, mandibular prognathism, accentuated supraorbital ridges, jaw cysts and a broad nasal root), skeleton (spina bifida occulta, fused, absent or cervical ribs, kyphosis, scoliosis, cervical and thoracic vertebral fusion, bridging of sella turcica, frontal and temporoparietal bone 'bossing', spina bifida occulta, shortened 4-5th metacarpals, epithelial-lined cysts of the jaws (N Engl J Med 1960; 262:908, ibid, 314:700cpc)

Nevus A pigmented tumor of the skin and/or mucosae; nevi are considered hamartomas and contain spindle-shaped melanocytes **MELANOCYTIC NEVUS** The most common nevus, which is subdivided into 1) **Compound nevus**, composed of nevus cell nests at the dermal-epidermal interface and dermis 2) **Intradermal nevus**, composed of nevus cell nests confined to the dermis 3) **Junctional nevus**, composed of nevus cell nests confined to the dermal-epidermal interface and 4) **Spindle and epithelioid cell nevus of Spitz**; see Blue nevus, Giant hairy nevus, Halo nevus; Cf Lymph node inclusions

Newcastle's disease A self-limited unilateral follicular conjunctivitis caused by an avian paramyxovirus which inhibits the oxidative burst in phagocytes, inducing the release of pyrogenic cytokines; spontaneous recovery follows 1-2 weeks of illness; the Newcastle agent causes a fatal pneumoencephalitis in fowl

New drug application see NDA

New Jersey vesicular stomatitis virus An enveloped RNA rhabdovirus with a single-stranded negatively coiled genome that replicates in infected host cell cytoplasm, first identified in the 1920s with a reservoir in wild animals, eg swine in Georgia, spider monkeys in Central America Clinical 60% of exposed subjects develop disease after a 1-2 day incubation, with fever, chills, malaise, myalgias, nausea, vomiting and pharyngitis; despite the name, oral vesicles are relatively uncommon Prognosis Spontaneous resolution in one week

New Orleans asthma see Yokohama asthma

'New scientist' A PhD scientist who has recognized the changing atmosphere in research; the modern scientist is no longer able to sustain a career in research by merely doing benchwork, but must also be part businessman, communicator, 'grantsman' and must be financially and politically adept, computer-literate and have strong interpersonal skills; Cf 'Lab rat'

New York City medium MICROBIOLOGY A growth medium containing hemolyzed equine erythrocytes, horse serum, yeast extract, vancomycin, colistin, amphotericin and trimethoprim, which is used to identify ***Neisseria gonorrheae*** allowing better recovery of organisms than that obtained with the Thayer-Martin medium; NYC medium also supports the growth of mycoplasma and ureaplasma

New York Heart Association classification A functional classification (table) of cardiac failure, that serves to stratify patients accorrding to severity of disease and the need for (and type of) therapeutic intervention (Criteria Committee of the New York Heart Association, Inc: Diseases of the Heart and Blood Vessels, 6th ed, Little Brown, Co, Boston 1964)

NewYork Heart Association

I	Asymptomatic heart disease
II	Comfortable at rest but symptomatic with normal activity
III	Comfortable at rest but symptomatic with less than normal activity
IV	Symptomatic at rest

New Zealand mice Two strains (New Zealand black NZB and New Zealand white NZW) of inbred mice that are used to study autoimmunity; NZW mice are asymptomatic; NZB mice develop autoimmune hemolytic anemia and low titers of antinuclear antibodies, spontaneously activated B cells, defective T cells and defects in DNA repair; when NZW are crossed with NZB, the progeny develop an autoimmune syndrome with severe immune complex disease, glomerulonephritis, lupus cells and high titers of anti-nuclear antibodies; thus the F_1 generation of NZB/NZW mice serves as an animal model for autoimmune disease and lupus erythematosus

Nexin A 150 kD protein that is integral to axonemic structures in cilia and flagella; see Cilia, Dynein

Nexus Site of electrical connection between two cells; see Neuromuscular junction; Cf Gap junction

NF see National Formulary

NF-AT Nuclear factor of activated T cells see Immunophilins

NGF see Nerve growth factor

NGU Non-gonococcal urethritis

NHL Non-Hodgkin's lymphoma see there

NHTSA National Highway Traffic Safety Administration; see MVA

Niacin test MICROBIOLOGY Niacin (nicotinic acid) plays a key role in the oxidation-reduction reaction in mycobacterial metabolism; although all ***Mycobacterium*** species produce nicotinic acid, ***M tuberculosa, M simiae*** and ***M szulgai*** produce the greatest amount; lesser amounts are produced by ***M africanum, M bovis, M marinum*** and ***M chelonei***, ss ***cheloni*** and ***M chelonei***, ss ***abscessus***; differences in nictonic acid production form the basis of a test allowing speciation of positive mycobacterial cultures

NIAID National Institute of Allergy and Infectious Diseases A branch of the National Institute of Health Director A Fauci; NIAID coordinates activities related to the therapy of AIDS

Nick MOLECULAR BIOLOGY A single-stranded break in double-stranded helix of nucleic acids, usually DNA; 'nicked sites' are characterized by increased mobility

Nickase A restriction endonuclease that introduces a break in one strand of the double-stranded DNA

'Nickel and dime' lesions A fanciful descriptor for the annular, waxing and waning maculopapular lesions seen at the mucocutaneous borders at the mouth and nasolabial folds in protracted untreated secondary syphilis, more common in dark-skinned subjects; these lesions may coincide with anogenital condylomata lata Note: Nickels are US coins with a value of $.05, dimes are worth $0.10

Nick translation MOLECULAR BIOLOGY A method used to prepare a radioactive 'probe' of a segment of DNA of interest, where the polymerase and 5'→ 3' exonuclease activities of DNA polymerase I are allowed to occur simultaneously Technique ***Escherichia coli*** DNA polymerase I is added to a solution containing a) A duplex DNA molecule of interest to be used as a 'probe' and b) A radioactive or 'hot-labelled' nucleotide containing either a purine or pyrimidine labeled with ^{32}P; the DNA polymerase both 'nicks' the DNA (acting as a 5'→ 3' exonuclease and 'mends' the double-stranded DNA (acting as a 3'→5' polymerase) using a ^{32}P-labelled nucleotide in the repair process; once a probe is radioactive or labelled, it may then be placed in a hybridization fluid containing a Southern-blotted nylon or nitrocellulose membrane containing the DNA segment of interest and allowed to anneal with its 'mirror-image'

NICODARD National Information Center for Orphan Drugs and Rare Diseases; see Orphan disease, Orphan drug

Nicotine 1-methyl-2-(3-pyridyl) pyrrolidine SUBSTANCE

ABUSE A toxic pyridine liquid alkaloid found in cigarette smoke; urine levels of nicotine in smokers 0.616-18.480 µmol/L (US: 0.1-3.0 mg/L) and in nonsmokers < 0.431 µmol/L (US: < 0.07 mg/L); nicotine is a highly toxic and rapidly acting natural insecticide, which may cause human intoxication by inhalation, skin absorption or ingestion, either the result of accidental exposure or suicidal ingestion **Clinical** Transient central nervous system stimulation followed by depression or paralysis, accompanied by nausea, salivation, abdominal pain, vomiting, diarrhea, cold sweats, headache, vertigo, confusion, incoordination, slowing of the pulse rate, dyspnea with potentially paralysis of the respiratory musculature and intense vagal stimulation which may cause transient or permanent cardiac arrest; death occurs within 1-4 hours of ingesting a fatal adult dose (> 60 mg) **Treatment** Emesis, gastric lavage, atropine (*Nicotiana tabacum* stimulates the cholinergic receptors); see Conicotine, Nicotine gum, Passive smoking, Smokeless tobacco, Smoking

Nicotine replacement therapy SUBSTANCE ABUSE The use of nicotine gum (Nicotine polacrilex chewing gum) and transdermal nicotine patches to alleviate or attenuate the symptoms of nicotine withdrawal; non-smoking nicotine replacement must be supplemented by behavioral intervention and training to minimize recidivism; transdermal patches are two-fold more effective than placebos and may be more effective than nicotine gum, currently the only approved replacement therapy in the US (Mayo Clin Proc 1990; 65:1529, 1619)

Nicotine gum Nicotine polacrilex A masticant that slowly releases nicotine, ameliorating the effects of tobacco withdrawal and the intensity of relapse factors, eg weight gain (J Am Med Assoc 1990; 264:1564)

NIDDM see Non-insulin-dependent diabetes mellitus

Night blindness Nyctalopia Defective vision in reduced illumination, often implying defective rod function with delayed dark adaptation and perceptual threshold; it is either congenital and stationary with myopia and degeneration of the disc, eg retinitis pigmentosa, hereditary optic atrophy or progressive and acquired with retinal, choroidal or vitrioretinal degeneration, eg cataract, glaucoma, optic atrophy, retinal degeneration and, the 'classic' cause of nyctalopia, vitamin A deficiency

Nightmare Pavor nocturnus Fearful dreams most commonly affecting children during REM (rapid eye movement) sleep and accompanied by hyperactivity of the autonomic nervous system **Treatment** None

'Night soil' Human feces used as a fertilizer for ground crops (tubers, vegetables, berries), which serves as a vehicle for various parasites, commonly, *Ascaris lumbricoides* in the Western hemisphere, the eggs of which remain viable for long periods) and *Clonorchis sinensis* in the Orient

Nightstick fracture FORENSIC MEDICINE A solitary ulnar fracture occurring when the arm is raised to parry the blow of a nightstick, which may be used by some police and security guards

Night sweats Nocturnal, often drenching diaphoresis, a clinical finding described as characteristic of terminal Hodgkin's disease, tuberculosis, trypanosomiasis and giant cell (temporal) arteritis

NIHL see Noise-induced hearing loss

NIH National Institutes of Health A group of agencies of the US government located in Bethesda, Maryland that funds and directs government-sponsored medicine-related research activities in the US, directed by Bernadine P Healy, MD, which has an annual budget of $8 x 10^9 (Science 1991; 252:1242n&v); Cf INSERM

NIH scoring system IMMUNOLOGY A technique for typing the human leukocyte anti-gens HLA-A, -B, -C, -DQ and -DP, devised at the National Institutes of Health, which uses a 150X inverted microscope, giving a value of 1 for every 10% of cells lysed, detected by active exclusion of a dye, trypan blue (table)

NIH scoring

Score	% Lysis	Interpretation
1	0-9%	**Negative**
2	10-19%	± Negative
4	20-39%	± Positive
6	40-79%	Positive
8	80-100%	**Positive**

NIHL see Noise-induced hearing loss

Nikethamide A central nervous system stimulant formerly used in emergency situations in respiratory failure; direct supportive measures, eg mechanical ventilation and maintenance of cardiovascular function are more useful and this agent has been abandoned

Nilutamide RU 23908 An antiandrogenic agent used to prevent the potentially fatal flare-up reaction that may occur in early treatment of metastatic prostatic carcinoma; see Disease flare-up

NIMH National Institute of Mental Health

9 + 2 pattern Nine plus two arrangement A configuration of microtubules characteristic of eukaryotic cilia and flagella, in which a pair of central tubules is surrounded by nine peripheral doublets of microtubules; see Cilia

Ninhydrin Triketohydrindene CLINICAL TOXICOLOGY An oxidizing reagent that reacts with amino acids and proteins that is used to screen urine specimens for the presence of and semiquantify α-amino acids, as it yields colored compounds

Ninth day erythema Milian's erythema A erythematous dermatopathy of historic interest related to the use of arsenicals to treat syphilis

NIOSH see National Institute for Occupational Safety and Health

Nipple appearance CYTOPATHOLOGY A 'succulent' nuclear protrusion of blasts seen in papanicolaou-stained cerebrospinal fluid, a finding which in combination with prominent nucleoli is characteristic of leukemic involvement of the central nervous system; see Nuclear blebbing; Cf 'Tit' sign

Nipple discharge Serous and/or serosanguinous discharge from the breasts that is most common in peri- and post-menopausal women, caused by a variety of lesions, eg benign intraductal papilloma (nipple adenoma), ductal ectasia and Paget's disease of the breast as well as advanced ductal carcinoma of the breast

Nit An empty louse egg shell, deposited by ***Pediculus capitis, P corporis*** and ***Phthirus pubis*** ('crabs')

Nitrates NO_3-bearing compounds are a major component of explosives and fertilizers; when drinking water is obtained from wells contaminated by runoffs from nitrogen-fertilized fields (EPA standards for well water allow a maximum 10 ppm or 10 mg/L of nitrate), nitrates are converted in vivo to nitrites, and may cause fatal methemoglobinemia in newborn infants and, less commonly, in adults deficient in glucose-phosphate dehydrogenase Note: Nitrates may be converted in the stomach to N-nitrosamines, a potent gastric carcinogen; Deionizers, desalination, reverse ionization, ion exchange and distillation remove nitrates in the drinking water; in-line charcoal filters do not (see Nature 1991; 350:223); see Blue people, Monday death, Nitroglycerin

Nitric oxide ENVIRONMENT A gas byproduct of high temperature combustion, eg internal combustion engines which upon exposure to light results in NO_2 formation, a highly irritating smog gas and a major contributor to the Greenhouse effect PHYSIOLOGY Nitric oxide (NO) has been recently identified as a neurotransmitter;it is released when glutamate binds to the NMDA receptor, allowing the entry of calcium ions, which combine with calmodulin, activating nitric oxide synthase (NOS), releasing NO into the synaptic space; once in the post-synaptic neuron, NO activates guanylyl cyclase, which generates cGMP, which in turn initiates a phosphorylation cascade; NO (formerly, endothelium-derived relaxing factor) is a potent locally-acting vasodilator requiring L-arginine as a substrate that is generated by NOS present in blood vessels, cytotoxic macrophages, adrenal gland and brain (Nature 1990; 347:768) and other tissues; in the stomach, it is released by non-adrenergic, non-cholinergic nerves, resulting in a reflex relaxation of the stomach to accommodate increased volume of food and fluids (Nature 1991; 351:477); excess NO may be neurotoxic and play a major pathogenic role in neurodegenerative disorders including Huntington's and Alzheimer's diseases; NOS has sequence homology with cytochrome P450 reductase, an enzyme intimately involved in the hepatic metabolism of drugs (Science 1991; 252:1788n&v)

Nitroblue tetrazolium test see NBT

Nitrogen balance CLINICAL NUTRITION A crude indicator of the adequacy of nutrition is the protein lost during a 24-hour period, calculated by urinary excretion of nitrogen products produced by the urea cycle; usually 0.5 g/day of dietary protein is adequate to maintain an appropriate nitrogen balance; in a negative nitrogen balance, loss exceeds intake, a situation seen in aging, burns and protein-losing enteropathy Note: In the induction phase of chemotherapy, a 'physiologic' negative balance occurs due to massive lysis of malignant cells; a positive balance is typical of growth periods, ie in the young, in pregnancy and in convalescence from burns

Nitrogen mustard(s) ONCOLOGY A family of alkylating agents used primarily to treat malignant lymphoma, in the MOPP regimen for stage III and IV Hodgkin's disease, in acute lymphocytic leukemia, topically for mycosis fungoides; all mustards have a $-N(CH_2CH_2Cl)_2$ group and enter the cells via the choline transport system; tumor cells may develop mustard resistance through enhanced repair of alkylated DNA or thiol-mediated mustard inactivation **Toxicity** Gastrointestinal (nausea, vomiting), myelosuppression with pancytopenia, alopecia, local tissue injury, diarrhea, diaphoresis

Nitrogen washout curve RESPIRATORY PHYSIOLOGY A measurement of the time required to eliminate N_2 gas from the lungs when breathing another gas (usually O_2), a clinical test of use in identifying the presence of poorly ventilated lung regions

Nitroglycerin Glycerol trinitrate An organic nitrate that serves as a short-acting agent for the treatment of anginal pain and congestive heart failure Side effects Headache, tachycardia, nausea and hypotension; other organic nitrates, eg ethylene nitrate and trinitrotoluene (TNT) are used to produce explosives

NK cell see Natural killer cell

NK receptor(s) A family of receptors for the tachykinin family of peptides, designated NK1 for substance P, NK2 for neurokinin A and NK3 for neurokinin B; see Substance P, Tachykinins

NMDA N-methyl-D-aspartate A chemical used in neurophysiology to probe a group of membrane proteins, designated 'NMDA receptors'

NMDA receptor(s) N-methyl-D-aspartate receptors (NMDA-R) A family of membrane-bound ion channels that open when NMDA as well as neurotransmitters, eg acetylcholine, glycine, GABA and glutamate are bound, regulating the strength and stability of excitatory synapses, allowing positively charged ions to flow into the neuron; NMDA-Rs mediate the slow component of excitatory post-synaptic potentials and play a key role in neural, synaptic and behavioral plasticity and may be pivotal in the development of opiate tolerance and dependence (Science 1991; 251:85); the NMDA receptors can undergo robust synapse-specific long-term potentiation, which is related to learning and memory (Nature 1991; 349:157) Note; NMDA-Rs are involved in pathological cerebral processes, in excitotoxic neuronal death due to cerebral ischemia and epilepsy; NMDA-R activation requires glycine acting at an allosteric site tightly coupled to the receptor; NMDA-R-activated ion flow in the hippocampus is inhibited by ethanol (perhaps through a mechanism of membrane 'fluidization'), thus explaining the central nervous system depression associated with intoxication; the NMDA-R is unusual as both chemical transmitters or a change in electric potential can activate the sodium, potassium and calcium ion channels

NMN Nicotinamide mononucleotide

NMR Nuclear magnetic resonance see Magnetic resonance imaging

NMR spectroscopy A technique that analyzes molecules by studying magnetic structure; the nucleus of each hydrogen atom (other molecules are involved but have a lesser contribution) acts as a magnet and sets up its own field and influences the fields of other, nearby atoms; by perturbing a field and observing the response, data is generated which, with the proper algorithms, allows structural analysis, and is a technique used in research to analyze three dimensional protein conformations; the 'dimensions' of NMR spectroscopy do not refer to physical dimensions, but rather how the data is collected and displayed **ONE-DIMENSIONAL NMR** A straight line of data is obtained, where a powerful magnet is used to align all the nuclear spins in the same direction; the sample is then bombarded with radiofrequency radiation turning the nuclear 'magnets' on their sides, rotating them around the axis of the applied magnetic field, causing the rotating (or 'precessing') nuclei to generate their own magnetic fields which are detected by the magnetic coil and analyzed; each molecule 'precesses' at a different 'resonance frequency', due to their bonding to other molecules; 1-D NMR provides enough information to solve the structure of simple molecules; with complex molecules, the NMR spectrum is too 'busy' to solve the structure **TWO-DIMENSIONAL NMR** Analysis of a series of 1-D NMR experiments, typically 1000 'runs', allowing examination of proton interactions; if the amino acid sequence is known, the information obtained in the 2-D NMR can be used to determine how a protein twists upon itself; 2-D NMR has a 'resolution' limit of proteins with 100 or fewer amino acids **THREE-DIMENSIONAL NMR** adds a step in which the spins of the precessing hydrogen ions interact with the spins of the precessing carbon ions, in a series of abbreviated 2-D NMR 'runs'; 3-D NMR has a 'resolution' limit of 150 amino acids **FOUR-DIMENSIONAL NMR** is expected to resolve proteins up to 300 residues in length Note: NMR analysis of protein conformation (ie three-dimensional structure) is preferred to X-ray crystallographic analysis, which requires a pure crystal of a protein that may require months to obtain (Science 1990; 249:411, 364); the advantage is that it allows the study of proteins in solutions and in non-crystalline states, which more closely simulate physiologic environments Method A sample is 'zapped' with a beam of electromagnetic energy, exciting nuclei of certain atoms, especially hydrogen to a higher energy state; when the beam is turned off, the excited molecules return to a ground state; as each of the molecules returns, it has a characteristic relaxation 'signature'; an increase in the relaxation time (Normal 0.154 msec) of fat's methylene (NH_2) component may be seen in metastases, but is not statistically significant; NMR spectroscopy and scanning tunnel microscopy offer new insights into the dynamics of protein molecules and protein-folding (Science 1989; 243:45)

NMS see Neuroleptic malignant syndrome

NNN medium Novy, MacNeal and Nicolle medium MICROBIOLOGY A growth medium for parasites, eg *Leishmania donovani* and *Trypanosoma cruzi*

Nobel prizes Physiology or Medicine (P&M), Chemistry (Chem, if applicable), Physics (Phy, if applicable); in brackets [], the value of the prize in that year **1991** (P&M) E Neher and B Sakmann, both German, both Max-Planck Institute; Development of the patch-clamp technique and discovery of ion channels in cell membranes **1990** (P&M) JE Murray and ED Thomas, both American, at Harvard and Fred Hutchinson (Seattle), respectively; Pioneer work in renal and bone marrow transplantation, respectively (Chem) EJ Corey, American, Harvard, Devising methods to synthesize complex molecules found in nature [$710 000] **1989** (P&M) JM Bishop and HE Varmus, both American, both at U California, San Francisco; Cellular and viral oncogenes [$475 000] (Chem) S Altman, Canadian-American, Yale, Connecticut; TR Cech, American U Colorado, Denver; RNA autosplicing [$475 000] **1988** (P&M) GB Elion and GH Hitchings, both Americans, both at Burroughs-Wellcome, North Carolina and Sir J Black, British, U London; Development of drugs essential for treating heart disease, peptic ulcers, gout and leukemia [$390 000] **1987** (P&M) S Tonegawa, Japanese, Massachusetts Institute of Technology; Generation of antibody diversity [$340 000] **1986** (P&M) R Levi-Montalcini, Italian-American and S Cohen, American; Nerve growth factor and Epidermal growth factor respectively (Phy) E Ruska, G Binnig, Germans and H Rohrer, Swiss; Electron microscopy [$290 000] **1985** (P&M) MS Brown, JL Goldstein, both American, both U Texas; Lipoprotein lipase and cholesterol metabolism (Chem) HA Hauptman, J Karle, both Americans; X-ray crystallography for analysis of biological molecules [$225 000] **1984** (P&M) C Milstein, Argentinian at Cambridge, GJF Köhler, Swiss at Basel; Monoclonal antibodies; NF Jerne, Dane at Basel; Theoretical groundwork in immunology (Chem) RB Merrifield, American, Rockefeller Institute; Protein analysis and drug development [$190 000] **1983** (P&M) B McClintock, American, Cold Spring Harbor; 'Jumping genes' [$190 000] **1982** (P&M) S Bergstrom, B Samuelsson, Sweden and JR Vane British; Prostaglandin synthesis (Chem) A Klug, South African, Cambridge; Structural analysis of viruses and subcellular particles [$157 000] **1981** (P&M) RW Sperry, DH Hobel, TN Wiesel, Americans; Brain research [$180 000]

'Nocebo' A negative placebo effect that may occur when patients in a clinical trial recognize (or think they recognize) that they are getting a placebo (ie, not receiving therapy), and fare worse due to the effect of negative suggestibility (Lancet 1991; 338:899); Cf Placebo

Nociceptors Nerve and reflex loops for reception and response to pain; receptors are periarticular and mucocutaneous

'No code' orders see Do not resuscitate (DNR)

NOD mouse Non-obese diabetic mouse A mouse strain with an inherited predisposition toward autoimmune disease resembling the human insulin-dependent diabetes mellitus (IDDM); both IDDM and NOD mice have similar genetic defects in HLA-DQ (human class II MHC) and I-A (the murine class II homologue); NOD mice lack a large segment of DNA in their MHC I-E region; in transgenic NOD mice, insertion of either I-E or correction of the I-A defect reduces insulinitis and prevents disease progression (Nature 1990; 345:722, 724, 727, 662n&v)

Nodes CARDIOLOGY The intrinsic pacemakers of the heart, the nodes are composed of neural tissue; the sinoatrial node (normal rhythm, 70/min) is located at the junction of the superior vena cava with the right atrium and conducts impulses by way of three Purkinje fiber tracts (the anterior internodal tract of Bachman, the middle internodal tract of Wenckebach and the posterior internodal tract of Thorel) to the atrioventricular node (normal rhythm, 45/min) located in the right posterior portion of the interatrial septum, which in turn is continuous with the bundle of His (normal rhythm, 35/min)

Nodovenous shunt A surgical decompression procedure used to reduce and eliminate the future development of lymphedema caused by lymphatic blockage, classically due to microfilariasis, in those patients who have 'failed' diethylcarbamazine therapy

Nodular adenosis A benign, well-circumscribed lesion of the breast that has features of both sclerosing adenosis and blunt duct adenosis

Noise Random variation in signals of the electromagnetic spectrum that carries no useful information from the source; Poisson noise is statistical fluctuation in the number of information carriers (photons, electrons), which appears as 'snow' in a cathode ray tube, a function of the statistical variation of the rays received by the detector and number of electrons produced by the photomultiplier; see White noise; Cf Chaos

Noise-induced hearing loss Reduction in auditory perception induced by loud sounds, inculpated in one-third of the 28 million hearing-impaired adults in the US, occurring with prolonged exposure to sound levels above 85 decibels, although there is a wide range (30-50 dB) of individual susceptibility to sound (J Am Med Assoc 1990; 263:3185)

Noise pollution The presence of noise and sounds in the workplace and environment that is annoying or excessive to the point of causing loss of productivity Prevention Active noise control

Noma Gangrenous stomatitis Cancrum oris An acute necrotizing, polymicrobial and ulcerating infection of the orofacial tissues seen in malnourished children, which rapidly erodes to deep tissue, exposing bone and teeth Microbiology Anaerobic fusospirochetes, eg *Borrelia vincenti* and *Fusobacterium nucleatum*, less commonly, *Bacteroides melaninogenicus* and filiform gram-negative bacteria Treatment High doses of intravenous penicillin; correction of dehydration and malnutrition

'No-man's land' HAND SURGERY A fanciful synonym for the fibrous sheath of the flexor tendons of the hand, specifically in the zone from the distal palmar crease to the proximal interphalangeal joint; any tendon injury to the distal forearm, wrist of hand could be a 'no-man's land' if a) the facilities and/or equipment is inadequate b) the operator is inexperienced or exhausted or c) the tendon is potentially damaged beyond salvage; see Rule of threes Note: A 'no man's land' is a belt of ground between the most advanced elements of opposing armies or an area controlled by neither side of conflict

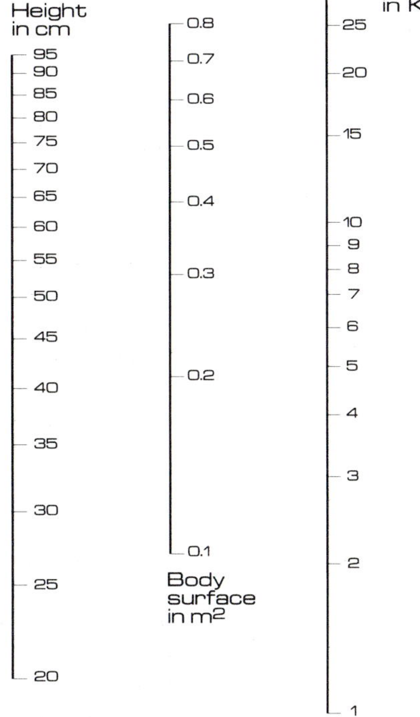

Nomogram for body surface area in children

Nomina Anatomica Although the vast majority of anatomic terminology is derived from classic roots, there is some disagreement on minutiae, more often related to loyalties to tradition, mentors or jingoism than to logic; the first system was established in 1895 by the German Anatomical Society, which held its first meeting in Basel, since known as the Basel Nomina Anatomica (BNA), which gave the names in Latin; the nations adopting the system then translated the terms into their own respective languages; the French were the first to break away from the BNA pack, as they felt that terms based on ancient gallic tradition served them better; the British left the BNA fold in 1933, as they felt the arbitrary anatomic positions were too rigid and did not reflect human anatomy, and therefore generated the 'Birmingham revision'; the Germans (who started it all) were the next to break away, and in 1937 delivered to the not-so-eagerly-awaiting-world, the Jena Nomina Anatomica; oddly, the same Americans who won the West, remained true to the original BNA; in 1955, the Fifth International Congress of Anatomists approved the Paris Nomina Anatomica, which comprises the 'State of the art' anatomic nomenclature, the details of the 12th Congress of Anatomists held in 1985, 'der letzte Schrei' in the scintillating world of anatomy is summarized in: Nomina anatomica:Nomina histologica:Nomina embryologica (Churchill-Livingstone, 1989)

Nomogram An alignment chart (figure, left) in which there are three or more abscissas, each measuring a specific para-meter and mathematically or empirically defined as having a relation to each other; the abscissas are placed parallel to each other on an open two-dimensional field; a straight line drawn when two of the parameters are known, allows determination of the value of the third (unknown) parameter)

Non-A non-B hepatitis see Hepatitis, non-A, non-B

Non-clathrin coated vesicles see Golgi-derived coated vesicles

Noncompliant patient A patient who does not conform to the prescribed program of medical therapy, as may occur in patients who are being treated with chronic dialysis (J Am Med Assoc 1991; 265:1579); see Patient compliance, Negligence (contributory); Cf 'Good' patient

Nondisjunction GENETICS The failure of homologous chromosomes or sister chromatids to separate during mitotic anaphase, an event resulting in one daughter cell receiving both copies of the entire chromosome, eg in Down syndrome, one daughter cell is trisomic for chromosome 21, ie has 47 (2n + 1) chromosomes, while the other daughter cell is monosomic, ie has 45 (2n - 1) chromosomes

Nonessential amino acids Any amino acid that can be synthesized by an organism from available substrates; Cf Essential amino acids

Nongonococcal urethritis (NGU) A condition causing dysuria, pyuria and symptoms similar to, but less intense than gonorrhea, most commonly caused by ***Chlamydia trachomatis***; NGU is more common in heterosexuals (14% had chlamydial isolates, homosexuals 5%) than gonococcal urethritis (12% versus 25% in homosexuals); other causes of NGU include ***Ureaplasma urealytica*** and ***Mycoplasma genitalium*** although NGU, defined as the presence of abundant neutrophils in the urine, often reveals no organisms

Non-Hodgkin's lymphoma see Working classification

Non-insulin-dependent diabetes mellitus (NIDDM) Adult-onset or type II diabetes mellitus A condition comprising 90% of diabetes mellitus; 80% of NIDDM patients are also obese (an association known as 'diabesity'), insulin-deficient and insulin-resistant; NIDDM is diagnosed when a) fasting glucose is 7.8 mmol/L (US > 140 mg/dl) on two or more occasions or b) when in a 75 g glucose tolerance test, the 2-hour and one of the other values (drawn at the 30, 60 or 90 minute intervals) are greater than 11.2 mmol/L (US > 200 mg/dl) **Treatment** NIDDM does not usually require exogenous insulin, although it may be required during 'crises'; see Glucose tolerance curve, MODY; Cf IDDM

Non-ionizing radiation Electromagnetic radiation, the photons of which have insufficient energy to ionize atoms, including sound, ultraviolet, visible and infrared light and radiowaves

Nonlinear analysis see Chaos

Non-operative cranioplasty see Head shaping

Nonparametric test STATISTICS A value, eg a median or percentile, or a statistical test, eg a rank-sum test that does not assume a specified mathematical form for the underlying distribution; results from nonparametric analysis have less statistical power but eliminate the need for specifying the mathematical form for the underlying distribution of data

Non-'participation' The non-acceptance of a physician of the fees paid by Medicaid, or less commonly in Medicare; nonparticipation is a key factor in lack of access of low-income Americans to adequate health care and is attributable to the low rate of reimbursement by Medicaid for the actual costs of the services rendered, delays in reimbursement and increasing costs of malpractice insurance; see Participation

Nonphotochromogen MICROBIOLOGY One of a group of atypical mycobacteria that produce a scant amount of pale yellow pigment; unlike the so-called 'photochromogens', exposure of nonphotochromagens to light does not intensify the color, a feature seen in ***Mycobacteria avium-intracellulare, M gastri, M haemophilum, M malmoense, M nonchromogenicum, M terrae*** and ***M triviale*** ; see MAIS, MOTT, Runyon group, Tuberculosis

Nonprotein nitrogen assay (NPN assay) LABORATORY MEDICINE A test measuring the non-protein nitrogen-bearing compounds in plasma (total nitrogen concentration 14.3-25 mmol/L in serum (US: 20-35mg/dl), including urea (45% of the total NPN), amino acids, ammonia, creatine, creatinine and uric acid; NPN has fallen into disfavor as an indicator of renal function, as it is non-specific, increasing in non-renal conditions, eg dehydration, gout, hepatopathy, high-protein diet, increased protein catabolism (or chemotherapy), muscle wasting diseases, corticoid therapy and prerenal and postrenal azotemia **Method** Protein was removed by precipitation and the remaining organic nitrogen was mixed with a catalyst and sulfuric acid and converted to NH_4HSO_4; the NH_3 released was measured directly

Non-reducing sugar A sugar that does not contain an aldehyde or potential aldehyde and will not reduce inorganic ions in solution

Non Q-wave infarction A subendocardial myocardial infarction (MI) in which the EKG pattern consists of a persistent abnormal ST-segment depression in all but the aVR lead (which shows ST-segment elevation), often accompanied by T-wave changes; most cardiologists diagnose a non-Q-wave MI when the clinical, enzymatic and radionuclear findings are consistent with MI, with or without the above EKG changes (N Engl J Med 1990; 322:743); see Thallium imaging

Nonsecretor see Secretor

Nonsense codon Stop codon A triplet of RNA nucleotides (UAA, UAG or UGA) on the mRNA that cause ribosomes to stop transcription

Nonsense mutation Null mutation A point mutation on a 'structural' gene, which results in the encoding of one of three nucleotide triplets or codons (ATT, ATC or ACT) that result in the transcription of corresponding stop codons (UAA, UAG or UGA) on the mRNA, which when detected by the translation machinery, terminates protein synthesis, effectively eliminating the gene's product and therefore its function; alternately, a stop codon may be present and a nonsense mutation results in an elongated protein product, as the appropriate stop codon no longer exists

Nonsense suppressor gene A gene that encodes a tRNA molecule that 'reads through' a nonsense (stop) mutation, resulting in the translation of an amino acid instead of protein chain termination

Nonsense syndrome Ganser syndrome Balderdash syndrome PSYCHIATRY A condition in which a person gives 'astonishingly' incorrect answers to simple questions; although this illness is considered to be factitious in nature, the 'nonsense symptom' may occur in hysteria, schizophrenia, or transiently in normal subjects under stress or when fatigued; Cf Factitious 'diseases'

Non-smoking tobacco see Smokeless tobacco

Non-specific esterase (NSE) α-naphthyl butyrate esterase An enzyme on the external face of the plasma membrane of alveolar macrophages and circulating monocytes; NSE is a common monocyte 'marker', the activity of which is inhibited by sodium fluoride, which does not occur in granulocytic esterase and inhibits gastric secretion and intestinal motility

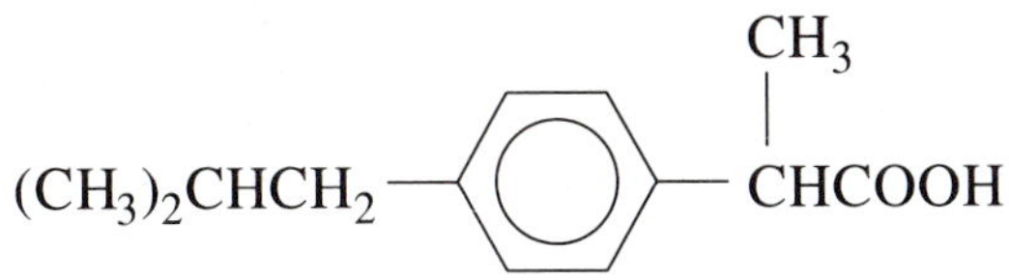

$$(CH_3)_2CHCH_2-C_6H_4-CH(CH_3)COOH$$

Ibuprofen

$$C_6H_4(COOH)(OCOCH_3)$$

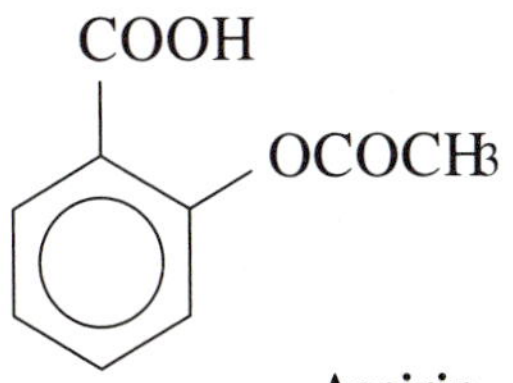

Aspirin

NSAIDs

Nonsteroid antiinflammatory drugs (NSAIDs) A family of weak organic acids that 1) Inhibit prostaglandin biosynthesis, by inhibition of cyclooxygenase, and to a lesser degree lipooxygenase and 2) Interfere with membrane-bound reactions, eg NADPH oxidase in neutrophils, phospholipase C in monocytes and G protein regulated processes; other responses that occur at high NSAID levels, eg interference with proteoglycan synthesis by chondrocytes, transmembrane ion flux, cell-cell interaction, unmask T cell suppressor activity (N Engl J Med 1991; 324:1716rv); other postulated activities include decreased production of free radicals and superoxides, which may interact with adenylate cyclase, altering intracellular cAMP levels, reducing vasoactive and nociceptive mediator release from granulocytes, basophils and mast cells Therapeutic uses of NSAIDs Rheumatoid arthritis, gouty arthritis, ankylosing spondylitis, osteoarthritis, serosal inflammation, Bartter syndrome and other inflammatory conditions Note: Although aspirin is an NSAID, many practitioners equate NSAIDs with the newer non-aspirin agents derived from propionic acid, indoles or pyrazolone or designated as fenamates, pyrrole alkanoid acid or oxicams Chemical classes of NSAIDs Carboxylic acid: Acetylated, eg aspirin (figure) or nonacetylated, eg sodium salicylate Acetic acid analogs, eg indomethacin, tolmetin, sulindac Propionic acid analogs, eg ibuprofen (figure), naproxen Fenamic acid analogs, eg mefanamic acid Enolic acid analogs, eg oxyphenbutazone, phenylbutazone and Nonacidic compounds, eg proquazone Side effects Rash, pruritus, edema, vertigo, drowsiness, tinnitus, aseptic meningitis, nausea, vomiting, gastric ulcers and potentially fatal gastrointestinal hemorrhage, jaundice, Stevens-Johnson syndrome, Henoch-Schönlein syndrome, fatal aplastic anemia, acute renal failure

Non-stress test OBSTETRICS An indirect non-invasive monitor of the well-being of a fetus, where the frequency of fetal movement, degree of heart rate acceleration and beat-to-beat variation of the heart rate are monitored to determine the 'health' of the placental vasculature; see Deceleration, Montevideo units; Cf Fetal heart monitoring

Non-traditional cancer therapy see Unproven methods of cancer therapy

Non-ulcer dyspepsia (NUD), Moynihan's disease A condition characterized by ulcer symptoms in the absence of gross ulceration; 30-60% of dyspeptics have no demonstrable macroscopic lesions Clinical Symptoms range from that of a classic duodenal ulcer (epigastric burning, 1-3 hours after meals, relieved by food or alkali) to functional indigestion (bloating, belching, fullness and nausea, not relieved by antacids and worsened by meals); fat intolerance is common ENDOSCOPY The duodenal mucosa demonstrates edema, erythema, petechial hemorrhage and erosions; Cf Dumping syndrome

Non-union A diaphyseal fracture that is a) Unhealed after more than nine months and b) Has no synovial pseudoarthrosis (a non-union in which a synovioid membrane forms, filled with synovioid fluid) Treatment Non-invasive electrical stimulation of bone (J Am Med Assoc 1989; 261:917)

NOR Nucleolus organizer region

NORD National Organization for Rare Diseases A private non-profit organization which a) Acts as a 'clearing house' of information for Orphan diseases (see there) and b) Facilitates communication among governmental agencies and the research community (eg locating patients for clinical trials); see NICODARD, Orphan disease, Orphan drug/product

Normal distribution F distribution STATISTICS A generic term for any member of the parametric family of probability distributions which have symmetric, bell-shaped curves of data points, eg gaussian distribution

Normality CHEMISTRY An obsolete term, which expresses the concentration of a solution as gram-equivalents of substance X per liter of solution; Cf Molality and Molarity

Normoblast An immature nucleated erythrocyte; in order of maturation, the erythroid series develop into pronormoblast, followed by mitosis, basophilic normoblast I (E2, followed by mitosis), basophilic normoblast II (E3), polychromatophilic normoblast (E4, followed by mitosis), polychromatophilic normoblast (E5), orthochromatic normoblast, reticulocyte, erythrocyte

Norplant Levonorgestrel A proprietary implantable contraceptive that prevents pregnancy by inhibiting ovulation and causing thickening of cervical mucus; Norplant consists of six cylinders filled with Levonorgestrol (a progestin) allowing five years of protection against unwanted pregnancy, with a 'failure rate' similar to fallopian tubal ligation and vasectomy; it should not be used in women with liver disease of any nature, a history of breast cancer or thrombotic tendencies Side effects Menstrual irregularities, headache, nervousness, nausea, vertigo and increased size of the ovaries and fallopian tubes, dermatitis, acne, weight gain, breast tenderness and hirsutism

'North American operation' CANCER SURGERY A term attributed to the pelvic surgery service at Memorial Sloan-Kettering Hospital in New York, referring to radical surgery for a 'frozen pelvis', consisting of radical en bloc resection of the uterus and urinary bladder; see 'Frozen pelvis'; Cf 'All-American' and 'South American' operations

Northern blotting MOLECULAR BIOLOGY A technique used to detect the presence of specific mRNA molecules; the RNA in a sample is denatured, eg with formaldehyde, to prevent hydrogen bonding between base pairs and ensure that the RNA is unfolded and linear; the sample is separated according to size by gel electrophoresis and transferred or 'blotted' on a nylon or nitrocellulose membrane, placed in a solution containing a labeled DNA 'probe' and then autoradiographed, a procedure similar to Southern blotting; see Blotting, Southern blotting

Norwalk agent(s) A group of parvoviruses (single-stranded DNA) that cause 'winter vomiting disease', first described in Norwalk, Ohio and inculpated in up to 40% of nonbacterial epidemics of gastroenteritis in the US, and is a frequent cause of traveller's diarrhea **Clinical** After a 1-2 day incubation, it may present explosively (keeping an entire community at the edge of its seat), often accompanied by nausea, vomiting, abdominal cramping, anorexia, malaise and myalgia, transmitted in an oral-fecal fashion, eg exposure to recreational swimming water or by ingestion of raw shellfish, cake-frosting, stored water on cruise ships; the Norwalk agent is difficult to identify as it doesn't grow in cell culture and there are no animal models; cDNA has been constructed and the amino acid sequence motif of the RNA polymerase has been identified (Science 1990;250:1580) **Prognosis** Spontaneous resolution without sequelae

Norwegian itch A severe variant of scabies most common in institutionalized persons, especially those with Down syndrome or either debilitated or immunosuppressed patients are covered by hosts of mites (***Sarcoptes scabei*** var homini) causing a psoriasis-like pachydermia, variably accompanied by thickened nails, generalized hyperpigmentation, eosinophilia and pyoderma with lymphadenopathy; see Seven-year itch

Nose coverage MALPRACTICE INSURANCE A component of a medical malpractice insurance policy in which a physician's liability is assumed by the previous malpractice insurance carrier, usually until such time as the physician has a new policy; the 'nose coverage' period is usually brief and may be extended as a courtesy by the insurance carrier when a physician moves to another state in the US; Cf Tail coverage

Nosocomial AIDS Acquired immunodeficiency syndrome that may occur in certain disadvantaged nations, where a hypodermic needle may be used and re-used; in the Soviet Union, two outbreaks of HIV-1 seroconversion occurred, infecting 58 and 23 children respectively (N Engl J Med 1990; 323:1844c)

Nosocomial infection An infection beginning three or more days after admission to a hospital; the microorganisms that cause nosocomial infection are a function of a) The underlying disease process, eg burns are associated with ***Pseudomonas aeruginosa***, diabetes mellitus with anaerobes, gram-negative bacilli and ***S aureus***, leukemia with enterobacteriaceae due to indwelling vascular accesses and post-operative wounds with ***S aureus***) and b) The organ system involved, often facilitated by an indwelling catheter, tracheostomy or other device

'Notch' HEALTH CARE POLICY A precipitous drop in health care benefits for individuals or families despite a marginal increase in incomes, where those with earnings above the 'notch' will not qualify for the benefits

Notching RADIOLOGY Small grooves on the anterior aspect of ribs seen on a plain chest film of children with post-ductal (ductus arteriosus) coarctation of the aorta, due to the 'tracks' from the pressure of collateral vessels on the ribs, which may be seen on a plain chest film

Notched nuclei see Buttock cell

Notch sign of Rigler RADIOLOGY A short, straight radiolucency best appreciated by tomography that penetrates a relatively well-circumscribed lung mass, first described as characteristic of malignancy, where the notch corresponds to the shadow of a feeder vessel penetrating the mass; since the notch sign is also seen in other conditions, eg granulomatous infections, the sign is of questionable usefulness

Notebook RESEARCH A book, that is generally bound with sewn pages in which a person performing bench research records, preferably dated and in ink, the nature of each experiment and all of the data that he collects from each 'run' of an assay, column chromatogram, gel electrophoretogram or other, either copied from instrument, or the actual tape or hard copy read-out from the instrument Note: Laboratory notebooks have been scrutinized in at least two cases of alleged fraud in science and thus may prove to be a research scientist's single most important 'accountability document'; see Raw data; Cf Log(book)

Notifiable diseases PUBLIC HEALTH A group of communicable diseases that a local, state or federal government wishes to maintain under surveillance in order to control and prevent the spread of infections; the US system of reporting notifiable diseases evolved from the Quarantine Act of 1878, which authorized the US Public Health Service to collect morbidity data on cholera, smallpox and yellow fever; each state in the US has its own list of notifiable infectious diseases and depends largely on reporting by the individual physician, where the completeness of reporting ranges from 6-90%; Infectious diseases that are 'notifiable' in most of the United States include amebiasis, anthrax, botulism, brucellosis, campylobacteriosis, chancroid, chickenpox/H zoster, cholera, diphtheria, encephalitis (unspecified), giardiasis, gonococcosis, invasive ***Haemophilus influenzae***, hepatitis (all forms), HIV-1 and HIV-2, Legionella, leprosy, leptospirosis, lymphogranuloma venereum, malaria, measles, meningitis (aseptic, ie presumed viral, and bacterial), meningococcal disease, mumps, pertussis, plague, poliomyelitis, psittacosis, rabies, Reye syndrome, Rocky Mountain spotted fever, rubella, salmonellosis, shigellosis, syphilis, tetanus, toxic shock syndrome, trichinosis, tuberculosis, tularemia, typhoid fever, typhus and yellow fever (J Am Med Assoc 1989; 262:3018); see Reportable occupational diseases

Notochord The vertebral column of the embryo, which is

composed of cartilage and eventually replaced by bone; vestigeal rests of the notochord persist in the adult as nucleii pulposi, which may rarely give rise to chordomas

Novacor A proprietary implantable cardiac ventricular assist device in the protocol stage, which may serve as a mechanical bridge while a patient in terminal cardiac failure is waiting for a heart transplant

Novelty diets see Diet, fad

Novobiocin MOLECULAR BIOLOGY An antibiotic that interferes with ATP-dependent gyrase (A type II topoisomerase that introduces negative supercoils into a relaxed closed circular molecule) by preventing ATP from binding to gyrase's B subunit

N-proCT N-procalcitonin A protein secreted by the parafollicular (thyroid C) cells, which is highly conserved among diverse species (from salmon to humans) and stimulates osteoblasts and inhibits osteoclasts; N-proCT may have a role in osteoporosis and is related to the calcitonin gene-related peptide; see C cells, CGRP

N protein A 25 kD protein of unknown function contained in small nuclear ribonucleic proteins (snRNPs) of neurons, which has been used to understand differences in RNA-processing in cells of different lineages

NPT Nuclear Non-Proliferation Treaty An international accord signed by 120 nations, pledging not to pursue development of nuclear weapons; see IPPNW, London club, Nuclear war

NRC Nuclear Regulatory Commission NUCLEAR MEDICINE A US government agency that licenses users of radioactive materials, sets limits of worker exposure and regulates the production, use and disposal of radioactive materials; 'NRC units' are used to quantify exposure to radioation, where the maximum allowable is 100 µCi/3 months or by bioassay

NSABP National Surgical Adjuvant Breast and Bowel Project A series of on-going multicenter clinical trials that are evaluating the effects of certain chemotherapeutic agents, eg tamoxifen and 5-FU in treating advanced carcinoma of the breast and large intestine

NSAID see Non-steroid anti-inflammatory drugs

NSE 1) see Neuron-specific enolase 2) see Non-specific esterase α-naphthyl butyrate esterase

NSILA Non-suppressible insulin-like activity An action displayed by acid-dissociable 7.5 kD serum complex with activity of insulin-like growth factor (IGF-I and IGF-II), somatomedins A and C; most NSILA is associated with a high molecular-weight protein (NSILP), which has significant homology with IgG's Fc fragment

NST see Non-stress test

5'-NT see 5'-Nucleotidase

NT-3 see Neurotrophin-3, Nerve growth factor familty

N-terminal The end of a protein or polypeptide that contains the free amine group, placed by convention at the left of a diagram

Nuclear blebbing An ultrastructural finding of unknown significance that is typical of malignant lymphocytes as seen in lymphomas, which consists of the loss of coherene of the nuclear membrane with the nucleoplasm (figure); nuclear blebbing has virtually no diagnostic utility, as prognostication and diagnosis of lymphoproliferative diseases are based on light microscopy, immunoperoxidase, flow cytometry and various methods of molecular biology; see Nipple appearance

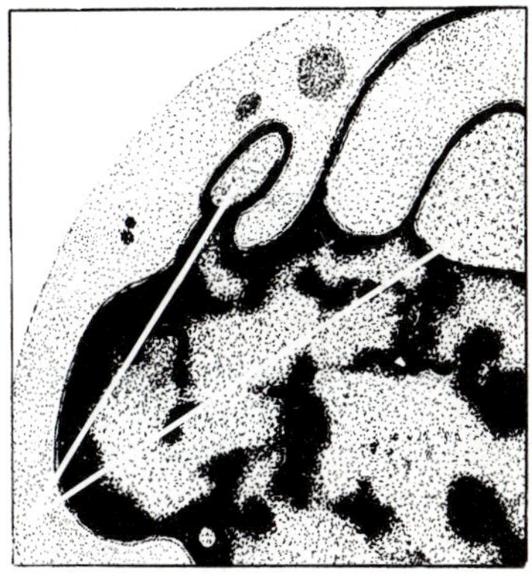

Nuclear blebbing

Nuclear contour index (NCI) A value obtained by measuring the complexity of the nuclear rim with a graphic digitalizer on an electron micrograph, allowing evaluation of the cerebriform cells of mycosis fungoides, a value which has no diagnostic, prognostic or therapeutic utility; see Nuclear blebbing;Cf Nuclear roundness factor;

Nuclear:cytoplasmic asynchrony see Maturational arrest

Nuclear:cytoplasmic ratio N:C ratio A crude parameter used in cytology and surgical pathology, where interphase, ie nondividing, nuclei are proportionately larger than their accompanying cytoplasm; the N:C ratio is usually increased in malignant cells

Nuclear dust PATHOLOGY Granular debris seen in any necrotizing process, corresponding to fragmented nuclei and, if infected, bacteria, as may occur in leukocytoclastic vasculitis or a ruptured abscess RENAL PATHOLOGY Rounded fragments of 1-3 mm in diameter basophilic debris derived from partially degraded hematoxylin bodies, classically described in focal proliferative glomerulonephritis seen in lupus erythematosus (WHO morphologic classification class III)

Nuclear envelope Nuclear pores A double-membrane envelope that separates the 'noble material' from the cytoplasm, communicating therewith by 70 nm in diameter pores; the outer nuclear membrane is contiguous with the endoplasmic reticulum

Nuclear family SOCIAL MEDICINE The core family unit, classically consisting of heterosexually oriented male and female partners and their direct genetic progeny; disintegration of this unit and its central role in society is widely held to be responsible for significant losses of mental equilibrium; Cf Extended family

Nuclear magnetic resonance see Magnetic resonance imaging, NMR

Nuclear medicine An area of medicine that uses radioisotopes for the diagnosis and treatment of disease, ie radiation oncology; diagnostic nuclear medicine encompasses in vitro assays of clinical specimens, eg immunoassays for various hormones, including human chorionic gonadotropin (β-HCG), insulin and thyroid-stimulating hormone (TSH) Note: Radioactive immunoassays are being increasingly replaced by enzyme-linked immunoassays, which are easier to perform, the reagents are more easily stored and do not have the problems inherent in using and disposing of radioactive waste; nuclear medicine also encompasses in vivo diagnostics in the form of scintillation counters to 'scan' various body regions for the presence of increased uptake of radionuclides, which when focal, implies primary neoplasia or metastases

Nuclear power plant Nuclear reactor; see Chernobyl, Radiation injury, Sellafield study, Three Mile Island; Cf ENVIRONMENT

Nuclear roundness factor (NRF) The degree to which a nucleus in cross section approximates a perfect circle; increased nuclear irregularity is often associated with aggressive cell growth, and may be used to grade epithelial malignancy; like the nuclear contour index, the NRF has little diagnostic, prognostic or therapeutic utility, and thus although the objective nature of the NRF makes it a candidate for computer-based imaging analysis, the wide variability of cell populations in malignancy and the existence of malignant 'bland cell' tumors, make the relatively primitive structural details provided less useful than functional analysis of a tumor's potential for aggression by measuring gene amplification, the loss of tumor suppressor genes, or DNA ploidy analysis

NUCLEAR WAR, BLAST EFFECTS

A	B	C	
1.3	140	750	Everything is flattened, 'moonscape'
4.8	70	460	Almost everything is flattened
7.0	35	255	Heavy construction is not flattened
9.5	20	150	Building walls blown away
18.6	7	55	Survival is possible

A Kilometers from 'ground zero' (blast epicenter)
B Air pressure, kg/m^2
C Wind velocity in kilometers/hour

Nuclear war The potential medical consequences of even a limited nuclear war would be devastating (N Engl J Med 1986; 315:905) Definitions **FIRE WINDS** Wind that is produced by air heated to one million degrees centigrade, which burns anything combustible, rising and sucking air into its vortex; the wind is most intense in metropolitan areas and less intense in rain **LD_{50}** The radiation dose that is lethal to 50% of those exposed (2.5-6.0 Gy), assuming that optimal care, ie transfusions, trauma and nursing care, antibiotics and nutrition is available; given that a nuclear war would destroy hospitals and blood donors, drugs or food would not be available, a lower radiation exposure eg 1.5 Gy to the marrow and 2.2 Gy to the body would be lethal **NUCLEAR CRASH** An economic crash that would follow a nuclear war; if 1% of the global nuclear arsenal targeted the US liquid fuel production and importation, 8% of the US population would die immediately; 60% would die of starvation in the next two years; it has been projected that post attack economies would be operating at 40% of pre-attack capacity for up to 25 years after a nuclear exchange (Science 1987; 236:1517) **NUCLEAR WINTER** A prolonged period of cold weather due to massive atmospheric soot injections in a full-scale nuclear 'exchange'; according to the TTAPS model, the midsummer land temperatures would decrease by 10-20°C in northern latitudes, to sub-freezing in the southern hemisphere, disrupt the monsoons and deplete the ozone layer (Science 1990; 247:166); see Disaster, TTAPS model

Nuclease A generic term for hydrolytic enzymes that cleave the phosphodiester bonds in the nucleic acids of DNA and RNA, which can be either exonucleases (EC 3.1.11-16) or endonucleases (EC 3.1.21-31); see Restriction endonuclease

Nucleated erythrocytes A finding that is normal in the peripheral blood of newborns, but distinctly abnormal in adults and seen in thalassemia major or leukoerythroblastic reactions Note: Birds normally have nucleated red cells

Nucleic acid A polymeric molecule that is either a double-stranded chain of DNA nucleotides (which carries the genetic information) or a single-stranded chain of RNA (which is pivotal in protein synthesis); the individual units of the nucleic acids are pyrimidine nucleotides (cytosine, which is present in both DNA and RNA, thymine, present in DNA and uracil, present in RNA), purine nucleotides (Adenine and Guanine, nucleotides shared by DNA and RNA); both nucleotides are linked to another nucleotide base and attached to a sugar (RNA and DNA chains each have a pentose sugar: D-deoxyribose for DNA and D-ribose for RNA), which is attached to the phosphate group; without the phosphate, the sugar and base together are called nucleosides; with one phosphate, it is a mononucleotide, eg AMP, a second phosphate dinucleotide, eg ADP and a third high energy phosphate added yields a trinucleotide, eg ATP; see DNA, mRNA, Purines, Pyrimidines, RNA, rRNA, tRNA

Nucleolin A 100 kD protein associated with intranucleolar chromatin and ribosomal particles that is thought to have a role in mRNA transcription and assembly of ribosomes

Nucleolini Small, spherical clumps of ribonucleoprotein in the nucleolus, which by electron microscopy appear as zones of fibrillar lucency surrounded by granular, electron-opaque rings; the size variability of the nucleolini is greater in malignancy than in benign conditions

Nucleolus An RNA-rich intranuclear region composed of ribosomes, strands of DNA that encode ribosomal RNA and the constellation of cognate enzymes; in general, cells with small or inconspicuous nucleoli are not actively dividing or producing proteins, in general, benign; nucleoli are usually basophilic and may reach considerable size in certain malignancies (breast and renal cell carcinoma, epithelioid sarcomas, immunoblastic and Hodgkin's lymphoma), the nucleolus may be eosinophilic and reach gargantuan proportions

Nucleoside analogs Molecules that structurally mimic nucleosides; the dideoxynucleoside family, eg dideoxycytidine, 2',3'-dideoxyinosine and 3'-azido-2',3'-dideoxythymidine, inhibits reverse transcriptase after anabolic phosphorylation and is used to treat retroviral infections, eg HIV-1; see Zidovudine (3'-azido-2',3'-dideoxythymidine)

Nucleosome A coherent aggregate of highly basic proteins that is associated with chromosomes, originally classified according to the proportion of the content of basic amino acids in each; the H1, H2A, H2B, H3, H4 classes of histones occur in all eukaryotes (H5 is a unique variant in avian erythrocytes); the histone complexes contain a 140 base-pair strand of DNA coiled around double cylinders of histones H2a, H2b, H3 and H4; nucleosomes are separated from each other by 'naked' 25-100 base pairs in length segments of DNA Note: The H1 histone can be removed with impunity and thus is considered extrinsic to the histone complex; histones allow tight organized packing of DNA while limiting DNase cleavage or 'attack'; see Histone

5'-Nucleotidase LABORATORY MEDICINE A hydrolytic enzyme that cleaves the phosphate from 5'ribonucleotide; elevation of 5'-NT is more specific than alkaline phosphatase in hepatobiliary disease and is highest in patients with posthepatic jaundice, intrahepatic cholestasis and infiltrative hepatic lesions

Nucleotide see Nucleic acid

Nucleus HISTOLOGY The cell 'organelle' that contains the genetic material (DNA) and the replicative and transcriptional machinery (RNA and binding proteins) necessary to copy the genomic information and encode the structural and functional proteins required for cell function NEUROANATOMY An aggregate of neuronal cell bodies sharing a common function, eg accessory nucleus, caudate nucleus, nucleus ambiguus ORGANIC CHEMISTRY The portion of a molecule that is the major determinant of chemical behavior, eg benzene ring, β-lactam ring, cyclopentano-perhydrophenanthrene in steroids

Nuclide An atom with a specific atomic number, mass number and energy level

NUD see Non-ulcer dyspepsia

Nude mouse A strain of laboratory mice that is hairless, thymusless (congenital thymic aplasia) and T cell-less, which must be raised in a gnotobiotic environment, and is of greatest use in studying graft-versus host disease

Null allele A segment of DNA that is not known to produce a protein product

Null cell A lymphocyte lacking T cell and B cell markers including lineage-specific cluster of differentiation (CD antigens and surface immunoglobulins, formerly known as a 'third population' cell, which comprise up to 20% of peripheral lymphocytes; null cells participate in antibody-dependent cell-mediated cytotoxicity and is the cell phenotype most commonly seen in childhood acute lymphocytic leukemia; null cells are of three types: a) Undifferentiated stem cells that later mature into T or B cells, b) Cells with labile IgG and a trypsin resistant high-affinity Fc receptor and c) Large granular lymphocytes (NK and K cells) Note: Null cell lymphoproliferative disorders demonstrate heavy and/or light chain rearrangements and thus null cell malignancies are often of B-cell origin; see ACDD, Large granular lymphocytes, Pan B cell markers, Pan T cell markers

Null DNA preparation A method used to determine the overlap of genes in various tissues; the mRNA from the tissue in question is allowed to react with non-repetitive DNA; the DNA that reacts is isolated, constituting the mDNA preparation; the DNA that does not react is the 'null' DNA; the 'null' DNA is then hybridized in excess mRNA from another tissue; the proportion of the mDNA that reacts serves to identify the proportions of genes expressed in the second tissue as well as the first tissue

NUREMBURG CODE The voluntary consent of the human subjects is absolutely essential. This means that the person involved should have legal capacity to give consent; the person should be so situated as to be able to exercise free power of choice, without the element of force, fraud, deceit, duress, over-reaching or other ulterior form of constraint or coercion, and should have sufficient knowledge and comprehension of the elements of the subject matter involved as to enable him to understand and make an enlightened decision. This latter element requires that before the acceptance of an affirmative decision by the experimental subject, it should be made known to him the nature, duration and purpose of the experiment, the method and means by which it is to be conducted, all inconveniences and hazards to be reasonably expected and the effects upon his health or person which may possibly come from his participation in the experiment. The experiment should be such as to yield fruitful results for the good of society, unprocurable by other methods or means of study and not random and unnecessary in nature... The experiment should be conducted so as to avoid all unnecessary physical and mental suffering and injury... The degree of risk to be taken should never exceed that determined by the humanitarian importance of the problem to be solved by the experiment.

Null hypothesis STATISTICS A hypothesis that assumes that if there are no differences between two populations (or sets of data) being compared, a statement of probabilities (P value) can be made

Null mutation see Nonsense mutation

Null phenotype The non-expression of a protein because its corresponding gene is defective or absent on both inherited haplotypes; most null phenotypes involve the red cell, eg blood group O, M-N-S-s-, Fy(a-b-), Jk(a-b-), Rh null (---/---); although the most common null phenotype is that of the ABO group O, which occurs in 45-to-55% of the population; null phenotypes are relatively uncommon; other null phenotypes include non-red cell proteins, as in non-expression of complement proteins ($C3_0$), transferrin (Tf_0) and haptoglobin (Hp_0)

Null syndrome see Rh/null syndrome

'Numb chin' sign A rare clinical finding that may be the first sign of carcinoma metastatic to the mandible

Numbers see Measurement

Number three ('3') sign A finding on a plain anteroposterior chest film which, when seen with rib notching, left ventricular hypertrophy and precordial systolic murmurs is suggestive of coarctation of the aorta

Nuremburg code BIOMEDICAL ETHICS An internationally sanctioned code of research ethics that was formulated in response to the revelations of the extent and brutality of the Nazi war crimes that forced experiments of little scientific value on concentration camp victims; the Nuremberg code establishes strict standards for scientific studies on human subjects based on the principles of autonomy and informed consent (see page 503 for wording); the Declaration of Helsinki is an extension of this code that was formulated in 1964 and revised in 1975; see Declaration of Helsinki, Geneva Convention, Institutional review board; Cf Unethical medical research

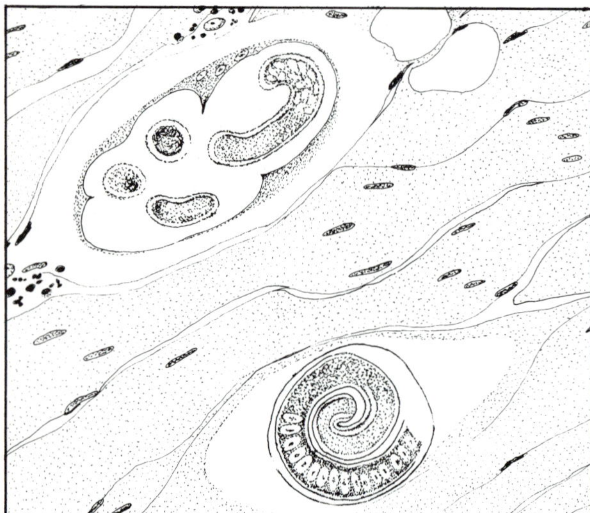

Nurse cell

Nurse cells A term that has been used in several different contexts HEMATOLOGY Macrophages of erythroblastic islands in the bone marrow, involved in erythrophagocytosis, iron storage and transfer PARASITOLOGY Histiocytes and other cells that serve as a 'nursery' for the bradyzoites of *Toxoplasma gondii*, affecting the immunocompromised or in infants PATHOLOGY Skeletal muscle cells (above figure) which the larvae of *Trichinella spiralis* modify to create an intracellular environment suitable for their own survival and later encystation

Nursemaid's elbow Subluxation of the head of the radius, caused by a longitudinal 'yank' on the forearm (by a nursemaid, nanny or caregiver), forcing the child's elbow into extension; the child's arm is immobile and the child is in pain; the subluxation is reduced by firm supination at 90° and extension, followed by immobilization with a posterior splint or a sling

Nursing home HEALTH CARE INDUSTRY A facility that is largely dedicated to the long-term care of the elderly; there are currently about 1.5 million nursing home residents in the USA, estimated to cost $34.7 billion (US); the probability of nursing home use increases sharply with age; 17% of those age 65-74 spend one or more years, as do 60% of those aged 85; 21% spend five or more years in a home and this use is up to two-fold greater in women than in men (N Engl J Med 1991; 324:595); see Geriatrics, Home health care; Cf Hospice

Nutcracker esophagus see Corkscrew esophagus

Nutcracker phenomenon A clinical finding in hemoglobin SC disease, in which left-sided renal hemorrhage causes infarction of renal papillae, due to increased pressure as the left renal vein passes between the aorta and the superior mesenteric artery; increased pressure causes renal medullary anoxia sufficient to sickle the red cells

Nutmeg liver A descriptor for a liver with chronic passive congestion, a hepatopathy that is secondary to cardiac decompensation and failure, the gross morphology of which has been fancifully likened to a cut nutmeg; if the congestion is severe, these changes may be accompanied by hemorrhagic necrosis Pathology Intense congestion with deep red, centrilobular zone, sharply demarcated from the pale tan peripheral zones corresponding to the liver plates due to stasis and concomitant fatty degeneration of the liver Histopathology Central veins are dilated and congested, the sinusoids are widened with extravasation of red cells, thickening of arterial walls and hepatocytic atrophy (shrunken eosinophilic cells with pyknotic nuclei) and fatty degeneration

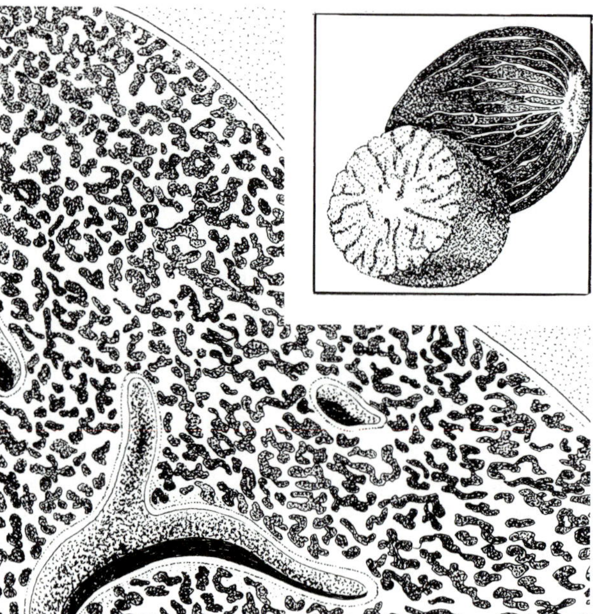

Nutmeg liver

Nutrient medium MICROBIOLOGY A generic term for any culture medium that provides the physical support and the essential nutrients required for the growth of microorganisms, usually carbohydrates, eg dextrose and protein eg birdseed or brain-heart infusion

Nutritional 'mumps' Chronic, asymptomatic bilateral enlargement of the parotid and/or submaxillary salivary glands that occurs endemically in a population suffering from multiple clinical signs of malnutrition including cachexia, hypoproteinemia, anemia, angular cheilosis, pellagroid hyperpigmentation

NZB/NZW see New Zealand mice

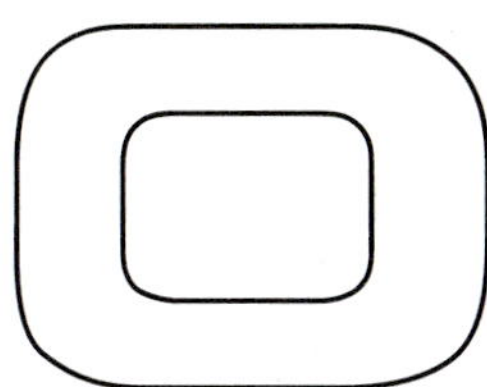

O Symbol for: Oxygen

o Symbol for: ortho-

O-11 10-(propoxy)decanoic acid) An analog of myristic acid that is highly toxic to trypanosomes and non-toxic to human cells, which has therapeutic potential in treating trypanosomiasis, for which the only agent available for treating end-stage (meningoencephalitic) disease is melarsoprol, which itself causes death in 5% of patients (Science 1991; 252:1851)

OAF Osteoclast-activating factor(s) A group of lymphokines, eg tumor growth factor α that mobilize calcium and are produced in excess in malignancy and rheumatoid arthritis, causing osteolysis-induced hypercalcemia

Oak leaf spots A descriptor for the size and shape of the pigmented cutaneous macules seen in patients with von Recklinghausen's disease and tuberous sclerosis

O antigen MICROBIOLOGY A bacterial lipopolysaccharide-protein antigen used for the serological classification of enteric bacteria, including ***Proteus*** species, forming the basis of the Weil-Felix test (used for the classification of ***Rickettsia*** species) and ***Shigella*** species for categorization of its 40 serotypes TRANSFUSION MEDICINE An oligosaccharide precursor for the A and B antigens of the ABO blood group, fucose-galactose-N-acetylglucosamine-glucose; see Bombay phenotype

Oasthouse disease 'Beer baby syndrome' A disorder characterized by increased α-hydroxybutyric acid in the urine and stools, which imparts a characteristic 'oasthouse' odor, described in methionine malabsorption (defective intestinal absorption of methionine and other amino acids); the gastrointestinal bacteria ferment the excess methionine into α-hydroxybutyric, α-ketobutyric and α-aminobutyric acids which are then absorbed and excreted Clinical Failure to thrive, seizures, hypotonia and edema; α-hydroxybutyric acid may also rarely appear in the urine of patients with phenylketonuria Note: An oasthouse is a building or kiln for drying hops, which are the ripe, dried pistillate catkins of a hop (***Humulus lupulus***) used especially to impart a bitter flavor to malt liquors

Oat cell carcinoma A histologic subtype of small cell carcinoma of the lung, characterized by a dense hyperchromatic oval nucleus, often with a vague central groove and minimal cytoplasm Ultrastructure Neurosecretory granules, containing hormones (ACTH, ADH, bombesin, calcitonin, CRF, estrogen, FSH, growth hormone, histaminase, HPL, LH, MSH, PTH, renin, serotonin) Clinical Highly aggressive with a 3-month survival without therapy, often accompanied by cerebellar degeneration (80% have metastasis to the brain) Molecular biology Homozygous loss of tumor suppressor gene on chromosome 3 Treatment Non-surgical; up to 85% respond to combination chemotherapy using CCNU, cyclophosphamide, doxorubicin, vincristine and etopoisde (VP-16); although extensive disease at time of discovery is often fatal within two years, 50% of those with limited metastases respond to therapy and 15-20% survive two years; radiotherapy may control bone pain, spinal cord compression, superior vena cava syndrome and bronchial obstruction; see Small cell carcinoma

Obesity A condition that is regarded as a premorbid addiction disorder, defined as 10% (or 20%) above an individual's standard weight; the ideal body weight is 21 kg/m^2 (the average American is 20% overweight, weighing 25.5 kg/m^2); the child is father of the man—an obese child is often an obese adult and the patterns may be established as early as three months of age (decreased energy expenditure in infants of obese mothers, N Engl J Med 1988; 318:461); in the past 20 years, there has been a 54% increase in obesity and a 98% increase in superobesity in children 6 to 9 years of age; obesity is classified according to 1) Anatomy a) Android ('beer-gut') obesity is more common in males, more central or truncal in distribution and places the subject at risk for diabetes mellitus b) Gynecoid obesity is more common in females, the fat is distributed in the lower abdomen and legs and is less commonly associated with atherosclerosis 2) Psychological profile 3) Age of onset, eg Juvenile, mature, during pregnancy or other 4) Type of tissue change, eg hyperplastic or hyperplastic-hypertrophic and 5) Primary or secondary a) Primary obesity is associated with HLA-B18 and is a component of Allström, Blount, Cohen, Carpenter, Laurence-Moon-Biedl, Prader-Willi and other eponymically-dignified syndromes b) Secondary or acquired obesity comprises the bulk of obesity Laboratory Obesity mimics the findings of non-insulin-dependent diabetes mellitus, including insulin resistance, increased glucose, cholesterol and triglyceride levels, decreased HDL and norepinephrine and depression of the sympathetic and parasympathetic nervous system; Co-morbid conditions associated with obesity Cardiovascular disease, thromboembolism, cholecystitis, cholelithiasis, abnormal gastrointestinal transit, poor wound healing, atelectasis, hepatic steatosis and fibrosis Treatment Diet, exercise, behavior modification; Cf Adipsin, Diets, Gastric 'balloon', Morbid obesity, Superobesity

'Obe-tension' A relatively common clinical association of obesity with hypertension; Cf Diabesity

Obitiatrist see 'Doctor Death'

OBS see Organic brain syndrome

'Observation' hip ORTHOPEDICS A condition characterized by transient focal osteolysis of the hip bones that may be accompanied by mild synovitis or osteoarthritis, which is either idiopathic or secondary to minor trauma and infection **Treatment** None, observation (hence the name) usually suffices

Obsessive-compulsive disorder (OCD) A condition that was once considered a rare, therapeutically-refractory neurosis; OCD affects 1-2% of the US population, has a neurophysiopathological component and may respond to certain tricyclic antidepressants (N Engl J Med 1989; 321:497) **Pathogenesis** The biological roots of OCD are extrapolated from avian studies by K Lorenz who hypothesized that certain bird behavior, eg nest-building, courtship and grooming were 'hard-wired' into the brain and, like OCD, repeated in exactly the same sequence **Treatment** Clomipramine is of use in one clinical form of OCD, trichotillomania and is of use in other forms of OCD (J Am Med Assoc 1990; 263:1896)

Obstetric hypercoagulability profile A battery of tests for a woman who may be at risk, eg repeated abortions for coagulopathic diatheses, which supplements the details provided by the obstetric screening profile, measuring in addition, proteins C and S, anti-thrombin III, lupus anti-coagulant, fibrinogen and plasminogen Note: Prothrombin time and partial thromboplastin time are measured on admission for delivery

Obstetric (screening) profile LABORATORY MEDICINE A battery of laboratory tests for a pregnant woman who is not known to have, or to be at risk for, conditions that might complicate labor and delivery, which includes CBC with white cell differential count, blood group, Rh typing and a Rh-Du test for all Rh negative women, antibody screening, measurement of rubella titers and hepatitis B surface antigen and syphilis serology

Obstructive hydrocephalus Hydrocephalus due to interference with the flow of cerebrospinal fluid, resulting in enlarged ventricles; obstructive hydrocephalus may be due to congenital aqueductal stenosis or atresia, eg Dandy-Walker syndrome, a complication of intracranial infection, violent birth trauma or transmitted in an X-linked recessive fashion; Cf Communicating hydrocephalus

Obstructive sleep apnea syndrome A clinical complex due to the pathophysiological response to anatomic defects of the nasopharynx, characterized by loud snoring, nocturnal oxyhemoglobin desaturation and disrupted sleep, accompanied by daytime hypersomnolence, related to the loss of the mechanisms designed to prevent death by asphyxiation **Clinical** Many symptoms are cardiovascular, eg apnea-induced arrhythmia, bradycardia, increased ventricular ectopic activity and hypertension and are associated with obesity, nasal obstruction,adenoidal and tonsillar hyperplasia, macroglossia, retrognathia, acromegaly and hypothyroidism **Treatment** Therapy should be individualized and may include surgery, eg uvulopalatopharyngoplasty is successful in 50% of cases (Mayo Clin Proc 1990; 65:1087, 1250, 1260); Cf Snoring; Cf Narcolepsy, Sleep disorders

Obturator sign RADIOLOGY A unilateral increase in the obturator muscle bulk, seen as a soft tissue bulge on the inner pelvis with medial displacement of the normal fat line, considered characteristic of infectious arthritis, which may be seen in trauma-induced hemorrhage

Occam's razor see Ockham's razor

Occipital horn Broad, calcified protrusions (occipital exostoses) that extend caudally from the base of the skull, characteristic of X-linked type IX Ehlers-Danlos syndrome, a morbid process, which like Menke's kinky hair disease is related to defective copper metabolism, resulting in secondary lysyl oxidase deficiency and by extension, collagen defects; other anomalies in type IX Ehlers-Danlos syndrome include hyperextensibility and facile bruisability of skin, a long thin face and neck, atrophic scars, cardiac murmur, medullary sponge kidney and polycystic kidneys, episodic syncope, borderline intelligence, hammer-shaped distal clavicle and saber shins (Radiology 1984; 152:665)

Occult blood LABORATORY MEDICINE Grossly inapparent hematochezia that often presages colonic adenocarcinoma may also be seen in amebiasis, heavy metal poisoning and acute gastrointestinal ischemia Note: Usually more than 50 cc/L is required to recognize blood in the stools, which is detected by either a) The guaiac method eg, Hemoccult II, a low-cost screening technique that uses a guaiac-impregnated paper to indirectly measure hemoglobin by semiquantitating hemoglobin's pseudoperoxidase activity; while sensitive, the guaiac method is nonspecific, since peroxidase activity is present in uncooked red meat, fish, uncooked fruits and certain cruciferous vegetables, eg broccoli and cauliflower; false guaiac positivity occurs in gastrointestinal bleeding at a distance, either 'north' eg gingiva, stomach or 'south', eg hemorrhoids of the colon and with drug therapy, eg iron therapy, aspirin, non-steroid anti-inflammatory drugs and topical iodine; false negative results may be due to improper storage of test slides, intermittent bleeding of lesion, hypervitaminosis C and degradation of hemoglobin by colonic bacteria; HemoQuant is more specific as it quantifies the conversion of heme to fluorescent porphyrins Note: These tests assume that the carcinoma has produced an ulcer and therefore is bleeding; 20-30% of patients with colorectal cancers have a negative fecal occult blood test

Occult infection An infection that is first recognized by secondary manifestations, eg elevated polymorphonuclear leukocytes in the circulation or fever of unknown origin, most often caused by a bacterial infection in an obscure site, eg an abscess of the subphrenic or other intraabdominal region

Occult primary malignancy (OPM) Occult cancer A malignancy of unknown origin that first manifests itself as a metastasis, often having a poor prognosis; OPMs are problematic as appropriate therapy requires that the primary malignancy be eradicated, and many remain obscure despite aggressive diagnostic work-up; certain malignancies metastasize to certain sites with greater than expected frequency (table, facing page) **Treatment** Up to 30% of patients with metastases arising from an occult primary adenocarcinoma may respond to chemotherapy (using mitomycin C, adriamycin and vincristine); poor therapeutic response is more common in men and in those with hepatic and/or infradiaphragmatic metastases (Am J Clin Oncol 1990; 13:55)

Occupational asthma A clinical complex that causes predominantly pulmonary symptoms in previously healthy subjects exposed to a noxious working environment; occupational asthma may affect 3% of the USA population, many of whom function adequately, despite the symptoms; the causative agent elicits an immediate hypersensitivity reaction, divided into low molecular weight substances, eg isocyanates, anhydrides, soldering metals, metal salts and wood dusts, which act as haptens and high molecular weight substances, eg plant dusts, laboratory animal danders, shellfish and enzymes; see Hypersensitivity pneumonitis, Monday morning sickness, Sick building syndrome

Occupational medicine The medical specialty concerned with disease or dysfunction arising from work-related injuries and/or exposure to noxious agents or stimuli; the most prevalent occupational afflictions include exposure to asbestos (resulting in asbestosis or asbestos-induced pleural plaque formation), noise (causing hearing loss), solvents, welding fumes, fiberglass (causing upper respiratory irritation and bronchitis, solvent intoxication and asthma), musculoskeletal dysfunction due to repetitive trauma, heavy metal intoxication, silicosis, toxic hepatitis, dysfunctional psychologic reactions to the workplace Note: Dermatoses are under-represented as an occupational disease as patients with work-related dermatopathies are most often seen by dermatologists (N Engl J Med 1990; 322:594); in the US, regulations regarding occupational safety are promulgated by the Occupational Safety and Health Administration (see OSHA) and the National Institute of Occupational Safety and Health (see NIOSH)

Ocher codon One of three mRNA nucleotide codons signaling chain termination (nonsense codons); ocher corresponds to UAA, see Amber, Opal, Nonsense suppressor

OCCULT PRIMARY MALIGNANCIES; Common primary sites

Bone Breast, bronchus, prostate, thyroid, kidney

Central nervous system Breast, bronchus, kidney, colon

Head and neck Carcinoma of the oropharynx, nasopharyngeal and thyroid; most are squamous cell carcinomas, others include adenocarcinoma, melanoma, rhabdomyosarcoma, oat cell, salivary gland and thyroid carcinomas

Liver Stomach, colon, breast, pancreas or bronchus

Lung Breast, colon, kidney, melanoma, sarcoma, stomach, testis, thyroid

Lymph nodes Axillary Breast, melanoma, lymphoma **Cervix** Naso- and oropharynx, thyroid, larynx, lymphoma **Inguinal** Urogenital tract, anus, melanoma, lymphoma **Supraclavicular** Bronchi, breast, stomach, esophagus, pancreas, colon, lymphoma

Ovary Stomach, colon

Serosal surfaces Bronchi, breast, ovary, lymphoma

Skin Melanoma, breast, bronchus, stomach or kidney

Ockham's razor CLINICAL DECISION-MAKING The simplest expression of scientific truth(s), named after William Ockham, a 14th century philosopher who held that '...*A PLURALITY MUST NOT BE STATED WITHOUT NECESSITY*...' ie theories should be expressed as simply as possible and when two theories exist to explain a similar phenomenon, the most parsimonious should prevail, ie be no more complicated than necessary

OCT see Oxytocin stress test

***oct*-1, *oct*-2** Vertebrate homeobox genes with roles in segmentation, anterior-posterior axis determination and cell type specification, which appear after the primitive streak stage of embryological development, and encode the Oct-1, Oct-2 and Oct-3 proteins, which up-regulate transcription by means of an octamer of amino acids known as the OCTA motif

***oct*-3** A vertebrate gene that encodes a transcription factor containing a POU-specific domain and a homeodomain, expressed in undifferentiated pluripotent cells of the early embryo and in primordial and female germ cells (Nature 1990; 345:686)

OCTA motif MOLECULAR BIOLOGY An eight base pair regulatory sequence of DNA that is a B-cell specific promoter of immunoglobulin genes; the transcription control elements (including the TATA box, the OCTA motif and the enhancer) of the immunoglobulin gene chains ensure that these chains will be synthesized within the B lymphocytes but not in other cells

Octreotide acetate Sandostatin, SMS 201-995 A somatostatin analog with high affinity for growth hormone (GH) that causes a marked decrease in serum GH and amelioration of symptoms in 70% of patients with acromegaly and is more effective than bromocriptine; octreotide also reduces the effects of TSH-secreting tumors, malignant or metastatic carcinoid, pancreatic endocrine (islet cell) tumors and theoretically, any tumor that has a high concentration of somatostatin receptors; when radiolabelled, octreotide may be used to localize somatostatin receptor-rich tumors (N Engl J Med 1990; 323:1246, Mayo Clin Proc 1991; 66:283)

Oculocerebrorenal syndrome of Lowe An X-linked recessive disorder that maps to chromosome Xq24-26 Clinical Congenital cataracts, cognitive impairment, renal tubular dysfunction (Fanconi syndrome), areflexia, hypotonia, glaucoma, corneal ulceration and idiopathic joint swelling Laboratory Proteinuria, increased muscle enzymes, α_2-globulin and high-density lipoprotein cholesterol Treatment Alkalinization of the urine, supplemental potassium, phosphate, calcium carnitine (N Engl J Med 1991; 324:1318)

OD see Overdose

ODD syndrome Oculodental dysplasia An autosomal dominant condition characterized by hypertelorism, microphthalmia, myopia, hypoplastic teeth, syndactyly, camptodactyly, visceral malformation and no mental retardation

Odor Numerous, relatively uncommon conditions may be associated with typical odors, often occurring in inborn

ODORS OF BIOMEDICAL INTEREST (Breath and urine smells)

Odor	Source
Acetone (Russet apples)	Chloroform, ethanol, isopropanol, ketoacidosis, lacquer
Acrid (pear-like)	Chloraldehyde, paraldehyde; *Bacteroides melaninogenicus*
Ammonia	Renal failure, uremia, N-ethyl morpholine
Bitter almonds	Cyanide
Burned chocolate	Infection by *Proteus* species
Cabbage	Methionine (see also Hops)
Campherous	1,8-cineole
Carrots	Circutoxin
Coal gas	Carbon monoxide
Disinfectants	Phenol, creosote
Eggs,rotten	H_2S, mercaptans, disulfuram (Antabuse)
Ether-like	Ethylene chloride
Fecaloid, putrid	Infection by *Clostridium* species
Fishy	Vaginal infection by *Haemophilus gardnerella*, 'rice-water' choleric stools; di-N-butylamine, diethylamine, hepatic failure
Floral (sweet, fruity)	Diabetes, acetone, ethyl- and isobutyl- /acetate, phenyl methylethyl carbinol
Fruity/alcohol	Amyl nitrate, ethanol, isopropanol
Garlic	Arsenic, phosphorous, selenium, tellurium, thallium, malathion, parathion, DMSO (dimethyl-sulfoxide)
Grape juice	Infection by *Pseudomonas* species
Halitosis	Oral infections
Hop-like	Oasthouse disease (α-hydroxybutyric acid)
Maple syrup	Maple syrup urine disease
Mint	Menthone
Mothballs	Camphor-products
Mousy/musty	Phenylketonuria
Musty basement	Infection by *Streptomyces* and *Nocardia* species
Musty (fish, raw liver)	Hepatic failure, zinc phosphide, pentadecanolacetone
Odorless urine	Acute tubular necrosis
Peanuts	RH-787 (Vacor, see Vacor diabetes)
Pungent	Ethylchlorvynol; formic acid
Putrid	Dimethyldisulfide
Rancid fish	Tyrosinemia
Rotting fish	Trimethylaminuria
Shoe polish	Nitrobenzene
Sour and pungent	Ethyl acrylate, 2-methyl-5-ethyl pyridine, propionic acid, 2,4-pentanedione
Sweaty feet	Glutaric acidemia, type II, isovaleric acidemia
Sweet and musty	Isobutylacrylate
and rancid	2,6 butanol
and sharp	Methylethylketone
Swimming pool	Hawkinsinuria
Tomcat urine	β-Methylcrotonylglycinuria
Violets	Turpentine
Wintergreen	Methylsalicylate

errors of metabolism (table, above)

Oedipus complex PSYCHIATRY The constellation of consequences (according to Freud) which result from the sublimation of a boy's psychosexual desire for his mother, likened to the Oedipus of Greek mythology who killed his father and married his mother Note: Oedipus' desire for his mother, Jocasta, was completely innocent, while her incest is regarded by some scholars as having been a conscious act; see Jocasta complex

OFAGE Orthogonal field alternation gel electrophoresis A technique that allows separation of large, chromosome-sized, ie 200-3000 kilobase pair segments of DNA, that would be used to compare the homology of related organisms; once the large segments are separated, they may be manipulated by Southern blotting (Nucleic Acids Res 1984; 12:5647); Cf Pulsed field gradient gel electrophoresis

Office of Management and Budget (OMB) An agency of the US federal government established in 1970 to evaluate, formulate and coordinate management procedures and program objectives within and among Federal departments and agencies, controlling administration of the Federal Budget, routinely providing the president with recommendations regarding budget proposals and relevant legislative enactments

Office of Scientific Investigation A body organized in 1989 under the auspices of the US National Institutes of Health, which is encharged with investigation of allegations of scientific misconduct and fraud by investigators who are receiving US federal grant monies

Office of Technical Assessment (OTA) An organization established by the US Congress in 1972 as a nonpartisan analytical support agency, which aids Congress to evaluate the impact of new technologies, anticipate, plan for their consequences on society and coordinate large-scale international research projects

Off-label use CLINICAL PHARMACOLOGY The use of a drug, eg tretinoin, an analog of vitamin A or medical device, eg injectable collagen to treat a condition for which it has not received approval by a regulatory agency, eg the US Food and Drug Administration, the penalty for which may be seizure, injunction and prosecution (J Am Med Assoc 1991; 266:11)

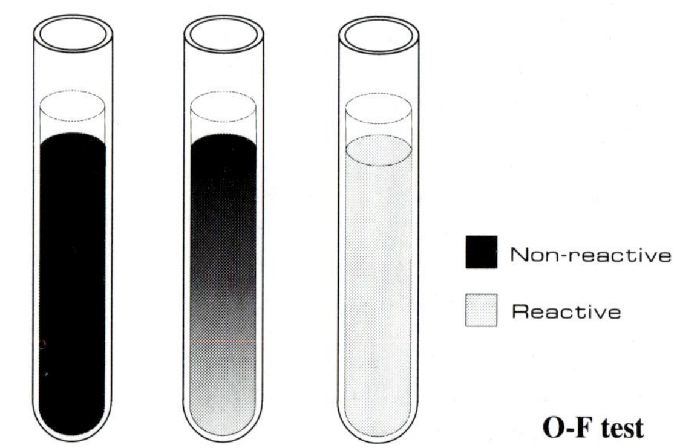

O-F test

O-F test Oxidative-fermentative test MICROBIOLOGY A test used to characterize the fermentative qualities of gram-negative rods, which detects the acid production by fermentative bacteria; two tubes are partially filled with different concentrations of fermentable sugars and a peptone (Hugh-Leifson medium), one of which is overlayed with sterile mineral oil, creating an anaerobic environment; oxidative bacteria (glucose oxidizer, eg *Pseudomonas aeruginosa*) produce acid only in the open tube exposed to atmospheric oxygen (figure, right); fermenting organisms (glucose fermenter, eg *Escherichia coli*) produce acid in both tubes and non-saccharolytic bacteria (non-saccharolytic, eg *Moraxella* sp) are inert

'oid-oid' disease DERMATOLOGY A uncommonly-used colloquialism for the combination of exudative disc**oid** dermatitis and lichen**oid** dermatitis

Oil(s) The relative health benefits of the different types of dietary fats is not clear and definitive studies have yet to be performed (J Am Med Assoc 1990; 263:3146), although it is known that the more saturated, ie the greater the number of double bonds in the carbon chain of the fatty acid, the greater is the risk for atherosclerosis; see Fish, Olive oil, Tropical oils; Cf Mineral oil

'Oil droplet' appearance A descriptor of the early lesions, often with a refractory rim seen in the fundus of children with galactosemia, which may develop into cataracts within the first few postpartum weeks

oil red O A histologic stain for detecting neutral fat (triacylglycerides); optimal results are obtained with frozen tissues, as the paraffin-embedding process requires a fat-dissolving xylene step, oil red O positivity serves to distinguish thecomas from fibromas and supports the diagnosis of renal cell carcinoma, when the surgical pathologist is confronted with a clear cell tumor of unknown origin; fat stains are of little use in distinguishing liposarcoma from other sarcomas as the former may be negative and the latter positive; oil red O positivity may occur in ceroid or lipofuscin-rich tissues, demonstrating a speckled pattern

Okadaic acid A specific inhibitor of protein phosphatases, PP1 and PP2, which inhibits T antigen, mimics the stimulation of glucose transport into adipocytes by insulin and increases macrophage production of prostaglandin E_2

Okazaki fragments MOLECULAR BIOLOGY Segments of DNA that are produced in discontinuous replication Background: DNA replication (duplication) is a synthetic process that occurs in the 5'-to-3' direction using the antiparallel strand as a template; while replication of the 3'-to-5' mother strand forms a continuous 5'-to-3' daughter strand, replication of the 5'-to-3' mother strand occurs in the same 5'-to-3' direction, but only in short (circa 1000 nucleotide) segments known as Okazaki fragments, in 'semi-continuous' replication, utilizing short RNA primers to begin the 5'-to-3' replication; linkage of the Okazaki fragments requires removal of the RNA, filling of the gaps and nick ligation (figure, right); see Replication

Okra sign A normal radiologic finding when the upper duodenal bulb is mildly twisted and filled with air, the cross-sectional view of which is fancifully likened to a transected okra (*Hibiscus esculentus*)

OKT4, **OKT8** see CD4 and CD8

'Oldest old' GERIATRICS Individuals who are older than 85, the fastest growing age group in USA and other developed nations; the expense of caring for the 'graying' population will become an enormous burden that may only begin to plateau in the year 2020; the two most costly non-fatal age-dependent diseases are dementia and osteoporosis, often associated with hip fractures (J Am Med Assoc 1990; 263:2335)

'Old man sleeping after dinner' Neurology A fanciful descriptor for the image evoked by a full-scale activation of the parasympathetic nervous system, which may be accompanied by bradycardia, bronchoconstriction resulting in noisy respiration, snoring, meiosis and increased salivation (drooling)

Old soldier's heart Da Costa syndrome Irritable heart A descriptive term for the predominantly cardiac symptoms of combat fatigue, seen in war-weary soldiers and consisting of precordial pain, dyspnea, exercise intolerance, mental and physical fatigue, dizziness, giddiness and palpitations, often precipitated by emotional and physical stress; see Combat fatigue

Old soldier/sergeant syndrome see Combat fatigue

Olestra Sucrose polyester A synthetic, no-calorie fat that has an appearance, taste and texture virtually identical to fat, but unlike the usual dietary fats composed of three fatty acids linked to a glycerol, it is composed of eight fatty acids linked to glucose and is too big for digestion by the body's enzymes

O-level An English examination taken at age 16 by the more academically able students, including those who intend to attend university, which has been replaced by the GCSE; see Polytechnic; Cf A-level

Olfactory hallucination Phantosmia The illusion of smelling a foul odor that is perceived to be either a)

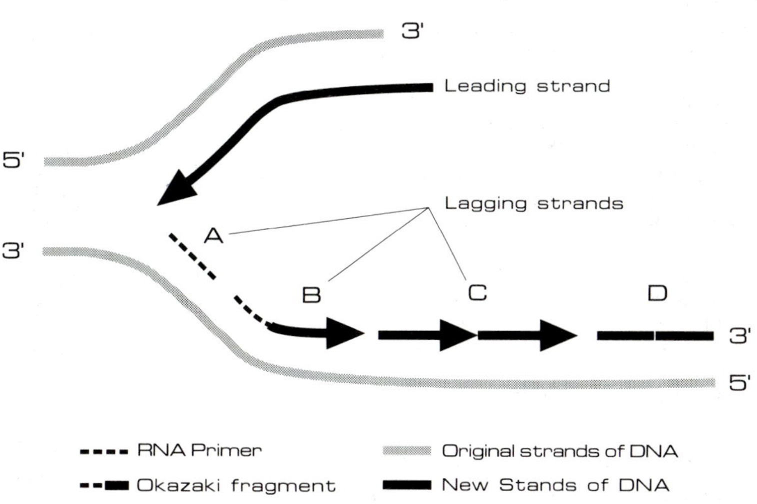

Okazaki fragments

Extrinsic, ie of non-self origin and which is mildly annoying but not a pervasive problem for the patient or b) Intrinsic, ie perceived to emanate from the patient's own sweat, flatus or halitosis and which may prove overwhelmingly disconcerting to the patient

Oligoclonal bands LABORATORY MEDICINE Multiple discrete bands in the γ region of cerebrospinal fluid electrophoresed on an agarose gel and stained with Coumassie blue; the finding, while non-specific, occurs in 90-95% of multiple sclerosis patients (corroborated by measuring myelin basic protein); oligoclonal bands may occur in other cerebral disease processes, to wit: Herpetic encephalitis, bacterial or viral meningitis (40-60% of cases have bands), carcinomatosis, toxoplasmosis, neurosyphilis (60% positive), progressive multifocal leukoencephalopathy, subacute sclerosing panencephalitis (90% have bands) and may appear transiently in Guillain-Barré disease, lupus erythematosus vasculitis, amyotrophic lateral sclerosis, spinal cord compression, diabetes, cerebrovascular events

Oligogene A gene which, when mutated, produces major phenotypic alterations, as it encodes segments of multiple structural genes; Cf Polygene

Oligohydramnios Oligoamnios A relative deficiency of amniotic fluid which occurs when the fetus swallows more often than usual, secondary to placental insufficiency, donor twin, urinary tract malformation

Olive oil CLINICAL NUTRITION A vegetable oil that contains the highest (77%) level of monounsaturated fatty acids of all cooking oils; some evidence has favored the use of olive oil for reducing cholesterol (N Engl J Med 1986; 314:436); in one study of polyunsaturated fat-supplemented diets, HDL_2 was 50% higher, HDL_3 was 7% lower (resulting in a 23.5% total increase in HDL levels) and the apo-B, 5.4% higher than those using predominantly monounsaturated fats (J Am Med Assoc 1990; 263:2462), data that contradicts some reports that olive oil is optimal in lowering cholesterol; nevertheless, the high olive oil consumption and relatively low incidence of cardiovascular disease in Italians suggests a cause-and-effect relation between the two Note: Olive oil is produced in Greece, Italy, Spain and Tunisia and graded as pure (refined to remove acid), Virgin (a natural olive oil with 1-3.3% acid) and Extra virgin (less than 1% acid); the US FDA (Food and Drug Administration) uses the terms Virgin (oil extracted after the first pressing) and Refined (extracted after a second pressing with chemicals added to reduce the acidity); Cf Fish oil, Tropical oils

Olive sign see Pyloric olive

Olympian brow Marked thickening of the bony prominence of the forehead, due to persistent or recurrent periostitis, a classic manifestation of late congenital syphilis

OMB see Office of Management and Budget

Omega-3 fatty acids Polyunsaturated fatty acids with a double bond between carbons 3 and 4; fish oils, eg eicosapentanoic acid, are predominantly omega-3 and thought to protect against atherosclerosis, acting to lower plasma LDL, increase HDL, alter production of prostaglandins and to decrease synthesis of leukotrienes and possibly also interleukin-1; see Fish; Cf Olive oil, Tropical oil

Omega loop GASTROINTESTINAL RADIOLOGY see Bird's beak sign MOLECULAR BIOLOGY A nonregular secondary protein structural motif composed of a segment of continuous polypeptide that traces a looped path in three-dimensional space; initially described as random coils, omega loops are often located on the protein's surface and thus assumed to have key roles in molecular function and biological recognition

Omega oxidation A metabolic pathway for short 8-12 carbon fatty acids in which the terminal methyl group is first oxidized to a hydroxyl group then to a carbonyl group, leading to the formation of a dicarboxylic acid

Omega protein Type I topoisomerase An enzyme first discovered in ***Escherichia coli*** that relaxes negative supercoils in DNA without leaving nicks in the double helix; see DNA supercoiling, DNA topology

Omega sign CLINICAL MEDICINE A sign seen in melancholia in which the patients have a furrowed brow due to sustained contraction of the corrugator muscle, which is often accompanied by Veraguth's folds, which are upward, inward peaking of the upper eyelids, a finding fancifully likened to the Greek letter omega

Omental cake see Pancake omentum

Omeprazole A drug that inhibits gastric secretion by altering the activity of the transmembrane proton pump, H^+/K^+-ATPase, which is the final step in acid secretion in the parietal cells of the stomach; omeprazole appears to be more effective than the H_2-receptor antagonists, eg cimetidine, ranitidine in treating duodenal and gastric ulcers, reflux esophagitis and Zollinger-Ellison syndrome (N Engl J Med 1991; 324:965rv)

OMS Organic brain syndrome

Omsk hemorrhagic fever A flavivirus infection occurring in the summer in the steppes of western Siberia causing hemorrhage and encephalitis Vector Tick (*Dermacentor pictus*) Clinical Abrupt onset with high fever, headache, myalgia and prostration of 1-2 weeks in duration, hemorrhage from all orifices, anemia, leukopenia, thrombocytopenia and albuminuria; the disease may also be biphasic, with the latter phase being more intense; Mortality 1-2.5% Treatment Supportive, symptomatic, analgesic

Onanism Coitus interruptus A term incorrectly equated to masturbation, but Onan's act was to spill his 'seed' on the ground during coitus with his brother's wife

Onchocerca 'dermatopathy' Several skin changes are described in onchocercosis, which may be shiny ('lizard skin'), spotted ('leopard skin') and thickened ('elephant skin')

Oncocyte Oxyphilic cell Hürthle cell An enlarged, pale eosinophilic epithelial cell filled with granular (mitochondria-laden) cytoplasm (figure, below), with a high ATPase and oxidative enzyme activity; oncocytes increase with age and starvation, thus implying that oncocytes are associated with degenerative phenomena; oncocytes and benign oncocytomas occur in bronchial, lacrimal, salivary, parathyroid and thyroid glands, the anterior pituitary and kidney; rarely, malignant oncocytomas occur in salivary glands, nasal cavity, paranasal sinuses, mediastinum and thyroid and the kidneys; renal oncocytomas are unique in that, unlike renal cell adenomas, they may become very large without being malignant and are considered by some authors to be renal cell carcinoma variants with a good prognosis (grade I tumors), which when the nuclei are atypical are designated as oncocytic renal cell carcinomas; other proliferations of oncocytes include oncocytic carcinoma of the pancreas, oncocytic carcinoid of the lungs, clinically similar to the 'garden variety' carcinoid and oncocytosis of the salivary gland, considered an age-related hyperplasia

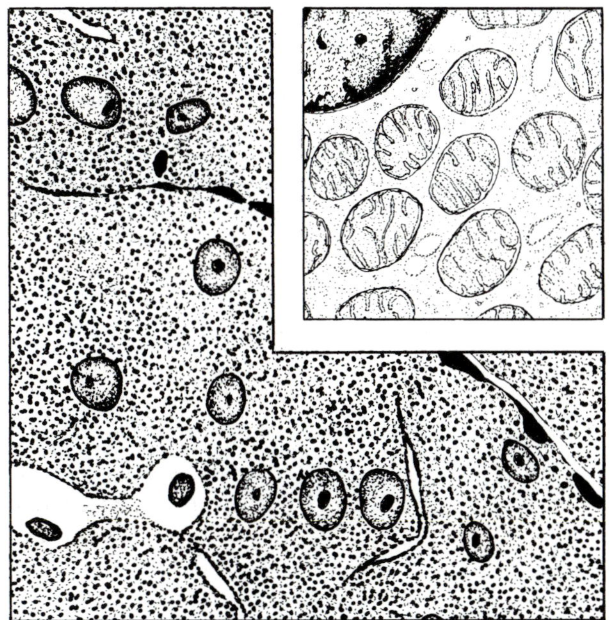

Oncofetal antigens ONCOLOGY Antigens that are expressed in the fetus during embryogenesis, but which are not produced in significant quantities in adults; oncofetal antigens may re-appear during malignant de-differentiation and include α-fetoprotein (AFP), which is elevated in 70% of hepatocellular carcinomas) and carcinoembryonic antigen (CEA), which is present in the fetal gut, liver and pancreas, non-specifically elevated in many benign or malignant processes in the adult, used to diagnose recurrence in patients with known colonic adenocarcinoma

Oncogene(s) A heterogeneous family of 'cancer genes' that are capable of inducing malignant transformation, which are derived from oncogenic RNA (oncorna-) viruses and from normal genes (proto-oncogenes); these genes are highly conserved in evolution and encode proteins vital to regulating gene expression or growth signal transduction; proto-oncogenes may undergo malignant transformation ('activation') by translocation, eg Philadelphia chromosome, gene amplification or by point mutation, eg K-*ras*; oncogenes are elucidated by either using the viruses that cause cancer (viral oncogenes or v-onc) in animals or by isolating tumorigenic genes from malignant cells; the human genome has more than 20 proto-oncogenes and cellular oncogenes (normal genes with tumorigenic potential); the presence of an oncogene is insufficient for carcinogenesis (Nature 1990; 346:756) as malignant transformation is a process that requires multiple genetic events or 'hits'; allelic loss is considered indicative of the presence of an anti-oncogene, eg the loss of 3p, 13q and 17p alleles occurs in various malignancies and may represent early transitional phases on the road to malignancy; oncogenes encode proteins of four types (table); see Proto-oncogene

Oncogene theory A carcinogenic theory that attributes malignancy to activation by radiation or carcinogens, of latent retroviral genes that are normally present within cells; once activated, the oncogenes 'drive' the cancer through synthesis of various hormones or possibly through assembly of a complete oncogenic virus; according to this theory, all cells have written in their genome the potential for malignancy

Oncogenic virus Any DNA virus, eg human papillomavirus or RNA virus, eg retrovirus that is capable of causing malignant transformation of cells

'Oncomouse' A proprietary transgenic mouse produced that carries human genes, which increases the mouse's susceptibility to cancer, serving as a tool for pharmaceutical and medical research; see Transgenic mouse

Oncornavirus An obsolete term for oncogenic RNA viruses and retroviruses

Ondansetron GR 38032F A selective antagonist of serotonin S_3 receptors, that is reported to be effective in controlling nausea and vomiting induced by cisplatin (N Engl J Med 1990; 322:810, 816), a chemotherapeutic agent (*cis*-dichloro-diamineplatinum) used to treat ovarian, testicular, urinary bladder, as well as head and neck cancers

Ondine's curse see Sleep apnea syndrome

One and one-half syndrome of Fischer NEUROLOGY A unilateral pontine lesion involving both the medial longitudinal fasciculus and the pontine paramedian reticular formation, causing the combination of ipsilateral gaze palsy and internuclear ophthalmoplegia on the contralateral gaze; the only remaining horizontal movement is abduction of the contralateral eye; the eyes are straight or exodeviated Etiology Focal lesions of the brain stem, eg multiple sclerosis, primary or secondary tumors, eg glioma, hemorrhage or infarction, arteriovenous malformations and basilar artery aneurysm

PROTEINS ENCODED BY ONCOGENES

1) Growth factors, eg *sis* oncogene encodes platelet-derived growth factor
2) Receptors
   a) Membrane receptors with protein-tyrosine kinase activity, eg *fms. erb*B, *neu* (*erb*-2), *ros*
   b) Intracellular receptor, eg *erb*A
3) Intracellular transducers a) Protein-tyrosine kinase, eg *src, yes, fps*(*fes*), *abl, met,* b) Protein-serine/threonine kinases, eg, *mos, raf,* c) Ras proteins, which encode guanine nucleotide binding proteins with GTPase activity, eg H-*ras,* Ki-*ras,* N-*ras* and d) Phospholipase, eg *crk*
4) Nuclear transcription factors, eg f*os, jun, myb, myc,* N-*myc,* p53, RB, *rel, ski*

One bone-two bone sign OBSTETRICS A simple method used in ultrasonography to differentiate the upper arm or thigh (one bone) from the forearm or lower legs (two bones) in fetal ultrasonographic evaluation

One-dimension gel quantification see Gel electrophoresis, Polyacrylamide gel electrophoresis

One-eyed vertebra RADIOLOGY A descriptor for the unilateral ('one eyed') destruction of a lumbar vertebral pedicle, fancifully likened to the one-eyed jack of a deck of Western playing cards, where the 'nose' is contributed by the spinous process; the one-eyed vertebra is a rare finding seen on a plain anteroposterior film in carcinoma metastatic to a vertebral body, 'classically' of breast origin

One gene, one enzyme theory A hypothesis of historic interest that held that one gene encoded a specific enzyme or other protein, a posit now known to be correct in principle, but naïve, in that one gene encodes a polypeptide chain and a complete protein requires the splicing out of intervening sequences (introns) of mRNA, which are derived from 'junk' DNA, prior to the translation of mRNA into a protein

One-hit theory A hypothesis stating that red cell lysis occurs if the damage to only one site on the membrane is sufficient to evoke complement activation

One-hit, two-hit model of Knudsen A hypothetical paradigm of mutagenesis explaining the disparity in the hereditary patterns in children with retinoblastoma, where one or two steps are required for cancerization; in brief, a malignancy may require homozygous mutated alleles; one mutated allele (the first 'hit) is inherited from a parent; the second allelic 'hit' may occur through environmentally-induced damage, initiating a tumor 'cascade' (Proc Natl Acad Sci (USA) 1971; 68:820); normal genes may also have antioncogenic properties; see Retinoblastoma, Tumor suppressor genes Note: While the one hit-two hit model of carcinogenesis is being increasingly validated, most tumors are far more complex and require multiple 'hits' before becoming metastatic malignancies; in transgenic mice, the expression of the oncogene v-*jun* is insufficient alone to produce tumors but requires wounding, which provides a second epigenetic 'hit' (Nature 1990; 346:756)

One, two, three sign The finding of massive but discrete lymph nodes in the right paratracheal, right and left hilar regions, seen in a plain chest film in sarcoidosis; the sign may be a technical artifact as the same patients seen by tomography demonstrate bilateral paratracheal involvement

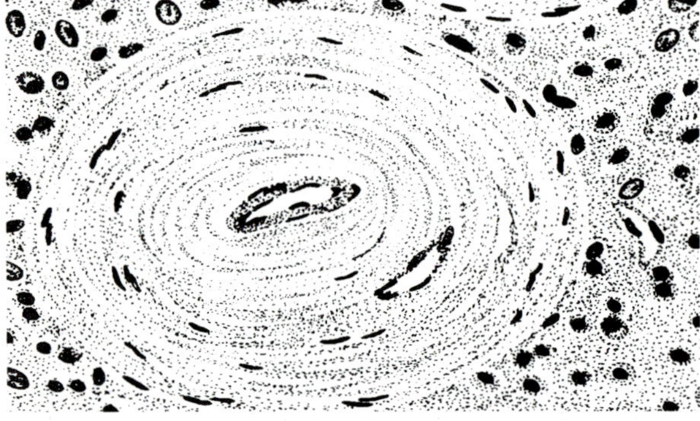

Onion skin changes, vessels

Onion bulb formation see Onion skinning

Onion skinning A pattern characterized by concentric laminations of differing radiologic or histologic densities, described in BONE RADIOLOGY Laminated periosteal reaction due to neo-osteogenesis, either benign, eg osteomyelitis, pulmonary hypertrophic osteoarthropathy, rickets or malignant, which may be coarse laminations, eg osteosarcoma or delicate laminations with periosteal layering, eg Ewing sarcoma HEMATOPATHOLOGY Concentric fibrosis of the splenic central and penicilliary arteries, characteristic of lupus erythematosus, most common in those with thrombocytopenic purpura HEPATIC PATHOLOGY Concentric lamellar fibrosis surrounding medium-sized bile ducts in the portal spaces of livers with sclerosing cholangitis, which may be accompanied by aggregates of lymphocytes with germinal centers and granulomas GASTROINTESTINAL PATHOLOGY Concentric perivascular arrangement of fibroblasts and loose collagen seen by the Masson trichrome stain in gastric inflammatory fibroid polyps MALIGNANT HYPERTENSION 'Onion skin' changes are descriptive of concentric arterial thickening (figure, above) with progressive luminal narrowing, due to hyperplasia of the smooth muscle cells and basement membrane reduplication, which may be accompanied by necrosis and fibrinoid deposits (necrotizing arteriolitis) and ischemic damage with renal involvement; similar changes may occur in the gall bladder, periadrenal fat, peripancreatic intestinal arterioles NEUROPATHOLOGY A term referring to the connective fibrous tissue surrounding the periaxon in Dejerine-Sottas disease, a neuropathy due to incomplete spinal cord injury specifically to the trigeminal nerve, characterized by hypalgesia or analgesia that spreads centrifugally in a laminated fashion; alternately in the peripheral nervous system; 'onion skinning' may also be due to repetitive myelination and demyelination, in large peripheral myelinated nerves in Charcot-Marie-Tooth and Roussy-Levy syndromes (onion-bulb formation, figure, facing page, low power above, ultrastructure, below)) OBSTETRICS Laminated pockets of myometrial gas, seen in septic abortions, especially due to ***Clostridium perfringens***; despite the severity of clinical disease, hysterectomy may not be necessary, if the uterine cavity is curetted and antibiotic therapy is adequate VASCULAR PATHOLOGY Perivascular collagen deposition as seen in lupus erythematosus, in necrotizing arteriolitis and in any stage of syphilitic obliterative endarteritis with proliferation of the endothelial cells with luminal narrowing

On-off phenomenon NEUROLOGY Marked period fluctuations in the response to L-Dopa therapy in Parkinson's disease; the term 'on-off' also refers to the waxing and waning of the parkinsonism itself (Science 1990; 247:574)

ONPG *o*-nitrophenyl β-D-galactopyranoside MICROBIOLOGY A substance used for determining the presence of β-galactosidase in bacteria (present in ***Escherichia coli***) causing the release of the yellow *o*-nitrophenol into the medium

Ontogeny recapitulates phylogeny EVOLUTIONARY BIOLOGY A postulate that holds that some stages in the development of an individual (ontogeny) repeat certain aspects in the evolutionary development of a species of organisms (phylogeny)

Onyalai A variant of idiopathic thrombocytopenic purpura described in males of the Bantu tribe, possibly related to vitamin C deficiency and characterized by periorbital hemorrhagic bullae

O'nyong-nyong A dengue-like alphavirus infection of East Africa Vector *Anopheles funestus* Clinical Abrupt onset of fever, frontal or retro-orbital headaches, an early generalized, blanching macular rash and severe arthralgias EKG Sinus bradycardia, ventricular ectopia, prolongation of P-R interval and flattened T waves Laboratory Pancytopenia, acidosis and hemoconcentration Treatment Symptomatic and supportive

Opal codon One of three mRNA stop codons (alternately known as 'nonsense' codons as they do not designate an amino acid); Cf Amber codon

OPD syndrome Otopalatodigital syndrome An X-linked dominant complex characterized by craniofacial deformity (frontal and occipital bossing, hypertelorism, small nose and mouth, partial anodontia, cleft palate), short trunk and bradydactyly

o, p'-DDD Minotane A therapeutic agent derived from insecticides that selectively destroys (by blocking mitochondrial activity and inhibiting steroid synthesis) both normal and neoplastic adrenal cortex (zona fasciculata

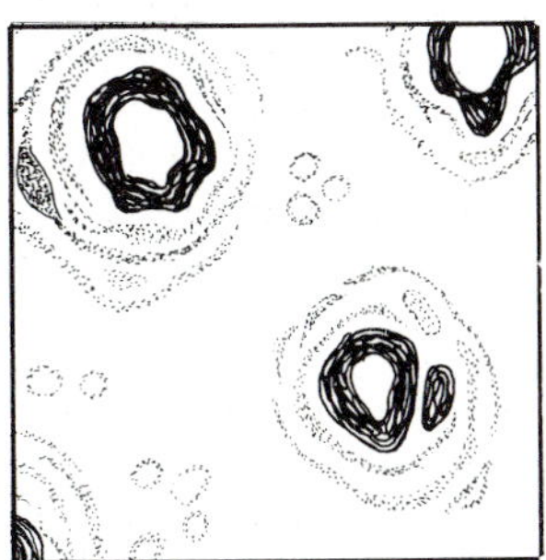

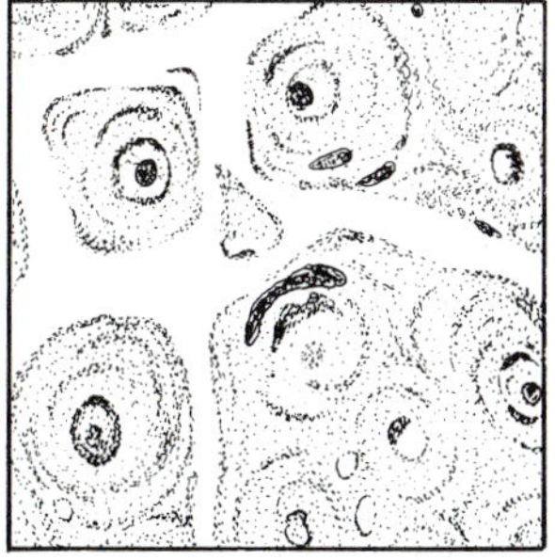

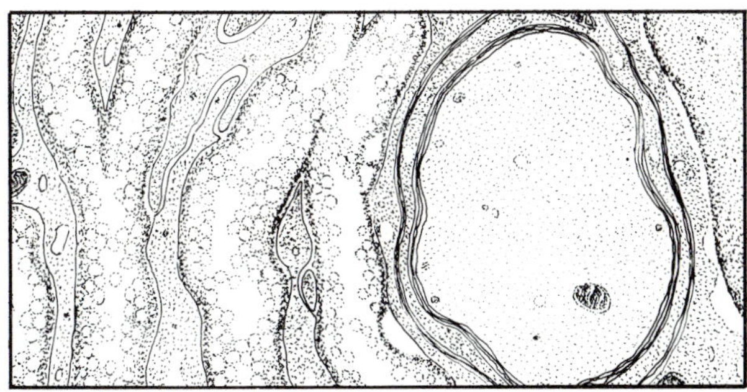

and reticularis); o,p'-DDD is used to treat adrenocortical carcinoma; the patients become hormonal 'cripples' requiring supplements of glucocorticoids and mineralocorticoids Side effects Anorexia, nausea, diarrhea, vomiting, skin rashes, gynecomastia, arthralgia and leukopenia

'Open face sandwich' domain A type of three-dimensional protein structural motif seen in the enzyme RuBisCO in which one surface is exposed to solvent, (Adv Protein Chem 1981; 34:167, Science 1988; 241:71); the enzyme initiates photosynthesis and is comprised of eight large and eight small subunits

Open heart surgery A surgical procedure in which the thoracic cavity is opened to repair, on an elective or emergent basis, conditions directly affecting the heart; the most commonly-performed elective open heart procedure is a coronary artery bypass graft, typically performed on an older white male; 15% of these procedures are limited to valvoplasty; factors adversely affecting the outcome of open-heart surgery include a subsequent need for reoperation, recent myocardial infarct, dialysis dependency, diabetes mellitus, congestive heart failure and a low ventricular ejection fraction (J Am Med Assoc 1990: 264: 2768); see Atherosclerosis, Coronary artery bypass graft; Heart-lung machine

Open protocol system CLINICAL PHARMACOLOGY An FDA-approved protocol that allows the use of drugs or other therapeutic agents outside of a controlled trial (and prior to approval of these agents by the FDA); open protocols may be indicated for patients with terminal disease for which there is no known cure or for a condition that has failed to respond to standard therapies; although drug efficacy data cannot be generated, as the cases are single and usually scattered among multiple health care institutions and care-givers, ie 'anecdotal' in nature, side effects and potential complications can be determined, and added to the pool of information weighed in whether to approve a therapeutic agent; see Compassionate IND protocol

Open reading frame (ORF) A long uninterrupted sequence of mRNA that begins with the start codon AUG, and ends with (but does not itself contain) a stop codon (UAG, UGA, UAA); most ORFs have been assigned to proteins, the remainder are called URFs or unassigned reading frames

Open system architecture COMPUTERS A design of a computerized information system that uses a network manager (a centralized electronic 'clearinghouse') to retrieve data and send it back to the requester; the OSA 'philosophy' circumvents many of the problems inherent in integrating the diverse elements of hospital information systems, since it allows each individual department, eg laboratories, pharmacy, finances and others to choose the hardware and software most appropriate for its needs; see Computer, Hospital information system, LAN

Opera glass hand see Main en lorgnette

Operating system COMPUTERS The software that allows a computer to respond to system commands and to run applications programs, eg word-processing, databases and other applications, eg Microsoft™'s MS/DOS is a standard disk operating system in the IBM and IBM 'clone' types of microcomputers

Operating team The participants in a sterile surgical operation that is performed under general (less commonly, local) anesthesia, divided into the scrubbed sterile members, including the surgeon, assistants to the surgeon (commonly understood to be licensed physicians, although other persons may fill this role in routine procedures) and a scrub nurse; the nonsterile team members include the anesthesiologist, a circulating nurse, a pathologist, should an intraoperative consultation be required and technical personnel to operate complicated devices, eg heart-lung machine or intraoperative blood salvage devices, used during the procedure

Operation Ranch Hand ENVIRONMENT A herbicide-spraying program carried out during the Vietnam conflict between 1961 and 1971 that used agent Orange (2,3,7,8-tetrachlorodibenzo-p-dioxin, TCDD, intracorporal half-life, seven years); the mean residual TCDD level in non-exposed Vietnam veterans is 5 parts per trillion (ppt), the mean in 'Ranch Handers', 49 ppt and in the highly exposed, 200-2000 ppt (MMWR 1988; 37:309; see WA Buckingham, Operation Ranch Hand: The Air Force and Herbicides in Southeast Asia, 1961, Washington DC, US Air Force, 1982); see Dioxin

Operator (gene) A segment of DNA adjacent to one or more structural genes, which controls the transcription of the genes by the presence or absence of repressor proteins

Operon The functional unit of transcription, which contains an operator, its cognate repressor protein and the gene that the operator-repressor dyad controls; see Transcription unit

Ophthalmologist A physician trained in the diagnosis and treatment of diseases of the eye who may prescribe drugs and perform surgery Education Twelve years (four years each of college or university, medical school and residency); Cf Orthoptist, Optician, Optometrist

Opiate A generic term for any natural (eg opium), semi-synthetic (eg morphine) or synthetic (eg fentanyl), usually alkaloid narcotic agent with opium-like activity

Opioid peptides Endogenous opiates A group of natural polypeptide neurotransmitters that are involved in the perception of pain, response to stress, regulation of appetite and sleep, memory and learning, which are derived from three precursor molecules (prodynorphin, proenkephalin A and proopiomelanocortin or POMC), giving rise to more than 20 endogenous opioids, all of which have the same amino terminal tetrapeptide (Tyr-Gly-Gly-Phe); presence of opioids in tumors may indicate neuroendocrine differentiation (N Engl J Med 1989; 317:1439)

Opium A narcotic first used by the Romans, extracted from the unripe seedpod of the poppy, *Papaver somniferum*; morphine was extracted from opium by a German pharmacist Sertuerner; other opiates later derived from opium include heroin and the less potent and less addicting codeine; see Heroin, Narcotics

OPLL Ossification of the posterior longitudinal ligament see Dagger sign

Opportunistic infection An infection caused by a microorganism, usually bacterial that is part of the normal 'flora', which becomes pathogenic when the host is immunocompromised by an unrelated disease, eg AIDS or diabetes mellitus

Opsin A transmembrane protein that is the major component in the photoreceptor, rhodopsin, which has seven membrane-spanning helices and interacts with the transducing G proteins; Cf Retinal

Opsonin Greek, to make appetizing A generic term for any substance or 'factor' that binds to red cells, bacteria or other exogenous agents, increasing their susceptibility to phagocytosis, including antibodies, complement proteins and basement membrane components, eg fibronectin;relative strengths of opsonins in humans: IgG3 > IgG1 > IgG2, C3b

Optical tweezers A tool in cell biology in which a beam of laser light is used to manipulate subcellular organelles, creating an optical trap or allow measurement of mechanical forces of motor molecules including myosin, kinesin and dynein

Optician A health care worker who grinds eyeglasses and fits contact lenses according to a prescription written by optometrists and (less commonly) by ophthalmologists Education One to two year apprenticeship or training program Note: Not all states in the US require licensing of opticians; Cf Ophthalmologist, Optometrist

Optochin test Ethylhydroxycupreine disc P disc test MICROBIOLOGY Optochin is a quinine derivative with detergent-like activity, causing selective lysis of ***Staphylococcus pneumoniae*** at low concentrations (less than 5 μg/ml), typically the zone of lysis around a 6 mm paper disc impregnated with optochin is 14 mm; lack of inhibition by optochin implies that the organism on the growth plate is not ***S pneumoniae*** ; Cf MIC

Optometrist A health care worker qualified to examine the eyes and related structures in order to identify abnormalities; optometrists prescribe eyeglasses and other visual aids, but are not qualified to establish a definitive diagnosis, prescribe drugs or perform surgery Education Six years (Two or more years of college education and four years of optometry school); Cf Ophthalmologist, Optician

Oral contraceptives see Contraceptives; Cf Norplant

Oral rehydration therapy PUBLIC HEALTH A treatment modality directed at correcting dehydration diarrhea; the most accepted form of administration is the 'dry pack' distributed by UNICEF and the WHO, which contains 3.5 g NaCl, 2.5 g $NaHCO_3$, 1.5 g KCl and 20 g of glucose to be dissolved in one liter of water, given per os; despite the relatively low cost, there may be economic barriers to the use of commercial rehydration solutions (J Am Med Assoc 1991; 265:1724); Cf Ringer's lactate

Orange book CLINICAL PHARMACOLOGY *APPROVED DRUG PRODUCTS WITH THERAPEUTIC EQUIVALENCE EVALUATIONS*; a document (Publication # 917-016-00000-3) produced by the US government printing office, listing the FDA-approved generic equivalents of brand-name drugs

Orange-ophilia CYTOLOGY An obsolete term for a vague attempt to form keratin on the part of some cells of poorly-differentiated epidermoid carcinomas; a peculiar variant is described in which the cytoplasm has a 'pumpkin orange' color, which is held by some to be relatively specific for squamous cell carcinoma of the head and neck region

Orange peel skin appearance see Peau d'orange appearance

Orange person syndrome A rare clinical condition caused by an overdose of rifampin, coloring the skin and body fluids a deep orange, accompanied by altered hepatic function (elevated bilirubin, alkaline phosphatase and transaminase levels) and pruritus (Cutis 1988; 42:175) Note: The skin of subjects ingesting excess carotinoids, eg 'carrot diet' may also have a deep orange hue, which is of merely cosmetic interest, as it resolves by appropriate dietary alterations; see Red man syndrome

Orcein HISTOLOGY A brownish material that contains fourteen different substances which arise when orcinol is oxidized in ammonia water; orcein is used to stain elastic fiber, chromosomes and before the availability of immunoperoxidase stains for hepatitis B antigens, was of use in identifying hepatitis B surface antigens in the tissue of chronic carriers Note: Orcein-staining for identifying hepatitis has been replaced by in situ hybridization

Oregon plan HEALTH CARE REIMBURSEMENT A legislative modification of the US State of Oregon's Medicaid program that has become a focus of debate on all aspects of the US national health policy, including access to limited services, costs, effectiveness, rationing of services and provision of basic care; the Oregon plan is an attempt to reconcile the finite financial resources with the virtually ceiling-less needs for health care; Oregon will fund a prioritized list of about 600 services, designed as a comprehensive health benefit package for the poor (who are covered under the auspices of the Medicaid program); priority services that are reimbursed include pneumococcal pneumonia, various acute infections and intoxications, heart failure and physical and sexual abuse, including rape; not covered under the plan is artificial insemination, acute tonsillitis, end-stage HIV disease and counseling for obesity (J Am Med Assoc 1991; 266:417, Am Med News 22/July/91)

Orf Ecthyma contagiosum A benign self-limited infection acquired by handling infected sheep and goat skins and flesh; in the immunocompromised patient, the lesion may be very large Agent Orf (Papova) virus, an agent similar to that which causes milker's nodes

ORF see Open reading frame

Organ bank A repository, usually shared by multiple hospitals for relatively long-term storage of certain tissues destined for transplantation, including acellular bone fragments, bone marrow and corneas; other major organs, eg heart, lung, liver, kidneys and pancreatic islets are not stored in organ banks as their viability is limited to 48-72 hours and require immediate transplantation; Cf UNOS

Organ brokerage TRANSPLANTATION The sale of an organ, eg a kidney by a living donor, or any commercial transaction for the obtention through coercion of an organ for transplantation (J Am Med Assoc 1991; 265:1302) Note: In the USA, medical centers involved in organ procurement traditionally rely on altruism as a source for organs, since the National Organ Transplant Act (Public law 98-507, 3 USC) makes it illegal to acquire, receive, or transfer any human organ for valuable consideration

Organ cluster transplantation A procedure used in primary upper abdominal malignancy affecting the biliary tract, duodenum or stomach with secondary involvement of the liver; the Pittsburgh group resected all or most of the stomach, liver, pancreas, spleen and major portions of the small and large intestine, filling the structural and functional void with an 'organ cluster graft' comprised of the liver, pancreas, duodenum and a portion of the jejunum; while seemingly 'heroic' in scope, 8 of the 10 were alive at 3 to 9 months with adequate hepatic and pancreatic function (Ann Surgery 1989; 210:374); Cf Heroic surgery

Organic acidemia A clinical presentation of 'inborn errors of metabolism', often first seen in infants who present with poor feeding, vomiting, tachypnea, acidosis, hyperammonemia, ketosis, ketonuria, irritability and convulsions or hypotonia and lethargy, findings that are otherwise suggestive of neonatal sepsis; diseases accompanied by organic acidemia include isovaleric and propionic acidemias, maple syrup urine disease, medium chain acyl dehydrogenase deficiency, glutaric, methylmalonic and formiminoglutamic acidurias

Organic brain syndrome Cerebral degeneration in the form of cortical atrophy with 'simplification' of myelinated tracts, a process that is usually irreversible, often age-related and associated with atherosclerosis; see Lacunar state, Multi-infarct dementia

Organic food(s) A broadly-defined category of comestibles that in the purest form, are grown without reliance on chemical fertilizers or pesticides; see Health food; Cf Enriched food, Fortified food, Refining

Organicism see Holistic medicine

Organoid A synthetic 'organ' that has some properties, eg angiogenic and secretory capacities of an organ; the first generation organoids are composed of Gore-Tex, collagen, heparin-binding growth factor-1 and endothelial cells with an inserted gene and have therapeutic potential as delivery systems for CD4 in the treatment of AIDS (Proc Nat Acad Sci 1989; 86:7928), Alzheimer's and other diseases; see Biohybrid artificial pancreas; Cf Liposome

'Organ' panel(s) Laboratory diagnosis-related groups A group of diagnostic tests that have been determined to be the most cost-effective, sensitive and specific for evaluation of a particular diseased organ, organ system or disease (JB Henry, *CLINICAL DIAGNOSIS AND MANAGEMENT*, 18th ed, WB Saunders, 1991); see Anemia panel, Bone/joint panel, Cardiac injury panel, Cardiac risk evaluation panel, Collagen disease and arthritis panel, Collagen disease/lupus erythematosus panel, Coma panel, Diabetic panel, Electrolyte/fluid balance panel, General health panel, Hepatitis (immunopathology) panel, Hypertension panel, Kidney panel, Liver panel, Metastatic disease panel, Neoplasm panel, Pancreatic panel, Parathyroid panel, Pulmonary panel, Thyroid panel, TORCH panel

'Organ recital' PSYCHIATRY The listing by a hypochondriac of a litany of complaints from multiple organs and organ systems; the physician may himself naively perpetuate the 'illness', as the patient is gratified by a relationship that can only be maintained as long as the subject is perceived to be sick; see Factitious 'disease', Munchausen syndrome; Cf Ulysses syndrome

Oriental flush complex A facial erythema seen in up to 80% of Orientals who drink alcohol, possibly due to an atypical isomer of alcohol dehydrogenase that causes rapid metabolism of ethanol and high acetaldehyde levels

Oriental sore A form of cutaneous leishmaniasis that occurs in a) The Near East Desert rodent hosts *Rhombomys opimus, Psammomys obesus* Vector Sandfly *Phlebotomus papatasii* or b) Mediterranean rim and subsaharan Africa Host *Procavia* species Vector *Phlebotomus longipes* Clinical Oriental sores begin as erythematous papules on the face or extremities 2-8 weeks after exposure; the papule later vesiculates, pustulates and ulcerates, the dry form is crusted, the wet form, oozing Treatment Most lesions spontaneously heal in six months, otherwise pentavalent antimony

ORIF Open reduction of an internal fracture

Origin LABORATORY TECHNOLOGY The point of application in a chromatogram or an electrophoretic gel of a specimen or sample MOLECULAR BIOLOGY The site of initiation of replication

'Original (antigenic) sin' IMMUNOLOGY The tendency to produce antibodies to an epitope or antigenic determinant that resembles a determinant on an antigen encountered previously, thus being similar to a secondary immune response; the term derives from the biblical story of Adam in the Garden of Eden, who fell from God's grace, committing the 'original sin' of eating a forbidden fruit, forever dooming humanity to inherit sin

Ornish regimen see Diet

Ornithinemia, type I HHH syndrome An autosomal recessive condition with hyperornithinemia, postprandial hyperammonemia and homocitrullinemia, of early childhood to late adulthood onset Clinical Vomiting, repeated neurological 'attacks' after high-protein meals, resulting in lethargy, ataxia, choreoathetosis or coma, with moderate to severe growth and mental retardation Pathogenesis Unknown, although ornithine decarboxylase or mitochondrial transport of ornithine is possibly involved Ultrastructure Bizarre, elongated mitochondria with crystalloid inclusions Treatment Protein limitation and dietary supplements with ornithine or arginine

Ornithinemia, type II HOGA syndrome A condition characterized by hyperornithinemia with gyrate atrophy (HOGA) of the choroid and retina causing a slowly progressive loss of vision, myopia and nyctalopia, decreased glutamate levels and minimal hepatic and renal tubular dysfunction; aside from the visual impairment, these patients are essentially asymptomatic; about 10% have proximal muscle weakness with variable histologic abnormalities of the type 2 skeletal muscle fibers Pathogenesis 10-20-fold elevation of ornithine and mild increases of lysine, glutamic acid and glutamine, due to deficiency of ornithine-δ-aminotransferase Treatment Dietary and metabolic manipulation are unsuccessful

Ornithine transcarbamylase deficiency see Hyperammonemia

Oroya fever An infection by *Bartonella bacilliformis*, the cutaneous or verrucous form was long known in Peru; the acute form was first recognized in 1870 during construction of the railway from Lima to Oroya, the bacterial nature of the condition was established by D Carrion, a medical student who inoculated himself with verrucous material and subsequently died therefrom Epidemiology Most common in northern South America, where the sandfly vector, *Phlebotomus verrucarum* flourishes Clinical The onset may be either insidious or abrupt and accompanied by high fever, chills, diaphoresis, headaches, changes in the mental status, brisk hemolysis causing marked anemia (0.5×10^{12}/L; US: 500 000/mm^3) and a leukemoid reaction, followed by myalgias, arthralgias, dyspnea, insomnia, angina, delirium (and if extreme, coma and death in 30% of cases), accompanied by thrombocytopenic purpura and lymphadenopathy; the verrucous form may follow Oroya fever or be the only sign of infection Treatment Chloramphenicol (to prevent the frequent complication of Salmonella), blood transfusion Prevention DDT spraying to eliminate sandfly vector

Orphan Annie eyes A descriptor for certain features of the fetal alcohol syndrome, characterized by hypertelorism, rounder and shorter palpebral fissures and exotropia, likened to the round, blank eyes of the 'Little Orphan Annie'

Orphan Annie (eye) nuclei SURGICAL PATHOLOGY A descriptor for the nuclei characteristic of the follicular variant of papillary carcinoma of the thyroid (figure, below), which are large, round-to-oval and cleared of chromatin, fancifully likened to the eyes of Little Orphan Annie, the heroine of a comic strip by the same name (below) created in 1924, in which all the protagonists, including the faithful dog Sandy, who punctuates her diatribes with a sympathetic 'arf-arf', Daddy Warbucks and his faithful man-servant Punjab have the same pupil-less eyes

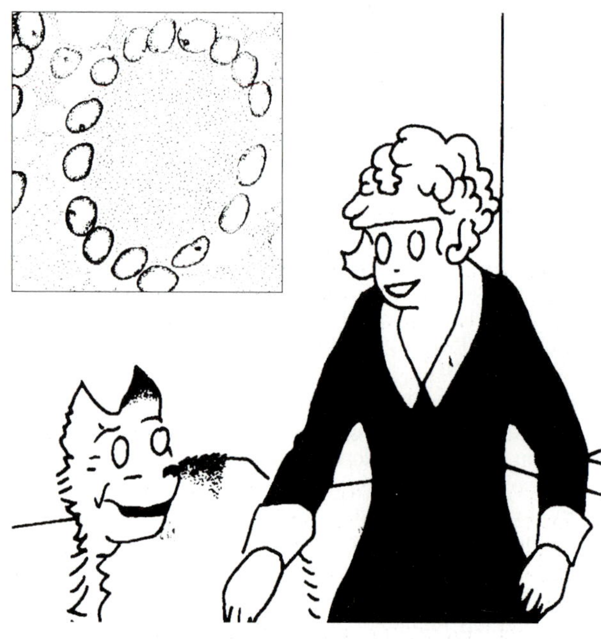

'Orphan' disease Any morbid condition affecting fewer

than 200 000 people in the USA, ie affecting less than 1/1000 people; because of the need for public information, a 'hotline' is available for professionals and family members of those with orphan diseases 1-800-999-6673; orphan diseases include acoustic neuroma, Addison's disease, ankylosing spondylitis, amyotrophic lateral sclerosis, autism, brain tumors, Charcot-Marie-Tooth, chronic fatigue syndrome, chronic granulomatous disease, Cornelia de Lange syndrome, craniofacial deformities, cystinosis, dizziness, dysautonomia, dystonia, epidermolysis bullosa, essential blepharospasm, 5p- syndrome, Friedreich's ataxia, glycogen storage disease, Guillain-Barré disease, graft-versus-host disease, histiocytosis X, Huntington's disease, ichthyosis, non-AIDS immune deficiencies, Klippel-Trenaunay syndrome, leukodystrophy, Lowe syndrome, Lyme disease, malignant hyperthermia, Marfan's disease, Ménière's disease, multiple sclerosis, mucopolysaccharidoses, narcolepsy, neuroblastoma, neurofibromatosis, Paget's disease, porphyria, Parkinson's disease, polycystic kidneys, Prader-Willi disease, retinitis pigmentosa, Rett syndrome, sarcoidosis, scleroderma, sickle cell disease, Sjögren syndrome, Sturge-Weber disease, TAR syndrome, Tay-Sachs disease(s), (Giles de la) Tourette syndrome, tuberous sclerosis, Turner syndrome, William syndrome, Wilson's disease; see NICODARD, NORD

Orphan Drug Act (Public Law 97-414) A US federal law designed to provide tax incentives, developmental grants and a seven-year marketing monopoly for companies developing drugs for Orphan diseases (see above); Some 'orphan drugs' have been very successful (PEG-ADA, for severe combined immunodeficiency, Enzon Corp; erythropoietin, for anemia in chronic dialysis, Amgen Corp; human growth hormone, Genentech), allowing up to $100 million in revenues (Science 1990; 248:678); Cf Pseudo-orphan drugs

Orphan drugs/products Drugs, biologics, medical devices and foods of potential or actual use in treating 'orphan' diseases, which are diseases often considered by the pharmaceutical and therapeutic industries to be too rare for developing commercially viable products; from a practical stand-point, only 1 in 10 000 agents 'screened' for therapeutic potential ever reach the marketplace (Science 1991; 252:1080); the US Orphan Drug Act (see below) enacted in 1983 provided an incentive for such development, resulting in a number of approved agents eg, α erythropoietin (used for the anemia of chronic renal failure), anti-thrombin III, botulinum toxin A (strabismus and blepharospasm), cromolyn sodium (mastocytosis), gancyclovir (CMV retinitis), inhalation pentamidine (*Pneumocystis carinii* prophylaxis in 'at risk' subjects), intravenous mitoxantrone (acute non-lymphocytic leukemia), intravenous rifampin (tuberculosis for those who cannot ingest the drug per os), selegiline (for Parkinson's disease that is refractory to L-dopa or carbidopa), teriparatide (to distinguish pseudo-hypoparathyroidism and hypoparathyroidism-related hypocalcemia), ucephan (chronic management of patients with uric cycle enzymopathies) NORD ☎ 1 (800) 999-6673; Cf Pseudo-orphan drug

'Orphan patient' A patient with primary hypochondriasis that has its psychodynamic origin in the unconscious gratifications of bodily symptoms and physical suffering that begins when a patient mistakenly assigns serious disease to normal bodily functions or to benign symptoms of trivial illnesses or to the somatic symptoms of emotional arousal; orphan patients are often treated by primary care physicians, because, although they would be better treated by psychiatrists, that would represent acknowledgement of a mental and not a physical disease; see 'Organ recital', Munchausen syndrome, Self-mutilation

ORT see Oral rehydration therapy

Ortet The single cell that is the precursor for a clone of cells

'Orthopedic shoes' A term coined by shoe manufacturers, not by the orthopedic community at large; such shoes may cause potential harm to a normal child's foot as they may be too stiff

Orthoptist A person who works under the supervision of an ophthalmologist, tests the strength of eye muscles and who teaches exercises designed to strengthen eye muscles and improve eye coordination, eg in patients with 'lazy eye' Education Three years (Two years of college and one to two years apprenticeship); see Ophthalmologist

Orthotist A person who fabricates, designs and fits orthopedic devices prescribed by a physician

Orthozyme CD5plus A proprietary anti-T cell immunotoxin composed of the A chain of the castor bean toxin ricin, conjugated to a murine monoclonal antibody, which targets the CD5 antigen present on 95% of peripheral T cells; this agent's ability to selectively deplete T cells, might translate into a therapy for recalcitrant graft-versus-host reactions (J Am Med Assoc 1991; 265:2041n&v); see Graft-versus-host disease, Magic bullet

OSA see Open system architecture

OSHA Occupational Safety and Health Administration An arm of US federal government, created in 1970 by the Williams-Steiger Act that recommends health and safety procedures and promulgates standards for the work place; OSHA is not empowered to enforce recommendations but may impose fines of $1-10 000 to non-complying facilities

OSI see Office of Scientific Investigation

OSMED Osteospondylomegaepiphyseal dysplasia An autosomal recessive form of chondrodystrophy, characterized by dwarfism, deafness and deformities of the external ear, saddle nose, thin hair, leathery skin, soft tissue calcifications, cleft palate and an achondroplasia-like pelvis

Osmiophilic Any intracellular substance or organelle that has affinity for the electron-dense osmium tetroxide, which fixes and stains cells for ultrastructural examination

Osmolality LABORATORY MEDICINE A measurement of the amount of osmotically effective solute per 1000 grams of solvent; serum osmolality is an often misused clinical test for evaluating hyponatremia, and is a test that is useful to a) Determine whether the serum water content deviates significantly from the norm and b) Detect the presence of foreign low-molecular weight substances in the blood, eg ethanol, methanol and isopropanil, sorbitol, mannitol, glycerin and INH; the most common cause of increased osmolality is ethanol (100 mg/dl increases osmolality by 22 mmol/dl) Quantification Freezing point depression vs dew-point (based on the colligative property of vapor pressure, equivalent to the total number of particles in a solution which equals the amount by which the dew point is depressed below ambient temperature; the disadvantage is that it doesn't measure ethanol, isopropanol, methanol, since the volatile (alcohol) adds to vapor pressure of the solution while decreasing same due to solute effect, resulting in a lower osmolality measured; contribution of toxic substances to serum osmolality, units in mOsm/kg of water: Methanol 33.7 mOsm/kg H_2O Ethanol 22.8 mOsm/kg H_2O, ethylene glycol 19.0 mOsm/kg H_2O, acetone 18.2 mOsm/kg H_2O, isopropanol 17.6 mOsm/kg H_2O, trichloroethane 9 mOsm/kg H_2O and others

Osmolarity The concentration of osmotically active particles in a solution (solute/liter of solution)

Osmolar gap The difference between the measured osmolality and the calculated osmolality; the measured osmolality is determined by freezing point depression (osmolality as solute/kilogram of solvent); the calculated osmolality (mOsm) is determined by the formula: 2 Na^+ (mEq/L) + BUN (mg/dl)/2.8 + glucose (mg/dl)/18

Osmotic diarrhea Increased volume and frequency of fecal flow caused by ingestion of a poorly absorbable solute (either a carbohydrate or divalent ion) or hypertonic material, resulting in a fecal osmolality higher than plasma osmolality; osmotic diarrhea may occur in: Antacid therapy, disaccharidase deficiency, magnesium sulfate ingestion and others, lactulose therapy, malabsorption (glucose-galactose, fructose or generalized), mannitol and sorbitol ingestion; see Chewing gum diarrhea

Osmotic fragility The susceptibility of erythrocytes to osmotic lysis; in hypotonic solutions, red cells behave as perfect osmometers, where the free water rapidly equilibrates, causing the cells to swell; since the membrane has limits on its extensibility, cells with weaker membranes are more susceptible to osmotic lysis, a susceptibility that is classically increased in hereditary spherocytosis, due to a wide variety of molecular defects, affecting spectrin, ankyrin, protein 4.2 or spectrin-actin interaction, hereditary elliptocytosis and erythrocytic 'senility'; osmotic fragility is decreased in jaundice, iron therapy, thalassemia, sickle cell anemia, following splenectomy and in 'target' erythrocytes; see Spherocytosis

Osteoarthropathy see Hypertropic pulmonary osteoarthropathy

Osteoblastic tumors Those tumors that produce substances with parathyroid hormone-like activity, including metastatic prostate carcinoma, osteoma, osteoblastoma, osteosarcoma, chondrosarcoma; see Hypercalcemia of malignancy

Osteocalcin A noncollagenous bone protein, the production of which is stimulated by vitamin D3 and inhibited by glucocorticoids (Science 1989; 246:1158)

Osteochondritis Combined inflammation of the bone and articular surface (usually aseptic); a legacy of the German school of medicine was eponymic immortalization of each joint, thus Freiberg's disease corresponds to osteochondritis of the metatarsal head, Haglund's disease (osteochondritis of the calcaneus), Köhler's disease (tarsal-navicular bones), Legg-Calve-Perthes disease (epiphyseal femoral head), Osgood-Schlatter disease (tibial tubercle), Panner's disease (humeral head), Sinding-Larsen-Johannson disease (patella), Thiemann's disease (metacarpal and metatarsal bones), Wegner's disease (osteochondritis with epiphyseal separation seen in congenital syphilis)

Osteoclast-like giant cell A multinucleated giant cell with abundant eosinophilic, finely granular or homogeneous cytoplasm containing up to one hundred uniform oval nuclei each measuring 5-7 μm with scattered small nucleoli and peripheral chromatin; osteoclast-like giant cells are often scattered among plump spindled mononuclear cells and may occur in benign and malignant conditions, including fibrous histiocytoma, histiocytosis X, in the mural nodules of mucin-producing ovarian carcinomas, hepatocellular carcinoma, Hodgkin's disease and tumoral calcinosis (Kikuyu's bursa)

Osteogenesis imperfecta (OI) A heterogenous group of autosomal dominant conditions with variable penetration due to a variety of defects, eg deletions, frame shifts, point mutations, rearrangements and substitutions in the genes responsible for collagen production, as well as glycine substitution and exon skipping (Nature 1990; 348:18n&v) Clinical OIs vary in presentation and may have thin bones, multiple fractures, blue sclera, deafness due to middle ear osteosclerosis, scoliosis, thin skin, visceral herniation, dentinogenesis imperfecta, vascular lesions

Osteopathy A school of medicine practiced predominantly in the USA that is based on Dr Andrew Tayor's theory of healing, first delineated in 1874, that holds that a normal body in a state of wellness is in correct adjustment and that disease represents a loss of coherency of structure and/or function and the inability to mount a normal defense against infection, malignancy, inflammation, toxins and other inciting agents; the difference between doctors of medicine (MDs) and doctors of osteopathy (DOs) was formerly greater than in the current environment, the chief distinction is that osteopaths rely more on 'manipulation' of various body parts; otherwise, DOs prescribe drugs and may train in the same teaching hospitals as MDs; there is a greater tendency for osteopaths to provide primary care, as general practitioners of medicine, gynecologists and pediatricians

Osteopetrosis A heterogeneous group of cortical and trabecular osteosclerotic disorders; the vertebral margins are often rounded, have deep indentations for the anterior and posterior veins and marked osteosclerosis, commonly associated with a central radiolucency, imparting a 'sandwich appearance; in the long bones, osteopetrosis is characterized by metaphyseal failure of molding, a finding also seen in van Buchem's endosteal hyperostosis, dysosteosclerosis and tertiary syphilis; in the murine model, osteopetrosis is autosomal recessive, has a limited bone remodeling capacity, has a marked decrease in mature macrophages and osteoclasts and is due to a mutation on chromosome 3 in the coding region of the macrophage colony-stimulating factor gene (Nature 1990; 345:442);see Marble bone disease

Osteoporosis A condition characterized by attenuation of bone, representing the most common morbid condition of the elderly female **Clinical** forms: Primary idiopathic osteoporosis or 'benign' osteoporosis is a rare autosomal dominant condition of early onset that is symptomatic in one-half of cases, radiographically mimicking the malignant form, but which is rarely pernicious clinically Primary involutional osteoporosis is divided into **TYPE I ('POSTMENOPAUSAL') OSTEOPOROSIS** A relatively common condition with a 6:1 female:male ratio, affecting those aged 50-75, characterized by decreased estrogen, accelerated trabecular bone loss, 'crush' fractures associated with abnormal PTH secretion and age-related decrease in response to vitamin D [1,25$(OH)_2D_2$] (N Engl J Med 1989; 320:277); 15-20 years after the onset of menopause, this form of osteoporosis may reach a 'burned-out' phase with no further bone loss **TYPE II ('AGE-RELATED') OSTEOPOROSIS** A less common condition with a 2:1 female:male ratio, affects those over age 70 and is characterized by trabecular and cortical bone loss (the elderly female typically suffers a 35% loss of cortical bone and a 50% loss of trabecular bone), affecting vertebral bodies and flat bones, resulting in hip fractures and wedge-type vertebral fractures, due to a) Decreased osteoblast function (reduced IGF-I, hGH and local regulators) b) A marked decrease in calcium absorption (to 50% of 'normal' with reduced vitamin 1,25$(OH_2)D_2$, possibly due to decreased activity of renal 1-α hydroxylase) and c) Other factors, including decreased clearance of parathyroid hormone's carboxyl (COOH) terminals and increased calcium resorption; calcitonin's role in this form of osteoporosis is unclear **Statistics** Age-related osteoporosis causes more than 10^5 fractures/year in the US (vertebrae 54%, hip 23%, distal forearm or Colles fracture, 17%); 25% of women older than 70 have evidence of vertebral fractures, as do 50% of women older than 80; 90% of femoral head fractures occur in those older than 70; one-third of women age 90 or older have had femoral head fractures, which is a significant risk for long-term institutionalization and in-hospital mortality; the annual cost of osteoporosis is \$6 x 10^9, USA (J Am Med Assoc 1989; 261:1025) Secondary osteoporosis is 'driven' by non-osseous 'axis' factors, which may be iatrogenic, surgical (early oophorectomy, orchiectomy, subtotal gastrectomy), drug-related (corticosteroids, anticonvulsants, heparin, L-thyroxine), endocrinopathic (hypogonadism, increased adrenocortical, parathyroid or thyroid activity), gastrointestinal (alactasia, malabsorption), bone marrow (mastocytosis, metastatic malignancy, multiple myeloma), collagenopathy-related, due to osseous disease (osteogenesis imperfecta, Marfan's disease, rheumatoid arthritis) and others, eg immobilization, chronic obstructive pulmonary disease **Risk factors for osteoporosis** Caucasian, elderly, female, thin habitus, immobilization, space travel (weightlessness), extreme exercise and/or amenorrhea, alcoholism, endocrinopathies (acromegaly, Cushing's disease, hypogonadism, hyperthyroidism, hyperparathyroidism) **Possible risk factors** Heredity, dietary calcium deficiency, smoking (which depresses osteoblastic activity), inadequate exercise, alcohol consumption, low calcium intake, exercise, small body frame, levels of serum and urinary calcium and creatinine; patients receiving physiological doses of levothyroxine may have decreased bone density (J Am Med Assoc 1991; 265:2688); obesity may exert a protective effect against osteoporosis, possibly due to adipose tissue converting androgen to estrogen, increasing osseous resistance to the lytic effects of parathyroid hormone and/or the fact that obesity increases skeletal loading, which by a piezoelectric mechanism, stimulates an osteoblastic response along the lines of stress **Pathophysiology** Estrogen acts on osteoblasts by a receptor, modulating the extracellular matrix, increasing procollagen type I and transforming growth factor-β mRNA, playing a key role in mineralization and remodeling Note: The 'classic' exercise-related osteoporosis may be more a function of aymptomatic disturbances of ovulation, ergo estrogen-related than of physical activity (N Engl J Med 1990; 323:1221) **Diagnosis** Bone densitometry **Treatment** Calcium supplements may not be equivalent in replacing bone calcium, with calcium citrate malate possibly being better than calcium carbonate; fluoride increases vertebral bone mass of cancellous bone type, but decreases cortical mineral density and increases skeletal fragility and is thus of no use in treating postmenopausal osteoporosis (N Engl J Med 1990; 322:802) **Prevention** The bone loss in the early post-menopausal period (< 5 years) is not affected by calcium supplementation (N Engl J Med 1990; 323:878); the use of estrogen for osteoporosis must be based on objective diagnosis of osteoporosis, eg single and dual photon absorptometry of the radius, lumbar spine and hip (Ann Int Med 1990; 112:96), given estrogen's potential for 'driving' proliferative changes of the endometrium; thiazides increase renal conservation of calcium; cyclic etidronate (a diphosphonate agent) reduces bone resorption by inhibiting osteoclast activity (N Engl J Med 1990 322:1265);

'Ostrich legs' see Champagne bottle legs

OTA see Office of Technical Assessment

OTC see Over-the-counter agents/drugs

OTC Ornithine transcarbamylase A mitochondrial matrix enzyme that catalyzes the conversion of ornithine and carbamyl phosphate to citrulline in the urea cycle; OTC is expressed in the liver and intestine and its mitochondrial activity is required for ammonia detoxification; OTC deficiency is X-linked with frequent de novo mutations or may be a mosaic; if completely absent it is usually lethal in the neonatal period; a milder form is characterized by transient potentially life-threatening hyperammonemia (N Engl J Med 1988; 319:999)

Othello syndrome Erotic jealousy A delusion of sposal

infidelity, a form of psychotic paranoia that is primary or more commonly, a symptom of organic 'psychopathies', which include senile dementia, cortical atrophy in boxers and alcoholics; Othello, Shakespeare's tragic hero murdered his wife, Desdemona, when Iago led him to believe her unfaithful

Otopalatodigital dysplasia Taybi disease An X-linked dominant condition, completely expressed in males and partially expressed in carrier females, characterized by conduction-type deafness, a distinct facies with prominent supraorbital ridges, a broad nasal root, flattening of the mid-face and a small jaw, digital abnormalities including short broad fingers; bone dysplasia with dislocation of the radial heads and/or hips, dwarfism, mental retardation*

Ouch-ouch disease see Itai-itai byo

Outcomes 'movement' HEALTH CARE ADMINISTRATION An increasingly organized trend in the US health care industry that assesses the results or outcome of various therapeutic modalities, analyzing efficacy and assuring quality in patient care; the 'movement' has been driven by a) The need for cost containment b) Competition in the medical marketplace for a 'fair' price of high quality services and c) Regional differences in the use of certain medical procedures, causing unnecessary and excess expense in high-use areas or sub-optimal care in low-use areas Note: The developing outcomes 'industry' is predestined to create new bureaucracies and introduce greater inefficiencies without reducing the cost of what is already the world's most expensive health care system (N Engl J Med 1990; 323:266ed)

'Outlier' LABORATORY MEDICINE Any value that lies far outside of the standard deviations of the mean that would encompass the entirety of a population being tested; see Trimming HEALTH CARE MANAGEMENT Any patient who has either an extremely long length of stay or who has incurred extraordinarily high costs Note: The inclusion of 'outliers' in calculations and the establishment of a mean introduces small but potentially significant statistical errors; see High mortality outlier

Output media Any floppy diskette, form, paper 'printout', 'hard copy' or device that displays in some readable format computer-processed data; see Computers

Ovalocytosis A condition occurring in up to 30% of certain ethnic groups in southeast Asia caused by a defective band 3 protein, in which there is increased affinity of erythrocyte membrane band 3 to ankrin, resulting in a marked increase in red cell rigidity; ovalocytosis may represent a form of evolutional defense, as ovalocytes are innately resistant to the parasites of *Plasmodium falciparum* (N Engl J Med 1990; 323:1530)

Ovarian vein 'syndrome' A clinical complex due to an enlarged and tortuous right ovarian vein with incompetence of the venous valves, typically seen in pregnancy, which is accompanied by hydronephrosis and pyelonephritis Clinical Intermittent right flank pain coinciding with menstruation, recurring urinary tract infection and exacerbation with progesterone Treatment Surgical

Overdose SUBSTANCE ABUSE Consumption of any therapeutic agent, drug or narcotic in excess of the dose required to produce the usually desired effects; overdoses are either accidental or suicidal and many agents has its own relatively characteristic clinical, diagnostic and therapeutic 'fingerprint'; see 'Designer' drugs, Heroin, 'Ice'

Overflow diarrhea Secretory diarrhea in which the fluid produced in the upper intestine exceeds the resorptive capacity of the lower intestine, classically seen in cholera, mediated by adenylate cyclase, which is locked in the 'on' position by the cholera toxin

Overflow proteinuria Persistent proteinuria without glomerular disease, characterized by excess production of filterable, low molecular weight proteins, exceeding the resorptive capacities of the renal tubules, eg increased lysozyme in myelomonocytic (M4) leukemia or Bence-Jones proteinuria; the condition is usually asymptomatic if the protein loss is less than 2.0 g/d

Overhanging ledge sign RADIOLOGY A descriptor for prominent chondro-osseous overgrowths commonly seen in the distal acral articulations of gouty arthritis, considered to be most common in those with concomitant diffuse idiopathic skeletal hyperostosis, see DISH

Overhead costs see Indirect costs

Overkill Excess nuclear (war) destructive capacity beyond that required to destroy a target, measured in 'units' of human mortality, where an overkill of 10 indicates a nuclear destructive capacity that is 10-fold greater than that necessary to destroy a given population; because of the image of senseless excess evoked by the word, overkill has become a mainstream colloquial term in medicine, as in diagnostic overkill or therapeutic overkill; see Nuclear war; Cf Chemical warfare

Overlap syndrome GASTROENTEROLOGY The presence of histologic features of both Crohn's disease (granulomas, well-preserved cytoplasmic mucin, lymphoid aggregates and edema) and ulcerative colitis (crypt abscesses, mucosal atrophy and regeneration and marked hyperemia) in the same colon biopsy specimen, precluding a specific diagnosis of either; significant overlap occurs in about 15% of the biopsies of these two conditions and some authors use the term 'indeterminate' syndrome NEUROLOGY see Parkinsonism plus syndromes RHEUMATOLOGY Overlap syndrome(s) are subtypes of connective tissue disease with features of two or more rheumatologic disorders, including lupus-mixed connective tissue disease overlap, rheumatoid arthritis-lupus overlap (1% of cases), scleroderma-polymyositis overlap (8-12% of cases) and lupus-polymyositis overlap (5-10% of cases) VASCULAR DISEASE A combination of systemic necrotizing vasculitis with features of polyarteritis nodosa and Churg-Strauss disease (allergic angiitis and granulomatosis), involving small and medium muscular arteries of the lung, causing hypertension and hypersensitivity

Overread see Underread

Over-the-counter drug (OCD) A therapeutic agent that does not require a physician's prescription, which the

US Food and Drug Administration feels can be safely self-prescribed by non-physicians; 300 000 OTC medications are available in the USA, which contain 700 different active ingredients and generate $7.4 x 10^9$ in annual sales Note: The 'opposite' of an over-the-counter drug is a prescription drug; 'under-the-counter' is a colloquial adjective for any illicit product

Overuse syndrome SPORTS MEDICINE Chronic trauma caused by repetitive forces on the musculotendinous apparatus and chondro-osseous tissues, causing inflammation, pain or dysfunction of the involved joint(s), bones and ligaments, and potentially avulsion fractures

'Overvalued procedure' Any of a group of surgical procedures, for treating non-malignant conditions, eg cholecystectomy that the US Congress has considered to be 'too expensive' and has targeted for budget cuts from Medicare reimbursement; see Resource-based relative value scale

Ovolacteal vegetarian see Lacto-ovo vegetarian

Owl eye appearance A 'classic' descriptor for inclusions seen by light microscopy in cytomegalovirus (CMV) infection, in which the markedly enlarged CMV-infected epithelial cells have massive eosinophilic intranuclear inclusions which may be half the size of the nucleus and surrounded by a clear halo (thus mimicking the inclusions of herpes simplex), clearly delineating the inclusions from the nuclear membrane; CMV-infected cells may also have smaller basophilic inclusions in the cytoplasm, which may correspond to viral capsid proteins; CMV-infected tissues often demonstrate necrosis and chronic inflammation Note: the term 'Owl eye nuclei' has also been applied to the caterpillar cell of rheumatic heart disease, when the latter is viewed longitudinally

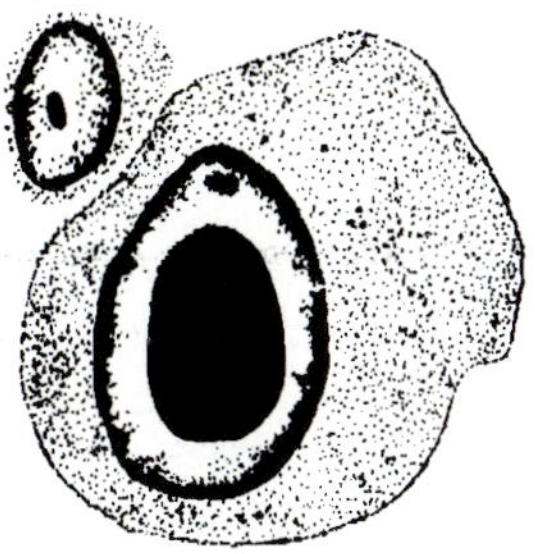

Owl eye appearance

Ox eye Buphthalmos A progressively enlarged eye most commonly seen in children with congenital glaucoma; over time, the head of the optic nerve undergoes cupping and atrophy, resulting in blindness

8-oxo-7-hydrodeoguanosine (8-oxodG) GERONTOLOGY A modified guanosine residue that is formed when DNA suffers oxidative damage, which is a key player in mutagenesis, carcinogenesis and in the aging phenomenon; the presence of 8-oxodG on one strand is permissive to base pairing by either dAMP or dCMP; incorporation of potentially mutagenic dCMP or dAMP nucleotides is followed by transient inhibition of chain extension in the 3' direction of the modified base(s) (Nature 1991; 349:431); see 'Garbage can' hypothesis, Oxygen radicals

Oxygen dissociation curve Oxygen saturation curve PHYSIOLOGY A curve that describes the relationship between hemoglobin oxygen saturation and tension; defined by a sigmoid curve which reflects the interaction of the four hemoglobin molecules involved in oxygen uptake, transport and release; a 'right shift' of the curve indicates decreased hemoglobin affinity for oxygen, as in decreased pH, ie acidosis, increased temperature and PCO_2, while a 'left shift' indicates increased oxygen affinity with increased pH, decreased temperature, decreased 2,3 DPG and PCO_2; see 2, 3 DPG

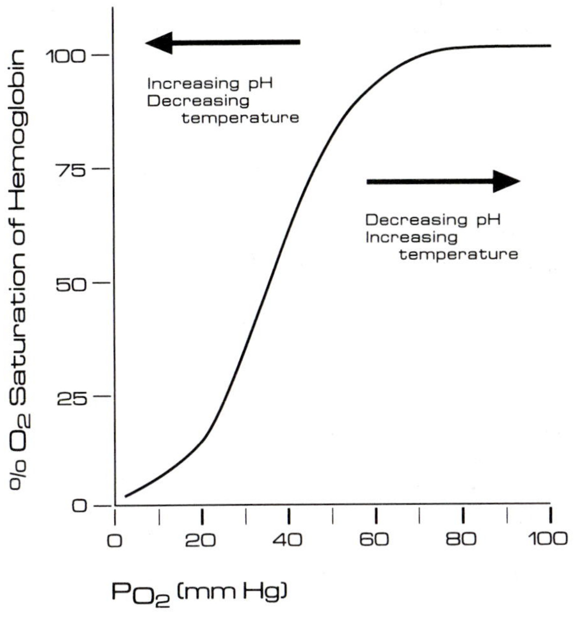

Oxygen dissociation curve

Oxygen free radicals A family of highly reactive, toxic molecules that appear when electrons are added to oxygen in the presence of hydrogen ions; one electron yields superoxide anion radical, a second electron yields H_2O_2 and a third electron yields hydroxyl radical; free radicals are produced in vascular endothelium and in neutrophils by membrane phospholipid catabolism and are generated in the reperfusion phase after myocardial infarction; the free electrons have reactive affinity for unsaturated fatty acids and sulfhydryl amino acids, attacking cells by breaking protein strands, damaging membrane lipids, destroying lipid cross-links and causing fatty acid oxidation; under normal circumstances, cytochrome oxidase prevents destruction of adjacent molecules; free radicals may be eliminated ('scavenged') by catalase, glutathione reductase, superoxide dismutase, vitamin E; during ischemia, xanthine dehydrogenase (which produces uric acid) is converted into xanthine oxidase producing free radicals from oxygen and hypoxanthine; see Free radicals, Respiratory burst

Oxygen paradox MUSCLE PHYSIOLOGY A phenomenon seen when chronically hypoxic muscle is exposed to normal oxygen levels; the muscle cells 'overdose' on oxygen and die, an effect thought due to oxygen radicals; Cf Calcium paradox

Oxygen saturation curve see Oxygen dissociation curve

Oxygen toxicity Tissue and molecular damage due to the effects of oxygen free radicals in cellular and extracellular micro-environments; oxygen toxicity occurs in older subjects, in shock and in inflammation; the toxic effects of atmospheric oxygen on strict anaerobic bacteria are not fully clarified, possibly related to the lack enzymes, eg superoxide dismutase, catalases and peroxidase, capable of metabolizing free radicals and are incapable of growth in greater than 0.5% ambient oxygen; to reduce the oxidation-reduction or 'redox' potential of a medium, reducing agents such as thioglycolate and L-cysteine may be added to the anaerobic transport medium; see Anaerobes

Oxytocin

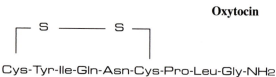

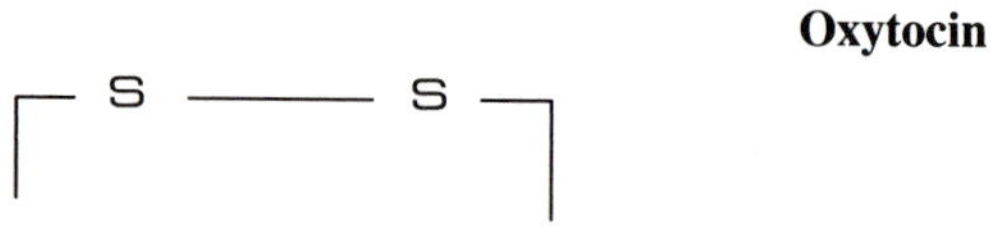

Oxytocin stress test OBSTETRICS A clinical test for evaluating the fetus' ability to 'weather' labor that uses oxytocin, an eight-residue hypothalamic polypeptide released into the posterior pituitary (of both mother and fetus) that induces and stimulates labor; oxytocin is titrated so that three contractions occur in 10 minutes; if three 'decelerations' occur within 10 minutes, the fetus is considered 'at risk' for labor-related complications and should be delivered as soon as possible Note: Because uterine contraction causes a decreased uteroplacental blood flow (see Deceleration), a clinically controlled 'trial of labor' should be performed in women at high risk for uteroplacental insufficiency; such 'at-risk' pregnancies include women with chronic obstructive lung disease, diabetes mellitus, underlying heart disease, hypertension, narcotic addiction, post-term pregnancy, preeclampsia, sickle cell anemia; a positive OCT is characterized by consistent late decelerations and ample indication for an expedient delivery; Cf Fetal heart monitoring, Non-stress test

Ozena Ozaena A mucopurulent nasal discharge in chronic atrophic rhinitis, seen in long-standing systemic disease, eg iron-deficiency anemia or chronic local infection, described in southern Europe; the etiologic role of ***Klebsiella ozaenae*** is speculative as this organism is sensitive to broad-spectrum antibiotics, while ozena is refractory to antibiotic therapy

Ozone ENVIRONMENT There are two types of ozone (O_3); **'GOOD' OZONE** or the ozone layer covers the earth's upper atmosphere and blocks the wavelengths of ultraviolet light (UV-B and UV-C) that cause DNA damage; 'good' ozone is being depleted at a rate of 4-5% per decade, and will result in an extra 200 000 deaths in the next 50 years through sun-induced malignancies (Science 1991; 252:204n&v); the recent increasing incidence of malignant melanoma, has been attributed to the destruction of the ozone layer, although atmospheric models have not confirmed this posit (Mayo Clin Proc 1990; 65:1368ed); depletion of 'good' ozone is largely attributed to CFC accumulation in the atmosphere after release from air conditioners, spray cans and manufacturing plants that produce electronics and plastics; CFCs break down in the atmosphere, releasing chlorine, catalyzing ozone destruction **'BAD' OZONE** is bluish gas with a slightly pungent odor (which at high levels causes tracheobronchitis, pulmonary edema and hemorrhage) formed in the lower atmosphere through complex photochemical reactions involving volatile organic compounds and nitrogen oxides, the internal combustion engine, photocopiers and laser printers; ozone is used as an oxidizing agent in organic chemical production, as a food disinfectant and as a bleaching agent; the federal guidelines from the US Environmental Protection Agency, are 0.12 ppm of ozone as an hourly peak, a level which has not been met in 62 US cities, including Denver, Los Angeles and New York City; see CFCs, Greenhouse effect, Montreal protocol

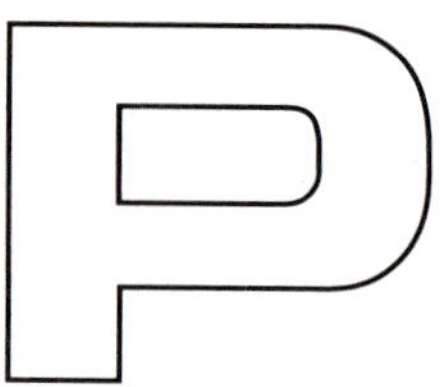

P

P Symbol for: Inorganic phosphate; phosphate; phosphorus; polarization; pressure; probability; proline

p Symbol for: Atomic orbital with angular momentum; para-, pico-, pressure; proton; sample proportion (binomial distribution in statistics); the short arm of a chromosome

P The three Ps The association of pituitary adenoma, pancreatic neoplasia and parathyroid adenoma in Multiple endocrine neoplasm, type I (Wermer syndrome)

p21*ras* protein(s) A family of 21 kD membrane-associated proteins encoded by the c-***ras*** gene that bind to guanine nucleotides, which have a low intrinsic GTPase activity and are thought to be involved in the growth-promoting signal transduction pathway

p24 antigen The 24 kD core antigen of the human immunodeficiency virus type 1 (HIV-1), which is held responsible for AIDS; p24 is the earliest marker of HIV-1 infection, and is detectable days to weeks before seroconversion to anti-HIV-1 antibody production; screening for the p24 antigen does not help identify anti-HIV-1 seronegative or blood donors with 'silent' infections (N Engl J Med 1990; 323:1308, 1312)

p41 PARASITOLOGY A 41 kD polypeptide that is preferentially expressed at the end of maturation in the asexual blood stage of ***Plasmodium falciparum***, with 60% amino acid homology with the vertebrate enzyme, aldolase and which has aldolase activity

P_{50} The oxygen tension at which hemoglobin is one-half (50%) saturated, a value equal to 26 torr (mm Hg) in normal red cells; the P_{50} value is obtained from the midpoint of the oxygen dissociation curve and does not reflect the shape of the curve; with increased oxygen affinity, P_{50} decreases, resulting in a 'Left shift' (see there) of the dissociation curve; a high P_{50} indicates decreased oxygen affinity of the hemoglobin Note: Hemoglobin is almost fully saturated with a partial pressure of oxygen (PO_2) of 85 torr; see Oxygen dissociation curve

p53 A nuclear (tumor-suppresing) phosphoprotein encoded by the proto-oncogene *p53*, which is located on chromosome 17p13; in its native or 'wild' form, p53 inhibits cell growth control and transformation and its normal role is in activating the transcription of genes that suppress cell proliferation, thus acting as a tumor suppressor protein; inactivation of the p53 gene by mutation leads to transformation (Science 1990; 249:1046, 1049); in clinically aggressive human papillomaviral infection, the E6 viral protein binds to p53, preventing its activity (Science 1990; 248:76); p53 is either low or defective in most lung cancers, colorectal carcinoma and in bladder cancers and in the last-named is detectable in urine specimens (Science 1991; 252:706); loss of p53 is a late event in the multistep process in tumor development and may coincide with the transition from benign to malignant growth; the p53 oncogene is thought to be involved in one-half of colorectal, one-third of breast and some small cell carcinomas of the lung and in tumors of the bone and brain, and is mutated in all patients with the Li-Fraumeni syndrome; p53 is an allelic gene that is normally present in pairs, one of which is lost in tumor formation; in the majority of tumors with an allelic deletion, the remaining p53 allele has a missense mutation; the wild-type (normal) p53 gene product acts as a tumor suppressor, a single amino acid substitution may abrogate its tumor suppressive activity, as all mutated p53s thus far isolated are characterized by a loss of tumor-suppressing activity, increased transforming ability and increased ability to bind to heat shock protein hsp70 (Science 1990; 250:113) Note: Tumor production requires that a mutation (deletion, point mutation or rearrangement), commonly affecting a 'CpG island' be present in both alleles, while one wild-type or non-mutated is sufficient to prevent cancer formation (Science 1990; 250:176); p53 mutations differ according to the affected site, including transitions, transversions and base pair mutations, which may reflect differences in etiological contributions of both exogenous and endogenous factors to carcinogenesis (Science 1991; 253:49); p53 is the most commonly altered gene in human tumors, identifiable in up to one-half of all malignancies, and an important first step in the tumorigenic process, as exemplified by the Li-Fraumeni cohort in which there is an inherited mutation of the p53 gene (Nature 1990; 348:747), which is followed within 10 to 30 years by various malignancies; see Li-Fraumeni syndrome; the native p53 protein is thought to control the entry of the cell into the S phase; see Tumor suppressor genes

P170 A 170 kD plasma membrane-bound glycoprotein encoded by the MDR (multidrug resistance) gene, composed of sugar residues and a protein chain that traverses the cell membrane 12 times, forming a 'gated' transmembrane pore, using ATP-derived energy to export various drugs from the cytoplasm to the extracellular space; since most of the drugs actively exported are hydrophobic and arrive in the cell by passive diffusion across the membrane, the amount of drug required to reach therapeutic levels in the face of an active exporting system such as P170 may be enormous, reaching levels that are toxic to non-tumorous cells; leukemic blast crises are characterized by increased expression of P-glycoprotein in leukemic cell membranes; see Multidrug resistance gene

$P210^{bcr/abl}$ see Philadelphia chromosome

P450 A protein complexed to cytochrome oxidase, which has a peak spectrophotometric absorption at 450 nm and forms the terminal portion of the electron transport system in adrenal mitochondria and hepatic microsomes; P450 is responsible for hydroxylation of phenobarbital, increasing water solubility and hydroxylation of polycyclic aromatic hydrocarbons for conjugation with glucuronate or sulfates

PAAC Physicians Association for AIDS Care

PAC Papular acrodermatitis of childhood or Gianotti-Crosti syndrome; Political action committee; Premature atrial contraction; Pulmonary artery catheterization

Pacemaker syndrome A relatively common (up to 20% are affected) complication of implanted pacemakers, characterized by vertigo, syncope, dyspnea, weakness, decreased exercise tolerance, postural hypotension, palpable hepatic and jugular vein pulsations Etiology Alternating atrioventricular asynchrony in which the atrium contracts against closed valves, raising venous pressure or the ventricle contracts before the blood has arrived, causing transiently inadequate cardiac output Treatment Dual chamber pacing pacemaker and antiarrhythmic agents

Pacemaker theory CELL BIOLOGY A hypothesis that attempts to explainthe aging process, postulating that certain organs have a predetermined lifespan, the functions of which deteriorate with age in the form of immunosenescence (75% decrease in T cell activities, increase in autoantibody formation and increased risk of infection and malignancy) and neuroendocrine changes (altered carbohydrate metabolism and sleep patterns)

Pachydermoperiostosis (Pdp) A condition characterized by induration of the skin in the natural folds, accentuation of the creases of the face and scalp, clubbing of the fingers and periostosis of the long bones; hereditary Pdp is known as the Touraine-Solente-Gole syndrome;

acquired Pdp appears in later life and may be associated with bronchogenic carcinoma; Cf Hypertrophic (pulmonary) osteoarthropathy

Pachydermy A non-specific term for leathery subcutaneous induration due to an accumulation of inelastic connective tissue, as in acromegaly or due to accumulation of protein-rich mucin, collagen and fibroblasts, as occurs in myxedema

Package insert CLINICAL PHARMACOLOGY A paper accompanying a prescription drug that contains full product information, including the indications for its use, forms of administration and side effects; see Advertising

Packaging MOLECULAR BIOLOGY The process of folding or compacting and insertion of the long (estimated 3 billion base pairs in length) DNA molecule into a smaller and more efficient space or region, eg formation of chromosomes and nucleosomes; Cf Protein folding

Packed red cells TRANSFUSION MEDICINE A concentrated unit of erythrocytes prepared from a unit of whole blood by removing most of the plasma, yielding a volume circa 200 ml, of which 80% of the volume is red cells and 20% plasma; 'packed units' are stored at 4°C in plastic bags for up to 42 days, using CPDA-1 (citrate-phosphate-dextrose-additive) solution; these units should be used for active bleeding, excess intraoperative blood loss, low 'pre-op' or 'post-op' hematocrits, chronic anemias, eg sickle cell anemia, thalassemia, chemotherapy for cancer, dialysis, blood exchange; see CPDA-1, Quad pack, Single unit transfusion, Storage lesions, Whole blood

Packed unit see Packed red cells

Packing LABORATORY TECHNOLOGY *noun* The solid material, usually beads of varying porosities that form the solid (stationary) phase in column chromatography *verb* The process of adding the solid material, eg pouring of the beads, into a chromatographic column OTORHINOLARYNGOLOGY see Nasal packing

Packing ratio MOLECULAR BIOLOGY The length of DNA divided by the length of the unit that contains it, which may be as great as 7000; because of DNA's complexity, it cannot be directly packaged, but rather requires hierarchies of organization; the FIRST PACKING LEVEL is that of DNA wound into beadlike particles, giving it a packing ratio of 6; the SECOND PACKING LEVEL is the coiling of the 'beaded strings' into a helical array, constituting a 30 nm fiber found in both interphase chromatin and mitotic chromosomes, yielding a packing ratio of 40; the THIRD AND HIGHEST PACKING HIERARCHY is determined by the packing of the fiber itself, which is modified by accessory proteins and has a ratio of 1000 or more

'Pack-years' A crude indicator of a person's cigarette consumption, calculated as the packs of cigarettes smoked per day, multiplied by the length of consumption in years; eg two packs of cigarettes smoked per day for 20 years is 40 pack-years, which is associated with a relative risk (RR value) of 60 for suffering a smoking-related malignancy

'Pacmen' A highly colloquial term coined by US legislators for hidden liabilities that the government must pay in the future, eg rising costs of health care, potentially rising to hundreds of billions (US) of dollars; Pacman is one of the first video games to be popularized, a game in which little 'mouths' gobbled up dots on the game board

Padded dash(board) 'syndrome' A vanishingly rare form of trauma, most commonly affecting the right front seat occupant ('passenger side' in many countries) in an automobile accident when he/she is restrained by a lap-type safety belt; in an abrupt stop, the passenger's body is thrown forward at the waist and the hyperextended neck strikes the dashboard at the level of the thyroid cartilage **Clinical** Respiratory distress due to upper airway obstruction, due to a hematoma, fluid accumulation, aspiration of saliva, fluids, subcutaneous emphysema, fractures of cartilage, accompanied by pain on deglution Note: Shoulder restraints and air bags in automobiles appear to have virtually eliminated this form of motor vehicle-related trauma

Padlock sign RADIOLOGY An uncommon finding by computed tomography in which a mass density is accompanied by adjacent ring enhancement, representing eccentric cavitation in a solid intracranial lesion; while characteristic of higher grade astrocytomas, abscesses and metastases, it is also seen in craniopharyngioma, meningioma, prolactinoma (with cystic changes) and tuberculosis and thus hasf little diagnostic specificity

PAF see Platelet activating factor

PAGE see Polyacrylamide gel electrophoresis, SDS-PAGE

Paget's disease of bone A condition largely affecting older Northern European males that is most common in the lumbosacral spine, pelvis and skull **Laboratory** Very high alkaline phosphatase **Complications** Cardiac failure due to arterio-venous shunting; osteosarcoma and other sarcomasoccur in 1-25% **Histopathology** Low-power microscopy reveals a classic 'mosaic' pattern of thickened, poorly mineralized and osteoclastic bony trabeculae, later demonstrating abnormal hyperplasia, increased vascularity, prominent and scalloped cement lines, osteoblasts and osteoclasts; osteoid is not prominent and is poorly mineralized **Ultrastructure** Measles virus-like intranuclear inclusions are a constant feature **Treatment** Calcitonin, usually of salmon origin; most of the 25% of cases that develop anti-salmon antibodies respond to human calcitonin; alternate therapies include diphosphonates, mitrimycin and surgery for decompressing critical cranial structures, or hip replacement if necessary; see Mosaic bone

Paget's disease of the breast A 'weeping', eczematoid erosive lesion of the nipple first described by Sir James Paget in 1874 that is almost invariably associated with underlying intraductal breast carcinoma (carcinoma in situ, ductal type), and when accompanied by a palpable mass implies an invasive carcinoma **Histopathology** Large clear epithelial cells with atypical nuclei located in the basal layer, often arranged in oligocellular clusters **Differential diagnosis** Bowen's disease, malignant melanoma Note: Paget's cells may imbibe melanin granules (a process known as cytocrinia), resulting in the misdiagnosis of melanoma **Prognosis** Survival hinges on aggressiveness of the underlying duct cell carcinoma, or less commonly on lobular carcinoma: Cf

Intraepidermal carcinoma

Paget's disease, extramammary A disease that is similar morphologically to Paget's disease of the breast, but less often associated with underlying malignancy; the condition arises from skin adnexae, visceral malignancy or rarely, de novo, appearing in the scrotum, perineum and labia majora and is more often mucin-positive than Paget's disease of the breast

PAI see Plasminogen activator inhibitor

Pain NEUROLOGY The sensation of marked discomfort that is either sharp and well-localized (conducted along A-delta fibers) or dull and diffuse (conducted along C nerve fibers; Brodmann's area 24 appears to be a catchment region for pain, and thus the cortex is selectively activated in response to pain; the parietal and limbic regions of the cortex appear to respond to the location and intensity of the pain and the limbic region regulates the emotional response to pain (Science 1991; 251:1355); therapy for recalcitrant pain (post-surgery, burn and terminal cancer patients) is often inadequate due to the care-givers' fear of opiate addiction, in those with terminal cancer, the analgesia may be administered more frequently as opiates in these patients appear to be less addicting, possibly due to an alteration in the endorphin receptors or processing of endorphins (Sci Am 1990; 262:27); see Gait control theory, Patient controlled analgesia

'Pain and suffering' see Malpractice, damages

Painful bruising syndrome A psychosomatic trauma-induced condition of unknown etiology, described in emotionally-labile women that appears on the legs, face and trunk, characterized by recurring painful ecchymoses with a ladder-like morphology, accompanied by syncope, nausea, vomiting, gastrointestinal and intracranial bleeding

Painful crisis One of the 'crises' common in sickle cell anemia where 'sludging' of sickled red cells causes capillary stasis and infarction, resulting in incapacitating musculoskeletal pain or 'referral'-type organ pain, hemoptysis, hematuria, melena and central nervous system symptoms; painful crises occur at a rate of 0.8 episodes/year in sickle cell disease, 1.0 per year in sickle-β-thalassemia and 0.4 per year in hemoglobin SC-β thalassemia; this frequency is translated into a 'pain rate', which is a measure of disease severity that correlates with early death in patients with sickling anemias (N Engl J Med 1991; 325:11); hemolytic 'crises' consist of rapidly evolving anemia, leukocytosis, jaundice and fever

Painful fat syndrome An atypical, chronic and symmetric swelling and tenderness of the legs, more commonly affecting adolescent females; the lipedema is painful on pressure, is non-pitting and fancifully likened to pigskin

Painful heel An idiopathic affliction of older men causing tenderness of the heel associated with focal edema and in one-half of cases, calcaneal spur formation Prognosis Persistent pain or spontaneous resolution

Painful red leg syndrome Erythromelia Increased sensitivity to skin temperatures above 32°C; individual patients often become symptomatic at an exact temperature, with focal vasodilation and a burning sensation Treatment Aspirin; secondary erythromelia may occur in hypertension or polycythemia vera

Pain rate see Painful crisis

'Paintbrush' hair A descriptor for fragile, beaded and longitudinally split hair shafts seen in trichorrhexis nodosa, a common condition caused by hair dryness resulting from 'excess' hair care (too frequent shampooing, combing and brushing); Cf Flag sign, Pili torti, Woolly hair syndrome

Paired helical filaments (PHF) NEUROPATHOLOGY Structures that are the main constituents of the neurofibrillary tangles of Alzheimer's disease, composed of 210 nm filaments of predominantly A68 protein wound into a helix; PHFs are relatively insoluble, may be composed of ubiquitin and occur in Down syndrome, Hallervorden-Spatz disease, lead encephalopathy, lipofuscinosis, subacute sclerosing panencephalitis, tuberous sclerosis, in neurites surrounding amyloid-rich senile plaques and in neuropil threads; see A68 protein, Neurofibrillary tangles, Senile plaques

PAJAMA experiment(s) A series of experiments carried out by A Pardee, F Jacob and J Monod that led to the concept of repressor proteins as regulators of gene expression, which act at specific sites along the DNA, designated as operators (Nobel prize, 1965, Science 1988; 239:1545)

Pale body A well-circumscribed, pale eosinophilic cytoplasmic inclusion, thought to be characteristic of fibrolamellar carcinoma of the liver (Cancer 1980; 46:1448)

Pale cells A non-specific descriptor for cells with homogeneous, lightly eosinophilic cytoplasm, occurring in a) Lung Cells in sclerosing hemangioma which have an appearance midway between type II pneumocytes and stromal connective tissue cells, b) Liver Hepatocytes with a 'washed-out' appearance caused by hypertrophy of the endoplasmic reticulum, as seen in barbiturate intoxication and c) Lymph nodes Plasmacytoid CD8-positive T cells that are scattered or arranged in clusters in T cell lymphoproliferative disorders, eg immunoblastic lymphadenopathy (IBL), angioimmunoblastic lymphadenopathy and IBL-like T cell lymphoma

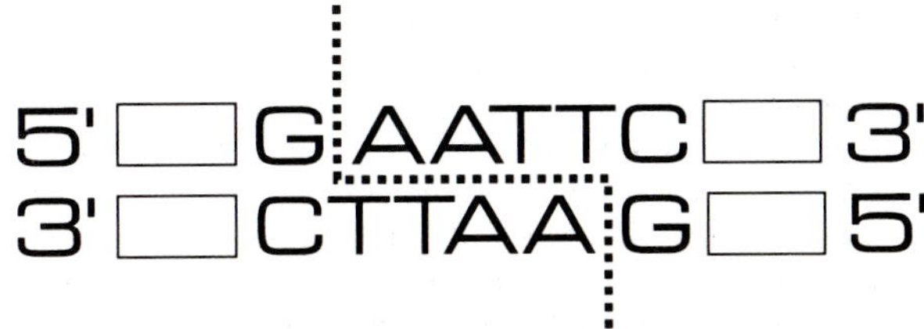

Palindromic site of restriction endonuclease (*Eco*RI) cutting

Palindrome Greek, Reading the same, backward and forward MOLECULAR BIOLOGY A sequence of duplex DNA with dyad symmetry, ie a sequence that is the same when either strand is read in a defined direction, eg the 5' to 3' direction; inverted repeats of double-stranded DNA are located opposite each other on contiguous strands of DNA and the axis of symmetry can be drawn to separate the inverted repeats; this symmetry allows formation of hydrogen-bonded hairpin loops and stem-and-loop structures; experimental denaturation of palindromic regions may lead to the formation of semistable cruciform loops capable of interacting with binding proteins (it is uncertain whether cruciform loops exist in vivo); palindromic DNA renatures rapidly and comprises up to 5% of eukaryotic DNA, representing recognition sites for regulatory proteins, eg the lac operon; restriction endonucleases usually cut double-stranded DNA through segments with dyad symmetry, as shown in the accompanying figure (dashed line indicates the cleavage line of the *Eco*RI)

Palindromic rheumatism A form of monoarthritis that may precede rheumatoid arthritis Clinical Intermittent recurring (more than 5 attacks in 2 years) episodes of intense gout-like pain and joint inflammation, more common in middle-aged men, affecting the knee, wrist or dorsum of hand, accompanied by transient subcutaneous nodules; although the condition is distinct between patients, each attack tends to follow the same pattern in the individual patient Laboratory Non-specific elevation of erythrocyte sedimentation rate and acute phase reactants

Palisading Picket fence arrangement French, palisade, a fence made of pales, forming an enclosure or defense A commonly used descriptor for a light microscopic appearance in which elongated and compressed, usually epithelial cells are perpendicular to a surface, eg a basement membrane, an appearance that has been described in chondroblastoma (bone), oligodendroglioma (brain), ulcerative colitis-related dysplasia (colon) due to the vertical arrangement of tall, crowded goblet cells with pseudopalisaded hyperchromatic nuclei, seen lining branched colonic glands), endocervical adenocarcinoma (endocervix), malignant epithelial mesothelioma (lung), rheumatoid pannus (joint), ameloblastoma (oral cavity, also known as a 'tombstone' pattern, which may also be seen in primordial cysts and odontogenic keratocysts), mucinous cystadenoma and mucinous cystadenocarcinoma (ovary) and basal cell carcinoma (skin, see figure); the term also refers to the arrangement of ***Corynebacterium*** species, more commonly described as having a 'Chinese character' appearance

Palliative surgery A therapeutic modality carried out in the face of hopelessly incurable malignancy, justified to reduce the severity of symptoms and improve the quality of life, relieving pain (cordectomy), hemorrhage (cystectomy for bleeding urinary bladder), obstruction (colostomy or gastroenterostomy) or infection (amputation of a necrotic and malodorous tumor-ridden breast or extremity); see 'Heroic' surgery, Mutilating surgery

Palliative therapy Any treatment of a terminally-ill patient intended to alleviate pain and suffering, without performing aggressive ('heroic') procedures; palliative therapy recognizes the incurable nature of a pernicious process and seeks, through various modalities, eg surgery and radiotherapy, to reduce or shrink tumor masses compressing vital structures, seeking to increase a patient's 'quality time' before death; see Karnovsky scale; Heroic therapy

PALS Periarteriolar lymphoid sheath The layer of lymphocytes surrounding the central arterioles in the spleen (alternately known as 'white pulp'), comprising the bulk of splenic lymphoid tissue; the PALS is composed of T cells surrounding the central arteriole, which are in turn surrounded by B cells; in the unstimulated state, the B cell zone consists of a primary follicle; following stimulation, a central germinal center is evident

PAM Pulmonary alveolar macrophage; see Primary acquired melanosis; see Primary amoebic meningoencephalitis

Panagglutination see Polyagglutination

Pan-B cell marker(s) Hematology Surface antigens that are present on all normal B lymphocytes; CD19 is considered the best pan-B cell marker, which may replace identification of surface immunoglobulins as an indicator of B cell lineage; other surface antigens included under the rubric of pan-B markers are CD20 and CD24; see Pan-T cell markers

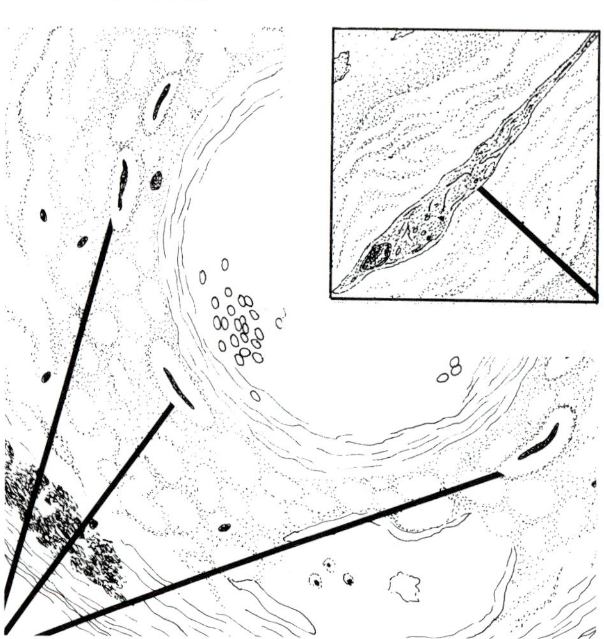

Pancake cell

Pancake cell A flattened compressed endothelial cell seen in intravascular fibrous atherosclerotic plaques that stain intensely with actin (N Engl J Med 1986; 314:488) and which appears to play a role in atherosclerosis (figure, above)

Pancake omentum An omentum that has undergone marked thickening and induration secondary to diffuse infiltration by malignancy, usually of epithelial origin, most commonly, by advanced ovarian cystadenocarcinoma, but also by carcinoma of the colon, stomach or pancreas; the omental 'cake' is seen by computed tomography (CT) as a flattened layer of tumor separating the small or large intestine from the anterior abdominal wall; Cf 'Policeman of the abdomen'

Pancreatic cholera syndrome(s) A group of clinical complexes characterized by diarrhea caused by endocrine tumors of the pancreas, most commonly VIPoma (vasoactive intestinal peptide-producing pancreatic tumor, see WDHA) Note: VIPoma-induced diarrhea is a diagnosis of exclusion, given its incidence of one case per million population per year, but should be considered when diarrhea of unknown origin with a volume of greater than one 1 liter/day is prolonged for more than four weeks and causes hypokalemia, salt and water depletion

Pancreatic endocrine tumors (PET) A group of tumors comprising a small proportion of pancreatic neoplasms, including APUDoma, islet cell tumor and nesidioblastoma, most commonly found in the body and tail, the sites of the greater concentration of islets of Langerhans; although PETs appear in 0.5-1.0% of unselected autopsies, the prevalence of functional, hormone-producing tumors is less than $1:10^5$; the tumors are named according to the predominant hormone being produced, eg gastrinoma, glucagonoma, VIPoma, PPoma and others, although most tumors produce more than one hormone Histopathology Four patterns have been described: Solid, gyriform, glandular and nondescript Prognosis Most PETs are indolent and a ten-year survival is the norm after initial resection; more aggressive lesions may respond to chemotherapy, eg streptozocin; see WDHA syndrome, Zollinger-Ellison syndrome

Pancreatic panel LABORATORY MEDICINE An abbreviated and cost-effective battery of chemical assays of use in detecting pancreatitis, which includes amylase, lipase, calcium and glucose; Cf Organ panel

Pancreatic polypeptide PP A 36-residue polypeptide of unknown function secreted by the pancreatic islet 'F' cells in various animal species

Pancreatic rest A focus or foci of ectopic pancreatic tissue that may have all the histological components of a normal pancreas (including acini, ducts and islets of Langerhans), which remains in the upper gastrointestinal tract after embryogenic steps including rotation of the ventral anlage and its fusion with the dorsal anlage; pancreatic rests occur in multiple sites in the midgut, eg stomach, small intestine and 'classically' finding in Meckel's diverticulum, and rarely occur in the liver, mesentery and omentum, simulating metastatic adenocarcinoma

Pancreatic sufficiency A term coined in reference to patients with cystic fibrosis (and probably equally applicable to diabetics with adequate insulin production) who have sufficient exocrine pancreatic function to allow normal digestion without enzyme supplements, a finding in patients who have milder disease and are older when diagnosed, who have lower levels of sweat chloride, milder respiratory disease, normal growth and a better prognosis (N Engl J Med 1990; 323:1517); see Cystic fibrosis

Pancreatic transplantation (PT) A procedure designed to halt the progression of diabetic neuropathy (N Engl J Med 1990; 322:1031) and achieve complete glycemic control; pancreatic transplantation requires that a large segment or the entire pancreas be harvested, thus donors are often cadaveric; PT is often combined with renal allograft transplantation, necessitated by diabetic nephropathy; because of the limited access to the procedure, recipients must be as 'perfect' (immunologically, as well as clinical stable), as possible; the most common exclusionary criterion is the presence of cardiovascular disease; one-year survival of patients is 93% (Mayo Clin Proc 1990; 65:475, 483, 496); one-year graft survival is 50-80%; when a living HLA-matched donor undergoes hemipancreatectomy, the donor's insulin secretion and glucose control deteriorates (whether clinical diabetes mellitus develops in the donor is uncertain, N Engl J Med 1990; 322:898, J Am Med Assoc 1991; 265:510); Cf Biohybrid artificial pancreas, Islet cell transplantation

Pancytopenia A disorder of peripheral blood arising in the bone marrow, characterized by hypoplasia or aplasia of normal hematopoietic precursor cells, ie marrow hypoplasia with abnormal precursor cells as in hypoplastic myelodysplasia; pancytopenia occurs in aplastic anemia (drug-related, especially common in chemotherapeutic agents used to treat malignancy, radiotherapy, toxins), marrow replacement by hematopoietic, lymphoproliferative and metastatic malignancy, storage diseases, osteopetrosis, myelofibrosis, hypersplenism (congestive splenomegaly, hematopoietic malignancy, storage diseases, sarcoidosis, malaria and kala-azar), infection (fungemia, septicemia, tuberculosis) and megaloblastic anemia

Pandemic An epidemic affecting a large number of people at the same time and in many different communities; well-described pandemics include a) AIDS b) Cholera Seven pandemics have been described, the most recent of which occurred from 1961 to 1981 c) Influenza which was uncommon until 1889, after which time (for unknown reasons) influenza pandemics have occurred about every 10 years, where new immunotypes are related to antigenic changes in the surface glycoprotein, hemagglutinin and neuraminidase that protrude from the viral envelope d) Syphilis The syphilitic or 'great pox' pandemic swept through Europe in the 1500s and is thought to have been more virulent than 'modern' syphilis e) Yersinia pandemics were first described in Egypt, 542 AD, spreading to Turkey and Europe; a second began in Asia minor and Africa in the early 1300s, causing the Black Plague, killing one-fourth of Europe; a third occurred in Europe in the pre-industrial age and a fourth pandemic is in progress, which began in China in 1860 and migrated by ship to India, Asia, Brazil and California

Panic attack(s) PSYCHIATRY Recurrent episodes of unpredictable, sudden and intense apprehension or fear, often accompanied by a somatic component including dyspnea, palpitations, chest pain, choking or smothering sensation, vertigo, a sensation of unreality, paresthesia, hot and cold flashes, faintness and trembling; fear of dying, 'going crazy' and being trapped are virtually universal components and while an attack is occurring, the subjects are disinclined to appear in public and thus also suffer from transient agoraphobia; panic attacks affect 3.6% of the adult population in the US (J Am Med Assoc 1991; 265:742), they are transient and fall short of the criteria required to diagnose 'Panic disorder'

Panic disorder A psychogenic complex affecting 1.5% of the US population characterized by recurrent and unpredictable episodes (panic attacks) of sudden, intense apprehension, fear and autonomic nervous system hyperactivity Clinical Dyspnea, palpitations, chest pain, a sensation of choking, dizziness, loss of reality sense, paresthesias, hot and cold flashes, sweating, faintness, trembling, a fear of dying or of 'going crazy'; the fear of an attack in public may result in functional agoraphobia; those with panic disorders have an 18-fold greater incidence of suicidal ideation than a mentally 'fit' population (N Engl J Med 1989; 321:1209) Note: Panic attacks and panic disorder differ only in degree and frequency and the potential transient nature of panic attacks

PANIC VALUES

ANALYTE	SI UNITS	US UNITS
Calcium	< 1.65 mmol/L	< 6.6 mg/dl
	> 2.22 mmol/L	> 12.9 mg/dl
Glucose	< 2.6 mmol/L	< 46 mg/dl
	> 26.9 mmol/L	> 484 mg/dl
Potassium	< 2.8 mmol/L	< 2.8 mEq/L
	> 6.2 mmol/L	> 6.2 mEq/L
	> 8.0 mmol/L if hemolyzed	
Sodium	< 120 mmol/L	< 120 mEq/L
	> 158 mmol/L	> 158 mEq/L
CO2	< 11 mmol/L	< 11 mMol
plasma	> 40 mmol/L	> 40 mMol

Panic values Critical values Laboratory results from patient specimens that must be reported immediately to the clinician, which are often of a nature requiring urgent therapeutic action (table, above); other 'critical' values include parameters from a) Hematology, eg blasts or sickle cells on a peripheral smear, possibly indicating leukemia or sickle cell anemia b) Microbiology, eg positive gram stain or culture from blood, serosal fluids or cerebrospinal fluid, acid-fast stain or positive mycobacterial culture results c) The blood bank Incompatible cross-match and positive serology for VDRL; the panic values differ in each laboratory and the route by which the communication occurs is at the discretion of the laboratory director (J Am Med Assoc 1990; 263:704); see Decision levels

Pannus A reticulated membrane of granulation tissue, typical of the chronic prolifero-destructive phase of rheumatoid arthritis in which immune complexes form at the synovial membranes, evoking a non-specific immune response by macrophages, which produce interleukin-1, fibroblast-activating factor, prostaglandins, platelet-derived growth factor, substance P and others, resulting in global destruction of chondro-osseous tissues Histopathology Exuberant synovitis that covers the articular surface and which may be accompanied by edema, causing fusiform swelling and erythema of the overlying joints with vaguely palisaded histiocytes; with time, the pannus fills the joint space, causing subchondral demineralization and cystic resorption, due to the release of enzymes and fibrous ankylosis Note: Pannus formation also occurs in the fibrovascular proliferative response to *Chlamydia trachomatis* infection of the cornea and conjunctiva, as well as in tuberculous synovitis

Panspermy hypothesis A naive theory of historic interest that posited that life originated from some place, prior to the origin of the solar system, traveled through space and was deposited on various planets in the form of heat-resistant spores; see Spontaneous generation

P antigen An antigen related to ABH blood group that is located on the red cell surface and composed of three sugars (galactose, N-acetyl-galactosamine and N-acetyl-glucosamine), containing P antigens, P_1, P_2, P^k and p, of which P^k and p are rare; the relatively rare anti-P_1 antibody produced by P_2 individuals may produce clinically significant hemolysis; the anti-P_1 antibody can be neutralized with echinococcal hydatid cyst fluid, serving to identify this IgM molecule; a 'biphasic' autoanti-P antibody occurs in patients with paroxysmal cold hemoglobinuria, fixing complement at 4°C, hemolyzing the erythrocytes at 37°C

Pan-T cell marker(s) A group of cell surface antigens that are present on all normal T lymphocytes, including CD2 (formerly, OKT 11/Leu 5), a 50 kD molecule found only on T cells, corresponding to the sheep erythrocyte rosette marker and CD7 (formerly, Leu9), a 41 kD molecule that may also be found in T cell acute leukemias and rare early acute myeloid leukemia; other surface antigens regarded as pan-T markers are CD1 (peripheral T cells and cortical thymocytes), CD3 (mature T cells) and CD5; see Pan-B cell markers

Panzerherz German, armored heart A synonym for pericardial calcinosis, a rare complication of chronic pericarditis

PAO Peak acid output PHYSIOLOGY A measurement of maximum hydrogen ion (H^+) production by the gastric parietal cells, defined as the sum of the two highest consecutive 15-minute acid outputs after pentagastrin or histamine stimulation, multiplied by 2; PAO indirectly quantifies the number of functional parietal cells and has a normal value of 10-60 mmol/hr, which is similar to MAO; see BAO

PAP 1) PEROXIDASE-ANTIPEROXIDASE TECHNIQUE Immunoperoxidase method A method for identifying antigens in tissues, using monoclonal antibodies and 'amplification' steps to detect an antigenic 'signal' Method: The tissue is fixed, eg with formalin, washed with trypsin to block the tissue's endogenous peroxidase, incubated with non-human serum to block nonspecific antibody binding, incubated with a monoclonal antibody raised against the antigen to be tested (which is coupled to an enzyme, eg peroxidase that is covalently bound to the Fc end of the monoclonal antibody); the tissue is then incubated with a substrate (H_2O_2 and diaminobenzidine); if the antigen is present in the tissue, the substrate will be digested, resulting in a color change that is measured by a spectrophotometer, see ABC 2) PRIMARY ATYPICAL PNEUMONIA see Interstitial pneumonia 3) PULMONARY ALVEOLAR PROTEINOSIS

Papain A proteolytic enzyme of broad specificity derived from *Carica papaya* that is used in a) IMMUNOLOGY Papain, used in early work to delineate immunoglobulin structure, digests immunoglobulin into two antibody (Fab) fragments and a crystallizable (Fc) fragment; see Fab fragment, Fc fragment, Pepsin TRANSFUSION MEDICINE Papain, ficin and other enzymes can be used to modify rec cell antigens, enhancing the reactivity of some antigen-antibody systems, eg Rh and Kidd and abolishing the reactivity of others, eg M, N, Fy^a and Fy^b, thus aiding in the identification of antigens that may cause hemolytic transfusion reactions

Papanicolaou ratio see Maturation index

Papanicolaou test Pap smear GYNECOLOGY A cytologic sampling from the uterine cervix and endocervix that serves to detect dysplasia and squamous cell carcinoma of the cervix; while the 'Pap smear' continues to be the 'gold standard' method for early detection of this cancer, various factors prevent this simple procedure from detecting the theoretical 100% of these potentially curable malignancies, including sampling error, insufficient time devoted to screening and fatigue by the histotechnologist performing the screening; the Pap test commonly also suffers from lack of clinical information, poor patient compliance, inadequate follow-up and poor reproducibility (J Am Med Assoc 1989; 261:737); cytologic sampling from the vaginal vault is used for evaluating a woman's hormonal status, see Maturational index; named after G Papanicolaou, the test's creator

Paper chromatography A form of partition chromatography that allows separations based on differences in the rate of diffusion, solubility of solute and the nature of the solute, where the stationary phase is a filter paper and the mobile phase is a solvent containing a molecule of interest; paper chromatography was formerly used to fractionate a) Sugars, which are now separated by column chromatography b) Amino acids, which are currently analyzed by ion-exchange chromatography and c) barbiturates, which are now separated by thin-layer or gas-liquid chromatography or high-performance liquid chromatography

Paper money skin A descriptor for the small randomly scattered subcutaneous blood vessels found on the upper arms in hepatocellular failure as well as the healed lesions of pyoderma gangrenosum, so-named as the finding has been fancifully likened to the fine hair-like threads seen in US paper currency, which is so designed to reduce counterfeiting of paper currency

Papillary and solid epithelial neoplasm of the pancreas (PSENP) A distinct low-grade pancreatic carcinoma that is most common in young females, which measures 5-15 cm, and is accompanied by hemorrhage and necrosis; certain histologic features suggest that it may represent a primitive endocrine tumor Histopathology Low mitotic activity, hyaline globules, foam cells Prognosis Excellent with adequate resection

Papillary necrosis A complication of acute pyelonephritis, consisting of uni- or bilateral lesions of one or more pyramids, with a white-gray discoloration of the pyramid tips Histopathology Coagulation necrosis with preservation of the outlines of the tubules Etiology Diabetes mellitus, sickle cell anemia, analgesics (aspirin and phenacetin), ischemia and pyelonephritis related to obstruction

Papillary ring A radiologic manifestation of papillary necrosis of the kidneys, seen by contrast studies of the upper urinary tract, in which debris from necrotic medullary tissue and pyramids fills the cup-shaped calices

Pa-ping A condition described in mainland China, clinically similar to hypokalemic periodic paralysis (periodic attacks of truncal and limb paralysis) caused by ingesting barium salts, resulting in hypokalemia by blockage of the potassium channels in skeletal muscle, preventing the efflux of potassium from the intra- to the extracellular fluid space

Papovavirus A family of small icosahedral double-stranded DNA tumor viruses, eg SV40 and polyomavirus that induces both benign and malignant neoplasms; papovavirus infection may be either 'permissive' or 'non-permissive'; monkey cells are susceptible to permissive infection, within which papovavirus reproduces, causing lysis; rodent cells are 'non-permissive' and early viral proteins (T antigens) cause the cell to undergo transformation, which is permanent if the viral genome becomes integrated into the host's genome or transient if the cell rids itself of the viral genome

Para-Bombay phenotype TRANSFUSION MEDICINE A variant of the Bombay phenotype of the ABO blood group, in which the individuals have an Se (secretor) gene allowing the formation of blood groups A and B and its expression in secretions, but not allowing the formation of A and B red cells, given the absence of the H gene Note: In the Bombay phenotypes, an individual lacks the H gene and its product, fucosyl transferase and thus cannot express blood groups A or B on the red cells or in secretions; Cf Bombay phenotype

Parachute-related injury Unanticipated complications of jumping out of aircraft for business or pleasure; in the military, the mortality is 1/51 000 jumps and the annual rate of attrition through incapacitation is 0.4%, which has been reduced by modern parachute design and larger canopies; the most common non-fatal injuries are vertebral, lower extremity (see Cavalry fracture) and facial fractures; the amount and intensity of injuries is a function of wind speed, weight of the diver and his state of physical fitness

Parachute reaction Anterior propping reaction PEDIATRICS Protective abduction of the arms, extension of the elbows and wrists and spreading of the fingers, which is a normal defense reflex, elicited when an infant is held in ventral suspension and is tilted abruptly forward toward the floor, seen between the 7th and 9th months of age, a response that is asymmetrical in infants with hemiparesis and may be the first manifestation of cerebral palsy

Parachute valve complex of Shone A cardiac malformation tetrad comprised of a 'parachute' mitral valve (chordae tendinae of both of the leaflets of the mitral valve inserted into the left ventricular papillary muscle causing obstruction of the blood flow), supravalvular stenosis, subvalvular aortic stenosis and variably present coarctation of the aorta

Paracrine glands see Glands

Paradigm An example, hypothesis, model or pattern; in the usual context, a paradigm refers to a widely accepted explanation for a set or constellation of biomedical (or other) phenomena, which becomes accepted when data accumulates to corroborate aspects of the paradigm's theory, as occurred in the 'central dogma of molecular biology' (which held that only DNA could give rise to new strands of DNA and the only way in which proteins could be encoded was by mRNA transcription from DNA and protein translation from the mRNA transcript); a 'paradigm shift' represents an early decay or incipient collapse in the paradigm that occurs when new data accumulates, which partially invalidates the previously-accepted the theory or which is completely at odds with the paradigm, as occurred when it became evident that RNA could give rise to DNA by way of retroviral reverse transcriptase, which contradicted the tenets of the 'central dogma', see there

Paradoxic effect MICROBIOLOGY A biological variable that affects the interpretation of the minimum lethal concentration of an antibiotic, in which the proportion of surviving bacteria increases with an increased concentration of antibiotics, a phenomenon that is most common in cell wall active agents; see Minimum bactericidal concentration

Paradoxic embolism Emboli that occur when thrombotic material passes through right-to-left cardiac shunts, circumventing the filtering effect of the pulmonary vessels and passes to the general circulation, potentially causing cerebral abscess Clinical Meningeal irritation (stiff neck, drowsiness, fever and headache), focal signs including aphasia, hemiplegia, jacksonian convulsions, increased intracranial pressure and coma

Paradoxic hypertension A hypertensive episode that develops two to three days following surgery in older patients operated for coarctation of the aorta, associated with abdominal pain due to increased pressure in visceral arteries that had, prior to the procedure functioned at lower pressure; the 'jolt' of pressure requires intense antihypertensive medication, without which intestinal ischemia is a serious potential consequence

Paradoxic (overflow) incontinence Constant or intermittent dribbling of urine due to chronic overdistension of the bladder (volume from 1000 to 3000 ml, normal, circa 500 ml), with attenuation of the muscle; this may be confused (and therefore is paradoxic) with pure stress incontinence;

'Paradoxical movement' NEONATOLOGY A misnomer for the respiratory movement of newborns, whose breathing is entirely diaphragmatic; with inspiration, the anterior thorax draws inward and the abdomen protrudes;in the neonate, 'paradoxic breathing' is normal

'Paradoxical nasal obstruction' see Nasal cycle

Paradoxic pulse CARDIOLOGY A decrease of greater than 10 mm Hg in the systolic blood pressure upon inspiration, a finding which like the Kussmaul sign (an abnormal increase instead of a normal fall in jugular venous pressure with inspiration) is strongly suggestive of cardiac tamponade (impaired diastolic filling of the heart due to increased intrapericardiac pressure), clinically characterized by air hunger, mild cyanosis and visible distension of neck veins

'Paradox of the lek' EVOLUTIONARY BIOLOGY A phenomenon described in a vast array of animals (frogs, fish, birds, mammals, man), in which the female selects a mate from a group or 'lek' (which one author facetiously likened to a 'singles bar'), based on elaborate mating displays and other intangible or paradoxical factors (Nature 1991; 350:33)

Paraffin section SURGICAL PATHOLOGY A stained section of tissue mounted on a glass slide and examined by light microscopy; in contrast to the 'frozen section' in which a tissue is examined within minutes of its removal from a patient, 'permanent section' tissues are fixed in formalin and bathed in a series of solutions (in order, formalin, 70% alcohol, 95% alcohol, 100% alcohol, xylene) that dry the tissue and allow its infiltration with paraffin, an optimal embedding material for histologic evaluation of tissue; see Hematoxylin and eosin; Cf Frozen section

Paraganglioma A neural crest tumor that is more common in women that occurs in the head and neck; 2-9% of those in the carotid body, vagal body and jugulotympanic region are malignant; 25% of laryngeal paragangliomas are malignant Criteria for malignancy Central necrosis of zellballen, invasion of vascular spaces and lymph nodes and increased mitotic activity; see Zellballen

Parahemophilia Coagulation factor V deficiency A condition characterized by mild bleeding or petechial hemorrhage or menorrhagia that is either congenital, due to the autosomal recessive defect in the gene for factor V or acquired due to the development of IgA or IgG antibodies to factor V Laboratory Increased partial thromboplastin time and prothrombin time Treatment Fresh plasma

Parallel interface COMPUTERS A port that transmits or receives byte-sized blocks (8 bits) of data at a time; see Computers, Modem

Parallel tracking CLINICAL THERAPEUTICS A recently devised mechanism by which promising therapeutic agents are made available in the USA at an early stage of the drug development process (without interfering with the necessary research studies) to those who are not eligible to participate in clinical trials because of geographic or entry criteria; the research or clinical trials of the drug proceed on one 'track' while the drug is being used for treatment (outside of trials) on a separate or 'parallel track'; although the treatment IND regulations focus on the early availability of experimental drugs to patients with life-threatening situations, the parallel tracking plan, still being developed by the combined efforts of the FDA, NIAID, NAPO (National AIDS Program Office) and drug companies, is aimed at speeding clinical testing and marketing approval of potentially useful new drugs (from the Clinical Trials Office of the NIAID, Rockville, Maryland, Science 1990; 250:1505n&v)

Paralogous An adjective for a protein product that is encoded by genes located at multiple separate loci and/or on different chromosomes

Paralytic ileus GASTROENTEROLOGY Functional 'obstruction' of intestinal flow, often following abdominal surgery; other causes of 'paralytic' ileus include electrolyte abnormalities, eg hypokalemia, drugs including phenothiazine, narcotics, gram-negative sepsis, circulating catecholamines, diabetic ketoacidosis, mesenteric vascular disease, porphyria, retroperitoneal hemorrhage, spinal and pelvic fractures; see Gastroparesis

Paramedic A health professional certified to perform advanced life support procedures, eg intubation, defibrillation and administration of drugs under the direction of a physician; paramedics function in urgent care situations provided from an emergency vehicle or air service; in contrast, an emergency medical technician (EMT) is only certified to perform basic life-support maneuvers

Parana hard skin syndrome An autosomal recessive form of pachydermy of unknown pathogenesis, described in a small geographic region around Parana, Brazil, characterized by rapidly progressive induration of the skin at all joints, retarding growth and 'freezing' the articulations in semi-flexed positions, later resulting in pulmonary insufficiency due to constriction of the thoracic cage and death, which may be associated with mental retardation (Lancet 1974; 1:215)

Paraneoplastic cerebellar degeneration A rare affliction of patients with 'female' cancers, eg breast, ovary, endometrium, associated with cerebellar symptoms of nystagmus, dysarthria and appendicular and gait ataxia that may precede clinical evidence of cancer by months or years Histopathology Extensive Purkinje cell loss, perivascular and leptomeningeal inflammation Pathogenesis Unclear, possibly an autoimmune reaction to two Purkinje cell antigens, CDR62 and CDR34, by an antibody designated anti-Ro (N Engl J Med 1990; 322:1844); see Purkinje cell antibodies

Paraneoplastic syndrome(s) A variegated family of comorbid conditions due to the indirect (remote or 'biologic') effects of malignancy, which may be the first sign of a neoplasm or its recurrence; paraneoplastic syndromes occur in more than 15% of all malignancy, are due to the production of hormones, growth and other as-yet unidentified 'factors', often regressing with adequate treatment of the primary tumor; the range of expression is broad and includes tumor-related cachexia, hormonal effects, neuromuscular disease, eg peripheral neuropathy, myopathy, central nervous system and spinal cord degeneration and inflammation, leukemoid reaction, reactive eosinophilia, peripheral 'cytoses or 'cytopenias, hemolysis, disseminated intravascular coagulation, thromboembolism, thrombophlebitis migrans, renal dysfunction, nephrotic syndrome, uric acid nephropathy, gastrointestinal symptoms (anorexia, vomiting, protein-losing enteropathy, malignant hepatopathy), bullous mucocutaneous lesions, acquired ichthyosis, acanthosis nigricans, dermatomyositis, tylosis, lactic acidosis, hypertrophic pulmonary osteoarthropathy, hyperlipidemia, hypertension, hyperamylasemia and amyloidosis; see Ectopic hormones

Paraneoplastic pemphigus An uncommon autoimmune complex rarely seen in malignancy, especially lymphoproliferative disorders caused by autoantibodies against desmoplakin I, bullous pemphigoid antigen and other epithelial antigens Clinical Persistent and painful erosions of the oropharynx and vermilion border and severe pseudomembranous conjunctivitis, confluent erythema of the skin of the upper trunk (N Engl J Med 1990; 323:1729)

Parasitic limbs PEDIATRICS Duplicated extremities seen in arthrogryposis, which are medial, retroflexed, small, immature and have no clinical evidence of innervation; this rare congenital malformation is subdivided into myogenic and neuropathic forms, the latter of which may be associated with spina bifida or the segmental absence of anterior horn cells

Parathion An acetyl-cholinesterase-inhibiting organophosphate insecticide and nerve poison that forms a stable covalently-bound complex with a serine residue at acetylcholinesterase's active site; acute intoxication is characterized by nicotinic and muscarinic effects which, when severe, may cause respiratory failure within minutes; chronic intoxication may cause demyelinating neuropathy and axonal degeneration Treatment Atropine

Parathyroid panel LABORATORY MEDICINE A battery of tests that has been determined to be the most 'efficient', ie cost-effective, in evaluating calcium and phosphate metabolism, including measurement of calcium, phophate, magnesium, alkaline phosphate, total protein levels, albumin, creatinine and urinary calcium; see Organ panel

Parathyroid 'squeeze' test ENDOCRINOLOGY A clinical test consisting of massaging or gentle compression (squeezing) of the side of the neck that is thought to harbor a parathyroid adenoma, which will respond by increasing serum parathyroid hormone

Paratope IMMUNOLOGY The sum total of the points of contact between an antigen's epitope and an immunoglobulin's hypervariable regions; whereas most of the 120 amino acid positions of the light and heavy chains in the variable regions have < 10% variability, amino acid positions 29-34, 49-52 and 91-95 on the light chain and positions 30-34, 51-63, 84-90 and 101-110 on the heavy chain are veritable 'hot-spots', having 20-60% variability in the amino acid sequence; this variability confers high specificity, defined as an idiotype, and the ability to recognize the vast number of antigenic epitopes; Cf Epitope, 'Hot spots', Idiotype

Parental age see Paternal age

Pareve NUTRITION A food product that is completely devoid of animal-derived products, often equated to the term 'non-dairy'; see Vegan

Parite An intra-arterial fibrous plaque in atherosclerosis, which may display dystrophic calcification

Parking-lot crystals A fanciful descriptor for the parallel, almost herringbone angulation of the crystalloid material seen by electron microscopy in the degenerated mitochondria of 'mitochondrial myopathies'; see Ragged red fiber disease

Parkinson's disease A progressive neurologic disease

characterized by tremors and rigidity followed by inhibition of voluntary movement, a shuffling gait due to neuron degeneration in the substantia nigra and focal loss of dopamine production and, with time, severe mental deterioration; MPTP, a toxic contaminant during the production of certain 'designer drugs', causes a clinical picture mimicking Parkinson's disease; the selective destruction of the dopamine neurons is the direct result of its metabolite, MPP^+ (1-methyl-4-phenylpyridium), an effect reversed by brain-derived neurotrophic factor (Nature 1991; 350:230, 195) **Treatment** L-dopa is effective in early disease, as it is transported to the brain and converted into dopamine, but with time, loses efficacy; 'brain-graft' surgery has proven disappointing in treating parkinsonism, although the related modality, fetal nerve graft (mesencephalic dopamine neurons from 8-9 week fetuses) may prove effective (Science 1990; 247:529), as may be deprenyl, a monoamine oxidase inhibitor that blocks the chemical conversion of MPTP to MPP^+; see BDNF, MPTP, Fetal-brain tissue grafting

Parkinsonism-plus syndromes A generic term for typical Parkinson's disease-like complexes that are accompanied by other neurologic disease, including concomitant impairment of ocular movement, orthostatic hypotension, cerebellar ataxia or dementia; these conditions include olivopontocerebellar degeneration with ataxia, parkinsonism-amyotrophic lateral sclerosis overlap, parkinsonism-dementia (normopressure hydrocephalus, gait disturbance and urinary incontinence), progressive supranuclear palsy with ophthalmoplegia, Shy-Drager syndrome with orthostatic hypotension, striatal degeneration

Paroxysmal atrial tachycardia (PAT) A cardiac arrhythmia initiated by a premature atrial beat conducted through a tract initiated in the AV node; once the ventricle contracts, an echo atrial beat is stimulated via a retrograde tract, resulting in a reverberating re-entry phenomenon, which results in an atrial rate of 180-300 beats/minute; PATs in infants may be life-threatening and result in fatal congestive heart failure; PATs in older children may be secondary to fever, are usually less than 24 hours in duration and relatively benign **Treatment** Simple vagal stimulation, eg carotid sinus massage, an ice bag, breath-holding; if intense, cardioversion or prolonged digoxin therapy

Paroxysmal cold hemoglobinuria (PCH) A disease that 1) Rarely is 'paroxysmal' clinically 2) Not always precipitated by the cold and 3) Does not always cause hemoglobinuria; PCH comprises 2-5% of autoimmune hemolytic anemias and is caused by IgG (Donath-Landsteiner) antibodies that react at $< 15°C$ and are directed against the ubiquitous P antigen on red cells; PCH was first described by Donath and Landsteiner in 1904 in a patient with tertiary syphilis who developed paroxysmal fever, chills, headache and diffuse corporal pain with hemoglobinuria; PCH may be transient and secondary to viral exanthemas of childhood **Clinical** After exposure to the cold, the patient experiences myalgia, abdominal cramping and headaches, hemoglobinuria, Raynaud's phenomenon, cold urticaria and occasionally jaundice **Laboratory** Positive direct Coombs test (using anti-C3 antiserum), anemia, hemoglobinuria, decreased haptoglobin, increased bilirubin and lactate dehydrogenase; the antibody is a non-agglutinating IgG that binds to red cells at cold temperatures and when warmed to 37°C, evokes complement-mediated hemolyses; the Donath-Landsteiner antibody elutes from the red cells in vitro, while the complement remains fixed, thus is a 'biphasic' hemolysin; anti-P reacts with all normal neutrophil antigens except for p and P^k Prevention Maintain the body warm **Treatment** If PCH is chronic, corticosteroids or immunosuppressive therapy

Paroxysmal myoglobinuria see Periodic paralysis

Paroxysmal nocturnal hemoglobinuria (PNH) An acquired hemolytic disease due to the proliferation of an abnormal clone(s) of myeloid stem cells, the progeny of which are highly susceptible to complement-mediated membrane damage, due to a deficiency in the 70 kD delay accelerating factor (DAF); when susceptible erythrocytes are exposed to activated (by classic or alternate pathways) complement, the afflicted red cells bind more C3b than normal; membrane-bound C3b is a positive feedback signal for the alternate complement pathway via factors B and D, resulting in generation of more C3b; C5 convertase and the C5-9 membrane attack complex are activated, resulting in intravascular hemolysis Note: DAF is also absent in platelets and myelocytes from these subjects, making them equally sensitive to complement-mediated lysis **Clinical** Thrombotic tendencies, increased susceptibility to infections; PNH may evolve into aplastic or sideroblastic anemia, myelofibrosis or acute myelogenous leukemia **Laboratory** Leukopenia, thrombocytopenia, dimorphic red cell population, iron-deficiency, decreased leukocyte alkaline phosphatase, decreased erythrocyte acetylcholinesterase alterations of the properdin (alternate pathway of complement lysis) Negative direct Coombs test and increased susceptibility of erythrocytes to complement-mediated hemolysis

Parrot beak syndrome of Waardenburg An autosomal disease with clinical features of Apert and Crouzon syndromes with a typical facies characterized by a parrot-beaked nose, jaw hypoplasia, antimongoloid slant of the eyes, hypertelorism, deformed ears, hydrophthalmos, acrocephalysyndactyly and cleft palate, as well as leukoderma, musculoskeletal contractions of the elbows and knees, congenital heart disease, pseudohermaphroditism, autosomal dominant and recessive; other parrot noses have been described Rubenstein-Taybi disease and Pierre Robin disease; see Bird face

Parrot fever Bird fancier's lung Psittacosis, an infection of birds by ***Chlamydia psittaci*** may cause asymptomatic infection, an influenza-like disease or serious pneumonia in humans who are exposed to feathers, tissues or droppings from a wide variety of birds, which may be sick or carriers of ***C psittaci*** **Clinical** Most cases are asymptomatic; symptomatic cases require a 1-2 week incubation, which is followed by chills, moderate to high fever, slow pulse, severe headache and myalgias, anorexia, nausea, vomiting, arthralgia and mental clouding; pneumonic symptoms are less common with production of minimal mucoid sputum mixed with hemorrhage, and if severe, accompanied by hypoxia and cyanosis Treatment Tetracyclines

Parrot syndromes JM Parrot was transiently honored with two 'Parrot syndromes' 1) Syphilitic osteochondritis (1871) and 2) Failure to thrive (1877)

Parsimony principle see Ockham's razor

Part A One of the two components of the Medicare reimbursement system of the USA, which consists in the compulsory hospital insurance financed by contributions from employers, employees and participants; 'part A' pays for the costs of hospitalization, but does not pay the physicians' fees; see Medicare, Part B, TEFRA

Part B A component of the Medicare reimbursement system that provides supplementary payments for medical services and supplies that are not covered under part A; part B is voluntary, covers physicians' fees and individual provider services and is financed in part by monthly premiums paid by the enrollees and in part by the US federal government; see Medicare, Part A, Participation, TEFRA; Cf Medicaid

Partial thromboplastin time Activated partial thromboplastin time (aPTT) A one-stage coagulation test that is sensitive to deficiencies of antihemophilic factors; aPTT is prolonged in deficiencies of factors V, VIII, IX, X, XI, XII, Fletcher factor, high-molecular weight kininogen, lupus inhibitors and heparin

Partial twinning A group of rare congenital anomalies of cloacally-derived structures, including focal doubling of the alimentary tract beginning at Meckel's diverticulum and extending to the anus, doubling of the bladder, vagina, penis, sacrum or lumbar vertebrae

Participation HEALTH CARE INDUSTRY A neologism for a formal agreement between Medicare and health care providers, ie hospitals and physicians, in which the provider(s) agrees to 'accept assignment', ie accept Medicare's fees as payment in full for any health care services rendered; 48% of US physicians participate, ranging from 20% participation in Idaho to 83% in Alabama, differing in specialties from 72% by nephrologists to 37% by anesthesiologists (Am Med News 10/Jun/91); non-participating providers may charge more for the same services but must submit the bills directly to the patient; participation also refers to the acceptance of an insurance or health plan's established or calculated fee as the maximum amount collectable for the services rendered

Partition chromatography Normal phase chromatography A chromatographic technique in which the distribution of substances in the mobile liquid phase and a stationary liquid phase (which is immobilized on a porous solid, eg a filter paper or on a starch column) is a function of the solubility of the compounds in the two different phases; Cf Reversed phase chromatography

'Partnering' A term of some utility (Science 1990; 250:1643), coined in reference to a recently-observed phenomenon that transcription factors from different classes of molecules, ie those having different structural motifs, could cross-hybridize to form chimeric dimers

Party wall appearance The apparent but not actual sharing of plasma membranes by distinct and separate cells within glands; the 'party wall' effect is described in canalicular adenoma of the salivary glands and in gastric glands with inflammatory atypia in regeneration and is not thought to have neoplastic potential

Parvovirus A small icosahedral single-stranded DNA (class II) virus that is capable of either autonomous intracellular replication or requires that the host cell be co-infected with an adenovirus

Parvus et tardus CARDIOLOGY A small arterial pulse with a delayed systolic peak that may be associated with an anacrotic 'shoulder' on the upstroke of the carotid pulse, a pattern seen in older patients with severe aortic stenosis

'Passenger or driver' controversy The presence of a particular lesion and a specific microorganism in a host cell or tissue with such regularity that it is unclear whether the microorganism (or lesion) is an epiphenomenon, ie a 'passenger' or whether it is pathogenically linked to the lesion, ie a 'driver'; this debate often arises when analyzing scar cancers, or in the common association of human papillomavirus types 16 and 18 with carcinoma of the uterine cervix

Passive-aggression PSYCHIATRY A personality disorder in which the patient expresses personal conflicts through retroflexed anger in the form of covert obstructionism, procrastination, stubbornness and inefficiency; the term was first used by US military psychiatrists during World War II and is part of DSM-III parlance, known in Europe as 'passive sociopathy'; 0.9% or more of the population exhibits passive-aggressive or passive-dependent behavior; the defenses include turning against oneself (a form of sado-masochism), denial, rationalization and hypochondriasis Prognosis for normalization of these individuals is poor; of 73 passive-aggressives followed for 11 years in one series, only 9 were symptom-free, the remainder had persistent psychiatric difficulties, abused alcohol or were clinically depressed; Cf 'Anal-retentive'

Passive anaphylaxis A 'borrowed' anaphylactic reaction that occurs when an organism is exposed to antigens after having been injected with preformed antibodies to the antigen of interest that were 'raised' in another organism; see P-K test

Passive immunity A 'borrowed' and transient immune resistance to various organisms, seen in neonates as a result of the passive transplacental transfer of IgG of maternal origin

Passive smoking (PS) Involuntary 'smoking' by non-smokers who breathe ambient air containing the same carcinogens inhaled by a cigarette smoker; PS is estimated to cause an estimated 2500-8400 excess annual cases of smoking-related malignancy (in the USA); mere physical space separation allows significant reduction in exposure to non-smokers; 'mainstream' smoke is directly inhaled by the smoker, while 'sidestream' or environmental smoke is produced by the smoker, but absorbed more by non-smokers who don't have the benefit of a filter; passive smokers are exposed to dimethylnitrosamine (a potent carcinogen), benzo(a)pyrene and carbon monoxide (CO), acrolein, arsenic, benzene, cyanide, formaldehyde, nitrosamines, radionuclides and others); levels of nicotine in unventilated areas may exceed industrial threshold limit levels (> 500 μg/mm^3); air zones with CO levels of greater than 30 ppm cause a passive smoker to have CO blood levels equivalent to having smoked five or more cigarettes; prolonged exposure to 30 ppm may cause carboxyhemoglobin levels sufficient to impair visual discrimination and cause psychomotor impairment; it has been suggested that 'common courtesy' rules on the part of smokers is insufficient to reduce PS and thus legislation may be necessary to reduce these risks to PS victims (J Am Med Assoc 1990; 263:2208); exposure to three hours/day of PS is reported to be associated with a three-fold increase in cancer of the uterine cervix (J Am Med Assoc 1989; 261:1593); in children, neonates and fetuses, PS is inculpated in poor pulmonary function, bronchitis, pneumonia, otitis media and middle ear effusions, asthma, lower birth and adult weights and heights, sudden infant death syndrome (SIDS) and poor lung (and physical) development, and a higher perinatal mortality (related to placental vascular disease including placenta previa and abruptio placentae); these children are themselves more likely to become smokers and are at increased risk for developing cancer in a dose-related manner, in all sites 50% higher than expected, and up to two-fold greater in non-Hodgkin's lymphoma, acute lymphocytic leukemia and Wilm's tumors; PS by children with cystic fibrosis adversely affects growth and health, resulting in increased hospital admissions and poor performance in pulmonary function tests (N Engl J Med 1990; 323:782); 17% of lung cancer in non-smokers is attributed to high levels of exposure to cigarette smoke during childhood and adolescence (N Engl J Med 1990; 323:632); see Conicotine

Passive transport The movement of solutes across biological membranes by simple diffusion down a concentration gradient, which requires neither energy expenditure nor carrier molecules

Passover phenomenon see Harvest Moon phenomenon

PAS stain HISTOLOGY The periodic acid Schiff reaction results from periodic acid-induced oxidation of hydroxyl groups on hexoses and hexosamines to aldehydes, which then react with a Schiff base, forming a magenta-colored complex; many substances and cells are PAS-positive, including neutral mucosubstances (positive in esophageal, gastric and anal glands), fungi, parasites, ceroid, polysaccharides, glycogen (staining will disappear with amylase treatment), glycolipids and glycoproteins; the PAS stain is optimal for delineating basement membranes and reticulin, for demonstrating the intracytoplasmic crystals in alveolar soft part sarcoma and the bacteria-like inclusions in the macrophages of Whipple's disease, as well as Paget's disease and Gaucher's disease in which PAS demonstrates glucocerebroside

Pass-through phenomenon ENDOCRINOLOGY LABORATORY MEDICINE In the copper reduction test used for glucose determination, when > 11 mmol/24 hour specimen (US: 2.0 gm/24 h) is in the urine, the reagent strip undergoes a rapid transition through the entire spectrum of color changes and to the unwary, simulates the strip's original color and might be interpreted as being negative, resulting in discontinuation of insulin therapy

Pasteur effect The inhibition of certain metabolic pathways by increased oxygen, causing oxidative phosphorylation, yielding increased ATP, which inhibits phosphofructokinase, resulting in decreased glycolysis and a decrease in lactic acid accumulation

Pasteurization Heat 'sterilization' of food products, devised by Louis Pasteur to destroy the bacteria responsible for spoilage of wine and beer, for which it continues to be used; pasteurization of milk requires heating to 62C for 30 minutes or to 80° C for 15-30 seconds (flash pasteurization), temperatures that destroy all potential pathogens

PAT 1) see Paroxysmal atrial tachycardia 2) Preadmission testing A battery of tests required prior to hospital admission for elective therapy, eg cataract extraction or cholecystectomy, which serve to establish baseline values and parameters; in a community hospital setting, a typical PAT battery includes a CBC ('complete blood count') and leukocyte differential count, prothrombin and partial thromboplastin time, a multichannel analysis of blood chemistries, a complete urinalysis, an electrocardiogram and a chest film

Patch and cut repair MOLECULAR BIOLOGY A mechanism of DNA repair, in which a damaged segment of DNA is excised by the DNA ligase only after the segment has been repaired by a DNA nuclease

Patch-clamp technique Voltage clamp technique NEUROPHYSIOLOGY A technique in which a micropipette is used to remove by suction, a minuscule (0.5 μm in diameter) patch of plasma membrane that bears one or only a few ion channels; the patch is clamped and the potential of the ions flowing across the patch is measured, thus evaluating the effect on the membrane potential of the closing and opening of single channels and measurement of the different ion compositions of solutions on either side of the membranes; this simple technique resulted in the discovery of ion channels in cell membranes and has provided vast information about the cell and nerve physiology; its co-developers, E Naher and B Sakmann of the Max-Planck Institute were awarded the 1991 Nobel prize (Science 1991; 254:380n)

Patching IMMUNOLOGY Aggregation on the surface of a lymphocyte of membrane receptor proteins that have been cross-linked by lectins and antibodies, a step that precedes 'capping' and internalization of antigen-antibody complex for processing of the antigen and presentation of the antigen in the context of a major histocompatibility complex; see Capping

Patch testing An epicutaneous patch test devised in 1895 by Jadassohn to measure contact (delayed-type) sensitivity, which consists of applying a patch with a low dose of a potentially allergenic substance to an unexposed body part and observing the site 1-2 days later; the skin of modern man is subjected to numerous organic and inorganic chemicals including toxins, carcinogens, irritants and allergens; up to 5% of the general population has dermatitis and 7% or more of dermatology practice consists in management of allergic contact dermatitis;

50% of occupational absenteeism is related to contact dermatitis (Mayo Clin Proc 1989; 64:415rv)

Patent A document that grants an inventor in terms of a determined number of years, the exclusive right to make use of and sell his invention; the duration of US patents is 17 years with an extension for up to eight years (if the product was in the regulatory approval process, eg FDA); when a commercial product is invented in academics, the holder(s) of the patent is required to share income with various departments in the university; at Harvard, the patent holder(s) retain 25-35%, the department where the holder(s) works retains 30-40% (one half for the holder(s)' research activities, one half for the department), the dean and president retain 20% and 15% respectively, for their own technology transfer funds and for use in teaching (for review of the US Patent and Trademark Office, see Science 1991; 253:20n&v)

Paternalism LEGAL MEDICINE The practice of interacting with a patient as a father to a child, ie carrying out acts intended to benefit the child that may either limit his freedom or be contrary to his wishes; the principle is subdivided into a) **WEAK PATERNALISM**, in which the person is substantially incompetent or very young and b) **STRONG PATERNALISM**, in which the person is competent and may fully realize the impact of a decision made for him; strongly paternalistic acts, eg medicating a dying Christian Scientist (see Christian Science), is an issue with considerable legal impact, as forcing therapy against a patient's wishes may result in the criminal charges of assault and battery against the medical team; Cf Doctor-patient interaction

Paternity testing FORENSIC MEDICINE A battery of tests required to determine, with reasonable or absolute certainty, a child's genetic parents **DIRECT EXCLUSION OF PATERNITY** 1) The child has a genetic marker that is absent in the mother and not present in the father; in complex systems where a child lacks all paternal antigens, the putative father is excluded or 2) The child is an 'amorph', ie does not express a gene present in both mother and father **INDIRECT EXCLUSION OF PATERNITY** 1) A gene is present in the child that can be transmitted only by a male, and which the putative father does not have 2) The child is homozygous for markers not seen in a parent or 3) The parent is homozygous for a marker not seen in the child (paternity is excluded); indirect exclusions are accepted when confirmed by a second method by another laboratory Note: Genetic markers are used in 'classic' paternity testing, but those of very high or very low frequencies are of limited value in differentiating among individuals, although very low frequency genetic markers are used to determine statistical likelihood of paternity; genetic markers include red cell antigens (M-N, S-s, Rh-C-c, Rh-E-e, K-k, Fy^a-Fy^b, Jk^a-Jk^b), various erythrocyte enzymes (adenosine deaminase, glucose-6-phosphate dehydrogenase) isomers, HLA antigens, immunoglobulin allotypes and non-immunoglobulin serum proteins; since the late 1980s, DNA 'fingerprinting' has become the legally accepted way of establishing or excluding parentage, using the 'Jeffries' probe; the issue of parentage comprises the majority of court cases in India and the CCMB of Hyderabad has patented its own DNA probe based on the repetitive GATA sequence isolated from the poisonous snake, the banded krait

Paternal age Although increased maternal age is associated with chromosome defects in the progeny, often occurring in trisomies, there is also an increased incidence of certain conditions in children born to older men, including achondroplasia (N Engl J Med 1986; 314:521), Klinefelter syndrome and Marfan's disease; paternal chromosomal abnormalities occur in 2.6% of habitual abortion and most are translocations, occurring at a ten-fold greater rate than normal (Fertil and Steril 1978;29:414); see Maternal age

Pathergy see Necrosis

Pathologists' disease Any lesion that is defined as malignant by histological criteria, which is detected as an incidental finding and which in clinical practice is regarded as a non-aggressive lesion, not requiring treatment, eg pancreatic endocrine carcinoma or well-differentiated adenocarcinoma of the prostate Note: The concept of 'benign malignancy' appears to require re-evaluation, as 16% of stage A1 carcinomas of the prostate, traditionally regarded as a 'pathologist's tumor', followed for 10 years progress to higher stages and require therapy (Urology 1990; 36:210)

Patient 'Bill of Rights' (and responsibilities) A statement developed by the American Hospital Association that delineates the treatment that a person has a right to expect while he is a patient in a hospital and the behavior that is expected of the patient with respect to his own therapy, follow-up and conduct while in the hospital

Patient compliance The strictness to which the patient adheres to the physician's regimen, diet, treatment and whether the patient returns for re-examination, follow-up or treatment; poor patient compliance with a prescribed plan of therapeutic action may result in complications that are beyond the physician's control and must be documented to prevent legal action by the patient or his estate, should non-compliance prove fatal

Patient-controlled analgesia (PCA) A method that allows patients to self-administer intravenous narcotic-analgesic drugs via a programmable pump, a modality of use in managing post-operative pain and for patients in the latter stages of terminal cancer, allowing them to obtain pulse doses above baseline level and a degree of autonomy over one's own pain medication; see Pain

Patient dumping see Dumping

Patient 'mix' The demographics of a patient population being served by a hospital, classified according to disease severity, see Case-mix index or according to socioeconomic parameters

Patient-physician relationship A formal relation that exists between the physician and the patient, often equated to medical 'duties' that the physician must perform in a professionally acceptable manner Note: Mere conversation with a patient may be sufficient in the eyes of a court to establish such a relation; in this regard, referral of a patient to a specialist or termination of a relation must be documented, or it may be considered 'abandonment'; Cf Doctor-patient interaction

'Patient zero' A French-Canadian airline steward, whose promiscuity linked him epidemiologically to 40 of the first 248 men to be diagnosed of what had been called gay-related immune deficiency (GRID), a disease now known as AIDS; 'patient zero' died of terminal renal failure, and had had four episodes of ***Pneumocystis carinii*** pneumonia; the true 'patient zero' is unknown as earlier cases of AIDS are being discovered from sera that were stored for decades from patients who had died of unusual immunodeficiency syndromes; the earliest presumed case of AIDS in the USA occurred in a 15 year-old male homosexual who died in the St Louis City Hospital in 1968 with florid lymphogranuloma venereum, culture-confirmed chlamydial infection, lymphopenia, CMV, Epstein-Barr virus, Herpes simplex infection (and HIV-1 by Western blot), depletion of the lymphoid tissue, anergy to tuberculosis and histoplasmin, a positive Frei test and Kaposi sarcoma (J Am Med Assoc 1988; 260:2085); an earlier 'patient zero' was an unmarried Manchester seaman who probably acquired the infection in voyages to Africa in 1955-57 and died of a puzzling immunodeficiency (Lancet 1960; 2:951), whose stored serum proved to be HIV-1 positive by the polymerase chain reaction (Lancet 1990; 336:51)

Pavor nocturnus Nightmare

PBC see Primary biliary cirrhosis

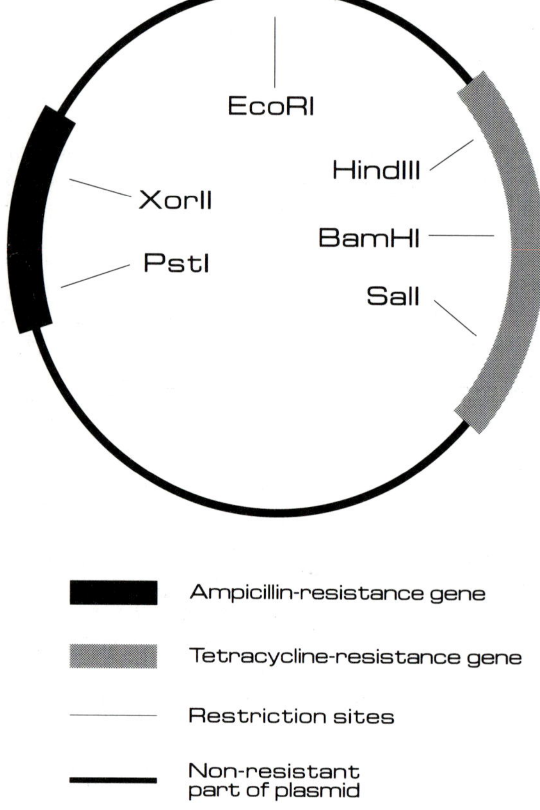

pBR 322 MOLECULAR BIOLOGY A circular plasmid widely used as a cloning vector for amplifying a segment of DNA of interest; pBR322 is itself a recombinant DNA molecule and has unique restriction endonuclease sites (*Eco*RI, *Hind* III, *Bam* HI, *Sph* I, *Sal* I, *Xma* III) in the tetracycline resistance gene and restriction endonuclease sites (Pst I, Pvu I) in the ampicillin resistance gene, sites which allow rapid identification (screening) of bacteria bearing these colonies

PC Personal computer, Professional corporation

PCA see Patient-controlled analgesia

PCB Polychlorinated biphenyl(s) ENVIRONMENT A family of chemicals that were widely used in industry for fluid-filled capacitors and transformers, hydraulic tanks, plasticizers, resins and carbonless copy paper; the commercial products, known in the US as aroclors are complex mixtures of PCB homologs and isomers and are highly persistent in the environment; PCBs were banned in 1979 due to their toxicity **Pathophysiology** PCBs induce increased steroid hydroxylase and cytochrome oxidase activity, as well as increased drug turnover by inducing endoplasmic reticulum **Clinical, acute** PBC poisoning Chloracne, hyperpigmentation and meibomian gland dilatation; biodegradation of PCBs is limited to molecules with less than five chlorides; anaerobic organisms, eg DCB1 have been identified in sediment from the Hudson river (which passes between New York and New Jersey, both active producers of industrial waste including PCBs) reduce the highly chlorinated PCBs into mono- and dichlorobiphenyls which are then more easily degraded by aerobic bacteria Note: Bacterial dechlorination of PBCs may be accelerated by adding an electron donor, eg vitamin C, exposing PBC to sunlight and maintaining the contaminated soil well hydrated (Science 1988; 242:752); see Yucheng disease, Yusho disease

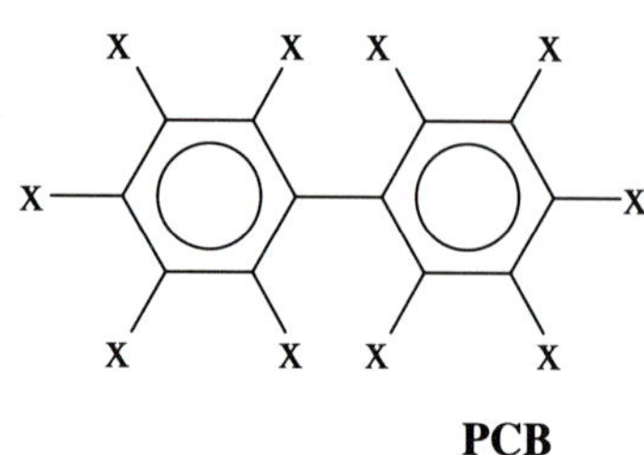

PCDD Polychlorinated dibenzo-p-dioxins see Dioxin

PCDF Polychlorinated dibenzofuran(s) see Dioxin

P cell Pacemaker cell A specialized ovoid-to-stellate, 5-10 µm in diameter myocyte found in clusters in the sinus node of the heart, which has few mitochondria, little sarcoplasmic reticulum and myofibrils and is thus assumed to be an electrical rather than a contractile cell; Cf T cells

PCH see Paroxysmal cold hemoglobinuria

PCO see Polycystic ovaries

P-component CARDIOLOGY One of the two components of amyloid detected by electron microscopy; the major component is fibrillary and has a characteristic periodicity; the minor or P-component, appears as stacks of pentagonal doughnut-like structures with a hollow core, forming short rods, similar to the histiocytosis X body (external diameter, 9 mm, internal, 4 mm); the P-component circulates as a soluble serum protein and is of unknown significance

PCP 1) see Phencyclidine 2) see *Pneumocystis carinii* pneumonia

PCR see Polymerase chain reaction

PCTA see Percutaneous transluminal coronary angioplasty

PDGF see Platelet-derived growth factor

PDGF-B protein Platelet-derived growth factor-B protein A protein with homology to the v-*sis* oncogene product; PDGF-B protein residues 105-144 are responsible for conformational alterations in receptor interaction and may be related to the greater transforming potency of the B protein chain (Science 1990; 248:1541); PDGF-B protein may have a role in atherosclerosis, a disease of large and medium-sized arteries characterized by focal thickening of the inner vessel wall; growth-regulatory molecules may be involved in intimal proliferation and accumulation of smooth muscle cells, which in turn is responsible for the vasoocclusive lesions of atherosclerosis, as the PDGF-B chain is present within macrophages at all phases of atherosclerosis (Science 1990; 248:1009);

P-disc see Optochin disc

PDR Physicians Desk Reference A book published annually (Medical Economics, Oradell, NJ) that lists the approximately 2500 therapeutic agents that in the USA require a physician prescription; the book is divided into seven color-coded sections *White* Manufacturers' index, containing the company addresses and list of products *Pink* Product name index, an alphabetical listing of the drugs by brand name *Blue* Product classification, where drugs are subdivided into therapeutic classes *Yellow* Generic and chemical name index *Multicolored* Photographs of the most commonly prescribed tablets and capsules *White* Product information, a reprint of the manufacturers' product inserts and *Green* Diagnostic product information, a list of manufacturers of diagnostic tests used in office practice and the hospital; Cf Over-the-counter drugs

Peach pit appearance A fanciful descriptor for the 70-85 µm eggs of *Hymenolepis diminuta*, in which the six-hooked oncosphere is surrounded by a membrane separated by a large space from the outer shell, a space likened to the peach flesh itself

'Peak E' 1,1'-ethylidenebis[tryptophan] A novel amino acid recently identified in and held responsible for the eosinophilia-myalgia syndrome, so designated as it causes a peak or spike on the paper or 'hard copy' when analyzed by high-performance chromatography (Science 1990; 250:1707); see Eosinophilia-myalgia syndrome

'Peak' Peak level Therapeutic drug monitoring The maximum serum level of free or unbound drug, a value used to monitor antibiotic therapy where success depends on high levels of antibiotics in the infected site(s), while maintaining the drug below toxic levels, as is required to avoid nephro- and ototoxicity in aminoglycoside therapy; the 'peak' is usually measured about one-half hour after an oral dose of a drug; Cf Trough levels

Pearl index Obstetrics A formula that facilitates comparison of the efficacy of the method of contraception, calculated as the pregnancy rate in population divided by 100 years of exposure (table); see Condoms, Morning-after pill, Norplant, RU 486

Pearly An adjectival descriptor of the opalescent sheen seen in the colonies of *Bordetella pertussis*

Pearl index (pregnancies/100 years of use)

Physiologic 15-30/100 years Coitus interruptus, natural family planning (rhythm or safe period), eg calender method, evaluation of cervical mucusa or temperature

Chemical 15-20/100 years Contraceptive sponges

Barrier methods 2-20/100 years Intrauterine devices, condoms

Hormonal 1-3/100 years

Surgical << 1/100 years Ligation of fallopian tubes, ligation of vas deferens

Pear-shaped bladder see Tear-drop bladder

Pea soup stool A descriptor for the khaki-green, slimy stools typically seen in the third week of typhoid fever at which point the patients are in a 'toxic state' and at greatest risk for intestinal perforation and hemorrhage; similar stools occur in enteropathic *Escherichia coli* infections of infants

Peau d'orange appearance Pigskin A widely-used adjectival descriptor for any bosselated, rugose surface, usually of the skin with deep, pin-point dimpling that was first likened by French authors to the skin of an orange; the 'classic' peau d'orange change occurs in the skin overlying breast cancer Ophthalmology A fundo-

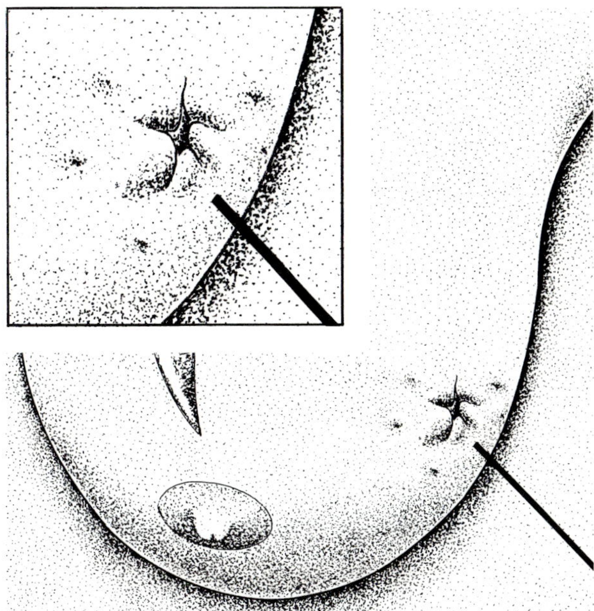

Peau d'orange change, skin

scopic finding corresponding to diffuse, rugose hyperpigmentation of the retinal epithelium in patients with angioid streaks RADIOLOGY One of three radiologic patterns of monostotic fibrous dysplasia, which is described as delicately increased trabeculation with increased opacity and peau d'orange-like mottling of edges of the osseous lesion; monostotic fibrous dysplasia may also appear as a small unilocular radiolucency with sharp borders or as a poorly-circumscribed, radiopacity with innumerable, delicate trabeculations that blends with adjacent normal bone SKIN Peau d'orange-like changes of the skin are classically seen in advanced duct cell carcinoma of breast, in which there is subcutaneous 'puckering'(figure, page 537) accompanied by dermal edema, desmoplastic induration, superficial bossellation, erythema, local tenderness that may be accompanied by ulceration; peau d'orange skin changes may also be seen in 1) Eosinophilic fasciitis, characterized by diffuse leathery induration of the skin with deep furrows, seen in advanced disease with thickened collagen bundles in the lower third of the reticular dermis, entrapment of the eccrine glands, hyalinization, inflammation and induration of the fibrous septae 2) Thrombophlebitis of the superficial veins of the breast (Mondor's disease), in which the skin is dimpled by compressible vessels 3) Erysipelas Group A streptococcal infection, characterized by sharply demarcated, raised and painful skin lesions, occurring in patients who are very sick and febrile with cellulitis of the lower legs arising in fissures between the toes in tinea pedis 4) Myxedema, appearing as 'doughy' puckering and thickening in the skin due to deposition of glycosaminoglycans with accentuation of the follicular orifices in a background of non-pitting plaques and nodules 5) Traumatic fat necrosis, most common in the breast with minimal trauma and which may present with fixation of the skin to the fascial planes 6) Plaque stage of mycosis fungoides 7) Pyogenic granuloma, characterized by a bosselated mucocutaneous surface overlying a lesion that is neither pyogenic (purulent), nor a granuloma, but rather is a florid proliferation of vessels or a granulation tissue reaction

Pectin(s) A heterogeneous family of highly-branched, highly-hydrated and glucuronic acid-rich polysaccharides derived from fruit and used to produce gelling agents

Pediatric AIDS Children who acquire HIV perinatally have a very poor prognosis, often becoming symptomatic (lymphoid interstitial pneumonia, encephalopathy, recurrent bacterial infection and candida esophagitis) within the first year; the five-year mortality is about 50% (N Engl J Med 1989; 321:1791); see AIDS

Pediatric fibromatoses see Fibromatoses

Pediatric trauma score (PTS) EMERGENCY MEDICINE A triage tool that has no advantage over the easier-to-learn Revised Trauma Score; the PTS measures six parameters (weight, airway, systolic pressure, central nervous system status, open wound and skeletal trauma) J Am Med Assoc 1990; 263:69, N Engl J Med 1991; 324:1477)

Pedigree Clinical genetics An ancestral chart of the blood relatives and mates of a patient (index patient) with a disease or hereditary characteristic of interest (figure)

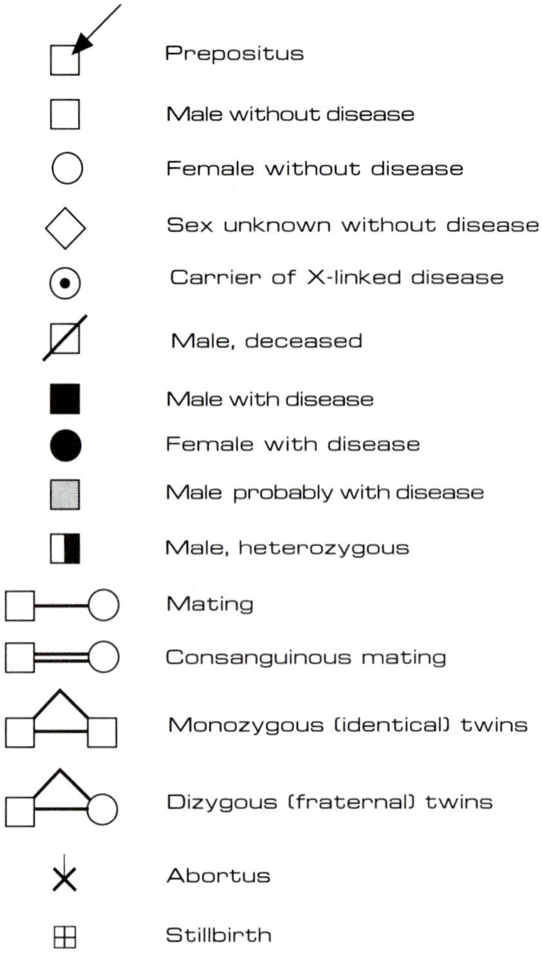

Prepositus
Male without disease
Female without disease
Sex unknown without disease
Carrier of X-linked disease
Male, deceased
Male with disease
Female with disease
Male probably with disease
Male, heterozygous
Mating
Consanguinous mating
Monozygous (identical) twins
Dizygous (fraternal) twins
Abortus
Stillbirth

Pedigree symbols

Note: The name is of Latin derivation, pes for foot and grus for crane, as a pedigree chart has an appearance likened to that of a crane's foot

PEEP Positive end-expiratory pressure A therapeutic modality that consists in the active (interventional) maintenance of a slightly positive pressure in the tracheobronchial tree during assisted pulmonary ventilation, such that the alveoli are not allowed to completely collapse between breaths; PEEP is of greatest use in adult respiratory distress syndrome (ARDS) and is generated by attaching an airflow threshold resistance device to the expiratory port of the non-rebreathing valve of a manual or mechanical ventilator, allowing a decrease of airway pressure to a plateau level Disadvantages Increased intrathoracic pressure results in decreased cardiac output and may cause alveolar rupture and possible pneumothorax; forms of PEEP Prophylactic PEEP The pressure is maintained at 1-5 cm H_2O, preventing atelectasis, while increasing the functional residual capacity above closing volume Conventional PEEP The pressure is maintained at 5-20 cm H_2O and is indicated where an inhaled oxygen fraction at 0.6 cannot maintain the PaO_2 above 60 Torr High PEEP The pressure is maintained at 20-50 cm H_2O

and is of use in marked hypoxia, as may occur in severe pulmonary edema

Peeping Tom 'syndrome' see Sexual deviancy

Peer review The objective evaluation of a physician's or scientist's performance by colleagues, which may take the form of either 1) Peer review of articles for publication in official organs of communication, ie journals (see J Am Med Assoc 1990; 263:1317-1440) or 2) Review of the quality, necessity and appropriateness (suitability) of care provided by an individual physician, ie Peer review organizations (PROs), which in the US contract with the Health Care Financing Administration

Peer reviewed journal (PRJ) ACADEMIA A professional journal that only publishes articles that have been subjected to a peer review process, which entails sending the manuscript to physicians or scientists with expertise in an area related to the subject matter in the article; because the 'submission-to-acceptance' ratio may be 5:1 or more, PRJs are rightly regarded as elitist and canonical, ie certifying original thought and medical progress; acceptance of articles in such journals is considered an indicator of appropriate scholarship for an academician seeking career advancement (J Am Med Assoc 1991; 266:2830c); Cf Throwaway journal

Peer review organization see PRO

PEG 1) Percutaneous endoscopic gastrostomy GASTROENTEROLOGY A method of placement of an enteric feeding tube that avoids the costs and morbidity of surgical intervention to achieve the same goal (J Am Med Assoc 1991; 265:1426) 2) Polyethylene glycol THERAPEUTICS An inert long-chain synthetic molecule that may be attached to various proteins making them invisible to the immune system; multiple PEGs have been attached to ADA (adenosine deaminase), one of the enzymes responsible for SCID, allowing long-term survival of the molecule within the body; PEG has been attached to hemo globin, and has potential as a transport vehicle for artificial blood (Science 1990; 248:305c); in the management of surgical patients, PEG has been used to mechanically purge the large intestine in preparation for surgery

Peg cells see Hobnail cells

Peg teeth Incisors with a barrel-shaped deformity, which when accompanied by a central notch are known as Hutchinson's teeth, a 'classic' finding in congenital syphilis that may also be seen in Williams (elfin-facies) syndrome, anhidrotic, hipohidrotic and the Robinson types of ectodermal dysplasia

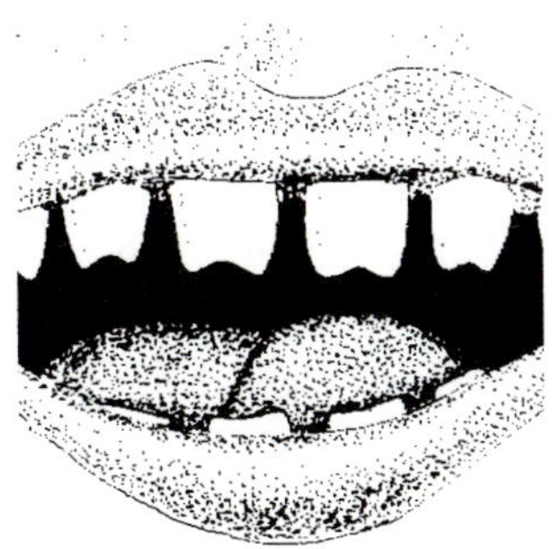

Peg teeth

PEH see Pseudoepitheliomatous hyperplasia

Peliosis hepatis An enlarged liver characterized by multiple cavernous blood-filled cysts related to the use of contraceptives and androgenic steroids and occasionally associated with malignancy and tuberculosis; a distinct form, known as bacillary peliosis hepatis has been described in HIV-positive subjects, see Bacillary angiomatosis

Pellagrous 'boot' A sharply-demarcated erythema affecting the acral portion of the leg or arm (pellagrous 'glove'), a clinical manifestation of severe niacin deficiency that may be exacerbated by sun exposure; a vesiculo-bullous variant of niacin deficiency known as Casal's necklace occurs in the head and neck **Histopathology** Dermal edema, superficial collagen degeneration, chronic perivascular inflammation and hyperkeratosis; see Ds (the three Ds)

Pellet The aggregated membrane-derived materials, fragmented organelles and macromolecules at the bottom on a centrifuge tube; Cf Button

Pelvic floor SURGICAL ANATOMY A well-defined region that is bordered anteriorly by the pubis and posteriorly by the sacrum, laterally by the ischial and iliac bones, superiorly by the peritoneum and inferiorly by the levator ani and coccygeus muscles, the last-named forming the pelvic diaphragm; pelvic organs include the uterus and adnexae, anteriorly, the bladder, posteriorly the rectum and neurovascular tissues; see North American operation, Frozen pelvis

Pelvic inflammatory disease (PID) GYNECOLOGY An imprecise term for the intense pain due to direct extension of a lower genital tract infection (often sexually-transmitted) along the mucosa, first causing asymptomatic endometritis, followed by acute salpingitis and increasing symptoms as it spreads into fallopian tubes that become engorged with pus (pyosalpinx) and purulent leakage into the peritoneum; PID is accompanied by leukostasis, fever, chills, nausea and vomiting, extreme tenderness of the uterine cervix and adnexae **Epidemiology** PID appears to be more common in those non-caucasians, of low education levels, who begin sexual intercourse earlier and who have increased coital activity; PID is reported to be three-to-four-fold more common in IUD users and in those who douche three or more times/month (J Am Med Assoc 1990; 263:1936); ectopic pregnancy is seven-to-ten-fold more common in PID; 500 000 cases of PID are reported/year in the US, 50% of which are due to *N gonorrhoeae*, less commonly, *Chlamydia trachomatis*; 15% of those with gonococcal cervicitis develop PID **Clinical** Severe pain, peritonitis, low-grade fever **Complications** Fallopian tube scarring, infertility

Pencil-in-cup sign Mortar-and-pestle sign RHEUMATOLOGY A tapering of the convexity and exaggeration of the opposite concavity (figure, page 540) in the distal phalangeal articulation(s), which is accompanied by osteoporosis and seen in the atrophic neuropathic arthropathy of both severe psoriatic and rheumatoid arthropathy

'Penciling' A descriptor for the marked resorption of the distal phalanges (acro-osteolysis), a radiologic finding typical of scleroderma that may be idiopathic or which may also occur in severe burns accompanied by soft tissue contractures, 'black toe' disease (ainhum), hyperparathyroidism, neural leprosy, lupus erythematosus, neuropathic disease, eg diabetes mellitus, tabes dorsalis,

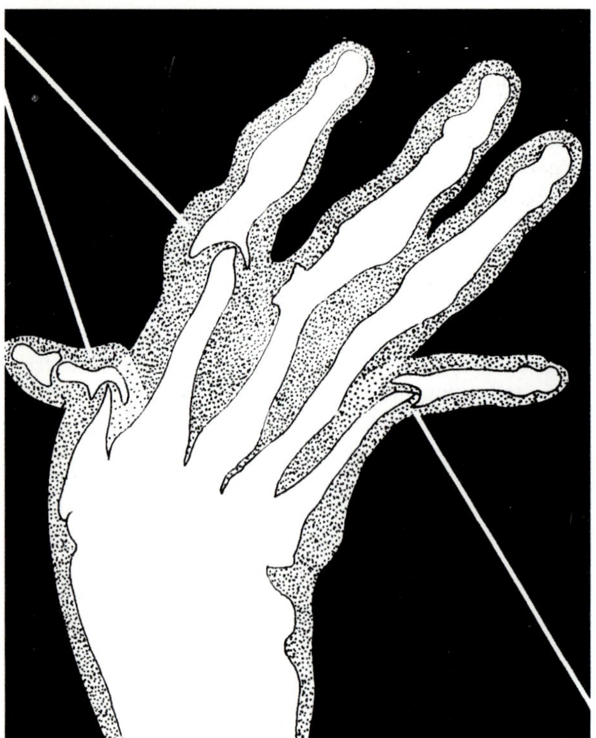

Pencil-in-cup sign

progeria, psoriatic arthritis, exposure to polyvinylchloride, Reiter syndrome and sarcoidosis; Cf Spade deformity

Pencil-point thinness Marked attenuation of the cortex of long bones, seen in advanced scurvy of young children

'Pencil pusher' A derogatory colloquialism for any low-level bureaucrat, eg in an academic center, hospital, regulatory or reimbursement agency

Penem A member of the β-lactam group of broad-spectrum antibiotics, which act on the bacterial cell wall and lyse bacteria that are in the resting phase, thus contrasting with penicillins that kill only those bacteria which are in the growth phase by inhibition of cell wall synthesis

Penetrance Penetration The disruption of a surface, as in penetrating, eg gunshot wounds, hospital-acquired penetration contact due to infected 'sharps', or forcible penetration in rape GENETICS The degree to which a genotype will be phenotypically expressed when the genes for a condition are present in full complement, which in a single gene trait, requires one allele with the gene of interest in an autosomal dominant condition or both alleles (homozygosity) in an autosomal recessive condition

Penguin gait A fanciful descriptor for the waddling gait of patients with muscular dystrophy in whom there is marked exaggeration of the lumbar lordosis, a rolling of the hips from side to side in the stance phase of each forward step (in order to shift the weight of the body), exaggerated lateral tilting and rotation of the pelvis to compensate for the weakened gluteal muscles accompanied by overuse of the trunk and upper extremities during ambulation

Penicillinase-producing *Neisseria gonorrhoeae* (PPNG) Any of a number of strains of *N gonorrhoeae*, many of which have penicillinase-producing plasmids; PPNG are common in non-caucasian illicit drug abusers, prostitutes and their sexual partners (J Am Med Assoc 1989; 261:2357); other penicillinase producers include *Staphylococcus aureus*, which comprise the majority of penicillinase producing organisms, *Haemophilus influenza* and *Escherichia coli* Note: 21% of *N gonorrhoeae* isolates are resistant to penicillin, tetracycline, cefoxitin, spectinomycin (2.2% PPNG, 1.0% plasma-mediated tetracycline-resistant *N gonorrheae*, 16.8% chromosome-mediated, ie non-plasmid-mediated antibiotic resistance) Treatment Ceftriaxone (J Am Med Assoc 1990; 264:1413); see Methicillin-resistant *Staphylococcus aureus*

Penicillin binding protein (PBP) An enzyme required for the synthesis of the bacterial cell wall; the PBP gene is mutated in some strains of β-lactam-resistant pneumococci, resulting in excess enzyme production, circumventing penicillin's negative action on cell wall synthesis (J Am Med Assoc 1991; 265:14n&v)

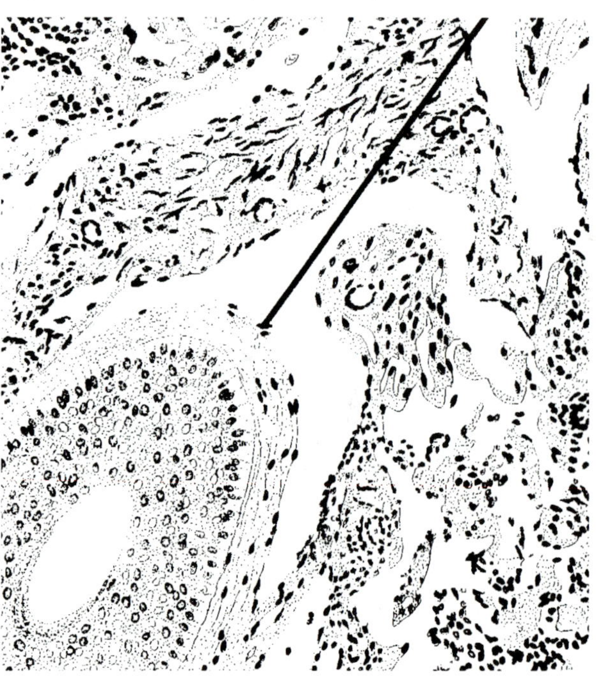

Peninsula (promontory) sign

Peninsula sign A histopathological finding seen in the patch (early) stage of Kaposi sarcoma, in which pre-existing vessels and/or hair follicles (figure, above) jut into widely dilated, jagged, thin-walled neoplastic vascular spaces, which are lined by attenuated endothelial cells that surround pre-existing superficial and periadnexal vascular plexuses

Penn State heart An artificial heart that was designed to serve as a 'bridge', prior to transplantation of a permanent heart; the longest survival with this heart was 13 months; all recipients of this heart have died; see Jarvik-

7, Ventricular assist device

Pentamidine isoethionate A second-line agent used to treat *Pneumocystis carinii* pneumonia in AIDS patients who do not respond to trimethoprim-sulfamethoxazole; Optimal prophylactic administration is by aerosol, reducing the episodes of *P carinii* by 65% (N Engl J Med 1990; 323:769) Adverse reactions Potentially severe, including arrhythmia, azotemia, hypotension, sterile abscesses at the injection site, pancreatitis, diabetes mellitus and dose-related, potentially life-threatening hypoglycemia (J Am Med Assoc 1988; 260:345)

Penta-X syndrome see XXXXX syndrome

Pentraxin family A group of circulating glycoproteins with cyclic pentameric symmetry that includes C-reactive protein complement C1 and serum amyloid P (N Engl J Med 1990; 323:508)

PEPCK Phosphoenolpyruvate carboxykinase A protein that governs the rate-limiting step in gluconeogenesis; transcription of the PEPCK gene and subsequent gluconeogenesis is increased by glucocorticoids and adenosine 3',5'-monophosphate and decreased by insulin, all three molecules for which the gene has recognition sites (Science 1990; 249:533)

Pepper commission (plan) A \$86 x 10^9 health plan approved by a US Congressional committee (named after Representative Claude Pepper who chaired the committee before he died), intended to provide a) either job-based or public health insurance-based access to medical coverage for all Americans and b) provide home and community-based care and three months of nursing home care to people of all ages; Cf Catastrophic health insurance (N Engl J Med 1990; 323:1005)

Pepper syndrome Massive metastatic involvement of liver by neuroblastoma resulting in the 'peppering' of the hepatic parenchyma by innumerable small dark aggregates of tumor cells, described by W Pepper (Am J Med Sci 1901; 121:287), giving rise to one form of 'blueberry infant'

Peppermint stick candy bones A fanciful descriptor for the radiologic appearance of some cases of osteopetrosis, in which the defect in osteoclastic activity is intermittent, giving rise to radiodense and radiolucent bands, most often in the bony pelvis, paralleling the iliac crest

Peptide map BIOCHEMISTRY A two-dimensional 'fingerprint' of a protein that has been first digested with an enzyme, eg trypsin, followed by thin-layer chromatography in one direction (dimension) and electrophoresis at pH 6.5 in the other direction (Proc Nat Acad Sci [USA] 1990; 87:26)

Peptide T A short polypeptide present in HIV-1's envelope that had been proposed as having potential for treating AIDS and later discarded prior to reaching the investigational new drug stage fo development

Peptide YY A 36-residue peptide produced in the distal ileum and proximal colon that is released by fatty foods and thought to be involved in secretion of pancreatic enzymes

Peptone A variable in length, hydrolyzed mixture of short polypeptide chains that are not precipitated by ammonium sulfate, which may be used in commercial preparations of culture media in the microbiology laboratory

Per capita consumption (foods, US) The average American has become more obese, as measured by triceps skin thickness, but is apparently eating better; between 1963-1980, he decreased his animal fat consumption by 39%, butter by 33%, tobacco by 27%, milk by 24% and eggs by 12%; in addition, he increased his consumption of vegetable oils by 58% and fish by 22%, changes that are in part responsible for the 53% decrease in atherosclerosis-related death and a 38% decrease in cerebrovascular accidents (both of which peaked in 1968)

Per cutaneous transluminal coronary angioplasty (PCTA) CARDIOLOGY A technique of interventional angiography introduced in 1977 for treating coronary arteries stenosed by atherosclerosis and by 1990, an estimated 150 000 PCTA procedures are performed annually in the USA; PCTA consists of balloon expansion of one or more stenosed coronary arteries and is indicated for single and multivessel disease, stable and unstable angina and acute infarction; up to 90% of PCTA procedures are successful under optimal conditions, with re-stenosis occurring in 30%, although it is unclear whether PCTA's long-term outcome is better than coronary artery bypass (J Am Med Assoc 1989; 261:2109rv); when PCTA is compared to tissue plasminogen activator (TPA) combined with heparin and aspirin therapy after an acute myocardial infarction, coronary arteriography, PCTA is indicated only in those cases with demonstrable ischemia (TIMI-II data, N Engl J Med 1989; 320:618); a 60-70% success rate in renovascular hypertension due to atherosclerosis and 90% success in fibromuscular hyperplasia have been reported in renal arteries treated with transluminal angioplasty Note: PCTA is associated with a 3-7% risk of in-hospital coronary closure, a complication that may be prevented by using a balloon-expandable, flexible metallic coil-type coronary artery stent (Mayo Clin Proc 1991; 66:268); see Coronary artery bypass surgery, Excimer laser therapy; Cf Balloon valvoplasty

Per diem Latin, by the day *Adjective* The practice by hospitals of charging 'daily' rates, where the expenses incurred on a daily basis are averaged over the entirety of the hospital's census; those who utilize few services will in a sense 'subsidize' those with more expensive and/or extensive and complicated hospital stays *Noun* A temporary employee, eg a nurse, who receives a higher hourly salary but does not get the benefits enjoyed by salaried employee, eg vacation and pension plan

Perfluorodecalin see Artificial blood

Performing arts medicine A developing subspeciality of occupational medicine that formally addresses the medical complaints of those who perform for a living, by playing a musical instrument, singing, or dancing; in the USA, an estimated 200 000 earn their livelihoods from the performing arts (130 000 as instrumentalists, 20 000 as vocalists, 50 000 as 'others'), of whom 50% (more often women) have had complaints that threaten or force them to retire themselves from their profession; the most common problems are those of the muscle-tendon unit, which range in severity from mild pain to complete incapacitation, related to a combination of relatively repetitive movements of a limited number of muscles and the awkward position required to hold the instrument and/or weight of the instrument; other clinical disorders include overuse 'syndromes', nerve impingement and facial dystonia Treatment Rest; β-adrenergic agents for performance anxiety (N Engl J Med 1989; 320:221rv)

Perforating collagenosis, reactive An autosomal recessive condition of early childhood onset characterized by recurring umbilicated papules due to an ill-defined collagen defect

Perforin A 70 kD monomeric protein present in specific secretory granules of natural killer cells and cytotoxic T cells which in the presence of calcium, inserts itself into a target cell membrane, forming a self-associating polymer, seen by electron microscopy as a 5-20 nm annular transmembrane 'doughnut' which, once inserted into a membrane, is stable, allowing critical ions to diffuse out of a cell, hastening its demise; see Membrane attack complex, Porin

Perfusion TRANSPLANTATION The intravascular irrigation of an isolated organ with blood, plasma or physiological substance, eg University of Wisconsin solution, for the purpose of either studying its metabolism or physiology under 'normal' conditions or for maintaining the organ as 'fresh' as possible, while transporting the donated organ for transplantation; see Slush preparation

Pericardial 'knock' CARDIOLOGY A loud third heart sound occurring when the ventricular filling is abruptly stopped at the end of the early diastolic pressure dip, ie at the end of the rapidly filling phase of the ventricles; classically associated with severe constrictive pericarditis, the pericardial knock has a relatively high pitch, often increases in intensity with inspiration and coincides with the nadir of the 'y' descent of the jugular venous pulse

Perineal pearls NEONATOLOGY Cysts filled with viscid green-white mucoid material, located in the anterior perianal region, occasionally extending to the scrotum, a finding pathognomonic for imperforate anus

Periodic paralyses A group of conditions characterized by centrifugal 'attacks' of paralyzing, focal or systemic weakness of hours to days in duration, accompanied by a loss of deep tendon reflexes, refractoriness of muscle fibers to electrical stimulation, profound changes in potassium levels, variable cardiac arrhythmias and complete recuperation between attacks; rest following vigorous exercise may evoke an attack in a group of muscle fibers without changing the systemic potassium levels **NORMOKALEMIC PERIODIC PARALYSIS** a) Primary or hereditary A condition with attacks of childhood onset that may disappear by middle age; exposure to cold may provoke attacks and over time, result in vacuolar myopathy; the attacks may be provoked by high carbohydrate, high sodium diets during periods of excitement and may respond to oral potassium b) Secondary or acquired A condition associated with thyrotoxicosis, hypokalemia or potassium wasting by the kidneys or the gastrointestinal tract or due to accidental ingestion of absorbable barium salts that block potassium channels, reducing the egress of potassium from the muscles, evoking systemic hypokalemia or hyperkalemia, which may be associated with renal or adrenal insufficiency **HYPERKALEMIC PERIODIC PARALYSIS** An autosomal dominant variant of muscular dystrophy caused by a defective gene on chromosome 17, which encodes the α subunit of a sodium channel in muscle cell membranes, closely linked to the growth hormone gene GH1 (Science 1990; 250:1000) Clinical Early onset, most intense in males in whom paralytic attacks follow strenuous exercise, affecting the legs and eyelids; hyperkalemia may be prevented by acetazolamide; with time, the severely afflicted develop persistent weakness and dystrophic changes in muscle **HYPOKALEMIC PERIODIC PARALYSIS** An autosomal dominant condition of late onset that is more intense in males and occurs following strenuous exercise or carbohydrate meals, affecting the extremities, respiratory and cardiac muscle, potentially causing ventricular tachycardia and premature ventricular contractions Treatment Potassium chloride, acetazolamide; the severely afflicted may develop persistent weakness and dystrophic changes in muscle Differential diagnosis (all forms of periodic paralysis) Carnitine palmityl transferase deficiency and glycogen storage disease, type V

Periodic acid-Schiff stain see PAS stain

Periodontal disease DENTISTRY Gingival disease with chronic inflammation, extension of infection into the periodontal ligaments and alveolar bone destruction; periodontal disease is the most common cause of loss of teeth in adults, the result of combined bacterial infection and impaired host response; 300 different bacterial species occur in healthy mouths, most of which are gram-positive, eg actinomyces and streptococci; in gingivitis, the oral flora changes, streptococci are reduced, actinomyces increased and other organisms appear including ***Fusobacterium nucleatum, Lactobacillus, Veillonella*** and ***Treponema*** species; periodontal disease is associated with ***Actinobacillus actinomycetemcomitans*** in juvenile and ***Bacteroides gingivalis*** in adult periodontitis (***B gingivalis*** implanted subgingivally in primates produces bone loss and periodontitis, Science 1988; 239:55); other organisms implicated in periodontal disease include ***B intermedius, B forsythus, Selenomonas sputigena, Eikenella corrodens*** and spirochetes Note: Alveolar bone destruction, the bête noire of periodontitis, is the combined result of bacterial products (collagenases, proteases, leukotoxins, low molecular weight metabolites and bacterial lipopolysaccharide) and a host defense gone awry (alteration of fibroblast response and collagen synthesis, release of lytic enzymes, lymphotoxin, prostaglandins and osteoclast activating factor); leukocyte disfunction predisposes those with certain conditions to periodontitis, including Chediak-Higashi disease, Crohn's disease, cyclic neutropenia, diabetes mellitus, Down syndrome and the lazy leukocyte syndrome (N Engl J Med 1990; 322:373) Differential diagnosis Hypophosphatasia, histiocytosis X, leukemia and vitamin C and/or vitamin D deficiencies

Perioperative blood salvage see Intraoperative blood salvage

Peripheral (reparative) giant cell granuloma Giant cell epulis Osteoclastoma ORAL PATHOLOGY A sessile or pedunculated gingival or alveolar process mass, more common in the young female mandible (age 5-15, female:male ratio, 2:1), possibly induced by trauma, eg tooth extration **Radiology** Superficial erosion and peripheral cuffing of the bone **Histopathology** Unencapsulated ingrowth of fibrous tissue, capillaries and osteoclast-like giant cells are thought to arise from a fusion of proliferating endothelial cells **Differential diagnosis** Giant cell tumor of bone, hyperparathyroid-induced 'brown' tumor **Treatment** Curettage, but not (as was formerly practiced on occasion) extraction of the teeth

Peripheral nerve sheath tumor(s) (PNST) Schwannoma A group of tumors that are thought to arise in the neural sheath; three lesions have received the 'peripheral nerve sheath' adjective a) **PERIPHERAL NERVE SHEATH GANGLION** A rare, tender mass in the nerve, accompanied by pain and/or numbness, most commonly located within the popliteal nerve at the head of the fibula, demonstrating central degenerative myxoid changes, implying a reactive process, rather than a true neoplasm b) **PERIPHERAL NERVE SHEATH MYXOMA**, see Neurothekeoma and c) **MALIGNANT PERIPHERAL NERVE SHEATH TUMOR** or Malignant schwannoma Note: Because a direct link to the Schwann cell has proven elusive, the term schwannoma is less commonly used than the more noncommittal PNST

Peritoneal dialysis A therapeutic modality used for clearing toxic substances from the body in patients who are in terminal renal failure, which may be 1) **INTERMITTENT PERITONEAL DIALYSIS** A treatment modality requiring up to eight hours per session, making it only practical for home therapy or 2) **CONTINUOUS AMBULATORY PERITONEAL DIALYSIS** (CAPD) A treatment modality in which the patient exchanges 1.5-3.0 liters of sterile dialysate containing hypertonic glucose, three to five times/day, requiring 30-40 minutes per session, a therapy that is ideal for diabetics in renal failure who have poor venous access, as insulin may be delivered in the dialysate **Side effects** CAPD results in hyperlipidemia and obesity due to the high glucose of the dialysate and sclerosing peritonitis; long-term failure may be due to peritoneal infections, eg candidiasis and phaeohypomycosis (***Fusarium*** species); peritoneal dialysis is slower than hemodialysis for clearance of low molecular weight solutes (20-25 ml/min versus 150 ml/min for urea), but provides better clearance for higher weight substances; see 'Middle molecules'

Perivascular pseudorosette see Rosettes, Homer-Wright

PERLA Pupils equal, reactive to light and accommodation A common clinical acronym for normal oculomotor functions

Perleche French, to lick one's lips Angular cheilosis A condition characterized by inflammation, exudation, maceration and fissuring at the angles of the lips, caused by multiple etiologies, including decreased vertical dimension in the edentulous elderly with loss of alveolar bone, 'sagging' of cheeks due to myotonia (see Bloodhound face), sialorrhea, candidiasis, ariboflavinosis (with glossitis, keratitis and seborrhea-like dermatitis), malnutrition and streptococcal infection

Permanent section see Paraffin section

Permanent vegetative state Persistent vegetative state

Pernicious vomiting of pregnancy see Hyperemesis gravidarum

Pernio see Chilblains

Peroxisomal diseases A heterogeneous group of diseases in which peroxisomes are either lacking or markedly reduced in numbers; these patients have metabolic defects in all major biosynthetic peroxisomal pathways, failing to synthesize lipids or oxidize long-chain fatty acids; these metabolic defects cause a marked increase in plasma levels of very long chain fatty acids, especially C26:0 and C26:1 (hexacosanoic acid), increased trihydroxycoprostanic acid and increased pipecolic acid (an intermediate in lysine catabolism) and increased bile acid precursors with defective activity of peroxisomal acyl CoA:dihydroxyacetonephosphate acyltransferase in platelets and fibroblasts; peroxisomal diseases include Zellweger's cerebrohepatorenal syndrome, rhizomelic chondrodysplasia punctata, neonatal adrenoleukodystrophy, infantile Refsum disease and hyperpipecolic acidemia

Peroxisomal proliferators A group of chemicals that evoke a marked proliferation of hepatic peroxisomes and hepatic hyperplasia, including industrial plasticizers, herbicides and hypolipemic drugs that lower-triglycerides and cholesterol but which may not have clinical utility given their hepatotoxicity in rodents (Nature 1990; 347:645)

Peroxisome A membrane-bound cell organelle that contains the enzymes necessary for synthesizing hydrogen peroxide (H_2O_2), including D-amino acid oxidase, catalase and urate oxidase

Persistent vegetative state (PVS) Cognitive death A persistent loss of upper cortical function that may follow acute, eg infections, toxins, trauma or vascular events or chronic, eg degenerative events; in PVS, the patient is bed ridden and his nutritional support is completely passive, either parenteral or via naso-gastric tube; PVS patients do not require respiratory support or circulatory assistance for survival and are in a state of chronic wakefulness without awareness which may be accompanied by spontaneous eye opening, grunts or screams, brief smiles, sporadic movement of facial muscles and limbs; while the eyes blink upon stimulation, they do not do so in response to visual threats; some patients chew or clamp their teeth; urinary and fecal incontinence is universal; recovery generally occurs within the first month if at all; beyond the 3rd month, recovery is rare; maintaining the estimated 5-10 000 US patients in a PVS costs $2-10 000/month each person, or a total of $120 to $1200 million/year (in the USA alone) Note: The US record for longevity in the PVS is since October 1951 (Am Med News, 7/Jan/91); the ethical and medicolegal issues being raised by these patients are considerable (J Am Med Assoc 1990;

263:426); see Advanced directives, DNR, Harvard criteria, Living will, Quinlan; Cf Procurement

Persister phenomenon Persistance phenomenon MICROBIOLOGY A technical artefact that occurs in antibiotic susceptibility testing, where a percentage of organisms persist on the culture plate, simply because they are not in the growth phase at the time of testing, resulting in a 'red herring' that might be misinterpreted as representing bacterial resistance to an antibiotic; if these organisms are subcultured and retested, less than 0.1% of the inoculum persists (Ann Int Med 1982; 97:339)

Personality testing PSYCHOLOGY Any of a number of psychological tests, including the individual Rorschach inkblot test or the multiple choice California Psychological Inventory that is designed to objectively measure certain facets of an individual's personality and among other claims, to predict his ability to function in the work-place; it is felt by some experts in the field that personality testing is of little benefit and is poorly predictive of future behavior (Nature 1990; 348:671ed)

Personal physician A physician who assumes responsibility (or who in a court of law, is held to be responsible) for a patient's care; in the US, this role was formerly carried out by a 'general practitioner' who often had a decades-long relationship with the patient and his family; in the current environment of specialization and subspecialization, the personal physician may be in any field, although the role is often carried out by a physician with board certification in family practice or in internal medicine, and who is specialized in gastroenterology or cardiology: Cf Private patient

pERT see Phenol-enhanced reassociation technique

Perversion injuries Traumatic lesions induced by deviant sexual activities, most commonly involving the anus and rectum or lower urogenital tract, consisting of the tearing of tissues, with resultant infections, caused by various devices ranging from high pressure hoses per rectum to various objects or body parts designed to stimulate or enhance sexual arousal; see Sexual deviancy

PEST hypothesis A theory of historic interest that held that proteins with a short intracellular half-life (< 2 hours) contained one or more regions rich in proline, glutamic acid, serine and threonine (amino acids abbreviated as P, E, S and T), generally PEST regions are flanked by clusters with positively charged amino acids; it was thought that the PEST amino acids 'marked' proteins for early degradation (Science 1986; 234:364), a hypothesis that has been replaced by the 'N-end rule', see there

Pesticide Any agent for annihilating ambient arachnids, antagonistic arthropods, abominable animals or pugnacious plants, eg fumigants, fungicides, herbicides and insecticides; most pesticides are highly toxic and potentially fatal given their high arsenical or organophosphate content and store in adipose tissue given their lipid solubility; see Intermediate syndrome

PET see Pancreatic endocrine tumor

Petaloid globules A descriptor for the serrated flower petal-like degenerated elastic fibers seen by light microscopy in the benign tumor, elastofibroma, best visualized by elastin stains, eg Gomori or Verhoeff stains

Pet-associated disease Humans have for millenia domesticated a vast menagerie of animals, usually vertebrates and often mammals, for companionship or amusement; the human-pet dyad may cause morbidity in man when either a) The animals act as vectors for various microorganisms, eg dogs (rabies), cats (toxoplasmosis) and parrots (psittacosis) or when b) The animals attack the owner (colloquially known as 'turning'), an event that is relatively common in animals not bred for domestication, eg coyotes, lions, pythons and weasels; given the often unusual clinical presentations that characterize pet-associated illness, a detailed anamnesis is imperative to establish a diagnosis (Am Fam Prac 1990; 41:831); see Cat, Dog, Fish-tank granuloma

PET scan Positron emission transaxial tomography NUCLEAR MEDICINE A non-invasive imaging modality that uses radionuclides to detect biochemical and pathological abnormalities in living tissues, most commonly used to evaluate the cerebral cortex **Technique** A positron-emitting radionuclide, eg ^{11}C, is administered parenterally, travels a short distance, encounters an electron, the positron's antimatter counterpart, resulting in an annihilating reaction producing a pair of γ rays emitted in virtually opposite directions to each other, detected by a rotating array of detectors and a three-dimensional image of the spatial distribution of the annihilations generated by a computer Note: Positrons are short-lived particles that do not exist in nature and positron-emitting substances must be generated in a linear accelerator, the β-emitting substance is 'tagged' to a molecule, eg glucose and injected into the blood stream, where it travels to the brain; changes in regional blood flow can be measured in 'real time' for the analysis of various cognitive processes (Science 1990; 248:1556); PET scans may be used to evaluate AIDS-related neuropathology (response to AZT by local increase of glucose metabolism), dementia (focal neuronal loss, gliosis, allowing differentiation among Alzheimer's disease, Huntington's disease, multi-infarct dementia, tardive dyskinesia), epilepsy (localization of seizure focus, making surgical therapy viable), malignancy (gliomas, residual tumor, pituitary adenomas), Parkinson's disease (decreased dopamine), psychiatric disease (depression, schizophrenia), radiopharmaceutical analysis and cardiac disease (detection of coronary arteriosclerosis and ischemia)

Peter Pan and Wendy complex PSYCHIATRY A marital dyad composed of a narcissistic and/or unfaithful husband who devotes considerable time to studies, sports or extramarital liaisons and a depressed long-suffering wife; see Wendy dilemma

Peter Pan face A descriptor for the wrinkled, dehydrated and hairless facies of a subject with 'classic' hypopituitarism

Peter Pan syndrome(s) Clinical complexes named after the 'boy who would not grow up' ENDOCRINOLOGY Peter Pan syndrome is a state of physical immaturity due to a hypothalamic defect with underdeveloped secondary sexual characteristics that occurs in male children with microphalus and decreased height PSYCHOLOGY The Peter Pan 'syndrome' is a state of unconscious postponement of maturity, characterized by magical thinking, narcissism and chauvinism

Petit mal epilepsy Absence attack epilepsy NEUROLOGY A form of epilepsy characterized by episodic arrest of sensation and voluntary activity **Clinical** Transient loss of contact with the environment, decline in school performance **Diagnosis** A three-minute hyperventilation test may elicit an 'absence' **Treatment** Trimethadione, ethosuximide; Cf Grand mal seizure

Petit syndrome see Triad, Petit's

Petri dish A universal accoutrement of the microbiology laboratory devised by RJ Petri (1852-1921) while he was an assistant to R Koch in Berlin, which consists of two flattened clear glass or plastic plates, one larger than the other, allowing ease of examination of bacterial cultures, while preventing environmental contamination; this simple container was as instrumental as the gram stain in revolutionizing microbiology and the study of infectious disease

Petrified man syndrome Generalized myositis ossificans A rare idiopathic disease in which the interstitial tissues undergo extensive fibrosis and ossification; the lesions first appear in late childhood as firm tumor masses that later extend to globally to involve muscle, tendons, ligaments, fascia, aponeuroses and skin; tragically, the patients may find employment in circus 'freak' shows; in general, glossal, diaphragmatic, laryngeal and perineal musculature is spared and patients die of respiratory infections as the intercostal muscles may becom petrified; Cf Parana hard skin syndrome, Stiffman syndrome

PETT Positron emission transaxial tomography see PET

Peyote Magic mushrooms SUBSTANCE ABUSE A trivial name for mushrooms of the genus ***Psilocybe***, which contain the psychotropic agents, psilocybin and psilocin **Clinical** Minutes after ingestion, euphoria, hallucinations, tachycardia, mydriasis, rarely also fever and seizures

PF4 Platelet factor-4 A platelet-derived protein present in α granules and secreted therefrom during platelet aggregation as a high molecular weight tetramer associated with chondroitin sulfate; PF4 is involved in immune modulation, chemotaxis and inhibition of bone resorption and angiogenesis (Science 1990; 247:77)

PFGE see Pulsed field gel electrophoresis

P-glycoprotein see P170

PHA Phytohemagglutinin IMMUNOLOGY A lymphocyte mitogen that is used in vitro to measure lymphocyte-mediated cytotoxicity; PHA is mitogenic for T cells (lymphocytes), stimulating CD4 ('helper') T cells more than CD8 ('suppressor') T cells; PHA is a weaker mitogen for B cells; the degree of response in the respective cells can be measured based on the amount of IL-2 the cell produces

Phaedra complex The libidinous desire of a stepmother for a stepson; since the two are not genetically related, a sexual liaison is not incestuous; Phaedra of Greek mythology married Theseus but was attracted to his son Hippolytus who rejected her advances; the spurned Phaedra then had Theseus kill the son; Cf Jocastra complex

Phage typing A technique that characterizes certain strains of bacteria after initial speciation, in a fashion analogous to DNA 'fingerprinting', using bacteriophages (viruses capable of lysing bacteria)

Phagocytic index (PI) A measurement of nonspecific hyperreactivity of the immune system, manifested by an increased clearance of colloidal carbon, which is accelerated in graft-versus-host disease; see Splenic index

Phakomatoses Greek Phakos, lens Neurocutaneous syndromes A group of inherited conditions, many of which are autosomal dominant, that result in the disordered growth of ectodermal tissues, causing distinctive skin lesions and tumors and/or malformations of the nervous system and/or retina **ATAXIA-TELANGIECTASIA** of Louis-Bar An autosomal recessive disorder characterized by cerebellar ataxia, oculomotor apraxia, telangiectasias of bulbar conjuncta, skin of ears and skin folds (appearing by age three) and sinopulmonary infections; with time, the telangiectasias extend to the butterfly region of the face; most patients die in adolescence **BASAL CELL NEVUS SYNDROME** see Nevoid-basal cell carcinoma syndrome **NEVUS SEBACEOUS** of Jadassohn A clinical condition characterized by a congenital solitary lesion most often present in the scalp which, when large, may be associated with internal derangements including intracranial masses, seizures, mental retardation, skeletal abnormalities, pigmentary changes, ocular lesions and renal hamartomas; 10% of the skin lesions develop into basal cell carcinoma **STURGE-WEBER DISEASE** Encephalotrigeminal angio-matosis A disease characterized by congenital capillary hemangiomas of the head and neck, following normal developmental milestones, mental retardation may ensue, caused in part by the sluggish flow of blood through the pial vessels and venous hemangiomas in the leptomeninges and fronto-parietal cortex with ipsilateral port-wine nevi, 'Tram-track' radiopacities on the skull caused by calcification of the cerebral cortex **TUBEROUS SCLEROSIS** Bourneville-Pringle disease An autosomal dominant disorder (50% arise de novo) **Clinical** Convulsions, seizures, mental retardation, skin lesions (adenoma sebaceum, associated with sebaceous gland atrophy, angiofibromas, dermal fibrosis with dilated capillaries, shagreen patches), cardiac rhabdomyomas, pulmonary fibrosis, bronchiolarhematomas, bilateral tubular adenomas of the kidneys, pancreatic cysts, angiomyolipomas, myxedematous glossitis, spina bifida **Neuropathology** Astrocytic gliosis, which evokes lesions likened to 'candle wax drippings' **VON HIPPEL-LINDAU DISEASE** An autosomal dominant condition with retinal hemangioblastoma, increased erythropoietin production and cerebellar hemangioblastoma **Clinical** Ataxia, headache, papilledema, angiomas of the liver, kidney, renal adenomas, papillary cystadenomas of the epididymis, pancreatic cysts, adrenal pheochromocytomas Note: 25% develop renal cell carcinoma **VON RECKLINGHAUSEN DISEASE** A relatively common (1/3500) autosomal dominant condition **Clinical**

Neurofibromas, cafe au lait spotting of the skin, scoliosis, gliosis, glioblastoma multiforme, ependymoma, meningioma and schwannoma, 5-10% sarcomatous degeneration, spina bifida and glaucoma; see Neurofibromatosis

Phallotoxin A toxic, heat-stable cyclic heptapeptide derived from poisonous mushrooms, eg *Amanita phylloides, A verna, A virosa, Galerina autumnalis, Cenocybe filaris* and others, which with other cyclopeptides is responsible for 90 to 95% of the 100 annual (USA) deaths caused by poisonous mushrooms Clinical Stage 1 Abrupt onset of abdominal pain, nausea, cramping, vomiting, diarrhea with blood and mucus Stage 2 Apparent recovery with increasing liver enzymes Stage 3 1-3 days post-ingestion Hepatic, cardiac and renal failure, coagulopathies, seizures, coma and death Treatment None

Phantom RADIOLOGY A mass or dummy that approximates tissues in its physical properties that may be used to calibrate or determine the dose of radiation being applied to a tissue

Phantom bone disease see Disappearing bone disease

Phantom limb syndrome Chronic intense pain localized to the site of an amputated or denervated limb; 60-70% of amputees have a phantom limb sensation; 10-15% have phantom limb pain (syndrome); the degree of pain is often a function of the amount of pre-amputation pain; the pain is often refractory to treatments that include excision of amputation neuroma, rubbing, electrical stimulation, peripheral nerve or spinal blocks, narcotics and sympathectomy Note: Lord Nelson (1758-1805) lost his right arm when his fleet attacked Tenerife, and suffered until his death with phantom limb symptoms (Proc Roy Soc Med 1970; 63:299)

Phantom tumor A well-circumscribed accumulation of fluid in the interlobular spaces seen on a plain chest film which may occur in congestive heart failure

Pharmacist A person qualified by a graduate degree in pharmacy, who is licensed by the state to prepare, dispense and provide control over controlled drugs, usually having the title of RPh (registered pharmacist); Cf Pharmacologist

Pharmacologic dose CLINICAL PHARMACOLOGY A supraphysiological dose of a substance, eg mineralocorticoids, that are normally present in the body, in order to produce a 'pharmacologic' effect

Pharmacologic phlebotomy CRITICAL CARE MEDICINE The use of morphine in pulmonary edema to reduce the fluid load in the pulmonary vessels by pooling the blood into the capacitance vessels

Pharmacologist A person who has an advanced degree in pharmacology (MA or PhD), and is qualified to conduct research and evaluation of drugs and therapeutic agents, pharmacokinetics and effects; Cf Pharmacist

Pharmacologic stress imaging (PSI) CARDIOLOGY An increasingly popular alternative to the exercise stress test used in evaluating patients with coronary artery disease, allowing risk stratification; PSI is of use in those subjects who cannot perform an adequate exercise stress test; in PSI, dipyridamole is infused intravenously, producing marked coronary arteriolar vasodilation, leaving the peripheral arterioles relatively intact; dipyridamole also prevents cell uptake of adenosine, potentiating the agent's vasodilatory effect; in the myocardial regions perfused by normal coronary arteries, blood flow increases in the endocardial and epicardial layers, indicating a normal coronary artery reserve; in coronary artery stenosis, there is diminished uptake and clearance of intravenously administered ^{201}thallium, resulting in an initial ^{201}thallium defect that is followed by a delayed redistribution in images viewed two to four hours after injection; the side effects induced by dipyridamole are immediately reversible with aminophylline (J Am Med Assoc 1991; 265:633rv); Cf Treadmill stress test

Pharyngeal arches EMBRYOLOGY A series of primitive structures that appear in the fourth to fifth week of the embryo, and give rise to major structures of the head and neck; the first pharyngeal arch, dorsal aspect gives rise to the maxillary process, incus malleus, muscles: masseter, temporal, pterygoid, anterior digastric, mylohyoid, tensor tympanicus, palatine; the first pharyngeal arch ventral aspect gives rise to the mandibular (Meckel's) process, trigeminal, mucosa of tongue; the second pharyngeal arch (of Reichert) gives rise to the stapes, styloid, temporal, stylohyoid, stapedius, posterior digastric, auricular, facial 'mimic' musculature; the third pharyngeal (hyoid) arch gives rise to the stylopharyngeal and glossopharyngeal nerve; the fourth and sixth pharyngeal (thyroid) arche(s) give rise to the cricothyroid pharyngeal laryngeal musculature; the fifth arch never fully develops; Cf Aortic arches

Pharyngeal clefts EMBRYOLOGY Primitive structures seen in the five-week embryo, only one of which, the dorsal aspect of the first pharyngeal cleft, gives rise to the external auditory canal; the second, third and fourth pharyngeal clefts undergo atrophy and are covered by the second pharyngeal arch

Pharyngeal 'facelift' Palatopharyngoplasty A 'tuck and tighten' surgical procedure for the soft palate and pharynx, which eliminates redundant mucosa in an attempt to reduce the noise level in those who snore; see Obstructive sleep apnea syndrome, Snoring

Pharyngeal pouches A series of embryonic structures that appear simultaneously with the pharyngeal arches and clefts consisting of outpouchings along the lateral wall of the pharyngeal gut that have been likened to the gills or branchia of amphibians and fish; this progenitor tissue gives rise to various structures of the pharynx; the First pouch gives rise to the middle ear and eustachian tube, the second pouch to the palatine tonsils, the third pouch to the inferior parathyroids and thymus, the fourth pouch to the superior parathyroids and the fifth pouch to the ultimobranchial body in the thyroid gland

Pharyngeal structure Any structure including bone, cartilage, lymphoid tissues, muscles, nerves, and spaces that migrates to its respective place during early embryogenesis under the baton of the primitive pharynx (pharyngeal arches, clefts and pouches), each giving rise to specific structures

Phase 1, 2 and 3 studies CLINICAL PHARMACOLOGY A series

of clinical trials that address the safety and efficacy of an 'investigational new drug' (IND) that is being 'sponsored' by a pharmaceutical company with the purpose of bringing the product to the marketplace **Phase I Early clinical pharmacology stage** Involves 20-80 subjects and should generate enough data to allow a properly controlled trial; FDA's review at this point ensures that subjects are not exposed to unreasonable risks **Phase 2 Later clinical pharmacology stage** Involves several hundred patients with the first controlled clinical studies with the purpose of generating enough data to a) at least suggest (if not prove) that the drug actually works and b) demonstrate the most common side effects **Phase 3 Final clinical pharmacology stage** Involves several thousand patients, the expanded clinical trials which should generate enough information to establish both the drug's effectiveness for specific indications and identify populations at special risk from its use; both phase 2 and 3 are meant to ensure that the scientific design would create the data necessary to meet premarket approval of the drug; NDA (new drug applications) were often rejected because the data from the phase 2 and 3 trials revealed study design flaws, forcing the sponsor to repeat work, which has been largely eliminated by the '1987 rewrite' of the IND status Note: Occasionally, an agent's benefit is so obvious, eg zidovudine (AZT) that the need for phase 3 studies, a stage immediately preceding an official NDA, may be obviated;see Compassionate investigational new drug, IND, NDA, Treatment IND

Phase contrast microscope A microscope that converts the differences in refractive index into variations of light intensity, allowing visualization of structural details in situ within living cells; see Microscopy

Pheasant hunter's toe An acute attack of podagra (gouty arthritis of the toe), that follows long walks typical of pheasant hunting, a sport of the wealthy, who were most commonly afflicted by gout

Phencyclidine (PCP) 'Angel dust' Substance abuse A recreational hallucinogen with significant side effects, causing neurologic dysfunction, with schizophrenia-like behavior, analgesia, dysarthria, nystagmus, ataxia, seizures, delirium, coma, as well as gastrointestinal symptoms, increased blood pressure and temperature and depressed pulmonary function; a PCP receptor has been identified and when bound by certain ligands, eg PCP and MK-801, results in neuronal vacuolization and loss of mitochondria in the posterior cingulate and retrosplenial cortices of the rat brain; in utero exposure to PCP results in high levels in the fetus (in experimental rats), due to immaturity of enzyme clearance systems

Phenol-enhanced reassociation technique Molecular biology A method that identifies seven DNA clones (pERT clones) mapped to band p21 of the X chromosome, one of which, pERT87 is defective in 7% of patients with Duchenne's and Becker's muscular dystrophy, resulting in short protein products of a defective gene

Phenome Phenotype

Phenotypic suppression The suppression of a phenotypic mutation during translation of a DNA sequence into mRNA, or during translation of the mRNA transcript into a protein, eg misreading in the presence of 5-fluorouracil, an agent that inhibits thymidylate synthetase

Phenylpropanolamine (PPA) An 'over-the-counter' drug used in nasal decongestants, cough medication and diet control aids; there are few side effects, although PPA has been reported to short-lived, low-grade increases in systolic and diastolic blood pressure (J Am Med Assoc 1989; 261:3267)

Phenytoin-induced gingival overgrowth see PIGO

Phenytoin lymphadenopathy A phenytoin-induced condition characterized by generalized lymphadenopathy, rashes, fever and a slight increase in the incidence of lymphoma Histopathology Effacement of lymphoid follicles, mixed cell infiltrate of immunoblasts, plasma cells, eosinophils and necrosis; some cases have progressed to malignant lymphoma, although the association with phenytoin therapy may be a 'passenger' phenomenon; see Pseudopseudolymphoma

Pheochromocytoma 10% tumor A paraganglioma of adrenal medulla, 10% of which are associated with systemic disease, including von Recklinghausen's disease, von Hippel-Lindau syndrome, Sturge-Weber disease and MEN IIa and IIb; pheochromocytomas may produce ACTH, calcitonin and VIP Clinical The pheochromocytoma triad (headaches, sweating attacks and tachycardia) in a hypertensive patient has a 94% specificity and 91% sensitivity for the diagnosis of pheochromocytoma; absence of all in a hypertensive patient completely excludes pheochromocytoma); other symptoms include nervousness, anxiety, tremor, facial pallor, nausea and/or vomiting, fatigue, chest or abdominal pain, weight loss Laboratory Increased vanillylmandelic acid (VMA), metanephrine, free catecholamines, MHPG, dopamine and homovanillic acid (HVA) Diagnosis Measure free norepinephrine and 3,4-dihydroxyphenylglycol in urine (N Engl J Med 1988; 319:136) or the traditional 24-urine collection for metanephrine and VMA (ibid; 319:1417c)

Pheromone A hormone released by an organism that is capable of evoking, in a member of the same species, a physiological response that is usually related to mating, eg those that block olfaction in pregnant mice and those that determine sexual orientation of ***Saccharomyces cerevisiae***

Philadelphia chromosome A small acrocentric chromosome from the distal long arm of chromosome 22 that is transferred to the long arm of chromosome 9 [t(9;22)(q34;q11)] in 95% of cases of chronic myelogenous leukemia (CML); the Philadelphia chromosome (PC) is often associated with a better prognosis (44-month survival versus 15-month survival in PC-negative CML, Science 1960; 132:1947); it may also be present in acute lymphocytic (5-20% of cases) and non-lymphocytic leukemias and is generated in a pluripotent stem cell (appearing in myeloid, erythroid, megakaryocytic and lymphoid lines) by a reciprocal translocation, resulting in juxtaposition of the c-***abl*** gene on chromosome 9 with a gene of unknown function, with a ***bcr*** (breakpoint cluster region) on chromosome 22; the resulting hybrid ***abl/bcr*** gene encodes $P210^{bcr/abl}$, a phosphoprotein unique to CML that resembles v-*abl* as it has disregulated protein-tyrosine kinase activity; when the hybrid gene is inserted into a retroviral vector, used to infect bone marrow, then transplanted into irradiated syngeneic mice, CML is induced in the mice (Science 1990; 247:824); see P210$^{bcr/abl}$

Philadelphia cream cheese appearance A fanciful descriptor for the caseating necrosis seen in tuberculosis, which has a whitish color and 'paste-like' consistency

Phlebodynia Vein pain A hysterical reaction of uncertain validity, which affects women and is accompanied by malaise, headache and mild fever; see Factitious disease(s)

Phlebothrombosis see Thrombophlebitis

Phocomelia An intercalary-type of congenital skeletal limb deformity, due to the idiopathic absence of the radial elements of a limb bud; in complete phocomelia, the hand is directly attached to the shoulder or the foot to the pelvis; see Thalidomide

Phonosurgery OTORHINOLARYNGOLOGY A surgical procedure performed on the vocal cords and adjacent tissue with the purpose of improving the timbre, tone and quality of the voice; Cf Uvulopalatopharyngoplasty

Phorbol ester

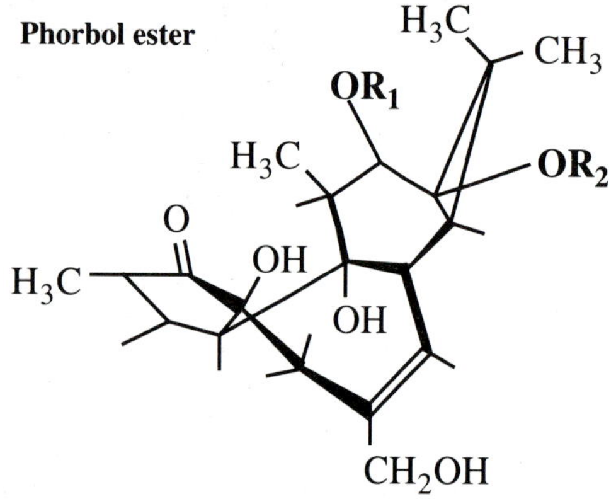

Phorbol ester(s) A family of potent tumor-promoting esters (figure), eg TPA, derived from the alcohol phorbol obtained from croton oil, which evoke various responses in cultured cells including increased cell growth, synthesis of macromolecules and prostaglandins, alteration of cell morphology and membrane permeability; see TPA

Phosphatidylinositol 4,5 biphosphate (PI) An inositol phospholipid present at the cytoplasmic leaflet of the plasma membrane that is hydrolyzed by phospholipase C, yielding 1,2 diacylglycerol and the water soluble inositol 1,4,5-triphosphate (both of which are 'second messengers'), which diffuses to the surface of the endoplasmic reticulum, opening a calcium-specific channel, evoking a specific cell response

Phosphoenolpyruvic acid (PEP) A high-energy compound, which upon dephosphorylation degrades to pyruvic acid and contributes a high-energy phosphate, leading to the synthesis of ATP from ADP

Phospholipase A_2 (PLA_2) A family of enzymes that hydrolyze the 2-ester bond of L-glycerophospholipids; since some forms of PLA_2 catalyze the release of arachidonate, which precipitates the inflammatory 'cascade', it is of interest to produce molecules that mimic PLA_2's active sites, sites that have recently been resolved by crystallography (Science 1990; 250:1563)

Phospharamidon A neutral protease inhibitor that prevents the conversion of 'big' endothelin, the pre-pro endothelin into endothelin-1, by inhibiting the action of the endothelin converting enzyme and causes a slow lowering of blood pressure in hypertensive rats; see Endothelin

Phosphorus binders A group of orally-administered agents, eg calcium acetate, which increase gastrointestinal excretion of phosphorus in patients with chronic renal failure (N Engl J Med 1989; 320:1110)

Phosphorylation PHYSIOLOGY The process of adding a phosphate group to a protein, eg phosphorylation of a receptor by a protein kinase, an activity that serves to regulate receptor-mediated transcription of target genes (Science 1990; 250:1740)

Phossy jaw OCCUPATIONAL MEDICINE An effect of chronic occupation-related poisoning by elemental or yellow phosphorus causing mandibular necrosis **Clinical** Early symptoms of toothache and sialorrhea, loosening of the teeth, pain and mandibular swelling are followed by bone necrosis and recalcitrant sinus tracts; the current OSHA levels of 0.1 mg/m^3 averaged over an 8-hour shift are below the toxic levels that would cause this complication

Phot A unit of light intensity equal to 1 lumen/cm^2; Cf Photon

Photoactivators Ingested substances that enhance the deleterious effect of light, including PUVA, tetracycline, psoralens (celery, parsnips, figs and parsley); see PUVA

Photoaging Functional deterioration of sun-exposed regions, resulting in skin wrinkling, altered texture, discoloration, decreased epidermal thickness, basophilic degeneration of the dermis with loss of collagen and dermal vessels and epithelial atypia and dysplasia; most of the changes of photoaging are reversed by retinoin

Photobleaching see Fluorescence recovery after photobleaching

Photodynamic therapy A therapeutic modality in which tumor cells that concentrate a photosensitizer, eg a hematoporphyrin derivative, are destroyed by exposure to light at an appropriate wavelength, a modality of potential use in treating superficial, low-grade or in situ transitional cell carcinoma of the bladder; in one small study, 47% had complete tumor eradication (N Engl J Med 1987; 317:1251)

Photomultiplier tube (PMT) An electronic tube that amplifies the signal of electrons from incident radiation, which is an integral component of spectrophotometers

Photon A quantum of light energy equivalent to hv (h x v), where h is Planck's constant (6.625 x 10^{-27} erg-s) and v is the frequency of light measured in cycles/s; Cf Phot

Photoprotection Protection of cells from ultraviolet light-induced damage by exposing the cells to light in the high UV-A and low UV-B (310-370 nm) range, which either inhibits cell synthesis or activates a heat shock protein-like response Note: UV-C (200-290 nm) is damaging to DNA and amino acids, UV-B ranges from 290-320 nm and UV-A from 320 to 400 nm; Cf Sunscreen

Photoreactivation The process of repairing ultraviolet light-induced damage to DNA, which consists of cyclobutyl linkage of thymine residues (dimerization), which is repaired by four enzymes: ultraviolet-activated endonuclease (initiation, responsible for 80% of the defects), exonuclease, DNA polymerase and DNA ligase

Photoreactive keratectomy (PRK) A procedure in which an excimer laser is used to ablate and sculpt the cornea to exact specifications; in myopia, the cornea is flattened by 'shaving' 10-20 microns of corneal tissue from the center and tapering to the edges; in early therapeutic trials, the 20-40 seconds in duration procedure has been most successful in those with myopia of less than 5 diopters; the only reported complication is glare, and preliminary data suggests that PRK will be a better procedure than radial keratopathy, the other method of refractive surgery; marketing of the lasers for PRK awaits approval by the US Food and Drug Administration, anticipated by 1993 (Am Med News 28/Dec/90); see Refractive surgery

Phthisis bulbi A condition characterized by advanced degeneration and disorganization of the ocular globe, accompanied by retinal necrosis, atrophy, softening and shrinkage, thickening of the sclera with permanent scarring and loss of function; phthisis bulbi occurs in retinoblastomas or in untreated purulent endophthalmitis and may be accelerated by intraocular surgery; phthisis bulbi may predispose the retina to malignant melanoma

PHS see Pulmonary hemorrhagic syndromes

Phycomycosis see Mucormycosis

Phylloides tumor Cystosarcoma phylloides SURGICAL PATHOLOGY A breast tumor characterized by fleshy, leaf-like papillary projections of epithelial-lined stromal tissue extending into cystic spaces, which is most common in perimenopausal women; phylloides tumors range from the bland, benign and banal, histologically similar to typical fibroadenomas to the aggressive, characterized by florid stromal cellularity that mimics sarcomas; metastases occur in 3-12% of cases, with the stromal component spreading to bone and lung in contrast to lymph nodes, which are the usual catchment site for epithelial breast malignancies

Phylogenetic tree A dcertainiagrammatic representation of the development of a species based on select criteria; the traditional phylogenic classification is based on differences in an array of physical characteristics, eg types of feathers, skeletal anatomy, form of reproduction, or for lower organisms, the types of biochemical reactions an organism can produce, pigment production, or metabolic requirements; more recently, it has become apparent that classifications based on the relatedness of DNA and amino acid sequences of certain proteins, eg those of the respiratory path-way in mitochondria, are more valid, and allow determination of the point in evolution where one species diverged from another; see Urkingdom

Phrygian cap deformity An abnormal angulation or kinking of the distal portion of the gall bladder fundus (figure, below), due to a transverse fibrous septum of presumed congenital nature, often associated with cholelithiasis Note: Phrygian caps are conical, bent in front and were called the 'Cap of Liberty' during the French revolution for their symbolic significance, as they were worn in Phrygia, a country of ancient Asia minor by slaves who had won their freedom

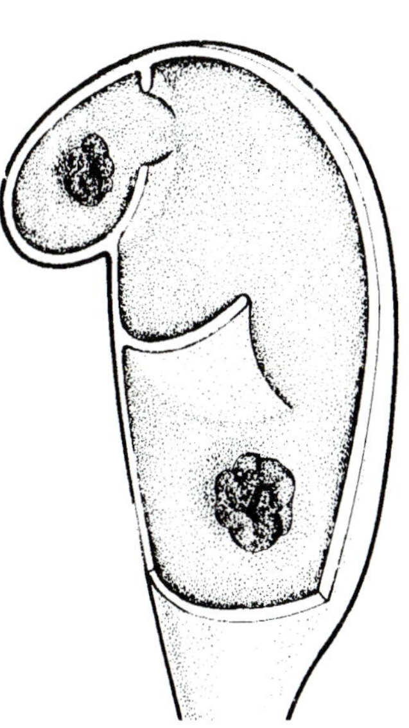

Phrygian cap deformity

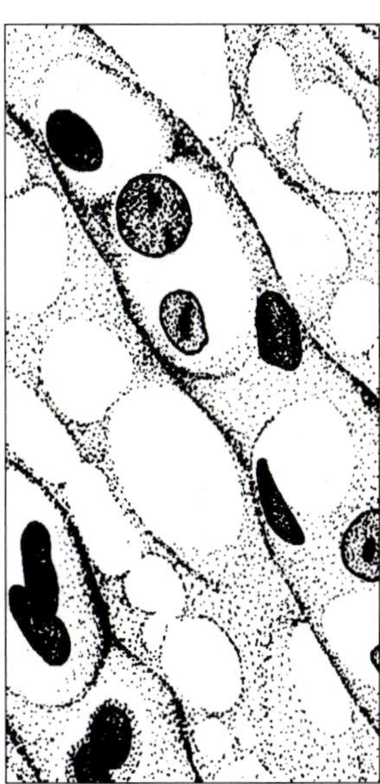

Physaliferous cells

Physaliferous cells Vacuolated mucin-filled cells, with a soap bubble-like appearance (figure, above) that are arranged in cords, sheets and nests, and divided by thin fibrous trabeculae; physaliferous cells are characteristic of chordomas, which are locally aggressive tumors that arise from remnants of the fetal notochord, most commonly developing in the sacrococcygeal region of women (male:female ratio, 3:1) during the fifth decade of life; the clinical course is marked by frequent recurrences Prognosis 40% develop metastases; many ultimately prove fatal; see Soap bubble

Physical fitness A state of physical well-being and higher-than-average exercise tolerance; stay-ing 'in shape' substantially reduces mortality rates (after adjusting for age, smoking habits, cholesterol, systolic blood pressure, fasting blood glucose and parental history of coronary vascular disease); cardiovascular mortality is 3.5 times greater in men and 10 times greater in women who are in the least fit quintile of a population; cancer mortality is five-fold greater in unfit men and 15-fold greater in unfit women (J Am Med Assoc 1989; 262:2395); see Exercise, Obesity

Physical map GENETICS A map of a chromosome or genome in which the distances are measured by methods other than through gene recombination

Physical restraints see Restraints

Physical status classification A classification of a subject's physical condition by the American Society of Anesthesiologists, which stratifies patients undergoing a surgical procedure into categories of relative risk for suffering complications during an operation or in the immediate post-operative period (table, below)

PHYSICAL STATUS CLASSIFICATION

Class 1 The patient has no organic, physiologic, biochemical or psychiatric disturbance; the pathologic process for which the operation is to be performed is localized and does not entail a systemic disturbance, eg inguinal hernia repair in a robust male

Class 2 The patient has mild to moderate disturbance caused either by the condition being treated surgically or by a physiopathological derangement, eg mild cardiac disease, mild diabetes mellitus, chronic bronchitis, essential hypertension

Class 3 The patient has severe systemic disease or derangement of any cause, which may defy classification, eg severe cardiac disease, angina or status post-myocardial infarction, severe diabetes with vascular complications, moderate to severe pulmonary compromise

Class 4 The patient has severe systemic disease that is already life-threatening, which may not be corrected by surgery, eg organic heart disease, with signs of severe cardiac insufficiency, advanced pulmonary, hepatic, renal or endocrine insufficiency

Class 5 The patient is virtually moribund, with little chance of survival who is submitted to an operation in desperation, eg ruptured aortic aneurysm, major cerebral trauma with rapidly increasing intracranial pressure

Emergency operation E A designation for any of the above classes, when the operation 'goes sour', eg an incarcerated hernia with strangulation would become a class 1E (RD Dripps, Introduction to Anesthesthesia The Principle and Practice, 6th ed, WB Saunders, Philadelphia, 1982 Note: This is found in an abbreviated form in Mayo Clin Proc 1991; 66:155)

Physician assistant (PA) An individual who is qualified to perform a wide variety of medically-related tasks under a physician's supervision, including taking a patient's history, performing physical examinations and autopsies Education Two post-graduate years beyond college or university, training as a pathologist assistant, physician assistant or surgeon assistant, and designated as PA-Cs; physicians assistants may then subspecialize for a one-to-two year period in various fields including neonatology, pediatrics, emergency medicine, occupational medicine and others

Physician expert witness A principal actor in the drama of malpractice litigation, defined by an adaption of the Council of Medical Specialty Societies (table, facing page) Note: It is considered unethical to link expert witness fees to the outcome of the case, as there is a potential for introducing bias (Bull, Am Coll Surgeons 1989; 74:6)

Physician 'glut' An excess of physicians that will theoretically develop in North America by the end of the 20th century; in 1970 there were 326 000 physicians; 706 000 are anticipated by the year 2000 with 271 physicians/10^5 population (another projection places this number as 176/10^5 J Am Med Assoc 1991; 265:2369) Note: It is unclear whether the predicted glut will materialize in the US; if it does, it is unlikely to cause massive physician unemployment, as new physician roles are being created in a high-technology, litigation-prone society, including new specialties, eg geriatrics, medical informatics and molecular therapy, and the creation of new roles in medicine, eg medical ethicists, quality assurance specialists, physician-bureaucrats, physician-lawyers and others (N Engl J Med 1991; 324:536) Note: An overabundance of physicians has been present in some European and South American countries for nearly a decade, where some physicians reportedly supplement their incomes performing various menial tasks; Cf Manpower shortage

'Physician invulnerability syndrome' The self-maintained delusion by some physicians that they are not susceptible to the same diseases as their patients, since the physician has made a 'contract' with a higher Being, and is ensured an aura of protection; this 'condition' results in self-treatment by the physician for potentially pernicious conditions, treatment delays, denial of mental or physical illness, abuse substance (eg alcohol, drugs) dependency and an unwillingness to bother colleagues who have the required expertise necessary to properly treat their medical illness

Physician office laboratories see POL

Physician profile HEALTH CARE INDUSTRY The list of a physician's fees by procedure, compiled by a 'third-party payer', ie an insurance company or Medicare, by a hospital or by his own staff in order to control his reimbursements and monitor his income

Physician shortage area A region (usually rural and/or of lower income, as in the inner city) where very few physicians practice medicine, in which there may be less than one physician per 5000 population Note: The dialog about physician shortage areas is usually in the context of the US and other developed nations; in some African countries, there may be 1 physician per 10^5 or more people; see Physician glut; Cf Manpower shortage

Physician's desk reference see PDR

pI Isoelectric point CLINICAL CHEMISTRY The pH at which a determined protein has a net charge of zero, the result of a combination of all the different side chains and their degrees of association; the higher the pI, the more cathodic is the protein on an electrophoresis run at a pH of 9.4

PI Principal investigator The chief architect of a grant application, who is often the person with the creative ideas, although he may not do the actual 'bench work',

PHYSICIAN EXPERT WITNESS

Recommended qualifications The physician expert witness should

a) Have a current, valid and unrestricted license to practice medicine in his state of practice

b) Be a diplomate (board-certified) or board-eligible in the specialty deemed relevant to the case

c) Be familiar with the clinical practice of the specialty involved in the case and

d) Be prepared to document the time he spends as an expert witness; see 'Hired gun'

Recommended guidelines for behavior of a physician expert witness He (she) is expected to be impartial and be neither advocate nor partisan in the legal proceedings; he should

a) Review the medical information relevant to the case and testify in an unbiased fashion

b) Review the standards of practice prevailing at the time of the event's occurrence

c) Provide the basis from which his testimony is derived, ie testimony based on experience or that derived from the medical literature

d) Receive compensation that is reasonable and reflects the time and effort spent in preparing the case

(which explains why the PI is often the last author listed on a publication); the PI is responsible for maintaining the budget, guiding the research team, travelling to symposia and lecturing on his group's research, organizing the publications for the experimental question in the grant proposal and reaching the conclusions based on the obtained data

PI system see Phosphoinositide system

Piano playing NEUROLOGY A fanciful descriptor for the finger movements secondary to the loss of position sensation, in which the patient seeks to discover exactly where his fingers are in space by periodic movement, a feature of the autosomal recessive Dejerine-Sottas disease, a severe peripheral sensorimotor neuropathy of infantile onset, which is accompanied by delayed ambulation and later loss of ambulation, becoming wheelchair-bound by early adulthood; these movement are often accompanied by truncal ataxia and choreic hand movements); 'piano playing' also refers to intermittent flexion and extension of the hands seen in tardive dyskinesia, a complication of chronic therapy with antipsychotic drugs, eg phenothiazines, butyrophenones

Piblokto ANTHROPOLOGY A transient hysterical reaction in Eskimo women, in which the subjects rip off their clothes in sub-zero weather, emitting animal and bird sounds, followed by amnesia for the event, a reaction that is postulated to stem from long-standing repression of the personality of the Eskimo female, whose status is that of property; Cf Koro, Zombie

Pica Ingestion of unusual substances with no known nutritional value, which is often associated with iron-deficiency anemia; the substance(s) ingested may aggravate the iron deficiency, as in geophagy, where the clay eaten acts as a ferro-chelator; other pica ingestants include laundry starch, ice (pagophagia) and newsprint; pica also occurs in zinc, copper and certain vitamin deficiencies, but evidence for a causal relation remains scanty; occasional cases of pica may be directly explained by the effect of the ingestant, such as caffeine from coffee grounds and nicotine from cigarette butts; Pica is a genus of magpies, birds famed for their omnivorous nature; like the magpie, a person or animal with pica craves or eats anything, often indigestible non-comestibles; see Geophagy

Pick-up sticks pattern CYTOLOGY A fanciful descriptor for the haphazard arrangement of epithelial cells seen in the cervical epithelium in reparative atypia

Picket fence fever pattern A descriptor for a saw-tooth pattern of often very high temperature peaks, a finding considered characteristic of pyogenic hepatic abscesses, which is accompanied by chills, sweating, nausea, vomiting, anorexia and pain

Picket fence arrangement see Palisading

Pickwick syndrome A complication of extreme obesity, in which there is marked cardiovascular compromise, with decreased tidal and expiratory reserve volumes, alveolar hypoventilation, hypoxia, cyanosis (and hypercapnia, if severe and prolonged), dyspnea, polycythemia, cardiac hypertrophy, pulmonary hypertension and edema, congestive heart failure and extreme somnolence; oxygen therapy is potentially fatal as it would remove the chemoreceptor drive of respiratory movement Note: The disease complex is named for the fat boy, Joe, in Charles Dickens' Pickwick papers; Cf Morbid obesity

Picture frame appearance A descriptor for monostotic involvement by Paget's disease of the bone where an isolated vertebral body is enlarged, centrally osteoporotic and surrounded by a rim of osteosclerotic cortex, involving the anterior and posterior margins as well as the vertebral end-plates; despite its increased radiologic density, the bone is more prone to fractures

Picture frame area BURN PHYSIOLOGY A limited zone of tissue directly beneath the advancing dermal edge, which contains the 'machinery' necessary for wound contraction and repair; excision of this rim of cells effectively stops epithelialization of burn wounds; the epithelial cells within the 'picture frame' are large, stellate and pale

Picture puzzle appearance see Jigsaw puzzle (cells, contour, model, tumor)

PID see Pelvic inflammatory disease

PIE Pulmonary interstitial emphysema, an uncommonly used acronym, given the potential for confusion with the PIE syndrome

Piebaldism Partial albinism A rare condition characterized by patchy amelanotic plaques (focally reduced or absent melanocytes) occurring on the forehead, scalp, thorax, elbows and knees, associated with a white forelock; Woolf syndrome is diagnosed when in addition, the scalp skin changes are accompanied by heterochromic irides, deafness and mental retardation

Piecemeal necrosis Necrosis of the liver cell plate in which a chronic inflammatory cell infiltrate is in direct contact with hepatocytes actively undergoing condensation and fragmentation (apoptosis); piecemeal necrosis imparts a 'ragged' low-power appearance to the usually lobular pattern of the limiting plate; piecemeal necrosis is a required histologic feature in cirrhosis and chronic active hepatitis and may be seen in primary sclerosing cholangitis

Piedmont fracture An isolated fracture located precisely at the distal third of the radius, named after a case presented by the Piedmont Orthopedic Society of North Carolina; current thinking holds that open reduction and fixation be performed when only one of the two forearm bones was fractured, since closed reduction results in a high incidence of non-union

PIE syndrome Pulmonary infiltrates with eosinophilia A disease complex characterized by intense, nonspecific symptoms accompanied by chronic relapsing fever, cough and dyspnea, seen in association with chronic eosinophilic pneumonia; PIE has been subdivided into: a) Simple PIE or Löffler syndrome b) Tropical eosinophilia, which may be associated with microfilarial infections and parasites, including ***Ascaris lumbricoides*** and ***Toxocara canis*** and c) Secondary chronic pulmonary eosinophilia, associated with allergic bronchopneumonia related to aspergillosis, bronchocentric granulomatosis, allergic angiitis and granulomatosis (Churg-Strauss syndrome), drugs (nitrofurantoin, sulfonamide) and infections (parasitic, fungal and bacterial)

Piezoelectric sensing Background: Piezoelectric crystals are those that produce a partial separation of electrical charge when they are deformed, such that equal, but opposite charges arise at the opposite surfaces of the crystal; all known crystals have a natural vibration, known as a resonant or fundamental frequency, which is a function of their chemical composition and each vibration causes the crystal to oscillate; when the crystal is piezoelectric (as is quartz), the resonance results in an oscillating electrical field; the piezoelectric effect has been used to measure antigen-antibody reactions, DNA-RNA interactions, and may be of use in clinical toxicology (Diag & Clin Testing 1990; 28:2/21)

PIF see Prolactin-inhibiting factor

Pig RADIATION SAFETY A (whiskey) shot glass-sized lead-shielded receptacle that is used to transport and store radioactive material in clinical or research labratories, substantially reducing a radioisotope's γ radiation; the origin of the term pig is uncertain, although certain relatives of the word pig suggest possible roots a) A pig is 1/8 of an English (250 pounds) ton, a unit of weight of cast iron b) A pig is an ingot of molten metal (often lead, but also iron and copper) fed from channels called sows and c) A derivation from the old English 'pygg' for a crock or jar, that later evolved to pig

Pig(s) As vectors for human infections: Bacteria ***Brucella suis*** Parasites ***Entamoeba polecki, Fasciolopsis buski,*** sarcocystosis, ***Taenia solium, Trichinella spiralis*** Viruses Swine influenzae

Pigbel The New Guinean name for enteritis necroticans, related to poorly cooked pork infested by type C ***Clostridium perfringens***, that may be consumed in orgiastic 3-4 day pork-eating 'marathons'; pigbel is endemicin the New Guinea highlands, affecting in particular those children with a poor immune response to clostridial toxins, low levels of proteases and a protein-poor diet that is high in sweet potatoes, which contain trypsin inhibitors Pathogenesis The trypsin-sensitive 'B' toxin of ***C perfringens***, type C (an organism isolated from 70% of the villagers) is not degraded given the relative trypsin insufficiency and intestinal parasitosis by ***Ascaris lumbricoides***, which secretes a trypsin inhibitor Clinical A 24-hour incubation is followed by intense abdominal pain, vomiting, bloody diarrhea and shock Mortality Up to 40% Histopathology Local infarction, edema, hemorrhage, neutrophil infiltration; one-half require resective surgery (N Engl J Med 1984; 311:1126c)

Pigeon breast appearance Anterior displacement of the sternum, adjacent cartilage and anterior rib cage due to abnormal pulling by respiratory musculature on soft bone, enlargement of the costochondral junctions and flattening of the thorax, a finding characteristic of advanced vitamin D-induced rickets

Pigeon breeder lung A form of hypersensitivity pneumonitis due to inhalation of protein from bird sera, excreta, and feathers, which evokes a type III or hypersensitivity reaction that may be followed by a type IV or granulomatous reaction; see Farmer's lung, Hypersensitivity pneumonitis

Pigeon toe Ding toe, In-toeing ORTHOPEDICS A deformity of the leg that first develops in childhood and is characterized by medial rotation of the forefoot (metatarsus varus) and medial tibial or femoral torsion, in which the bones are medially rotated; the resulting deformities require orthopedic correction

Piggie back devices CRITICAL CARE MEDICINE A device used in critically ill patients to optimize the intravenous delivery of fluids and drugs that need to be infused at different rates; in these devices, the reservoir and the valve controlling the rate of delivery are separate, while the delivery port itself, eg an intravenous access line may be shared

Pigmented neuroectodermal tumor of infancy Melanoameloblastoma Melanotic progonoma Retinal anlage tumor Pigmented ameloblastoma A tumor of neural crest origin affecting infants under 6 months of age that may rarely occur in adults, which may be located in the anterior maxilla, oral cavity and skull, and less commonly in the mediastinum, thigh, forearm and epididymis Clinical Locally aggressive, 15% recurrence rate, rarely metastatic Histopathology Small pseudoglandular nests of cells and alveolar (cup-like) formations lined by neuroglial cells with abundant cytoplasmic melanin in a dense collagenous matrix Laboratory Increased urinary vanillylmandelic acid; see Pseudonym syndrome

Pigmented villonodular synovitis ORTHOPEDICS A monoarticular morbid condition most often affecting the knee (less commonly, the ankle, hip and shoulder) of young adults characterized by a proliferation of yellow-brown hemosiderin-laden spongy tissue **Histopathology** Papillary projections in a background identical to nodular tenosynovitis **Treatment** Excision and with recurrence, re-excision **Differential diagnosis** Fibrosarcoma, synovial sarcoma, incontinentia pigmenti

PIGO Phenytoin-induced gingival overgrowth A hyperplastic process induced by phenytoin's direct stimulatory effect on gingival fibroblasts, resulting in increased collagen synthesis, a phenomenon seen in 10-30% of phenytoin-treated patients; Cf Phenytoin lymphadenopathy

Pi granules Lamellations of flattened perinuclear osmiophilic material in benign tumors of the peripheral nervous system, which are of unknown significance; see Myelin figures

Pigskin appearance Moroccan leather appearance A descriptor for the finely bosselated surface of the renal cortex after removing the capsule, where the papular elevations correspond to sclerotic hyalinized, hypertrophied arterioles, typically seen in benign nephrosclerosis; the 'pigskin' descriptor also refers to the taut, shiny, non-pitting and painful skin of patients with lipemia, usually affecting the lower extremities, see Painful fat syndrome

'Pigtail' 'Spaghetti' TRANSFUSION MEDICINE A regional colloquialism for the plastic tubes clamped off at 5 cm intervals that are connected to transfusion bags, and used for serological testing, in order to determine donor-recipient compatibility prior to transfusion

Pigtail catheter A drainage catheter with side holes, used for draining clear non-viscid or coagulable collections of bile, urine or pancreatic fluids; the 'pigtail' is inefficient in draining abscesses from solid organs, but may be used for perihepatic abscesses

PIH see Prolactin-inhibiting hormone

Pilgrim plant A nuclear power station in Massachusetts from which 'soft' epidemiologic data appear to some workers to support the controversial data from the Sellafield study, which in turn suggests that there may be an increased incidence of leukemia in those exposed to low levels, ie < 500 mrems/year of radiation Note: Data from France, a country that derives a great part of its energy from nuclear reactors, does not appear to confirm these studies; see Sellafield; Cf Three Mile Island

Pili torti A hair shaft defect (figure, right), most commonly affecting ash-blondes, where the hair is grooved and flattened at varying intervals and twisted on its axis; the defect is usually recognized by age 2-3, the hair having a 'spangled' appearance; pili torti is a component of Menke's disease (see Kinky hair, which is associated with mental retardation, either autosomal dominant or recessive); Cf Ringed hair, Woolly hair

Pili torti

'Pill' esophagitis Mucosal injury of the esophagus caused by per os medication, eg aspirin, nonsteroidal anti-inflammatory drugs, anticholinergics, iron-preparations, potassium chloride, tetracycline and quinidine **Clinical** Prolonged 'cancer-like' symptoms including retrosternal pain, progressive stricture, hemorrhage and perforation

'Pill hypertension' A form of hypertension affecting women who have an intrinsic predisposition for increased blood pressure, which is due to increased circulating angiotensinogen induced by estrogens in oral contraceptives

Pilot's wheel appearance see Mariner's wheel appearance

Pimp, Pimping ACADEMIA A practice in which persons in power ask esoteric questions of junior colleagues with the sole (but unexpressed) purpose of publicly demeaning them, most often occurring on ward rounds with a chief of service in a university hospital; the interrogating 'pimper' is theoretically interested in correct answers; the 'pimpee', usually a medical student, in self esteem, although correct answers to the questions gain neither credit for nor relief from this form of harassment; pimping serves to establish a 'pecking order' among the medical staff, suppress spontaneous or intellectual questions or pursuits, create an antagonistic atmosphere and perpetuate medical student abuse (J Am Med Assoc 1989; 262:2541-2; 263:1632c); Cf Pumping

PIN Penile intraepithelial neoplasia

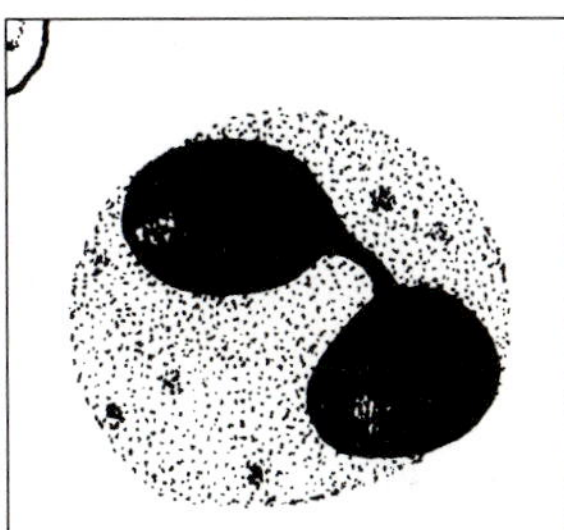

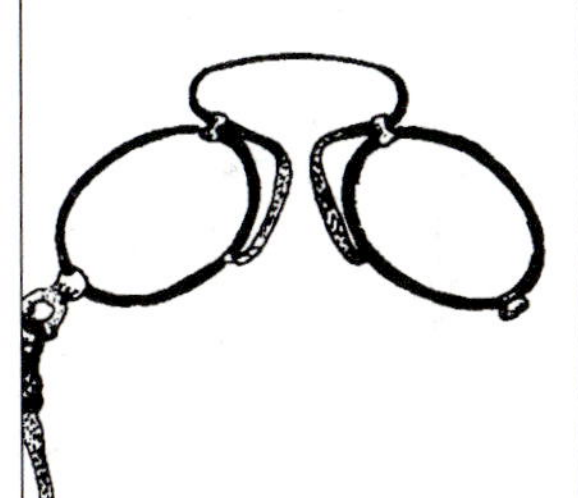

Pince-nez appearance

Pince-nez neutrophil Pelger-Huët anomaly HEMATOLOGY A descriptor for the polymorphonuclear leukocytes that fail to develop normal nuclear lobes, which are 'arrested' as a bilobed, peanut- or barbell-shaped nucleus with clumped dark chromatin, fancifully likened to pince-nez spectacles, a deformity that may also be seen in lymphocytes and monocytes; the condition is either autosomal dominant and asymptomatic or acquired (pseudo-Pelger-Huët anomaly) and associated with hematopoietic malignancies, eg mycosis fungoides, leukemia and preleukemia

Pincer (finger)nail An idiopathic excess tranverse curvature of the nail bed that is associated with intense pain and loss of soft tissue at the fingertips

Pine tree appearance see Christmas tree appearance

'Ping-pong' chromatography A variant of affinity chromatography that may be used to purify enzymes capable of forming covalent bonded intermediates **Method** A solution with the enzyme is poured into the chromatography column, allowed to link to its cognate substrate, which has been permanently bonded to the column's stationary phase and, then eluted by breaking the covalent bond, repeated in a simple two-phase, 'ping-pong'-like fashion

'Ping pong' infection A descriptor for the epidemiology of sexually-transmitted *Trichomonas vaginalis* infection, where a person is treated with antibiotics during the incubation period of his/her sexual partner's infection by the same organism; the partner later becomes symptomatic after the patient has responded to antibiotics, resulting in an infection that 'bounces' back and forth from the treated to the untreated partner, in a fashion likened to a ping-pong ball; *Trichomonas vaginalis* affects 3 million women in the USA and is more common in those with multiple partners, affecting at least 70% of prostitutes; β-hemolytic streptococcus may also have a 'ping-pong ball' pattern of infection

'Ping-ponging' HEALTH CARE INDUSTRY The practice of repeated passing of a patient from physician A to physician B and back again for the purpose of overcharging the patient's reimbursement agency, eg Medicaid or less commonly, private insurance company; see Family ganging, Medicaid mill

Ping-pong mechanism BIOCHEMISTRY A sequence of events that may occur in a catalytic reaction, where one substrate molecule is bound and a product molecule is released; a second substrate molecule is bound, releasing the metabolized product that was bound on the previous pass and so on, eg cleavage of polypeptide chains by a serine protease, or a transaminase-type reaction, where the enzyme transfers an amino group from an amino acid to a ketoacid, yielding a ketoacid where the amino acid was originally and a ketoacid where the amino acid was

Pink disease Acrodynia A form of chronic mercury intoxication of historic interest that occurred in infants given teething powder containing elemental mercury **Clinical** Pruritis, red-pink discoloration of cold, clammy skin, especially on the acral parts and on the buttocks, irritability, weight loss, photophobia, conjunctivitis, fever, leukocytosis, albuminuria and hypotonicity; Cf Mercury, Minamata disease

Pinkeye Acute contagious conjunctivitis by *Haemophilus aegyptius* or *H ducreyi*; 'Pinkeye' has been obfuscated by the lay person, who may use the term for any condition in which the eyes are pink, eg bilateral bacterial or viral conjunctivitis, 'misuse' of the eyes, ie smoke-filled rooms, chronic alcoholism, dissipated life style, severe iritis and closed angle glaucoma; see Red eye

Pink noise Random variation in an audio signal, ie sound that carries no useful information about the source; pink noise has an equal amount of energy in each octave band; Cf Chaos, White noise

'Pink puffer' A descriptor for a patient with chronic obstructive pulmonary disease, severe emphysema, having increased residual lung capacity and volume, decreased elastic recoil, decreased expiratory flow rate and diffusing capacity and a ventilatory/perfusion (V/Q) mismatch secondary to emphysema-related destruction of blood vessels **Clinical** Hyperventilation, shortness of breath Note: Arterial blood gases (PaO_2 and $PaCO_2$) are usually normal because of the compensatory hyperventilation Note: 'Pink puffers' may be clinically indistinguishable from 'Blue bloaters'; see Chronic obstructive pulmonary disease

Pink tag TRANSFUSION MEDICINE A label attached to units of packed red blood cells in compliance with the California State Blood Labeling Regulations that serves to identify units that are ABO group B Note: Color coding of packed units (group A is yellow, group O is blue and group AB is white) is not required by the US Food and Drug Administration, although the 'California system' has been adopted in certain regions in the US

Pink tetralogy of Fallot PEDIATRIC CARDIOLOGY A clinical variant of Fallot's tetralogy (ventricular septal defect, dextroposition of the aorta, pulmonary artery stenosis and right ventricular hypertrophy), in which the pulmonary stenosis is moderate and a balanced shunt across the ventricular septum allows a normal pink skin color and adequate oxygenation of hemoglobin, in contrast to the usual patient who is cyanotic and has 'blue' skin due to persistent oxygen desaturation

Pink tooth of Mummery Chronic perforating hyperplasia of the pulp A rare event consisting in internal resorption of a tooth, initiated by inflammatory hyperplasia of the pulp, usually not associated with caries; the condition may appear as a pinkish area on the crown, and because the lesion is effected by osteoclasts, is known as an osteoclastoma; if detected early, 'root canal' therapy can salvage the tooth, otherwise it must be extracted

Pinkus' tumor Fibroepithelioma A polypoid variant of basal cell carcinoma, commonly located on the back **Histopathology** Superficial with long, thin branching and anastomosing stands of basal cell carcinoma embedded in a fibrous stroma

Pinkus lymphoma A morphologic variant of T-cell lymphoma, in which the nuclei have a popcorn-like multilobated appearance, but do not differ in clinical behavior

'Pinky-printing' see Thumb-printing

Pinta A chronic infection by *Treponema carateum* that is virtually identical to syphilis, but not nonvenereal in transmission; pinta is endemic to Central and South America and is transmitted by direct muco-cutaneous innoculation, resulting in psoriasiform maculo-papular lesions, which without treatment over time cause acral cutaneous atrophy; Cf Yaws

Pinwheel pattern A low-power light microscopic pattern in which short fascicles of fibroblast-like or endothelial-like cells radiate from a central point bearing a vessel, as seen in sclerosing hemangioma; Cf Cartwheel pattern, Storiform pattern

'Pioneer' bacteria The first wave of bacteria to invade dentinal tubules in pre-clinical caries, which is followed by decalcification of the tubules, a process allowing more bacteria to penetrate the tubules, thus forming a true nidus of infection; see Periodontitis, Plaque

Pioneer neuron NEUROEMBRYOLOGY Subplate neurons appearing in the mammalian telencephalon, corresponding to the first post-mitotic neurons of the developing brain; these cells form an axonal pathway, facilitating the orientation of axonal projections, forming a neuronal scaffold which traverses the internal capsule and invades the thalamus in early fetal life; once the adult pattern of axonal projections is complete, the subplate cells disappear (Science 1989; 245:978); pioneer neurons are also required for the formation of embryonic peripheral nerves (ibid 1989; 245:982)

PIP Postinflammatory polyposis Pseudopolyposis 'Bridged' masses seen in the intestinal lumen in Crohn's disease and ulcerative colitis that are considered benign, nonspecific sequelae to inflammation of the mucosa

PIP$_2$ see Phosphatidylinositol 4,5-biphosphate

Pipestem calcification A fanciful term referring to the tubular mineralization of arteries typical of extensive atherosclerosis, which may cause pseudohypertension given their non-distensibility

Pipestem fibrosis A descriptor for the histological appearance of the hepatic portal spaces, characterized by hyaline thickening and tortuosity, accompanied by portal vein fibrosis, seen in chronic hepatic involvement (Symmer 'cirrhosis'), by ***Schistosoma mansoni*** and ***S mekongi***, which is not true cirrhosis, as the native architecture is preserved, but which may be associated with secondary hypertension

Pipestem ureter A thickened and fixed, aperistaltic ureter that course in a stiff pencil- or pipestem-like fashion from the kidney to bladder in advanced tuberculosis of the urinary tract

PISA see Primary idiopathic sideroblastic anemia

'Pistol shot' pulse Duroziez sign, see Water hammer pulse

***pit*-1 gene** A member of a large family of genes encoding proteins containing a homologous region known as the POU domain; pit-1 is present early in mammalian embryogenesis and encodes the Pit-1 protein, a pituitary gland-specific factor that activates the transcription of growth hormone and prolactin promoters (Nature 1990; 347:528); mutations in the pit-1 gene in mice result in a dwarf phenotype and lack of certain pituitary cells (Pit-1 protein is normally detected in somatotrophic, lactotrophic and thyrotrophic cells°; see POU-domain family

Pitting A splenic function in which intracytoplasmic inclusions, eg Howell-Jolly bodies or siderotic granules are removed from circulating red cells; coincident with removal of the inclusion, a fragment of erythrocyte membrane is also eliminated

Pittsburgh brain stem score CRITICAL CARE MEDICINE A scale used to determine the clinical status of a victim of cerebral trauma which measures carinal, corneal, 'doll's eye' reflex, eyelash and ice water caloric reflexes, Cf Glasgow scale

Pittsburgh criteria TRANSPLANTATION A democratic multifactorial system for selecting recipients of cadaveric kidneys, based on the University of Pittsburgh's transplantation experience; criteria for selecting recipients of a limited resource (transplant organs) is based on: *1) WAITING TIME* More time yields more points, to a maximum of 10 *2) QUALITY OF ANTIGEN MATCH* Two antigens each at A, B and DR histocompatibility loci, two points are given for each antigen matched to a maximum of 12 *3) PRESENCE OF PREFORMED RECIPIENT CYTOTOXIC ANTIGENS*, expressed with a panel of reactive antibody number; 10 points is given if the patient is sensitized and forms antibodies to the antigens of most of the human population *4) MEDICAL URGENCY* A rarely used criterion that is awarded when access sites for dialysis are exhausted *5) LOGISTIC FACTORS* Ease and rapidity of transplantation; points are given if the donor organ was nearing the end of its viable storage, ie > 24 hours post-removal, to a maximum of 6 points (J Am Med Assoc 1987; 257:3073); see Procurement, Transplan-tation; Cf Rationing

Pittsburgh pneumonia agent *Legionella micdadei* An often intracellular bacteria that is a frequent contaminant of hot and cold water supplies, which may cause bronchopneumonia with consolidation and a fibrinopurulent exudate, fever, pleuritic pain and cough, most often affecting immunosuppressed children; see Legionnaire's disease

Pituitary apoplexy A symptom complex accompanying hemorrhage or infarction of a pituitary adenoma, or irradiation of the pituitary gland **Clinical** Sudden headache, loss of vision, shock and ophthalmoplegia **Treatment** Replacement hormones

Pituitary dwarfism see Growth hormone-deficient dwarfism

PiZZ The most common variant allele in α_1-antitrypsin deficiency; the common normal allele is PiMM; see α_1-antitrypsin deficiency

'Pizza pie' appearance A descriptor for the fundoscopic appearance of the variegated retinal hemorrhage seen in cytomegalovirus retinitis, fancifully likened to a pizza pie with 'extra cheese' (J Am Med Assoc 1989; 262:3337)

P-K test Passive transfer test of Prausnitz-Küstner IMMUNOLOGY A clinical assay that measures allergic responsiveness to foreign proteins **Method** Serum from an allergic individual is injected intradermally into a non-allergic subject; the injection site is subsequently re-exposed ('challenged') with serum containing the antigen, which evokes a local anaphylactic reaction due to the release of IgE **Clinical** Urticaria, rhinitis, vasculitis, mononuclear infiltrate Note: The test originated from Küstner, who was allergic to fish; whose serum caused the passive allergic reaction in his friend Prausnitz's skin, resulting in a typical wheal-and-flare reaction

PKU Phenylketonuria

Placebo effect The usually beneficial effect that an inactive or inert substance, ie a placebo, has on a patient's clinical course; up to 30% of patients with conditions having psychologic underpinnings may report clinical improvement when medicated with a placebo; diseases that may respond to placebos, eg angina, arthritis, hypertension and post-operative pain, may also respond to biofeedback; the well-described analgesic effect of placebos may be mediated by endorphins; see

Biofeedback, 'Halo' effect, Hawthorne effect; Cf 'Nocebo'

Placental lactogen see Human chorionic somatomammotropin

Placental site trophoblastic tumor (PSTT) GYNECOLOGIC PATHOLOGY A rare uterine neoplasm of gestational tissue occurring in women of reproductive age, presenting as a 'missed' abortion, which ranges from microscopic to massive in size and from 'timid' to highly aggressive that actively secretes hPL (human placental lactogen) **Histopathology** Proliferation of monomorphic intermediate trophoblast cells that separate myometrial fibers either singly or in sheets **Prognosis** 10% mortality

Plague An epidemic infection by ***Yersinia pestis*** (described by Yersin in 1894 in Hong Kong); during plague epidemics, mortality may approach 100%; the marked aggression of the bacterium is linked to mutations in the genes encoding the proteins Yop-1 and invasin **Clinical** forms Bubonic (90% of cases), septicemic, pneumonic and, as a complication of any of the above, plague meningitis

Plakoglobulin An 85 kD protein of the adhering junctions of epidermal cells that forms part of the antigen complexes in pemphigus foliaceus and pemphigus vulgaris

'Plantibodies' Plant-derived antibodies, first produced in tobacco which may have a function in human research and applications, having the theoretical advantage of being less immunogenic than mouse antibodies

Plaque CARDIOLOGY An early lesion of atherosclerosis that may be found in subjects of any age in the large to medium-sized vessels DENTISTRY An indurated accumulation of polysaccharides and bacteria including ***Lactobacillus acidophilus*** and ***Streptococcus mutans***; see Periodontitis DERMATOLOGY A flat, solid, elevated skin nodule measuring more than one centimeter in diameter that is formed either by extension or coalescence of papules and may be seen in lichen amyloidosis, lichen simplex chronicus, lichen planus and psoriasis; a 'plaque' stage occurs in certain skin tumors, eg the second stages of both Kaposi sarcoma and mycosis fungoides NEUROPATHOLOGY Plaques or 'shadow plaques' Multiple, usually well-circumscribed, irregularly-shaped and sharply demarcated lesions in both the gray and white matter corresponding to foci of demyelinization, seen in the brain of patients with multiple sclerosis; Cf Senile plaques

Plaque (-forming) assay Plaque technique IMMUNOLOGY One of a group of in vitro methods that semiquantify either a) The amount of infective particles, ie bacteria or viruses in a solution, a technique known as a 'plaque assay', in which host cells are mixed with a potential pathogen in a gel and the number of cleared spaces, representing lysed host cells are counted or b) The amount of lymphocytes actively producing antibodies, known as 'Jerne's plaque technique', in which lymphocytes from an animal sensitized to the red cells of one species are mixed with those red cells in a gel; addition of complement results in lysis by the antibody-producing lymphocytes, evidenced by a cleared red space on the agar Method The test cells (usually spleen cells) are suspended on an immobile support medium in the presence of sensitized, antigen-coated erythrocytes; after incubation, the spleen cells are presumed to have had enough time to produce sufficient antibody directed against the antigen(s) on the red cells, allowing enough time for that antibody to diffuse through the medium; addition of complement to the milieu results in complement-mediated hemolysis, yielding a clear zone around the lyzed red cells; plaque-forming cell assays may be direct, indirect or 'reversed'

Plasma A clear yellow fluid that comprises 50-55% of the blood volume, consisting of 92% fluid, 7% protein and less than 1% of inorganic salts, gases, hormones, sugars and lipids; fibrinogen- and coagulation factor-depleted plasma is termed 'serum'

Plasma cell dyscrasias A group of lymphoproliferative diseases characterized by the presence of a monoclonal proliferation of plasma cells, which range in clinical behavior from the innocuous extramedullaryplasmacytoma and premalignant solitary plasmacytoma of bone to multiple myeloma; Cf Monoclonal gammopathy of undetermined significance, Myeloma

Plasma cell leukemia A neoplastic increase in circulating plasma cells; histopathologic criteria: Nuclear vacuolization, monotonous sheets of cells, > 20% leukocytes must be plasma cells or the absolute number of plasma cells in the peripheral blood must be > 2×10^9/L (US: > 2000/mm^3) **Clinical** Most cases are well advanced at the time of diagnosis, displaying massive tissue infiltration and marrow replacement at the time of diagnosis with a poor prognosis **Differential diagnosis** Reactive plasmacytosis, which may be associated with agranulocytosis, burns, chronic granulomatous disease, collagen vascular disease, exanthematous lesions, hypersensitivity reactions, non-malignant hepatic disease, nonmyelomatous malignancy, sarcoidosis, syphilis, subacute bacterial infection, streptococcal sepsis, typhoid, viral infection (especially infectious mononucleosis)

Plasma membrane Cell membrane

Plasmanate A proprietary form of plasma protein fraction that is approximately 90% albumin by volume, which is of occasional use as a volume expander; see Albumin, Colloid solutions; Cf Crystalloid solutions

Plasmapheresis A therapeutic modality in which the blood is drawn from a patient, the cells centrifuged, the plasma removed and discarded (or rarely, used to prepare certain blood-derived products), resuspended in an appropriate fluid, either albumin or albumin in saline and then readministered to the patient; the removal of one plasma volume (circa 2500ml) is sufficient to effect a 65% reduction in the amount of a toxin or deleterious (auto)antibody in the circulation (two volume exchanges reduce the undesired substance by another 20%); plasmapheresis is of therapeutic use in the hyperviscosity syndrome, myasthenia gravis, Eaton-Lambert syndrome, Goodpasture syndrome, post-transfusion purpura, acute Guillain-Barré syndrome, and is of use in reducing the amount of toxins in the circulation, eg paraquat, methylparathion, mushroom (***Amanita phylloides***); see Hemapheresis

Plasma R binder protein see R binder protein

Plasmid EXPERIMENTAL BIOLOGY An extrachromosomal

genetic particle present in some bacteria, consisting of a circular segment of double-stranded DNA that is capable of autonomous replication, ie independent of the bacterium's replicative machinery; R plasmids are a special type that carry genes enabling the host bacterium to resist the otherwise destructive effects of antibiotics, heavy metals, ultraviolet radiation and bacteriophages; plasmids are of great use in recombinant DNA technology, serving as vectors for transporting 'engineered' segments of DNA of interest into bacteria to increase the copy number of the DNA for the purpose of creating radioactive 'probes' or for sequencing, a function that has been partially replaced by the polymerase chain reaction, see pBR322, PCR (polymerase chain reaction); Cf Cosmid, YAC cloning

Plasminogen activator inhibitor-1 (PAI-1) An endogenous inhibitor of plasminogen activators that modulates vascular fibrinolytic potential by converting plasminogen into an actively-degrading enzyme, plasmin; a relative increase in PAI-1 is associated with thrombosis, a finding corroborated in transgenic mice bearing with PAI-1 (Nature 1990; 346:74); PAIs are lowest in subjects with high consumption of fruits, vegetable and root vegetables (J Intern Med 1990; 227:267), thus having potential currency as a barometer of health

Plastic bronchitis Fibrinous bronchitis An uncommon condition that may affect any age group, which is characterized by the production of large inspissated casts of the bronchial tree, often associated with allergic bronchopulmonary aspergillosis, bronchiectasis and cystic fibrosis **Clinical** Dyspnea, wheezing, cough, fever and occasionally, hemoptysis (Mayo Clin Proc 1991; 66:305)

Plaster cast lung A lung characterized by extensive pulmonary consolidation, most common in ***Klebsiella pneumonia*** infection, in which each lung weighs up to 1500g and is covered with fibrinopurulent exudate and copious slimy, mucoid pus

Plastic induration of the penis Peyronie's disease A condition characterized by unilateral fibrosis of the fascial sheath of one or both of the corpora cavernosa, leading to curvature and painful erection **Histopathology** Scar tissue formation and rarely, ossification of the penile shaft

Plastic pleurisy see Dry pleurisy

Plasticizer TRANSFUSION MEDICINE Any inert chemical, eg DEHP di-2-(ethylhexylphthalate), which gives the otherwise rigid polyvinyl chloride (PVC) plastic blood collection bags their favorable physical characteristics; because DEHP leaches out from the plastic into the blood and there is some evidence that suggests there may be toxic and potentially carcinogenic effect, it is being replaced by other agents, despite the fact that DEHP increases blood shelf life

Plate atelectasis RADIOLOGY Segmental atelectasis that is characterized by linear shadows of increased density at the lung bases that are horizontal, measure 1-3 mm in thickness and a few cm in length, and are typically seen after abdominal surgery or in pulmonary infarction

Plateau MICROBIOLOGY A phase in the growth cycle of bacteria in culture, in which the nutrients are sufficient to sustain growth and the cells dying are equal in number to those being produced de novo

Plateau development PEDIATRICS A form of disease progression that occurs in infants who reach their normal developmental milestones in the first few months or years of life, later slowing to a 'plateau' and finally begin a slow, inexhorable deterioration until death in early childhood; plateau development is characteristic of children with AIDS, Tay-Sachs disease and certain 'Floppy infant' syndromes

Platelet activating factor (PAF) A phospholipid synthesized by hematopoietic (leukocytes and macrophages) and endothelial cells that causes platelet aggregation, secretion of amines, neutrophil aggregation and enzyme release and increase in vascular permeability; PAF mimics both the physiologic and immunologic effects of some IgE-mediated events of anaphylaxis and cold urticaria, may have a role in endotoxic shock, the pathogenesis of gastric ulcers and a role in ovulation via arachidonic acid metabolism (Science 1989; 243:381), PAF is inactivated by phospholipases that cleave the substituted glycerides

Platelet aggregation	ADP	Epinephrine	Thrombin	Collagen	Ristocetin
Bernard Soulier	N	N	(N/-)	N	▼▼▼
Glanzmann	▼▼	▼▼▼	▼▼▼	▼▼▼	N
von Willebrand	N	N	(N/-)	N	▲▲▲
Storage pool disease	▼▼	▼▼	▼▼	▼▼	▼▼

Platelet aggregation studies LABORATORY MEDICINE A battery of assays (table,above) that measures the response of platelets to various aggregating substances eg ADP, epinephrine, thrombin, collagen, ristocetin and arachidonic acid, which is determined by an increase in optical density of stirred, platelet-rich plasma; normal platelets exhibit a primary and secondary phase response when exposed to collagen and ADP; platelet aggregation studies are used to diagnose coagulopathies due to platelet membrane defects

Platelet antibodies see Platelet antigens

Platelet antigens **Transfusion medicine** A group of antigens found on the surface of platelets that may elicit the production of platelet antibodies and be responsible for neonatal alloimmune thrombocytopenia and post-transfusion purpura, most commonly occurring as a reaction to the $P1^{A1}$ antigen in $P1^{A1}$ antigen-negative recipients; other platelets antigens causing purpura include Pl^{A2}, HLA-A2 and Bak^{a}

Platelet-derived growth factor (PDGF) A 32 kD dimeric protein that is a potent connective tissue mitogen, stimulating proliferation of fibroblasts, intimal smooth muscle (PDGF-like substances are autocrine stimulators of smooth muscle cell proliferation in early atherogenesis, N Engl J Med 1988; 318:1498) and some specialized epithelia, eg lens (Science 1988; 242:777) via tyrosine-specific phosphorylation; other PDGF activities include vasoconstriction, chemotaxis, activation of intracellular enzymes, eg glycogen synthetase and phosphatidylinositol turnover, Ca^{++} fluxes, increased transcription of certain genes and changes of the cytoskeleton; the PDGF system is involved in atherosclerosis and fibroproliferative pathology, eg pulmonary fibrosis, glomerulonephritis, myelofibrosis, keloid formation and in carcinogenesis; the PDGF dimer is composed of A or B chains, differing in their transforming abilities and has 3 isoforms, AA, AB and BB, recognized by two different PDGF receptors Note: PDGF's BB homodimer of PDGF has sequence homology with the v-sis oncogene

Platelet-derived growth factor receptor (PDGF-R) A 180-190 kD membrane glycoprotein with five immunoglobulin-like extracellular domains and a kinase insert in the cytoplasm, which mediates all PDGF's activities; PDGF-R and related receptors (CSF-1 and c-kit proto-oncogene) require a conformational change in the receptor protein before signal transduction occurs (Science 1989; 243:1564rv); a second 120 kD PDGF-R is encoded by a gene on chromosome 4q11 (ibid 1989; 243:800); see Immunoglobulin-like domains

Platelet transfusion A therapeutic modality for increasing circulating platelets (table, below); concentrates of platelets are obtained by a low speed ('light') centrifugation of a unit of whole blood, which yields 40-70 ml of platelet-enriched plasma containing 3 to 4 x 10^{11} platelets, a quantity sufficient to raise an 'average' adult patient's platelet levels by 10 x 10^9/L (US: 10 000/mm^3); platelets are optimally stored t 20-24°C with gentle agitation and should be transfused within 5 days of harvesting; patients with immunological lability should receive platelets from a single donor; see Platelet antigens

Platelet transfusion guidelines for transfusing one unit of (random-donor) platelets/10 kg body weight in 24 hours

Platelet count < 20 X 10^9/L (US: < 20 000/mm^3)

Platelet count < 40 X 10^9/L in active hemorrhage

Platelet count < 50 X 10^9/L in neonates, or patients with documented coagulopathies, recurrent fever, severe infections or patients receiving drugs that may cause platelet dysfunction

Platelet count < 100 X 10^9/L that is present prior to 'bloody' surgery, eg cardiopulmonary bypass or less than 48 hours after surgery

Bleeding time greater than twice the upper limit of normal

(J Am Med Assoc 1988; 259:2415)

Playboy bunny sign A fanciful descriptor for a normal hepatic vein junction, when seen by ultrasonography, where the inferior vena cava forms the bunny's 'head', the middle and lateral hepatic veins the 'ears'; the variably present right vein forms the optional 'pipe'

Pleated sheet see β-pleated sheet

Pleitrophin A heparin-binding growth factor (formerly, HBGF-8) that is structurally unrelated to the seven members of the HBGF family of polypeptid cytokines; pleiotrophin is mitogenic to fibroblasts in culture, promotes neurite outgrowth, is developmentally expressed and is highly expressed in the brain, uterus and is also found in other sites, including gut, muscle, lung and skin (Science 1990; 250:1690)

Pleomorphic adenoma see Mixed tumor

Pleomorphic xanthoastrocytoma NEUROPATHOLOGY A rare variant astrocytoma of the cerebral cortex and leptomeninges, which affects children and young adults Histopathology Marked cellular pleomorphism, bizarre giant cells, prominent lipid-laden macrophages and mitotic activity without necrosis Immunoperoxidase Positive for glial fibrillary acidic protein (GFAP) Prognosis Relatively good, despite the tumor's aggressive histological appearance

Pleotypic response The constellation of metabolic processes involved in initiating cell division, including membrane transport, synthesis of DNA, RNA and proteins and protein degradation

Plethysmography A technique that measures the changes in the volume of an organ, limb or the body **IMPEDANCE PLETHYSMOGRAPHY** is used to diagnose acute venous obstruction or vascular insufficiency of an extremity by measuring the change in limb volume with each arterial pulse and during cuff occlusion of the venous flow from the limb, the manipulation of which allows evaluation of either the arterial or venous flow **WHOLE BODY PLETHYSMOGRAPHY** measures the volume of gas in the lungs, including that which is trapped in poorly communicating air spaces, which is of particular use in chronic obstructive pulmonary disease and emphysema

PLEVA Pityriasis lichenoides et varioliformis acuta DERMATOLOGY An idiopathic papulovesicular disease with successive waves of lesions of the trunk and extremities Histopathology Spongiosis, dyskeratosis, parakeratosis and extravasation of red cells

Pleural 'tag' A radiographic 'knob' said to be seen in the periphery of one-fourth of patients with bronchoalveolar carcinoma but not with other pulmonary carcinomas (Am Rev Resp Dis 1982; 125:74)

Ploidy analysis LABORATORY MEDICINE A technique in flow cytometry that evaluates the chromosomal content of cells, a parameter of aggression in malignancy; in general, diploidy, ie the presence of two haploid sets of chromosomes, is a normal or near-normal state, while anaplastic and aggressive tumors are more often aneuploid or hyperdiploid; ploidy analysis is of use in prognosticating cancer of the bone (osteosarcoma), breast, colon, endometrium, lymphoma and ovary; in breast carcinoma with positive lymph nodes, survival is poor in the face of aneuploidy or hypertetraploidy; in lymph node-negative cases, 93% survived four years (or more) if the number of malignant cells in the S growth phase was < 7.0%; 71% survived if the S phase fraction was > 12% (N Engl J Med 1990; 322:1045); in osteosarcoma, near-diploid tumors have a low rate of relapse; hyperdiploid tumors have a high relapse rate in the early follow-up period; the same 'rule' (diploid, good prognosis, aneuploid, poor prognosis) applies to transitional cell carcinoma of the bladder, ovary and endometrium (88% of diploid and 57% of nondiploid tumors undergo progression (Mayo Clin Proc 1990; 65:643) Aggressive intermediate and high grade lymphomas, are often in the S (synthesis) phase of the growth cycle; aneuploidy is more common (40% of these tumors displayed aneuploidy in one study) in high-grade (ie aggressive) lymphomas than in low grade (15% aneuploidy) lymphomas; see Flow cytometry

Plowshare-like growth SURGICAL PATHOLOGY A descriptor for the ingrowth of aggressive dysplasia as it extends laterally beneath benign epithelium; plowshare-like growth may also occur when benign epithelium grows beneath regressing dysplasia, a far less common clinical event; Cf Bulldozing pattern, Stabbing pattern

PLP Parathyroid hormone-like protein see Hypercalcemia of malignancy

'Plucked bird' appearance An appearance classically described in children with Hutchinson-Gilford progeria, characterized by alopecia, midfacial cyanosis, atrophy of subcutaneous fat, sculptured nose with a 'beaked' tip, a disproportionately large head, prominent eyes and scalp veins, nail and dental dystrophy, micrognathia, xeroderma, pyriform thorax, a horse riding stance, thin limbs, stiff joints and osteoporosis

Plucked chicken skin appearance DERMATOLOGY Innumerable ('pebbly') 1-3 mm in diameter, yellow-white papules coalescing into patches, a characteristic finding in pseudo-xanthoma elasticum; a similar lesion may be acquired in those exposed to Norwegian salt-peter

Plume ENVIRONMENT A 'feather-like' extension of contaminated ground water into an aquifer from the site of the initial in-ground dumping of toxic chemicals, which extends for a variable, usually downgradient distance of up to ten miles; the speed of the spread is a function of the soil's porosity, frequency of rainfall and whether water is being added or removed from the aquifer by human sources; removal of a plume is virtually impossible and it may require decades to centuries before the contaminated soil is washed clean of the pollutant

Plump hilus sign of Fleischer RADIOLOGY An increased prominence of the hilar vasculature on the side most affected in acute pulmonary thromboembolism on a plain chest film

Plus strand The strand of a nucleic acid of viral origin that has a virtually identical base pair sequence to that of the corresponding mRNA of viral origin; see Minus strand

PML see Progressive multifocal leukoencephalopathy

PMLE see Polymorphous light eruption

PMNs Polymorphonuclear leukocytes, Neutrophilic granulocytes

PMR Proportionate mortality ratio PUBLIC HEALTH A statistic that allows the comparison of two or more populations without requiring knowledge of the population at risk for a morbid condition

PMS Premenstrual syndrome(s) A group of disorders characterized by affective, behavioral and somatic symptoms that consistently occur during the luteal (second) phase of the menstrual cycle, resolving with the onset of menstruation and vaguely linked to the fall in estrogen and progesterone from luteal peaks; although PMS was assumed to be a progestational endocrine dysfunction, the use of mifepristone, an antiprogestational agent to induce menses and luteolysis, did not affect the severity or duration of a PMS 'attack' (N Engl J Med 1991; 324:1174, 1208ed) **Clinical** PMS affects 10-30% of menstruating females and is characterized by several days of mental or physical incapacitation of varying intensity, insomnia, headache, emotional lability (anxiety, depression, irritability, loss of concentration, poor judgement, mood swings and tendency towards violence, evoked by environmental cues), acne, breast enlargement, fullness or tenderness, abdominal bloating with edema, craving for salty, sweet or 'junk' food **Treatment** No therapy has proven to be consistently effect, including progesterone (J Am Med Assoc 1990; 264:349)

PMT 1) Gynecology Pre-menstrual tension see PMS 2) Instrumentation see Photomultiplier tube

PNET Peripheral neuroendocrine or neuroepithelial tumor

Pneumatosis cystoides intestinalis (PCI) An uncommon disorder with multiple, variably-sized submucosal blebs of gas in the small intestine, large intestine and stomach that may percolate into the mesentery and omentum; 20% of PCI is related to COPD and respiratory distress, the rest are sporadic and asymptomatic, seen as an incidental radiologic finding on a plain abdominal film; PCI has been described in peptic ulcer disease, intestinal obstruction, intestinal bypass surgery for morbid obesity, mesenteric vascular occlusion, acute necrotizing enterocolitis, inflammatory bowel disease, perforated diverticulitis, collagen vascular disease, cystic fibrosis, diabetes mellitus, appendicitis, Whipple's disease, abdominal trauma (extrinsic or the result of endoscopy), ingestion of caustics, parasitosis, tuberculosis, lymphoproliferative disease **Pathogenesis** Uncertain; hypotheses include the mechanical percolation of gas pockets into tissue spaces, tissue invasion by bacteria with subsequent gas production and fermentation of carbohydrates in the intestinal lumen

Pneumocystis carinii (PCP) An opportunistic microorganism affecting immunocompromised hosts, especially those with AIDS, as well as those with leukemia, lymphoma, organ transplantation, corticosteroid therapy, cytotoxic drugs and the elderly (N Engl J Med 1991; 324:246); the uptake of *P carinii* into macrophages is mediated by a macrophage mannose receptor, a surface glycoprotein of the 'high mannose' type (Nature 1991; 351:155); the initial episode of PCP requiring hospitalization carries a 53% mortality; 63% die within a year of the first episode; 75% of those who survive the first hospitalization for PCP survive one or more years (J Am Med Assoc 1991; 266:89) **Diagnosis** Gomori-methenamine silver (GMS) staining of histologic slides Note:

Although *P carinii* has been traditionally regarded as a parasite with a thick-walled cyst containing six-to-eight round sporozoites that develop into trophozoites, it may actually be a fungus, given the location of certain major genes and its wall composition (N Engl J Med 1991; 324:263ed)

PNS Peripheral nervous system

Pocket dosimeter RADIOLOGY A small ionization chamber worn by those who are occupationally exposed to ionizing radiation and which semiquantifies incident X-rays; Cf Film badge

'Pocket shot' SUBSTANCE ABUSE Injection of heroin, cocaine or other substance of abuse into the 'pocket' in the neck located lateral to the sternocleidomastoid muscle and above the clavicle in an attempt to directly inject the internal jugular vein; given the relative lack of dexterity, the abuser may cause an apical pneumothorax or hydrothorax, often left-sided as most people are right-handed, in addition to an abscess related to non-sterile needles; Cf Skin 'Popping'

Podiatry The field of health care dedicated to the diagnosis and treatment of anatomic or traumatic diseases of the foot; podiatrists (chiropodists) are graduates of a four-year education program that follows a college or university education; podiatrists are examined and licensed by a state's medical board, carry a title of Doctor of podiatric medicine (DPM) and treat foot disease by medicine or surgery

POEMS syndrome Crow-Fucase or Takatsuki syndrome A multisystem disease characterized by the acronym of POEMS for Polyneuropathy (distal symmetric progressive weakness, paresthesias and reduced nerve conduction velocity), Organomegaly (hepatosplenomegaly, lymphadenopathy), Endocrinopathy (hirsutism), Monoclonal gammopathy (myeloma and focal osteosclerosis) and Skin lesions (hyperpigmentation, hypertrichosis, pachydermia and Terry nails)

Point mutation MOLECULAR BIOLOGY A change in one of the nucleotides on the double-stranded DNA molecule; because of the so-called 'degeneracy' of DNA (where 60 different triplets of DNA nucleotides encode only 20 amino acids), there is considerable margin for error, ie many point mutations are 'silent'; point mutations can be detected by single-strand conformation polymorphisms (Genomics 1989; 5:874) and direct sequencing of the DNA after using the polymerase chain reaction; see Degenerate code, Frame shift mutation

Poison A generic term for any substance that alters a cell's or organism's metabolism, evoking biochemical and histologic changes presaging irreversible cell damage and death; many toxins are removable by hemodialysis or peritoneal dialysis, eg sedative-hypnotics (chloral hydrate, ethanol, ethylene glycol, methanol, barbiturates, meprobamate), non-narcotic analgesics (acetaminophen, aspirin, phenacetin), amphetamines, heavy metals (arsenic, lead, mercury), other metals (calcium, lithium), halides, alkaloids (quinine, strychnine), anilines, carbon tetrachloride, ergotamine, isoniazid, nitrofurantoin, phenytoin, theophylline; other compounds are poorly removed by dialysis, including amitriptyline, anticholinergics, antidepressants, atropine, benzodiazepines, digitalis, hallucinogens, heroin, methaqualone, phenelzine, phenothiazines, propoxyphene

POISON TOXICITIES

Minimum lethal dose, mole/kg	
Botulinum toxin A	3.3×10^{-17}
Tetanus toxin	1.0×10^{-15}
Diphtheria toxin	4.2×10^{-12}
Agent Orange	3.1×10^{-9}
Curare	7.2×10^{-7}
Strychnine	1.5×10^{-6}
Cyanide	2.0×10^{-4}

Poison ivy A highly allergenic plant that owes this property to the chemical urushiol found in this and other plants eg mango, japanese lacquer tree and cashews; the most common urushiol-bearing plants in the USA are poison ivy (*Toxicodendron radicans*), located in the eastern US, poison oak (*T diversilobium*), located in the West and poison sumac (*T vernix*), located in the South Note: Urushiol may be carried by smoke from burning plants, potentially causing tracheitis and pulmonary edema in highly-sensitive individuals Note: Urushiol may remain active on unwashed clothing, causing reactions months to years after exposure **Treatment** Varying success is reported

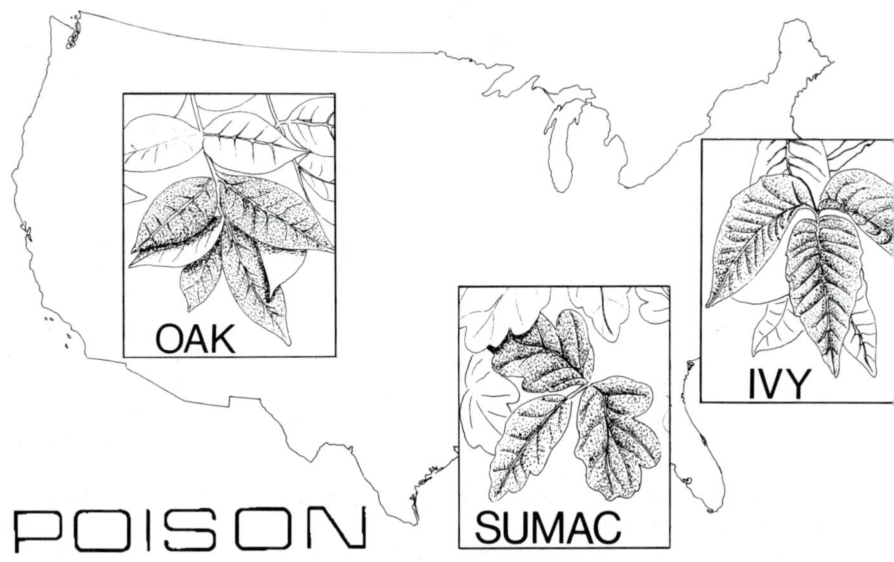

with desensitization therapy

Pokeweed mitogen A carbohydrate-binding lectin isolated from ***Phytolocca americana*** that stimulates the growth and proliferation of B-cells in culture, resulting in production of cytoplasmic or supernatant immunoglobulin; Cf Concanavalin-A, Lectins, Phytohemagglutinin

Pokkuri Japanese see Sudden unexplained nocturnal death

POL Physician office laboratory A small laboratory in a physician's office that has an abbreviated menu of tests that can be performed while the patient is still in the office, in order for the physician to make recommendations to a patient about his state of health and therapy; there has been an increasing tendency in the USA for private physicians to maintain such laboratories, driven by the increased reimbursement (from the 1984 Deficit Reduction Act, supported by the Health Care Financing Agency), convenience and evolving technologies, which allow sophisticated techniques to be performed in a small working space by a staff having little formal laboratory experience; POLs had, because of their small size and the simplicity of methodologies, been exempt from the stringent restrictions imposed on larger laboratories, but have been criticized by some for occasionally producing unreliable results, as POLs may bypass quality control procedures that comprise a large part of the reagent and labor costs borne by larger laboratories; to rectify the situation, the US government formulated the Clinical Laboratories Improvement Act (CLIA), requiring that POLs meet minimum federal certification criteria, including performance of quality control of specimens, maintaining standards for the personnel performing the tests and successful completion of periodic proficiency testing; CLIA regulations exempt those POLs that perform only 'waivered' tests, which either employ methods so simple and accurate as to render the likelihood of error negligible, or tests that pose no reasonable risk of harm to the patient even if performed incorrectly, eg 'dipstick' results, fecal occult blood, microhematocrit, microscopic analysis of pinworms, urinary sediment and vaginal wet mounts, qualitative ovulation tests and urine pregnancy tests; see CLIA

pol Polymerase see DNA polymerases

pol A structural gene of retroviruses that encodes reverse transcriptase, the other two structural genes are gag and env; see HIV-1, HIV-2, Retrovirus

Poland syndrome An autosomal dominant condition characterized by unilateral hypoplasia of skeletal muscle in the shoulder and breast region, affecting the pectoralis major, serratus anterior and latissimus dorsi) accompanied by ipsilateral syndactyly, described by Poland in 1841

Polar body The non-functional haploid daughter of a reduction division; prior to ovulation, the egg in the graafian follicle undergoes reduction division; one-half of the chromosomal complement, a haploid set is allocated to the mature, or secondary oocyte, the other haploid of 23 chromosomes becomes a small daughter, the first polar body; when the sperm penetrates the egg, a second reduction division occurs, a second polar body is formed which also degenerates; Cf Graafian follicle

Polar cap see Capping

Polarization A technique in which fluids and tissues are analyzed for the presence of crystals or crystalline material with an intrinsic ability to change the direction of light passing through them; when the polarizing lenses are crossed, no light can pass through and the field is black; the '+' and '-' adjectives refer to the change in the pathway of the light when a compensator (prepared from a glass slide with streaks cut in clear cellophane tape) is used; anisotropic crystals appear whitish and are not equal in different directions, thus having 'double' polarizing power or birefringence; anisotropism occurs in urate crystals (birefringence refers to polarization at a refractive index of one); without a compensator, the field is dark except for birefringent crystals of monosodium urate, calcium pyrophosphate, talc, cholesterol, and oval fat bodies; with the compensator added, the field is red and the crystal is either yellow or blue according to the orientation of the crystals; see Microscopy

Polarization microscopy see Microscopy

Polar leprosy A designation for either of the two extreme forms of leprosy; polar tuberculous leprosy has a relatively good prognosis, few organisms are present in the tissue and the body is capable of reacting with granuloma formation; polar lepromatous leprosy is substantially more aggressive with numerous lesions, an intense tissue load of organisms which blatently ignore the effete host defense, progressive papulo-nodular lesions and diffuse cutaneous induration; see Borderline disease, Leonine face

'Policeman of the abdomen' A fanciful synonym for the omentum, so designated as it was once thought that it had an intrinsic ability to move within the peritoneal cavity to sites of infection or inflammation; what little movement does occur with the omentum is due to diaphragmatic excursion, intestinal peristalsis and postural changes (rather than an intrinsic ameboid movement); the omentum's immune role is modest and, at most, acts as a repository for macrophages; Cf Pancake omentum

Polio(myelitis) vaccine(s) Two vaccines are available in the US for preventing poliomyelitis; both are highly effective and have a 95% 'take' rate of protection; the per os live attenuated Sabin vaccine is preferred by many workers to the subcutaneous inactivated (killed) Salk vaccine Complications Vaccine-related paralysis occurs in 1 of 2.6 million administrations of polio vaccines Contraindications Pregnancy, immunocompromise; see Vaccine

Political action committee (PAC) A 'special interest' group, often based in Washington DC, that distributes literature, lobbies for and makes contributions to politicians in order to influence decisions in the US Congress and Senate; eg A PAC organized by the American Medical Association will lobby for equitable changes in malpractice law, or firearms hobbyists will lobby against gun control

'Polka dot' pattern A descriptor for the multiple, small, circular patches involving a few hair shafts, seen in early scalp involvement by the superficial dermatophytic fungus *Trichophyton tonsurans*, which is an endothrix-type infection

Polle syndrome see Munchausen-by-proxy syndrome

Pollyannaism A descriptor for one of the postures in adoctor-patient relationship, in which the doctor (a 'Pollyanna') wears a facade of joviality and exudes unrealistic optimism in the face of terminal illness, disregarding the usual anxiety experienced by the patient, a posture that has been widely criticized; Pollyanna is the key character in Eleanor Porter's novel by the same name, who always looked on the positive side of any situation, however disastrous it might have been

Poly A see Polyadenylation sequence, Poly(A) tail

Polyacrylamide gel electrophoresis (PAGE) RESEARCH A type of high-resolution zone electrophoresis performed on a cross-linked polyacrylamide gel, which forms a component of the SDS-PAGE and disc gel electrophoretic procedures; see SDS-PAGE

'Polyadenomes en nappe' A descriptor for gastric polyposis that may cause hypoproteinemia in Menetrier's disease

Polyadenylation sequence MOLECULAR BIOLOGY An oligonucleotide segment of DNA that signals RNA polymerase II in ribosomes to terminate mRNA transcription; in thalassemia, poly A (AATAAA) is the signal leading to the premature cleavage of the β globin gene transcript and addition of the poly-A track; in some patients with hemoglobin H disease with a defective α^+ thalassemia gene, a point mutation changes the polyadenylation signal to AATAGA, resulting in an incorrectly processed and prematurely degraded RNA transcript

Polyagglutination Panagglutination TRANSFUSION MEDICINE Agglutination of red cells by serum that contains antibodies, autoagglutinins or alloagglutinins; the erythrocytes have altered membranes and are inappropriately agglutinated by anti-A or anti-B reagent serum, related to altered glycoproteins, eg T, Tn and Cad; polyagglutination may also occur with acquired B antigens and in HEMPAS and may be due to contamination of the serum by detergents, silica or metallic cations

Poly(A) tail MOLECULAR BIOLOGY A segment of 20-200 adenylic acid residues attached to the 3'-end of eukaryotic mRNA that is thought to increase mRNA's molecular stability by increasing its resistance to nuclease; see Transcription unit

Polybrene TRANSFUSION MEDICINE A polyvalent cation used to reduce the electrostatic repulsion (zeta potential) between erythrocytes, thereby enhancing the detection of weak agglutination when testing red cells for potential donor-recipient transfusion reactions; see Zeta potential

Polychlorinated biphenyls see PCBs

Polychromatophilia A combination of hemoglobin's affinity for acid stains and RNA's affinity for basic stains, eg Wright-Giemsa stain, a normal finding in young red cells with residual RNA; polychromatophilia of erythrocytes may occur in blood loss, hemolysis, anoxia, pulmonary disease, renal cell carcinoma, polycythemia vera and secondary polycythemia, eg living at high altitudes, massive obesity, chronic obstructive pulmonary disease, ectopic erythropoietin production by tumors, including hepatomas, pheochromocytomas and uterine leiomyoma

Polyclonal antibodies A bouquet of immunoglobulins produced by multiple, usually non-malignant clones of cells that have been summoned to arms by an antigen, which may elicit multiple clonal expansions, each responding to a different epitope on the antigen; see Epitope, Idiotype; Cf Monoclonal antibodies

Polycystic kidneys A variety of classifications exist for cystic diseases of the kidneys; since none is completely satisfactory or based on either pathogenesis or etiology, a pragmatic approach is to classify these lesions based on gross morphology which correlates reasonably well with clinical presentation and presumed hereditary transmission (table); see Multilocular cyst of the kidney

Cystic disorders of the kidneys

Renal dysplasia A relatively common, often acquired condition presenting in infancy as unilateral or bilateral and segmental, focally irregular cystic kidneys, related to mesenchymal immaturity and accompanied by obstruction

Infantile polycystic kidneys An uncommon autosomal recessive condition first seen in infants with massively enlarged kidneys and aberrant bile duct formation

Adult polycystic kidneys A common (1-2:1000 in the general population) autosomal dominant condition located to a gene on chromosome 16 affecting adults with large bumpy kidneys, cysts in the liver, lung and pancreas and berry aneurysms of the brain

Medullary sponge kidneys A relatively common bilateral condition of uncertain pattern of heredity, affecting adults with inability to concentrate urine, hypercalcemia, nephrolithiasis, pyelonephritis, distal renal tubular acidosis and cystic dilation of the collecting ducts; renal function and lifespan may be normal

Uremic medullary sponge kidney A rare inherited condition first seen in young adults as bilateral corticomedullary junction cysts and functional tubular defects, Fanconi syndrome and uremia

Polycystic liver disease A condition characterized by multiple millimeter to centimeter in diameter cysts lined by cuboidal epithelium; the hepatic disease is often obscured by the accompanying adult polycystic renal disease; 40% of the affected livers also contain von Meyenburg's complexes

Polycystic ovaries (PCO) Stein-Leventhal syndrome An idiopathic condition affecting 3.5-7.0% of females that is the most common endocrinopathy causing familial hirsutism **Clinical** Obesity, hirsutism, galactorrhea, secondary amenorrhea following dysmenorrhea, acne vulgaris (Br J Dermatol 1989; 121:675), increased luteinizing hormone and an increased risk of endometrial carcinoma related to unopposed estrogenic stimulation **Pathogenesis** Idiopathic; some cases have been associated with central nervous system trauma or injury in childhood **Diagnosis** Palpation, ultrasonography, increased prolactin, and functional testing with nafarelin, a gonadotropin-releasing hormone agonist that causes a male pattern response, suggesting that PCO has defective regulation of 17-hydroxylase and C-17,20-lyase (N Engl J Med 1989; 320:559); see HAIR-AN syndrome

POLYCYTHEMIA VERA

A CLINICAL

A1 Increased erythrocyte mass (male > 36 ml/kg, female > 32 mg/kg

A2 Arterial O_2 saturation > 92% (close to normal)

A3 Splenomegaly (which occurs in 75%)

B LABORATORY

B1 Thrombocytosis > 400 X 10^9/L (most cases)

B2 Leukocytosis > 12 X 10^9/L, in absence of fever or infection

B3 Increased alkaline phosphatase

B4 Increased vitamin B_{12} > 666 pmol/L (US > 900 pg/ml)

Polycythemia vera HEMATOLOGY A malignancy due to the expansion of an abnormal pluripotent stem cell population with increased erythropoietin-independent erythropoiesis and megakaryopoiesis **Laboratory** Increased leukocyte alkaline phosphatase, increased platelets, basophils, increased vitamin B_{12}, vitamin B_{12} binding capacity (transcobalamin I and III), decreased erythropoietin and stainable iron in the bone marrow; 15-20% of cases resolve in a so-called 'spent' phase with marrow fibrosis **Prognosis** 40% die of thrombosis and hemorrhage; others are at increased risk of myeloproliferative disease, with 5-15% of patients developing acute leukemia or myeloid metaplasia, or less comonly, acute leukemia of the FAB-M6 type **Diagnosis** Polycythemia vera requires that either all of 'A' criteria are present or two 'A' criteria and two 'B' criteria are present (table, facing page) **Treatment** Simple phlebotomy yields a 14-year survival; ^{32}P yields a 12 year survival and chlorambucil, a 9 year survival; the latter two may inducer secondary leukemia; hydroxyurea may be used for long-term treatment

Polydrug therapy see Polypharmacy

Polyembryoma A very rare, highly aggressive ovarian germ cell tumor of young adults characterized by numerous embryoid bodies resembling normal presomite embryos, invariably associated with malignant teratoma; see Embryoid bodies

Polyendocrine deficiency syndrome Polyglandular autoimmune syndrome Two, often overlapping endocrinopathies characterized by gonadal failure, possibly secondary to hypothalamic defects with vitiligo and autoimmune adrenal insufficiency (80% of cases have autoantibodies) TYPE I Autosomal recessive, of late childhood onset with hypoparathyroidism, mucocutaneous candidiasis, alopecia, pernicious anemia, malabsorption and chronic active hepatitis TYPE II OF SCHMIDT Autosomal dominant, of adult onset with Addison's disease and either autoimmune (Hashimoto's) thyroiditis or insulin-dependent diabetes mellitus; these conditions are HLA-linked in an as-yet unclear fashion

Polygenes A group of genes that controls a phenotypic feature, eg weight, pigmentation or eye color

Polykaryon Obsolete for 'multinucleated giant cell', which is composed of fused epithelioid macrophages

Polykarysomes Herpetic giant cell A cell with multiple nuclei, due to cell fusion induced by infection with Herpes simplex that may be seen in a Tzanck preparation (smear of fluid obtained from a skin vesicle)

Polyketide(s) A large class of naturally-occurring products including antibiotics, eg erythromycin, pigments, eg tylosin and immunosuppressants (Science 1991; 252:675) that are synthesized by fatty acid synthase-like activity

Polymerase chain reaction (PCR) MOLECULAR BIOLOGY A method for synthesizing large quantities of a segment of DNA starting from minimal amounts of less than 1 μg (theoretically as little as one copy of DNA); PCR exponentially 'amplifies' a double-stranded target DNA sequence that has been inserted between two oligonucleotide primers through multiple amplification cycles (figure), one step of which occurs at a high temper-

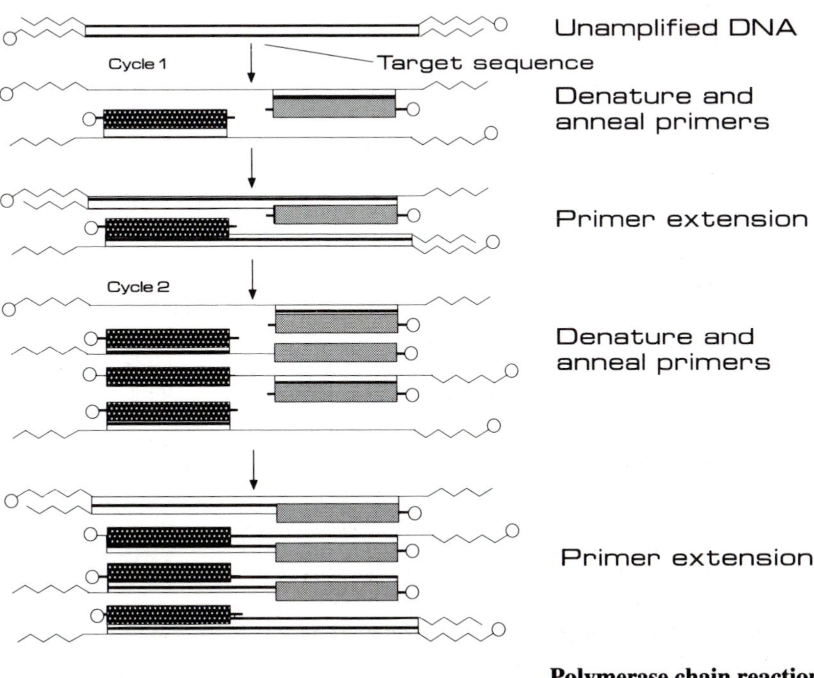

Polymerase chain reaction

ature, inactivating DNA polymerase, requiring that this enzyme be added at the beginning of each synthetic (amplification) cycle; the PCR allows the synthesis of millions of copies of a DNA segment of interest within 6-8 hours and is used for prenatal diagnosis (sickle cell anemia), detection of HIV-1, gene rearrangements in lymphoproliferative disorders and determination of fetal sex; once a DNA segment has been amplified, it is then evaluated by conventional DNA techniques Sensitivity In detecting leukemia in bone marrow, a biopsy has a 65-75% sensitivity, Southern blot analysis of gene rearrangement, 98-99% sensitivity and polymerase chain reaction, 99.999%; the PCR was developed by workers at Cetus corporation (Science 1985; 230:1350) and has revolutionized DNA diagnostics (Science 1988; 239:487)

Polymorphism GENETICS The presence in a population of two or more allelic variants appearing as different phenotypes or which result in genetic changes detectable by restriction fragment length polymorphism analysis, eg alleles of α_1-antitrypsin and the Rh blood groups MOLECULAR BIOLOGY see Restriction fragment length polymorphism

Polymorphous light eruption (PMLE) DERMATOLOGY An abnormal skin reaction to sunburn range ultraviolet B (290-320 nm) light that is more common in young adults, 4-24 hours after exposure to light, appearaing as papular, papulovesicular, plaque or diffuse erythematous lesions; the classic PMLE lesion is a plaque in which patchy lymphocytic infiltrates mimic the lesions of early lupus erythematosus **Treatment** Antimalarial drugs, eg chloroquine

Polymyalgia rheumatica RHEUMATOLOGY A relatively common affliction of the middle-aged population with a 2:1 female:male ratio, characterized by myalgia and arthralgia of the neck and proximal 'girdle' muscles, which is most prominent in the morning and after periods of rest; systemic symptoms are vague and include low-grade fever, malaise, weight loss and a moderately elevated erythrocyte sedimentation rate, which may be associated with other inflammatory, connective tissue disorders and malignancy, most commonly giant cell (temporal) arteritis

Polymyositis RHEUMATOLOGY A condition defined by the presence of four or more of the following criteria: 1) Symmetrical proximal muscle weakness 2) A characteristic skin rash (A scaling violaceous rash on the hands elbows and knees and a heliotrope rash on the eyelids, which is more typical of the often-associated dermatomyositis 3) Increased 'muscle' enzymes, eg the MM band of creatinine phosphokinase in the serum 4) A characteristic electromyographic pattern (insertional activity, normal conduction velocity, fibrillation potentials and motor unit potentials of increased frequency and decreased duration) and 5) Typical histopathology (T cell inflammation in the muscle fascicles, degenerating and regenerating muscle fibers and the presence of 'skip' areas of non-involvement) **Treatment** Corticosteroids; if the disease is recalcitrant, methotrexate and radiotherapy may occasionally be effective (Mayo Clin Proc 1990; 65:1480rv)

Polymyositis/dermatomyositis complex An 'overlap' syndrome in which polymyositis and dermatomyositis have multiple features incommon, including proximal distribution of muscle weakness, chronic 'round cell' inflammation, presence of an IgM rheumatoid factor, myopathic changes, spontaneous electrical discharges by electromyography and clinical response to corticosteroids

Polyoma virus A small icosahedral, double-stranded DNA virus belonging to the papovavirus family, which may be used to induce tumors in mice under experimental conditions

Polyp A generic term for any elevated 'tumor' mass, commonly understood to be epithelial in nature, which is often neoplastic; polyps are of greatest interest in the colon, female genital tract, nasopharynx and stomach **COLON** Colonic polyps are usually epithelial and either acquired or hereditary **Acquired polyps** are adenomatous or tubular in morphology, increasing in frequency with age; although often asymptomatic, larger polyps may announce their presence by bleeding, causing a change in bowel habits or if large enough, form a leading 'front' of an intussusception; histologic distinction between adenomatous polyps ('tight' round glands) and villous adenomas (finger-like fronds of elongated glands) has little practical importance, as both have malignant potential, ranging from 10 to 70%; periodic colonoscopy and polypectomy yields a three-fold reduction in subsequent cancer (Int J Cancer 1990; 46:159) **Hereditary polyps** are often epithelial and may be associated with clinical syndromes that overlap with each other a) Familial polyposis coli A premalignant, autosomal dominant condition presenting in early adulthood with hundreds to thousands of colonic polyps, related to the loss of the normal repression of DNA synthesis in the entire colonic epithelium; adenocarcinoma occurs in 70-100% of patients, prevented by prophylactic colectomy b) Gardner syndrome An autosomal dominant condition with premalignant polyps of the entire gastrointestinal tract; most patients develop colonic carcinoma; other neoplasms occurring in these pateints include biliary tract carcinoma, osteomas of the mandible, skull and long bones, soft tissue tumors (fibromas, lipomas), sebaceous cysts and rarely, neoplasia of the thyroid and adrenal glands and c) Turcott syndrome A rare autosomal recessive condition associated with brain tumors (medulloblastoma, glioblastoma) Other polypoid lesions of the colon include hamartomas, hyperplastic polyps, juvenile and retention polyps, which have little if any neoplastic potential a) Chronkhite-Canada syndrome A non-hereditary condition characterized by diffuse gastrointestinal polyposis, accompanied by alopecia, nail atrophy, cutaneous hyperpigmentation, weight loss, protein-losing enteropathy, electrolyte imbalance and malnutrition b) Peutz-Jeghers syndrome An autosomal dominant condition with hamartomas of the entire gastrointestinal tract, predominantly of the small intestine, focal Paneth cell hyperplasia, melanin spots in buccal mucosa, lips, and digits, intussusception and bleeding; colonic adenocarcinomas, when seen in these patients arise in adenomatous and not in hamartomatous polyps; some cases of Peutz-Jeghers disease may be associated with Sertoli cell tumor and annular tubules, see SCTAT **FEMALE UROGENITAL TRACT** Endometrial polyps appear to represent circumscribed foci of cystic glandular hyperplasia of the endometrium and may cause abnormal bleeding, or give rise to endometrial carcinoma, although this is uncommon; when smooth muscle is also present, they are designated as adenomatous polyps Differential diagnosis Polypoid smooth muscle tumors, benign and malignant; see Müllerian mixed tumor **NASOPHARYNX** Nasal polyps Inflammatory ('allergic') polyps of the nasal cavity are not true neoplasms, but rather are considered a reaction to inflammation or allergy; instead of the focal epithelial proliferation characteristic of true polyps, there is edema and chronic inflammation (eosinophils, plasma cells and lymphocytes) in these often bilateral, recurring intranasal lesions **SKIN** Squamous polyps and fibroepithelial polyps or 'skin tags' are benign prolapses of upper dermis onto the skin surface, which have no neoplastic potential **STOMACH** Gastric polyps are confusing, as it is often (incorrectly) assumed that the common colonic polyps are analogous to gastric polyps; hyperplastic polyps (designated as type I and II polyps by Japanese authors) comprise 75% of all gastric polyps and are usually benign Note: The occasionally used synonym, hamartomatous polyp is incorrect, as this term is best reserved for Peutz-Jeghers syndrome polyps; neoplastic polyps (Japanese type III and IV polyps) are single large, sessile or pedunculated, often antral tumors with atypical, mitotically active, pseudostratified glands analogous to neoplastic colonic polyps, which are thought to arise in intestinal metaplasia; the incidence of malignant degeneration, although low (3.5%), is twice that of gastric hyperplastic polyps; other gastric polyps are similar to colonic polyps and include hamartomatous polyps and juvenile (retention-type) polyps

Polypharmacy CLINICAL PHARMACOLOGY The use of mutiple drugs to treat one or a limited number of conditions, most commonly seen in elderly patients; in the US, very few proprietary and generic drugs are available as 'cocktails' (mixtures of two or more drugs); instead, most drugs are dispensed as single-agent formulations, which is widely thought to allow better titration of dosages and optimal control of each agent while minimizing the toxic effects; indications for increasing the number of drugs to treat a patient include a) The patient has multiple conditions b) The drugs are synergistic with each other and c) The disease is refractory to an accepted, single-agent therapy; see Therapeutic drug monitoring

Polypoid cell see Popcorn cell

Polyprotein A large protein, eg pro-opiomelanocortin (POMC) that is translated from a polycistronic mRNA molecule and is a precursor for a number of smaller polypeptides and proteins that are enzymatically cleaved from the mother molecule after translation; see Alternative splicing

Polyspecific anti-human globulin (AHG) Coomb's reagent TRANSFUSION MEDICINE A reagent containing antibody to human IgG and C3d that may also contain anti-C3b, anti-C4b and anti-C4d; commercially available Coomb's reagent has little activity against IgA and IgM heavy chains, but may react with these immunoglobulins as it may have antibodies reactive against the kappa and lambda light chains; polyspecific Coomb's reagent is used in the blood bank for routine red cell compatibility tests, alloantibody detection and direct antiglobulin test

Polytechnic ACADEMIA An institution of higher education created in Britain in the 1960s with the intent of providing vocational education and, more recently, applied research, in contrast to the British universities, which were dedicated to academics and pure research; because the polytechnics had been viewed as low-quality universities, the effort to merge the two educational systems (Nature 1991; 351:257n), has resulted in a deletion of the term polytechnic from the British system of higher education; as 1992, these institutions will be designated as Universities

Polytene chromosome MOLECULAR BIOLOGY A form of DNA rearrangement occurring in vivo in which segments of DNA are amplified (duplicated) up to 1000 copies and arranged into identical parallel arrays of DNA; the molecular basis (and 'logic') for the multiple repeated gene copies within a presumably linear gene is unknown

Polyunsaturated fatty acid A fatty acid with two or more double-bonded carbons; see Fatty acids, Fish oil; Cf Tropical oils

Polyvinyl chloride CLINICAL TOXICOLOGY A chemical that has a boiling point of -13.5°C (ie, is a gas at room temperature); the vinyl chloride monomer ($H_2C{=}CHCl$) is converted to polyvinyl chloride (PVC) by heating the liquid form at 40-70°C; in 1980, 2 1/2 million metric tons of PVC was produced in the USA, 87% of which was consumed by the soft plastics industry; other uses of PVC include colorants, lacquers, lubricants, tubing, packaging and biomedical devices; the acute and chronic interstitial lung disease seen in PVC intoxication is the result of the *bis*(2-ethyhexyl)phthalate (DEHP), an agent for 'plasticizing' vinyl chloride polymers and which has narcotic effects and causes acroosteolysis, PVC-induced hepatitis, soft-tissue changes, Raynaud-like phenomenon, hepatic hemangiosarcoma at doses as low as 250 ppm, brain tumors, poorly-differentiated large cell carcinomas and adenocarcinoma of the lungs; the current OSHA limit of this potentially explosive gas is 1 ppm over eight hours; Cf PCBs, Plasticizers, Toxic dumps

POMC see Pro-opiomelanocortin

Pompholyx Intense pruritus of the palmoplantar surfaces of possible psychogenic origin, possibly related to increased autonomic nervous system activity, which is more common in warm weather, characterized by crops of vesicles and bullae that may evolve into eczema; see Factitious dermatitis

Pontiac fever Pontiac disease A non-pneumonic epidemic infection by *Legionella pneumophila* serogroup 6 (and other *Legionella* species) first described in Pontiac, Michigan in 1968 **Clinical** After a 24-48 hour incubation, fever, headaches, myalgia, cough, occasionally diarrhea and neurological signs, with complete resolution within one week (N Engl J Med 1988: 318:571); Cf Legionnaire's disease

Pool The total quantity of a substance, material or resource in a 'universe', as in a microenvironment, eg metabolic pool, a population group, eg donor pool, or gene pool

PoP Plaster of Paris, gypsum

Popcorn An adjectival descriptor for a radiological or pathological finding that simulates the solitary kernels of 'popped corn'

Popcorn calcification Popcorn densities BONE A descriptive term for clusters of small scalloped radiolucencies with sclerotic margins seen predominantly in the epiphysis and metaphysis of the actively growing knee and ankle of children with osteogenesis imperfecta (figure); the popcorn appearance is thought to be due to fragmentation and disordered maturation of the physis with an irregular or defective growth plate, resulting in severe growth retardation LUNG A descriptor for the puffed and lobulated appearance that is typical of a well-circumscribed calcified solitary hamartoma, which is seen on a plain anteroposterior chest film and b) Multiple 'popcorn' nodularities are suggestive of pulmonary histoplasmosis and may be seen on a plain chest film SYNOVIUM The popcorn morphology refers to rounded multilobulated masses seen in the peri-articular region in synovial chondromatosis or in enchondromas, which serve to differentiate these from the radiologically similar low-grade chondrosarcomas

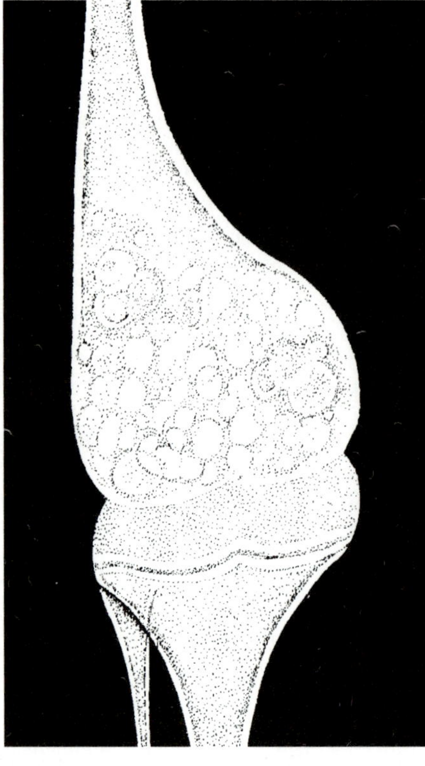

Popcorn calcifications

Popcorn cell Polypoid cell A Reed-Sternberg cell variant with a lobulated 'cloverleaf' nucleus, bubbly nucleoplasm, a small acidophilic nucleolus and a small rim of cytoplasm seen in lymphocyte-predominant Hodgkin's disease; similar 'Reider'-like cells occasionally occur in T-cell lymphoma and Pinkus tumor; see Reed-Sternberg cell

'Popeye' appearance A fanciful descriptor for the clinical changes seen in the Landouzy-Déjérine type of limb-girdle dystrophy, so named for the thinness of the upper arms with pseudohypertrophy of the forearm, a disease further accompanied by involvement of facial muscles, 'winging' of the scapula, incomplete eye closure, inability to whistle or to raise the arms above the head

'Popeye syndrome' Brachial entrapment syndrome An acquired condition seen in older men who do heavy work with their arms; the muscular hypertrophy of the forearm compresses the brachial artery with resultant forearm fatigue and paresthesias Note: Both this and the previous use of the 'Popeye' adjective refer to a comic strip sailor whose strength is attributed to the ingestion of spinach

Popliteal pterygium syndrome An autosomal dominant condition of neonatal onset and variable penetration and clinical expression Clinical A fibrous cord extends from the heel to the ischial tuberosity, limiting leg movement, which is accompanied by syndactyly, bone malformation, club feet, cleft lip and palate, crytporchidism and absence of labia majora

POPOP 1,4-Bis-2-(5-phenoxazolyl)benzene and PPO 2,5-diphenyloxazole Two organic liquid scintillation fluids used to detect β radiation in a radioimmunoassay; POPOP, a secondary fluor and PPO, a primary fluor absorb a sample's weak β radiation and emit flashes of light that are amplified 10^6 to 10^8-fold by a photomultiplier, which passes the signal to a scintillation counter; see Quenching, RIA

Popsickle panniculitis Inflammation of adipose tissue due to localized exposure to the cold, first described in a young child secondary to the ingestion of a 'popsicle', a frozen snack food that is licked; the reaction is attributed to the more saturated nature of fats in children (N Engl J Med 1970; 282:966cr)

Porcelain doll face The puffy, pale facies described in adults with myxedema, due to accumulation of glycosaminoglycans; in other skin regions, there is a greater amount of anchoring of the deep dermis to the surface, resulting in a 'pitted' appearance, termed 'Peau d'orange' changes

'Porcelain' gallbladder An extensively calcified and indurated galbladder that appears in a background of acutely exacerbated chronic cholecystitis and cholelithiasis; although extremely rare, the porcelain gall bladder is of interest as up to 20% develop carcinoma

Porcelain white appearance Indurated enamel-like fibrous plaques seen on the genitals and trunk with follicular plugging, characteristic of lichen sclerosis et atrophica

Porcupine cell tumor see Lymphoma, Large cell lymphoma with filopodia

Porin NEUROPHYSIOLOGY A voltage-gated membrane channel in the outer membrane of gram-negative bacterial walls that is arranged in a lattice of trimers of elliptical cylindrical walls of β protein sheet (Nature 1991; 350:167), serving as a diffusional pathway for molecules that are one-plus kilodaltons (kD) in size, including waste products, nutrients, antibiotics and bacteriophage receptors; a similar protein is present in the outer membrane of mitochondria, allowing passage of 10 kD molecules, especially when positively-charged; see VDAC (voltage-dependent anion-selective channel); Cf Perforin

'Pork barrel' funding Earmarking RESEARCH FUNDING The practice by the US Congress of attaching the costs of 'pet projects' to certain government spending packages; although the science community is opposed to bypassing the peer-review process (the usual conduit for obtaining federal funds); in the awarding of grant monies, as a limited number of groups benefit from unfair funding practices, at the cost of many potentially more deserving candidates, a university may nevertheless employ lobbyists in order to circumvent peer-review (Science 1988; 241:769ed, ibid 242:846c)

Porphin The parent molecule of porphyrins that is comprised of a tetrapyrrole ring

Portacaval shunt A surgical procedure that diverts blood away from the portal venous system, reducing portal hypertension, the cause of the most feared, and potentially fatal complication of cirrhosis, ie bleeding from esophageal varices; portacaval shunts divert blood around the liver into the inferior vena cava and may themselves cause morbidity due to hepatic failure or hepatic encephalopathy; the procedure of choice is thought by some workers to be a portacaval H-graft shunt, which facilitates the control of ascites, provides immediate portal decompression, control of variceal bleeding and provides the option for future restoration of portal circulation, if hepatic failure or encephalopathy develop

Porter-Silber chromagens Glucocorticoids detected by the Porter reaction (phenylhydrazine and sulfuric acid are added to urine), which are 21-carbon molecules with dihydroxyacetone side-chains with a peak absorption at 410 nm, including 11-deoxycortisol, cortisol, cortisone and some 17-hydroxicorticosteroids; the accuracy of the Porter-Silber reaction can be improved by extractions in organic solvents and purifying the urine extracts by chromatography; many drugs, eg chlorpromazine, meprobamate, reserpine and spironolactone interfere with the Porter reaction, causing a false elevation, while the test may be unreliable in neonates with congenital adrenal hyperplasia due to the production of abnormal (and measured) steroids

Port-wine nevus Nevus flammeus Flat hemangioma A common congenital neurovascular malformation, appearing as deep red-purple macular lesions, corresponding to cutaneous angioma(s), often located in the ophthalmic branch of the trigeminal nerve; when located on the meninges, the malformation may be confined to the occipitoparietal pial vessels, where sluggish blood flow predisposes to hypoxia of the underlying cortex **Clinical** 5% of patients with port-wine stains suffer from convulsions, mental retardation, hemiparesis or hemianopsia contralateral to the lesions; port wine nevi may occur in the normal population, eg Mikhail Gorbachev, or may be a component of various syndromes, eg Klippel-Trenaunay, Beckwith-Wiedemann, Cobb, Rubenstein-Taybi and trisomy 13 syndromes **Histopathology** Densely-packed, dilated capillaries in the dermis and subdermis **Treatment** Flashlamp-pulsed tunable argon dye laser, which is most effective if administered before age seven, often requiring more therapeutic sessions in facial lesions (N Engl J Med 1989; 320:416)

Port wine urine A descriptor for the transparent, red urine seen in myoglobinuria due to traumatic injury to muscle, intense, prolonged and/or violent exercise, eg marathon-running and karate; in contrast, hemoglobinuria with red cell casts is a turbid red color

Port-wine stools see Currant jelly stool

Positional cloning MOLECULAR BIOLOGY A time-consuming method for cloning a gene whose product is unknown, which entails a series of complex steps, including chromosomal location of the gene responsible for the disease by linkage analysis

Positive feedback see Feedback

Positive predictive value STATISTICS The number of true positives divided by the sum of true positives (TP) and false positives (FP), a value representing the proportion of subjects with a positive test result who actually have the disease, also known as the 'efficiency' of a clinical assay, defined by the accompanying formula: Note: In predictive values, as with prevalence, as the frequency of a disease decreases, the number of false positive tests increases; Cf Negative predictive value, ROC (receiver operating characteristic)

Positron emission transaxial tomography see PET scanning

Post-datism see Post-term pregnancy

'Post-doc' Post-doctorate fellow A person who has completed the academic and/or research activities required for the completion of his PhD (doctor of philosophy), or less commonly, MD (doctor of medicine), and who is pursuing research (often for a two-to-five year period) in the laboratory of an established scientist Note: The term also commonly refers to the activity itself, as in, *'...to do a post-doc'*

Posterior cord/column syndrome A neurologic complex due to the loss of vibration and position sense below a cord lesion, accompanied by tingling in the affected regions, with preservation of the perception of pain and temperature; since these lesions interrupt the central projections of the dorsal root ganglia cells, they may mimic tabes

Post-mortem PATHOLOGY A colloquialism for a post-mortem examination of a body, alternatively autopsy, necropsy; types of autopsies **BIOPSY ONLY** A minimalist post-mortem examination, in which, although the prosector has permission to enter body sites, and fully examine the organs, he may only keep fragments ('biopsies') for histologic examination **CHEST ONLY** An autopsy in which the family members have only given permission to examine the lungs and heart, in anticipation of identifying an occluding thrombus in the coronary arteries or finding massive pulmonary thromboembolism **COMPLETE** A complete autopsy in which the chest, abdominal and cranial cavities are examined **HEAD ONLY** A postmortem examination in which the pathology of interest is presumed to reside entirely in the cranial cavity **NO HEAD** An autopsy examining the chest and abdominal cavity without violating the cranial cavity; Cf Psychological autopsy

Post-operative erythroderma see Post-transfusion graft-versus-host disease

Post-operative headache A variably present post-operative complication occurring in the hours after recovery from general anesthesia, which may be due to a caffeine withdrawal state (Anesth Analg 1991; 72:449)

Post-operative psychosis A symptom complex said to occur after a surgical procedure, especially those requiring general anesthesia; although this is not considered a true clinical entity, surgery may uncover an underlying psychosis or cause anxiety with psychophysiologic, somatopsychic and psychosocial components

Post-partum depression Post-partum 'blues' A stress reaction occurring in women after delivery, characterized by depression, fatigue, irritability, insomnia (from the third to tenth days postpartum) and if extreme in degree, may result in infanticide

Post-partum renal failure Post-partum hemolytic uremic syndrome (PP-HUS) An idiopathic condition with a poor prognosis, characterized by renal failure, microangiopathic hemolytic anemia, thrombocytopenia and disseminated intravascular coagulation beginning from several days to ten weeks after a normal pregnancy and delivery; PP-HUS may be preceded by hypertension, proteinuria or preeclampsia Clinical Vomiting, diarrhea, flu-like illness may precede the oliguric or anuric phases of acute renal failure accompanied by hemolysis and coagulopathy; complete recuperation of renal function occurs in only 10% Histopathology Fibrinoid necrosis of vessel walls (similar to the changes seen in malignant hypertension), glomerular ischemia, fibrin thrombi in the afferent arterioles and glomeruli and subendothelial deposits of fibrin and C3 Treatment No therapy is consistently effective, although early diagnosis, control of hypertension and early dialysis may have a role in prevention; see TTP-HUS

Post-partum thyrotoxicosis Hyperactivity of the thyroid gland that is temporally linked to delivery, appearing as de novo Graves' hyperthyroidism, recurrent Graves' hyperthyroidism (characterized by high radioiodine uptake) and painless thyroiditis with hyperthyroidism (with low radioiodine uptake); these endocrinopathies are often mild and transient, possibly caused by the unmasking of associated autoimmune phenomena Treatment If necessary, propranolol

Post-perfusion lung Pump lung A clinical complex seen immediately after cardiovascular surgery Clinical Fever, dyspnea, cyanosis, hypotension and pulmonary edema, caused by anoxia, traumatic hemolysis of erythrocytes due to shearing against pump hardware, turbulence and possibly anaphylactic reaction against various materials (proteins and other allergens) in the tubing, congestive heart failure, acute renal tubular necrosis and urinary tract infection Pathology The lungs are dark red, heavy, congested and hemorrhagic Treatment Antibiotics, corticosteroids Prognosis Relatively guarded

Post-perfusion syndrome A clinical complex seen in 2% of patients who have undergone cardiac surgery, occurring 3-7 weeks after cardiopulmonary bypass, which resembles infectious mononucleosis or infectious hepatitis and is attributed to viruses transfused with the blood at the time of surgery; although it is characterized by fever, splenomegaly, lymphadenopathy, a maculopapular rash, anemia and atypical lymphocytes, the syndrome is benign and resolves spontaneously without therapy; Cf Post-resuscitation syndrome

Post-pill amenorrhea GYNECOLOGY Failure to resume menstruation within three months after discontinuation of oral contraceptives; amenorrhea of greater than 6 months occurs in 0.2% and in 15% is accompanied by galactorrhea; the work-up and treatment is similar to the usual type of amenorrhea, and thus this 'disease' is probably not a distinct entity

Post-polio syndrome A progressive late-onset disease occurring years after an attack of acute poliomyelitis, most often affecting previously involved muscles, characterized by muscle weakness, fasciculations and atrophy Histopathology 'Type grouping' of muscles, which is due to a denervation-renervation sequence; PPS is often benign and may reach a plateau phase; see Type grouping

Post-resuscitation syndrome (PRS) EMERGENCY MEDICINE A clinical complex seen in 'arrested' patients in whom cardiopulmonary resuscitation is delayed, characterized by protracted reduction in cardiac output despite normal blood pressure, due to a combination of cardiac pump failure, microthromboembolism (due to intravascular obstruction, causing increased systemic vascular resistance and disseminated intravascular coagulation) and vasospasm (multi-organ failure); the pulmonary insufficiency in PRS is due to relative respiratory dysfunction; cerebral ischemia contributes to PRS by triggering dysrhythmia, renal shutdown and pulmonary edema; PRS results from 'autointoxication' occurring when reperfused hypoxic tissues release kinins, bacterial endotoxins, endogenous pyrogens and other toxins; Cf Post-perfusion syndrome

Post-splenectomy 'syndrome' Hematologic findings that follow splenectomy, most prominently affecting the erythroid series, as the spleen is responsible for 'pitting' and 'culling' effete or defective red cells or those with inclusions Laboratory Increased lifespan of red cells, codocytes (target cells), schistocytes, Howell-Jolly bodies (nuclear chromatin remnants) and transient thrombocytosis

Post-term pregnancy OBSTETRICS A gestation that is correctly dated by Naegele's rule and is of greater than 42 weeks in duration; 12% of gestations are undelivered at 42 weeks and 7% at 43 weeks; the longer the delay before delivery, the greater is the mortality (0.7% at 40 weeks, 2.2% > 42 weeks); post-mature infants have increased mortality and morbidity since a) they are bigger and b) the placenta has planned obsolescence and undergoes fibrosis and infarcts after 40-42 weeks Clinical Absent lanugo, attenuated vernix caseosa, long finger- and toenails, abundant scalp hair, pale, parchment-like or desquamating skin and increased alertness Note: Most 'post-datism' is merely due to miscalculation of the last menstrual period; Cf Pre-maturity

Post-transfusion graft-versus-host disease A complex similar or identical to post-operative erythroderma, seen in immunocompetent blood recipients Clinical High fever, dermatitis, severe diarrhea, hepatic dysfunction and pancytopenia

Post-transfusion infection see Transfusion reactions

Post-trauma stress disorder (PTSD) A psychogenic complex related to intense mental stress secondary to trauma or armed conflict, defined as one or more of the following; symptoms relating to re-experiencing a traumatic event or symptoms related to avoiding the stimuli associated with the trauma or numbing of general responsiveness or symptoms related to increased arousal with long-term psychologic 'scars' (J Am Med Assoc 1990; 263:1227); PTSD is similar to the 'Vietnam syndrome', although in the latter conflict, moral guilt was reportedly placed on some of the combatants by nonparticipants, which is believed by some to have prevented the ex-soldiers from successfully resolving the issues of 'man's inhumanity to man'; this form (PTSD) of 'shell shock' occurs in less than 1% of the general population, 15-35% of Vietnam veterans, 30-50% of those exposed to natural disasters and up to 80% of those exposed to man-made disasters, eg Bhopal (J Am Med Assoc 1990; 264:2781); Cf Battle fatigue

Pot SUBSTANCE ABUSE A common synonym for marijuana

Potassium ion channels Cell physiology A group of transmembrane proteins found in excitable and other cell types, including thymocytes and T cells, which have a wide range of functional diversity; potassium channels are classified according to differences in biophysical (kinetics, conductance, sensitivity to voltage and second messengers) and pharmacologic properties and whether the channels are homo- or heteromultimeric, ie whether all the transmembrane channels in the complex are formed of the same or of different chains (Nature 1990; 345:530, 535, 475n&v); potassium channels can be activated by intracellular second messengers (eg arachidonic acid in cardiac muscle, Science 1989; 244:1174); see Ball-and-chain model, Voltage-gated channels

'Potato chip' desquamation Peripheral elevation of partially desquamated flecks of the superficial keratinized corneal layer of the skin, which follows the resolution of the erythematous lesions in staphylococcal scalded-skin syndrome, morphologically likened to potato chips or potato crisps

'Potato chip' operation(s) A highly colloquial term for the multiple, increasingly proximal, partial amputations of the lower extremities in the face of dry gangrene, the result of vasculo-stenotic occlusions in peripheral atherosclerosis, most often occurring in elderly patients with diabetes mellitus; since the patients are often disinclined to consent to a full above-the-knee amputation, which is the definitive therapy for occlusive, severely ischemic atherosclerosis, the vascular surgeon is forced to amputate in sequence, one or more toe(s), the midfoot, the foot, the leg below-the-knee and finally perform an above-the- knee amputation; the sobriquet for these operations derives from an advertisement for potato chips (potato crisps) that claimed that one potato chip was never enough

'Potato' liver A fanciful term for a liver punctuated on the surface and in the parenchyma by large indurated nodules of macronodular cirrhosis as seen in Wilson's disease

Potato node(s) RADIOLOGY A descriptor for the enlarged hilar and mediastinal lymph nodes seen in sarcoidosis

Potato nose A deformity inherited in an autosomal dominant fashion characterized by a bulbous proboscis and developmental visual field defect; Cf 'WC Fields' nose

Potato tumor A descriptor for a carotid body paraganglioma arising at the angle of the jaw causing a massive tuberoid tumor of young adults Pathology The tumor is firm, oval, highly vascular and composed of tumor cell nests; see Zellballen

Potency TRANSFUSION MEDICINE The degree of 'antigenicity' or the intensity of agglutination that may be elicited by different alloantigens; potency is a value that can be calculated by comparing the frequency of an antibody anti-X, in the population to the frequency of the alloantigen, X of interest, multiplied by the opportunity for immunization; the potency of the Kell antigen is equated to 1, Rh D is seven-fold more potent than Kell and Rh e is one-tenth as potent as the Kell

'Potomac fever' A 'disease' that may affect those who are temporarily in a position of power in Washington DC (the US capital), eg elected politicians or appointed health professionals, who bask in the glamor and 'glitz' of Washington and who, when defeated in elections or replaced, are disinclined to return to the 'dreary' hinterlands from whence they came Note: The Potomac River courses through the middle of Washington

Pouchitis' Acute inflammation of intestinal mucosa seen in an ileal reservoir that may extend transmurally, occurring as a late complication of restorative proctocolectomy, possibly due to obstruction and stercoral ulceration (N Engl J Med 1989; 321:1416c)

POU-domain gene family A family of genes including pit-1, which encode transcription factors, characterized by a 60 amino acid region similar to the classic homeodomain and a 76 amino acid region or POU-specific domain responsible for regulating cell-specific developmental events; see pit-1, Homeobox, Homeotic genes

POU-domain proteins A family of homeodomain proteins that transcriptionally activate cell-specific genes, participate in cell fate and are thought to act during embryogenesis through either stable activation of genes responsible for specific developmental pathways or for transient activation that occurs during highly specific developmental periods (Science 1990; 249:1300)

'Pour' plate MICROBIOLOGY A culture plate that contains both a nutrient agar and an inoculum of bacteria added to the agar while it is cooling, although pour plates had been used in the past to incubate β-hemolytic streptococci and microaerophlic bacteria, most culture plates used in the modern microbiology laboratory are prepared commercially, and thus this relatively unsophisticated test is no longer commonly used

Pouter pigeon breast deformity see Chicken breast deformity

Poverty SOCIAL MEDICINE An ill-defined term referring to an income level that is insufficient to provide for basic human needs of food, clothing, shelter and health care; in the US, a person at the poverty level is eligible for Medicaid and food assistance programs; see Engel's phenomenon, 'Fourth World, Homeless(ness), Medicaid

Powder-burn spots Mulberry spots A pattern of endometriosis consisting of multiple tiny puckered foci of hemorrhage, surrounded by minute stellate scars and varying fibrosis

Powder 'tattoo' FORENSIC PATHOLOGY A geographically-shaped lesion caused by a gun fired at close range, where the still-burning gunpowder embeds in the skin and cannot be wiped away, a finding of use in determining whether clothing was worn overlying an entry wound; Cf 'Stippling'

Power stroke see Rowboat model

Power 'take-off' lesion OCCUPATIONAL MEDICINE Avulsion of the loose skin of the scrotum and penis caused by moving parts from factory or farm equipment that may engage a trouser leg and twist upward; the skin may be torn from the glans penis (which is spared) and extend to the coronal sulcus

PPF Plasma protein fraction CLINICAL THERAPEUTICS A blood-derived colloid preparation that contains at least 83% albumin, providing volume expansion without risk of hepatitis or HIV-1; PPF, or albumin may be administered in the face of large-scale loss of colloid, eg hypovolemic shock, burns, retroperitoneal surgery; given its high cost, there is little justification for using albumin-based volume expanders when equivalent agents exist; futhermore, albumin infusions may rapidly increase the intravascular oncotic pressure, drawing large quantities of water from tissues into the vascular space, potentially causing cardiac overload; albumin may also evoke hypotensive episodes by releasing of vasoactive kinins and massive infusions of albumin decrease synthesis of plasma proteins including α, β and γ globulins, fibrinogen and the coagulation factors

PPLO Pleuropneumonia-like organism *Mycoplasma pneumoniae* An organism that induces asymptomatic respiratory infection or inflammation of the upper respiratory tract, including tracheitis and pharyngitis; *M pneumoniae* spreads by aerosol and causes up to three-fourths of all 'closed population' (military 'boot' camps, boarding schools and college) pneumonias, affecting ages 5-20 Clinical Headache, malaise, myalgia, low-grade fever, cough, chest tenderness Complications Erythema multiforme, Raynaud's phenomenon, cold agglutinin-induced hemolysis; less commonly neurologic, cardiovascular, musculoskeletal defects Treatment Erythromycin, tetracyclines

PPNG see Penicillinase-producing *Neisseria gonorrhoeae*

PPO HEALTH CARE INDUSTRY see Preferred provider organization INSTRUMENTATION 2,5-diphenyloxazole A fluor used for liquid scintillation counting; see POPOP

PP-oma An pancreatic polypeptide-producing islet cell tumor, 40% of which are malignant, characterized by hypercalcemia, hyperglycemia, hypomagnesemia and muscular weakness; Cf Gastrinoma, Islet cell tumors, Pancreatic endocrine tumors, WDHA syndrome, Zollinger-Ellison syndrome

PPRC Physician Payment Review Commission

P protein A regulatory protein that reactivates glutamine synthetase after inactivation through adenylation; Cf Protein P

PPS see Prospective payment system

'P' pulmonale Cardiology A sharply peaked P wave in an electrocardiogram (EKG) seen in chronic obstructive pulmonary disease (COPD), most prominent during exacerbation of clinical disease, although it is a relatively non-specific finding; other EKG findings in COPD include a right axis shift, early R waves in the precordial leads V_1 and V_2 and net negativity in V_5 and V_6

PQQ Pyrroloquinoline quinone A quinoprotein that may function as a vitamin-like growth factor; mice fed a PQQ-deficient diet grow poorly, do not reproduce, become osteolathyritic, have friable skin and have low quality collagen,with decreased cross-linking of collagen and elastin and decreased lysyl oxidase (Science 1989; 245:850)

Pravistatin A cholesterol-lowering agent, currently in European clinical trials that inhibits HMG-CoA (3-hydroxy-3-methyl coenzyme A) reductase, the rate-limiting enzyme of cholesterol synthesis; pravistatin decreases a) Lathosterol (a major cholesterol precursor, the level of which reflects the rate of cholesterol synthesis) by 63% b) LDL cholesterol by 39% and c) Total cholesterol by 26%; cholesterol reduction is due to increased LDL receptors on hepatocytes (N Engl J Med 1990; 323:224)

Praziquantel An anti-parasitic agent that is the current drug of choice for treating schistosomiasis (*S haematobium, S japonicum*), parasitic flukes (*Trematoda*, eg *Clonorchis sinensis, Opisthorchis viverrini, Paragonimus buski, Heterophyes heterophyes, Metagonimus yokogawai*) and tapeworms (*Hymenolepsis nana* and *Taenia solium*) Side effects Drowsiness, headache, nausea, backache, abdominal discomfort

Pre-admission testing see PATs

Prealbumin see Transthyretin

Prebiotic soup see Primordial soup

Precancer see Premalignancy

Precautions INFECTIOUS DISEASE A term implying that the isolation of an infected patient is optional but not mandatory; in practice, when a patient is designated as requiring 'precautions', both he and his specimens (body fluids and waste products) are handled with increased circumspection by his care-givers, as the term carries the implication that he is infected with a contagious or dangerous organism, eg hepatitis B or HIV-1; the Centers for Disease Control discourages identifying any specimen with 'precautions' or 'infectious' labels, ostensibly reasoning that all patient specimens should be handled as potentially infected; Cf Isolation; Reverse precautions

Precipitin An antibody that interacts with an antigen forming a precipitate that sediments out of solution

Precision LABORATORY MEDICINE A measurement of the reproducibility of a test or assay, ie its capability of producing the same results when the same assay is performed on the same specimen under the same conditions; a set of data with high precision has a low standard deviation and a low coefficient of variation, analogous to a tight cluster of arrows seen in target practice Note: Accuracy is defined as the correctness of results

Precocious puberty ENDOCRINOLOGY The appearance of secondary sexual characteristics before age 8 in girls and age 9 in boys; if the precocity results from activation of the hypothalamic-pituitary axis, it is designated as complete or true precocious puberty; if the precosity is secondary to ectopic production or autonomous secretion of end-organ hormones, it is designated as incomplete precocious puberty (table)

Precocious puberty

I True or complete precocious puberty (affects both sexes in a similar fashion)

a. Idiopathic

b. Constitutional or familial

c. Central nervous system disease, eg tumors (hypothalamic and pineal gliomas, craniopharyngiomas, germinomas, hamartomas of the tuber cinereum), as well as encephalitis, abscesses, cysts, sarcoidosis, tuberculosis

d. McCune-Albright syndrome

e. Hypothyroidism

f. Virilizing syndromes, eg Congenital adrenal hyperplasia

II INCOMPLETE PRECOCIOUS PUBERTY

Male Due to gonadotropin-secreting tumors, eg hepatoma, Leydig cell tumor, excessive androgen production or premature Leydig cell and germinal cell maturation

Female Due to ovarian follicle cysts or estrogen-producing neoplasms, eg granulosa cell tumor

Pre-eclampsia see Eclampsia

Predictive value of a positive test see Positive predictive value

Predictive value of a negative test see Negative predictive value

Pre-embryos see in vitro fertilization

Preferred provider organization (PPO) Health care industry A form of managed health care in which a limited number of health providers (physicians, hospitals and others) provide services to a defined group of clients for a negotiated fee-for-service rate that is below the 'market value' for the service(s); PPOs offer incentives to the clients for using their contracted physicians, where the PPO physicians are paid in full, while the non-PPO physicians are not and the client must pay the difference in the professional fees, eg 10-30% (allowing the client freedom of choice at a price); the number of PPOs has risen from 25 in 1982 to 506 in 1986; physician-sponsored PPOs have an average of 240 physicians; hospital-sponsored PPOs have 430 physicians (J Am Med Assoc 1990; 263:2635)

Pregnancy-related conditions see Chorea gravidarum, Herpes gestationalis, Melasma, Pregnancy 'tumor', Pruritus gravidarum, PUPPP; Cf Postpartum-related conditions

Pregnancy-specific β_1 glycoprotein SP-1 A protein of unknown function produced by the trophoblast that can be detected from the 16th day of pregnancy in the maternal serum and amniotic fluid, which shares sequence homology with the carcinoembryonic antigen family and contains repeating domains, conserved disulfide bridges and a β-sheet structure typical of proteins produced by the immunoglobulin gene superfamily (Biochemistry 1990; 29:2845)

Pregnancy 'tumor' Granuloma gravidarum Angiogranuloma An exuberant, pyogenic granuloma-like inflammatory response of pregnant gums to an overhanging margin of tooth filling or crown with excess calcium buildup, which appears in the first trimester in 0.5-2.0% of pregnancies, grows until delivery and regresses spontaneously without therapy, although it may re-appear with subsequent pregnancy; hypertrophic gingivitis is far more common than the pregnancy tumor and is seen in 7-20% of pregnancies

Preleukemia Myelodysplastic syndrome A group of clonal expansions of marrow stem cells characterized by dysmyelopoiesis, a complex of structural and functional abnormalities including abnormal cell morphology, ineffective hemopoiesis and chromosome defects, eg aneuploidy and pseudodiploidy; preleukemic states include acquired idiopathic sideroblastic and non-sideroblastic anemias, pancytopenia with hypercellular marrow and paroxysmal nocturnal hemoglobinuria, which may progress to acute non-lymphocytic leukemia Note: Certain genetic disorders have an increased tendency to develop leukemias, including hematologic diseases (Kostmann syndrome, Fanconi syndrome), anomalies of either sex chromosomes (Klinefelter and Turner syndrome) or autosomal chromosomes (ataxia-telangiectasia, Bloom syndrome and Down syndrome); acquired states predisposed to leukemias include bone marrow injury by drugs, eg chlorambucil, chemicals, eg benzene and radiation and myeloproliferative disease (agnogenic myeloid metaplasia, chronic myeloid leukemia, idiopathic thrombocytopenic purpura and polycythemia vera)

Prelymphoma A group of conditions characterized by often monotonous aggregates of lymphocytes and a known tendency to evolve to lymphoma and should thus warrant close clinical follow-up; prelymphomas include pseudolymphoma of the orbit and small intestine, lymphomatoid granulomatosis (an angiocentric lung disease with lymphoma-like extrapulmonary involvement), angioimmunoblastic lymphadenopathy, lymphoid interstitial pneumonitis Note: Lymphomas may occur in a background of chemotherapy, radiotherapy, connective tissue disease, monoclonality and immunocompromise, both congenital and acquired

Premalignancy Any of a group of lesions with a tendency to undergo malignant degeneration; precancers of epithelial origin may be a) Glandular, eg adenomatous hyperplasia (endometrium) and adenomatous polyps (colon, stomach) that evolve towards adenocarcinoma of their respective organs or b) Squamous, eg dysplasia of the uterine cervix or other urogenital mucosae; precancerous lesions of mesenchymal origin include prelymphoma and 'presarcoma' (an ad hoc coinage), the latter of which may be due to a variety of predisposing factors, eg osteosarcoma may arise in Paget's disease of bone, irradiation, hereditary multiple exostoses, polyostotic fibrous dysplasia, enchondroma and Mafucci's enchondromatosis; osteosarcoma may be induced under experimental conditions by various types of trauma, including chemical, eg turpentine, mechanical, eg local pressure, indwelling foreign bodies and ischemia, eg vessel clamping Note: Some of the histologic changes of epithelial premalignancy may be reversed by supplementing the diet with vitamin B_{12} and folate (J Am Med Assoc 1988; 259:1525), as well as vitamins C, A and E; Cf Preneoplastic state(s)

Preneoplastic states

Chromosome breakage syndromes Bloom syndrome, Fanconi syndrome

Genodermatoses Albinism, dyskeratosis congenita, epidermodysplasia verruciformis, polydysplastic epidermolysis bullosa, Werner syndrome, xeroderma pigmentosa

Hamartomatous syndromes Multiple exostoses, neurofibromatosis, Peutz-Jegher syndrome, tuberous sclerosis, von Hippel-Lindau syndrome

Immunodeficiency syndromes Ataxia-telangiectasia, Wiskott-Aldrich syndrome, X-linked agammaglobulinemia

Premature ovarian failure Cessation of menses before age 40, accompanied by elevated serum gonadotropin levels, often idiopathic, due to a deletion of a fragment of the long arm of chromosome X (46,XX,del(X)(pter-q21.3:q27-qter), or secondary to known causes including ovarian receptor antibodies, viral infections, cytotoxic drugs and irradiation

Prematurity OBSTETRICS The constellation of clinical findings in an infant delivered before 37 weeks of gestation (37 weeks from the first day of the last menstrual period) who is often also immature; morbid conditions associated with prematurity include anemia due to low iron and vitamin E, bronchopulmonary dysplasia, intraventricular hemorrhage, especially in the very low birth weight infants, permanent neurological sequelae and retinopathy **Interventions** Weight gain is faster and neurological development is improved, eg increased dopamine, norepinephrine and epinephrine in the urine of premature infants treated with stroking, taped messages from parents, soft music, low lighting, reducing incubator time and shortening the length of intensive hospital-based care; see Low birth weight; Cf Post-term pregnancy

Premelanosome An oval structure with a dense, grainy matrix and 'cross-striations', which comprises a pathognomonic ultrastructural criterion for melanocytes (figure, right, schematically enlarged 100 000x), which serves to confirm the diagnosis of melanoma; in practice, most melanomas

Premelting MOLECULAR BIOLOGY A phenomenon affecting double-stranded nucleic acids, eg DNA and DNA-RNA hybrid molecules, in which the two chains begin to dissociate at temperatures far below that at which complete disassociation occurs; see Breathing

Premenstrual syndrome see PMS

Pre-mRNA Pre-messenger RNA, Nuclear messenger RNA precursor A term which in the usual context refers to the 'primary RNA transcript', a messenger RNA molecule that is the direct transcription product or mirror image of a DNA 'template', which is an immature mRNA molecule containing intervening sequences (introns) that are not part of a mature mRNA, which is destined to be translated to form a cognate protein; introns are removed by splicing in a two-step process occurring in the spliceosome, where cleavage occurs at the 5' site and a guanosine residue at the 5' end of the intron is covalently joined to the adenine residue near the 3' splice site in a recognition element, known as the branch point sequence; in the second step, the 3' end of the pre-mRNA is cleaved and joined to the exons forming mature mRNA; some pre-mRNA molecules may be spliced at different sites resulting in the production of different proteins from one pre-mRNA molecule; see Alternative splicing; Cf hnRNA

Prenatal tests, fetal OBSTETRICS Laboratory tests and assays used to detect genetic and/or congenital fetal anomalies that would compromise the infant's well-being and quality of life to such a degree that the parents might prefer an abortion; these tests include measurement of α-fetoprotein levels in the mother's serum or amniotic fluid, chromosomal analysis, ultrasonography, chorionic villus biopsy (performed on or after the 8th to 10th gestational weeks, risk of spontaneous abortion or miscarriage, 1.0-1.5%), amniocentesis (performed on or after the 16th gestational week, risk of spontaneous abortion or miscarriage, 0.5%); diseases detected include α_1-antitrypsin activity, thalassemias, defects of sex and autosomal chromosomes including trisomies, deletions, mosaicisms, fragile X syndrome, hemophilia, neural tube defects (anencephaly, spina bifida), polycystic renal disease, Tay-Sachs disease; Cf Wrongful birth

Prenatal testing, maternal see Obstetric (screening) profile

Preneoplastic state(s) A broad group of congenital condi-

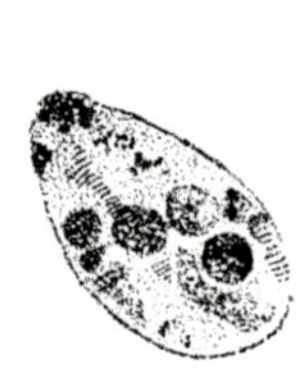

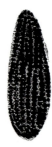

Premelanosomes

tions that predispose to development of malignancy (table); see Fragile X syndrome, Hereditary neoplasms, Premalignancy

Prenylation MOLECULAR BIOLOGY A post-translational modification of protein involving the addition of unit(s) of isoprene (C_5H_8); the function of which is unclear; activation of the Ras protein requires prenylation (Cell 1989; 57:1167); isoprenoids may help anchor proteins to cell membranes (Science 1990; 247:318,320)

Preproprotein An inactive precursor of a secretory protein, which is both a preprotein, ie a secretory protein that still has an attached 'signal sequence' of amino acids, and a proprotein, ie protein that is 'activated' by removing an oligopeptide

Pressure dressing A misnomer for an occlusive, but pressure-less wound dressing that stabilizes and partially immobilizes a region of skin, used in burns

Pressure pants An intermittent pneumatic leg compression device used to reduce the incidence of deep and proximal vein thromboses (J Am Med Assoc 1990; 263:2313), of use in preventing post-surgical venous thrombosis seen in general, prostatic, orthopedic and neurosurgery; pressure pants may be a viable substitute for pharmacological anticoagulation and is as cost-effective as warfarin which incurs daily laboratory costs for monitoring coagulation parameters; Cf MAST (Military anti-shock trousers)

Pressure ulcer Bedsore A decubital ulcer appearing on dependent sites, usually on the lumbosacral region, most common in the bed-ridden elderly, seen in 2-24% of nursing home residents and associated with an increased mortality, divided into *STAGE I* Nonresolving erythema with no break in skin *STAGE II* Erythema with superficial interruption of skin, abrasions or vesiculation *STAGE III* Full-thickness loss of skin with serosanguinous drainage *STAGE IV* Full-thickness loss of skin and invasion of deeper tissue (J Am Med Assoc 1990; 264:2905) **Treatment** A 'cocktail' of recombinant platelet-derived growth factor, proteases and cell-adhesion molecules has been reported to induce healing of wounds that have been recalcitrant to years of therapy (Science 1991; 252:1065n)

Prevalence EPIDEMIOLOGY The cases of a disease divided by the total number of subjects in the population; Cf Incidence

Prevascular phase ONCOLOGY A stable, relatively non-aggressive phase in tumor development that may persist for years, characterized by limited tumor growth; the prevascular phase has been studied in carcinoma of the breast, melanoma, urinary bladder and uterine cervix and may be 'switched' by an unknown mechanism to a 'vascular phase', which is characterized by the presence of angiogenic molecules, rapid tumor growth, bleeding and metastatic potential; semiquantification of the number of vessels (marked by immunoperoxidase staining of tissue with antibodies to factor VIII antigen) in a tumor may serve to identify tumors that have entered a vascular phase (N Engl J Med 1991; 324:1); see Metastasis

Priapism An uncommon condition characterized by prolonged and usually painful penile erection occurring in the absence of sexual excitement or desire; 60% of cases are idiopathic, the rest are due to a vast palette of diseases including drugs (anticoagulants, antihypertensives, corticosteroids, neuroleptics, tolbutamide, papaverine) leukemia, pelvic infection, pelvic malignancy, sickle cell anemia, substance abuse (alcohol, cocaine, marijuana, methaqualone), scorpion bites, penile or spinal cord trauma **Clinical** Painful, prolonged erection with a tense and congested corpora cavernosa, constituting a urologic emergency **Mechanism** Accumulation of highly viscous, hypoxic blood in the corpora cavernosa, due to a physiologic obstruction of venous blood **Prognosis** Without surgical decompression, interstitial edema and fibrosis of the penile shaft ensue, causing impotence Priapus is the Greek god of fecundity, born of Bacchus and Venus, who has a macrophallus

Pribnow box MOLECULAR BIOLOGY A highly-conserved-in-evolution 'consensus' sequence of six DNA nucleotides (TATAAT) that is located about 10 base pairs upstream (in the 5' direction) from bacterial promoter regions and separated by 5-8 base pairs from the initiation site for RNA polymerase

Price fixing HEALTH CARE INDUSTRY The reaching of an agreement or understanding with competitors of what a provider of goods or services will charge for those services or goods; it is considered unethical in the free market economy of the USA for two physicians to discuss fees for services; in order for a physician to ascertain a 'fair market' price for his services, he may hire a consultant who will use a variety of conversion factors for the value of that service in his region

Prick test A clinical test for immediate hypersensitivity, in which a diluted allergen is droppered on the skin and a sterile needle is used to 'prick' the epidermal surface; the reaction is then compared to that obtained with standardized mast cell secretogogues, eg compound 48/80, codeine and histamine; in contrast to the intradermal test, in which the very low concentrations of the allergen are allowed to penetrate below the epidermis, the prick test is more rapid, simpler and causes less discomfort for the patient, can be used to test infants and false positive results are rare, although false negative results are more common; both evoke increased production of IgE antibodies

Prickly heat see Miliaria

Primaquine PARASITOLOGY An oral 8-aminoquinoline antimalarial drug effective in treating relapses of clinical malaria, acting against the hepatic but not erythrocytic stages of ***Plasmodium vivax*** and ***P ovale***; it is a potent oxidant, causing hemolysis in glucose-6-phosphate dehydrogenase deficient patients, the so-called 'primaquine sensitivity syndrome' **Toxicity** Per os, no systemic effects; parenterally, potentially profound hypotension

Primary acquired melanosis A condition first seen in the middle aged population as a unilateral, diffuse brown pigmentation of the conjunctiva which may: a) Remain stationary or regress b) Slowly enlarge, but remain benign or c) Undergo malignant degeneration (17% of cases), where melanocytic atypia is a significant predictor of malignancy Note: Secondary acquired melanosis may be caused by acanthosis nigricans, keratomalacia, metabolic disease (Addison's disease, pregnancy), radiation, toxins (arsenic, thyroxin), trachoma, vernal conjunctivitis, xeroderma pigmentosum

Primary aebic meningoencephalitis (PAM) An intracranial infection caused by free-living amoebae, including *Naegleria* (*N fowleri, N grubei*), *Acanthamoeba, Hartmanella, Entamoeba histolytica* and others Clinical PAM may be acute and purulent, causing meningoencephalitis in young healthy persons swimming in stagnant artificial fresh water lakes, typically caused by *Naegleria* species; the inflammation and hemorrhage is most intense along the olfactory tract, inculpating the cribriform plate as the portal of entry via the nose; the prognosis is poor; the few survivors were treated to parenteral amphotericin B and miconazole and oral rifampicin, and had major sequelae; PAM may also be subacute with a granulomatous tissue reaction, which is more common in immunocompromised hosts

Primary autonomic dysfunction (PAD) A heterogeneous group of autonomic system dysfunctions characterized by hypoadrenergic postural hypotension with blunted vasomotor response to norepinephrine upon standing, decreased sweating, heat intolerance, gastrointestinal symptoms, impotence, urinary and fecal incontinence PAD type I is characterized by low plasma levels of norepinephrine PAD type II or Shy-Drager disease is further characterized by parkinson-type cerebral degeneration Differential diagnosis Postural hypotension may also be due to cerebral and spinal cord lesions, eg degeneration, infection, trauma and tumors and peripheral neuropathy, eg alcohol, amyloidosis, diabetes mellitus, porphyria and toxins

Primary biliary cirrhosis (PBC) A disease of adult women ages 30-65 Clinical Fatigue, pruritis, steatorrhea, hepatic osteodystrophy, renal tubular acidosis and a four-fold increase in hepatocellular and breast carcinoma; 80% of PBC also have autoimmune or connective tissue disease, including autoimmune thyroiditis, scleroderma, rheumatoid arthritis and Sjögren or sicca syndrome Histopathology (table) Laboratory 20-50-fold increase in alkaline phosphatase, IgM and antimitochondrial antibodies (of the 8 known antimitochondrial antibodies, M2 is most commonly associated with PBC); anti-SS-A/Ro antibodies occur in 20% of cases Treatment Liver transplantation (N Engl J Med 1989; 320:1709), colchicine, an agent that is both anti-fibrotic and anti-inflammatory and ursodiol, a non-toxic bile acid (N Engl J Med 1991; 324:1548); see Ursodiol

Primary care The least specialized level of medical care, often rendered by a 'primary' physician, who may be a general practitioner, family physician, internist, pediatrician, obstetrician or emergency room physician; primary care includes examination of a patient in a medical, behavioral and social context as well as performing preventive, diagnostic and therapeutic activities; most of a person's need for medical attention may be provided in a primary care situation and it is a point of entry into higher levels of health care; Cf Hospital-based medicine, Medical specialties, RAPERs, Secondary care, Surgical specialties, Tertiary care

Primary fluor A fluor, eg PPO, that is excited by radiation and which emits a flash of light in a scintillation device; see POPOP, Secondary fluor

Primary granules Primary lysosomes see Azurophilic granules

Primary hypertension Essential hypertension

Primary idiopathic sideroblastic anemia (PISA) Refractory anemia with excess blasts Acquired refractory sideroblastic anemia diGugliermo disease A pre-malignant symptom complex of older patients, often related to radio- or chemotherapy, 10-30% of whom later develop acute non-lymphocytic leukemia; PISA is a pluripotent stem cell defect characterized by ineffective erythropoiesis with a slight decrease in red cell survival, mild maturational impairment of all hematopoietic cell lines, coupled with a defect in iron metabolism, resulting in iron accumulation Clinical Pallor, fatigue, weakness, dyspnea and palpitations on exertion Laboratory 'Dimorphic' anemia with hypochromic-microcytic and macrocytic features; 40% of the erythroblasts are ring sideroblasts, anisocytosis, basophilic stippling, reticulocyte with impaired heme synthesis, decreased delta ALA synthetase and protease activity Prognosis Average survival: 20 months

Primary intention see Wound healing

Primary response The response that the immune system displays when it is first exposed to an antigen; Cf Secondary response

Primary RNA transcript see Pre-mRNA

Primary sclerosing cholangitis see Sclerosing cholangitis

Primary structure see Protein structure

Primary biliary cirrhosis Histopathology

Stage I Ductal hepatitis (triaditis) with florid, asymmetrical destruction of septal and interlobular bile ducts surrounded by a dense infiltrate of CD4 T lymphocytes and granulomas

Stage II Florid bile duct proliferation, with atypical bile ducts with irregular lumens, diffuse portal fibrosis and mononuclear cells in triads the 'periportal stage'

Stage III Fibrosis with portal-to-portal 'bridging' and nodule formation

Stage IV Cirrhosis or end-stage disease which is difficult to distinguish from other cirrhoses, although the absence of bile ducts corroborates the diagnosis

Primary tumor A neoplasm that in clinical parlance is regarded as malignant, arising in one site and capable of giving birth to metastatic or secondary tumors; see Metastasis; Cf Tumor of unknown origin

Primase A DNA-dependent RNA polymerase that synthesizes RNA 'primers' (4-12 nucleotide segments of RNA), which are required starting points for replicating the lagging antiparallel strands in DNA replication; once the primase adds the primers, DNA polymerase elongates the RNA primers with new DNA Note: The RNA-DNA complexes (known as Okazaki fragments) on the lagging strand of replicating DNA meet the next RNA primer, DNA polymerase clips out the 5' end RNA and fills in the gap; the last step is carried out by DNA ligase which joins the fragments; see Okazaki fragments

'Primed' cell A lymphocyte that has recognized an antigen and represents the theoretical starting point for an immune recognition 'cascade' Note: The 'primed' cell corresponds to the Y cell of the woefully naive 'XYZ cell theory' of immunology

Primer A short segment of RNA that is the starting point for synthesis of the lagging (antiparallel) strand of DNA in DNA replication; see Primase

Priming NEUROLOGY A type of implicit, nonie, conscious (not procedural, semantic or episodic) form of human memory that acts to improve identification of words and perceptual objects (Science 1990; 247:301)

Primordial soup Prebiotic ooze The Gemisch of simple organic molecules that was theoretically present in the primitive (circa four billion years ago) oceans and contained the synthetic building blocks for macromolecules and eventually living cells

'Prince Charles looking to the left' A fanciful descriptor for the eggs of the dwarf tapeworm, ***Hymenolepis nana***; the eggs measure 25 x 35 µm, have a smooth shell surrounding an oncosphere with six hooks, which distinctly 'look towards the left'; the oncosphere is contained within a tough inner envelope marked by two auricle-like polar thickenings, from each of which arise four-to-eight thread-like polar filaments; ***H nana*** is an intestinal cestode of worldwide distribution, but more common in temperate and subtropical regions; heavy intestinal infestations are due to auto-infection Treatment Niclosamide

Prion 'Slow spongiform encephalopathy virus' An unconventional infectious particle composed entirely of protein (with attached carbohydrate), which is the smallest known infective particle and is implicated in three diseases of man (Creutzfeldt-Jakob disease, kuru and Gerstmann-Straussler syndrome) and four diseases of animals (scrapie of sheep and goats, bovine spongiform encephalopathy, transmissible mink encephalopathy and chronic wasting disease of captive mule deer and elk); prions do not evoke inflammation or the production of specific antibodies and are resistant to the usual modalities that inactivate viruses, eg formalin, heat, nuclease digestion, radiation and ultraviolet radiation; prions contain a unique 28 kD hydrophobic glycoprotein particle, PrP that autopolymerizes into fibrillary amyloid-like (by electron microscopy) structures, existing in 2 isoforms: PrP^C, found in the normal brain and transiently expressed during development and PrP^{Sc} which is associated with cerebral degeneration, including Alzheimer's disease and scrapie, the primary amino acid sequences of both are identical; the gene encoding the PrP proteins is located on the short arm of chromosome 20 and is widely expressed in normal brains and the prions are composed largely of abnormal isoform(s) of the prion protein, generated through point mutations of the prion gene, one of which occurs in Libyan Jews with Creutzfeldt-Jakob disease (CJD), suggesting that some cases of CJD may be autosomal dominant with variable penetration (N Engl J Med 1991; 324:1091, Science 1991; 252:1515rv); transfer of a mutated prion gene into transgenic mice evokes a spongiform encephalitis with gliosis, confirming a cause-and-effect association between mutated prions and encephalopathy (Science 1990; 251:1587, 1509rn)

PRISM Pediatric risk of mortality CRITICAL CARE MEDICINE A prognostic scoring system for pediatric populations that derives from the PSI (physiology stability index), which assesses 34 physiological variables, assigning each a score of 1 to 5 based on the severity of derangement of the parameter on admission to the pediatric ICU; see Prognostic scoring systems

PRIST Paper radioimmunosorbent test An in vitro test that quantifies serum IgE; the range of IgE is broad (0.1-215 IU/mL) and differs with age; Cf RAST

Pritikin diet A high complex carbohydrate, low protein, low fat (<10%of caloric intake) and cholesterol diet that severely restricts caffeine, salt and sugar, which was formulated by a Mr N Pritikin after he was diagnosed of coronary artery disease in 1958; his first total cholesterol was 7.25 mmol/L (US: 280 mg/dl) in 1955; at the time of his death (due to complications of a well-differentiated lymphocytic lymphoma) in 1985, his cholesterol was 2.4 mmol/L (US: 94 mg/dl); post-mortem examination revealed mild cardiac hypertrophy and widely patent coronary arteries (N Engl J Med 1985; 313:52c); see Diet

Privacy Act of 1974 A federal statute (PL 93-579) reaffirming a US citizen's fundamental right to privacy, protecting him from misuse and unnecessary transfer of information by the federal government Note: Such legislation is extremely problematic in tracking persons with fatal communicable infection eg AIDS, as the essence of the Privacy Act is that a citizen's right to privacy overrides the public's rights for safety, an apparent contradiction of the principles of democracy Note: At least one state has overcome this particular dilemma by declaring AIDS a sexually-transmitted disease

Private antigen IMMUNOLOGY An HLA antigen that is determined by a single allele, eg HLA-B27 TRANSFUSION MEDICINE An antigen of very low frequency, found on the erythrocytes of less than 0.1% of the population, eg Peters (Pt^a); Wright (Wr^a), Batty (By), Hey, Good, Bishop (Bp^a), Box (Bx); Cf Public antigens

Private patient A patient whose care is entrusted to one physician who usually has had a long-term relation with the patient, and who is often directly reimbursed for his services by a 'third party' payer or by the patient; Cf Personal physician

prn Latin *pro re nata*, as needed

PRO Peer review organization An independent physician group, often organized in each state of the US that works with the US Federal Government to oversee health care provided to Medicare patients; PRO physicians review a percentage of Medicare patient medical records before, during and after hospitalization to ensure that the care given is medically necessary, provided in the appropriate setting and of a quality that meets accepted professional standards; PROs may review certain procedures prior to hospitalization to assess their necessity, eg carotid endarterectomy, cataract extraction, cholecystectomy, major joint replacement for degenerative joint diseases, coronary artery bypass with graft, peripheral revascularization therapy, hysterectomy, inguinal hernia repair, prostatectomy and pacemaker insertion

Proalbumin A protein precursor of mature albumin that has an extra hexapeptide at the amino terminal, which is cleaved as a final step in the Golgi apparatus; proalbumin defects may be either structural, eg proalbumin Christchurch and proalbumin Lille or functional, eg proalbumin Pittsburgh; Cf Prealbumin

Probability (p) STATISTICS The likelihood that an event will occur by chance; the lower the p value, the less likely it is that two sets of data occurred in a random fashion, ie the greater the likelihood that the two events are associated, while the higher the p value, the greater is the likelihood that the events are random associations; in verbal communication, there is a wide difference in interpretation of adjectives used for probability; when health professionals were surveyed, events that were regarded as 'certain' had a 95-99% chance of occurring, 'very likely' events occurred in 85-89%, 'probable' 64-77%, 'likely' 63-73%, 'frequent' 36-63%, 'not unreasonable' 23-47%, 'possible' 21-43%, 'unlikely' 10-20% and 'improbable' 10-13%; these adjectives are thus of little use in scientific communication (N Engl J Med 1986; 315:740c)

Probe Hybridization probe MOLECULAR BIOLOGY A DNA segment measuring up to several hundred base pairs in length that spans the region of a gene's point mutation or gene rearrangement; probes are labeled with ^{32}P or ^{35}S, or alternately, with a nonradioactive biotinylated tag and hybridize to their 'mirror image', forming dimers of DNA, DNA-RNA and RNA-protein; probes are used in molecular biology to identify the presence of a segment of DNA or RNA of interest in cells and tissues; see *in situ* hybridization

Problem-oriented medical record A formally organized medical record in which each of a patient's conditions or complaints are addressed individually, often organized by the acronym of SOAP (subjective criteria, objective criteria, assessment and plan); see Hospital record, Medical record, SOAP

Pro bono A non-reimbursed service (health care, legal) rendered to those who cannot afford to pay professional fees

Procedure manual LABORATORY MEDICINE A periodically updated manual that delineates in a step-by-step fashion, each of the diagnostic procedures performed by a clinical laboratory, explained with sufficient detail so that it may be performed by a person unfamiliar with the technique; alternately, a procedure manual may delineate contingency plans in case of an emergency; the procedure manual is often the focus of attention by inspecting and accreditating agencies as they are a mark of the quality of a laboratory's work and its degree of organization; Cf Logbook, Notebook

Processing BIOCHEMISTRY The synthetic and modification steps that are required for the maturation of various compounds, eg the primary RNA transcript that is processed to form functional mRNA or a protein that is processed by post-translational modifications, including cleavage of peptide bonds, formation of disulfide bonds, hydroxylation, phosphorylation and attachment of prosthetic groups LABORATORY MEDICINE The sum total of the steps that a clinical specimen passes through from the time of its arrival to the laboratory until the generation of a final report, which includes entering the specimen's relevant data in a log-book (usually performed by computer) and actual performance of the requested test

Procolipase see Colipase

Proconvertin Obsolete for coagulation factor VII

Procurement TRANSPLANTATION The process of obtaining organs for transplantation; the ideal donor of multiple organs destined for transplantation is a (recently) brain-dead patient with unimpaired circulation; the procurement process is costly and prior to activation of a 'procurement team', it must be established that the donor meets 1) Physical criteria, eg young age, state of previous excellent health prior to the trauma that left the donor in a persistent vegetative state, absence of history of substance abuse 2) Legal criteria, ie that appropriate permission for organ donation has been obtained from next-of-kin and 3) Laboratory criteria, which consists of a battery of serological tests, including IgG and IgM ELISA tests for HIV-1, HTLV-I, hepatitis A, hepatitis B, hepatitis C, RPR (for ***Treponema***); once these criteria are met, the 'team' may charter a small private jet and fly to the donor's hospital; once the donor's thoraco-abdominal cavity is opened, it is packed with a 'slush' preparation (ice and lactated Ringer's solution), which reduces the organs' activities to a metabolic 'ground zero'; the 'team' then organizes itself into 3 to 5 'sections', with each section poised to remove one organ block, eg the liver, pancreas, kidneys (which count as one block), heart-lung block or heart and lungs as separate blocks; there may thus be up to 10 people in the donor's body cavity during the procurement process; once the 'team' is ready, the aorta is cannulated and clamped above the heart; at this critical step (known as 'cross-clamping'), the 'clock' starts, after which time each organ block has an allowed 'cold ischemia time' before it becomes suboptimal for transplantation, which is 4 to 6 hours for the heart-lung block, 20 hours for the liver and pancreas, and 72 hours for the kidneys; after 'cross-clamping', the vena cava is cut and the donor's blood is exsanguinated and a perfusate (the 'Wisconsin solution') is gravity-fed into each organ via the aorta and arteries; the organs are then removed by each 'section' and placed in containers filled with 'slush' preparation, maintained at near 0°C, and then transported to their respective recipients; see Slush preparation, Wisconsin solution

Prodrug CLINICAL PHARMACOLOGY A drug ingested in the inactive form that is transformed into an active form by in vivo metabolic reactions

Proenkephalin A molecule generated by selective post-translational proteolysis from pro-opiomelanocortin (POMC), yielding met- and leu-enkephalins as well as the opioids, octapeptide and heptapeptide; proenkephalin production is increased in seizures and its gene may be the target of the heterodimeric complex of the proto-oncogenes, c-*fos* and c-*jun* (Science 1989; 246:1622)

Profession An occupation requiring intense preparation in a body of erudite knowledge that is applied in the service of society, has a system of self-governance and in which success is measured by accomplishments in serving society and/or furtherance of knowledge in the field rather than personal gain; see Learned profession, 'Yellow professionalism'

Professional corporation (PC) A legal entity in which each of the shareholders is a member of the same profession; many individual physicians in the US belong to a professional corporation that numbers from one individual to a dozen or more professionals; the advantages of incorporation include corporate ownership of equipment, tax and investment advantages, health benefits, leasing of transportation vehicles and limitation of malpractice liability

Professor A faculty member of the highest academic rank at an institution of higher learning, who professes special knowledge in an occupation requiring skill; in the USA, the 'pecking order' in academic science and medicine is based on a) Permanence of a position, ie whether it is 'tenured' and b) Rank, which in increasing order of peer recognition begins at instructor, assistant professor, associate professor and (full) professor, who is at the pinnacle; professors have attained national or international reputation for academic excellence, are among the most accomplished in their field, are eminent researchers, influential and able teachers and, if applicable, outstanding clinicians; see 'Chair'; Cf Chair

Professorial rounds A permutation of patient rounds that forms part of the teaching activities at an academic health care facility, in which the clinical, radiological and pathological data from one or a limited number of patients are presented; although the format of these 'rounds' varies, it intended to be a socratic dialog between a discussor at a podium and his junior and senior colleagues, serving to evaluate the steps made in arriving at the diagnosis, how to treat the patient(s) and to share the professor's experience; Cf Clinico-pathological conference, Grand rounds, Rounds

Profile EPIDEMIOLOGY A cross-sectional aggregation of health care data applied to any segment of the population being served or the individuals or groups providing the service and the statistics obtained therefrom; there are thus patient, physician and hospital profiles LABORATORY MEDICINE A panel of screening tests used to establish a baseline of normalcy for either a certain population, eg Executive profile or for a limited group of analytes, eg Lipid profile; see Organ panels

Profilin PHYSIOLOGY A 15 kD protein present in platelets and neutrophils that regulates the length of actin filaments, which is involved in altering the cell shape in carcinogenesis and thrombogenesis; profilin may mediate many of the intracellular events that follow binding of growth signal proteins to their cognate extracellular receptors, transferring signals from the cell surface to the nucleus; profilin may prevent phospholipase C (PLC) from catalyzing PIP_2 until PLC is phosphorylated by tyrosine kinase activated by growth factor-receptor interaction (Science 1991; 251:1231, 1181ed)

Progeria(s) A group of conditions characterized by markedly premature aging of childhood onset, in which morbid conditions usually seen in the elderly appear during puberty and death from 'old age' occurs by 20; several congenital conditions are associated with progeria Cockayne syndrome An autosomal dominant condition characterized by dwarfism, microcephaly, 'salt and pepper' choroidoretinitis, optic atrophy, cerebral calcifications, mental retardation, intention tremor, tottering gait, deafness, small trunk, long extremities, attenuated subcutaneous fat, sexual infantilism, hepatosplenomegaly, atherosclerosis and early death Hutchinson-Gilford syndrome A disease complex first manifest in infancy, characterized by poor growth, early onset atherosclerosis, periarticular fibrosis, attenuated subcutaneous fat, dwarfism, small face, beaked nose, baldness, parchment-like skin with brownish discoloration, poor dentition, poor muscle development and early death

Progenote The hypothetical precursor organism that is postulated to be ultimate 'stem organism', prior to the divergence of life forms into archaebacteria, prokaryotes and eukaryotes; see Urkingdom

Progestin A generic term for any natural or synthetic compound with progesterone-like activity

Progonoma see Pigmented neuroectodermal tumor of infancy

Prognostic scoring system Any of a number of analytic systems that attempt to predict outcome(s) and identify patients and clinical situations in which the potential value of intensive care is low, while the burden of therapy is high, providing a numerical prediction of patient mortality (J Intensive Care Med 1990; 5:33); see APACHE II, MPS, PRISM, SAPS and TISS

Programmed killing EMBRYOLOGY Selective destruction of the neurons that are overproduced in early brain development; although the neuroembryologic mechanism for this overproduction is unclear, the A68 protein may act as a target, marking cells for deletion

Progressive multifocal leukoencephalopathy (PML) A lesion of the central nervous system characterized by demyelinization, intranuclear viral inclusions in oligodendrogliocytes, scattered bizarre giant astrocytes, reactive fibrillary astrocytes, patchy cortical loss with scant inflammation; PML occurs in immunocompromised hosts, eg AIDS and is caused by papova (DNA-type) usually JC virus, rarely also by BK virus and is associated with AIDS (J Am Med Assoc 1990; 264:79cr)

Progressive transformation of germinal centers (PTGC) A lymphoid lesion characterized by enlargement of germinal centers in a background of follicular hyperplasia and effacement of the relatively sharply defined boundary between the germinal center and the mantle zone; 'transformed' germinal centers are composed of small round lymphocytes admixed with scattered immunoblasts and histiocytes and are most common in young males, appearing in a single, asymptomatic and enlarged lymph node; although it may occur in patients with nodular lymphocyte-predominance Hodgkin's disease (Verh Anat Ges 1975; 69:19), it is thought to be neither neoplastic nor a harbinger for future lymphoid malignancy (Am J Surg Pathol 1984; 8:725); see Germinal centers; Cf Regressively transformed germinal centers

Prohormone convertase(s) A family of enzymes that 'clip' functional hormones out of larger parent proteins, eg chopping out hormones at sites of dibasic amino acids

Projectile vomiting Violent and 'explosive' vomiting without antecedent nausea, or vomiting that occurs at the peak of maximum inspiration without the usual rhythmic hyperactivity of the respiratory muscles associated with 'retching' (diaphragmatic spasms that precede vomiting); projectile vomiting is associated with increased intracranial pressure, classically occurring in meningitides of young children

Prolactin A pituitary hormone with several molecular forms, eg 'big' and 'little' prolactin that is under inhibitory control by the hypothalamus; male and female hormone levels are similar, ranging from 1-25 ng/ml and have diurnal variation, peaking 4-5 hours after the onset of sleep; prolactin is increased in 70% of those with pituitary tumors (57% with > 100 ng/ml and 100% with > 300 ng/ml have pituitary tumors); prolactin is also increased in cirrhosis, empty sella syndrome, hypothyroidism, renal failure, MEN-I and with drug therapy (α-methyldopa, cimetidine, phenothiazine, verapamil, hormones, eg estrogen, growth hormone, thyroid-releasing hormone, psychotropic drugs) Quantification Radioimmunoassay

Prolactin-inhibiting hormone Dopamine

Proliferative breast disease(s) (PBD) A group of benign breast lesions characterized by proliferation of epithelial cells in the terminal ductal-lobular unit of the breast, which have a two-to-fivefold increased incidence of malignancy; PBD tends to occur in first degree relatives of patients with breast cancer; the susceptibility locus has been located at D17S74 (Science 1990; 250:1715); see D17S74, Sclerosing adenosis: Cf Mammary dysplasia

Proliferative phase The early or preovulation half of the menstrual cycle, initiated by the small peak in follicle-stimulating hormone; this phase, also known as the follicular phase, begins in the late luteal phase of the previous menstrual cycle under the influence of ovarian estrogen; the endometrium undergoes regeneration in preparation for implantation of an egg, if it becomes fertilized; during proliferation, the cervix becomes more vascularized, the os widens and the cervical mucus increases in volume, elasticity and undergoes arborization; see Ferning

PROM 1) Premature rupture of membranes OBSTETRICS The leakage of amniotic fluid prior to the onset of labor, an event occurring in 10% of term pregnancies and 15-20% of pre-term pregnancies, which is associated with increased mortality and morbidity; the etiology of PROM is unknown, but may be due to the combined action of bacterial or internal enzymes **Complications** Fetal infections, eg congenital pneumonia or septicemia and fetal wastage **Treatment** Deliver baby within 36 hours 2) Programmable read-only memory COMPUTERS A ROM chip that may be updated and altered by special equipment, eg ultraviolet light or electronic signals, which is not ordinarily accessible to the unskilled user, and therefore functions exactly as a ROM chip

Promiscuity MOLECULAR BIOLOGY The ability of a molecule with a conformational specificity, eg a receptor, enzyme or antibody, to bind to various non-specific ligands, substrates or antigens

Promiscuous DNA Segments of DNA that are postulated to have been 'shamelessly' transferred through transpositions between mitochondria, chloroplasts, nuclei and other organelles early in the evolution of primitive life forms

Promontory sign see Peninsula sign

Promoters MOLECULAR BIOLOGY The site on the DNA double helix where RNA polymerase attaches and initiates transcription; in the classic operon, the promoter is located adjacent (usually upstream) to the operator ONCOLOGY see Tumor promoters

Promoter mutation A mutation that affects the promoter region on the DNA, acting to a) Increase the efficiency of the initiation of transcription, through an increase in RNA polymerase binding to the initiation site, an 'Up' mutation, b) Decrease transcription, by decreasing RNA polymerase binding to the initiation site, a 'Down' mutation or c) Create a new promotion site

Promoter sequence A sequence of proviral DNA (DNA of retroviral origin that has become integrated into host DNA), which directs the RNA polymerase to a specific initiation site; promoter sequences, like the enhancer sequences are located within the long terminal repeats flanking proviral DNA; see LTR

Promotion see Tumor promotion

Proofreading Editing MOLECULAR BIOLOGY A generic term for any activity that allows correction of errors that occur during replication, transcription, translation or other processing of genetic information, eg that displayed by the α and delta DNA polymerase complexes in eukaryotic cells, in which mismatched double-stranded DNA, ie incorrectly hydrogen-bonded bases are removed by the 3'→5' exonuclease activity of DNA polymerases

Pro-opiomelanocortin (POMC) A 31 kD pituitary prohormone gene product released by corticotropin-releasing factor, which by post-translational processing, gives rise to different active peptides in the brain and gut including pituitary hormones (ACTH, α-, β- and γ-MSH), endogenous opiates (β-endorphin and enkephalin), α- and β-lipotropin

ProPAC Prospective Payment Assessment Commission HEALTH CARE FINANCING An independent body of experts in the US that recommends adjustments in the 'weight' and classification of the diagnosis-related groups, so that they reflect changes in costs of procedures and changes in technology and diagnosis; see DRGs

Properdin see Alternate pathway

Proposition 64 Ballot proposition 64 A proposal made in the early 1980s in a California State legislative referendum that AIDS was a disease of sufficient health risk to warrant quarantining of anyone infected with the human immunodeficiency virus (HIV-1), banning AIDS patients from providing health care, teaching in public schools or handling food; it was not passed (Science 1986; 234:277); see 'Informed'

Proposition 65 Ballot proposition 65 Safe Drinking water and Toxic Enforcement Act of 1986 CLINICAL TOXICOLOGY A state law passed in California requiring the government to list all the chemicals known to cause cancer or reproductive toxic effect; 12 months after having been so listed, people may not be exposed (occupational, water and environmental exposures) unless previously warned; 20 months after such listing, the substance may not be discharged into any actual or potential source of drinking water (J Am Med Assoc 1988; 260:951); see 'White-out'

Proposition 99 Ballot proposition 99 SUBSTANCE ABUSE A state law passed in California that increases the taxes imposed on tobacco products, 'earmarking' the funds for various anti-smoking activities, including education, treatment, research and protection of wildlife resources

Prosector's wart Cutaneous tuberculosis of historic interest that occurred on the hands of ungloved pathologists (prosectors) who performed autopsies on cases of tuberculosis, resulting in hyperkeratotic nodules due to direct tuberculin innoculation

Prospective payment system (PPS) The system of reimbursement for hospital and physician services, based largely on flat rates per admission calculated for each of 470 diagnosis-related groups that was introduced to force hospitals to become more efficient (Mayo Clin Proc 1990; 65:1171) Note: Coincident with the introduction of the PPS, the peer review organization system of quality and appropriateness of care was established; early conclusions on the PPS form of reimbursement are that it has not affected the mortality of hospital patients, has provided mechanisms for improving the quality of care, but has increased the likelihood that patients will be discharged from a health care facility with clinical 'instability' (J Am Med Assoc 1990; 264:1989); see DRGs

Prostatic carcinoma 106 000 new cases of prostatic adenocarcinoma are diagnosed annually in the US, causing 30 000 annual deaths; 35-50% of men > 70 years of age have prostatic carcinoma, although the behavior of prostatic carcinoma is difficult to predict, commonly, it remains occult and those with this cancer die of natural deaths; flow cytometry of tumor cells allows partial prediction of tumors most likely to progress, as DNA ploidy analysis reveals that diploid tumors (as elsewhere in the body)have a significantly better prognosis then aneuploid or aneuploid-tetraploid tumors (Mayo Clin Proc 1988; 63:103); although early stage A1 prostatic adenocarcinoma is traditionally regarded as a 'pathologist's tumor' not requiring treatment, a 10 year followup indicates that 16% progress to stages requiring therapy (Urology 1990; 36:210) Note: Prostatic carcinoma is more common and more aggressive in American blacks than whites; see PSA (prostate-specific antigen)

'Prostate years' A colloquialism of little utility for age 60 or older, when men begin to become symptomatic for urinary retention due to prostatic hyperplasia or, less commonly, adenocarcinoma

Prospect Hill virus A Bunyavirus related to Hantaan virus; see Korean hemorrhagic fever

Protein A MICROBIOLOGY A component of the *Staphylococcus aureus* cell wal, which, like protein G, binds to the Fc fragment of all four subclasses of immunoglobulin G; protein A has proven to be a useful reagent for identifying immunoglobulins and immune complexes

Protein A, B, C MOLECULAR BIOLOGY Three proteins associated with heterogeneous nuclear or nonribosomal RNAs from the HeLa cell line; nuclease treatment releases a 40S particle with these proteins which contain modified amino acids of unknown function, di- and trimethylarginines, located exclusively in nucleus

Proteins A, B, C, D HEMATOLOGY Anti-coagulants whose names derive from the immunologic characterization of the vitamin K-dependent clotting proteins into 4 groups (A-D); three of the names are of historic interest and no longer used, as protein A has become factor IX, protein B has become prothrombin and protein D has become factor X; protein C in current use

Protein B see above

Protein blotting see Immunoblotting

Protein C HEMATOLOGY Autoprothrombin II-A A 62 kD vitamin K-dependent serine protease with 2 sulfide-bonded glycoprotein chains that is converted to an active serine protease by thrombin and accelerated in this activity by protein S; protein C is a potent anticoagulant, which inactivates coagulation factors V and VIII:C, enhancing fibrinolysis (thrombolysis) by neutralizing the major inactivator of tissue plasminogen activator; protein C deficiency is either autosomal dominant of variable penetration or acquired, due to disseminated intravascular coagulation, warfarin therapy, hepatic disease and postoperatively; may fall to lless than 40% normal (4.8 μg/ml) are often symptomatic, causing recurrent venous thromboses; protein C production is orchestrated by the binding of thrombin to thrombomodulin on an endothelial cell receptor, switching it to the activated form; protein C increases tissue plasminogen and neutralizes the inactivator of plasminogen activator (fibrinolysis) and inactivates anticoagulation on Va and VIIIa using protein S as a cofactor; homozygous deficiency (< 1% normal protein C) presents as neonatal purpura fulminans (ischemic necrosis) with massive venous thrombosis and a syndrome mimicked by coumarin-induced skin necrosis; the homozygous form is treated acutely by factor IX and chronically by anticoagulation

Protein D see Proteins A-D involved in coagulation, above

Protein domain see Domain

Protein F Fusion protein VIROLOGY A 70 kD glycoprotein that is thought to be integral to mounting an appropriate immune response to respiratory syncytial virus; Cf Protein G

Protein folding The constellation of processes required for a protein to be converted from a simple polypeptide chain to a functional molecule with a three-dimensional configuration; see Protein structure

Protein fractionation A generic term for any technique for separating proteins, including centrifugation, chromatography, electrophoresis or precipitation

Protein G BACTERIOLOGY A component of the group G streptococcus cell wall that binds to the Fc region of all four subclasses of immunoglobulin G and which may be responsible for successful host defense against this organism VIROLOGY Attachment protein A 90 kD glycoprotein on the surface of and integral to the immune reaction to respiratory syncytitial virus (RSV); antigenic differences in the G protein are responsible for differences in RSV strains; Cf Protein F

Protein kinase C (PKC) A phorbol ester receptor encoded by an α gene on chromosome 17, a β gene on chromosome 16 and a γ gene on chromosome 19; PKC mediates multiple intracellular processes, acting by signal transduction, resulting in hormone secretion (calcitonin, catecholamines, insulin, growth hormone, steroids) and enzymes (amylase, pepsinogen), release of neurotransmitters, mediation of inflammation (release of histamine and serotonin and generation of superoxide) and anabolic effects (lipogenesis and gluconeogenesis); PKC is also involved in cell differentiation and tumor promotion; PKC is an intracellular enzyme with a protein kinase-like domain at the carboxyl terminal that is activated by extracellular signals received at the cell membrane receptors; phospholipase C-dependent hydrolysis of inositol phospholipid (especially phosphoinositol-4,5-*bis*-phosphate) into two second messengers: diacylglycerol (DAG) and inositol tris-phosphate (IP3, which mobilizes calcium from intracellular stores); DAG activates and lysosphingolipids inhibit protein kinase C (J Am Med Assoc 1989; 262:1826)

Protein-losing enteropathy A condition characterized by excess transmucosal efflux of plasma proteins from the intestinal lumen, due to increased permeability caused by mucosal cell damage, inflammation-induced ulceration or leakage from lymphatic vessels secondary to obstruction Etiology Paraneoplastic syndromes, gastric carcinoma, nontropical sprue, ulcerative colitis, congestive heart failure, constrictive pericarditis, superior vena cava thrombosis, pulmonic artery stenosis Histopathology Inflammation, mucosal ulceration Treatment Treat underlying cause

Protein M M antigen MICROBIOLOGY One of 55 serotypes of a protein located on the fimbriae of group A streptococci which has antiphagocytic properties and contributes to the streptococcal virulence; see LPSTGE

Proteinquake A functionally important movement of proteins, which like an earthquake, relieves the strain at a focus of the chain, with a return to an equilibrium state Note: A protein may assume a large number of conformational substates that have the same secondary structures, but different super-secondary structural substates causing a protein to perform its function at different rates; the existence of states and substates in proteins implies that there are two types of motion in proteins, ie equilibrium fluctuations (defined by the mathematics of chaos and equilibrium thermodynamics) and major conformational twists or 'quakes'; see Protein folding, Protein structure

Protein R GASTROENTEROLOGY A group of related 60 kD cobalamine-binding proteins found in gastric juice, milk, plasma, saliva, so designated as they all are rapid migrants on serum electrophoresis; see R-binding proteins

Protein S HEMATOLOGY A 69 kD vitamin K-dependent binding protein that is a cofactor for activated protein C (so named as it was discovered in Seattle); protein S exists as an active single chain protein or as an inactive disulfide-linked dimeric protein; when protein S is present with phospholipid, it enhances factor Va inactivation by protein C and binds C4b-binding protein; autosomal dominant protein S deficiency is clinically and therapeutically similar to heterozygous protein C deficiency and is characterized by pulmonary thrombosis, deep vein thrombosis, thrombophlebitis; protein S is quantified by Laurell rocket electrophoresis, which does not distinguish between the active free protein and the inactive complement C4b-bound protein S; the functional assay is based on protein C's lack of anticoagulant activity in the absence of protein S IMMUNOLOGY see Vitronectin

Protein-sparing CLINICAL NUTRITION The addition of carbohydrates and fats to a low-protein diet in order to minimize protein catabolism

Protein structure The conformation of protein, which is a function of its amino acid sequence and the bonds that are allowed to be formed with itself and other molecules within its sphere of activity **PRIMARY PROTEIN STRUCTURE** That structure of a protein that is a direct function of the sequence of amino acids **SECONDARY PROTEIN STRUCTURE** That structure of a protein that results from folding along one axis of the molecule, as in the formation of an α helix, due to the formation of hydrogen bonds along the length of a chain; see Super secondary structure **TERTIARY PROTEIN STRUCTURE** The three-dimensional conformation of a polypeptide chain folded upon itself, which is thought to result from the interaction of the side chains of amino acids, which may be immediately adjacent to each other or located across a chasm of intramolecular space **QUARTENARY PROTEIN-STRUCTURE** A protein structure that results from the interaction between individual polypeptide chains, or discrete by related proteins **QUINARY PROTEIN STRUCTURE** Any transient interaction of multiple, unrelated proteins; see Domain

Protein 'suicide' Protein inactivation CLINICAL GENETICS A molecular defect seen in a lethal variant of osteogenesis imperfecta, in which one of the three collagen chains (proα_1[I]) is markedly shortened, resulting in procollagen molecules incapable of forming a viable triple helix; the concept of protein suicide may help explain the greater than expected effects of certain seemingly innocent genetic defects

Proteinuria Loss of protein in the urine; normally, about 150 mg/day of protein is lost in the urine, one third of which is albumin, one third is Tamm-Horsfall glycoprotein and the remainder is divided among actively secreted proteins including retinol binding proteins, β_2-microglobulin, immunoglobulin light chains and lysozyme; in absence of disease, large proteins are retained due to their size, while the smaller proteins are actively resorbed *PROTEINURIA CAN BE CLINICALLY DIVIDED INTO A 1) GLOMERULAR PATTERN* Proteinuria due to a loss of the fixed negative charge on the glomerular capillary wall, allowing albumin and other large ($\geq$ 68 kD) molecules to leak into Bowman's space, seen in glomerulonephritis and nephrotic syndrome **Laboratory** Decreased albumin, anti-thrombin, transferrin, prealbumin, α_1-acid glycoprotein and α_1-antitrypsin *2) HEMODYNAMIC PATTERN* Proteinuria due to rheostatic changes elsewhere in the body, causing a loss of variably-sized protein (20 to 68 kD) molecules, seen in transient proteinuria, congestive heart failure, fever, seizures, exercise *3) OVERFLOW PATTERN* Proteinuria due to tissue or cell destruction elsewhere in the body, overwhelming the kidney's capacity to excrete certain proteins, as occurs in Bence-Jones proteinuria and myoglobinuria *4) TUBULAR PATTERN* Proteinuria due to renal tubular dysfunction with loss of normally filtered low molecular weight ($\leq$ 40 kD) molecules **Laboratory** Decreased β_2-microglobulin and lysozyme, as occurs in Fanconi syndrome, Wilson's disease, interstitial nephritis, antibiotic-induced injury and heavy metal intoxication

Protein X see pX protein

Protein Y see Ligandin

Protein Z A 44 kD vitamin K-dependent plasma protein that is a secondary cytoplasmic bilirubin-binding factor of unknown function; see Ligandin; Cf Z protein

Proteoglycan A high-molecular weight glycoprotein that is located on the plasma membranes of mammalian cells and in the extracellular matrix and separated according to differences in the core proteins and the composition of the linear polysaccharide chains or glycosaminoglycans, linked by covalent bonds to serine residues in the core proteins Note: Tumorigenesis is in part related to aberrant production of proteoglycans; see Basement membrane, Extracellular matrix; Cf Integrin family, Laminin

Proteoliposome A vesicular artificial organelle prepared from phospholipids, proteins and enzymes, that may be of use as a pharmacologic delivery system

Proteosome A hydrophilic multimeric conglomerate of outer membrane meningococcal proteins that is mitogenic for B cells, a property that makes these structures attractive as possible carriers and adjuvants (non-specific immune stimulators) for newer generations of vaccines through enhancement of immunogenicity; Cf Liposome

Proteus syndrome A rare disease, characterized by acral gigantism, plantar hyperplasia, hemangiomas, lipomas, varicosities, linear verrucous epidermal nevi, macrocephaly, cranial hyperostosis, pachydermy and hypertrophy of the long bones Proteus of Greek mythology tended Neptune's flock of seals and had the gift of prophesy; in order to escape the constant badgering of those interested in the future, he often changed himself into other forms, including wild animals or raging fire; see 'Elephant man'

Prothrombin complex concentrates (PCC) HEMATOLOGY Commercial products, eg FEIBA (Factor VIII inhibitor by-passing activity), which contain nonactivated factors IX, in addition to II, XI and X, which may be used to ameliorate the intensity and duration of joint and soft tissue bleeding in hemophiliacs who produce factor VIII inhibitors; PCC are 50% effective in staunching hemorrhage; factor IX concentrates are prepared by adding cold ethanol or ether to citrated plasma, which is then added to either calcium phosphate or ion-exchange resins (eg DEAE-Sephadex), allowing elution of a protein with therapeutic levels of vitamin K-dependent factors II, IX and X, and factors VII, protein C and protein S

Protist see Progenote, Urkingdom

Proton pump PHYSIOLOGY An ATP-dependent H^+ ion transporter assumed to be present in the membranes of lysosomes and vacuoles, which maintains a low pH (4.5-5.0) inside these organelles; proton pumping is also required in the electron transport chain, where an NADH (or FADH) is oxidized to NAD^+ (or FAH^+), releasing two electrons and a proton; Cf Na^+/H^+ antiporter, Na^+/K^+ ATPase

Proton NMR spectroscopy Water-suppressed proton NMR spectroscopy A laboratory technique that averages the methyl and methylene line widths in the NMR spectra of plasma lipoproteins; this technique was reported (N Engl J Med 1986; 315:1369) to be a valid cancer screen in asymptomatic subjects, a finding not confirmed in subsequent studies (ibid 1990; 322:949, 953, 1002)

Proto-oncogene A cellular gene that is homologous to a retroviral oncogene, in that it has latent transforming potential; proto-oncogenes include c-*erb*, c-*fos*, c-*jun*, c-*myb*, c-*myc*, c-*mos*, c-*raf*, c-*ras* and these act in normal growth and differentiation, as well as in the induction and/or maintenance of malignancy (N Engl J Med 1987; 317:955); proto-oncogenes coupled to control elements are capable of transforming normal fibroblasts into tumorigenic cells; slow retroviruses, which themselves lack viral oncogenes become tumorigenic when inserted in DNA adjacent to proto-oncogenes; many specific chromosomal translocations seen in human tumors occur at or near the proto-oncogene site and some proto-oncogenes may be 'amplified' in malignancy; proto-oncogenes are thought to become tumorigenic if the gene itself is altered, producing an abnormal gene product, or if there is an increase in the amount of the gene product, due to either gene amplification or changes in the control elements, eg there is increased expression of proto-oncogenes after cellular insults, eg CMV infection results in activation of c-*fos*, c-*jun* and c-*myc* (Science 1990; 247:561)

Protothecosis Infection by a ubiquitous, unicellular, alga-like organism that reproduces by endosporulation; human infection is rare, occurs in immunocompromised hosts, and is due to *Prototheca wickerhamii* or *P zopfii*, which cause chronic papulonodular skin lesions, wound infections, disseminated skin infections and lymphadenopathy **Treatment** Amphotericin B

Proud flesh A curious term for the exuberant granulation tissue seen in a poorly healed wound, which is characterized by florid, 'geographic' scarring on the skin surface, related to a defect of union of interrupted tissues by 'second intent' healing; see Keloid, Wound healing

Provirus A virus that is stably inserted in a host cell's genome, and is transmitted vertically to the host's progeny at the time of cell division

Proximal carcinogen A chemical or physical agent that (hypothetically) initiates the first (induction) step in a carcinogenic cascade

Proximity effect The increased catalytic response observed when an enzyme's substrate is brought more proximate to the enzyme's reactive sites

Prozac see Fluoxetine

Prozone phenomenon IMMUNOLOGY A false negative reaction seen when measuring antibodies by immune precipitation caused by a massive antibody excess, which inhibits the precipitation reaction Note: Since the reaction is optimal at an antigen-antibody ratio of 1:1, if there is strong reason to believe that a sample contains the suspected antibody (and may be displaying a prozone phenomenon), the sample should be serially diluted to prevent the specimen being reported as negative

PRP antigen Polyribosyl-ribitol capsular polysaccharide A cell wall component of ***Haemophilus influenzae*** that has intrinsic antiphagocytic activity, thus endowing ***H influenzae*** with a unique pathogenic mechanism; protective immunity against ***H influenzae*** requires opsonization with type-specific antibodies; the production of anti-PRP antibodies is poor until children reach age two and thus they may be susceptible to more than one episode; see Hib vaccine

PRP-D Polyribosylribitol-diphtheria toxoid see Hib

Prune belly syndrome of Eagle-Barrett Complete congenital absence of abdominal musculature, imparting a rugose, prune-like appearance to the flaccid abdominal wall; 97% occur in males and are accompanied by genitourinary anomalies, eg bilateral cryptorchism, hypoplastic and dysplastic kidneys; affected females have uterine abnormalities; although considered an X-linked disease, no chromosome defect has been identified, and this disease complex may represent a 'sequence' initiated by in utero urethral obstruction, causing urinary tract anomalies (megaureters, megabladder, patent urachus or urachal cyst); other findings include Potter's facies, talipes, hip dislocation, musculoskeletal and cardiac defects Treatment Corsets, excision of redundant tissue Prognosis Oligohydramnios may arise in utero, causing fatal fetal pulmonary hypoplasia, 20% are stillborn, 50% die in infancy

'Pruned tree' appearance A descriptor for a pulmonary arteriographic pattern seen in relatively central pulmonary thromboembolism

'Prune juice' discharge A descriptor for the dark brown vaginal discharge characteristic of a hydatidiform mole likened to the juice of stewed prunes (dried plums)

Prune juice sputum A descriptor for the dark-brown hemorrhagic sputum seen in well-developed pneumococcal pneumonia; Cf Rusty sputum

Pruritus gravidarum A condition affecting 1:300 pregnancies, beginning in the third trimester, first appearing on the abdomen later extending to the entire corporal surface Treatment Antihistamines; see Pregnancy-related conditions; Cf PUPPP

PSA Prostate-specific antigen A 34 kD glycoprotein serine protease secreted exclusively by the prostate epithelium that is responsible for lysis of the seminal coagulum; PSA is increased in 30-50% of patients with benign prostatic hypertrophy and in 25-92% of those with prostatic carcinoma; PSA is more sensitive than prostatic acid phosphatase (PAP) as a serum marker of prostatic carcinoma; PSA/PAP positivity is 63%/12% in stage A, 71%/22% in stage B, 81%/38% in stage C and 88%/67% in stage D (Diag & Clin Test 1990; 28:16); serum PSA levels can be monitored for recurrent prostatic adenocarcinoma, but because PSA is also elevated in acute prostatitis and to a lesser degree, in benign prostatic hypertrophy, serum PSA levels are not a cost-effective screening modality for prostatic cancer (Mayo Clin Proc 1990; 65:1118); prostatic cancer is present in 22% of those with PSA levels above 4.0 μg/L, and 60% of those with levels above 10 μg/L (N Engl J Med 1991; 324:1156)

Psammoma bodies Psammoma, Greek. sand Calcospherites, 'Corpora amylacea' Round laminated, 20-100 μm in diameter calcified masses (figure below) that may represent degenerated papillary clusters of cellular debris that are especially common in benign prostatic hypertrophy; and may occur in benign and malignant epithelial neoplasms, eg papillary carcinomas of the thyroid, ovary, endometrium, pancreas and kidney, meningiomas, benign 'sugar tumor' of the lung, mesothelioma, mesothelial cell hyperplasia, bronchoalveolar carcinoma; ovarian serous cystadenoma and dystrophic calcification of matrix vesicles and desmoid tumors

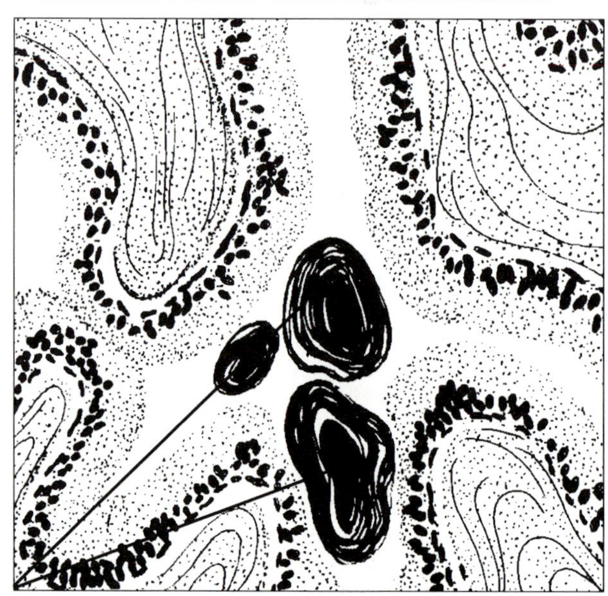

Psammoma bodies

Pseudoacanthosis nigricans A disease of obese darkly-pigmented adults, characterized by hyperpigmented patches Treatment Weight loss *TRUE ACANTHOSIS NIGRICANS* occurs in subjects of any size and color in a background of malignancy

Pseudoachondroplasia(s) A heterogeneous group of often autosomal dominant conditions, the most common of which is pseudoachondroplastic spondyloepiphyseal dysplasia Clinical Early onset with decreased limb growth (irregular 'mushroomed 'metaphyses, small, irregular and fragmented epiphyses, short bowing diaphyses), flattened vertebrae, lumbar lordosis, scoliosis, kyphosis, 'spatula' ribs, hypermobility of major and acral joints, short hands and feet, contractures of the hips and knees, waddling gait and early onset of osteoarthrosis *TRUE ACHONDROPLASIA* has more prominent truncal shortening, but is otherwise clinically similar

Pseudoalleles Two or more closely linked genes that in complementation studies behave as alleles, which may be separated by cross-over studies

Pseudoallergy An adverse, nonimmunologic, anaphylaxis-like reaction of sudden onset, that is often associated with food ingestion, which may be due to an anaphylactoid reaction, intolerance, eg psychogenic response, metabolic defect, eg enzymatic deficiency, tyramine, see cheese reaction and toxicity, eg tetrodotoxin *TRUE ALLERGIES* to comestibles are hypersensitivity reactions caused by mast cell release of IgE, in children, most commonly due to eggs, milk, peanuts, other nuts, fish, soy beans and shrimp

Pseudoaneurysm see False aneurysm

Pseudoangina see 'Heartburn'

Pseudoarthrosis ORTHOPEDICS Non-union of two fractured ends of long bones where the bone is covered by fibrous tissue or fibrocartilage; in the most extreme cases, the false joint is surrounded by a bursal sac containing synovial fluid; congenital pseudoarthroses, while rare, most often occur in von Recklinghausen's disease or in osteogenesis imperfecta; acquired pseudoarthrosis usually follows trauma, far less commonly, tumor-related osteolysis and fibrous dysplasia

Pseudoatrophy, cerebral Apparent decrease in the volume of cortical tissue, as seen by computerized tomography due to changes in cerebrospinal fluid production and alterations in the blood-brain barrier with secondary decrease in the interstitial fluid of the brain, resulting from steroid therapy (N Engl J Med 1984; 311:656cpc) *TRUE CEREBRAL ATROPHY* is irreversible

Pseudoautosomal region A small terminal region of homologous DNA sequences that is shared by mammalian sex chromosomes, which pair and recombine during male meiosis; in this region, alleles are freely exchanged between X and Y chromosomes and inherited as if they were autosomal; genes in this region are present in two doses in both males and females, but in the female escape inactivation; two genes are located in the X-Y pseudoautosomal region; MIC2 and encodes a cell-surface antigen and granulocyte-monocyte colony-stimulating factor (GM-CSF, Nature 1990; 345:734); Cf X chromosome inactivation

Pseudo-Bartter syndrome Hypokalemic-hypochloremic alkalosis, hyperactivity of renin-angiotensin-aldosterone system with increased aldosterone, normotension, pressor inactivity of angiotensin II, increased urinary prostaglandin E and atrionatriuretic peptide, due to furosemide therapy (N Engl J Med 1987; 316:167c) *TRUE BARTTER SYNDROME* has a similar laboratory 'signature' but is caused by enlarged juxtaglomerular apparatus

Pseudobubo Massive inguinal lymphadenopathy caused by ***Calymmatobacterium granulomatis***, the granuloma inguinale agent, characterized by soft subcutaneous fluctuant masses with overlying ulcers Note: Bubo is a generic term for any massively enlarged lymph node, visible in accessible regions (axillary or inguinal), and thus there is no 'true' bubo; the bubo of ***Chlamydia trachomatis*** (agent of lymphogranuloma venereum), has been anointed with various adjectives, including climatic bubo, Frei's bubo, nonvenereal bubo, strumous bubo and tropical bubo; syphilitic bubos have been adjectivally dignified as bullet bubo, primary bubo and venereal bubo; ***Haemophilus ducreyi*** (chancroid agent) causes the chancroid bubo and virulent bubo; the most famed of all is that of the bubonic plague, the 'malignant' bubo

Pseudobulbar palsy Spastic bulbar paralysis A disease of middle age resulting in dysarthria, dysphonia, dysphagia, drooling, bilateral facial weakness and is remarkable for the highly variable psychiatric component, in which the patients may lack emotional expression (simulating apathy or severe depression) or become enmeshed in trivialities or have inappropriate responses to environmental cues, also known as the 'Laughing sickness' for the characteristic pathologic laughing or crying Etiology The brains of these patients often demonstrate multifocal infarction, most commonly due to atherosclerosis, less commonly, to infections, trauma and degeneration Treatment Antibiotics Prognosis Guarded *TRUE BULBAR PALSY* results from weakness or paralysis of the muscles supplied by the lower brainstem motor nuclei (V, VII, IX-XII) and may be of sudden onset, caused by diphtheria and poliomyelitis or more indolent with atrophy of the same muscles

Pseudocapsule An investment of fibrous tissue partially surrounding a variety of neoplasms, especially of mesenchymal origin *TRUE ENCAPSULATION* implies a benign or at least a proliferating process that is circumscribed enough to allow complete removal; penetration of a tumor capsule is a notorious source of recurrence in otherwise low-grade carcinomas

Pseudocarcinomatous hyperplasia see Pseudoepitheliomatous hyperplasia

Pseudo-Chediak-Higashi anomaly A microscopic finding in Wright-Giemsa-stained peripheral blood smears in occasional patients with acute myelomonocytic and chronic myelogenous leukemia, seen as large, round, pink erythrocyte-like inclusions found in myeloblasts and promyelocytes; by ultrastructure, the inclusions correspond to abnormal peroxidase-positive granules that lack azurophilia due to absence of sulfated glycosaminoglycans *TRUE CHEDIAK-HIGASHI* inclusions are present in neutrophils and correspond to giant and abnormal azurophilic granules seen in Chediak-Higashi disease, a condition with increased susceptibility to pyogenic infections, photophobia, albinism, hepatosplenomegaly, lymphadenopathy and early death

Pseudocholera infantum see White stool diarrhea

Pseudocholinesterase (PChe) An enzyme present in the liver and plasma that rapidly metabolizes succinylcholine, a short-acting (5-10 minutes) neuromuscular blocker used in anesthesia; succinylcholine's duration of action is controlled by its rate of metabolism by PChe; certain subjects have congenital PChe variants with prolonged neuromuscular blockage with 'usual' doses of succinylcholine, which can be identified by the 'dibucaine' number; PChe activity may be decreased in various acquired conditions, including hepatic disease (hepatitis, cirrhosis, metastasis), malnutrition, acute infections, anemia, myocardial infarcts, malignancy, pregnancy, cytotoxic drugs, acetylcholinesterase inhibitors and dermatomyositis *TRUE CHOLINESTERASE* corresponds to acetylcholine cholinesterase; see Dibucaine number

Pseudochylous effusion A milky-white pleural effusion mimicking chylothorax, associated with high lipid levels (cholesterol or lecithin-globulin complexes) and seen in chronic pulmonary effusions, as in tuberculosis, rheumatoid arthritis or empyema; *TRUE CHYLOUS EFFUSIONS* are composed largely of chylomicrons originating from intestinally absorbed triglycerides Note: 1.5-2.5 liters of protein-rich (> 3.0 g/dl) chyle is produced and passes daily through the thoracic duct, which, when interrupted, causes chylothorax; 50% of cases of true chylothorax is due to tumor invasion of the ducts, 75% of which are related to lymphomas; 25% of cases are trauma-related with either open or closed wounds; most of the remaining cases of chylothorax are idiopathic

Pseudoclaudication A symptom complex affecting patients with lumbar spondylosis, defined as unilateral or bilateral discomfort or pain, paresthesia and weakness in the lower extremities evoked or exacerbated by walking and relieved by rest, sitting or flexing at the waist, caused by compression of the cauda equina, spinal stenosis or may be due to congenital narrowing of the spinal canal, best diagnosed by magnetic resonance imaging *TRUE CLAUDICATION* is a vascular event that persists despite rest or flexing of the waist and is recognized by the characteristic trophic changes of the extremities and loss of peripheral pulses in the lower extremities

Pseudoclue cell A squamous cell seen by the Papanicolaou technique (smear of vaginal and cervical cells) that is overlaid, ie pseudo-infected with Döderlein bacteria (which are normal flora of the external female genitalia) *TRUE CLUE CELLS* are squamous cells infected by ***Gardnerella (Hemophilus*** or ***Corynebacterium) vaginalis***

Pseudocoma A state mimicking acute unconsciousness with intact self-awareness, occurring in a) Organic disease states, eg 'locked-in syndrome' b) Psychogenic unresponsiveness, due to catatonic states, eg schizophrenia, severe depression, hysterical reactions or in frank malingering or c) Near-death experiences, for which there is no acceptable explanation *TRUE COMAS* are characterized by complete unresponsiveness during a coma state and for complete amnesia of events occurring while comatose

Pseudocroup see Laryngismus stridulus

Pseudocryptorchidism Retractile testis A testicle characterized by hyperactive cremasteric reflex drawing the organ into the inguinal canal, caused by cold temperature, fear and genital manipulation, occurring most prominently around age 5; Cf Migrating testis **Diagnosis** The pseudocryptorchid testis can be pushed into the scrotum *TRUE CRYPTORCHIDISM* refers to an undescended testis, which in the absence of spontaneous descent, should be surgically corrected before two years of age, as these patients are at an increased risk for germ cell neoplasm

Pseudo-Cushing syndrome A clinical complex seen in young obese subjects, characterized by truncal obesity and purple striae and increased urinary cortisol levels that fall short of those typical of Cushing syndrome **Treatment** Reduce weight, psychotherapy *TRUE CUSHING SYNDROME* has demonstrable increases in hypothalamic, or pituitary or adrenal hormones of either endogenous or exogenous origin

Pseudocyesis PSYCHIATRY A symptom complex affecting women with a strong and unfulfilled desire for children, resulting in amenorrhea, morning sickness, induration of breasts and increased abdominal girth; see Pseudopregnancy; Cf Sympathy 'pregnancy'

Pseudocyst PARASITOLOGY Macrophages laden with ***Toxoplasma gondii***, most often seen in the brain, typical of AIDS neuropathy *TRUE CYSTS* refer to a reproductive 'structure' with daughter cells within the cytoplasm PATHOLOGY A dilated space lined by neither epithelium nor mesothelium, classically seen in the pancreas as unilocular spaces lined by fibrous tissue, often following multiple bouts of acute pancreatitis or in the ultrarare hereditary pancreatitis TRUE EPITHELIAL CYSTS of the pancreas include 1) Dysgenic cysts associated with polycystic kidneys 2) Retention cysts, in which tumors, stones or inflammatory strictures cause prolapse of the ductal epithelium with cystic dilatation 3) Dyschylic cysts associated with cystic fibrosis and the most common 4) Cysts arising in pancreatic carcinoma

Pseudodementia Dementia-like symptoms due to psychological impairment, eg depression; pseudodementia is characterized by cognitive impairment of short duration, with preservation of attention and ability to concentrate and variable performance in tests with similar levels of difficulty; it is often transient, common in the elderly and may be due to chronic intoxication by prescribed drugs (anticholinergics, barbiturates, benzodiazepines, butyrophenones, corticosteroids, digitalis, IMAO and tricyclic antidepressants) or due to depression (caused by physical and emotional deprivation, accompanied by apathy, akinesia and anxiety); pseudodementia also occurs in normal pressure hydrocephalus, Creutzfeldt-Jakob, Huntington's, Parkinson's, Pick's and Wilson's diseases and endocrinopathy; Cf Pseudoatrophy, cerebral *TRUE DEMENTIA* is progressive and may demonstrate cortical atrophy by computed tomography and magnetic resonance imaging

Pseudodiabetes Defective carbohydrate metabolism secondary to chronic renal failure (uremia), with reduced glucose tolerance (rapid post-prandial rise and delayed return of glucose to normal), mild baseline hyperglycemia and insulin 'resistance'

Pseudo-Du cell TRANSFUSION MEDICINE An erythrocyte that has an Rh blood group that is Du-like in agglutination reactions; testing of the family's red cells reveals an Rh group 'c' allele in the trans position, which suppresses expression of a normal Rh 'D' antigen; see Du cell

Pseudoeosinophilia CYTOLOGY A red color shift in Papanicolaou-stained vaginal and cervical squames, seen when these cells are infected with coccoid bacteria *TRUE EOSINOPHILIA* of cervical squames is secondary to estrogen effect

Pseudoepidemic MICROBIOLOGY A cluster of bacterial 'infections', often by unusual organisms, that are reported as positive by the microbiology laboratory from patients who are not clinically ill; pseudoepidemics are caused by contamination of culture plates, ambient air or other common 'factor' in the environment, eg tap water, and have been described with *Mycobacterium gordonae, M avium* complex, *M scrofulaceum* and *Aeromonas hydrophilus*, each of which may also cause clinical disease, further complicating delineation of the nature of these conditions

Pseudoepitheliomatous hyperplasia Pseudocarcinomatous hyperplasia A nonspecific epithelial proliferation corresponding to reactive hyperplasia of stratified mucocutaneous epithelia, seen overlying infections (abscesses, *Blastomyces dermatitidis*, granuloma inguinale), granular cell tumors, inflammation (adjacent to ulcer margins and scars), burns and irritation Histopathology Acanthosis, irregular downgrowth of the rete pegs, pointed epidermal masses, with horn-pearl formation and florid mitotic activity, occasionally extending below the level of the sweat glands *TRUE CARCINOMA* usually has prominent cellular atypia and invasive 'fingerlets' of malignant cells that spread beyond subepithelial tissues, although very well-differentiated squamous cell carcinoma, eg verrucous carcinoma spread along a broad base

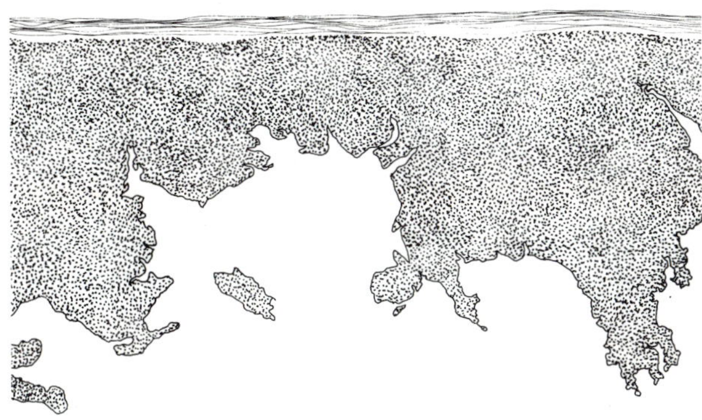

Pseudoepitheliomatous hyperplasia

Pseudofracture Looser zone A thin radiolucent line that mimics a true fracture and which is quasipathognomonic for osteomalacia in the adult, characterized by complex bony lesions typical of advanced renal failure

Pseudo-Gaucher cell A Gaucher-like histiocyte with normal β-glucocerebrosidase activity and abundant, crumpled tissue paper-like linear cytoplasmic deposits of various materials, including cerebroside, seen in conditions where the rate of cell destruction outstrips the macrophages' capacity to phagocytose cerebrosides and other membrane components; pseudo-Gaucher cells occur in chronic myelogenous leukemia, acute lymphocytic leukemia, hereditary neutrophilia, Hodgkin's disease, infectious mononucleosis, idiopathic thrombocytopenic purpura (in the spleen), thalassemia, congenital dyserythropoietic anemia, type II aplastic, hemolytic and iron-deficiency anemias, hereditary neutrophilia, post-necrotic cirrhosis, rheumatoid arthritis and vitamin E deficiency *TRUE GAUCHER CELLS* have a crumpled tissue paper-like cytoplasm replete with glucocerebroside, due to glucocerebrosidase deficiency

Pseudogene A DNA sequence that has a sequence similar to that of a known gene, but which itself does not encode a protein or portion thereof, thus also known as 'junk' DNA; pseudogenes may represent duplicated genes that are no longer active due to a non-functional mutational 'drift' in sequence

Pseudoglioma A term introduced in the ophthalmologic literature late in the last century to designate a heterogeneous group of pathologic entities that may be confused with retinoblastoma (thus the term 'pseudoretinoblastoma' would be more appropriate); pseudogliomatous lesions include 1) Leukokoria Coat's disease, diktyoma, incontinentia pigmenti, metastatic retinitis, Norrie's disease, persistent hyperplastic primary vitreous, retinal dysplasia, retrolental fibroplasia, secondary retinal detachment, toxocara endophthalmitis and 2) Retinal lesions Chorioretinal lesions that are either endophytic, eg retinal hamartomas, myelinated nerve fibers, colobomas, retinochoroiditis or exophytic larval, angiomatous or proliferative conditions

Pseudo-goiter see Modigliani syndrome

Pseudogout Chondrocalcinosis An arthropathy more common in elderly females, characterized by deposition of calcium pyrophosphate dihydrate (CPPD) crystals in large joints (knees, shoulders, hips), due to either local overproduction of pyrophosphate or a deficiency of phosphatase Histopathology Acute synovitis, followed by osteoarthritis; microscopic examination of synovial fluid reveals 'Coffin lid' crystals, which may be seen in other arthritic conditions including gout, osteoarthritis and rheumatoid arthritis *TRUE GOUT* usually affects smaller joints of older men who have increased uric acid levels and urate crystals in the joints; patients may also have diabetes mellitus or hypertension Polarized light microscopy Crystals with weak positive birefringence

Pseudogynecomastia An enlarged breast with hyalinized stroma, containing abundant small nerve fibers and occasionally multinucleated fibroblasts, seen in young males with neurofibromatosis see Gynecomastia

Pseudohermaphroditism Sex-reversed individuals whose

genotype is discordant with their phenotype; XX pseudohermaphroditic 'males' are first recognized when they complain of infertility; XY pseudohermaphroditic 'females' are missing a critical fragment of the Y chromosome that would otherwise result in 'maleness'; see X chromosome inactivation **FEMALE PSEUDOHERMAPHRODITISM** A condition caused by a relative excess of androgen in utero, resulting in a phenotypic male with genital ambiguity and/or virilization in a genotypic (46, XX) female Etiology 1) Adrenogenital syndrome Defects of 21-hydroxylase, 11 β-hydroxylase or 3 β-hydroxysteroid dehydrogenase, delta 5-4 isomerase deficiency, resulting in increased androgenic intermediates 2) Maternal ingestion of progestins or androgens and 3) Maternal virilizing tumors, eg luteoma of pregnancy; see Hermaphroditism, Intersex, Virilization **MALE PSEUDOHERMAPHRODITISM,** A condition caused by a relative deficiency of androgen in utero, resulting in a phenotypic female with ambiguous genitalia in a genotypic (46, XY) male Etiology 1) Gonadal defects Testicular regression syndrome, persistent müllerian duct origin, Leydig cell agenesis and defects in testosterone synthesis 2) End-organ defects Testicular feminization or androgen insensitivity syndrome, incomplete androgen insensitivity syndrome and 5-α reductase deficiency; see Hermaphroditism, Testicular feminization

Pseudo-Hirschsprung's disease Colonic inertia in children of possible psychogenic origin without histologic evidence of defective myoenteric innervation *TRUE HIRSCHSPRUNG'S DISEASE* is characterized by the absence of ganglion cells in Auerbach's and Meissner's plexuses

Pseudo-Hurler syndrome Mucolipidosis, type III A dysostotic syndrome of early childhood onset, characterized by a markedly reduced height, coarse, gargoyle-like facies, corneal clouding, mild retinopathy, mild mental retardation, joint stiffness and claw-hand deformity, due to a defect in phosphotransferase activity Note: For other Hurler-like syndromes, see Gargoylism *TRUE HURLER SYNDROME* (mucopolysaccharidosis, type IH) is due to deficient α-L-iduronidase with accumulation of dermatan sulfate and heparan sulfate in various tissues

Pseudohyperaldosteronism Liddle syndrome An autosomal dominant condition characterized by increased resorption of sodium by the distal renal tubules, potassium wasting (causing hypokalemic alkalosis) and hypertension, clinically mimicking primary aldosteronism Treatment Potassium chloride and triamterene to prevent potassium wasting *TRUE HYPERALDOSTERONISM* is due to hyperplasia, an adenoma or rarely, an adrenocortical carcinoma of the adrenal cortex, especially the zona glomerulosa

Pseudohyperhypoparathyroidism see Pseudohypohyperparathyroidism

Pseudohyperkalemia LABORATORY MEDICINE An in vitro phenomenon seen in megakaryocytic hyperplasia, thrombocytosis, leukocytosis or myeloproliferative disease, where rapid clotting of blood releases potassium from erythrocytes Laboratory Serum potassium is elevated; plasma potassium is normal

Pseudohyperparathyroidism see Hypercalcemia of malignancy

Pseudohypertension Sphygmomanometric cuff pressure that is higher than the actual blood pressure, due to markedly calcified ('pipestem') brachial arteries, most common in the elderly who have extensive atherosclerosis Diagnosis Osler's maneuver, which is a bedside method for assessing the palpability of the radial or brachial pulse distal to a point of presumed occlusion; Cf Hypertension, Small cuff syndrome, White coat hypertension

Pseudohyphae Elongated blastospores with focal constrictions ('link sausage' appearance) that are seen in *Candida* species *TRUE HYPHAE ARE A) NONSEPTATE* and include Zygomycetes, eg *Absidia, Mucor* and *Rhizopus* *B) SEPTATE, I) HYALINE TYPE* Dermatophytes, *Aspergillus, Geotrichum, Trichosporon* and *Pseudoallescheria* boydii *OR SEPTATE, II) DEMATIACEOUS TYPE* *Cladosporium, Curvalaria, Drechslera, Exophila, Phialophora* and others

Pseudohypoaldosteronism A heterogeneous group of salt wastage syndromes due to defects in the distal renal tubules, colonic mucosa, salivary and sweat glands, resulting in salt loss in the face of normal adrenocortical and renal function, due to a hyperactive renin-angiotensin system **TYPE I PSEUDOHYPOALDOSTERONISM** A familial disease of infant onset, characterized by salt-wasting, hypotension, increased plasma renin and aldosterone, hyperkalemia, hyponatremia, dehydration and metabolic alkalosis, clinically accompanied by vomiting, failure to thrive and periodic cyanosis when exposed to increased environmental temperatures Treatment Salt supplements **TYPE II PSEUDOHYPOALDOSTERONISM** An acquired condition due to the so-called 'distal chloride shunt', first seen in older children or adults, characterized by hypertension, hypervolemia, low-to-normal aldosterone, hyperkalemia and metabolic acidosis Treatment Salt restriction and diuretics *TRUE HYPOALDOSTERONISM* is either an isolated event or associated with hypocortisolism; the most common cause is decreased renin secretion (hyporeninemic hypoaldosteronism, seen in the elderly with renal failure, associated with diabetes mellitus, interstitial nephritis or multiple myeloma), deficiency of 18-hydroxylase or focal destruction of the adrenal cortex, resulting in hypereninemic hypoaldosteronism Laboratory Hyperkalemia, metabolic acidosis Treatment Correct primary defect, supplementary mineralocorticoids

Pseudohypohyperparathyroidism A clinical entity that is a combination of congenital end-organ resistance to parathormone (pseudohypoparathyroidism) and osteitis fibrosa cystica, seen in hyperparathyroidism, which may be related to differences in the transduction of the bone remodeling response, ie divergence of parathormone secretion and expression of parathyroid hormone receptor Note: Use of the term is discouraged as it lends to confusion; Cf Pseudopseudohypoparathyroidism

Pseudohyponatremia Spuriously low sodium levels due to either a) Intrinsic properties of a patient sample, as in hyperproteinemia (displacement of plasma water or due to the cationic nature of monoclonal proteins which bind sodium), hyperlipidemia or hyperviscosity or 2) Analytic factors, which occur while preparing samples for flame photometry or indirect potentiometry

Pseudohypoparathyroidism Albright's disease A hypoparathyroid-like state (hypocalcemia, hyperphosphatemia) due to end-organ resistance (by both bone and kidney with loss of renal tubule response to parathyroid hormone) to parathyroid hormone (with increased parathyroid hormone secretion, parathyroid gland hyperplasia), despite excess parathormone secretion in response to hypocalcemia by a normal or hyperplastic parathyroid gland; the condition is associated with a secondary hypocalcemia-induced increase in parathyroid function (administration of pharmacologic doses of parathyroid hormone normally results in increased urinary phosphate excretion and elevated cyclic AMP, but not in pseudohypoparathyroidism); the pattern of heredity is unclear, the male:female ratio is 2:1; skeletal changes include a rounded face, dental dysplasia, dry course hair, mental retardation **PSEUDOHYPOPARATHYROIDISM, TYPE I** is more common, autosomal dominant or X-linked; there is an inadequate cAMP response to parathormone **PSEUDOHYPOPARATHYROIDISM, TYPE II** is due to inadequate end-organ response to increased cAMP levels; children with type II are short and stocky with a rounded face, brachydactyly, tetany, foci of bony demineralization, osteitis fibrosa Treatment Both forms respond to vitamin 1,25 $(OH)_2D_3$; see Pseudopseudohypoparathyroidism *TRUE HYPOPARATHYROIDISM* is most commonly a sequela of thyroidectomy; more rarely, idiopathic or associated with athymia (DiGeorge syndrome) Clinical Electrolyte abnormalities (decreased calcium, increased phosphorus), which results in neuromuscular hyperexcitability, causing Chvostek sign, Trousseau sign, cramps, convulsions, dyspnea, photophobia, lethargy and ectopic calcification of the basal ganglia, cornea and soft tissue

Pseudohypophosphatasia A complex characterized by clinical and radiological features of vitamin D-resistant rickets and phosphoethanolaminuria, with increased pyridoxal 5'-phosphate (vitamin B_6 cofactor), caput membraneceum, osteopathy of the skull and long bones, failure to thrive, muscle hypotonicity; in one case, the tissue changes were non-specific, affecting the liver, bone and kidney, with normal alkaline phosphatase isoenzyme activity accompanied by defective phospholytic activity against the usual bone targets (N Engl J Med 1969; 281:604)

Pseudoidiopathic hypoparathyroidism Hypoparathyroidism described in one young adult with the laboratory parameters of idiopathic hypoparathyroidism and normal serum levels of a defective parathyroid hormone, resulting from a defect in peripheral conversion from prohormone or from a defect in peripheral activation of a secreted parathyroid hormone precursor; Cf Pseudohypoparathyroidism

Pseudoinclusion An ultrastructural finding in the nuclei of malignant epithelial cells, in which a 'bleb' of cytoplasm prolapses into the nucleus; Cf Nuclear blebbing

Pseudoincontinence The inability to retain urine, due to difficulty in reaching the toilet, advanced arthritis or other physical handicaps, causing anger and frustration in impaired persons *TRUE INCONTINENCE* only occurs with advanced or sudden spinal cord compression; overflow incontinence is secondary to peripheral (preganglionic or somatic afferent) defects in voiding

Pseudoinfarct An electrocardiographic Q wave inversion that mimics the EKG findings of myocardial infarction, which may be seen in Wolff-Parkinson-White syndrome, cardiac amyloidosis and hypertrophic cardiomyopathy, and is due to elongation and partial stretching of the nerve fibers *TRUE MYOCARDIAL INFARCTION* classically causes abnormalities of the Q wave (an EKG 'marker' for necrosis, often seen at the corresponding cardiac leads), an upward ST-segment displacement (a marker for injury) and an inverted T wave (a marker for ischemia)

Pseudoinfectious proctitis Noninfectious inflammation secondary to anal-erotic activity including trauma and erosion by inserted vibrators, bottles, eggs and other objects, allergic response to lubricants used in anal intercourse (cooking oil, suntan lotions, medicinal creams) and reactions due to toxins; Cf Sexual deviancy

Pseudoinsomnia Subjective difficulty in falling asleep that is described in 10% of those who claim to suffer from insomnia, despite objective observations to the contrary; see Insomnia, Sleep disorders

Pseudoinvasion A histologic finding that mimics the invasion of normal tissue by malignancy, consisting in penetration of nerves by benign processes, eg proliferating ductules in vasitis nodosa, normal and hyperplastic prostate, fibrocystic disease of the breast and normal pancreas; see Lymph node inclusions *TRUE INVASION* see Metastases; Cf Prevascular phase

Pseudoisochromic plates Colored plates that are comprised of variably-sized dots of different colors and used to classify color blind individuals with protanopsias and deuteranopsias (defective color vision for red and green); standard plates include the Ishihara atlas and Hardy-Rand-Rittler plates (J Am Med Assoc 1987; 258:841)

Pseudoisoenzyme One of two or more variant conformational forms of an enzyme, all of which have the same primary structure *TRUE ISOENZYMES* differ in primary and secondary structure

Pseudo-Kaposi sarcoma Kaposiform dermatitis A condition that clinically mimics Kaposi sarcoma, which is seen in the arteriovenous hemangiomas or arteriovenous fistulas of Klippel-Trenaunay disease Histopathology Proliferation of capillaries and fibroblasts, extravasation of erythrocytes and deposition of hemosiderin in dermis *TRUE KAPOSI SARCOMA* has, in addition to the above, microscopic features, demonstrates spindling of malignant cells with occasional cellular atypia and formation of slit-like spaces; see Peninsula sign

Pseudo-lecithin cholesterol acyl transferase deficiency see Lecithin cholesterol acyl transferase

Pseudolymphoma A form of lymphoid hyperplasia characterized by a relatively monotonous population of lymphocytes, seen in the breast, gastrointestinal tract, lung, mediastinum, orbit, salivary gland, skin, soft tissue, thyroidand other sites; pseudolymphomas, in contrast to lymphomas, are polyclonal, have well-preserved nodal architecture, intact cortical germinal centers of variable size and shape, little or no infiltration of the capsule or pericapsular fat by lymphocytes, active phagocytosis in the germinal center (nuclear 'dust' within histiocytes), inflammatory cell infiltration between germinal centers, mitotic activity confined to germinal centers, no alteration of the reticular framework; these lesions occur in younger patients, are smaller than lymphomas and may present in patients with concomitant lymphoma or in those who later develop lymphoma; see Phenytoin lymphadenopathy

Pseudomembrane Spiderweb membrane A thin and adherent, gray-white exudative lamination of the oropharynx extending from the tonsils to the contiguous soft and hard palates and pharynx, the removal of which causes hemorrhage; the pseudomembrane is composed of necrotic debris and neutrophils and is classically seen in diphtheria, causing a bull-like neck, pseudomembranes may also occur in shigellosis, staphylococcal infections, ***Clostridium perfringens***, ***C difficile*** and less commonly in viral infections of the oropharynx

Pseudomembranous bronchitis see Plastic bronchitis

Pseudomembranous candidiasis see Thrush

Pseudomembranous colitis An acute, often severe diarrhea that follows antibiotic therapy with ampicillin, clindamycin, metronidazole and others which eliminate the patient's native bacterial flora, resulting in superinfection by *Clostridium difficile*, rarely by ***Streptococcus aureus*** and other bacteria, which produce a *Clostridium sordelli*-like toxin, resulting in a Schwartzman-like reaction; the condition may occur in 'compromised' hosts or the elderly, in a background of colonic obstruction, leukemia, major surgery, uremia, spinal injury, colonic carcinoma, burns, infections, shock, heavy metal poisoning, hemolytic-uremic syndrome, cardiovascular ischemia, Crohn's disease, shigellosis, necrotizing enterocolitis and Hirschsprung's disease Clinical Mild diarrhea to fulminant disease with fever, dehydration and shock HISTOLOGIC CLASSIFICATION, STAGE I Early focal and superficial epithelial necrosis that may extend into the lamina propria with increased eosinophils, neutrophils and cytoclastic debris STAGE II Dome-shaped necrotic plaques distended by mucin and neutrophils at the base, covered by a fibrin plaque, necrotic tips of villi, debris and neutrophils, the 'volcano lesion'; the intervening mucosa is relatively normal STAGE III Little architecture is preserved; mucosal recovery is uncommon Note: There is no 'membranous' colitis

Pseudomyxoma peritonei A condition characterized by poorly-circumscribed gelatinous masses filled with malignant mucin-secreting cells; 45% of pseudomyxomas arise from the ovary, usually in a mucinous cystadenocarcinoma, which has prognostic significance, eg mucinous ovarian cystadenocarcinomas of undetermined malignant potential ('borderline' tumors) have a usual 10-year survival of 95%, but when associated with pseudomyxoma, the 10-year survival falls to 40%; 29% of cases of pseudomyxoma peritonei are due to the uncommon mucin-producing carcinoma of the appendix; the material must be differentiated from mucinous spillage into the peritoneum by a benign mucocele of the appendix; pseudomyxoma may also be due to various mucin-secreting carcinomas, rarely to ovarian fibroma and teratoma

Pseudoneuritis see Pseudopapilledema

'Pseudonym' syndrome(s) A disorder with more than five actively used aliases, including a) Agnogenic myeloid metaplasia (AMM), a disease for which the pathogenesis is poorly understood, the etiology unknown, the prognosis uncertain and the therapy ineffective; synonyms for AMM include myelofibrosis with myeloid metaplasia, splenic myelosis, osteomyeloreticulosis, aleukemic myelosis and primary myelofibrosis Note: Secondary myelofibrosis may occur in acute leukemia, lymphoma, metastases and hairy cell leukemia and b) Pigmented neuroectodermal tumor of infancy, also known as retinal anlage tumor, benign melanotic progonoma, pigmented epulis of infancy, melanotic adamantinoma, congenital melanocarcinoma and melanoameloblastoma

Pseudo-obstruction, acute colonic Ogilvie syndrome, Nontoxic megacolon Massive colonic dilatation without mechanical obstruction, possibly due to a sympathetic nervous system defect, causing chronic peristaltic paralysis, affecting the cecum, right colon, distal small intestine, less commonly, the esophagus and stomach Clinical Initially painless abdominal distension with nausea, pain relieved by vomiting and diarrhea and intermittent symptoms extending over years; the condition may be congenital, as in hereditary hollow viscus myopathy, acquired (diabetes mellitus, hypothyroidism, collagen vascular diseases, myotonic dystrophy, parkinsonism, multiple sclerosis, amyloidosis, trauma, surgery, inflammation (pancreatitis), infections, radiation therapy, malignancy, cardiovascular (myocardial infarct), neurologic, respiratory (pneumonia), metabolic (alcoholism, hypokalemia and other electrolyte imbalance, uremia), muscular dystrophy, familial dysautonomia (Riley-Day syndrome), porphyria, dysproteinemia, drug-related (phenothiazines, tricyclic antidepressants, ganglion blockers, clonidine, narcotics, anticholinergics) Treatment Decompression of the intestine, correction of electrolyte imbalance or cecostomy; see Paralytic ileus

Pseudo-orphan drug An orphan drug for which there is active commercial interest in the pharmaceutical industry, as the drug has potentially broader applications than those that fall under its 'orphan drug' status, eg human growth hormone received 11 distinct orphan disease applications from four different manufacturers, and thus would not be considered an 'orphan' product in the spirit of the legislation designed to provide a financial incentive to companies developing therapies for patients with truly rare ('orphan') diseases, eg porphyria *TRUE ORPHAN DRUGS* are those formulated with the specific understanding that the number of potential users is small and will probably always be so, eg cysteamine for treating patients with the very rare nephropathic cystinosis, a true orphan disease (Science 1991; 251:1159ed); see Ophan disease, Orphan drug

Pseudopapilledema OPHTHALMOLOGY A papilledema-like condition that mimics a swollen optic disc, consisting in a 'heaping up' of nerve fibers and glial tissues, associated with hypermetropia or farsightedness (due to axonal crowding at the disc) or drusen (hyaline material in the prelaminar nerve, fancifully known as 'rock' crystals) *TRUE PAPILLEDEMA* is progressive and is characterized by dilatation of veins, hemorrhages and exudates

Pseudoparaproteinemia An increase of transferrin to two-fold or greater than normal 2-4 g/L (US: 200-400 mg/dl), as a reaction to severe iron-deficiency anemia; because transferrin exists in only one molecular species and migrates as a 'tight' band in the β region in serum electrophoresis, it mimics paraproteinemia *TRUE PARAPROTEINEMIA* is any 'spike' on a gel electrophoresis or serum, which must be 'worked-up' to determine whether it corresponds to a monoclonal gammopathy, either benign or malignant

Pseudopelade of Brocq Alopecia cicatrisata A dermatopathy characterized by scattered, geographically-shaped alopecic patches; early disease is characterized by mild perifollicular erythema, upper dermal mononuclear inflammation and scaling, which is followed by smooth atrophic atrichous patches, a stage indistinguishable from end-stage lichen planopilaris, also mimicking circumscribed scleroderma and discoid lupus erythematosus; pseudopelade may be an isolated entity or associated with lichen planus, lichenoid dermatopathies and the Graham-Little syndrome

Pseudo-Pelger-Huët anomaly A morphology of granulocyte nuclei with a rounded, hyposegmented pince-nez appearance and coarse chromatin, due to a dissociation between cytoplasmic and nuclear maturation; these cells appear transiently in acute myelogenous leukemia, agnogenic myeloid metaplasia, chronic myeloid leukemia, erythroleukemia, infectious mononucleosis, aplastic and Fanconi anemias, malaria, response to myelotoxins, marrow metastases; therapy of the underlying condition causes a regression of the anomaly *TRUE PELGER-HUEANOMALY* is an autosomal dominant condition with characteristic bilobed neutrophils; heterozygous subjects with this condition are asymptomatic, although homozygosity for the Pelger-Huët gene may be lethal

Pseudoperoxidase see Occult blood

Pseudopodagra An intensely painful great toe, due to trauma, degenerative arthritis, psoriatic arthritis, calcium pyrophosphate dihydrate disease ('pseudogout'), rheumatoid arthritis, Reiter syndrome or infection *TRUE PODAGRA* corresponds to the classic gouty great toe

Pseudopolyp An 'island' of preserved colonic mucosa, surrounded by an ulcerated 'sea' of hemorrhagic mucosa, which is a finding most characteristic of ulcerative colitis that may be seen in nonspecific inflammatory bowel disease, bacterial dysentery, amebiasis due to *Entameba histolytica* and schistosomiasis; *TRUE POLYS* in the colon arise from the mucosa, and represent neoplastic proliferations, most commonly designated as adenomatous polyps or villotubular adenomas, which have a tendency, with time to undergo malignant transformation, see Polyps

Pseudoprecocity Isosexual pseudoprecocity occurs in female children and consists of signs of sexual maturation induced by functional ovarian tumors, eg juvenile type of granulosa cell tumor, due to increased estrogens and/or androgens **Clinical** Development of breasts, pubic and axillary hair, stimulation and development of the internal and external secondary sex organs, irregular uterine bleeding and a whitish vaginal discharge, acceleration of somatic and skeletal growth, and occasionally clitoromegaly *TRUE PRECOCITY* is accompanied by progesterone production and ovulation; see Precocity

Pseudopregnancy EXPERIMENTAL BIOLOGY A state that may be induced in laboratory rodents by sterile 'coitus' or stimulation of the cervix with a glass rod, which causes a neuroendocrine response, release of prolactin and retention of the corpus luteum, resulting in a pregnancy-like state without carrying a fertilized product(s); see Pseudocyesis; Cf Sympathy pregnancy

Pseudopseudolymphoma Paracortical lymphoid hyperplasia with proliferation of immunoblasts, associated with phenytoin therapy, see Phenytoin lymphadenopathy Note: Long-term phenytoin therapy has been associated with a slight increase in lymphoma

Pseudo-pseudohypoparathyroidism A rare genetic condition with the skeletal manifestations of pseudohypoparathyroidism, in the face of normal calcium and phosphorous levels; both the 'pseudo-' and the 'pseudo-pseudo' forms may occur in the same kindred implying that in the latter, a mechanism of an end-organ (renal tubule) resistance to parathyroid hormone is present; see Pseudohypoparathyroidism

Pseudopuberty A clinical finding in male infants with Leydig cell tumor associated with growth of pubic hair and penile enlargement *TRUE PUBERTY* is in addition to the above, further characterized by spermatogenesis

Pseudo-Reed-Sternberg cells Histiocytoid cells mimicking the diagnostic cells of Hodgkin's disease are seen in a variety of benign and malignant lesions, of a) Epithelial origin Thymoma, carcinoma of the breast and lung, b) Mesenchymal origin Proliferative myositis, malignant fibrous histiocytoma, c) Hematopoietic origin Infectious mononucleosis, cytomegalic inclusion virus, rubeola, AIDS, multiple myeloma, megakaryocytic hyperplasia, mycosis fungoides, nodular lymphoma, mixed cell type and poorly differentiated type lymphoma and d) Malignant melanoma *TRUE REED-STERNBERG CELLS* are the *sine qua non* requirement to establish the diagnosis of Hodgkin's disease and are abundant in lymphocyte-depleted Hodgkin's lymphoma; the 'classic' Reed-Sternberg cell is large (15-45 μm), binucleated or bilobed, often arranged as a 'mirror image', the chromatin is condensed at the periphery at the nuclear membrane; nucleoli are 'owl-eyed' ie dark and large surrounded by a clear halo (figure, page 590), the cytoplasm is abundant and amphophilic; the mononuclear variant cells, although non-diagnostic, may represent early Reed-Sternberg cells and the bi- and multinucleated form may be a cell of terminal differentiation **Ultrastructure** Large nuclei, dispersed chromatin, large nucleoli, abundant polyribosomes Immunoperoxidase Classic Reed-Sternberg cells express Ki-1 (CD30), Leu-M1 (CD15), Ia-like antigen and peanut lectin receptors

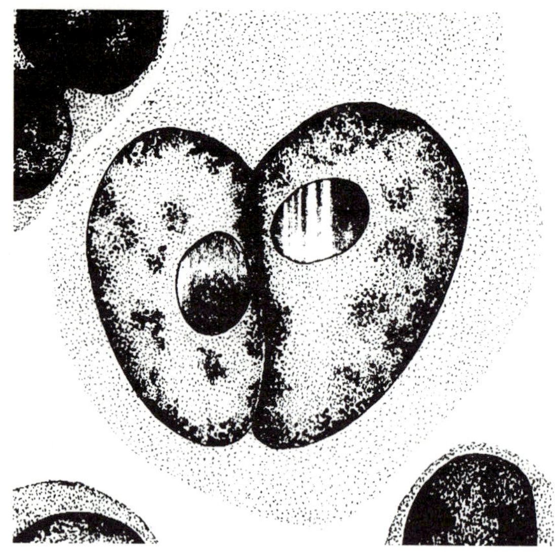

Reed-Sternberg cell

Pseudorheumatoid nodule A deep dermal granuloma annulare involving the eyelid, eyebrow, episcleral and orbital tissues; Cf Rheumatoid nodule

Pseudorosette A gliovascular structure seen by low-power light microscopy in ependymomas, in which blood vessels are surrounded by radiating, tapering processes of tumor cells oriented toward the vessel wall, best demonstrated by cell smears obtained fresh during surgery; pseudorosettes are more common in ependymomas than the 'classic' ependymal rosettes and may also be seen in Merkel cell tumors and Ewing sarcoma; see Rosettes of Homer-Wright and Flexner-Wintersteiner

Pseudosarcoma A tumor mimicking a mesenchymal malignancy, the significance of which differs according to the site of origin ORAL CAVITY Pseudosarcoma is preferably known as spindle cell carcinoma, a variant of squamous cell carcinoma SOFT TISSUE Pseudosarcomatous fasciitis is preferably known as nodular fasciitis UROGENITAL TRACT Pseudosarcoma is a small, sessile and/or friable 'tumor' with marked cellularity and mitotic activity that bleeds easily and occurs at the site of recent surgery to the bladder, prostate or in the vagina, representing a florid inflammatory response to a locoregional insult; Cf Inflammatory pseudotumor *TRUE SARCOMAS* are malignant mesenchymal tumors of soft tissues and the musculoskeletal unit, which affect all ages and have a broad range in prognosis

Pseudosilence see Silent ischemia

Pseudotabes An uncommon pattern of distal primary sensory neuropathy, occurring in long-standing diabetes mellitus characterized by shooting pains, most prominent at night, cutaneous hyperesthesia, impotence and neurogenic bladder, loss of superficial and deep sensation, painless ulceration of the feet, loss of tendon reflex, causing marked joint deformity, Romberg sign and occasionally Argyll-Robertson pupils *TRUE TABES DORSALIS* occurs in tertiary syphilis, develops 10-20 years after primary infection and is clinically characterized by impaired vibratory and position sense in the feet and legs, absent knee and ankle reflexes, a Romberg sign, ataxia, urinary incontinence and 'lightning' pains

Pseudothrombocytopenia A laboratory phenomenon caused by clumping of platelets in a blood collection tube containing an inappropriate anticoagulant; specimens for platelet counts should be collected in lavender topped tubes containing calcium EDTA

Pseudotuberculosis CLINICAL MEDICINE An innocuous mimic of the radiologic features of tuberculosis, described in one young woman whose braided hair fell into the field of an antero-posterior chest film, mimicking the radiologic appearance of tuberculosis (N Engl J Med 1985; 313:1227c) INFECTIOUS DISEASE Human infection by ***Yersinia pseudotuberculosis*** which causes acute mesenteric lymphadenitis, an infection that mimics acute appendicitis, characterized by abdominal pain and fever RESEARCH An infection of experimental mice by *Corynebacterium pseudotuberculosis* and *C kutscheri*, which cause non-specific signs of weakness and respiratory distress, possibly progressing to systemic abscess or less commonly, granulomas in the kidneys, myocardium or liver; the virulence of this condition is such that once an experimental colony of rodents is infected, it must be destroyed

Pseudotumor A non-specific descriptor for any well-circumscribed mass, including gastric inflammatory fibroid polyps, a bolus of helminths, eg ***Strongyloides*** species, as seen in Uganda, an 'amyloidoma' or an endometrioma *TRUE TUMORS* may be benign or malignant and are invested with a replicative capacity that may ('benign') or may not ('malignant') be under autoregulatory control

Pseudotumor cerebri Benign intracranial hypertension A cerebral complex caused by increased intracranial pressure with normal cerebrospinal fluid, diagnosed by 1) Presence of bilateral papilledema and objective evidence of increased intracranial pressure 2) Absence of focal neurological symptoms or signs 3) Absence of an extracranial cause of papilledema 4) Normal cerebrospinal fluid Clinical Most common in young obese women with dysmenorrhea of ovarian origin, causing visual defects (loss of acuity, diplopia and blind spots), headaches, nausea, vomiting, vertigo and tinnitus Etiology Anemia, leukemia, hyper- or hypovitaminosis A, lead intoxication, levothyroxine therapy, nalidixic acid, poliomyelitis, Guillain-Barre disease, Schilder syndrome, menarche, pregnancy, galactokinase deficiency, chronic hypoxia, allergies, post-cerebral trauma, corticosteroid therapy for rapid reduction of cerebral edema or withdrawal of steroids, chronic hypocalcemia with hypoparathyroidism with primary adrenal insufficiency, thyroid replacement, endocrinopathies (Addison's or Cushing's diseases), contraceptive use, tetracycline (in infants), intracranial venous occlusion and inflammation

Pseudotumor of the lung Inflammatory pseudotumor of the lung A generic term for a solitary radiologic lung mass, composed of aggregates of foamy histiocytes, plasma cells, lymphocytes, fibroblasts and collagen that are most often evoked by resective surgery or less commonly, infections; Cf Lymphomatoid granulomatosis

Pseudotumor of the orbit Inflammatory pseudotumor of the orbit An idiopathic proliferation of the lymphoid tissues surounding the ocular orbit **Clinical** Pain, exophthalmos, limitation of eye movement, lid erythema, edema, myositis, perineuritis, scleritis, dacryoadenitis; the lesion may be histologically impossible to differentiate from a true lymphoma, which then requires molecular studies to determine a lesion's clonality **Differential diagnosis** Dacryoadenitis, orbital myositis, vasculitis, sclerosing pseudotumors, lipogranuloma, epithelioid cell granuloma, xanthogranuloma

Pseudotumor of soft tissue A non-specific term for reactive proliferations or repair phenomena that measure less than 2 cm in greatest dimension, including hematomas, circumscribed fat necrosis, nodular fasciitis, foreign body granulomas, xanthogranulomas, proliferative myositis, myositis ossificans

Pseudo-Turner syndrome Noonan syndrome A congenital condition with a heterogeneous presentation that mimics some of the clinical findings of Turner syndrome; Noonan syndrome affects both sexes, and is characterized by short stature, webbing of the neck, developmental delays, pectus carinatum or pectus excavatum, cubitum valgum, congenital heart disease (pulmonary valve stenosis, atrial septal defect and others), a characteristic facies (hypertelorism, epicanthus, an anti-mongoloid palpebral slant) and gonadal defects ranging from severe to apparently normal *TRUE TURNER* (45, X0) syndrome affects 1:3000 live female births (95% of fetuses with this anomaly spontaneously abort, 25% of Turner syndromes have 45, X/46, XX mosaicism **Clinical** Lymphedema of the hands, feet and neck, webbing of the neck, congenital heart disease (Coarctation of the aorta and idiopathic hypertension), gastrointestinal telangiectasia, urogenital malformations and primary amenorrhea due to rudimentary ('streak') ovaries

Pseudouridine A chemically altered nucleoside found in tRNA

Pseudovitamin An organic substance that does not meet the accepted definition (see below) of a required human vitamin; representation of these substances as vitamins is widely regarded as being misleading, as the implication that they have natural curative effects is based on no known scientific principles; the US consumer spends an estimated $\$10^9$ annually on pseudovitamins, which have been divided into three broad categories 1) Metabolites, including a) Intermediate metabolites, eg orotic acid ('vitamin B_{13}') b) Substances whose metabolism requires B vitamins (eg choline, inositol, methionine) and c) Substances which are B vitamins for nonvertebrate organisms (para-aminobenzoic acid, a B vitamin for certain bacteria ('vitamin B_x') and carnitine, a B vitamin for mealworms ('vitamin B_t') 2) Pharmacologic substances, allegedly capable of favoring certain metabolic processes in humans, but which produce little (if any) objective improvement, eg bioflavinoids ('vitamin P') and 3) 'Snake oil remedies' that meet the legal definition of fraud, which include pangamate ('vitamin B_{15}'), laetrile ('vitamin B_{17}') and gerovital ('vitamin H_3') ***TRUE VITAMINS*** are organic accessory food factors that usually remain in food after removal of the basic elements including carbohydrates, fats, proteins, minerals, water and fiber, and are a) Necessary in trace amounts (daily intake in milligram to microgram quantities) and b) Essential as the body either does not produce them or does so in insufficient quantities

Pseudovitamin D resistant rickets Autosomal recessive vitamin D deficiency An inherited disease of bone and calcium metabolism characterized by the signs and symptoms of rickets, hypocalcemia, low-to-normal plasma phosphate and increased parathyroid hormone; the disease is subdivided into type I Defective (25-hydroxy-cholecalciferol 1-α-hydroxylase) that converts 25-(OH)- to 1,25-$(OH)_2$ vitamin D and which responds to exogenous 1,25-$(OH)_2$ vitamin D therapy and type II Associated with end organ defects and refractoriness of renal tubules, intestinal mucosa and bone

Pseudo-Whipple's disease A condition that mimics Whipple's disease seen in ***Mycobacterium avium-intracellulare*** infection in AIDS, which also occurred in a case report of infection by ***Corynebacterium equi***, agent of a suppurative pneumonia in young horses, isolated from the central nervous system of a young homosexual male with AIDS-related complex (N Engl J Med 1986; 314:1577c)

Pseudo-von Willebrand disease Platelet-type von Willebrand disease (vWD) An autosomal dominant condition similar to type IIB vWD, with moderately severe symptoms **Laboratory** Prolonged bleeding time, decreased plasma von Willebrand factor (vWF) and factor VIII levels, increased ristocetin-induced platelet aggregation, absence of large vWF multimers and presence of those same multimers in platelets; the nature of the defect is unknown but may involve platelet glycoprotein IB

Pseudoxanthoma elasticum of Grönblad-Strandberg A rare and progressive condition affecting the connective tissue of the skin, cardiovascular system, joints and eyes **Clinical** An early change is the lax, yellow and redundant 'plucked chicken skin' that coalesces into plaques, becoming thickened, grooved, leathery and inelastic, likened to 'Moroccan leather', involving the head, neck, trunk and upper legs, eye (angioid streaks of the optic fundus, bilateral hemorrhage and exudates into Bruch's membrane, degenerative changes impairing vision, optic pigmentation and chorioretinitis), cardiovascular system (murmurs, hypertension, congestive heart failure, intermittent claudication, angina, vessels with poor peripheral pulses, vascular occlusion), cerebral visceral and gastrointestinal hemorrhage; four types of pseudoxanthoma elasticum are described, of which the autosomal recessive type I is the most common, while the remainder differ according to the severity of skin, vascular and joint involvement

Psoas sign RADIOLOGY The loss of the sharp delineation of the psoas muscle border, which is normally seen on a plain erect abdominal film, a finding that may indicate the presence of intra-abdominal or retroperitoneal pathology, eg retroperitoneal hemorrhage in trauma victims or florid acute inflammation in a child with ruptured appendicitis

Psoralens A class of furocoumarins that is used as a drug to treat psoriasis and other skin conditions and is used as a nucleic acid probe as it covalently crosslinks nucleic acids between opposing strands of DNA,where the planar psoralen intercalates into the double helix and UV light (320-400 nm) induces a single cyclobutane addition with a pyrimidine base; Cf Photo-reactivation

PSS Progressive systemic sclerosis

PSTAIR MOLECULAR BIOLOGY A sixteen-residue polypeptide contained within the maturation promoting factor, which is necessary and sufficient to initiate mitosis by causing a transient surge in intracellular calcium (Science 1990; 247:327); see Mitotic spindle

Psychiatric evaluation The American Psychiatric Association's Diagnostic and Statistical Manual (DSM-III) produced in 1980, has helped standardize the language of mental illness, by describing psychiatric patients in terms of five 'axes'

Psychiatric evaluation parameters

Axis I Specific syndrome, eg depression, neurosis

Axis II Specific personality disorder, eg dependency, social development, reading or language disorder

Axis III Medical or physical conditions that may contribute to disease

Axis IV Psychosocial stressors, eg marital status

Axis V Highest level of adaptive function within the past year, eg functioning in the workplace

'Psychic energizers' THERAPEUTICS A colloquial synonym for antidepressant drugs that elevate mood, motivation and increase in quality of life

Psychic surgery HEALTH FRAUD A practice associated with 'spirit healing' in rural areas of the Phillipines, in which certain persons are alleged to act as mediums for healing forces, allowing them to perform painless surgery using their fingers and unsterile tools without violating the skin surface; psychic surgery is a form of prestidigitation, in which the tissues allegedly removed actually correspond to animal parts, eg chicken intestines or minerals, 'kidney stones' which are pebbles or volcanic rocks; see Unproven cancer therapy; Cf Psychosurgery

Psychoactive drugs SUBSTANCE ABUSE Pharmacologic agents that provide pleasure or ameliorate pain, potentially causing physical dependence and tolerance, which is the tendency to increase the drug's dose in order to achieve the same effect; use of non-prescribed psychoactive agents may be 'social'/casual or consist of frank addiction, which in descending order of addictive potential include cocaine and 'crack', amphetamines, opiates, nicotine, alcohol, benzodiazepine, barbiturates, cannabis, hallucinogens and caffeine

Psychogenic syndromes Anxiety-related conversion reactions that are caused by various endogenous or exogenous stresses, including hysterical reactions, psychogenic chest pain, psychogenic polydipsia, psychogenic purpura, psychophonasthenia and the 'women who fall' syndrome, a conversion reaction to aggressive or erotic impulses; Cf Factitial 'diseases'

PSYCHOLOGICAL TESTING

Perceptual-motor integrity are designed to rule out an organic (structural or physiologic, ie treatable) cause for the subject's behavior, including the Bender visual-motor Gestalt test, which can be administered from ages 5-adult, evaluating personality conflicts, ego structure and function and organic brain disease

Intelligence quotient tests are the most commonly used tests in the US, and have been devised by David Wechsler, including the Wechsler Preschool and Primary Scale of Intelligence (WPPSI, ages 4-6; 1949), Wechsler Intelligence Scale for Children-Revised (WISC-R, ages 5-15; 1974) and the Wechsler Adult Intelligence Scale (WAIS-R, ages 16 to adult; 1981); another commonly used IQ test is the Stanford-Binet that evaluates individuals from age 2 to adult

Potential achievement The Vineland Social Maturity Scale evaluates the capacity to function independently, administered to those up to age 25

'Projective' tests evaluate the sense of reality, eg the Rorschach ink-blot test, which requires considerable skill in administration, but yield the greatest insight into personality conflicts, ego structure and function, defensive structure and affective integration; other projective tests include the Thematic Apperception Test (TAT), Children's Apperception Test (CAT) and the 'Draw-a-person' and 'Draw-a-family' tests

Psychological autopsy An autopsy that analyzes the cause(s) of death, examining both the body and the circumstances (natural or unnatural) that led to death; in the 'usual' death, a person suffers from a known set of morbid condition(s) and dies as a natural consequence of the terminal progression of those conditions(s); in 'unnatural' death, eg homicide or suicide, determination of nosology is more difficult and requires analysis of circumstances preceding death; the 'psychological autopsy' focuses on the deceased's intentions relating to his own death; data gathered by the investigation team include 1) Life history, eg previous suicide attempts 2) Psychological data, eg indices of depression or agitation, recent loss of appetite or interest in life 3) Communicated information, including indications of morbid thoughts, eg '...I can't go on' 4) Nonpsychological details provided by the scene of death indicating attention to details that would ensure death, eg two bottles of the same medication used for overdose (Bull Suicidol July, 1968 pp 39-45) Note: Psychological autopsies are of interest to both insurance companies and beneficiaries of the deceased, as life insurance policies are often written so that the estate of someone who commits suicide will not collect death benefits; Cf Homicide, Suicide

Psychologic testing A group of tests used to determine a subject's intelligence quotient (IQ), 'normalcy' and future potentials (table, facing page)

Psychoneuroimmunology A developing field that is a hybrid of several disciplines, which studies the complex bidirectional interactions between the immune and the central nervous systems, where neuroendocrine system modulates immune function and CNS-immune system interactions appear to influence psychosocial dynamics; there are over thirty well-studied overlaps between the two systems in terms of shared cells and moderating substances (J Neurosci Res 1987; 18:1rv)

Psycho-organic 'syndrome' A petroleum solvent-induced neurological dysfunction characterized by fatigue, memory loss, loss of concentration and emotional lability, occurring after 5-10 years of regular exposure to solvents, eg styrene, toluene, affecting painters, degreasers, plastics and chemical workers (N Engl J Med 1990; 322:675)

'Psychosocial oncology' A field predominantly peopled by psychologists, which formally attempts to sway the course of advanced and/or metastatic malignancy by helping patients develop a positive' attitude; some 'soft' data suggest that the psyche may have an enhancing effect on the immune defenses; in one study of patients with metastatic breast cancer, those undergoing psychotherapy lived 19 months longer than controls and reported less anxiety and pain than the control group (Lancet 1989; 2:888) Note: Because of the difficulty in performing these studies and the often anecdotal nature of the data, the field may be regarded as 'fringe science' by traditional oncologists

Psychosomatic disease see Psychogenic 'syndromes'

Psychosurgery Neurosurgery to alleviate psychiatric symptoms, a technique first used in 1890 by G Burckhardt; psychosurgical procedures include topectomy (removal of pieces of cerebral cortex, weighing 20 g for pain to 50 g for fulminant schizophrenia), lobectomy and leukotomy (popularized by W Freeman during World War II), which consisted of thrusting an icepick-like device through the eye socket and wiggling the handle to rupture myelinated tracts); one author felt that the greatest success was achieved in patients who were older, female, black and those in simpler occupations; use of the Freeman procedure peaked in the late 1940s, and its decline coincided with the availability of the first generation of psychoactive drugs; tools used in modern psychosurgery to induce selective tract destruction include radioactive ^{90}yttrium implants in the substantia innominata, as well as cryoprobes, coagulation, proton beams and ultrasonic waves; psychosurgery is not commonly performed, as it must be established that the patients are unresponsive to all other therapy and that the condition is chronic, ie of greater than three years duration; significant improvement is reported in 60% of carefully selected patients, while in 3%, the symptoms worsen after the procedure; the measurable intelligence quotient may actually increase as there is a better ability to concentrate and memorize, while distraction has been cut to a minimum Complications occur in about 1% and include infections, hemorrhage and seizures; Cf Psychic surgery

Psyllium A grain of the plantago family with a high soluble fiber content that provides dietary bulk, acting as both a laxative and an agent to lower cholesterol; because psyllium contains a common aeroallergen, it may evoke an allergic reaction (anaphylaxis, rhinitis and asthma) in health care professionals who handle psyllium-based laxatives and later ingest them in food products (N Engl J Med 1990; 323:1072c)

PTAH stain of Mallory Phosphotungstic acid hematoxylin stain A stain used in histology to delineate various structures, including collagen (colored red), fibrin (blue), muscle (deep purple with well-defined cross-striations) and nuclei (blue); other structures including nerve, mitochondria, bone and elastin are well-visualized by the PTAH method

PTCA see Percutaneous transluminal coronary angioplasty

PTE Pulmonary thromboembolism

PTGC see Progressive transformation of germinal centers

PTHrP Human parathyroid hormone-related peptide PTH-like hormone A 453-residue protein first identified in malignancy that is both present in mammalian milk and apparently required for lactation and for transplacental transportation of calcium (Mayo Clin Proc 1990; 65:1408); see Hypercalcemia of malignancy

PTP laser Potassium-titanyl-phosphate laser A device attached to a flexible endoscope in otorhinolaryngology, which can be adjusted to vaporize, coagulate or cut (J Am Med Assoc 1990; 263:2670); see Lasers

PTSD See Post-trauma stress disorder

Public antigen Supratypic antigen TRANSFUSION MEDICINE An antigen present on the red cell surface of more than 99.9% of a population, the presence of which is determined by an indirect antiglobulin test (Coombs); these 'high frequency' antigens include Js^a, Lu^a, Ge, Ve, At^a, Cr^a, En^a, Gy^a, Hy, Jr, Jo^a, Ok^a, Ve; common (but not public) antigens are Lewis, P, MNSs, Ii, Kk and Duffy Note: Antibodies to public antigens are problematic in the blood bank as it is difficult to find a transfusable unit that is negative for antigen

Public Health Service The bureaucracy responsible for administering all health-related services of the US government, including the Centers for Disease Control, Food and Drug Administration, National Institute of Mental Health and the National Institutes of Health (which includes the National Library of Medicine and the National Cancer Institute)

Public idiotype determinant IMMUNOLOGY A recognition site or paratope present on an immunoglobulin that is shared by multiple other immunoglobulins despite their origin from different clones, also known as cross-reacting idiotypes

Public specificity The property in a human leukocyte antigen (HLA) in which the epitope is identical on multiple HLA molecules; in contrast, a private antigen is a highly-specific epitope recognized by few members of the immunoglobulin superfamily; see also Splits

Publication bias SCIENTIFIC JOURNALISM The tendency on

the part of investigators to submit, and for some reviewers and editors to accept for publication, manuscripts based on the direction or strength of a study's findings, meaning that negative results (being rather less 'interesting') are less likely to be published (J Am Med Assoc 1990; 263:1385); publication bias is divided into **PRE-PUBLICATION BIAS**, resulting from ignorance, laxity and lack of enterprise (on the part of those who would potentially perform the study) and a double standard created by peer review and informed consent **PUBLICATION BIAS**, as defined above and **POST-PUBLICATION BIAS**, resulting from editorials, reviews and meta-analyses (J Am Med Assoc 1990; 263:1392)

Puddle sign A method for detecting low quantities of ascitic fluid by having the patient on the hands and knees and bobbing the belly from below; in contrast, the lower limits of detection of ascites in the supine patient is 1-1.5 liters; in the supine patient, a 'blubbery' fluid wave is detectable by striking a flank on one side and palpating the 'splash' on the other side

PUFAs Polyunsaturated fatty acids see Fatty acids

Puff see Chromosome puff

Puffer fish A Japanese fish delicacy, some of the organs (intestine, ovaries and skin) of which contain tetrodotoxin, the most powerful known poison, which blocks the neuromuscular junction, causing numbness, motor weakness, ataxia and respiratory failure; a similar neuromuscular blockage can be evoked by the toxins from the blue ringed octopus; see Tetrodotoxin

Puffy tumor of Pott A fluctuant swelling overlying the frontal bones, when they affected by osteomyelitis, which is accompanied by a subperiosteal (pericranial) abscess, often secondary to chronic frontal sinusitis; the causative organism in children is often hematogenous in origin and in adults due to direct, traumatic origin Organisms *Staphylococcus aureus*, β-hemolytic streptococci and anaerobes Diagnosis Clinical, 'hot' lesion by ^{99m}Tc scanning; the tumor was first described by Pott in 1760 in association with tuberculosis

PUGH syndrome OPHTHALMOLOGY A clinical association characterized by the acronym of PUGH: Pseudouveitis, glaucoma and hyphema with neovascularization of iris and occlusion of the central retinal vein

'Pugilistic stance' FORENSIC MEDICINE A 'defensive' (fgure, right) or fetus-like position seen in badly burned bodies, which is induced by charring and contraction of musculature, and occurs regardless of whether or not the person was alive at the time of the fire Note: In a court of law, it is of interest to determine if a person died by being burned to death, which for many, is one of the 'ultimate horrors'; in a juried trial, a lawyer attempting to establish that the deceased party died in agony, may show the jury a photograph of the victim's charred body, doubled in a fetus-like crouch, inferring that the person died in pain; the jury may react by awarding the victim's estate multimillion-dollar settlement Note: A person who was alive at the time of a fire and died in the fire almost invariable has soot and carbon in the tracheobronchial tree

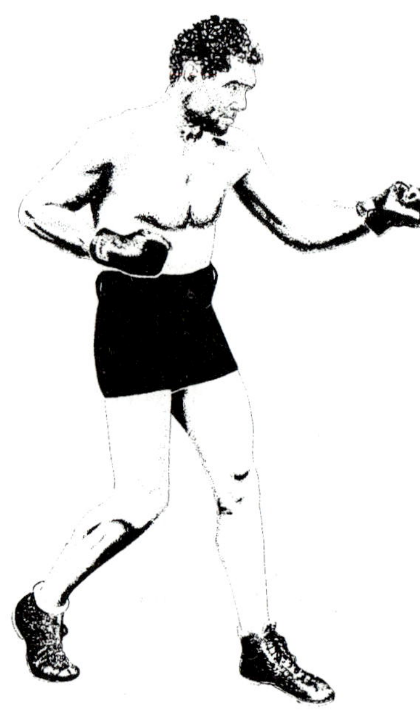

Pugilistic stance

Pulmonary alveolar proteinosis (PAP) A rare disease with a male:female ratio 2.5-4:1, most common in ages 30-50; although idiopathic, more than 50% of cases have been exposed to dusts, chemicals, eg busulfan, infections, eg nocardiosis, CMV, *Pneumocystis carinii*, toxins, eg aluminum and antimony; PAP may be idiopathic, associated with immune compromise or thymic aplasia Clinical Dyspnea, cough, fever, chest pain Radiology Symmetric bilateral 'bat wing'-like alveolar infiltrates, less commonly, unilateral patchy infiltrates Histopathology Uniform filling of alveoli by periodic acid Schiff-positive needle-shaped lipid-rich frothy material that may progress to intraalveolar deposition of granular material (figure, right), with complete preservation of alveolar architecture Ultrastructure Surfactant-like laminated material accumulates in necrotic alveolar macrophages Pathogenesis Excess phospholipid production by type II pneumocytes or defective pulmonary macrophage clearance of phospholipids (at the Mayo Clinic, 'Pulmonary alveolar phospholipoproteinosis' is preferred by some authors Treatment Bronchoalveolar lavage (BAL) with saline or heparin and acetylcysteine for removal of phospholipids, is required in more than one-half of patients; without BAL, there is progressive dyspnea and deterioration of pulmonary functions, a higher mortality and the risk of superinfections, especially with *Nocardia*, which

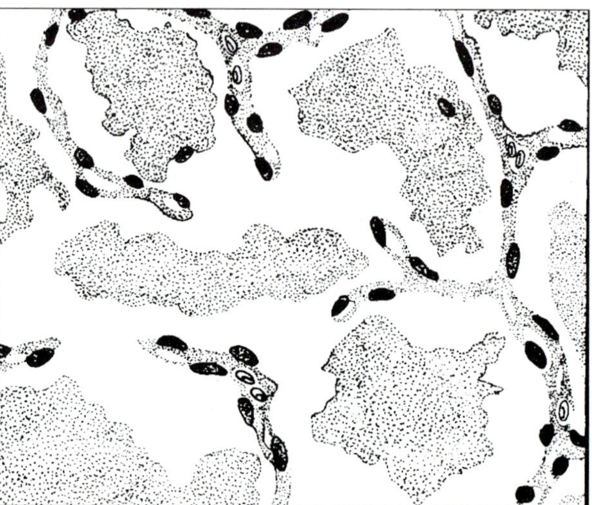

Pulmonary alveolar proteinosis

may be related to the enhanced growth of certain organisms secondary to the increased content of phospholipids

Pulmonary 'burns' Pulmonary parenchymal destruction caused by inhalation of irritating gases, including synthetic nitroso- compounds, eg burning mattresses, polyvinyl chloride containing hydrochloric acid and plastics, which generate toluene di-isothiocyanate: the combination of the toxins and intense heat affects the tracheobronchial tree causing pulmonary edema, congestion, parenchymal hemorrhage, epithelial desquamation and pulmonary necrosis

Pulmonary function tests see Pulmonary panel, Lung volumes

Pulmonary hemorrhagic syndrome(s) A generic term for nonneoplastic and noninfectious pulmonary pathology that presents with hemoptysis, including Goodpasture syndrome, idiopathic pulmonary hemosiderosis and the hemorrhagic vasculitides including hypersensitivity angiitis and Wegener syndrome

Pulmonary hypertension Chronic hypertension of the pulmonary arteries, defined as a mean pulmonary arterial pressure of greater than 20 mm Hg, or at altitudes over 5000 meters, above 25 mm Hg, corresponding to 'wedge' systolic/diastolic pressures of greater than 30/20 mmHg (normal: 18-25/12-16 mmHg); pulmonary hypertension (PH) is often secondary to stasis of blood in the peripheral circulation and is divided into passive PH and secondary forms (table, above): the major effect of PH is the increased work required of the right ventricle which, when prolonged, predisposes the patient to right ventricular failure, syncope, precordial pain and sudden death; PH may be idiopathic or secondary to Eisenmenger's complex, the respiratory failure of cystic fibrosis and chronic obstructive lung disease, with inhibition of endothelium-dependent pulmonary arterial relaxation due to depressed synthesis of nitric oxide or endothelium-derived growth factor (N Engl J Med 1991; 324:1539); in contrast to arterial PH is venous PH, which is defined as a pulmonary venous or left atrial pressure above 12 mmHg which, when acutely elevated above 20-30 mmHg, results in pulmonary edema

Pulmonary interstitial fibrosis see Jo-1 syndrome

Pulmonary panel A battery of cost-effective tests used to evaluate the functional reserve capacity of the lungs in patients who have a clinical diagnosis obstructive or restrictive lung disease; the panel measures CO_2 content, $PaCO_2$, PaO_2, pH, O_2 saturation, a/A ratio; Cf Organ panels

Pulmonary-renal syndrome A heterogeneous group of multisystem diseases, eg Goodpasture's and Wegener's diseases, which have prominent pulmonary and renal components and microangiopathic vasculitis **Clinical** Asymptomatic pulmonary infiltrates or pulmonary hemorrhage with episodic cough, hemoptysis, dyspnea and widespread alveolar infiltrates on chest films; renal involvement is characterized by microscopic hematuria, red cell casts and increased creatinine **Histopathology** Segmental necrotizing glomerulonephritis or glomerular crescent formation; rapid clinical deterioration occurs when more than 50% of the glomeruli have crescents (Mayo Clin Proc 1990 65:847)

Pulmonary Hypertension

Passive pulmonary hypertension, characterized by systemic congestion due to mitral stenosis, left ventricular failure, left atrial myxoma, anomalous drainage of the pulmonary circulation

Hyperkinetic pulmonary hypertension, where there is increased blood flow through the lungs due to congenital heart defects

Vaso-occlusive pulmonary hypertension, due to recurring vessel obstruction, seen in intravenous drug abuse and pulmonary thromboembolism

Vasoconstrictive pulmonary hypertension, associated with hypoxia, alveolar hypoventilation (mitral stenosis, coarctation of aorta, Eisenmenger's complex, ventricular septal defect and e)

Secondary pulmonary hypertension, which comprises 10-20% of cases, treated by addressing the underlying disease, including unilateral renal artery stenosis, coarctation of the aorta, primary aldosteronism and pheochromocytoma

Pulmonary sequestration An uncommon (1:1000 adult lobectomy specimens) congenital anomaly characterized by misplaced lung parenchyma, which lacks normal communication with the main tracheobronchial tree that may be intralobar or extralobar (table)

LUNG SEQUESTRATION	Intralobar	Extralobar
Separate pleura	No	Yes
Location	Posterior basilar	Above or below diaphragm
Age of onset	50% > 20 years	60% < one year
Symptoms	Recurrent pneumonia	Respiratory distress
Laterality	60%, left	90%, left
Male:female ratio	1:1	4:1
Other defects	Uncommon	> 50%, eg diaphragmatic defects, tuberous sclerosis
Bronchial communication	Uncommon, small	None
Arterial supply	Systemic; single aorta	Systemic; multiple, small
Venous drainage	Inferior pulmonary vein	Systemic; azygous and hemiazygous

Pulposus see Herniated disk 'syndrome'

Pulse NUCLEAR MEDICINE 1) A brief exposure to a radioisotope, in order to label a substance and follow its path through a metabolic labyrinth 2) A discharge of electric current produced by radionuclides in an ionization chamber or scintillation counter

Pulse-chase experiment A technique in cell biology to study a physiologic or metabolic process, in which the incorporation of a radioactive substance and its subsequent metabolism is followed as it moves through various cell compartments and disappears from the system; a 'pulse' of a radiolabeled molecule, eg an amino acid, a nucleoside or a phosphate ion is added to the cell and allowed to incorporate into a molecule of interest, followed several minutes later by flooding the extracellular milieu with 'chase' of unlabelled molecules while measuring the radioactive changes

Pulsed field gel electrophoresis MOLECULAR BIOLOGY A technique that is used to separate segments of DNA from several hundred to several thousand kilobase pairs in length, allowing the construction of a full-scale molecular map of ***Escherichia coli***, yeasts and the human major histocompatibility complex; pulsed-field electrophoresis fills a resolution gap that had previously existed between molecular cloning experiments that allowed analysis of a relatively small number of DNA base pairs and meiotic linkage allowing analysis of megabase segments of DNA

Pulseless disease Takayasu's arteritis An idiopathic segmental inflammation of the aorta and major branches, with narrowing of ostia (with 'tree-barking' of the vascular intima) of innominate, left carotid and subclavian arteries, visual disturbances, a 'reverse' coarctation with a thick-walled aorta, adventitial fibrosis, perivascular lymphocyte and plasma cell aggregates, possibly causing thrombosis Pathogenesis Unknown, possibly allergic; the disease affects young women, especially of Africa and Asia, causing weak acral pulses of the upper extremities, renovascular ischemia with hypertension, fever, arthritis, myalgia, pleuritis, pericarditis and rashes Laboratory Increased erythrocyte sedimentation rate and gammaglobulins Histopathology Chronic inflammation and fibrosis of the arterial wall, in particular affecting the branches of the aorta, causing a loss of pulse in the upper extremities (Acta Soc Ophthalmol Jap 1908; 12:554)

Pulse-temperature dissociation Background: The pulse rate increases 15 to 20 beats per minute for each degree increase in a fever above 39°C; a lower than normal increase in pulse rate or relative bradycardia is not uncommon and occurs in burns, drug fever, hepatitis, intoxication (eg trinitrotoluene, TNT), legionnaires' disease, malaria (blackwater fever), myocardial infarction, psittacosis, typhoid fever, yellow fever; relative tachycardia is far less common, but is typical of clinically silent pulmonary embolism, diphtheria and clostridial infections

Pulsus alternans CARDIOLOGY A pulse pattern in which the heart beats occur at regular intervals but in which there is rhythmic attenuation of the pulse pressure heights; sustained pulsus alternans may result from severely depressed left ventricular function, accompanied by an altered blood flow in the aorta, left ventricular and systolic pressures and often a third ventricular sound

Pulsus paradoxus CARDIOLOGY A marked decrease in the pulse amplitude during normal quiet inspiration or a decrease in the systolic pressure by greater than 10 mm Hg, a characteristic finding in cardiac tamponade, but less common in constrictive pericarditis, quantifiable by a sphygmomanometer; pulsus paradoxicus also occurs in superior vena cava obstruction, asthma, pulmonary embolism, shock or post-thoracotomy

Pump lung see Postperfusion lung

Punch-drunk syndrome Dementia pugilistica NEUROLOGY A complex that was reported to affect up to one-half of all professional boxers in the pre-safety era (J Am Med Assoc 1928; 91:1103); this condition is currently thought to affect 10-20% of professional boxers, and is regarded as being the cumulative effect of recurrent brain damage and progressive communicating hydrocephalus; the dysfunction is due to extrapyramidal and cerebellar lesions, that translate into dysarthria, ataxia and tremors, as well as pyramidal lesions, which cause mental deterioration and personality changes including rage reaction and morbid jealousy ('Othello syndrome'); early disease is characterized by unsteadiness of gait (with leg dragging), confusion, hand tremors, slowing of movement, head nodding, and eventually, parkinsonism; boxers' brains may demonstrate cortical atrophy that roughly correlates with the severity of dementia, accompanied by enlarged ventricles (normopressure hydrocephaly), a cavum septum pellucidum, loss of Purkinje cells, neuronal degeneration, gliosis of the substantia nigra, neurofibrillary tangles (especially of the medial temporal cortex, the amygdaloid nucleus and the hippocampal gyrus) Note: Other sports including steeplechasing, soccer, rugby, wrestling are not immune from blow-related dementia (J Am Med Assoc 1984; 251:2676, ibid, 1986; 255:2475); see Boxing

Punched-out An adjectival descriptor for rounded, well-circumscribed often multiple lesions that may be seen in various organ sites Note: When 'punched-out' lesions have scalloped borders, some authors prefer the adjective, 'cookie cutter' GASTROENTEROLOGY Punched-out lesions seen in the stomach by endoscopy usually correspond to benign gastric ulcers, which are well-demarcated with a sharply-defined wall and have a smooth base; Cf Heaped-up OPHTHALMOLOGY Single or multiple defects in coloboma of the optic fundus, due to malclosure of the embryonic fissure, leaving a multi-layered defect in the retina, retinal pigment epithelium and choroid, exposing the underlying sclera RADIOLOGY Rounded, sharply demarcated, cyst-like spaces without sclerotic margins, characteristic of multiple myeloma of the diploe of the skull, causing sharply demarcated 'holes', resulting from osteoclast-activating factor secretion in the plasma cells; punched-out bony defects also occur in well-circumscribed mutilating sarcoidosis of the small hand bones, chronic gouty arthritis as chondro-osseous lesions that communicate with the urate 'crust' through defects in the cartilage, childhood hypophosphatasia, leukemic foci in the skull and tuberculosis

Punctuation 'Punctuation marks' MOLECULAR BIOLOGY Those sequences of nucleic acids that are not themselves part of the structural portion of mature mRNA transcripts, but which provide instructions for the initiation and termination of transcription, likened to the heiroglyphic code of many languages that provide the lector with the 'hinting' for proper understanding of the written word; Cf Editing

Puppet children Angelman syndrome A congenital condition due to a reciprocal deletion of imprinted maternal loci at chromosome 15q11-13 (Am J Med Genet 1989; 32:285), resulting in repetitive ataxic seizures, fancifully likened to the jerking movements of marionettes

PUPPP Pruritic urticarial plaques and papules of pregnancy An erythematous papule and plaque-forming eruption seen late in the third trimester in up to 75% of primigravidas, which does not recur in subsequent pregnancies Histopathology Edema, chronic perivascular inflammation Treatment Topical steroids; see Pruritus gravidarum

Pure red cell aplasia PRCA A type of anemia caused by selective depletion of erythroid cells **ACUTE PRCA** Aplastic crisis A condition often preceded by viral gastroenteritis, pneumonitis, primary atypical pneumonia, mumps, viral hepatitis, pregnancy and drug toxicity Clinical General malaise, pallor and other symptoms of a chronic, compensated hemolyzing process Treatment The only consistently effective modality is discontinuance of an inculpated drug, if one can be identified **CHRONIC PCRA** MAY BE A) CONGENITAL Diamond-Blackfan disease A condition that is due to a decrease in erythrocyte stem-cells with decreased colony-forming units and burst-forming units and a poor response to erythropoietin Treatment Transfusions, corticosteroids OR B) ACQUIRED 30-50% of chronic acquired PRCA is associated with thymoma, other associations include rheumatoid arthritis, lupus erythematosus, chronic active hepatitis, hemolytic anemia and chronic lymphocytic leukemia

Pure white cell aplasia HEMATOLOGY Severe neutropenia, which is analogous to pure red cell aplasia which is either a) Associated with thymoma and hypogammaglobulinemia, and responds to plasmapheresis or b) Associated with other immune diseases eg Goodpasture's disease and responds to antithymocyte globulin or high-dose intravenous immuno-globulin

Purge LABORATORY MEDICINE To flush a gas out of a system or replace one atmosphere with another, as in gas-liquid chromatography

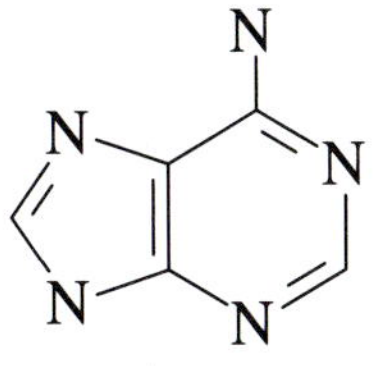

Adenine 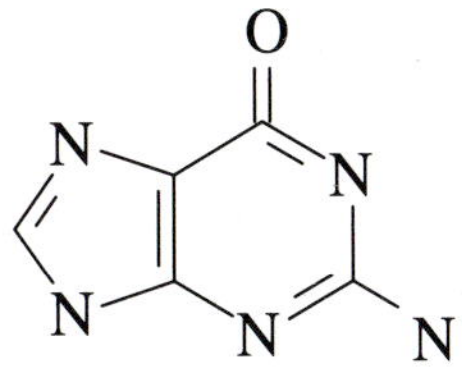 **Guanine**

Purine BIOCHEMISTRY One of 'building block' molecules (adenine and guanine) for ribonucleic acids, which is attached (or 'base pairs') to pyrimidine bases, each of which is separated from its nearest neighbor by a phosphate-sugar backbone, linked to each other with phosphodiester bonds, either with a single strand of ribose, forming ribonucleic acid (RNA), or with a double strand of deoxyribose, forming deoxyribonucleic acid (DNA); under normal conditions, adenine will only form a dimer with thymine (for DNA) or uracil (for hybrid RNA-DNA molecules) and not with a purine; see DNA forms; Cf Pyrimidine

Purine analogs CLINICAL PHARMACOLOGY A family of agents that mimic the chemical structure of purine and therefore act in pathological conditions in which there is increased production of DNA, acting through competitive inhibition with guanine and adenine; purine analogs have a broad range of therapeutic applications, and include azathioprine, a potent immunosuppressant, 6-mercaptopurine, a chemotherapeutic used to treat childhood acute lymphocytic leukemia and 6-thioguanine, used to treat the far less common childhood acute myeloid leukemia; other purine analogs include acyclovir and the xanthine oxidase inhibitor, allopurinol; see 6-MP

Purine nucleoside phosphorylase deficiency An autosomal co-dominant condition caused by defective purine metabolism and accumulation of deoxyGTP, with resultant immune dysfunction by inhibition of ribonucleotide reductase, and blockage of cell division, causing a predominantly T cell immune dysfunction Clinical Recurring opportunistic infections of the lungs, skin and genitourinary tract, autoimmune hemolytic anemia, bone marrow hypoplasia Laboratory Decreased T cells, increased urine and serum uric acid, increased inosine and guanosine; Cf Adenosine deaminase deficiency

Purple glove syndrome A clinical complex resulting from intravenous injection of phenytoin, in which there is discoloration, edema and blister formation of the hand (or acral part distal to an intravenous injection site); the edema evoked may cause ischemic necrosis, necessitating amputation Note: Phenytoin is alkaline and requires the use of propylene glycol as a stabilizer and tends to crystalize

Purple people 'syndrome' A condition affecting psychiatric patients receiving long-term, high dose chlorpromazine therapy, causing purple-gray discoloration on sun-exposed parts (later progressing to a permanent blue-black color), corneal and lenticular opacifications, due to accumulation of a photoactive metabolite of chlorpromazine, an aliphatic phenothiazine once widely used to treat schizophrenia, bipolar disease and psychoses Side effects Pseudodepression, extrapyramidal reaction eg tardive dyskinesia, autonomic nervous system effects eg urinary retention, weight gain, amenorrhea-galactorrhea and infertility, agranulocytosis and hypercholesterolemia

Purple top tube see Lavender top tubes

'Purple urine bag syndrome' A rare 'condition' in which the urine in a bag from a catheterized patient turns an intense purple hours to days after catheterization, an event most common in elderly women, due to infection of the urine by *Providentia stuartii* which has indoxyl sulfatase-like activity, converting urinary indoxyl sulfate into indigo (J Clin Microbiol 1988; 26:2152)

'Pushing glass' see 'Glass pusher'

Putrefaction FORENSIC PATHOLOGY Whole body decomposition, accompanied by tissue autolysis and gas production, which is the postmortem result of combined bacterial overgrowth and enzymatic digestion, occurring within one week in air, two weeks in water, eight weeks buried in soil or not at all, when buried in the marshes; see Adipocere, Bog bodies, 'Floaters'

PUVA 8-methoxy-psoralen with ultraviolet-A (λ 320-400 nm) therapy A therapeutic modality used for treating severe psoriasis; PUVA therapy causes Irregular hyperpigmented macular lesions with increased melanocytes and histological epithelial atypia; those receiving > 260 therapeutic sessions have an 11-fold greater risk of squamous cell carcinoma than those receiving < 160 sessions of PUVA (J Invest Dermatol 1988; 91:120); in one study, invasive squamous cell carcinoma in patients with psoriasis exposed to high levels of PUVA was reported to be over 200 times more common (predominantly of the male genital regions) that the unexposed population; those with low-level PUVA exposure had a greater than ten-fold increase in cancer risk (N Engl J Med 1990; 322:1093)

PV see Polycythemia vera

PVC 1) ENVIRONMENT see Polyvinyl chloride 2) CARDIOLOGY Premature ventricular contraction A condition characterized by premature, widened, bizarre QRS complexes which are not preceded by a P wave; PVCs are common in young subjects and are of no significance, but may be caused by anxiety, fever, various drugs and stimulants; they require investigation in underlying heart disease, if the PVCs increase with exercise, absence of intervening sinus rhythm, R-on-T phenomenon (see there) and if the patient is aware of the arrhythmia (which may be palpated as a 'skipped beat or 'tickle'); PVC's with a variable contour are considered multifocal; when the PVCs have identical contours, they are classified as unifocal, but may occur in a background of underlying heart disease, increasing the risk for cardiac death; PVCs are associated with drug toxicity (digitalis, quinidine and tricyclic antidepressants) and are an indication for discontinuing therapy

PVS see Persistent vegetative state

PWM see Pokeweed mitogen

pX protein A 16.5 kD protein encoded by hepatitis B virus (HBV) that indirectly transactivates viral and cellular genes by forming a protein-protein complex with cellular transcriptional factors CREB and ATF-2, subverting their native DNA binding specificities, such that pX-CREB and pX-ATF-2 bind to the HBV enhancer element, thus possibly explaining HBV's role in acute and chronic liver disease as well as hepatocellular carcinoma (Science 1991; 252:842); see Hepatitis

Pygmalion complex PSYCHIATRY The making over of one individual to suit the needs or desires of another; alternatively, high expectations for normal behavior and/or activities in patients with various impairments, eg physically- or mentally-impaired children, or severely demented elderly subjects (J Am Geriatr Soc 1990; 38:797); the term derives from GB Shaw's Pygmalion, in which a Cockney flowergirl is converted into an elegant woman by a professor of linguistics

Pygmies A tribe of Black Africans who are short in stature, partly due to a 50% reduction of high-affinity growth hormone binding protein, the amino acid sequence of which is homologous to the cell membrane's growth hormone receptor, resulting in a primary deficiency of insulin-like growth factor (IGF-I) or somatomedin C (N Engl J Med 1989; 320:1705)

Pyloric olive PEDIATRICS An abdominal mass palpated in early infancy that corresponds to a 'knot' of hypertrophied peripyloric smooth muscle and mucosal edema seen in pyloric stenosis, which is most common in first-born male infants, 7 weeks of age **Clinical** Non-bilious projectile vomiting, dehydration ('old man' appearance) **Laboratory** Metabolic alkalosis, hypokalemia and hypochloremia **Treatment** Rehydrate, lay open seromuscular layer (Fredet-Ramstedt pyloromyotomy); see Pyloric string sign

Pyloric string sign PEDIATRIC RADIOLOGY Elongation and narrowing of the pyloric passage as seen in an upper gastrointestinal radiocontrast series in a child with hypertrophic pyloric stenosis; Cf Pyloric olive, Tit sign

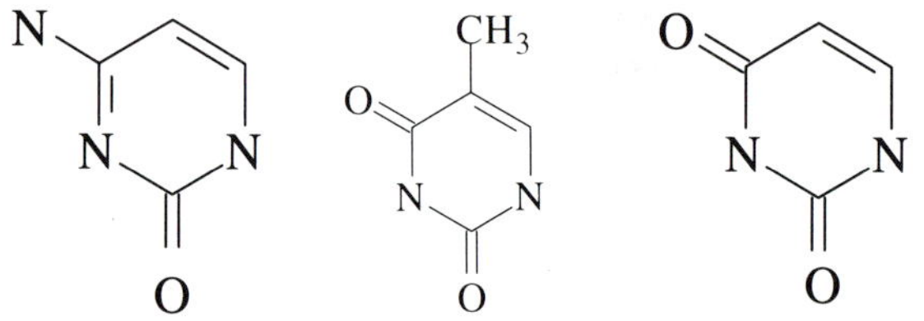

Cytosine **Thymidine** **Uracil**

Pyrimidine BIOCHEMISTRY One of 'building blocks' for ribonucleic acids, which is attached in chains of other pyrimidine or purine bases, each of which is separated from its nearest neighbor by a phosphate-sugar backbone, either with a single strand of ribose, forming ribonucleic acid (RNA, which integrates uracil and cytosine pyrimidine bases), or with a double strand of deoxyribose, forming deoxyribonucleic acid (DNA, which integrates thymidine and cytosine bases); under normal circumstances, pyrimidines only pair with purines, and not with pyrimidines, ie cytosine only pairs with guanine and thymidine with adenine (DNA) and uracil only pairs with adenine (RNA); see DNA forms; Cf Purines

'Pyramid' system GRADUATE MEDICAL EDUCATION A system used in highly-competitive and prestigious US teaching hospitals, which limits the number of resident physicians who graduate from highly-selective residency programs of post-graduate education, eg neurosurgery, by having a larger number of positions available for the first years of training than in the final years; while this places considerable stress on the resident, it is felt to ensure that only the best possible candidates graduate from the most prestigious programs; see Residency; Cf 'Match'

Pyroglobulin A type of myeloma protein that irreversibly precipitates at 56°C, unlike the Bence-Jones protein(s) typical of myeloma that re-dissolve as the temperature is increased above 56°C

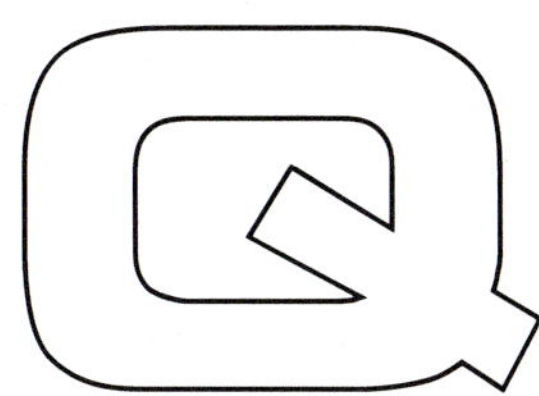

Q Symbol for: Glutamine; metabolic quotient; quantity of electric charge; ubiquinone

q Symbol for: Electric charge, long arm of a chromosome

QA Quality assurance Quality assessment A formal and systematic set of activities that provides a continuous audit against an established standard of quality and which provides a vehicle for correcting deviations from that standard so that a product maintains its quality; the four elements of quality assurance are: 1) Verifying process integrity 2) Assessing a product's quality against a standard 3) Accountability and 4) Liability for failure; for health professionals, quality assurance takes the form of continuing medical education, peer review, specialty, state licensing boards and utilization review; see Peer review organization, Quality control

QALE Quality-adjusted life expectancy PUBLIC HEALTH A model for clinical decision-making in which each stage of a health-state is correlated with life expectancy, eg in carotid artery disease, a patient may be a) In his usual state of health b) Alive with disability or c) Dead; each stage correlates the risk of instituting a therapeutic modality with the statistical potential for improved quality of life (J Am Med Assoc 1990; 263:2917, N Engl J Med 1990; 323:2504); Cf Karnovsky scale

QALY Quality-adjusted life-years see QALE

Q band GENETICS Fluorescent bands that appear at constant sites when chromosomes are stained with quinacrine, a fluorescent dye which inserts or intercalates into the DNA helix; because the bands fade with time, other chromosome stains are usually preferred; see Banding; Chromosome analysis

QC see Quality control

Q cycle A 'short loop' of electron transport occurring on the inner mitochondrial membrane, in which ubiquinone cycles between fully oxidized quinone, fully reduced quinone and the semiquinone intermediate that carries a single electron

Q fever An acute zoonotic rickettsial disease due to the globally-distributed *Coxiella burnetii* Reservoirs Cattle, sheep, goats and sundry small marsupials Vector Ticks, other arthropods Note: *C burnetii* is highly infectious, one organism may aggressively multiply and thus be sufficient to cause a clinical infection **Clinical** Abrupt onset of high fever, headaches, myalgia, malaise, hepatic dysfunction, patchy interstitial pneumonitis, fibrinous exudate, which may resolve without treatment; Q fever may cause an atypical pneumonia, rapidly progressive pneumonia or be an incidental finding in the background of a systemic febrile illness; the convalescent period may be prolonged but has a low mortality **Epidemiology**, pattern 1 Sylvatic Tick 'shuttle' between kangaroos and other marsupials Pattern 2 Human affected by aerosols from asymptomatic cattle, sheep, goats **Treatment** Tetracycline, chloramphenicol Note: The term 'Q fever' was coined by Derrick, a public health officer in Queensland, Australia, who in 1935 investigated a small outbreak of febrile illness, which he called Q or 'Query' fever

Q-switched laser pulse(s) DERMATOLOGY Bursts of energy obtained from the deep-red wavelength of the ruby laser, where energy is allowed to build up in the laser before discharge, resulting in power 'zaps' of high energy that penetrate several millimeters into the dermis and selectively damage melanin and which have been found to be useful in removing tattoos, especially those with black-blue pigment (colored tattoos respond less well); 72% of amateur tattoos respond with lightening or disappearance, 23% of professional tattoos are effectively treated (J Am Med Assoc 1990; 263:2633)

Q10 effect PHYSIOLOGY The effect that environmental temperature has on corporal metabolism, so as the body temperature rises, there is an increase in the rate constant for chemical reactions, and for every ten degree-Centigrade increase in temperature, there is a two-to-threefold increase in the reaction rate, accounting for a 10-13% increase in heat production for each degree centigrade rise in body temperature (DW Wilmore, The Metabolic Management of the Critically Ill, Plenum Press, New York 1977); see Pulse-temperature dissociation

Quaalude see Methaqualone

Quackery False representation of a substance, device or therapeutic system as being beneficial in treating a medical condition, eg 'Snake oil' remedies, establishing the diagnosis of a disease state, or in maintaining a state of good health, see Vitamins, 'Vitamins' ; Cf Holistic medicine

Quack Shaman One who impersonates a physician; a term that arrived to English in the 1500s from 'Quacksalver', for one who hawks or 'quacks' about his miraculous cures or 'salves'; the term had currency in the USA during that country's western expansion in the late 1900s, when very little or no training was required to open one's own 'surgery'; see Unproven forms of cancer therapy

Quad pack Quadruple pack TRANSFUSION MEDICINE A plastic blood collection bag that has three attached 'peripheral' bags allowing the sterile collection and separation of a unit of whole blood (usual volume, 500 ml)

into four 125 ml aliquots, which because they are sterile have a normal shelf life; the host bag may be used to collect plasma (approximately 220 ml), while each mini-unit bag can be further divided into four microunits; therefore one unit of blood may be used to transfuse up to twelve 20 ml aliquots, as may be required for neonates; see 'Cow method'

Quadrilemmal body A crystalloid structure seen within mitochondria that is composed of four sets of parallel lines, seen by electron microscopy within the abnormal mitochondria of Ragged red fiber disease; this structure is probably equivalent to 'Parking lot' crystals

'Quadruple' syndrome A congenital complex characterized by cleft palate, popliteal webbing, lip pitting and genital malformations; see Popliteal pterygium syndrome

Quality-adjusted life expectancy see QALE

Quality assurance see QA

Quality control (QC) LABORATORY MEDICINE A series of mechanism(s) used to determine the accuracy, reliability and consistency of data, assays or tests, often in the context of laboratory medicine, where QC consumes 10-20% of reagent and labor costs; tests performed by accredited clinical laboratories are delineated in their 'procedures manual' which contains the appropriate QC methods, usually requiring standardized solutions containing glucose, cholesterol, electrolytes and other substances that are either commercially available or obtained by pooling specimens from subjects known to be normal for the parameter being measured; see Multirule procedure; see QA

Quality of life The degree to which a person is able to function at his usual level of activity without, or with minimal compromise of routine Note: 'Quality', which can be objectively measured by the Karnovsky or by the QWB scales is one of the most significant factors weighed in the decision of whether or not to aggressively treat a fulminant terminal cancer, since a three month prolongation of a poor quality of life might be considered a Pyrrhic victory; see Karnovsky scale, QALE

'Quality' time SOCIAL MEDICINE Background: In the 'typical' North American family unit, both parents often hold full-time (40 hours/week) jobs and may relegate the task of raising their children to baby-sitters or day-care centers, seeing them one or two hours daily, and then, may be too busy with household chores to interact with them; the term stems from the philosophy espoused by some mental health care workers, that this lack of meaningful interaction during a child's critical formative years may be compensated for by assuring that the contact a parent has with his offspring be (high) 'Quality' time; see 'Supermom'; Cf Latchkey children

Quantal analysis NEUROPHYSIOLOGY A technique used to understand the nature of synaptic transmission at the neuromuscular junction in which 'quanta' or discrete packages of a neurotransmitter, eg acetylcholine are released from a presynaptic site, evoking a post-synaptic response; while the quantal model is largely correct, such a binomial (all-or-nothing) distribution is a gross simplification as synaptic responses are graded along the dendrites and are not identical in all sites (Nature 1991; 350:344, 271); see Long-term potentiation

Quarantine EPIDEMIOLOGY Restriction of freedom of movement allowed those with or presumed to have been exposed to a highly communicable disease, with the purpose of preventing its further dissemination; see Notifiable disease, Proposition 64

Quartan fever The fever pattern characteristic of infection by *Plasmodium malariae* in which fever spikes appear every third day (day one, day four, day seven and so on) in a background of low-grade fever; Cf Tertian fever

Quarter moon sign RADIOLOGY A descriptor for a collection of barium seen in an upper 'GI' series, which is relatively typical of benign gastric ulcers, which is produced by an overhanging fold of mucosa surrounding the ulcer mouth; benign ulcers often have a smooth inner margin with the concavity towards the lumen (figure), a finding that contrasts with that of malignant ulcers, which are more commonly characterized by an inner ulcer margin that is rugose with a convexity toward the gastric lumen; see Meniscus sign of Carmen Note: There has been an accelerating trend in the past decade in the US for gastroenterologists to perform the entire work-up for gastric symptoms, and at the same time as the endoscopic examination of the gastric mucosa, take a biopsy of areas that appear to be abnormal, which is widely regarded as being a more efficient and definitive diagnostic modality than an upper GI series

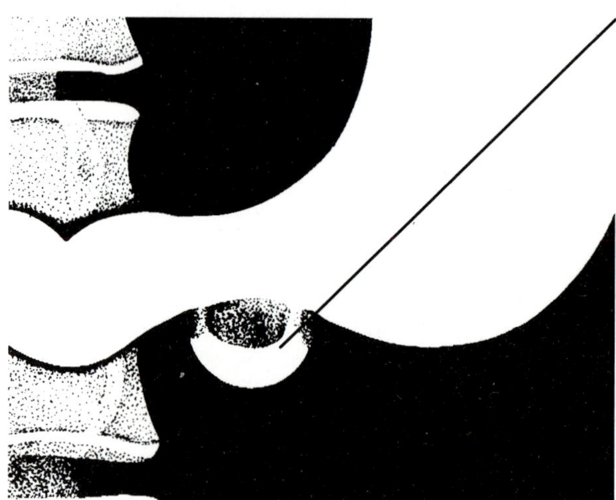

Quarter moon sign

'Quasimodo syndrome' A clinical complex characterized by severe kyphoscoliosis, dyspnea with associated hypoxia and altered sleep pattern (parasomnia), fancifully likened to the symptoms suffered by V Hugo's Quasimodo, the Hunchback; see Hunchback

Quasi-species A mixed population of viruses that have multiple variant nucleic acid sequences, eg human immunodeficiency virus-1 (HIV-1), which are somewhat distinct from the usually isolated forms

Quaternary syphilis The fourth chronobiological stage of syphilis, which follows tertiary syphilis, and is characterized by necrotizing, spirochete-laden encephalitis, which may be accompanied by evidence of end-stage HIV-1-induced anergy and/or loss of cell-mediated immunity against treponemal antigens); quaternary syphilis is a rare clinical entity, but may be seen as AIDS patients, who appear to be more susceptible to neurosyphilis (N Engl J Med 1987; 316:1569; N Engl J Med 1988; 319:1549c)

Quellung MICROBIOLOGY Swelling of encapsulated bacteria, eg *Hemophilus influenza, Streptococcus pneumonia, Neisseria* species and *Klebsiella* species; the reaction is based on the alteration of the refractory index, when the organisms are with a species-specific antiserum incubated with the patient specimen Technique A drop of *H influenzae* type b antiserum is mixed with a drop of the patient's specimen and a small loopful of 0.3% methylene blue; if the patient specimen has the bacterium, the blue-stained organisms are surrounded by a cleared 'halo' (an apparent swelling) which actually corresponds to antigen-antibody complex formation at the surface of the organism

Quenching INSTRUMENTATION Any interference with the transfer of energy in a liquid scintillation counter, eg non-specific absorption of light in a sample 'cocktail' prior to its arrival at the photomultiplier tube, which results in an incorrectly decreased value; quenching may be a) Chemical-type (due to impurities which absorb energy from the excited solvent) or b) 'Color'-type (due to photon absorption impurities), corrected for by adjusting the light pulse ratios and by internal or external standardization and occurs in counting β but not γ radiation; see POPOP, RIA

Queuing theory A mathematical model that analyzes the flow of resources (equipment, personnel, widgets etc) and attempts to optimize their utilization by simulating situations that have characteristics of the resources waiting in a line, ie 'Queuing' (N Engl J Med 1990; 323:604; Worthington DJ J Oper Res Soc 1987; 38:413)

Questionable cancer therapy see Unproven cancer therapy

'Quick and dirty' (Q&D) Crude but effective A survey, laboratory procedure or any type of test using the tools at hand to crudely answer an experimental question; although 'Q&D' techniques are of inadequate methodologic rigor to allow statistical analysis, they produce results on which reasonable conclusions may be drawn prior to performing a more definitive study with appropriate controls and recording of data

Quick-blot MOLECULAR BIOLOGY A method for selective mRNA or DNA immobilization from whole cells, allowing rapid quantitative analysis of small volumes of cultured cells (DNA 1983; 2:243); see Dot blot, Slot blot

Quickening OBSTETRICS A subjective feeling experienced during early pregnancy, that occurs around the 16th gestational week, likened to the 'fluttering of a bird' and which corresponds to the mother's first awareness of fetal movement; Cf Lightening

'Quicker-and-sicker' HEALTH CARE INDUSTRY A colloquialism criticizing the prospective payment system (PPS) form of health care reimbursement practiced in the US; under the PPS, the hospital is 'penalized' if a patient is not discharged in a pre-determined time period, based on the patient's diagnosis-related group (DRG) disease of admission; the attending physician is more likely to 'efficiently' discharge a patient with clinical instability, ie 'quicker-and-sicker'; since the introduction of the PPS, there has been a 43% increase in patients who have been discharged with unstable conditions, including temperature > 38.3°C, new incontinence, chest pain, dyspnea, tachypnea, confusion, heart rate > 130/min, systolic pressure < 90 mm Hg or diastolic pressure > 105 mm Hg, bradycardia and premature ventricular contractions (J Am Med Assoc 1990; 264:1980) Note: Despite an increase of patients discharged with established parameters of 'instability', there is little increase in subsequent mortality; see High mortality outlier, July phenomenon

Quick-freeze technique ELECTRON MICROSCOPY A method by which subcellular particles, eg the cytoskeleton, can be viewed in a relatively native state; the cells are gently treated with a non-ionic detergent (Triton X-100) which dissolves the plasma and organelle membranes as well as the cytosol; the remainder of the cell contents are frozen within milliseconds with liquid helium (-269°C), allowing no time for the formation of ice crystals or for structural distortion of the cytoskeleton; while the preparation is still frozen, the water vapor is drawn off in a vacuum; the remaining protein fibers are then spray coated with a thin layer of platinum and are ready for conventional electron microscopy; see Lyophilization

Quick section see Frozen section

Quick-stop mutants Temperature-sensitive mutants of *Escherichia coli* that immediately stop replicating once the temperature reaches 42°C; quick-stop mutants are also defective in initiating replication cycles

'Quiet zone' PULMONARY PATHOPHYSIOLOGY The terminal airways contribute little to the total airflow resistance (most resistance is contributed by bronchioles > 2 mm in diameter), thus although a disease process may begin in small airways, it may be clinically silent, ie a 'quiet zone' until it affects the larger airways

Quinlan, Karen Ann A young woman who lapsed into a persistent vegetative state in 1975 after ingesting an unknown quantity of tranquilizers and alcohol; this engendered the landmark 'right-to-die' legal cases in which her parents received permission by the New Jersey Supreme Court (Re: Quinlan, 70 N.J. 10 (1976)) to remove therapeutic support (a respirator) in 1976; following removal of life support modalities, she 'lived' another nine years, ultimately dying of pneumonia; Cf DNR, Euthanasia, It's over, Debbie

Quinolones Fluoroquinolones A family of antimicrobial agents, including ciprofloxacin, norfloxacin and ofloxicin that are absorbed orally and are active against a broad spectrum of bacteria; the quinolones target bacterial DNA gyrase (topoisomerase II, an enzyme that introduces negative supercoils in the DNA molecule and separates the interlocked DNA molecule, binding directly to the DNA-gyrase complex, antagonizing virtually all

DNA-related activities; bacterial resistance to quinolones is rare and entails mutations to alter the gyrase itself; quinolones are active against virtually all aerobic bacteria, including bacteria resistant to other antibiotics; these agents have been approved (in the US) for and are effective in treating genitourinary and prostatic infections as well as sexually-transmitted disease, as well as gastrointestinal and respiratory tract infections; despite the slightly higher cost of these agents, they may prove less expensive if they replace parenteral agents Side effects Minimal, confined to gastrointestinal discomfort and vague central nervous system symptoms (N Engl J Med 1991; 264:384rv)

Quinoproteins A unique class of bacterial oxidoreductases that utilize pyrroloquinoline quinone (PQQ) as a cofactor; see PQQ

Quinsy Peritonsillar abscess A late stage anaerobic infection that began as an aerobic pharyngitis (Vincent's angina), which consists of marked pharyngeal pain, dysphagia, low-grade fever, inflammation and medial displacement of the tonsil; usually quinsy is unilateral; bilateral lesions may cause partial pharyngeal obstruction Microbiology Most intraoral infections are polymicrobial mixtures of aerobes and anaerobes Treatment Oral penicillin or a broad-spectrum antibiotic active against *Fusobacterium necrophorum*

Qui tam lawsuit A lawsuit that attempts to recuperate monies paid by the US government to an individual who is convicted of fraudulent use of funds; qui tams originated in the False Claims Act of 1863, written during the US Civil war and were intended to give private citizens, facetiously known as 'whistle blowers', a financial incentive for reporting fraud, since in successful lawsuits, the citizen was entitled to 30% of the recuperated money; the existence of qui tams adds a powerful disincentive for committing scientific fraud, especially since by law, the damages paid are trebled, thus a National Institutes of Health grant of several hundred thousand dollars might prove to be lucrative for the plaintiff, even though in theory the plaintiff is 'altruistically' suing for damages on behalf of the United States government; US scientists are concerned that questions of scientific misconduct will be decided in a court of law by a jury of laymen (who would be more swayed by the trial's theatrics than the science being presented before them) rather than by a jury of peers (Science 1990; 249:734ed); see Fraud in science

Q value The total energy per atom released in a nuclear reaction, when the radionuclide is reduced to a ground state

'Q wave infarct' A myocardial infarct affecting the entire myocardial thickness, ie transmural, of the heart; most Q wave infarcts result from thrombotic occlusion of the proximal coronary arteries, often associated with hemorrhage into an ulcerated fibrous plaque; 'non-Q wave infarcts' are due to microthrombosis by platelet 'plugs', associated with low flow and multivessel coronary artery stenoses; EKG findings include prominent and prolonged (greater than 0.04 sec) Q waves, a 30% decrease in the R wave amplitude, prominent peaked T waves (indicating epicardial damage) and a hyperacute ST elevation; Cf Non-Q wave infarction

QWB scale Quality of well-being scale (developed by R Kaplan, UCSD) A list of 30 symptoms that determines the value people place on alleviation of those symptoms, quantifying treatment cost per 'quality life year', by examining the age of onset, the number of years of expected remaining life, the frequency of use of a particular procedure for a morbid condition, the efficiency of the treatment for the symptoms and the treatment cost (Am Med News 16/Mar/90); Cf Karnovsky scale, Quality of life

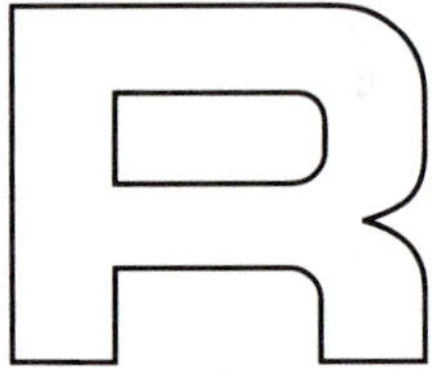

R Symbol for: Arginine; resistance; Roentgen

r Symbol for: recombinant; ribose; ring chromosome

Rs of research The three Rs of research Raw data, Reagents, Responsibility, the triad of 'materials' traditionally shared by scientists; in the current environment, several groups may be actively pursuing the same line of investigation, eg identifying a potentially important gene or protein, selfless cooperation is said to be facing extinction (Science 1990; 248:952); the phrase derives from nineteenth century rural America when schoolchildren learned the 3 Rs: Reading, 'Riting and 'Rithmetic; Cf 'Safari' research

RA Rheumatoid arthritis

RAA system Renin-angiotensin-aldosterone PHYSIOLOGY The RAA system is the major actor in humoral control of blood pressure and volume; renin is a proteolytic enzyme produced in the juxtaglomerular apparatus (as well as in the brain and endothelial cells) in response to decreased kallikrein, reducing the blood pressure, renin cleaves angiotensinogen, yielding the prohormone decapeptide, angiotensin I (A-I) that is then cleaved forming A-II, A-II is a potent vasoconstrictor, stimulating aldosterone synthesis and which in the central nervous system causes a dipsogenic response; the RAA system is activated by congestive heart failure, cirrhosis, edema, nephrosis, protein loss, malignant hypertension, renal artery stenosis; renal vasoconstriction is increased and renin and aldosterone secretion is decreased in those at risk for hypertension (N Engl J Med 1991; 324:1305) Note: Minor actors in the control of blood pressure include atrial natriuretic peptide and the kallikrein-kinin system, prostaglandins, (especially PGE_2), arginine and vasopressin

Rabbi Bergman see Towers nursing home

Rabbit curve R precipitation curve IMMUNOLOGY A symmetrical precipitation curve that is seen when an antigen is tested against its antiserum, the curve is broad and is typical of both rabbit and human antigen-antibody reactions, the latter is an 'H curve'

Rabbit ear appearance A descriptor for two elongated, finger-like structures joined at a base CARDIOLOGY A rabbit ear pattern occurs in a variant QRS wave, allowing the differentiation of ventricular tachycardia from the relatively innocent supraventricular tachycardia, in which the left 'ear' spike is higher than the right MICROBIOLOGY A rabbit ears appearance may be seen in either a) The characteristic acute angular budding of arthrospores seen by light microscopy in the imperfect fungus *Trichophyton* or b) The piroplasts of *Babesia microti* (figure) which tend to form packets of twos and threes of intracytoplasmic parasites within circulating erythrocytes

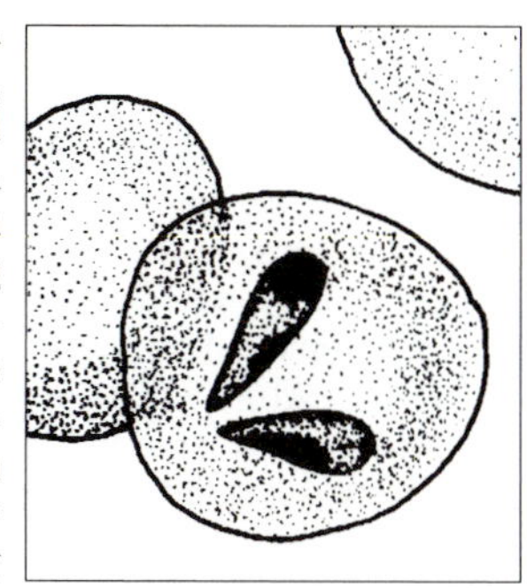

Rabbit ear appearance

Rabbit fever Tularemia

Rabbit ileal loop test A technique used to identify enterotoxins produced by serotypes of *Escherichia coli* and *Salmonella* species, in which the supernatant from these organisms in culture is inoculated into a ligated segment of ileum, which responds by 'locking' the intestinal adenylate cyclase into the 'on' position, increasing secretion of fluids into the loop of intestine (Infect Immunol 1973; 7:873)

Rabbit nose A descriptor for nose twitching and wrinkling by children with allergic rhinitis, which relieves pruritus or increases air passage; the characteristic upward rubbing of the nose ('allergic salute') may result in a groove formation at the tip of the nose

'Rabbit' stool A descriptor for the small rounded, mucus-covered fecal 'pellets' produced in irritable bowel syndrome

Rabbit syndrome NEUROLOGY A symptom complex characterized by focal perioral tremors and nose twitching that may be seen in parkinsonism as a late side effect of antipsychotic drug therapy; unlike tardive dyskinesia, the symptoms of rabbit syndrome respond well to antiparkinsonian agents (Clin Neuropharmacol 6 Supplement 1983; 1:S9-S26); see Tardive dyskinesia

Rabies A viral infection caused by a bullet-shaped 180 x 80 nm virion containing single-stranded RNA; after intramuscular 'injection' by an animal bite, the virion crosses the neuromuscular junction and infects the nerve, spreading centripetally into the central nervous system and centrifugally into the salivary glands of lower animals Rabies encephalitis in mammals may be either a) Furious, due to increased irritability of the central nervous system, accompanied by fever, hyperesthesia, anorexia, aggression; immediately prior to death, the afflicted mammal may run for hours until it collapses in complete paralysis or b) Paralytic, in which sialorrhea is followed by collapse Epidemiology Human rabies is rare--four cases have occurred within the US since 1980 (MMWR 1991; 40:132), although a number of other cases occurred outside of the US and developed once the subjects arrived; laboratory-confirmed disease in mammals is relatively common; of 5606 cases in 1985 (estimated to be 10% of actual number of animals infected), skunks accounted for 46%, raccoons 26%, bats 15%, cattle 4%, foxes 3%, dogs 2%, cats 2%, rabies may be transmitted person-to-person by inhalation or corneal transplant, but not from human bites Histopathology Cerebral edema, congestion, mild perivascular 'round cell' infiltration of the gray matter of the brainstem and spinal cord, marked loss of Purkinje cells, Babe's microglial nodules in the pons and medulla; Negri bodies are present within neurons and are most prominent in the hippocampus, medulla oblongata and cerebellum

RAC Recombinant DNA Advisory Committee A National Institute of Health (USA) committee involved in approving 'gene therapy', comprised of scientists and members of the public; the first RAC approved recombinant gene experiment involved insertion of a marker gene into terminally ill patients with malignancy to track the progress of tumor-infiltrating lymphocytes (TILs); planned therapies under consideration by the RAC include insertion of therapeutic genes for AIDS, cancer and adenosine deaminase deficiency; see Adenosine deaminase, TIL

Race An ethnic classification, subdivided in the US into five categories, according to origin: 1) White, not Hispanic (Europe, North Africa, Middle East); 2) Black, not Hispanic (Africa); 3) Hispanic; 4) American Native (Indians, Eskimos); 5) Asian and Pacific Islanders; stratification by race is of interest in several areas of medicine for a number of specific reasons CLINICAL MEDICINE Some HLAs are more common in certain racial groups and may be associated with particular diseases, thus helping to diagnose and manage difficult cases PUBLIC POLICY The Civil Rights Act of 1964 mandated equality in employment and educational policy and knowledge of race favors minority candidates TRANSFUSION MEDICINE Certain red cell antigens may be relatively uncommon in a particular race and knowledge of race reduces the labor required to find a suitable unit for transfusion TRANSPLANTATION Human leukocyte antigens (HLA) differ somewhat according to race and may be used to identify potential recipients for organ transplants

RA cell see Rheumatoid arthritis cell

Raccoon eyes appearance Black eyes A descriptor for bilateral periorbital accumulations of blood or other substances, likened to the nocturnal North American omnivore, *Procyon lotor*; this Panda bear-like appearance is classically described in periorbital hematomas, often associated with anterior-posterior displacement-type automobile accidents or basilar fractures; less commonly, the descriptor is applied to the periorbital purpura due to skin infiltration in primary amyloidosis, as a spontaneous event, or after prolonged eye-strain Note: Children with allergic rhinitis have a clinical appearance known as 'bags under the eyes'

Rachitic rosary see Rosary

Racquet cells A descriptor for variant 'strap' cells seen in rhabdomyosarcoma, which have a vaguely globose swelling at one end, tapering into elongated wispy cytoplasm, occasionally bearing the diagnostic cross-striations

Racquet fingernail An asymptomatic defect of the thumb in which the distal phalanx is shorter and wider than normal, resulting in a shorter and wider than normal nail with a loss of its curvature; racquet nails may occur as an autosomal dominant 'condition' or in tertiary hypoparathyroidism due to erosion of the underlying bone; Cf 'Clubbing'

rad A quantity of ionizing radiation (X-rays and γ rays) corresponding to an energy absorption of 100 ergs/g of tissue; the rad as a unit was 'retired' in 1985 and has been replaced by the gray (Gy), where 1 Gy equals 100 rads; Cf Roentgen

Radial immunodiffusion IMMUNOLOGY A simple method for quantifying serum proteins, eg apolipoproteins, complement proteins and immunoglobulins **Method** A gel with incorporated antibody has multiple wells cut in it; standard antigens and an unknown are droppered into the wells and the diameter of the reaction of the unknown is plotted on a curve and compared semiquantitatively with the standards; see Ring test, Spur

Radial keratotomy see Refractive surgery

Radial unit model NEUROEMBRYOLOGY A hypothesis explaining how the immense number of neurons in the cerebral cortex arise from progenitors lining the cerebral neocortex and are then distributed to appropriate layers of distinct cytotechtonic areas; according to this model, the ependymal layer of the embryonic ventricle consists of proliferative units providing a primitive map of the prospective areas; the proliferative units are transported via glial guides to the growing cortex in the form of ontogenetic columns, the final number of neurons dedicated to each column is modified by interacting afferent 'messages'; this model is supported by data provided by ultrastructure, immunocytochemistry, receptor autoradiography and kinetics of cell proliferation

Radiation hybrid mapping MOLECULAR BIOLOGY A technique for constructing high-resolution, contiguous maps of chromosomes, consisting in a statistical method that depends on X-ray-induced breakage of chromosomes to determine the distances between DNA markers (Science 1990; 250:245); Cf Pulsed field electrophoresis

Radiation The combined processes of emission, transmission and absorption of highly energetic waves and particles on the electromagnetic spectrum Types Alpha (α) **RADIATION** 2 protons and 2 neutrons, eg plutonium, radon; α radiation travels 15 cm in air and is stopped by a piece of paper; its role in soft tissue malignancy is well-established, see Radium Dial company, although its relation in epithelial malignancy is less certain; it is present in cigarette smoke and has been postulated to have an additive effect to the known carcinogens in tar **Beta β RADIATION** Electrons, eg strontium-90, tritium (^{3}H); β radiation travels at the speed of light, is stopped by wood and thin metals and is carcinogenic to skin **Gamma γ-RADIATION** Electromagnetic waves, eg cobalt-60; γ radiation is stopped by several feet of heavy concrete or 10-40 cm of lead and induces malignancy, inducing mutations at the glycophorin A locus in survivors of atomic blasts; 183/10^5 excess deaths in survivors of the Hiroshima and Nagasaki blasts, with a 13-fold increase in non-lymphocytic leukemia (peaking at 6 years post-blast), thyroid nodules and tumors (peaking at 15-20 years post-blast) and multiple myeloma 6-fold increase (peaking 30 years post-blast) Note: After radiation exposure, high-dose potassium iodide may be used to functionally block the effect of thyroid irradiation (J Am Med Assoc 1987; 258:629, 649) *CYTOPATHOLOGY* Radiation induces marked cellular atypia, elongation or 'spindling', cytoplasmic vacuolization, multinucleation, nuclear hyperchromasia and nuclear membrane wrinkling; the differences in pathology among organs is slight *COLON* Ulceration, necrosis, bleeding, eosinophilia *HEMATOPOIETIC TISSUE* Lymphopenia, followed by granulocytosis, followed by granulocytopenia, thrombocytopenia, erythroid hypoplasia and aplasia *LYMPH NODES* Lymphocyte depletion, hemorrhage and fibrosis *MUSCLE* Fibrosis, Zenker's degeneration *PROSTATE* Glandular atrophy, squamous metaplasia, cellular and fibromuscular atypia *SKIN* Atrophy, Epilation, erythema, fibrosis, eventually, soft tissue necrosis; see Acute radiation injury, Nuclear war

Radiation pneumonitis A condition caused by exposure of lung tissue to radiation, a common complication of therapy for mediatinal tumors, including malignant lymphoma, Hodgkin's disease, breast and esophageal carcinomas, the frequency of which is a function of the dose and the amount of tissue exposed to radiation **Incidence** Radiologic evidence of pneumonitis occurs in 65% of those whose lung fields have been irradiated, although clinically evident pneumonitis occurs in 6%, 2% of whom die from radiation pneumonitis **Histopathology** Alveolar septal thickening by collagen and basement membrane material, alveolar proliferation, desquamation of atypical cells within the alveolar septum, hyaline membrane formation and pulmonary vascular changes, protein leakage, interstitial infiltration and reduction of alveolar volume; other radiation 'syndromes' include radiation arthropathy, radiation carditis, radiation cytitis, radiation dermatitis, radiation enterocolitis, radiation fibromatosis, radiation hepatitis and radiation nephritis

Radiation sickness see Acute radiation injury syndrome

Radiator theory ANTHROPOLOGY A theory proposed by Dean Falk that attempts to explain how the human brain evolved from a 500 gram chimpanzee-like brain to the current size of about 1400 gram in less than 2 million years (a very short time span in evolutionary biology); Falk argues that the emissary veins are a crucial network that cools the brain in hyperthermia, thus being likened to a radiator, and may have been the crucial preadaption required for the increased size of the brain, given that the substantial differences between the configuration of the vascular systems of humans and non-human primates (Science 1990; 250:1339)

Radical neck dissection The most commonly performed major operation for head and neck malignancy, most of which are squamous cell carcinomas; the neck is opened laterally, the majority of the sternocleidomastoid muscle is removed, as are the regional cervical lymph nodes, the jugular vein, the spinal accessory nerve, the submaxillary gland and most of the parotid gland; a 'radical neck' may be combined with a partial resection of the mandible and tongue, depending on the lesion's topography; the term 'modified radical neck dissection' is ill-defined as there is a spectrum of what can be called 'modified'; some operators merely preserve the spinal accessory nerve, while others spare all functional tissue, including the sternocleidomastoid muscle and the jugular vein; Cf Commando operation, 'Heroic' surgery, Mutilating surgery

Radical scavenger see Free radical scavenger

Radioactive decay Those changes that occur in the nucleus of a radioactive isotope, which result in the liberation of neutrons, protons and electrons

Radiofrequency current CARDIOLOGY A level of electrical energy (31 watts or more), delivered through a large-tip electrode for ablation of the accessory ventricular conduction pathway in the Wolff-Parkinson-White syndrome, a therapeutic modality that produces better results than that of high energy direct current (N Engl J Med 1991; 324:1605, 1612), which generates more than 2000 volts, producing a combination of light, heat, barotrauma and an intense electrical gradient

Radioimmunoassay see RIA

Radioimmunoprecipitation assay (RIPA) A technique that is similar to Western blotting as it identifies antibodies to specific viral components and requires an electrophoretic separation step **Method** Disrupted. purified virus previously grown in culture with a radioactive amino acid is co-incubated with a test sample which may contain an immunoglobulin with specificity against the viral antigen; the immunoglobulins in the test sample are then subjected to polyacrylamide gel electrophoresis

Radiomimetic drug An immunosuppressive drug, eg an alkylating agent, that is used to treat malignancy, which has effects on nucelic acid, eg DNA mimicking those of ionizing radiation

Radiosensitivity The relative susceptibility of cells and tissues to irreversible damage by radiation, which either prevents mitosis or the completion of normal metabolic processes; lymphoid, hematopoietic and gonadal tissues are highly susceptible to radiation damage, while terminally differentiated tissues, eg bone, cartilage, muscle and peripheral nerve are relatively radioresistant; some malignancies, eg lymphoproliferative, gonadal malignancies, classically, seminoma and small cell carcinoma of the lung seem to 'melt away' with radiotherapy, whereas others, eg glioma, melanoma, renal cell carcinoma and sarcomas, are notoriously radioresistant

Radiothor An over-the-counter 'patent' medicine containing radium-226 and radium-228 in water, formulated in 1925 and produced until the early 1930s in the US; radium emits α radiation and can only penetrate short distances, but in that distance produces considerable damage; Radiothor was a self-medication claimed to be an endocrine system 'tonic' and of use in treating impotence and chronic diseases including anemia, rheumatism, multiple sclerosis, gout and others; the 'mild radium therapy' era collapsed when one of its chief proponents and users died of massive radium intoxication (J Am Med Assoc 1990; 264:614); see Health fraud, Quackery

'Radish' bacillus A trivial name for ***Mycobacterium terrae*** and the related ***M triviale***, members of Runyon group III (nonphotochromagens) mycobacteria, which are isolated from soil, vegetables (hence, 'radish') and milk and are essentially nonpathogenic

Radium Dial Company A defunct company in Illinois that in the 1920s highlighted clock faces with radium-laced luminescent paint; the workers, mostly women, often licked the tips of their paint brushes to bring them into a point, making their job easier and at the same time ingesting significant doses of radium (a rare radioactive element in the uranium decay series with a half-life of 1622 years); over time, these women developed severe osteoporosis and mesenchymal tumors including malignant fibrous histiocytoma and osteosarcomas; Cf Radiothor

Radon Radon-222 PUBLIC HEALTH A naturally occurring radioactive gas in the decay chain of uranium-238 to lead-206 that has a half-life of 3.8 days, decaying into two solid α particle-emitting daughters; radon exposure is associated with a relative risk of 12.7 due to lung cancer in non-smoking uranium miners (J Am Med Assoc 1989; 262:629) and is associated with an increased risk of leukemia, childhood malignancy, myeloid leukemia, renal cell carcinoma, melanoma and prostatic carcinoma in adults (Lancet 1990; 335:1008, 1292); 13 000 annual excess cases of lung cancer in the US are attributed to radon gas exposure, an effect that is synergistic with cigarette smoking; long-term exposure to 150 Bq/m^3 is held to be equivalent to smoking 1/2 pack of cigarettes/day; concentrations of radon gas in the home above 4 pCi/L (or 0.15 Bq/L) are felt to require active remediation, ie forced ventilation

RAEB see Refractory anemia with an excess of (myelo)blasts

raf MOLECULAR BIOLOGY A regulatory proto-oncogene that encodes a ubiquitous cytoplasmic protein kinase, which is a target for multiple growth factors and has a central role in signal transduction; the Raf kinase promotes cell proliferation that depends on growth factor receptors and membrane-associated oncogenes; the *raf* gene is an essential signal transducer that acts downstream of serum growth factors, protein kinase C and the *ras* oncogene (Nature 1991; 349:426); with the related *rif*, *raf* modulates hepatic levels of α-fetoprotein (AFP), acting in a 'trans' conformation, regulating AFP production via mRNA; increased expression of *raf* causes radioresistance in human laryngeal carcinoma, while reduced expression of c-*raf*-1 modulates tumorigenicity and radioresistance of squamous cell carcinoma (Science 1989; 243:1354)

RAG-1, **RAG-2** Recombination activating genes A pair of adjacent (8 kilobases apart) genes encoding proteins that synergistically activate V(D)J recombination; RAGs are thought by some workers to correspond to V(D)J recombinase (Science 1990; 248:1517)

Ragged red fiber disease (RRFD) A form of mitochondrial myopathy, defined by histopathology, which consists of extensive cell destruction at the skeletal muscle cell periphery with vacuolated fibers which are 'ragged' under high power, best viewed by the Gomori trichrome stain Ultrastructure Abnormal enlarged mitochondria with degenerated cristae and unique crystal-like inclusions ('parking-lot crystals'), accompanied by various defects in the mitochondrial electron transport chain, including mitochondrial ATPase, NADH-coenzyme Q reductase, cytochrome oxidase b and cytochrome oxidase c; RRF occurs in the skeletal muscle of mitochondrial encephalomyopathy (see MERRF), AIDS patients treated with AZT as a cytotoxic form of myopathy mediated by MHC Class I-restricted cytotoxic T cells (N Engl J Med 1990; 322:1098) Note: The ragged red fibers may occasionally be more basophilic ('blue') than red, may be seen in other mitochondrial myopathies and in the rare mitochondrial lipid glycogen disease

'Raggedy Ann syndrome' see Chronic fatigue syndrome

Ragocytes see Rheumatoid arthritis cells

RAIDS see Refrigerator 'AIDS'

'Railroad' nystagmus Opticokinetic nystagmus NEUROPHYSIOLOGY A normal bilateral optical response to objects moving slowly across a field of vision, which is considered a combination of pursuit and refixation saccades; this response may be calibrated by varying the size and speed of the moving objects and has been likened to the constant refixation of the eyes that occurs when people view fixed objects while seated in a moving train; Cf 'Seesaw' nystagmus

Railroad track appearance A descriptive term for parallel, relatively straight lines, radio-opacities or radiolucencies of varying length; when the parallel lines are curved, the descriptor 'Tramline' or 'Tram track' is a more valid adjectival descriptor NEPHROPATHOLOGY The railroad track appearance refers to parallel thickening and splitting of the glomerular capillary basement membrane due to subendothelial deposition of immune complexes, mesangial matrix and neutrophilic debris between the glomerular basement membrane and the vascular endothelium causing a double contour by light microscopy, a classic finding in type I and occasionally in type II membranoproliferative glomerulonephritis and cryoglobulinemia, which is best seen by silver and periodic acid-Schiff (PAS)-stains; the outer 'track' of the double contour corresponds to the original basement membrane that is continuous and easily recognized; the inner basement membrane 'track' is discontinuous and of variable thickness; Cf Crescent formation, Tram track appearance

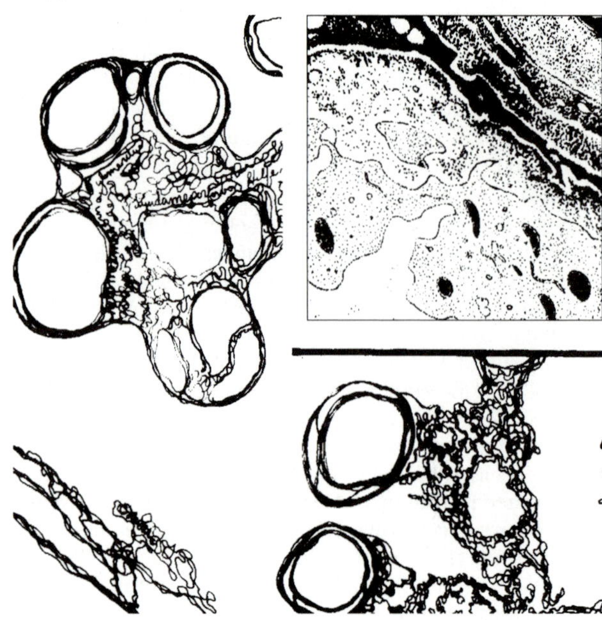

Railroad track appearance

Railroad track scars GASTROENTEROLOGY A descriptor for the macroscopic changes seen in the late fibrosing stages of Crohn's disease in which longitudinal mucosal lesions heal in parallel tracks, perpendicular to the length of the colonic lumen PLASTIC SURGERY A scar with obvious cross-hatched stitch marks due to poor repair, excess tension on the skin or to a delay in suture removal, which should be ideally removed on the third to fifth days (except when the sutures overlie highly mobile sites); some body regions, eg trunk, sternum and proximal extremities are more susceptible to cross-hatching

'Raining down' DERMATOPATHOLOGY A descriptor applied to 'dropping' of fascicles and individual nevus cells from the epidermis into dermis, a morphological feature of the benign Spitz's nevus, which aids in differentiating this from malignant melanoma

Raji cell IMMUNOLOGY A B lymphoblastic cell line that was originally obtained from a Burkitt's lymphoma that is used to detect immune complexes; the Raji cell has minimal or no surface immunoglobulin, low avidity Fc receptors and a high density of C3 receptors, making it ideal for detecting levels of background circulating immunoglobulins in serum, of use in diagnosing Waldenström's disease and immune complex disease; other methods for detecting immune complexes include the solid phase C1q, conglutination, polyethylene glycol precipitation of high molecular weight immune complexes

Râles French, rattle CLINICAL MEDICINE A term for the crackling or bubbling, discontinuous sounds or vibrations, which may be heard by auscultation in various diseased lungs, including those with bronchitis, pneumonia, atelectasis, pulmonary edema, heart failure, bronchiectasis and tuberculosis

RAM Random access memory COMPUTERS Temporary, immediately available computer memory that disappears upon loss of power, which contrasts to the a) Permanent 'software memory', stored on magnetic media, eg floppy disks or hard disks and b) Permanent 'hardware memory', stored on ROM (read-only memory) chips; RAM available to microcomputer users has risen from 16 kilobytes in the late 1970s to 128 Megabytes, a capacity which allows simulated manipulation of three-dimensional structures, eg for the design and advanced modeling of complex drugs or DNA-protein interactions

Raman effect That which occurs when a beam of incident light causes rotational and vibrational transitions in molecules, resulting in exiting scattered light that has a different frequency than the in-coming light

Raman spectroscopy A method for studying proteins in their native state by X-ray crystallography that records the spectrum of light scattered by a transparent medium at a right angle to the incident beam of monochromatic light; a peak or 'frequency shift' in the scattered light corresponds to vibration or rotation of the scattering molecules, providing information that is similar and complementary to that provided by infrared spectrophotometry; see X-ray crystallography

RAMI see Rate-adjusted mortality index

Ram's horn sign see Shofar sign

Ranch hand see Operation Ranch Hand

Rancidity Deterioration of fat-containing foods, resulting in an unpalatable (rancid) taste and unpleasant odor due to oxidation of the unsaturated fatty acids and hydrolysis of triglycerides into mono- and diglycerides, glycerol and free fatty acids; Cf Maillard reaction

RAND corporation A nonprofit organization engaged in research and analysis on issues of public welfare and national security, supported by monies from US government, philanthropies and foundations; the publications generated under RAND's aegis include breast feeding in developing nations and issues of cost containment, health care policy and quality assurance

Random walk Haphazard movement of a particle, eg Brownian movement or fluctuation of a molecule's three-dimensional configuration that is attributable to intrinsic vibration or chaos; see Breathing, Chaos; Cf Fractal analysis

Ranitidine see H_2 blockers

Rapamycin A drug isolated from a soil fungus on Rapa Nui on the Easter Islands, which has immunosuppressive activity, and although structurally similar to FK506, its activity differs, acting to suppress B and T cell proliferation, lymphokine synthesis and T cell response to IL-2; the desired immune response with rapamycin is achieved at levels 1/8 of the levels required of FK506 and 1/100 the levels of cyclosporin; see Cyclosporin, FK506

Rape FORENSIC MEDICINE An aggressive act that is considered to be sadistic rather than sexual in nature **Diagnosis** Detection of choline periodate (Florence test) with its characteristic rhomboid crystal as a marker for ejaculate is still being used in detection of rape, although isolation of DNA fragments with polymerase chain reaction is far more valid, as it serves to identify the perpetrator; because of the legal implications and logistical problems that the 'chain of evidence' may incur, investigation of rape in the US is a costly procedure; sexually transmitted infection occurs in about 40% of rape victims and the agents include *Neisseria gonorrhoeae*, cytomegalic inclusion virus, *Chlamydia trachomatis*, herpes simplex, *Treponema pallidum* and HIV-1 (N Engl J Med 1990; 322:713) **SPOUSAL RAPE** is that by the marital partner, against the latter's will **STATUTORY RAPE** is that where local or state law decrees that one of the partners has not reached adult status, ie is 'underage'; see Rape-trauma syndrome

RAPER(s) A commonly used acronynm for radiologists, anesthesiologists, pathologists and emergency room physicians, a group of board-certified medical specialists who are almost invariably hospital-based; because RAPERs generally do not practice their specialty outside of a medical facility, the health care reimbursement organizations and regulatory agencies in he USA have found it convenient to consider all RAPERs in a category separate from other physicians who 'compete' for patients and have other expenses not incurred by RAPERs

Rapeseed oil syndrome see Toxic oil syndrome

Rape-trauma syndrome An acute stress reaction to a life-threatening situation in which sexual assault was attempted or successful, divided into psychological phases Phase I Disorganization; onset 2-3 weeks post-attack; the victim blames herself for having provoked the attack Phase II Long-term reorganization, often the victims are left with residual chronic anxiety, phobias, hypochondriasis, loss of self-esteem or depression

'Rapture of the deep' Nitrogen narcosis A neurological response to increased nitrogen gas dissolved in the blood that occurs in scuba divers, resulting in causing euphoria, apathy, loss of judgement, which is most common at depths below 20 meters **Prevention** Use of helium-oxygen gas; see Caisson's disease

Rapunzel syndrome A fanciful term for the symptoms of a massive trichobezoar caused by trichotillomania and trichophagia, seen most commonly in mentally retarded or deranged females **Clinical** Epigastric pain, bloating, nausea and vomiting **Radiology** A mass lesion, usually gastric with 'strands' of hair extending into the upper small intestine **Laboratory** Hypochromic microcytic anemia, the hair acts as an iron chelator **Treatment** Surgery; see Bezoar Note: Rapunzel was a maiden with long hair in a fairy tale written by Jacob Grimm

RAR-alpha Retinoic acid receptor-α see Differentiation therapy

Rare disease see Orphan disease

Rare earths Any of a group of oxides of widely distributed, but relatively scarce minerals, corresponding to the fifteen elements with atomic numbers from 57 to 71, including erbium, gadolinium, lanthanum, neodymium, some of which have properties making them useful as crystals in lasers; see Lasers; Cf Trace minerals

RARS Refractory anemia with ringed sideroblasts see PISA

***ras* gene(s)** A family of oncogenes and proto-oncogenes, first identified in a rat sarcoma, which encode oncoproteins or proto-oncoproteins; *ras* genes (c-*ras*, H-*ras*, K-*ras*, N-*ras* and v-*ras*) encode 21 kD proteins ($p21^{ras}$) with roles in the transduction of growth signals, binding guanine triphosphate (GTP) and catalyzing its hydrolysis to guanine diphosphate (GDP); ras proteins acquire cell-transforming potential with 'activating' amino acid substitutions at positions 12, 13 or 61 due to point mutations on the *ras* gene, located at 11p13; c-*ras*, the cellular proto-oncogene encodes a highly conserved 21 kD membrane-bound protein with a low GTPase activity; a point mutation in c-*ras* yields v-*ras* with impaired GTPase activity and inhibited 'off switch', resulting in sustained activation, possibly of a calcium channel (Science 1990; 250:1743); the ras oncoprotein is an extracellular signal for cell growth received by a transmembrane receptor protein, which induces a GDP-for-GTP exchange with the intracellular ras proteins, resulting in a GTP-ras protein complex required for ras protein function; in neoplasia, this complex is 'locked' in the new conformation and, lacking intrinsic GTP-hydrolytic capacity, is left in the 'turned-on' or neoplastic position (Science 1990; 247:939); *ras* is required for the activity of other oncoproteins, including tyrosine kinase and such growth stimulants as the tumor-promoting phorbol ester; *ras* genes are the most highly conserved oncogenes and are expressed in cancer of the bladder, colon, lung, pancreas, prostate, stomach, in T-cell malignancy, acute myelogenous leukemia and melanoma; *ras* expression in the NIH3T3 tumor cell line is associated with an increased intrinsic resistance to ionizing radiation; cell-activating point mutations (at various sites in the DNA) of *ras* genes are common in some adenocarcinomas, eg pancreatic (90% have a K-*ras* mutation), colorectal (50% mutated) and thyroid (50% mutated) carcinomas, but are rare in breast and ovarian malignancy; presence of a point mutation on the K-*ras* codon 12 in pulmonary adenocarcinoma indicates a relatively poor prognosis, despite a lower clinical stage at time of diagnosis (N Engl J Med 1990; 323:561); see $p21^{ras}$

***ras* activation** Increased expression of the *ras* oncogene, which precedes clinical disease (Science 1990; 248:1101); when rats are exposed at birth to a carcinogen, nitrosomethylurea; high resolution restriction fragment length polymorphism analysis of a polymerase chain reaction-amplified *ras* sequence revealed H-*ras* and K-*ras* two weeks after the carcinogen treatment but two months before the onset of neoplasia; the oncogenes remain latent until the rats are exposed to estrogens, which is then followed by the development of mammary carcinoma; activated *ras* oncogenes occur in carcinomas of the lung, colon and pancreas as well as in well-defined precancerous lesions eg adenomas and myelodysplasia; progression to more malignant stages of disease requires activation of other oncogenes or deletion of growth suppressor gene; see Ruffling

Raspberry tongue A descriptor for the characteristic enanthema of scarlet fever, in which the tongue is bright red with edematous white papillae; Cf Strawberry tongue

'Raspberry' tumor A fanciful synonym for an intraductal papilloma of the breast, a pink, lobulated and cystic tumor attached to the walls of dilated ducts; the intraductal papilloma may simulate malignancy both clinically, as it often presents with hemorrhage of the nipple and pathologically, due to complexity of the cellular proliferation and loss of the myoepithelial cell layer

RAST Radioallergosorbent test A 'solid phase' radioisotopic method for detecting specific allergenic IgE antibodies in serum, similar to an agglutination test; the allergen-antigen complex is bound to an insoluble cyanogen-bromide activated paper disk and the patient's serum is added; sera containing the antibodies in question will complex to radioactive IgE; RAST correlates reasonably well with bronchial provocation testing; rare false positive RAST results from allergies to ragweed/grass, although RAST is neither more sensitive nor specific than skin testing, it avoids the risk of sensitization and anaphylaxis inherent to in vivo testing; see Mail-order medicine

Rat The rat, especially the Norway rat (*Rattus norvegicus*) has and continues to perform a yeoman's service in experimental medicine and biology; in the mid-nineteenth century, it was used for anatomy, physiology and nutrition; in the current experimental environment, rats have been inbred to select for desired feature(s), and strains exist that are of use for studying immunogenetics, transplantation, cancer-risk assessment, cardiovascular disease and behavior; 'rat work' is less expensive that working with larger mammals and rats have a shorter breeding time (Science 1989; 245:269rv), and are preferred by many to mice (which may be too small); Cf *Caenorhabditis elegans,* Guinea pig, Zebrafish; rats are vectors and/or reservoirs of disease, including Bunyavirus, the black plague and rat-bite fever

Rat-bite fever An acute febrile illness usually acquired from a rat bite which inoculates either *Streptobacillus moniliformis*, agent of Streptobacillary rat-bite fever, see Haverhill fever or *Spirillium minor*, agent of Spirillary rat-bite fever, see Sodoku

'Rat-bitten' kidneys A descriptor for kidneys with a renal cortex with one or more small jagged rat-bite-like umbilications on the surface after removing the capsule, which corresponds to one or more infarcts caused by arterionephrosclerosis

Ratchet phenomenon CELL BIOLOGY A term referring to terminal differentiation of cells, as occurs in adipocytes and peripheral neurons, which is a complex structural and functional process representing a point of 'no return'; for normal cells, dedifferentiation or 'simplification' is virtually impossible, while return to a more 'primitive' state is highly characteristic of malignant cells Note: A ratchet is a wrench that functions in only one direction

Rate-adjusted mortality index (RAMI) The expected in-hospital mortality rate based on actual in-hospital rates for diagnoses, grouped by their diagnosis-related group (DRG) code and adjusted for age, race, sex, the presence of co-morbidities and the principle operative procedure(s); increased RAMI values imply that the patient is more severely ill ***ab initio*** (J Am Med Assoc 1991; 265:374)

Rate-limiting step The slowest phase of a reaction, eg the step in a multi-enzyme cascade that sets the pace of the reaction

Rationing HEALTH CARE POLICY Allocation or distribution of a scarce product, commodity or service; the rationing of medical services is a major issue in the USA, in an era of mounting deficits and limited resources; the US health care system is the costliest in the world, consuming 11.3% of the gross national product and at the same time, is unequally distributed (J Am Med Assoc 1991; 265:105); legislative bodies are becoming increasingly involved in the dialog of how to implement a palatable form of health care rationing; see Health care rationing, Oregon plan

Rat tail tapering RADIOLOGY *BRONCHI* A descriptor for the abrupt loss of the normal arborization of the bronchus in bronchography as occurs in intraluminal neoplasms, in particular squamous cell carcinoma Note: This sign is rarely evoked in the era of computed tomography *HEART* A descriptor for a smooth progressive narrowing to a point of maximal stenosis of the left anterior descending coronary artery, seen by angiography; Cf Bridging *PANCREAS* A descriptor for relatively abrupt narrowing of the pancreatic duct in endoscopic retrograde cholangiopancreatography (ERCP), a finding suggestive of pancreatic adenocarcinoma

Raw data Notebook Data that is directly obtained from instrument read-outs, which has not been subjected to calculations, statistical analysis or classification; in research, it is critical to collect raw data consistently, ie in the same place and in a logical and ordered sequence, especially for those receiving US government grant monies, as raw data may be viewed as governmental property, subject to public scrutiny; see Notebook, Rs (three) of Research; Cf Fraud in science

Raw milk see Unpasteurized milk

RBC Red blood cell or erythrocyte

RBE see Relative biological effectiveness

RB gene Retinoblastoma gene A tumor suppressor gene located on chromosome 13q14 that encodes a 105 kD nuclear phosphoprotein with DNA-binding activity that regulates cell growth and is expressed in normal tissues and is phosphorylated during the S and G2-M phases of the cell cycle; some RB gene mutations encode in a protein that binds poorly, if at all to the regulatory site; malignancy is facilitated if the defect is homozygous; expression of normal RB protein in tumors is associated with a 60% five-year survival, while heterogeneous or decreased expression of the RB gene product is associated with a less than 30% survival (N Engl J Med 1990; 323:1467); RB gene defects are also seen in sarcomas, carcinoma of the breast and bladder and in small cell carcinoma of the lung; see Retinoblastoma, Tumor suppressor genes

R binder protein (RBP) One of two (the other is transcobalamin II) major extracellular vitamin B_{12} transporters that facilitate the absorption of the vitamin B_{12}/intrinsic factor complex by the intestinal mucosa and its subsequent transport to the liver; RBP may be increased in hepatocellular carcinoma and polycythemia vera; the 'R' designation refers to the rapid electrophoretic mobility of both transcobalamin I and transcobalamin III; transcobalamin II and RBP are immunologically identical but differ in the carbohydrate composition; congenital deficiency of RBP is extremely rare and may cause a multiple sclerosis-like clinical picture; Cf S protein

RBRVS see Resource-based relative value scale

RCA Red cell agglutination

RCF Relative centrifugal force

RDA see Recommended daily allowances

RDW Red blood cell distribution width An estimate of erythrocyte anisocytosis, which is a parameter generated by automated red cell counters, eg the Coulter counters and the Technicon H-6000, which is an aid in determining the cause of a given anemia (table)

RED CELL DISTRIBUTION WIDTH (RDW)

RDW	MCV	DISEASE STATE
Normal	▼	α or βthalassemia
▲	▼/N	Iron deficiency, hemoglobin H, S-β
▲	Normal	Aplastic anemia
▲	▲	Megaloblastic anemia (folate, vitamin B_{12} deficiencies)
N/▲	▲	Liver disease, myelotoxins, chronic lymphocytic and myelocytic leukemias, sickle cell anemia, hemoglobin SC, sideroblastic anemia, myelofibrosis, chemotherapy, mixed iron and vitamin B_{12} deficiency

MCV Mean corpuscular volume

Reactivation A generic term for the restoration of a cell or molecule's functional activity after photochemical, ultraviolet light or ionizing radiation-induced damage

Reactive hypoglycemia Plasma glucose measuring < 2.8 mmol/L (US: < 50 mg/dl) with symptoms of adrenergic neural activation, eg weakness, palpitations, tremor, sweating and hunger occurring after a meal or following oral glucose loading, caused by compensatory insulin hypersecretion

Reactive leukocytosis see Leukocytosis

Reactive marrow A nonspecific descriptor for a polyclonal response of the bone marrow to a local or systemic 'insult', often inflammatory in nature; marrow reactivity may be confined to one cell line, as in reactive granulocytosis, reactive mast cell hyperplasia or reactive thrombocytosis Note: The polyclonal nature of certain reactive hyperplasias, eg reactive histiocytosis, reactive lymphocytosis and reactive plasmacytosis may be difficult to distinguish from their malignant counterparts

Read MOLECULAR BIOLOGY The obtention of specific information from one nucleic acid's 'script' for the production of a) A complementary strand, as in transcription of mRNA from DNA, b) A duplicate strand, as in replication of DNA or c) A similar message, written in a different 'language', as in the translation of a protein from a mature mRNA transcript

Reading frame A segment of processed and mature mRNA that is capable of being translated into a polypeptide

Read-through The continuation of a) Transcription of DNA by RNA beyond the normal termination signal, due to the inability of the RNA polymerase to recognize the terminator or b) Translation of an RNA into a protein beyond the normal stop codon

Reagent red cells TRANSFUSION MEDICINE Commercially available erythrocytes that have common antigens (Rh-D, Rh-C, Rh-E, Rh-c, Rh-e, M, N, S, s, P_1, Le^a, Le^b, K, k, Fy^a, Fy^b, Jk^a, Jk^b) on their surfaces; these antigens are the ones most often implicated in potentially fatal hemolytic transfusion reactions, when they are transfused into patients having these antibodies in their serum; the presence of antibodies in the recipient's serum is detected by a 'major cross-match'

Reagin An obsolete generic term for IgE, referring to a) IgE as an initiator of the immediate hypersensitivity reaction and b) IgE as a non-specific antibody produced in syphilis that is directed against phosphatidylglycerol (cardiolipin) and measured by the VDRL slide flocculation test and RPR card agglutination, which may have a high false positive rate, see Biological false positivity; given the two unrelated uses of reagin, the term should be deleted from the medical vocabulary

'Real-time' imaging Visualization of a dynamic process within microseconds after its occurrence, a modality requiring very rapid information processing, ie as the process occurs, as in 'B' mode ultrasound; some ultrafast computers in computed tomography allow quasi-real time imaging Note: Certain imaging modalities such as fluoroscopic angiography and other fluoroscopic procedures are intrinsically 'real-time' but are not designated as real time

Reanneal MOLECULAR BIOLOGY The renaturation of DNA under experimental conditions, where complementary single strands are of 'self' origin, in contrast to an annealing reaction where the complementary single strands forming the duplex molecule are of different sources, ie hybrid molecules; see High-stringency hybridization, Low-stringency hybridization

Rearrangement see Gene rearrangement

Rebound insomnia Increased insomnia of greater duration than the baseline, which may appear if long-term therapy with hypnotics is abruptly stopped, an effect that is most intense with short-acting agents; see Insomnia

RecA protein(ase) A 38 kD protein with DNA-dependent ATPase activity that is pivotal in gene recombination and SOS repair; see SOS repair

Receptor An integral membrane-bound protein with a highly specific recognition or target site; when a ligand, eg an antigen, drug, hormone or virus binds to its respective receptor, the cell responds by activating a membrane-bound enzyme producing 'second messengers'; in the gastrointestinal tract two such activation pathways exist: 1) The adenylate cyclase/protein kinase pathway A pathway that is activated by cholera toxin, secretin and vasoactive intestinal peptide (VIP) and 2) The calcium-inositol-protein kinase C pathway, which is activated by acetylcholine, bombesin, cholecystokinin and substance P; the chief mechanism for down-regulating the number of receptors on a cell surface is endocytosis, ie internalization of the receptor-ligand complex, forming a receptosome Note: Many oncogenes encode proteins with receptor activity, including *fms* (which encodes colony-stimulating factor), *erb*B (which encodes epidermal growth factor receptor) and *erb*A (which encodes a thyroid hormone receptor in the nucleus); see Cyclic AMP, G proteins, Protein kinase C, Second messengers

Receptosome A receptor-ligand-laden coated pit that has budded from the cytoplasmic surface; reduction of receptor sites in this fashion serves to down-regulate the activity of a particular substance, eg low-density lipoprotein and lysosomal enzymes

Recertification Recredentialing GRADUATE MEDICAL EDUCATION A process that is currently in the planning stages in the USA, which will ultimately require physicians to prove periodically, eg every 7-10 years that they have maintained their medical knowledge and skills at a high level or standard of practice; this process is viewed as potentially providing a means of cost containment; how implementation of the recredentialing process would occur is uncertain and may include reexamination by the physician's specialty board or monitoring of the physician's methods for managing patients (J Am Med Assoc 1991; 265:752)

Receiver operating characteristic see ROC

Recognition A highly-specific binding interaction that occurs between macromolecules, eg antibody recognition of an antigen or that of tRNA with aminoacyl-tRNA synthetase

Recombinant DNA technology MOLECULAR BIOLOGY The constellation of techniques that comprise 'gene engineering', in which a gene producing a protein of interest from one organism is spliced into the genome of another organism, eg a phage DNA integrated into a plasmid is inserted into a 'carrier' bacterium; recombinant DNA technology entails three general steps: 1) Use of restriction endonucleases to obtain a fragment of DNA of interest 2) Joining or splicing the 'passenger' DNA fragment into a'vector' DNA and 3) Insertion of the recombinant hybrid molecule into an actively reproducing host cell, which generates multiple copies of the inserted gene per cell Note: Proteins produced in this manner are assigned a prefix of 'r', eg rIL-2 to indicate interleukin-2 produced by recombinant techniques in yeasts or bacteria; recombinant products are pure and lack the complications of animal-derived proteins, eg severe immune responses or potential mortality from human-derived products, eg human growth hormone that carried the risk of Creutzfeld-Jakob syndrome; see Genetic engineering, pBR322, Polymerase chain reaction

Recombinant pharmacology MOLECULAR THERAPEUTICS An emerging field in which recombinant DNA techniques are used to produce DNA-derived biological products for use in disease or to enhance a desired biologic function; such products include: α- and γ-interferons, interleukins, tissue plasminogen activator, epidermal, fibroblast, platelet-derived and transforming growth factors, erythropoietin, granulocyte-macrophage-colony stimulating factor, growth hormone, insulin, luteinizing hormone, superoxide dismutase, tumor necrosis factor and factor VIII (N Engl J Med 1990; 323:1800); see Biological response modifiers

Recombination A normal meiotic process in which the genes from two genetically distinct individuals are mixed, resulting in progeny that differ from both parents; recombination occurs in the form of crossing-over in humans and conjugation, transduction and transformation in lower organisms; see Recombinant DNA technology

Recombination repair see Sister chromatin exchange analysis

Recombination signal sequence (RSS) A DNA oligomeric 'motif' that is a necessary and sufficient signal for directing the recombination of immunoglobulins, consisting of a dyad-symmetric heptamer, an AT-rich nonamer and a spacing region of either 12 or 23 base pairs; RSSs flank all recombinationally competent V, D and J gene sequences; see RAG-1, V(D)J recombination

Recommended daily allowance (RDA) CLINICAL NUTRITION A guideline of essential nutrients that are recommended by the Food and Nutrition Board of the National Research Council for daily ingestion in an idealized normal person engaged in averge activities in a temperate environment for optimal nutrition, here in a 'standardized' 70 kg man: Vitamin A 1000 µg; vitamin D 5 µg; vitamin E 10 mg; vitamin C 60 mg; thiamine 1.2 mg; riboflavin 1.4 mg; niacin 16 mg; vitamin B_6 2.2 mg; folacin 400 µg; vitamin B_{12} 3 µg; Mineral: Calcium 800 mg; phosphorus 800 mg; magnesium 350 mg; iodine 150 mg; iron 10 mg; zinc 15 mg; the RDA must be adjusted upward during increased activity, body growth and size, pregnancy, lactation and environmental factors; the RDA are designed for a state of wellness and are poorly applicable in the sick, traumatized and burned

Reconstructive surgery A generic term for any surgical procedure that attempts to restore a tissue close to its original structure, as in cosmetic reconstructive surgery following a mastectomy or to its original functional state, or in a colostomy 'take-down', restoring a normal fecal flow; Cf Mutilating surgery

Recoverin A 23 kD cyclase protein that is central to the response of the eye to light and dark which has a key role in the recovery of the dark state; when recoverin is stripped of the calcium that binds at the so-called 'EF hand' sites, it activates guanylate cyclase, promoting the resynthesis of cylic GMP, which in turn opens the cation channels that were closed by light, thus restoring the dark state of the rod or cone (Science 1991; 251:915)

Red bag A red plastic bag that conforms to the standards required for the disposal of non-'sharp' and potentially infectious biohazardous waste by health care facilities; to 'Red-bag' is, by extension a verb Note: The fouling of beaches, along the Northeastern US coastline in the summer of 1988, with biological waste including blood collection tubes with viable HIV-1, resulted in stringent guidelines for disposal of all human-derived waste, requiring that it be placed in red bags for either 'in-house' incineration or transportation to landfills; see Biohazardous waste

'Red bone' A microscopic descriptor for dense, avascular bone seen in advanced otosclerosis which is markedly eosinophilic by the hematoxylin and eosin stain

'Red book' A publication generated by the committee on infectious diseases of the American Academy of Pediatrics, which contains the recommendations and immunization schedules for all licensed vaccines, information on hepatitis B control, hemophilus and measles, treatment of tuberculosis, guidelines on AIDS, recommendations and information on sexually-transmitted disease and infection control in day-care settings and hopitals, and is updated every 4 to 5 years

Red bugs Chiggers Microscopic chelicerate arthropods that pierce the skin producing intensely pruritic hemorrhagic and papular lesions

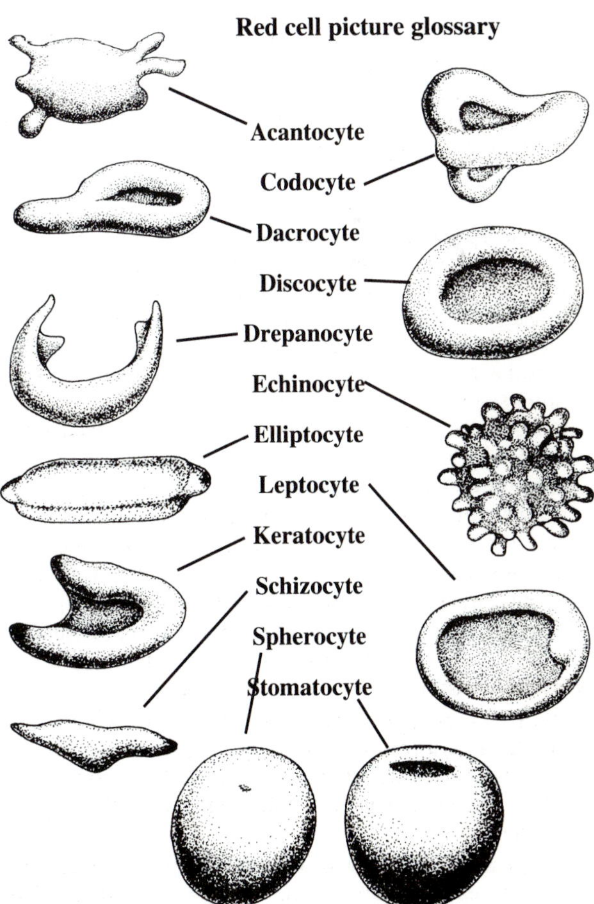

Red cell distribution width see RDW

Red cell fragmentation 'syndrome' A traumatic hemolytic condition caused by mechanical intravascular destruction of red cells by either a) Cardiac valve disease or prosthetic valves, accompanied by low serum haptoglobin, hemosiderinemia and defective red cells, eg schistocytes or b) Microangiopathic hemolytic anemia, which occurs in malignant hypertension, thrombotic thrombocytopenic purpura and disseminated carcinomatosis

Red cell 'flicker' MEMBRANE PHYSIOLOGY Thermally excited undulation of the red cell membrane that may be seen by phase-contrast microscopy; measurement of these undulations provides an estimate of erythrocytic elasticity, which may be markedly altered by alcohol ingestion, cholesterol loading and cross-linking agents

Red cell preservative(s) TRANSFUSION MEDICINE A medium designed to maintain a unit of packed red cells in a fluid state until the time of transfusion; the now-obsolete acid citrate dextrose (ACD) and citrate phosphate dextrose (CPD) allowed the units to be stored for 21 and 28 days respectively; the current generation of blood preservatives, citrate phosphate dextrose with adenine (CPDA) and additive solution (ADSOL) lengthen the viable shelf-life of packed red cells to 35 and 42 days respectively

Red Cross, American A relief agency founded in 1881 under a US congressional charter that fulfils American obligations in certain international treaties, serving members of the armed forces, veterans and families, aiding disaster victims, providing blood services, service opportunities and training of hospital volunteers Headquarters: Washington DC Budget: $796 million Staff: 20 200

Red Cross, International International Red Cross and Red Crescent Movement An international Geneva-based organization with circa 150 members, which 'endeavors to prevent and alleviate human suffering wherever it may be found, to protect life and health and to ensure respect for the human being; the organization is comprised of the International Committee of the Red Cross and the League of Red Cross (LRC) and Red Crescent Societies; the LRC is similar to that of the American Red Cross, with which it is directly affiliated and plays a major role in coordinating international disaster relief, providing care for refugees outside of conflict areas, health education, blood services and coordinates education efforts and pre-disaster planning; Cf Medicins sans Frontieres

Red degeneration Carnous degeneration A type of necrosis seen in uterine leiomyomas/fibromas that is thought to occur more commonly in pregnancy Histopathology Aseptic necrosis, autolysis, hemorrhage and acute inflammation

Red diaper 'syndrome' A rare form of gastroenteritis of early infancy caused by ***Serratia marcescens***, which produces a red pigment Treatment Sulfasalazine and gentamicin

Red eye An inflamed eye caused by conjunctivitis evoked by allergens, bacteria, viruses and air-born irritants or which is related to episcleritis, corneal ulcer (infectious or traumatic), uveitis, glaucoma (acute or chronic), cellulitis and others; Cf Pink-eye

Red fiber see Red muscle

'Red flag' LABORATORY MEDICINE An indicator, eg an asterisk that is generated when an analyte's value falls 'out of range', ie above or below a laboratory's predetermined values for normal; Cf Decision level, Panic value SCIENTIFIC JOURNALISM An article appearing in a peer-reviewed scientific journal which, when published, reaches startling conclusions that are likely to appear in the lay news media, eg Washington Post, New York Times, which are reported less for their scientific value than for their sensationalist impact (Science 1989; 243:733); 'Red flags' in medical journalism have included articles on the significance of vitamin C and the common cold (Proc Natl Acad Sci 1971; 68:2678, pancreatic cancer due to coffee consumption (N Engl J Med 1981; 304:603) and validation of the homeopathic principle (Nature 1988; 333:816); while a major component of journalistic excellence is newsworthiness, editors of major legitimate journals dislike 'red flag' papers as any erroneous conclusions reached by the paper's author(s) may compromise the journal's credibility; see 'Media epidemic'

Red gum disease Erythema toxicum neonatorum A benign relatively common condition that affects 4-77% of all neonates in the first week after delivery, consisting of intraoral erythema, generalized macules, papules and occasionally pustules associated with tissue eosinophilia; the condition was first described in ancient Mesopotamia between the Tigris and the Euphrates rivers Treatment Unnecessary; spontaneous resolution

Red 'hepatization' A descriptor for the pathological changes in the lung seen in well-developed lobar pneumonia, which is red (due to extravasation of erythrocytes) and liver-like (firm, carnose and dense due to the accumulation of fibrin), as well as friable due to the incipient necrosis

'Red herring' An unusual clinical, radiologic or pathologic finding that should be ignored in the context of a patient's disease presentation; the herring is a smoke-cured fish (***Clupidae rubis***) with a potent odor that has long had currency for training dogs to follow a scent along the ground, although the persistence of the odor may lead the tracking dog astray; by analogy, a 'red herring' is any detail that might side-track the diagnostician, which should be ignored; Cf 'Zebras'

'Red hot throat' A nonspecific descriptor for an erythematous, acutely inflamed oropharynx that may occur in various infections, including ***Streptococcus pyogenes, Neisseria gonorrheae, Corynebacterium diphtheriae, Bordatella pertussis*** and ***Haemophilus influenzae*** as well as various viral infections

Red infarct Focal necrosis that occurs in tissues with dual circulations, eg liver and lung, which is the direct result of venous thrombosis

Redlich's encephalitis see von Economo's encephalitis

'Red-lining' The practice of denying certain services to individuals in a municipality based on geographic differences that have been delineated by red lines on a city map; 'red-lining' is a practice common in real estate and was attempted in an area of San Francisco in a way that would have denied health benefits to AIDS patients; the responsible health maintenance organization was fined $250 000

Red man syndrome A centripetal maculopapular erythema of abrupt onset accompanied by hypotension that may occur after rapid intravenous infusion of vancomycin for gram-negative septicemia in neutropenic patients, resulting in a release of histamine causing flushing or cardiac arrest; the rash may involve the head and neck ('red neck' syndrome) or large areas of the body, and affect females ('red person' syndrome, J Am Med Assoc 1986; 55:2445c) and resolves spontaneously in minutes to hours (N Engl J Med 1988; 319:1053) Note: The designation 'Red man syndrome' has also been applied to rifampin overdose (Scot Med J 1975; 20:55); since this condition causes an orange discoloration, the term Orange person syndrome appears preferable, although both may act by a similar mechanism

Red mouth disease An infection of trout and salmon by *Yersinia ruckerii*

Red muscle CELL PHYSIOLOGY One of the two main types of skeletal muscle, which corresponds to the 'dark' meat of chickens and contains abundant mitochondria and myoglobin; these fibers, also known as 'slow-twitch' fibers, contract and fatigue more slowly than white fibers and generate ATP by aerobic catabolism of glucose and fats, utilizing myoglobin-bound oxygen; see White muscle

Red neck syndrome see Red man syndrome

Red neuron A histopathologic finding in infarcts of the central nervous system; 6-12 hours after the onset of ischemia, neurons are swollen and display nuclear disintegration, the cell bodies are triangular with a dark blue nucleus and dense bright pink cytoplasm, resulting in myelin sheath disintegration, cell death, loss of astrocytes and oligodendrocytes

'Red nose syndrome' see WC Fields' nose

Red nucleus Nucleus ruber NEUROANATOMY A prominent egg-shaped mass in the tegmentum of the midbrain that extends from the caudal limit of the superior colliculus and receives deep cerebellar fibers from the superior cerebellar peduncle and some fibers from the frontal cortex and projects to the tegmentum, forming the rubroreticular tract, to the caudal region becoming the rubrospinal tract and to the lateral ventral nucleus of the thalamus

'Red out' A homogeneous red-orange color seen by gastrointestinal endoscopy when the intestinal mucosa is directly covering the endoscope's lens, allowing only the passage of light across the blood vessel-rich mucosa; red-out can be corrected by a puff of air to push the mucosa away from the visual field

Red pulp A histologically distinct zone of the spleen that is separated from the white pulp by the marginal zone of lymphocytes; the red pulp is composed of Billroth's cords, a non-endothelialized region of slow passage of circulating red cells, where local hypoxia, low pH and low glucose cause stress on senescent, damaged or otherwise effete erythrocytes (table); see White pulp

RED PULP FUNCTIONS

Conditioning Readying of reticulocytes for the rigors of circulation, ieremoval of up to 30% of the membrane and pitting of the last few residual mitochondria

Culling Macrophage-induced removal of red cells erythrocytes from the microcirculation which have defective membrane proteins, crystallized cytoplasm or other defects

Pitting Removal of erythrocytic inclusions, including: Howell-Jolly bodies (residual DNA), Heinz bodies (precipitated hemoglobin) and parasites (malaria, leishmaniasis)

Reutilization of iron After hemolysis, iron is stored in the macrophages

Red pulp disease(s) A generic term for any infiltrative process of the spleen that preferentially affects the red pulp, including chronic myelogenous leukemia, heavy chain disease, iron deficiency, hairy cell leukemia, malignant histiocytosis, rheumatoid arthritis; Gaucher's disease completely effaces the splenic architecture and histiocytic lymphoma affects both the red and white pulp; see White pulp diseases

'Red tape rationing' Limitation of access to a service through inconvenience, where 'red tape' is the paperwork generated in a bureaucratic system, which forms a major impediment to efficiency; in the US health care industry, the amount of red tape required to justify a person's admission to hospital, treatment or continued hospitalization in the face of complications becomes enormous and has been viewed as a form of health care rationing by 'red tape'

Red tide A body of sea water with high concentrations of dinoflagellates, in which massive algal proliferation imparts a reddish color to the sea surface, described in the gulf of Maine (USA); under optimal salinity, temperature and nutrient conditions, the marine algae, *Gonyaulax catanella* and *G tamarensis* proliferate, producing saxitoxin (a potent neuromuscular toxin that blocks voltage-dependent sodium channels in neurons), which is concentrated in clams and shellfish (but not in lobster and finned fish); birds and mammals feeding on these shellfish rapidly develop neuromuscular blockade with intense centripetal paresthesias, nausea, vomiting, diarrhea, later vertigo, numbness of the face and scalp, sensory loss, dysphagia, dysarthria and intention tremor; if severe, intoxication may cause flaccid quadriplegia or respiratory paralysis (death); treatment is supportive Note: Not all red tides are toxic and some outbreaks of 'red tide disease' occur without the red tide; *Gymnodinium breve* causes red tide off Florida and the region surrounding the Gulf of Mexico, but evokes milder neurotoxic reactions, including paresthesias, abnormal temperature sensation, ataxia, nausea, vomiting and diarrhea; Cf 'King-Kong' peptide

'Red tide' INFECTIOUS DISEASE A colloquial phrase from the 1950s that died in the 1960s, referring to the fact that many bacterial infections were gram-negative, ie 'red', an observation attributed to the virtually indiscriminate use of the first widely available antibiotic, penicillin (which is most effective against gram-positive coccal bacteria) for every conceivable infection, resulting in a relative increase in the incidence of infections by gram-negative bacteria, which are pink by the gram stain, causing a 'red' shift; this imbalance shifted towards equilibrium with the availability of aminoglycosides, which are more effective against gram-negative bacteria

Reducing atmosphere A humid atmosphere rich in oxidizable gases including hydrogen, hydrogen sulfide, nitrogen, ammonia and methane that is thought to have existed on the primitive earth of 4.5 billion BC; Cf Primordial soup

Reducing sugars Disaccharides that are linked with an aldehyde or ketone group and the hydroxyl group of another nonreducing sugar, eg galactose, lactose, glucose, maltose, fructose and pentose; reducing sugars are formed by action of amylase on starch and measured by reduction of phosphomolybdate, ferricyanide or 3,5-dinitrosalicylate; the presence of reducing sugars suppresses β hemolysis, therefore should not be used in tests for identifying streptococci; assays for reducing sugars may be false positive by the copper reduction test, in the presence of uric acid, creatinine, homogentisic acid, nalidixic acid and probenecid

Reductionism A philosophy that higher levels of (often arbitrary) complexity can be understood through reduction to their simplest components; see Lumping; Cf Splitting

Red urine disease(s) Those clinical conditions associated with red urine (a term of little diagnostic utility), which include hematuria secondary to glomerulonephritides, bladder tumors, foreign bodies or calculi, infection, inflammation, thrombosis and conditions that may be diagnosed by examining the urinary sediment; less common causes of red urine include trauma-related myoglobinuria or hemoglobinuria, congenital erythropoietic porphyria, porphyria cutanea tarda, acute intermittent porphyria, pyrrolinuria, ingestion of beets, phenol sulfonphthalein, fuchsin, aniline dyes in candy and food, anthraquinolone laxatives if the urine is alkaline, desferroxamine, rifampin, isoniazid and under unusual circumstances, aspirin

Re-entry CARDIOLOGY A common cause of paroxysmal atrial or supraventricular arrhythmia, which is coupled to premature ventricular depolarization; for re-entry to exist, there must be a one-way complete block in conduction, coupled to tissues, eg scar tissue that responds more slowly to electrical impulses arriving from 'the other end'; once begun, re-entrant arrhythmias are self-sustaining; re-entry may be ordered (ie the circuit for the re-entry is constant) or random (the re-entry circuits are variable in duration and location)

Re-entry tear VASCULAR SURGERY The most distal intimal tear seen in a dissecting aortic aneurysm, a point that is presumed to be the site where the blood returns to the circulation

Reference range LABORATORY MEDICINE A set of values established as reasonable maximums or minimums for a given analyte; in order for a laboratory to produce accurate results, ie control its quality, it must be certain that the normal results are consistent and fall within the range of 'normalcy' and that abnormal results fall outside of that reference range, which is usually two or more standard deviations above or below a laboratory's mean; most laboratories pool sera from patients who have 'normal' values for the analyte being measured; in establishing the reference range 1) The reference subjects should be normal, healthy and, if indicated, subdivided into various age-groups, sex, occupation, ethnic origin or other parameter 2) The laboratory should use a consistent protocol, in which the precision, reliability and accuracy are delineated, preferably on the same instrument; the sample should be obtained under 'standard' conditions, ie pre- or post-prandial, similar volume, where each test tube has a standard amount of anticoagulant and thus differences in volume would yield differences in coagulation studies 3) The range for the reference value should be broad enough to encompass the vast majority of normal subjects 4) The statistical methodology and decisions for 'tail cutoffs' must be clearly and logically delineated 5) The range must allow for updating of patient pool, new clinical data and new methodologies; Cf Decision levels, Panic values

'Referral' North American colloquialism for a patient who has been referred for a second opinion or therapy to a specialist or subspecialist with greater expertise, as the patient has a disease or condition that the primary or referring physician is incapable of or does not wish to treat

Referral center see Tertiary care

Referral center bias Any skewing in morbidity or mortality statistics based on data generated from referral centers, which may not be representative of the entire population (Mayo Clin Proc 1990; 65:1185); see 'Institutional effect'

Referred pain Pain that is localized to a region other than that which is the site of disease, eg pain from a myocardial infarct is classically referred to the jaw and upper arm

Refining CLINICAL NUTRITION The processing of a food substance to extract a component of interest, usually referring to the refining of sugar; health and natural food advocates are highly critical of this process and tout beet sugar, molasses and honey to be far superior to refined or 'white' sugar, although the nutritive value of the 'virgin' products in terms of trace minerals and vitamins is minimal; see 'Health' food, Organic food

Refractive surgery OPHTHALMOLOGY A surgical technique performed on the cornea, which corrects myopia by changing the cornea's conformation; two procedures are currently available **RADIAL KERATOTOMY** A procedure in which a diamond knife (cost of equipment, $2500) is used to make incisions at the edge of the cornea, flattening it, but weakening its overall structure and **PHOTOREACTIVE KERATECTOMY**A technique that is still regarded by insurance carriers as investigational, ie not reimbursed by insurance carriers; in photoreactive keratectomy, an excimer laser (cost of equipment, ranges from $300 to 500 000) cuts concentric circles in the cornea, 'photoshaving' the center of the cornea, imparting a more homogenous consistency

Refractory anemia with excess blasts see PISA

Refrigerator 'AIDS' (RAIDS) A laboratory artifact consisting in an inversion of the ratio of T helper to T suppressor cells (T4:T8 or CD4:CD8 ratio), which occurs when flow cytometric specimens are refrigerated prior to analysis, causing a relative decrease in the CD4+ T cells (N Engl J Med 1983; 309:435c); see AIDS, Helper:suppressor ratio

Refugee A person who, owing to a well-founded fear of being persecuted for reasons of race, religion, nationality, membership in a particular social group or political opinion is compelled to live outside of the country of his nationality; refugees may also be those fleeing from war, civil disturbance and violence of any kind; a permutation is that of an 'internally displaced' person who moves within the borders of one country for the same, above-mentioned reasons; the mortality rate of refugees is 60-fold greater than that of a similar non-displaced population, is highest in children and is due to measles, diarrhea-related illnesses, acute upper respiratory tract infections, malaria and is in part related to the virtually endemic protein-energy malnutrition and micronutrient deficiencies that characterize the refugee state (J Am Med Assoc 1990; 263:3296); see Amnesty International, Red Cross; Cf Disaster, Homeless-(ness), Torture

Regan isoenzyme A variant alkaline phosphatase first identified in a patient name Regan, a young caucasian male who died from bronchogenic carcinoma metastatic to the lymph nodes, adrenal glands, spleen, kidney and brain; the Regan isoenzyme is a heat-stable, L-phenylalanine-sensitive carcinoplacental enzyme, similar to placental alkaline phosphatase in electrophoretic mobility which occurs in circa 5% of carcinomas as well as occasionally in normal subjects

Regeneration PHYSIOLOGY The sum total of activities leading to regrowth of cells and tissues; tissues with a high rate or potentially high rate of regeneration, include bone marrow, gastrointestinal tract, liver and skin; 'stable' populations with a low rate of regeneration include the adrenal gland, kidney, liver, lymph nodes, pancreas, thyroid gland; neural tissue and cartilage are regarded as non-regenerative

Regionalization The subdividing of a broadly available service, eg a blood bank, into quasi-autonomous regional centers that are able to make decisions and provide better and/or faster service to hospitals and health care facilities that are located the greatest distance from a 'centralized' service's hub

Regression see Linear regression

Regression line STATISTICS A line that defines the amount of change in one variable per unit change in the other; see Linear regression

Regressively transformed germinal centers SURGICAL PATHOLOGY A finding of uncertain significance in which germinal centers in lymph nodes are small, have onion-skin-like layering, are devoid of lymphocytes and composed of dendritic reticulum cells, vascular endothelial cells and hyalinized PAS-positive intercellular material; see Germinal centers; Cf Progressively transformed germinal centers

Regulated waste Waste products that must be handled in a specified fashion in accordance with governmental regulations; regulated waste can be divided into **1)** **BIOHAZARDOUS WASTE** Potentially dangerous infectious agents, often originating from health care facilities and/or research laboratories; these waste products place a relatively small or confined group of people at risk for infection during the time necessary for the infectious agent to desiccate or otherwise become inactive; see Biohazardous waste, 'Sharps' **2)** **RADIOACTIVE BYPRODUCTS** from clinical and research laboratories or power stations that emit radiation ranging from low-level and virtually innocuous α particles to high-level γ-radiation emitting products that must be stored decades or centuries in specialized vaults and **3)** **NON-BIODEGRADABLE CHEMICALS**, including heavy metals, dioxins, halogenated biphenyls, terphenyls, naphthalenes, dibenzodioxins and related products that are toxic to biological systems in very low (parts per million or parts per billion) concentrations, originating from a vast array of manufacturing processes, which unlike biohazardous waste, create problems from the 'cradle to the grave', requiring special precautions during manufacture, storage, shipping, consumption and disposal; since many of these chemicals are lipid-soluble, they may store for long periods in the adipose tissues of workers handling these products

Regulator gene R gene A gene that encodes a DNA-binding protein repressor that controls an operator site on the DNA

Regulatory agency A generic term for any organization or body of a federal, state or local government that creates and enforces rules concerning the delivery of a service; see Environmental Protectional Agency, OSHA (Occupational Safety and Health Administration)

Regulatory proteins MOLECULAR BIOLOGY Proteins that were first discovered in bacteria, which bind to specific regulatory sites in DNA and are crucial in controlling transcription; the structural motifs and chemical modifications that convert the inactive to active forms of regulatory proteins, eg chain cleavage, methylation and phosphorylation, are similar at all levels of phylogenic differentiation

Rehydration solution Any fluid that is used to treat severe bacterial (eg, *Vibrio cholerae*, *Escherichia coli*) or viral (eg, Rotavirus) diarrhea; these conditions are rarely accompanied by systemic disease other than the severe prostration inherent in massive fluid loss, and are usually the result of intestinal cyclic AMP cyclase having been been locked into an 'on' position, which causes a flushing phenomenon that responds only to time and appropriate fluid replacement (antibiotics are rarely useful); two types of solutions are available, glucose-based, which increases intestinal resorption of fluids and electrolytes, and rice-syrup-based solution, which in addition decreases the stool output, and therefore would appear to be the agent of choice (N Engl J Med 1991; 324:517)

Reimbursement Payment by a third-party, eg an insurance company, to a hospital or other health care provider for services rendered to an insured person (beneficiary)

Rejection An immune reaction evoked by allografted organs; the prototypic rejection occurs in renal transplantation, which is subdivided into three clinico-pathologic stages: **HYPERACUTE REJECTION** Onset within minutes of anastomosis of blood supply; the kidneys are soft, cyanotic with stasis of blood in the glomerular capillaries, segmental thrombosis, necrosis, fibrin thrombi in glomerular tufts, interstitial hemorrhage, leukocytosis, erythrocyte stasis, mesangial cell swelling, deposition of IgG, IgM, C3 in arterial walls **ACUTE REJECTION** Onset 2-60 days after transplantation, with interstitial vascular endothelial cell swelling, interstitial accumulation of lymphocytes, plasma cells, immunoblasts, macrophages, neutrophils; tubular separation with edema/necrosis of tubular epithelium; swelling and vacuolization of the endothelial cells, vascular edema, bleeding and inflammation, renal tubular necrosis, sclerosed glomeruli, tubular 'thyroidization' **CHRONIC REJECTION** Onset is late (often more than 60 days after transplantation, and frequently accompanied by acute changes superimposed, increased mesangial cells with myointimal proliferation and crescent formation; mesangioproliferative glomerulonephritis; see Cyclosporin A, FK 506, Graft-versus-host disease

Rejuvenation solution TRANSFUSION MEDICINE A solution that may be used to salvage outdated O-positive and O-negative red cells, which can then be glycerolized and frozen for future use; one such solution, PIPA,contains pyruvate, inosine, phosphate and adenine, which after a one-hour incubation at 37°C, 'restores' ATP and 2,3-diphosphoglycerate (2,3-DPG) levels to 150% of the levels at the time of donation; see Red cell preservatives, Storage lesion(s)

Relapse Recrudescence of a malignancy, often leukemia; in acute lymphocytic leukemia, the most common sites of relapse are bone marrow, testes and central nervous system; aggressive treatment of these sites (eg intrathecal) at the time of initial diagnosis is held responsible for the relatively high cure rate in leukemia; 80% of children and 50% of adults with a relapse of acute lymphocytic leukemia may achieve a second, albeit short-lived remission and some may be cured; see Bone marrow transplantation, Chemotherapy, Cyclophosphamide, Remission

Relapsing fever Cabin fever, vagabond fever, bilious typhoid, fowlnest Epidemic borreliosis (*B recurrentis, B hemisi, B turicatae, B parkeri* and others) is louse-born (*Pediculus humanis*) **Clinical** History of recent outdoor camping, fevers with 'negative' blood cultures, Jarisch-Herxheimer-like hypotensive 'crises' following therapy with antibiotics and thrombocytopenia Endemic borreliosis is transmitted by ticks (*Ornithodoros* spp) that inject borrelia during a blood meal **Clinical** Abrupt onset of high fever, headache, photophobia, nausea, vomiting, myalgias, arthralgias, abdominal pain, a productive cough and minimal respiratory distress; late relapses typically involve the central nervous system (meningismus, peripheral neuritis, cranial nerve paralysis) **Treatment** Tetracycline, erythromycin, chloramphenicol

Relapsing polychondritis An uncommon condition characterized by inflammation and cartilaginous degeneration, beginning about age 40 **Clinical** Fever, vasculitis and arthropathy **Diagnosis** Three or more of the following symptoms (in descending order of frequency): Auricular chondritis with ear drooping, non-erosive arthritis, nasal chondritis with saddle nose deformity, upper respiratory obstruction, audiovestibular symptoms and cardiovascular disease, eg aortic insufficiency **Prognosis** 74% five-year and 55% ten-year survival

Relative biological effectiveness (RBE) RADIATION BIOLOGY The ratio of the effect that one form of ionizing radiation has on a biological system to that of an identical dose of a different form of ionizing radiation, a value of interest since equal doses of different types, eg neutrons, γ and X-rays, of ionizing radiation do not produce equal biological effects, eg if 6 Gy of X-rays and 4 Gy of neutrons are lethal to a biological system, then the RBE is 1.5; the former standard used to compare different radiations was 250 kV X-rays, chosen at the time of standardization, as it was the only level widely available Note: Although this value is firmly entrenched in the literature, it suffers from problems of comparison

Relative bradycardia see Pulse-temperature dissociation

Relative tachycardia see Pulse-temperature dissociation

Relative value scale see Resource-based relative value scale

Relative risk see Risk

Relaxation MOLECULAR BIOLOGY Any conversion of a system to a state requiring less energy, eg the conversion of a supercoiled DNA molecule to a non-twisted form or the return of muscle to a ground state; Cf Protein folding

Relaxed helix A double-stranded circular DNA molecule in which the supercoils have been reduced in number by a topoisomerase

Relaxin An insulin-like polypeptide that is produced by the corpus luteum and relaxes parturition-related ligaments at the symphysis pubis and sacroiliac junctions, and softens the uterine cervix during pregnancy

Releasing factor Releasing hormone

Relman's criteria see Authorship

'Relman revision' MEDICAL JOURNALISM A modification by former editor of the New England Journal of Medicine (NEJM), Arnold S Relman, MD, of the Ingelfinger rule of medical journalism, which required a news media 'blackout' until the time an article is published in the NEJM; Relman modified the Ingelfinger rule to allow early release of critical information with great potential impact on patient management prior to formal publication in the NEJM (Am Med News 11/Mar/91); see Embargo arrangement, Ingelfinger rule; Cf Clinical alert

rem Roentgen-equivalent in man A unit of absorbed radiation, approximately equal to a rad or 0.01 Seivert; see Gray, Sievert

REM see REM sleep

Remission ONCOLOGY The regression of symptoms or lesions in a malignancy, most commonly referring to the disappearance of a lympho- or myeloproliferative tumor by radio- or chemotherapy and amelioration of clinical symptoms, which may be temporary, partial or complete; a complete remission of long enough duration, eg two years in childhood lymphocytic leukemia, is termed 'permanent remission' or cure, the goal of therapy for all malignancies; leukemia therapy hinges on a) Induction of remission, which is attainable in more than 90% of children and 50% of adults with acute lymphocytic leukemia, using a combination of vincristine, prednisone and doxorubicin b) Central nervous system (CNS) prophylaxis The first site of relapse in most children is the CNS, an event largely prevented by 24 grays (2400 rads) of prophylactic radiotherapy, often in combination with intrathecal methotrexate Note: When parenteral vincristine and intrathecal methotrexate are administered in the same therapeutic session, there is a real danger of inadvertent switching of syringes and intrathecal administration of vincristine, an error that is well-described in the world literature and universally fatal, regardless of how quickly intrathecal 'washout' begins and c) Maintenance Continuation, consolidation or intensification (oftherapy); in acute lymphocytic leukemia, standard maintenance regimens include cycles of methotrexate, 6-mercaptopurine and 'pulses' of remission-inducing agents; see Cure; Cf Relapse

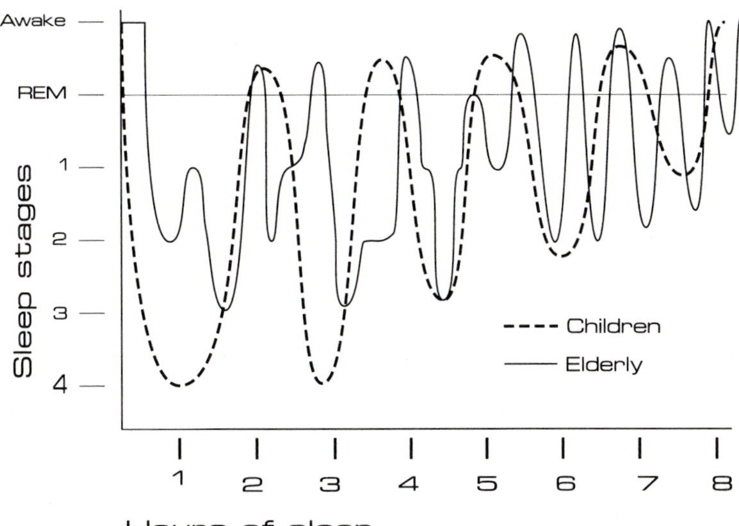

Remnant removal disease see Hyperlipoproteinemia, type III

REM sleep Rapid eye movement sleep A segment of the normal sleep cycle in which the usual high-amplitude slow brain waves seen by EEG are replaced by rapid eye movement, rapid, low-voltage irregular EEG activity, a pattern similar to that seen in an awake and alert subject, also known as paradoxical or desynchronized sleep, which is further characterized by loss of skeletal muscle tone due to an increase in activity of the reticular inhibiting area of the medulla and clusters of large phasic potentials originating in the pons (pontogeniculooccipital spikes); in the fetus, REM sleep predominates and may switch to the cyclical pattern as early as two days after birth (figure above demonstrates an increase in volatility of sleep with age); see Insomnia, Sleep disorders

'Re' mutant(s) INFECTIOUS DISEASE A family of mutant gram-negative bacteria that lack all or most of the polysaccharides in the terminal and core regions of the endotoxins; survival in non-immunized patients with gram-negative septicemia correlates with the levels of anti-'Re' lipopolysaccharide antibodies

Renal agenesis A rare disease of infants characterized by bilateral renal agenesis, low-set floppy ears, a broad, flat nose and pulmonary hypoplasia; these infants die within hours after birth; infants with unilateral renal agenesis have normal lung development and are asymptomatic in the neonatal period

'Renal' glycosuria A relatively common (1:500) autosomal recessive condition in which glycosuria occurs without hyperglycemia, is unrelated to diet, the subjects are asymptomatic, have a normal glucose tolerance test and utilization and storage of carbohydrates, but may become transiently ketotic in stress or pregnancy

Renal panel see Kidney panel

Renal tubular acidosis (RTA) A condition caused by functional defects in the distal renal tubules, with loss of

Renal tubular acidosis (RTA)

Type I RTA is the 'classic' distal RTA, due to a selective defect in distal tubule acidification, resulting in a pH gradient defect with hyperchloremia (with persistent bicarbonate excretion), hypokalemia , moderate metabolic acidosis and an inappropriately high (> 6) urinary pH

Type II RTA is due to defective proximal tubule acidification; when the blood pH is decreased, tubular acidification occurs normally; when plasma bicarbonate normalizes, type II RTA wastes bicarbonate, causing metabolic acidosis, hyperchloremia and hypokalemia, which may be accompanied by the Fanconi syndrome; these patients are prone to osteopenia and rickets

'Type III RTA' is a designation formerly applied to infants with renal bicarbonate wasting, now thought to be a subtype of type I RTA

Type IV RTA corresponds to generalized (nonselective) distal RTA, which is due to aldosterone deficiency or antagonism; hyperchloremia, hyperkalemia, metabolic acidosis and salt wasting

ability to form ammonia and to exchange hydrogen cations; the glomerular filtration rate is normal with persistent metabolic acidosis and hyperchloremia, there is marked decrease in urinary excretion of acid **Laboratory** Acidic urine with acidosis, low bicarbonate excretion, poor ammonium clearance and increased clearance of potassium (table)

Renaturation The reforming of a molecule's native configuration after it has been altered by environmental pressures, eg high salt or temperatures

Renin PHYSIOLOGY highly-specific aspartyl proteinase with one substrate, angiotensinogen; renin is secreted by the granular cells of the juxtaglomerular apparatus in response to a reduction in renal perfusion pressure and converts angiotensinogen to angiotensin I (a decapeptide), which is the precursor of angiotensin II (an octapeptide) and angiotensin III (a heptapeptide), the latter two of which are potent vasoconstrictors, stimulating thirst and increasing aldosterone production; renin secretion is increased in tumors, malignant hypertension, during increased secretion of CRF (corticotropin-releasing factor), Cushing's disease **Treatment** Estrogens and vasodilators; see Hypertension

Renovascular hypertension (RVH) Systemic hypertension due to renal artery obstruction by atherosclerosis, fibroplastic disease, aneurysms and embolism; see Goldblatt kidney; RVH has a wide range of effects, causing hemorrhage in the cerebellum, pons, internal capsule and basal ganglia **ESSENTIAL HYPERTENSION** The kidneys display granularity of cortical surface, and are hisstologically characterized by hyaline atherosclerosis in afferent glomerular capsular arteries, which later become tortuous, thick-walled and narrowed, thus becoming a source of chronic ischemia, which is accompanied by 'piecemeal' necrosis of glomeruli **MALIGNANT HYPERTENSION** The kidneys grossly display 'Rat-bite' scars, and are histologically characterized by arterionephrosclerosis and glomerular capillary necrosis with thrombosis (necrotizing glomerulonephritis), as well as 'flea-bitten' kidneys, with acute glomerular rupture with pinpoint fibrinoid necrosis (hypertensive arteriolitis), petechial hemorrhages on cortical surface, fibrinoid necrosis of the distal interlobular 'onion-skinned' arteries and afferent arterioles with thrombosis, juxtaglomerular apparatus hyperplasia (also seen in acute and chronic glomerulopathies, hypertension, diabetes mellitus and polycystic kidney disease) **Treatment, medical** Empirical, as a function of the severity of disease and a patient's individual response to the available agents, which include diuretics, β-adrenergic blockers, vasodilators and angiotensin-converting enzyme **Treatment, interventional** Percutaneous transluminal angioplasty of the renal artery, 60-70% success rate in atherosclerosis; 90% success rate in fibromuscular hyperplasia

Reovirus A family of naked (non-enveloped), 1-4.0 kilobase double-stranded RNA viruses, which includes orthoreovirus, orbivirus and rotavirus. which are uncommon causes of gastroenteritis, rhinopharyngitis, occasionally hepatitis and rarely, encephalitis, pneumonia and Colorado tick fever; see Rotavirus

Repeats see Repetitious DNA

Repertoire The array of molecules (or capabilities) that are inherent, but not necessarily expressed in a system, a term most commonly used in immunology, referring to the broad responsiveness to specific antigenic signals that both B and T lymphocytes have as a result of the different combinations of genes (variable, diversity, joining) that can be spliced together to create the exquisitely specific immunoglobulins (B cells) or T cell receptors (T cells)

Repetitious DNA Repetitive DNA Segments of DNA that are similar in sequence to each other; 'highly repetitious' segments of DNA, are short (5-10 nucleotides) oligomers, virtually identical in sequence to each other and present in thousands to millions of copies per genome, usually as non-functional or 'spacer' DNA; these short, identical DNA fragments, also known as simple sequence DNA, comprise 10-15% of the genome;'intermediate repeats' are moderately repetitious segments of DNA comprising 25-40% of the genome, ranging from 150-300 nucleotides to 6000 nucleotides in length, known as SINES or LINES for short or long interspersed elements and are present in up to several hundred copies per genome; the repeated DNA that encodes rRNA, tRNA and histones is known as Tandem repeat DNA

Replicating fork MOLECULAR BIOLOGY A Y-shaped region in a replicating DNA molecule where there is separation of the parent strands of DNA and synthesis of daughter chains; see Okazaki fragments, Replicating bubble

Replication The process of synthesizing a daughter DNA molecule from a parent DNA 'template', which for the double-stranded DNA typical of eukaryotes, occurs during the S phase of the cell cycle in a bidirectional fashion; the DNA is unwound from histones, separated by a helicase into single connected strands of DNA from which a leading and continuous daughter strand of DNA grows in the 3' ➔ 5' direction, mediated by DNA polymerase; the lagging and discontinuous daughter strand uses the opposite parent DNA strand as a template, also grows in the 3' ➔ 5' direction and requires the action of a DNA polymerase, a primase and a ligase to join the short daughter strands, known as Okazaki fragments; see Lagging strand, Leading strand, Meselson-Stahl experiment, Okazaki fragments

Replication bubble(s) Replication eye(s) MOLECULAR BIOLOGY One of multiple transiently expressed bead-like structures that are seen by electron microscopy along a segment of double-stranded DNA, corresponding to multiple sites of simultaneous DNA replication, where each of the bubbles corresponds to growing forks of daughter DNA with replication of double-stranded DNA occurring in both directions simultaneously; see Replicating fork

Replicon The functional unit of replication, which contains an initiator locus, the site where RNA polymerase binds and produces an RNA primer known as an initiator and a replicator locus, the replication initiating site

Reportable occupational disease Reportable event PUBLIC HEALTH A generic term for an occupational or environmentally-related morbid condition that a local, state or federal government wishes to maintain under surveillance; each of the United States has occupational diseases of particular interest, which often overlap, including asbestosis, bronchitis and acute pulmonary edema due to fumes and vapors, byssinosis, caisson's disease, coal worker's and other pneumoconioses, heavy metal, lead, pesticide and radiation poisoning, intoxication with acid, alkali, antimony, benzene, beryllium, cadmium, chlorinated hydrocarbons, chlorine, chromium, Freon™, hydrogen cyanide, manganese, mercury, petroleum products, other solvents and sulfur dioxide), pulmonary fibrosis, silicosis (J Am Med Assoc 1989; 262:3041); non-occupational events that require reporting to central health authorities include AIDS, child abuse, drug addiction, venereal disease, (gunshot or stab) wounds; for reportable infectious disease, see Notifiable disease

Reporter gene A gene, the phenotype of which is relatively easy to monitor, that may be used to study promoter activity at different points in an organism's development; in recombinant DNA technology, reporter genes may be attached to a promoter region of interest

Reproductive history OBSTETRICS A set of four numbers that may be used to define a woman's obstetric history eg 4-3-2-1, would mean four term infants delivered, three preterm infants, two abortions, one child currently living; since this system leads to confusion, it is recommended that only parity and gravidity be used, supplemented with gestational information where relevant

Reptation LABORATORY TECHNOLOGY The movement of a substance in a snake-like fashion; reptation occurs in the high-voltage gel electrophoresis of large DNA molecules, and refers to the loss of the sieving effect, which introduces drag to molecules that is proportional to their length, thereby allowing separation of molecules according to size; at a certain length of molecule, the sieving effect falls off, and molecules begin to migrate at similar speeds, regardless of size, and 'reptate' through the ge; see Field inversion electrophoresis

Reptilase time HEMATOLOGY The time that reptilase, an enzyme from ***Bothrops atrox*** venom, requires to cleave fibrinopeptide A, a value that is increased in hypofibrinogenemia < 0.8 g/L (US <80 mg/dl), dysfibrinogenemia and disseminated intravascular coagulopathy, but not by heparin-induced coagulopathy

Reserve cell hyperplasia GYNECOLOGIC CYTOLOGY A proliferation of cuboidal subcolumnar cells under the squamocolumnar junction of the uterine cervix; reserve cells appear early in the cervix of infants and are thought to be the cell at risk for malignant degeneration in squamous cell carcinoma of the uterine cervix

Residual bodies Aggregates of undigested granular or coarsely laminated material seen by electron microscopy within lysosomes in a wide variety of clinical conditions, including sea-blue histiocytosis, granular cell myoblastoma and in changes associated with aging, eg lipofuscin deposition

Residency A period of formal graduate medical education that consists of on-the-job training of medical school graduates, which is sponsored by and takes place in a teaching hospital; residencies often follow a one-year internship, are from two to six years in duration and precede a fellowship; a completed period of residency is required for certification by specialty boards; see Fellowship, GME, Internship; Cf CME (continuing medical education)

Residue Amino acid residue BIOCHEMISTRY The functional portion of a monomeric 'unit' that is present in a polymer, which lacks the atoms removed during the polymerization process, analagous to a building block without the mortar; amino acid residues in polypeptides include a removed hydrogen atom, a hydroxyl group or a molecule of water, depending on the amino acid's position in the chain

Res ipsa loquitur Latin The facts speak for themselves A legal doctrine that helps a plaintiff recuperate damages despite circumstances under which it would be impossible for him to prove negligence, eg permanent comatose state following a routine cesarian section or a sponge left behind during surgery; *res ipsa loquitur* is evoked whenever damages would not have occurred in the absence of negligence or had the person in charge (of the patient's management) used 'due' care; see Malpractice

Resolution The minimum distance or degree of separation between two points that can be identified as distinct, defined in terms of light microscopy (also known as 'resolving power') or electron microscopy, X-ray diffraction patterns, electrophoresis, chromatography or other separation procedures

Resource(s) The components of a system, eg equipment, space and labor that are available to perform a task of any nature, a term that has currency in the parlance of clinical laboratory bureaucrats

Resource-based relative value scale (RBRVS) HEALTH CARE ADMINISTRATION A scale that was developed by W Hsaio et al at Harvard University, which ranks physicians' services by the labor required to deliver those services; the RBRVS was sponsored by the Health Care and Financing Administration (HCFA contract 17-C-98795/1-03), in an effort to address the inequalities of physician reimbursement (J Am Med Assoc 1988; 260:2347-2438, N Engl J Med 1988; 319:835) and its data is based on the current procedure codes (CPT codes) for the services paid by Medicare and may ultimately be used by Medicare, the major health insurance intermediary in the US to determine which procedures are or are not overpriced (Am Med News 7/Dec/90); see CPT codes, DRGs, Overrated procedures

Respirator brain NEUROPATHOLOGY Global necrotic softening of the cerebral cortex, seen in 'brain dead' bodies that have been kept 'alive' by means of mechanical support; Cf Coma dépasse

Respiratory burst An abrupt increase in the consumption of oxygen,which is followed by a sequence of metabolic events occurring in neutrophils and mononuclear cells prior to bacteriolysis, designed to produce microbicidal oxidants by partial reduction of oxygen; the respiratory burst is activated by the same stimuli (contact with ingestible particles or high concentrations of chemotactins) that evoke neutrophil degranulation; the initial event in the respiratory burst is a one electron reduction of O_2 to O_2^- (superoxide) by membrane-bound oxidase; the H^+ liberated in the accompanying hexose monophosphate shunt reaction combines with the oxygen, forming H_2O_2; see Oxygen free radicals

Respiratory chain complex(es) A group of proteins encoded by the mitochondrial structural genes that are responsible for the oxidation-reduction reactions in mitochondria Complex I catalyzes the oxidation of NADH by coenzyme Q (ubiquinol) and is composed of seven subunits Complex II catalyzes the oxidation of succinate by coenzyme Q Complex III catalyzes the oxidation of reduced coenzyme Q (ubiquinol) by cytochrome c Complex IV catalyzes the oxidation of reduced cytochrome c by oxygen itself Complex V corresponds to ATP synthase, which consists of two subunits

'Respiratory syndrome' A relatively specific immune response to high-dose rifampin therapy, characterized by a flu-like complex, dyspnea and wheezing, leukopenia and thrombocytopenia; other hypersensitivity reactions caused by rifampin include flushing, fever, pruritus without rash, urticaria, eosinophilia, hemolysis and interstitial nephritis-induced renal failure

Respondeat superior A legal doctrine that holds an employer responsible for an employee's wrongful act; the application of respondeat superior requires that there be proof of a 'master-servant' or controlling relation; since this doctrine does not absolve the employee of liability, both the injured party and the employer may sue the employee for negligence; see also 'Captain of the ship', 'Deepest pockets', Malpractice

Restless leg syndrome A clinical complex characterized by nocturnal cramping of the anterior calf, restlessness, a feeling of heaviness, painful paresthesia and tingling of the legs with uncontrolled twitchings, interfering with sleep; the condition is usually idiopathic, but may occur in uremic polyneuropathy and hypercalcemia or may be associated with sleep disorders Treatment Home remedies, eg hot baths, creams and cotton stockings may be as effective as the commonly prescribed clonidine, alternation of chemically unrelated substances (benzodiazepines, opiates, L-dopa) or transcutaneous electrical nerve stimulation (J Am Med Assoc 1991; 265:3014q&a)

Restraint Any device used to restrict the free movement of patients with behavioral problems, who may cause harm to themselves and others, most commonly used in the elderly with dementia; physical restraints include chairs with locking lap trays, wrist and ankle cuffs, belts and Posey vests, which are used for from 25 to 85% of nursing home patients; pharmacologic restraints include anxiolytic, neuroleptic, sedative or hypnotic agents, which are used on 11 to 72% of patients, especially if the patients are physically abusive (J Am Med Assoc 1991; 265:1278)

Restriction endonuclease A bacterial enzyme that recognizes short (4-6) oligonucleotide sequences, known as 'restriction sites' and cleaves double-DNA wherever such sequences occur; the restriction sites are usually inverted repeats or palindromes, ie they are the same on each chain when they are read in the same direction, leaving a short 4 to 6, single-stranded 'sticky' end of DNA at each site of scission Note: Bacteria do not digest themselves as they have an intrinsic methylase that adds methyl group to one of the nucleotides within the restriction site, preventing autocleavage; see *Eco*RI, *Hin*dIII

RESTRICTION ENDONUCLEASES

Name	Cleavage site	Organism
BamHI	G/GATC*C	*Bacillus amyloliquifaciens*
EcoRI	G/AA*TTC	*Escherichia coli* RY13
HindIII	A*/AGCTT	*Haemophilus influenza* Rd
PstI	CTGCA/G	*Providentia stuartii* 164
SmaI	CCC/GGG	*Serratia marcescens* Sb
XhoI	C/TCGAG	*Xanthomonas hocicola*

/ Point of cleavage
* Base modified by a specific methylase

Restriction fragment length polymorphism see RFLP

Retained antrum syndrome A rare complication resulting from the inadequate resection of the distal antrum and pylorus during antrectomy and a Billroth II gastrojejunostomy; in its new location, the retained antrum's pyloric glands are bathed in alkaline secretions, stimulating gastrin release from antral and pyloric cells, resulting in *de novo* peptic ulceration

Reticulate (initial) body MICROBIOLOGY A stage of development of *Chlamydia trachomatis*, where multiple perinuclear lobated 2-6 µm gray-brown masses have lost the dense acidophilia characteristic of the preceding elementary body; see Intermediate body

Reticulin The loose fibroconnective stromal support tissue of the bone marrow; reticulin increases with age, marrow reticulin ranges from 0-1+ (few discernible fibers) in normal subjects to 4+; a coarsened collagen fiber network is characteristic of myelofibrosis

Reticulocyte count The enumeration of immature erythrocytes or reticulocytes is a simple means of evaluating the rate of red cell production Note: Because of delayed or premature release of erythrocytes from the bone marrow and different rates of cell maturation, correlation of peripheral reticulocytes with erythrocytic hyperplasia is not absolute but adequate for most purposes Principle Residual RNA in immature red cells is stained with a supravital dye, eg brilliant cresyl blue*

Retin-A see Retinoic acid

Retinal 11-*cis*-retinal A light-absorbing retinal pigment that absorbs visible light at 400-600 nm, resulting in an isomeric transition of the 11-*cis*-retinal moiety to a trans-retinal conformation causing a G protein-mediated depolarization event

Retinal anlage tumor see Pigmented neuroectodermal tumor of infancy

Retinol Vitamin A

Retinitis pigmentosum A group of heterogenous autosomal dominant retinal degenerations affecting 1:3500 of the population, characterized by nyctalopia and progressive centripetal loss of the visual fields progressing to blindness by middle age, caused by one or more point mutations in the rhodopsin gene located on the long arm of chromosome 3 (N Engl J Med 1990; 323:1302)

Retinoblastoma A neoplasm affecting 1:15-30 000 infants, 10-20% of which are hereditary; 70% of retinoblastomas are unilateral and arise *de novo*; bilateral tumors are associated with germ cell neoplasms and occasionally other tumors including osteogenic sarcoma and Ewing sarcoma Pathogenesis Retinoblastoma cells are deficient in tumor growth factor-β_1 receptor, a protein that inhibits cell growth; the defective retinoblastoma gene was identified by RFLP analysis, maps to chromosome 13q14 and encodes a tumor suppressor protein Histopathology Primitive dark blue cells classically arranged in Flexner-Wintersteiner rosettes Note: The tumor arises when both alleles have been inactivated; mRNA expression of 'retinoblastoma gene' is also absent in 60% of small cell carcinomas of the lung and 75% of pulmonary carcinoids; see One-hit, two-hit model, RB gene, Rosettes

Retinoblastoma susceptibility gene see RB gene

Retinoic acid (RA) A morphogenic molecule involved in vertebrate development, which in conjunction with precursor retinoids, is thought to specify positional identity on an axis during embryological development and regeneration in a dose-dependent and graded fashion; RA affects development of chick limb buds, the floor plate of the neural tube and may produce cleft palate in mice; seven retinoic acid receptors have been identified, explaining the broad range of RA effects (Nature 1990; 345:766n&v, 815, 819); RA is used to treat cystic acne, actinic keratosis, psoriasis, photoaging and oral leukoplakia; it is contraindicated in pregnant women, see below

Retinoic acid embryopathy A teratogenic complex induced by a vitamin A-derived product resulting in a 26-fold increase of congenital malformations, including microtia, anotia, cleft palate, cardiac (conotruncal and aortic arch), neural crest, craniofacial, thymic defects, hyperostoses, retinal and optic nerve abnormalities, central nervous system malformations, premature closure of the epiphyseal plates; an identical embryopathy occurs with 'megadose' ingestion of vitamin A

Retinopathy, hypertensive A condition induced by prolonged hypertension, subdivided into Grade I Arteriolar narrowing due to vasoconstriction, and intimal hyalinization (arteriolosclerosis) Grade II As with grade I with more extensive vascular thickening, which imparts a copper (column of blood still visible) or silver (no longer visible) 'wire' appearance, with 'nicking' of the veins where they are crossed by arteries Grade III In addition to grade II lesions there is hemorrhage (flame-shaped or splinter type), within the nerve fiber layer, commonly around the optic nerve head and macula, exudates, edema (containing lipid, protein and fibrin) and marked nicking; the characteristic 'macular star' consists of whitish-gray spots with fluffy borders and 'cotton-wool' spots (minute whitish superficial disciform retinal nerve fiber-layer infarcts) with 'cytoid' bodies (globular, acidophilic masses, the center of which is either more acidophilic or occasionally basophilic), measuring 10-20 μm and corresponding to swollen ganglion cell axons Grade IV As above, accompanied by edema of the optic disk Note: Retinal detachment may occur in grades III and IV

Retirement 'syndrome' PSYCHIATRY Acute or chronic maladjustment to retirement (a non-working state), most common in those who had no extracurricular activity except their chosen field of labor Clinical Irritability, apathy, asthenia, increased alcohol consumption, nonspecific autonomic nervous system complaints

Retort tube appearance A descriptor for fallopian tubes affected by acute pelvic inflammatory disease with hyperemia and fibrin deposition; the lumen is filled with pus and the fimbriae are sealed Note: A retort is a vessel used for distillation with an elongated tapering cone attached to the receptacle containing the fluid to be distilled

Retraction balls, axonal NEUROPATHOLOGY Eosinophilic and argentophilic swelling of axons, occasionally seen at the proximal and distal ends of severed nerve fibers undergoing Wallerian degeneration, which is thought to represent extruded axoplasm; retraction balls are seen in the early stages of cerebral hemorrhage or infarcts; retraction balls with brainstem necrosis are characteristic of methotrexate leukoencephalopathy

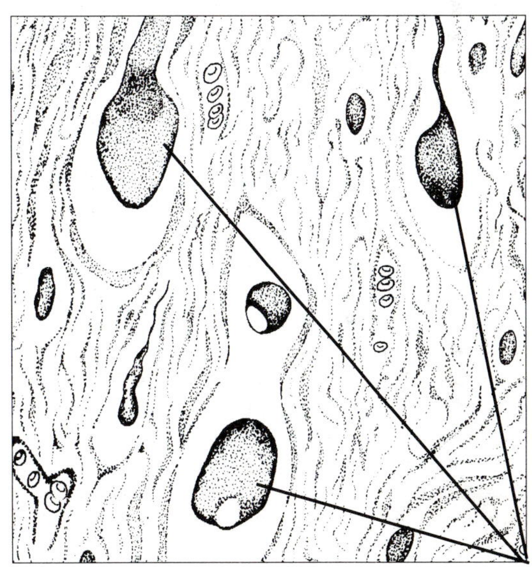

Retraction balls

Retroposition RNA-mediated transposition of genetic material; Cf Transposition

Retroposon A mobile segment of genetic information, eg a retrovirus that transposes by way of an RNA intermediate

Retrovir see Zidovudine

Retrovirus An RNA virus with two copies of an 8500 base pair plus-stranded RNA genome that is capable of inserting and efficiently expressing its own genetic information in a host cell's genome, by transcribing its own RNA into DNA that is integrated into the host genome; retroviruses are the focus of major research efforts due to their relation to human T cell lym-

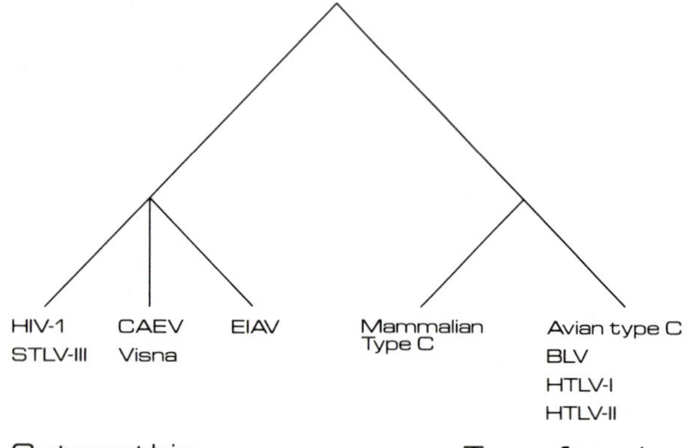

photrophic viruses and human immunodeficiency virus (HIV-1, see figure for relatedness among the various retroviruses); these viruses are widely used in research to introduce foreign DNA into a cell of interest and could theoretically be used to introduce a missing or defective segment of DNA into a cell line or organism for therapeutic purposes; the only approved use of retroviruses in humans is to 'mark' tumor infiltrating lymphocytes in experimental cancer therapy (Science 1989; 246:983; 240:1427rv); see HIV, HTLV, Rous sarcoma virus

Reverse CAMP test MICROBIOLOGY An assay that is identical in principle to the CAMP test, which identifies *Clostridium* species, where a known group B β-hemolytic streptococcus is used and if positive, the arrowhead points toward *C perfringens*; Cf CAMP test

Reverse discrimination The denial of employment or admission to a professional school or employment position based on the fact that the applicant is not of a minority race; since the US Civil Rights Act of 1964, many organizations have been required to accept applicants from underprivileged socioeconomic strata or previously discriminated-against racial groups; this led to a two-tiered system in which the presumed-to-be-advantaged racial group was often required to meet higher academic standards, while the 'hurdle' was often lowered on behalf of the underprivileged; in the Bakke decision of 1978, a caucasian applicant was allowed admission to medical school after he proved 'reverse discrimination'

Reverse '5' sign A finding on a plain antero-posterior film of an infant with hypoplastic left heart syndrome, in which the enlarged right atrium corresponds to the hip of the '5' and the superior vena cava corresponds to the shoulder of the '5'; see Baby Fae heart

Reverse genetics MOLECULAR BIOLOGY Any of a number of procedures for identifying mutant genes when a mutant phenotype is known but the responsible gene product(s) or linked markers are not; in 'forward' or traditional genetics, both the gene product, eg a defective protein and the amino acid sequence are often known before the search for the gene itself begins; in 'reverse genetics', identification of the gene is far more difficult, since the gene product is unknown at the time the search for the gene begins; one approach is to create a cDNA library from a cell that does not carry the disease in question, then perform 'subtraction' Southern blots, an extremely arduous technique that was successful in identifying the defective protein in chronic granulomatous disease; see Candidate gene method, Gene scanning

Reverse paternity testing FORENSIC MEDICINE The evaluation of a biological specimen alleged to originate from a crime victim or missing person, in order to determine whether that person is the child of parents with known genetic markers; the most commonly used marker is HLA-DQ-α, although any genetic marker, eg GmKm haplotyping, protein polymorphisms and red cell antigens may be used

Reverse 'precautions' A group of infection control procedures, including sterilization and isolation used to protect a patient (rather than the care providers or other patients) who is immunocompromised, either as a congenital condition, eg combined variable immunodeficiency syndrome or an acquired condition, eg bone marrow irradiation in preparation for marrow transplantation; 'reverse precautions' are required when the absolute neutrophil count falls below 0.5 x 10^9 (US: 500/mm^3); see Gnotobiotic environment

Reverse T_3 3,3',5'-Triiodothyronine rT_3 One of the conversion products of T_4 (thyroxine), the level of which reflects the rate of peripheral conversion of thyroid hormones of T_4 to T_3; normal rT_3 levels 0.15-0.77 mmol/L (US: 10-50 ng/dl); most circulating thyroid hormone is T_4; 35% is monodeiodinated to T_3, 15-20% is metabolized to tetraiodothyroacetic acid and the remainder is converted to rT_3; although rT_3 has little or no metabolic activity, an increased rT_3 level in patients with non-thyroidal disease indicates that the patient is not functionally hypothyroid; see Euthryoid sick syndrome

Reverse 3 sign(s) A pair of radiologic findings in the gastrointestinal tract, referring to either a) Broadening of the duodenal loop with a 'puckering' around the ampulla of Vater, classically associated with pancreatic adenocarcinoma at the head of the pancreas, seen in barium studies of the upper gastrointestinal tract or b) Indentation of the cecum on a plain abdominal film in acute appendicitis; Cf Figure 3 sign

Reverse transcriptase MOLECULAR BIOLOGY An RNA-dependent DNA polymerase that is capable of copying genomic RNA into DNA, catalyzing the synthesis of DNA using retroviral RNA as a template; reverse transcriptase has three enzymatic activities; a) The single-stranded RNA molecule copies itself, b) The retrovirus then forms a double-stranded DNA-RNA hybrid genome, transcribing a complementary strand of DNA opposite the RNA template, a polymerase activity; the strand of RNA is then removed by reverse transcriptase's ribonuclease H function; once the DNA is freed of the RNA, the polymerase portion of the molecule then synthesizes a second strand of DNA (Science 1991; 252:31); reverse transcriptase was first identified in oncogenic viruses, and homologous enzymes with similar activities have been found in bacteria, insects, eg *Drosophila* and mammals; the enzyme is a widely used molecular research tool, and used to make cDNA (complementary DNA) clones from mRNA

Reverse transcription The copying of single-stranded retroviral RNA into double-stranded DNA catalyzed by reverse transcriptase, an enzyme so designated as it is the reverse of the usual direction of tanscription from DNA to RNA, see Central dogma, HIV, Retrovirus

Reversion The change of a mutated nucleic acid to its state prior to mutation

Revici method A form of alternative cancer therapy that is based on Revici's theory that '...A DISEASE CAN BE DUALISTIC, WITH A PREDOMINANCE OF ONE GROUP OF LIPIDS (STEROLS) OR THE OPPOSITE (FATTY ACIDS), ONE ANABOLIC AND CONSTRUCTIVE, THE OTHER CATABOLIC AND DESTRUCTIVE...'; according to this theoretical framework, the control of disease requires determination of the nature of a biological imbalance and providing the substance that corrects it; the method is alleged to detect catabolic or anabolic processes by urinary pH; catabolic therapeutic agents include fatty acids, magnesium, selenium and sulfur; anabolic agents include caffeine, iron, lipols, lithium, zinc; the method has no demonstrable efficacy and is based on no established scientific principle (CA—A Journal for Clinicians 1989; 39:119); see Unproven methods of cancer therapy

Reviewer SCIENTIFIC JOURNALISM A recognized expert in a field who reviews a manuscript for publication in a major scientific or medical journal and either recommends its acceptance to the journal or advises its rejection based on various criteria; most reviewers rejected an average of 1.5 manuscripts for various reasons, some 'zealots' may find some merit in virtually all the manuscripts they review, while others, the 'assassins', reject most of the manuscripts they recieve (Science 1991; 251:1424n&v); Cf Authorship, Publication bias

Revised trauma score (RTS) EMERGENCY MEDICINE A triage tool that measures physiological parameters including the Glasgow coma scale, systolic blood pressure and respiratory rate; when used in the pediatric population, prediction of survival was more accurate with the RTS than with the pediatric trauma score (J Am Med Assoc 1990; 263:6); see Triage

Revolving door 'syndrome' PSYCHIATRY SOCIAL MEDICINE A cyclical pattern of short-term readmissions to the psychiatric units of health care centers by young adults with chronic psychiatric disease; this syndrome first appeared in the USA in the 1970s with the implementation of strict(er) criteria for civil commitment of mentally disturbed patients, which arose from a concern about the potential for causing harm to oneself or to others; because more people with major mental illness are no longer hospitalized, and theoretically are well-controlled with drug therapy, eg tricyclic antidepressants, these persons may commit minor crimes and be imprisoned, resulting in 'criminalization' of persons with psychiatric disease Note: 30-40% of the general prison population and homeless people in the USA suffer from psychiatric or addictive disease (Psychiatr J Univ Ottawa 1988; 13:154); see Homeless(ness)

Reye syndrome A potentially fatal condition characterized by acute encephalopathy and fatty degeneration of the liver that is linked in a dose-dependent manner to the use of aspirin in children during viral infections (J Am Med Assoc 1988; 260:657) **Clinical** Vomiting, hepatic dysfunction, minimal neurological impairment often preceded by viral upper respiratory tract infections or varicella **Histopathology** 'Fine-droplet' fatty liver **Ultrastructure** Megamitochondria with distended and fragmented cristae and flocculated matrix **Laboratory** Increased transaminases, glutamine and ammonia in cerebrospinal fluid, hypoglycemia and metabolic acidosis **Treatment** None universally accepted Note: 'Stage migration' has occurred in Reye syndrome, as milder cases are being diagnosed, and it is increasingly recognized as a relatively 'benign' condition; see Lovejoy's classification, Will Rogers phenomenon

RF see Rheumatoid factor(s)

R factor HEMATOLOGY see R binder protein INFECTIOUS DISEASE Resistance factor An enzyme (chloramphenicol acetyltransferase) that inactivates chloramphenicol by 3-O-acetylation, which is produced by R-plasmids in both gram-negative and gram-positive bacteria, including ***Enterobacteriaceae, Haemophilus influenza, Neisseria gonorrhoeae*** and ***Streptococcus pyogenes*** Note: Other mechanisms for antibiotic resistance include membrane impermeability, alteration in intracellular target sites, alteration or overproduction of a target enzyme, active pumping out of a substrate and auxotrophic forms which bypass inhibitory steps; see Methicillin-aminoglycoside resistant ***Streptococcus aureus***

RFLP Restriction fragment length polymorphisms Restriction site polymorphism MOLECULAR BIOLOGY Local variations in the DNA sequence of individual humans or animals that may be detected by restriction endonuclease enzymes (which 'cut' the double-stranded DNA whenever they recognize a certain highly-specific oligonucleotide sequence or 'restriction' site); these individual variations or polymorphisms in the DNA sequences occur approximately 1 per 200-500 base pairs and cause the genome to be cut at different sites, yielding fragments of different length that are unique to each individual (the likelihood of two people having the same RFLPs is estimated to be $1/10^9$), but nevertheless normal; these different fragments may then be identified by electrophoresis as larger restriction fragments migrate more slowly; although the differences in fragment lengths may be linked to chromosomal loci for a certain disease (Am J Hum Genet 1980; 32:314), these point 'mutations' rarely translate into functional defects as a) Not all genes are 'structural', ie do not encode functional protein b) DNA is 'degenerate', ie obeys the law of DNA conservation, in which 64 different DNA codon sequences encode in only 20 amino acids, 3 stop codons and 1 start codon, thus allowing for multiple 'silent' errors and c) All individuals carry 5-10 potentially lethal mutations under normal circumstances Note: Single base pair substitutions can either create or abolish restriction endonuclease sites, as will tandem repeats; RFLPs are useful genetic markers as they help identify the inheritance pattern of a gene of interest; if one is able to locate a RFLP that has the same heredity pattern as a genetic condition, then the gene responsible for that disease can be localized, thus one must find a DNA sequence closely associated or linked to a disease of interest; RFLP analysis is of use in identifying genes associated with autosomal dominant inherited neurologic diseases, including Huntington's disease located on chromosome 4, myotonic dystrophy on chromosome 19 and Duchenne's dystrophy on chromosome X; in allogenic bone marrow transplant recipients, RFLP analysis is of use in documenting chimerism, allograft failure, recurrent leukemia or in identifying a secondary lymphoproliferative malignancy; an alternative method for investigating clonal populations is based on differences in DNA methylation patterns that exist between active and inactive alleles of two X-linked genes

RF-S A factor present in human S phase cells that activates DNA replication and which contains a homologue of Schizosaccharomyces pompe p34*cdc2* kinase that is responsible for control of DNA synthesis (Science 1990; 250:786); see p34*cdc2*

RGD family A group of proteins that are present in the extracellular matrix that have cell adhesion functions, mediated by the 'RGD' tripeptide, Arginine-Glycine-Aspartic acid (designated as RGD by the single letter code for amino acids); RGD proteins include collagens, fibrinogen, fibronectin, glycoprotein IIb and IIIa, LFA-1 with Mac-1 and VLA1-5 on leukocytes, laminin, osteospondin, thrombospondin, vitronectin, von Willebrand factor, together with their respective receptors; the RGD family constitutes a versatile recognition system providing cells with anchorage by interaction of surface receptors with cytoplasmic proteins (talin, ankyrin, actin, vinculin, fibroconnexin) and extracellular proteins (fibronectin, collagen, vitronectin and others), traction for migration and signals for growth, phagocytosis, polarity, position, cell differentiation, platelet aggregation and complement binding; see Integrins

R gene see Regulator gene

Rh Rh system A group of 7-10 kD erythrocyte membrane-bound antigens that are independent of phosphatides and proteolipids; the Rh system is very complex and much of its genetics and role in red cell structure and function are not understood; Rh^+ and Rh- refer to the presence or absence of the erythrocyte-bound antigen D; Rh 'antigen' is actually a composite of multiple antigens, including Rh-C (c, C, CG, C^w), Rh-D (D, D^u, D^w), Rh-E (e, E, E^w), Rh-G, Rh-LW, Rh-Ne^a and Rh_{null}; Frequency of the Rh antigens in Caucasians: Rh-e, 98%; Rh-D, 85%; Rh-c, 80%; Rh-C, 70%; Rh-E, 30%; unlike the ABO blood group, antibodies against the D antigen are not formed naturally, ie in the absence of exposure, thus an Rh- subject with circulating anti-D antibodies has been exposed to the D antigen by previous transfusion or pregnancy; exposure to the D antigen is of concern in obstetrics as the mother's anti-D antibody is an IgG, which crosses the placenta, potentially causing hemolytic disease of the newborn (titer > 1:16 at the eighth month usually indicates maternal formation of alloantibodies, evidenced by stomatocytes in the maternal blood) Note: 300 µg of anti-D (RhoGAM) immunoglobulin 'neutralizes' a 30 ml feto-maternal hemorrhage containing 15 ml of Rh-bearing red cells; see Rh immune globulin

Rhabdovirus A family of single-stranded RNA viruses that includes the rabies virus and causes vesicular stomatitis

Rheumatic fever The late non-purulent sequelae of upper respiratory tract infection by streptococcus group A; the diagnosis is based on major criteria (carditis, chorea, erythema marginatum, polyarthritis and subcutaneous nodules) and minor criteria (arthralgia, fever, history of previous rheumatic fever, or evidence of cardiac involvement, laboratory parameters of increased acute phase reactants, anti-streptolysin O titers, C-reactive protein and erythrocyte sedimentation rate), as delineated by Jones and subsequently modified; see 'Chinese menu disease'

Rheumatoid arthritis An autoimmune inflammatory arthropathy defined by the 1987 revised criteria (table, below), which requires that criteria 1-4 be present for more than six weeks; the 'revised criteria' yield a 91-94% sensitivity and 89% specificity (Arthritis Rheum 1988: 31:315)

RHEUMATOID ARTHRITIS (Revised criteria)

1) Morning stiffness in and around joints lasting at least one hour before maximum improvement
2) Soft tissue swelling ('arthritis') of three or more joints observed by a physician
3) Swelling (arthritis) of the proximal interphalangeal, metacarpophalangeal or wrist joints
4) Symmetric swelling (arthritis)
5) Rheumatoid nodules
6) Presence of rheumatoid factor
7) Roentgenographic erosions and/or periarticular osteopenia

Rheumatoid arthritis cell RA cell An atypical neutrophil containing 1-20 dense, black 0.5-2.0 µm in diameter cytoplasmic inclusions (figure, facing page) containing IgM rheumatoid factor, IgG, complement and fibrin, which is seen by phase contrast microscopy in wet synovial fluid preparations in patients with rheumatoid arthritis; RA cells comprise 5-100% of the neutrophils of patients with rheumatoid arthritis but are relatively non-specific and may be seen in other connective tissue diseases, including septic arthritis and gout

Rheumatoid factors (RF) A group of often polyclonal IgM (rarely also IgG or IgA) antibodies that are directed against the Fc portion of denatured IgG; RFs are produced by synovial neutrophils in 80% of patients with rheumatoid arthritis; RFs are non-specific and may be seen in infections (bronchitis, kala azar, leprosy, subacute bacterial endocarditis, syphilis, tuberculosis, viral), hepatic disease (biliary obstruction, cirrhosis, fatty liver, granulomas, neoplasia and viral hepatitis) and others (diabetes mellitus, idiopathic pulmonary fibrosis, osteoarthritis, paraproteinemia, Raynaud's disease, sarcoidosis and Sjögren syndrome) and are present in 3% of the normal healthy population; RFs may cause immune complex deposits which activate complement and release leukocytic hydrolases from neutrophils, causing tissue injury **Histopathology** Fibrinoid necrosis in small blood vessels Laboratory Detection of RFs is not standardized; the tests may be based on erythrocyte agglutination (Rose-Waaler test), latex agglutination (Singer-Plotz test), nephelometry, fluorescence immunoassay and enzyme-linked immunosorbent assay (ELISA)

Rheumatoid nodule A mass on tendons, tendon sheaths, periarticular tissue, serous membranes (pleural, pericardium), meninges, cardiac valves, kidneys, lung parenchyma, skin, spleen, synovium, vessels and viscera, seen in 20% of patients with rheumatoid arthritis, similar nodules occur in lupus erythematosus and rheumatic fever **Histopathology** Vaguely geographic area of central necrosis, (containing collagen, lipids, nucleoproteins, acid mucopolysaccharides, serum proteins and immunoglobulins), surrounded by successive rims of fibrinoid degeneration, fibrosis and palisaded histiocytes

Rheumatoid pneumonitis A clinical form of diffuse interstitial pulmonary fibrosis that occurs in 2% of patients with rheumatoid arthritis, which is accompanied by a varying degree of pulmonary compromise; rheumatoid pneumonitis may result from the rare coincidence of two uncommon conditions, ie rheumatoid arthritis and interstitial pneumonia, the latter of which may be induced by gold therapy, exposure to an environmental toxin or related to smoking

Rh immune globulin (RhIg) An Rh immune globulin concentrate used to prevent the maternal immunization against the infant's Rh group D antigen; one commonly used product, RhoGAM, contains 300 mg of antihuman immunoglobulin/vial, sufficient to 'neutralize' a feto-

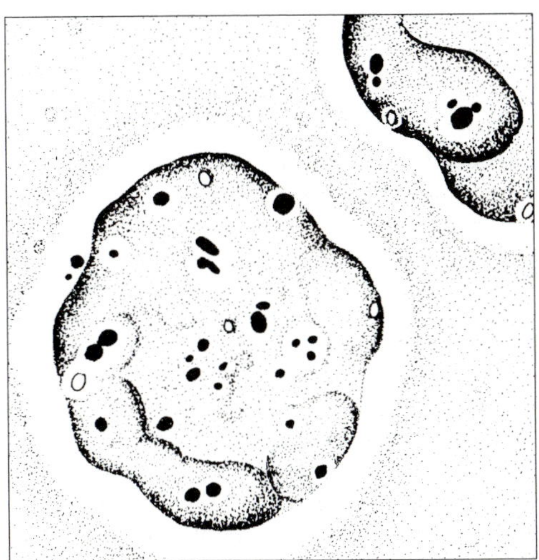

Rheumatoid arthritis cell

maternal hemorrhage of 15 ml of red cells; RhIg is indicated when the mother is Rh negative or has anti-RhD antibody titer of > 1:4; see Hemolytic disease of the newborn

Rh_{null} TRANSFUSION MEDICINE A rare Rhesus system phenotype found on erythrocytes in which there is complete non-expression of Rh antigens, resulting from either the more common regulator type defect, consisting in homozygous inheritance of the gene $X^{o}r$ or inheritance of an amorphic gene (---/---); both Rh_{null} phenotypes are associated with decreased red cell survival and stomatocytosis due to a membrane defect; Rh_{null} expression is enhanced by concomitant presence on the red cell surface of blood groups M, -N, -En^a and depressed by -S, -s, -U

Rhinophyma see WC Fields nose

Rhodopsin A member of a family of receptors bearing seven transmembrane helices coupled to G proteins

RhoGAM see Rh immune globulin

Rhomboid crystals A descriptive term for a) The characteristic membrane-bound, rod-shaped crystalloid structures with 10 nm periodicity seen by ultrastructure in the malignant polygonal cells of alveolar soft part sarcoma and b) The notched cholesterol crystals obtained from joint fluid in patients with diverse chronic inflammatory or chronic degenerative arthropathies

rho termination factor MOLECULAR BIOLOGY A protein that interacts with a growing mRNA chain in bacteria, terminating transcription of an operon

Rhythm methodGYNECOLOGY The contraceptive method sanctioned by certain religious bodies in which unprotected intercourse is allowed shortly after a menstrual period or before the onset of the next period; the rhythm method is widely recognized to be the least effective form of contraception, resulting in 20 pregnancies/100 woman-years; see Contraceptives, Pearl index

RIA Radioimmunoassay IMMUNOLOGY LABORATORY MEDICINE A method that measures either an antigen or antibody based on competitive inhibition of labeled antigens on the binding of unlabeled antigens to specific antibodies, the uptake of which displays a characteristic sigmoid curve; RIA allows measurement of minimal amounts of immunogenic substances, including enzymes and hormones and is of great use in research as it is relatively easy to design an assay to detect the analyte(s) of interest; RIAs are being phased out of the clinical laboratory in favor of enzyme assays, which eliminate the regulatory and disposal problems inherent in maintaining radioactive materials on-site; see POPOP, Quenching; Cf ELISA

Ribavirin (1-β-5-D-ribofuranosyl-1,2,4-triazole-3-carboxamide) A synthetic nucleoside analog that restricts the synthesis of viral proteins, interfering with capping of the mRNA of a variety of viruses; ribavirin is approved for aerosol treatment of severe respiratory syncytial virus infection in the pediatric population (N Engl J Med 1991; 325:24)

Ribbon cell SURGICAL PATHOLOGY An elongated eosinophilic variant of the 'strap' cell seen in pleomorphic rhabdomyosarcoma; see Strap cell

Ribbon ribs A descriptor for ribs with marked costal hypoplasia or attenuation, a finding characteristic of trisomy 13-15 and trisomy 18 syndromes, and may be seen in neurofibromatosis, Gorham's angiomatosis, hyperpara- thyroidism, osteodysplasia, osteogenesis imperfecta, poliomyelitis, rheumatoid arthritis and scleroderma

Ribonuclease An endonuclease that catalyzes RNA hydrolysis, cleaving its 3',5' phosphodiester bonds **Ribonuclease III** hydrolyzes double-stranded RNA **Ribonuclease A** catalyzes RNA yielding mono and oligonucleotides with 3'-pyrimidine termini **Ribonuclease D** removes excess tRNA nucleotides from precursor tRNA, forming the 3'-terminus of this molecule **Ribonuclease H** (RNase H) removes the RNA molecule that is a template for the first strand of DNA; RNase H is of interest to AIDS researchers as a possible target for a new family of anti-HIV-1 drugs (Science 1991; 252:88); see HIV-1, Reverse transcriptase **Ribonuclease P** is a ribozyme of bacterial origin that cleaves an oligonucleotide from precursor tRNA at the 5'-end of mature RNA; Cf RNA polymerase

Ribonucleoprotein A molecule with RNA covalently bound to protein; see snRNPs (small ribonucleoproteins)

Ribonucleotide reductase A heteromultimeric enzyme which is needed by all proliferating cells to catalyze the *de novo* synthesis of deoxyribonucleotide precursors for DNA

Ribosomal lamellar complex (RLC) Granulofilamentous body An ultrastructural finding consisting of hollow cylindrical structures composed of ribosome-studded spirals and concentric lamellae (see figure, Hairy cell leukemia, page 272); RLCs were first described as pathognomonic for hairy cell leukemia, but also occur in chronic lymphocytic leukemia, acute myelogenous leukemia, lymphosarcoma, multiple myeloma, Waldenstrom's macroglobulinemia,adrenocortical adenoma, paraganglioma and other conditions

Ribosomal RNA(s) A family of single-stranded nucleic acids that range from 100 to 3000 base pairs in length, assemble in heteromultimeric forms and which serve as 'docking stations' for messenger RNA and nascent polypeptide strands

Ribosome A nucleoprotein-rich organelle that is critical to the translation of a mature mRNA transcript into a protein; the ribosome holds mRNA in place while its message is read, holds protein in place during chain elongation and serves as a docking station so that tRNA can contribute a cognate amino acid specified by the mRNA

Ribozyme A catalytic RNA that is capable of breaking and forming covalent bonds and functions as an enzyme, cutting and splicing along an 'internal template', acting at restricted 'wobble' base pair sites (J Am Med Assoc 1988; 260:3030rv); T Cech observed that pre-ribosomal RNA could cut and splice itself, thus acting as molecular 'scissors', while S Altman found that transfer RNA could be cut by another separate piece of RNA in conjunction with a protein, observations for which Cech and Altman were awarded the 1989 Nobel prize in Chemistry; the existence of self-splicing RNA molecules raises the question of whether the first inherited molecule in the 'primordial soup' was RNA rather than DNA; modified ribozymes may have potential as anti-HIV-1 therapeutic agents as a ribozyme with a hammerhead structural motif has been isolated that reduces the level of HIV-1 gag RNA expression (Science 1990; 247:1222)

Rib-tip syndrome Sharp episodic pain at the costal margin, caused by hypermotility of the anterior end of the costal cartilage of (usually) the tenth rib, secondary to trauma

'Rib-within-a-rib' appearance A descriptor for the parallel lines seen in the ribs by a plain chest film due to subcortical osteoporosis in pateints with severe chronic thalassemia

Rice bodies Orthopedics Numerous elongated and indurated oval-to-rounded rice-like masses composed of collagen types I, III and V in ratios of 40/40/20 (the same ratio as the synovial membrane), which that a common mechanism exists for 'rice body' formation, eg synovial ischemia; rice bodies may occur in the joints of patients with rheumatoid arthritis, lupus erythematosus, septic arthritis, tuberculous bursitis and synovial chondromatosis; Cf Joint 'mice'

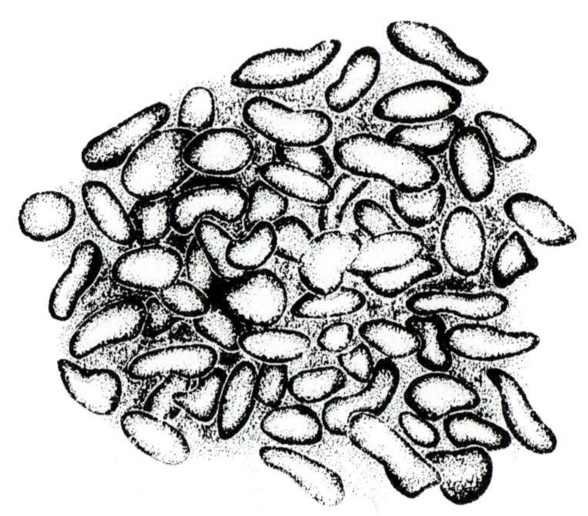

Rice bodies

Rice water stools Clear and watery diarrhea with a vaguely fishy odor, that is admixed with flecks of mucus, fancifully likened to the appearance of water from boiled rice, an appearance classically seen in cholera; cholera stool is low in protein and isotonic with the plasma, corresponding to a 'secretory' diarrhea in which adenylate cyclase is locked in the 'on' position by enterotoxins produced by *Vibrio cholera* and by some strains of *Escherichia coli*; at early postmortem examination, the intestines are stiff and non-distensible and fancifully likened to 'iron rods' due to the antemortem metabolic acidosis and loss of potassium; see Cholera cot

Ricin A toxic vegetable poison from the castor bean plant (*Ricinus communis*) which causes agglutination and fulminant hemolysis at very high dilutions ($1/10^6$) Clinical Abdominal pain, nausea, cramps, convulsions, dehydration, hemolysis, cyanosis, renal failure (oliguria, hematuria) and circulatory collapse; see also Magic bullet Note: Ricin poisoning was implicated in some KGB 'executions' during the Cold War, as with Georgi

Markov, a Bulgarian defector

RID see Radial immunodiffusion

Rider's bone Post-traumatic myositis ossificans (heterotopic bone formation) seen on the upper femur of equestrians in relation to the adductor muscles

Rift valley fever A dengue-like viral disease spread by mosquitoes in floods, causing fatal enzootic hepatitis in ruminants (sheep, cattle) and occasional human epidemics, by direct contact; the agent is a genus of the phlebovirus genus of the Bunyaviridiae family Clinical Abrupt onset with a biphasic fever curve, headaches, prostration, myalgias, anorexia, nausea, vomiting, conjunctivitis, lymphadenopathy; fatalities are related to hemorrhagic fever or encephalitis Mortality 5-20%

Right middle lobe syndrome see Middle lobe syndrome

Right shift see Oxygen dissociation curve

'Right to die' movement Background: The potential for lawsuits in medically 'hopeless' health care situations is enormous and in the US, physicians often feel compelled to attempt what they perceive to be futile resuscitations and other duties in order to maintain the vital functions of an elderly body with machinery that is 'rusted beyond repair'; the 'right to die', and to do so with dignity, is rapidly becoming a fundamental freedom in the USA, and in civilized countries, engendering such organizations as the Hemlock Society; see Advanced directives, 'Doctor Death', DNR, Euthanasia, 'It's over Debbie'; Cf Persistent vegetative state

Rigid loop sign One or more non-motile, crescent-shaped segments of edematous small intestine which have been 'paralyzed' in position, ie not changing regardless of whether the film has been taken in the upright and decubitus position, a finding seen in a plain abdominal film in mesenteric venous occlusion

Rigid spine syndrome(s) A heterogeneous group of early onset muscle dystrophies, eg X-linked Emery-Dreifuss syndrome, in which muscular atrophy begins by early adolescence, often accompanied by multiple contracture of the spinal musculature and other muscle groups

Rigor mortis Post-mortem corporal rigidity PATHOLOGY The rigid contraction of skeletal muscles that is first seen in the jaw 2-4 hours after death, later appearing on the trunk and extremities, reaching its peak at 48 hours, disappearing in the same order of its development; the rapidity of onset of rigor mortis is related to environmental factors, including temperature, occurring more rapidly in hot weather and may begin earlier if there was increased muscular activity prior to death, eg convulsions, strychnine poisoning, sunstroke and tetanus; rigor also occurs in cardiac and smooth muscle, affecting vessels and the gastrointestinal and urogenital tracts Pathogenesis After death, intracellular glycogen is depleted, ATP falls and the pH rises precipitously; rigor begins at ATP levels of 85% normal and disappears as the levels fall below 15%

Rimantidine An antiviral agent that is a structural analog of amantadine and estimated to be 75% effective in preventing influenza A disease during community epidemics, although it is only partially effective as therapy and post-exposure prophylaxis for influenza A, since drug-resistant strains rapidly appear (N Engl J Med 1989; 321:1696); see Canyon region

Rim pattern Peripheral rim pattern, Shaggy pattern An immunofluorescent pattern that is arranged peripherally along the nuclear membrane, due to the deposition of antibodies directed against double-stranded DNA, deoxyribonucleoprotein and histones; high antibody titers (> 1:200) are often present in the sera of patients with lupus erythematosus and may be seen in other connective tissue diseases: see Antinuclear antibodies; Cf Speckled pattern

Rim sign GASTROINTESTINAL RADIOLOGY An opacification of the margin of a congenital choledochal cyst seen by a plain abdominal film GYNECOLOGIC RADIOLOGY An attenuated annular radiopacity seen in the pelvis by infusion urography corresponding to cystic pelvic mass(es), usually of ovarian origin; a similar finding may occur in benign unilateral pelvic masses with a smooth serosal contour, eg fibroma-thecoma and cystadenofibroma ORTHOPEDIC RADIOLOGY see Snowcap sign PEDIATRIC RADIOLOGY An annular, attenuated periadrenal radiopacity occurring in the rare cases of neonatal hemorrhage in this region, seen by high-dose excretory urography UROLOGIC RADIOLOGY A series of connected, overlapping physaliferous rims seen in the nephrogram phase of selective renal angiography of advanced hydronephrosis, where the attenuated curved vascular tissue surrounds dilated calices of the renal pelvis

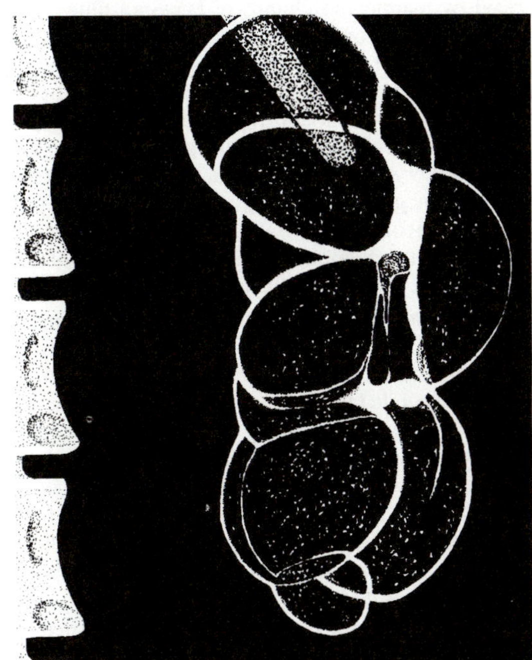

Renal rim sign

RIND Reversible ischemic neurological disability A variant of a transient ischemic attack defined as an ischemia-induced focal loss of neurologic function of abrupt onset, the disability from which is greater than 24 hours but less than 3 weeks induration; Cf Multi-infarct dementia, Transient ischemic attack

Ring abscess A descriptor for the histological appearance of an abscess seen in infective endocarditis which consists of a central focus of neutrophils, necrosis and bacteria, surrounded by fibroblasts and fibrosis, frayed cardiac muscle fibers and 'round' inflammatory cells, including plasma cells and lymphocytes

Ringbindenfibern see Ringed fibers

Ring chromosome Cytogenetics An anomalous chromosome in which there is a break near the end of each arm of the chromosome with joining of the broken tips to themselves; phenotypic expression is a function of the amount of lost material; when the X chromosome is involved, r(X), may result in a Turner-like syndrome

Ringed fibers Peripheral myofilaments that are reoriented and encircle the other myofibers of the same bundle; there are thus central, longitudinal fibers, surrounded by fibers, which to the German eye, mimic the back of a 'spiral' notebook, ergo the alternative term, Ringbindenfibern; these fibers show no evidence of phagocytosis nor regeneration and are a subtle histological marker for myotonic dystrophy

Ringed hair Pili annulati A rare inherited developmental anomaly of the hair shaft that has no known clinical significance characterized by alternating bands of light and dark hair due to air cavities within the shafts themselves; Cf Pili torti; Woolly hair disease

Ringed sideroblast A pathologic erythroblast characterized by marginated clumps of Prussian blue-staining granules corresponding to iron-loaded mitochondria, seen in the bone marrow or in the peripheral smears of red cell maturational disorders accompanied by ineffective erythropoiesis and hyperferremia, eg acquired idiopathic sideroblastic anemia, pyridoxine-responsive anemia, dyserythropoietic anemia, lead intoxication and certain hemoglobinopathies; up to 50% of cases with ringed sideroblasts eventually develop leukemia, including acute monocytic leukemia, myelomonocytic leukemia and erythroleukemia

Ring enhancement A finding in the brain by computed tomography (CT) imaging, consisting of a radiolucent zone surrounded by a faint radiodense rim, which in turn is surrounded by a second radiolucent zone outside of the rim, where the rings correspond to regional edema, hypervascularity and hypercellularity with early ingrowth of fibroblasts; although ring enhancement per se is non-specific, it is considered typical of early cerebral abscesses, but may also be seen in various brain tumors; intravenous contrast material may be used to enhance faint radiodense 'rings'

Ring, esophageal A partially encircling intraluminal mass in the esophagus, also known as Schatzki's ring, is actually a web; to be semantically correct, a ring is composed of mucosa, submucosa and muscle (which the esophageal ring lacks); the literature is sparse on the clinical and pathological differences between the esophageal rings and webs, and the distinction may be of little practical use; see Webs

Ringer's solution A physiologic, ie isotonic, saline solution containing sodium chloride and potassium chloride at 0.9%

Ringer's lactate solution A standardized sterile physiologic solution containing calcium chloride, potassium chloride, sodium chloride and sodium lactate, which contains 1.35 mmol/L calcium, 4 mmol/L potassium and 130 mmol/L sodium (US: 2.7 mEq/L calcium, 4 mEq/L potassium and 130 mEq/L sodium), that is used as a topical irrigant and as a crystalloid solution for restitution of fluid volumes

Ring form MICROBIOLOGY A characteristic appearance of erythrocytes infected by *Plasmodium* species; the trophozoite 'rings' are globose, have a central vacuole, a red chromatin mass and blue cytoplasm; with maturation, the 'rings' evolve to an ameboid form

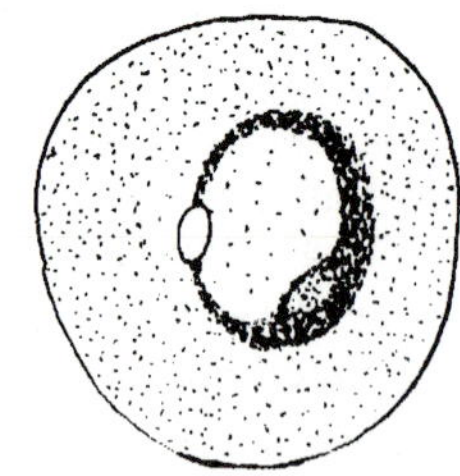

Ring form

Ring formation see Ring enhancement

Ring granuloma see Doughnut granuloma

Ring, mesangial see Mesangial ring

Ring-shaped nuclei Cells of the myeloid series, eg mature polymorphonuclear granulocytes (neutrophils) in which the lobes of the nuclei are connected by an attenuated bridge composed of nuclear material; ring-shaped nuclei may be a subtle cytologic marker for chronic granulocytic or neutrophilic leukemia (Am J Clin Pathol 1986; 86:748)

Ring shadows A descriptor for the annular thickening of the bronchial walls seen by a plain chest film in bronchiectasis, which is identical to 'tram-track shadows'

Ring sign UROLOGIC RADIOLOGY Annular filling defect(s) seen in the renal calices by intravenous pyelography, which result from necrotic sloughed papilla, see Papillary necrosis Analgesic abuse, Sickle cell anemia, Obstructive uropathy

Ring test IMMUNOLOGY A simple precipitin test, where antigen is layered over an antibody solution and the amount of precipitation at the interface is measured; see Radial immunodiffusion

Ringworm Tinea corporis Dermatophytosis A superficial fungal infection by *Trichophyton rubrum, T mentagrophytes, Microsporium canis* and *M gypsum*, rarely also *Epidermophyton*; in children, *T canis* is the most common agent; the trivial name derives from the lesion's characteristic onset as a scaly plaque spreading centrifugally with central clearing **Differential diagnosis** Nonfungal dermatopathies, including erythema annulare, the 'herald patch' of pityriasis rosea and eczematous lesions **Treatment** Most lesions resolve without therapy; otherwise, miconazole, and if severe, griseofulvin

RIPA see Radioimmunoprecipitation assay

Ripple effect see Signal event

Rippling effect A descriptor for the layered angiographic appearance of blood vessels in the cortical sulci peripheral to a cerebral abscess through which the blood flows in an undulating pattern; other cerebral lesions differ in that they may be associated with gyral edema or with neovascularization

Rippling muscle disease A disorder of adolescent onset that is usually autosomal dominant, occasionally sporadic, which results when local compression of a muscle evokes myoedema, followed by longitudinal contraction of a muscle, moving transversely across the muscle in a 10-20 muscle fascicle wave fancifully likened to 'plucking a chromatic scale on a harp'; while superficially resembling myotonia, the entity is electrically silent and clinically benign

'**Rip van Winkle syndrome'** Pathological hypersomnia; see Narcolepsy, Sleep disorders

RISA 1) Radioactive iodinated serum albumin 2) Radioimmunosorbent assay A radioisotopic technique for detecting low levels of IgE; Cf RAST

RISC chip Reduced instruction set computer chip COMPUTERS A 'smart' chip currently under development that uses different algorithms and modern ultramicrocircuitry design to provide greater and more efficient computing power, while reducing the number of instructions required for each task; RISC chips are being planned for the next generation of microcomputers in a joint venture between the IBM and Apple computers and already are found within laser printers

Risk EPIDEMIOLOGY The probability of suffering from a particular disease **ABSOLUTE RISK** The number of persons suffering from a disease when the exposed population is known with certainty **RELATIVE RISK** An estimate of persons suffering from a disease, based on an extrapolation of the persons presumed to be exposed to a predetermined factor; see Epidemiology

Risk assessment TOXICOLOGY The process by which new chemical substances are evaluated for their potential impact on human health, a process that entails determining the substance's toxicity and the number of people exposed to the substance; see Ames' test, Toxicity testing

Risk management The constellation of activities (planning, organizing, directing, evaluation and implementation) involved in reducing the risks of injury to patients and employees and reducing property damage or loss within health care facilities; risk management in its various forms, including non-medical liability is estimated to cost 15% of the US federal government budget, ie between \$60 and \$175 x 10^9 annually

Ristocetin An antibiotic that induces platelet aggregation *in vitro*; the ristocetin cofactor assay quantifies the ability of von Willebrand factor in plasma to agglutinate platelets in the presence of ristocetin; in the absence of ADP, calcium and fibrinogen are required for platelet aggregation, a period designated as 'ristocetin time', which is prolonged in afibrinogenemia, dysfibrinogenemia, heparin therapy, idiopathic thrombocytopenic purpura, infectious mononucleosis, acute leukemia, Glanzmann's disease and storage pool diseases; in Bernard-Soulier disease, there is no aggregation due to the lack of a membrane receptor; in von Willebrand's disease, aggregation does not occur without normal plasma; see Platelet aggregation

Risus sardonicus A fixed 'sarcastic' grimace and anxious expression with drawing up of the eyebrows and corners of the mouth due to spasms of the masseter and other facial muscles, accompanied by rigidity of the neck and trunk muscles with arching of the back, a clinical finding in generalized tetanus, due to a neurotoxin produced by ***Clostridium tetani***, a soil contaminant with a 7-10 day incubation period, having up to a 90% mortality in the unvaccinated or susceptible populations, eg urban narcotic addicts; the classic spasms of risus sardonicus (trismus, spasmus caninus) may be elicited by external stimuli and may also be seen in strychnine poisoning, hysteria, catalepsy Note: The caricature of this grotesque facial expression is that seen on Batman's arch enemy, the Joker

Ritalin see Methylphenidate

RITARD model Removable intestinal tie adult rabbit diarrhea model An animal model for studying the pathogenesis of diarrhea induced by ***Vibrio cholerae*** toxin (Infec Immun 1983; 41:1175)

River blindness Onchocerciasis A disease of littoral regions in tropical Africa and Latin America, affecting an estimated 30 million people, the earliest immunogenic marker for ***O volvulus*** infection is designated OV-16 (Science 1991; 251:1603) Agent ***Onchocerca volvulus*** Vector Blackfly, genus ***Simulium*** Clinical Although the adult may reach 0.5 m in length and travels under the skin causing pruritic bumps and scarring, it is the microfilaria that are most problematic, as they plug the lymphatic channels, causing elephantiasis and blindness (punctate keratitis, pannus formation, corneal fibrosis, iridocyclitis, glaucoma and optic atrophy) Prevention Pesticides to eliminate blackflies, while impractical are often used Treatment Ivermectin, 1-2 doses/year, which inhibits reproduction of the parasites and paralyzes the microfilaria, appears to be the current first line therapy, alternatively, diethylcarbamazine; see Ivermectin

RLC see Ribosomal lamellar complexes

RNA editing Any natural alteration of the gene expression that occurs at the level of messenger RNA, by a variety of mechanisms, including insertion, deletion or substitution of nucleotides in an RNA molecule (Nature 1991; 349:434, 370); see editing

RNA hybridization see Hybridization

RNA ligase An enzyme integral to RNA splicing, which catalyzes the formation of phosphodiester bonds

RNA-recognition motif see RRM

RNA polymerase(s) A family of enzymes that copy strands of RNA from a DNA template; RNA polymerase I synthesizes pre-rRNA, is present in the nucleolus and when digested, yields three cleavage products: -28S, 5.8S and 18S; RNA polymerase I is capable of transcribing the DNA from any species, provided that a species-specific transcriptional protein is attached, usually 'upstream' of the gene segment to be transcribed; RNA polymerase III synthesizes RNA outside of the nucleolus, including tRNAs and 5S rRNA; type III RNA polymerase, like type I RNA polymerase requires a species-specific activating protein; Cf Ribonucleases, Ribozymes

RNA splicing The process in which the non-translating

portions or introns from the primary transcript of DNA are removed and the exons are joined together, forming an mRNA transcript from which proteins will be transcribed

hnRNA see Heterogeneous nuclear RNA

RO-1 The basic grant for the individual researcher, awarded by the National Institute of Health (USA), which averages $200 000; there were 4600 new RO-1s in 1990

Roaches see Cockroaches

Robertsonian translocation Centric fusion CLINICAL GENETICS A chromosomal anomaly seen in 4% of Down syndrome children, consisting of a balanced translocation, where a segment from the long arm of 21 is translocated to another chromosome, most commonly to chromosome 14 t(14q21q); three of the six possible resulting genotypes are viable: One is completely normal, one is genotypically abnormal, but phenotypically normal, ie the chromosomes are translocated but normal and one case expresses Down syndrome, ie both genotypically and phenotypically abnormal; The risk of repetition of a Robertsonian-type Down syndrome is 10-15% for a maternal carrier and 5% for a paternal carrier of the translocation

'Robin Hood syndrome' Reverse cerebral steal Reduction of blood flow to relatively well-oxygenated tissue by vasoconstriction, 'freeing' the available blood for ischemic and hypercapneic tissues; the adjectival sobriquet of 'Robin Hood' derives from the legendary English folk hero, who allegedly stole from the rich to give to the poor, allegorically similar to this condition; in the usual 'steal' syndrome blood flow is robbed from oxygen-poor tissues by oxygen-rich tissues

ROC Receiver operating characteristic Clinical decision making A curve that describes the relationship between a true positive fraction and a false positive fraction for a diagnostic procedure that can take on multiple values (figure, below); the ROC curve describes a graph in which the horizontal axis represents the false positive fraction and the vertical axis represents the true positive fraction (Semin Nuc Med 1978; 8:299); the curve plots false positives versus false negatives; each point reflects the strategy of calling all results for a given value positive or negative where a binary disease status exists (presence or absence of disease, eg myocardial infarct if CK-MB is elevated, or no myocardial infarction if CK-MB is not elevated) Note: ROC analysis is a viable alternative to the possibly over-simplistic Four-cell decision matrix, see there

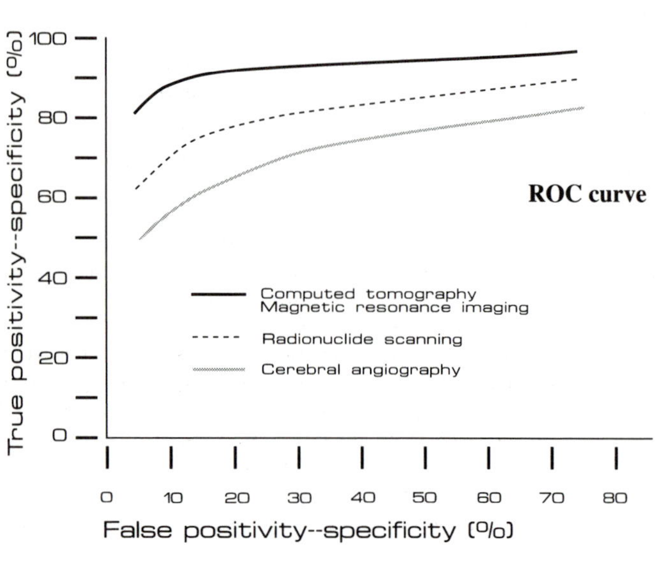

True positivity--specificity (%)

Computed tomography
Magnetic resonance imaging
Radionuclide scanning
Cerebral angiography

False positivity--specificity (%)

ROC curve

Rocio encephalitis An epidemic viral infections occurring in Brazil that is similar to Japanese encephalitis and is maintained in wild birds and transmitted by mosquitoes

Rockefeller University Founded in 1901 as the Rockefeller Institute for Medical Research on a 15-acre campus in Manhattan, the 'Rock' supports 600 regular faculty and post-doctoral investigators, 125 graduate students and 975 support staff on an annual budget of $100 million; there are 45 laboratories with a broad range of research, one-third of which concentrate on mechanisms of cancer; other interests include neuroscience, viruses and immunology; 19 Nobel laureates have been associated with the University and two of its students have won the Nobel prize; Cf Howard Hughes Medical Institute, Salk Institute, Whitehead Institute

Rocker bottom feet Congenital vertical talus, pes valgus A rigid flatfoot deformity caused by a malpositioned navicular bone at the neck of the talus; the ankle is in severe equinus and the forefoot in dorsiflexion, ie rocker bottom-like, accompanied by contraction of the talonavicular, deltoid and calcaneal cuboidal ligaments, the peroneus brevis and triceps surae muscles Rocker bottom feet occur as isolated deformities or may accompany trisomy 18 and 13 Treatment Early, manipulation and plaster correction of the forefoot into plantar flexion, inversion and adduction; 'benign neglect' represents malpractice as this deformity requires triple arthrodesis when ignored

Rocker bottom shadow A horizontal, broad, curved soft tissue radiodensity that partially overlies the heart, extends into the hilum, corresponding to the thymus, seen in a plain antero-posterior chest film in neonatal pneumomediastinum, and derives its name from old wooden cradles; see Spinnaker sail sign

Rocket electrophoresis of Laurell A one-dimensional enzyme immune assay in which an antigen-bearing fluid is electrophoresed through agarose containing antiserum to the antigen of interest (figure, facing page); rocket electrophoresis is used to quantify von Willebrand factor levels in the blood and derives its name from the sharp projectile-like immunoprecipitin spike

Rocky Mountain spotted fever A exanthematous disease first described in Indian squaws in the Bitterroot Valley, Montana, located in the Rocky Mountains, which is more common in the eastern US from April to October and may occur in large cities, eg, New York (N Engl J Med 1988; 318:1345) Agent ***Rickettsia rickettsii*** Hosts Furry woodland creatures (rodents *et al*) Vectors Wood (*Dermacentor andersoni*) and dog (*D variabilis*) ticks Pathogenesis Endothelial damage activates platelets, fibrinolysis and the intrinsic and extrinsic coagulation pathways (N Engl J Med 1988; 318:1021) **Clinical** One-week incubation, followed by a discrete pale, blanchable centrifugal maculopapular rash, which may be dusky in color. hence the alias, 'black measles', persistent headache, fever, occasionally with coughs and râles, myalgia, malaise, splenomegaly; nausea, vomiting, abdominal pain, central nervous system symptoms (delirium, stupor, ataxia, meningismus), myocarditis, EKG abnormalities, thrombocytopenia, multiple coagulopathies, renal failure and shock **Laboratory** Weil-Felix test is positive for antibodies to OX-19 and OX-2 **Treatment** Tetracycline, chloramphenicol **Prognosis** Mortality 3 to 10%; greater in blacks and those over age 40

Rod cell NEUROPATHOLOGY A modified microglial cell that increases in size and number in paretic dementia (tertiary syphilis) as well as in subacute encephalitides, eg encephalitis lethargica, cerebral trypanosomiasis (*T gambiense*); rod cell-like changes are also seen in normal astrocytes in acute toxic insults; the bipolar forms, which are normally perpendicular to the surface, proliferate and increase in size, the nuclei elongated, the cytoplasm loses its trabeculation and is best visualized with a basic aniline dye or Prussian blue, due to rod cells' accumulation of iron

Rodent ulcer A deeply invasive basal cell carcinoma of long duration with induration of ulcerated walls

Roe *vs.* Wade SOCIAL MEDICINE, OBSTETRICS A 'landmark' legal case that was presented before the US Supreme Court in 1973, which abortion; the decision was based on the concept that 1) The constitutional right to privacy is broad enough to encompass a woman's right to an abortion and 2) The state's interest to abridge that constitutional right is related to the stage (in trimesters) of pregnancy Note: The 1989 US Supreme Court decision in the Webster case appears to represent a partial retreat from a legal environment that facilitated abortions, and to some, signal a return to political conservatism (N Engl J Med 1989; 321:1200); see Mexico City policy, Webster decision; Cf Amsterdam strategy, ZPG

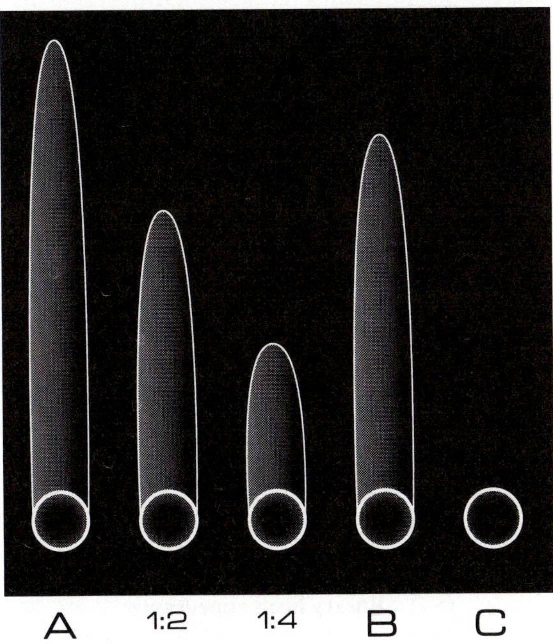

A Serial dilutions of a positive control at 1:1, 2:1 and 4:1dilutions
B Unknown or patient specimen
C Negative control

Roentgen A unit of dose exposure to X- and gamma-radiation, corresponding to the amount of radiation capable of producing an electrostatic unit of positive and negative ions when passing through 1 cc of dry air at standard temperature and pressure (2.58×10^{-4} of ions/kg air); Cf Gray, Rad, Rem

'Roentgen-hangover' see Acute radiation injury syndrome

Rolfing ALTERNATIVE MEDICINE A deep massage therapy developed by IP Rolf that seeks to 'realign' the body by altering the tone of myofascial tissues, facilitating 'structural integration'; rolfing is philosophically similar to chiropractic, in that inaccurate or poor posture is thought to be detrimental to a person's health, energy, mental and physical efficiency, and like chiropractic, the claims of therapeutic success are uncertain as large double-blinded studies have not been performed Note: It is probable that the highly individualized nature of these therapies precludes valid statistical studies of their efficacy; see Chiropractic

'Roller ball surgery' GYNECOLOGY A colloquialism for laser surgery of uterine leiomyomas, which are benign tumors composed of dense stroma that markedly deform the endometrium, and may make successful pregnancy impossible by preventing normal endometrial expansion; in this technique, the tumors are 'shelled out' by rolling the tumors while cutting with the laser

Rolling circle replication MOLECULAR BIOLOGY The mechanism by which bacteriophages efficiently reproduce; after injection of the phage chromosome into a host bacterium, the phage directs protein synthesis, using the host's reproductive machinery, first reproducing in the relatively inefficient 'theta' mode; after several rounds of theta reproduction, the phage chromosomes switch to the sigma or 'rolling circle' mode, in which the circle extends a tail; the replication machinery then hooks directly onto the tails, allowing continuous phage production; once the enzyme terminase recognizes the cos sequence of nucleotides at the end of the viral chromosome, it closes the circle and begins another round of replication

ROM 1) Range of motion ORTHOPEDICS The arc of an articulation's movement, potentially limited by musculoskeletal defects 2) Read-only memory COMPUTERS A silicon chip that contains permanent instructions, including entire routines or programs that cannot be erased or altered by the microprocessor; Cf PROM, RAM

'Roman bridge' A descriptor for a histological hallmark of in situ carcinoma of the breast of cribriform type, which consists of curved 'bars' of well-differentiated, bland malignant cells without an intervening fibrovascular core, which span two or more points of a duct (see figure, page 632); this appearance has been fancifully likened to the voluptuous architecture typical of the public works of the Roman empire Note: This 'soft' histopathological criterion for malignancy is most often confused with intraductal epitheliosis of the breast

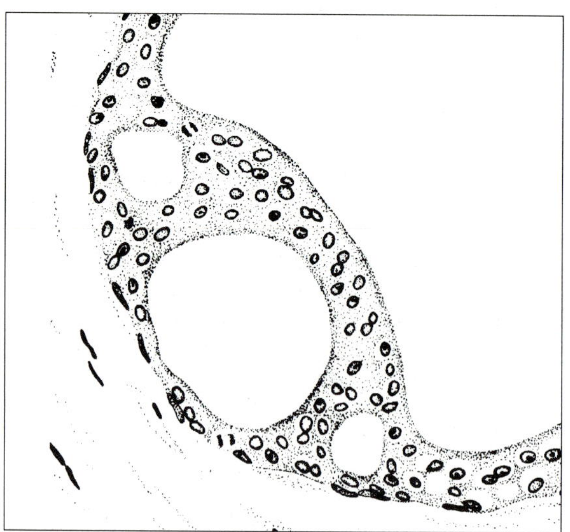

Roman bridge appearance

Roman fever Antiquated for malaria

Romanovsky stains HISTOPATHOLOGY A group of eosin-methylene blue stains, eg Wright-Giemsa and Leishman that are used for peripheral blood smears; the red cells are stained lilac and bacteria or parasites, platelets, lymphocytes, red to purple

R-on-T phenomenon CARDIOLOGY A premature ventricular depolarization that is so early in the cardiac cycle that it falls on the apex of the preceding T wave, potentially presaging ventricular tachycardia or fibrillation; the EKG finding of an 'R-on-T' is considered an indication for the intensity of anti-arrhythmic therapy eg lidocaine

'Room temps' TRANSFUSION MEDICINE Blood bank argot for antibodies that agglutinate at room temperature, and which have minimal potential for causing transfusion reactions Note: Most antibodies of clinical importance, ie those capable of inducing transfusion reactions, occur with IgG antibodies that agglutinate at 37°C; Cf Cold agglutinin disease

Rooming-in NEONATOLOGY The placing of a newborn in the same room as the mother in the early post-partum period, which is thought to foster maternal-fetal bonding and facilitate breast-feeding (Acta Paediatr Scand 1990; 79:1017); see Bonding, Rooting

'Root canal' DENTISTRY A colloquialism for the complete therapy of a tooth with well-advanced decay that is no longer superficial enough for a simple amalgam filling to be adequate permanent therapy; a 'root canal' consists of opening, cleansing and sterilizing the root canal, closing and filling it with an impervious material, preventing future infection and covering with a porcelain cap

Rooting NEONATOLOGY The searching for the mother's nipple by the neonate, which is often accompanied by grunting, opening of the infant's mouth and sucking; this reflex of early infancy is elicited by touching the baby's cheeks and by the smell of milk

Rope sign NEUROLOGY An acute angulation between the chin and larynx due to weakness of the hyoid muscles, resulting in posterior displacement of the hyoid bone, and narrowing the hypopharyngeal passage

Rope's test see String test

ROSC Return of spontaneous circulation

'Rorschach proglottid' A descriptor for the broad, short gravid proglottids of ***Diphyllobothrium latum***, which have been fancifully likened to the appearance of certain Rorschach ink blots; Cf Zipper proglottid

Rorschach test Rorschach technique of projective assessment Ink blot test A type of personality testing in which 10 ink blots are presented to a subject for his interpretation of what he sees in the 'picture' (figure, right); the test generates an enormous amount of data, much of which requires subjective interpretation; first used in 1921, the 'ink blot test' reached its peak of popularity in the 1950s but continues to have currency among psychologists; see Psychological testing

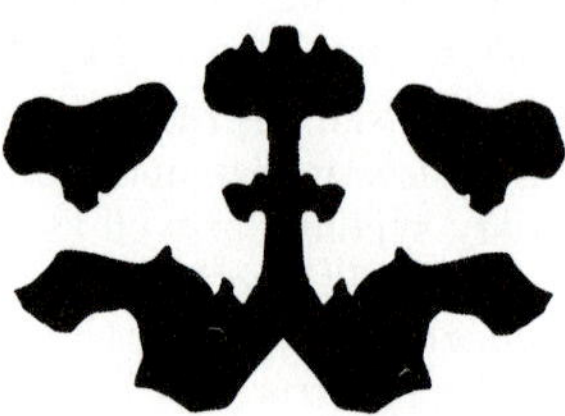

Rorschach ink blot

Rosary An adjectival descriptor of occasional use in medicine, referring to periodic expansions or densities arranged in a linear fashion, likened to a string of beads used to count prayers, especially the Roman Catholic 'Rosary', a devotion consisting of meditation on the five sacred mysteries during recitation of five decades of Ave Marias, each of which begins with a paternoster and ends with a Gloria

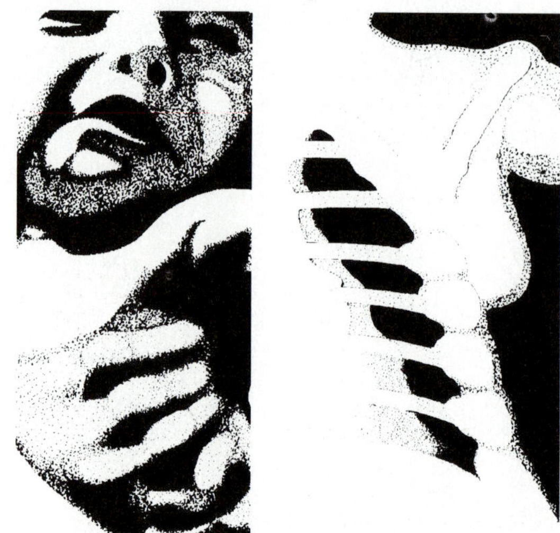

Rosary bead appearance

Rosary, rachitic Bulbous widening of the costochondral junction due to softened epiphyses seen in infants with vitamin D-deficient rickets (figure, above); the 'rachitic' rosary may also be seen in congenital neonatal hypophosphatemia, childhood hypophosphatasia and in adenosine deaminase deficiency

Rosary, scorbutic Bulbous enlargement of the costochondral junction, similar to the rachitic rosary except that the angulation of the scorbutic 'beads' is sharper than in rickets as it is due to subluxation of the sternal plate

Rosary bead appearance COLONIC RADIOLOGY A descriptor for the exaggerated haustral contractions seen in barium studies of the irritable bowel syndrome, often accompanied by constipation, pain and hardened, dehydrated and pelleted or rabbit-like stools

Rosary bead esophagus see Corkscrew esophagus

Rosebud hands A combination of bony and soft tissue syndactylism seen in Apert's craniocephalosyndactyly syndrome, which may be further accompanied by scaphocephaly, premature closure of the cranial sutures and mental retardation, facial deformities including hypertelorism, a high forehead, bulging eyes, short nose, synostosis of the vertebral bodies and carpo-tarsal syndactyly or lobster-claw feet

Rosenthal classification A numerical notation system used as an alternative for phenotyping the Rh blood groups Note: although the classification is more logical, it is unlikely to replace the Race-Fisher and Weiner systems that are firmly entrenched in the blood banking literature

Rosenthal's disease Factor XI deficiency, Hemophilia C

Rosenthal fibers NEUROPATHOLOGY Small elongated eosinophilic processes seen by light microscopy in the astrocytes of chronic degenerative neural diseases, eg Alexander's disease, multiple sclerosis and spongioblastoma, as well as in cerebellar astrocytomas

Rose spots INFECTIOUS DISEASE Transient 1-5 mm in diameter reddish macules that blanch on pressure, are located on the lower chest and upper abdomen and are related to bacterial emboli in cutaneous vessels accompanied by focal aggregates of dermal macrophages; rose spots classically occur in *Salmonella typhi*-induced typhoid fever during the first week of disease, coinciding with the onset of splenomegaly

Rosette A term for a garland-like arrangement of structures, cells or bodies around a central point or blood vessel, usually seen by light microscopy HEPATOLOGY Liver cell 'rosettes' correspond to hepatocytes that deviate from their usual trabecular pattern, divided into cholestatic rosettes, a response attributed to biliary obstruction and consequent cholestasis and regenerative rosettes, seen in a background of severe chronic active hepatitis, acute and chronic inflammation IMMUNOLOGY **E ROSETTES** Nonimmune rosettes The spontaneous clustering of sheep erythrocytes around T-cells; Erythrocyte rosettes are formed by lymphocytes with abundant CD3 receptors, which are 'pan-T' cell markers **EA ROSETTES** Eythrocyte-antibody rosettes Clusters of sheep erythrocytes around monocytes and macrophages sensitized with sheep erythrocyte hemolysin, which occurs when the Fc portion of the hemolysin molecule attaches to the Fc receptor on the surface of the M cell **EAC ROSETTES** Erythrocyte-antibody-complement rosettes Cell clusters formed by B cells, monocyte and macrophages when sheep erythrocytes have been sensitized with a heterophile antibody in the presence of complement NEUROPATHOLOGY **EPENDYMAL ROSETTES** Structures that recapitulate features of the normal ependymal cavity, which have a small central rounded-to-elongated lumen, optional cilia and blepharoplasts (distinct basally oriented granular corpuscles in the cytoplasm) **FLEXNER-WINTERSTEINER ROSETTES** Structures which are pathognomonic for well-differentiated retinoblastomas, consisting of 'bland' nuclei arranged around a fibrillary background of axonal material **HOMER-WRIGHT ROSETTES** Perivascular pseudorosettes A 'classic' finding in neuroblastomas, characterized by a ring of tumor cells arranged in 'garlands', surrounding a central space filled with pale-staining neuro-fibrillary material, packed around a delicate fibrovascular core (figure, below); the tumor cells themselves have scant, poorly-defined cytoplasm, the nuclei have coarse but evenly dispersed chromatin, may have marked mitotic activity (olfactory neuroblastomas demonstrate low mitotic activity) Note: Esthesioneuro-blastomas have been subdivided into tumors with true rosettes (neuroepitheliomas), tumors with pseudorosettes (neuroblastomas) and those that don't form rosette-like structures (neurocytomas), the last being a distinction of questionable usefulness

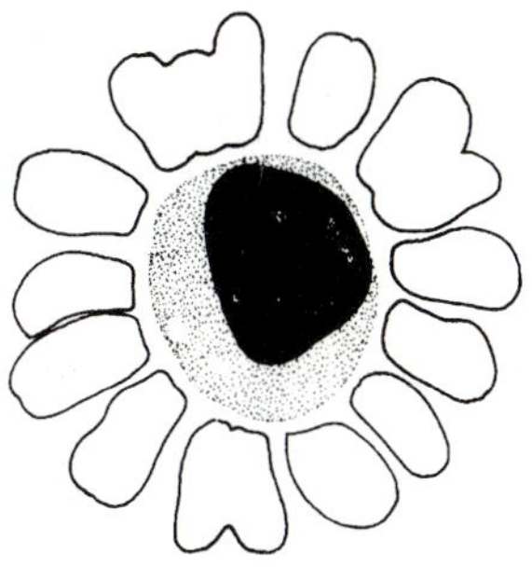

E rosette

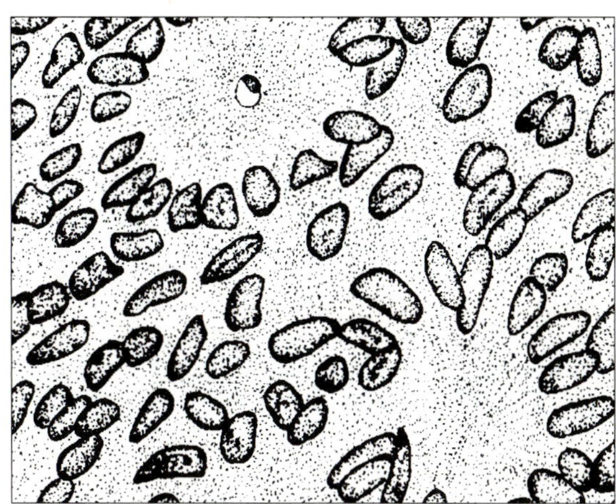

Homer-Wright rosettes

Rosette blisters DERMATOLOGY Annular arrangement of sausage-shaped bullae around an eschar on the trunk, genitalia and legs in idiopathic linear IgA dermatosis, an eruption with variable pruritus, most common in infants **Immunofluorescence** Liner IgA, occasionally C3 **Treatment** Sulfapyridine or corticoids; most cases spontaneously resolve within 2-4 years

Rosette test NEONATOLOGY A screening test for detecting significant fetomaternal hemorrhage, where an indicator cell forms easily-identified rosettes around individual

Rh-D fetal cells that may be present in the Rh-negative mother; this qualitative test can detect a 10 ml or greater fetomaternal hemorrhage and should be followed by a quantitative test, eg the Kleihauer-Betke test

Rose-Waaler Test IMMUNOLOGY A specialized anti-immunoglobulin test with sheep erythrocytes sensitized with a subagglutinating dose of rabbit anti-sheep erythrocyte IgG; when rheumatoid factor is present in test serum, it combines with the membrane-bound IgG, causing agglutination; the Rose-Waaler is less commonly used as most rheumatoid factor tests use latex particles to establish agglutination

Rosewater syndrome An X-linked form of male pseudohermaphroditism characterized by gynecomastia, sterility, increased testosterone, estrogen and gonadotropins; see Pseudohermaphroditism

Rose windows Circular pores or fenestrations with wedge-shaped slits covered by a thin diaphragm, located in the capillary walls of endocrine glands, eg pancreatic islet cells, which may be seen by electron microscopy and freeze fracturing techniques; the name derives from the circular windows filled with tracery, used in Gothic architecture

Rotating crystal technique A method for determining the three-dimensional conformation of a substance, which consists of analyzing the X-ray diffraction patterns of a single purified crystal of a molecule of interest, which is mounted and rotated around multiple axes, providing multiple diffraction spots that can be used to resolve the molecule's secondary structure

Rotavirus An encapsulated double-stranded RNA viral member of the reovirus family, which measures 70 nm in diameter and is a major agent of epidemic and endemic gastroenteritis, usually causing mild disease, which may be severe in children under age two due to intense vomiting; see Astrovirus, West-to-East phenomenon

Rotator cuff SURGICAL ANATOMY The musculotendinous covering of the shoulder joint, which is delineated anteriorly by the subscapularis muscle, superiorly by the supraspinatus muscle and posteriorly by the infraspinatus and teres minor muscles; degenerative change of the rotator cuff tendons is considered a normal aging process,especially affecting the supraspinatus tendon at the zone of Codman, due to susceptibility of its vascular supply; see Frozen shoulder, Milwaukee shoulder syndrome

Rouleaux Stacks of erythrocytes, likened to stacked coins; rouleaux formation occurs with increased plasma fibrinogen and globulins, increased sedimentation rate due to dextran and monoclonal gammopathies (multiple myeloma, Waldenström's disease), cryoglobulinemia, sarcoidosis and cirrhosis; rouleaux formation, which interferes with identification of weak antigen-antibody reactions in the blood bank, can be reduced *in vitro* by adding saline or other low-ionic strength solution; see LISS

'Round' cells A generic term referring to relatively small (10-20 μm) leukocytes with (usually) a single round-to-oval nucleus; round cells include lymphocytes, monocytes, plasma cells and occasionally epithelioid histiocytes

'Round cell' tumors SURGICAL PATHOLOGY Tumors that are composed of relatively monotonous sheets of cells with bland round-to-oval, relatively basophilic nuclei, clumped chromatin, scanty cytoplasm, and often have a 'primitive' appearance; round cell tumors are often poorly differentiated, defy classification of embryologic lineage by routine histological examination and may require an array of special studies including a) Immunoperoxidase stains to detect the presence of intermediate filaments or hormone production b) Electron microscopy to identify dense core granules or premelanosomes and c) Molecular studies to detect amplification of genes, as in the T cell receptor's β chain; tumors that may present with a round cell appearance include lymphomas, undifferentiated carcinomas, neuroendocrine tumors, and amelanotic melanomas

Rounds Bedside visits by a physician (or other health professionals) in order to evaluate treatment, assess the current course and to document the patient's progress or recuperation; see Professorial rounds, SOAP; Cf Grand rounds

Rous sarcoma virus (RSV) A single-stranded RNA virus that causes sarcoma in chickens, and which is the prototypic acute transforming retrovirus; RSV's genome contains *gag* (which encodes a structural protein in the viral core), *pol* (which encodes reverse transcriptase) and *env* (which encodes envelope glycoprotein) and V-src (the viral oncogene responsible for RSV's in vivo and in vitro oncogenic potential); Cf HIV, Retrovirus

Roux-en-Y procedure GENERAL SURGERY Any of a group of surgical procedures in which a Y-shaped anastomosis includes the small intestine; the distal resected end is implanted into an organ, eg bile ducts (choledochojejunostomy and portoenterostomy), esophagus (esophagojejunostomy) and pancreas (pancreaticojejunostomy), while the proximal end is implanted into the small intestine further 'downstream' to prevent reflux

R plasmid see Plasmid

RPR test Rapid plasma reagin test, see Reagin

RQ Respiratory quotient see Pulmonary function tests

RRM RNA-recognition motif An 80-residue polypeptide in the A protein of the U1 small nuclear ribonucleoprotein particle (snRNP); the RRM is a hallmark of an RNA-binding protein, and contains two ribonucleoprotein consensus sequences, RNP-1 and RNP-2 and structurally consists of a four-stranded anti-parallel β sheet with two α helices (Nature 1990; 348:515, 485ed)

16S rRNA A ribosomal RNA molecule that is essential for protein synthesis and present in thousands of copies per cell

RS-61443 A chemical derived from mycophenolic acid that inhibits guanosine synthesis and by extension, T cell proliferation, as well as B lymphocyte proliferation; RS-61443 is synergistic with cyclosporine in ameliorating chronic rejection in transplants and is thought to act by reducing chronic vascular rejection; see Cyclosporin, FK506

RSS see Recombination signal sequence

RS3PE syndrome Remitting seronegative symmetrical synovitis with pitting edema A subgroup of patients with rheumatoid arthritis with sudden onset, seronegativity for rheumatoid factors **Treatment** Aspirin, Nonsteroid anti-inflammatory drugs **Prognosis** Excellent (J Am Med Assoc 254:2763)

RSV 1) Respiratory syncytial virus A 'pediatric' virus that causes 55 000 annual hospitalizations and 2000 annual deaths in children Note: A vaccine is under development that marries RSV's F glycoprotein, which induces cell-to-cell fusion and G glycoprotein, which controls viral attachment and penetration 2) see Rous sarcoma virus

rT_3 see Reverse T_3

RTA see Renal tubular acidosis

rt-PA recombinant tissue Plasminogen activator

Rubber hose appearance see Garden hose appearance

'Rubbia effect' ACADEMIA Increased governmental funding for a field of research area after it has netted a Nobel prize (or acquired prestige for other reasons), as occurred in Italy's Instituto Nazionale per Fisica Nucleare, an agency that for many years had had a miniscule budget that was increased exponentially when physicist Carlo Rubbia won the Nobel prize in Physics (Science 1985; 228:1508)

Rubella German measles, Röteln, Third disease; Cf Rubeola

Rubella syndrome see Congenital rubella syndrome

Rubeola A term that is best avoided as it has been applied to both measles and rubella; Cf Rubella

RU 486 Roussel-UCLAF 38486, Paris 11β-(4-dimethyl-amino phenyl)-17β-hydroxy-17α-(prop-1-ynyl)-estra-4,9-dien-3-one), Mifepristone POPULATION CONTROL A 19-norsteroid antiprogesterone abortifactant that acts by receptor competition with high-affinity binding to both glucocorticoid and progesterone receptors; a single 600 mg oral dose of RU-486 blocks progesterone, which would otherwise enable the uterus to accept the incoming fertilized egg; RU 486 is then followed within 36-48 hours by a prostaglandin analog (gemeprost or sulprostone), which induces uterine contraction and expulsion of the egg Efficacy 96% Incomplete expulsion 2.1% Persistent pregnancy 1%, hemostasis defects 0.9% (N Engl J Med 1990; 322:645) Side effects Minimal pelvic pain, fatigue, nausea, headache

Ruffled border The convoluted cytoplasmic membrane of actively resorbing osteoclasts; ruffling is increased by parathyroid hormone, which stimulates bone resorption and is inhibited by calcitonin, which decreases resorption of calcium and phosphate; ruffling therefore acts to increase the active cell surface; Cf Moat

Ruffling A component of cell motility, which is observed by fibroblasts in tissue culture, corresponding to the trailing edge of the cell; in contrast to the leading edge, in which actin-rich lamellipodia move forward and establish themselves in new territory, the ruffled edges swing over top of the cell and stay behind in the previous zone; see Lamellipodia

Rugger jersey spine appearance A descriptor for a pattern of osteosclerosis which is most marked in the vertebral end plates adjacent to joint spaces, fancifully likened to a 'Rugger jersey', seen in those with secondary hyperparathyroidism (renal osteodystrophy); the changes may also be seen in renal tubular disease, including Fanconi syndrome, renal tubular acidosis, vitamin-D-resistant rickets, chronic glomerulonephritis, diabetes mellitus and hypertension Note: In uremic osteodystrophy, the alternating bands of increased and attenuated radiological density of vertebral bone do not affect the cortex

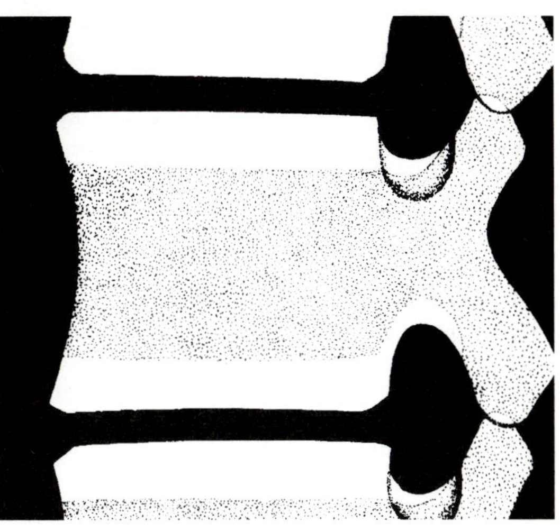

Rugger jersey appearance

Rule of nine A method for rapidly assessing the extent of burns on the skin surface, which determines the amount of fluid required as replacement therapy; the head and arms each represent 9% of the skin surface, the anterior or posterior surface of the legs represent 9% each, the anterior and posterior truncal skin represent 18% each and the inguinal area 1% (figure) Caveat: The rule does not apply to children, as the head is proportionately larger, and comprises 19% of the surface area of infants, for whom the 'palm of the hand' rule is used, where an area the size of the infant's palm is equivalent to 1% of the body surface

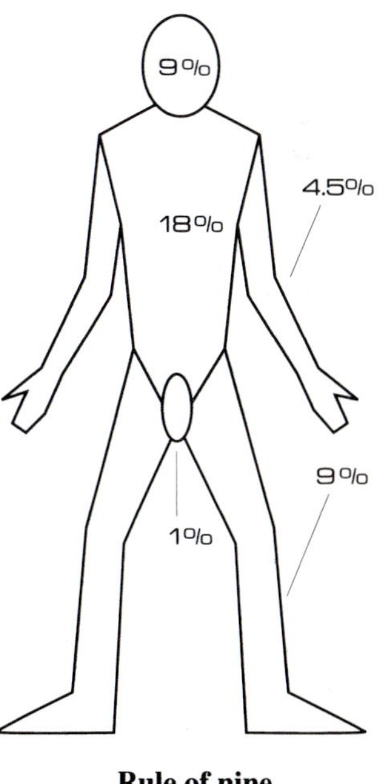

Rule of nine

Rule of the forceps OBSTETRICS A simple rule that serves as a reminder of which handle of the forceps should be used on which side of the patient: Left blade, left hand and left side of mother; Right blade, right hand and right side of mother

'Rule of rescue' HEALTH CARE REIMBURSEMENT The perceived duty to save endangered life whenever possible; this rule directly conflicts with the cost-effectiveness approach which attempts to implement a fair allocation of limited resources, by providing the most health care services for most people (J Am Med Assoc 1991; 265:2218); see Coby Howard, Health care rationing, 'Squeaky wheel' effect; Cf Oregon plan

Rule of thirds FLUID PHYSIOLOGY Body water comprises approximately two-thirds of the total body weight (more in children, lesser amounts in adults); one-third is extracellular, two-thirds is intracellular; of the extracellular fluid one-third is intravascular, two-thirds is interstitial; of the intravascular fluid, one-third is intracellular and two-thirds is plasma

Rule of threes HAND SURGERY Two guidelines for staged reconstructive surgery of the hand, used to determine whether a digit should be amputated: 1) Of the five tissues in the hand (bone, joint, coverage, muscle and nerve), if three or more require reconstruction, amputation should be considered, unless the thumb (which must be salvaged at all costs) or entire hand is involved and 2) The number of staged operations should be no more than three, as the functional defects remaining after more surgery may outweigh the benefits; see No-man's land

Rules of two see Meckel's diverticulum

'Rum fits' SUBSTANCE ABUSE Generalized alcohol withdrawal-related convulsions presenting as status epilepticus seen in chronic alcoholics 12-48 hours after a major decline in blood alcohol levels **Clinical** Hypocapnia and hypomagnesemia have a postulated but unproven role; one-third of cases progress to delirium tremens; Cf 'Cold turkey'

Rumination 'syndrome' Merycism Regurgitation of nonacidic food 10-15 minutes after deglution; the patient either expectorates or chews and re-swallows the food; rumination may occur in those with emotional and intellectual defects, and in children is associated with failure to thrive or marasmus; rumination may respond to biofeedback, although some patients may regard it as pleasurable, frustrating therapeutic efforts Note: Ruminators may perform publicly, 'regurgitating' colored handkerchiefs and other sundry novelties

RUNYON GROUPS

Group I Photochromogens Yellow when exposed to light *M kansasii, M simiae, M marinum, M asiaticum*

Group II Scotochromogens Pigmented when grown in the dark *M scrofulaceum, M gordonae, M xenopi, M flavescens*

Group III Non-pigmented organisms *M africanum, M avium-intracellulare, M bovis, M haemophilum, M malmoense, M terrae, M triviale, M gastri, M ulcerans, M nonchromogenicum, M shimoidei*

Group IV Rapid growers *M fortuitum, M cheloni cheloni, M cheloni abscessus, M smegmatis, M phlei, M vaccae, M thermoresitibile*

RYE CLASSIFICATION (Hodgkin's disease)

Lymphocytic predominant 10%of cases, more common in young adult males, often early, low stage disease without 'B' symptoms Five-year survival: 90%

Nodular sclerosing 40% of cases, more common in young adult females, usually early, low stage disease with or without 'B' symptoms Five-year survival: 70%

Mixed cellularity 40% of cases, more common in young adult males, often stage II-III disease with or without 'B' symptoms Five-year survival: 50%

Lymphocyte-depleted 10% of cases, more common in older adult males, usually stage III-IV disease with or without 'B' symptoms Five-year survival, 30%

Running Long-distance running SPORTS MEDICINE The energy expended during running is a function of the time the foot applies force to the ground during each stride, thus running distance X at high speed consumes the same amount of energy as running the same distance at a slower speed, even though the rate of energy consumption is higher (Nature 1990; 346:265); excess training may evoke myocardial infarction, possibly related to carnitine-like deficiency; amenorrhea acts to conserve energy in female distance runners, who despite consumption of 200 cal/d less than control subjects, do not lose the expected 5 kg/year, as amenorrhea (which commonly occurs in females who run long distance) is characterized by very low levels of progesterone (a hormone that raises the basal metabolism by 10%); the decrease of testosterone in male runners is thought to be a similar adaption to decreased available energy; see Exercise, Exercise-associated amenorrhea; Cf Blood doping

Runt disease Runting syndrome IMMUNOLOGY An experimental graft-versus-host disease that was induced in Billingham and Brent's experimental mice, characterized by weight loss, splenomegaly, diarrhea, anemia, leukemia, lymphoid atrophy, hepatic necrosis, infections, which in newborn mice is invariably fatal

Runyon groups A classification of MOTTs (***Mycobacterium*** species other than ***M tuberculosis***), many of which have been isolated from dust, soil, tap water and other innocuous sites (table, left); see MAIS, MOTT, Tuberculosis

Rust *vs* Sullivan see 'Gag rule'

Rusty lungs Brown induration of the lungs due to accumulation of hemosiderin-laden macrophages; see Heart failure cells

Rusty sputum A descriptor for the characteristic sputum produced in pneumonia caused by ***Streptococcus pneumoniae*** and ***Klebsiella pneumoniae***; which is composed of bacteria, hemorrhage, mucus and sloughed necrotic tissue

r-value Correlation coefficient A widely used statistical method that determines the relatedness (to a maximum of +1) or unrelatedness (to minimum of -1) of two series of data, allowing calculation of values in a scattergram, so that linearity or degrees of total randomness can be determined

RVS see Resource-based relative value scale

Ryanodine receptor A calcium channel of the sarcoplasmic reticulum, the gene for which, RYR, maps to chromosome 19q13.1, a locus close to genetic markers that map near the malignant hyperthermia susceptibility locus (Nature 1990; 343:559), and therefore the RYR gene is thought to play a role in this condition; see Malignant hyperthermia

Rye Classification A widely-accepted classification that divides Hodgkin's disease into four distinct clinicopathological categories (table, facing page)

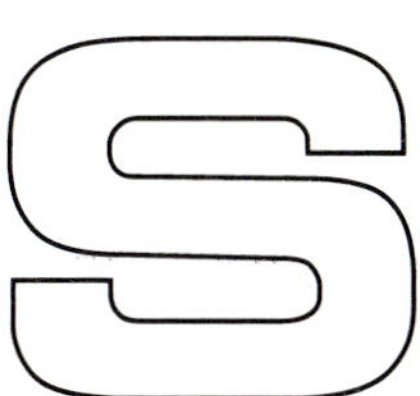

S Symbol for: entropy; mean dose/unit cumulated activity; period of DNA synthesis in the cell cycle; serine; standard deviation; substrate; Sulfur; Svedberg unit; mathematical sum

s Symbol for: Distance; sedimentation coefficient; second (time); standard deviation

Ss A mnemonic for the risk factors that have been implicated in of nasopharyngeal carcinoma: Smoking, spirits, sepsis, sunlight, syphilis, spices (and Epstein-Barr virus)

S1 fragment That portion of the myosin molecule that remains after trypsin and papain digestion; the S1 fragment binds to actin fibers and has an intrinsic unidirectional polarity

S1 nuclease protection analysis A method used in molecular biology to identify specific mRNA transcripts, in which mRNA fragments are mixed with a specific radioisotopic-DNA probe; if the mRNA of interest is present, it will hybridize to the DNA, joining at the corresponding base pairs; addition of S1 nuclease to the mixture, then digests all the non-paired or single-stranded RNA or DNA in the solution

S4 sequence PHYSIOLOGY A structural motif with basic amino acids at every third or fourth position that acts as a voltage sensor in voltage-dependent sodium, calcium and potassium channels; mutation of the S4 gene, alters the voltage-dependency of the channels (Nature 1991; 349:305)

S-100 IMMUNOHISTOCHEMISTRY An acidic heterodimeric protein composed of α and β chains that was first isolated from brain and is present in normal tissues, including neural crest, myoepithelium, breast ducts, sweat and salivary glands, skin, serous acini of bronchial glands and schwann cells, as well as in malignant melanomas and neurofibrosarcomas (Mayo Clin Proc 1990; 65:164)

S-100 fraction MOLECULAR BIOLOGY A sub-cellular fraction containing ribosomes, tRNA, and amino acyl-tRNA synthetase, obtained by ultracentrifugation at 100 000*g*, and is of use in studying the mechanics of amino acid incorporation into proteins; see Microsomes, Ultracentrifugation

SAAB assay Selected and amplified binding site imprint assay MOLECULAR BIOLOGY A technique for examining a gene's protein-recognition site that is applicable to any purified or partially purified protein or cloned gene, which identifies the DNA sequences necessary for protein binding (Science 1990; 250:1104)

Saber sheath trachea A non-motile deformity of the intrathoracic trachea in which the coronal diameter of the trachea is less than one-half of the sagittal diameter; the lateral tracheal walls are thickened and there is an abrupt transition of shape to a curve at the thoracic outlet, best appreciated by antero-posterior tomography and considered characteristic of chronic obstructive pulmonary disease

Saber shins A descriptor for the thickened, anteriorly-bowed (with possible lateral bowing) tibial cortex, caused by chronic periostitis which spares the epiphysis, first described in latent congenital syphilis, which may also be seen in advanced acquired syphilis; non-progressive, bilateral and symmetrical anterior bowing of the tibia and fibula may be seen in achondroplasia, type IX Ehlers-Danlos syndrome, enchondromatosis, fibrous dysplasia, excess fluoride ingestion during pregnancy,

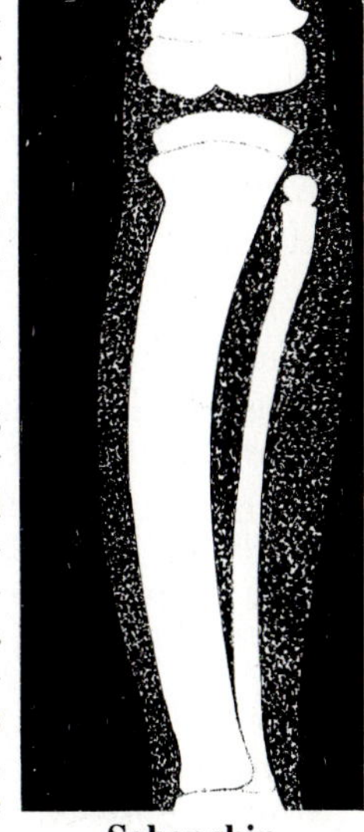

Saber shin

hyperparathyroidism, hyperphosphatasia, neurofibromatosis, osteogenesis imperfecta, osteomalacia, osteomyelitis, rickets, thanatophoric dwarfism and Weismann-Netter syndrome

Sabot heart Coeur en Sabot PEDIATRIC CARDIOLOGY A heart with a boot-like radiologic silhouette, in which the tip of the 'boot's toe' corresponds to an elevated cardiac apex, while the broad 'foot' portion corresponds to an increased prominence of the left cardiac border resulting from right cardiac hypertrophy; the sabot change classically occurs in well-developed Fallot's tetralogy (infundibular pulmonary stenosis, interventricular septal defect, right cardiac ventricular hypertrophy and a dextraposed, therefore overriding, aorta)

Saccharomyces cerevisiae see YAC cloning

Saccharopinuria Scally-Carson Syndrome An autosomal recessive condition characterized by abnormal lysine metabolism due to inactivity or absence of aminoadipic semialdehyde-glutamate reductase Clinical Moderate mental retardation, spastic diplegia, short stature and excretion of excess saccharopine, lysine and citrulline in the urine

Sacrifice RESEARCH *Verb* A euphemism for the killing of laboratory animals after an experiment's completion or as part of an experimental protocol that requires examination of internal organs or obtention of tissue or fluids for various analyses

Sacrum A name borrowed from the Egyptians who thought the bone was sacred to Osiris, their god of resurrection and agriculture; briefly Osiris' brother and enemy, Seth, chopped him up into pieces, one of which was close to the scrotum, the organ of rejuvenation and fertility (J Am Med Assoc 1987; 257:2061)

SAD Seasonal affective disorder 'Winter blues' A clinical complex characterized by photolabile depression that is most prominent during the winter; an uncertain number of SAD patients respond to high intensity light, which acts to alter their circadian rhythm, a therapy that is most effective in the morning; a light intensity of 10 000 lx viewed at very close range may be required to reset the biological clock (Sleep 1990;13:267); Cf Melancholia, Melanocholy

Saddle back curve A descriptor for the febrile curve seen in trench fever, where 3-5 days of high temperature are followed by 3-5 days of low temperatures, occurring in up to eight waves before resolution; a similar fever curve may also occur in bartonellosis, chinkungunya and Colorado tick fever; Cf Camelback curve, Pulse-temperature dissociation

Saddle bag scrotum Aarskog syndrome A scrotal fold that overhangs the penis, inherited in an X-linked recessive fashion and accompanied by faciogenital dysplasia, short stature and facial defects

Saddle embolus A large thrombus lodged at an arterial bifurcation, where the blood flows from a large bore vessel to a smaller one; the 'classic' saddle embolus occurring at the bifurcation of the pulmonary arteries in fatal pulmonary thromboembolism (PTE) due to centrally-migrating venous embolus, is distinctly uncommon; in the more typical case of PTE, the emboli are more peripherally located than the pulmonary arteries

Saddle nose Marked depression of the nasal root, classically described as a late manifestation of congenital syphilis-induced rhinitis and frontal periostitis, which destroys adjacent bone, cartilage and potentially also the nasal septum; the saddle nose deformity has also been described in AIDS embryopathy, Christ-Siemans-Touraine syndrome, deletion syndromes, fetal trimethadione syndrome, Laron-type dwarfism, leprechaunism, multiple epiphyseal dysplasia, type III, OSMED syndrome, relapsing polychondritis, thanotophoric dwarfism, Wegener's granulomatosis and a variety of conditions that are further characterized by gargoyle-like facies

Sado-masochism see Sexual deviancy

SADR Severity-adjusted death rate A calculated rate of mortality based on the severity of a morbid condition, a statistic of use in determining the appropriate reimbursement from Medicare Note: In the current economic environment in the US health care industry, a patient's 'allowable', ie reimbursed length of stay is determined by disease severity; see Case-mix index, DRGs, Medicare

'Safari study' 'Helicopter research' A clinical or epidemiologic research project that is conducted by foreign scientists who have used local contacts to gain access to a population group and obtain samples that are then analyzed in the home laboratories of the visiting scientists, who neither make the data available to the host investigators, nor include them as authors in the reports, despite their contributions (Science 1990; 250:199n&v); see Rs of research

Safe blood TRANSFUSION MEDICINE Packed red cells and blood products obtained from subjects with no known risks for exposure to transfusion-transmissible microorganisms (TTM), eg malaria, human immunodeficiency virus (HIV-1) which have been fully tested and are negative for the presence of TTM by a direct assay of viral products, eg detection of hepatitis B surface antigen, by an indirect assay of exposure to viruses, eg antibodies to hepatitis C virus and HIV-1 and 'surrogate' assays, eg measurement of transaminases, which are non-specific indicators of hepatic inflammation; 'safe' blood carries an estimated 1:61 000 chance of containing HIV-1 (which is undetectable as the patients are in a 'window period' prior to the production of antibodies to HIV-1); see Blood shield laws, Euroblood, Surrogate markers

Safe harbor rules HEALTH CARE INDUSTRY A broad term for any series of guidelines promulgated by the US government after specific legislation is enacted; because of the broad wording and vagueness of certain laws, it is often unclear what are considered to be legal or illegal activities regarding conflicts of interest, eg self-referral to health care facilities in which the physician has a financial interest or other questionable buisiness or ethical practices (Am Med News 23/Sep/91); the guidelines thus serve to define those practices ('safe harbors') that are fully accepted in the eyes of the law

Safe sexual activities SAFE SEX GUIDELINES A group of guidelines for the relative safety of various sexual activities in terms of the potential for transmitting infection,

SEX GUIDELINES

Safe sexual activities Mutual masturbation (male or female), social kissing (dry), body massage, hugging, body-to-body contact (frottage), light sado-masochistic activities (without bruising or bleeding)

Possibly safe sexual activities (for which insufficient data is available, which should be considered with caution) French (wet) kissing, vaginal or anal intercourse with a condom, fellatio interruptus, cunnilingus, urine contact ('water sports', ie urination on sexual partner)

Unsafe sexual activities (the risk increases with multiple partners) Vaginal or anal intercourse without a condom, manual-anal intercourse ('fisting'), oral-anal contact (anilingus, 'rimming'), fellatio totalis (oral-semen contact), blood contact, sharing of sex toys

(from DG Ostrow, in KK Holmes, et al Sexually Transmitted Diseases, 2nd ed, McGraw-Hill, New York, 1990 and 'AIDS Information for Physicians', Med Soc of New Jersey, 1989)

in particular HIV-1 (table, above), which is of use in advising patients; see Sex industry, Sexual deviancy, Sexually-transmitted disease

Safety PUBLIC HEALTH The condition of being secure or safe from undergoing or causing injury, harm or loss; any activity or element in the environment for which the risks of its use and disposal are considered acceptable is considered to be safe; see Small parts standards

'Safety net' hospital A public hospital in the US that provides health care to all patients, regardless of their ability to pay for the services provided; public hospitals provide a disproportionate share of high-cost services, including trauma surgery, burn therapy, genetic counseling, hemodialysis, psychiatric services, imaging analysis, cardiac catheterization, surgery and organ transplantations Note: Because of the crumbling financial infrastructure and increasing loss of revenue in the US inner cities, many 'safety net' facilities are being forced to close, potentially leaving those live in these areas without adequate health care facilities

Safety pin appearance A descriptor for a morphology in which an elliptical structure demonstrates bipolar staining with central attenuation HEMATOLOGY A descriptor for the erythrocytes of thalassemia MICROBIOLOGY The safety pin morphology is a typical light microscopic finding in *Bacter-oides fragilis*, a gram-positive anaerobe with a centrally cleared zone corresponding to vacuoles, *Chilo-mastix mesnili* Lemon-shaped cysts which have a cyclostomal fiber and peripheral staining, *Calymmatobacterium granulomatis*, the gram-negative coccobacillary agent of granuloma inguinale; the name refers to the arrangement of the Donovan bodies located within the macrophages, visualized by hematoxylin and eosin (purple), silver stain (brown-black) and Wright-Giemsa stains and ***Yersinia*** species, especially ***Y pestis*** (bubonic plague), best seen with the Wayson (carbol fuchsin-methylene blue) stain as large coccobacillary forms

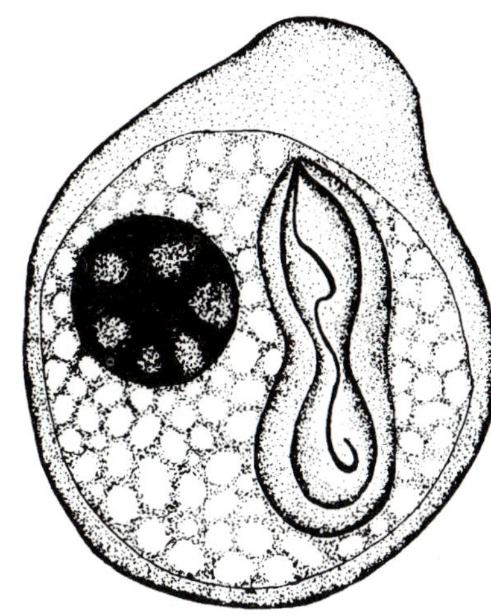

Safety pin appearance

Sagging rope sign PEDIATRIC ORTHOPEDICS A thin opaque curved line (figure, below) in the upper femoral metaphysis, which in the anteroposterior (or posterior) view extends laterally from the inferior border of the femoral neck, is within the femoral neck for a distance, often reaching the superior border of the femoral neck; the 'sagging rope' is typical of, but not invariably present in Perthes' disease and occurs whenever ischemia and growth are simultaneous, indicating damage to the epiphyseal growth plate and may be seen in (spondylo-) epiphyseal dysplasia, achondroplasia and cretinism (J Bone J Surg (Br) 1981;63B:43)

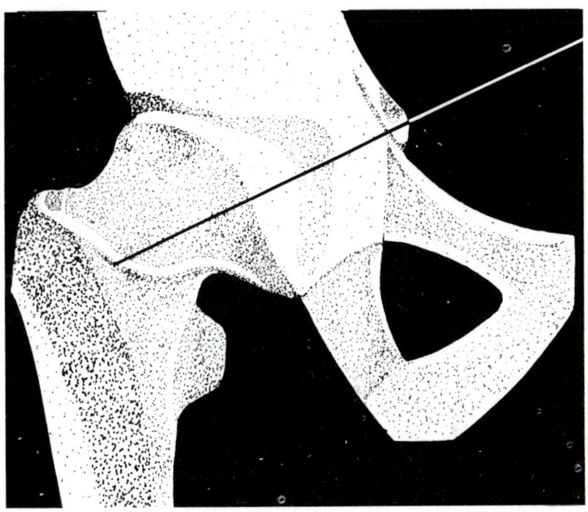

Sagging rope sign

Sago spleen Tapioca spleen A descriptor for the rounded, translucent masses of amyloid that replace lymphoid follicles in splenic amyloidosis

SAIDS Simian acquired immunodeficiency syndrome A retrovirus group D-induced infection in the rhesus monkey (***Macaca mulatta***) with AIDS-like features including CD4 lymphocyte depletion, opportunistic infections and neoplasms, severe weight loss, multifocal granulomatous encephalitis Note: SIV has little sequence homology with HIV, but is similar to the hamster A-type particle; see HIV-1, HIV-2, Retroviruses, SIV

Sailor's skin see Solar elastosis

Sail sign RADIOLOGY A sharply demarcated triangular radiopacity seen in the mediastinum of 10% of normal children, which corresponds to the thymus and disappears on inspiration, see Rocker-bottom shadow

Sail vertebra A hook or wedge deformity of an upper lumbar vertebra, thought to be due to physical stress, which may be seen in early-onset hypothyroidism, achondroplasia, Morquio, Hurler and Hurler-like syndromes, metatropic dwarfism and spondylometaphyseal dysplasia

Saint disease(s) In the Dark and Middle Ages (AD 476 to circa AD 1400), all disease was considered a visitation from God to punish one for various sins and one prayed to certain saints to rid oneself of the disease (table, right)

Saints' diseases (obsolete)

St Agatha's disease	Mastitis
St Aignon's disease	Tinea
St Anthony's dance	Chorea
St Appolonia's disease	Toothache
St Arman's disease	Pellagra
St Avertin's disease	Epilepsy
St Avidus's disease	Deafness
St Blaizes' disease	Tonsillitis
St Claire's disease	Conjunctivitis
St Dymphna's disease	Insanity
St Erasmus's disease	Colic
St Fiacre's disease	Hemorrhoids
St Francis' disease	Erysipelas
St Gervasius' disease	Rheumatism
St Gete's disease	Cancer
St Giles' disease	Leprosy
St Guy's dance	St Vitus dance
St Hubert's disease	Rabies
St Ignatius disease	Pellagra
St Job's disease	Syphilis
St Kilda's disease	Colds, infection
St Louis' disease	Encephalitis
St Main's disease	Scabies
St Martin's disease	Alcoholism
St Mary sickness	Ergotism
St Mathurin's disease	Psychosis
St Modestus's disease	Chorea
St Paul's evil	Epilepsy
St Roch's disease	Bubonic plague
St Sebastian's disease	Plague
St Sement's disease	Syphilis'
St Valentine's disease	Epilepsy
St Vitus's dance	Sydenham's chorea
St Zachary's disease	Mutism

St Anthony's fire A term of Middle Age vintage for paresthesia and erythema, which may have been due to 1) **ERYSIPELAS** An acute infectious dermatitis by group A streptococci due to streptococcal pharyngitis ('strep throat'), less commonly caused by other coccal organisms; erysipelas is most common in the very young and very old, often occurring on the face in a 'butterfly' pattern with orbital edema, an 'angry' red color that may become vesiculobullous in advancing margins and be accompanied by fever Treatment Antibiotics 2) **ERGOT POISONING**, in which the name referred to the skin color, secondary to peripheral vasospasm, vasomotor depression and weak adrenergic antagonism at α-adrenergic, serotonin and tryptamine receptors and 3) **HERPES ZOSTER**

St Helenian cellulitis A condition described on the island of St Helena of possibly viral origin with a male:female ratio of 1:3 Clinical Intense burning pruritus of the legs with erythematous vesicles, accompanied by headache, rigors and pulmonary edema

St Louis encephalitis (SLE) A summer-fall infection, first described in an epidemic in St Louis, Missouri in 1933, caused by an arbovirus Vector *Culex* mosquito Clinical Vague flu-like prodrome, followed by severe headaches, stiff neck, loss of deep tendon reflexes, blurring of vision, hyperthermia, confusion and delirium Neuropathology Edema, hemorrhage, lymphocytic infiltration, degeneration and gliosis Mortality 20%; Cf California encephalitis, Eastern and Western equine encephalitides

St Vitus' dance Sydenham's chorea Rapid, involuntary movement of the face, causing grins, grimaces, contortions and tics, extremities, causing erratic flailing and if unilateral, hemichorea, hands, causing repeated partial fisting of the hands or a 'milkmaid's grip' and the togue, in which the muscular fasciculation has been likened to a 'bag of worms'; Sydenham's chorea is a major criterion for the diagnosis of rheumatic fever by the Jones' criteria, and develops after a latency period of several weeks-to-months

Salaam convulsions A spasm of early infancy onset that occurs 20-100 times/day, disappears by age two or evolves into grand mal seizures with significant mental retardation, described by neurologist Dr West, who likened his son's lightning-quick bobbing of the head and flexion and extension of the trunk and arms to the Arab genuflexion of greeting and prayer

Salaam movements Violent jackknife-like movements seen in unclassified seizures, intermittent ictal events

***Salicornia bigelovii* Torr** GLOBAL NUTRITION A seed crop plant that may be grown in salt water, which was developed from a wild halophyte; *S bigelovii* yields high-quality oil, containing 30% protein and 30% unsaturated fatty acid-rich oil; this crop may be a viable substitute for soybean oil and is of potential use in cultivation in 'marginal' regions of the world (Science 1991; 251:1065)

Salicylism CLINICAL TOXICOLOGY Acute symptoms resulting from aspirin (salicylate) overdose, causing a severe metabolic acidosis and a large anion gap; in the early phase, salicylates stimulate respiration through central mechanisms, decreasing $PaCO_2$ and plasma bicarbonate levels; salicylates interfere with mitochondrial metabolism, and when the mitochondria degenerate, cause a release of unmeasured organic acids, increasing the anion gap

Saline abortion see Abortion

Salivary gland inclusion disease Obsolete synonym for Cytomegalic inclusion virus

Salk Institute A facility for biomedical research built in 1960 from monies provided by the 'March of Dimes' in the mold of Jonas Salk, the creator of the polio vaccine; from 1973 to 1987, the Salk Institute was second only to the Cold Spring Harbor Laboratory in production of 'most cited papers' (Science 1990; 249:361), see Citation impact

Salla disease An autosomal recessive condition first seen and most common in the Salla region of northeast Finland Clinical Moderate-to-severe psychomotor retardation, coarse facies, clumsiness, slow speech, spasticity, ataxia Laboratory Patients excrete and store 10-30-fold normal quantities of N-acetyl-neuraminic acid (NANA or sialic acid) Histopathology Hematopoietic (Salla) cells have abundant NANA-filled vacuoles (lysosomes), due to the defective egress of sialic acid from the lysosomes

Salmon patch/lesion An adjectival descriptor for various mucocutaneous lesions with a flesh-red color likened to that of the large soft-finned anadromous table fish of the Northern Atlantic (*Salmo salar*) or of rivers tributary to the northwestern Pacific coastline of Canada and USA (*Oncorhynchus* species); Salmon patches are seen in 1) Tuberculous sclerosis Papular, dark pink eruptions of the face, especially at the nasolabial folds, first appearing in childhood, becoming more prominent post-pubertally 2) Macular hemangioma or nevus simplex Small pale pink, ill-defined macules corresponding to focal ectatic vessels on the glabella, eyelids, upper lip and neck in 30-50% of normal neonates, that are more prominent with crying or temperature changes; the face lesions fade with time, but the nuchal and posterior occipital lesions may persist, but if covered with hair are not a cosmetic problem 3) Boston exanthema A discrete nonpruritic 0.5-1.5 cm papule seen on the face, upper chest and rarely, the extremities, caused by an enterovirus, echovirus 16; the appearance of the salmon patch in Boston exanthema coincides with defervescence of clinical disease 4) Nevus flammeus Birth mark A single lesion, most commonly seen on the forehead, eyelids, nape of neck that may be autosomal dominant 5) Progressive syphilis-related interstitial keratitis A reddish corneal discoloration due to neovascularization (J Am Med Assoc 1989; 262:2921) 6) Sickling hemoglobinopathies A descriptor for the discoloration seen in the ocular fundus, see Sea fan appearance

SALT Skin-associated lymphoid tissue; see MALT

Salt and pepper appearance An adjectival descriptor for an appearance in which minute hyperpigmented lesions or radiopaque 'granules' are admixed with equally-sized hypopigmented lesions or radiolucent granules

Salt and pepper choroidoretinitis OPHTHALMOLOGY Focal or diffuse mottled whitish lesions admixed with variably-sized pigmented deposits in the optic fundus of congenital rubella (German measles) and Cockayne's progeria syndrome, which are not associated with visual impairment; a 'salt-and-pepper' appearance is also described in the peripheral retinal fundus in both women carriers and in early stages in men with X-linked diffuse total choroidal vascular atrophy

Salt and pepper chromatin URINARY CYTOLOGY Small granules of chromatin separated by translucent nucleoplasm, characteristic of benign urothelial (transitional) cells Note: In contrast, malignant urothelial cells have coarsely clumped chromatin and do not allow passage of light

Salt and pepper pattern RADIOLOGY Punctate and granular decalcification alternating with focal mineralization, classically seen in the skull of primary hyperparathyroidism; these lesions are rarely seen as the disease does not often evolve to this advanced stage

Salting-out LABORATORY TECHNOLOGY A decrease in a protein's solubility in a solution of high ionic strength by increasing the concentration of neutral salt in the solution, which causes a partial dehydration of the protein through the competition between the proteins and the salt ions for the solvating water molecules

Salvage chemotherapy A treatment modality used when a patient with malignancy has 'failed' in one or more chemotherapeutic regimens; Salvage therapy is problematic as the patients may already be in poor condition with fulminant clinical deterioration, have large bulky aggressively growing tumors and multi-drug resistances; salvage therapy is used in Hodgkin's and non-Hodgkin's lymphoma and small cell carcinoma; see Heroic therapy

Salvage pathway ONCOLOGY Any metabolic pathway using substrates that are not the usual biosynthetic intermediates for a product, eg 1) The salvage of free purines from the hydrolysis of nucleotides for the generation of new nucleotides, or 2) The secondary pathway of nucleotide synthesis, in which thymidylate is produced by thymidine kinase from thymidine, rather than the usual path in which deoxyuridylate is methylated by thymidylate synthetase into thymidylate, a pathway utilized by patients with megaloblastic anemia; see Leukovorin 'rescue'

SAM 1) Self-assembly monolayer PHYSICAL BIOCHEMISTRY A model system formed of long-chain alkanethiolates that are deposited on a metal film allowing the study of protein-organic surface interactions, which is of use in understanding the mechanisms of protein adsorption in protein chromatography, immuno-diagnostic and other clinical assays, biomaterials and cell adhesion (Science 1991; 252:1164) 2) Substrate adhesion molecules MOLECULAR BIOLOGY see RGD family 3) Systolic anterior motion CARDIOLOGY An anomalous movement of the anterior leaflet of the mitral valve that appears to strike the interventricular septum in early diastole, seen in patients with idiopathic hypertrophic subaortic stenosis and obstruction

Same-sense mutation A specific type of silent (DNA) mutation caused by a simple point mutation that gives rise to a different triple of DNA nucleotides being transcribed into a 'synonym' codon, resulting in the incorporation of the same amino acid into the growing polypeptide, as would have been incorporated by the original, non-mutated triple of DNA nucleotides; since the protein is unchanged, same-sense mutations are 'silent'; see Degenerate code, Silent mutation

Sampling error An 'error' that occurs in a diagnostic work-up, in which insufficient, inadequate or non-representative material was obtained for analysis, referring in particular to biopsy material, or, less commonly to cytological samplings Note: In establishing a diagnosis from a biopsy material, the clinician and the pathologist wage a silent war; the clinician or radiologist who obtains the material justifies his parsimony, as the dictum of 'the larger the piece of tissue obtained', the greater are the complications', is often true; while the latter realizes that the rule of 'the bigger, the better' is crucial to establishing histological patterns and in minimizing tissue artefacts; 21- and 22-gauge 'skinny' needles guided by computed tomography in expert hands may be sufficient to minimize sampling error

Sanctuary sites ONCOLOGY Those regions of the body (central nervous system and testes) where leukemic cells are relatively protected from the cytolytic effects of systemic chemotherapy; before the sanctuary concept was appreciated, more than one-half of patients with leukemia had central nervous system involvement within 2 years of remission, an event that is prevented by prophylactic radiotherapy (1800-2800 cGy) and intrathecal methotrexate; see Remission

Sandal keratoderma DERMATOLOGY Lesions of the soles of the feet seen in pityriasis rubra pilaris, accompanied by scaly erythematous patches which later become fissured and hyperkeratotic

'Sanded' nuclei A descriptor for globose granular hepatocytic nuclei that are replete with hepatitis B core particles

Sander's disease Paranoia

Sandfly Tropical sandfly A small (3 mm), hairy insect (figure, right) with a stinging persistent bite that is a vector for bartonellosis, leishmaniasis and sandfly fever New world sandfly, *Lutzomyia longipalpis* and other species are vectors for bartonellosis (*B bacilliformis*) and leishmaniasis (*Leish-mania mexicana*, *L braziliensis*) Old world sandfly, *Phlebotomus papatasi* is the vector for the Oriental button (*Leishmania tropica*) New and Old world sandflies can be vectors for kala-azar (*Leishmania donovani*)

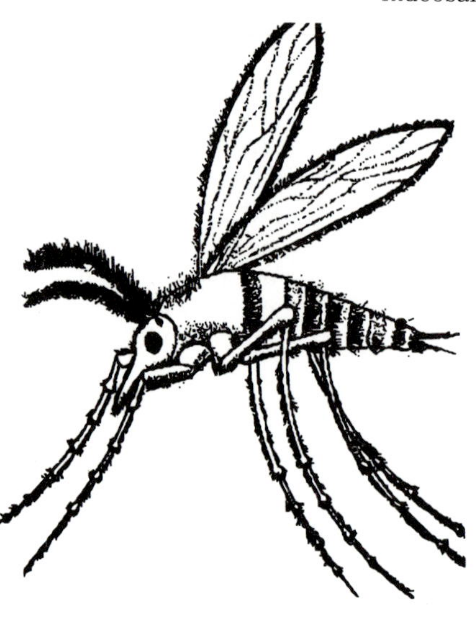

Sandfly

Sandfly fever Phlebotomus fever An acute, self-limited viral infection caused by five distinct serotypes of Arbovirus, occurring in the Mediterranean rim countries, eastern Africa and Central Asia during dry hot weather Clinical Abrupt onset of high fever, headache, ocular pain, photophobia, vomiting, dysgeusia, arthralgia and occasionally aseptic meningitis

Sandoglobulin see Human immune globulin

Sandpaper skin A descriptor for ´1) The coarse, bumpy, cool, pale, hypotrichous skin characteristic of hypothyroidism and 2) The skin surface in scarlet fever with indurated hair follicles; sandpaper mucosa refers to the bright bumpy, intraoral erythema of scarlet fever that desquamates with the resolution of infection

'Sandwich' methodology IMMUNOLOGY A descriptor for a technique that allows identification of an antigen or antibody by 'sandwiching' a molecule of interest, X between two other standardized molecules (Y and Y´) that either recognize molecule X immunologically or serve as immune recognition sites Principle The first layer is the tissue- (or latex bead-bound) antigen; the second layer corresponds to the first antibody (AB1), raised in (for example) a rabbit against the bound antigen; AB1 is placed in a solution and bathes the bound antigen; if AB1 does not recognize the antigen, it will be washed off; the second antibody, AB2, is an anti-rabbit antibody, the variable end of which recognizes the constant region of AB1; the final layer of the sandwich is an indicator or detector molecule that is attached to the constant region of AB2, and consists of an enzyme or a radioactive or fluorescent marker; Cf Avidin-biotinylated complex; see Immunoperoxidase method

Sandwich vertebrae RADIOLOGY A descriptor applied to the increased density of the vertebral end-plates with normal bodies and preservation of intervertebral spaces, classically described in osteopetrosis; Cf Rugger jersey

Sandy patch A descriptor for aggregates of calcified submucosal schistosoma (usually S mansoni) ova, which may be seen in the rectum; see Circumoval bodies, Pipe stem fibrosis

Sanger sequencing Dr F Sanger delineated methods for determining the sequence of DNA and proteins **1) SANGER (DNA) SEQUENCING** dideoxy method is an enzymatic method for sequencing DNA Method: A single strand of DNA to be sequenced is hybridized to a 5'-end-labeled deoxynucleotide 'primer'; four separate radiolabeled (^{32}P) reaction mixtures are prepared in which a 'primer' is elongated using a DNA polymerase; each mixture contains all four possible deoxynucleotide triphosphates, in addition to one of the four possible (^{32}P radiolabeled) dideoxynucleotide triphosphates, in a ratio of 1:100; since the latter have no 3' hydroxyl groups, the chain will not be elongated when these residues are added to the chain, and reactions with these residues end prematurely; each mixture is then denatured and separated by electrophoresis **2) SANGER (PROTEIN) SEQUENCING** A method for determining the amino acid sequence of large polypeptides, in the first step, proteolytic enzymes are used to break the peptide bonds only between selected amino acids, resulting in a number of smaller polypeptide fragments; these fragments are then separated according to their migration speeds in a solvent on chromatographic paper; since the speed of migration differs according to the solvent, 90° rotation and repetition of the electrophoresis produces a characteristic 'fingerprint' for each polypeptide; the fingerprinted spot is then removed and the amino acid sequence of each fragment is then determined by biochemical means; the entire protein's sequence is then determined by fitting together overlapping sequences in a coherent fashion; the latter Sanger sequencing method has been supplanted by Erdman's method for sequencing proteins

San Joaquin valley fever Coccidioidomycosis

S antigen Soluble antigen An incomplete viral form produced in the early stages of some viral infections

SAO Sham feeding-stimulated acid output A stimulatory test used to evaluate the adequacy of vagotomy in patients requiring the same for gastric ulcer disease (normal: SAO ranges from 10 to 0% of the peak acid output); see BAO, MAO, PAO

Sao Paulo typhus Brazilian form of Rocky mountain spotted fever

SAP(s) Sphingolipid activator proteins A family of small 8-13 kD heat-stable proteins required for sphingolipid hydrolysis; the genes for SAP-1 and SAP-2 are located on chromosome 10 on the same locus; **SAP-1** activates hydrolysis of cerebroside sulfate, GM1 ganglioside and globotriaosylceramide by arylsulfatase A, acid β-galactosidase and α galactosidase; SAP-1 deficiency results in accumulation of cerebroside sulfate and other glycolipids, causing a clinical disease with features of metachromatic leukodystrophy **SAP-2** activates hydrolysis of glucosylceramide, galactosylceramide and sphingomyelin by β-glucosylceramidase, galactosylceramide β-galactosidase and sphingomyelinase respectively; SAP-2 deficiency was reported in a case with variant Gaucher's disease **SAP-3** activates hydrolysis of ganglioside GM2 by β-N-acetylgalactosaminidase A and is deficient in the AB variant of GM2 gangliosidosis

Saponin(s) A group of water-soluble, surface acting plant glycosides that are detergents at high dilutions and are potent hemolytic agents

SAPS Simplified acute physiology score; see Prognostic scoring systems

SARA see Sexually-acquired reactive arthritis

Saranac A fresh-air tuberculosis sanatorium, built in 1884 near Lake Saranac in the Adirondack mountains of New York; when effective anti-tuberculosis drugs (streptomycin 1944, isoniazid 1951 and others) became available, the raison d'être of this and other anti-tuberculous 'Magic mountains' ceased to exist; see Single disease hospital

Sarcoma botryoides Greek, botrios, grapelike Embryonal rhabdomyosarcoma A sarcoma that is most common in young children, 90% of which occur in girls under age five, usually located on the anterior vagina, occasionally in the urinary bladder or nasopharynx **Pathology** Superficial grape-like bosselations **Histopathology** Dense superficial cellular ('cambium') layer which overlies loose myxoid stroma **Treatment** Wide local excision Extrapelvic spread often indicates a poor prognosis

Sarcoplasmic masses 'Smudgy' masses of eosinophilic sarcoplasm devoid of normal striations typically seen by light microscopy in myotonic dystrophy, which is further characterized by cords of nuclei and atrophy of type I muscle fibers

Sargramostim Recombinant GM-CSF A biological response modifier licensed in 1991 that accelerates myeloid recovery in patients with lymphomas and acute lymphoblastic leukemia, whose bone marrow has been suppressed by chemotherapy and/or radiation; because of the limited number of patients who might benefit from sargramostim (estimated 3000 to 5000 autologous bone marrow transplants), it has received an 'orphan' status **Side effects** Mild rash, diarrhea, asthenia, malaise (J Am Med Assoc 1991; 265:2315); see G-CSF, GM-CSF

SART Standard acid reflux test An assay that evaluates esophageal pH for reflux esophagitis, utilizing standard stress maneuvers; Cf BAO, MAO

SAS syndrome Supravalvular aortic stenosis; see Elfin face syndrome of Williams

Sashimi see Sushi

Satellite A common adjectival descriptor for lesions, masses, patterns or radiologic densities that surround a central point

Satellite abscess A characteristic multifocal lesion of nocardiosis, in which there is slow, indolent extension of 'daughter' abscess nodules from a central focus of purulent necrosis, each surrounded by an incomplete fibrotic layer

Satellite bags TRANSFUSION MEDICINE A series of plastic bags attached via tubes in a closed system to a 'mother' bag used for the donation, allowing sterile separation of blood components

Satellite bodies GENETICS Discrete masses of chromatin attached to the short arm of an acrocentric chromosome, which not seen in the Y chromosome; Cf Double minutes

Satellite cells Cells adjacent to the basement membrane with oval-to-elongated nuclei and a thin rim of cytoplasm containing a few mitochondria, seen in the myocytes of Duchenne's muscular dystrophy **Histology** Oligodendrogliocytes that surround neurons in the gray matter

Satellite colonies see Satellite phenomenon

Satellite DNA Segment(s) of highly-repeated eukaryotic DNA that differs from the bulk or 'main band' DNA, and may be separated therefrom by ultracentrifugation using a cesium chloride density gradient, resulting in a smaller, 'satellite' band of DNA fragments

Satellite infections Minigranulomas seen in atypical mycobacterial infections, eg fish tank granuloma, swimming pool granuloma)

Satellite nodules DERMATOLOGY Minute tumor cell nests, measuring circa 0.05 mm in diameter that are present in the reticular dermis, panniculus or in vessels in malignant melanoma, which are separated from the melanoma itself; melanomas with satellite nodules have a four-fold worse prognosis than melanomas of similar thickness without satellites (Cancer 1987; 53:2183)

Satellite phenomenon BACTERIOLOGY 1) The growth of colonies of some species of *Haemophilus* (*H influenza, H parainfluenza, H hemolyticus*) in the vicinity of Staphylococci, the latter of which produce a growth factor V (NADP); Cf CAMP test, Reverse CAMP test 2) The growth of minute, symbiotic, thiol- or vitamin B_6-dependent mutant bacteria in the vicinity of group A Streptococcus 3) The ability to hydrolyze casein and other components of growth media, causing a satellite-like transparency of an otherwise translucent growth medium, allowing differentiation among various aerobic actinomycetes, eg *Actinomadura, Nocardia* and *Streptomyces* species

Satellite RNA A low weight (5S to 8S) RNA that may associate with rRNA in plants

Satellite virus A virus that co-infects with a pathogenic virus, eg tobacco necrosis satellite virus, adenovirus-associated virus

Satellitism The rimming of neutrophils by platelets in the peripheral blood, a phenomenon that may evoke spurious thrombocytopenia by automated platelet counters, which may be associated with cryoglobulinemia, hypergammaglobulinemia, immune complexes or use of an EDTA anticoagulant during collection of the blood

Saturated fatty acid A fatty acid lacking double bonds in the alkyl chain; most natural saturated fatty acids contain an even number of double bonds and those with less than ten carbons are liquid at room temperature

Saturation A satiated state BIOCHEMISTRY A state in a macromolecule, in which the maximum amount of ligands are bound to recipient sites CHEMISTRY The maximum amount of a solute that can be permanently dissolved in a solution under a defined set of conditions ORGANIC CHEMISTRY Presence of only single bonds on the carbon molecules

Saturday night special FORENSIC MEDICINE A colloquial term attributed to the Detroit police department, referring to an easily purchased and inexpensive, often 38-caliber, revolver that is used for 'crimes of passions', often occurring on Saturday night

Saturday night palsy Alcoholic neuropathy A group of transient neuromuscular defects affecting a subject who falls in a stuporous state in an unnatural position, classically after an alcoholic 'binge', or overdose of sedatives; the palsies may affect 1) The legs, causing a partial transient deficit known as neurapraxia, affecting the peroneal nerve with a greater motor than sensory loss, with recuperation within six weeks, which may be due to the axon's inability to re-establish a membrane potential rather than actual disruption of the axon or 2) The arms due to compression of the radial nerve against a hard edge or surface

Saturnine gout Chronic lead intoxication A gout-like complex secondary to imbibition of 'moonshine' whiskey distilled in copper tubing joined with lead solder that may present with interstitial nephritis, reduced glomerular filtration rate and hypertension Note: Although in the current environment, excess lead exposure is more common in the lower socioeconomic strata, eg children in inner cities, workers who repair automobile radiators and others Note: Gout was historically a disease of the upper class, who continue to be heavily-exposed through leaded drinking crystal; fine port contains 89 μg/L of lead before decanting into leaded crystal, rising to 5,331 μg/L after four months of storage and 21,530 μg/L after five years of storage (Lancet 1991; 337:141); see Moonshine; Cf Pheasant hunter's toe

Sausage link fundus

Saturn's ring OPHTHALMOLOGY A whitish ring surrounding the cornea and blue sclera seen in osteogenesis imperfecta

Satyr ear A congenital abnormality of the auricle where the helix lacks the usual rolled contour and the tubercle is unusually prominent, coming to a vague point; satyrs are minor deities of Greek mythology with pointed ears, horns, a van Dyck beard, a male torso and the body and legs of a goat, who serve Bacchus, the god of fertility, roaming the countryside and having multiple sexual encounters (J Pediatr 1982; 100:250)

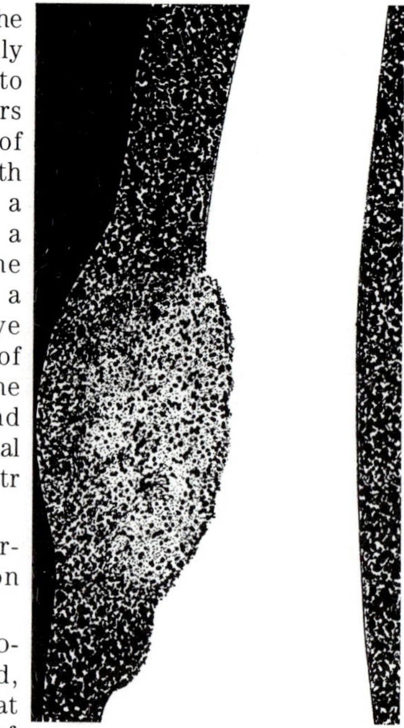

Saucerization

Satyriasis Male hypersexuality, see Don Juan syndrome

Saucerization ORTHOPEDICS A flattened, disciform defect that parallels the shaft of long bones (figure), which may be seen on a plain film, punctuated by microcalcifications, that is considered to be typical of fibrosarcoma with bony involvement

Sausage link pattern OPHTHALMOLOGY A descriptor for the marked dilatation and tortuosity of retinal veins that are focally segmented at arteriovenous crossings (figure, below), seen in the optic fundus in grade II hypertensive retinopathy, in non-proliferative diabetic retinopathy and, is classically described in Waldenström's macroglobulinemia or hyperviscosity syndrome

Sausage toes A fanciful descriptor for edematous tenosynovitis of the toes, which may be seen in non-specific arthritis, as well as in Reiter's syndrome and psoriatic arthritis

'Savannah syndrome' A term of uncertain origin that explains the North Americans' mania for maintaining a lawn as a primal human instinct to clear forest and vegetation, imposing his sense of order on the environment

Savant Idiot savant An individual who lacks the ability to reason abstractly but has a remarkable overdevelopment of a skill, eg mathematical or calendar 'calculation', memory, mechanical ability or talent in music and the visual arts; most savants are male and have IQs above 40 (thus 'idiot' is incorrect, as that now obsolete term referred to those with an IQ under 25); they may be blind and autistic; the savant's talent may appear and disappear virtually overnight; the pathogenesis is unclear but may be related to a dichotomy of function between the right and left brain

Sawfish pattern CARDIOLOGY A descriptor for the jagged systolic narrowing of the left anterior descending coronary artery when seen by angiography, a finding considered characteristic of hypertrophic cardiomyopathy (Circulation 1982; 66:800); Cf Bridging

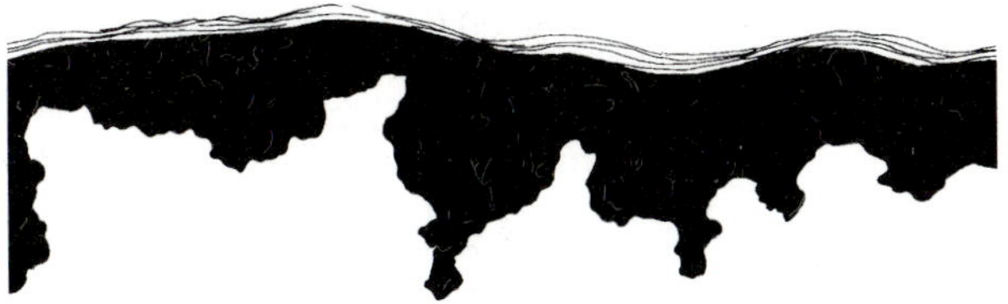

Saw tooth pattern

Saw-tooth pattern DERMATOPATHOLOGY A histopathologic appearance corresponding to a jagged and thickened dermal-epidermal junction, classically described in lichen planus (figure, above) RADIOLOGY A jagged radiocontrast column seen by barium studies of the colon in ischemic colitis, exudative enteropathy, cathartic colon, necrotizing enterocolitis due to congenital megacolon (Hirsch-sprung's disease) and rarely in diverticulosis, a pattern atttributed to a combination of edema and erosion of the mucosa

Saxitoxin

Saxitoxin A potent paralyzing neurotoxin first isolated from the Alaskan clam (*Saxidomus giganteus*) that binds to the cell membrane's sodium channel, blocking depolarization at the neuromuscular junction, increasing sodium permeability; the toxin is heat stable, water soluble and rapidly absorbed from the gastrointestinal tract; as few as six clams may be fatal; see Conotoxin, Red tide

SBE Subacute bacterial endocarditis

SBLA syndrome see Li-Fraumeni syndrome

SBT 1) Serum bactericidal titration see Minimum bactericidal concentration 2) Symplastin bleeding time

SC disease Sickle-hemoglobin C disease A hemoglobinopathy affecting circa 1:800 US blacks, characterized by a marked increase in infections, eg bacterial meningitis and Salmonella osteomyelitis due to a defect in the alternate (properdin) complement pathway; other effects of SC disease include 1) Osteoporosis, which result in the formation of 'fishmouth vertebrae' 2) Nephropathy, with poor renal concentration, acidification and increased glomerular filtration rate Note: Juxtamedullary erythrocytes traverse the hyperosmolar medulla, sickle and cause papillary necrosis, which is more common in SC disease than in sickle cell anemia 3) Retinopathy, which occurs in 75% of SC disease in contrast to 15% of patients with the usual form of sickle cell anemia; fundoscopic findings include a 'black sunburst' pattern, due to increased glycolysis in the end-arteriolar system and a 'seafoam' pattern, a proliferative retinopathy **Laboratory** Reticulocytes comprise 5-25% of the peripheral erythrocytes; the 2,3 DPG and factor VIII are increased, the osmotic fragility is decreased; red cells have a 'holly-leaf' or navicular configuration

SCAB Single-chain antigen binding protein(s) Unique manufactured polypeptides that link the variable sequence of an antibody's light chain (VL) to the variable sequence of an antibody's heavy chain (VH); SCABs could be produced from any monoclonal antibody, have the advantage of smaller size and reduced immunogenity of the heavy chain constant region and are of potential use in chemical separations, biosensors, imaging and therapy of malignancy, cardiovascular disease and others; see Abzymes

Scabies A condition caused by the 'itch' mite, *Sarcoptes scabei hominis*, which most commonly affects children, is transmitted by direct contact, causes an intensely pruritic linear eruption corresponding to the tracks of the burrowing beasts; the pruritus results in excoriation and secondary pyoderma, often located in the head and neck with sparing of the palmoplantar regions **Treatment** Lindane lotion, benzene hexachloride

Scaffold Any structural matrix that provides the physical support for a functional system, but which participates little in the system's activity

Scalded skin syndrome Staphylococcus scalded skin syndrome, Toxic epidermal necrolysis A vesiculo-bullous dermatopathy that resembles a second-degree burn, characterized in the early stages by erythema, followed by exfoliation, variably accompanied by painful movement of involved areas, anorexia, nausea, diarrhea and vomiting; SSSS/TEN in infants may be due to an epidermolytic toxin produced by group 2 staphylococci, often phage types 71 and 55 and initially has a high mortality that drops to 5%; SSSS/TEN in adults may be due to exposure to drugs, eg sulfonamide, phenylbutazone, salicylate, penicillin and barbiturates or chemical, eg acrylonitrile exposure, and has a mortality rate of 30-40%

Scalenus syndrome see Thoracic outlet syndrome

Scaling PERIODONTICS The removal of dental plaque (an early lesion predisposing to periodontitis) and 'tartar' or calculus from the crown of a tooth and root surfaces; see Periodontal disease

Scalloping Scallop sign BONE RADIOLOGY A descriptor for a semilunar erosion at the ulnar aspect of the distal radius, seen in patients with advanced rheumatoid arthritis, caused by spontaneous rupture of the digital extensors; the 'scallop' is often more prominent as it may be rimmed by an osteosclerotic margin CHEST RADIOLOGY A descriptor for tethering of the visceral to parietal pleura, seen in pneumothorax that arises in previous lung disease GASTROINTESTINAL RADIOLOGY A descriptor for the appearance of candidal esophagitis, in which there are irregular serrations seen by a barium 'swallow study'

SCAN Suspected child abuse or neglect PEDIATRICS A potential case of child abuse, which in the US is a delicate issue, as a false accusation of child abuse opens the physician to the charges of 'defamation of character', while ignoring signs of abuse is moral malpractice; strong indicators of abuse include trauma of any type in a child under one year of age and an infant who arrives dead to a health care facility; see Battered child syndrome, Infanticide

Scanner COMPUTERS An input device that measures differences in light absorption on typed pages, which is used in conjunction with optical character recognition software, allowing direct entry of written text into a computer's work processing environment; scanners may also be used to input line drawings and photographs that may be subsequently manipulated in a desktop publishing environment INSTRUMENTATION A device that measures the differences in chromatic or radioactive intensity on a two-dimensional matrix, eg electropherogram or chromatogram, for the purpose of quantitative analysis of various substances

Scanning electron microscope (SEM) An electron microscope with limited diagnostic utility that creates a three-dimensional image of a cell or tissue's surface, by analyzing the pattern of deflection of primary and secondary electrons; see Microscopy; Cf Scanning tunnel microscopy

'Scanning power' SURGICAL PATHOLOGY The lowest magnification (20x to 25x) power used in diagnostic pathology, which allows surveying of tissues and pattern recognition; see Microscopy; Cf High power field

Scanning speech NEUROLOGY A slurring of phonation associated with cerebellar defects, in which there is inappropriate rate, range, force and direction of voluntary movements

Scanning tunnel(ling) microscope (STM) A powerful 'microscope', developed by Binnig and Rohrer (Nobel prize, Physics, 1986) that produces high resolution, three-dimensional images of atomic and subatomic particles on various surfaces, where the instrument's tip scans a sample, atom by atom, combining high spatial resolution with spectroscopic analysis; unlike other microscopes, STM uses neither incident light nor radiation, and thus does not require lenses, light or electron sources, but rather uses the electrons from the surface as the only source of radiation Technique An ultrafine needle is brought several billionths (10^{-9}) of a centimeter from the surface being analyzed, at which distance, the voltage must be maintained at very low levels to prevent electrons from jumping the gap between the needle and the surface being analyzed; because electrons are not in motion, classical physics does not apply; the process is rather explained by the quantum mechanical effect of 'tunnelling', which allows a faint current to pass from the needle to the surface and back as it scans the surface's atomic landscape, producing a three dimensional image of organic and inorganic surfaces and biological molecules, including bacteriophage particles, circular DNA and native double-stranded DNA (Nature 1990; 346:294); Cf Scanning electron microscope

Scar-cancer A cancer that is often located in the pulmonary apices and associated with pre-existing scars, wounds or inflammation, eg healed tuberculosis, infarcts, abscess cavities, bronchiectasis and metallic foreign bodies, eg bullets; 80% of scar cancers are adenocarcinomas, 15% are squamous cell carcinomas with the rest being of other histopathological types; it is unclear the effect, if any, that scarring has on either the pathogenesis or prognosis of cancer, and whether the scar is merely an epiphenomenon; see Passenger/driver controversy

Scarlet fever A reaction due to pharyngitis by Streptococcus group A, which produces an erythrogenic toxin, consisting of an oral enanthema ('raspberry' tongue, 'strawberry' tongue), generalized blanching erythema (sparing the palmoplantar region and mouth with circumoral pallor) and linear petechiae, known as Pastia's lines

Scarlett O'Hara 'syndrome' A coinage of uncertain origin that refers either to 1) Pretentious eating habits when a person is in the public eye or 2) A peer-group accepted eating 'disorder' in which, given the need for young female socialites to attend multiple dinners, dances and parties often in short time periods, the women may self-induce emesis as a form of weight control; the 'syndrome' derives its name from Scarlett O'Hara, the fictional heroine in the American Civil War novel, *Gone with the Wind*, who engorged herself prior to public meals rather than appear unlady-like Note: Pathological over-eating behind closed doors without serving a social purpose is known as the 'Binge-purge syndrome'

Scar-sarcoidosis Sarcoidosis arising in a scar, a rare condition that may engender a similar controversy to Scar cancer

Scatter factor A 62 kD heterodimeric cytokine joined by disulfide bonds that is secreted by certain fibroblasts, enhancing the movement, dissociation and scattering of epithelial cells; the single-stranded 30 kD peptide has significant sequence homology with hepatocyte growth factor/hepatopoietin A

Scattergram A plot of data points in a two-dimensional coordinate system that is used to determine whether there is a correlation between the two variables on the X and Y axes(figure, facing page, is a linear regression of data points correlating the serum levels of calcitriol and physical activity with bone density

SCD Sudden cardiac death

SCEA see Sister chromosome exchange analysis

S cell Secretin-producing endocrine cells in the mucosa of the upper small intestine; see Secretin

SCF Stem cell factor A hematopoietic growth factor that is a product of the SI gene in mice and which is a ligand for c-*kit*, a proto-oncogene of the tyrosine kinase receptor family, expressed during embryogenesis in those cells associated with the migratory pathways and targets of melanoblasts, germ cells, hematopoietic stem cells and possibly also the brain and spinal cord (Nature; 1990; 347:667)

'Scheduled' drugs see Controlled drug substances

SCID mice A mouse model for AIDS, which may be used to study the interaction of anti-HIV drugs or immune-enhancers in an in vivo system, without the ethical dilemma that is posed in human testing of substances with unknown effects; the SCID mouse model is also used to study tumor interactions in immune compromised hosts

Schistosomes PARASITOLOGY Phylum Platyhelminthes, Class Trematoda In its various guises, the genus *Schistosoma* is estimated to infect 200 million world citizens, killing 800 000 annually, the morbidity of which is related to an exuberant tissue reaction to the eggs, as the organisms themselves do not replicate within the host; see Circumoval body, Pipestem fibrosis, Swimmer's itch

Schizocytes Schistocytes Helmet cells HEMATOLOGY Fragmented erythrocytes that arise from either an intrinsic increase in cell fragility or from intravascular rugosities that traumatize the cells; schistocytes are a non-specific finding that may be associated with hemolysis, trauma, prosthetic heart valves, megaloblastic and microangiopathic anemias, disseminated intravascular coagulation, hemolytic uremic syndrome and thrombotic thrombocytopenic purpura; Cf Selenoid cells

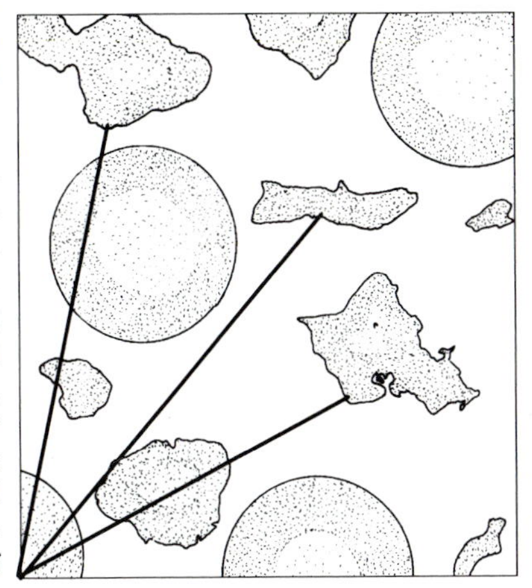

Schizocytes

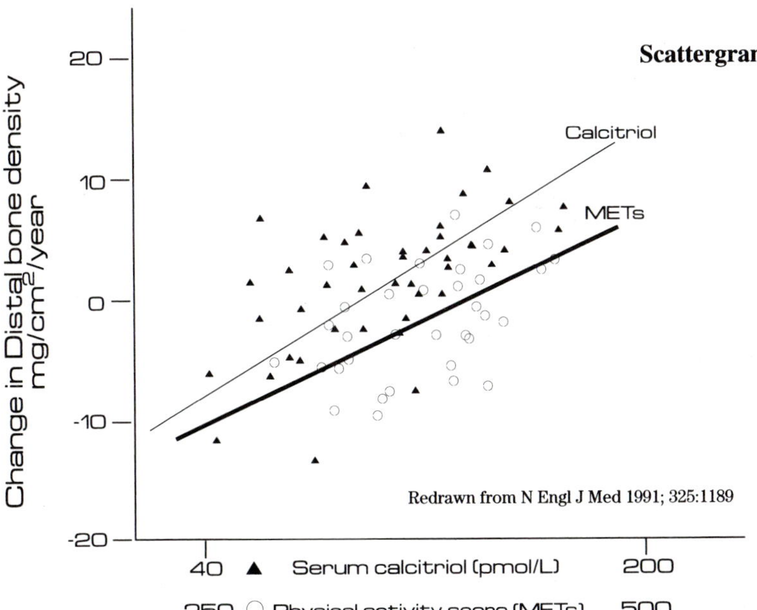

Scattergram

'Schlepper' German, tugboat, tractor MOLECULAR BIOLOGY A colloquial term for any molecule, eg a carrier protein that combines with a poorly- or non-antigenic molecule, eg a hapten, enhancing its immunogenicity and mediating its transporation through the cell or body

'School of fish' appearance A non-specific descriptor for a light microscopic pattern characterized by multiple, discrete oval-to-elongated structures arranged in long roughly parallel fascicles ANATOMIC PATHOLOGY A variant arrangement of the fascicles of malignant cells in malignant fibrous histiocytoma, more commonly known as a 'storiform pattern' MICROBIOLOGY The light microscopic arrangement of the gram-negative bipolar-staining coccobacillus *Haemophilus ducreyi* (Chancroid agent)

Schwannoma A tumor of Schwann cells that is thought to arise from the neural crest; by convention, the 'benign schwannoma' is preferably known as neurilemmoma and the 'true' or malignant schwannoma is designated simply as schwannoma; although it is the most common malignancy of peripheral nerves, it is poorly understood and because of the difficulty in establishing the schwann cell as the schwannoma's cell of origin, there is a justification in the equivalent term 'malignant peripheral nerve sheath tumor' Histopathology Few intracytoplasmic filaments, abundant cytoplasmic processes, layered basal lamina, numerous granular lysosomes Pathogenesis In one schwannoma tumor line, a potent glial mitogen was isolated that is an epidermal growth factor, an autocrine growth factor as well as a mitogen for astrocytes, Schwann cells and fibroblasts (Nature 1990; 348:257)

SCID see Severe combined immune deficiency

Scimitar syndrome A rare vascular anomaly, more common in women that may present in early childhood, the pulmonary veins of which drain into the inferior vena cava, appearing as a curved (scimitar-shaped) radio-opacity adjacent to the right cardiac border Clinical Asymptomatic or fever, dyspnea, recurring pneumonia, chest pain and wheezing Pathology Right lung and right pulmonary artery hypoplasia, dextrocardia, anomalous origin of pulmonary arteries from the aorta to right lung, anomalous venous drainage of right lung into the inferior vena cava and anomalous right diaphragm Treatment Surgical, pneumonectomy or correction of cardiac 'plumbing' defects; Cf Sequestration complex

Scintillation The sporadic emission of quanta of light by fluorescent substances, eg POPOP, after radioactive excitation; scintillation forms the basis of the radioimmunoassay, is detected using a solid or liquid fluor, which may be mixed in a 'cocktail' to enhance the detection of the flashes of light; see POPOP, Radioimmunoassay

Scirrhous Greek skirrhos, gypsum An adjectival descriptor for the dense stroma of certain carcinomas that produce abundant connective tissue; scirrhous induration or 'desmoplastic reaction' is highly characteristic of ductal carcinoma of breast and may be seen in pancreatic adenocarcinoma

Scirrhous carcinoma A term recently deleted from the pathology literature that refers to the 'classic' invasive ductal carcinoma of the breast, in which there is marked induration with 'chalky streaks' due to increased deposition of elastin fibers, often accompanied by microcalcifications detectable on mammography

SCIWORA Spinal cord injury without radiological abnormality Serious spinal cord damage and disruption of tracts in the absence of a fracture, an event that occurs most commonly in children Mechanisms Flexion, hyperextension, longitudinal distraction and ischemia causing complete and severe partial cord lesions Treatment Regional stabilization, neurosurgical exploration

Sclerosing adenosis SURGICAL PATHOLOGY A form of hyperplasia of the glandular component (adenosis) of the breast that may be confused with carcinoma, which consists of an indurated, often small multinodular lesion that is more cellular in the center with florid myoepithelial proliferation (immunoperoxidase stain reveals abundant actin); sclerosing adenosis lacks trabecular formations, necrosis and cellular pleomorphism, which are histological findings of carcinoma; malignant degeneration in sclerosing adenosis is rare but well-described; see Fibrocystic disease, Proliferative breast disease(s); Cf Mammary dysplasia

Sclerosing cholangitis An idiopathic bile duct inflammation with cholestasis, often associated with other autoimmune diseases, eg Crohn's disease, ulcerative colitis and Addison's disease Clinical Jaundice, pruritis, portal hypertension Radiology Endoscopic retrograde cholangiography reveals beading and narrowing of the affected biliary tract Laboratory Increased alkaline phosphatase Histopathology Periductal fibrosis and inflammation, portal edema, fibrosis, bile duct dilatation or focal obliteration and loss of bile ducts, copper deposition, cholestasis and with time, evolution into primary biliary cirrhosis (N Engl J Med 1991; 324:186); see Primary biliary cirrhosis

Sclerosing epithelial hamartoma Desmoplastic trichoepithelioma A benign hair follicle tumor that is more common on the face of young (< age 30) females Histopathology Compressed epithelial nests, focal calcification, and dermal fibrosis Treatment Excision

Sclerosing hamartoma with tubular adenoma see Sclerosing metanephric hamartoma

Sclerosing hemangioma A term that is used in 1) PULMONARY PATHOLOGY for an often benign lesion of adult females characterized by a well-circumscribed, slowly growing mass of polygonal cells thought to arise from type II pneumocytes with a variably present mesenchymal stroma and 2) DERMATOPATHOLOGY for what is now known as 'benign fibrous histiocytoma' or less commonly as dermatofibroma and nodular fibrosis

Sclerosing lipogranuloma A rare lesion of the penis, scrotum and vulva, described in adults and thought to be due to autoinjection of exogenous paraffin Histopathology Fat necrosis, histiocytes, foamy macrophages, giant cells, fibrosis and hyalinization

Sclerosing lymphangitis An idiopathic condition characterized by firm cord-like subcutaneous masses encircling the penis at the coronal suture that resolve in 2-6 weeks Histopathology Dilated lymphatics with sprouts of endothelial cells and thickened, fibrotic vessel walls

Sclerosing metanephric hamartoma A lesion of children under two years of age that is presumed to precede Wilm's tumor, histologically characterized by the presence of blastemal and tubular elements in a fibrous stroma, subdivided into simple sclerosing hamartoma, simple tubular hamartoma and sclerosing hamartoma with a central adenoma, which is considered to be an early Wilm's tumor; Cf WAGR syndrome, Wilm's tumor

Sclerosing peritonitis Extensive peritoneal fibrosis that occurs in response to asbestos, silica in intravenous drug abusers, in patients with carcinoid syndrome or those receiving β-blockers Pathogenesis Unknown, possibly related to inhibition of the release of lysosomal enzymes or due to mesenteric panniculitis Clinical Intestinal obstruction due to massive peritonial adhesions

Sclerosing retroperitonitis Ormund's disease A rare idiopathic proliferation of fibrous tissue in the retroperitoneum that encases the ureters, potentially causing renal failure, and which may evoke fibrous proliferation elsewhere, including sclerosing cholangitis and mediastinitis, Riedel's thyroiditis, pseudotumor of the orbit and generalized vasculitis

Sclerosteosis syndrome An autosomal recessive condition of children leading to deafness with bony overgrowth and occlusion of cranial foramina, accompanied by an asymmetrically enlarged mandible, syndactyly and onychodysplasia

Sclerotic bodies Mycology Thick-walled, 4-12 μm in diameter, round, chestnut-brown structures with a 'copper penny' appearance, seen in chromoblastomycosis, which correspond to an intermediate fungal form that is midway between yeasts and hyphae that reproduces under acidic conditions in a muriform fashion, ie multiplying by forming vertical and horizontal septations

Scombroid intoxication A histame-reaction that results from eating spoiled fish in the Scomberesocidea family (saury, skipjack, maki-maki, dolphin, tuna, bonito, seerfish, butterfly kingfish, mackerel); these fish have free histamine in their muscle that is decarboxylated when infected by *Proteus* spp; if the infection is intense, oral antihistamines or even activated charcoal may be needed to ameliorate the systemic effect of the histamine (N Engl J Med 1991; 324:716); see Fish; Cf Ciguatera poisoning

Scotch™ tape test MICROBIOLOGY A method used in the clinical laboratory for 1) Retrieval of eggs from the perianal region in children infected with pinworm

(*Enterobius vermicularis*) and 2) Observing fungi in a fashion that is similar to their 'native' conformation in culture; a piece of transparent adhesive tape is touched to a colony of fungi; the tape is then adhered to a glass slide with a dropper of lactophenol blue

Scotty dog sign RADIOLOGY A fanciful descriptor for the normal appearance of lumbar vertebra when viewed obliquely, where the pedicle, the transverse process, the superior articular process and the inferior articular process form the eye, nose, ear and front legs respectively; spondylolysis will demonstrate a fracture through the dog's neck (figure, below); Cf Dog ear sign

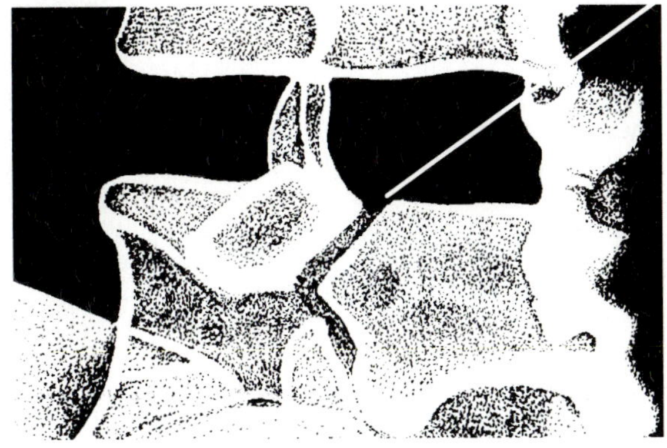

Scotty dog sign

Scout films RADIOLOGY Any preliminary film taken of a body region prior to a definitive imaging study, eg a scout chest film prior to performing computed tomography of the chest; 'scouts' serve to establish a baseline and are used prior to angiography, computerized tomography or magnetic resonance imaging

sCR1 soluble Complement receptor type 1 A recombinant DNA product that binds activated C3b and C4, promoting their inactivation by complement factor I; in rats, sCR1 significantly reduces hypoxia-induced myocardial injury, which is in part due to complement activation (Science 1990; 249:146)

'Scrambled egg' appearance OPHTHALMOLOGY A fanciful descriptor for the changes of the optic fundus seen in Best's autosomal dominant vitelliform degeneration; initially, there is a smooth sharply demarcated yellow-orange egg-yolk-like macule with little loss of visual acuity, affecting children and adolescents; later, the lesion degenerates, becoming scrambled-egg-like, resulting in retinal pigmentation, chorioretinal atrophy and visual impairment

Scrapie A prion-induced infection, once thought to be due to slow viruses, which causes fatal neurologic degeneration in sheep and goats, who scrape (ergo scrapie) themselves on rocks and other surrogate back-scratchers; the scrapie agent is one of the family of transmissible spongiform encephalopathies, which are thought to integrate themselves into the cell membrane, possibly as replicable glycoproteins; see Bovine spongiform encephalopathy, Kuru, Prion, Slow virus

Screening MOLECULAR BIOLOGY The use of a low-stringency radiolabeled or biotinylated hybridization probe to detect gene segments of potential interest from genomic or complementary DNA library; see Cloning PUBLIC HEALTH A process in which a large population group is evaluated for the possible presence of a morbid condition by measuring clinical parameters, eg blood pressure (to detect hypertension), sigmoidoscopy (colon cancer), radiologic parameters, eg mammography (breast cancer) or laboratory parameters, eg blood cholesterol (coronary artery disease), guaiac-positive stools (colon cancer) or 'pap' smears of the uterine cervix (cervical cancer); screening tests in general have high sensitivities and low specificities allowing detection of most patients with a morbid condition, while having the acceptable disadvantage of a high rate of false positivity Note: Because screening assays achieve their intended goal in detection, albeit in an inelegant and inefficient manner, they have been fancifully termed 'shotgun' tests as both obtain the desired effect while sacrificing finesse; see Cancer screening

Screwdriver teeth see Peg teeth

Screw-worm *Cochliomyia hominivorax* A fly that lays eggs in the open wounds of livestock; once hatched, the larvae feed on living flesh and may kill a calf via its umbilical cord wound within days; the screw-worm has recently migrated from its indigenous regions of the Western hemisphere to Libya where 1989 saw 1900 cases in cattle and 30 confirmed human cases; the US Agency for International Development felt that if not eradicated before it established a 'beachhead' in Africa, the screw-worm could devastate marginal livestock regions of Africa, and in the 1991 growing season, indicated that the pest had been corralled

SCRIMP technique PATHOLOGY A method by which a reasonably valid working diagnosis of the findings of a postmortem examination can be rendered in rapid time, consisting of SCRaping pathological tissue(s), and IMPrinting it on a glass slide (Hum Pathol 1983; 14:93) Note: The paperwork normally inherent in a postmortem examination often delays the generation of a final report for up to three or months in the US; hence the potential utility of such a simple technique

Script CLINICAL MEDICINE, PSYCHOLOGY The verbal component of patient communication which recognizes that different phrases may have the same meaning but the order, choice of the words or the manner in which they are said can either stimulate or inhibit communication

Scrotal tongue Grooved tongue Congenital lingual furrows that are a component of Melkerson-Rosenthal syndrome or may be seen in Down syndrome, which are attributed to sucking and mouth breathing; the finding has no pathological significance and is only of interest as food particles get stuck and are later colonized by oral bacteria, eliciting halitosis Treatment Brush teeth and tongue

Scrolls A descriptor for the ultrastructural morphology of mast cell granules, which may also rarely occur in variant chronic myelogenous leukemia with basophilia, a structural feature supporting a common origin of mast cells and basophils; the nature of the granular material is unknown

Scrub nurse A nurse (or technician) who participates in a sterile surgical operation, preparing sterile supplies and passing them to the surgeon, assisting the surgeon during the procedure, accounting for needles, sharps, sponges and other supplies used during the operation, and teaching any new (and qualified) personnel details of operating room protocol; see Circulating nurse, Operating team, Physician assistant

Scrub typhus Japanese river fever, Kedani fever A disease caused by a ***Rickettsia tsutsugamushi*** Vector Chiggers (the larval stage of the mite, ***Leptotrombidium deliensis***, or ***Trombicula pseudoakamushi***), inhabitants of scrub vegetation that feed on host rodents Clinical 1-3 week incubation; after scarring of the inoculation papule, there is abrupt onset of high fever, with a pulse-temperature dissociation, headache, malaise, cardiac dysfunction with minor changes in the electrocardiogram, eg T wave inversion, a pale pink, centrifugal maculopapular rash, lymphadenopathy and interstitial pneumonia Diagnosis Proteus OX-K antigen seropositivity Treatment Tetracycline, chloramphenicol, ciprofloxin

SCTAT Sex cord tumor with annular tubules A rare ovarian tumor with clinicopathologic differences that depend on the tumor's association with Peutz-Jegher syndrome **SCTAT WITH PEUTZ-JEGHER SYNDROME** is a small, bilateral, multifocal and calcified lesion that is rarely functionally active, with some cases being associated with adenoma malignum of the cervix **SCTAT WITHOUT PEUTZ-JEGHER SYNDROME** is often large, unilateral, focal, rarely associated with adenoma malignum; 40% secrete estrogen and 20% of cases behave in a malignant fashion Histopathology Sharply circumscribed, rounded epithelial nests composed of ring-shaped tubules, likened to atrophic testes; also simple and complex ring-shaped tubules with a pattern between a granulosa cell tumor and Sertoli cell tumor

Sculptured nose A thinned, sharply chiselled nose with atrophy of the subcutaneous adipose tissue seen in the Hutchinson-Gilford progeria syndrome, see also 'Plucked bird' appearance

Scurvy line see Trümmerfeld zone

'Scut monkey' UNDERGRADUATE MEDICAL EDUCATION A highly colloquial and demeaning term that generally refers to a medical student who has been relegated to the bottom rung of a team involved in patient management team in a university-affilitated health care facility, and performs so-called 'scut' work; see Extern, Medical student abuse, Pimping

Scut work Menial, non-patient care-related activities that are often passed to medical students (externs) or interns, although they are actually the responsibility of other health-care workers; the array of 'scut' details is vast and includes obtaining supplies, performing ward paperwork, going to the pharmacy, laboratory and emergency room with specimens or paperwork, acting as an orderly, cleaning the nurses station, going for pizza and so on; scut duties are often cited as a subtle form of 'medical student abuse'; see Medical student abuse, Pimping

SDAT Senile dementia, Alzheimer type, see Alzheimer's disease

SDBT see Senile dementia, Binswanger type

SDS-PAGE Sodium dodecyl sulfate-polyacrylamide gel electrophoresis LABORATORY TECHNOLOGY A technique for determining a polypeptide chain's molecular weight, where short proteins are dissociated with SDS at a neutral pH, minimizing the protein's net charged, in the presence of mercaptoethanol which breaks the protein's disulfide bonds, yielding random coils of polypeptides that have the same charge/mass ratio, which are then separated by the gel's sieving effect as a function of molecular weight; see Polyacrimide gel electrophoresis

Sea blue histiocyte A histiocyte with abundant light sea blue-staining granular cytoplasm when stained with a 'Romanovsky' stain; the color is due to degradation moieties of complex lipid, seen in lipid storage disease, due to alterations in glycoprotein metabolism or in aging; these cells are often autofluorescent, and are positive with the periodic acid Schiff, sudan black and Prussian blue stains; sea blue histiocytes are non-specific and may be seen in 1) Congenital lipid storage defects, eg Wolman's disease (lipase defect with increased triglycerides and esters), cholesteryl ester storage disease, adult Niemann-Pick disease, Tay-Sachs disease and hyperlipoproteinemia 2) Acquired benign conditions, eg hypochromic anemia, SC disease, post-necrotic cirrhosis, rheumatoid arthritis, vitamin E deficiency, chronic granulomatous disease, ceroid histiocystosis of the spleen in idiopathic thrombocytopenic purpura and 3) Acquired malignant conditions, eg Hodgkin's disease, chronic myelogenous leukemia, polycythemia vera, erythroleukemia and myelodysplasia

Sea blue histiocyte syndrome An autosomal recessive condition with abundant sea-blue histiocytes causing organomegaly and compromised function, resulting in hepatosplenomegaly, thrombocytopenia and masses in the skin, lungs, gastrointestinal tract, nervous system

Seabright Bantam 'syndromes' Background: The Seabright Bantam rooster has feminine-in-appearance tail feathers that result from a defective end-organ response to androgenic hormones accompanied by a 100-fold increase in aromatase activity, which converts androgens to estrogens; 'Seabright Bantam', then, is a generic adjective for clinical complexes that are caused by defective end-organ responses to structurally and functionally normal hormones, including ADH-resistant diabetes mellitus, growth hormone resistance syndrome of de Morsier, testosterone resistance syndrome (Morris' syndrome), pseudohypothyroidism (parathormone resistance) and Savage's follicle-stimulating hormone resistance syndrome, while the human equivalent of the Sebright Bantam rooster is due to an overproduction of estradiol and causes gynecomastia (N Engl J Med 1991; 324:317cr)

Sea fan appearance OPHTHALMOLOGY A fanciful descriptor for the splayed vessels seen in proliferative retinopathy in sickling hemoglobinopathies (hemoglobin SC and sickle-thalassemia) that may be accompanied by salmon-patch pigmentation, vascular tortuosity and occlusion and arteriovenous anastomoses

Sea foot see Immersion foot

Sea gull pattern see Gull wing pattern

Sealed envelope appearance A descriptor for the high-power light microscopic appearance of *Pneumocystis carinii*, when stained with Gomori-methenamine silver (GMS), which is seen in lung biopsies and pulmonary cytology specimens; the envelope's 'flap' corresponds to the organism's folded membrane, serving to differentiate these from the often similar erythrocytes and non-specific debris

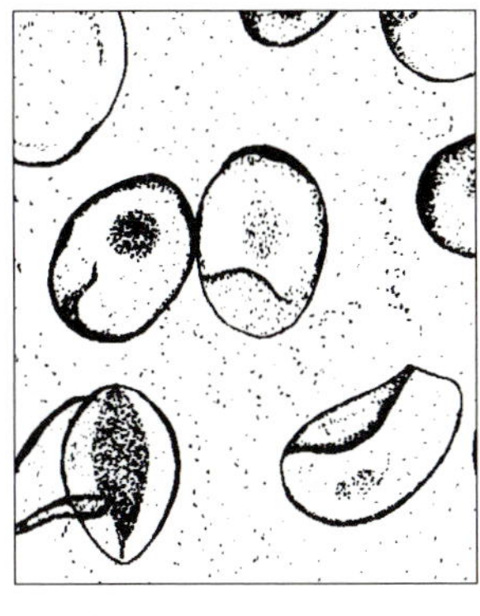
'Sealed envelopes'

Seal finger A monoarticular infection of the finger with digital puffiness occurring in coastal Scandinavia and Canada, generally in those working in wildlife and marine-related professions, possibly due to fastidious micrococcal bacterial infection Treatment Tetracycline

Seat belt (use) laws PUBLIC HEALTH Legislation that is being increasingly enacted in developed nations, requiring the use of safety belts in motor vehicles; following enactment of these laws, the use of seat belts doubles to 60%, the fatalities and critical injuries per automobile accident are reduced from 10 to 15% (J Am Med Assoc 1991; 265:1409)

Seat belt syndrome Contusion of anterior abdominal wall caused by lap seat belts, which may produce lumbar spine fractures with horizontal splitting of the vertebral body and posterior arch, trauma to bowel, vessels, spleen and liver; in the US, lap-type safety belts are only found in the front seats of older automobiles, although they contiue to be used in the back seats; Cf Dashboard fracture, Padded dash(board) syndrome

Seattle committee BIOMEDICAL ETHICS A group comprised of members of the community in Northwestern USA that met on a regular basis in the late 1960s to decide the relative 'social worth' (thereby 'playing God') of patients in need of hemodialysis, which at the time was limited in availability; a typical 'God committee' was composed of a clergyman, a banker, two physicians, a housewife, a labor leader Note: The dilemmas inherent in making decisions regarding allocation of limited life-saving resources has become a major ethical and budgetary battleground in the US; see Health care rationing, 'Rule of rescue', Social worth

Seborrhea petaloides DERMATOLOGY A condition characterized by garland-shaped lesions of seborrheic dermatitis appearing on the face, trunk and proximal extremities, most commonly seen in the obese

Secondary care Health care provided by a specialist in a non-high technology situation, eg in a private office or specialty care that is provided in a community hospital, to a patient who has been referred by a primary care physician, for special studies, eg cardiac stress test, computed tomography or special procedures, eg cholecystectomy, endoscopic polypectomy; secondary care facilities include general acute care hospitals or specialized outpatient facilities that treat 'garden variety' diseases, for which the risks of therapy are minimal, well-defined and length of hospitalization is short and uncomplicated; Cf Primary care, Tertiary care

Secondary deficiency A nutritional deficiency state that is not due to the lack of ingestion of an essential nutrient, ie a primary deficiency, but rather the result of either an increased requirement for that substance, eg iron in pregnancy, or decreased availability or 'wastage' of the nutrient, as in proteinuria in a nephrotic syndrome

Secondary diabetes Diabetes mellitus that occurs by a pathogenic mechanism other than the usual type I and II diabetes; secondary diabetes mellitus may result from pancreatitis, pancreatic carcinoma, pheochromocytoma, hemochromatosis or acromegaly or by use of drugs known to impair glucose metabolism, eg corticosteroids

Secondary fluor A fluor, eg POPOP, that is used in a scintillation device to shift the wavelength of light emitted by the primary fluor to a longer wavelength, for which the photomultiplier has a greater sensitivity; see Primary fluor, Quenching, RIA

Secondary granules see Lysosomes; Cf Primary granules

Secondary intention see Wound healing

Secondary malignancy A malignant neoplasm that is directly attributed to environmental toxins, physical agents and radiation, or which arises in the background of another malignancy treated by radiotherapy or chemotherapy; the most common post-therapeutic secondary cancers are acute non-lymphocytic leukemias, including acute myelogenous leukemia, acute promyelocytic leukemia, acute monocytic leukemia, erythroleukemia and preleukemia; chromosomal changes in secondary leukemias include loss of the entire (or long arms of) chromosomes 5 (-5 or -5q) and 7 (-7 and -7q); survival in spontaneous ANLL is 30% at 12 months, survival in post-therapeutic (secondary) ANLL at 12 months is 10% (J Am Med Assoc 1990; 264:1006); the peak incidence of secondary malignancy occurs 5years after chemotherapy is first administered; in ovarian carcinoma, there is a 12-fold increased risk for future malignancy in those treated with chemotherapy; radiotherapy does not produce an additive effect; the most leukemogenic chemotherapeutic agents in one study were chlorambucil and melphalan, and as combined therapies, doxorubicin and cis-platin (N Engl J Med 1990; 322:1); in Hodgkin's disease, there is a nine-fold increase in secondary leukemia in those treated with chemotherapy compared to radiotherapy; after six cycles of chemotherapy the risk increases to 14, the incidence peaks 5-8 years after initiating chemotherapy; the most inculpated agents are procarbazine and mechlorethamine, the risk doubled in those with splenectomy (N Engl J Med 1990; 322:7); children treated with alkylating agents have relative risk of 4.7 for future bone sarcomas, while those treated radiotherapy have a 2.7 risk for bone sarcoma, increasing to a 40-fold risk when doses to the bone exceed 6000 rad PRIMARY-SECONDARY MALIGNANCY DYADS include 1) BREAST CARCINOMA Removal of the axillary 'tail' lymph nodes, begets angioedema that may induce angiosarcoma 2) GERM CELL NEOPLASIA Radiotherapy or chemotherapy to sensitive tissue in teratomas may 'activate' non-germ line tissue, giving rise to sarcomas, as well as other tumors, including nephroblastoma, neuroblastoma and adenosquamous carcinoma 3) RETINOBLASTOMA Fatal secondary sarcomas occur in 10% of hereditary retinoblastomas treated with chemotherapy and radiotherapy, but not in non-hereditary retinoblastoma (N Engl J Med 1988; 318:581) Physical agents causing secondary malignancy include 1) Radiation (actinic or radiotherapeutic)to the head and neck causing secondary basal cell carcinomas; latent period to secondary neoplasm 3-65 years 2) Chronic irritation (Marjolin's ulcer) causing skin cancer or chronic injury, eg heat-induced squamous cell carcinoma (Kairo cancer, Japan; Kang cancer, China; Kangri cancer, Kashmir; 'peat moss' cancer, Ireland) 3) Scar-induced malignancy, eg malignant fibrous histiocytoma arising in sites with metal objects or shrapnel or malignancy induced by mechanical trauma, a relation which in humans is anecdotal and 4) Ischemia and squamous cell carcinoma adjacent to varicose veins

Secondary malignant fibrous histiocytosis A tumor of mesenchymal tissues that appears to be the most common malignancy inducible by external forces; malignant fibrous histiocytoma has beenassociation with other tumors, eg chordoma (Am J Clin Pathol 1984; 82:738), or may be induced by radiation, eg to the cervix for cancer, long term foreign bodies, eg scrapnel in bone or induced in rats by chemical, eg injections of 4-hydroxyaminoquinolone-1-oxide

Secondary obesity Obesity that is a symptom of other conditions including central nervous system disease (defects of the hypophyseal-hypothalamic axis, intracranial leukemia and other lesions), congenital (Alström-Hallgren, Bloumant, Carpenter, Cohen, Lawrence-Moon-Biedl, Prader-Willi and Vasquez) syndromes and endocrinopathies (hypothyroidism, insulinoma, Cushing syndrome, polycystic ovary disease, pituitary dwarfism); see Morbid obesity, Obesity,

Secondary (immune) response The enhanced immune response of an organism when it is re-exposed to an antigen, after it has had sufficient time to generate an immune recognition 'cascade'

Secondary structure see Protein structure

'Second genetic code' A term coined (Nature 1988; 333:117) to describe the sites on transfer ribonucleic acid (tRNA) that determine which amino acids will be joined by aminoacyl tRNA synthetase (AAS); the correct attachment of amino acids to specific tRNAs is critical for accurate translation of genetic information from nucleic acid to protein; the 'first' genetic code deciphers the rules governing insertion of specific amino acids in response to the sequence of the mRNA and is the result of alignment of aminoacyl-tRNAs along the mRNA template by base pairing between the tRNA anticodon and the template's codons; because tRNA molecules must interact interchangeably with the protein synthesis apparatus, they all have similar secondary and tertiary structures, but within this framework, variation must exist so that each tRNA is recognizable to its cognate AAS; the 'second genetic code' implies a common set of rules governing tRNA recognition by the various AASs, which appears to be unlikely, and the term 'tRNA identity' better describes the features of the tRNA molecule that make one tRNA recognizable to its cognate AAS and prevents its recognition by other AASs (Science 1988; 240:1591ed) Note: The 'first' genetic code is the double helix of DNA that opens temporarily to encode a chain of complementary mRNA and contains the message for the correct order of amino acids to be assembled into proteins; the second step toward protein production requires that tRNA and attached amino acids line up in the order specified by the mRNA; it had been unclear how a particular tRNA and its synthetase (the enzyme which links tRNA to a specific amino acid) recognized each other, as tRNA molecules are virtually identical, a mystery that was partly solved by X-ray crystallography of tRNA and its respective synthetase (Science 1989; 246:1135, 1122)

'Second-look' operation A second surgical procedure in the same site, usually the abdomen, with the intent of continuing therapy that could not be completely performed for various reasons during the first operation GENERAL SURGERY A second-look operation is performed in the gastrointestinal tract to re-examine questionably viable segments of small intestine 24-48 hours after an initial massive resection for ischemia, with the hope that sufficient small intestine (at least 30%) remains viable, thereby circumventing the 'short bowel syndrome' GYNECOLOGIC ONCOLOGY A second-look operation is a laparotomy performed for an ovarian carcinoma that was initially deemed inoperable, and later re-examined to determine whether radio- and/or chemotherapy were successful in reducing the size of the tumor to allow a debulking procedure or to determine whether therapy may be discontinued or requires modification after 10-12 courses of chemotherapy SURGICAL ONCOLOGY Second-look procedures are performed in colons previously resected for adenocarcinoma and monitored by carcinoembryonic antigen (CEA) levels; an elevation of CEA greater than 35% above the patient's established baseline is suggestive of metastasizing recurrence; at operation, less than one-half prove to be resectable

Second messenger CELL PHYSIOLOGY A substance released from the cytoplasmic face of a receptor after a ligand interacts with its cognate receptor on the cell's external surface and elicits a response from a G protein; these substances, eg cyclic AMP, inositol 1,4,5-triphosphate (IP3) and 1,2-diacylglycerol (DAG), in turn mediate various intracellular activities; IP3 acts on the endoplasmic reticulum, releasing calcium which binds to calcium-binding proteins, troponin and calmodulin, the latter of which undergoes an activating conformational change; the calcium-calmodulin complex then activates: adenylate cyclase, cAMP phophodiesterase, Ca^{++}-Mg^{++}-dependent ATPase, glycogen phosphorylase and myosin kinase, resulting in various physiologic effects; DAG acts on protein kinase C, increasing the secretion or production of hormones, enzymes, neurotransmitters, vasoactive compounds and other molecules; see 1,2-Diacylglycerol, G Proteins, PIP_2, Protein kinase C

Second opinion Formal or informal advice from a second health professional as to the correctness of a diagnosis and the appropriateness of a suggested therapy; second opinions are sought 1) By the beneficiary of a health insurance policy; second opinions are often encouraged by insurance companies, especially when a surgical procedure is recommended, as a second physician may not recommend the procedure, thus reducing the insurance company's costs and 2) By the patient, who may either not trust the rendered diagnosis or proposed therapy or who prefers to corroborate the first opinion for his own peace of mind

Second order reaction A chemical reaction, the velocity of which is proportional to either the product of the concentrations of the reactants or to the square of the concentration of one of the reactants

Second-set rejection IMMUNOLOGY An accelerated allograft rejection seen in patients who have already rejected one transplanted organ, as are patients who have been fancifully termed 'liver eaters'

'Second-wind' phenomenon INBORN ERRORS OF METABOLISM A substrate-dependent variation of exercise tolerance, in which previously fatiguing exercise can be performed with relative ease, after a period of rest; in muscle phosphofructokinase deficiency (Tarui's disease), the 'first' wind is extraordinarily short since muscle glycolysis is impaired due to an inability to generate pyruvate, the oxidative fuel required to provide normal aerobic power; in these patients, exercise capacity depends on availability of alternate fuels, eg free fatty acids to meet requirements for oxidation in muscle during exercise; high carbohydrate meals in these patients exacerbate their exercise intolerance by inhibiting lipolysis, depriving the muscle of their energy source (N Engl J Med 1991; 324:364) RHEUMATOLOGY A surge of subjective 'energy' that occurs after a short rest period, typical of the mid-afternoon fatigue seen in rheumatoid arthritis

Secretin A 27-residue helical peptide structurally similar to gastric inhibitory polypeptide (GIP), vasoactive inhibitory polypeptide (VIP) and glucagon produced by the S cell in the upper small intestine (and brain), released by acid, bile or fat into the intestinal lumen, stimulating the release of water and bicarbonate from the pancreas, neutralizing gastric acid, stimulating intestinal motility and the release of bile and gastric acid and inhibiting gastrin; since secretin releases gastrin from gastrinomas, secretin stimulation tests are of diagnostic utility in the Zollinger-Ellison syndrome

Secretogogue An agent that increases gastrointestinal electrolyte and fluid secretion by increasing adenylate cyclase activity or by increasing calcium in the cytosol; secretogogues include bacterial endotoxins (cholera exotoxins, shiga toxins and others), hormones (calcitonin, glucagon, secretin, vasoactive inhibitory polypeptide and others), detergents (bile acids, fatty acids and hydroxy fatty acids), laxatives and others (food allergies and resultant mast cell degranulation)

Secretors TRANSFUSION MEDICINE Background: ABO blood group antigens, Le^a and Le^b are not intrinsic to erythrocytes but are produced in other tissues, possibly in the intestinal epithelium and adsorbed from the plasma onto red cell glycosphingolipids; the presence of Lewis antigens on red cells depends on whether the subject has inherited one Le or two le genes, which encode fucosyl transferase, adding a fucose to the ABO blood group type I oligosaccharides; those subjects who also inherit the dominant Se(H) gene, producing an antigen, Le^b; subjects with ABO blood groups, A_x and B_x who don't secrete A or B substance; 80% of the normal subjects are 'secretors', ie ABH antigens are present in their secretions; see Lewis system

Secretory carcinoma, breast see Juvenile carcinoma

Secretory carcinoma, endometrial A well-differentiated variant of endometrial carcinoma in which the cells have vacuolated or clear cytoplasm, thus resembling normal secretory endometrium **Prognosis** Similar to well differentiated endometrial carcinoma **Differential diagnosis** Clear cell carcinoma, Arias-Stella reaction, and endometrial hyperplasia with increased secretion

Secretory component see Secretory piece

Secretory phase see Luteal phase

Secretory piece A short polypeptide chain carried by dimeric IgA that is added to IgA when it is secreted by the intestinal luminal cells, which is thought to confer protection against proteolytic digestion

SED Spondyloepiphyseal dysplasia see Pseudoachondroplasia

Seder syncope A vasovagal collapse induced by the horseradish (active ingredient, isothiocyanate) used in the celebration of the Judaic Passover Seder, a symbolic meal that commemorates the bitterness of Jewish slavery in ancient Egypt (J Am Med Assoc 1988; 259:1943); see Spicy food, Sushi syncope

Sedimentation equilibrium A laboratory method used for separating a substance and calculating its molecular weight, which consists of sedimentation by ultracentrifugation, allowing the centrifuge to spin at speeds low enough and for a long enough period of time to establish an equilibrium for the solute between sedimentation and diffusion

'Seed and soil' hypothesis A theory based on Sir James Paget's study of women dying of breast cancer, in whom metastases were relatively common to the liver and brain and uncommon in other organs; Paget postulated that certain tumors were predisposed to spread to certain sites based on the host's ability to support the growth of those particular tumor cells; Paget's theory contrasts with Ewing's 'mechanical theory' of tumor spread, in which tumor colonization is held to be related to the pattern of blood flow away from a malignancy; both theories are partially correct and not mutually exclusive; in terms of 'soil', the host tissue may produce mitogenic factors, eg acid-fibroblast growth factor and hematopoietic factors, general inhibitors which encourage the cells to stay and grow, eg transforming growth factor-β, tumor necrosis factor-α or organ-specific inhibitors, currently being elucidated; support for the mechanical theory lies in non-specific production of angiogenesis factors, and specific routes of metastases, eg Batson's plexus which is the route of prostatic metastases to the bone (N Engl J Med 1990; 322:605, Paget, Lancet 1889; 1:571); a third facet of the hypothesis is the 'seed' itself, in which there is structural and functional tumor cell heterogeneity that allows the cells to work synergistically to create an environment for distant spread of malignancy, eg tumors implanted in nude mice will not metastasize unless implanted in the appropriate organ; see Metastasis

Seed calculi Innumerable small oval concrements that may form in a markedly hydronephrotic renal pelvis in ureteropelvic obstruction

SEER The Surveillance, Epidemiology and End Results program A database maintained by the National Cancer Institute, Bethesda, Maryland, which is comprised of 11 population-based registries throughout the US, and represents about 10% of the US population; the SEER is of use in evaluating trends in malignancies and other morbid conditions

'Seesaw' nystagmus Torsional-vertical ocular oscillation NEUROLOGY A clinical finding in which one eye moves up while the other moves down, seen in bitemporal hemianopia due to sellar or parasellar mass lesions, a movement is fancifully likened to the up and down bobbing of a children's seesaw; Cf 'Railroad' nystagmus

SEIR equations A standard epidemiological model for infectious diseases, based on the acronym, Susceptible-exposed-infectious-recovery, representing categories into which a susceptible population is divided; the SEIR model may be an over-idealization of epidemiology while more realistic models demonstrate chaos (Science 1990; 249:499)

Selectin(s) A family of cell adhesion molecules (CAMs) or glycoproteins that are critical to interactions between endothelium and cells in the circulation (Nature 1991; 349:196n&v) Homing receptor selectin gp90mel, LAM-1, LEC-CAM-1 A glycoprotein expressed on leukocytes that facilitates their binding to endothelium during lymphocyte recirculation through peripheral lymph nodes and neutrophil egress from the circulation to sites of inflammation; see CD62; see Adhesion receptors

Selective molecules Any large family of molecule that provides specificity to the involved 'reactants', including cadherins, enzymes, immunoglobulins, integrins and selectins

Selective termination OBSTETRICS Selective abortion of one or more products of a 'higher multiple' gestation for various indications, eg chromosomal or physical abnormalities Note: For the clinical and ethical implications, see Obstet Gynecol 1988; 71:289; see Interlocking

Selective thermophotolysis A therapeutic modality in dermatology that 'bleaches' certain skin lesions, eg port-wine nevi and tattoos (lesions with preferential light absorption) by using a short-pulsed CO_2 laser that delivers ultrashort 'zaps' of laser energy; see Lasers

Selegiline L-deprenyl A selective monoamine oxidase type B inhibitor, which in combination with L-dopa, is reported to be useful for early symptomatic treatment of parkinsonism (Arch Neurol 1991; 48:31)

Selenium A trace mineral which when deficient, has been implicated in various clinical conditions, eg the dilated cardiomyopathy of Keshan disease, which is attributed to a defect in the function of glutathione peroxidase, without which there is increased platelet aggregation due to impaired free radical salvage or in the catalytic function of type I deiodinizing thyroxine-activating enzyme (Nature 1991; 349:438); see Keshan disease

Selenoid 'cells' Half moon cells Erythrocyte ghosts caused by mechanical shearing which occurs when red cells are abnormal, young or the plasma is hyperlipemic

Self-bougienage A therapeutic modality in which a patient auto-introduces a 44-46-F Maloney dilator tube to treat benign recurrent esophageal strictures; most of one small cohort of subjects with dysphagia prior to the initiation of self-bougienage were asymptomatic during the 3-year follow-up period (Mayo Clin Proc 1990; 65:799)

'Selfish' DNA see Junk DNA

Self-mutilation PSYCHIATRY Auto-destructive acts affect an estimated 1:1500 population; most self-mutilation is psychogenic in origin, related to physical confinement, deprivation, depression, often related to childhood experiences and the acts may be performed as a form of 'self-cleansing' to cauterize the 'pain of living'; self-mutilation is also an integral component of certain hereditary conditions, eg Lesch-Nyhan syndrome and Cornelia de Lange syndrome and is attributed to imbalances of neurotransmitters

Self-referral HEALTH CARE INDUSTRY The referral of patients to a facility, eg radiologic imaging center, in which the referring physician has a commercial interest; self-referral has two major impacts on medical care, 1) Ethical Conflict of interest, ie whether the diagnostic procedure ordered is appropriate and 2) Financial Increased cost of health care delivery, as the mean cost of imaging per episode of care is 4.4 to 7.5-fold higher for self-referring physicians (N Engl J Med 1990; 323:1604); see Fee-splitting, 'Safe harbor' rules; Cf Referral, Second opinion

Self restriction see MHC restriction

Sellafield study An epidemiologic study that attempted to address the statistical finding of increased incidence of childhood leukemia in the region of the Sellafield nuclear 'reprocessing' plant; four children of fathers exposed to more than 100 mSv (1 rad = 10 milliSieverts) developed leukemia, inculpating a genetic event (the so-called 'Gardner effect') below the accepted exposure level of 50 milliSieverts/year that passed to the fetus via the sperm (Br Med J 1990; 300:423); while meticulously performed, the statistical power of the study is weak and in mice, the offspring produced with irradiated spermatogonia had no increase in leukemia (Nature 1990; 345:671c); furthermore, in France, where 75% of electricity is produced by nuclear power plants, there is no increase in leukemia (ibid, 1990; 347:755); in those occupationally exposed to low levels of radioactivity (Oak Ridge National Laboratory, USA), the radiation-cancer dose response is ten-fold higher than previous estimates and the incidence of leukemia two-fold greater (J Am Med Assoc 1991; 265:1397); living near such facilities does not appear to increase mortality (J Am Med Assoc 1991; 265:1403) Summary The data is complex, the levels of secondary exposure are unknown and the effects of low-level exposure to radiation uncertain; see Pilgrim plant

Semiconservative replication see Meselson-Stahl experiment

'Semilethal' A mutant gene that is lethal if it is present in the homozygous state, or a mutation that when present at full 'genomic strength' is lethal to less than 100% of a population with the mutation

Seminoma see Germ cell tumors

Semi-starvation neurosis PSYCHIATRY A pre-anorexia nervosa state that most commonly affects subjects who, as children had been described as being 'good girls', who have perfectionist tendencies and demonstrate the effects of long-term caloric restriction including fatigue, weakness, apathy, passivity, withdrawal and regression; see Anorexia nervosa

Semisynthetic A chemical compound derived from a natural substance that is subjected to one or more synthetic steps to impart desired qualities, eg natural penicillin has a β-lactam ring and a thiazolidine ring; one derivative of the parent molecule, 6-aminopenicillanic acid, when obtained from *Penicillium crysogenum* grown in a side chain-depleted medium yields semisynthetic penicillins, which incorporate specific precursors in culture that have desired properties

Senescence, cellular Background Normal cells, eg human diploid fibroblasts and others have a finite proliferative lifespan, at the end of which the cells remain alive in an arrested state, known as replication senescence, which occurs after about 60 cell divisions, with the cell being arrested at the G1/S boundary of the cycle; senescent arrest is similar to terminal differentiation as it involves repression of proliferation-promoting genes and either expression of antiproliferative genes or through activity of post-transcriptional factors, eg loss of telomere sequences; 'escape' of cells from biological aging is rare and occurs in immortal cell lines and in neoplasia; senescent cells are larger and less motile, have an enlarged nucleus and an increased content of RNA, protein, glycogen, lipids and lysosomes (Science 1990; 247:1129); senescence is a state due to the presence of inhibitor(s) preventing entry into the S phase; one such inhibitor is $p110^{Rb}$, a retinoblastoma protein that is non-phosphorylated in quiescent and senescent diploid fibroblasts; fusion of these cells with cells bearing oncogenes (SV40 T antigen, adenovirus E1A and HPV) results in phosphorylation of $p110^{Rb}$ and initiating the S phase in quiescent cells (Science 1990; 249:666) Note: Quiescent cells cease proliferation, enlarge, senesce and die; senescence is postulated to occur via either 1) An error catastrophe model, with accumulation of random damage and mutations of DNA with loss of proliferative capacity, accompanied by intracellular build-up of poorly metabolized detritus ('garbage'), in particular lipofucsin and/or 2) A genetically programmed model ('pacemaker' theory), in which immortality is, virtually by definition, characteristic of malignant cells; senescence may be driven by a gene on chromosome 1 (Science 1990; 247:707); see Geriatrics, Gerontology

Senile dementias Progressive neurodegenerative disease(s) that may be divided into two groups of approximately equal size 1) Primary neuronal degeneration or what has become known as Alzheimer's disease (see note, below) and 2) Vascular degeneration due to atherosclerosis, resulting in a lacunar state; computed tomography and magnetic resonance imaging studies indicate that ischemia of the periventricular white matter may be responsible for a significant number of senile dementias, disconnecting the relatively intact cerebral cortex, resulting in true subcortical dementia or Binswanger type dementia (J Am Med Assoc 1987; 258:1782) Note: The widely extant practice of equating dementia occurring at any age (an event that is common in those older than seventy) with Alzheimer's disease is incorrect, in that Alzheimer's original description referred to PRE-senile dementia, which occurred in the fourth and fifth decades; Cf Alzheimer's disease, Lacunar state, Multi-infarct dementia, Pseudodementia

Senile osteoporosis see Osteoporosis

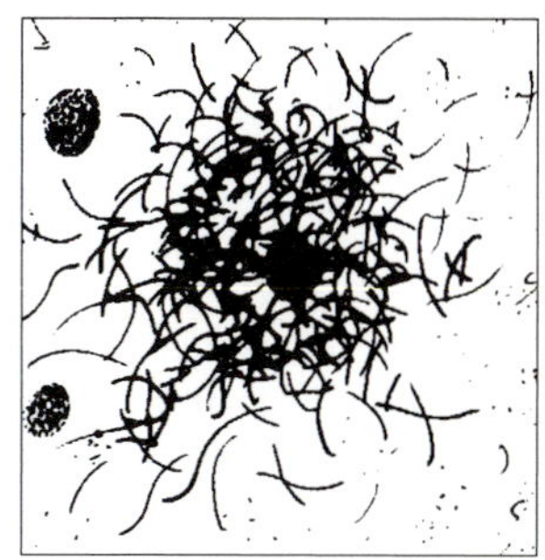

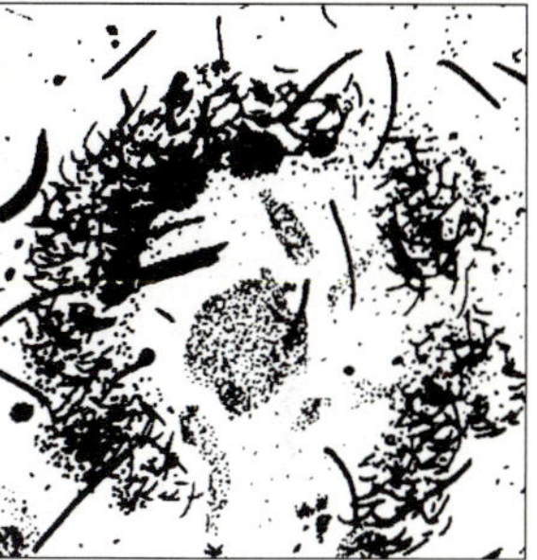

Immature Senile plaque Mature

Senile plaque Neuritic plaque A neuropathological finding consisting of a core of extracellular amyloid surrounded by a spherical mass of dilated cholinergic, argyrophilic neurites (axons/dendrites), confined to the grey matter (neocortex, hippocampus, amygdala, less commonly, the basal ganglia and elsewhere; neuritic plaques are relatively specific for and a constant finding in Alzheimer's disease; see Paired helical filaments

Sensitivity STATISTICS The degree to which a test or clinical assay is capable of confirming or at least supporting the diagnosis of a disease X, ie the analyte is appropriately abnormal in a subject with the disease; sensitivity is determined by the simple ratio of those who have a positive test result and the disease (true positives), divided by the sum of those with positive test results and the disease (true positives) and those with negative results who have the disease (false negatives), multiplied by 100 to yield a percentage; sensitivity then, represents the proportion of subjects with a disease which a test is capable of detecting

Sensitizer A substance that increases the susceptibility to a stimulus including light, eg a photosensitizer or to immune responsiveness, eg an adjuvant or allergen

Sentinel clot An adherent blood clot or prominent blood vessel, seen by upper gastrointestinal endoscopy in two-thirds of peptic ulcers that have previously hemorrhaged, occurring when a lateral defect in the arterial wall protrudes as a plug of fibrin above the ulcer base

Sentinel loop RADIOLOGY A dilated segment of jejunum seen in the left upper quadrant in an upper gastrointestinal radiocontrast 'series', which although non-specific, is considered characteristic of acute pancreatitis; Cf Colonic cut-off sign

Sentinel node Signal node of Virchow An isolated, enlarged often left-sided supraclavicular lymph node, classically associated with metastatic gastric carcinoma, which when found, indicates that the malignancy is non-resectable; Cf Mary Joseph nodule

Sentinel pile The swelling at the lower end of a chronic anal fissure, palpable as an anal mass, which may be the first or most prominent manifestation of a fissure, hence, a 'sentinel'

Sephadex A proprietary group of cross-linking dextrans used in gel electrophoresis

Sepharose A proprietary group of agarose gels used in electrophoresis

Sepsis syndrome A systemic response to infection, defined as hypothermia < 35°C (96°F) or hyperthermia > 39°C (101°F), tachycardia (> 90/minute), tachypnea (20 breaths/minute), a clinically evident focus of infection or positive blood cultures, one or more end organs with either dysfunction or inadequate perfusion, cerebral dysfunction, hypoxemia (PaO_2 < 75 mmHg), increased plasma lactate or unexplained metabolic acidosis, oliguria (< 30 mL/hour) and a leukocyte count of < 2.0 x 10^9/L or > 12.0 x 10^9/L (US: < 2000/mm^3 or > 12 000/mm^3); the sepsis syndrome is one of the most common causes of adult respiratory distress syndrome (Crit Care Med 1989; 17:389)

Septic shock A clinical condition identical to the sepsis syndrome with an added component of hypotension (systolic blood pressure < 90 mm Hg or loss in the baseline systolic pressure of greater than 40 mmHg)

Septo-optic dysplasia sequence of de Morsier An idiopathic condition characterized by incomplete early morphogenesis of the anterior midline brain, causing hypothalamic defects, hypoplasia of the optic chiasma and absence of septum pellucidum Clinical Pendular nystagmus, visual impairment, secondary hypopituitarism, sexual precocity and aberrant retinal vasculature Treatment Growth hormone replacement

Sequenase MOLECULAR BIOLOGY A proprietary enzyme preparation used in DNA sequencing, which derives from the bacteriophage T7 DNA polymerase that has been modified to optimize the properties for sequencing

Sequenator An instrument for the semi-automated or automated determination of a sequence of amino acids in a protein (Edman sequencing) or nucleotides in a segment of DNA (Sanger sequencing), the latter of which is known as a 'gene machine'; see Human genome project, Sequencer

Sequence MOLECULAR BIOLOGY Noun A heteromeric chain of similar, but not identical molecules, eg nucleotides or amino acids Verb to determine the sequence (order of arrangement) of a sequence; see Chromosome walking PEDIATRICS A pattern of multiple congenital anomalies arising from a single early primary defect followed by a 'cascade' of secondary and tertiary defects; the Pierre-Robin sequence is caused by primary mandibular hypoplasia, which results in a tongue that is too small for the oral cavity and which drops back (glossoptosis), blocking closure of the posterior palatal shelf, resulting in a high arched U-shaped cleft palate; a sequence then, is a set of clinicopathologic consequences of the aberrant formation of one or more early embryologic structures; sequences are divided into 1) Malformation sequences due to poor formation of tissues 2) Deformation sequences, related to unusual forces acting on normal tissues and 3) Disruption sequences in which there is a breakdown of normal tissue; examples of sequences include athyroidotic hypothyroidism sequence, DiGeorge sequence, early urethral obstruction sequence, bladder exstrophy sequence, cloacal extrophy sequence, holoprosencephaly sequence, jugular lymphatic obstruction sequence, Kartagener syndrome sequence, Klippel-Feil sequence, laterality sequence, meningomyelocele, anencephaly, iniencephaly sequence, occult spinal dysraphism sequence, oligohydramnios sequence, Rokitansky sequence, septo-optic dysplasia (de Morsier) sequence, sirenomelia sequence

Sequence homology see Homology

Sequencer DNA sequencer A fully automated DNA sequencing device, known as HUGA (Human genome analyzer), produced by a Japanese consortium that contributed various technologies; because of the need to duplicate sequences for damaged genomic fragments, and as a form of quality control, HUGA's raw speed of 108 000 base pairs/day is reduced to 20-30 000 base pairs (Nature 1991; 351:593n&v)

Sequencing MOLECULAR BIOLOGY The act of determining the primary order of nucleotides (DNA sequencing), eg Maxam-Gilbert method or amino acids (protein sequencing), eg Edman or Sanger techniques; see Maxam-Gilbert sequencing, mini-protein (Edman) sequencing, Sanger sequencing

Sequence tagged site map see STS map

Sequential model see Induced fit model

Sequestration complex A pulmonary abnormality in which an aberrant pulmonary lobe is separated from the pulmonary parenchyma by its own pleura and own vascular supply arising directly from the aorta; the venous drainage is by the azygous or hemiazygous veins; the complex is frequently associated with diaphragmatic hernias and gastrointestinal malformations; the lung tissue may be normal or chronically inflamed Pathogenesis Defective embryogenesis in an abnormal accessory tracheobronchial bud from the foregut Note: Early closure of the normal lung bud would give rise to an intralobar lesion; see Pulmonary sequestration and table, page 595;Cf Folded lung, Scimitar syndrome, Trapped lung

SERC Science and Engineering Research Council The principal source of funds for academic research in Britain Budget 1991: 400 million pounds; see MERC; Cf INSERM, NIH

Serial interface COMPUTERS A connection port to a computer that transfers information in bits, which is slower than transfer of information in bytes; Cf Modem, Parallel interface

Serial murder FORENSIC PSYCHIATRY A series of homicides

in which a single person (or small group) selects victims based on a shared characteristic or, less commonly, at random; serial killers share various historical and behavioral patterns, including arsonal tendencies, compulsivity, drug and/or alcohol-abusing parents, evidence of biochemical and/or genetic abnormalities, history of sexual assault, drug or alcohol abuse, cruelty to animals, interrupted or absence of 'bliss of childhood', are often the victims of cruel parenting and products of difficult or unwanted pregnancy, masks of sanity, ritualistic behavior, search for help and feeling of powerlessness (to prevent the killing), history of perinatal head trauma, severe memory disorders, neurological impairment, 'pathological' lying, sexual deviancy and suicidal tendencies (J Norris, Serial Killers, Doubleday, New York, 1988)

Serial passage The repeated transfer of subpopulations of a pathogenic organism, eg the BCG strain of ***Mycobacterium tuberculosis***, through a series of animals, tissue culture cells or growth media, with the purpose of attenuating the pathogen's aggression while maintaining its immunogenicity

Serine proteases A family of proteolytic enzymes that have a similar three-dimensional conformation and an active site with a serine residue, forming an ester between the serine's hydroxyl group and the carboxyl group of a catalyzed peptide bond; serine proteases include coagulation cascade enzymes (vitamin K-dependent factors II, VII, IX and X, and factors XI and XII) as well as trypsin, chymotrypsin

'Serious misconduct' A euphemism in the science community for overt and/or intentional act(s) of fraud or fabrication of research data; misconduct in science includes simple 'correction' of data points in an assay, eg trimming, but becomes 'serious' when there is a deliberate attempt to deceive colleagues, as truth-telling is expected of scientists; see Fraud in science

Seroconversion The change of an immune status from that of non-production of a particular antibody, often being directed against an antigen of viral origin, eg HIV's p24 and p41 or hepatitis B's surface antigen (HBsAg) or e antigen (HBeAg), to a state of detectable production

Serotonin 5-hydroxytryptamine PHYSIOLOGY A molecule secreted by activated platelets that has a vasodilating effect on normal human coronary arteries; damage to the vascular endothelium, as occurs in coronary artery disease results in an unopposed serotogenic vasoconstriction and ischemia; serotonin thus appears to be a major actor in acute coronary artery disease, myocardial infarction and angina (N Engl J Med 1991; 324:641, 648)

Serotonin hypothesis A postulate that holds that schizophrenia and many of its related symptoms are due to multiple defects in serotonin metabolism

Serpentine cords A descriptor for the end-to-end arrangement of certain mycobacteria eg ***M tuberculosis*** and ***M bovis***, which, with the acid-fast stain, have a beaded appearance by high-power light microscopy

Serpiginous tract The descriptor for a twisted, vermiform radiolucency surrounded by a sclerotic rim, seen in long bones in pyogenic osteomyelitis (organisms include streptococci, staphylococci and ***Brucella*** species) or in infarction accompanied by intramedullary calcification

Serpiginous ulcer SEXUALLY-TRANSMITTED DISEASE A relatively uncommon clinical variant of the transient genital ulcer seen in chancroid (***Hemophilus ducreyi***), characterized as a single large rapidly-spreading shallow ulcer of the inguinal region Note: Psoriatic lesions have also been described as having a serpiginous pattern of extension

Serpin family A group of 52-65 kD serine protease inhibitor proteins (antithrombins), which are present in low (< 20 mg/dl) levels in the serum (table)

SERPINS

α_2-antiplasmin

Antithrombin III, which inhibits activated serine protease enzymes including thrombin, IXa, Xa and XIa

Heparin cofactor II, a protein having significant homology with antithrombin III and which in the presence of heparin (and dermatan sulfate) forms a 1:1 complex with thrombin, inactivating it

Plasminogen activator inhibitor-I (PAI-I), which inactivates tissue plasminogen activator

PAI-II, a urokinase inactivator

Serum The fluid component of blood from which the coagulation factors have been removed; Cf Plasma

Serum protein electrophoresis see SPEP

Serum response element (SRE) A small regulatory element that flanks the c-*fos* gene that is a primary nuclear target and the site of action for two signal transduction pathways, one of which activates protein kinase C (PKC) and the other which transmits signals in a PKC-independent pathway; SRE function requires binding of a protein designated as a serum response factor that acts at two different sites, explaining the specificity of the two signal transduction pathways (Science 1991; 251:189)

Serum sickness An immune response seen after re-exposure to an antigen to which an organism has been previously sensitized; immediately after exposure, there is antigen excess; from days 5-14, small antigen-antibody complexes accumulate in the vessels, causing the lesions of serum sickness; by the second week, antibodies predominate, forming larger antigen-antibody complexes that are catabolized by the reticuloendothelial system Clinical The soluble circulating immune-complexes result in urticaria, fever, adenopathy and occasionally arthritis; see Immune complex disease, Zone of equivalence

Serum spreading factor(s) Two plasma glycoproteins, weighing 65 kD (vitronectin) and 75 kD, respectively that mediate the attachment, spreading and differentiation of various cells, and which are inculpated in metastases; see Vitronectin

Servant see *Respondeat superior*

'Service' patient SOCIAL MEDICINE A patient who has become the ward of a health care facility, often by default as they have no insurance and a medical condition requiring long-term surveillance or care; service patients are generally cared for by house staff physicians and reimbursement for such patients is often relegated to those programs, eg Medicaid, that reimburse nominal amounts for services provided; see Homeless(ness), 'Safety net' hospitals; Cf Private patient

Setting sun sign PEDIATRICS A clinical finding consisting of inferior ocular deviation, characteristically seen in severe infantile hydrocephalus (occasionally also occurring in subdural hematomas) that is often accompanied by the 'cracked-pot' sign, prominence of the scalp veins, thinned and shiny skin, a high-pitched cry and optic nerve atrophy due to nerve and chiasm compression

Seurat spleen A descriptor for the punctate pattern of the extravasation of radiologic contrast material seen in a ruptured spleen, fancifully likened to the painting style of the French impressionist, Georges Seurat (1859-1891)

Seven-day fever A rodent-born infection by the spirochete, *Leptospira heptomadis* that has been reported in Japan and Europe and causes jaundice and fever; Cf Five-day fever

Seventh day disease Neonatal infection by *Clostridium tetani*, most common in the developing nations where contaminated instruments are used to cut the umbilical cord and dress the wound; by the end of the first week (the usual incubation period), the infant becomes irritable, spastic and tetanic **Mortality** Untreated *C tetani* infection may have a 70% mortality

70s, the rule(s) of A mnemonic for tumors of the central nervous system (CNS): 70% are primary CNS neoplasms, 70% of primary neoplasms are glial, 70% of primary glial tumors are astrocytomas and 70% of these are high grade **Children** 70% of tumors arise in the posterior fossa, 70% of those occurring before age 2 are medulloblastomas and 70% of supratentorial tumors are craniopharyngiomas **Adults** 70% are in the hemispheres, 70% of those in the pineal region are germinomas, 70% of those in the pituitary gland are adenomas, of which 70% are chromophobe

Seven-year itch Obsolete for scabies, which afflicted Napoleon's troops in epidemic proportions during the Russian campaign; see Scabies

Severe combined immune deficiency (SCID) A heterogeneous X-linked or autosomal recessive condition that is more common in blacks with onset in the first few months of life; this group of immunodeficiency syndromes is characterized by dysfunctional T- and B-lymphocytes **Clinical** Morbiliform rash, hyperpigmentation, severe recurring, often pulmonary infections (*Candida, Pneumocystis carinii*, cytomegalic inclusion virus, Epstein-Barr virus, herpes virus and varicella), failure to thrive and early death **Immunology** Combined humoral (hypo- or agglobulinemia) and cellular immune defects (absent response to T-cell mitogens, eg phytohemagglutinin), T- and B- cell lymphopenia, deficient IL-2 production (N Engl J Med 1990; 322:1718cr); SCID is subdivided according to defects in adenosine deaminase (ADA) and purine nucleoside phosphorylase (PNP, although it is also considered a variant of Nezelof's disease) enzymes and a defect in a DNA-binding protein required for the expression of HLA genes **Treatment** Bone marrow transplant; gene therapy and enzyme replacement in ADA deficiency are in the experimental protocol stage; see Adenosine deaminase deficiency, 'Bubble boy', Purine nucleoside phosphorylase, SCID mice

Severely debilitating illness A condition in which there is major irreversible morbidity, eg blindness or neurological degeneration, eg Alzheimer's or Parkinson's diseases; see Illness, Life-threatening illness

Sex chromosomes The human sex chromosome is composed of a pseudoautosomal region, corresponding to the site of recombination between the X and Y chromosomes and the sex chromosome specific regions; between these two regions, ie in the boundary zone, the sex chromosomes differ, with the Y chromosome having an Alu sequence (Nature 1990; 337:81, ibid; 344:663); see H-Y antigen, Testis-determining factor, X-chromosome inactivation, XIST

Sex cord-stromal tumors SURGICAL PATHOLOGY *OVARY* Tumors that comprise 5% of all ovarian neoplasms (one-half of which are fibroma-thecomas), and differentiate toward sex cords and/or specialized ovarian tissue, in the form of 'female' (ie, granulosa and theca) cells, male (ie, Sertoli and Leydig) cells or indifferent elements; classification of ovarian sex cord-stromal tumors (table) is based on morphology rather than hormonal status and ancillary studies, eg immunoperoxidase and immunohistochemistry) TESTES Tumors of Leydig and Sertoli cells comprise circa 5% of all testicular neoplasms, 10% of which behave in a malignant fashion; Cf Germ cell tumors

SEX CORD TUMORS (Int J Gynecol Pathol 1982; 1:101)

Granulosa-stromal cell tumors

a) Granulosa cell tumor, adult and juvenile types
b) Thecoma-fibroma group: Thecomas (typical and luteinized), fibromas, cellular fibromas and fibrosarcomas
c) Stromal tumors with a minor sex cord component
d) Sclerosing stromal tumor
e) Unclassified

Sertoli-stromal cell tumors

a) Sertoli cell tumors
b) Leydig cell tumors
c) Sertoli-Leydig cell tumors Well-, intermediate or poorly-differentiated or with heterologous elements

Gynandroblastoma

Sex cord tumor with annular tubules

Unclassified

Sex guidelines see Safe sexual activities

Sex 'industry' Any of a group of activities related to purchase of sexually-related services, especially involving direct contact of orogenital mucosae; the sex industry has always functioned with a 'tolerable' baseline of sexually-transmitted disease, which has drastically changed since the advent of the AIDS epidemic, as in certain underdeveloped countries, the sex industry is intimately linked to tourism and a young teenager's body may provide sustenance for his/her entire family, at a salary far below the cost of an adequate supply of the condoms necessary to prevent the transmission of human immunodeficiency virus; see AIDS, Condoms, HIV, Safe sexual activities, Sexual deviancy, Sexually-transmitted diseases

Sex-linked disease Inherited chromosome X-linked conditions, which are carried by the mother and expressed by the son, eg Fabry's disease, pyruvate kinase deficiency, G6PD deficiency, Xg^a blood group, factor VIII and factor IX deficiencies; see Testis-determining factor

Sex-reversed individuals see Pseudohermaphroditism, Sexual reassignment

Sexual anhedonia Sexual dysfunction in males where the erection and ejaculation are normal but without pleasure during orgasm, which may be psychogenic or secondary to drug abuse, eg cocaine Treatment Psychiatric, detoxification

Sexual deviancy Sexual excitement to the point of erection and/or orgasm when the object of that excitement is considered abnormal by the society in which it is practiced **ANAL INTERCOURSE** Sodomy, 'Buggery' Insertion of penis, other parts of the anatomy or sex toys per rectum, practiced by 14.3% of men and 18.6% of women Note: The sexual transmission efficacy of hepatitis B virus is 8.6-fold greater than HIV-1 in insertive anal intercourse in homosexuals (N Engl J Med 1990; 264:230) **BESTIALITY** Sexual intercourse with animals **BONDAGE AND DOMINANCE** A form of sado-masochism in which one partner is tied, hand-cuffed or otherwise restrained in one position while the other partner assumes castigatory and/or authoritative roles and performs a variety of 'punitive' erotic acts **COPROPHILIA** Sexual arousal obtained by manipulating fecal material **CROSS DRESSING** Wearing of clothes that are designed to be worn by those of the opposite phenotypic sex, an activity that is regarded as mildly deviant, and then, only when it becomes the person's dominant costume **CRUISING'** Engaging in multiple anonymous sexual encounters with multiple partners, usually in a male homosexual context **EXHIBITIONISM** Lady Godiva syndrome Public display of genitalia **FISTING** Insertion of the fisted hand into the rectum of a sexual, usually male partner **FROTTAGE** Full body contact between partners without sexual penetration (a non-deviant activity that contrasts with the following entry) **FROTTEURISM** 'Bakerloo' syndrome Sexual arousal from rubbing against those of the opposite sex in crowds (Bakerloo is a subway line in London) **'GERBILING'** The insertion of live gerbils or other small rodents in the anus as a form of eroticism, given that the hypoxia causes the animals to suffer preterminal convulsions which is perceived as pleasurable **'GOLDEN SHOWER'** Urination on the sexual partner(s) prior to engaging in sexual activities, most often homosexual **PÆDERASTY** Homosexual child molestation **PÆDOPHILIA** (US: Pedophilia) Heterosexual child molestation, defined as a six-month or longer period of recurrent, intense sexual urges and sexually-arousing fantasies involving sexual activity with prepubescent(s) (younger than age13); the pædophile must in addition have acted on the urges or be markedly distressed by them (J Am Med Assoc 1989; 261:602rv); Cf Pedophilia **PARAPHILIA** Recurrent intense sexual urges and fantasies in response to sexual objects or situations which are not part of normative arousal patterns, eg clothing fetishes **PEDOPHILIA** Sexual arousal with feet and shoes; Cf Pædophilia **SADO-MASOCHISM** A form of erotic deviancy in which the sexual dyad is composed of a partner who is sexually aroused while inflicting pain and another who is aroused while receiving pain; the term derives from the French novelist, Count Donatien-Alphonse-Francois de Sade who inflicted pain and wrote about it and Leopold von Sacher-Masoch, a German novelist who enjoyed pain and wrote about it **SCOPTOPHILIA** Voyeurism or 'peeping Tom-ism'; see Child abuse, Safe sex guidelines **WATER 'SPORTS'** see above, 'Golden shower'

Sexual differentiation see Hermaphroditism, Hirsutism, Müllerian ducts, Precocious puberty, Pseudoprecocious puberty, Testis-determining factor, Virilization, Wolffian ducts, XXX, XXY, XXXY, XYY syndromes

Sexuality The human sexual response, which is a function of external cues for heterosexual or homosexual orientation and the ability to produce and respond to gonadotropin-releasing hormone, which when disrupted leads to infertility; by age 13, 7.6% of US whites and 15.3% of US blacks have had sexual relations; by age 20, 65% and 85%; see Homosexuality, Transsexuality

Sexually-acquired reactive arthritis A polyarthritic complex occurring in HLA-B27-positive subjects triggered by sexually-transmitted *Chlamydia trachomatis* (Br Med J 1978; 1:605)

Sexually-transmitted diseases (STD) Infections (and tumors) that are transmitted by direct genital and orogenital contact; most common sexually-transmitted agents in USA: *Chlamydia trachomatis* 3-5 million cases (estimated in 1990, MMWR 1990; 39:53); type 2 herpes simplex 2-3 million (1990); *Neisseria gonorrhoeae*, 720 000, 25 300 penicillin-resistant (1988); *Treponema pallidum*, primary and secondary syphilis, 40 117 (1988) 357 congenital cases (New York City) STD agents *C trachomatis, Hemophilus gardnerella*, hepatitis B virus, herpes simplex, human immunodeficiency viruses (HIV-1 and HIV-2), human papilloma viruses (HPV), *Treponema pallidum, Mycoplasma hominis, N gonorrhoeae*, streptococcal species, *Trichomonas vaginalis, Ureaplasma urealyticum* SEXUALLY-TRANSMITTED NEOPLASIA Dysplasia and squamous cell carcinoma of the uterine cervix, penis and anus often arise in a setting of previous HPV infection; HPV types 16 and 33 are implicated in penile intraepithelial neoplasm; HPV types 6, 11 and 42 are implicated in condyloma acuminata, but are not related to malignancy; many male sexual partners of women with cervical intraepithelial neoplasia, cervical flat condylomas, condyloma acuminatum or variants of intraepithelial neoplasia

Sexual maturity rating Tanner staging A system for objectively determining sexual maturity, correlating chronologic age with a group of anatomic parameters, determining the degree of adolescent maturation; the most commonly used system was delineated by Tanner (Growth at Adolescence, Blackwell, Oxford, 1962); in females, five stages of maturation are recorded for pubic hair and breast development; in males, five stages are recorded for pubic hair, growth of the penis and testicles (Arch Dis Children 1966; 41:454)

Sexual reassignment The surgical conversion of a person's external (secondary) sexual characteristics to those of the opposite sex *MALE-TO-FEMALE CONVERSION* entails bilateral orchiectomy, penectomy, vaginoplasty and estrogen therapy *FEMALE-TO-MALE CONVERSION* is only partially successful and entails mastectomy, hysterectomy and androgenic hormone therapy Note: The male:female ratio of reassignment procedures is estimated at 3 to 7:1 Complications of reassignment are in part a function of whether therapy occurs in a legitimate medical environment, eg breast carcinoma associated with excess estrogen supplementation (J Am Med Assoc 1988; 259:2278) or whether reassignment is self-performed, eg illicit silicon injections (N Engl J Med 1983; 308:764), which may cause high fever, dyspnea, thoracic pain, acute respiratory failure with bilateral pulmonary interstitial infiltrates, airspace consolidation and Swiss cheese-like vacuolization of the dermis and macrophages (Arch Sex Behavior 1978; 7:337, 1986; 15:187)

Sexual stimulants No drug has proven effective in increasing libido and sexual performance, although several agents are believed by some to have this effect; see Aphrodisiac, Yohimbine

S factor One of two DNA-binding factors that help RNA polymerase I to initiate and transcribe the appropriate pre-rRNA genes; the B factor binds directly to DNA, 150 nucleotides upstream from the initiation site and this binding is markedly enhanced by the S factor; see Initiation complex; Cf Factor S

SGA Small for gestational age; see Low birth weight

SH2 region, **SH3 region** Src homology regions A group of highly conserved non-catalytic domains typical of proteins with intracytoplasmic tyrosine kinase activity, present in Abl, Fps, Src and tensin (Science 1991; 252:668)

Shadow casting RESEARCH A technique in electron microscopy for studying the surfaces of cells and intracytoplasmic regions, which may be carried out after freeze fracturing the region of interest, the fractured surface is sprayed with metal ions at a fixed angle, resulting in the decreased deposition of metal ions on sites that are at obtuse angles from the spray

Shadow cell A pale lightly pink cell, often devoid of a discernable nucleus DERMATOPATHOLOGY A pale, lightly eosinophilic anuclear keratinocyte with a central clearing seen in the center of pilomatrixomas (calcifying epithelioma of Malherbe), more common in older lesions where the characteristic basaloid cell component may be absent HEMATOPATHOLOGY A descriptor that may be applied to any cell that doesn't stain, ie is negative by the immunoperoxidase stain in tissues or in cytologic specimens, serving as vague tissue landmarks

Shadow plaque NEUROPATHOLOGY A 'classic' finding in the nervous system of patients affected by multiple sclerosis, which corresponds to an area of vague demyelination, which may be seen by gross examination, figure, below); other histological features of multiple sclerosis include myelin-axonal dissociation, where there are preserved axons without myelin, and accumulation of sudanophilic lipids resulting from myelin catabolism; see Multiple sclerosis

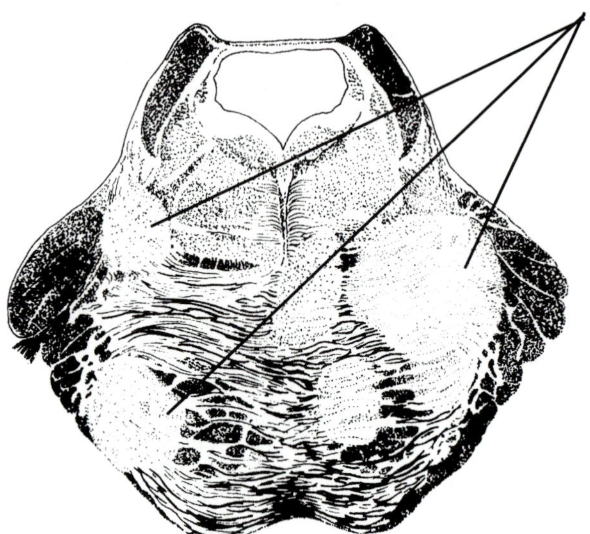

Shadow plaques

Shaggy heart sign A descriptor for the 'ragged' appearance of the cardiac contour seen in a plain chest film in occasional patients with *Bordetella pertussis* (whooping cough) infection; when seen during the paroxysmal stage; the shagginess is due to densities that obscure the cardiac borders (figure, facing page) and correspond to peribronchial thickening and infiltration of the basal triangle extending laterally from the hilum to the flattened and lowered diaphragm

Shagreen patch Indurated flesh-colored clusters of closely-set papules likened to shagreen that are present on the back and lumbosacral region, seen in tuberous sclerosis and other mucocutaneous lesions, including adenoma sebaceum in a 'butterfly' pattern, hypopigmented macules, gingival and periungual fibromas Note: Shagreen is an untanned leather prepared from the skin of horses, camels and others, covered with round granulations by pressing small seeds into the grain or hair side, scraping off the rugosity when the hide dries and soaking it to cause the compressed or indented portions of the skin to swell in relief and then dyed a bright color, often green; Cf Butterfly rash

Shaken baby 'syndrome' see Whiplash-shaken baby syndrome

Shaker Physiology A *Drosophila melanogaster* mutant

that shakes under ether anesthesia; the shaker gene encodes a structural component of a voltage-dependent potassium channel protein; see Potassium ion channels

Shake stability test see Foam stability test

Shaman A 'medicine man' from an aboriginal society whose healing ability derives from trance-like or 'supernatural' states; see Ethnomedicine

Sham feeding A clinical method for determining the completeness of vagotomy; food is smelled, seen and chewed, but not swallowed; acid output is measured by aspirating acid secretions via a nasogastric tube; acid production induced by sham feeding of greater than 10% of pentagastrin-stimulated peak acid output (PAO) implies intact vagal innervation

Shark skin appearance; see Shagreen patch

'Sharps' Any sharp object, eg syringe needles, scalpel blades, broken test tubes and glass that may contain potentially infected human blood, fluids and tissues; 'sharps' are a form of biohazardous waste that requires special handling given their ability to penetrate plastic and cardboard receptacles designed for the disoposal of human wastes and tissue; see Biohazardous waste, Regulated waste

'Shaving cream' appearance FORENSIC PATHOLOGY A descriptor for the bubbly or foamy material that oozes from the nostrils and mouth of narcotic addicts who have overdosed and died in frank pulmonary edema; Cf Mushroom of foam

SHBG Sex hormone binding globulin ENDOCRINOLOGY A β-

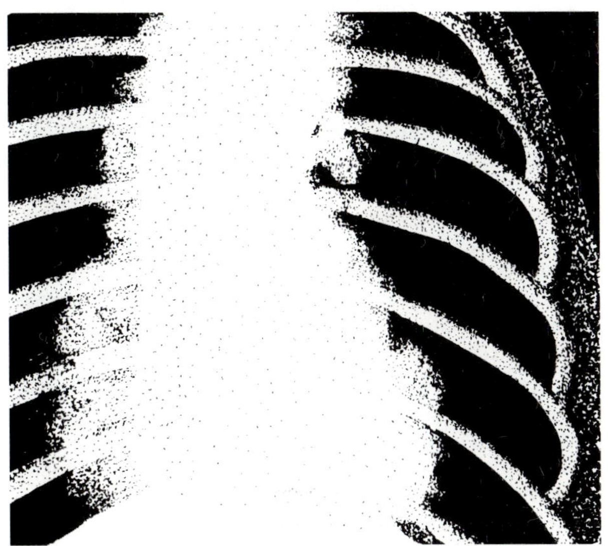

Shaggy heart appearance

globulin synthesized in the liver that binds testosterone, estradiol and other steroids containing a 17-β hydroxy substitution; natural sex hormones may be displaced from their binding site on SHBG by synthetic steroids, eg methyltestosterone and norgestrol, either by intent or inadvertently

Sheaf appearance see Wheat sheaf appearance

Sheath A tubular covering, shell or protective layer that may be formed around a) Axons, sheathed by schwann cells, although it is unknown how many cells a schwann cell sheathes b) Bacteria, either individually or when arranged in chains or c) Cells when being examined by flow cytometry; see Flow cytometry

Shelf life A term borrowed from business, which in the hospital environment refers to the length of time that a blood product or therapeutic agent may be stored under appropriate conditions before it must be discarded, which in transfusion medicine ranges from 24 hours for washed red cells to ten years (or more) for frozen red cells

'Shelf' sign RADIOLOGY A flattened horizontal mass often accompanied by mucosal irregularity that may be seen by barium enema in colonic adenocarcinoma

Shell nail see Spoon nail

'Shell shock' see Post-traumatic stress disorder

Shelter A building that often has a barracks-like atmosphere that houses abused women and their children, homeless persons or other disenfranchised population, providing them a place to sleep, food and clothing but little privacy

'Shelterization' SOCIAL MEDICINE An adaptive response by those living in shelters for the homeless in the USA, characterized by increased passive behavior and a decrease in personal hygiene (Hosp Community Psych 1990; 41:521); Cf Homeless, Institutionalization 'syndrome'

Shepherd's crook deformity A rarely observed prominent curving of the proximal femoral shaft, likened to the hooked staff used by the shepherds of yore, described in polyostotic fibrous dysplasia, chondrosarcoma and Paget's disease of the bone, characterized as a marked softening of femoral neck, associated with cortical thickening, accentuated trabeculation and unilateral shortening of the leg

'Sherlock Holmes' test A test for occult blood that removes iron from heme yielding fluorescing porphorins Note: The sobriquet derives from the fictional Sherlock Holmes who used a test of uncertain nature to confirm a reddish stain as being blood

Shift reticulocytes The finding of reticulocytes in the peripheral circulation longer than the usual 24 hours after their release from the marrow, resulting in a false elevation of the reticulocyte count, which is a common finding in severe anemia

Shift work OCCUPATIONAL MEDICINE A job in a hospital, company, factory, eg automobile, petrochemical or textile factory or other business that is open, and often operating at full staff 24 hours per day; the first 8-hour (day) shift begins at 0600-0900; the second (evening) shift begins at 1400-1700 and the third (night or 'graveyard') shift begins at 2200-0100; 20% of US employees work in a non-diurnal pattern, ie evening and night shifts and because of the relative unpopularity of the 'off' hours, are constantly being 'rotated', such that the workers must continually readjust their schedules; 20% of the population is relatively intolerant of shift work, as it requires abrupt changes of the circadian rhythm; diabetes and epilepsy are exacerbated by shift work and autonomic dysfunction is common as are increased fatigue-related accidents, increased risk of cardiovascular and gastrointestinal disease, infertility and long-term poor adjustment (insomnia); the circadian rhythm may be 'switched' by exposure to bright light at night and darkness during the day (N Engl J Med 1990; 322:1253, 1306); see Circadian rhythm, Insomnia, Jet lag

Shiga neurotoxin An exotoxin produced by ***Shigella dysenteriae*** type 1 that is responsible for neurotoxicity, enterotoxicity and cytotoxicity, which is structurally similar to the cholera toxin (composed of 1 A and 5 B subunits) and to ricin (a toxin of higher plants); the A subunit inhibits protein synthesis by enzymatic inactivation of the 60S ribosomes in a fashion analogous to that of ricin's protein inhibition; Shiga-like toxins(formerly designated as 'vero' toxins) are produced by ***Shigella*** species and ***Escherichia coli*** and are inculpated in enteropathogenic ***Escherichia coli*** and enterohemorrhagic ***E coli*** infections as well as in the hemolytic-uremic syndrome; see EHEC, EPEC

Shiley heart valve Björk-Shiley 60 degree Converso-Concave prosthetic heart valve An artificial heart valve manufactured from 1979 until 1985, when it was withdrawn from the market for strut fractures; 85 000 Shiley valves had been sold worldwide, transplanted into an estimated 23 000 patients in the US and Canada; strut fractures of the valve, first noted in 1976, are associated with a 0.02-0.3% annual death rate, with 800 deaths apparently re;ated to valve failure; physicians who implanted the valves have been advised to tell their patients, or they too become legally liable should valve failure occur; the manufacturer has begun an aggressive program for identifying and warning the valve recipients of their potential risk (Am Med News 26/Dec/90)

Shine-Delgarno sequence MOLECULAR BIOLOGY A segment of mRNA that includes part or all of the 5'-AGGAGGU-3' leader sequence, which pairs with the 16S ribosomal RNA, ensuring the proper alignment of the AUG start codon for the initiation of translation of proteins

Shingles Herpes zoster A term from Latin, Cingulum, girdle, related to the band-like involvement of neurocutaneous tissues seen in this condition

Shin 'splints' Innocuous pain over the antero-lateral aspects of the tibial bone that is relieved by rest, elevation and exposure to cold temperatures

Shiny coin appearance A fanciful descriptor for aggregates of basic calcium phosphate crystals seen by phase contrast microscopy; Cf Snow ball appearance

'Shiny Schultz' OBSTETRICS A form of placental 'delivery' that follows delivery of the infant, in which the placenta slips through the vagina with the (shiny) fetal surface showing; the blood and clots are within the pocket formed by the placenta; Cf 'Dirty Duncan'

SHIP Steroid hydroxylase inducer protein A labile, as yet uncharacterized protein that is thought to regulate some of ACTH's long-term effects by stimulating the transcription of the P450 enzymes involved in cortisol synthesis

Shipyard conjunctivitis Epidemic keratoconjunctivitis described in factory workers thought to be caused by adenoviruses

Shmita-salmonellosis Shmita is the Judaic practice of letting the land lay fallow every seventh year (as per biblical injunction, Exodus 23:10, Leviticus 25:1, 18, Deuteronomy 15:1); since the land is not being farmed on the seventh year, food is purchased from gentiles; one report (J Am Med Assoc 1983: 250:2470c) implicated the use of human fertilizer ('night soil') in the salmonellosis due to this religious practice; see Judaism, practice of

SHML see Sinus histiocytosis with massive lymphadenopathy

Shmoos A descriptor for ***Saccharomyces cerevisae*** yeast forms that are inhibited in cell division by an α factor present in the culture medium; in contrast, the α yeast forms of ***S cerevisae*** are not inhibited in cell division when exposed to α factor, due to a nonrandom gene rearrangement that allows the yeasts to change from 'male' to 'female' mating phenotypes; the term was coined by yeast geneticists who likened the yeasts' appearance to that of minor characters in the 'Li'l Abner' comic strip by Al Capp

Shock A condition characterized by clinical signs and symptoms caused by a cardiac output below that required to fill the arterial tree with blood of sufficient pressure to provide organs and tissue with adequate blood flow (after Simeone, 1964); shock is classified based on separate but related mechanisms of cardiac dysfunction (pump failure), decreased volume (loss of blood or extracellular fluid) or changes in arterial resistance or venous capacity

Shock lung Post-traumatic respiratory insufficiency, traumatic 'wet lung' CRITICAL CARE MEDICINE A condition affecting the lungs, in which a change in pulmonary compliance and oxygenating capacity, results in an adult respiratory distress syndrome-like (ARDS-type) picture with defective aeration of the lungs, due to multiple factors, including aspiration of gastric contents, atelectasis, cerebral injury (affecting respiratory rate), interstitial edema, microembolism, oxygen toxicity, sepsis, oxygen toxicity or fulminant meningococcemia; see Adlt respiratory distress syndrome

Shofar-blowing emphysema Painful interstitial emphysema of the head and neck, caused by blowing the Shofar, a difficult wind instrument that requires considerable intraoral pressure (the 'embouchure' of wind instrument players), made more difficult by the blower's lack of practice and underdeveloped buccal musculature, resulting in percolation of the air into the neck Note: The Shofar is a ram's horn trumpet that was blown by the ancient Hebrews in battle and still blown at the time of 'high' Jewish holidays, ie before and during Rosh Hashanah and at the end of Yom Kippur or Yom teruah, the 'Day of blowing' (J Am Med Assoc 1983; 250:2470c); see Judaism, practice of

Shofar sign RADIOLOGY A descriptive term for a stomach that has been deformed by the chronic changes of Crohn's disease, in which a relatively normal gastric fundus and body funnel into a gastric antrum has been converted into a stiffened tube with superficial rugosities and sluggish peristalsis, when viewed by an 'upper GI' radiocontrast study, imparting an appearance fancifully likened to the sacramental Shofar (ram's horn, see above) of Jewish high holidays, an appearance identical in import to the far more commonCrohn's disease of the terminal ileum, where the small intestinal stiffening has been likened to a garden hose Note: Transverse line in figure indicates the usual length of a shofar

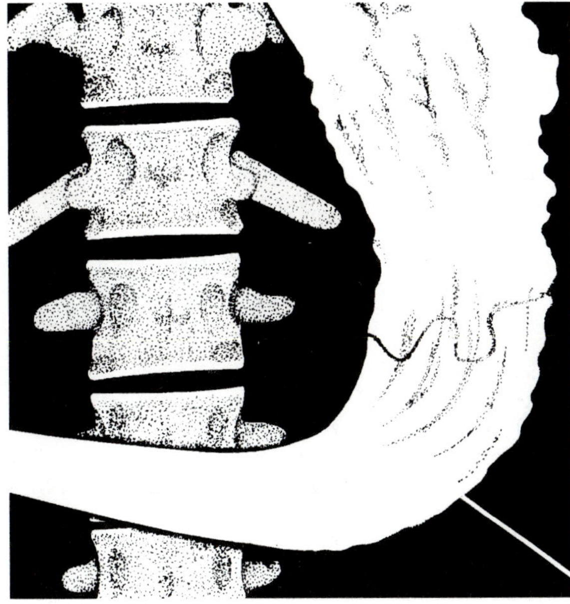

Shofar (ram's horn) sign

Shooter bone Myositis ossificans of the deltoid muscle of soldiers evoked by repeated trauma caused by the recoil of a rifle's butt against the upper anterior arm

'Shooting gallery' SUBSTANCE ABUSE A location, often an abandoned building in a depressed urban area, where intravenous drug abusers congregate, purchase and inject ('shoot') heroin and cocaine; shooting galleries are unique to the US and are places of relative camaraderie in which addicts may share needles, often contaminated by HIV (Am J Public Health 1990; 80:150); see Needle exchange programs, 'Pocket shot', 'Skin popping'

Short bowel syndrome A post-surgical syndrome that follows large segmental resections of the small intestine, causing complex nutritional imbalances and/or malnutrition; massive small intestinal resection may be required in a) Multiple congenital atresias or stenoses of the neonatal intestine; when the loss is significant, diarrhea and malabsorption may appear shortly after birth; barium studies reveal a malrotated colon and markedly shortened small bowel; if the infant survives the first few months, intestinal function improves and b) Massive resection of gangrenous small intestine due to mesenteric arterial occlusion (see 'Second look' operation), traumatic interruption, volvulus or Crohn's disease; excess resection results in inadequate small intestinal digestion and absorption of nutrients, minerals and vitamins, causing hypovitaminosis and malnutrition, anemia (both hypochromic and megaloblastic anemias), diarrhea, electrolyte imbalances and marked increase in oxalates (derived from bile salt detergents that pass into the circulation, inundating the kidneys with oxalates that crystallize in the renal tubules, causing the renal failure typical of the short bowel syndrome), lactic acidosis, osteopenia and steatorrhea; up to 70% of the absorptive surface may be lost and tolerated; if the patient survives the surgery, the residual tissue undergoes adaptive hyperplasia of the absorptive villi, an increase in absorptive cells and an increase in small intestinal caliber; after stabilization and temporary parenteral nutritional support, oral feeding must be initiated as soon as possible to stimulate the adaptive response Treatment High in 'quality' protein (essential amino acids) diet, middle chain triglycerides, vitamins and minerals

'Shorting' A form of health care fraud committed by a pharmacy in which fewer pills or lesser amounts of a drug are dispensed than is specified on the physician's prescription form; Cf 'Kiting'

Short interspersed repeated elements (SINE) A family of short, 70 to 300 base pair, repeated segments of DNA that includes the Alu sequence family, which are present in up to 100 000 copies in the human genome, which are not currently known to have a function; Cf Junk DNA, LINE

Short leg syndrome see Long leg syndrome

Short-loop feedback PHYSIOLOGY The hypothalamic hormones are schematically represented as an 'axis' consisting of two circuits, the hypothalamic-pituitary loop (short loop) and the pituitary-end organ loop (long loop); see Loops

Short rib-polydactyly syndrome (SRPS) A complex characterized by short stature and short horizontal ribs, divided into **TYPE I SRPS** An autosomal recessive condition with polydactyly, metaphyseal irregularities of long bones, small iliac bones, transposition of great vessels, and pulmonary hypoplasia and **TYPE II SRPS** of Majewski A condition characterized by a narrow thorax, polysyndactyly, cleft lip, malformed ears, ambiguous genitalia, epiglottic and laryngeal hypoplasia, glomerular cysts and absent gallbladder

Shoshin beri-beri A fulminant form of beri-beri, ie thiamine deficiency, largely of historical interest Clinical Cardiac dilatation, cardiomegaly, tachypnea, shallow breathing, cyanosis and, due to pyruvate accumulation, cardiovascular collapse, hepatomegaly and mydriasis Note: Thiamine is responsible for oxidative decarboxylation, in its absence, the orange-colored methyl glyoxal and pyruvate accumulate, resulting in myocardial toxicity

Shotgun FORENSIC MEDICINE A sports weapon, popularized by water fowl hunters, which is widely regarded as the most efficient 'execution' weapon for moving targets; death by shotgun is rare in civilized countries, given the strict gun control laws; in the USA, homicide and suicide by shotgun is not uncommon; the shot or pellets spread out in a relatively consistent fashion, such that the distance from the muzzle in meters is approximately equal to three times the diameter of the target, thus a 60-70 cm in diameter spread of shot pellets corresponds to a muzzle range of two meters, a value of some forensic use for determining the proximity of an alleged perpetrator of a crime; while short-term, a victim might survive certain shotgun wounds, massive infection secondary to multiple perforations in an abdominal blast entails prolonged recuperation, if the surgeon is successful in salvaging the intestine Note: When new, shotguns have a full 'choke', a narrowing at the end of the barrel to ensure that the shot (pellets) remain closely clustered in their trajectory; when the barrel is shortened by cutting, creating a 'sawed-off' shot-gun, the trajectory of the pellets is shorter, the spread of the shot much wider and devastation to the body more complete; see Cookie cutter wounds, Execution wounds

'Shotgun approach' A diagnostic method or technique in which every conceivable parameter is measured in order to detect all possible clinical or laboratory nosologies, however remote the possibility a rare disease is present; in the USA, not considering a potentially treatable disease in a difficult case may result in potentially costly litigation and thus physicians may in the face of such cases resort to the 'shot-gun method', an often-criticized result of practicing 'defensive medicine', increasing the cost of health care without improving patient management; Cf Screening

Shotgun experiment 'Shotgunning' MOLECULAR BIOLOGY A crude but effective method used to identify a specific gene associated with a disease, which consists in non-specifically cloning all the fragments that result from a restriction endonuclease digest of the entire genome of an organism known to contain a gene of interest, yielding a constellation of fragments known as a gene bank or gene library, which is followed by an identification step, consisting in screening for the desired gene; Cf 'Quick and dirty'

Shotty lymphadenopathy A non-specific descriptor for clusters of multiple small, contiguous and indurated lymph nodes that may be palpated in the inguinal, cervical and other regions in children with viral infections, which, when palpated in adults is characteristic of syphilis, and may be seen in carcinoma metastatic to lymph nodes

'Shoulder' OBSTETRICS A descriptor for the gently-sloped acceleration rhythm seen on a paper printout of the fetal heart monitor that either precedes or follows a typical deceleration, in contrast to the usual 'acceleration' (a short-term increase in the heart rate above baseline) occurring in response to fetal movement; see Deceleration

Shoulder-hand syndrome A clinical complex characterized by shoulder pain, swelling, stiffness, vasomotor symptoms of the arm and hand, cutaneous edema and induration, affecting those over age 50 as a complication of myocardial infarction, or less commonly, a cerebrovascular accident or head trauma, a condition that is thought due to reflex sympathetic stimulation; some patients later develop adhesive capsulitis, sclerodactyly and limitation of motion of the extremity with patchy regional demineralization; see Rotator cuff

Shoulder pad sign Enlargement of the glenohumeral joint due to peri-articular accumulation of amyloid in primary or secondary (multiple myeloma) amyloidosis, appearing as a regional soft tissue density

Shoulder pointer 'syndrome' SPORTS MEDICINE A simple separation or 'sprain' of the acromioclavicular joint is commonly associated with contact sports (eg football, wrestling, karate, hockey) as well as non-contact sports due to dislocations or strain, eg swimming, gymnastics without joint instability

Shredded appearance A descriptor for the morphology of skeletal muscle that has been exposed to extreme heat or cold, resulting in necrosis with irregular transverse bands of dense material separated by lighter areas **Mechanism** Sudden over-contraction of muscle Note: The shredded appearance may also be seen in myotonic dystrophy or as an artefact of fixation; see Contraction band necrosis, Wavy changes

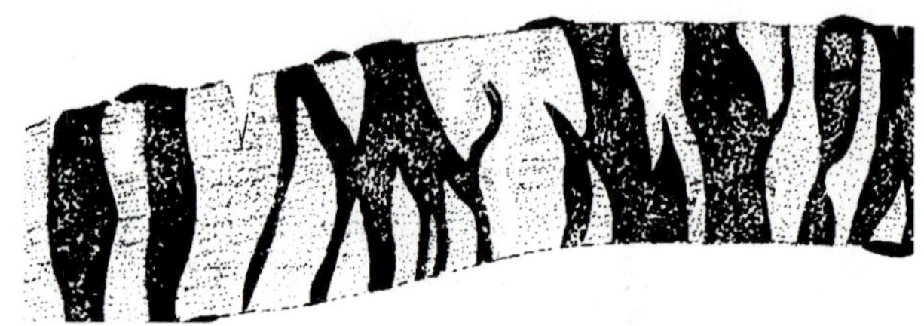

Shredded appearance, muscle

Shredded cassette appearance A descriptor for the morphology of colonies of ***Erysipelothrix rhusiopathiae*** (erysipeloid agent), likened to the 'confused' tangled strands of a partially broken audiocassette

Shrewmouse profile A fanciful descriptor for the facies of children seen after ankylosis of the jaw following scarlet fever, an extremely incommon clinical event

'Shrinking field' technique RADIATION ONCOLOGY A method used in radiotherapy for treating a large mediastinal lymphoid malignancy, in which the treatment field is decreased in size (shrunken) as the tumor responds or 'melts'; see Mantle port

Shrinking lungs Elevation of the diaphragm due to pleural adhesions, plate-like atelectases and chronic fibrosis, a finding described as typical of lupus erythematosus; shrinking lungs are radiological and pathological findings that may not translate into clinical disease

Shrinking pleuritis with rounded atelectasis see Folded-lung syndrome (N Engl J Med 1983; 308:1466cpc)

Shunt nephritis Glomerulonephritis described in about 4% of infants with infected (cerebral) ventricular-atrial shunt **Clinical** Weight loss, lethargy, fever, hypertension, arthralgia, lymphadenopathy, hepatosplenomegaly and a frank nephrotic syndrome, largely due to the delay in recognizing the infection **Laboratory** Anemia, hematuria, azotemia; the most common bacteria isolated are *Staphylococcus epidermidis* and *S albus* **Treatment** Antibiotics, possibly also high dose prednisone **Prognosis** One-half of cases resolve with therapy, one-fourth have persistent urine abnormalities; the remainder die of the neurological defects that necessitated the ventricular shunt

Shunts PEDIATRIC CARDIOLOGY While bypass of the pulmonary circulation (shunting) is a normal physiological process in utero, it becomes abnormal upon delivery of the infant; shunts are of two types a) Those in which already oxygenated blood in the left heart passes back into the right heart (left-to-right) and b) Those which partially bypass the lungs, with venous blood directly entering the systemic circulation (right-to-left shunt) **LEFT-TO-RIGHT SHUNT** *ACYANOTIC SHUNT* The right and left sides of the heart communicate by an atrial or ventricular septal defect and patent ductus arteriosus; the blood flows from the region of highest (left heart) to lowest (right heart and systemic circulation) pressure, as occurs in ventricular septal defects and corrected L-transposition of the great arteries; since the blood does not bypass the pulmonary circulation, it is well-oxygenated **Clinical** The plethora of blood causes pulmonary congestion and hypertension that becomes significant when the pulmonary blood flow is 1.5-2.0-fold greater than the systemic flow with diastolic overloading and cardiac dilatation, which without correction results in cardiac failure, a late complication is bacterial pneumonia related to stasis within the pulmonary circulation **RIGHT-TO-LEFT SHUNT** *CYANOTIC SHUNT* There is a variable degree of pulmonary circulation bypass accompanied by obstruction of blood flow into the pulmonary circulation; right-to-left shunts include Fallot's tetralogy (ventricular septal defect, pulmonary valve stenosis, overriding or dextroposed aorta and secondary right ventricular hypertrophy), transposition of the great vessels, tricuspid valve atresia, truncus arteriosus and total anomalous return of pulmonary veins; the pulmonary blood flow is less than in left-to-right shunts **Clinical** Cyanosis with limited exercise tolerance, neurological damage and compensatory polycythemia; as children, these patients are often very sick and by adolescence, may suffer acquired coagulopathies

Shuttle A short cyclical metabolic pathway in which reducing elements are passed from the cytoplasmic NADH to the electron transport system within the mitochondria by way of molecular intermediates

Shuttle vector MOLECULAR BIOLOGY A self-sufficient DNA molecule that is capable of replicating in a variety of hosts, including yeasts and bacteria

Shy bladder Vesica Pudica A psychoneurologic reflex, more common in men, characterized by the inability to initiate urinary flow in public places

SI Systeme International d'unites The international system for standardization of units of measurement, which is a refinement and extension of the metric system, which is based on a) Seven basic units: m meter (length), kg kilogram (mass), s second (time), A ampere (electric current), K Kelvin (thermodynamic temperature), cd candela (luminous intensity), mol mole (amount of a substance) and b) Units that derived from the first group: N newton (force), J joule (energy) and L liter (volume) Note: The SI sanctions l for liter; because this may be confused with number 1, L is often substituted in the USA, a convention adopted by the author; the USA is also the only country that has not yet converted entirely to the SI system of reporting laboratory values; for most analytes, the conversion is simple; in hematology, the number of cells (red cells, white cells, and platelets) in a cubic millimeter (mm^3) are converted to those present in one liter, multiplied by 10^6; in chemistry, the units are converted from milligrams/deciliter to millimoles/liter and most analytes have a 1:1 ratio with SI units; some values are transformed into SI units by using a conversion factor, with appropriate adjustment for the types of units (table)

SI (common US to SI conversions)

	CF*	Final units
Acetone	172.2	mmol/L
Albumin	10.0	mmol/L
Alanine aminotransferase	0.482 U/L	Karmen units
Bilirubin	17.10	µmol/L
Calcium	0.2495	mmol/L
Cholesterol	0.0258	mmol/L
Creatinine	88.40	µmol/L
Glucose	0.0555	mmol/L
Hemoglobin	10.0	g/L
Iron	0.1791	µmol/L
Lipoproteins (LDL)	0.2586	mmol/L
Lipoproteins (HDFL)	0.2586	mmol/L
Magnesium	0.4114	mmol/L
Phosphate	0.3229	mmol/L
Potassium levels, mg	0.2558	mmol/L
Protein	10.0	g/L
Trioiodothyronin (T3)	0.1536	nmol/L
Triglycerides	0.0113	mmol/L
Urea nitrogen	0.3570	mmol/L, urine

*CF Conversion factor

SIADH Syndrome of inappropriate antidiuretic hormone secretion ENDOCRINOLOGY A clinical complex characterized by excess vasopressin (ADH) secretion despite low plasma osmolarity, water retention and dilutional hyponatremia **Etiology** SIADH occurs in untreated Addison's disease, ACTH deficiency, hypopituitarism, ectopic hormone production in carcinomas (oat cell, bronchogenic, pancreatic, uterine, bladder and prostatic), lymphoproliferative disorders, mesothelioma, thymoma, central nervous system disease (trauma, infection, chromophobe adenoma, metastases), pulmonary disease (pneumonia, tuberculosis, use of positive-end-expiratory pressure (PEEP) ventilatory support, drugs (chlorpropamide, vincristine) and others, eg porphyria and AIDS **Clinical** Hypervolemia, hypouricemia, often reduced creatinine **Diagnosis** Hyponatremia, natriuresis (urinary sodium > 20 mEq/L with decreased BUN), absence of clinical symptoms of volume depletion, decreased maximum urinary dilution, normal renal and adrenal function **Treatment** Corticosteroids as they suppress vasopressin secretion (N Engl J Med 1989; 321:492)

Sialadenoma papilliferum A rare, benign exophytic tumor of the salivary gland Histopathology Papillary exophytic overgrowth of both the intercalated duct epithelium and surface squamous epithelium

Sialidosis, type I see Cherry-red spot myoclonus syndrome

Sialidosis type II A hereditary condition characterized by coarse facies and dysostosis multiplex which has been divided into a congenital form with ascites, hydrops fetalis, gargoyle-like facies, visceromegaly, mental retardation, myoclonus, tonic-clonic seizures, cherry-red spots, hearing loss, defect of neuraminidase, usually with a partial defect of β-galactosidase; the infantile and juvenile forms may be less severe Histopathology PAS-positive inclusions in lymphocytes, bone marrow, neurons and Kupffer cells

Sialyl-Lewis X A molecular determinant present on myeloid cells and on some tumor cells (Science 1990; 250:1132), which serves to explain the vasculotropism of some invasive tumors; see ELAM-1

'Siamese' twins Conjoined gestational products resulting from a failure in division of the yolk sac or due to delayed monovular separation, an event estimated to occur in 1:200 000 term deliveries, most of which are joined at the chest (thoracopagus), the prognosis is a function of adequacy of surgical separation Note: The most famous Siamese twins, Chang and Eng Bunker, were born in Siam (now Thailand) in 1811, married the Yates sisters in North Carolina in 1843, respectively fathered 10 and 12 children and died at age 62, within hours of each other

Sicca complex Symptoms related to generalized drying of mucosae, affecting a) Eyes, causing xeroconjunctivitis due to decreased tears, thick, 'ropy' secretions on the inner canthus, foreign body (tired, itchy and sandy) sensation and decreased visual acuity and b) Mouth Xerostomia with decreased salivation due to lymphocyte infiltration and duct obstruction, with soreness, adhesion of food to mucosa, 'cracker' sign, angular cheilitis, lingual fissuring and acceleration of caries; the sicca complex is most often associated with Sjögren syndrome and may also occur in amyloidosis, hemochromatosis, hyperlipoproteinemia type IV and V, sarcoidosis, vitamin C and A deficiency, scleroderma and other collagen vascular diseases

'Sick building' syndrome Tight building syndrome PUBLIC HEALTH A group of symptoms that are two to three-fold more common in those who work in large, energy-efficient buildings, associated with an increased frequency of headaches, lethargy and dry skin Clinical manifestations fall in a number of categories (table, right)

Sick cell 'syndrome' Redistribution of sodium between the intracellular and extracellular compartments without changes in the total body sodium, occurring in severely ill patients and presumed to be due to the inefficiency of the Na^+/H^+ antiporter

Sickle cells Drepanocytes The fragmented scythe-shaped cells that result from the formation of 'tactoids' within erythrocytes of 'sickling' hemoglobins; hemoglobin exists in two conformations, the 'R', relaxed or oxygenated form and the 'T', tense or deoxygenated form, which readily transform, one to the other, depending on the oxygen conditions; deoxygenation of hemoglobin S causes it to polymerize into rigid, rod-like fibers (tense form), which upon curvilinear alignment, give rise to the classic sickle cell shapes Note: T is in part related to the uncoupling of the spectrin-based membrane skeleton from the lipid bilayer (Science 1991; 252:574); see Spectrin, Tactoid

Sickle cell disease A congenital hemoglobinopathy that affects 0.15% of Black children in the US, caused by a point mutation on the gene that encodes β hemoglobin, resulting in a defective functioning of hemoglobin, causing the erythrocytes to 'sickle' under low oxygen conditions; sickle cell anemia was first described in a West Indian student (Arch Int Med 1910; 6:517), and most cases in blacks have been traced to a family in the Krobo tribe in 1670; other sickle cell anemias occur in Greece, Italy, Israel, Saudi Arabia and subcontinental India, and in addition to hemoglobin S, which causes the classic sickle cell anemia, are due to other hemoglobin defects, in which sickling plays a key role in producing clinical disease, including hemoglobin SC disease, hemoglobin SD disease and β thalassemia

Sickle cell 'prep' A laboratory test used to screen for sickle cell anemia, where sodium metabisulfite is used to desolubilize hemoglobin S to the crystallized deoxygenated form, causing the cells to sickle

Sickle chest syndrome A complication of sickle cell anemia caused by intravascular 'sludging' of circulating cells Clinical Chest pain, dyspnea and fever due to

Sick building syndrome(s)

Hypersensitivity pneumonitis Allergic alveolitis An allergic response to various microorganisms including water-borne amoeba, known as Humidifier lung, see there

Allergic rhinitis and asthma, related to dust mites

Infections, causing miniepidemics, eg Legionnaire's disease, Pontiac fever and Q fever by airborne organisms of low pathogenic potential that thrive in stagnate water and are disseminated through poorly-maintained air conditioning systems

Skin eruptions, due to fiberglass, mineral wool or other particles; those who wear contact lenses in these environments may suffer corneal abrasions and lens damage

Mucous membrane irritation syndromes, including dry throat, cough, tightness in chest, sinus congestion and sneezing due to tobacco smoke, janitorial solvents and cleaning materials, eg chlorine, reactions to photochemical or other toxins, eg in laser printers due to the styrene-butadiene toners (N Engl J Med 1990; 322:1323c) and ozone production by photocopiers

Pseudoepidemics related to 'mass hysteria'

thromboses in the terminal pulmonary arteries Prognosis Guarded

Sickle particles A descriptor for the curved bacteria-like structures seen by high-power light microscopy in the macrophages of Whipple's disease in the myocardium, lung, spleen, liver, pancreas, mesentery, retroperitoneum, soft tissue, lymph nodes, adrenal glands and brain

Sick Santa 'syndrome' OCCUPATIONAL MEDICINE The sum of the infectious diseases afflicting those who seasonally don St Nicholas garb, exposing themselves to infected aerosols; other Santa-related symptoms include frostbite (Salvation army Santas), psychological (repressed anger), neuromuscular symptoms (prolonged periods in uncomfortable positions, eg holding children on the knees)

Sick sinus syndrome A diffuse cardiac conduction system disease characterized by a pathologically slow or erratic rate of sinus depolarization due to impaired automaticity; a 'sick sinus' is more common in the elderly and, if severe, may be symptomatic with dizziness, palpitations, exercise intolerance, syncopes and cerebral dysfunction associated with a combination of persistent sinus bradycardia (30-60/min) and supraventricular tachyarrhythmia, thus the trivial synonym, 'brady-tachy' syndrome Treatment Verapamil, diltiazem or pacemaker

SIDA Syndrome d'immunodeficience acquise, French for AIDS Note: The other Romance languages, ie Italian, Portuguese and Brazilian and Spanish use an equivalent acronym for AIDS

Siderophilins A family of 80 kD monomeric non-heme iron-binding glycoproteins, eg transferrin and lactoferrin that bind two iron ions in conjunction with two carbonate ions

SIDS Sudden infant death syndrome Definition from 2nd Intl Conf on SIDS, World Health Organization *'SUDDEN AND UNEXPECTED DEATH OF AN INFANT WHO WAS WELL OR ALMOST WELL PRIOR TO DEATH WHICH REMAINS UNEXPLAINED AFTER AN ADEQUATE AUTOPSY'* Frequency of SIDS in different ethnic groups, USA Asian 0.5/1000; caucasian 1.3/1000; black 2.9/1000; American Indian 5.9/1000; SIDS is more common in premature male infants under six months of age; the parents are more commonly in lower socioeconomic strata, narcotic addicts, cigarette smokers or unwed mothers Histopathology Non-specific, possibly related to a preterminal asphyxiating event, as petechiae occur on the thymus, epicardium and pleura; one fatal event misinterpreted as SIDS is involuntary smothering (see the Ballad of Moll Magee, WB Yeats) by an exhausted mother who 'co-sleeps' with the infant Laboratory No consistent abnormalities; a potential cause of SIDS is the fungus ***Scopulariopsis brevicaulis*** that grows well on the plastic covering of baby mattresses, producing toxic heavier-than-air trihydride gases (phosphine, arsine, stibine) that may concentrate at the child's head; since they don't move well at this age, the infants may 'smother' from the gas (Lancet 1990; 335:670c); in some cases reported as SIDS, the infants are found lying face down in soft polystyrene foam-filled cushions, apparently dying of rebreathing type suffocation (N Engl J Med 1991; 324:1858)

Siemann An International System (SI) unit of conductivity that measures the quantity of electricity transferred across a unit area per unit of potential gradient in a unit of time

Sievert (Sv) The International System (SI) unit of radioactive biological effectiveness; 1.0 Sv = 100 rem; see Gray, Rad; Roentgen

'Sieving' GASTRIC PHYSIOLOGY A theory that attempted to explain how food passes from the stomach to the duodenum; it had been assumed by some that lighter, partially digested particles would flow as the central portion of a parabolic 'column' into the duodenum, a theory that was later modified to include mechanical and size factors, where particle transit time is directly related to fluid viscosity and velocity and inversely related to particle density and diameter

Sieving Molecular sieving; see Gel filtration chromatography, Reptation

Sigma factors MOLECULAR BIOLOGY Accessory proteins that aid RNA polymerase in recognizing specific DNA 'promoter' sites to be transcribed, which results in a 'bind-release-bind' sequence fancifully likened to Tarzan swinging from the vines; once the RNA polymerase hits a sigma factor, by analogy, a tree trunk, transcription begins

'Sigmoid' esophagus see Bird's beak sign

Sigmoid kinetics The rate behavior of an enzymatic reaction that yields a sigmoid (S-shaped) curve for a plot of reaction velocity versus substrate concentration, a curve typical of allosteric enzyme-substrate systems, which demonstrate cooperative interaction

Sigmoidoscope A device for examining the sigmoid colonic mucosa, divided into rigid and flexible sigmoidoscopy; because of its simplicity, the rigid sigmoidoscope is of use in examining the anorectum and distal sigmoid; for higher lesions, the flexible sigmoidoscope reduces patient discomfort, has a two to four-fold greater diagnostic yield than rigid sigmoidoscopy and has a useful 'reach' of 60-70 cm, allowing rapid evaluation, photography and biopsies of the large intestine; as the bowel preparation is minimal, electrocoagulation polypectomies are ill-advised, given the danger of explosion due to the various gases in this region (J Am Med Assoc 1990; 264:89rv); Cf Flatulence

Sigmoid septum An angulated deformity of the aorta seen in idiopathic hypertrophic subaortic stenosis

Signal event An event, usually man-made, in which there is a tremendous 'signal', often in the form of a 'disaster', eg Love canal or the Libby Zion case, which engenders multiple 'ripple' effects of legislation and 'landmark' legal cases, due in part to a popular outcry against prevailing policies that were inadequate or incapable of addressing the event Note: Such events may result in legislative overreaction and the 'solution' may spawn a host of unanticipated ethical dilemmas

Signal hypothesis The theory explaining the mechanism by which secretory proteins are selected for export by the rough endoplasmic reticulum (RER), according to which, the mRNA encoding the secretory protein contains a 'signal sequence' immediately downstream from the start codon; the mRNA's translation is initiated by free ribosomes in the cytosol, which synthesize a hydrophobic N-terminal oligomeric 'signal peptide'; once the signal peptide leaves the ribosome, it binds to a receptor on the RER, around which a transmembrane pore develops, through which the nascent protein extrudes and becomes glycosylated; finally the mature protein is transported via the Golgi apparatus to its final intra- or extracellular destination

Signal peptide see Signal sequence

Signal recognition particle (SRP) MOLECULAR BIOLOGY A multi-unit 11S cytoplasmic protein with a key role in exporting nascent proteins from the cytoplasm of mammalian cells; SRP is constructed of six discrete polypeptides (P9, P14, P19, P54, P68 and P72) linked to a 300-nucleotide RNA sequence that recognizes a secretory protein's 'signal sequence', allowing transportation of the protein from the site of production at the tRNA into the lumen of the endoplasmic reticulum for future extracellular secretion; termination of SRP action requires its dissociation from its receptor, the energy contributed by GTP hydrolysis (Science 1991; 252:1171)

Signal sequence MOLECULAR BIOLOGY A prehormone's NH_2 terminal amino acids that are critical for the transfer from its site of synthesis in the cytoplasm to the endoplasmic reticulum; the signal peptide binds the polyribosome complex (mRNA, ribosomes and nascent proteins) to the endoplasmic reticulum; after cleavage of the signal peptide, the protein becomes either a prohormone or a hormone; although there is no homology among the different signal sequences, they have one or more positively charged amino acids near the N-terminus, followed by 6-12 hydrophobic residues; since the signal sequences are not found in the mature proteins, they are thought to be cleaved from the protein while it is being translated

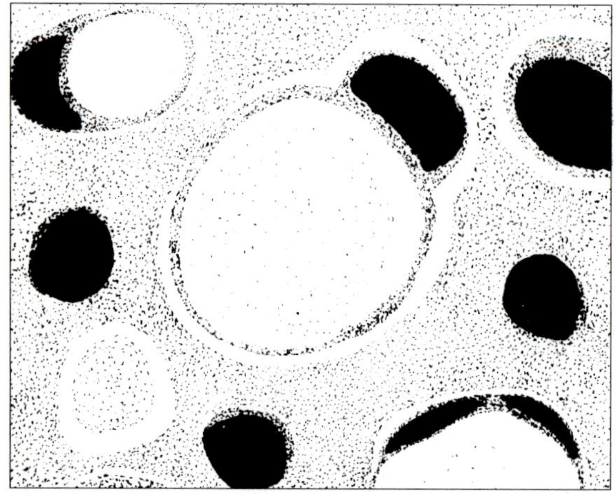

Signet ring cells

Signet ring cell An almost invariably malignant cell in which there is copious clear cytoplasm flattening a hyperchromatic nucleus to one side (figure, above), having an appearance fancifully likened to that of a signet ring; malignancies composed predominantly of signet ring cells often carry a worse prognosis; most signet ring carcinomas occur in the stomach, but occur in carcinomas of the breast, colon, gall bladder, lung, nasal cavity, prostate and thyroid (medullary carcinoma), urinary bladder, as well as mesotheliomas, rhabdomyosarcoma, balloon cell melanoma, oligodendrogliomas, myxoid angioblastomatosis, myxoid liposarcoma, lymphomas (eg, signet ring cell lymphoma) and is a morphology typical of normal fat cells and oligodendrogliocytes

Signet ring cell lymphoma(s) see Lymphoma

Signet ring form A morphologic descriptor for the trophozoite form of *Plasmodium falciparum*, seen by light microscopy in a peripheral blood smear, which are often accompanied by Schüffner's dots

Signet ring sign RADIOLOGY Hypodense 'rings' corresponding to the thickened bronchioles in bronchiectasia, which may be seen by high-resolution computed tomography of the lungs (Mayo Clin Proc 1989; 64:1284), corresponding to the Ring and Tramtrack signs of bronchiectasia seen on plain films of the chest

Significance STATISTICS A measure of the deviation of data from a statistical mean, defined by a probability (p) value, where a p of 0.05 indicates a 5% possibility or 1 chance in 20 that a data set will differ from a mean and 19 chances in 20 that the data set will not

Significant other see Most significant other

Silencer motif MOLECULAR BIOLOGY A 6-12 base pair segment of DNA present within the immunoglobulin light chain that binds to enhancer proteins, preventing upregulation (enhancer activity) of non-B cells

Silent angina see Silent ischemia

Silent carrier state The presence of a genotypic abnormality that is not detected in the phenotype, eg silent carrier state in α thalassemia in which the defect in globin chain synthesis is so mild that it is inapparent Note: Crossing of a silent carrier with a person bearing the α thalassemia trait results in hemoglobin H

Silent ischemia CARDIOLOGY Myocardial hypoxia that is not associated with the usual manifestations of crushing precordial anginal pain, which occurs in 15-30% of acute myocardial infarctions that have objective evidence of myocardial ischemia by EKG (ST-segment depression), radionuclide angiography or echocardiography, associated with coronary artery vasospasms or atherosclerosis (Mayo Clin Proc 1990; 65:374); ischemic silence has potentially grave consequences, as future hypoxia cannot be prevented *TYPES OF 'SILENCE'* **TRUE SILENT ISCHEMIA** The nociceptive pathways have a marked decrease in sensitivity to pain, as occurs in diabetes mellitus, also known by the misnomer of 'silent angina' (as 'angina' implies pain), present in 10-20% of patients with both coronary artery disease and diabetes mellitus resulting in significant coronary artery spasms **'PSEUDOSILENCE'** The patient either i) Denies the pain, recognizing both its import and that myocardial ischemia would have an immediate impact on his lifestyle or ii) Recognizes the pain but attributes it to something else, ie heartburn (J Am Med Assoc 1990;

264:1132); patients with 'silent' ischemia have more significant three-vessel disease, more severe stenosis of the left anterior descending coronary artery and lower ventricular ejection fractions; they require coronary artery bypass or percutaneous transluminal coronary angioplasty (see PCTA) therapy three times more often and have a six-fold greater incidence of myocardial infarction than those with typical ischemia; Cf Angina, Total ischemic burden

'Silent killer' Silent lesion A medical condition that may progress to very advanced stages prior to manifesting itself in the form of clinical disease or at the time of diagnosis; most silent killers are malignant, so-named for their vague symptoms, and have often metastatized by the time of diagnosis; silent killers include ovarian cancer, in which there is a slow increase in abdominal girth, lower abdominal malaise and dyspepsia, carcinoma of the tail of the pancreas, brain tumors, especially of the frontal lobe and malignant melanoma, which may involute at the primary site

Silent mutation Isocoding mutation Any mutation that does not cause a detectable phenotypic effect; since 95% of the DNA thus far sequenced does not encode proteins (infelicitously known as 'junk' DNA), silent mutations are 20-fold more common than those with detectable effects; as a further means of ensuring phenotypic fidelity, the 'degeneracy' of nucleic acid codons is such that point mutations may impact on multiple different codons, and may still be transcribed and translated into a correct amino acid; see Degenerate code, Same-sense mutation

Silicon A gray-black semiconducting metal that is naturally present in silicates and which is used as 'doped' crystals in electronic semiconducting devices, eg COMPUTERS

Silicon chip COMPUTERS A wafer of silicon with microcircuitry etched on its surface, comprising the 'highway' upon which information travels in a microprocessor, see Computers, Microprocessor

Silicone A polymer composed of a repeating unit -R_2Si-O- in which R is a simple hydrocarbon; silicones are widely used in medicine given their stability, water repellency and inert nature, one of which, polydimethylsiloxane, is a prosthetic material enclosed in plastic bags of various sizes and shapes for use in plastic surgery to impart cosmetically acceptable contours to soft tissues, most commonly used in women for breast augmentation and in men for chin augmentation; the complications of such implants in trained hands are minimal and are confined to rupture of the bags and/or fibrosis (J Am Med Assoc 1989; 261:350); subcutaneous, often illicit, injection of silicone for breast enlargement without the enclosing bag (reportedly performed in transsexual males) may be associated with high fever, diffuse arthritis, renal failure, dry cough, hemoptysis, diffuse bilateral pulmonary infiltrates with patchy ill-defined airspace consolidaton, acute pneumonitis, hypoxemia, alveolitis (alveolar macrophages with silicone inclusions, neutrophils, eosinophils), diminished pulmonary functions (decreased total lung and ventilatory capacities, forced expiratory volume and PO_2) and granuloma formation (Am Rev Respir Dis 1987; 135:236)

Silicosis OCCUPATIONAL MEDICINE Exposure to silica dust (potteries, foundries, sand pits and construction) is associated with emphysema, compromised respiratory function and pulmonary fibrosis **Radiology** Bilateral symmetrical interstitial fibrosis, hilar lymphadenopathy with 'eggshell' calcification; unlike asbestos, it is a non-manufactured product, has received less media attention and its workers less financial compensation for undue exposure (J Am Med Assoc 1989; 262:3003)

Silo-filler's disease Silo-filler's lung OCCUPATIONAL MEDICINE A toxic gas-induced pneumonitis and bronchiolitis caused by inhalation of nitrogen oxides in freshly filled grain silos, often coupled to asphyxia; once grains are in storage, plant nitrates are fermented by microbes to NO_2 and N_2O_4, peaking 1-5 days after storage; nitrogen dioxide reaches the terminal airways, forming highly irritating nitrous and nitric acid, causing a chemical pneumonitis and massive pulmonary edema **Clinical** Cough, light headedness, dyspnea, hemoptysis, choking; forms of presentation include a) Collapse and sudden death b) Acute alveolar damage with pulmonary edema c) Early and reversible bronchiolitis obliterans and d) Late and irreversible bronchiolitis obliterans (Mayo Clin Proc 1989; 64:291, 368) **Differential diagnosis** Mycotoxicosis, an allergic reaction, see Farmer's lung **Treatment** High doses of corticosteroids may prevent the bronchiolitis obliterans common in heavily exposed survivors Note: A similar condition occurs in ice hockey players (J Am Med Assoc 1990; 263:3024c)

Silver Spring monkeys A group of primates used by a grant-funded psychologist for research related to rehabilitation of stroke victims, which required total denervation, performed on the monkeys by dorsal rhizotomy; because animals will treat deafferented limbs as foreign, they chewed off fingers and/or removed bandages; after allegations of cruelty to the monkeys and unsanitary conditions (Nature 1991; 351:93c), the local police removed the animals to protective custody (Science 1981; 214:1218); the monkeys became a rallying point for animals' rights activism; although the researcher had his animals returned, and all the charges against him were dismissed, the research was suspended Note: As of 1991, the last two monkeys of the original 17 Silver Spring monkeys seized by the police were aging, alive and still providing data on renervation phenomena (Science 1991; 252:1857, 1789n&v)

Silver syndrome Russell-Silver syndrome A clinical complex attributed to absence of insulin-like growth factor II, causing intrauterine growth retardation, hemihypertrophy, low birth weight and height, increased urinary gonadotropins (with resultant precocious puberty), occasional cafe au lait-type pigmentary changes, incurved fifth finger, syndactyly of toes, triangular face and pouting mouth; 10% develop Wilm's tumor **Treatment** Growth hormone

Silver wire appearance A descriptor for the fundoscopic appearance of grade IV arteriolosclerotic retinopathy, in which the arterial wall becomes completely opaque so the blood column is not seen and the light is completely reflected, yielding a white 'line', likened to a silver wire, regardless of whether the lumen is occluded; patency of the vessel is best determined by fluorescein angiography; Cf Copper wire appearance

Simian crease Simian fold A dermatoglyphic pattern appearing as a single deep transpalmar crease (figure, below) formed by the fusion of the proximal and distal palmar creases, classically seen in trisomy 21, that may be seen in trisomies 13 and 9 and in the fetal trimethadione syndrome; see Dermatoglyphics; Cf Triradius

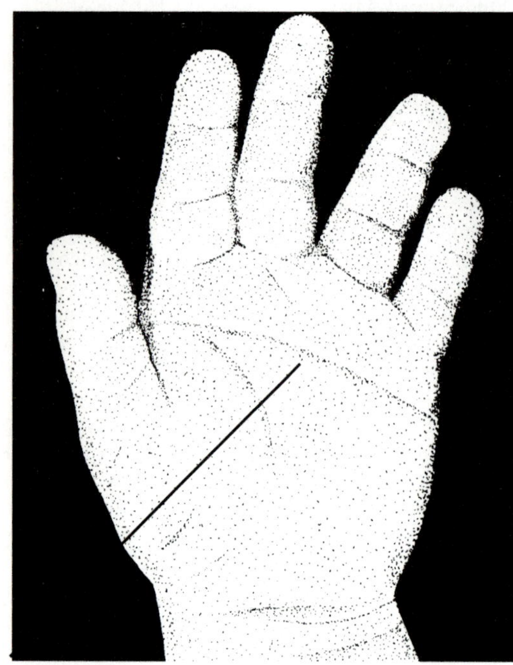

Simian crease

Simian virus 40 see SV-40

SIMM Single in-line memory module COMPUTERS An add-on memory board used in the Macintosh family of microcomputers to increase the random access memory (RAM), up to 64 megabytes or more, an amount required for complex molecular modeling; see Computers, RAM

SINE see Short interspersed repeated elements

Sine wave CARDIOLOGY An electrocardiographic finding described in severe hyperkalemia where the 'P' wave disappears and the QRS complex and 'T' wave merge in an oscillating pattern; a sine wave therefore constitutes a medical emergency, requiring immediate therapy, both short-term (calcium gluconate, sodium bicarbonate and glucose infusion) and long-term (cation-exchange retention enema)

Singapore foot Tropical term for superficial pedal mycosis

Singer-Nicholson model see Fluid-mosaic model

Singer's node Laryngeal polyp A non-inflammatory stromal reaction common on the anterior third of the vocal cord, seen in those who misuse their voices, eg singers, disk jockeys **Histopathology** Edema and myxoid degeneration of subepithelial tissue Note: The lesion has no premalignant potential; Cf Noise-induced hearing loss

Single breath imaging see Spiral computed tomography

Single copy DNA Non-repetitive DNA Unique DNA sequences that occur only once in a haploid genome, which correspond to structural genes and introns

Single disease hospital A health care facility serving patients suffering from a disease with no known therapy; single-disease hospitals had been built for leprosy, tuberculosis (for which the number of sanatoriums and hospitals in the US peaked in 1925 at 536 facilities) and mental illness (from 1880 to 1950); as therapy becomes available, single disease hospitals lose their raison d'etre and close; in AIDS, 4% of all US hospitals provide care for 32% of all AIDS patients, raising the question of whether 'AIDS-only' hospitals may serve a function; historically, patients in single-disease facilities receive sub-optimal care since often the only change in their status was death (N Engl J Med 1990; 323:764); see Saranac

Single letter designation see Amino acids

Single photon emission computed tomography see SPECT

Single unit transfusion (SUT) TRANSFUSION MEDICINE A therapeutic 'agent' that has long been controversial, since if a single unit of packed cells suffices as therapy, it is thought by some workers that the transfusion may not have been indicated at all; SUTs were once popular as 'tonics' for older patients with low-grade anemias, most of whom respond to iron supplements and vitamins; transfusion services generally frown upon SUTs, and without justification, a SUT represents malpractice; see Transfusion 'trigger '

Sinobronchial syndrome Kartagener syndrome; see Cilia

Sinus histiocytosis with massive lymphadenopathy Rosai-Dorfman disease A clinical condition most common in young blacks, characterized by massive bilateral cervical lymphadenopathy (one-fourth of SMHL is extranodal, affecting periorbital tissues, upper respiratory tract, skin and central nervous system, but does not involve the bone marrow or spleen), fever, leukocytosis, elevated erythrocyte sedimentation rate and polyclonal hyperimmunoglobulinemia **Pathology** The lymph nodes are matted, yellow with effaced architecture and display florid sinusoidal infiltration by histiocytes that are positive by the immunoperoxidase stain for S-100 **Prognosis** Uncertain; most cases resolve spontaneously, although some cases have been aggressive, and ultimately, fatal

Sinus of Morgagni syndrome Cranial nerve syndrome A clinical complex characterized by unilateral deafness, pain in the sensory zone of the mandibular division of the trigeminal nerve, immobility of the ipsilateral palate, and trismus, due to invasion by a malignancy, often a squamous cell carcinoma arising in the lateral nasopharynx

SIR Silent information repressor MOLECULAR BIOLOGY A protein that suppresses transcription of silent DNA copies at the mating locus of a haploid yeast gene

Sirenomelia Mermaid syndrome A heterogeneous dysplastic complex that may be inherited (caudal regression syndrome) or teratogenic in nature, characterized by multiple anomalies, including fusion (symmelia) of the lower extremities with external leg rotation, musculoskeletal atrophy and clubfoot, imperforate anus, unilateral or bilateral agenesis of the kidneys and/or genitalia, focal agenesis of the lumbosacral spine and various viscera Note: Some anomalies may be incompatible with life

SIRS a) Soluble immune response suppressor b) see Subcutaneous insulin-resistance syndrome

sis An oncogene isolated from the simian sarcoma virus, present in human cells as a proto-oncogene encoding platelet-derived growth factor-like protein, SIS, which evokes proliferation of smooth muscle cells, epithelial cells and fibroblasts, providing a link between normal growth-controlling pathways and the unregulated growth of cancer cells

Sister chromatid(s) A pair of metaphase chromosomes or nucleoproteins that are joined at a centromere

Sister chromosome exchange analysis GENETICS A technique used to monitor environmental damage resulting from increased exposure to chemicals, toxins and ultraviolet light, which consists in a dark repair of thymine dimers, where undamaged segments are exchanged for damaged segments between homologous duplex molecules; sister chromatid exchanges are increased in chromosome damage syndromes, eg Bloom syndrome and in cells from normal individuals when exposed to chromosome damaging conditions; Cf Ames test, Chromosome breakage syndromes

Sister Mary Joseph nodule A non-ulcerating periumbilical nodule that is a metastatic mass originating from an adenocarcinoma of the stomach, colon, ovary or pancreas, which may be the first mass detected in gastric carcinoma, and is a marker for a poor prognosis; 20% remain of unknown origin at the time of autopsy (J Am Acad Dermatol 1984; 10:610); Sister Mary Joseph was the superintendent of St Mary's Hospital in Rochester, Minnesota and as Dr WJ Mayo's surgical assistant was credited with recognizing the poor prognosis of this lesion

Sisyphus reaction PSYCHIATRY A state characteristic of a stress-driven type 'A' person, who obtains no gratification from accomplishing the difficult goals he places upon himself, a complex likened to Sisyphus of Greek mythology who angered Zeus and was made to roll a boulder up a hill, and each time he came close, but never quite made it to the top; see 'Anal-retentive', 'Toxic core', Type A personality

SIT Serum inhibition titration test Schlichter test A serial dilution assay for determining both the optimal antibiotic and its proper dose in treating certain bacterial infections; see MIC (minimum inhibitory concentration)

Site-directed mutagenesis CELL PHYSIOLOGY An experimental technique in which amino acids are substituted in a protein of known function to determine the location of a particular activity, eg receptor binding or ion channel activity

Sitophobia Fear of eating due to the unpleasant symptoms of nausea, vomiting and abdominal pain that occur after eating; sitophobia is characteristic of chemotherapy-induced anorexia, and may occur in Crohn's disease and chronic mesenteric artery insufficiency, and differs from anorexia nervosaas there is an appetite, but it is curtailed by the anticipated emesis and nausea

SIV Simian immunodeficiency virus A primate lentivirus that is the closest relative to HIV-1 and HIV-2; SIV and HIV both have a lentiviral morphology, tropism for CD4 lymphocytes and macrophages and use the CD4 molecule for a receptor, extra genes (*tat, rev, vip, vpr* and *nef*) that are not found in other retroviruses, typical cytopathologic changes and the ability to cause chronic disease after a long latency period; the study of AIDS may be facilitated by the recently identified clone of SIV, SIVmac239, which produces an AIDS-like disease in monkeys (Science 1990; 248:1109); see Retroviruses, SAIDS; Cf HIV-1, HIV-2

'Sixth disease' Roseola infantum; Cf Fifth disease

'Skimming' HEALTH CARE INDUSTRY A form of 'reverse dumping', in which insurance companies actively enroll, and hospitals actively seek the healthiest, wealthiest and best-insured segment of the population, since healthy people are less likely to use the services they are paying for, and the wealthy and well-insured pay their bills; skimming thus increases the profits for the insurance companies and health care facilities (N Engl J Med 1988; 319:1086); Cf Dumping

'Skimping' HEALTH CARE INDUSTRY Delaying or denial of services to members of a prepaid or 'capped' health plan as a means of controlling costs (since the monies received by the health plan remain constant, providing 'extra' services is more costly to the plan), eg delaying cataract surgery or reducing the frequency of costly procedures to levels below those considered appropriate by other practitioners and health care facilities; see Capitation

Skin adnexal tumor (SAT) SURGICAL PATHOLOGY A family of tumors derived from the primitive ectoderm, which develops into eccrine and apocrine sweat glands, sebaceous glands and hair follicles; most SATs are benign, eg eccrine cylindroma, keratoacanthoma syringoma, trichoepithelioma, although malignant SATs are not uncommon and include extramammary Paget's disease, sweat gland carcinoma PROGNOSIS Most SATs respond to wide local excision

Skin graft Autologous skin, donated skin or surrogate skin that is used to cover skin sufaces with third degree burns; one innovation in covering burn wounds is culturing of the patient's own cells into confluent sheets of keratinocytes to cover exposed areas; despite the theoretical advantages, autologous skin may not 'take', due to the lack of type IV collagen 7-S basement membrane binding sites and anchoring fibrils (J Am Med Assoc 1988; 259:2566); see Split thickness graft; Cf Artificcial skin, 'Spray-on' skin

'Skinny' needle A 22-gauge needle used for percutaneous, often radiologically-guided biopsies or aspiration cytology specimens obtained from radiologically-identified masses of the breast, lung and sites of difficult access; when positive, skinny needle biopsies avoid the co-morbidity associated with open biopsies; contrarily, negative results may result from sampling errors and should be followed by open biopsy if the lesion is suspected as potentially malignant Note: Small bore needles are 20-22-gauge; large bore needles are 14-18-gauge; see Interventional radiology

Skin 'popping' SUBSTANCE ABUSE Lubrication of needles with oral secretions prior to intradermal injection of narcotics; the resultant subcutaneous abscesses may be infected with ***Eikenella corrodens***, an inhabitant of the oral cavity; Cf 'Pocket shot'

Skin 'tag' Acrocordon Fibroepithelial polyp DERMATOLOGY A benign polypoid skin tumor that is more common in adults, may first appear as multiple lesions during pregnancy or as an epiphenomenon of malignancy of undetermined significance (Dtsch Med Wochenschr 1988; 113:323)

Skin window of Rebuck IMMUNOLOGY An in vivo method for studying host response to antigenic stimuli, in which a sterile glass coverslip is placed over superficially abraded skin; after 3-4 hours, most of the cells picked up on the coverslip are neutrophils; at 12 hours, 'round' cells, eg lymphocytes, plasma cells and monocytes and at 24 hours, monocytes and macrophages

'Skip' lesion Any lesion in which normal, ie pathologically not involved, tissue is interspersed with tissue affected by the pathological condition; skip lesions are described in 1) Metastatic malignancy, see below 2) Polyarteritis nodosa, referring to the interspersed 'skipping' or sparing of vessels and 3) Crohn's disease, referring to the interposition of the involved (and uninvolved) segments of the terminal ileum that are separated from segments of relatively normal small or large intestine, seen both radiologically and by gross examination Note: The 'characteristic' skip lesions occur in only 20-25% of Crohn's disease

Skip metastases The metastatic spread of a malignancy in which contiguous regions are skipped, although distant foci are present, thus implying a poor prognosis; skipping is typical of lymphatic permeation of a lymphoproliferative disease, eg Hodgkin's disease; skipping is also described in rare cases of osteosarcomas with multiple discrete and separate tumor nodules in the same bone, but located at a distance; transarticular skipping of osteosarcoma may occur via the periarticular venous anastomoses

Slab A block of gel used for an electrophoretic separation of proteins or nucleic acids

'Slam bang' technology A colloquialism for any diagnostic or therapeutic modality with effects that are so dramatic in early clinical trials on small cohorts that the technology is readily accepted, eg renal lithotrypsy, without waiting for the usual lag period required to accumulate data from large cohorts

s-Laminin NEUROPHYSIOLOGY A laminin-like protein found in the extracellular sheath surrounding myocytes that is thought to act as a homing signal for the ingrowth of regenerating motor neurons (s for synapse); see Laminin

Slant culture MICROBIOLOGY A bacterial culture that is grown on a solid (ie, agar-based) growth medium that has been poured in a test tube and allowed to solidify at a slanted angle; slant cultures are prepared with various chemical substrates, eg triple iron agar for the purpose of providing both aerobic (when the inoculum is 'streaked' on the agar surface) and anaerobic (when the inoculum is 'stabbed' deep into the agar) environments, allowing identification of specific reactions that are characteristic of a particular bacterial species

Slanted palpebral fissures A characteristic facial anomaly seen in Aarskog, Apert, Coffin-Lowry, Cohen, Conradi-Hünermann, DiGeorge, femoral hypoplasia-unusual facies, 5p-, Jarcho-Levin, Miller, Miller-Diker, Nager, Opitz-Frias, partial trisomy 10q, Pfeiffer, rhizomelic chondrodysplasia punctata, Rubenstein-Taybi, Säthre-Chotzen, Sotos, Treacher-Collins, trisomy 9 mosaic, trisomy 9p, trisomy 20p, XXXXX and XXXXY syndromes

Slapped cheek appearance A well-circumscribed, intense facial erythema of sudden onset that is followed by an erythematous maculopapular rash of the entire body, characteristic of 'fifth disease' (erythema infectiosum), due to parvovirus B19; see Fifth disease, B19

Slavic type of Wilson disease A predominantly neurologic form of Wilson's disease of later (adolescent) onset with normal ceruloplasmin levels

SLE 1) St Louis encephalitis 2) Systemic lupus erythematosus; see Lupus erythematosus

Sleep apnea syndrome Ondine's curse Marked alveolar hypoventilation during sleep despite normal blood-gas levels while awake, due to a failure of autonomic ventilation, resulting in sleep apnea, as well as increased cardiac arrhythmias and hypertension; the condition most often affects the severely obese (due to tonsillar hyperplasia, relative micrognathia and central apnea, with loss of the ventilatory drive in the medulla), but may follow bilateral cordotomy in the cervical region, used to control intense midline or perineal cancer-related pain (through severance of the spinothalamic tract through a ventrolateral incision into the second cervical segment) or may rarely occur in infants; primary hypoventilation is secondary to a loss of central nervous system chemoreceptor response, which affects men, age 20-60 Note: Ondine was a mythological water nymph who exhausted her human lovers; according to one victim, '*...ALL OF THE THINGS MY BODY ONCE DID BY ITSELF, IT DOES NOW ONLY BY SPECIAL COMMAND...I HAVE TO SUPERVISE FIVE SENSES, TWO HUNDRED BONES, A THOUSAND MUSCLES...A SINGLE MOMENT OF INATTENTION, AND I FORGET TO BREATHE...HE DIED, THEY WILL SAY, BECAUSE IT WAS A NUISANCE TO BREATHE*'—J Giraudoux, Ondine, 1939; see Narcolepsy, REM sleep

Sleep disorder(s) The field of 'dyssomnology' is becoming a medical subspecialty practiced by 'clinical polysomnographers', who have divided sleep disorders into a) Insomnias Disorders in initiating and maintaining sleep b) Hypersomnias Disorders of excessive somnolence, eg narcolepsy, sleep deprivation and obstructive sleep apnea c) Disorders of the sleep-wake schedule, eg jet lag and shift work and d) Dysfunctions associated with sleep, sleep stages or partial arousals, eg night terrors and enuresis (Mayo Clin Proc 1990; 65:857, 861); see

Insomnia, Pseudoinsomnia; Cf Shift work

Slice RADIOLOGY Colloquial for a collimation scan interval in computed tomography or equivalent in magnetic resonance imaging

Sliding filament model A (validated) model that explains muscle contraction as a telescope-like action, mediated by the hydrolysis of ATP, with the sliding of thick myosin filaments by means of pivoting (myosin) heads past the thin actin filaments; when viewed by electron microscopy, the muscle's A band decreases in thickness

Sliding hernia One of two types of hiatal hernias (esophagus), characterized by axial displacement of the esophago-gastric junction into the thoracic cavity through the esophageal hiatus, which, invested with its own peritoneal cloak, slides in and out of the thoracic cavity in response to changes in intra-abdominal and intrathoracic pressures; the paraesophageal hiatal hernia is partially fixed at the fundus and the stomach 'rolls' into the chest, and when extreme, becomes an 'upside-down' stomach

Slim disease The name for AIDS in Uganda, where clinical disease is characterized by extreme weight loss (hence, 'slim' disease), fever, a pruritic maculopapular rash, malaise, chronic diarrhea, respiratory infections and oral candidiasis; Kaposi sarcoma and lymphadenopathy are relatively less common than in the AIDS described in developed nations (Lancet 1985; 2:849)

'Slippery slope' A term that has been used as an adjective, eg slippery slope abuse, for patient-related decisions that are at the extreme periphery of certain issues, the ethical impact of which has been incompletely explored, and which themselves raise moral questions that are even more at the ethical 'edge' than the original issue (N Engl J Med 1990; 322:1881); such a slippery slope might occur if all surgeons were compelled to undergo periodic HIV testing, and they responded by demanding that all patients be tested as well

'Slip, slap, slop' DERMATOLOGY An abbreviated health care advisory of Australian origin for reducing the risk of ultraviolet light-induced skin damage and malignancy, where patients are advised to slip on a tee-shirt, slap on a hat and slop on some sunscreen

Slit lamp OPHTHALMOLOGY A low-power microscope with a specialized illuminating system for examining the anterior segment of the eye, allowing visualization of transparent and nearly transparent ocular fluids; the slit lamp is of particular use in dendritic keratitis, foreign bodies of the cornea and in tumors of the iris

Sloan-Kettering affair see the 'Mouse incident'

Slot blot analysis MOLECULAR BIOLOGY A rapid method for semiquantitating DNA (eg for detecting gene amplification) in a solution by electrophoresis, which differs from 'dot' blot analysis only in that the well in the agar is a 'slot' rather than a punched-out hole, a 'dot'; see 'Quick and dirty' methodology

'Slow channel' calcium antagonists (SCCA) CLINICAL PHARMACOLOGY A family of drugs used to manage angina, which attenuate vascular contractility and resistance by reducing the entry of calcium into myocardial and vascular smooth muscle cells; SCCAs, eg verapamil, are most effective for Prinzmetal's vasospastic angina, but are also of use in angina pectoris; since some SCCAs may decrease myocardial contractility or atrioventricular conduction, these agents cannot be used with impunity in patients with concomitant congestive heart failure, bradycardia or atrioventricular blocks

Slow channel syndrome An autosomal dominant neuromuscular dysfunction of early onset, characterized by weakness and atrophy of the proximal, cervical and shoulder girdle muscle groups, due to slow closure of acetylcholine receptor ion channels, resulting in prolongation of the end plate potential and accumulation of calcium in the post-synaptic region, where the excess calcium is 'toxic', destroying junctional folds and acetylcholine receptors

'Slow code' BIOMEDICAL ETHICS A response to a call for emergency cardiopulmonary resuscitation (CPR, a 'code') in which the usual celerity in not exercised and the full therapeutic armamentarium is not utilized; 'slow codes' have emerged as a form by which a physician may bypass the paperwork required for a legally acceptable 'Do not resuscitate' order, when the patient is in a hopelessly terminal state and the physician believes that aggressive CPR efforts would be futile; see Advance directives, DNR

Slow reactive substance(s) of anaphylaxis see SRS-A

Slow twitch fibers see Red muscle

Slow viruses A group of viruses that may cause fatal infectious encephalitides after prolonged latency periods; slow viruses were formerly divided into conventional and unconventional viruses, a division that is no longer valid, as unconventional 'viruses' are now recognized as a group of organisms composed entirely of subverted cell proteins known as prions; conventional slow viruses include measles, a paramyxovirus, which causes subacute sclerosing panencephalitis, rubella, which causes the rare progressive rubella panencephalitis and papovavirus, which causes progressive multifocal leukoencephalopathy; some soft data have implicated slow viruses in the pathogenesis of insulin-dependent (type I) diabetes mellitus and Paget's disease of the bone Slow viruses are usually inactivated by sodium hypochlorite (bleach), ethanol iodine and autoclaving; see Prions

Slush preparation TRANSPLANTATION An isotonic solution consisting of sterile saline crushed in ice, combined with lactated Ringer's solution; slush preparations are used to maintain the heart, lungs, kidneys, liver and other large organs destined for transplantation at the lowest possible metabolic rate (ie, the lowest possible temperature above freezing), while transporting them from the donor to the recipient; in the earliest stages of procurement, the icy slush is poured into the donor site (of a 'brain-dead' patient), cooling the organs to the maximum at the time of 'cross-clamping', at which time the organs are perfused with the so-called 'Wisconsin' solution; the slush solution is then transported with the organ to the recipient; see Procurement, UNOS, Wisconsin solution

Slutsky affair RESEARCH ETHICS Alleged misrepresentation of data that was published by a cardiologist in California;

has been suggested that 10% of his publications were based on completely unreliable information (J Am Med Assoc 1990; 263:1416) and one-half of the remainder were possibly invalid; see 'CV-weighing', 'Serious misconduct'

SMA see Spinal muscle atrophy

Small airways disease A non-infected, obstructed state that is largely confined to the small airways or bronchioles (< 2 mm in diameter), most often seen in smokers, accompanied by inflammation, initiated by inhaled irritants and accompanied by hypersecretion and lesions of the small airways, including fibrosis, ulceration, metaplasia and proliferation of smooth muscle fibers Note: The functional changes of COPD (chronic obstructive pulmonary disease) are thought to be due to small airways disease rather than chronic bronchitis

Small 'blues' IMMUNOLOGY A technical artifact due to incomplete mixing of the specimens in histocompatibility testing, seen as acellular debris in the HLA test wells due to excess trypan blue mixed with protein, producing blue 'blobs'

Small capacity syndrome One of the post-gastrectomy syndromes characterized by early satiation, which may result in significant weight loss and malnutrition; see Dumping

'Small' cell A cell measuring 9-14 μm with a faint or indistinct rim of cytoplasm and an oval-to-elongated nucleus with relatively dense chromatin, thought to be of neuroendocrine origin, due to the presence of cytokeratin and secretory granules; when a vague 'crease' in the nucleus is also present, the descriptor 'oat cell' may be used; small cells are classically described in the small cell carcinoma of the lung, see below, and may appear in the breast, nasopharynx, bladder, cervix Note: Non-epithelial lesions with small cells include sarcomas (Ewing sarcoma, rhabdomyosarcoma of alveolar and embryonal types, granulocytic sarcoma, reticulum cell sarcoma and liposarcoma), Wilm's tumor, neuroblastoma, lymphoma, plasmacytoma

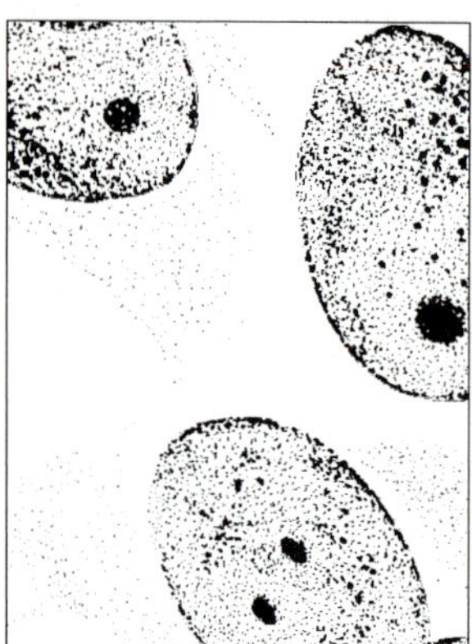

Intermediate small cell

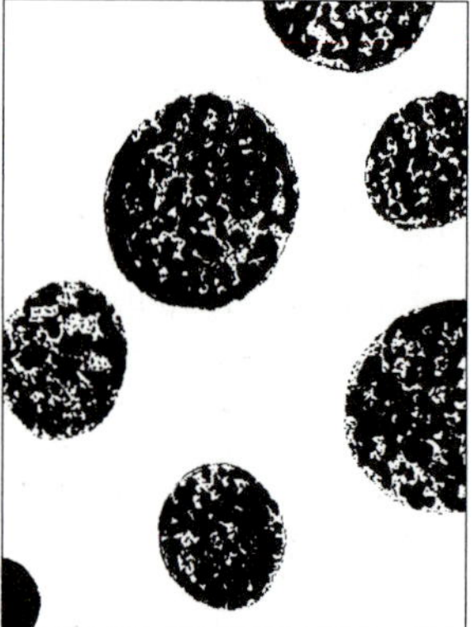

Oat-type small cell

Small cell carcinoma A highly aggressive malignancy, usually of the lung that arises in the proximal bronchus and spreads early to the hilum and mediastinal lymph nodes MOLECULAR BIOLOGY Small cell carcinoma, like all malignancy, is a multigene event, in which recessive tumor suppressor genes are lost and oncogenes are activated and the chromosome defects include multiple genomic 'hits' including a 3p deletion (3p(14-23) and/or translocations to chromosomes 17 and 8), a defective retinoblastoma gene (located in 13q14) and 17p deletions Note: 3p changes also occur in 25% of non-small cell carcinomas **Histopathology** Small cell carcinoma of the lung is subdivided into intermediate cell (below, left) and mixed cell (58%) types and lymphocyte-like (oat) cell type (below, right), which comprises the remaining 42%; these cells are 'decorated' by the immunoperoxidase method with antibodies to Leu-7, HNL-1 antigens, neuron-specific enolase and chromogranin **Treatment** The best results are with combination chemotherapy (cyclophosphamide, doxorubicin, vincristine, VP-16 and cisplatin), which causes some regression in 90%, complete regression in 50%; 5% survive five years; radiotherapy evokes an objective reduction in tumor bulk in 80-90% of cases **Prognosis** Without treatment, 3 month survival

Small cuff syndrome A form of pseudohypertension in which the cuff used to measure the blood pressure is disproportionately small and both the systolic and diastolic pressures are 'hypertensive' (Clin Pediatr 1966; 5:579); Cf Pseudohypertension, White coat hypertension

Small left colon syndrome A rare cause of distal colonic obstruction, described in infants with abdominal distension, 40% of whom are offspring of type I diabetic mothers; the large intestine is small from the anus to the splenic flexure with normal ganglion cells, due to a transient delay in development

Small nuclear ribonucleoproteins see snRNP

Small parts standard PUBLIC HEALTH A series of mandates promulgated by the US Consumer Product Safety Commission, requiring that toys marketed to children under age three be free of small parts and other potential hazards, given the tendency of this age group to perform a 'taste test' on virtually all non-comestibles (J Am Med Assoc 1991; 265:2848)

Smallpox A disease of historic interest; the variola virus probably appeared in the first agricultural settlements (10 000 BC) and typical lesions are present on the mummy of Ramses V (1160 BC); smallpox was well-established in post-Roman Europe and sailed with 'los conquistadores' to the New World, devastating native populations; E Jenner used vaccination, a technique of Turkish origin, reducing the then-prevalent mortality of 20% to less than 1%; before vaccination, smallpox killed 500 000/year in Europe and caused 1/3 of acquired blindness; the last case occurred in Somalia in 1977 and the smallpox battle was declared as won by WHO resolution 33.3 in 1980; the last smallpox stocks (held at the Centers for Disease Control in Atlanta and at the Research Institution for Viral Preparation in Moscow) will be destroyed in 1993 after the virus has been completely sequenced, and has not been destroyed previously as both superpowers were concerned that the other might use the agent for biological warfare (Nature 1991; 348:666)

'Small round cell tumors of infancy' A group of tumors

that are characterized by a similar histologic pattern that may require special studies, eg immunoperoxidase, ultrastructure and in situ hybridization to delineate the cell of origin and (by extension), the optimal therapeutic modality; these tumors include Ewing sarcoma, neuroblastoma, rhabdomyosarcoma, non-Hodgkin's lymphoma and the 'Askin tumor', a diagnosis of exclusion

Small stomach syndrome see Dumping syndrome, early

Small syndrome An autosomal recessive variant of Coat's disease characterized by loss of visual acuity, nerve deafness, hypomimia, muscular dystrophy and mild mental retardation

Sm (anti-Smith) antibodies A family of antibodies that are relatively specific for systemic lupus erythematosus (SLE) that react with polypeptides found in U1, U2 and U4/6 small nuclear ribonucleoproteins (snRNPs), which have a critical role in the splicing of pre-mRNA; Sm antibodies are present in 29% of cases of SLE and unlike antibodies to double-stranded DNA, do not increase with clinical exacerbation of SLE; see Antinuclear antibodies

'Smart' card MEDICAL RECORDS An identification card, often of credit card size, containing patient information ranging from 250 bytes of information (a 'dumb' card), allowing only simple identification to 2 megabytes of information, with large files; 'smart' cards are in the early implementation stage in some Japanese hospitals and will solve many of the problems inherent in the paper form of medical records

'Smart chip' see RISC chip

'Smart' terminal A computer terminal with its own central processing unit, allowing both input and output of data, thus having the capacity for free-standing operation; Cf 'Dumb' terminal

Smiling face appearance Monkey face appearance A fanciful descriptor for the characteristic morphology of the trophozoite form of *Giardia lamblia*, in which the 'eyes' correspond to the nuclei

SML see Smoldering myeloid leukemia

Smog ENVIRONMENT An acronym of smoke and fog; smog has little in common with fog as smog results from the combustion of various, often synthetic materials with the production of noxious volatile byproducts; smog mortality increases substantially when smoke and sulfur dioxide (SO_2) levels exceed 750 $\mu g/m^3$ Clinical Dyspnea, acute exacerbation of chronic obstructive pulmonary disease; subjects exposed to smog may present with asthmatiform symptoms (wheezing and markedly increased respiratory effort) or if the smog is intense, marked cyanosis (PaO_2 < 50 mmHg; $PaCO_2$ 50-100 mmHg), accompanied by congestive heart failure, obstructive lung disease and anoxic cor pulmonale Note: Air pollution was first described in 1661 and elevated to an art-form by industrialization; the first major smog 'attack' occurred in the 1930s in Belgium's Meuse valley (63 inhalation deaths), caused by high concentrations of sulfur dioxide, sulfuric acid and fluorides; the December 1952 smog attack of London caused an estimated 4000 excess deaths, attributed to sulfur dioxide Note: The most smog-laden cities in the world are Mexico City and Athens, in the USA, Denver and Los Angeles; see Bhopal, Yokohama asthma

Smokeless tobacco A chewed (chew) or snorted (snuff) tobacco product that is popular among athletes, the indigent and native Americans and tragically among children (up to 17% of 5 year-olds in certain regions have tried smokeless tobacco); 'chew' is used by an estimated 12 million Americans and is directly linked to oral cancer; 30 000 new cases of oral cancer occur annually in the US with 40% mortality; see below entries

Smoker profile The number of smokers internationally has increased by 75% in the last 20 years; 10^9 smokers consume up to an estimated 10^{12} cigarettes annually (J Am Med Assoc 1990; 263:3312); the US per capita cigarette consumption rose from 54 in 1900, peaked at 4500/year in 1968 and declined to 3200/year in 1988; the tobacco-industry 'loses' up to 2.5 million smokers/year, 2.1 million to health-related 'attrition', ie quitting, 400 000 to smoking-related death; the peak age of initiation of habitual smoking is 16; in the People's Republic of China, 400/year were consumed in 1953 and 1900/year by 1988 , a trend that has continued to increase *EDUCATION* 8.3% of physicians smoke (national average, 30%), under age 30, 4.5% of US physicians smoke; 18.4% of college-educated people are smokers, in contrast to 34.2% of high school drop-outs (J Am Med Assoc 1989; 261:56); smoking adolescents have a higher absentee rate, lower grade-point average and lower achievement test scores; the education-addiction disproportion is expected to accelerate; by the year 2000, 40% of high school dropouts will smoke versus 5% of college graduates *RACE* 34% of adult blacks are smokers, 28% of whites, 27% of hispanics; in the US,(J Am Med Assoc 1990; 264:1505, 1575)

Smoker 'syndrome' see Smoking

Smoking An addictive habit causing the most preventable form of cancer, lung carcinoma, which accounts for 25% of all cancer deaths; the annual lung cancer death rate has risen from $2/10^5$ in the 1930s to nearly $50/10^5$/year in 1985, translating into 152 000 new cases in 1988 and 139 000 deaths in the US *ECONOMIC COSTS OF SMOKING* Direct costs due to smoking have been estimated to be circa \$16 x 10^9 annually in the US, due to hospitalization, and the indirect costs, circa \$35 x 10^9, due to lost productivity, earnings, disability, prematurity; the cost of smoking to the entire population is \$200 per capita and by an arcane calculation, it has been estimated that one cigarette reduces life span by 5 minutes; smoking-related fires kill 1500 and injure 4000/year in the US; smokers suffer an *EXCESS MORTALITY OF 350 000/YEAR, RELATED TO MALIGNANCY* In addition to lung cancer, smokers have a five-fold increase in laryngeal, oral and esophageal cancer; 30% of bladder cancer and 30% of pancreatic carcinoma is thought to be smoking-related; there is a 1.5-fold increase in gastric, hepatobiliary and renal malignancies and leukemias; there is a persistant increase in the risk of leukemia and myeloma for those who quit smoking later in life, implying the occurrence of a permanent malignant change in the stem cells (J Natl Cancer Res 1990; 82:1832) *HEART DISEASE* Coronary artery disease, atherosclerosis (J Roy Soc Med 1990;

83:146), aortic aneurysms, cor pulmonale, strokes and infarcts Note: The relative risk of myocardial infarction of 3.6 in smoking women declines and plateaus to 1.2 within 3 years of smoking cessation (N Engl J Med 1990; 322:213) *NON-MALIGNANT LUNG DISEASE*, eg emphysema, chronic bronchitis and markedly (10-15-fold) increased incidence of interstitial fibrosis; other derangements seen in smokers include *ALTERED DRUG METABOLISM* and delayed absorption of alcohol *GASTROINTESTINAL TRACT* Peptic ulcer, esophageal reflux, cirrhosis (which is possibly a statistical artefact, as smokers may also be alcoholics) Note: Some anecdotal reports imply that ulcerative colitis may be ameliorated by smoking *HEMATOLOGY* 4.8% of smokers have hematologic parameters that fall in a range of anemia, while 8.5% of non-smokers fall in the same range (J Am Med Assoc 1990; 264:1556) *INFECTIONS* The higher incidence of bacterial infection in smokers may be due to increased mucosal adherence of bacteria (Indian J Med Res 1989; 89:381) *OBESITY* Heavy smokers are more often obese than lighter smokers and in the face of abrupt smoking cessation, experience more intense cravings, implying that there may be a physiological difference in heavy smokers (J Am Med Assoc 1988; 260:1581) *OSTEOPOROSIS* and fractures of the wrist, hip and vertebrae, possibly related to reduced endogenous estrogens that occur in menopause, early lower levels of all estrogens in the luteal phase may explain why some series report a reduced incidence of breast cancer in smokers TOBACCO PROMOTION EXPENDITURES 1975 $491 x 10^6; 1981 $1547 x 10^6; 1988 $3274 x 10^6 (MMWR 1990; 39:261) TOXINS Tobacco contains hundreds of toxins which act in concert to induce malignancy, with nicotine and tars being the most stongly implicated carcinogens, although ^{210}Polonium and α radiation may play supporting roles Laboratory Smokers have increased hematocrit, high conicotine levels, increased albuminuria in type I diabetic smokers (J Am Med Assoc 1991; 265:614), and decreased high-density lipoprotein levels in children exposed to passive cigarette smoke (Circulation 1990; 81:586)

Smoking cessation Cessation of cigarette smoking is followed by an average weight gain of 2.8 kg in men and 3.8 kg in women; 10-15% of ex-smokers gain 13 or more kg (N Engl J Med 1991; 324:739); most withdrawal therapies, eg hypnosis, psychotherapy, group counseling, exposing smokers to patients with terminal lung cancer and nicotine chewing gum are consistent only in their inefficacy (J Am Med Assoc 1989; 262:3011, N Engl J Med 1988; 318:15); 10% of depressed and 18% of non-depressed subjects are able to quit (J Am Med Assoc 1990; 264:1541) and cessation in the severely depressed causes exacerbation of depression (J Am Med Assoc 1990; 264:1546); see Chronic obstructive lung disease, Emphysema, Passive smoking, Smokeless tobacco

'Smoking gun' A metaphor referring to the definitive confirmation of a cause-and-effect relation; in the legal system, the act of homicide can only be absolutely confirmed if the perpetrator is found alone with the victim(s), holding a 'smoking gun', a phrase adopted in medicine for determining the etiology of a disease, where the statistical strength and design of a study produces evidence so compelling, that the cause-and-effect relation is likened to that of a 'smoking gun'

'Smoky' The US Army code name for the test detonation of a thermonuclear device in August 1957 in which soldiers were exposed to radioactive fallout; two decades later, the participants were found to have a significant increase in the incidence of leukemia (J Am Med Assoc 1980;244:1575); the relation of radiation to polycythemia vera remains controversial; see Bravo; Cf Operation Ranch Hand

Smoldering myeloid leukemia An indolent form of multiple myeloma that meets all the criteria of myeloma without producing significant anemia; a case may 'smolder' for 20 years, eventuating into osteolytic lesions, hypercalcemia and renal insufficiency, potentially with a survival of five or more years; smoldering leukemic conditions include preleukemia, refractory anemia with excess blasts (RAEB) and subacute myeloid leukemia; most cases have an established malignant clone and are accompanied by refractory 'cytopenias, and cellular dysfunction; 'smoldering' states have an indolent course with infections, hemorrhage and occasionally blast transformation ; see Preleukemia

Smooth muscle antibodies IMMUNOLOGY IgM or IgG autoantibodies present in the serum of approximately 60% of patients with chronic active (autoimmune) hepatitis, 30% of patients with biliary cirrhosis and which may be transiently elevated in low titers in various viral hepatitides and in biliary cirrhosis

SMR 1) Standardized mortality ratio 2) Sexual maturity rating

Smudge cell HEMATOLOGY Red-purple nuclear debris with clumped chromatin and rounded nucleolar remnants, representing degenerated lymphocytes and nucleated erythrocytes (figure, right); Cf Basket cells; similar cells are characteristic of the karyorrhectic lymphocytes of acute and chronic lymphocytic leukemia LIVER PATHOLOGY A smudge cell is an enlarged basophilic hepatocyte replete with adenoviral particles PULMONARY PATHOLOGY Smudge cells are diffusely basophilic, streaked cytomegalovirus-infected alveolar and bronchial cells with an indistinct nuclear:cytoplasmic 'frontier' due to vacuolization of the nuclear membrane

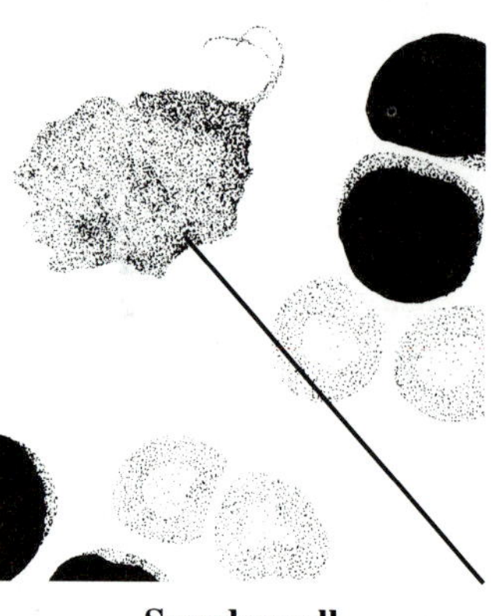

Smudge cell

'Snake oil' remedies HEALTH FRAUD Any of a group of substances that are claimed (without substantial evidence) to be effective in treating a wide variety of medical conditions; in the classic sense, these therapies were sold by 'quacks' in the late 1800s in the 'wild' western United States, prior to the stringent control of the pharmaceutical industry, which is currently operates under laws and regulations promulgated by the US Food and Drug

Administration, and contained alcohol, herbs, narcotics and various other, often inactive, ingredients; see Food and Drug Administration, Pseudovitamins, Unproven cancer therapies

Snake skin see Cathartic bowel

SNOMED Systematized nomenclature of medicine

SNOP Systematized nomenclature in pathology

Snore Snoring A harsh buzzing noise evoked in a sleeping person attributed to the vibration of a redundant soft palate; snoring increases with age, affects 60% of men, 40% of women and has been associated with a two-fold increased risk for high blood pressure, coronary ischemia and stroke (Br Med J 1987; 294:16), as well as alcoholism, arthritis, asthma, daytime drowsiness, depression, diabetes mellitus, insomnia and obesity, but as an isolated symptom does not require treatment; snoring may be reduced by using a nasal dilating agent (Arch Otolaryngol, Head Neck Surg 1990; 116:462) Note: The loudest recorded snore is 88 dB; see Obstructive sleep anpea syndrome; Cf Sleep disorders, Uvulopalatopharyngoplasty

'Snorting' SUBSTANCE ABUSE The preferred method for consumption of cocaine; the powder is placed in a spoon or on a horizontal surface, one nostril is held closed and the cocaine is 'sniffed', often with a drinking straw; with prolonged use, the nasal cartilage may perforate due to repeated ischemic episodes related to cocaine's intense vasoconstriction; Cf Cocaine, Crack

Snow ball appearance A descriptor for the scanning electron micrographic appearance of the crystalloids seen in the synovial sediment of arthritic joints afflicted with basic calcium phosphate crystal disease(s); Cf Shiny coin appearance

'Snowcap' sign ORTHOPEDICS A descriptor for a broad radiopaque band covering up to two-thirds of the articular surface in ischemic necrosis of the femoral head due to various conditions that compromise the epiphyseal vascular supply; after the initial structural failure causing a sclerotic 'snowcap', a thin subchondral fracture 'rim' appears as this portion of the femoral head collapses, giving rise to a 'step' formation; the snowcap is non-specific and may occur in prolonged ischemia of the femoral head due to anemia, hemophilia, endocrinopathy, congenital disease and malignancy

Snowflake cataract A fanciful descriptor for punctate subcapsular lens opacifications that may rapidly evolve to a cataract in young patients with diabetes mellitus

Snowman sign PEDIATRIC CARDIOLOGY A rounded, figure of eight-like cardiac contour seen on a plain anteroposterior chest film of infants with total anomalous drainage of the pulmonary veins accompanied by dilatation of the common pulmonary vein and supracardiac drainage; the unique contour is produced by the dilated left ventricle and superior vena cavae and left innominate vein; a similar appearance may be secondary to a prominent thymic shadow

Snow Mountain agent A Norwalk agent-like virus that evoked an acute shellfish-related miniepidemic of gastroenteritis that occurred at a ski resort, characterized by a 1-4 day duration, watery diarrhea, vomiting and abdominal cramping (Am J Epidemiol 1987; 126:516)

snRNPs Small nuclear ribonucleoproteins A family of 100 to 300 nucleotide in length RNA molecules that form RNA-protein complexes in the eukaryotic nucleus, some of which are involved in RNA processing; the U series of snRNPs contains 2 classes of proteins; one class ('shared proteins') is found in all snRNPs, regardless of the U RNA species and consists of proteins designated as B, B', D, E, F and G; the second class, U ('unique') proteins are unique to snRNPs, and contain specific RNA, eg U1-U7 that may be autoantibody targets in lupus erythematosus

Snuff see Smokeless tobacco

Snuffbox ANATOMY A triangular depression on the dorsal pollicar aspect of the hand when the thumb is fully extended, bordered laterally by the extensor pollicis brevis and abductor pollicis longus tendons and medially by the tendon of the extensor pollicis longus; the sobriquet 'Tequila triangle' refers to the snuffbox's use when drinking tequila, a Mexican inebrient

Snuffles Profuse, mucopurulent and hemorrhagic nasal discharge containing viable *Treponema pallidum*, seen in infants with early congenital syphilis

'Snurposome' see Spliceosome

Snurps see snRNPs

SOAP A mnemonic for the data that should be included in a problem-oriented medical record and in each entry in a patient's progress notes during hospitalization, including *SUBJECTIVE DATA*, supplied by the patient or family *OBJECTIVE DATA*, ie physical examination and laboratory data *ASSESSMENT*, a summary of significant (if any) new data and *PLAN OF DIAGNOSTIC OR THERAPEUTIC ACTION*; see Hospital chart, Medical record

Soap bubble A commonly used descriptor for dilated smoothly-contoured cyst-like or ballooned, occasionally loculated space(s); see Physaliferous BONE RADIOLOGY An expansile, often eccentric, vaguely trabeculated space with a thin, sclerotic, sharply defined margin, characteristic of an aneurysmal bone cyst (lesions that are neither aneurysmal, nor true cysts, but rather are filled with blood and not invested with a coherent membranous lining); other bone lesions with soap bubble-like expansions include giant cell tumor, osteosarcoma, solitary bone cyst, non-ossifying fibroma, fibrous dysplasia, metastatic carcinoma, chondromyxoid fibroma, the 'combined' stage of Paget's disease of the bone, expansile mandibular lesions of cherubism, metastatic renal cell carcinoma Note: The radiological finding of multiple 'punched-out' lytic lesions of bone, including multiple myeloma, angiosarcoma and ameloblastoma have also been described as soap bubble-like GASTROINTESTINAL RADIOLOGY A descriptor for the physaliferous air spaces seen in an abdominal plain film in gas-producing bacterial abscesses MICROBIOLOGY A morphologic descriptor of *Pneumocystis carinii*; see 'Sealed envelope' appearance NEUROPATHOLOGY A descriptor for the microscopic appearance of *Cryptococcus neoformans* when stained with India ink, most prominent in the Virchow-Robin space

Soap, calcium A descriptor for the chalky, white-to-pale yellow, rounded lenticular precipitates caused by enzyme-induced fat necrosis, which cover the peritoneum and pancreas, classically associated with acute pancreatitis, seen on gross examination of the abdominal cavity

Soap colitis see Chemical colitis

SOB Shortness of breath

SOB medium A bacterial growth medium designed to quantify bacteria in water, waste water, dairy products and foods, composed of NaCl, KOH and $MgSO_4$, bactotryptone and yeast extract

'Social disease' An obsolete euphemism for sexually-transmitted disease, see there

Socialized medicine A health care system in which a) The entire population's health care needs are met without charge or at a nominal fee and b) The organization and provision of all medical services are under direct governmental control; by extension, physicians and other health care providers are government employees and

Social medicine A field of medicine that studies the impact of the collective behavior of organized society on individuals belonging to various, often disadvantaged subgroups within the society; see Engel's phenomenon, Homeless(ness), Latch-key children, Supermom

Social Security amendments of 1983 The federal legislation that provided for the implementation of the current US health care reimbursement system in which payments are based on diagnosis-related groups (DRGs); the reimbursement is divided into a 'service' component, ie hospital-related costs, known as 'part A' and a 'professional' or physician component, known as 'part B', controlled by peer and utilization review; see DRGs, Part A, Part B

'Social worth' MEDICAL ETHICS The value of a person's life to society; the criteria for a person's 'social worth' are nebulous, but there is an increasing need for society to delineate objective criteria that facilitate decisions on who is entitled to receive limited (ie, less than infinite), potentially life-saving medical resources; any system of rules that determines the relative value of one person's life versus another's depends on 1) The criteria used for selection and 2) Who is empowered to make these decisions, ie who has the right to 'play God'; a particular patient may be excluded based on a) constituency factors, including geography, age and ability to pay for a life-saving procedure b) progress of science, ie if the therapy is experimental, then the patient should not have other underlying disease and c) prospect of success, ie the treatment should be reserved for those patients most likely to benefit from the therapy; see Pittsburgh criteria, Seattle committee

Socratic method MEDICAL EDUCATION An 'alternative' curriculum or philosophy for teaching medical students that differs from the traditional curriculum in that instruction is in the form of problem-solving and testing of hypotheses; students taught by the Socratic method score lower in standardized examinations (which test fact-based knowledge) and higher in oral examinations (J Am Med Assoc 1991; 265:2373), which test the ability to reason and logically analyze patient management scenarios

SOD see Superoxide dismutase

Sodium azide MICROBIOLOGY A substance added to a transport medium of laboratory specimens, eg urine for the culturing of bacteria that prevents oxidative phosphorylation and bacterial overgrowth

Sodium-calcium exchanger A membrane protein with a critical role in myocardial contractility, which regulates free cytosolic calcium ions; the exchanger depends on an electrochemical sodium gradient for its energy and undergoes conformational changes as it moves ions (Nature 1991; 349:621); Cf Na^+/H^+ antiporter

Sodium pump see Na^+/K^+-ATPase

Sodoku Rat-bite fever A disease caused by ***Spirillum minor***, a gram-negative flagellated microaerophilic bacterium found in the saliva of 10% of healthy laboratory and wild rats; two-to-three weeks after exposure, the inoculation site becomes ulcerated, purulent and scarred, accompanied by lymphadenitis, fever that may recur cyclically for months and then spontaneously resolve, myalgias and a purple maculopapular rash, which spreads from the inoculation site to the entire body Treatment Penicillin, tetracycline; Cf Haverhill fever

'Sofa pillow' liver see Hepar lobatum

Soft A colloquial adjective for either a) That which does not have statistical significance, ie the statistical 'p' value is not < 0.05, as in 'soft' data or 'soft' risk factors; Cf Fragile data b) That which is socially regarded as relatively innocuous, as in 'soft' drugs, eg nicotine or alcohol where dependence is often considered psychological or c) That which is based on objective data, as in 'Soft' sciences

'Soft' risk factors Those risk factors that place a subject at increased risk for suffering a morbid process, but which do not reach statistical significance, eg 'soft' risks for atherosclerosis, including sedentary life style, obesity, type A personality, use of oral contraceptives, hyperuricemia, high carbohydrate intake; vide sopra, 'Soft'

'Soft' sciences A term applied to fields of study in which accrual of objective and reproducible ('hard') data is virtually impossible as these fields examine societal phenomena and dynamics that are most amenable to philosophical interpretation; the major soft sciences are anthropology, economics, psychology, sociology and more recently, social medicine

Soft tissue sarcoma(s) A family of malignancies that arise from mesenchymal tissues, including bone (osteosarcoma), cartilage (chondrosarcoma), fat (liposarcoma), muscle (rhabdomyosarcoma), nerve (malignant schwannoma), smooth muscle (leiomyo-sarcoma) and stroma (fibrosarcoma); other tumors of uncertain histogenesis, presumed to be of mesenchymal origin are traditionally classified as soft tissue sarcomas, including alveolar soft part sarcoma, epithelioid sarcoma, malignant fibrous histiocytoma and synovial sarcoma; the sites of predilection and age of presentation differ according to the tumor; under age 10, lipoblastoma and rhabdomyosarcomas are most common; between ages 15-40, alveolar soft part, epithelioid and synovial sarcomas are common; between ages 25-60, fibrosarcoma and malignant schwannoma are common and after age 45, liposarcoma and malignant fibrous histiocytoma predominate Note: The behavior of soft tissue sarcomas is a function of histologic aggression, as measured by cellularity, differentiation and pleomorphism, mitotic activity and presence of necrosis Differential diagnoses Pseudosarcomas, which are either a) Mesenchymal and non-malignant soft tissue lesions including fibrous histiocytoma and fibromatoses and b) Non-mesenchymal and malignant, most commonly spindle cell squamous carcinoma of the oral cavity, anaplastic carcinoma and malignant melanoma; most soft tissue tumors reveal clonal chromosomal aberrations, eg Ewing sarcoma and primitive neuroectodermal tumor are associated with t(11;22); poor prognostic markers in neuroblastoma include 1p- and double minute chromosomes; in mesothelioma 1p-, 3p-, -22, noncomplex karyotype; in synovial sarcoma t(X;18), see N Engl J Med 1991; 324:436

Software The sequence of programmed instructions required to operate a computer, including assemblers, compilers, programs, routines and translators; software is commonly understood to be any program that is available commercially or through networks that can perform certain tasks, which in the microcomputer environment, include word processing programs, databases, spreadsheets, graphics and desktop publishing; see Computer; Cf Hardware

Soft X-rays Long wavelength, low-frequency X-rays of low penetrance, eg Grenz radiation

Solar elastosis Degeneration of the subdermal elastic tissue by prolonged actinic exposure, causing wrinkled 'sailor's skin', predisposing the skin to various skin-based malignancies including basal and squamous cell carcinoma and malignant melanoma

Soldier's heart see Old soldier's heart

Soldier's plaque A descriptor for the pearly white, thickened, non-adherent, epicardial 'plate' that occurs in healed chronic pericarditis

Solenoid structure Molecular biology A configuration of DNA formed during DNA condensation in the eukaryotic nucleus; the solenoid structure consists of histones wrapped with supercoiled DNA, known as nucleosomes, connected to each other by linker DNA, having an ultrastructural appearance likened to beads on a string; see Histone

Sol-gel A liquid-crystal cytoskeleton composed of hollow microtubules oriented toward the cell's center, with microfilaments located in the cell periphery; 'sol-gel movement' is a characteristic ameboid locomotion by unicellular eukaryotes and tissue macrophages, which move by extension and retraction of long pseudopods changing constantly from a fluid-like sol to a semisolid gel state

Solid-state tumorigenesis A phenomenon described in experimental rodents, in which inert plastics elicit soft tissue sarcomas, occurring with a characteristic frequency, latency period and histopathologic type; given the broad experience with artificial silicone breast implants, biomechanical prosthesis and other long-term indwelling devices, the phenomenon is not thought to occur frequently in humans

Solid waste management The constellation of methods used to eliminate civilization's 'detritus', including burial in landfills, recycling, ie reuse, with the refuse serving as raw material for newly manufactured products and incineration, the heat from which may be used as a source of energy; Cf Biohazardous waste, Hazardous waste, Regulated waste

Solitary congenital nodular calcification Dermatology A skin lesion seen on the extremities or head and neck region in which the epidermis is acanthotic and hyperkeratotic, with calcified subcutaneous masses of unknown significance

Solitary hunter 'syndrome' see 'Lone wolf'

Solitary rectal ulcer(s) syndrome (SRUS) A disease of young adults, more common in females with irregular bowel habits, thought to be related to an internal rectal prolapse associated with an abnormal perineal descent Etiology Idiopathic or related to laxative abuse or anal intercourse Clinical Hematochezia, variably accompanied by anal or abdominal pain, passage of mucus per rectum, excess straining on defecation, with a 'flap valve' effect where the puborectalis muscle fails to completely relax, creating a high pressure zone, potentially resulting in rectal prolapse; the ulcers average 2 cm in diameter and are close to the anal verge Treatment Stool softeners; when SRUS is accompanied by rectal prolapse, rectopexy may be required

Solve-rate Forensic medicine The percentage of homicides for which the killer is identified with reasonable certainty, a value that differs according to country, availability of effective homicidal weapons, permissiveness for crimes of passion, substrate of violence, abuse substance subculture, size of community, social inequities and other intangibles; in the US, the solve-rate ranges from 55% to 85%

Somatization disorder(s) Briquet syndrome A group of conditions characterized by symptoms suggesting organ dysfunction(s) that are not supported by laboratory or clinical parameters; the symptoms are often vague, do not appear to be under voluntary control and may fulfill some psychological need Clinical The patients are sickly (or believe themselves to be), have pseudoneuralgias (visual defects, dysphagia, loss of voice, urinary retention, convulsion, seizures), gastrointestinal symptoms (colicky pain, nausea, vomiting), dysmenorrhea, loss of libido, pain (back, genitalia and joints), cardiopulmonary symptoms, including dyspnea, palpitations and chest pains; see Factitious diseases

Somatomammotropins A group of hormones, eg growth hormone 21.8 kD, prolactin 22.5 kD and placental lactogen 21.8 kD that share intrinsic lactogenic and growth-promoting activity, despite a wide difference in sequence similarity or 'homology' (growth hormone and prolactin have 16% 'homology', while growth hormone and placental lactogen have 83% 'homology')

Somatomedin see IGF-I, IGF-II (insulin-like growth factors)

Somatomedin(s) ENDOCRINOLOGY A generic term for a group of low (7-10 kD) molecular weight growth factors released from the liver and kidney by growth hormone that produce insulin-like effects on target tissues and lead to increased incorporation of sulfate in collagen; somatomedins include epidermal growth factor, fibroblast growth factor, sex steroids, thyroid hormones, erythropoietin, tropic hormones and 'factors' with multiplication-stimulating activity and non-suppressible insulin-like activity

Somatomedin C see Insulin-like growth factor-I

Somatostatin NEUROPHYSIOLOGY A 14-residue neuropeptide secreted by the brain that inhibits the secretion of growth hormone, thyroid releasing hormone and insulin, and stimulates glucagon secretion, as well as the delta cells of pancreatic islets and gastrointestinal tract cells, inhibiting secretogogue-mediated changes in ion transport, gastrin and gastric acid secretion, increasing intestinal transit time and stimulating sodium and chloride absorption in the ileum and colon; somatostatin is a paracrine hormone that acts as an 'off' switch in the gastrointestinal tract, and has a 'yin-yang' relation with bombesin, which acts as an 'on' switch; see Bombesin

Somatostatinoma Delta cell tumor A somatostatin-producing tumor of the pancreatic islet delta cells, more common in the pancreatic head and tail that may rarely affect the duodenum, characterized by decreased gastric acid secretion and metastasis to liver and bone

Somatostatinoma syndrome A paraneoplastic syndrome caused by ectopic somatostatin secretion Clinical Vomiting, hypochlorhydria, abdominal pain, diarrhea, malabsorption, weight loss, cholelithiasis and defective glucose control, causing secondary diabetes mellitus Laboratory Increased somatostatin (which being an inhibitory hormone, evokes 'reactive' decrease in insulin and glucagon), decreased gastrin, steatorrhea, anemia

Somatostatinoma triad A trilogy of symptoms considered to be typical of patients with gallstones, diabetes mellitus and diarrhea

Somatostatin-receptor imaging A unique technique for localizing and semiquantifying endocrine and neuroendocrine tumors, eg carcinoids, chemodectomas and pancreatic endocrine tumors, including gastrinomas and insulinomas, by using a radiolabeled analogue of somatostatin (octreotide) and detecting the uptake with either a gamma-camera or by single photon emission computed tomography (SPECT, N Engl J Med 1990; 323:1246)

Somatotropin Growth hormone

Somatotropin release-inhibiting hormone A hormone produced and released from the anterior hypothalamus in response to various stimulants, eg high circulating glucocorticosteroids, which inhibits the release of both growth hormone and thyroid stimulating hormone

Somogyi effect Rebound hyperglycemia A phenomenon described in diabetics in whom hyperglycemia occurs as a counter-regulatory overcompensation to nocturnal hypoglycemia (Bull St Louis Med Soc 1938; 32:498); the Somogyi effect may cause the clinician to increase the dose of insulin (in order to compensate for the 'physiological' nocturnal hyperperglycemia), which exacerbates the rebound hypoglycemia, when in fact, the insulin dose should be lowered; see Dawn phenomenon, Glucose tolerance test, Subcutaneous insulin-resistance syndrome

SOP see Standard operating procedure

Sorbitol A polyhydroxyl alcohol or polyol synthesized from glucose by aldose reductase in nerve tissue, produced in excess in diabetics; sorbitol may be further metabolized to fructose, which together cause increased osmotic pressure, intracellular edema, schwann cell swelling, anoxia and nerve demyelination and thus are implicated in diabetic neuropathy; Cf Advanced glycosylation endproducts

Sorbonne The University of Paris (formerly, the Sorbonne) began as a theological school attached to the cathedral of Notre Dame du Paris and was founded by 1253 by Robert de Sorbon; the Sorbonne had a stormy history, often taking the 'wrong' side in delicate political issues, and was closed by convention in 1790 and as such no longer exists; of the 13 campuses of the University of Paris, Paris I, III and IV campuses may be considered 'the Sorbonne' as they are housed in the original Sorbonne site in the Latin Quarter (Nature 1990; 346:136n&v)

Sorting signal(s) MOLECULAR BIOLOGY Amino acid sequences that are encoded in a polypeptide or which are added after translation to indicate the direction of a protein's flow through the cell

SOS box A 20 base pair operator sequence present in *Escherichia coli*, which binds the LexA repressor, activating many genes involved in repair of ultraviolet light-induced damage

SOS repair Mutation repair MOLECULAR BIOLOGY An error-prone repair system that functions when ***Escherichia coli***'s DNA is damaged by bond-breaking physical agents or toxins; after the 'insult', a group of genes are activated, including the ***recA*** gene, which encodes RecA protein, lysing certain DNA-binding proteins including the LexA repressor; the LexA repressor binds to the repressor site, activating transcription of proteins involved in repair; although SOS repair is 'sloppy', it restores DNA damaged by thymine starvation, chemicals, eg mitomycin C and ultraviolet light, preventing cell death, hence SOS, after the international Morse code signal for maritime distress; see Thymine dimer

South African porphyria Porphyria variegata

'South American' operation A radical surgical procedure for a 'frozen' pelvis, consisting of en bloc resection of the uterus and rectum; Cf 'All-American' and 'North American' operations

'Southern blindness' see SC disease

Southern blotting A method for detecting the presence of and optimally manipulating specific DNA sequences previously separated by gel electrophoresis delineated by EM Southern (J Mol Biol 1975; 98:503) Southern blot hybridization technique 1) DNA is extracted from cells

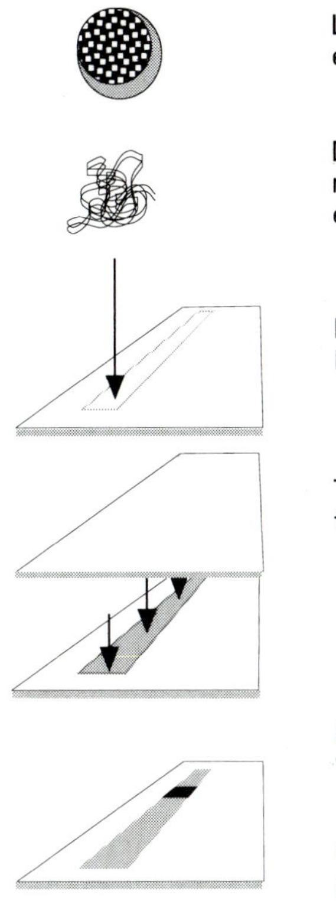
Lyse cell(s) and extract DNA
Digest DNA with restriction endonuclease
Electrophorese lysate
Transfer DNA to membrane
(nylon or nitrocellulose membrane)
Incubate membrane with probe
(Radioactive or biotinylated probe)
Wash, perform autoradiography

Southern blot hybridization

2) DNA is digested with a restriction endonuclease, cutting the DNA into fragments several hundred to thousand base pairs in length 3) The fragmented DNA is separated by size with agar gel electrophoresis 4) A nitrocellulose or nylon membrane is placed on the gel 'slab' and bathed in an alkaline buffer solution, which denatures the DNA, separating it into single strands 5) A layer of dry blotting material, often paper towels is placed on top of the membrane, creating an osmotic pressure gradient sufficient to transfer the separated DNA fragments from the delicate gel 'slab' onto the membrane; this step is the 'Southern transfer' per se Note: The transfer may also be effected by vacuum 6) The presence of DNA fragments of interest is then determined by bathing the membrane in a 'hybridization' fluid continuing either a ^{35}S or ^{32}P-radiolabeled or biotinylated 'probe' (figure, above); if the DNA fragment of interest is present, the probe binds to the single strand of DNA and is detected by autoradiography, or by substrate digestion if the probe is biotinylated (illustration)

Southwestern blot A technique that combines the principle of Southern hybridization, which identifies DNA fragments, with 'Western' immunoblotting, which identifies proteins of interest; a protein is hybridized to its cognate membrane-bound single-stranded DNA molecule, usually the gene that encodes the protein, eg an enhancer or regulatory factor (J Biol Chem 1990; 265:8725); the method is of greatest use for identifying transcription-related proteins located in the nucleus

SP-1 see Pregnancy-specific β-1 glycoprotein

SP1 Stimulatory protein 1 An RNA polymerase II transcription factor that contains a zinc-finger domain required for DNA binding; SP1 binds to a guanine and cytosine-rich sequence of DNA lying 200 base pairs or less upstream of the start sites for RNA synthesis and may be a general promoter-binding factor required for activating various genes

Space sickness Space adaption syndrome The effects of space travel on human physiology include motion sickness, occurring in 67% of astronauts, in 13% of whom it is severe Clinical The condition begins in the vestibular system of the inner ear, causing 'sensory confusion', resulting in vertigo, which is accompanied by nausea, vomiting, gastrointestinal dysmotility, malaise, diaphoresis, sialorrhea, yawning, anorexia, hyperventilation (resulting in hypocapnia with vasodilation of the lower extremities and pooling of blood), causing postural hypotension and syncope; prolonged space flight is associated with osteoporosis and disuse atrophy of muscle and may be punctuated with various inconveniences, eg the in-flight waste management systems fail on most space flights

Spade deformity CARDIOLOGY A finding by contrast ventricular angiography, likened to a playing card spade, appearing in focal concentric apical left cardiac ventricular hypertrophy, confined to the ventricular apex, seen at end-diastole in the right anterior oblique ventriculogram and in two-dimensional echocardiography; the deformity may be accompanied by 'giant' negative T waves on electrocardiography

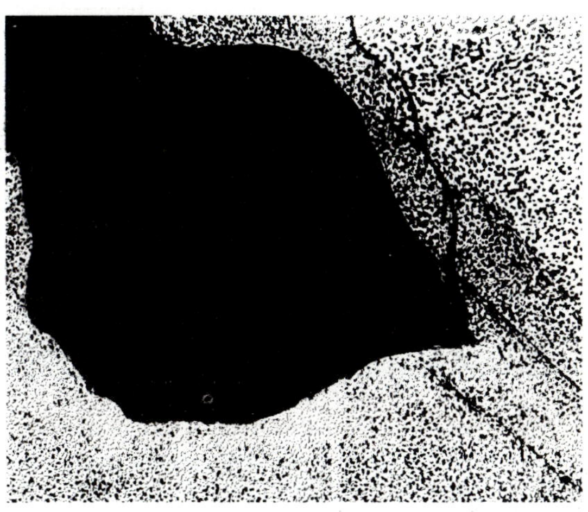

Spade deformity

Spade hand A descriptor for the progressive cylindrical carpal thickening seen in pachydermoperiostosis; Cf Rosebud hand

Spade-like configuration A descriptor for the radiologic appearance of enlarged terminal tufts of the distal phalanges typical of acromegaly; Cf Penciling

'Spaghetti' see 'Pigtail'

'Spaghetti tumor' SURGICAL PATHOLOGY A descriptor for

the growth pattern of the relatively indolent endolymphatic stromal myosis, a uterine stromal tumor that is clinically characterized by abnormal uterine bleeding, pelvic pain and uterine enlargement **Pathology** The cut surface is yellow-orange with bulging polypoid projections, fancifully likened to rigatoni in a melted cheese sauce; mitotic activity is a marker for aggressiveness in uterine stromal tumors; at one end of the spectrum is the mitotically inactive uterine stromal nodule, at the other, stromal sarcomas, which may have more than ten mitotic figures/ten high power fields; the spaghetti tumor usually has less than five mitotic figures/ten high power fields **Prognosis** 85% 15-year survival, despite metastases

Spanish fly A substance that has been held by some members of the lay public to have aphrodisiac qualities, which is prepared from the hemolymph or coelomic fluid from the blister beetle, *Lytta vesicatoria*, member of the family Meloidae; when applied to mucocutaneous surfaces, it causes erythema, urticaria and vesiculation; per os, it causes gastrointestinal irritation, nausea, vomiting, diarrhea, cramping and collapse; as little as 60 mg of this highly nephrotoxic agent may be fatal; the active component is cantharidin, a rubifacient; ammonia may partially ameliorate the pruritus induced by the blister fluid and corticosteroids may relieve the pain

Sparse fur mutation A murine model for ornithine decarboxylase deficiency, characterized by abnormal skin and hair and ornithine decarboxylase deficiency, due to a single point mutation

Spasmodic torticollis see Wry neck

Spasmus caninus see Risus sardonicus

Spastic colon Spastic colitis; see Irritable bowel syndrome

Spatula ribs Broad flattened ribs typical of pseudoachondroplasia, see there

Specialist A person who has a recognized expertise in something; in the usual medical context, a specialist is board-eligible or board-certified in a recognized area of medicine, eg pathology, pediatrics or psychiatry, has undergone a formal residency training program of three or more years and is entitled to sit for the closure ('specialty board') examination in that field; Cf Subspecialty

Specialty board An organization, recognized and approved by the American Board of Medical Specialists in conjunction with the American Medical Association's Council on Medical Education and the American Dental Association, that certifies, through standardized examinations that a physician has achieved a sufficient knowledge base to practice his chosen specialty; see Board certification, Peer review, Residency; Cf State board

'Species-ism' A neologism coined by animal rights activists, for some of whom the use of animals in research is a crime akin to sexism and racism, implying that animals are equivalent to humans as sentient beings; see Animal rights activism, Animal Welfare Act

Specific gravity A measure of the solutes in a fluid, a value that reflects the kidney's ability to concentrate urine: if a random urine specimen has specific gravity greater than 1.023, the kidney's ability to concentrate is assumed to be normal; specific gravity is tested by refractometry, which measures the ratio of the velocity of light in air to the velocity of light in a solution; specific gravity increases in the syndrome of inappropriate secretion of antidiuretic horme (SIADH), uncontrolled diabetes mellitus, proteinuria, eclampsia and obstructive uropathy and decreases in renal tubular damage, chronic renal insufficiency, diabetes insipidus and malignant hypertension

Specificity BIOCHEMISTRY The degree of an enzyme's selectivity for a substrate IMMUNOLOGY The avidity of an antibody for an antigen PHYSIOLOGY The degree of a ligand's affinity for a receptor STATISTICS The number of true negatives in a series of data (usually in the context of laboratory tests designed to detect the presence of a disease), divided by the sum of the number of true negatives and false positives, representing the proportion of subjects without a condition which a test will designate as negative; see Efficiency

Speckled lentiginous nevus Nevus spilus DERMATOLOGY A form of lentigo simplex that presents at birth, arising secondary to a junctional nevus with maturation of the cells in the dermis

Speckled oral leukoplakia Any white flecked or nodular lesion on an atrophic erythematous base that is seen in erythroplasia, thus being a combined leukoplakia and erythroplasia

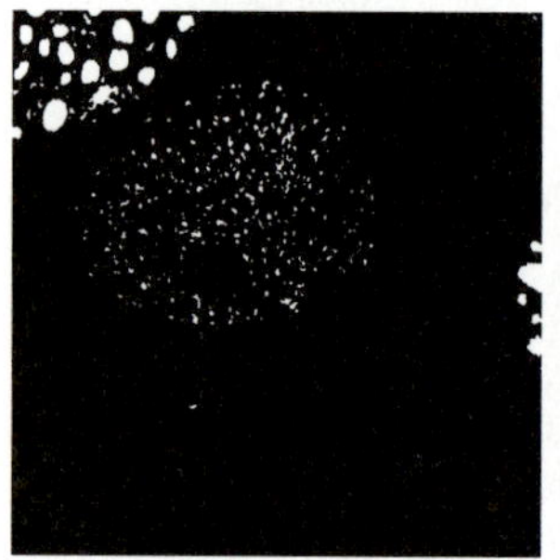

Fine speckles

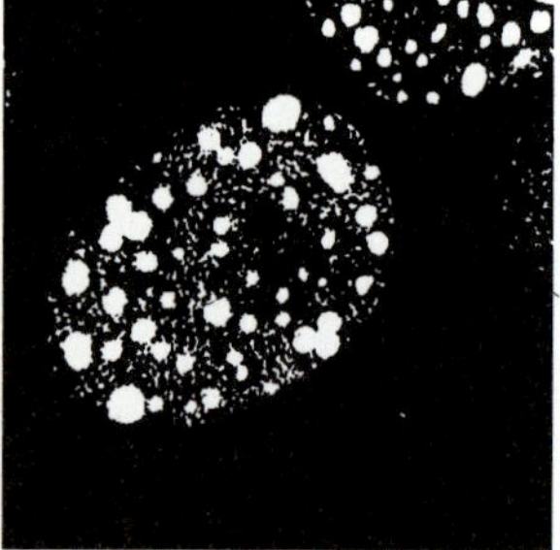

Coarse speckles

Speckled pattern RHEUMATOLOGY An immunofluorescence pattern that may be seen when the human epithelial cell line HEp-2 is stained with serum from patients with various connective tissue diseases; speckled patterns are most common in lupus erythematosus, but may also be seen in mixed connective tissue disease, the sicca and Sjögren syndromes, polymyositis, rheumatoid arthritis and drug-induced immune reactions; the 'speckled' pattern is the least specific, most common and variable of immunofluorescent patterns and is subdivided into 1) Fine or true 'speckles', due to anti-centromere staining, most commonly seen in mixed connective tissue disease 2) Coarse 'speckles', most commonly due to antibodies to nonhistone nuclear proteins: nRNP, Sm, SS-B/La and Scl-70 and c) Large 'speckles', 3-10/nucleus, which occur in IgM antibody to class H3 histones, typical of the undifferentiated connective tissue disease; see Antinuclear antibodies

SPECT Single photon emission computed tomography A non-invasive technique for reconstructing cross-sectional images of the distribution of radiotracers, used to evaluate the central nervous system (acute ischemic episodes, epileptic foci, vascular dementia and Alzheimer's dementia), myocardial perfusion and detect subtle changes in bone metabolism; although SPECT was reported before computed tomography and magnetic resonance imaging (Radiology 1963; 80:653), its clinical application was delayed until the development of suitable radiopharmaceuticals, eg rubidium-82, iodine-123, technetium-99m, thallium-201 and instrumentation, ie adaption of the Anger scintillation camera to rotate around the patient; SPECT analysis of thallium distribution in dynamic studies of cardiac function reduces the subjectivity inherent in interpretation of thallium scans; thallium-201 SPECT is less sensitive, specific and accurate than rubidium-82 PET in imaging myocardial perfusion for those with coronary artery disease (J Nucl Med 1990; 31:1899) Note: Positron emission tomography provides similar information as SPECT at the higher cost of positron decay radionuclides (J Am Med Assoc 1990; 263:561)

'Spectacle' sign A well-circumscribed osteosclerotic rim at the sphenoids, which imparts a bespectacled appearance to the skull on a plain film in patients with idiopathic hypercalcemia

Spectrin A dimeric and tetrameric fibrous protein arranged in a filamentous network, anchored to the cytoplasmic face of the erythrocyte membrane and held responsible for the red cell's shape, and which is defective in spherocytosis; see Band 3.1, Ghost, Spherocytosis

'Speedballing' SUBSTANCE ABUSE A form of intravenous drug abuse in which cocaine and heroin are injected either sequentially or in tandem

SPENP Solid and papillary epithelial neoplasm of the pancreas; see Papillary and solid epithelial neoplasm

SPEP Serum protein electrophoresis A screening method for determining protein 'homeostasis'; serum proteins are divided into prealbumin/albumin, α1 and α2, β and γ zones; regions of the protein electrophoresis are increased or decreased in certain conditions, or variable in the presence of gene polymorphism (table, right)

S peptide A peptide derived from the S protein of *Bacillus subtilis*

Sperm antibody An antibody directed against the sperm heads or tails; sperm antibodies were initially reported to occur in 15-20% of infertile women; newer methods using higher titers as 'cut-offs' for positivity have shown that 3% of infertile males and 2-9% of infertile females produce antibodies to sperm Note: The higher the titers, the more likely the couple will remain infertile without some form of interventive action, which includes intercourse with a condom so that the woman's immunologic memory is allowed to 'decay', sperm washing and insemination (SWIM method) and corticosteroid therapy

Spermatocytic seminoma A distinct variant of seminoma that comprises 5% of all seminomas, which occurs in old men and old dogs Pathology Gelatinous masses with highly pleomorphic, bizarre and mitotically active cells that are not associated with teratomas Prognosis Excellent, some tumors have a sarcomatous component, whereupon the clinical course is aggressive with metastases Treatment Orchiectomy

Spermicides A contraceptive method with a relatively high contraceptive failure rate of 11.9 per one hundred woman-years; the forms of administration include foams, creams and sponges; most contain the surfactant nonoxynol 9, an agent that reduces the risk of sexually-transmitted diseases as it is also bactericidal and viricidal; the incidence of toxic shock syndrome is slightly increased in sponge users (one per two million sponges); spermicides are not associated with teratogenesis or trisomies (N Engl J Med 1987; 317:474, 478), although some 'soft' data suggest limb reduction defects; see Contraceptives, IUDs, Litogens, Pearl index, RU 486

SPF rating Sunburn protection factor rating PUBLIC SAFETY A system promulgated by the US Food and Drug Administration that provides a ratio ('X'/1) between the length of time that a person may be exposed to solar radiation covered with a particular sunscreen than without the agent, which corresponds to a multiplication factor ranging up to 30 or 40; the SPF rating suffers from a number of flaws, including the lack of experimental model and that solar radiation is at a peak for circa four hours/day, and it is widely felt that any SPF rating above 15 is of little use; see Malignant melanoma, Sunscreen, Tanning salons, Ultraviolet radiation

'Spherical pneumonia' A rounded radiologic focus of often streptococcal pneumonia that may mimic a pulmonary or mediastinal mass

Spherocytosis HEMATOLOGY A condition characterized by an increase in osmotic fragility and autohemolysis of globose red cells due to defects in erythrocyte membrane proteins Hereditary spherocytosis is an uncommon (1:5000) autosomal dominant condition Clinical Anemia, intermittent jaundice, splenomegaly, gallstones, leg ulcers, which is due to defects or absence

SERUM PROTEIN ELECTROPHORESIS

	Abnormality	Clinical conditions
↓	Prealbumin	Decreased functional hepatic mass, inflammation, malnutrition
↓	Albumin	Inflammation, malnutrition, malignancy, increased extracellular volume, burns
↑	$\alpha_1$antitrypsin	Inflammation, hepatocellular injury
↓	$\alpha_1$antitrypsin	Deficient allele
V	$\alpha_1$antitrypsin	Polymorphism of α_1-antitrypsin
↑	α_2-macroglobulin	Selective proteinuria in age extremes
↑	$\alpha_2$haptoglobulin	Inflammation
↓	$\alpha_2$haptoglobulin	Hemolysis, hepatosplenic sequestration
↑	$\beta_1$transferrin	Iron deficiency, estrogens
↓	$\beta_1$transferrin	Malnutrition, burns, inflammation
V	$\beta_1$transferrin	Polymorphisms of transferrin
↓	$\beta_1$lipoprotein	Hypercholesterolemia
↑	$\beta_2$complement C3	Chronic inflammation, bile obstruction
↓	$\beta_2$complement C3	Complement activation
V	$\beta_2$complement C3	Polymorphism of C3
↑	β_2 IgA	Malignancy, infection of mucosal surfaces, rheumatoid arthritis, ethanol, cirrhosis
↑	γ region band	Monoclonal antibody, polyclonal stimulation

of *A) SPECTRIN* The most common defective protein in hereditary spherocytosis, that either fails to form head-to-head tetramers or binds incorrectly to ankyrin or band 4.1 protein *B) 4.1 PROTEIN* and *C) ANKYRIN* due to a defective gene on chromosome 8 (N Engl J Med 1990; 323:1046); acquired spherocytosis may be the first manifestation of a delayed hemolytic reaction (eg transfusion of ABO incompatible blood) or seen in hypersplenism secondary to cirrhosis or chronic infections

Spheroid NEUROPATHOLOGY A local axonal dilatation filled with degenerated organelles, seen by light microscopy as a rounded, eosinophilic and granular mass at the edges of infarcts, in axonal dystrophies and in degenerating or regenerating axons

Spheroid body myopathy A rare, slowly progressive, autosomal dominant neuromuscular disease affecting type I muscle fibers, which by electron microscopy displays spherical heterogenous bodies with fine fibrillar and amorphous granularity

Spherophakia-brachymorphia Weill-Marchesani syndrome A complex characterized by myopia, subluxation of the lens, glaucoma, brachydactyly, brachycephaly

Sphingolipidoses A group of inborn errors of sphingolipid metabolism in which lysosphingolipids accumulate, inhibiting protein kinase C activity in signal transduction, cellular differentiation and in tumor promotion; sphingolipidoses include Fabry's disease (increased globotriaosylsphingosine and galabiosylsphingosine), Gaucher's disease (glucosylsphingosine), Krabbe's disease (galactosylsphingosine), metachromatic leukodystrophy (sulfogalactosylsphingosine, sulfolactosylsphingosine), Niemann-Pick disease (sphingosylphosphorylcholine), as well as GM1 gangliosidosis, GM2 gangliosidoses, which includes Tay-Sachs and Sandhoff diseases and GM3 gangliosidosis or sphingolipodystrophy Note: For many 'inborn errors of metabolism', the defective chromosomal region has been identified, eg the defect in Tay-Sachs disease maps to chromosome (C) 15q, the defect in Sandhoff's disease maps to 5q and that for metachromatic leukodystrophy maps to 22q

Sphinx neck appearance see Webbed neck

Spicy food Comestibles that are marinated in and/or contain chili peppers, mustards with horseradishes or other spices that evoke a desired intraoral sensation that crosses pain with pleasure, which, when intense may elicit an autonomic nervous system response, including diaphoresis; the most commonly used 'spicy' condiment is hot pepper containing capsinoids, which in mild hot (chili) sauce contains nordihydrocapsaicin and N-nonanoic acid (synthetic vanillylamide); moderate hot sauce contains homodihydrocapsaicin; very hot sauce is high in capsaicin and dihydrocapsaicin, which is effective in dilutions of 1:100 000; 'hot' mustards owe their gustatory effects to horseradish, the active ingredient of which is isothiocyanate, a component of wasabe, a mustard used to season Japanese food (see Sushi syncope), and in religious ceremony (see Seder syncope); it is unclear whether hot foods are carcinogenic, as capsaicin is mutagenic by the Ames assay (a bacterial screen for carcinogens) and may cause colon cancer in rats; in contrast, capsaicin is also an antioxidant, and therefore also has anti-carcinogenic properties; oxidized capsaicin also binds to and inactivates the 'j' form of cytochrome P-450 enzyme, which is thought to activate certain mutagens, including nitrosamine and polycyclic aromatic hydrocarbons; spicy foods have been traditionally denied to gastric ulcer-prone individuals, although jalapeños placed in direct contact with the gastric mucosa cause neither ulcers nor hemorrhage (J Am Med Assoc 1988; 260:3473)

Spider angioma Nevus araneus A superficial spider-like cluster of capillaries composed of a central 'feeder' vessel and multiple minute tortuous and dilated radiating vessels with a peripheral erythema; when the involved vessel is large, it may pulsate and blanch on pressure; while classically due to increased circulating estrogens as seen in pregnancy and alcoholic cirrhosis, spider angiomas may occur in chronic hepatic congestion secondary to constrictive pericarditis and may be a normal birthmark in children

Spider cell Spiderweb cell GYNECOLOGIC CYTOLOGY An uncommon variant epithelial cell seen in cervical metaplasia in papanicolaou-stained smears, morphologically similar to those described in rhabdomyomas (see below) and in 'sugar' tumors PULMONARY PATHOLOGY see Sugar tumor SURGICAL PATHOLOGY A variably-sized undifferentiated mesenchymal cell with a small central, acidophilic and stellate mass connected by thin striations to the cell periphery, containing vacuolated cytoplasm and fibers radiating toward the nucleus Note: Although the larger 'spider' cells are typical of myxomas and myxoid liposarcoma and 'spiderweb' cells are typical of rhabdomyomas and pleomorphic rhabdomyosarcomas, in practice the distinction is arbitrary and of little utility as immunoperoxidase stains and ancillary studies are used to determine the tumor's cell of origin

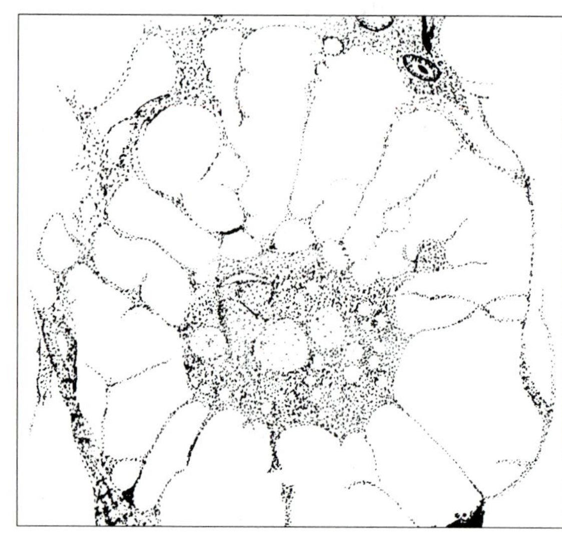

Spider cell

Spider(-like) colonies MICROBIOLOGY A descriptor for the morphology of the colonies of *Actinomyces israeli* seen under low power microscopy; Cf Medusa head colonies

'Spider' dystrophy Macroreticular dystrophy A branching arachnoid pigmentary pattern seen in an autosomal recessive form of retinal pigment dystrophy of the epithelium, appearing as bilateral, symmetrical lesions that do not affect vision

Spiderweb cell see Spider cell

Spiderweb membrane see Pseudomembrane

Spike LABORATORY MEDICINE A sharp peak seen in the β or γ region in serum or urine protein electrophoresis, most commonly occurring in malignant lymphoproliferative disorders, eg multiple myeloma or Waldenstrom's disease, which may also be seen in monoclonal gammopathy of undetermined significance; a spike indicates monoclonality unless proven otherwise, but may not be seen if the immunoglobulin production is normally very low, as in IgD and IgE myelomas, as the spike may be obscured by the curves corresponding to more abundant IgG, IgA and IgM; see Umbrella effect NEUROLOGY A sharply-defined depolarization on an electroencephalogram RENAL PATHOLOGY Needle-like deposition of basement membrane material within the mesangial matrix, seen in early membranous glomerulonephropathy, best visualized by the periodic acid Schiff stain Note: Membrane deposition is usually idiopathic but may be secondary to drugs, eg gold therapy, infections, eg syphilis, connective tissue disease, eg lupus erythematosus, renal vein thrombosis and malignancy VIROLOGY A projection on the surface of the virus that may be seen by electron microscopy, corresponding to either hemagglutinin or neuraminidase, present on the coat of influenza viruses

Spike-and-dome contour CARDIOLOGY A descriptor for the carotid arterial pulse curve seen in idiopathic hypertrophic subaortic stenosis (IHSS), which rises abruptly and falls during midsystole (spike), later rising a second time at a slower rate during late systole (dome); the jugular pulse in IHSS is characterized by a prominent a (atrial) wave; see Hypertrophic cardiomyopathy, Spade deformity

'Spike and wave' pattern An electroencephalographic pattern seen in petit mal absences, occurring as symmetric and synchronous, three or more per second discharges with an abrupt beginning and end Note: Slower spike and wave pattern occurring at 2.5 or less discharges per second is more common in the Lennox-Gestaut syndrome

Spike potential(s) ELECTROMYOGRAPHY Single rapid (100-200msec) voltage 'transients' that occur spontaneously in smooth muscle cells, when the cells have resting membrane potentials above the spike potential threshold, as occurs in the lower esophageal sphincter

Spina bifida Rachischisis posterioris A lesion due to defective fusion of the vertebral arch that normally occurs at the 21-29 somite stage in the fifth fetal week LABORATORY Increased α-fetoprotein levels; occult spina bifida affects up to 10% of adults (seen at tertiary care centers); see A-fetoprotein, Multivitamins

Spinal muscle atrophy (SMA) A heterogeneous group of conditions that selectively affect the α motor neuron, characterized by degeneration of the anterior horn cells with associated muscle weakness and atrophy, affecting an estimated 1:20 000 newborns; despite the clinical heterogeneity of the SMAs, the defect of all forms lies in a mutation of chromosome 5q11.2-13.3 (Nature 1990; 345:823); SMAs have been arbitrarily subdivided into type I Acute or infantile onset form of Werdig-Hoffman, type II Intermediate form (onset in childhood), type III Juvenile onset form of Kugelberg-Welander and type IV Adult onset form

Spinal shock A clinical complex caused by trauma to the vertebral column and spinal cord, appearing as a transient (3-6 week in duration) loss of reflex activity due to functional or anatomic interruption of the corticospinal tracts, occurring into two phases *1) ARREFLEXIA*, characterized by complete 'failure' below the lesion, including tetraplegia, paraplegia, overflow incontinence, paralytic ileus, gastric atony and depression of cremasteric reflex, followed several weeks later by *2) HYPERREFLEXIA*, ie exaggeration of reflexes with flexor spasms and autonomic dysreflexia, bladder distension, diaphoresis, hypertension and bradycardia; certain reflexes, eg anal 'wink', bulbocavernosus and cremasteric reflexes, full penile erection, reflex leg withdrawal and Babinski sign, are retained after complete spinal cord transection since these reflexes don't require higher levels of control Note: In obstetrics, 'spinal shock' refers to an idiopathic post-partum vasomotor collapse that follows spinal anesthesia, secondary to various stressants of delivery, including acute blood loss, electrolytic imbalance, adrenocortical insufficiency, pre-eclampsia, anesthesia itself and amniotic fluid embolism

Spinal vasculature steal syndrome A clinical complex characterized by arteriovenous malformation of the spinal cord, causing spinal cord compression, that may respond to ligation of the 'offending' artery

Spina ventosa A fusiform expansile lesion of short diaphyseal bones, especially phalangeal bones with cortical and trabecular destruction and 'ballooning' of the cortex without a sclerotic reaction; spina ventosa was first described in tuberculosis, also occurring in congenital syphilis (Spina ventosa luetica)

Spindle A structure consisting of microtubules, which is responsible for the alignment and movement of chromosomes during cell division; see MTOC

Spindle see Mitotic spindle

Spindle and epithelioid cell nevus Spitz nevus, Juvenile 'melanoma'

Spindle cell carcinoma An often aggressive and undifferentiated carcinoma composed of sweeping fascicles of elongated epithelial cells of transitional, squamous, undifferentiated or rarely glandular origin that mimics a sarcoma both clinically (presenting as a soft tissue mass) and pathologically (having bizarre fibroblast-like cells with atypical mitotic figures); spindle cell carcinomas have received the confusing synonyms of pseudosarcoma and carcinosarcoma and are most commonly seen in the oral cavity (male:female ratio, 10:1), as a variant of the squamous cell carcinoma, which is well-described in the larynx, upper respiratory and upper gastrointestinal tracts, thyroid gland and rarely in the female genital tract; one-fourth of patients with malignant pseudosarcomas had had previous regional radiotherapy Ultrastructure Aggregates of keratohyaline, bundles of tonofilaments, scant and poorly developed desmosomes and rare premelanosomes Treatment Surgery

Spindle cell lipoma A benign tumor of adipose tissue, most common in the neck and shoulders of adults, of interest as these tumors may be confused with myxoid liposarcomas by the novice and can be distinguished therefrom by the absence of a plexiform vascular pattern and lipoblasts

'Spinnaker sail' sign A descriptor for a displaced thymic shadow seen by a plain chest film in a neonate with a unilateral pneumomediastinum, fancifully likened to a fully-blown spinnaker sail; bilateral pneumomediastinum in the neonate is fancifully designated as the 'angel wings' sign; see Rocker bottom sign

Spinnbarkeit German, stretchability The 'stretchability' of cervical mucus, or the length that strands of cervical mucus reach before breaking (at least 6 cm), a reaction that parallels the 'ferning' reaction, peaking on the 14th day of the menstrual cycle; see Ferning; Cf String test

Spiral annulets see Ring fibers

Spiral computed tomography Helical scanning A recently-developed permutation of computed tomographic imaging (CT) based on 'slip-ring' technology, in which a large image volume is acquired by continuous rotation of the detector, scanning images at a speed of 10 mm/second, allowing the acquisition of a 25 cm three-dimensional 'gapless' block of radiologic information in a single breath; it has been predicted that spiral CT will have a major impact on radiocontrast studies of cerebral vasculature and the gastrointestinal tract, body regions that are less well studies because of the two-dimensional nature of the images and the prolonged acquisition time; the information obtained with spiral CT scanning is markedly superior to the single 'slice' images from the current generation of CT imagers and, in the future, these latter machines are likely to be relegated for use only in patients who cannot hold their breath (Diag Imaging 1991; 13:98); Cf High-resolution computed tomography

Spironolactone bodies Rounded, eosinophilic intracytoplasmic inclusions that may be observed in the zona glomerulosa of the adrenal cortex of patients receiving spironolactone Ultrastructure Whorls of endoplasmic reticulum or myelinoid figures with central lipid core; similar inclusions have been identified in adrenal adenoma, adrenogenital syndrome, Conn's disease, pheochromocytoma and paraganglioma (Arch Pathol Lab Med 1975; 99:416); see Lamellar bodies

'Splashback' FORENSIC PATHOLOGY Protrusion of tissue from a bullet's entrance wound, resulting from the kinetic energy imparted by the bullet; although the tissue surrounding the entrance wound closes over, the gases expanding after the bullet find the path of least resistance for escape, leaving via the entrance wound, pushing out fragments of subcutaneous tissue

Splenic flexure syndrome A condition caused by swallowed gas that passes often only as far as the transverse colon, producing abdominal distension and discomfort that is relieved by defecation or passing of flatus

Splenic index A parameter used to evaluate the extent of experimental graft-versus-host disease; the ratio of the spleen to body weight is relatively constant and increased in graft-versus-host disease; the index is not suitable for humans; see Phagocytic index

Splenosis The autotransplantation of splenic tissue to unusual sites after open splenic trauma, eg automobile accidents, gunshot or stab wounds; the splenic pulp implants appear as red-blue nodules on the peritoneum, omentum, and mesentery, morphologically similar to multifocal pelvic endometriosis; Cf Hypersplenism

Splice junction MOLECULAR BIOLOGY A segment of DNA involved in RNA splicing, defined by the GU dinucleotide at the 5' end of the intron, known as the donor or left junction and an AG dinucleotide at the 3' acceptor or right junction of the intron

Spliceosome MOLECULAR BIOLOGY A nuclear structure that folds pre-mRNA into a substrate and splices out the intervening sequences or introns of RNA (which are not translated into proteins) from mRNA precursors and splices together the exons (which are translated into proteins), forming a mature mRNA molecule; because eukaryotes are rich in nonprotein-encoding introns, the spliceosome function is essential to gene expression in eukaryotic cells; by affinity chromatography, it appears that the minimum components of a spliceosome are four small nuclear ribonucleoproteins (snRNPs U1, U2, U5 and U4/6), which are required for the proper folding of the RNA, splicing it into a mature messenger RNA; snRNPs aggregate together on the chromosomes as particles ranging from 1 to 20 μm in diameter, designated as 'snurposomes' (Science 1991; 252:1499); other spliceosome components as well as a number of different proteins that have been designated as PRPs (for pre-RNA processing); the release of mRNA from the spliceosome requires the presence of an RNA helicase-like protein PRP22 (Nature 1991; 349:487); other proteins, eg PRP16 an RNA-dependent ATPase are transient in their interaction with the spliceosome (ibid; 349:495); see DEAD-box proteins Note: U6 is widely conserved across species from yeast to human and may be the most critical component of a spliceosome, as experimentally-induced U6 mutations either prevent spliceosome formation or interfere with the splicing process (Science 1990; 250:404); see Transcription unit

Splicing MOLECULAR BIOLOGY The cutting and rejoining of strands of a linear molecule, eg DNA, RNA or protein GENE SPLICING is an experimental procedure in which a segment of DNA is covalently inserted into a 'host' molecule or vector, creating a 'recombinant' DNA molecule PRE-MRNA SPLICING A vital cell process that is intrinsic to eukaryotic cells, consisting in a two-step phosphotransferase reaction requiring ATP hydrolysis, in which certain segments of template-derived RNA known as introns (intervening sequences that do not encode proteins) are excised and the exons (sequences of RNA that encode proteins) are joined, by action of a 'spliceosome'; the mature mRNA is then translated into a protein; pre-mRNA splicing is site-specific and requires precise sequence recognition at the intron boundaries or splice junction PROTEIN SPLICING A phenomenon by which two or more proteins can be generated from a single primary translation product, by a process known as alternative splicing, while a second product is formed upon rejoining of the two ends (Science 1990; 250:651)

Splinter hemorrhage(s) Small linear subungual hemorrhages that are red when fresh and brown when aged, located at the distal third of the nailbed Pathogenesis The blood 'leaks' into the avascular squames under the fingernails due to microemboli and/or increased capillary fragility; although splinter hemorrhages are characteristic of acute and subacute bacterial endocarditis, they are more commonly due to trauma, occur in up to 10% of normal subjects and in 40% of patients with mitral stenosis; splinter hemorrhages are also described in the retinal disk in papilledema, most commonly due to retinal vein occlusion or subarachnoid hemorrhage

Split gene A gene composed of multiple segments of DNA that encodes polypeptides (exons), separated by segments of non-polypeptide encoding DNA (introns), which are excised or spliced out, forming a transcript from which a cognate protein is transcribed; see Exon, Intron, Spliceosome

Split hand/foot see Lobster claw deformity

Split papule A skin nodule with a central linear erosion seen adjacent to the mouth or nose in secondary syphilis

'Splits' IMMUNOLOGY A designation for HLA antigens that were first described as private antigens and subsequently shown to be public antigens; the new status is indicated by a parenthesis enclosing its old status; see Private antigen, Public antigen

Split thickness graft A 'thin' skin graft (0.25-0.35 mm in thickness) that includes the epidermis and a minimal amount of dermis; split-thickness grafts have the advantage of more rapid availability of donor sites for further engraftment, more rapid vascularization, longer post-transplantation survival in the recipient site and are of greatest use in contaminated skin sites, burn sites and sites with poor intrinsic vasculature; thick split-thickness grafts are more resistant to trauma, result in less contraction and allow some degree of sensation but survive poorly in the recipient site; see Skin graft; Cf Artificial skin, Spray-on skin

'Splitting' ACADEMIA The division of a well-defined morbid condition into ever smaller subtypes, eg subdividing Laurence-Moon-Biedl-Bardet syndrome into the Laurence-Moon and Bardet-Biedl syndromes, a practice known as 'hair-splitting' Note: Although ostensibly the purpose of splitting is to identify subgroups of patients with a better or worse prognosis or response to therapy, the real (and rarely admitted) purpose may be to generate publications of greater volume than value, which increases the bulk of writer's curriculum vitae without adding substantively to scientific knowledge; Cf 'Lumping' RENAL PATHOLOGY see Railroad track appearance

Spoked wheel pattern A pattern of chromatin clumping seen at the periphery of the nucleus in basophilic normoblast (pre-erythrocyte) and plasma cells

Sponge kidney see Polycystic kidneys

Spongiform pustules Kogoj's microabscess Subcorneal aggregates of neutrophils typical of psoriasis

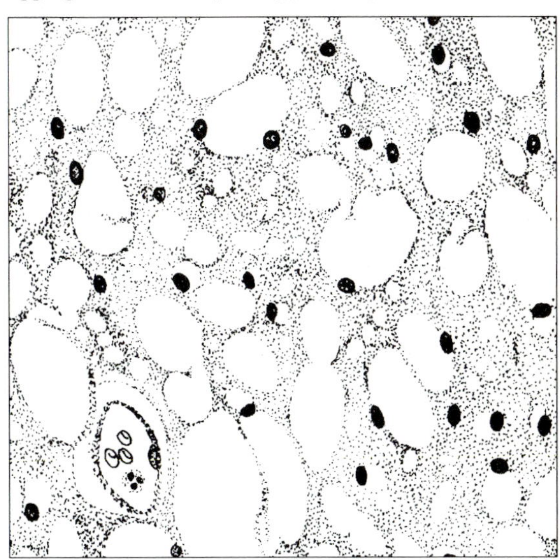

Spongy degeneration

Spongy degeneration of Van Bogaert-Bertrand, Canavan's disease An autosomal recessive condition characterized by diffuse vacuolization of the deep cerebral cortex, predominantly affecting the white matter, but also the gray matter, caused by hydropic degeneration of the glial cells and myelin Clinical Onset in early infancy with hypotonia and poor head control, optic atrophy and blindness, mental retardation, rigidity, hyperreflexia, seizures and progressive macrocephaly; death occurs by age 2-5 Histopathology Cortical and subcortical vacuolation which produces the spongy appearance; Cf Leukodystrophy Note: Degenerative and spongiform gliotic reactions may in some cases be due to an abortive retroviral infection, as in defective production of the viral env (envelope) protein (Nature 1990; 346:181, Proc Nat Acad Sci 1989; 86:2021)

Spontaneous pneumothorax A condition affecting an estimated 17 000/year in the USA, which may be idiopathic or secondary to underlying pulmonary disease, eg chronic obstructive pulmonary disease, most commonly occurring in previously healthy males, age 20-40, secondary to rupture of subpleural blebs Clinical Sudden onset of chest pain, with dyspnea proportionate to the size of the pneumothorax; tension pneumothorax, while rare, may compromise the circulation by a ball-valve mechanism Treatment Suction followed by water seal drainage Prognosis 30% recur on the same side, a tendency that may be reduced by intrapleural tetracycline (J Am Med Assoc 1990; 264:2224); 10% occur de novo on the opposite side

Spontaneous remission of malignancy A rare clinical event; Everson and Cole catalogued 241 cases as of 1966 (Spontaneous Regression of Cancer, WB Saunders), and defined spontaneous regression of cancer as the partial or complete disappearance of a histologically-confirmed malignancy in absence of treatment or with treatment deemed inadequate to sufficiently alter its natural course; malignant melanoma comprises 10% of the cases of spontaneous regression of malignancy, with the caveat that in melanoma the primary lesion may involute or completely disappear only to resurface as a fulminant and aggressive malignancy after the reporting of a complete cure

Spooning A descriptor for a hand deformity in patients with chorea, in which the outstretched hands, slightly flexed wrists and metacarpophalangeal joints slightly hyperextended demonstrate a distinct concavity

Spoon nail A rare acquired nail dystrophy seen in bronchiectasia in which the nail bed is atrophic and the nail has a 'hollowed' appearance; see Clubbing

Sporotrichoid infection see Swimming pool granuloma

Sporozoite surface protein-2 see Malaria vaccine

Sport CLINICAL GENETICS A phenotypic trait that appears de novo in an individual and is subsequently inherited by his progeny, thought to be related to a spontaneous mutation or an environmental mutagen acting on the egg or sperm; Cf Lysenkoism

Sports 'anemia' A red cell mass that falls in the mild anemic range, which is typical of 'endurance' athletes; this relative increase in plasma volume appears to be a physiological response to the repeated and transient dehydration that occurs in long races; a 'normal' hematocrit would be detrimental to muscle action and predispose the athletes to life-threatening thrombotic events, thus making 'blood doping' a potentially dangerous practice

Sports medicine A subspecialty of occupational medicine that is usually practiced by orthopedic surgeons or by rehabilitation medicine physicians, which is involved in the care of those who spring, sprint, splash, bash or bogey, for play or profit; see Anabolic steroids, Boxing, Exercise, Exercise-associated amenorrhea, Running; Cf Performing arts medicine

Spot *Noun* A focus on a chromatogram or electrophoretic gel containing a substance of interest *Verb* To apply a minute amount of material to a chromatographic or electrophoretic support prior to performing the procedure

Spotted bone disease Osteopathia condensans disseminata An autosomal dominant condition characterized by multiple small foci of osteosclerosis in the spongiosa of the pelvis, metaphysis of long bones, tarsal and carpal bones; often associated with subcutaneous bony nodules

Spotted leg 'syndrome' A condition characterized by patches of subdermal atrophy secondary to diabetic vasculitis, most common below the knee in older diabetics; the affected skin is smooth, shiny and hyperpigmented due to hemosiderin deposition and increased melanin

Spotted pigmenti nevi A variant of intradermal nevi that is located adjacent to eccrine ducts and enveloped by nevus cells

S pouch of Parks A surgically created reservoir used to preserve anal continence in ulcerative colitis after total colectomy; the terminal ileum is aligned in an S-shape, incised and sewn over, anastomosing the pouch to a cuff of anorectal musculature, thereby creating a continent rectum; surgical procedures with a similar function include the lateral internal reservoir and the J pouch

Spousal benefits SOCIAL MEDICINE Those benefits, including health care insurance and life insurance that are provided to the spouse, ie husband or wife of an employee; in the US and other developed nations, these benefits are being extended to unmarried partners, including those of the same sex (Am Med News 15/Apr/91)

'Spray-on' skin A polymeric material for covering superficial second-degree burn wounds; it is no longer used as it is contraindicated in deep second- and third-degree burns, where it would have been most useful, due to increased superficial infections and non-adherence; see Artificial skin, Split-thickness graft

Spreadsheet An electronic matrix of rows and columns that allows for user-defined entry of data in either an alphabetical or numerical fashion and its simultaneous manipulation Note: The most popular spreadsheet program in the IBM-PC microcomputer environment has been Lotus 1-2-3

SPROM Spontaneous premature rupture of membranes; see PROM

S protein MICROBIOLOGY A large protein cleaved from subtilin, a protein derived from ***Bacillus subtilis*** PHYSIOLOGY Cobalamin (vitamin B_{12})-binding proteins, eg intrinsic factor and transcobalamin II; S protein was named for its relatively slow electrophoretic mobility; Cf R protein

Sprue syndrome see Celiac sprue, Tropical sprue

Spur IMMUNOLOGY A sharply curved projection from a precipitation line that is characteristic of 'partial identity' between two antigens when examined by Ouchterlony's two dimension-double immunodiffusion technique, which indicates that there is cross-reactivity of the antigens with the antibody (figure, facing page, bottom)

Squamocolumnar junction The zone of transition from squamous epithelium to secretory and glandular epithelium; squamocolumnar junctions occur in the nasopharynx, esophagogastric junction and anus, as well as the uterine cervix where it is the site of initiation of cervical squamous cell carcinoma; the junction migrates external to the os after vaginal delivery and migrates internally in the postmenopausal endocervix

Squamous eddies DERMATOPATHOLOGY Whorls and 'waves' of eosinophilic, flattened squamous cells arranged in an onion-peel fashion, typical of irritated seborrheic keratosis, simulating either the keratinization of the follicular infundibulum, seen in the proliferating trichilemmal cyst/tumor or the squamous pearls of well-differentiated squamous cell carcinoma; Cf Horn pseudocyst, Squamous pearl

Squamous odontogenic tumor A relatively uncommon oral lesion composed of nests of benign squamous epithelium lying in a fibrous stroma, with a round-to-triangular radiolucency at the neck of the tooth's root, most often first appearing in the adolescent female, causing pain and loosening of the teeth Treatment Simple excision

Squamous pearl Horn pearl Keratin pearl A compact round cluster of curved and flattened keratinocytes that have glassy, pale pink laminations, most characteristic of well-differentiated squamous cell carcinoma that may be seen in keratoacanthoma and in synovial sarcoma; when seen in papanicolaou-stained smears of the cervix and vagina, keratin pearls are indicative of estrogenic effect ; Cf Horn pseudocyst, Squamous eddies

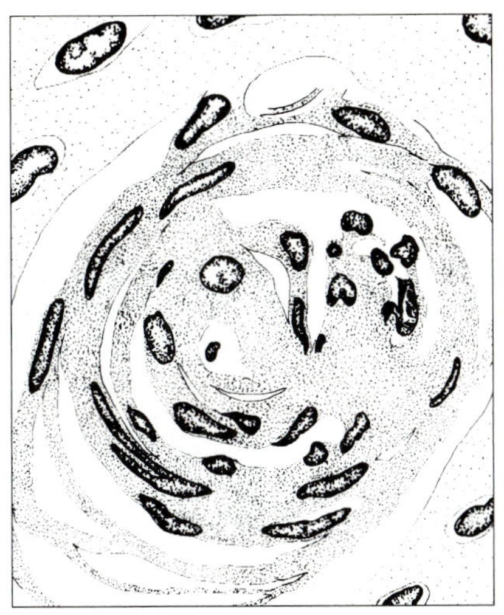

Squamous pearl

Square root sign CARDIOLOGY A pressure contour seen by cardiac catheterization, consisting of an elevation of the right ventricular diastolic pressure with early filling and a subsequent plateau, which is a finding suggestive of chronic constrictive pericarditis

Square wave CARDIOLOGY An abnormal blood pressure response to the Valsalva maneuver (increased diaphragmatic pressure against a closed glottis, increasing intrathoracic pressure to 40mm Hg), seen in left ventricular failure, where the blood pressure increases at the onset of the Valsalva maneuver (VM), remains elevated until the VM is released after which the blood pressure abruptly drops to baseline without 'overshooting' the baseline pressure, accompanied by little change in the pulse pressure and without tachycardia Note: Normal subjects respond to VM with a slow decrease in blood and pulse pressure and increase in heart rate; when VM is stopped, the return to normal is accompanied by an 'overshooting' of the baseline

Square wave jerk(s) NEUROLOGY Brief, intermittent and horizontal ocular oscillations, arising from the defects in the primary gaze position, most common in cerebellar disease

'Squaring' RADIOLOGY A descriptor for the sharp demarcation of the lower patella, seen after multiple hemarthroses in hemophiliacs

Squat jump 'syndrome' SPORTS MEDICINE A transient clinical complex caused by intense and violent exercise, first described secondary to the 'squat-jump', a form of calisthenic, resulting in myoglobinuria with swelling of the quadriceps, proteinuria, hematuria and hemo-globinuria

Squatting PEDIATRICS A position assumed by a child with cyanotic congenital heart disease, classically in Fallot's tetralogy, in the face of acute hypoxia; squatting relieves the exertion-induced dyspnea by decreasing the right-to-left shunt and increasing the systemic vascular resistance and pulmonary blood flow; adults with Fallot's do not squat as they know their exercise tolerance level

'Squeaky wheel' effect The effect of placing a problem, complaint or 'injustice' in an appropriate forum or advertising it in such a way as to produce the greatest stridency, causing it to garner enough sympathy and support to be addressed, regardless of the principle of fair-play; this principle resulted in the US government-sponsored reimbursement of experimental autologous bone marrow transplantation for patients with advanced breast cancer (cost $125 000 per patient), which equals the cost of 2000 screening mammograms; since '*...THE SQUEAKY WHEEL GETS THE OIL...*', decisions may be made for a small but vocal minority rather than for the broader interests of society, addressing private patient concerns rather than public health needs and short-term expenditures rather than long-term savings (J Am Med Assoc 1991; 265:3300); see Rule of rescue; Cf Signal event

SQUID imaging Superconducting quantum interface device imaging SQUIDs are the most highly sensitive (detecting magnetic fields $1/10^9$ that of the earth's gravity) low-'noise' amplifiers in existence; SQUIDs are used in biomagnetic imaging to measure the magnetic flux created when electrical energy flows through neurons; SQUIDs may be connected to a network of superconducting antenna coils designed to measure magnetic flux and housed in a helium-filled dewar (a metal container with an evacuated space between the walls that may be silver coated to prevent the transfer of heat) to maintain a low (-269°C) temperature; optimal imaging requires a room that shields out all radio and sound waves and placement of the sensor as close as possible to the body; the magnetic signals are detected, amplified, filtered, processed and displayed on a computer; SQUIDs cost $2-3 million and are

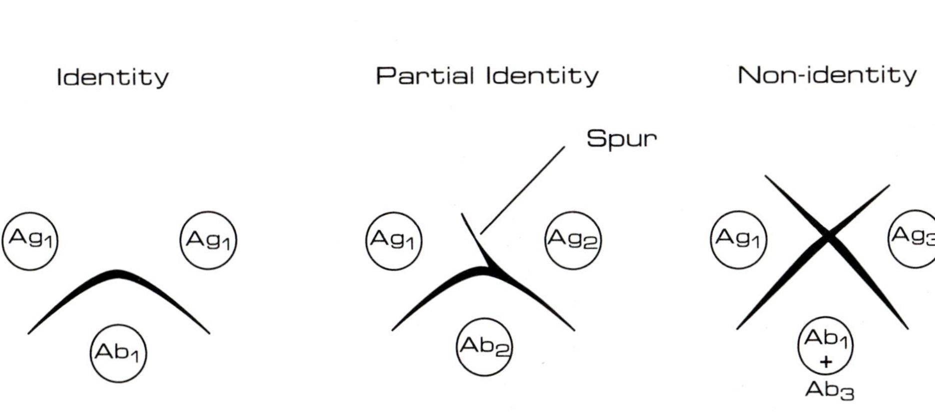

Double immunodiffusion, spur

of potential use for diagnosing epilepsy, stroke, migraines, language disorders, schizophrenia, motor and sensory defects and cardiac arrhythmias (J Am Med Assoc 1990; 263:623); see Imaging

Squiggle Tilde A symbol (~) used to designate a high-energy (usually phosphate) bond

Squiggly cells HEMATOPATHOLOGY A colloquial term for a variant cell of no known diagnostic or prognostic significance seen in Lennert's diffuse mixed cell lymphoma and occasionally in T cell lymphomas

Squirting papilla DERMATOPATHOLOGY A histopathologic feature of psoriasiform lesions, characterized by intermittent 'regurgitation' of fluid and leukocytes at the head of the papilla, seen in psoriasis and pityriasis rubra pilaris

SR 4233 An agent with anti-neoplastic potential, ingested in a non-toxic form and metabolized into a selectively tumoritoxic form, releasing DNA-damaging oxygen free radicals into the oxygen-depleted environment typically inhabited by tumor cells that have outgrown their blood supply and survive in low-oxygen conditions

src The Rous sarcoma virus-derived oncogene that provided the first evidence that cancer could be induced by introducing a gene into a normal cell; c-*src* is a proto-oncogene encoding a 60 kD tyrosine-kinase protein kinase ($pp60^{c\text{-}src}$) that is located in the plasma membrane, possesses tyrosine kinase activity, and phosphorylates the tyrosine residues of other proteins, thus being a generalized growth-promoting signal; *src*-family proteins interact with cellular proteins via an N-terminal unique region or by a conserved SH2 region; see SH2

Src homology region(s) see SH2/SH3 regions

SRIF see Somatotropin release inhibiting hormone

SRP see Signal recognition particle

SRS-A Slow reacting substance of anaphylaxis IMMUNOLOGY The group of cysteinyl leukotrienes, LTC_4 and LTD_4 (LTE_4 is also involved but is a lesser actor), polyunsaturated 20-carbon fatty acids derived from arachidonic acid and platelet-activating factor and released from mast cells during anaphylaxis; SRS-As cause slow sustained and potent smooth muscle contraction, bronchoconstriction (1000-fold more potent than prostaglandins or histamine) and increased capillary permeability, platelet aggregation, proteolysis of the basement membrane components, providing chemotaxis for eosinophils and neutrophils; are potent bronchoconstrictors, stimulate mucus secretion and increase the permeability of postcapillary venules; SRS-As (especially LTC_4 and LTD_4) are increased in asthmatics and involved in immediate hypersensitivity, with bronchoconstriction, and cardiac depression

SRUS see Solitary rectal ulcer syndrome

SRV-1 A type D simian AIDS virus that infected a macaque colony in California, the genome of which shares little in common with HIV-1, although the genes are similar, and include an **LTR** (long terminal repeat), ***gag*** (inner shell protein), ***pol*** (polymerase), ***env*** (envelope) and an *orf* (open reading frame) between the *gag* and *pol* that encodes a viral protease; see SAIDS, SIV, Retrovirus

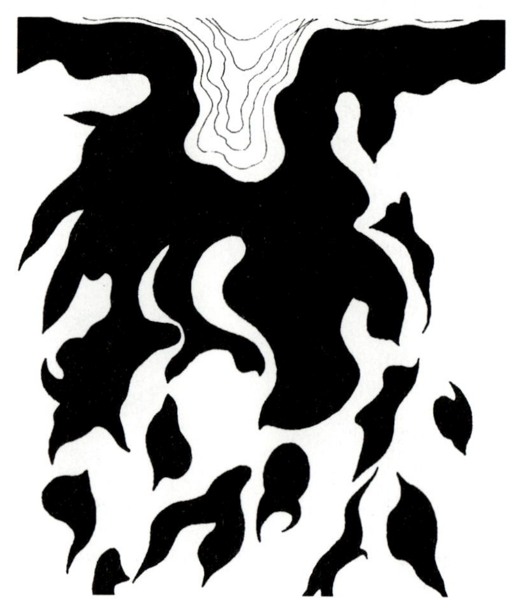

Stabbing invasion

SRY The protein encoded by the 14 kilobase *sry* (sex-determining region of the Y chromosome) gene in humans (Nature 1990; 348:448, 445, 452) that corresponds to the long-elusive testis-determining gene on the Y chromosome (Tdy); the homologous mouse protein is designated Sry; the *sry* gene is sufficient to assign 'maleness', as corroborated by its insertion into female transgenic mice, which develop into phenotypic males (Nature 1991; 251:117, 96); see X chromosome inactivation

SS-A Ro A cytoplasmic antigen against which 25% of patients with lupus erythematosus and 40% of those with Sjögren syndrome have circulating antibodies; Cf Antinuclear antibodies

SS-B La A cytoplasmic antigen against which patients with lupus erythematosus and Sjögrens syndrome have circulating antibodies; anti-SS-B antibodies are thought to be associated with a better prognosis in lupus and lower anti-nuclear antibodies, see there

SSB protein Single-stranded (DNA) binding protein A heterotrimeric polypeptide protein that binds single strands of DNA, involved in constructing an active growing fork in DNA replication in bacteria; SSB acts on the T antigen and topoisomerases to unwind DNA, facilitating access of replication proteins, stimulates the activity of polymerases and has a critical role in DNA excision repair (Nature 1991; 349:539)

Ssc1p, Ssc2p, Ssc3p, Ssc4p Heat shock proteins in yeasts

SS disease Sickle cell anemia due to homozygous hemoglobin S

SSPE see Subacute sclerosing panencephalitis

SSSS SSŚ syndrome see Staphylococcus scalded skin syndrome

SS syndrome see Streptococcal-sex syndrome

Stab MICROBIOLOGY *Verb* To inoculate a semisolid bacterial growth medium, usually in a 'slant' tube by using a jabbing motion, usually performed in conjunction with streaking, which combines anaerobic ('stab') and aerobic ('streak') conditions in the same test tube, as used by the triple sugar iron agar tubes; Cf Streak

'Stabbing' invasion SURGICAL PATHOLOGY A pattern of tumor infiltration in which jagged, finger-like strands of malignant epithelial cells invade subepithelial tissue (see figure, facing page), classically seen in the 'garden variety' of squamous cell carcinoma, which is often accompanied by a brisk inflammatory reaction; Cf 'Bulldozing' invasion

Stab cells HEMATOPATHOLOGY Immature, bilobed or not yet fully segmented polymorphonuclear leukocytes that are increased in the peripheral blood in acute infection; see Left shift

Stacked coin appearance GASTROINTESTINAL RADIOLOGY A descriptor for the incomplete filling and parallel spiculation of the plical folds seen in radiocontrast studies of the small intestine (most striking in the jejunum given the prominence of plical folds), corresponding to thickening of the wall by either intramural hemorrhage or hematoma formation, related to anticoagulants, blood dyscrasia, trauma, Meckel's diverticulum, endometriosis or infiltration of the intestinal wall, as in lymphoma; Cf Rouleaux

Staff privileges Admitting privileges The rights that a health professional has as a member of a hospital's medical staff, including hospitalization of his private patients, a seat on committees in the hospital, and participation in decisions relevant to the hospital's future; physicians receive staff privileges when they meet certain standards set by the medical staff and board of trustees, eg board certification, experience and subspecialty expertise, in exchange for which the physician performs certain duties without pay, including teaching, providing emergency care or clinic services Note: Most physicians in the US are private practitioners who usually have staff privileges in more than one hospital; Cf Hospital-based physician, RAPERs

Stage migration see Will Rogers phenomenon

Staggered cut MOLECULAR BIOLOGY A type of scission of the DNA double helix, classically produced by restriction endonucleases, in which there is an overhanging single-stranded tail of four to six nucleotides comprising the 'sticky' ends; see Restriction endonuclease, 'Sticky' ends

Staghorn calculus A concrement with broad arborescence that fills (and forms a radiologically visible 'cast' of) the renal pelvicaliceal system (figure, right) often composed of magnesium ammonium phosphate, concentrated in the urine by urea-splitting bacteria, including *Proteus* species and some staphylococci, inducing urine alkalinization and mineral precipitation; staghorn calculi may also occur in hyperparathyroidism

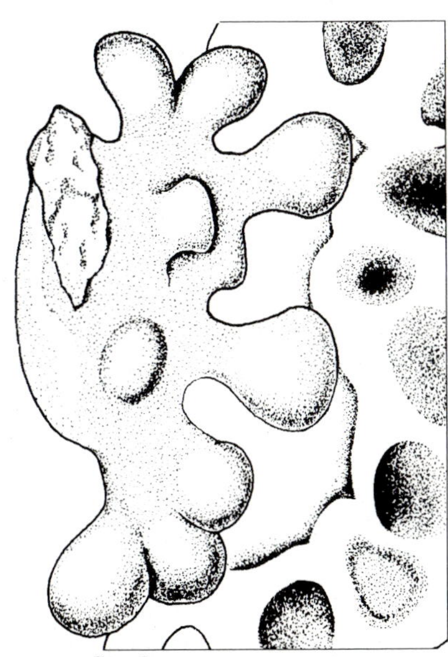

Staghorn concrement

Staghorn pattern ANATOMIC PATHOLOGY A pattern seen by low-power light microscopy, consisting of multiple sharply-branched and jagged vessels, classically seen in hemangiopericytoma, which may also be seen in Kaposi sarcoma, as well as synovial sarcoma, mesenchymal chondrosarcoma, leiomyosarcoma, leiomyoma and myofibromatosis; see Promontory sign

Staging ONCOLOGY An evaluation or 'work-up' of a patient to determine the severity and extent of a disease in order to guide therapy, which is required since each stage has a relatively standard treatment; as an example, stage 1 carcinomas often respond to simple resection, but usually require other modalities including radiotherapy and/or chemotherapy in higher stages; staging is performed for malignancy and occasionally, other conditions eg AIDS; for most malignancies, there are four stages, ranging from the early and well-circumscribed stage I to the aggressive, metastatic and preterminal stage IV; epithelial malignancies are staged according to a tumor's direct extension or depth of invasion, lymph node involvement by tumor and presence of metastases; staging in lymphoid neoplasia requires determination of lymphoid region and bone marrow involvement, presence of transdiaphragmatic spread and presence of clinical symptoms, eg night sweats; see B symptoms, Dukes classification, FIGO, TNM classification

Stagnant loop syndrome see Blind loop syndrome

Stain HISTOLOGY A series of dyes used to selectively color tissues or cells for microscopic examination; hematoxylin and eosin (H & E) colors the nuclei blue (basophilic) and the stromal or support tissue a light pink (acidophilic or eosinophilic) and is by far the most commonly used stain for examination of tissues removed during surgery; other stains of occasional use in diagnostic pathology include acid-fast stain for mycobacteria, Bodian stain for myelin, congo red for amyloid, Fontana-Masson stain for melanin, gram stain for bacteria, Grimelius stain for tumors of neural crest origin, eg APUDoma and carcinoid, Masson's trichrome stain to differentiate between muscle and collagen, periodic acid Schiff stain for complex carbohydrate and mucosubstances and Prussian blue stain of iron

Staircase pattern LABORATORY MEDICINE A descriptor for a pattern seen when a multimeric protein is separated into lanes in an electrophoretic gel, where each step corresponds to a different length of proteins, as seen in von Willebrand factor multimers; see Rocket electrophoresis

Staircase ventilation A form of delivery of positive end-expiratory pressure (PEEP) used in early cardiac arrest, where the lungs are prevented from full collapse (exhalation) in order to 'recruit' collapsed or fluid-filled alveoli, thereby increasing arterial PO_2; since a prolonged increase in intrathoracic pressure can both stop a weakly beating heart and (by distending the stomach) predispose to regurgitation, PEEP is 'stepped-down' as quickly as possible; see PEEP, Step-down therapy

Staircase vertebra A broad, flattened vertebral body with prominent articular facets and spinal processes, seen on a plain antero-posterior film in spondylometaphyseal dysplasia, an autosomal dominant condition with short trunk, short stature and osseous defects

Standard conditions Standard temperature and pressure (STP) A temperature of 0°C and a pressure of 1 atmosphere (760 mm Hg); Cf Standard state

Standard deviation (SD) Square root of the variance A statistical measure of the dispersion of a set of values about a mean, where a graphic representation of the data points is described by a curve with Gaussian distribution, ie bell-shaped; in a Gaussian distribution curve, ± 1 SD includes 68% of the data points, ± 2 SD includes 95.45% of the data and ± 3 SD includes 99.73% Note: SD cannot be determined when two (or more) relatively distinct populations are mixed, eg glucose values of normal subjects and diabetics, as each population can be accurately defined under a single peaked distribution curve Note: WS Gosset published his observations and statistical methods under the nom de plume of 'Student'; his methods were delineated in the seminal paper, '*The Probable Error of a Mean*', which has been designated as the Student '*t*' test

'Standard drink' A unit used in clinical medicine to evaluate alcohol consumption; one standard drink is equal to 44 ml (a 'shot') of 40% alcohol by volume, also known as 'hard' liquor (gin, vodka, whiskey) or 150 ml of 12% alcohol by volume, eg wine or 360 ml of 5% alcohol by volume, eg beer

Standard of care A level of competence in performing medical tasks that is accepted as reasonable and reflective of a skilled and diligent health care provider, which obliges a physician to confine his practice of medicine only to those areas of his expertise; such standards may be delineated by a hospital's medical staff bylaws or the standards published by a specialty college, eg the American College of Obstetricians and Gynecologists; the term has legal ramifications, as any deviation from a 'standard' may be considered to be an act of negligence; since a jury of laypersons cannot be expected to evaluate these standards; in a court of law, the defendant and plaintiff may call upon 'expert witness(es)' specialized in the appropriate field or involved in a germane area of research, who may quote extensively from the literature, defending or refuting the claim that the 'standard' has been adhered to; see Malpractice

Standard operating procedure (SOP) A technique, method or therapeutic modality that is performed 'by the book', using a standard protocol that has met a set of internally or externally defined criteria; see Procedures manual

Standard state A thermodynamic 'reference' state—temperature 25°C; pressure 760 mm Hg; system components present in a defined reference state, ie at neutral pH and 1.0 molar concentration; see Standard conditions

Standing orders Instructions for patient management that are to be followed (usually by the nursing staff) on a regular and consistent basis, unless instructed to the contrary, eg standing orders for medications or changing of wound dressings

'Stanford syndrome' see Indirect costs

Staphylococcal scalded skin syndrome Ritter syndrome A disease of low mortality affecting infants in hospital nurseries, due to exfoliatin produced by *Staphylococcus aureus*, phage group II, type 71, which evokes an enzymatic degradation of the upper granular layer of the epidermis Clinical Prodrome of malaise, fever, irritability, generalized erythema and tenderness of skin surface, followed by midepidermal bullae formation; Cf Toxic epidermal necrolysis, Toxic shock syndrome

'Starch blocker' A crude bean-derived amylase inhibitor that was marketed as a means of allowing one to eat in excess without gaining weight, a claim not corroborated by well-designed studies; the purified amylase inhibitor may be effective in improving glucose tolerance in diabetes mellitus (Mayo Clin Proc 1986; 61:442)

Starch gel electrophoresis A high-resolution zone electrophoresis that uses a hydrolyzed starch support matrix

Starch granuloma see Talc granuloma

'Starry Night' sign A descriptor for the capillary phase pattern in arteriography of a traumatized spleen that demonstrates focal or diffuse small rounded shadows corresponding to stasis of contrast material in the marginal splenic sinusoidal circulation, fancifully likened to the sky seen in Vincent van Gogh's 'Starry Night', painted in 1889 at St Remy-de-Provence

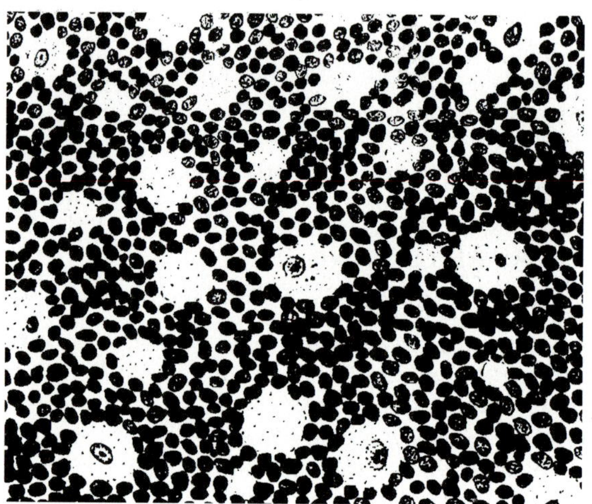

Starry sky sign

Starry sky pattern Hematology A descriptor for a pattern seen in lymph nodes by low-power light microscopy consisting of multiple holes corresponding to lymphoblasts or phagocytosing histiocytes lying within a sheet of relatively monotonous lymphocytes (figure, above), an appearance likened to stars in the sky, a pattern classically in Burkitt's lymphoma, less commonly in other immature lymphomas, granulocytic sarcoma, mediterranean lymphoma, lymphoblastic leukemia, as well as in benign conditions including idiopathic thrombocytopenic purpura and lymphoid hyperplasia MICROBIOLOGY A 'starry sky' pattern is described in the cytoplasm of infected cells with abundant immunostained *Chlamydia trachomatis* NEPHROLOGY A 'starry sky' pattern may be seen by immunofluorescence in acute post-infectious glomerulonephritis due to the finely granular deposition of C3 and immunoglobulin in the capillary walls and mesangium

Start codon MOLECULAR BIOLOGY Initiator codon The mRNA trinucleotide, AUG, which is the signal for initiating protein synthesis, recognized by methyonyl-tRNA; Cf Stop codons

Starvation CLINICAL NUTRITION A condition resulting from prolonged global deprivation of food, occurring in abnormal environmental conditions, eg during war or famine, or in normal society through wilful neglect of others, eg children, the handicapped or elderly by parents, family, care-givers or guardians or by self-neglect in the elderly, mentally feeble or those who irrespective of means, choose to live in apparent poverty; without food and water, the body loses 4-5% of its total weight/day and few survive beyond 10 days; when water is provided, a starving person may survive up to 60 days Clinical Hypovitaminoses, malnutrition, decreased subcutaneous fat with thin, dry and hyperpigmented skin stretched over bone prominences, atrophy of organs, marked attenuation of the gastrointestinal tract, with an enlarged concrement-laden gall bladder; see Minnesota experiment MICROBIOLOGY A state in bacterial colonies, in which either nutrients are actively withheld for experimental expediency or there is depletion of nutrients through consumption

Starvation diabetes Transient glucose intolerance accompanied by glycosuria that occurs when a person ingests carbohydrates after prolonged starvation, an effect attributed to suboptimal glycogen synthesis and storage

Starvation diet see Diet, very low calorie

Starvation stools Watery green feces that develop when a subject is maintained on a clear-liquid starvation-type diet; see Diet (Starvation)

Starzl's criteria see Pittsburgh criteria

'Stat' CLINICAL MEDICINE *Adverb* Immediately LABORATORY MEDICINE *Noun* A specimen, often from the critical care unit or emergency room, that is given priority in the clinical laboratory in order to measure various analytes with immediate potential impact on patient management; 'stats' may include, requests for blood glucose levels, hematocrit, electronic leukocyte differential count, certain enzyme levels, prothrombin time, partial thromboplastin time, BUN and creatinine; Cf 'Stats'

State board An organized body in a sovereign state of the US that oversees the activities of the licensed physicians and health care professionals in that state, assuring that a high standard of practice by the physicians (and others) is maintained and that the use of controlled drug substances is appropriate and without impropriety; Cf Specialty board

State boards Examinations administered by a (US) state board of medical examiners in order to license a physician in a particular state; these examinations play an ever-decreasing role in state medical licensure, as these bodies now rely on standardized national examinations for assessing a physician's knowledge of medicine ; see FLEX exam

Station OBSTETRICS The level of descent of the presenting part in the pelvis in a vaginal delivery; full engagement of the presenting part at the iliac spines is considered station 'zero'; two methods are used to determine fetal station; the more traditional determination of station divides the long axis of the birth canal above and below the ischial spine, where -3 corresponds to a presenting part at the pelvic inlet and +3 corresponds to a presenting part that has reached the perineum; an alternate system starts above and below the ischial spine, measuring five levels, each being one centimeter; given the potential for confusion, the two systems for classifying obstetric stations are not interchangable during a delivery (and two different systems probably should not be used in the same health care facility)

'Stats' Colloquial for statistics; Cf 'Stat'

'Statue of Liberty' position ORTHOPEDICS The mandatory position for the hand (when standing) after reconstructive and corrective hand surgery or after traumatic injury; while sitting, the hand may be rested with the elbow on the table, as long as the hand is above the level of the heart, in order to prevent accumulation of edema that might compromise the arm's blood supply

Status asthmaticus An imprecisely-defined clinical entity of prolonged duration in which there is decreased response by asthmatics to drugs for which they had previously been sensitive; urgent care specialists consider status asthmaticus as the failure to respond to three therapeutic interventions with adrenergic bronchodilators in the emergency department; patients in status asthmaticus are invariably hypoxemic and require hospital admission for monitoring of arterial blood gases and pH Treatment Hypercapneic patients should be rehydrated, given oxygen, large doses of aminophylline and methylprednisone; high-dose intramuscular triamcinolone is more effective than low-dose prednisone (N Engl J Med 1991; 324:585); steroids prevent early relapse of acute asthma as long as they are continued (ibid 1991; 324:788)

Status fibrosus Fibrous transition of muscle caused by pressure from an adjacent compressing tumor, a reactive process that is distinct from muscle fibrosis, which may be either congenital, affecting the vastus intermedius of the quadriceps in children or acquired in adults, related to intradermal injections of penicillin, pentazocine or other drugs that cause local irritation

Status thymolymphaticus A 'condition' described in the late 1940s and 1950s as pathological thymic hypertrophy, which was treated with radiotherapy; it later became apparent that the thymus undergoes normal physiological hypertrophy, reaching a maximum of 15-25 grams at puberty, involuting thereafter; those who received radiotherapy for status thymolymphaticus are at an increased risk for thyroid and breast malignancy; 36 years after irradiation, the incidence of breast cancer was two-fold that of age-matched siblings, with an adjusted rate ratio of 3.6 (N Engl J Med 1989; 321:1281) Note: Radiotherapy was at one time used for a vast array of conditions, eg hypertrophy of tonsils, acne, eustachian tube dysfunction, facial hemangiomas, pertussis, tinea capitis and others

Statute of limitations LEGAL MEDICINE Background: In a lawsuit for negligence against a physician(s) or hospital, the plaintiff has two or three years (depending upon the state in the USA) in which to file a claim for damages; the time period begins either from the moment the act occurred or from the moment the plaintiff discovered that the act was negligent; for children, this period usually begins after he/she reaches age 21 or 18 (or younger if they are considered 'emancipated minors', by virtue of marriage or financial independence)

STD see Sexually-transmitted diseases

Steakhouse syndrome A clinical complex caused by plugging of the lower esophago-gastric sphincter with a large, poorly chewed bolus of food, usually meat, often steak, accompanied by intense epigastric pain that resolves spontaneously if the food passes into the stomach Predisposing factors Alcohol imbibition, edentulousness; Cf Cafe coronary, Sushi syncope

Steal syndrome(s) Vascular steal syndromes Symptom complexes that appear when arterial stenoses reduce regional oxygenation and compromised organs and tissues 'steal' blood from adjacent regions; steal syndromes are adjectivally designated by the affected artery, eg aorticoceliac steal syndrome or subclavian steal syndrome and may involve the mesenteric, pulmonary, subclavian, renal-splanchnic, spinal, subclavian and thyroid-cervical arterial systems; vascular steal syndromes are most commonly due to 1) Atherosclerosis 2) Therapy, eg coronary (artery) steal syndrome, a potential effect of the use of vasoactive agents for chronic anginal pain, which cause an increase of blood flow to well-vascularized regions with normal oxygenation and a decrease of blood flow to the stenosed and nonreactive vessels or 3) Malformations, eg intracranial steal syndrome, in which increased blood flow into a cerebrovascular malformation is accompanied by progressive neurological disability due either to compression or flow of the blood away from the underlying cerebral cortex; Cf 'Robin hood' syndrome

Steely hair syndrome see Kinky hair syndrome

Steeple sign see Gothic arch sign

Steering wheel 'syndrome' A blunt chest injury affecting an automobile driver in a 'head-on' collision; the heart bears the brunt of the injury with contusion of the anterior epicardium and myocardium, compression of the heart between the sternum and vertebral column and sudden increases in intrathoracic pressure, potentially rupturing cardiac structures, including the ventricular septum, chordae or the free wall Note: Only 20% of major blunt chest injury victims have elevated creatinine phosphokinase and thus the index of suspicion should be high; Cf Dashboard fracture, Padded dash(board) syndrome, Whiplash

Stem cell(s) Any primitive cell that is capable of dividing and giving rise to both primitive daughter cells like itself and cells capable of undergoing differentiation; in adults, the stem cell capability of the early embryo is lost except in the bone marrow where it is retained by the hematolymphoid precursors; these cells are divided into the most primitive and undifferentiated (pluripotent) cells and the partially differentiated (unipotent) cells; in mice, the 'ultimate' stem cell (ie the most primitive cell capable of reconstituting the entire hemato-lymphoid system) subset is negative for lineage differentiation (eg granulocyte, macrophage and others) markers and bears the cell surface differentiation antigen, Thy-1 and an antigen designated as the stem cell antigen-1 or Sca-1 Note: Mature blood cells require cytokines that induce growth or division, eg IL-3 and colony-stimulating factors and differentiation, eg macrophage-granulocyte inducer-type 2; these cytokines act in a programmed fashion, where the interactions determine the balance of mature and immature cells in normal hematopoietic development

Step-down therapy CARDIOLOGY Downward 'titration' or reduction by stages of the doses and agents used to control blood pressure; the 'steps' in the control of blood pressure range from thiazide diuretics, β blockers or converting enzyme inhibitor (mild hypertension, diastolic < 100 mg Hg) to hydralazine, prazosine, minoxidil, guanethidine or furosemide (severe hypertension, diastolic pressure > 120 mHg); Cf 'Staircase' ventilation

Step formation see Snowcap appearance

Stepladder configuration GASTROINTESTINAL RADIOLOGY A pattern seen by a barium enema of the ascending colon, in which rigid fibrosis causes transverse linear fissures intersecting with gullies of contrast material lying in deep longitudinal ulcers, a finding described in regional enteritis (Crohn's disease), when radiocontrast 'spills' past the constricted and narrowed terminal ileum, imparting a 'railroad track' appearance on gross examination; see Garden hose appearance, String sign RHEUMATOLOGY A descriptor for the consecutive subluxations in the cervical spine seen in rheumatoid arthritis, variably accompanied by narrowing of the intervertebral disk space

Stercoral ulcer A colonic ulcer that develops in elderly or mentally-retarded patients with intractable constipation secondary to pressure of impacted fecal material and sluggish mesenteric arterial circulation

Stercoroma A tumor-like fecal mass in the rectum

Stereo drawings Background Three-dimensional (3-D) analysis of complex molecules allows determination of their 'signature' in terms of reactive or binding sites and is having an increasing impact on the design of new therapeutic agents; stereo images appear with relative frequency in major scientific journals; to view the image in stereo, either: 1) Hold the figure 10 cm from the eyes without glasses, focus on a distant object, lower the eyes to the drawing and re-focus on the middle image, giving the right-handed (correct) form or 2) Hold the page at about 20 cm, allow the eyes to 'cross', then re-focus on the middle image for the exotic left-handed stereoisomer (Science 1986; 233:623c); see Protein structure

Stereotactic radiotherapy A therapeutic modality using heavy charged particles (protons or helium ions), photons (γ radiation) or a linear-accelerator to treat intracranial lesions that are inaccessible to conventional neurosurgery; the intent of stereotactic radiotherapy is to induce local endothelial proliferation with vascular wall thickening, occluding the malformation, while sparing adjacent cerebral tissue; a beam of mono-energetic heavy particles such as helium has the advantage of 1) Delivering a very high dose of radiation to a tissue depth known as the 'Bragg ionization peak' 2) A sharper lateral edge and 3) Minimal amounts of secondarily excited, ie radioactive particles; stereotactic radiotherapy effectively reduces symptoms in inaccessible arteriovenous malformations, but has a long latency between therapy and response and suffers a 12% risk of serious neurologic sequelae (N Engl J Med 1990; 323:96); see Gamma knife

Steric hindrance A physicochemical barrier that prevents or attenuates a reaction or a conformational response

Sterilization A process that destroys pathogens, by a) Autoclaving Pressurized moist heat, 121.5°C x 30 minutes b) Dry heat sterilization at 129.8°C x 2 hours and c) Gas sterilization with ethylene oxide (used for equipment that cannot withstand high temperatures, which has the disadvantage of being carcinogenic, expensive, explosive and irritating to mucosal membranes; see Disinfection

STEROID CELL TUMOR CLASSIFICATION

Stromal luteoma Benign tumors that produce estrogen, rarely androgens

Leydig cell tumor Most (82%) are benign, one-half produce excess androgens and they are subdivided into i) Hilus cell tumor and ii) Non-hilus cell tumor

Steroid cell tumor of adrenal cortical type, a tumor that may cause Cushing syndrome

Steroid cell tumor, not otherwise specified, the most common group, no age predilection, cell of origin unclear; one-fourth are clinically malignant (greater than 7 cm in diameter, with cystic degeneration and necrosis)

Steroid cell tumor A tumor also designated 'lipid cell tumor', a term less preferred by RE Scully, the most widely-read scholar of ovarian pathology, as lipid in various ovarian tumors is not uncommon (table, above); see Lipid cell tumor

Steroid receptor superfamily CELL PHYSIOLOGY A group of structurally similar hormone receptors located adjacent to the nucleus that are involved in signal transduction; the binding of a ligand to the receptor is thought to induce an allosteric change allowing the receptor-hormone complex to bind to a DNA response element in the promoter region of a target gene, modulating gene expression; these receptors have a critical role in neuroendocrine and signal transduction leading to growth, morphogenesis, homeostasis and proliferation (Nature 1990; 347:645, 709); steroid receptor superfamily ligands include glucocorticoids, mineralocorticoids, progesterones, estrogens, estrogen-related 1 hormone, estrogen-related 2 hormone, androgens, ecdysone, retinoic acid, vitamin D_3 and thyroid hormone, as well as the viral oncogene product, v-erbA, and a protein implicated in hepatocellular carcinoma

Sticky end Cohesive end MOLECULAR BIOLOGY An oligomer of complementary COOH- and NH_2- termini from the opposite ends of segments of double-stranded DNA, that result from a 'staggered cut', usually by a restriction endonuclease; sticky ends may be used as points of insertion of DNA into various cloning vectors; see Restriction endonuclease, Staggered cut

Stiff baby syndrome An autosomal dominant complex of variable penetration characterized by increased startle reflex and virtually continuous motor activity by electromyography, choking, vomiting and dysphagia, which may improve with age; Cf Floppy infant syndrome(s)

Stiff heart 'syndrome' CARDIOLOGY A non-specific term for ventricular pump failure due to restrictive heart disease **Clinical** Chest pain, exertional dyspnea, increased venous pressure, extra-diastolic murmurs, hepatomegaly, ascites and edema **Etiology** Idiopathic or related to amyloidosis, constrictive pericarditis (irradiation, mycosis, trauma and tuberculosis), hemochromatosis and myocardiopathies of various etiologies; Cf 'Stone' heart

Stiff lung syndrome see Adult respiratory distress syndrome

Stiff man syndrome A rare motor dysfunction disorder with a 2:1 male:female ratio **Clinical** Stiffness of axial and appendicular muscles with intermittent superimposed painful muscle spasms precipitated by emotional or physical stress, accompanied by lower back pain, hyperlordosis, motor and gait abnormalities, diaphoresis and tachycardia **Etiology** Unknown, variously thought to be idiopathic, autosomal dominant or the most probably autoimmune, given the presence of antibodies against glutamic acid decarboxylase (Nature 1990; 347:151) and pancreatic islet cells; it is associated with epilepsy, insulin-dependent diabetes mellitus and other organ specific autoimmune disorders, eg myasthenia gravis, thyroiditis and adrenalitis **Diagnosis** Simultaneous video-electroencephalographic-surface electromyography demonstrates continuous motor unit activity in the afflicted muscles while the muscle is at rest (Mayo Clin Proc 1990; 65:960) and abnormal activity of small gamma motor neurons **Treatment** Cortisol if there is adrenocortical dysfunction, benzodiazepines, plasma exchange (Mayo Clin Proc 1989; 64:629rv;1991; 66:300)

Stiff neck syndrome see Wry neck

Stiff skin syndrome A non-progressive autosomal dominant condition of uncertain origin characterized by accumulation of hyaluronidase-digestible material, possibly a variant of mucopolysaccharidosis, with focal indurations of the skin, renal concrement formation, joint enlargement, diabetes mellitus and duodenal ulcers

Stillbirth Fetal death prior to complete extraction or expulsion from the mother of a product of conception, irrespective of the duration of pregnancy; death is indicated by the lack of evidence of life or movement once the separation occurs

Stimulation test A generic term for any clinical assay that evaluates the synthetic reserve capacity of a substance of interest, providing information on whether the production of the hormone is maximal; stimulation tests include the metapyrone test for adrenal hypofunction and the maximum acid output (MAO) assay in Zollinger-Ellison syndrome; Cf Suppression test

Stippling An adjectival descriptor for a punctate appearance or, in radiology, white granularity in a radiolucent background, which, parenthetically is a term that is similar, if not identical to the more graphic adjectival descriptor of 'salt-and-pepper' BONE RADIOLOGY Punctate calcifications in epiphyseal ossification centers, which may occur in congenital calcific chondrodystrophy, cretinism, ischemic necrosis (osteochondrosis), multiple epiphyseal dysplasia, pituitary gigantism, sclerotic osteopetrosis and sclerotic osteopoikilosis COLONIC ENDOSCOPY A pattern of fine granularity of the mucosa described as being most characteristic of early ulcerative colitis ESOPHAGEAL ENDOSCOPY A pattern seen in esophagitides due to corrosive agents, reflux, infections, eg candidiasis and radiation HEMATOLOGY see Basophilic stippling RENAL RADIOLOGY A pattern seen in papillary transitional cell carcinomas with incomplete filling of the pelvi-caliceal system due to tumoral replacement in the intravenous pyelogram

Stochastic process CLINICAL DECISION-MAKING A method for problem solving that is defined by the laws of probability, ie randomness, where every step is uncertain and the solution is by trial and error; Cf Aunt Millie approach, Heuristic process

Stoichiometry The study of the quantitative (mass, volume, moles) relations that chemical compounds in reacting systems have with each other

Stocking-and-glove distribution NEUROLOGY A pattern of peripheral nerve disease characterized by a relatively sharply-demarcated loss of pain, touch, temperature, position and vibration sensation, accompanied by weakness, muscular atrophy and loss of tendon reflexes, eg the 'stocking' pattern of distal diabetic polyneuropathy is characterized by waxing and waning paresthesias that worsen at night

'Stomach virus' A colloquial lay term for any gastroenteritis of presumed viral origin that may be accompanied by diarrhea, fever and possibly also nausea, vomiting and abdominal pain; viral gastroenteritis is commonly caused by enteroviruses, rotavirus and possibly also astroviruses

Stomatocytes Stomos, Greek, Mouth Cup-shaped erythrocytes that are prominent in Rh_{null} disease, which may be seen in acute alcoholism, hepatopathies, an artefact seen in red cells stored in a hypotonic solution, or related to various red cell membrane defects, ameliorated with splenomegaly

Stomatocytosis An autosomal dominant condition characterized by increased osmotic fragility of red cells, autohemolysis, splenomegaly and mild anemia that is partially corrected by splenectomy

'Stoned' 'Wasted' SUBSTANCE ABUSE A colloquial expression for a state of quasi-stupor of varying intensity that may be induced by various abuse substances, eg heroin, marijuana and alcohol Note: Those who abuse sustances generally prefer to stay in a state of pleasant euphoria, or 'high'; a commonly used hierarchy of 'street' terms (in the USA) for the subjective sensations that occur during a session of substance abuse begins with a low-level 'buzz', followed by a 'high', as the intensity of the drug's effect increases, after which the abuser is 'stoned' which when extreme, is referred to as being 'wasted'; 'High'; Cf 'Bad trip'

'Stone' heart CARDIOLOGY Irreversible ischemia-induced cardiac rigor mortis, in which the heart undergoes global spastic contraction in systole; the anoxia rapidly depletes glycogen and ATP, causing death; a heart of stone is exceptionally rare and is most common in severe heart disease (New York Heart Association class IV); see Rigor mortis; Cf Stiff heart 'syndrome'

'Stones, bones and groans' A facetious, but accurate clinical triad seen in hyperparathyroidism, where prolonged elevation of parathyroid hormone and end-organ response thereto results in disseminated calcium deposition (stones), osteoporosis (bones) and gastrointestinal symptoms including nausea, vomiting, anorexia and weight loss and recalcitrant peptic ulcers (groans)

Stop codon Terminator codon Any one of the three triplets (UAA, UGA and UAG) of nucleotides on a messenger RNA molecule, which when translated, stops the elongation of the chain of polypeptides; see Codon; Cf Degenerate code, Start codon

Storage disease(s) A group of diseases often designated 'Inborn errors of metabolism', in which a defective or functionally absent enzyme causes organ dysfunction through accumulation of precursor substances derived from metabolism of glycogen, amino acids, often contained within lysosomes; each has a relatively distinct pattern of organ involvement, eg in glycogen storage disease, the overload substrates compromises the liver, skeletal muscle and cardiac muscle; see Brancher and Debrancher disease

Storage lesion TRANSFUSION MEDICINE The constellation of changes occurring in a unit of packed red cells during storage; from the time of collection to the time of transfusion, pH decreases from 7.6 to 6.7; ATP falls from 100% to 45%; 2,3 DPG decreases to less than 10% of original levels (replenished within 24 hours of transfusion); potassium rises from 4.2 to 78.5 mmol/L (US: 4.2 to 78.5 mEq/L); ammonium rises to 470 μmol/L (US: 800 μg/dl); sodium falls from 169 to 111 mmol/L (US: 169 to 111 mEq/L); free hemoglobin in the plasma rises from 82 to 6580 mg/L (US: 8.2 to 658 mg/dl) and the levels of labile proteins, eg complement, fibronectin and coagulation factors have fallen to negligible levels Note: The physiologic effects of storage lesions are negligible in the absence of a previous compromise of the patient's (recipient's) status; see Red cell preservatives

Storage pool disease(s) A group of platelet disorders due to deficiencies of platelet granules, divided into a) α granule storage pool disease, see Gray platelet syndrome and b) Dense granule deficiency or delta-storage pool disease **Clinical** Moderate bleeding **Laboratory** Prolonged bleeding time, decreased platelet ADP content and serotonin levels Note: Dense granules are also deficient in Chediak-Higashi, Hermansky-Pudlak, TAR and Wiskott-Aldrich syndromes **Treatment** Hemostasis with platelet transfusions, cryoprecipitate and desmopressin acetate (DDAVP), which release von Willebrand factor from storage sites, the first-line treatment of choice

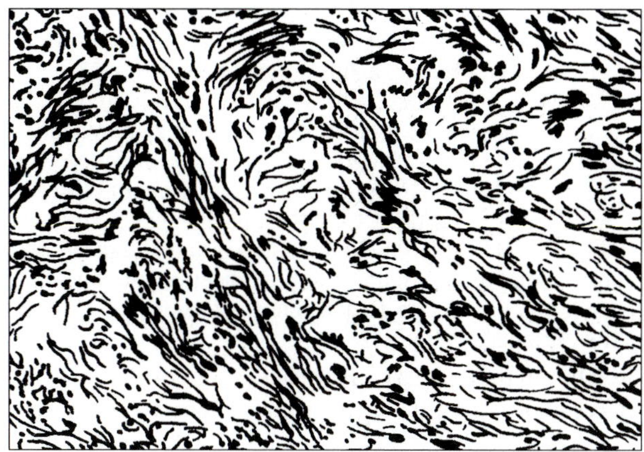

Storiform pattern

Storiform pattern Storia, Latin, woven hemp, mat A pattern seen by low-power light microscopy, characterized by loosely-arranged whorls of elongated, spindled fibroblast-like cells; although highly non-specific, the pattern is most often seen in fibrohistiocytic lesions and may appear in benign tumors, eg dermatofibroma, giant cell tumor of tendon sheath, in tumors of low malignant potential, eg atypical fibroxanthoma, dermatofibrosarcoma protuberans and in frankly malignant tumors, eg malignant fibrous histiocytoma; the storiform pattern may also be seen in non-histiocytic lesions, including nodular fascitis, leiomyoma, leiomyosarcoma, schwann cell tumors and spindle cell carcinoma; see Cartwheel pattern, Pinwheel pattern

Stork leg see Champagne bottle legs

Stork marks NEONATOLOGY Capillary 'nevi' seen as focal 'spots' on the face and neck; the lesions usually fade within the first year or two of life, but may persist on the neck

'Stormy' fermentation MICROBIOLOGY The descriptor for a turbid reaction of *Clostridium* species in litmus milk with coagulation and gas production

Straddle lesion A complex injury of the perineum, usually due to a fall in which the point of impact is between the legs (as in falling on a fence), accompanied by major trauma to the posterior urethra, extravasation of blood and urine through Buck's fascia, often extending into the scrotum, perineum, central tensor and anterior abdominal wall under Scarpa's fascia Note: Straddle-type bicycle injuries in young females may mimic the changes seen in sexual assault

Straight back (and flat chest) syndrome A physiologic variant 'condition' due to a loss of the normal thoracic kyphosis, which reduces the anteroposterior chest diameter, making the pulmonary artery and right hilum more prominent, displacing the heart to the left, giving the false impression of cardiomegaly; a straight back is associated with atrial septal defects and scoliosis and may cause mild pulmonary vein obstruction and dilatation evoking a harsh late systolic ejection murmur, which is asymptomatic unless the findings are misinterpreted by the examiner, in which situation, an otherwise healthy individual may become a cardiac 'cripple'

Strangulated hernia Prolapse of a loop of intestine into a hernial sac with vascular compromise and with time, infarction of the entire prolapsed loop; Cf Incarcerated hernia

Strap cell SURGICAL PATHOLOGY An elongated eosinophilic cell with vague cross-striations classically seen in rhabdomyosarcomas of intermediate differentiation; 'strap' cells may also be seen in teratomas with rhabdomyosarcomatous differentiation Note: The 'strap cell' described in inflammatory pseudotumors lacks cross-striations

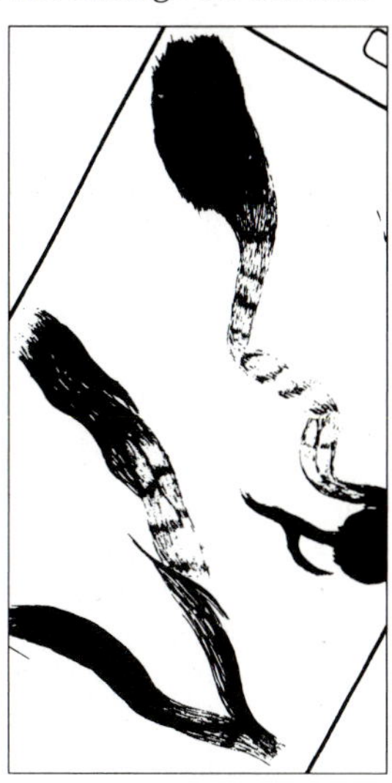

Strap cells

Strap muscles Colloquial for the small, flat infrahyoid muscles inferior to the hyoid bone which include the sternohyoideus, omohyoideus, sternothyroideus, thyrohyoideus and levator glandulae thyroideae

Strawberry A descriptor applied to any relatively round, dark red or occasionally dark green mass or lesion, punctuated by light-colored dots, mimicking the fruit, *Euonymus americanus*

Strawberry angioma A nasopharyngeal hemangioma, which when it affects children, may cause airway obstruction; rarely, if the blood volume flowing into a hemangioma is large, arteriovenous shunting may cause cardiac decompensation Note: Giant angiomas with thrombocytopenia, are eponymically dignified as the Kassabach-Merritt syndrome

Strawberry cell A morula-type plasma cell with red-purple cytoplasm, punctuated by minivacuoles of polyclonal immunoglobulins, seen in the perivascular cuff of 'round cells' in chronic African trypanosomiasis

Strawberry cervix Colpitis macularis A descriptive term for the quasi-pathognomonic colposcopic appearance of subepithelial punctate petechiae seen in the uterine cervix infected by the sexually-transmissible *Trichomonas vaginalis*, variably accompanied by 'Double hairpin' capillaries; see Strawberry mucosa

Strawberry foot rot An actinomycetales, *Dermatophilus congolensis*, which infects sheep, causing pustular dermatitis

Strawberry gallbladder A descriptor for the appearance of the mucosa seen in the relatively common cholesterosis of the gallbladder, where aggregates of cholesterol/lipid-laden histiocytes overlie an erythematous or verdant mucosa, occasionally causing a giant cell reaction

Strawberry hemangioma Strawberry mark Strawberry nevus A raised irregular, bright-red capillary hemangioma or reactive proliferation of small subdermal vessels first seen in infancy, that expands aggressively for several years then involutes or disappears (90% are no longer visible by age seven) Histopathology Abundant closely packed and mitotically active spindled cells in spaces with relatively little blood Treatment Excision if necessary or high dose prednisone

Strawberry mark see Strawberry hemangioma

Strawberry mucosa GYNECOLOGY A lesion identical to the strawberry cervix, characterized by edema, erythema and spotting of tiny blisters, due to infection of the female genital mucosa, vaginal wall, portio and urethral meatus, usually caused by *Trichomonas vaginalis* and seen by colposcopy in up to 92% of women infected with *T vaginalis*, often accompanied by yellowish and/or purulent discharge, vulvar itching and a fish-like odor (J Am Med Assoc 1989; 261:571) Histopathology Intense superficial polymorphous cell infiltration by neutrophils, lymphocytes, plasma cells

Strawberry nevus see Strawberry hemangioma

Strawberry spots Small erythematous spots seen by endoscopy of the large intestine infected with *Entamoeba histolytica*

Strawberry tongue A characteristic enanthema of the tongue, characterized by hypertrophy of the fungiform papillae, accompanied by changes of the filiform papillae in a bright red background; the tongue is classically seen in scarlet fever, but also occurs in Kawasaki's disease (mucocutaneous lymph node syndrome), toxic shock syndrome and in the early stages of yellow fever

Straw consumer A term that is a variant of 'straw man', ie an imaginary person who has been created to serve a particular purpose (in its original form, a straw man was made by farmers to scare away crows, ie a 'scarecrow'), or alternately, a proposition or hypothesis created for the sake of argument; a straw consumer, then, is an imaginary consumer of health care (or other) services, who would have opinions on potentially controversial issues, eg the practice of HIV-infected dentists or surgeons

Straw Peter syndrome A neurologic complex affecting children, more commonly boys, who are purposelessly hyperactive, impulsive, aggressive and have a short attention span with minimal cortical dysfunction Treatment Methylphenidate Struwwelpeter was a character in a poem about a frenetic, unruly and unkempt boy Note: This syndrome is possibly the same as the Attention-deficit hyperactivity syndrome, see there

Streak MICROBIOLOGY *Verb* To inoculate a semisolid bacterial growth plate by running a culture loop across the medium in three different directions or in a 'slant' tube performed in conjunction with stabbing, which provides anaerobic ('stab') and aerobic ('streak') conditions in the same test tube; Cf Stab

'Streaked' tonsils Striated yellow-orange discoloration caused by aggregates of lipid-laden macrophages in the tonsil, as well as in the thymus, lymph nodes, bone marrow and gastrointestinal tract; streaked tonsils are seen in about 80% of patients with Tangier's disease, an entity characterized by hepatosplenomegaly and peripheral neuropathy Laboratory Very low cholesterol and HDL, both due to complete deficiency of apolipoproteins I and II

Streak ovaries Clinical genetics Thin, rounded fibrous gonads with an attenuated cortex, medulla and hilum typical of the histologically infantile ovaries of Turner (45, XO) syndrome; oocytes are invariably absent in adult streak ovaries as their development requires granulosa cell activity that doesn't occur in absence of a second X chromosome; primary ovarian tumors in streak ovaries are rare given the virtual absence of germ cells Note: Turner syndrome patients are at an increased risk for endometrial carcinoma, a complication attributed to neoplasia 'driven' by replacement estrogen, rather than the chromosomal defect

Stream see Downstream, Upstream

Street virus A virus, eg rabies, that is in its natural or genetically unmodified form, and which may be obtained from domestic and wild animals

'Strep throat' A generic term that may be applied to virtually any infectious erythema of the oropharynx and tonsils; although the name implies a bacterial origin (streptococcal throat) and is usually treated with antibiotics, it is most commonly due to viruses, eg Epstein-Barr virus and cytomegalic inclusion virus and less commonly due to streptococci, diphtheria, tularemia, toxoplasmosis, brucellosis, salmonellosis and tuberculosis; true streptococcal pharyngitis has a 2-4 day incubation period, pain on swallowing, headache, malaise, fever, anorexia; children may also suffer nausea, vomiting and abdominal pain Physical examination Extreme hyperemia covered by punctate or confluent yellow-gray exudate with edema, lymphoid hyperplasia, causing an estimated 30 million cases annually; the organism's virulence is related to the M protein, against which a vaccine is under development (Science 1989; 244:1487)

Streptococcal sex syndrome A rare recurrent erythroderma resulting from post-coital *Streptococcus agalactiae* bacteremia, related to poor lymphatic drainage in women who have had perineal radiotherapy or lymph node excision for malignancy (J Am Med Assoc 1987; 257:3260)

Streptokinase A fibrinolytic enzyme used to lyse thrombi in early myocardial infarction, with the purpose of minimizing or reducing the size of the infarct in arterial occlusions and in pulmonary thromboembolism; streptokinase has an efficacy similar to that of tissue plasminogen activator and urokinase; see tPA

Stress fracture A fracture resulting from repeated, relatively trivial trauma to the bone, affecting runners (fibula or tibia), soldiers (metatarsal bones), jack-hammer operators (metacarpal bones) and office workers (coccyx)

Stress testsee Treadmill exercise

Stress ulcer(s) Stress-driven individuals are thought to be prone to peptic ulceration, a posit supported by animal models; these ulcers have been subdivided according to presumed etiology **ACTIVITY ULCER** A type of gastric erosion that is produced when rats are placed in a running wheel with only one hour of food per day **EXERTION ULCER** Gastric ulceration that is associated with excessive and unexpected forced activity, eg a rotating cage keeps the rodents constantly running and the gastric juices flowing to the maximum **RESTRAINT ULCER** An ulcer that appears in rats within hours of being placed in a very confined spaces, especially when the ambient temperature is lowered **SHOCK ULCER** Gastric ulceration in humans that is related to burns, eg Curling's ulcer, ischemia, neurologic injury, eg Cushing's ulcer, sepsis or trauma; see Executive monkey, 'Toxic core', Type A personality

'Stretch marks' Pregnancy striae Purplish 'stripes' seen on the lower abdomen, thighs, on the iliac crests and breasts in pregnancy and in corticosteroid excess, which become whitish after birth but do not disappear

Striction The reduction of the total volume of two substances when mixed, due to solute-solvent interaction

Stringent factor An enzyme that synthesizes ppGpp and pppGpp, which regulate the rate of RNA synthesis in the stringent response, a decrease in RNA synthesis that occurs in wild bacteria after removal of an essential amino acid

String of beads sign GASTROINTESTINAL RADIOLOGY A descriptor for the radiologic findings in small intestine obstruction, where the 'beads' correspond to pockets of gas oriented in an oblique line, a function of the amount of fluid and the intensity of peristalsis; although characteristic of mechanical obstruction, this sign may also be seen in adynamic ileus due to inflammation PULMONARY RADIOLOGY A descriptor for distribution of sarcoid granulomata along the pulmonary septae

String of pearls sign RADIOLOGY A descriptor for the multiple arterial dilatations and strictures seen in fibromuscular dysplasia, a condition affecting small and medium-sized arteries including the renal and extracranial cephalic vessels

String sign GASTROINTESTINAL RADIOLOGY COLON A linear fraying of the barium column with luminal stenosis, spasm, ulceration and scarring, seen in the terminal ileum in long-standing Crohn's disease that is rarely also seen in ulcerative colitis; grossly, the affected intestine is thickened, rigid and has been fancifully likened to a 'Garden hose' ESOPHAGUS An elongated, narrowed and straight single, occasionally dual channel(s) of contrast as seen in well-developed hypertrophic pyloric stenosis

String test Rope's test RHEUMATOLOGY A bedside test for determining the viscosity of synovial fluid, or 'quality' of the mucin clot in synovial fluid, which is a reflection of hyaluronidate polymerization; the further a drop of synovial fluid falls before separating ('stringing effect'), the greater the fluid's viscosity, ergo the more normal; a few drops of synovial fluid are added to 10 ml of diluted (2-5%) acetic acid and the length of the 'strand' formed between drops of fluid is measured; a decrease in the strand length implies chemical deterioration due to inflammatory (sepsis, gout, rheumatoid arthritis), but not degenerative joint disease; see Spinnbarkeit UROLOGY A macroscopic method for determining active spermatogenesis; the testicle is bisected, forceps are used to grasp the parenchyma and visually note the separation of the strands of fibers

Stripping BIOCHEMISTRY Hydrolysis of amino acid from an aminoacyl-tRNA MOLECULAR BIOLOGY Separation of ribosomal proteins from ribosomes PATHOLOGY Removal of the renal capsule at the autopsy table in order to evaluate the renal surface, which may demonstrate lesions of hypertension; see Flea-bitten kidneys, Rat-bitten kidneys SURGERY Removal of the renal capsule from the kidney and pedicles in order to interrupt the lymphaticorenal fistulas, thereby treating the intractable chyluria induced by ***Wuchereria bancrofti*** (N Engl J Med 1990; 323:552c)

Stroke Apoplexy A condition that is the leading cause of disability in the USA (500 000 new victims annually, 20-30% of whom are left with severe residua) and the third leading cause of death (20-30% early mortality); a stroke is characterized by abrupt loss of consciousness due to either hemorrhage or vascular occlusion of cerebral blood vessels, leading to immediate paralysis, weakness and speech defects Etiology The predisposing factors of cigarette smoking and hypertension are more predictive of carotid atherosclerosis than are serum lipid and lipoprotein levels (Mayo Clin Proc 1991; 66:259); the residua of a stroke may be either temporary, see Transient ischemic attack or permanent, causing an Alzheimer's dementia-like complex due to a 'shower' of small infarctions, see Multi-infarct dementia or with large losses of cerebral tissue, may result in a lacunar state, see Ètat lacunaire Pathophysiology After an arterial occlusion, infarction of the cerebral tissue (core region) irrigated by the occluded vessel is inevitable, unless the clot is lysed immediately; an adjacent or penumbral region surrounding the core region may be salvaged if the collateral circulation is adequate; the ischemia-induced damage is explained by the glutamate cascade model, which may be 'dissected' for examining treatment options Prevention Systolic hypertension is a major cause of strokes; low-dose chlorthalidone therapy reduces the incidence (5-year absolute benefit) of strokes by 30 events/1000 participants and major cardiovascular events by 55 events/1000 (J Am Med Assoc 1991; 265:3255)

'Stroke belt' Southeastern USA, a region with a high incidence of hypertension in the black population, among whom the blood pressure is 10 mm Hg systolic and 6 mm Hg diastolic higher than in similar subjects in Colorado (J Am Med Assoc 1991; 265:2957c); the 'stroke belt' phenomenon remains an epidemiologic conundrum of uncertain origin variously attributed to differences in geography, intensity of skin color, diet or other factors

Stromal 'crumbling' Fragmentation dense stromal cellularity, a non-specific histologic feature of dysfunctional uterine bleeding, seen in a specimen from an endometrial curettage

Stromalysin-3 A member of the secreted matrix metalloproteinase family, which degrades the extracellular matrix and has been identified in the (desmoplastic) stroma of invasive, but not in situ carcinoma of the female breast; such stromal factors are thought to be responsible for invasion in epithelial malignancy: gene expression, ie transcription of this and other matrix metalloproteinases may be induced by diffusible factors, eg platelet-derived growth factor, fibroblast growth factor, transforming growth factor-α and cytokines, providing a mechanism by which malignant cells may effect the next step in their progression (Nature 1990; 348:699)

Structural gene Any segment of DNA that is transcribed into messenger RNA and translated into a polypeptide or protein

Structural protein A protein that is a structural, eg collagen, intermediate filaments and microtubules, rather than a functional component of a cell

Struma ovarii The presence of mature thyroid tissue as the predominant tissue in an ovarian teratoma, potentially causing clinical hyperthyroidism; 5-10% of struma ovarii become malignant, the only absolute criterion for which is the presence of metastasis

Struvite concrements Triple phosphate stones Renal concrements composed of magnesium ammonium phosphate, $Mg(NH_4)(PO_4)\text{-}6H_20$, formed in the renal pelvis, potentially giving rise to a Staghorn calculus, and in the urinary bladder by action of urea-splitting bacteria, eg *Proteus, Pseudomonas, Klebsiella* and *Staphylocccus* species; struvite stones appear as coffin-lid crystals in alkaline urine

Strychnine A highly toxic rodenticide (that is less than effective in this regard as rats avoid its bitter taste), that elicits central nervous system hyperactivity, causing painful, recurrent tonic motor seizures, muscle tightness and cramping, risus sardonicus, followed by marked flaccidity, decorticate posturing and death; strychnine may be ingested by humans with suicidal or homicidal intent; symptoms appear at doses as low as 15 mg, death occurs with doses above 60 mg, through Renshaw cell inhibition and terminal respiratory paralysis Treatment Control seizures with diazepam and phenobarbital; for muscle relaxation, curare and succinylcholine

STS see Serological tests for syphilis

ST-segment depression see Silent ischemia

STS-map Sequence-tagged site map MOLECULAR BIOLOGY A means (Science 1989; 245:1434) for standardizing communication among the research groups involved in constructing the 3 billion base pair human genome map; the STS proposal is not an alternative to the current strategies for mapping the human genome, but rather redefines the end product; since all DNA mapping strategies use cloned segments of DNA as landmarks, regardless of whether they are 'contig' maps, restriction maps, polymorphism maps or whether the landmarks are sequences that hybridize in situ to a particular chromosomal band, the STS protocol calls for all mapping groups, regardless of whether they are searching for a gene or sequencing an entire chromosome (J Am Med Assoc 1989; 262:2353), to also sequence a short tract of DNA from the clone that defines the landmark; this then allows both 'little science' and 'big science' laboratories, to participate in the Human Genome project; the goal is to construct an STS map with landmarks every 10^5 bases within the first five years of the Human genome project; see cDNA library, Human Genome project

Stucco keratosis A form of seborrheic keratoses, which is gray-white and symmetrical, measuring 1-3 mm in diameter, that occurs on distal extremities Histopathology Hyperkeratosis with a church-spire-like extension of papillae Treatment Removal by scraping

Student's elbow Bursitis of the olecranon related to prolonged resting of the elbows on table tops, classically seen in students

Student's '*t*' test A statistical test that determines whether the mean value of 'set A' data differs significantly from that of 'set B' data; the *t*-test may be performed after an '*F* test' Note: WS Gosset, ex of Oxford, was employed by a brewery in Dublin in 1899 and was responsible for interpreting barley data; his employer preferred that his statistical methods be published under a pseudonym and he chose 'student'; see Standard deviation

STUMP Smooth muscle tumor of undetermined malignant potential; see Borderline tumors

Stump 'blowout' Leakage of the blind end (the 'stump') of a duodenum that has been partially resected for ulcer; the leak may be due to technical error or suture line failure, especially in a previously scarred or edematous duodenum; complications of leakage include peritonitis, hepatic bed abscess, pancreatitis and external fistula formation with electrolyte derangement

Stump carcinoma A carcinoma arising at the gastric 'stump' that remains after a subtotal (Billroth I or II) gastrectomy; it is unclear whether patients with gastric resection are at increased risk for future carcinoma of the stomach, and the reported incidence of gastric stump carcinoma ranges from no increase in some studies to a two-to-three-fold increase in others; if the association is real, the incidence of carcinoma accelerates 15-20 years after surgery and may be related to reflux gastritis, which induces dysplasia and cancer, bile reflux or hypochlorhydria which facilitates the colonization of bacteria that release carcinogen(s); the incidence of stump carcinoma may be related to the bile reflux seen in Billroth II resections (N Engl J Med 1988; 319:195), or due to chronic infection by ***Helicobacter pylori*** (ibid, 1991; 325:1127, 1132, 1170ed) Note: It is possible that there is an increased incidence of gastric carcinoma in patients with gastric ulcers, even in the absence of surgery

'Stunned' myocardium Transient (hours to days in duration) postischemic contractile abnormalities seen after myocardial reperfusion begins in acute myocardial infarction (J Am Med Assoc 1990; 264:455c); Cf Hibernating myocardium

Stuttering A defective speech pattern most often characterized by staccato repetition of the first phoneme of a spoken phrase, which is thought to be of environmental origin, although a vague genetic component may be present Note: Stutterers in history have reportedly included Moses the Prophet, Aristotle, Lewis Carroll, Churchill, Darwin, Marilyn Monroe and Jimmy Stewart

Stuttering (disease pattern) An adjectival descriptor for intermittent progression of disease, characterized by a staccato pattern of deterioration, eg multiple sclerosis or a stroke in evolution

Sty External hordeolum Inflammation of Moll's or Zeis' sebaceous gland, most often of staphylococcal origin; when Meibomian glands are inflamed it is known as an internal sty

Subacute myelo-optic neuropathy (SMON) A neuron dysfunction complex that begins with diarrhea and abdominal pain and is followed by sensory and motor disturbances of the lower limbs, ataxia, impaired vision, convulsion and coma

Subacute necrotizing encephalomyelopathy of Leigh An autosomal recessive condition of neonatal onset Clinical Swallowing and feeding difficulties, hypotonia, weakness, ataxia, peripheral neuropathy, external ophthalmoplegia, impaired hearing and vision and convulsions Pathogenesis Defective mitochondrial membrane-bound electron transfer system (respiratory chain) proteins, specifically in the mitochondrial electron transport complex IV, eg cytochrome C oxidase

Subacute sclerosing panencephalitis of Dawson (SSPE) A slow virus-induced inflammation evoked by the measles virus or by measles vaccines; the long latency period of months to years may be due to the slow development of hypersensitivity or autoimmune response Clinical Onset often occurs in childhood, with mental dysfunction, dyskinesia, myoclonus, hypotonia and emotional lability; it is usually fatal within 1-3 years Histopathology Perivascular mononuclear and plasma call infiltration in gray and white matter, neuronal degeneration, intranuclear and intracytoplasmic inclusions in neurons and glial cells Ultrastructure Tubular intranuclear and cytoplasmic inclusions of Dawson Electroencephalogram Suppression of the normal rhythm, punctuated by bursts of high-voltage slow and sharp waves Laboratory Paretic gold curve with markedly elevated immunoglobulins in the cerebrospinal fluid Treatment None; Cf Prions

Subclavian steal syndrome A cerebrovascular insufficiency syndrome caused by stenosing or occlusive atherosclerosis of the left subclavian artery, proximal to the origin of the vertebral artery, which reverses the blood flow to the vertebral artery, supplying the brainstem, 'stealing' the blood from the brain by the posterior cerebral circulation to supply collateral circulation in the arm causing both cerebral and brachial ischemia, decreased peripheral pulse and a bruit over the stenotic vessel; subclavian stealing may also occur in congenital vascular malformations, after neurosurgery, Takayasu's disease, thrombosis, trauma and tumors; see Steal syndromes; Cf 'Robin Hood syndrome'

Subcloning A type of cloning in which a segment of DNA of interest that has already been cloned, isolated and 'chopped' with a restriction endonuclease, is subjected to a second round of cloning in an appropriate receptor

Subcutaneous insulin-resistance syndrome (SIRS) Insulin-resistance in insulin-dependent diabetese mellitus that is attributed to an insulin-specific protease present in the subcutaneous tissue, the existence of which is increasingly controversial; if SIRS does exist, it is very rare (N Engl J Med 1986; 315:147); see Dawn phenomenon, Somogyi effect

Suberosis A form of hypersensitivity pneumonitis caused by exposure to cork dust and fungus, eg *Penicillium* fungus; see Farmer's lung; Hypersensitivity pneumonitis

Subfertility A term referring to a male condition in which semen parameters are below the lower limits of normal on two or more occasions; criteria used include: volume less than 1.5 ml, sperm density less than 20 million/ml, sperm viability less than 60%, motility less than 2 (on a scale of 1 to 4) and greater than 60% abnormal forms; subfertile semen may also demonstrate hyperviscosity, sperm agglutination, polyspermia and/or hematospermia; Cf Anti-sperm antibodies, Infertility

Subglottic webs see Laryngeal web

Submersion syndrome Near drowning A symptom complex due to prolonged submersion without death Clinical Tachypnea, mild hyperthermia, restlessness, vertigo, confusion, nausea, vomiting, shock, accompanied by pulmonary congestion and edema and depending on the water temperature, hypothermia; see Drowning; Cf Muddy lung

Subphrenic interposition syndrome of Chilaiditi A condition caused by the interposition of the colon between the liver and diaphragm, which is most commonly symptomatic in children, and improves with age Clinical Abdominal pain, vomiting, anorexia, constipation, abdominal distension (bloating) Treatment Avoidance of 'gassy' foods

Subspecialty A field of sub-specialized expertise, eg interventional radiology in a specialty, eg radiology that requires one or two years of a fellowship training period beyond residency in an officially recognized training program, at the end of which an examination may be required; some subspecialties may be approached from different fields, pediatric oncologists are usually pediatricians, but may also be oncologists; see Fellowship; Cf Specialty

Substance A term that is now less commonly used than the equally nebulous term, 'factor', which refers to any poorly-characterized molecule or group of molecules of plant or animal origin that have some discernible effect either in vivo or in an in vitro system Note: Since by this definition, virtually any molecules or class of agents could be regarded as a 'substance', it has become a less preferred term in scientific parlance

Substance abuse An activity that may be defined as a) The use of illicit, potentially addicting drugs, eg cocaine b) The misuse of prescribed drugs with stimulatory or depressant activities on the nervous system, eg amphetamines or barbiturates or c) The habitual use of commercially-available substances that are known to have a wide variety of deleterious effects in addition to the desired effects, eg alcohol and tobacco Statistics (National Institute on Drug Abuse, USA, 1988 household survey) two million teenagers had tried illicit drugs, 600 000 used cocaine in the survey year; habitual use of cocaine in most developed nations has increased exponentially; 12% of employed 20-40 year-olds and 5 000 000 women of child-bearing age regularly use illicit drugs; USA, 1986: 18 200 000 used marijuana at least once/month, 5 800 000 used cocaine at least once/month Substance abuse among resident physicians (J Am Med Assoc 1991; 265:2069) and medical students (J Am Med Assoc 1991; 265:2074) Rehabilitation Self-help organizations include Alcoholics Anonymous, Cocaine Anonymous, Narcotics Anonymous; see Alcohol, Cocaine, Crack, Ice, Marijuana

Substance Fa Cortisone **Substance G** Adrenosterone **Substance H** Histamine **Substance P** An 11-residue neuropeptide belonging to the tachykinin family, which is produced by alternative splicing of mRNA, stored in secretory vesicles of the brain and gastrointestinal tract that binds to a receptor designated NK1 (Science 1990; 247:958); substance P conveys the sensation of pain and noxious stimuli (heat, pressure, caustic chemicals) to the central and peripheral nervous system, causing nonmyelinated or thinly myelinated fibers to discharge; substance P closes potassium channels, increases cell polarizability, responses to all stimuli and cell sensitivity to endogenous opioids (enkephalins and adenosine-mediated neurotransmitters); substance P bridges the nervous and immune system, as it promotes inflammatory responses, activating macrophages, recruiting inflammatory cells, increasing the expression of substance P receptors in the endothelial cells in the sites of inflammation, eg large intestine in colitis, joints in rheumatoid arthritis, lungs in asthma, skin in psoriasis and nervous system in nerve trauma; substance P also causes smooth muscle contraction, vasodilation, stimulation of salivary gland secretion, extravasation of plasma, secretion of prostaglandins, oxygen-free radicals and IL-1, potentiating IL-1-induced fibroblast proliferation; prevention of substance P release may help explain the benefits of corticoids in attenuating immune reactions (Science 1990; 249:625rn); see CP-96345, Tachykinin **Substance Q** Deoxycorticosterone **Substance S** 11-deoxycortisol

Subungual exostosis Subungual or periungual trabecular bone formation appearing as a solitary mass on the dorsal aspect of the distal phalanx of the great toe, most common in young females

'Subway chart' A complex set of data generated from positron emission tomography (PET) scanning of the macaque brain which has multiple centers for a specific function and a far greater number of circuits connecting the centers; van Essen of the California Institute of Technology found 32 cortical areas involved in some aspect of vision and 305 circuits connecting these areas Note: As the technique of PET scanning matures in the human, subway charts may be developed

Succimer An oral agent that may be used to treat severe lead poisoning in children above 2.17 µmol/L (US: 45 µg/dl) (J Am Med Assoc 1991; 265:1802); see Lead, Saturnine gout

Succotash CLINICAL NUTRITION A vegetable preparation containing corn (low in lysine, an essential amino acid) and beans (low in tryptophan, another essential amino acid), thereby providing adequate dietary protein, a food of use in developing nations

Sucrose density gradient A gradient prepared with various concentrations of sucrose ranging from 5% to 25%, used to separate particles and molecules by mass or chain length of the molecule Note: 'Density' is a misnomer retained by convention, as the technique is more properly known as zonal centrifugation, see there

SUD Sudden unexpected death; see Sudden unexplained nocturnal death

Sudan Black B stain A stain with affinity for phospholipids and sterols, used in histology to identify fat; in hematology, both specific and azurophilic granules in cells of the myeloid series are positive, as are the leukemic cells in some acute myeloid leukemias (AML), which by the French-American-British classification, includes AML M1 (promyeloblastic leukemia, 3% of blasts stain with Sudan Black B—SBB, as well as with peroxidase—Px and ASD chloroacetate esterase—CAE), AML M2 (myeloblastic leukemia with maturation, > 85% of blasts stain with SBB/Px/CAE), AML M3 (promyelocytic leukemia, > 85% of blasts stain with SBB/Px/CAE), AML M4 (myelomonocytic leukemia, 20% of blasts stain with SBB/Px/CAE)

Sudden death FORENSIC MEDICINE Precipitous demise of any type, most commonly due to cardiovascular disease, caused by ischemia, arrhythmia, shock (aortic dissection), congestive heart failure, accompanied by hypoxia, polycystic disease of the heart, familial endocardial fibroelastosis and Kawasaki's disease, the latter of which more commonly affecting children; sudden death is more common in alcoholics, nulliparous women and in those with major psychiatric diseases; other causes of sudden death include anaphylaxis and 'cafe coronary', poisons (carbon monoxide, hydrogen sulfide, cyanide, nicotine, organophosphate pesticides), gastric rupture due to Hirschsprung's disease, ulcers, septicemia, obstruction, bezoars, cardiovascular and cerebrovascular lesions Note: The most common pathology seen in a sudden death is pulmonary edema

Sudden unexplained nocturnal death (SUND) An idiopathic condition occurring in young, previously healthy, Southeastern Asian males (Bangungut in Filipinos, Lai tai in Thais, Pokkuri in the Japanese) Histopathology Patchy intense loss of myoglobin from myocardium, with interstitial myoglobin deposition; the condition is thought to be due to an anomaly in the conduction system coupled with 'culture shock' and relocation-related stress in emigrants, as the peak incidence (25 reported cases/year) of SUND coincided with the peak influx of refugees from Southeast Asia (MMWR 1988; 37:568); in Thailand, SUND is associated with endemic distal renal tubular acidosis (Lancet 1991; 338:930)

SUDS Sudden unexplained death syndrome, see above

Sugar cane workers lung see Bagassosis, Farmer's lung

Sugar coating A descriptor for the gray-pink plaque-like elevations of the cerebellar folia, characteristically seen with medulloblastoma

Sugar icing appearance see Zuckerguß

Sugar substitutes CLINICAL NUTRITION A group of carbohydrates, eg fructose, sorbitol and xylitol, of potential use as replacements of the usual dietary sugars (glucose and sucrose) in diabetics, as these molecules do not require insulin for certain steps in their metabolism; the potential advantage is less than optimal, in that the diabetic liver converts a significant portion of fructose and its metabolites into glucose; see Artificial sweeteners

Sugar tumor A benign, sharply defined, but nonencapsulated lung tumor (figure, below) characterized by exuberant vascularity and round, polygonal glycogen-filled clear cells with well-defined borders, which are surrounded by hyalinized boundaries with focal calcifications and 'spider' cell formation; the sugar tumor is thought to be of neuroendocrine origin, given the presence of neurosecretory granules and ultrastructural appearance of the endoplasmic reticulum

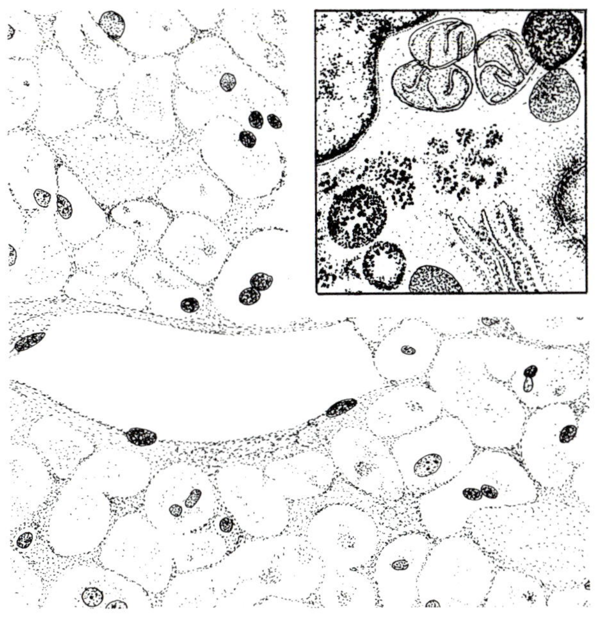

Sugar tumor

Suicidal behavior(s) PSYCHIATRY Covert or completed acts indicating that suicide is being or has been considered; these behaviors include suicidal ideation, attempted suicide or inappropriate euphoria in a person who had previously suffered severe depression Physical examination is often non-contributory, although transverse linear scarring at the wrists may indicate previous suicidal attempts or unusual scars suggestive of self-mutilation may be associated with depression; see Psychological autopsy

Suicide A form of death that is illegal in most societies; an estimated one in one hundred people think about suicide annually; many consult a non-psychiatric physician in the six months prior to the act *AGE* The rate rises with age, with peaks in adolescence and college (age 15-25), later increasing in older subjects; suicide is more frequent in adolescents who abuse psychoactive drugs *MANNER OF DEATH* Most successful suicide in the USA is by firearms Men: Firearms 46%, hanging 22%, gas 16%, poison 10% Women: Poison 41%, strangulation 17%, gas 15%, drowning 10%, firearms 8.5%; in 1970 45% of females died by poison, 32% by firearms; In 1980 poisoning decreased to 20%, firearms increased to 55%, with regional differences (Mayo Clin Proc 1990; 65:13) Physician suicide rate is the highest of any professional; female physicians are thought by some workers to be three times more likely to autodestruct than other female professionals *PREDISPOSING CONDITIONS* Mental illness, especially depression, but also schizophrenia; 15% of those with affective disorders die by suicide; 10-15% of alcoholics kill themselves, accounting for one-fourth of all suicides (the suicide rate in alcoholics is 500-fold greater than in the general population, often by firearms J Am Med Assoc 1990; 263:3051); other 'at-risk' conditions include AIDS, cancer, spinal cord injuries, seizure disorders and Huntington's disease; one half of suicide victims are unmarried, whites commit suicide twice as frequently as blacks *ANNUAL INCIDENCE* 28 000 (USA), 12/100 000; from 1950 to 1980, the male rate increased 305% and female 67%; from 1955-77, suicides jumped 230% in the 15-24 age group (J Am Med Assoc 259:356); suicide is attempted more often in women, but more often successful in men (male:female ratio, 4:1); 1980, young white males, 20.2/100 000, white females, 5/100 000 *SUCCESS RATE* Suicide attempt:success ratio is 5:1; in North America, there are seasonal peaks in suicides in March and September, with most occurring at home; the bodies are often discovered by family or friends

Suicide substrate BIOCHEMISTRY A substrate that is not normally recognized by an enzyme, which has become altered so that it reacts with an adjacent site on the enzyme, covalently linking to an active site on the enzyme, inactivating it

Sulfites Sulfiting agents (Sulfur dioxide, sodium sulfite, sodium or potassium bisulfite or metabisulfite) have been used to prevent discoloration of fruits and vegetables, eg coleslaw, potatoes and avocados served in public places, as in salad bars or are added to packaged foods, eg canned seafood, grapefruit juice, beer and wines; although well-tolerated by most people, up to 5% of asthmatics may be sensitive to sulfites (possibly related to low levels of sulfite oxidase), reacting with nausea, diarrhea, bronchospasm, pruritus, edema, hives, potentially anaphylactic shock and death; some drugs used for asthma may contain sulfiting agents, potentially exacerbating the problem

'Sulfur' granules A descriptor for the 1-2 mm firm yellow-white nodules lying within a partially encapsulated suppurative mass that may be punctuated by sinus tracts extending to the skin from the tonsils, uterine cervix, peripelvic tissue and lungs in infection by *Actinomyces israeli* Histopathology Basophilic clumps of filamentous, branching actinomycotic bacteria, acute inflammation and necrosis; the yellow color is due to foamy macrophages and tissue response to invasion; in actinomycosis (figure, below), the bacteria are within macrophages; in nocardiosis, the bacteria are extracellular; cultures often reveal mixed organisms including streptococci and fusiform bacteria Note: Up to 85% of pelvic actinomycosis in females is related to an intrauterine device that has been in place for three or more years

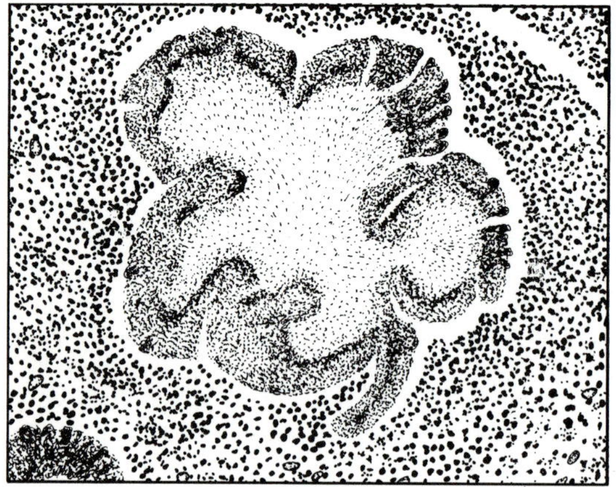

Sulfur granule

Sumatriptan An agonist of serotonin (5-HT) that binds to the 5-HY1D receptor, causing vasoconstriction of the cranial vessels, as well as blocking the extravasation of plasma; sumatriptan is reported to be effective in treating acute migraine, a condition that has been pathogenically-linked to intracranial vasodilation, resulting in a reduction in headaches, clinical disability, nausea and photophobia **Side effects** Tingling, dizziness, hot flushes (J Am Med Assoc 1991; 265:2831)

Summer itch Hydroa aestivale Hutchinson's prurigo DERMATOLOGY A rare variant of polymorphous light eruption (PMLE) that appears before puberty on covered areas of the skin, which is characterized by small papules topped by a vesicle; with time, the lesions, undergo lichenification and scarring; phototesting with ultraviolet-B light may elicit a PMLE-like reaction; see Polymorphous light eruption

Summit lesions see Mushroom lesions

Sump syndrome Biliary obstruction and food reflux in patients with previous choledocoenteric anastomosis, a condition fancifully likened to a sump pump (Gastroenterology 1987; 92:781)

Sunblock An opaque substance, usually formulated from zinc or titanium oxides, which is designed to completely prevent solar radiation from reaching the skin; Cf Sunscreen

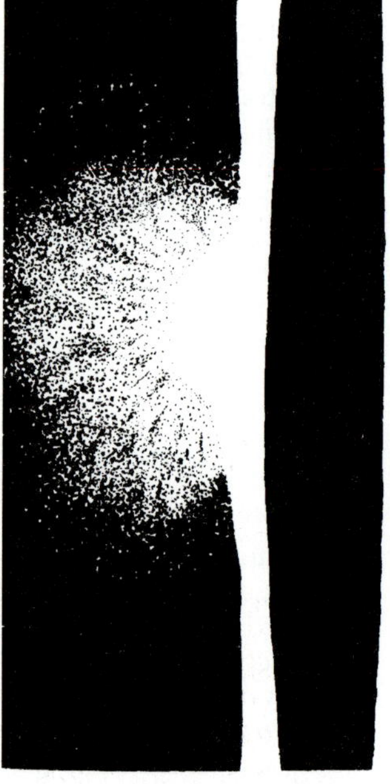

Sunburst pattern

Sunburn protection factor see SPF rating

Sunburst pattern 'Sunray' pattern RADIOLOGY A descriptor for the appearance of a periosteal reaction, in which dense filiform spiculations are perpendicular to the periosteum, classically seen in osseous infiltration by the common or 'garden variety' osteosarcoma, but uncommon in parosteal osteosarcoma, as this latter tumor evokes a minimal periosteal reaction; the adjective 'sunburst' also refers to the irradiating spiculation of the ileal bone around the acetabulum in Voorhoeve syndrome (osteopathia striata)

SUND see Sudden unexplained nocturnal death

Sunday morning palsy see Saturday night palsies

Sunflower cataract Sonnenblumenkatarakt A descrip-tive term for the radiating orange-tinted anterior capsular and subcapsular opacities in the lens due to copper deposition, seen in adolescents with Wilson's disease; the vision is not affected

'Sunk' costs LABORATORY MEDICINE Costs in equipment, reagents and dedicated supplies that have already been incurred, and which should not be included in future budget or financial considerations; in general, sunk costs are monies lost when a certain technique is no longer used or becomes obsolete

SUN/PUN Serum urea nitrogen/plasma urea nitrogen; see BUN

Sunscreen A transparent substance, eg oxybenzone, and dioxybenzone, that absorbs or scatters UVB (ultraviolet B) light (J Am Med Assoc 1991; 265:3217); these products may be combined with 5% para-aminobenzoic acid to yield commercial products that maximize UVA absorption, which induces the desired browning effect due to increased melanine production, while minimizing UVB absorption; the ability to block UV light is rated on the poorly standardized SPF (sunshine protection factor) scale, which ranges up to a maximum of 40; Cf Melanoma, Tanning salon, Ultraviolet light

Superantigens IMMUNOLOGY A family of antigens that combine with class II major histocompatibility complex (MHC) proteins, forming ligands capable of interacting with a large number of T cell α-β receptors, a level of interaction that requires only a specific Vβ element, inducing a brisk response from T cells with the appropriate Vβ complex; whereas most antigens are capable of stimulating the proliferation of no more than 1% of T cells, superantigens markedly stimulate proliferation of CD4 T cells in mixed lymphocyte cultures, 'recruiting' up to 10% of the T cells by binding to the variable β region (Vβ) of the T cell receptor and to the α-1 domain of the HLA-DR of the major histocompatibility complex (MHC), interacting with T cells in a unique geometric conformation (Science 1990; 248:685, 705), polyclonally activating T cells, independently of the T cell receptor's α chain, regardless of the peptide binding in the T cell receptor's pocket; superantigens have been identified in bacteria, eg toxic shock syndrome toxin-1, produced by ***Staphylococcus aureus*** (Nature 1990; 346:471) and in mice, encoded by either the *mls* gene of the mouse mammary tumor virus (Nature 1991; 349:524) or by its open reading frame, ORF (ibid, 1991; 350:203); the p30 superantigen encoded by the *gag* gene from the murine leukemia virus causes the mouse acquired immunodeficiency syndrome (Science 1991; 252:424); see Mls antigens

'Superbug' MICROBIOLOGY An organism which, when ingested by macrophages, is either not digested or is resistant to phagocytosis; superbugs include *Mycobacterium leprae, Leishmania* species (which reproduce within the endocytic vesicles) and *Legionella* species (which inhibit intravesicular phagosomal acidification, turning off the system designed to destroy it)

Supercoiling see Superhelix

Superconductivity A physical phenomenon destined to have broad applications in medicine, especially in information systems, once a superconductor becomes available that operates closer to room temperature; the temperature at which superconductivity could be induced had been stagnant at 20° Kelvin until the mid-1980s, but it is currently obtained in liquid nitrogen; optimal 'high-temperature' superconductors contain a combination of yttrium oxide, barium carbonate and copper oxide; superconductivity is characterized by 1) zero resistivity (sharp drop in electrical resistance by several orders of magnitude) and 2) Meissner effect (a metal in a constant magnetic field cooled below its superconductivity transitional temperature has zero magnetism filed in its interior, seen as a large negative magnetic susceptibility below the transitional temperature); the physics of superconductivity is poorly understood

Superfecundation OBSTETRICS Fertilization of a second ovum by a second sperm after one has already been fertilized; see Higher multiples, Twin; Cf Superfetation

Superfemale see XXX syndrome

Superfetation OBSTETRICS Fertilization and subsequent development of a second ovum after the first has already been implanted in the uterus; serving as a theoretical explanation for the difference in times of delivery of fraternal 'twins'; Cf Superfecundation

Superfund ENVIRONMENT A \$1.6 x 10^9 fund created by the US Congress in 1980 and administered by the Environmental Protection Agency (EPA) that was intended to be a five-year 'crash' program to clean up thousands of leaking toxic dump sites in the USA; during the first five-year plan, very little was achieved beyond the realization that the pundits had vastly underestimated the magnitude of the environmental contamination, and that many US citizens were living near dumps contaminated with dioxin, PCBs, heavy metals (lead, mercury and arsenic) and other toxic chemicals; in 1986, the Superfund program was renewed under the Superfund Amendments and Reauthorization Act that provided \$8.6 x 10^9 and gave the EPA the 'muscle' to enforce regulations and to fine those who criminally release toxins; see Environmental Protection Agency, Toxic dump site

Supergene A segment of DNA containing linked genes that are protected from cross-over exchanging of DNA and are thus transmitted intact from one generation to the next

Superhelix MOLECULAR BIOLOGY A structure that results when a circular double-stranded DNA, eg SV40 virus or polyomavirus is twisted on its axis, converting it into a figure eight or multiple looped chains; a twist in the opposite direction of that of the DNA's double helix is designated as left-handed, negative or underwound, a twist in the same direction as the double helix is termed right-handed, positive or overwound; replication and packaging of DNA in all organisms requires supercoiling, which is described by three parameters: 1) Linking number, which corresponds to the number of times the double helix crosses over on itself 2) Twist, which is related to the frequency and periodicity of the winding of one strand around the other, which under normal physiological conditions occurs every 10.6 bases for right-handed DNA and 3) Writhe, which relates to the pathway in space of the axis of the double helix

Superinfection An infection that occurs when the native flora of a body region are substantially reduced, often by antibiotic therapy, allowing invasion by opportunistic organisms, as occurs in pseudomembranous colitis or vaginal candidiasis

Superinfection 'immunity' The finding that two related organisms, eg plasmids, cannot successfully invade a host cell simultaneously

Superior mesenteric artery syndrome An uncommon condition caused by compression of the superior mesenteric artery Etiology Loss of cushioning regional adipose tissues (that maintain an appropriate arterial angle), seen in excess weight loss, rapid growth in children without corresponding gain of weight, in those with an asthenic habitus or in patients fixed in a hyperextended position by spinal injury or surgery Clinical Postprandial epigastric pain, distension, nausea, abdominal cramps, weight loss Diagnosis Distension of the proximal duodenum by barium studies and narrowing of the angle between the aorta and the superior mesenteric artery as seen by aortography or sonography Treatment The syndrome is a diagnosis of exclusion that often responds to conservative therapy including adoption of a postprandial knee-chest position while prone, smaller meals and an elemental diet

'Supermom' SOCIAL MEDICINE A colloquial term of recent vintage, but uncertain derivation, for a woman who raises children, performs the household duties expected of a 'domestic engineer' or housewife and works a full-time job; the supermom 'syndrome' is poorly studied, but appears to be very common, as 60-70% of US women of child-bearing age are in the workforce, a significant minority of whom are single-parent heads of household; supermoms suffer from a combination of external and largely uncontrollable stresses related to motherhood, as well as internal and self-induced stresses of attempting to perform their regular jobs well or even advance in a career, coupled to the tedium of household tasks; see Latchkey children, 'Quality' time

Superobesity see Morbid obesity

Superoxide anion $O_2{\cdot}^-$ A highly-reactive free radical that forms when a molecule of oxygen gains an electron, as occurs in inflammation or ionizing radiation; $O_2{\cdot}^-$ readily combines with protons, other superoxide anions and hydrogen peroxide, forming various toxic and reactive species; $O_2{\cdot}^-$-induced damage is implicated in age-related degenerative phenomena, see Garbage can hypothesis; $O_2{\cdot}^-$, is mutagenic and may have a major role in the carcinogenic 'cascade'; see Free radicals*

Superoxide dismutase An enzyme present in all aerobes that catalyzes the reaction $O_2{\cdot}^- + O_2{\cdot}^- + 2H^+ = H_2O_2 + O_2$, which serves to protect the organism against the havoc wreaked by oxygen free radicals; see Antioxidant therapy

Super-secondary structure A protein structural motif, eg a β barrel or β meander, which lies between a formal secondary structure, ie α-helix or β-pleated sheet and a formal tertiary structure, ie a domain; see Protein structure

'Superwoman' syndrome(s) A clinical complex that may affect any female with more than two X chromosomes, which tends to be more pronounced with more X chromosomes; see XXX, XXXX and XXXXX syndromes

Suppression test A clinical test or assay, eg dexamethasone suppression test, that is used to determine whether a substance (hormone or protein) being produced in excess is under the control of regulating or releasing factor(s), and therefore responsive to a feedback loop or whether the excess production is autonomous, and not under feedback control; Cf Stimulation test

Suppressor gene see Tumor suppression

Suppressor T cells A complex group of $CD8^+$ T lymphocytes that suppress the immune response by decreasing the activity of the T helper (CD4) cells against both endogenous (self) antigens and exogenous antigens; see Cytotoxic T cells, Helper cells, T cells, T cell receptor

Suppressor tRNA A transfer RNA molecule that is transcribed from a suppressor gene, which cancels the effect of a mis-sense or nonsense mutation by pairing directly with a nonsense (stop) codon, leading to the incorporation of a 'correct' amino acid

Supratypic antigen see Public antigen

Supravital stain A stainJanus green B, neutral red and thioflavin T, eg that is used to examine living cells by light microscopy, allowing visualization of various dynamic processes in situ; supravital stains may be injected into a cell and metabolized in a particular site, then removed, fixed and further evaluated, and are of use in detecting phagocytosis within macrophages and in examining mitochondria

Surfactant A mixture of dipalmitoyl-phosphatidylcholine and other lipids and proteins lining the alveoli, without which the alveoli would collapse upon expiration in accordance with the laws of Laplace; surfactant is produced by type II pneumocytes and secreted as lamellar bodies into the amniotic fluid; fetal surfactant production begins by the 20th week of gestation, but is only adequate to consistently ward off respiratory distress syndrome on or after the 35th week; see L/S ratio

Surfactant replacement therapy Intratracheally administered bronchoalveolar fluid derived from calves (98% lipids, comprised of 90% phospholipid, especially dipalmitoyl-phosphatidylcholine and 2% apoproteins), which elicits a marked improvement of gas exchange when used in premature infants; in very low birth weight infants, the improvements in pulmonary function are not statistically significant (J Pediatr 1990; 116:295); prophylactic bovine surfactant administered intratracheally decreases the need for neonatal respiratory support and improves the survival rates of premature infants, especially in those under 30 weeks (N Engl J Med 1991; 324:865, 910ed)

Surfactin An oligopeptide linked to a fatty acid with detergent properties that is released by ***Bacillus subtilis*** and causes hemolysis

Surfer's rib A sports injury caused by the 'lay-back' maneuver in surfing, which results in an avulsion of the first rib at its muscular attachments Clinical Pleural hemorrhage, brachial plexus injury (potentially, syncope and sudden death), decreased arm pulses seen by arteriography

Surge Any increase in the flow of a substance above a relatively constant baseline COMPUTERS A sudden increase in amperage (flow of electrons), that has potential for damaging current-sensitive electronic equipment; surges are rare and most often occur when a power station temporarily shuts down, and another takes over; lightning-related surges are distinctly uncommon REPRODUCTIVE PHYSIOLOGY An abrupt increase in luteinizing hormone (LH) secretion Background: LHRL (luteinizing hormone-releasing hormone) is normally secreted in episodic bursts resulting in cyclical peaks of LH; LHRH bursts are increased by estrogens and decreased by progesterone and testosterone and increase in frequency until the end of the follicular phase, at which time a surge of LH signals the onset of endometrial secretion in preparation for a fertilized egg

'Surgical' specialty A specialty of health care in which interventional procedures constitute a significant component of patient management; surgical specialties include obstetrics and gynecology, ophthalmology, otorhinolaryngology, surgery (cardiothoracic, colorectal, general, neurologic, orthopedic, plastic) and urology; Cf Hospital-based medicine, 'Medical' specialty, Primary care

Surgicenter HEALTH CARE INDUSTRY An ambulatory surgical facility in the US, in which minor or 'same day' surgical procedures, eg removal of cysts or skin lesions, are performed

'Surplus lines' company MALPRACTICE INSURANCE A medical malpractice insurance carrier that insures physicians at premium rates several times higher than the rates charged by the 'standard lines' malpractice insurance carriers, which routinely impose large deductibles; they do not advertize their 'products' nor have fixed premium rates; a physician applies to surplus-lines carriers if he has been denied coverage by other carriers, often after having lost his standard coverage due to various reasons including unfavorable claim and 'pay-out' history, governmental or hospital disciplinary action, or after allegations of drug abuse, sexual harassment or Medicare fraud; the typical surplus-line applicant is age 45-55 and is board-certified in neurosurgery, plastic surgery, obstetrics and gynecology, orthopedic surgery, family practice, otorhinolaryngology or general surgery; non-board certified physicians and foreign medical graduates are no more likely to require 'surplus-lines' coverage than board-certified and US medical graduates (J Am Med Assoc 1989; 262:1335)

Surrogate marker(s) LABORATORY MEDICINE A parameter or group of parameters measured in order to detect a pathologic condition when a more specific test doesn't exist, is impractical or is not cost-effective; surrogate testing is used for a) Non-A, non-B hepatitis, measuring alanine aminotransferase and antibodies to hepatitis B core antigen (anti-HBc) and b) Human immunodeficiency viral infection, using p24 antigen levels in serum in pg/ml (< 31 pg/ml is considered negative), level of CD4 T cells/mm^3 (N Engl J Med 1991:324:137) and the helper:suppressor(CD4:CD8) ratio of T lymphocytes

Surrogate motherhood True surrogate motherhood is that in which a woman carries a gestational product that is not her own genetically, where one haploid set of genes is contributed by the genetic or natural father and the second haploid is contributed by the genetic mother (who for various reasons, eg hysterectomy, uterus didelphys or other reasons, cannot carry fertilized ovum); in the usual scenario, the diploid product is fertilized in vitro and implanted in the uterus of the surrogate mother; legal issues regarding true surrogacy are relatively simple, at least theoretically, since the gestational mother is performing a service (usual fee, $10 000) in carrying an egg that is not her own genetically; a permutation of this theme, with vastly distinct legal implications, is 'partial surrogacy' in which a genetic father's haploid chromosome complement, ie the sperm is used to artificially inseminate the egg of a woman (the genetic father's wife may be infertile for various reasons) who is both the gestational mother and the genetic or natural mother and who agrees to carry the conceptus to term, at which time the genetic father and his infertile wife retain the newborn infant; the difficulty arises if at the time of delivery the woman carrying the fetus wishes to retain the child, which is, in a sense one-half 'hers'; see Artificial reproduction, Baby M

Surrogate parent A person who plays the role of a child's parent while the child is in the hospital

Surrogate parenting see Artificial reproduction

Survival analysis STATISTICS A component required for critical interpretation of data from clinical trials that uses life-tables with cumulative survival rates, forming a distribution or set of probabilities of a person under a therapeutic protocol of surviving certain time intervals

Survivor syndrome see Concentration camp syndrome

Susceptibility theory An attempt to explain the non-random ('skipping') lymph node involvement at the time of diagnosis in Hodgkin's disease, postulating that Hodgkin's disease is multifocal ab initio, but only some lymphoid regions are susceptible, ie provide suitable environments for the maintenance of malignant cells; Cf Skip metastasis

Sushi A popular Japanese delicacy prepared from raw fish that may be a vector for parasites, including ***Anasakis*** (most commonly, ***A simplex*** of subfamily Anisakinae, order Ascaridida), Contracecum and Phocanema (***Pseudoterranova decipiens***), which often affect sushi made from mackerel caught in early spring **Endoscopy** Edema, gastritis, erosion **Clinical** Myalgia, abdominal pain **Radiology** Thread-like larvae may be seen in radiocontrast studies **Treatment** Endoscopic removal Notes: 1) Fishes used for preparing sushi that are known to harbor parasites include ceviche or South American cod, green herring (Netherlands), Pacific pollack, Pacific red snapper and squid 2) Other raw fish dishes of parasitic potential include sashimi, gravlax, pickled herring, lomi lomi and lox (cold-smoked salmon) 3) Other organisms present in sushi include ***Dioctophyma renale, Heterophytes, Strongyloides***, trematodes (paragonimiasis, ***Nanophyetus salminicola***), ***Metagonimus yokogawai***, cestodes (***Diphyllobothrium latum***) and ***Vibrio parahemolyticus*** 4) Preventive measures: Cooking to 60°C for 10 minutes, or blast-freezing to -35°C for 15 hours or to -23°C for 7 days *FREEZING FOR 24 HOURS, SALTING, SMOKING AND PICKLING ARE NOT CONSISTENTLY TO EFFECTIVELY KILL PARASITES* (N Engl J Med 1990; 322:1011); irradiation is not legal

Sushi syncope A transient condition caused by ingesting a bolus of wasabe, a very 'hot' mustard (active ingredient: isothiocyanate) used to flavor sushi; the index case had a transient myocardial infarct-like attack with diaphoresis, pallor, confusion and vasomotor collapse (J Am Med Assoc 1987; 258:218c); see Seder syncope, Spicy food

Suspended heart 'syndrome' A radiologic finding in which the heart appears as if suspended in the mid-thorax, ie cardio-thoracic 'separation', when viewed in a left oblique and occasionally in the right oblique position; the 'syndrome' is accompanied by low T waves in the II lead and a prominent S-T depression in the III lead and has no known clinical significance

Sutton's law MEDICAL DECISION-MAKING A guideline evoked to temper the enthusiasm of externs (US medical students in their third and fourth years of school) who want to 'work up' an acute abdomen for porphyria, metastatic medulloblastoma or other esoterica; the 'law' is attributed to the noted bank robber, Willie Sutton, who, when asked why he robbed banks, reportedly replied, '...that's where the money is'; to apply Sutton's law then, is to search for the most likely cause of a symptom, ie to go where the 'money' is; see Hoofbeats; Cf Red herring, 'Zebras'

SV-40 Simian virus 40 A small icosahedral, double-stranded DNA papovavirus, which, like the JC virus, may cause progressive multifocal leukoencephalopathy; SV-40 is of interest as it was the first molecule in which DNA superhelicity was identified and it may be used to transform cells in vitro as a form of 'permissive' infection, eventually leading to host cell lysis

Svedberg (S) A unit of sedimentation coefficiency or 'buoyancy', equal to 10^{-13} seconds (rate of dispersion), determined by ultracentrifugation; S provides an estimate of a substance's molecular weight, and was named after Svedberg, who won the 1926 Nobel prize for inventing the ultracentrifuge

Sverdlovsk A Soviet industrial city in the Ural mountains that became a focus of international interest in 1979 through an epidemic of anthrax, which was alleged by some US officials to have been due to a leak in a secret military lab involved in the testing and/or manufacture of biological warfare (prohibited by a treaty signed by the Superpowers in 1975); although cutaneous anthrax responds well to high-dose penicillin, if the spores are inhaled or ingested, the mortality reaches 75%, making anthrax a theoretically ideal biological weapon; of the 96 victims, 64 died during the outbreak; the official Soviet explanation, accepted by American epidemiologists, is that the outbreak was related to tainted spore-infected meat sold by private butchers (Science 1988; 240:383); see Biological warfare

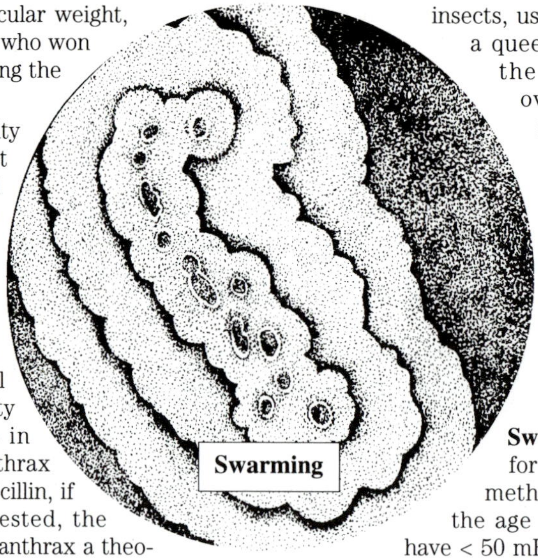

Swainsonine A plant alkaloid with anti-tumor growth activity, inhibiting synthesis of β 1-6-branched carbohydrate, which serves as a recognition site for endothelial receptors, facilitating retention of tumor cells in the microvasculature; swainsonine is being studied for potential use in human malignancy (J Am Med Assoc 1990; 263:2289c)

Swamp fever Synonym for 1) Equine infectious anemia, a viral infection of horses, transmitted by hematophagous arthopods, causing weakness, recurrent fever, marked anemia and muscular atrophy 2) Malaria 3) Marsh fever A water-born infection (Vector *Rattus rattus*) by the spirochete, *Leptospira grippotyphosa*, which causes fever, general malaise and aseptic meningitis

Swan neck A descriptor for a thin curved neck, resulting from muscular atrophy characteristic of myotonia dystrophica, which may be accompanied by 'myopathic facies' (see 'Hatchet' face), myotonia, dysphagia, frontal baldness, testicular atrophy and cataracts; a variant of the gracile swan neck is described in the Modigliani syndrome

Swan neck deformity RENAL PATHOLOGY A descriptor for the shortened and attenuated initial segment of a dissected proximal convoluted renal tubule seen by light microscopy in patients with De Toni-Fanconi syndrome RHEUMATOLOGY A descriptor for the hyperextended proximal interphalangeal joint and compensatory flexion of the distal interphalangeal joints caused by shortening of the extensor tendon, classically seen in rheumatoid arthritis, which may also be seen in lupus erythematosus, Jaccoud's (post-rheumatic fever) arthritis, psoriatic arthritis, scleroderma and camptodactyly; Cf Boutonniere deformity

Swan syndrome see Blind spot 'syndrome'

Swarming CLINICAL TOXICOLOGY A mass of hymenopteran insects, usually bees that are in transit with a queen, which may sting a person by the hundreds, causing a toxic overdose of yellow jacket venom resulting in gastrointestinal symptoms, headache, fever, syncope, and less commonly, seizures, renal failure, vasomotor collapse and death MICROBIOLOGY A descriptor for a light overgrowth of *Proteus mirabilis* or *P vulgaris* on MacConkey agar, that is likened to ocean waves (figure, left), resulting from *Proteus* motility

Swarming

Sweat chloride test A diagnostic test for cystic fibrosis; the Gibson-Cooke method is performed preferably after the age of two months; normal subjects have < 50 mEq/L (mean, 18 mEq/L) and those with cystic fibrosis have > 60 mEq/L (average, 100 mEq/L) of chloride in the sweat; the test is also positive in Addison's disease, adrenogenital syndrome, diabetes insipidus (nephrogenic type), fucosidosis, glucose-6-phosphatase deficiency type of glycogen storage disease, malnutrition, nephrotic syndrome or may be incorrectly positive through a technical error

Sweat gland tumor see Skin adnexal tumors

Swedish porphyria Acute intermittent porphyria

Sweet clover disease A cattle coagulopathy caused by rumination on clover with a vitamin K inhibitor (Can Vet Rec 1922; 3:74; N Engl J Med 1984; 311:645); see Warfarin

Swimmer's ear Recurrent external otitis caused by *Pseudomonas aeruginosa*, due to prolonged swimming, more common in hot, humid climates

Swimmer's itch Cercarial dermatitis caused by exposure to nonhuman schistosomes present in the sediment of fresh water lakes frequented by ducks; although the organism cannot complete its life cycle in the human, repeated cutaneous exposure elicits a hypersensitivity reaction consisting of papular erythematous rash with edema and pruritus; a similar eruption may also occur with non-infective contact exposure to human schistosomes, including *S haematobium* and *S mansoni*

Swimmer's view RADIOLOGY A patient position that allows optimal visualization of the lower cervical spine

Swimming pool granuloma An indolent skin infection clinically mimicking spirotrichosis with cellulitis, lymphadenitis and joint infections, caused by atypical mycobacteria, *M marinum* or *M kansasii* after percutaneous inoculation with contaminated fresh or salt water, developing into a solitary nodule at sites of abrasion (elbows, knees and feet), later becoming indurated and ulcerated, resembling cutaneous tuberculosis, occasionally developing satellite lesions; Cf Fish tank granuloma

Swimming suit distribution see Bathing trunk distribution

Swine influenza vaccine 'affair' PUBLIC HEALTH A misadventure that occurred in the USA in 1976, as an overreaction to the fear of a major human epidemic; the incident began with a 'signal event' in which two unusual viruses were identified in pigs in New Jersey, with a related mini-epidemic among military recruits; in response, the Centers for Disease Control (CDC) in Atlanta recommended the manufacture and administration of vaccine before the onset of the 'flu season' the following winter; 50 million received the vaccine, 1000 people suffered vaccine-related Guillain-Barré syndrome; the anticipated epidemic did not materialize and virtually no cases of swine influenza occurred in humans; the unused vaccine was destroyed and $84 million was paid in claims to the Guillain-Barré victims; the affair caused a transient erosion in the public's confidence in the CDC, which has played a pivotal role in worldwide epidemiology; see CDC

'Swinging heart' CARDIOLOGY A fanciful synonym for the electrocardiographic (EKG) findings in electrical alternans, in which there is a regular alteration in the direction and/or amplitude of one or more components of the EKG reading, eg simultaneous oscillation of the P waves, QRS complexes and T waves (total electrical alternans); these features are highly characteristic of cardiac tamponade (J Louisiana State Med Soc 1990; 42:5)

Swiss agammaglobulinemia IMMUNOLOGY An autosomal recessive form of severe combined immunodeficiency (SCID), which has a high mortality in early infancy due to a combination of severe diarrhea, malabsorption with disaccharidase deficiency and villar atrophy; the defective cellular and humoral immunity makes these patients susceptible to a menagerie of opportunistic pathogens, including *Candida albicans*, cytomegalovirus, measles, *Pneumocystis carinii* and varicella, as well as graft-versus-host disease Pathogenesis Decreased T and B cells at the stem cell level Laboratory Anemia, lymphopenia, elevation of liver enzymes, electrolyte imbalance secondary to chronic diarrhea Treatment Aggressive antibiotic therapy, gammaglobulins; HLA-matched bone marrow transplantation may effect permanent remission; see Adenosine deaminase deficiency

Swiss cheese A popular adjectival descriptor used in various medical specialties for a gross appearance, microscopic pattern or radiologic field punctuated by multiple variably-sized, sharply demarcated cystic spaces

'Swiss cheese' brain An artefact that may be seen in brains that have been inadequately infiltrated with formalin, coupled with invasion of the non-quite-fixed brain by gas-forming *Clostridium* organisms (figure, below left)

'Swiss cheese' breast A non-specific term for multiple, variably sized spaces lined by ductal epithelium, which may be seen in various benign breast diseases, including blunt duct adenosis, fibrocystic disease and epitheliosis (papillomatosis)

'Swiss cheese' endometrium A descriptor for the histopathology of cystic glandular hyperplasia, which may be seen in the menopausal endometrium, in association with increased estrogen from persistent follicles, granulosa-theca cell tumors of the ovaries, adrenocortical hormones or from exogenous estrogen therapy; these endometria usually present with postmenopausal bleeding; by light microscopy there are increased epithelial and stromal elements with large dilated swiss cheese-like glands lined by a one-cell layer of epithelium (figure, below middle)

'Swiss cheese' hemangioma A descriptor for the radiological pattern of ossification described as typical musculoskeletal hemangiomas

'Swiss cheese' histiocytes Mononuclear-phagocytic cells seen in mucopolysaccharidosis type VIII, characterized by granular cytoplasm filled with variably-sized, well-circumscribed storage vacuoles

'Swiss cheese' liver A descriptor for the liver in peliosis hepatis, which is punctuated by multiple 0.2 mm or less in diameter blood-filled lacunae, which are often devoid of endothelial lining, and thought to represent distended sinusoids or central or portal veins

'Swiss cheese' lung A descriptor for the multicystic appearance of a plain chest film in an infant with cystic

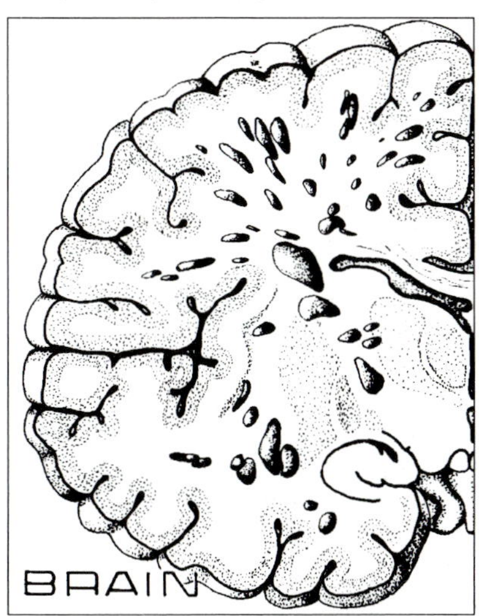

'Swiss cheese' brain

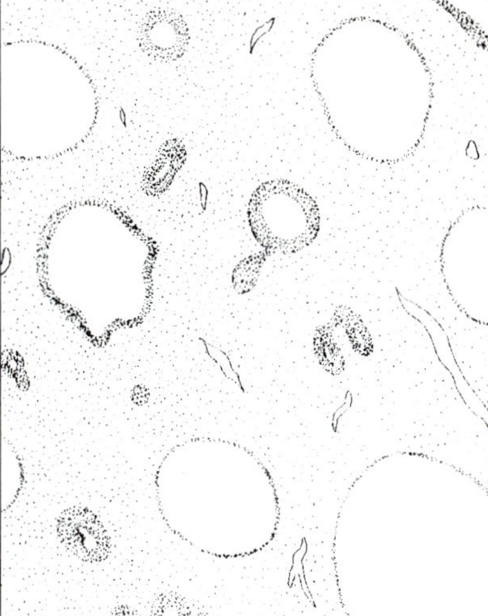
'Swiss cheese' endometrium

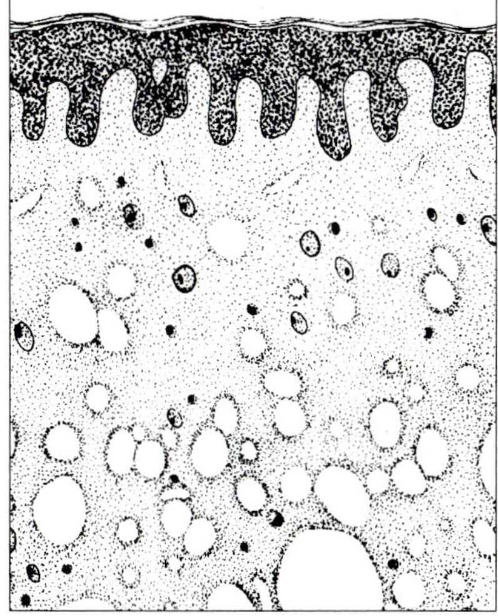
'Swiss cheese' skin

adenomatoid malformation, where the involved area is overexpanded and the mediastinum is shifted towards the normal lung; the infant presents with respiratory distress of the newborn and may require an emergency lobectomy or pneumonectomy depending on the extent of the lesion

'Swiss cheese' platelets A descriptor for giant platelets with vacuolated granular spaces, accompanied by thrombocytopenia, increased bleeding time and an abnormal platelet aggregation response to ADP and collagen

'Swiss cheese' polyp GASTROENTEROLOGY A descriptor for the low-power light microscopic findings in the juvenile retention polyp, a hamartomatous (not precancerous) lesion of the colon, where the polyp's dilated glands are filled with mucus; retention polyps may be first recognized by rectal bleeding and treated by simple excision

'Swiss cheese' skin A descriptor for the histology of paraffinoma or oil granuloma due to cutaneous injection of lipid-rich substances, resulting in variably-sized, swiss cheese-like fibrotic cavities (figure, page 709) filled with lipids, scattered foamy histiocytes and a foreign body type giant cell reaction, without birefringence; this condition may be seen in factitial panniculitis induced by autoinjection of mineral, cotton seed oil and other oils or in illicit injection of silicone, see Silicone, Transsexuals

'Swiss cheese' skull see Punched-out lesions

'Swiss cheese' ventricular septal defect A variant of ventricular septal defect in which there are multiple serpentine defects in the ventricular muscle, making surgical closure difficult

'Swiss roll' technique SURGICAL PATHOLOGY A method for examining the maximum amount of tissue from a flat organ; the tissue is rolled 'a la burrito' and then sectioned perpendicular to the length of the specimen; the technique is of greatest use for examining the stomach and placenta, and derives its name from a popular pastry

Swiss type of hereditary persistence of fetal hemoglobin A laboratory finding without clinical significance characterized by an inherited increase in red cells containing hemoglobin F, first identified in Swiss army personnel

Swiss type immunodeficiency see Swiss agammalobulinemia

Switch defect disease see Hyperimmunoglobulin-M disease

Switching HEMATOLOGY The change in expression of the β-like hemoglobin genes during the transition from the embryonic to the fetal and adult stages in erythrocytes; activation and high-level expression of these genes is directed by a locus control region located 5' to the ε gene; expression of the adult β gene requires progressive silencing of early (ε, γG, γA and δ) genes, which is probably mediated by stage-specific factors binding to sequences flanking the genes (Nature 1991; 350:252) IMMUNOLOGY Class switching see V(D)J recombination

SWOG Southwestern Oncology Group

Symbiotic psychosis A psychological disorder of questionable validity that may affect young children after a normal infancy and following a precipitating event, eg birth of a sibling; characterized by attacks of panic-like anxiety accompanied by marked regression of social behavior and intellectual development; in the most extreme form, the symbiotic child physically clings to the mother and others in an almost indiscriminate fashion; speech regression may occur and become garbled or jargonistic, ultimately leading to a state of secondary autism that may respond to therapy

Sympathy pregnancy Couvade A 'condition' in which a man simulates some of the features of pregnancy, predominantly gastrointestinal symptoms of anorexia, morning sickness, constipation, diarrhea, toothaches and mood swings, either as a cultural phenomenon, eg practiced by primitive tribes, eg the Tchambulis of New Guinea, in an attempt to symbolically share the suffering(s) of a pregnant woman; in 'civilization', couvade is not a formally practiced custom, and thus 'male pseudopregnancy' is regarded as a benign, self-limited neurosis occurring in the husband of a pregnant woman; see Pseudocyesis; Cf Pseudopregnancy

Symport A transmembrane carrier protein that simultaneously binds and transports two substances in the same direction, eg the transport of sodium and glucose into the cell; in contrast, antiport systems are characterized by simultaneous transport of two compounds to the opposite face of a membrane

Synapsin(s) A class of nerve terminal specific cytoskeletal proteins (neuropeptides) that bind to synaptic vesicles; the four synapsins thus far identified are synapsins Ia and Ib and synapsins IIa and IIb, together comprising 0.62% of the neuron's protein, generated by alternative splicing of two different genes; the synapsins have been implicated in the short-term regulation of neurotransmitter release from nerve endings and in the development of synapses, connecting synaptic vesicles to the active zone (Nature 1991; 349:697)

Synaptic plasticity NEUROPHYSIOLOGY Malleability present in most neurons in various forms, including presynaptic inhibition, homosynaptic depression, presynaptic facilitation and modulation of transmitter release by tonic depolarization of the sensory neuron (Science 1990; 250:1142); activation of a neuron receptor, eg NMDA receptor may directly alter synapse plasticity (Nature 1991; 349:154); endogenous nitric oxide is responsible for synaptic plasticity in the cerebellum (ibid 1991; 349:326); see Nitric oxide

Synaptophysin A 38 kD transmembrane glycoprotein isolated from neurons, which spans the synaptic vesicular membrane four times, the carboxy terminal of which is the binding site for various cell factors; synaptophysin is a marker for neuroendocrine differentiation and is produced in neuroblastoma, ganglioneuroblastoma, ganglioneuroma, pheochromocytoma, paraganglioma, as well as carcinoids, medullary thyroid carcinoma and pancreatic endocrine tumors

Syncytial giant cell hepatitis An acute and chronic hepatitis described in adults characterized by multinucleated giant cells arranged in a syncytial or rosette pattern, bridging fibrosis and cholestasis, containing viral particles by ultrastructural examination, thought to be induced by paramyxovirus (N Engl J Med 1991; 324:455); see Giant cell hepatitis

Syndactyly Fusion of the fingers, which may be cutaneous, due to bridging soft tissues, or osseous, due to bone fusion of varying severity; in general, only soft tissue syndactylism is treated, without which ostosis develops at the articulations with loss of function; syndactyly is seen in congenital syndromes including Apert, Bloom, Carpenter, cryptophthalmus, Cohen, Conradi-Hünermann, Cornelia de Lange, EEC, Escobar, Goltz, Holt-Oran, Jarcho-Levin, Langer-Giedion, Meckel-Gruber, Miller, oculodentodigital, oral-facial-digital, partial trisomy 10q, Pfeiffer, Poland sequence, popliteal web, Robert, Saethre-Chotzen, Smith-Lemli-Opitz and triploidy syndromes; Rosebud hands

Syndrome X CARDIOLOGY Microvascular angina A condition characterized by anginal pain without detectable atherosclerotic lesions within the coronary arteries, a condition thought to represent 1 to 15% of patients with anginal pain Note: Atherosclerosis of a degree sufficient to explain angina is seen in 85% of angiograms ENDOCRINOLOGY A clinical complex in older adults with truncal obesity, characterized by hyperinsulinemia, insulin resistance, decreased glucose tolerance or type II diabetes mellitus Laboratory Decreased HDL-cholesterol and increased triglycerides (N Engl J Med 1989; 320:702,733; 322:229); Cf Diabesity

Synergism Cooperative interaction between two or more components in a system, such that the combined effect is greater than the sum of each individual constitutent **BACTERIAL SYNERGISM** An effect inferred but unproven in anaerobic infections, where there are three or more different species of both aerobic and anaerobic bacteria in an infected site, and the virulence of the lesion is a function of the number of species involved; examples of bacterial synergism include Meleny's cutaneous ulcer (*Staphylococcus aureus* and microaerophilic streptococci), Ludwig's angina and Vincent's angina; see Anaerobes **PHARMACOLOGIC SYNERGISM** An approach to recalcitrant bacterial infections or virulent malignancies in which the therapeutic agents each affect different pathways or steps in a metabolic pathway, making the treatment more efficient, eg penicillin and an aminoglycoside; see Combination chemotherapy

Synergistic necrotizing cellulitis A form of necrotizing fasciitis characterized by involvement of skin, subcutaneous tissue, fascia and muscle, where the lesions are usually located on the legs or the perineum, arising in a perirectal abscess; predisposing factors include diabetes mellitus, obesity, advancing age and cardiorenal disease Clinical Small skin ulcers that ooze a red-brown fetid liquid fancifully termed 'dishwater pus', surrounded by gangrenous patches punctuated by preserved islands of normal-appearing skin, pain, tenderness, tissue gas, systemic toxicity and bacteremia; Fournier's disease is a special type arising in the scrotum

Synexin A protein that causes calcium-dependent aggregation of chromaffin granules and promotes the fusion of these granules during exocytosis

Synonym codon Synonymous codon Any of a number of triplets of adjacent RNA nucleotides (codons) that are translated into the same amino acid, eg the messenger RNA codons UUA, UUG, CUU, CUC, CUA and CUG all are translated into the same amino acid, leucine; this redundancy of codons, also known as 'degeneracy', allows point mutations to occur in the genome or during transcription without the host cell being penalized by the loss of a critical structural protein; see Codon, Degenerate code, Same-sense mutation, Silent mutation

Synonym syndromes see Pseudonym syndrome

Synovial sarcoma SURGICAL PATHOLOGY A mesenchymal malignancy that comprises up to 10% of all soft tissue tumors, most common in young (age 20-40) males, occurring in the knee, ankle, foot or other joints Pathology The tumor ranges from firm and calcified to friable and necrotic, and has a 'biphasic' histologic pattern, characterized by variable interspersed bands of spindled and epithelioid cells; the material within the gland-like spaces is mucicarmine-positive, PAS (periodic acid Schiff)-positive/diastase-resistant tumor that is strongly reactive for keratin stains, thus causing the uninitiated to misdiagnose these lesions as adenocarcinomas; monophasic synovial sarcoma mimics fibrosarcoma, malignant schwannoma and leiomyosarcoma Prognosis 50% five-year survival; extensively calcified tumors have a higher (84%) five-year survival

SYR Sex-determining region of the Y chromosome see Testis-determining factor

Syringoma A sweat gland tumor that is most common in pubertal females, located on the eyelids, neck, upper anterior chest and vulva appearing as multiple flesh-colored to yellowish papulonodules Histopathology The dermis is replete with small ducts, cysts and solid comma-shaped cords or strands of epithelial cells; Cf Cylindroma

Systemic angioendotheliomatosis see Angiotrophic lymphoma

Systemic idiopathic fibrosis A condition characterized by retroperitoneal fibrosis of unknown etiology that may extend to the anterior chest wall Clinical Backache, fever, nausea, vomiting, constipation, anemia, oliguria, anuria, peripheral vascular insufficiency; fibrosis-induced ureteral compression may lead to urinary retention and renal failure

Systemic immunoblastic proliferation A recently described condition caused by proliferation of immature lymphocytes Clinical Dyspnea, rash, hepatosplenomegaly, lymphadenopathy and a tendency to develop into immunoblastic lymphoma; Molecular analysis reveals gene translocations

Systemic mastocytosis see Mast cell

System manager The person encharged with coordinating the electronic flow of data from various departments in a hospital or laboratory information system, who often serves as a first rung 'trouble shooter' should any problems arise in the system

Syzygy Fusion of two organs, each of which retains a clear histological distinction, eg Spleno-gonadal fusion

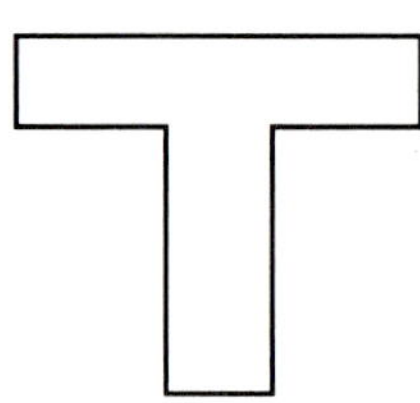

T Symbol for: Absolute temperature; tera-; tesla; threonine; thymidine; thymine; time; translocation; tritium; tocopherol; twisting number

t Symbol for: transfer (RNA); variable (statistics)

T-200 Obsolete for CD45 or Leukocyte common antigen

T1 antigen see CD5

T3 antigen see CD3

T_3 thyrotoxicosis Hyperthyroidism in which T_3 (triiodothyronine) but not T_4 is elevated; these patients are clinically heterogeneous and lack distinctive signs and symptoms, comprising about 4% of those with hyperthyroidism due to Graves' disease, toxic nodular goiter and thyroid adenomas and a higher percentage of hyperthyroidism in regions with lower levels of iodine

T4 antigen see CD4

T_4 thyrotoxicosis Hyperthyroidism in which T_4 (thyroxine) but not T_3 is elevated, which occurs in patients with iodine-induced thyrotoxicosis and in euthyroid patients who are sick for other reasons, see Euthyroid sick syndrome

T7 assay see Free thyroxine index

T8 antigen see CD8

T12 assay see Free thyroxine index

TA-AB Techoic acid antibody assay MICROBIOLOGY A test that measures the titers of antibody to techoic acid, a constituent of the Staphylococcal cell wall; 90% of patients with *S aureus*-induced endocarditis have increased TA-AB levels and the assay is used to diagnose *S aureus* osteomyelitis, culture-negative endocarditis, to determine response to therapy and to detect possible relapse

Tabby A mutant gene that is responsible for a form of ectodermal dysplasia with anhidrosis in male mice, an animal model for the X-linked human disease, hypohidrotic ectodermal dysplasia, which causes hyperpyretic crises in children; post-natal injection of epidermal growth factor in tabby mice elicits growth of dermal ridges and functional sweat glands and may have the same effect in some humans with ectodermal dysplasia (Nature 1990; 345:544); Cf EEC syndrome

Tabby cat pattern see Thrush breast appearance

Tabun Dimethyl-phosphoramidocyanidic acid A potent cholinesterase inhibitor (lethal dose of 0.01 mg/kg) that had currency during the first World War as a chemical weapon; Tabun and the use of related 'nerve gases' was banned by the Geneva protocol of 1925; see Chemical warfare; Cf Zyklon B

Tac antigen see CD25

Tâche blanche Tache, French, spot INFECTIOUS DISEASE A small whitish hepatic abscess that may be seen in bacteremia PATHOLOGY A focal fibrotic spot on the epicardium of the elderly, which is of no known significance

Tâche noire A blackened cutaneous ulcer at the site of a tick bite, the initial lesion of boutonneuse fever (*Rickettsia conorii*) and scrub typhus (*R tsutsugamushi*)

Tachykinin A family of widely-distributed biopeptides that shares the COOH-terminal sequence Phe-X-Gly-Leu-Met-NH_2 and includes substance P, neurokinins A and B, neuropeptide K and neuropeptide-γ; tachykinins cause vasodilation, gastrointestinal and urogenital smooth muscle contraction and stimulation of salivary gland secretion; tachykinin receptors are designated as NK1, NK2 and NK3; see Substance P

Tactile agnosia NEUROLOGY An impairment of tactile object recognition, which is a subtle, nondisabling disorder caused by unilateral damage to parietotemporal cortices that may be severe in left cerebral infarctions; tactile agnosia should be distinguished from astereognosis, a complex somatosensory disorder and tactile aphasia (Mayo Clin Proc 1991; 66:129)

T activation TRANSFUSION MEDICINE Removal of an N-acetyl residue (sialic acid) by bacterial neuraminidase, which exposes hidden antigenic epitopes, against which there are natural antibodies in the circulation of most adults, resulting in polyagglutination; T activation can be detected by using aged blood, cord sera or by treating the cells with 2 mercaptoethanol (2-ME) to destroy the IgM antibodies

Tactoid HEMATOLOGY A birefringent fluid crystal-like structure composed of 21 nm in diameter fibers of deoxygenated hemoglobin that distort and decrease the deformability of erythrocytes in sickle cell anemia; these structures consist of seven intertwined double-stranded molecules that form both tactoids and spherulites by a 'double nucleation' model (Nature 1990; 345:833) Note: tactoids are not true crystals since they are arranged in one-dimensional stacks; see Sickle cells, Spectrin

Tactoid bodies NEUROANATOMY Rudimentary structures of sensory nerve differentiation, seen as oligocellular whorls of flattened cells, which may be recapitulated by malignant schwannomas

Tadpole cell CYTOLOGY An uncommon cell seen in epidermoid carcinoma of the uterine cervix that is elongated and club-shaped with one broad end that tapers to a narrow end, and has an eccentric, rounded hyperchro-

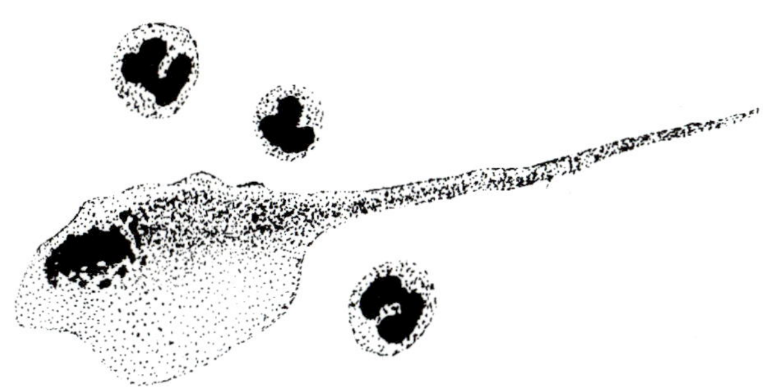

Tadpole cell

matic nucleus or nuclei within often keratinized cytoplasm; the related 'spindly' cell, which is tapered at both ends, may also be seen in epidermoid carcinomas of the cervix, as well as of the lungs

Tadpole sign ULTRASONOGRAPHY A comma-shaped 'shadow' that is located below a malignancy, which is of lesser sonographic density directly beneath the center of a tumor than at the edges; 'tadpoles' appear in malignant masses and have ragged margins, related to necrotic tissue, which is a poor conductor of ultrasonic waves; Cf Tennis racquet sign

Taffy candy 'syndrome' CARDIOLOGY A fanciful descriptor for the clinical symptoms that result from elongation of the anterior leaflet of the mitral valve, which may be idiopathic or be associated with rheumatic fever and myocardial infarction

Taffy pulling effect Marked elongation of a structure, likened to stretched taffy candy or chewing gum CARDIOLOGY Marked elongation and thinning of the anterior mitral leaflet's chordae associated with mitral valve regurgitation, which may later rupture SURGICAL PATHOLOGY Spindled, darkly basophilic streaks and strands due to the extreme delicacy of the nuclear chromatin; although this 'crush artefact' is highly characteristic of pulmonary small (oat) cell carcinomas, it may also be seen in lymphomas and chronic inflammation

TAH Transfusion-associated hepatitis

TAH-BSO Total abdominal hysterectomy-bilateral salpingo-oophorectomy

Tail Any elongated, usually terminal component of an organism, cell, molecule, statistic or other component in a system that slowly arrives to a baseline

Tail coverage MALPRACTICE INSURANCE An umbrella of malpractice insurance protection that a physician is obliged to retain until the 'statute of limitations' (a period of two to three years) has been completed, which covers malpractice claims that may be initiated after a physician has moved to another state or retired (the so-called tail period); the cost of 'tail coverage' is equal to at least one year of malpractice premium coverage and may be multiples thereof Note: In the USA, malpractice insurance costs from $2000 to $200 000 per annum, a fee that is a function of location (Florida, California and New York State are highest) and the relative risk for lawsuit in a specialty; the standard 'claims-made' malpractice insurance policies are less expensive, but do not cover tail periods; see Malpractice, Statutes of limitations Cf Nose coverage

Tailing LABORATORY TECHNOLOGY The diffusion of a 'spot' of a substance of interest at the trailing edge in a chromatogram or electrophoretic gel, which contrasts to the sharply-demarcated leading edge

Tailings ENVIRONMENT The residual sandy waste remaining after extraction of uranium from mined ore; tailings were used as landfill in one site in the Western US under homes and public buildings, resulting in high gamma-radiation exposure to inhabitants and required removal by the Environmental Protection Agency

Tail sign see Comet tail sign

'Take' TRANSPLANTATION IMMUNOLOGY The adherence of a free skin graft occurring between days three and five of the transfer of skin; if the graft 'takes', it is pink indicating neovascularization; the thinner the graft, the more likely it will 'take', as long as it contains dermis; 'take' also refers to the prolonged survival of any transplanted organ that passes the hyperacute (vascular) and chronic (immune-mediated) phases of rejection

Talc granuloma A foreign body giant cell reaction seen in: 1) The peritoneum, body cavities or tissues or elsewhere, due to contamination by surgical glove lubricants, eg talc, lycopodium, mineral oil rice or corn starch, or by cellulose fibers from disposable gauze pads, drapes, gowns and other paper products 2) Various organs, commonly the lungs of intravenous drug abusers, where the substance of abuse, usually a white powder, has been 'cut' with starch or talcum powder; the granulomas measure 14-50 µm in diameter and are located in eccentric patches of connective tissue and fibrous septae; the lungs show mild medial hypertrophy of the pulmonary arteries, but are not associated with pulmonary hypertension and 3) In patients using talc in the subepithelial tissues of external genitalia, causing talc granulomata of the vagina, cervix, uterus, tubes, urethra and bladder

Talin A 235 kD protein that comprises 3-8% of the platelet's protein, which with vinculin, attaches actin filaments to the platelet's plasma membrane

Talk and die 'syndrome' A form of presentation in acceleration-deceleration brain injury that, like a progressive subdural hematoma, has a latency period (here, 48-72 hours) until death; the condition is no longer invariably fatal as early treatment of cerebral edema reduces mortality

TAMI studies Thrombolysis and angioplasty in myocardial infarction studies A series of multi-center clinical trials designed to examine the role of angioplasty, urokinase, heparin and prostacyclin in the management of acute myocardial infarction (J Am Med Assoc 1990; 263:2629); see CASS, TIMI studies

Tamoxifen ONCOLOGY A widely preferred agent used to treat early estrogen receptor-positive breast carcinoma; meta-analysis indicates that tamoxifen reduces breast cancer mortality by 20% in women over the age of 50, while conventional chemotherapy reduces mortality by 25% in those under age 50; estrogen receptor-negative patients may respond to 5-fluorouracil and methotrexate with leucovorin rescue; prophylactic tamoxifen may be of use in postmenopausal women at high risk for breast carcinoma (J Nat Cancer Inst 1990; 82:1310ed)

T & A see Tonsillectomy and adenoidectomy

Ts and Blues SUBSTANCE ABUSE A pair of drugs with some currency as recreational drugs of abuse, which produce a euphoric state likened to that evoked by heroin at a lower cost; pentazocine ('T'), a narcotic analgesic, is mixed with pyribenzamine, an antihistamine dispensed as blue tablets (Blues), which together are heated and injected in mutiple 'sets'; when used during pregnancy, 35% of the infants suffer neonatal withdrawal syndrome and growth retardation (J Repro Med 1986; 31:236)

T & S see Type and screen

Tandem repeat A sequence of oligonucleotides present in native DNA in multiple copies and adjacent to each other, ie in tandem; tandem repeats include the genes for 45S pre-rRNA, 5S rRNA, various tRNAs and the histone family of DNA-related proteins; the repeated segments are virtually identical to each other, are arranged in a head-to-tail fashion and are separated by 'spacer' segments of varying lengths of DNA; see Repetitive DNA, Telomere; Cf Junk DNA

Tangier disease A rare autosomal recessive condition due to deficiency in α-lipoprotein, first described on Tangier Island in the Chesapeake Bay, Maryland **Clinical** Lymphadenopathy, hepatosplenomegaly, mild proximal peripheral neuropathy, intermittent diarrhea and corneal opacification **Laboratory** Absent high-density lipoprotein, low cholesterol (< 120 mg/dl), decreased phospholipids, normal to increased triglycerides **Pathology** Enlarged yellow-orange tonsils, lymphoid tissues and rectal mucosa, due to massive storage of cholesteryl esters in foamy macrophages in the bone marrow, lymph nodes, thymus, spleen, liver, skin, jejunum, schwann cells and tonsils **Prognosis** Usually benign, rarely coronary artery disease

'Tango and cash' SUBSTANCE ABUSE A form of heroin available on the street market for illicit drugs in the Northeastern USA that is 'cut' with fentanyl, providing its users with more 'bang for the buck', resulting in a number of fatal overdoses; since fentanyl is relatively inexpensive to produce and results in a greater 'high', this combination may increase in popularity (J Am Med Assoc 1991; 265:2962c)

'Tanned' red cells IMMUNOLOGY Red blood cells that have been treated with a 1:20-40 000 dilution of tannic acid, which allows them to act as antigen carriers, enhancing the visualization of antigen-antibody reactions, eg hemagglutination; protein binding to erythrocytes is strengthened by adding a covalent binder eg toluene di-isocyanate

Tanner stages see Sexual maturity rating

Tanning devices PUBLIC HEALTH Beds or booths fitted with ultraviolet (UV) light bulbs that emit ultraviolet-A, and lesser amounts of ultraviolet-B radiation, homogeneously delivering maximal light in the minimum time; the desire for a 'healthy' tan' has spawned an industry in the US that is serviced by poorly-regulated tanning salons; 58% of subjects in one study (MMWR 1989; 38:333) reported injury at commercial tanning facilities; 37% were injured at home, with damage to a) Eyes Corneal injury 85%, unspecified 13% and combined corneal and retinal injury 3% b) Skin Photoaging, first and second degree burns c) Degeneration of dermal blood vessels and d) Non-specific dysfunction of the immune system

T antigen(s) MOLECULAR BIOLOGY A group of 90 kD proteins present in the nucleus that bind tightly to DNA, playing a pivotal role in viral DNA transcription and replication during the lytic cycle; the T antigen is involved in the transition from early to late transcription, as occurs when the SV 40 virus invades the cell; the three sites binding T antigen are close to the initiation site for RNA synthesis and a local increase in T antigen decreases the transcription of T antigen's gene; see T proteins, Cf T cell antigens TRANSFUSION MEDICINE An antigen present on the surface of all red cells that is 'hidden' (thus known as a cryptantigen) from the immune system by an N-acetyl neuraminic acid residue; when this residue is removed by a bacterial infection, polyagglutination may occur, as all subjects except infants intrinsically produce antibodies that react with the exposed T antigen, although the hemolytic potential of the antigen is unclear; see T activation

t antigen 'Little t' An antigen related to the T antigen of the SV40 virus, with which it shares N-terminal sequence homology

Tapioca pudding appearance see Sago spleen appearance

Tapir nose A descriptor for a collapsed nose with a 'reversed ski jump' appearance caused by ulceration and destruction of the nasal septum, a classic finding in espundia, an infection caused by *Leishmania braziliensis*; tapirs are nocturnal ungulates of tropical America, Sumatra and Malaya, related to horses and rhinoceri

Tap water infection An infection by an organism contaminating drinking water, which are responsible for either true enteral infections or pseudoepidemics, in which the tap water contaminates a step in the culture of bacteria; tap water organisms include bacteria, eg *Aeromonas hydrophilus* (often associated with gastrointestinal tract and wound infections), *Legionella pneumophila, L dumoffi* (N Engl J Med 1991; 324:109) and other *Legionella* species, *Mycobacterium chelonae*, amoebae (eg *Acanthamoeba hatchetti, Filamoeba nolandi* and *Hartmanella* species), *Giardia lamblia,* a diplomonad flagellate, Pittsburgh pneumonia agent (*Tatlockia micdadei*), *Pseudomonas pickettii* (J Am Med Assoc 1991; 265:981), *Rhodococcus* (*Gordona*) *bronchialis* (N Engl J Med 1991; 324:104) and others of undetermined clinical significance (J Am Med Assoc 1990; 263:2924) Note: Some organisms are thermophilic, and colonize hot water supplies, eg *Legionella pneumophila, M xenopi, M kansasii*, while others are cryophilic, eg *Mycobacterium avium, M chelonae abscessus*

Taq polymerase *Thermus aquaticus* polymerase, an enzyme that revolutionized retrieval of minute amounts of DNA from a specimen, see Polymerase chain reaction

TAR Transactivation response protein The HIV-1 tat gene product that transactivates viral gene expression and is essential for HIV-1 replication; TAR inhibits the production of an interferon-induced 68 kD protein kinase (Science 1990; 247:1216)

Tardive dyskinesia NEUROLOGY A late complication seen in 20% of young adults receiving long-term neuroleptic therapy, consisting of abnormal and irreversible involuntary movements of the face, trunk and extremities; tardive dyskinesia paradoxically disappears with resumption of therapy; see 'Piano playing', Rabbit syndrome

Target An adjectival descriptor for any lesion or radiologic finding in which there are three or more relatively well-circumscribed, concentrically-arranged annular patterns or radiodensities

Target cells CYTOLOGY Metaplastic endocervical cells seen in papanicolaou-stained smears containing inclusions within vacuoles, characteristic of cells infected with *Chlamydia trachomatis* HEMATOLOGY Helmet cells, Codocytes Red cells with peripheral and central distribution of hemoglobin related to a) A relative decrease in hemoglobin (Hemoglobins C or S or thalassemia, the first of which are accompanied by crystal formation or rarely, deficiency anemia, post-splenectomy and acute blood loss b) A relative increase in the membrane itself as occurs in lecithin-cholesterol acyl transferase deficiency or obstructive jaundice or c) Related to a transient change in pH

Target fibers Transversely sectioned muscle cells stained with nicotinamide adenine dinucleotide-tetrazolium reductase (NADH-TR) which have a central inactive zone devoid of membrane-bound organelles surrounded by a dense reactive rim, in turn surrounded by a zone of normal sarcoplasm; target cells occur in 20-30% of denervated muscle, often affecting type I muscle fibers

Target follicle HEMATOPATHOLOGY A descriptor for the concentric layering of mature lymphocytes in the mantle zone around germinal centers, seen by low-power light microscopy in the hyaline-vascular form of Castleman's disease (angiofollicular lymphoid hyperplasia)

Target lesion DERMATOLOGY A lesion typical of erythema multiforme (EM) in which a vesicle is surrounded by an often hemorrhagic maculo-papule; EM is often a self-limited dermatosis of acute onset that resolves within 3-6 weeks, and has a cyclical pattern; EM lesions are 'multiform' and include macules, papules, vesicles and bullae and may be idiopathic or follow infections, drug therapy or occur in immunocompromised hosts

Target sign GASTROINTESTINAL RADIOLOGY A smoothly-contoured radiopacity with both central and peripheral radiolucency, seen in pedunculated colonic polyps, when viewed en face by double contrast (air-contrast) barium studies; the 'eccentric' target sign is seen in gastrointestinal diverticuli where a small amount of radiocontrast enters the pouch and is surrounded by the radiopaque body of the diverticulum PULMONARY RADIOLOGY A descriptor for circumscribed pulmonary aspergillomas or foci of necrotizing bronchopneumonia seen in a plain chest film; Cf Coin lesions

Target sequence A short segment of recipient DNA that is the target for transposon insertion; the sequence undergoes self-replication and the transposon is inserted between the two target sequences; see Transposon

Targett A low frequency antigen of the Rh system, the presence of which may cause a depression in D antigen expression

TAR RNA Transactivation response RNA A segment of RNA located at the 5' end of the untranslated leader region of all viral messenger RNAs; inversion of TAR RNA eliminates transactivation and point mutation of the segment reduces its activity; HIV-1's Tat protein binds the TAR region and may be involved in HIV's pathogenicity (Science 1990; 249:1281)

Tarsal tunnel syndrome A carpal tunnel syndrome-like complex caused by post-traumatic fibrosis, abductor hallucis hypertrophy, tenosynovitis or fascial band entrapment by the posterior tibial nerve Clinical Pronounced plantar surface and toe causalgia that may irradiate to the calf, paresthesias, cyanosis, coldness and numbness Treatment Massage, steroid injection, weight reduction or surgical decompression of the compartment

TAR syndrome An autosomal recessive disease of perinatal onset characterized by thrombocytopenia with absent radius Clinical Profound thrombocytopenia, purpura with amegakaryocytosis in bone marrow and bilateral aplasia of the radii and thumbs; up to two-thirds of patients have leukemoid reactions, occasionally anemia and eosinophilia, cardiovascular disease, eg atrial septal defect, Fallot's tetralogy, cutaneous and renal anomalies Prognosis One-half die in the first year of life due to intracranial hemorrhage

Tart cell A segmented neutrophil that has retained some nuclear fragments in its evolution towards becoming a full-fledged LE (lupus erythematosus) cell; tart cells retain the chromatin clumps, nucleoli and nuclear membrane

TAT MOLECULAR BIOLOGY TAT protein see *tat* gene PSYCHOLOGY Thematic apperception test A projection-type psychological test that evaluates a child's sense of reality, personality traits and gives insight into his fantasies; see Psychological testing

TATA see Tumor-associated transplantation antigen

TATA box MOLECULAR BIOLOGY A highly conserved oligonucleotide (thymidine-adenine-thymidine-adenine) sequence that is present in many frequently and/or rapidly transcribed genes, eg hemoglobin, histone, U6 and 7SK genes, and required for efficient transcription; the TATA sequence is located in a fixed site 25-35 nucleotides upstream (5' direction) from the TATA box and is recognized by and responsible for positioning of RNA polymerase II (RpII), which in turn is responsible for processing and transcribing mRNA; Cf CCAAT box, Pribnow box

TATA protein see TFIID

***tat* gene** A gene present in retroviruses eg HTLV-I, HIV-1 that encodes the Tat transactivating protein, which enters the nucleus, stimulates viral proliferation, possibly via a viral promoter, in turn activating other retroviral genes; the *tat* gene is oncogenic and induces mesenchymal tumors in experimental systems Note: Tat alone is capable of activating cells, suggesting the existence of an as-yet unidentified cellular analog of an activating protein

Tatlockia micdadei A new designation for *Legionella micdadei*, an organism which has previously had other aliases including Pittsburgh pneumonia agent and the TATLOCK strain

Tattoo A relatively permanent form of cutaneous decoration that may range from simple, often small dark-colored insignias, messages or symbols that may be performed by amateurs in prison to elaborate multi-colored animals, objects or scenes performed by more skilled workers under relatively sterile conditions; tattoo pigment is dermal and periadnexal in distribution, similar to argyrosis; the pigments are either a) Permanent, eg carbon, vermillion, India ink and Prussian blue, some of which may be removed by laser surgery or b) Nonpermanent, eg cinnabar and aniline; see Laser surgery

Tattooing TRAUMATOLOGY The complex skin abrasions and wounds filled with debris, glass and dirt, that result from being dragged along a road, often occurring in pedestrian victims of automobile accidents; treatment requires adequate debridement and often wound healing by second intent

tau Kendall's tau STATISTICS A non-parametric measure of correlation between a known fact and a set of variables, ranging from +1.00 to -1.00, which is used where parametric statistical distortions arise from data distributed in a non-normal fashion or in the presence of extreme outliers of data points

Tau protein(s) A group of 55-62 kD microtubule-associated phosphoproteins (MAPs), first isolated from the brain that have major sequence homology with MAP2; the different sequences of the MAP family are generated by alternative splicing of transcripts; tau proteins migrate in the β-γ region in an electrophoretic gel, are encoded by chromosome 21, are induced during neurite outgrowth, and regulate microtubule assembly, limiting growth and shrinkage of dynamic microtubules, co-localizing with the microtubules, increasing tubulin polymerization, decreasing the rate of microtubular depolymerization, possibly facilitating generation of spirals from the α-β dimer in microtubules, are prominent in Alzheimer's neurofibrillary tangles and are the main antigen of the paired helical filaments that accumulate in the degenerating neurons of Alzheimer's disease; the Tau 69 protein may correspond to A68; see A68

Tautomerism An equilibrium between two or more distinct isomeric forms of a molecule, eg an enzyme

Taxol A chemotherapeutic agent that acts on microtubules, inducing tubulin polymerization and formation of stable and non-functional microtubules (vinca alkaloids and colchicine cause microtubule depolymerization); taxol evokes a response in some refractory neoplasms, evoking a positive response in one-third of cisplatin-resistant ovarian carcinoma, as well as malignant melanoma and non-small cell carcinoma of the lung (J Natl Can Inst 1990; 82:1247); taxol is a complex molecule obtained from the bark of the yew tree, a native of old-growth forests in the Northwest US, which has antineoplastic potential, taxol is controversial as an enormous amount of ancient forest trees are required to both complete clinical trials and if successful, to market the drug (Science 1991; 252:1780n&v)

Taxon The group or category of an organism, which is classified according to characteristics that it has in common with other similar organisms; classic taxonomy is based on phenotypic differences between organisms and divided according to a hierarchy of kingdom, phylum, class, order, family, genus, species and, if applicable, subspecies and/or strain, with subdivisions between categories, eg suborder and superfamily Note: It is being increasingly recognized that taxonomy must be based on features that are more scientifically valid than the subjectiveness inherent in phenotyping, eg comparison of DNA sequence similarity ('homology')

TB see Tuberculosis

TBG Thyroxine-binding globulin

TBI Total body irradiation

TBT see Transcervical balloon tuboplasty

TCA suicide see Tricyclic antidepressants

TCBS agar Thiosulfate-citrate-bile salt-sucrose agar MICROBIOLOGY The preferred 'recovery' medium for *Vibrio cholera*

TCDD 2,3,7,8-Tetrachlorodibenzo-p-dioxin see Agent Orange, Dioxin

TCE 1,1,1-Trichloroethylene $CHCl=CCl_2$ ENVIRONMENT A volatile chlorinated hydrocarbon that boils at 88°C and is highly soluble (1000 ppm) in water; TCE was formerly used as a degreasing agent and disposed of by pouring into the ground, thus becoming a major ground water contaminant that is detectable in 'plumes' up to 10 km from its original dump site and often present in 'Superfund' toxic dumps; some microorganisms co-metabolize TCE when using methane, propane or toluene as sources of oxygen Toxicity: Peripheral neuropathy, carcinogenic in rats Note: Chloral hydrate, a TCE metabolite is used as a sedative, a questionable practice given its known toxicity (Science 1990; 250:359c); see Bioremediation, Plumes, Superfund, Toxic dumps, 'White-out'; Cf Dioxin, PCBs

T cell T lymphocyte The T (thymus-drived) cell is the most complex cell of the immune system, given 1) The diversity of T cell types, including T cells with activator, cytotoxic, delayed hypersensitivity and suppressor activities 2) The wide range of cytokines, growth factors and immune modulators produced by activated T cells; see Biological response modifiers 3) The complexity of T cell interaction with exogenous and endogenous antigens, eg mediation of delayed hypersensitivity, graft-versus-host disease and 4) The complexity of T cell maturation in thethymus; 50-70% of circulating leukocytes are myeloid; the rest are lymphocytes, of which T cells (defined as having 'pan T cell' markers, CD2 and CD7 and other T cell markers including CD1, CD3 and CD5) comprise 70-85%, while the B cells comprise 15-30%; T cells respond to an antigen via an antigen-presenting cell, which engulfs and processes extracellular antigen (bacterial, viral or other), which is then transported to the cell surface and complexed with the 'self' MHC class II molecule, a process known as MHC restriction

T cell Transitional cell CARDIOLOGY A specialized myocyte that is found in clusters in the sinus node; T cells are intermediate in size, structure and organization between the P cells (see there) and normal atrial myocytes and connect with either of these cells; perinodal T cells surround the sinus tract and are thought to 'bundle' impulses leaving the sinus node and to filter premature ectopic atrial impulses; see P cells

T cell immunodeficiency syndromes (TCIS) A group of immunodeficiency states arising from partial or absolute defects in T cell function; TCIS are generally more severe than B cell defects, have no effective therapy and are characterized by recurrent opportunistic infections, eg by *Pneumocystis carinii*, cutaneous anergy, growth retardation, a decreased life span, wasting or 'runting', diarrhea, increased susceptibility to graft-versus-host disease, potentially fatal reactions to live viral or BCG vaccinations and an increased incidence in malignancy; TCIS include DiGeorge syndrome (thymic hypoplasia), Nezeloff syndrome (cellular immunodeficiency with immunoglobulins) and T cell defects, eg absence of inosine phosphorylase and purine nucleoside phosphorylase deficiency

T cell lymphoma (TCL) A malignant proliferation of T cells that is diagnosed by detecting rearrangement of the T cell receptor's β chain, which may be 'driven' by Epstein-Barr and other viral infections (table, below) MOLECULAR BIOLOGY TCLs have a characteristic chromosomal translocation t(8;14)(q24;q11), with a chromosome 8 breakpoint 3 kilobases in the 3' direction from the c-*myc*, a cellular proto-oncogene, and a chromosome 14 breakpoint, 36 kilobases in the 5' direction from the constant region gene of the T-cell receptor α-chain, resulting in a gene rearrangement on chromosome 8 and the functional Jα segment on chromosome 14, suggesting that the translocation is simultaneous with the T-cell receptor rearrangement, catalyzed by the same systems involved in joining V-J, this is thus similar to the c-*myc* translocations linked to immunoglobulin loci in B-cell malignancies; 18% of one series of 303 lymphomas were T cell lymphomas, 73.% were B cell lymphomas and 8% were indeterminant lymphomas Note: The clinical presentation, histology and immunology of TCL is heterogeneous and one-half are extranodal at the time of presentation (table)

CLASSIFICATION, T CELL LYMPHOMAS

Small lymphocytic lymphoma or well-differentiated lymphocyte-like lymphoma (circa 13%, T cell lymphomas)

Convoluted cell lymphoma or poorly-differentiated lymphocytic lymphoma (52%)

Immunoblastic sarcoma or 'histiocytic' lymphoma (19%)

Mycosis fungoides/Sezary syndrome, composed of cerebriform cell (11%)

Lymphoepithelial cell (Lennert"s) lymphoma (5%)

Cutaneous TCL Epidermotropism, paracortical proliferation in the lymph nodes and periarterial proliferation in the spleen, aggregates of epithelioid cells, prominent vascular channels; often resistant to chemotherapy and radiotherapy

T cell maturation The thymic microenvironment is required for early T-cell differentiation and most migrations of thymic precursor cells occur in the embryonic and early postnatal period; the cells are processed, become competent and are exported to peripheral lymphoid compartments, divided into a conceptual stage I The earliest T cells (10% of thymic lymphocytes) have a CD2 (T11) rosetting marker and non-T stem-cell markers, including CD38 (T10) and transferrin (T9); the cells then acquire a thymocyte antigen, CD1a (T6) that reacts with Langerhans cells and CD4 (the 62 kD MHC class II-restricted antigen) and CD8 (the 76 kD MHC class I-restricted antigen) Stage II 70% of thymocytes express CD4, CD8, CD1a and CD38; with maturation CD1a is lost and cells acquire antigens defined by pan-T markers (CD3 and CD11) and segregate into CD4 (helper phenotype) and CD8 (suppressor phenotype) T cells Stage III Immunocompetence is acquired in the thymus, as defined by the CD3-associated antigen Ti, maturing with exportation; the CD4 and CD8 cells lose CD38 and express increased CD5 and CD3; CD4 T cells represent 55-70% and CD8 T cells represent 20-35% of circulating T lymphocytes

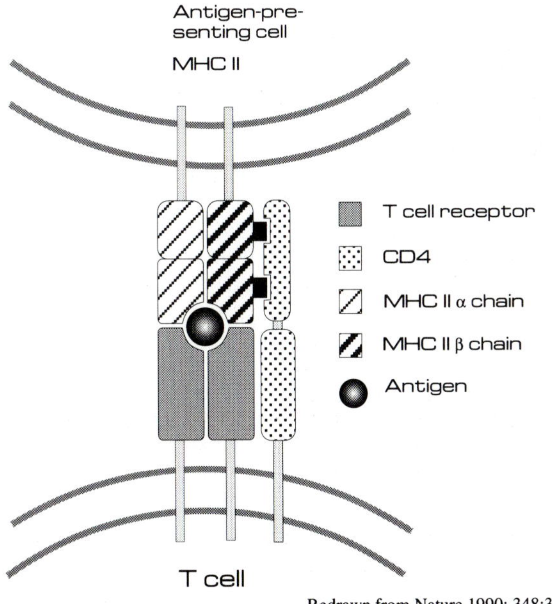

Redrawn from Nature 1990; 348:393

T cell receptor on CD4 lymphocyte

T cell receptor (TCR) A disulfide-linked heteropolymeric membrane-bound protein that is non-covalently complexed to five or more CD3 polypeptides (figure, above); the TCR-bearing average cell has a relatively low (20-40 000/cell) receptor density; TCR specificity is conferred by rearrangement of VDJC (V Variable, D Diversity, J

Joining and C Constant) genes, in a fashion analogous to that of the variable heavy and light immunoglobulin chains in B cells, see Gene rearrangement, which serves as a marker for clonality; the residues present at the V/αJ/α junction are critical to the early selection process, and as the stem cell matures, V, D, J and C exons are spliced together; TCR's α, β and γ genes are variable, while the delta and epsilon genes are constant, and are identified by complementary DNA techniques; TCR regulates signal transduction via a) the phosphatidylinositol pathway, inducing increased inositol phosphates and diacylglycerol, mobilizing cytoplasmic free calcium and activating protein kinase C, which then activates the b) tyrosine kinase pathway (Nature 1990; 348:66); TCR responds differently as a function of the ligand, allowing a 'fine-tuning' of T cell response to antigens (Science 1991; 2552:1308); see CD (cluster of differentiation)

T cell specificity see MHC restriction

T cell tolerance IMMUNOLOGY The deletion of T-helper, T-delayed hypersensitivity and cytotoxic T cell subsets under certain circumstances, which leads to tolerance of the suppressor T cells, which are, in turn, responsible for deleting either B or other T cells, directly suppressing cells that have been 'turned on' by T cells, thus being transferred, as a form of 'infectious' tolerance; high zone tolerance refers to the requirement by B-cells for high affinity B-cell receptors to multivalent antigens; low-zone tolerance is required for weakly immunogenic antigens that are not destroyed by T-suppressor cells, which are triggered at lower doses than T-helper, low zone tolerance is partial and only affects some lymphocytes

TCID Tissue culture infective dose VIROLOGY An objective measurement of a body fluid's infective potential, where serially-diluted aliquots of a fluid, eg plasma, are placed in cell cultures to detect growth and measured in units of TCID/ml plasma; the $TCID_{50}$ is that dose of virus that produces a toxic effect in 50% of test animals over a specified period of time

TDF see Testis-determining factor

TDM see Therapeutic drug monitoring

TDO syndrome Tricho-dento-osseous dysplasia An autosomal dominant condition characterized by kinky, curly hair, small defective teeth that fall out by late adolescence, osteosclerosis and craniosynostosis

TdT Terminal deoxynucleotide transferase An intracellular DNA polymerase that catalyzes the irreversible addition of 5'-deoxynucleotides to the 3' hydroxy- ends of DNA and is a marker for human T cell differentiation from the stem cell to the prothymocytic stages in the thymic cortex and medulla; TdT is detected by indirect immunofluorescence in immature T and B cells, in 1-5% of marrow cells, 60-90% of cortical thymocytes, various leukemias, eg T cell leukemia, in 90% of common acute lymphoblastic leukemias, 50% of acute undifferentiated leukemia, 30% of chronic myeloid leukemia in blast crisis, occasionally also in pre-B acute lymphoblastic leukemia but rarely in chronic lymphocytic leukemia

TEA Tetraethylammonium chloride An experimental potassium channel blocker used to study action potentials (Science 1990; 250:276)

Tea-drinker's disease Theism A caffeine-induced nervous condition that is uncommonly reported in the current environment, clinically characterized by congestion of cephalic vessels, excitement, and/or depression, pallor, cardiac dysrhythmia, hallucinations and insomnia (J Am Med Assoc 1887; 7:410)

Team approach see Medical team

Teardrop bladder TRAUMATOLOGY A descriptor for a markedly distended urinary bladder in which a trauma-induced hematoma surrounds the bladder base, lifting it out of the pelvis; external pressure narrows the bladder neck into an attenuated 'stem', while a broad base at the bladder's apex imparts a piriform configuration by excretory urography; other causes of a teardrop bladder include extensive pelvic lipomatosis, inferior vena cava occlusion, psoas muscle hypertrophy, and rarely pelvic lymphadenopathy

Teardrop cell Dacrocyte A deformed red cell that has squeezed through a reticuloendothelial system bearing increased connective tissue, seen in agnogenic myeloid metaplasia, myelofibrosis and other reticuloendothelial replacement disorders that compromise marrow space, causing splenic overload or loss of functional splenic tissue, including megaloblastic anemia, bone metastases, hereditary elliptocytosis and sickle cell anemia; see Red cell glossary

Teardrop fracture A fracture-dislocation type of compression fracture of the anterior aspect of the body of a cervical vertebra, caused by hyperflexive compressive forces that burst the vertebral body, separating and displacing a wedge-shaped fragment of bone from the antero-inferior margin of the vertebral body; the potential danger in these fractures is posterior displacement into the spinal canal causing cord compression; Cf Wedge fracture

Teardrop sign An elongated soft-tissue mass that prolapses into the maxillary antrum, which may be seen in a plain film of the face in blunt trauma to the anterior rim of the orbit, causing a 'blowout' fracture to the orbital floor

Teat and udder sign RENAL RADIOLOGY A fanciful descriptor for an appearance that may be seen in an excretory urogram when the kidney is affected by a mass lesion located at the cortico-medullary junction, where the papillae and short-stemmed calyces ('teats') are associated with a large displacing mass ('udder')

Technologist see Medical technologist

Technician A person with at least two years of formal college or university education in a wide range of laboratory techniques, who upon passing the appropriate examination written and administered by the American Society of Clinical Pathologists, carries the title of MLT(ASCP); technicians are empowered to perform clinical tests, but not to report the results without the approval of a medical technologist

Techoic acid antibody assay see TA-AB

Teflon Polytetrafluoroethylene A polymeric molecule that is resistant to organic solvents, has a melting temperature of 225°C, and has diverse medical applications including use in prosthetic articulations, vascular grafts and in low-temperature chemical reactions

TEFRA Tax Equity and Fiscal Responsibility Act of 1982 (Public Law 97-248) A US federal law that provided for key health care expenditure reforms, including risk-sharing contracts with health maintenance organizations and revision of reimbursement arrangements with hospital-based physicians, where the hospital's reimbursement from Medicare ('part A') is clearly separated from the professional component (or physician's services, 'part B'); TEFRA placed a ceiling or 'cap' on the annual operating revenues per inpatient Medicare case at each hospital; see DRGs, RBRVS

Telecanthus-hypospadias syndrome BBB syndrome An X-linked recessive condition characterized by hypertelorism, a broad nasal bridge, cleft lip and palate, cardiac defects, imperforate anus and hypospadias and mental retardation

Teleology A view of the physical universe that holds that all structures and functions in an organism have a purpose and confer an evolutionary advantage to the organism; according to Aristotle, the purpose of each component was invoked by a supernatural being Note: In order to dignify the heuristically logical argument that nothing evolves without a raison d'etre, while circumventing the mystical import of the concept, the ersatz term 'teleonomy' has been suggested, although teleology continues to be widely preferred

Telepathology An embryonic field that may eliminate the need for small rural hospitals to have an on-site surgical pathologist, which utilizes high-resolution video cameras and robot microscopes to transmit images of tissues and manipulate specimens to a center with multiple experts

'Telephone receiver' deformity PEDIATRIC RADIOLOGY A descriptor for the long tubular bones of infants with thanatophoric dwarfism; the bones are short, broad with metaphyseal flaring, occasionally display 'cupping' of the end-plates; afflicted bones have a rhizomelic distribution and are markedly curved at the ends; other bone anomalies in this condition include the Cloverleaf skull deformity, frontal bossing and H- or U-shaped vertebral bodies

Teleradiology A form of delivering expert radiology services by transmitting a digitalized image obtained by angiography, computed tomography, magnetic resonance imaging, positron emission tomography, sonography, thermography and other imaging devices via satellite or telephone circuits to radiologists who may be located hundreds of kilometers away; the major disadvantage is the time required for transmitting the image

'Telescoped' urine casts LABORATORY MEDICINE Molded proteinaceous material found in the urine sediment that contains all the possible elements found in renal disease, including red cells, leukocytes, hyaline, cellular and granular casts, fat and lipid; these casts are typical of lupus erythematosus, but may also be seen in other collagen vascular diseases and renal disorders (eg acute and chronic glomerulonephritis, the nephrotic syndrome and renal transplant rejection), subacute bacterial endocarditis, hyperviscosity syndrome, malignant hypertension, toxemia, heavy metal poisoning, multiple myeloma, amyloidosis and sickle cell disease; see Casts

'Telescoping' The 'compression' or overlapping of clinical or pathological features of a disease or lesion that is normally subdivided into chronological stages of progression

Telescoping fractures Those fractures seen in osteogenesis imperfecta where marked osteoporosis facilitates an axial compaction fracture with collapse, shortening and thickening of the long bones

'Television intoxication syndrome' A term that arose from a legal case in which a 'depraved heart' murder was attributed to the alleged perpetrator's suggestibility and loss of reality sense, resulting from his excess television viewing ('intoxication') Note: While the term has not been legitimized in the medical literature, it is heuristically logical that the 40-50 hours of weekly television (passive entertainment), viewed by children in the US, and elsewhere, would cause various unanticipated side effects; see 'Couch potato'

Telomere MOLECULAR BIOLOGY A 3-5 kilobase pair segment of DNA composed of variable (in number) tandem 'repeats' of the oligonucleotide sequence TTAGGG, which is added to the end of linear chromosomes by a nontemplate mechanism involving a multifunctional telomerase; the TTAGGG repeats were first described as 'junk' DNA, but are present in high copy numbers in the centromere and demonstrate marked evolutionary conservation among species, possibly preventing incomplete replication and chromosomal instability; telomeres are elongated in immortalized cells and increasingly shortened in normal cells undergoing senescence (Nature 1990; 345:458)

Template A mold or pattern used as a guide to form a copy of the original, as is the use of a DNA 'template' to produce a copy of itself or, through transcription into RNA, which subsequently matures into messenger RNA, which is a template for translation into proteins

Temporal lobe syndrome of Klüver-Bucy The functional loss of major portions of the temporal lobes and rhinencephalon (amygdala, hippocampus, uncus and hippocampal gyrus); this can be reproduced experimentally in monkeys by bilateral temporal lobectomy Clinical Visual agnosia, tendency to examine all objects orally and examine immediately all objects seen, loss of emotion, hypersexuality in the form of heterosexual, autosexual and homosexual activity and increased consumption of meat Histopathology Degeneration of myelinated fiber tracts in most communicating and projecting tracts in the face of minimal retrograde cellular degeneration; see Hypersexuality

Temporomandibular joint syndrome see TMJ syndrome

TEN see Toxic epidermal necrolysis

Tenascin A matrix protein composed of six identical 210 kD proteins, which is synthesized by the mesenchymal cells of the developing embryo and responsible for differentiation of epithelial tissues

Tennis elbow Lateral epicondylitis SPORTS MEDICINE A condition with no limitation of movement, swelling or pain when the articulation is moved passively, but which is painful when actively moved **Diagnosis** Active dorsiflexion of the wrist against resistance or firm fingertip pressure over the lateral humeral epicondyle produces sharp pain **Treatment** Rest, splinting and if necessary, local injection of corticosteroids; see Golf elbow

Tennis leg Exercise-induced rupture of calf muscles that may occur following any violent exercise in which the rapidly-moving body abruptly changes directions, including tennis, soccer, downhill skiing **Clinical** An audible snap may be heard in the popliteal space, accompanied by severe calf pain and hematoma, due to a rupture of the gastrocnemius muscle **Treatment** Immobilization in plantar flexion and physical therapy

Tennis racquet An adjectival descriptor for a relatively elongated cell, lesion, structure or radiological density that is globose at one end and elongated at the other, likened to the popular recreational device used in tennis

'Tennis racquet' appearance A descriptive term for the ping-pong paddle-like thickening of the mesangium in glomeruli affected by in Kimmelstiel-Wilson disease

'Tennis racquet' cell An uncommon variant rhabdomyoblast seen in sarcoma botryoides, a form of rhabdomyosarcoma affecting children

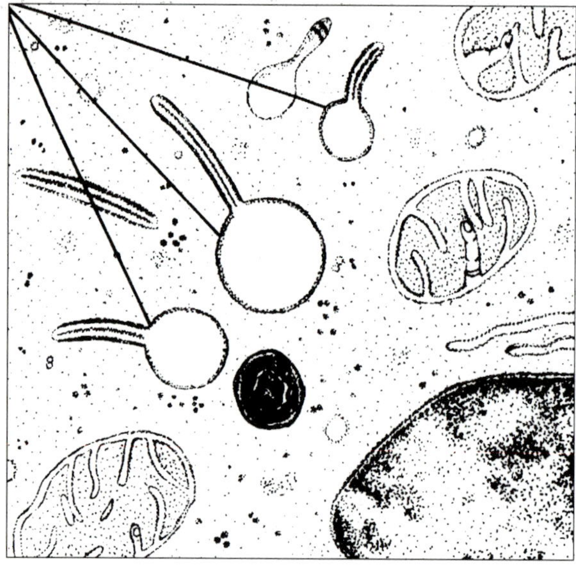

Tennis racquet granules

'Tennis racquet' granule Birbeck granule Langerhans' granule A subcellular particle with a pentalaminar 'handle' and bulbous terminal dilatation of uncertain significance that is seen by electron microscopy in the antigen-presenting Langerhan's cell and in histiocytes (figure)

'Tennis racquet' sign The descriptor for a finding in a 'blighted ovum' in which the ultrasonically empty gestational sac is compressed (the racquet's 'handle') and adjacent to a surrounding decidual reaction (the 'paddle'); Cf Tadpole sign

'Tennis racquet' spores MICROBIOLOGY A descriptive term for the morphology of the subterminal spores in the gram-positive *Clostridium tetani*, as well as in *C diphtheriae* (figure, right)

Teniposide An investigational drug for acute lymphoblastic leukemia used in early relapse, while the patient is still in the consolidation phase of chemotherapy or used in an attempt induction in patients who failed a first induction

Ten percent tumor A mnemonic for pheochromocytomas, as 10% are malignant, 10% are bilateral, 10% are extra-adrenal, 10% occur in children and 10% are associated with other systemic disease, including von Recklinghausen's disease, von Hippel-Lindau syndrome, Sturge-Weber disease and multiple endocrine neoplasia (MEN) IIa and IIb

TENS Transcutaneous electrical nerve stimulation A modality for controlling pain that utilizes low-level electric shocks to the skin; TENS effect is explained by the 'gate' theory of pain and is used to relieve pain of the lower back and neck, 'phantom' limb syndrome and amputation stump pain; in lower back pain, TENS may be no more effective than a placebo (N Engl J Med 1990; 322:1627; 323:1423c); Cf Biofeedback

Tensilon test A clinical test used in patients with known myasthenia gravis to distinguish between a myasthenic and cholinergic crisis; the short-acting cholinesterase inhibitor, Tensilon (edrophonium chloride), is administered with a syringe containing 10 mg; if one minute after 2 mg is injected, there is no change in muscle strength, then the remainder is injected; in a cholinergic crisis, the weakness will worsen and be accompanied by colicky pain and fasciculation of the eyelids; see Myasthenic crisis

Tensin(s) A pair of 150 kD and 200 kD actin-binding proteins that have phosphotyrosine-binding activity and may mediate signal transduction pathways in the cytoskeleton (Science 1991; 252:712)

Tension headache Cephalgia related to prolonged muscle contraction, which beginning as an occipital non-pulsatile, vise-like pain extending fronto-temporally, with 'tight' posterior cervical, temporalis or masseter muscles; tension headaches are most common in women who also suffer migraines and are related to postures requiring sustained contraction of the above muscles, exacerbated by stress

Ten/thirty (10/30) rule TRANSFUSION MEDICINE A clinical guideline (tansfusion 'trigger') for when to transfuse packed red cells, ie when the hemoglobin is below 100 g/L (US: 10 g/dl) and/or when the hematocrit is below

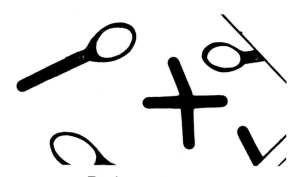

Tennis racquet spores

30%; with the advent of AIDS, clinical decisions to transfuse blood have become more conservative, and unless a patient is actively bleeding, hospital transfusion committees may sanction the lower '9/27' or '8/24' rules, since clinically stable patients often tolerate very low red cell masses without co-morbidity; see Single unit transfusion, Transfusion 'trigger'

Tenting CARDIOLOGY A term for the symmetrical 'peaking' of the 'T' wave on the electrocardiogram, which is associated with a lengthening of the P-R interval, typically seen in early hyperkalemia; with further increases of potassium, the P wave disappears and a sine wave appears INTERNAL MEDICINE A clinical sign consisting in light pinching of a patient's skin, which under usual conditions, springs back to a flattened position; a delay in flattening or tenting is characteristic of relatively severe dehydration and in the elderly whose dermal collagen and elastin have undergone age-related cross-linking

Tenure ACADEMIA A status granted to a person with a 'terminal' degree, eg doctor of medicine (MD) or doctor of philosophy (PhD), after a trial period, which protects him from summary dismissal; individuals in academics who hold positions on the 'tenure track' are expected to assume major duties in research, teaching and, if applicable, patient care, fostering through their activities, the academic 'agenda' of their respective departments; see Endowed chair, Lecturer, Professor; Cf 'Chair'

Teratogen Any agent that acts on a developing fetus, inducing structural abnormalities; maternal medications with known teratogenic effects include aminopterin (abortion, malformations), anticoagulants, anticonvulsants, cytotoxic drugs, mepivacaine (bradycardia, death), methimazole and propylthiouracil (goiter), ^{131}I (destruction of fetal thyroid), male sex hormones (methyltestosterone, 17-α-ethinyl-testosterone and 17-α-ethinyl-19-nortestosterone, masculinizing to female infants), tetracycline (hypoplasia and pigmentation of tooth enamel) and trimethadione (abortion, multiple malformations, mental retardation); female sex hormones act on genital structures causing masculinization with defective external female genitalia, transplacental carcinogenesis by DES; see Fetal warfarin syndrome, Fetal hydantoin syndrome, Thalidomide; Cf 'Litogen'

Teratogenesis The generation of malformations during the early development of the fetus, presumed to be due to any of a number of environmental toxins; major congenital malformations occur in 1:10 000 infants, 45% of which are de novo autosomal dominant or X-linked mutations that cannot be predicted (N Engl J Med 1989; 320:19); 'soft' data implies that some occupations are at an increased risk for fetal malformations, eg nursing (exposure to chemotherapy, hexachlorophene, anesthetics, eg NO_2, halothane), cosmetologists (hair spray, fingernail adhesives), chemical manufacturing and processing (various agents,especially petrochemicals), those in the petrochemical industry; see Bendectin, Crack babies, DES, Fetal syndromes, Sellafield studies and Thalidomide

Teratoma A tumor derived from the multipotent cells of one or more of the primitive embryologic layers (ectoderm, endoderm, mesoderm), which differs in prognosis according to the organ involved and degree of maturation of the tissues; teratomas are most common in the mediastinum, ovary and testicle, but may occur in the urogenital tract and various parenchymal organs **MEDIASTINAL TERATOMA** A tumor that may occur in both sexes, which are most commonly composed of mature epithelium, as well as neural, gastrointestinal, chondral and respiratory tissues and are almost invariably benign; mediastinal teratomas composed of immature elements are too rare for valid prediction of their future behavior **OVARIAN TERATOMA** A tumor that includes the common (20% of all ovarian neoplasms) mature teratoma, 98% of which are benign and the uncommon immature (malignant) teratoma, which is graded according to the amount of immature neuroepithelial tissue present (the greater the amount the worse the prognosis) and treated by surgery and multiagent chemotherapy **TESTICULAR TERATOMAS** are designated as A) ADULT TERATOMA, if all the cellular elements are mature B) IMMATURE TERATOMA, if areas reminiscent of the primitive tissues seen in Wilms' tumor (a 'prototypic' primitive tumor) are present or C) TERATOMA WITH MALIGNANT TRANSFORMATION, if a malignancy, usually a squamous cell carcinoma or adenocarcinoma, arises in an adult teratoma

Terminal COMPUTERS A peripheral component of a computer network that has a monitor, an input device, eg a keyboard and often an output device, eg a printer; a 'dummy' terminal allows simple accession of information; a 'smart' terminal is used for data entry and some forms of data manipulation MOLECULAR BIOLOGY The end of a) A protein, either the N-terminal or the COOH-terminal or b) A segment of a polynucleotide chain, either the 3' (upstream) end or the 5' (downstream) end of the molecule

Terminal bar CYTOLOGY The portion of the cell below and perpendicular to the cilia seen papanicolaou-stained smears of the ciliated columnar cells, which is thought to correspond to the sum of the belt desmosomes, actin filaments and other proteins aggregated at the apical end of the cells; teminal bars are seen in the normal respiratory epithelium, adenomas, adenocarcinoma, APUDomas, transitional and papillary carcinomas of the urinary bladder, synovial sarcomas and mesotheliomas

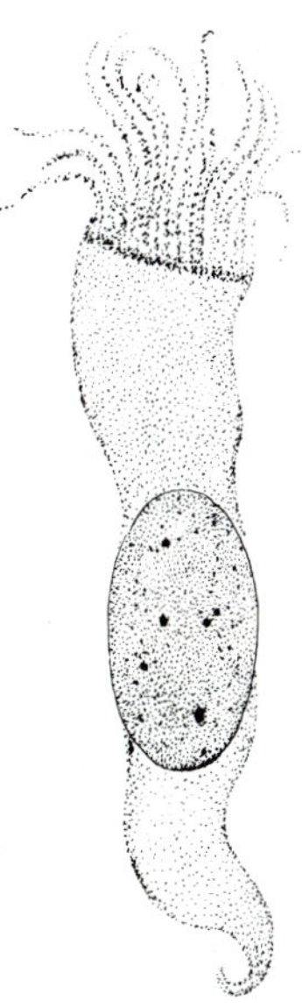

Terminal bar

Terminal cancer A malignancy that is expected to cause the patient's death within a short period of time, ie weeks to several months; patients with terminal cancers have one or more of the following features: no response to any form of therapy, tumor-related cachexia and marked weight loss, florid metastases to multiple sites or 'secondary' metastases, ie those arising from an already metastatic focus, marked jaundice (when the liver is replaced with malignancy), a need for constant pain medication and compression of vital stuctures of 'impossible' surgical access; terminal cancer patients are best treated with compassion and moral support administered by 'significant other(s)' in a hospice environment, although some patients may seek 'miracle' cures and undergo 'heroic' forms of surgery or actively seek unproven therapies for cancer; see 'Heroic' surgery, Hospice, Most significant other, Unproven therapies for cancer; Cf Spontaneous remission of cancer

Terminal duct carcinoma A low-grade malignant salivary gland tumor that is most common in the palate, which despite a uniform cell type, has a wide range of architectural configurations, including tubular, cribriform, solid and fascicular patterns **Prognosis** Recurrence 12%; loco-regional lymphoid metastases 10% **Treatment** Excision, post-operative radiation

Terminal repeat MOLECULAR BIOLOGY A segment of redundant oligonucleotides present at one or both ends of DNA; see Long terminal repeat; Cf Telomeres

Terminal reservoir 'syndrome' GASTROENTEROLOGY A potentially massive dilation of the descending and sigmoid colon, particularly common in the elderly, which is initially caused by voluntary suppression of defecatory urge; as the rectal stretch receptors degenerate, a vicious cycle of overextension and fecal impaction develops (Gerontology 1983; 29:181)

Termination MOLECULAR BIOLOGY The final step in a) Polypeptide synthesis, after which it is released by the ribosome or b) The transcription of mRNA from the DNA template by RNA polymerase, which ends with a termination or stop (UAA, UAG, UGA) codon; see Translation

Terpene(s) see Isoprenoid(s)

Terry-Thomas sign An increased space between the navicular and lunate bones seen in a frontal film of a wrist with subluxation of the carpal navicular bone, in which there is backward rotation of the proximal pole and forward rotation of the distal pole; this increased gap has been fancifully likened to the dental diastema of the late British comic actor, Terry-Thomas

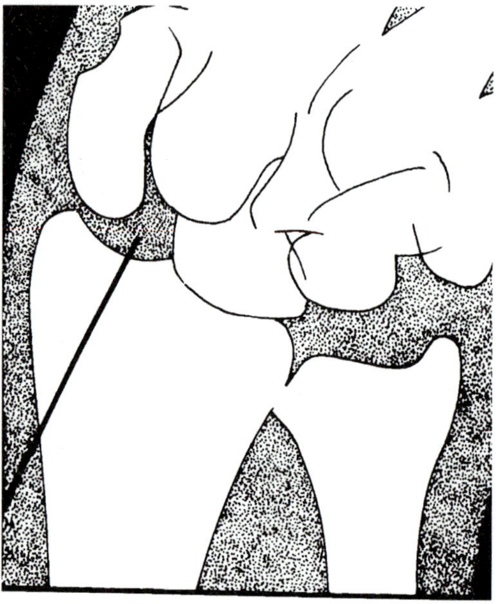

Terry-Thomas sign

Tertian fever A fever characterized by febrile paroxysms occurring every third day, as in the 48-hour febrile peaks in *Plasmodium vivax* malaria, also known as benign tertian malaria; malignant tertian fever is caused by the more virulent *P falciparum*, which in its most intense form may be fatal within days; Cf Quartan fever

Tertian malaria see Tertian fever

Tertiary care HEALTH CARE INDUSTRY The most specialized level of health care, which is administered to patients who have complex diseases and/or may require high-risk pharmacologic regimens or surgical procedures; patients who receive tertiary care are usually referred by either a primary care giver or by a specialist who recognizes that the therapy appropriate for a patient is beyond his ability or expertise to perform in his own environment; such care is provided in 'tertiary care centers', often university hositals, as it mrequires sophisticated technology, a team of specialists and often subspecialists, a diagnostic support group and intensive care facilities; tertiary care includes complex neurosurgery, transplantation and experimental oncology protocols; Cf Primary care, Secondary care

Tertiary center bias see Referral center bias

Tertiary structure see Protein structure

Testicular feminization syndrome Morris syndrome A pseudohermaphroditic state due to an X-linked testosterone receptor deficiency, which causes a poor end-organ response to androgens, giving rise to a blind vaginal pouch without uterine tissue; there is normal secretion of and response to müllerian inhibiting hormone, resulting in a phenotypic female with adequate secondary sex characteristics; although the gonads often harbor Sertoli cell adenomas, malignancy occurs in only 4% of cases of testicular feminization; therefore, unlike mixed gonadal dysgenesis in which malignancy is common in younger patients, in testicular feminization, it is better to preserve the gonads until after the pubertal growth spurt

Testicular malignancy see Germ cell tumors

Testis-determining factor (TDF) A protein encoded by a gene in the SYR region on the short arm of the Y chromosome (Nature 1990; 346:240, 245, 279), which is responsible for development of primary male organs; see X-chromosome inactivation; see X chromosome inactivation

Test of healing A therapeutic trial of H_2-blockers, eg cimetidine, ranitidine that is used in patients with a gastric ulcer, in whom a decrease in ulcer-type of pain is equated with therapeutic success; non-resolution of symptoms after 3-6 weeks of H_2-blocking therapy is considered an indication for endoscopy and endoscopic biopsy as the possibility of a gastric carcinoma must be ruled out

'Test-tube' baby A full-term gestational product resulting from in vitro fertilization of an egg that was implanted in a uterus and carried to term by either the genetic mother or by a surrogate (gestational) mother; the first successful test-tube baby was baby girl Brown born in 1978 (N Engl J Med 1990; 323:1200ed); see Artificial reproduction, Baby M, in vitro reproduction, Surrogate motherhood

Test tube rete pegs DERMATOPATHOLOGY A descriptor for the uniformly elongated rete pegs that are accompanied by edema and vascular congestion of the papillae, findings characteristic of psoriasis; see 'Squirting papillae'

Tetanospasmin A 150 kD neurotoxin produced by *Clostridium tetani* that is the most toxic substance known to man, causing profound muscle spasms due to tetanospasmin's blockage of the release of glycine (a neurotransmitter for group 1A inhibitory afferent motor neurons), resulting in unrestrained muscle firing and sustained muscular contraction, potentially causing lockjaw, dysphagia or acute respiratory failure by tetany of the diaphragm; see Poisons

Tetanus toxoid A small peptide fragment that selectively elicits helper immune response but not immune suppression; the tetanus is a highly effective vaccine for *Clostridium tetani* and most of the US population has received tetanus toxoid at 2, 4, 6 and 15 months (the 'primary' series), a 'booster' between ages 4-6 and (theoretically) should receive another 'booster' every ten years; in open 'dirty' wounds, booster shots are often given, as well as 250 units of tetanus immune globulin to 'cover' for possible clostridial contamination

Tetra-X syndrome see XXXX syndrome

Texas cattle fever Bovine babesiosis A now-eradicated tick-borne infectious disease of cattle caused by *Babesia bigemina*

T(-shaped) fracture Y-shaped fracture ORTHOPEDICS A type of intercondylar fracture of the distal femur that occurs in falls from a height with the feet extended, resulting in a violent impact of the femur on the tibial plateau; similar fall-related fractures may occur as the distal tibia impacts on the ankle or as an intercondylar fall-related fracture to the distal humerus; Cf Lover's heels

TFIIA, TFIIB, TFIID, TFIIE, TFIIF MOLECULAR BIOLOGY A group of initiation factors required for RNA polymerase II (RpII) to initiate transcription at promoter sites, which are assembled in a defined sequence; TFIID binds to the TATA box, an oligonucleotide sequence present in most promoters that is transcribed by RpII; after TFIID and TFIIA are bound to the promoter, TFIIB, RpII and TFIIE/TFIIF can be incorporated into the initiation complex; TFIID is a highly-conserved 37.7 kD polypeptide that is probably the polypeptide most central to the initiation of eukaryotic mRNA synthesis, binding to the TATA box promoter element, regulating the expression of most genes transcribed by RNA polymerase II; the C-terminal 181 amino acids of human TFIID have an 80% amino acid sequence similarity ('homology') with a similar protein in the yeast *Saccharomyces cerevisiae* (Science 1990; 248:1646) and are functionally interchangeable in vitro (Nature 1990; 346:291)

TGF Transforming growth factor(s) A group of distinct polypeptides that have been isolated from virus-transformed rodent cells, capable of altering cell phenotype, causing fibroblasts to lose anchorage-dependence and stimulating angiogenesis

TGF-α Transforming growth factor-α A 50-residue polypeptide synthesized by transformed cells, which has a 35% amino acid sequence similarity ('homology') with epidermal growth factor (EGF); both are angiogenic, but TGF-α is ten times more potent than EGF in stimulating cell growth

TGF-β Transforming growth factor-β A 25 kD homodimeric, regulatory peptide produced by various normal and neoplastic cells bearing TGF-β receptors; TGF-β is thus both autocrine and paracrine, opposing the action of endogenous cytokine, tumor necrosis factor, balancing the immune system; in epithelial and connective tissue, TGF-β recruits macrophages and fibroblasts, evoking collagen production and angiogenesis (capillary formation), forming granulation tissue, playing a role in wound healing; TGF-β inhibits cell proliferation and differentiation, inhibits neutrophil adherence, regulates other cytokines, stimulates extracellular matrix production (ECM) and is down-regulated by decorin (Nature 1990; 346:281); the inability to produce TGF-β or to respond to its inhibitory effect has a role in carcinogenesis; recombinant TGF-β (Genentech) may be of use in myocardial infarction (Science 1990; 249:61) Note: Because TGF-β1 elicits ECM production, anti-TGF may be useful in treating mesangial proliferative glomerulonephritis (Nature 1990; 346:371); TGF-β1 induces collagen I and III production in cirrhosis, corresponding to the elusive cirrhosis transforming growth factor, causing fibrosis; TGF-α production is increased in cirrhosis with regeneration (N Engl J Med 1991; 324:933)

THA 1) Total hip arthroplasty see Total hip replacement 2) Tetrahydroaminoacridine A long-acting acetylcholinesterase co-inhibitor administered with lecithin that was reported to ameliorate the symptoms of Alzheimer's disease, a claim that has not been substantiated (Br Med J 1990; 300:495, N Engl J Med 1990; 322:1272)

Thalidomide 2,6-dioxo-3-phthalimido-piperidine A drug that was first marketed as a sedative and sleeping aid, which was thought to have responsible for up to an estimated 12-15 000 cases of embryopathy, having this effect between days 45 to 55 of a human gestation; one dose is sufficient to cause birth defects, often resulting in phocomelia or 'flipper' extremities; the thalidomide tragedy is a chilling example of the effects of stereochemistry; L-thalidomide is a powerful tranquillizer; the D- form is teratogenic (Nature 1989; 342:631; see Chirality), possibly acting by causing lysosomal defects, as occurs in the Japanese quails, the animal model of thalidomide embryopathy; thalidomide has a new generation of indications, including the treatment of rheumatoid arthritis, photodermatitis, Behçet's disease, lupus erythematosus and graft-versus-host disease (J Am Med Assoc 1990;263:1497); it is also of use in treating the skin lesions of lepromatous leprosy (erythema nodosum leprosum, available in the USA as an investigational drug; other leprosy agents include clofazimine, rifampin and dapsone or diaminodiphenyl sulfone)

Thallium imaging CARDIOLOGY A myocardial perfusion technique in which the radionuclide thallium-201, is injected as a diagnostic adjunct to cardiac stress tests, with the purpose of detecting regional ischemia or infarcts TYPES STRESS IMAGING Images which identify perfusion defects during exercise REDISTRIBUTION IMAGING Images obtained after a 3-4 hour rest period to identify 'redistribution' of the isotope Note: In many regions of viable 'hibernating' myocardium, there are defects that appear during stress imaging and which do not disappear upon redistribution imaging, thus falsely simulating irreversible lesions; a minibolus of thallium-201 at 3-4 hours ('REINJECTION IMAGING') delineates areas that might have otherwise been considered non-viable (N Engl J Med 1990; 323:141); see Treadmill exercise test

THAM Tris(hydroxymethyl)aminomethane Tris buffer EMERGENCY MEDICINE An amine proton donor that is administered intravenously during early cardiopulmonary resuscitation to treat lactic acidosis; THAM is regarded by some to be a completely interchangeable substitute for sodium bicarbonate at the same dosages (in mEq), acting to neutralize fixed acids in tissues *ADVANTAGES* THAM is not a CO_2 donor, thus hyperventilation of an already compromised patient is not required in order to 'blow off' the CO_2 and it easily enters the intracellular spaces *DISADVANTAGES* THAM causes apnea, hypoglycemia, venous irritation, and because it is a powder requiring mixture, it would be difficult to use in a true emergency

Thanatophoric dwarfism Greek thanatophoric, death bearing Chondrodysplasia punctata dwarfism of Conradi-Hünerman n A form of dwarfism with a 2:1 male:female ratio, in which the infants are stillborn or die in the early neonatal period Clinical Hydrocephaly, megalocephaly with frontal bossing, chondrodystrophy, narrow thorax with respiratory difficulties, congenital heart disease, hypotonia and hyporeflexia (floppy infant), hypertelorism, cloverleaf skull, saddle nose, marked skeletal abnormalities with shortened deformed 'telephone receiver' long bones, affecting the epiphysis, causing micromelia, alteration of the foot, lenticular opacity, shortened extremities with curved fingers, H or U-shaped vertebrae and pulmonary hypoplasia resulting in short postnatal survival

Thaumatin A 207 single-chain protein that has a 100 000-fold greater affinity (on a molar basis) than dextrose for the human sweet taste receptor; see Artificial sweeteners

THBR see Thyroid hormone binding ratio

THCA see Trihydroxycoprostanoic acid syndrome

THC receptor The cannabinoid (marijuana) receptor has been identified and has characteristics of a G protein-coupled receptor found in the brain and neural cell lines which inhibits adenylate cyclase activity in a dose-dependent, stereoselective fashion (Nature 1990; 346:561); see Marijuana

Theca cell tumor A sex cord-stromal tumor of the post-menopausal ovary that is yellow, large and unilateral, composed of fascicles of lipid-rich spindle cells interspersed with collagen, reticulin fibers and hyaline plaques; thecomas and other estrogen-producing tumors, eg granulosa cell tumors may induce adenomatous hyperplasia of the endometrium or well-differentiated endometrial carcinoma in 3-20% of cases; see Sex cord-stromal tumors

Theine Obsolete for caffeine

Therapeutic drug monitoring (TDM) Pharmacokinetics The regular measurement of the serum levels of those drugs that require close 'titration' of doses in order to ensure that there are sufficient levels in the blood to be therapeutically effective, while avoiding potentially toxic excess; drug concentration in vivo is a function of multiple factors: 1) Patient compliance, ie whether the patient is actually taking the drug in the doses prescribed 2) Bioavailability, ie whether the substance enter the circulation, interacting with its cognate receptor(s), or whether it is ionized and 'free' or bound to a carrier molecule, often albumin 3) Pharmacokinetics, ie whether the drug has reached equilibrium, which requires four-to-six half-lives of drug clearance (a period of time for one-half of the drug to 'clear', either through metabolism or excretion, multiplied by four to six); the drug may a) interact with foods or other drugs at the site of absorption, eg tetracycline binding to cations or chelation with binding resins, eg bile acid-binding cholestyramine that also sequesters warfarin, thyroxine and digitoxin or interactions of various drugs with each other, eg digitalis with quinidine resulting in a three-fold decrease in digitalis clearance b) be poorly absorbed due to gastrointestinal hypermotility or large size of the molecule c) be lipid soluble, which affects the volume of distribution; a highly lipid-soluble substance has an enormous affinity for adipose tissue and a low tendency to remain in the vascular compartment (see Volume of distribution); d) undergo biotransformation, with 'first pass' elimination by hepatic metabolism, in which polar groups are introduced into relatively insoluble molecules by oxidation, reduction or hydrolysis; for elimination, lipid-soluble drugs require the 'solubility' steps of glucuronidation or sulfatation in the liver; water-soluble molecules are eliminated directly via the kidneys, weak acidic drugs are eliminated by active tubular secretion that may be altered by therapy with methotrexate, penicillin, probenecid, salicylates, phenylbutazone and thiazide diuretics Kinetics a) First order kinetics The elimination of a drug is proportional to its concentration b) Zero order kinetics Drug elimination is independent of the drug's concentration 4) Physiological factors a) Age Lower doses are required in both infants and the elderly, in the former because the metabolic machinery is not fully operational, in the latter because the machinery is decaying, with decreased cardiac and renal function, enzyme activity, density of receptors on the cell surfaces and decreased albumin, the major drug transporting molecule b) Induction of enzymes involved in a drug's metabolism may reduce the drug's activity; enzyme-inducing drugs include barbiturates, carbamazepine, glutethimide, phenytoin, primidone, rifampicin c)

Inhibition of enzymes involved in drug metabolism results in enhanced drug activity, prolonging the action of various drugs, including chloramphenicol, cimetidine, disulfiram (Antabuse), isoniazid, methyldopa, metronidazole, phenylbutazone and sulfonamides 5) Genetic factors play an as-yet poorly defined role in therapeutic drug monitoring, as is the case of the poor ability of some racial groups to acetylate drugs 6) Concomitant disease, ie whether there are underlying conditions that may affect drug distribution or metabolism, eg renal disease with decreased clearance and increased drug levels, or hepatic disease, in which decreased albumin production and decreased enzyme activity result in a functional increase in drug levels, due to decreased availability of drug-carrying proteins; therapeutic drug monitoring requires that a) The method measures what it is designed to measure, and not a bioinactive metabolite b) The turn-around time is reasonable enough to allow adjustment of dosages c) Tolerance to the drug does not develop d) Concentration of the drug in the serum is proportional to the concentration at the site of action, ie receptor and there is a correlation between the concentration in the serum and the therapeutic effect and e) The therapeutic range is well-defined, and the toxic and therapeutic ranges are close enough to require monitoring

Therapeutic index CLINICAL PHARMACOLOGY The ratio of a drug's toxic level to therapeutic level, calculated as the toxic concentration (TC) of a drug divided by the effective concentration, expressed as TC_{50}/EC_{50}, a point at which 50% of patients have a toxic reaction to the drug to be monitored; the lower the therapeutic index, the more difficult it is to titrate a drug's dose in a patient and the more imperative it is that the drug be monitored; see Apparent volume of distribution, First-order kinetics, Peak levels, Trough levels, Volume of distribution, Zero-order kinetics

Therapeutic privilege BIOMEDICAL ETHICS A paternalistic principle under which the truth is withheld from a patient owing to concern that if the details of a therapeutic procedure are fully delineated, the patient may choose to forego an operation that the physician believes to be in the patient's best interest or his only option for improved quality of life and/or survival; since therapeutic privilege assumes in part that the patient is something less than an autonomous, self-directed person, 'therapeutic privilege' is rarely invoked in the USA as a justification for surrogate decision-making, given the fear of litigation on the part of physicians; in the US, a physician's moral duty is to tell the truth, regardless of the potential harm that may result from a patient receiving too much information that he may be incapable of understanding; see Doctor-patient interactions, Paternalism

'Therapeutic privilege' doctrine LEGAL MEDICINE A doctrine with legal weight that protects the physician when faced with a patient who may be too emotional or apprehensive to fully and logically assess his needs for a therapeutic intervention; such situations may arise in emergencies, advanced age and dementia; when possible, the physician should obtain permission from the nearest relative; Cf Doctor-patient interaction, Informed consent, Paternalism

Therapeutic window The range of a drug's concentration in which the desired effect occurs, below which there is little desired effect and above which toxic effects appear; the therapeutic window differs among patients and may be determined empirically

Thermography A diagnostic technique formerly used to diagnose breast cancer, which detects the increased warmth of the skin overlying malignancy, a relatively non-specific finding that also occurs in mastitis; the technique was abandoned due to the unacceptably high rates of false positivity and false negativity; Cf Mammography, Xeroradiography

Thermomotor dissociation see Pulse-temperature dissociation

Thesaurocytes see Flame cells

'Thick' section A toluidine blue-stained section of a tissue that is embedded in a hardened epoxy resin, which measures from 0.5 to 1.5 μm in thickness and is cut from the same block of tissue as the 'thin' sections that are to be examined by transmission electron microscopy; examination of 'thick' sections by light microscopy allows rapid selection of the optimal tissue for ultrastructural studies Note: Sections for routine histologic examination by light microscopy are 5 to 8 μm in thickness and are embedded in paraffin; see Thin section

Thin-layer chromatography (TLC) LABORATORY MEDICINE A technique in which a thin layer of alumina, polyacrylamide gel, silica gel or starch gel is bonded to a glass or plastic plate and then bathed for 30-90 minutes in a solvent containing a substance of interest, allowing the substance to migrate by capillary action; if further identification of the substance is required, the 'spot' of drug may be scraped off for further analysis by gas-liquid chromatography; TLC is often used to 'screen' for the presence of drugs of abuse

Thin section A 0.05 μm thick section of epoxy resin-embedded tissue that is stained with a heavy metal, eg lead or uranium for examination by transmission electron microscopy; Cf Thick section

Thioredoxin A ubiquitous 12 kD protein that donates electrons to ribonucleotide reductase and has disulfide isomerase activity

Third-day blues see Postpartum 'blues'

'Third diabetic syndrome' A form of diabetes mellitus described in young black patients that is thought to differ from type I (insulin-dependent/juvenile onset) diabetes in that a) 30-40% have HLA-DR3 or HLA-DR4 antigen, in contrast to caucasians, 95% of whom express HLA-DR3 or -DR4 b) 40% have islet cell antibodies, versus 70-80% of whites c) Most patients are easily controlled by diet or oral anti-diabetes agents and d) the inheritance pattern appears to be autosomal dominant

'Third factor' see Natriuretic hormone

Third generation cephalosporins A group of broad-spectrum antibiotics including cefatoxime, ceftazidime, ceftriaxone and moxalactam that are structurally related to penicillins and used against penicillinase-producing bacteria; third generation agents have increased activity against enteric bacteria, are stable against the β-lactamases of *Haemophilus influenzae* and *Neisseria gonorrhoeae*, have a longer serum half-life than the first generation cephalosporins and thus can be administered twice per day, successfully cross the blood-brain barrier and are thus effective against gram-negative central nervous system infections **FIRST GENERATION CEPHALOSPORINS**, eg cephalothin, cephaloridine and cefazolin are effective against penicillinase-producing streptococci, pneumococci and staphylococci and active against important gram-negative pathogens, including *Escherichia coli*, *Klebsiella* and *Proteus*, having prophylactic currency in intra-abdominal surgical procedures and is of use in treating penicillinase-binding *Staphylococcus aureus* **SECOND GENERATION CEPHALOSPORINS**, eg cefamandole, cefoxitin and cefuroxime offer only minimal improvement over the first generation, although cefoxitin is of use in treating *Bacteroides fragilis* infections; 'serious' systemic infections are usually treated by third generation cephalosporins **FOURTH GENERATION CEPHALOSPORINS** do not exist and would need to be active against methicillin-resistant staphylococci and enterococci

Third party HEALTH CARE INDUSTRY A person or organization ancillary to the doctor-patient 'dyad', who/that participates in financing the services rendered, eg a health insurance carrier, or who acts as an administrative agent for processing and paying claims or for health care services provided, eg Blue Cross/Blue Shield, Medicare

Third sector see Voluntary sector

Third space A non-physiologic space into which fluids may pass in emergency clinical situations, the size of which cannot be calculated; the intracellular space comprises 65-80% of the body fluid volume and the extracellular space comprises the remaining 20-35%, of which 25-35% is plasma volume and 65-75% is interstitial volume; the 'third space phenomenon' is an emergency situation in which a derangement of 'Starling' forces allows sequestration of fluids into relatively nonfunctional extracellular 'compartments', eg within the lumen in intestinal obstruction, to the skin in burns, to the pleura or peritoneum in vascular rupture or ascites, or elsewhere; fluid replacement calculations are based on the first and second spaces, and are of little use in determining internal redistribution or 'parasitic losses' of fluid into third spaces; third space losses are treated with saline solutions or crystalloids and 'titration' with blood pressure Note: Starling forces are the sum of the positive intravascular oncotic pressure and the negative pressure provided by the venous flow, which act to maintain fluid in the vessels, minus the oncotic pressure in the interstitial space and the forward pressures of the blood as it is 'driven' into the capillaries, both of which act to pull fluid from the intravascular space

Thirteen-day fever Shanghai fever A typhoid-like *Pseudomonas* infection described in the tropics, characterized by fever, myalgia and diarrhea that resolves spontaneously without residua

Thomsonism ALTERNATIVE MEDICINE A health care philosophy of historic interest that was espoused by S Thomson (1769-1843), a farmer and 'endowed healer' from New Hampshire, who qualified the ancient Greek doctrine of disease being the imbalance of the four 'bodily fluids' (blood, phlegm, yellow bile and black bile) with the modifiers of hot and cold, wet and dry; Thomson concluded that cold was the ultimate pathological state and sought to cleanse the body, adding to the body's heat by using *Lobelia inflata*, as an emetic and enema (J Am Med Assoc 1987; 257:1632); see 'Holistic' medicine, Homeopathy, Hot-cold syndrome, Naturopathy

Thoracic inlet injury Traumatic injury to the base of the neck involving the superior mediastinal vessels (innominate, subclavian, proximal common carotid arteries and veins); damaged vessels in the thoracic inlet are surgically problematic as facile access is blocked by the clavicosternal 'shield'; although the correlation of anatomic defects with clinical symptoms is poor, adequate regional exploration and hemostasis in this region results in reduced mortality

Thoracic outlet syndrome Scalenus syndrome A condition caused by compression of the brachial plexus and subclavian artery between a cervical rib and the scalenus anticus muscle Clinical Unilateral paresthesia, myalgia, myasthenia and muscular atrophy, associated with vasomotor disorders, edema and thromboses, most commonly affecting women with osteoporosis, which may be also occur in pregnancy, trauma or overstretching Note: The thoracic outlet is a tight anatomic compartment containing vessels and nerves that are either resident, in or traverse through the space; compromise of this space causes specific 'syndromes', including cervical rib syndrome, scalenus anticus syndrome, costoclavicular syndrome, pectoralis minor syndrome and the first rib syndrome; although vascular compromise occurs in 90% of these syndromes, the symptoms are predominantly neurogenic

'Thorn apple' appearance A descriptor for the yellow-brown spherical ammonium biurate crystals with long irregular spikes, found in normal alkaline urinary sediment, structures that have been likened to thorn apples, the fruit of the jimsonweed, *Datura stramonium* (figure, right)

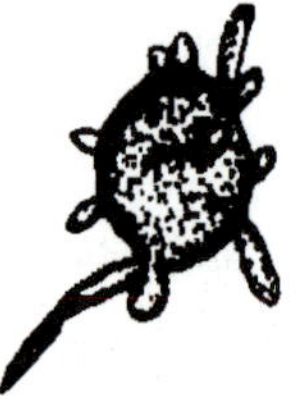

Thorn apple

Thorn sign RADIOLOGY A vaguely-defined spicular radiologic shadow (figure, facing page) that tapers medially from the lateral chest wall, which corresponds to a thickening of the minor fissure, most commonly seen in a right-sided pleural effusion; since the finding appears in most positions, the thorn sign should prompt a lateral decubitus film and ultrasonography to confirm the presence of pleural fluid

Thorotrast Thorium dioxide $^{232}ThO_2$ A radiocontrast medium that emits α particles, has a half-life of 400 years and is stored in the reticuloendothelial system; Thorotrast was first used in 1928, and was abandoned in 1947 with reports of Thorotrast-induced neoplasia; the prototypic Thorotrast-induced tumor is hepatic angiosarcoma, but cholangiocarcinoma and hepatocellular carcinomas are also related to throrotrast (rarely, all three tumors may occur in the same patient Cancer 1982; 49:2161), as can be leukemias, lymphomas, carcinoma of the lung, kidney and bladder, head and neck sarcomas, mesothelioma and malignant fibrous histiocytoma (NJ Med 1990; 87:47); see Radiothor, Radium Dial Company

3/B translocation syndrome A congenital complex due to translocation of a chromosomal fragment from chromosome 3 to a 'B' chromosome (chromosome number 4 or 5), which affects 40% of the progeny of female carriers, causing craniofacial and cardiac anomalies, cleft lip and palate; 15% of the children born to male carriers have the disease, but all are stillborn

Three-day fever Pappataci fever A dengue-like infectious disease described in the Balkans and elsewhere in Southern Europe, resulting from the injection of an unidentified virus by the sandfly, ***Phlebotomus papatasi***

Three Mile Island ENVIRONMENT A nuclear power plant near Pittsburgh, Pennsylvania that approached core meltdown in 1979 due to delayed recognition of equipment malfunction; no injuries occurred, but the incident resulted in a costly cleanup; see Chernobyl, Goiania; Cf Sellafield

'Three-piece suits' A colloquial and non-specific term for any businessman, which in the health care industry, includes 'medicrats' (MD/MPHs, ie physicians with a master's degree in public health, hospital administrators), financial officers, pharmaceutical representatives ('detail men'), and 'bean counters', who function within a medical center's bureacracy

Three Ts (agents) of parasitic myocarditis: Trichinosis, toxoplasmosis and trypanosomiasis

Threshold The limit at which point a physiological effect takes place, eg threshold of the renal tubules for the absorption of solutes and threshold of photoreceptors for light

Threshold limit value (TLV) OCCUPATIONAL MEDICINE The concentration of an airborne chemical or potentially toxic (measured in parts per million/cubic liter/hour exposure) or radioactive substance (measured in microcuries) below which employees may work over an eight-hour period without known adverse effect

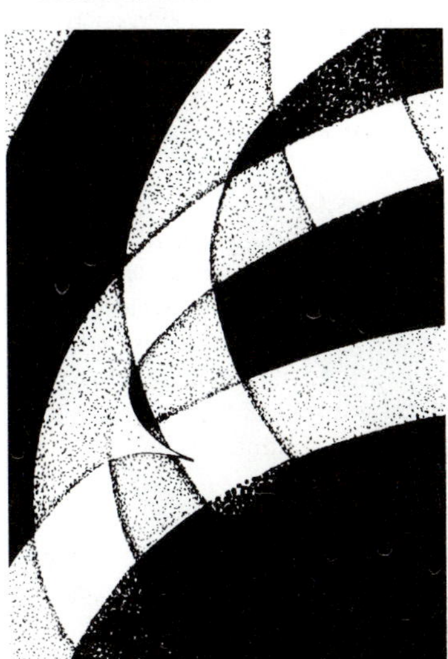

Thorn sign

Thrill CARDIOLOGY A palpable murmur correlating with zones of maximum intensity of auscultated sounds; rough lower sternal border thrills occur in ventricular septal defect, apical systolic thrills are associated with mitral valve insufficiency; diastolic thrills may be palpated in atrioventricular valvular stenosis

Thrombomodulin A 68 kD endothelial cell membrane receptor that mediates anticoagulation, binding thrombin and catalyzing its transformation into protein C activator Pro-C(a), which in the presence of calcium, causes a 30 000-fold increase in activated protein C; thrombomodulin and coumadin both inactivate protein C and in coumadin-induced necrosis, protein C is reduced; Pro-C(a) is constantly inactivating factors Va and VIIIa prior to indiscriminate intravascular coagulation

Thrombophlebitis Phlebothrombosis A term that arose when deep vein thrombosis was thought to occur either without inflammation (phlebothrombosis) or with inflammation (thrombophlebitis), a concept that has long since been abandoned, although the term thrombophlebitis continues to be used in reference to inflamed or infected thrombi, potentially giving rise to septic infarcts

Thrombopoietin(s) A group of proteins produced in a variety of tissues that regulate the quantity of megakaryocyte-committed stem cells, modulating the maturation and development of platelets

Thrombospondin A glycoprotein composed of three 145 kD subunits that is stored in the α granules of platelets and secreted at the site of vascular injury, binding to the arginine-glycine-aspartic acid oligopeptide or RGD sequence; thrombospondin mediates interactions of adhesive proteins with integrin receptors, binding platelets to cells at the glycoprotein-IV (CD36) receptor; it is present in platelets, fibroblasts, endothelial cells and in the extracellular matrix, where it binds to collagen V, fibrinogen and fibronectin and is increased in inflammation, wounding and stress Note: It may also bind erythroid stem cells to stromal regulatory cells in the formation of erythroblast islands; see Integrin family

Thrombosthenin see Actomyosin

Thrombotic thrombocytopenic purpura (TTP) A rare (1:10^6/year) disorder of the microcirculation most common in women age 20-50 **Clinical** Moschcowitz's pentad: Thrombocytopenia, splenomegaly, varying neurological signs, disseminated intravascular coagulation and fever, as well as pallor, jaundice, thrombosis, fibrin thrombi in renal vessels, heart, liver and spleen, epistaxis, cerebral, retinal and vaginal hemorrhage, neurologic defects, eg headache, confusion, aphasia, transient paresis, ataxia, sensory disturbances and coma, cardiac dysfunction, hepatomegaly and pancreatitis; TTP may be associated with lupus erythematosus, rheumatoid arthritis and Sjögren syndrome **Laboratory** Thrombocytopenia, usually < 50 000/mm^3, normal coagulation factors, decreased complement proteins, Coomb's-negative microangiopathic hemolytic anemia (often severe, 30% have decreased hemoglobin < 55g/L, US: < 5.5 g/dl) and reticulocytosis), schistocytes, burr cells, helmet-shaped erythrocytes, normoblasts and reticulocytosis, increased unconjugated bilirubin, increased plasma hemoglobin and hemosiderin, decreased haptoglobin and proteinuria **Pathogenesis** Platelet-aggregating factor and/or multimers of factor VIII:vWF (von Willebrand factor) induce TTP-related platelet agglutination, a phenomenon reversed by immunoglobulin therapy, implying absence of antibodies normally responsible for inhibiting platelet aggregation (Mayo Clin Proc 1989; 64:956) and decreased endothelial ability to stimulate prostaglandin G synthesis **Treatment** Cortico-steroids, aspirin, dipyridamole; if no response, plasmapheresis Note: TTP has been recently recognized to be a polar form of a condition, at the other end of which is hemolytic-uremic syndrome, see there, TTP-HUS

Thromboxanes A family of substances produced from arachidonic acid by cyclooxygenase, which generates prostaglandin G_2 that is subsequently converted by thromboxane (Tx) synthetase into the most biologically important product, TxA_2, which increases after vascular injury, eliciting a primary hemostatic response, inducing platelet aggregation and vasoconstriction; TxA_2 also inhibits platelet adenylate cyclase, reducing cAMP and mobilizing calcium; see Arachidonic acid

'Throw-away journal' A medical journal that is received gratis or by non-paid subscription, which contains (in general) non-peer-reviewed articles, often in the form of reviews; 'throw-aways' are in large part supported by advertising, and have an advertisement/article ratio that is significantly higher than that of their academic counterpart, the 'peer-reviewed journal (J Am Med Assoc 1991; 266:2830c); 'throw-aways' are broad in the scope of material covered, may provide adequate reviews of emerging areas and relevant updates, have abbreviated bibliographies and are often sponsored by the pharmaceutical industry; Cf Peer-reviewed journal

Thrush Pseudomembranous candidiasis A term first used by Pepys in 1665, that refers to an erythematous intraoral lesion overlaid by white, creamy patches, which correspond to necrotic debris, squames, fibrin, inflammatory cells, abundant fungal hyphae and bacteria

Thrush breast appearance Tabby cat, Tigroid appearance A descriptor for the patchy lesions of fatty metamorphosis of the cardiac subendothelium and papillary muscle most prominent in the left ventricle, which is related to caused by prolonged hypoxia, where the red-brown myocardium alternates with yellow bands of fatty degeneration; a similar lesion may be caused by diphtheria, see Flabby heart

Thucydides 'syndrome' MEDICAL HISTORY The Plague of Athens (430 to 427 BC) decimated Athens' population of 300 000 and probably signaled the end of Greek civilization, which had in two generations created or nurtured the basic pursuits of philosophy, history, tragedy, comedy and democracy; the Greek general, Thucydides, recorded the plague's clinical features, which are variously postulated to have been due to smallpox, bubonic plague, scarlet fever, typhus, measles, typhoid fever, ergotism or an influenza virus complicated by a toxin-producing noninvasive staphylococcus, ie a form of toxic shock syndrome (N Engl J Med 1985; 313:1027)

'Thumb' and 'little finger' signs A pair of radiologic findings seen on plain lateral films of the neck; the 'thumb' occurs in acute epiglottitis and corresponds to an edematous aryepiglottic fold (epiglottic shadow) with near-complete obliteration of the valleculae and pyriform sinuses, likened to an adult's thumb; the 'little finger' is used for comparison, where the epiglottic shadow is svelte, resembling an adult's little finger

'Thumbprinting' A finding in a barium study of the colon, which consists of multiple broad, sharply-defined short and rounded often symmetric indentations in the contrast column; although it is described in both a) Mesenteric artery ischemia or ischemic 'colitis' with infarction and intramural hematoma formation (often at the splenic flexure and descending colon) and b) Ulcerative colitis, 'thumbprinting' is non-specific and may be seen in pneumatosis cystoides intestinalis (due to indentation of the barium column by the mucosa-covered gas), pseudomembranous colitis, ***Entamoeba histolytica*** amebiasis, ***Escherichia coli*** O157:H7 enterocolitis (due to submucosal edema) and other infectious colitides, hemorrhage, Crohn's disease, endometriosis, hereditary angioneurotic edema, amyloidosis and malignancy (lymphoma, metastases); when the edema affects the mucosal folds of the small intestine, it is called 'Pinky printing'; thumbprinting in the markedly thickened folds of the gastric fundus and body in an upper gastrointestinal tract may occur in Menetrier's disease (giant hypertrophic gastritis); Cf Collar button lesion

Thymic wave sign A subtle radiopaque undulation caused by the costochondral junctions of adjacent ribs, seen by a plain antero-posterior chest film in a normal thymus; thymic tumors are more firm and thus are not indented by the ribs

Thymine dimer A focal defect in DNA formed after exposure to ultraviolet light, which consists of pairing of the thymine pyrimidines across the double helix, pre-

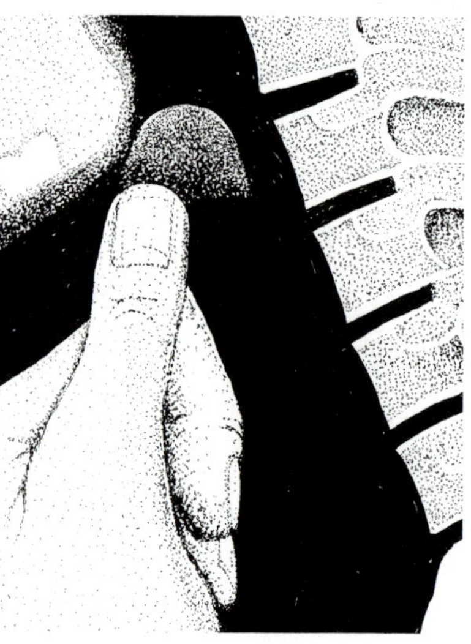

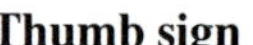

Thumb sign

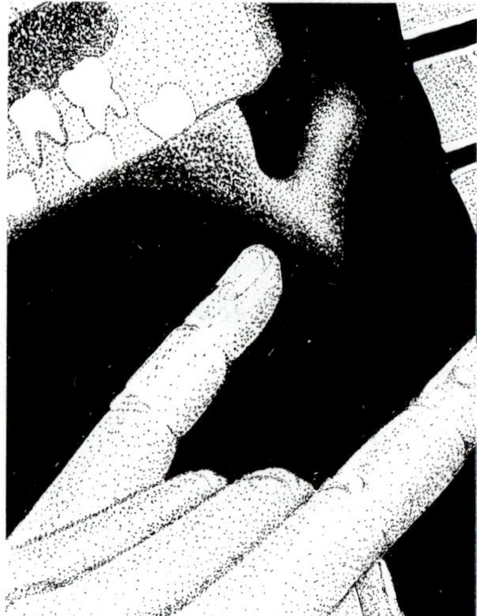

Little finger sign

venting DNA replication; it is not the dimer itself that is mutagenic, but rather the 'sloppy' repair mechanism, which is carried by the SOS repair system; ultraviolet light may also induce direct mutations into the DNA by base pair substitution (transversion) and 'frame shift' mutations in the form of duplications and deletions; see SOS repair

Thymoma A thymic epithelial cell neoplasm located in the anterior mediastinum, which is often first seen as an incidental finding on a plain antero-posterior chest film Clinical Thymomas may be associated with connective tissue disease (giant cell polymyositis, rheumatoid arthritis, systemic lupus, Sjögren's disease, dermatomyositis, polymyositis and scleroderma) skin disease (pemphigus vulgaris, lichen planus, alopecia areata), hematopoietic disease (erythrocytosis, erythroid hypoplasia, pernicious anemia, aplastic anemia), multiple myeloma, angioimmunoblastic lymphadenopathy, inflammation, eg granulomatous myocarditis, meningoencephalitis, thyroiditis, immunologic disorders (hypogammaglobulinemia, IgA deficiency, monoclonal gammopathy, mucocutaneous candidiasis), malignancy (internal malignancy, which occurs in up to 17% of cases and others including myasthenia gravis, adrenal atrophy, Cushing's disease, ulcerative colitis and Crohn's disease; the prognosis is a function of capsular invasion, mitotic activity, cytologic atypia, nuclear hyperchromasia Pathology Solid to cystic, yellow-gray, well-encapsulated and separated into lobules by connective tissue Histopathology Aggregates of plump-to-spindled epithelial cells, separated by fascicles of mature, activated lymphocytes Differential diagnosis Lymphoma

Thymosin alpha-1 Thymopoietin A thymic hormone that induces T cell helper function, stimulating lymphokine production, eg interferon, macrophage inhibiting factor, increasing the expression of Thy-1.2 and Lyt-1,-2,-3 markers on T cells, modulating TdT levels in thymocytes Normal levels: 1250-2250 pg/ml in newborns; 580 pg/ml in adults

Thymotaxin see β_2-microglobulin

Thymus The immune organ responsible for T cell production and maturation; the thymus weighs 10-35g at birth, increasing to 20-50 g by puberty, involuting to 5 g or less in the elderly; poor understanding of this age-related physiological hyperplasia resulted in 'therapeutic' irradiation to the head and neck region of some subjects in the early 1950s, some of whom subsequently (decades later) developed papillary carcinomas of the thyroid; see Status thymolymphaticus, T cell maturation

Thyroid crisis see Thyrotoxic storm

Thyroid hormone binding ratio 'T_3 and T_4 uptake' test A laboratory technique that analyzes the distribution of radiolabelled T_3 and T_4 in a serum sample, providing an indirect estimate of the free fraction of T_3 and T_4; the method entails addition of charcoal or a resin to a specimen, then quantifying the radiolabeled ('hot') T_3 bound to the matrix, expressed as a ratio of matrix-bound RIA value to the serum protein-bound RIA value, usually 33-50%; see Free thyroxine index

'Thyroidization' see Tubular thyroidization

Thyroid panel LABORATORY MEDICINE An abbreviated battery of serum tests used to detect the presence of functional abnormalities of the thyroid 'axis'; the panel measures T_3 (triiodothyronine), T_4 (thyroxine), FTI (free thyroxine index) and TSH (thyroid-stimulating hormone; see Organ panel

Thyrotoxicosis see T_3 thyrotoxicosis, T_4 thyrotoxicosis

Thyrotoxic storm A hypermetabolic state superimposed on hyperthyroidism, often occurring in Grave's disease, less common in toxic multinodular goiter and rarely in Hashimoto's disease ('Hashitoxicosis'); the symptoms of hyperthyroidism, eg weight loss, heat intolerance, myasthenia, poor mental concentration, diarrhea, diaphoresis and cardiac palpitations, may be triggered by infection, thromboembolism, surgery, physical or psychological trauma, parturition or withdrawal from thyroid-blocking drugs, into becoming a life-threatening hypermetabolic state, characterized by hyperthermia, tachycardia and cardiac, hepatic and cerebral dysfunction Laboratory Increased serum thyroxine (T_4) and tri-iodothyronine (T_3), decreased cholesterol Treatment Reduce the hypermetabolic state, inhibiting thyroid hormone release with iodine, blocking thyroid hormone synthesis with propylthiouracil and other anti-thyroid agents, blocking adrenergic neurotransmission with β-adrenergic antagonists and glucocorticoids to 'cover' for functional hypoadrenalism; see Euthyroid sick syndrome, Hashimoto's disease, Hashitoxicosis

Thyrotropin Obsolete for thyroid-stimulating hormone (TSH)

Throxine-binding prealbumin see Transthyretin

TI see Therapeutic index

TIA see Transient ischemic attack

TIBC Total iron-binding capacity LABORATORY MEDICINE A quantitative measurement of transferrin's ability to transport iron; in normal subjects, 33% of transferrin's sites are occupied by iron; in iron deficiency, pregnancy and viral hepatitis, 15% of transferrin's binding sites are occupied, therefore transferrin's capacity to bind iron or TIBC is increased; in iron-overload syndromes, eg hemochromatosis and hemosiderosis, transferrin has few sites available to bind iron and therefore the TIBC is decreased

TIBO Tetrahydroimidazobenzodiazopinone(s) A class of benzodiazepine-related compounds with anti-HIV (human immunodeficiency virus) activity that at low doses, reduce in vitro viral replication by inhibiting reverse transcriptase (Nature 1990; 343:470); TIBO's inhibition of reverse transcriptase is reported to be five times more potent than that of zidovudine

Tic Habit spasm A complex of multiple abrupt, coordinated involuntary movements, including eye blinking, facial gestures, shoulder shrugging, which the patients feel compelled to complete, which when controlled, may be followed by more intense and frequent 'rebound' contractions; tics are exacerbated by stressants and ameliorated by psychotherapy; Giles de la Tourette syndrome causes a severe form of tics affecting young males, age 2-15, characterized by intermittent compulsive vocalizations and movements (sniffing, barking, obscenities or obscene gestures) that may be more controlled with age; while no consistent anatomic abnormalities have been identified, the constancy of the presentation implies an organic nature of the condition; Cf Jumping Frenchmen of Maine syndrome

Tic douloureux Trigeminal neuralgia The most common cause for paroxysmal neuropathic pain of the fifth cranial nerve, which may be due to oral pathology or an acoustic neuroma; the latter condition should be ruled out if the tic is refractory to carbamazepine

Tick An arthropod of the Ixodidae family, which is a common vector of bacterial and viral infections, *Dermacentor andersoni* North America Vector for Rocky Mountain spotted fever (RMSF), Colorado tick fever, tularemia and tick paralysis, *D marginatus* Asia Vector for Russian spring-summer fever, tick-borne encephalitis virus, possibly also Congo-Crimean hemorrhagic fever virus and *Babesia* Reservoir for Omsk hemorrhagic fever virus, *D occidentalis* Pacific Coast North America Vector (presumed) for RMSF, Colorado tick fever, *D parumapertus* Southwestern USA Vector for RMSF, Colorado tick fever, *D variabilis* Eastern USA Vector for RMSF, tularemia, Colorado tick fever and tick paralysis; Asian and African ticks, vectors of Rickettsialpox *Ixodes dammini* Northern deer tick, vector of *Babesia microti*, see Lyme disease

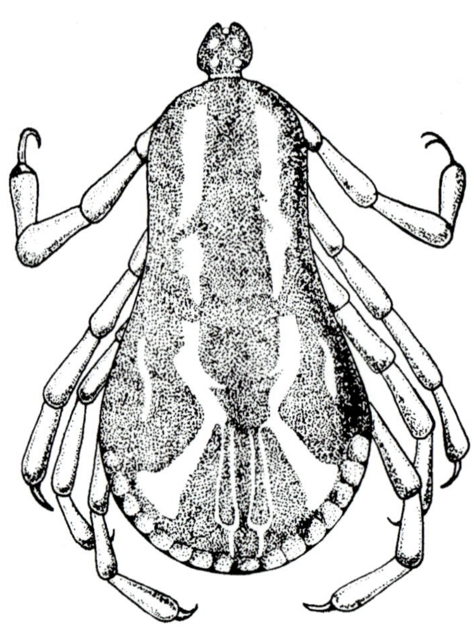

Tick

Tick-borne fever see Relapsing fever

Tick-borne hemorrhagic fever A group of diseases in which ticks are incriminated as vectors: Congo-Crimean hemorrhagic fever Vector *Hyaloma marginatum*; Kyasanur forest disease Vector *Haemaphysalis turturis*, *H spinigera*; Omsk hemorrhagic fever Vector, *Dermacentor pictus, D marginatus*

Tick paralysis A flaccid ascending quadriplegia that resembles Guillain-Barré syndrome, produced by the bite of certain pregnant ticks, eg Rocky mountain wood tick (*Dermatocentor andersoni*) and dog ticks, thought to be due to an unidentified toxin Treatment Tick removal

Ticlopidine An experimental platelet anti-aggregating drug that is reported to be useful in minimizing cerebral ischemia, stroke and the progression of diabetic retinopathy in patients at high risk for stroke Side effects Diarrhea, rash, gastritis or gastric ulcers, hemorrhage, thrombocytopenia, severe reversible neutropenia and a slight increase in cholesterol (N Engl J Med 1990; 323:1487c, Arch Ophthalmol 1990; 108:1577); see TIA

Tigering see Thrush breast appearance

'Tiger' substance A striated material of unknown significance, which is occasionally seen by light microsopy in the stroma of dysgerminomas and seminomas (Eur J Cancer 1965; 1:253)

'Tiger-top' tubes LABORATORY MEDICINE A sterile blood collection tube with a swirled red and black or green rubber stopper that is coated with silicone, has a gel on the bottom, can be directly centrifuged to separate red and white cells and, like yellow top tubes, are used to collect specimens for human immunodeficiency virus (HIV-1), retroviruses (HTLV-I and others), acetone, alcohol, urea nitrogen and creatinine

Tight junction CELL BIOLOGY A cell junction composed of thin bands that completely encircle a cell, in which the contributing plasma membranes of adjacent cells are directly apposed with virtually no intervening space between them; tight junctions are typical ultrastructural findings in epithelial cells, seen in adenomas, adenocarcinoma, APUDomas, transitional and papillary carcinoma of the urinary bladder, synovial sarcoma and mesothelioma; Cf Gap junction

Tigroid nuclei A morphology of the nuclei of skeletal muscle cells due to the resynthesis of contractile proteins, associated with denervation, target fiber formation and type group atrophy

Tijuana A city in Mexico that has occasionally served as a destination (as have other cities) for patients hoping to be cured of terminal malignancy by unproven cancer therapies offered in some 'clinicas' of self-proclaimed cancer specialists, who often describe their therapies as 'alternative', 'holistic' or 'natural', which are based on some form of 'metabolic therapy' (Questionable methods of cancer management--sSpecial communication, 13/June/90, American Cancer Society); see 'Metabolic therapy', Unproven methods of cancer therapy

TIL Tumor-infiltrating lymphocytes IMMUNOLOGY T lymphocytes with antitumoral activity that are isolated from a patient with cancer, tagged (for later identification) with neomycin-resistance gene and grown by culturing single cell suspensions obtained from tumors in tissue culture media

TIL therapy An experimental therapeutic modality in which antigen-specific tumor-infiltrating T lymphocytes (TILs) are isolated from biopsies of the patients with a malignancy and co-administered with interleukin-2; TIL therapy yields a 30% response rate in high-grade melanoma (N Engl J Med 1990; 323:570); Cf LAK/IL-2 therapy

Time of flight mass spectrometry (TOF-MS) LABORATORY MEDICINE A technique that measures the time required by an ion to travel from its source to a detector; at the start of the 'flight', all ions have the same kinetic energy, but separate according to their mass, such that the ions arrive at different times; TOF-MS can be used for measuring the mass and structure of ionized substances, especially for the identification of drugs and their metabolites; see Mass spectrometry

Times Beach ENVIRONMENT A city in the state of Missouri that was abandoned, by order of the US Environental Protection Agency in 1983, when dangerously high levels of dioxins were identified in the water and soil, which were the result of the spraying of dioxin-tainted oils (to control dust) on the roads and highways (Arch Environ Contam Toxicol 1988; 17:139); see Agent Orange, Chemical pollutants, Dioxin

TIMI studies CARDIOLOGY A series of long-term multicenter, multi-national, multi-agent studies designed to determine which of a number of early interventions would provide the best survival for myocardial infarctions; the TIMI Thrombolysis in myocardial infarction) trials have studied the effects of early thrombolytic therapy in recanalizing occluded coronary arteries, in limiting the size of the infarct and residual cardiac dysfunction, and reduction of mortality, analyzing various combinations of tissue plasminogen activator (tPA), heparin, aspirin and coronary arteriography followed by prophylactic percutaneous transluminal angioplasty; one study concluded that intravenous β-blockade with recombinant tPA is adequate therapy in uncomplicated myocardial infarcts (N Engl J Med 1989; 320:618); in one TIMI trial (Lancet 1986; 1:397), mortality was reportedly reduced by 47% if tPA was used within one hour, 17% if the therapy was delayed 3-6 hours and was reported to offer little advantage if therapy began six or more hours after the ischemic insult; see CAST, TAMI studies, tPA

Timolol maleate A β-adrenergic antagonist used as a topical solution, which causes a worsening of lipid profiles with an increase in triglycerides and low-density lipoprotein and decrease in high density lipoprotein (Arch Ophthalmol 1990; 108:1260)

TIMPs Tissue inhibitor of metalloproteinases A substance which under normal circumstances, inhibit collagenases; a TIMP has been identified in certain tumor cell lines that binds type IV collagenase, but does not inhibit it, possibly leaving it in a fully activated position

Tingible bodies HEMATOPATHOLOGY Variably-sized karyorrhectic nuclear debris present in and adjacent to macrophages in benign lymphadenopathies, often located in the germinal centers in toxoplasmosis, infectious mononucleosis, varicella and herpes zoster lymphadenopathy, cat-scratch disease and brucellosis

Tin tack appearance see Carpet tack appearance

Tinted spectacles sign PSYCHIATRY The wearing of dark-colored glasses under normal lighting conditions, in absence of photophobia or photosensitivity; 'soft' data suggests that this sign may sometimes be associated with an underlying psychoneuroses, as the scores for the symptom dimensions measured (anxiety and phobic anxiety, depression, global psychological distress, obsession-compulsion, paranoid ideation, psychotic behavior and somatization) were significantly higher in subjects who don 'shades' (J Roy Soc Med 1989; 82:606) Note: No rose-colored spectacles sign has been described

Tissue committee QUALITY ASSURANCE A committee in a hospital that reviews the appropriateness of all surgical procedures performed in the institution, correlating the pre- and post-operative diagnoses established by the surgeon and the diagnosis rendered by the pathologist; a tissue committee is a requirement for hospital accreditation in the US and serves as a mechanism to ensure that tissues are not removed unnecessarily, ie in the absence of a well-defined pathology

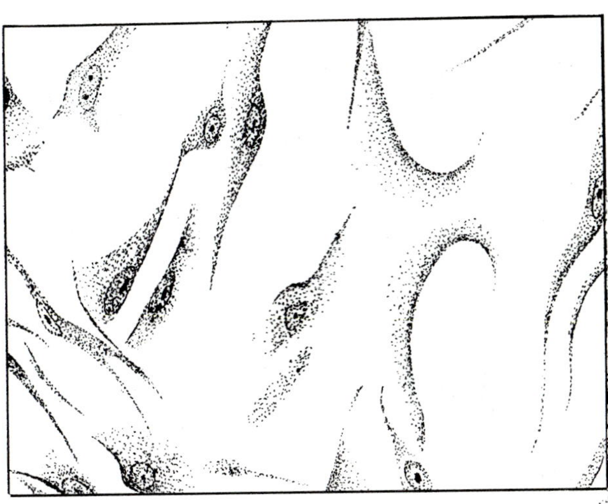

Tissue culture appearance

'Tissue culture' appearance SURGICAL PATHOLOGY A loose, haphazard arrangement of plump, spindled cells, usually fibroblasts that may have elongated cytoplasmic processes, typically seen in nodular fasciitis, a 'storiform' pattern that has been fancifully likened to that seen when normal fibroblasts are grown in culture media

Tissue culture infective dose see TCID

Tissue factor Obsolete for tissue thromboplastin

Tissue paper appearance see Crumpled tissue paper appearance

Tissue plasminogen activator see tPA

Titer The amount of a substance that can be manipulated by serial dilution; determination of 'titers' is of clinical use in determining a present infection or past exposure to an antigen or virus, where rising titers, ie presence of an antigen-antibody reaction at high dilutions of an antigen, indicate a developing disease, while falling titers indicate a resolving condition; see Antibody titers

'Title X' projects POPULATION CONTROL A US federal government-sponsored program for family planning clinics that was initiated under the Reagan Administration; under the recent 'Gag rule' resulting from a US Supreme Court decision, physicians have been interdicted from fully counseling women who are unintentionally pregnant; the wording of the decision has been interpreted as preventing physicians from offering these women nondirective counseling on pregnancy termination, as well as prenatal care, infant and foster care, and adoption, thereby representing governmental interference of the patient-doctor relationship; see 'Gag rule'

'Tit' sign Pyloric tit sign A radiologic finding in an upper gastrointestinal series of films of a child with hypertrophic pyloric stenosis, in which the completely obstructed antrum and adjoining pyloric canal simulate the voluptuous curves of a breast and nipple; the nipple becomes pronounced as the pyloric muscle unsuccessfully attempts to contract and push the barium beyond the markedly stenosed canal; rarely a normal peristaltic pouch may transiently increase in size, temporarily simulating the tit sign

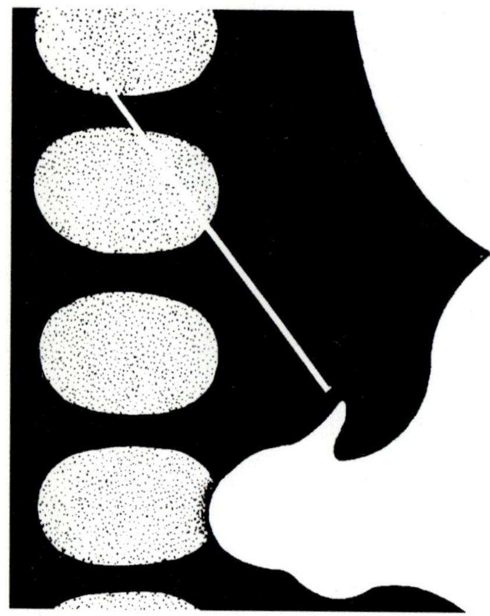

Pyloric tit sign

Titin Connectin A large myofibrillar protein present in the M and Z lines as well as in the A and I bands, that serves to align the myosin thick filaments during contraction

TKO selection GENETICS A tool for rapidly identifying genes that inhibit proliferation in a specific restrictive environment; this assumes that specific inhibition of a growth inhibitory gene conveys growth advantage, 'forward selecting' a desired inactivation event; TKO (technical knock-out) selection identifies thioredoxin as the mediator of a growth inhibitory signal in tumor suppression (Science 1991; 252:117)

TLC see Thin layer chromatography

TLV see Threshold limit value

T lymphocytes see T cells

Tm PHYSIOLOGY The maximum reabsorptive capacity for glucose in the renal tubules, which is between 11.2 and 13.2 mmol/L (US: 200-240 mg/dl); under usual circumstances, slightly prior to reaching the Tm, incomplete glucose reabsorption occurs, causing a 'splaying' in the response, a value designated as Km

TMJ Temporomandibular joint

TMJ syndrome Temporomandibular joint-myofascial dysfunction syndrome A complex neuromuscular disorder related to dental malocclusion, possibly exacerbated by trauma, psychological stress and grinding of teeth **Clinical** Nonspecific unilateral facial pain and spasms of the masseter muscle **Treatment** No therapy is consistently effective; modalities used with varying degrees of failure have included physical (moist heat) therapy, analgesics, soft diet and surgery, eg high intracapsular condylectomy

TMP-SMX see Trimethoprim-sulfamethoxazole

TNF see Tumor necrosis factor

TNM classification An international system for staging malignacy, formulated by the UICC (Union Internationale Contre Cancrum) that measures three major parameters: T for size or extent of the primary tumor, as determined by clinical exam, endoscopy, laparoscopy, biopsy or resective procedures, N for number of involved lymph nodes and M for presence or absence of metastases; TNM classification forms the basis of treating malignancy; lower case letters may precede the TNM formulation as a means of providing supplementary information, including aTNM (autopsy staging, for cancer diagnosed at advanced stage), cTNM (clinical-diagnostic staging), pTNM (post-surgical resection-pathologic staging), rTNM (retreatment staging), sTNM (surgical-evaluative staging)

Tn syndrome A chronic condition associated with polyagglutination of erythrocytes, characterized by severe thrombocytopenia, hemolytic anemia and leukopenia; red cells and platelets are deficient in T-transferase (UDPGal:GalNAc-β-3-D-galactosyltransferase), resulting in the inability to express the GPIb glycoprotein and expression of the cryptantigen, Tn, which reacts with naturally-occurring antibodies, causing global hemolysis and coagulation

TNTC Too numerous to count MICROBIOLOGY A colloquial abbreviation for a confluent 'lawn' of bacteria on a culture plate that may be seen in urinary tract infections, where confluence is approximately equal to 10^5 colonies

Toad fish see Puffer fish

Toad skin appearance see Cathartic colon

Toadstool motility see Umbrella motility

Toad test A bioassay of historical interest that used the South African clawed toad, ***Xenopis laevis***, to detect increased production of human chorionic gonadotropin; injection of plasma from pregnant human females induces the release of sperm in the toads

'Tobacco nodules' A descriptor for the appearance of organized perifollicular hemorrhages, ie Gamna-Gandy bodies that are seen in passive splenic hyperemia due to portal hypertension; these structures consist of iron- and calcium-encrusted collagen and fibrosis surrounding atrophic malpighian follicles

Tocol A generic term for a group of eight naturally-occurring fat soluble compounds with a 6-chromanol nucleus bearing two methyl groups and a branched isoprenoid chain with vitamin E activity, the most biologically active of the tocol family is D-α-tocopherol; see Vitamin E

Toddler's diarrhea PEDIATRICS A condition that is defined as the presence of unresolved diarrhea with mild malabsorption that persists after the resolution of acute gastroenteritis; toddler's diarrhea is considered by some workers to be a possible prelude to the irritable bowel

TNM classification for staging malignancy

T Tumor

T-is Carcinoma in situ
T-a Non-invasive
T-x Cannot be fully evaluated for non-specified reasons
T-0 Localized tumor
T-1 Lesion extends to muscle, eg bladder, colon, breast
 T-1a < 0.5 cm in greatest dimension
 T-1b < 1.0 cm in greatest dimension
 T-1c < 2.0 cm in greatest dimension
T-2 Invasion into muscle
T-3 Persistent induration of organ following resection
 T-3a Invasion to deep muscle
 T-3b Invasion through the organ
T-4 Tumor invasion or fixation
 T-4a Adjacent organ invasion
 T-4b Fixation to bladder or colonic wall; in breast, edema

N Nodes

N-0 No lymph node metastasis
N-1 One regional lymph node metastasis
N-2 Multiple, mobile regional lymph node metastases
N-3 Fixed regional lymph node metastaseis
N-4 Beyond regional lymph node involvement
N-X Lymph nodes, not evaluable

M Metastasis

M-0 No evidence of metastases
M-1 Distant metastases are present
M-X Distant metastases, not evaluable

Less used components of the TNM classification :

R Resective success

R-0 No residual tumor exists after resection
R-1 Microscopic residual tumor exists
R-2 Gross residual tumor is present after surgery

Pathological staging (pTNM Post surgical histopathology)

P Surgical specimen with histopathological changes
P-is Malignancy in situ
P-0 No tumor in specimen, or completely excised in situ malignancy
P-1 Malignancy confined to the lamina propria
P-2 Malignancy extending to less than half of muscle layer
P-3 Malignancy extending to more than half of muscle layer
P-4 Malignancy extending to more than half of muscle layer with infiltration of adjacent organs
P-X Malignancy, not evaluable

G Histopathological grading

G-0 No anaplasia seen
G-1 Low amount of anaplasia
G-2 Moderate amount of anaplasia
G-3 High amount of anaplasia
G-X Presence of anaplasia, not evaluable

syndrome Clinical Abdominal pain, vomiting, loose, malodorous stool, highly-irritating rash of the buttocks, dysuria and urinary urgency; the onset of illness may coincide with death, illness, family crisis or environmental stress

Todeserwartung German, awaiting death Social medicine A symptom complex affecting the elderly who have been relegated to nursing homes either by society or by progeny Clinical Hypochondriasis, hysteria, impulsiveness, loss of self-esteem, withdrawal from reality and obsession with death Therapy Displays of affection, household pets, involvement in child care; associated cortical atrophy and mental lassitude may be controlled by using video games for mental stimulation; see Geriatrics; Cf Elderly abuse, Melanocholia, 'Shelterization'

Toe-walking Orthopedics A defect in gait, where the patients walk on 'tip-toes' due to force of habit, congenital tight heel cords or cerebral palsy with mild spasticity

'Toke' Substance abuse To inhale a large air volume while smoking a substance of abuse, eg marijuana or 'crack', maintaining the lungs expanded with a slight Valsalva maneuver, in order to maximize the substance's absorption; Cf 'Snort'

Tokyo-Yokohama asthma see Yokohama asthma

Tolerance Immunology see Immunological (self) tolerance Instrumentation The accepted or standardized limit of allowable error in an instrument or analytic procedure Microbiology A poorly-understood phenomenon in which the minimum concentration of penicillin required to kill staphylococci is up to thirty-fold greater than the inhibitory concentration, values that are normally close to each other; see Methicillin-aminoglycoside resistant *Staphylococcus aureus*, Persister phenomenon Pharmacology An increase in dosage of a drug required to achieve the same effect, which is a function of increased metabolism, eg by hypertrophy of the endoplasmic reticulum or increased expulsion of the drug from a cell, eg by amplification of the multidrug resistant gene by a malignant cell, see MDR

Toluidine blue Pathology A metachromatic thiazin stain used for the 'thick' sections in ultrastructure, which is toxic by inhalation, ingestion and absorption, potentially causing hematuria secondary to hemorrhagic cystitis and methemoglobulinuria and thus should be avoided by those with glucose-6-phosphate deficiency

Toluidine method Laboratory medicine A technique in which *o*-toluidine, an aromatic amine, reacts with glucose in a hot acetic acid solution to produce colored derivatives, allowing the quantification of glucose, which gives similar results to those generated by the enzymatic methodology used in multichannel analyzers

'Tomato catsup' fundus A fanciful descriptor for the fundoscopic findings in cerebral lipidosis, Prader-Willi syndrome (characterized by hypertonicity, hyperphagia, neonatal obesity, small stature, hands and feet, mental retardation), Sturge-Weber's disease and Zellweger's cerebrohepatorenal syndrome (an autosomal recessive condition characterized by dysmorphia, hepatomegaly and increased long chain fatty acids) (Arch Opthalmol 1974; 92:69)

'Tomato effect' CLINICAL DECISION-MAKING Rejection of an effective treatment for a disease for illogical reasons, as may occur when conventional logic dictates that a drug should have no therapeutic value or is toxic, eg colchicine and aspirin (J Am Med Assoc 1984; 251:2387) Note: When the tomato (*Lycopersicon esculentum*), a New World plant from Peru was brought back by the Spanish explorers, it was an instant success with both the Italians (pommo d'oro, golden apple) and the French, who thought it an aphrodisiac (pomme d'amour, apple of love), but was relatively unpopular in the rest of Europe, as 'logic' held that the tomato was poisonous as it belongs to the deadly night shade family of plants, which includes belladonna and mandrake; this belief persisted until a tomato was eaten publicly in Massachusetts in 1820; the only known ill effect from tomatoes lies in herbal teas prepared from its leaves; see Herbal teas

'Tombstone' advertisement An advertising layout format in which the 'copy' is a white field with text surrounded by a black border, often carrying a message with a potentially negative impact; because of tobacco's adverse effect on health, one person proposed that the tobacco industry could exercise their right to advertise their products (a right guaranteed by the US Constitution), by using an ironic variant of tombstone advertising, which would carry only the product and its picture, eliminating the implication, through symbols or slogans, that the user's life would be improved through use of the product

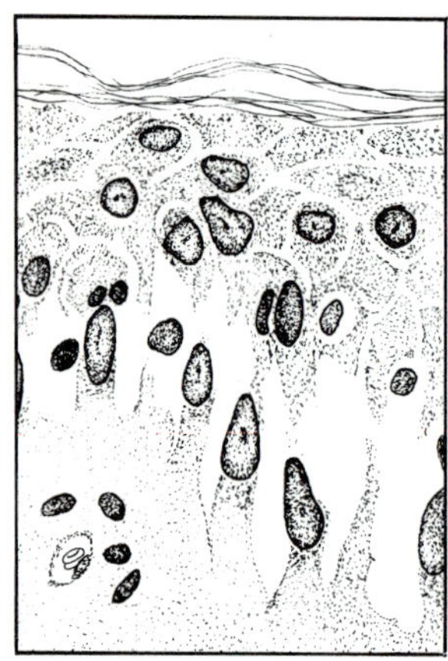

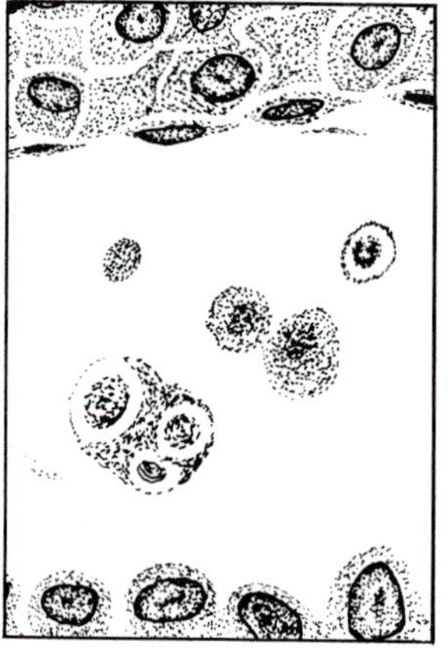

Tombstone appearance

Tombstone appearance DERMATOPATHOLOGY A fanciful descriptor for the multiple hobnail-like cells which have lost their intercellular bridges above and lateral to the basal layer of residual epithelial cells in pemphigus vulgaris; the above figure demonstrates early lesions on the left and later lesions on the right VASCULAR PATHOLOGY A descriptor for the bulging of epithelial-like endothelial cells into the vascular lumen in Kimura's disease; Cf Hobnail appearance

Tongue worm Pentastomid A blood-sucking invertebrate parasite that infests the nasal cavity of carnivores; human disease is caused by ***Armillifer armillatus*** (usual host, snakes) and ***Linguatula serrata*** (usual host, sheep and goats); pentastomiasis is global in distribution; linguliasis or Halzoun's disease is more common in the Middle East and results from eating poorly-cooked meat; the larvae cause pain, itching, sneezing due to transnasal migration, dysphagia, vomiting and lymphadenopathy; a large bolus of worms may cause fatal obstruction

Tonometer A device that measures the tension or partial pressure of a gas in a liquid, used in a clinical setting to standardize arterial blood gas measurement, equilibrating the blood with a known mixture of gas at 37°C, serving as a form of quality control in determining the levels of CO_2 and O_2 in patient specimens

'T on P' phenomenon CARDIOLOGY A electrocardiographic finding consisting of sinus tachycardia with prolongation of Q-T and a delayed T wave followed or overlapped by the succeeding P wave; the 'T on P' phenomenon is suggestive of alkalosis

Tonsillectomy and adenoidectomy (T&A) A simple surgical procedure that was commonly performed in the US in the 1950s by non-specialists for a wide variety of indications, including prophylactically, a trend that has completely reversed; in the current environment, the two procedures often performed as separate procedures for different indications, tonsillectomy for recurrent pharyngitis or peritonsillar abscesses and adenoidectomy for chronic or recurrent otitis media **Microbiology** Potential pathogens may be cultured from 80% of pediatric T&As and include α-hemolytic streptococci, ***Haemophilus*** species, ***Staphylococcus aureus*** and ***Streptococcus pneumoniae*** (Arch Otolaryngol Head Neck Surg 1988; 114:763); the relative risk for Hodgkin's disease in elderly subjects who had T&As as children is reported to be as high as a relative risk of 3.0, although the data is sparse (J Nat Cancer Inst 1987; 78:1)

'Toothache in the bones' A fanciful descriptor for the intense aching pain described in the diabetic foot with peripheral symmetric polyneuropathy

Toothpaste artefact NEUROPATHOLOGY An artefact seen in the spinal cord, which results from its suboptimal removal from the vertebral column, resulting in a 'telescoping' prolase of spinal cord white matter, which may be interpreted by the neophyte as a spinal cord infarct, which is a rare autopsy finding

Toothpaste sign A descriptor for a column of dense radiocontrast that has passed through a narrowed ureteral opening at the trigone and lies in a toothpaste-like fashion on the bladder floor; this finding may be caused by postoperative contraction of the vesical neck, as may occur intransureteral resections of the prostate, as well as in suprapubic and perineal surgery

Tooth sign Asymptomatic, vaguely dentate ossifications that are perpendicular to the patellar surface seen on an axial ('skyline') view of the patello-femoral joint, which, while associated with degenerative changes, are of themselves of no clinical significance **Differential diagnosis** Paget's disease of the bone and reactive sclerosis secondary to chronic osteomyelitis

Tophus The pathognomonic lesion of gout, which appears grossly as white chalky, pasty material composed of crystalline and amorphous urates, eg monosodium urate monohydrates, surrounded by mononuclear cells, fibroblasts and a foreign body-type giant cell reaction with epithelioid histiocytes; when preserved in alcohol or other non-aqueous solution, microscopy reveals bright anisotropic negatively birefringent crystals in compensated polarized light; tophi are most often periarticular but also occur in the tendon sheath, epiphyseal bone, subcutis, at the helix and antihelix of the external ear, in the renal pelvis and interstitium; with time, bony ankylosis may ensue, due to cartilaginous destruction, by local collagenase and prostaglandin E_2, synovial proliferation, pannus formation, subchondral osteolysis, bony overgrowth and fibrosis, demonstrating 'punched-out' lesions by radiology

Topoisomerase An enzyme that alters the topology of DNA, catalyzing the interconversion of one topoisomer to another, changes the amount of superhelicity and formation of DNA knots and catenations, requiring transient breaking and rejoining of the strands of DNA's double helix; type I topoisomerases produce a transient single break in the double helix, causing a relaxation of twisted helices (known as swivelases, untwistases); type II topoisomerases increase the double helix's winding number, increasing its superhelicity; see Superhelicity

TOPV Trivalent oral polio vaccine

TORCH(eS) PEDIATRICS Toxoplasma, other, rubella, cytomegalic inclusion virus, herpes (and syphilis) An acronym for a group of in utero infections that may induce major malformation in the fetus and cause prominent neurologic defects, eg seizures, hydrocephalus or microcephaly

TORCH panel PEDIATRICS A 'shotgun' serologic screen for diagnosing antenatal infection; the finding of increased IgM in the neonate implies in utero infection, which should be further characterized by measuring the IgM levels for specific organisms Note: The quantitative TORCH screen has a high rate of false positive and negativity TORCH agents TOXOPLASMOSIS, which causes periventricular microglial nodules,thrombosis and necrosis; obstruction of the foramina causes hydrocephalus; with prolonged survival, there is intracranial calcification, hepatocellular, adrenal, pulmonary, cardiac necrosis and extramedullary hematopoiesis RUBELLA which results in low birth weight, hepatosplenomegaly, petechiae and purpura, congenital heart disease, cataracts, microophthalmia and microcephaly; central nervous system symptoms include lethargy, irritability, dystonia, bulging fontanelles and seizures; see Congenital rubella syndrome CYTOMEGALOVIRUS which is associated with early hepatosplenomegaly, hyperbilirubinemia, neonatal thrombocytopenia, microcephaly and a mortality of 20-30%; later manifestations include mental retardation, deafness, psychomotor delays, dysodontogenesis, chorioretinitis, learning disabilities; an estimated 33 000 congenital cases occur per year in the USA, of which 10% are symptomatic HERPES SIMPLEX may cause prematurity; it becomes symptomatic after the first week of life; central nervous system symptoms include irritability, seizures, chorioretinitis, hydrocephalus, flaccid or spastic paralysis, opisthotonos, decerebrate rigidity and coma; in neonatal HSV infection, no deaths occur in those with localized disease, 15% die if encephalitis is present and 57% die if HSV is disseminated, potentially evoking disseminated intravascular coagulopathy (N Engl J Med 1991; 324:450) SYPHILIS (an optional 'TORCH') Congenital syphilis has increased to epidemic rates in the urban US since the mid-1980s; the clinical findsings are non-specific and include fever, lethargy, failure to thrive and irritability

Tori palati Benign osseous 'tumors' of the oral cavity that may be associated with malignancy, eg squamous cell carcinoma of the overlying epithelium; Cf Pseudoepitheliomatous hyperplasia

Torpedo A focal fusiform swelling of the axon of Purkinje cells, located in the first portion of the axis cylinder prior to the origin of collateral branches, often accompanied by swollen dendritic ramifications and patchy displacement of Purkinje cells, a typical pathologic finding in olivopontocerebellar atrophy of the granular layer of the cerebellum

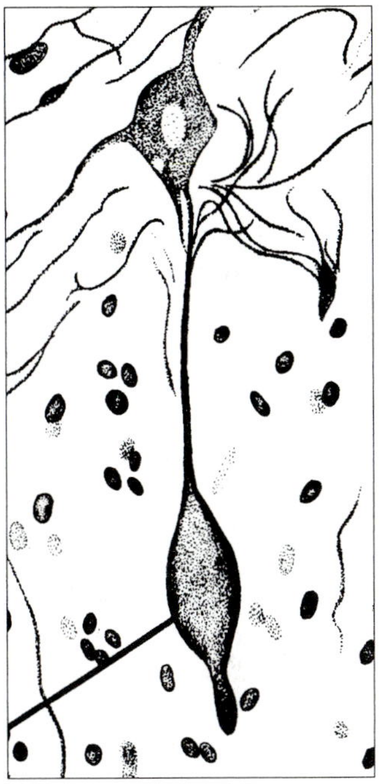

Torpedo

torr A unit of pressure corresponding to 1/760 atm or a pressure of 1 mmHg or 1.0 millimeter of mercury (133.3224 pascal) Note: Although pascal is the unit for pressure that is offically accepted by the International System, torr continues to be widely used by clinical workers who often measure blood pressures

Torsade de pointes CARDIOLOGY A form of polymorphic ventricular tachycardia with prolonged Q-T intervals that are initiated by a premature ventricular depolarization striking near the apex of a delayed T wave; torsades have irregular rates of 200-250/min with marked variability in amplitude and direction of a QRS wave that seems to twist (French torsade, twist) around an isoelectric baseline; torsades may spontaneously resolve or evolve to ventricular tachyarrhythmia and may be non-specific or due to drugs, eg adrenergics, antihistamine (J Am Med Assoc 1990; 264:2788), phenothiazine, procainamide, quinines and tricyclic antidepressants, electrolyte imbalance, eg hypokalemia, hypomagnesemia, central nervous system hemorrhage or trauma, long Q-T wave syndrome, liquid diet and underlying heart disease Treatment Isoproterenol

Tort reform bill A legislative package that had been proposed by the Bush Administration, with the purpose of reducing the health care costs inherent in an advanced free-market system and litigation-prone society, eg USA; the proposal calls for a $250 000 'cap' on non-economic ('pain and suffering') awards, and an end of lump sum payments and duplicate awards; see 'Defensive medicine', Malpractice

Torticollis see Wry neck

Tortoise shell nucleus Checkerboard nucleus A fanciful descriptor for polychromatophilic normoblast nuclei that are round with dark, coarse and eccentric chromatin and distinct parachromatin, a feature of use in differentiating these cells from lymphocytes in the bone marrow; the cytoplasm is pink and relatively abundant

Tort system A legal system in which wrongful acts may be tried by jury and awards given for (real or peceived) damages to a plaintiff, which is a key facet of American judicial system; it has been estimated that up to 2.6% ($\$117 \times 10^9$) of the US gross national product (GNP), is consumed by some form of direct or indirect legal fees, including payment of claims, administrative costs and attorney's fees; in contrast, Switzerland spends 0.8% of GNP on its legal system; Canada, Austria, France, 0.6%; West Germany, Italy 0.5%; Japan, Spain, Denmark 0.4% Note: There are 14 times more lawyers in the US than in Japan; see Malpractice

Torture The deliberate, systematic or wanton infliction of physical or mental suffering by one or more persons acting alone or on the order of any authority to force another person to yield information, to make a confession or for any other reason; methods of torture range from verbal threats and humiliation to bizarre displays of man's inhumanity to man including beating the soles of the feet ('falanga'), suspension from a rod by the hands and feet (la 'bandera'), submersion of the head in water (often soiled by excreta, 'submarino'), striking blows at the victim's head and ears ('telefono'), food and water deprivation, mutilation, forcing the victims to watch others being tortured or killed; the 'torture syndrome' is characterized by a wide range of residual effects, including extreme anxiety, insomnia, nightmares, phobias and suspicion; the long-term effects of torture have been termed 'post-traumatic cerebral syndrome', and are characterized by three or more of the following symptoms: impaired memory, headaches, intolerance of alcohol, sleep disorders, marital and emotional disturbances (J Am Med Assoc 1988; 259:2725); it is unclear whether the cerebral atrophy described as a terminal effect of torture is the result of multiple blows to the head; see Amnesty International, Refugee, Unethical medical research; Cf Boxing

Torulopsis glabrata A yeast-like mucosal saprobic fungus, with features of *Candida* and *Cryptococcus*; *T glabrata* may rarely cause an opportunistic infection in immunocompromised hosts Clinical Spiking fever, hypotension, urinary tract infection and fungemia Note: *Torulopsis* is closely related to *Candida* and may ultimately be integrated within the genus *Candida*, although *T glabrata* has only a yeast form

Torus fracture An incomplete fracture of the diaphysis of long bones with buckling of the cortex on the side opposite the fracture; in contrast, the 'greenstick fracture', is ruptured on the convex aspect of the bone

Total hip replacement A procedure that replaces the femoral head and its articular surface with a completely synthetic device, thus being a biomechanical solution for a biological failure; the first 'total hip' was replaced in 1962; in the USA of 1990, an estimated 120 000 are replaced annually, each costing $8500 Indications Advanced osteoarthritis and rheumatoid arthritis with disabling pain Complications Loosening of one or more of the synthetic components, dislocation, femoral head fracture, deep vein thrombosis, nerve damage and (rarely) infection (N Engl J Med 1990; 323:725rv)

Total ischemic burden CARDIOLOGY The sum total of all episodes of symptomatic and asymptomatic or 'silent' myocardial ischemia

Total knee replacement A procedure that substitutes a painful arthritic knee and its articular surface with a synthetic device; the first 'total knee' was replaced in the 1950s but the hinging design was primitive, resulting in high failure rates; these problems were solved by the 1970s by using an unlinked (non-hinged) knee articulation; the excess rigidity problem was solved by retaining and inserting the posterior cruciate ligament into the articular apparatus; an estimated 120 000 'total knees' are performed annually at a cost of $25-30 000 each Indications Advanced osteoarthritis and rheumatoid arthritis with disabling pain; in assessing the surgical candidates, the patient's age, weight and physical activity must be considered Complications Loosening of one or more of the synthetic components, dislocation, femoral head fracture, infection (very rare), deep vein thrombosis, nerve damage (N Engl J Med 1990; 323:801rv)

Total lymphoid irradiation Sequential radiation therapy to the 'mantle' and 'inverted Y' lymphoid regions, a combination of fields that may be used in extensive stage IV Hodgkin's and non-Hodgkin's lymphomas

Total parenteral nutrition see TPN

Totipotence The ability of a usually primitive cell to express the entire range of its genetic information and to give rise to a completely differentiated adult organism; Cf Stem cell

Tourniquet A cord or constrictive band used to reduce the blood flow to one or more extremity; because tourniquets, especially those using thin or narrow devices, worsen distal ischemia and may increase venous bleeding, direct compression of bleeding vessels is preferable to 'encirclement' for hemostasis; tourniquets continue to have some clinical currency in reducing the centripetal flow of toxins in snake and scorpion bites, and in reducing the cardiac load in acute congestive heart failure, as may occur in an acute myocardial infarct, where the tourniquets are rotated, simultaneously with other emergency measures, including oxygen, lasix, nitroprusside and nitroglycerine; when used, a tourniquet should be confined to the proximal portion of the extremity

Tourniquet paralysis An obsolete clinical complex caused by prolonged tourniquet compression of an extremity, resulting in loss of touch, light pressure, vibration and position sensation Note: Complete recuperation is usual within three months

Tourniquet test Capillary fragility test of Rumpel-Leede A clinical sign elicited when the sphygmomanometer cuff is left inflated for 15 minutes on the arm at a pressure midway between the systolic and diastolic pressures; 10 or more petechiae within a circle 2.5 cm in diameter is considered a positive result and may occur with thrombocytopenia of less than 70 x 10^9/L (US: 70 000/mm^3), nonthrombocytopenic purpura or scurvy

Towers nursing home A nursing home in New York that was the focal point of US Federal investigations for possible Medicaid fraud, and alleged physical abuse and starvation of elderly patients during the late 1960s and early 1970s (Facts on File, Vol 35:1028E1, Vol 38:232F1)

'Towns' ACADEMIA A colloquial term for the clinical faculty of a medical school, who are in relatively close contact with the community, ie work in the 'town', actively practice medicine, see patients and are less (if at all) involved in research activities; 'To practice medicine without books, is to sail the seas without charts...' Sir William Osler; Cf 'Gowns'

'Toxic core' PSYCHIATRY A component or 'factor' hypothesized to cause increased cardiovascular mortality in type A personalities; coronary artery disease-prone type A individuals have a cynical mistrust of others, are angry and repress marked hostility towards others; clinical data suggests that over time, the cardiovascular mortality is up to 4-to-7-fold greater in subjects with a 'toxic core' personality; see Type A personality

Toxic dump ENVIRONMENT Any site that is (or was) a repository for chemical pollutants, often placed there illegally, either in standard 50 gallon (circa 200 liter) drums or poured directly into the ground; of greatest concern with the thousands of identified toxic dump sites is the slow leaching of toxic chemicals (known as 'plumes') into the water table and aquifers, thereby contaminating drinkingwater; see Chemical pollutants, Environmental Protection Agency, Plumes, Superfund; Cf Regulated waste

Toxic epidermal necrolysis of Lyell A hypersensitivity reaction in adults that may represent an extreme form of erythema multiforme (EM), as it is associated with the same etiological factors as EM, including drug hypersensitivity, eg allopurinol, barbituates, carbamazepine, nonsteroid anti-inflammatory drugs (phenylbutazone and oxicam derivatives) and sulfonamides, including sulfamethoxazole-trimethoprim, infections, vaccination, radiotherapy and malignancy **Clinical** After a prodrome of fever, malaise, and erythema, subepidermal bullae develop, leading to epidemal sloughing **Complications** Dehydration, electrolyte imbalance or 'third space phenomenon', abscess formation, sepsis and shock **Treatment** Symptomatic therapy, as with second degree burns; Staphylococcal scalded skin syndrome

Toxic granulation HEMATOLOGY Large, irregular granules that are deep blue-violet by 'Romanovsky'-type stains, eg Wright-Giemsa stain and variably positive by the periodic acid-Schiff stain; these granules correspond to secondary autolysosomes with an increased membrane permeability, are seen in metamyelocytes, band or segmented neutrophils and lymphocytes and may be induced by rapid turnover of cell products and may be seen in leukemoid reactions and in infections, related to bacterial products; toxic granulations may also be seen in eclampsia, irradiation, hepatic disease and terminal cancer Note: Also seen in peripheral blood smears of patients with acute infections are 'toxic' cytoplasmic vacuolization, Döhle bodies and a 'left shift' of the myeloid series

Toxicity index see Toxicity testing

Toxicity testing ENVIRONMENT A component of risk assessment that is required by law in the USA for all new chemicals, for new purposes of old chemicals or for combinations of new and old chemicals; toxicity testing attempts to identify hazards, including adverse effects, cancer, nephrotoxicity and teratogenesis and to quantitate exposure-response relation (measured by LD_{50}, the chemical 'dose' that is lethal in 50% of the test animals, and ED_{50}, the 'effective dose' that causes a consistent change in 50% of tested animals); standard 'whole animal toxicity tests' determine acute, subacute, chronic, reproductive and developmental toxicity, and study ocular and skin irritation (Draize test), hypersensitivity, phototoxicity, toxicokinetics and behavioral changes; conventional animal testing for one agent costs $0.5-1.5 million (US) and may require the sacrifice of thousands of animals to put a chemical into production; the less expensive in vitro assays include the mutagenic bacterial or genotoxicity screen devised by Ames, cytotoxicity (total cellular-protein assay and the neutral red dye test), which measures inhibition of protein production (IC_{50}) and the chorioallantoic membrane test (CAM test, in which the shell of a fertilized chicken egg is removed, revealing the veined chorioallantoic membrane, the site of application of the test chemical (Sci Am 1989; 261/2:24); see Ames test, Risk assessment

Toxic megacolon An acute colitis with partial or complete colonic dilatation, which represents a severe life-threatening complication, and occasionally the presenting sign of ulcerative colitis and Crohn's disease **Clinical** High fever, abdominal pain, tachycardia and leukostasis **Treatment** Resection of diseased colon, salvaging rectal sphincter if possible; Cf Megacolon

Toxic oil syndrome An epidemic that centered around Avila, Spain, occurring from mid-1981 until mid-1983, as a result of ingestion of olive oil contaminated with rapeseed oil, the latter of which was intended for industrial use and contained aniline; clandestine factories attempted to chemically remove the aniline and sold the product as olive oil to low-income families **Clinical** Fever, pneumonia-like illness, followed by gastrointestinal disease, eosinophilia and a prolonged rash; late neurological sequelae included myalgias, motor deficits, major muscle group atrophy, carpal tunnel syndrome, contractures of the jaw and extremities; of the estimated 20 000 cases, 340 people died; see Yusho disease

Toxic shock-like syndrome (TSLS) 'Jim Henson's' disease An epidemic infection caused by a highly virulent, antibiotic-resistant strain of group A streptococcus, which begins as a mild skin infection or 'strep throat' and rapidly progresses to high fever, hypotension, focal vasodilatation and soft-tissue cellulitis of an intensity that may require amputation; most cases have occurred in patients lacking predisposing factors, and it is unknown whether TSLS is due to a new strain of bacteria or represents the reappearance of streptococcal toxin A, the toxin responsible for scarlet fever that has not been produced in streptococci since the 1940s) Note: TSLS was first identified by a group of infectious disease specialists, the 'Rocky Mountain Pus Club' (N Engl J Med 1989; 321:1) and was responsible for the death of Jim Hensen of the Sesame Street Muppets (Science 1990; 249:22rn)

Toxic shock syndrome (TSS) A disease caused by ***Staphylococcus aureus*** strains that produce the toxin, TSST-1 (toxic shock syndrome toxin-1, designated 1 in anticipation of a 2, which has not been identified), formerly, enterotoxin F or exotoxin C is a superantigen (Nature 1990; 346:471); these strains of ***S aureus*** exhibit lysogeny (presence of a temperate bacteriophage, the production of which is enhanced in Mg^{++}-depleted medium); superabsorbent tampons are divalent cation chelators and thus the intravaginal microbiological milieu favors growth of lysogenic strains; the early cases of TSS occurred in tampon users and most began as vaginal lesions; TSS may also arise in foreign bodies, eg sutures Clinical Abrupt onset of high fever (> 40°C), nausea, vomiting, watery diarrhea, which may occur during menstruation, followed by an intense blanching mucocutaneous erythema, desquamative palmo-plantar rash and cleavage of the basal layer of the epidermis; without therapy, the patients deteriorate, become lethargic and confused, develop capillary leakage, hypotension, adult respiratory distress syndrome, renal and multiorgan failure and frank shock; even with appropriate therapy (non-β-lactam containing antibiotics), mortality is 5-10%; 88% of genital and 53% of non-genital TSS have been linked to a single strain of ***Staphylococcus aureus*** (Proc Natl Acad Sci 1990; 87:229); see Superantigen

'Toxic' staring Fixed staring, abnormal behavior, altered mental status, delirium, aphonia and coma, classically described in typhoid fever; see Rose spots

Toxic state INFECTIOUS DISEASE A condition typically seen in the third week of typhoid fever at which point the patients are sickest, mentally disoriented and at greatest risk for intestinal perforation and hemorrhage; see Pea soup stool

'Toxic tort' A lawsuit that centers around a drug, chemical or other substance in the environment, that is either incriminated in a disease process, eg DES and thalidomide, or implicated by vague and/or 'soft' circumstantial evidence, eg Agent Orange, video display terminals; a criticism of the jury process in ;toxic tort' cases is that they require that the judges, lawyers and juries (who generally are not trained to interpret statistical data of any nature) evaluate the validity of scientific evidence and understand the limits of the techniques used and by extension, the statistical method used (Science 1988; 239:1508); see Litogen

Toxic vacuolization HEMATOLOGY Rounded 'empty' cytoplasmic spaces within neutrophils seen in gram-negative bacteremia and endotoxemia; see Toxic granulation

Toxoid IMMUNOLOGY A bacterial toxin or other antigen that has been treated with formaldehyde in order to decrease the substance's toxicity while preserving antigenicity; toxoids are used to prepare diphtheria and tetanus vaccines

Toxoplasmosis triad Typical histopathologic findings seen in lymph nodes infected with ***Toxoplasma gondii*** consisting of a) Monocytoid cells in the sinusoides b) Florid follicular hyperplasia c) Aggregates of epithelioid histiocytes

Toy balloon appearance A fanciful descriptor for the globular red-yellow retinal hemangioblastoma (balloon-like) seen by fundoscopic exam which has paired vessels (corresponding to the balloon's strings) to and from the lesion; Cf Balloon, Hot air balloon appearance

TPA 12-O-tetradecanoylphorbol-13-acetate A potent tumor promoter of the phorbol ester family that mimics diacylglycerol, which locks protein kinase C into the 'on' position; see Phorbol ester

tPA tissue-plasminogen activator A thrombolytic protease that converts plasminogen into plasmin, activating fibrinolysis, without affecting the circulating plasminogen or fibrinogen; tPA is commercially available in a recombinant form, r-tPA; other thrombolytic agents include urokinase, streptokinase and APSAC or anisoylated streptokinase plasminogen activatory complex; tPA has currency in reducing the mortality of myocardial infarction in the immediate post-ischemic period, although it may offer no advantage over other less expensive agents, with a patency rate of the infarct-related artery of 76% in the streptokinase-treated group and 75% in the tPA-treated group (N Engl J Med 1989; 320:817); thrombolytic therapy given in the first post-infarct hour reduces mortality by 47% and reduces mortality in pulmonary thromboembolism Physiology Plasminogen activation elicits formation of plasmin (a proteolytic enzyme that degrades fibrin, the main protein of the thrombus scaffold), modifying platelet function, degrading circulating fibrinogen and coagulation factors V and VIII, lowering the hemorrhagic 'threshold', which is potentially fatal in patients with central nervous system hemorrhage

TPH Transplacental hemorrhage

TPN Total parenteral nutrition Intravenous hyperalimentation CLINICAL NUTRITION A modality that attempts to provide all the body's need for nutrition without using the gastrointestinal tract; TPN is used for a) Correction of nutritional depletion in the face of inadequate oral intake and/or intestinal absorption, as in Crohn's disease, malignancy, pseudo-obstruction, radiation enteritis, short bowel syndrome, sprue and b) Conditions requiring bowel rest and nutritional restitution, eg non-specific colitides and associated growth retardation, enterocutaneous fistulas and pancreatitis; a typical TPN formulation provides 40 kcal/kg with 1-1.5 g/kg of calories provided by protein, two-thirds of the remainder by carbohydrates, one-third by lipids; 30

ml/kg of H_2O and appropriate electrolytes, trace elements and vitamins; TPN is used in children with diaphragmatic hernia, malrotation, esophageal atresia, tracheo-esophageal fistula, gastroschisis, volvulus, meconium ileus and omphalocele Complications (see table, below)

TPR 1) Temperature, pulse and respiration 2) Third-party reimbursement

TRAb Thyroid-stimulating hormone receptor antibodies Antibodies that are pathogenically linked to Graves' disease, which may be quantified by a) Bioassays that measure the ability of a patient's immunoglobulins to stimulate thyroid activity, eg increasing cAMP production in Fisher rat thyroid cells (FRTL-5), assays that are less sensitive than b) Radioreceptor assays that measure inhibition of binding of labelled TSH to its receptor; both assays confirm the diagnosis of euthyroid Graves' disease with ophthalmopathy and atypical hyperthyroid Graves' disease

Trabecular bars SURGICAL PATHOLOGY Rigid rows of malignant epithelial cells with their long axis perpendicular to the long axis of a 'bar', a histologic criterion supporting the diagnosis of ductal carcinoma in situ of the breast; see 'Roman bridges'

Trabeculation of the bladder A forme fruste of bladder diverticulosis caused by partial urinary obstruction at the bladder neck, which is often secondary to prostatic hypertrophy; the increased intravesicular pressure results in mucosal herniation and fibrous cords that spread haphazardly across the bladder, histologically characterized by squamous metaplasia, epithelial hyperplasia, chronic inflammation and occasionally transitional or less commonly, squamous cell carcinoma

Trace mineral Any of a group of metal ions that are essential for life, functioning as enzyme co-factors and playing critical roles in the organization of molecules, membranes and mitochondria; they are present in milligram or microgram amounts and maintained in a delicate balance between the Scylla of toxic excess and the Charybdis of deficiency, which may induce metabolic failure, an event most common in total parenteral nutrition; trace elements include arsenic, chromium, cobalt, copper, fluorine, iodine, iron, manganese, nickel, selenium, silicon, tin, vanadium, zinc (Science 1981; 213:1332)

COMPLICATIONS OF TPN

HEPATIC DYSFUNCTION Cholestasis, cholelithiasis, hepatic dysfunction, jaundice, hepatomegaly, micronodular cirrhosis, lipofuscinosis and steatosis (most common in TPN of premature infants)

RELATED TO INDWELLING INTRAVENOUS LINE Misplacement of the 'line', infections, eg Candida species, aspergillosis

METABOLIC DEFECTS Hyperglycemia (osmotic diuresis, hyperosmolarity), post-infusion hypoglycemia, hyperosmolar coma, ketoacidosis and other metabolic derangements, excess or deficiency of electrolytes, including Na^+, K^+, Cl^-, eg hyperchloremic acidosis and mineral imbalances, affecting Mg^{++}, PO_4 and Ca^{++} with hypercalcemia, accompanying pancreatitis, hypercalciuria and metabolic bone disease

NUTRITIONAL IMBALANCES General decrease in essential fatty acids, trace minerals (copper, chromium, molybdenum, tin, zinc) and vitamins, and increased triglycerides and cholesterol

'Tracks' SUBSTANCE ABUSE Linear scars on mucocutaneous surfaces that may be accompanied by intense venous sclerosis and edema of the extremities, a characteristic finding in long-term heroin addicts; Cf Skin 'popping'

Track sign A normal anatomic variant of the femur in which the linea aspera or pilaster (site of attachment of the major adductor and extensor muscles) is more prominent than usual and is located on the posterior midshaft, thus having a radiodense 'tube-within-a-tube' appearance that should not be confused with the Blade of grass sign of Paget's disease of the bone

Traffic see Sexual traffic

Traffic accidents see MVA

'Traffic light' diet A dietary regimen designed to reduce atherosclerosis and weight; see Diet

Trailer sequence MOLECULAR BIOLOGY An untranslated segment of mRNA nucleotides that follows the termination signal (stop codon) at the 3' end, which does not include the poly(A) tail

Trail-making test of Reitan A two-part psychomotor test for assessing motor speed and integration, in which multiple dots are connected to form various objects; like the Bender-Gestalt test, the 'Trail-maker' serves as a screening test to detect gross organic defects; see Psychological testing

Train track appearance see Railroad tracks; Cf Tram tracks

TRAM flap Transverse rectus abdominus musculocutaneous flap GENERAL SURGERY A rotated piece of tissue used as an alternative to a prosthesis in post-radical mastectomy reconstructive breast surgery; the operating time and the recovery period is longer, but the cosmetic result is often better

Tram track appearance Tramline calcification A descriptive term for parallel, curved lines, radio-opacities or radiolucencies of varying length (when the parallel lines are straight, 'railroad track' appears to be a more valid adjectival descriptor) NEURORADIOLOGY A descriptor for the parallel calcified enhancement of cortical vessels seen in tuberous sclerosis (Sturge-Weber syndrome), due to calcium and iron deposition seen on a plain skull film, see figure, page 740 RADIOLOGY, BONE A descriptor for the split cortical thickening with parallel neo-osteogenesis (endosteal splitting), seen in infarctions of long bones in sickle cell anemia RADIOLOGY, LUNG A descriptor for the parallel, thickened bronchial walls seen on a plain chest film in bronchiectasis; Cf Railroad track, Ring shadow

Trans-activation (trans-acting) locus Molecular biology A region of the DNA molecule affecting genes located on the opposite chain; Cf cis-activation

Transactivator see Transcription activator

Transaminase-type mechanism see Ping-pong mechanism

Transbronchial needle biopsy (TBNA) An endoscopic technique used to obtain cytopathological material from a submucosal endobronchial lesion or an accessible extrabronchial mass, if there is evidence of extrinsic compression; TBNA is of use in establishing the diagnosis of both diagnosing bronchogenic carcinoma, carcinoid, bronchogenic cyst, lymphoma, sarcoid, pneumonia and abscesses Complications Pneumothorax, hemomediastinum, hemorrhage, bacteremia and rarely, false-positive diagnosis of malignancy; up to 37% of malignancy can be diagnosed by TBNA (Mayo Clin Proc 1989; 64:158); see Bronchoalveolar lavage, 'Skinny needle' biopsy

Transcervical balloon tuboplasty GYNECOLOGY A procedure that is similar in principle to balloon angioplasty, which attempts to re-establish the patency of fallopian tubes, stenosed by the vicissitudes of endometriosis and salpingitis; tubal patency was re-established in one or both tubes in 92% of the 77 women in one study, 22 of whom became pregnant (J Am Med Assoc 1990; 264:2079); ballon tuboplasty offers an alternative to microsurgery or in vitro fertilization for women with 'mechanical' infertility, which is responsible for 25-30% of female infertility

Transcranial Doppler ultrasonography A non-invasive modality of bedside imaging of the intracranial cerebral circulation in critically-ill hospitalized patients and outpatients, used to diagnosis vasospasm, assess collateral circulation and stenoses, to confirm brain death and to monitor circulation in neurosurgical patients (Mayo Clin Proc 1990; 65:1350rv)

Transcription MOLECULAR BIOLOGY The copying of a strand of DNA to generate a complementary strand of RNA; usually only one of the strands of DNA's double helix is capable of providing information which, when transcribed into RNA is translatable into a cognate polypeptide chain; in eukaryotes, three different RNA polymerases are responsible for producing RNAs: RNA polymerase I (RP-I), which generates ribosomal RNA (rRNA), RP-II, which synthesizes messenger RNA (mRNA) and RP-III which generates transfer RNA (tRNA)

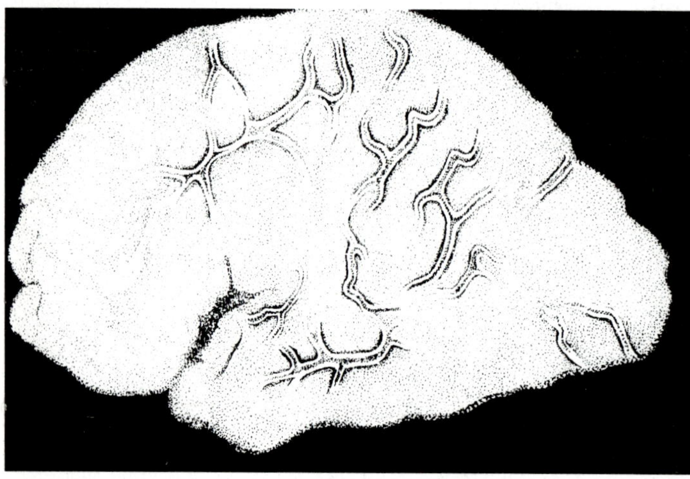

Tram track appearance

Transcription activator A protein that binds to DNA, activating its transcription machinery Note: Transcription requires a transcription activating protein in addition to RNA polymerase II, the TATA box and TATA factor, see TFIID; in eukaryotes, there are multiple 15- to 20- DNA base pair transcription activator-binding sites; once the activator is bound, a conformational change occurs, forming a pre-initiation complex (containing RNA polymerase, TFIIA, TFIIB, TFIID, TFIIE and TFIIF) at the transcription start site; DNA transcription activators are either 'universal' or activators that only function in some cells (Nature 1990; 346:329)

Transcription factors DNA-binding proteins that are necessary for gene activity, but don't participate directly in the regulation of gene activity; most of these factors have a positive effect on gene regulation and are involved in the organism's development

Transcription unit MOLECULAR BIOLOGY A DNA sequence (figure, facing page) that is transcribed into a coherent peptide, which is demarcated by flanking sequences; promoter elements are present -500 to -1000 nucleotides upstream (ie, in the 5' direction) of the transcription unit, closer to the beginning of the exon is the TATA box, located at -30 nucleotides, followed by the cap or initiation site (standardized as +1); from the cap to the ATG (start codon) is an untranslated portion of DNA; the exons are separated by introns, which are removed at the time the primary RNA transcript is processed, yielding mRNA; after the final exon is coded for, there follows an untranslated sequence, containing AATAAA separated 10-20 nucleotides from the poly(A) tail, followed by the termination site at the 3' downstream end and finally the flanking sequence

Transcutaneous electric nerve stimulation see TENS

Transdermal therapy CLINICAL PHARMACOLOGY The use of topical prolonged-release forms of drugs, eg nitroglycerin patches or testosterone replacement therapy (J Am Med Assoc 1989; 261:2525)

Transducer INSTRUMENTATION Any device that transforms one form of energy to another, eg a photocell that converts light into electrical energy; the transducer is the major component in ultrasonographic devices, containing both an emitting and receiving piezoelectric crystal

Transducin An 83 kD heterotrimeric G protein composed of Tα, Tβ and Tγ subunits that transduces a light signal into cells, mediating the light activation signal from photolyzed rhodopsin to cGMP phosphodiesterase; for GTP to bind to transducin, the Tγ subunit must have an attached farnesyl moiety (Nature 1990; 346:658)

Transducin family A family of eleven or more rhodopsin-related proteins that have sensory, neurotransmitter and hormone receptor functions, which includes β-adrenergic and muscarinic acetylcholine receptors; the transucin family members are membrane-bound, allowing

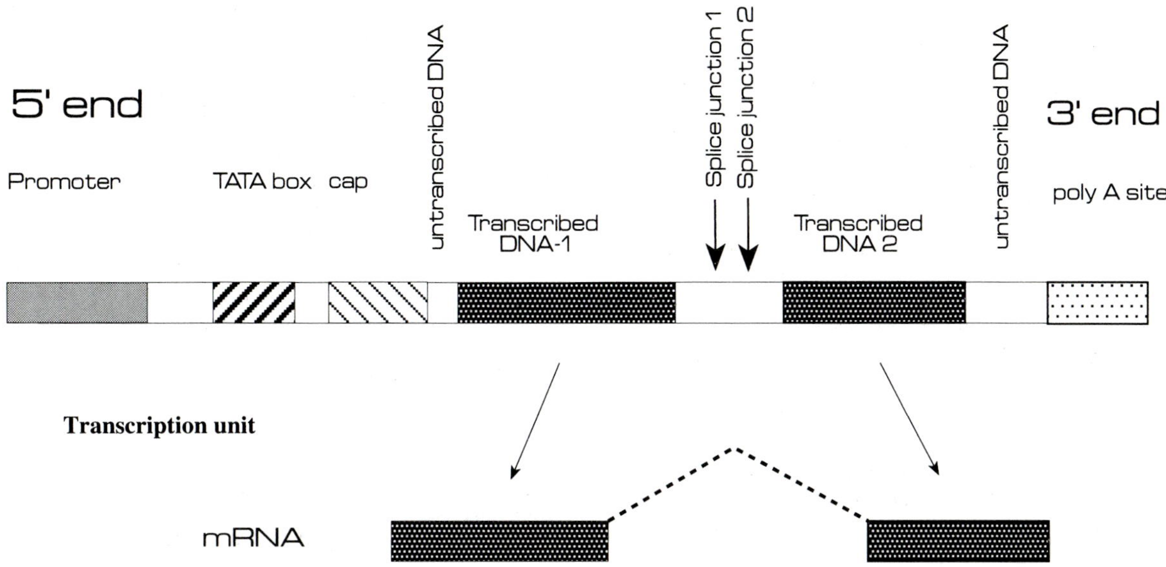

the cell to communicate with the external environment, have significant amino acid sequence homology and similarities in secondary and tertiary structures, including the presence of several transmembrane segments and share a common mechanism of action in that the intracellular signal occurs via G protein activation (Science 1991; 251:558)

Transduction A type of genetic recombination that occurs in bacteria, in which DNA is donated from one cell to another by means of a phage (a virus) or other vector; the most efficient transducing vectors are retroviruses (N Engl J Med 1990; 323:570)

Transesophageal echocardiography CARDIOLOGY An ultrasonographic imaging modality used to examine cardiac structure (valves, chambers and passages or inflow and outflow tracts) and function in which a transducer is placed immediately behind the heart in the esophagus and stomach; because there are no interfering air spaces or bone, the image is superior to that obtained with transthoracic echocardiography and is of particular use in evaluating the status of the endocardium, eg to identify vegetations on the cardiac valves (N Engl J Med 1991; 324:795); early devices were one-dimensional, using a horizontal plane beam, which made it difficult to visualize anterior and posterior structures and to depict contiguous long-axis and off-axis spatial relationships; this problem was resolved with the introduction of two (biplanar) and three (multiplanar) dimension devices (Mayo Clin Proc 1990; 65:1193rv); see Doppler color flow imaging, Echocardiography

'Trans' fatty acid (TFA) CLINICAL NUTRITION An unsaturated fat in which the carbon moieties on the two sides of the double bond point in opposite directions; minimal TFAs are present in animal fats; TFAs are abundant in margarines, frying fats and shortenings and are formed when polyunsaturated fat-rich vegetable and marine oils are 'hardened' by hydrogenation, producing fats with a firmness and consistency desired by both the food manufacturers and consumers; TFAs comprise 6-8% of the 120 g fat/day consumed per capita in developed nations; the recent trend away from consumption of tropical oils has resulted in an increased TFA consumption; the most abundant TFA is elaidic acid and its isomers, which are 18-carbon molecules bearing one double bond; in one study (N Engl J Med 1990; 323:439), increased dietary TFA resulted in increased total cholesterol and LDL-cholesterol and decreased HDL-cholesterol; the intensity of the lipid changes seen in a high TFA diet are as unfavorable as in a diet rich in saturated fatty acids Note: Oleic acid is a monounsaturated fatty acid with a cis configuration (carbon moieties lie on the same side of the double bond); most natural fats and oils contain only ***cis*** double bond; Cf Fish, Olive oil, Polyunsaturated fatty acid, Tropical oils, Unsaturated fatty acid

Transfection The extraction of double-stranded DNA from tumor cells to induce the phenotypic changes of malignancy in a second population of cells, which when performed in non-mammalian cells has been termed transformation

Transfer factor of Lawrence IMMUNOLOGY A substance derived from leukocyte lysates that is dialyzable, ie has a molecular weight of less than 10 kD, is produced by most mammals, elicits a delayed hypersensitivity reaction and stimulates lymphokine production; transfer factor may have some therapeutic currency in selected patients with Wiskott-Aldrich syndrome and mucocutaneous candidiasis and was once used with equivocal results to treat tuberculosis and leprosy

Transfer RNA (tRNA) A 70-80 residue RNA molecule that is encoded by tandemly repeated DNA and has a cloverleaf structure that binds an amino acid, transferring it to a growing polypeptide chain, and releasing the amino acid at the time the tRNA is transiently 'docked' to a ribosome via the complementary anticodon on the messenger RNA; the normal planar representation of transfer RNA folds back upon itself to allow the maximum stability through formation of multiple hydrogen intrachain bonds at the 'arms' of the cloverleaf; the segments of RNA that are not hydrogen-bonded are termed 'loops'; Cf Messenger RNA,

Ribosomal RNA, 'Second genetic code'

Transformation HEMATOLOGY see Blast transformation MOLECULAR BIOLOGY 1) The alteration of an organism's genome by insertion of DNA from another species, eg bacterial transformation, which follows recombination with an isolated fragment of DNA from a genetically distinct organism; plasmid DNA is most common DNA used to transforma bacteria; Cf Transfection 2) Malignant transformation The conversion of a cell to one with a malignant phenotype, either due to infection with an oncogenic virus or due to environmental factors

Transforming growth factor-beta see TGF-β

Transfusion-associated graft-versus-host disease (TAGVHD) A variant of graft-versus-host disease in which immunocompetent T lymphocytes are transfused to a recipient and attack the recipient's immune system; the risk factors for TAGVHD are poorly defined (N Engl J Med 1990; 323:315), but are thought to include those bone marrow graft recipients and those who have been otherwise immunocompromised by chemotherapy or malignancy Clinical Rash, abnormal liver function tests and severe pancytopenia; mortality of 84% within 21 days of transfusion; some underlying diseases, eg leukemia have a lower mortality than others Prevention Irradiation of cellular blood products with 15 Gy (1500 rad); up to 50 Gy can be used for most blood-derived products

Transfusion medicine Blood banking A field of subspecialization in either clinical pathology or internal medicine that is involved in patient management through administration of blood cells and blood products including fresh-frozen plasma and cryoprecipitate; transfusion medicine specialists wear many hats and must be versant in relevant areas of hematology, immunology and infectious disease, both clinically and from a laboratory standpoint, participate in establishing standards for use of these products in a health care facility, and address the legal aspects of transfusions; the major *LEGAL ISSUES OF TRANSFUSION MEDICINE* pivot around *A) WHETHER THE PRODUCT BEING TRANSFUSED IS SAFE*, ie not infected, especially with human immunodeficiency virus, see Blood shield laws and *B) WHETHER A PERSON HAS THE RIGHT TO REFUSE A MEDICALLY-APPROPRIATE AND POTENTIALLY LIFE-SAVING BLOOD TRANSFUSION*; in the US, the doctrines that protect personal freedoms regard blood transfusions as an 'assault' if the medical team administers blood against the will of a mentally-competent person, who is not pregnant, has no children and refuses transfusion on religious grounds Note: Transfusions are problematic when the recipient is a minor and the parent refuses to allow a transfusion (the courts can override this dilemma by intervening in the child's interest); the courts may also oblige a transfusion when the patient is a parent of minor children who would become wards of the state upon the patient's death through exsanguination; in the USA, the US Food and Drug Administration and the American Association of Blood Banks (AABB) set standards and provide guidelines in transfusion medicine; see AABB

Transfusion reaction(s) Any of a number of clinical complexes related to the transfusion of blood or blood products; the term may be simplistically viewed as any untoward response to non-self blood products, which elicit febrile reactions that are either minor, occurring in 1:40 transfusions, attributed to non-specific leukocyte-derived pyrogens, or major, occurring in 1:3000 transfusions, due to a true immune reaction, which are graded according to the presence of urticaria, itching, chills, fever and, if the reaction is intense, collapse, cyanosis, chest and/or back pain and diffuse hemorrhage Note: If any of these signs appear, or if the temperature rises more than 1°C, the transfusion must be stopped; most patients survive if less than 200 ml has been transfused in cases of red cell incompatibility-induced transfusion reaction; over 50% die when 500 ml or more has been transfused; the mortality of these reactions is approximately 1.13/10^5 transfusions Types (table, below)

TRANSFUSION REACTIONS

I IMMUNE, NON-INFECTIOUS TRANSFUSION REACTIONS

Allergic urticaria with immediate hypersensitivity

Anaphylaxis Spontaneous anti-IgA antibody formation, described in approximately 1:30 of subjects with immunoglobulin A deficiency, which occurs in circa 1:600 of the general population (total frequency: 1/30 x 500-700 = 1/15 000-21 000) Antibodies to red cell antigens, eg antibodies to ABH, Ii, MNSs, P1, HLA

Serum sickness Antibodies to the donor's immunoglobulins and other proteins

II NON-IMMUNE, NON-INFECTIOUS TRANSFUSION REACTIONS

Air embolism A problem of historic interest that occurred when air vents were included in the transfusion sets

Anticoagulant Citrate anticoagulant may cause muscle tremor and electrocardiographic changes

Coagulation defects Depletion of factors VIII and V, a dilutional effect that requires massive transfusion of 10 or more units before becoming significant

Cold blood In ultra-emergent situations, blood stored at 4°C may be tranfused prior to reaching body temperature at 37°C; warming a unit of blood from 4°C to 37°C requires 30 kcal/liter of energy, consumed as glucose; cold blood slows metabolism, exacerbates lactic acidosis, decreases available calcium, increases hemoglobin's affinity for oxygen and causes potassium leakage, a major concern in cold hemoglobinuria

Hemolysis A phenomenon due to blood collection trauma, a clinically insignificant problem

Hyperammonemia and increased lactic acid Both molecules accumulate during packed red cell storage and when transfused, require hepatorenal clearance, of concern in patients with hepatic or renal dysfunction, who should receive the freshest units possible

Hyperkalemia Hemolysis causes an increase of 1 mmol/L/day of potassium in a unit of stored blood, of concern in patients with poor renal function, potentially causing arrhythmia Iron overload Each unit of packed red cells has 250 mg iron, potentially causing hemosiderosis in multi-transfused patients

Microaggregates Sludged debris in the pulmonary vasculature causing adult respiratory distress syndrome may be removed with micropore filters

III INFECTIONS TRANSMITTED BY BLOOD TRANSFUSIONS

Viruses Cytomegalovirus, Epstein-Barr virus, hepatitis A-E, HIV-1, HIV-2, HTLV-I, HTLV-II Note: In the US, the highly-sensitive polymerase chain reaction estimates the probability that a screened donor will be positive for HIV-1 at 1:61,171; 95% percent upper confidence bound, 1:10,695 (N Engl J Med 1991; 325:1)

Bacteria Transmission of bacterial infections from an infected donor is uncommon and includes brucellosis and syphilis in older reports, while more recent reports include, Lyme disease and, Yersinia enterocolitica (MMWR 1991; 40:176) Note: Although virtually any bacteria can be transmitted in blood, it is usually due to contamination during processing rather than transmission from an infected donor

Parasites Malaria, filariasis, toxoplasmosis, Trypanosoma cruzi (J Am Med Assoc 1989; 262:1433), babesiosis

Transfusion 'trigger' The hematocrit and hemoglobin values at or below which packed red cells are usually ordered for transfusion by a clinician; in the current environment of potentially fatal transfusion-transmitted infections, the formerly used transfusion trigger of 10g hemoglobin and 30% (the '10/30 rule') is no longer acceptable as most patients, especially the elderly, may be stable and asymptomatic with hematoglobins far below 10 g and often respond to iron supplementation, as one of the smost common cause of anemia in this age group is iron deficiency

Transgenic animals see Transgenic organisms

Transgenic chicken An animal of value for both research and the poultry industry, in which genes are inserted using a replication-defective reticuloendotheliosis virus vector (Science 1989; 243:533)

Transgenic mice A mouse 'created' in vitro by transferring genes into the mouse embryo, serving as a useful model for studying autoimmune phenomena, oncogenesis, embyrology (Science 1989; 246:1265) and physiology; insertion of foreign genes may have consequences for the host, eg when PHT1-1 transgenic mice are homozygous for a transgene insertion, eg heat shock protein, hsp 70, the 'legless' mutation appears, in which the hindlimbs are shortened and the forelimbs have bone defects, accompanied by cerebral and craniofacial defects, which are not seen in heterozygotes; transgenic mouse models have been produced for hypoxanthine guanine phosphoribosyl transferase deficiency, sickle hemoglobin, which express the disease (Science 1990; 247:566) and others Note: It had been reported that transgenic mammals could be produced by simply fertilizing mouse eggs with sperm mixed in a DNA-containing milieu, a finding that could not be reproduced by other groups (Science 1989; 246:446)

Transgenic organisms An animal or plant that has been modified by insertion of foreign genes that express proteins of interest; transgenic technology is currently limited by the inability to direct the site of gene insertion, since a gene may be inserted in a position that results in activation of one of the host's structural genes

Transgenics A therapeutic modality in which genes of interest are inserted into an organism, compelling it to produce a protein that is either missing or desired; transgenics is in advanced planning stages for treating human disease and is already in use for treating conditions in commercial plants and animals

Transgenic sheep At Edinburgh's Animal Breeding and Research Organization (ABRO), transgenic sheep have been produced, serving as 'factories' for producing coagulation factor IX and α_1-antitrypsin; ABRO's sheep produce higher volumes of useful protein than transgenic mice; in ABRO's protocol, engineered stem cells are first grown in culture to determine whether the DNA of interest is successfully integrated before producing the whole animal (Science 1990; 249:124n&v)

Transient ischemic attack (TIA) NEUROLOGY A focal, abrupt ischemia-induced loss of neurologic function, accompanied by disability of less than 24 hours in duration (when the disability is greater than 24 hours, it is known as reversible ischemic neurologic disability or RIND); symptomatic TIAs often precede cerebral infarctions or strokes, typically occurring in older patients with marked cerebrovascular atherosclerosis, potentially affecting any cerebral vessel; despite clinical resolution, computed tomography scans demonstrate residual anatomic lesions in 15% of both RINDs and TIAs Prevention Low dose (30 mg) aspirin, a level at which '...*INHIBITION OF AGGREGATION CAUSED BY THE DIMINISHED PRODUCTION OF THROMBOXANE A_2 IN PLATELETS IS STILL COMPLETE, (BUT) THE PRODUCTION OF PROSTACYCLIN, WHICH HAS AN ANTIAGGREGATION EFFECT IS LITTLE AFFECTED IN THE ENDOTHELIAL CELLS*'; prostacyclin production is inhibited by the currently recommended higher doses of aspirin (N Engl J Med 1991; 325:1261)

Transition MOLECULAR BIOLOGY Any point mutation of DNA in which either a purine is substituted for another or a pyrimidine is substituted for another; Cf Degenerate code

Transitional panel see Metastatic disease panel

Transkaryotic implantation The alteration of the nuclei of implanted cells, eg fibroblasts by adding DNA sequences through stable or transient transfection, a technique that enhances the potential of gene therapy since a) The transfected cell line can be well-characterized prior to definitive transplantation, b) Different anatomic sites may be used for the transplantation and c) regulated expression of the gene of interest can be obtained

Translation MOLECULAR BIOLOGY The process whereby the genetic information on messenger RNA (mRNA) is 'decoded' and converted into a coherent protein, during which transfer RNA (tRNA) converges on ribosomes packaged as rRNA and, at the behest of mRNA, dispenses amino acids to a growing polypeptide chain; protein synthesis is divided into initiation, elongation and termination steps

Translocase A ribosomal enzyme that catalyzes the GTP-dependent translocation reaction in protein synthesis, shifting the tRNA-amino acid complex from the ribosome's A site to its P site, where it proffers the next amino acid to the growing polypeptide

Translocation 1) The activity of the translocase enzyme, see above 2) The *in vivo* transfer of a chromosomal segment to another, non-homologous chromosome; such a transfer may link two segments of otherwise silent DNA, resulting in a 'renegade' gene encoding a hybrid protein, eg $P210^{bcr/abl}$, a phosphoprotein unique to chronic myelogenous leukemia, which has deregulated tyrosine kinase activity, thus acting to 'drive' the neoplasm

Transluminal angioplasty see Percutaneous transluminal angioplasty

Transmembrane protein A protein that is fully integrated in the plasma membrane, characterized by a hydrophilic COOH extracellular domain, a hydrophobic 25-30 residue transmembrane region and a hydrophilic NH2 intracellular domain; see Fluid mosaic model

Transmission electron microscopy see Microscopy; Cf Scanning electron microscope, Scanning tunneling microscope

Transplantation The use of usually non-self tissue(s) to replace a malfunctioning organ; solid organ and hematopoietic precursor transplantations are being performed with increasing impunity in bone marrow, bone matrix, cardiac valves, heart, heart-lung, kidney, liver, pancreas, skin and intestine, largely due to the availability of agents, eg cyclosporin A and FK 506, which effectively battle the otherwise limiting complication of graft-versus-host disease Annual transplantations performed in the US (table, below); see Graft-versus-host disease, Liver transplantation, Lung transplantation, Pancreas transplantation, Procurement, Skin graft, UNOS

TRANSPLANTATION STATISTICS, USA

Site	Number‡	Cost/case*	Centers #
Middle ear	100 000*	$2 000	Most ENT
Cornea	28 000 *	$6 800	400
Kidney	9 340	$36 000	237
Heart	1 988	$110 000	154
Bone marrow	1 322 *	$95 000	72
Liver	2 524	$238 000	58
Pancreas	528	$35 000	86
Heart/lung	52/185	$165 000	82/77

‡1990 *1986 #Number of centers performing procedure

Transplantation antigens see MHC (Major histocompatibility complex)

Transplantation rejection The constellation of host immune responses evoked when an allograft tissue is transplanted into a recipient, which may be reduced by best possible matching of major histocompatibility antigens and ABO blood group and ameliorated by using various immunosuppressive agents, including cyclosporin, FK 506 and rapamycin; see Graft-versus-host disease

Transposition The DNA-mediated movement of genetic material within the genome; Cf Retroposition

Transposon Transposable elements A type of 'jumping gene' or segment of DNA that is capable of inserting itself into or excising itself out of a gene locus, an ability that is regulated by genetic, environmental and developmental factors; the tissue specificity and timing of transposon activity is pivotal in ontogeny; in maize (where transposons were first discovered by Nobel laureate Barbara McClintock) and by extension, in other organisms, the excision of transposons during development is controlled by the host (Science 1990; 248:1534); see 'Jumping genes'

Transsexuality A clinical condition in which a person has an irrepressible desire to belong to the opposite phenotypic sex, a desire that may be satisified by simple 'cross-dressing' or may be of such intensity to compel the person to seek sexual reassignment; see Sexual reassignment

Transthyretin A 55 kD homotetrameric protein composed of four 127-residue polypeptide chains that binds both thyroxine and retinol Serum levels: 0.15-0.36 g/L (US: 20-40 mg/dl); transthyretin is markedly decreased in malnutrition and in acute and chronic inflammation, and thus is considered a 'negative acute phase protein', which may be defective in autosomal dominant amyloidosis; because transthyretin migrates in front of albumin on a serum electrophoresis, it had been formerly termed 'prealbumin'; since the protein is 1) Structurally distinct from albumin 2) In murine systems, is a term that refers to other proteins migrating in the same electrophoretic regions, eg α_1-antitrypsin and 3) Potentially causes confusion with the term proalbumin, the more informative term, transthyretin has been substituted (Nomenclature committee of IUB, J Biol Chem 198X; 256:12); Cf Proalbumin

Transverse lie Shoulder presentation OBSTETRICS A non-cephalic, non-breech position, in which the fetus' long axis is perpendicular to that of the mother's, an event occurring in 1:300 births, due to lower uterine obstruction, eg placenta previa, intrauterine leiomyomas or an ovarian tumor in the cul-de-sac, or may occur in a multiparous uterus with a lax wall; 'transverse lies' are managed by cesarian section or, less commonly, gentle external version if the membranes have not ruptured; the risks of an internal version are unacceptably high and it is rarely performed

TRAP Tartrate-resistant acid phosphatase A 60 kD acid phosphatase isoenzyme that migrates in band 5, which is present in and relatively specific for the leukemic cells of hairy cell leukemia; weak TRAP staining occurs in infectious mononucleosis, chronic lymphocytic leukemia, lymphosarcoma, Sézary cells, osteoclastic bone tumors and Gaucher cells; the hydrolytic activity of some protein phosphatases towards certain phosphoproteins such as casein and histone is resistant to tartrate inhibition; see Hairy cell leukemia

Trapdoor scar PLASTIC SURGERY A descriptor for an unesthetic scar that puckers above the skin surface in a large healing 'horseshoe' avulsion flap, most commonly seen in automobile windshield injuries

Trapped lung A sequestered segment of lung seen in empyema, where a portion of a bacterially-infected lobe and visceral pleura 'fix' the affected lung in a partially collapsed position Note: Hippocrates was the first to recognize and drain an empyema, now a rare complication of bacterial pneumonia due to staphylococci, streptococci and gram-negative bacilli; Cf Folded lung, Scimitar syndrome, Sequestration complex

T ratio A statistical test used when a set of data (or study) has few data points (or subjects); the T ratio is of use in determining whether the results obtained are due to chance alone

Trauma score EMERGENCY MEDICINE A physiologic index measuring systolic blood pressure, respiratory rate and expansion, capillary refill, eye opening and verbal and motor responses, placing them on a scale of 2 to 16; the trauma score is a predictor of injury severity and the probability of survival; below a score of 12, a patient would benefit from transfer to a trauma center (J Am Med Assoc 1986; 256:1319), Cf Injury severity score

Traumatic tap A diagnostic lumbar puncture in which there is incidental hemorrhage due to violent movement by the patient or tearing of vessels, a risk inherent in the procedure, which is not indicative of true pathology within the cerebrospinal fluid; a traumatic tap is differentiated from subarachnoid hemorrhage by the absence of xanthochromia, decreasing erythrocytes in serial tubes and rapid coagulation of blood

Trauma X A euphemism for the physical signs of child abuse; see Battered child syndrome, Child abuse

Traveler's diarrhea Montezuma's revenge, Aztec two-step, Turkey trot, Dehli belly Most diarrhea in travellers is acquired orally and caused by the heat-stable and heat-labile toxins of *Escherichia coli* and *Shigella*; the intensity of infection depends on the quality of the water supply, previous host exposure and susceptibility; pathogens on cruise ships include *Shigella*, and *Salmonella* (the latter of which is an uncommon cause of traveller's diarrhea in developing nations as it grows best in animal protein, eg mayonnaise-based egg and macaroni salads), *Vibrio parahemolyticus*, less commonly, *Aeromonas hydrophila, Campylobacter jejuni, Plesiomonas shigelloides, V cholerae* (non-01), *V fluvialis* and *Yersinia enterocolitica*; parasites causing traveller's diarrhea include *Giardia lamblia* (causing the 'Trotskys' in travellers to Russia, boasting excursions unannounced by Inturist), *Entamoeba histolytica, Balantidium coli, Cryptosporidium species, Dientamoeba fragilis, Isospora belli* and *Strongyloides stercolrals*; viruses are less commonly implicated in traveller's diarrhea, but include Norwalk-like agents and rotavirus Treatment Rehydration, bismuth subsalicylate, narcotic analogs to slow the motility and trimethoprim-sulfamethoxazole if antibiotics are required Note: Prophylactic antibiotics are rarely indicated, and unless one travels to areas at high risk for a certain infection, most subjects are often advised to 'sit it out'

'Trawling' MOLECULAR BIOLOGY 1) Traditional DNA sequencing, which like the North sea fishing technique from whence the analogy, catches everything within range of the 'trawl'; chromosomal 'trawling' contrasts with Chromosome walking and Chromosome jumping, see there, in that there is no 'skipping' from one to another DNA segment 2) An activity of the endocytic microtubule network that constantly 'trawls' allowing certain receptors, eg transferrin to pass through the 'fishnet' while other receptors, eg epidermal growth factor receptor are trapped, forming a multi-vesicular body filled with a specific receptor 'cargo' (Nature; 1990; 346:335; 346:318)

Treadmill exercise test CARDIOLOGY The most commonly used clinical test for accurately assessing a person's risk of death from cardiovascular events; the treadmill exercise score is calculated as the duration of exercise in minutes − (5 x the maximal ST-segment deviation in millimeters during or after exercise) − (4 x the treadmill angina index, ie no angina during exercise = 0, nonlimiting angina = 1, exercise-limiting angina = 2); the results range from a score of 15 for a normal person at no known increased risk to -25 for those at highest risk (N Engl J Med 1991; 325:849); see Thallium imaging

Treadmilling An equilibrium state in muscle, in which the length of actin and microtubular polymers remains constant, as the rate of addition of monomers of actin or tubulin (which form microtubules) at one end of the molecule is equal to the rate of loss or degradation at the other end

'Treated' wood CLINICAL TOXICOLOGY Wood impregnated with preservatives, eg chromium-copper-arsenate, creosote, inorganic arsenicals and pentachlorophenol, to increase its useful life, preventing attack by insects, fungi and other organisms; chronic exposure to the fumes of burning wood or skin contact therewith may produce a combined heavy metal intoxication syndrome

Treatment-investigational new drug (TIND) A drug that is made available to patients who are very ill with life-threatening diseases, prior to the drug's official approval by the Food and Drug Administration; 1987 IND 'rewrite' makes a limited number of INDs available if there is a gap in the therapeutic arsenal, ie if there is no known and/or effective therapy for a particular disease which the TIND appears to effectively treat; the prolonged period of time required for the approval of new therapeutic agents is problematic in AIDS, as these patients may clamor for therapy, regardless of how minimal the positive effect; if a candidate TIND agent is very early in the testing process and the data available is scant, approval for TIND usage is unlikely and one turns to the 'compassionate use' clause (driven by the often desperate plight of AIDS patients) to allow the very ill to at least import their own therapeutics, however ineffective '...PRIMUM, NON NOCERUM...' (N Engl J Med 1989; 320:281); life-threatening diseases for which TINDs are used include AIDS, advanced congestive heart failure and refractory malignancy; agents that have been under TIND protocols include cytomegalovirus (CMV) immunoglobulin for transplantation of a CMV seropositive donor kidney into a seronegative individual, pentostatin (deoxycoformin) for hairy cell leukemia patients refractory to interferon-α; trimetrexate glucuronate, which is indicated for *Pneumocystis carinii* as it is reported to have a 1500-fold greater affinity for *Pneumocystis carinii*'s dihydrofolate reductase than does trimethoprim; see Compassionate IND, IND

Treatment-related malignancy see Secondary malignancy

Treatment window HEMATOLOGY A 4-6 day period during which a patient with factor VIII inhibitor-producing hemophilia A may respond to a bolus of factor VIII, which by complexing with the inhibitors may reduce their level to the point to allow hemostasis

Tree bark appearance A descriptor for intimal and subintimal plaques that encase the mouth of small aortic branches, due to obliterative endarteritis of vasa vasorum with ischemic destruction of the vascular media causing inflammation, neo-vascularization and fibrous scarring, leading to aneurysms and surface irregularities; although the appearance is typical of late syphilis, it may also be seen in Takayasu's disease, Reiter's disease and rheumatic heart disease

Treefrog hand appearance A fanciful descriptor for the broadened distal digits with elongated fingers seen in the otopalatodigital syndrome (Taybi syndrome), an X chromosome-linked disease characterized by a short stature, variable mental deficiency, cleft soft palate, microstomia and conduction-type deafness; Cf clubbing

Trembler mice A strain of mice that produces virtually no peripheral nervous system myelin when homozygous for the Tr mutation, despite which they have a normal lifespan (Science 1988; 241:344)

Trench fever Werner-His disease A rickettsia-like disease caused by ***Rochalimaea quintana***, transmitted by the feces of the body louse (***Pediculus humanus***) under crowded conditions of poor hygiene, well described in the trenches in World War I and in endemic form in underdeveloped nations Clinical Abrupt onset of paroxysmal fever, asthenia, chills, vertigo, headache, backache, quasi-pathognomonic pain on the shins, truncal rash, transient maculopapules and moderate leukocytosis; febrile relapse(s), see Saddleback curve Treatment Tetracyclines, broad-spectrum antibiotics, eradicate lice

Trench foot A condition first described in World War I in soldiers whose feet were damp and exposed to near-freezing temperatures for prolonged periods, causing acral vasoconstriction and heat loss; the resulting ischemia unchains a vicious circle of necrosis, endothelial damage, intravascular 'sludging' of cells, extravasation of protein and fluid, resulting in more ischemia; the prolonged cold is followed by vasodilation, burning pain and paresthesiae with the formation of hemorrhagic blebs or gangrene, accompanied by cellulitis, lymphangitis, swelling, thrombophlebitis and persistent hypersensitivity to cold with secondary Raynaud's phenomenon Histopathology Perivascular fibrosis, muscular hyperplasia and necrotizing vasculitis Treatment Slow warming of foot; if the tissue is warmed too rapidly, reactive hyperthermia, blistering and potentially thrombosis occurr Note: It may be of use pathogenically to separate trench foot from the virtually identical 'immersion foot', see there

Trench mouth see Acute necrotizing ulcerative gingivitis

Treponemal tests see Serological tests for Syphilis

Tretinoin A topically applied cream that reverses some of the effects of photoaging, both clinically (decreased skin wrinkling, improved skin texture and color) and microscopically (increased epidermal thickness, increased collagen and dermal vessels and 'erasing' epithelial atypia and dysplasia) Mechanism Unknown, possibly related to tretinoin's inhibition of collagenase, which degrades the anchoring fibril collagen; tretinoin therapy doubles the number of anchoring fibrils at the dermal-epidermal junction (J Am Med Assoc 1990; 263:3057); see Retinoic acid, Vitamin A

TRF Thryotropin-releasing factor, obsolete, see TRH

TRH Thyrotropin-releasing hormone A hypothalamic tripeptide(pyroglutamic acid-histidine-proline) which releases TSH after receptor attachment and activation of the cAMPase

Triad A trilogy of clinical or pathological findings, which are often initially described as (highly) characteristic for a disease, but which often ultimately prove to be relatively non-specific ASTHMA TRIAD ASA triad Nasal polyps, asthma and aspirin intolerance; variously considered to be inherited or due to environmental factors, related to aspirin's inhibition of cyclooxigenase in prostaglandin production CHRISTIAN'S TRIAD Lytic bony lesions, diabetes insipidus and exophthalmos A classically described, but observed trilogy of symptoms described in histiocytosis X CHARCOT'S TRIAD Nystagmus, 'scanning' speech and intention tremor A trilogy of clinical signs described as characteristic for multiple sclerosis which is non-specific and only occurs in advanced cases HEMOCHROMATOSIS TRIAD Hepatomegaly, diabetes mellitus and bronze cutaneous pigmentation LENNOX'S TRIAD Petit mal epilepsy, akinetic seizures and myoclonic jerks PETIT'S TRIAD Mydriasis, increased intraocular pressure and alteration of the retinal vessels due to autonomic nervous system activity RENAL CELL CARCINOMA TRIAD Pain, palpable mass and hematuria; seen in 10% of patients with renal cell carinoma SAINT'S TRIAD Hiatal hernia, cholelithiasis and diverticulosis TOXOPLASMOSIS TRIAD Marked follicular hyperplasia with active mitosis and phagocytosis, small granulomas composed of epithelioid histiocytes and distension of marginal and cortical sinuses by monocytoid B cells TROTTER'S TRIAD Hypoacusia, impaired soft palate movement, mandibular neuralgia, typical of eustachian tube malignancy WILSON'S TRIAD Chronic active hepatitis, Kayser-Fleischer rings of the iris, degeneration of the lenticular nucleus WATERHOUSE-FRIDERICHSEN TRIAD Meningococcemia, multiple petechial cutaneous hemorrhages and bilateral adrenal hemorrhages

Triaditis A generic and non-specific term for chronic inflammation of the hepatic portal triad

Triage EMERGENCY MEDICINE Triage, French, sorting A

method first used on the battlefield, in which the most extremely wounded were placed in an 'expectant' category, ie expected to die, and therefore not treated, while the limited medical personnel could attend to those most likely to survive; triaging, then is assessment of injury intensity and the immediacy or urgency for medical attention (table, below)

TRIAGE PRIORITIES

Highest priority Respiratory, facial, neck, chest, cardiovascular, hemorrhage, neck injuries

Very high priority Shock, retroperitoneal or intraperitoneal hemorrhage

High priority Cranial, cerebral, spinal cord, burns

Low priority Lower genitourinary tract, peripheral nerves and vessels, splinted fractures, soft tissue lesions

Trial and error method see Stochastic method

Triangular face A hypoplastic face with prominent zygomatic arches, sunken cheeks, down-turned mouth and brownish facial discoloration, characteristic of Mulibrey nanism, which has also been described in the Russell-Silver and Turner syndromes; Cf Hippocratic facies

Triangle of Codman RADIOLOGY A wedge-shaped periosteal elevation of bone seen on a plain film of the long bones, described as characteristic of Ewing sarcoma, which may also be observed in osteosarcoma, metastases to bone, hematomas, syphilis and tuberculosis

TRIC Tracoma-induced interstitial conjunctivitis

Triceps skin-fold thickness A value used to estimate corporal fat, measured on the right arm halfway between the olecranon process of the elbow and the acromial process of the scapula; Normal, males: 12 mm; females: 23 mm; Cf Mid-arm muscle mass

Trichrome stain A stain used in histopathology that colors collagen green, muscle red-purple and myelin brown; the stain is of particular use in determining the presence of muscle invasion in certain carcinomas, eg transitional cell carcinoma of the urinary bladder

'Trick' movements HAND SURGERY A series of movements that an active and highly-motivated person will perform to circumvent the limitations of musculoskeletal paralysis; these movements would never be performed under normal circumstances and thus are often bizarre and uncoordinated; the disadvantage is that prolonged 'trick'-type compensation may stretch various hand structures and may persist as a habit once the tendons have been surgically rerouted

Tricyclic antidepressant suicide A peculiar form of death that is thought to be more common in those who are receiving therapeutic antidepressant agents; most drugs of this family have three central rings and a short linear chain attached to the terminal nitrogen and are thus tertiary amines; TCAs were first used in the late 1950s to treat endogenous depression and revolutionized the

Tricyclic antidepressant

N

$CH_2CH_2CH_2N(CH_3)_2$

treatment of patients with severe ('decompensated') mental illness, allowing many to be de-institutionalized; TCAs are thought to act by central inhibition of the reuptake of biogenic amines; they are widely prescribed and represent the most common drug involved in suicide attempts by single, young females without previous history of autodestructive thoughts; the reported TCA overdose mortality of less than 15% includes the elderly and children (including accidental TCA overdoses) may in fact underestimate the true incidence, as up to 70% of TCA suicides are successful and never reach the hospital Clinical, overdose Parasympathetic disease with anticholinergic effects, including mydriasis, xerostomia, urinary retention, decreased peristalsis, cardiac disease (intractable myocardial depression, hypotension, ventricular tachycardia, fibrillation or heart block) and central nervous system disease (confusion, agitation, hallucinations, myoclonus and seizures, lethargy that may progress to coma and respiratory arrest) Laboratory TCA levels correlate poorly with the clinical status as circulating levels of the highly lipid-soluble TCA represent a minute portion of the body load, and TCA metabolites with similar clinical effects are not measured

Trident hand see Main en trident

Trident sign PEDIATRICS A clinical finding in Turner syndrome, consisting of a low hairline that extends in three vaguely defined vertical bands down the characteristically webbed neck, fancifully likened to a King Neptune's trident, a three-pronged spear

Trigeminy CARDIOLOGY A form of arrhythmia in which every third QRS wave is a ventricular premature depolarization or contraction; see PVCs

Trigger finger RHEUMATOLOGY A digit in which the flexor tendon passes through a fibro-osseous tunnel, the tendon sheath that extends from the distal palm to the distal finger joint; any fusiform swelling (congenital, edema or tenosynovitis) of the tendon or tendon sheath can cause a painful lock-snap sensation, leaving the finger or thumb in flexion or extension; the trigger finger is most common in women in their sixth decade, associated with de Quervain's disease and carpal tunnel syndrome as well as rheumatoid arthritis and collagen vascular disease; trigger digits in children may be idiopathic or associated with chromosomal defects; trigger or locked fingers may also be caused by a variety of fractures, tendinous or ligamentous lesions

Trigger points Local regions of increased tenderness that may occur in fibrositis, often located around the vertebrae medial to the scapula

Trigger thumb A congenital fixed flexion deformity of the thumb, related to a narrow flexor pollicus longus tendon sheath in the region of the metacarpophalangeal joint, a condition that may be present at birth or acquired later in life; if severe, trigger thumbs may require surgical correction

Trigger zone Relatively circumscribed regions adjacent to nerves, often in the head and neck, which when stimulated even with light touch, may elicit marked neuralgia accompanied by lightning pain; trigger zones include the lips and buccal cavity (evoking trigeminal neuralgia and tic douloureux), tonsillar or posterior pharynx (glossopharyngeal neuralgia) and in the muscles involved in the myofascial pain syndrome

Trihydroxycoprostanic acid (THCA) syndrome An autosomal recessive condition of neonatal onset characterized by hepatosplenomegaly, growth retardation, rickets, elevated THCA in serum and bile, histologically characterized by cholestasis, decreased number of interlobular bile ducts, portal fibrosis and cirrhosis

'Trilateral' retinoblastoma The rare (1:10^8 cases are estimated to occur annually) association of a bilateral retinoblastoma with a tumor of the pineal gland, a region known as the 'third eye' in lower animals, given the presence of afunctional photoreceptors **Clinical** Onset between 3 months and 15 years of age; most are fatal **Pathogenesis** Local inactivation of the retinoblastoma binding protein in the face of an intact retinoblastoma gene locus (Arch Ophthalmol 1990; 108:1145); see Retinoblastoma

Trimethoprim-sulfamethoxazole (TMP-SMX) One of the few effective, commercially-produced combination antibacterial available in the US, formulated as a 1:20 ratio of TMP to SMX; this broad-spectrum oral agent is effective in genitourinary, gastrointestinal and respiratory tract infections and is the antibiotic of choice in treating *Pneumocystis carinii* pneumonia, for which there is a failure rate of 5-20%; TMP-SMX is relatively non-toxic in non-immunocompromised patients, although it has been reported that 60% of those with AIDS have adverse side effects, including elevated liver function tests, neutropenia, thrombocytopenia, erythematous maculo-papular rash, rarely Stevens-Johnson syndrome, exfoliative dermatitis, nausea and vomiting Note: Trimethoprim-dapsone is thought to have fewer side effects of an intensity that would require changing to pentamidine therapy (N Engl J Med 1990; 323:776)

'Trimming' RESEARCH ETHICS A method used in science to 'correct' experimental data, eliminating the high and low values most in excess of the mean in an experimental 'run'; while these values are within the confines of statistical probability, they make the assay look sloppy on paper, and thus are 'trimmed'; trimming has long been considered a form of scientific misrepresentation (C Babbage, *REFLECTIONS ON THE DECLINE OF SCIENCE*, London, 1830); Cf 'Cooking, Fraud in science

Triple airway maneuver EMERGENCY MEDICINE A procedure used to clear the air passages of those with upper airway obstruction, where the mandible is moved forward and rescue breathing is performed through the mouth and the nose

Triple apical pulse CARDIOLOGY A double systolic pulse that is coupled with presystolic distension, an uncommon but characteristic finding by precordial palpation in hypertrophic cardiomyopathy

Triple-blinded study CLINICAL THERAPEUTICS A study in which the patients and researchers are unaware of whether a treatment (experimental drug) or placebo is being administered (ie 'double-blinded'); in addition, the team analyzing the data is unaware of which group's data they are evaluating, ie from the placebo or treatment arm of the protocol; although triple-blinding ensures that there are no post-trial bias(es) introduced into the study, it is rarely performed in practice; see Blinding, Double blinding

Triple bypass surgery see Coronary arterial bypass graft

Triple helix DNA MOLECULAR BIOLOGY An artificially-produced conformation of DNA that has a third strand of antisense DNA, designed to bind at specific oligonucleotide sequences on DNA's double helix; triple helix DNA is of considerable interest experimentally, and has therapeutic potential, given that in a properly designed triple strand, a site otherwise bound by a protein promoter or suppressor can be blocked and the corresponding gene either turned on or off; see Antisense DNA and RNA; Cf Achilles heel cleavage

Triple helix protein A polyprotein with a quaternary structural motif composed of three intertwined left-handed α helical proteins, wound in a right-handed helix, a conformation typical of collagen, which owes its strength and resistance to proteolytic digestion to the high number of covalent cross-linking bonds between adjacent tropocollagen molecules

Triple iron agar MICROBIOLOGY (TIA) A nutritionally-rich bacterial growth medium that may be used to direct the initial identification of gram-negative bacteria, especially *Enterobacteriaceae*; a bacterium's growth on TIA and the related KIA (Kligler iron agar), can be used to detect three characteristics of bacteria: The ability to produce gas by the fermentation of sugar, the generation of H_2S, which appears as a black precipitate and the fermentation of sucrose (TIA) or lactose (KIA)

Triple response of Lewis *A TRIAD OF TRANSIENT SKIN CHANGES* seen in immediate hypersensitivity when the skin is firmly stroked by a pointed object, characterized as *1) STROKE OR IMMEDIATE RESPONSE* due to the local release of prostaglandin, histamine, serotonin and bradykinin *2) FLARE* appearing as a red halo, due to vasodilation and *3) WHEAL* in which there is swelling and blanching of the stroke due to histamine release from mast cells, edema of intercellular junctions with protein and fluid accumulation

Triple stones see Struvite concrements

Triplet see Codon

'Triple threat' physician A rare (and claimed by some to be a vanishing) breed of physician who is 1) A world-class researcher or of a caliber sufficient to obtain self-supporting grants 2) A teacher with the skill of Socrates and 3) A clinician with active patient contact; see Professor, Socratic method

Triple X syndrome see XXX syndrome

Triploidy syndrome(s) see XXX and XXY syndromes

Tripod sign NEUROLOGY A nuchal-spinal sign in which the sitting position requires a rigid spine and both arms extended towards the back for support, typically seen in children with non-paralytic poliomyelitis

Triradius DERMATOGLYPHICS A pattern of whorls seen on the palms of children with trisomy 13 and 21, a finding of itself without pathological significance, which serves merely to support the usually obvious diagnosis of these trisomies

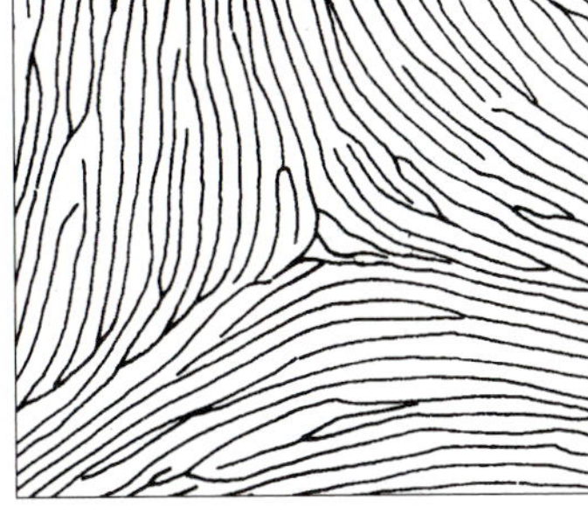

Triradius

Tris Tris(hydroxymethyl) aminomethane A substance used to prepare buffers (tris buffer) for biological systems at a desired physiologic pH range of 7.2 to 9.2

Triskelion see Clathrin

Triton 1) ^{3}H Tritium nucleus, a radionuclide consisting of one proton and two neutrons, which is a weak β-emitter with a physical half-life of 12.26 years 2) A family of proprietary nonionic, surface-active agents

Triton tumor An uncommon peripheral nerve tumor with muscular differentiation that is either benign, usually designated as neuromuscular hamartoma, or malignant; Triton tumors are most common in the head, neck and trunk, with a peak incidence at 35 years of age, often associated with von Recklinghausen's disease; the symptoms are typically neurologic and related to enlarging tumor masses Histopathology Scattered rhabdomyoblasts that may have cross-striations within malignant schwannoma-like stroma (figure, below); desmin and myoglobin may be seen by immunoperoxidase staining; Five-year survival is 12% Note: The name derives from a group of newts (Genus, *Amblystoma*) or small salamanders (Genus, *Triturus*) , trivially known as tritons, in which there is an intimate relation between limb degeneration and innervation, a phenomenon first described by JT Todd in 1823; although the presence of nerves is not an absolute prerequisite for limb regeneration (J Exp Zoo 1959; 140:101), the name triton was retained by pathologists as a tribute to the theory that motor nerves could induce endoneural cell differentiation into muscle cells; the salamanders in turn received their name from Triton, the son of Poseidon and Amphitrite, an inferior sea-deity who had the head and torso of a man and the tail of a dolphin

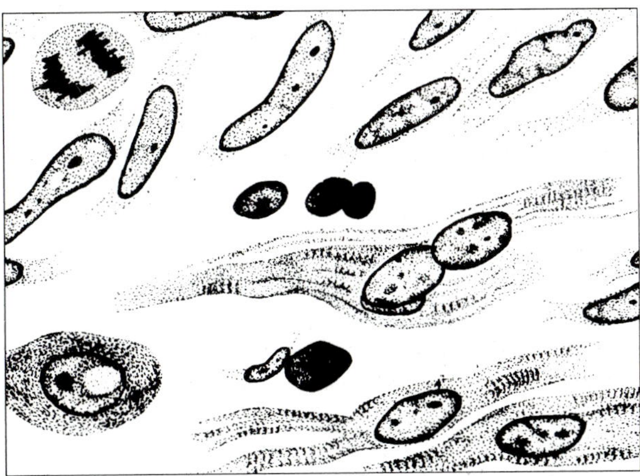

Triton tumor

Triton X-100 A proprietary quaternary ammonium surface-active salt, iso-octyl phenoxy polyethoxy ethanol; in low concentrations, Triton X-100 removes most of the plasma membrane except regions with a hexagonal arrangement; Triton X-100 is used as a surfactant, detergent, wetting agent and emulsifier

Trivial complaint A symptom, sign or lesion, usually identified by the patient, which is regarded as having no impact on the patient's well-being or the management of an unrelated medical condition Note: Given the litigious environment of the practice of medicine in the USA, defensive medicine all investigations of 'trivial complaints' must be documented in writing

Trivial name A popularized, working or common name for a organ, eg Bauchspeicheldrüse, German, pancreas, structure or molecule that is not based on standardized nomenclature or rules delineated by international bodies, eg Enzyme Commission, Nomina Anatomica and the International System

trk An oncogene that was first identified in colonic carcinoma, which encodes the 140 kD Trk protein, which structurally resembles those of tyrosine kinase receptors, probably corresponding to the high molecular weight nerve growth factor receptor; the Trk protein appears to process the intracellular signal after nerve growth factor binds to the extracellular receptor; trk is relatively specific and most prominently expressed on neurons of neural crest origin (Science 1991; 252:554); activation of the trk tyrosine kinase receptor may provide a mechanism for signal transduction by nerve growth factor (Nature 1991; 350:158)

Trojan horse 'effect' Any disastrous result of an anticipated gain; or, the masking of a dangerous agent within an innocent garb EPIDEMIOLOGY Any unanticipated vector of an organism or potential route of disease transmission, as Hagnaya wreathes as vectors for parasites or used rubber tire casings that provide ideal breeding sites for the northern Asian mosquito, *Aedes albopictus* which is a potential vector for Bunyaviridae and LaCrosse viruses (Science 1990; 250:1738) INFECTIOUS DISEASE HIV-1 causes a 'Trojan horse' type of infection, in which HIV-1 binds to the CD4 receptor, enters the cell and integrates itself into the host genome as a provirus, thus remaining hidden from the immune system, similar to the Trojan horse; upon lysis of the CD4 receptor-positive cells (helper T cells and macrophages), the virus is liberated and HIV-1 either re-enters the circulation or continues infecting other cells via the CD4 receptor

Trojan horse inhibitor LABORATORY METHODOLOGY A molecule that is introduced by affinity labeling into the active site of an enzyme, or other protein, with the purpose of delineating the enzyme's active site , as the 'Trojan horse' molecular mimic prevents the target-protein from performing its usual function

'Trolley car' policy An insurance policy that has multiple restrictive riders and clauses that essentially prevent the insured party from collecting benefits except under the most extraordinary circumstances, ie the policy-holder's being hit by a trolley car

Tropical eosinophilia A clinical complex that predominantly affects the lungs, which occurs in the Near and Far East due to a hypersensitivity response to filarial worms, eg *Brugia malayi* and *Wuchereria bancrofti* Clinical Malaise, wheezing, chronic productive cough with bilateral râles Histopathology The lungs display a polymorphous cell infiltrate, composed of eosinophils, 'round' cells, fibroblasts and eventually fibrosis Treatment Diethylcarba-mazine, Ivermectin

Tropical oils A family of cooking oils derived from palm and coconuttrees that differ from other vegetable oils in that like animal fats, they have a high content of saturated fatty acids and thus are thought to have significant atherogenic potential; see Fish (oil), Olive oil, Trans fatty acids

Tropical spastic paraparesis (TSP) A form of HTLV-I infection causing progressive lower extremity weakness, sparing the upper extremities and mental faculties; TSP occurs in the Caribbean, West Africa, the Seychelles Islands and Colombia and is thought to be identical to the HTLV-I-associated myelopathy described in the Japanese, a form of progressive leg paralysis; some of cases of 'multiple sclerosis' may correspond to TSP; see HTLV-I

Tropical splenomegaly syndrome Big spleen disease An idiopathic splenomegaly affecting malnourished children and adult females in malaria-endemic regions, eg New Guinea and Africa, which is thought to be a defective immune response to *Plasmodium malariae* Clinical Massive splenomegaly, asthenia, fatigue Laboratory Marked increase of IgM antibodies against *Plasmodium vivax*, decreased T-helper cells and CD4:CD8 (helper:suppressor) ratio Treatment Chloroquine

Tropical sprue An idiopathic malabsorption complex, described in the tropics, occurring either in miniepidemics or in Caucasians who have recently arrived to the region; it has been related to either subclinical deficiencies of certain nutrients (protein, folate, vitamin B_{12}, fats and sugars) or an as-yet unidentified pathogen, resulting in diarrhea-induced weakness that favors the overgrowth of coliform bacteria indigenous to the tropics Clinical Malaise, fever, anorexia, intermittent diarrhea, chronic malabsorption, which in the epidemic form first affects adults; prolonged malabsorption causes vitamin deficiencies, muscle wasting, muco-cutaneous pigmentation and edema Histopathology Lengthening of the crypts, broadening and shortening of villi, chronic inflammation and non-specific increase in lipids, seen in biopsies of the small intestine Treatment Folic acid, vitamin B_{12} and broad-spectrum antibiotics eg Tetracycline, luminal sulfonamides

Tropocollagen The basic polymeric structural unit of collagen, which is a triple helix of α collagens, which forms larger units of collagen fibrils and fibers

Tropoelastin 68 kD polypeptide composed of nonpolar amino acids

Troponin A 76 kD heterotrimeric minor protein present in the thin filaments of striated muscle, which has the combined functions of binding calcium and tropomyosin, inhibiting actomyosin ATPase and regulating muscle contraction

'Trough' THERAPEUTIC DRUG MONITORING The minimum serum concentration of a drug being administered over a prolonged period that has potential side effects, eg aminoglycoside antibiotics, which have well-known ototoxic and nephrotoxic effects; the trough levels are measured immediately prior to administration of the next dose, the level for which should be above the extrapolated minimum inhibitory concentration of the infecting bacteria, see MBC, MIC, Therapeutic drug monitoring; Cf Peak levels

Trümmerfeldzone Scurvy line A radiolucent band seen in the primary spongiosa of the metaphysis, corresponding to a zone of complete osseous disintegration susceptible to fractures Histopathology Immature fibroblasts, hyalinoid material and hemosiderin-laden macrophages; below this zone is an area completely free of hematopoietic cells, the 'Gerüstmark', composed of connective tissue

Trustworthiness MEDICAL ETHICS A moral principle in which a person both deserves the trust of others and does not violate that trust; trustworthiness is expected of physicians and the trustworthy physician has a duty to fulfil all voluntary commitments and responsibilities of an office or role, eg that of 'healer'; the physician is further expected to neither deceive or cheat another

Truth-telling see Therapeutic privilege

Trypan blue dye exclusion test CELL CULTURE A rapid laboratory test that determines the viability of cultured cells or determines the percent of cell lysis as a measure of cytotoxic activity of a tissue culture supernatant fluid; the trypan blue stain is excluded from cells by active transport and thus blue cells are dead cells

Trypanosomiasis, African The genus *Trypanosoma* causes African sleeping sickness, which cripples both the livestock in the region, and an estimated 50 million people are at risk for this hematogenous parasitemia a) *Trypanosoma brucei rhodesiense* Vector Tsetse fly Location East Africa Clinical Acute febrile syndrome, rapidly progressing to death, b) *T brucei gambiense* Vector Tsetse fly Location West Africa Clinical Chronic with central nervous system depression (sleeping sickness)

Trypanosomiasis, American *T cruzi* (Chagas' disease) Vector Reduviid (kissing) bug Clinical Acute, infants, malaise, fever, hepatosplenomegaly Chronic (or asymptomatic), altered cardiac conduction (the most common cause of congestive heart failure in South America), megaesophagus and megacolon Treatment Melarsoprol, a toxic agent used for end-stage meningoencephalitix disease or O-11 10-(propoxy)decanoic acid), a myristic acid analog that is highly toxic to and specific for trypanosomes (Science 1991; 252:1851)

Tryptophan-associated eosinophilic connective-tissue disease see Eosinophilic-myalgia syndrome

TSI see Triple sugar iron

TSLS see Toxic shock-like syndrome

TSP see Tropical spastic paraparesis

T-strain A mycoplasma that grows 'tiny' colonies (hence, 'T'), which had been assigned into a separate genus, *Ureaplasma* with one species, *U urealyticum*, an organism exclusive to humans that causes nongonococcal urethritis and is capable of metabolizing urea

Tsutsugamushi disease Japanese Tsutsuga, dangeous; mushi, bug see Scrub typhus

TTAPS model The 'nuclear winter' model that was generated by Drs Turco, Toon, Ackerman, Pollack and Sagan, who concluded that the consequences of even a limited nuclear exchange would result in a 'no-win' situation for any belligerent nation; their manuscript, which became known as the 'Blue book' was never published published, as one of the authors felt it had created so much dialog that multiple revisions were incapable of salvaging it in the original form; other authors support the theoretical possibility of the TTAPS model, which has been partially supported by data generated from the burning oil fields in Kuwait; see IPPNW, Nuclear war

t-test see Student's t-test

TTP-HUS A formerly separated combination of thrombotic thrombocytopenic purpura (TTP) and hemolytic-uremic syndrome (HUS), which are polar expressions of the same disease defined by a pentad consisting of features of TTP described by Moschcowitz, ie thrombocytopenia, microangiopathic hemolytic anemia, neurological abnormalities and fever as well as renal disease (J Am Med Assoc 1991; 265:91cr) Clinical Abrupt onset in children following a viral upper respiratory tract infection or may be associated with a verotoxin in *Escherichia coli*-induced gastroenteritis; the hemolytic-uremic component is less common in adults, but may occur in pregnancy, at parturition or during chemotherapy; spontaneously resolving renal failure occurs in 60% (10% progress to chronic renal failure); renal failure may be more common in *Escherichia coli* O157:H7 infections and these organisms were inculpated in 16% of those with HUS (N Engl J Med 1990; 323:1161) Laboratory Reticulocytosis, increased bilirubin and fibrin split products (without disseminated intravascular coagulation), reduced haptoglobin Treatment Most cases resolve spontaneously, others require high dose corticosteroids Note: A higher neutrophil count and/or bloody diarrhea on admission is thought to indicate a poor prognosis

Tuberculid A non-infectious skin lesion due to hypersensitivity to *Mycobacterium* species, divided into papulonecrotic tuberculid, which consists in symmetrical waves of sterile papules with central ulceration and obliterative vasculitis and lichen scrofulosorum, which consists of groups of tiny, sarcoid-like red papules

Tuberculosis A disease of antiquity, which was called the 'King of diseases' in Sanskrit; one million new cases of *Mycobacterium tuberculosis* develop per year worldwide, of which an estimated 10% of those in underdeveloped nations eventually die; 'smear'-positive cases in Africa (165/10^5), are more often clinically inactive than those in Asia where the rate is 110/10^5 US incidence: 9.3 cases/10^5 (white/hispanic 5.7/10^5, black 26.7/10^5, asian 49.6/10^5); in 1984, the previous trend of a decreasing incidence of tuberculosis in the US reversed itself during the mid-1980s, due to increases of *M tuberculosis* and *M avium-intercellulare* in AIDS patients (N Engl J Med 1991; 324:1644) Unique growth characteristics include arylsulfatase positivity in *M cheloni* and growth inhibition by thiophene-2-carboxylic acid hydrazide in *M bovis*; optimal growth temperature 32°C in *M marinum, M ulcerans, M haemophilum* and 42°C in *M xenopi*; all *Mycobacterium* species produce nicotinic acid, *M tuberculosis, M simiae* and *M szulgai* produce the greatest amount; lesser amounts are produced by *M africanum, M bovis, M marinum* and *M chelonei cheloni* and *M chelonei abscessus* Nitrate reduction *M tuberculosis, M kansasii, M szulgai, M flavescens, triviale, M fortuitum, M smegmatis; M szulgai* is a scotochrome at 37°C and photochrome at 25°C Growth media Lowenstein-Jensen, Middlebrook 7H10 Treatment PRIMARY DRUGS Isoniazid, ethambutol, rifampicin, streptomycin SECONDARY DRUGS Ethionamide, capreomycin, kanamycin, cycloserine, pyrazinamide, para-aminosalicylic acid; see MOTT, Runyon classification

Tubular complexes Tubuloreticular structures Intracellular inclusions of undetermined nature and significance, seen by electron microscopy, which consist of 800-1500 x 20-40 nm cytoplasmic masses of twisted, haphazardly arranged, undulating tubules that are contiguous with the cisternae of the adjacent endoplasmic reticulum; these structures are focally positive for acid phosphatase and terminal deoxynucleotidyl transferase (TdT) and occur in lymphocytes and endothelium in AIDS and other viral infections, Chediak-Higashi disease, collagen vascular disease, immunodeficiencies, B- and T-cell lymphoproliferative disorders, melanoma and sarcomas, and can be induced in vitro by a variety of tissue culture toxins; Cf Vesicular rosettes

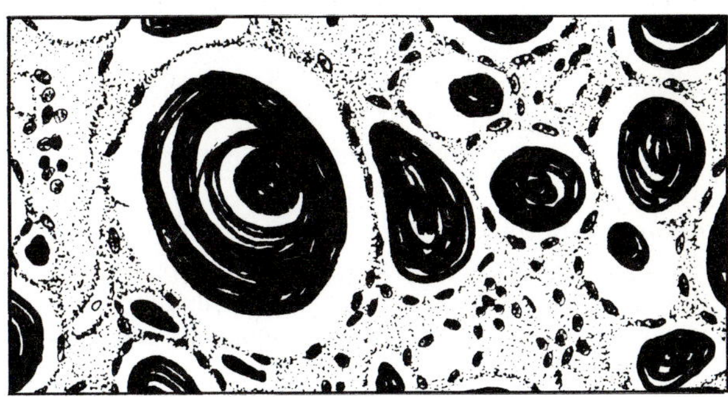

Tubular thyroidization

Tubular 'thyroidization' RENAL PATHOLOGY The filling of the renal tubules, especially the proximal convoluted tubules, with homogenous pale eosinophilic proteinaceous casts (figure, above), an appearance likened to colloid in thyroid acini, and a typical histologic feature of chronic pyelonephritis, less commonly seen in amyloidosis and ischemia; Cf 'Blocked pipe' appearance

Tubulin A heterodimeric protein composed of a 50 kD α and a 50 kD β chain arranged in repeating head-to-tail units, which form microtubules when warmed to 37°C in the presence of GTP; see Cilia, Flagella, MAPs, Microtubules, MTOC

Tufts Tufting SURGICAL PATHOLOGY A histologic finding consisting of microscopic papillary projections that rise from the epithelial lining in serous carcinomas of low malignant potential, which in addition demonstrate nuclear atypia, increased mitotic activity and absence of stromal invasion; see Borderline tumor

Tuftsin Leukocidin A phagocytosis-promoting tetrapeptide (Thr-Lys-Pro-Arg) derived from a leukokinin globulin, which represents residues 289-292 of the immunoglobulin Fc receptor; tuftsin is produced in the spleen and is chemotactic for neutrophils and macrophages, it stimulates phagocytic motility, enhances antigen processing and aids in oxidative metabolism

Tumbling motility MICROBIOLOGY A descriptor for the end-over-end motility characteristic of *Listeria monocytogenes*, when these organisms are incubated in nutrient broth at room temperature; when an inoculum of *L monocytogenes* is 'stabbed' in a test tube filled with semisolid medium, its mobility is restricted and it displays an 'umbrella' pattern of growth; see Umbrella growth

Tumor-associated antigens IMMUNOLOGY ONCOLOGY Molecules such as CA 19-9, CA-125 and CA 195 that may be associated with specific tumors, including lymphoma, carcinoma, sarcoma and melanoma; although the epitopes of these antigens may elicit cellular and/or humoral immune response against the tumor, this response is rarely adequate to defend the host against the tumor; tumor-associated antigens have been subdivided into *CLASS 1 ANTIGENS* Highly specific to a particular tumor and present in one or only a few individuals and not found in normal cells, eg Tumor specific transplantation antigen *CLASS 2 ANTIGENS* Present on a number of related tumors from different patients and *CLASS 3 ANTIGENS* Present on both normal and malignant cells but which are expressed in increased amounts in malignant cells Note: Class 2 antigens are of greatest potential use in developing clinically useful assays since they are present in many tumors and are rarely observed in normal subjects

Tumor doubling time ONCOLOGY A value of clinical interest that allows a relatively accurate prediction of tumor aggressiveness; although tumor doubling is less elegant than evaluating genomic events (recombination, point mutations and gene amplification) in determining tumor aggression, for specific tumor types, it is of prognostic value in determining growth of untreated tumors; tumor doubling times range from 8 to 600 days, depending on the cell and tumor type; see Gompertzian growth

Tumor initiator A carcinogen that interacts directly with a susceptible cell's DNA, evoking the first step in a theoretical two-step carcinogenic cascade, which may then be followed by the action of a tumor promoter

Tumorlet A nodular hyperplasia of spindled cells related to Kulchitsky's neuroendocrine cells, seen in the bronchial wall in patients with bronchiectasia or occasionally associated with carcinoid tumors

Tumor lysis syndrome see Acute tumor lysis syndrome

Tumor markers There is no circulating protein or metabolite that is consistently elevated in, or specific for any malignancy; at best, 'tumor markers' are relatively non-specific and cannot be used as screening tools, but may, under certain circumstances, be used to detect recurrence (through rising serum levels, eg carcinoembryonic antigen, CEA) in patients with known and treated malignancy; in clinical parlance, tumor markers include oncofetal proteins (α-fetoprotein, CEA) and tumor-associated antigens (CA-125, CA 19-9); several highly non-specific circulating molecules have been erroneously called 'tumor markers' including enzymes (CK-BB, acid phosphatase, alkaline phosphatase, galactosyltransferase, LDH, lysozyme, neuron-specific enolase), hormones (bombesin, calcitonin, β-hCG, HPL), metabolites (catecholamines, polyamines and sialic acid), proteins (binding proteins, ferritin and hormone receptors) and others (chromogranin A immunoglobulins, polyanions)

Tumor necrosis factor(s) (TNF) A molecule that mediates shock and tumor-related cachexia, divided into TNF-α and TNF-β; TNF-α (cachexin) is a 17 kD pluripotent protein cytokine produced primarily by monocytes and mast cells (Nature 1990; 346: 274), the 3' end of which has sequence homology with other biological response mediators, including lymphotoxin, IL-1, GM-CSF and interferons; TNF-α production is increased in a broad palette of clinical conditions including inflammation, sepsis, lipid and protein metabolism, hematopoiesis, angiogenesis, collagen vascular disease, terminal chronic heart failure (with activated renin-angiotensin system; N Engl J Med 1990; 323:236), host resistance to viruses and parasites, eg severe falciparum malaria (N Engl J Med 1989; 320:1586), in children dying of severe infectious purpura and in malignancy; corticosteroids inhibit TNF-α biosynthesis **Short-term side effects** Fever, headache and hypotension **Long-term side effects** Cachexia, chills, fatigue, anorexia and thrombocytopenia; in rodents, high TNF levels cause piloerection, diarrhea and a poorly-groomed appearance Note: Endotoxemia is a TNF-induced event with a shock-like clinical picture with interstitial pneumonia, vascular plugging by neutrophils, acute tubular necrosis, gastrointestinal tract, adrenal gland and pancreatic ischemia and hemorrhage **Laboratory** Hemoconcentration, metabolic acidosis, hypoglycemia and hyperkalemia

Tumor necrosis factor receptor A 461 amino acid receptor protein with a cysteine-rich extracellular domain that shares sequence similarity to neural growth factor receptor and to an open reading frame from the Shope fibroma virus (Science 1990; 248:1019)

Tumor promoter Cocarcinogen A substance, often lipid-soluble, that has no intrinsic carcinogenic potential, but which when applied repeatedly, is capable of amplifying the cancer-inducing effects of other substances, ie initiators; the classic tumor promoter is phorbol ester and its derivatives isolated from *Croton flavens*, which is a potent and specific activator of protein kinase C; high-fat diets are 'promotional', eg linoleic acid-rich corn, safflower and sunflower oils are promoters, but olive oil is not; see Antipromoter

Tumor promotion The theoretical second stage in a two- or multi-step carcinogenic sequence, which follows an 'initiation' step and requires that the tumor promoting substance(s) be applied in a repeated or continuous fashion

Tumor seeding The spillage of tumor cells and their subsequent growth into tumor 'colonies'; tumor seeding is often of greater theoretical than actual importance, but has been described in malignant cell spillage from an operative field, and along needle biopsy tracts, as potential complications of diagnostic or therapeutic procedures

Tumor suppressor gene A growth-regulatory gene that encodes a protein capable of suppressing malignant transformation; in most malignancies, multiple steps are necessary before these genes are either inactivated by mutation or lost; the p53 gene on chromosome 17p13 is mutated or inactivated in all histologic types of lung cancer (Science 1989; 246:491); other tumor suppressor genes include RB, DCC, NM23, ras and tyrosine kinase gene on chromosome 3; see DCC gene, One-hit, two-hit model, p53, Promoter, RB gene, TKO selection

Tunnel effect GASTROENTEROLOGY Visualization of only the open end of the stainless steel tube used in rigid sigmoidoscopy, see Sigmoidoscopy

Tunneling The transfer of a particle, eg an electron, across a potential energy barrier without the particle passing the barrier; see Scanning tunneling microscopy

Tunnel vision NEUROLOGY Concentric constriction of the visual fields, which is thought to be secondary to degeneration of the cells of the calcarine cortex, a symptom characteristic of chronic methylmercury poisoning, that may also be accompanied by multiple scotomata, diminished auditory acuity and changes in mental status; another organic cause of tunnel vision occurs in infarction of the sensory relay nuclei of the thalamus with relative sparing of the occipital lobes; see Mercury

'Tunnel vision' PSYCHIATRY A concentric constriction of both visual fields, where the absolute size of the visual fields tends to be the same regardless of the distance from object being viewed, a finding typical of hysterical reactions or hypersuggestibility states,

Turban tumor DERMATOPATHOLOGY A variant form of cylindroma, a sweat gland tumor that arises on the scalp, appearing as a large red-pink, usually hairless tumor with a bosselated surface that has been fancifully likened to a turban, occasionally growing to 50 cm in maximum size Histopathology The tumor cells are arranged in a pattern fancifully likened to a child's jigsaw-puzzle, see 'Jigsaw puzzle' tumor

Turbidity test A test for sickle cell anemia based on the decreased solubility of hemoglobin S in dithionate, which is less accurate than the sodium bisulfate or sickle cell test; see Sickle cell test

Turbidimetry A laboratory technique that semiquantifies a substance in suspension, based on the decrease in forward light transmission by the suspension; Cf Nephelometry

TURP Transurethral resection of the prostate

Tuskeegee study BIOMEDICAL ETHICS A prospective study of 431 black males in Tuskeegee, Alabama with seropositive latent syphilis of greater than three years duration that was begun in 1932 to examine the long-term effects of untreated syphilis; although the study provided information on the ultimate fate of syphilis, ie hypertension and cardiovascular disease were more common than central nervous system disease, the latter affecting 4% of survivors, a figure far lower than previously reported (Arch Int Med 1964; 114:792), a public outcry was raised against nontreatment of a disadvantaged minority solely on the basis of 'scientific curiosity' and the study was stopped in 1972, decades after penicillin had become available; see Unethical medical research

TWAR agent MICROBIOLOGY A fastidious strain of *Chlamydia psittaci* (the name derives from the first two isolates, which had been designated TW-183 and AR-39); TWAR may cause outbreaks of community-acquired pneumonia and is thought to be a relatively common cause of upper and lower respiratory tract infections, as the TWAR antibody occurs in 20-45% of normal adults, it is assumed to be transmitted person-to-person and may be fatal in the elderly Clinical Acute pneumonia in young adults, pharyngitis and laryngitis Treatment Tetracycline

T wave alternans CARDIOLOGY A series of fluctuations in the overall length of the T wave that are consistently increased in a wide variety of conditions, including coronary artery occlusion, hypothermia, Prinzmetal's angina and the long Q-T syndrome; T wave alternans is predictive of the risk for ventricular fibrillation and is preferable to assessing the potential for fibrillation by provocative tests (Science 1991; 252:437)

'Tweedledee and Tweedledum syndrome' see Folie à deux

Tween A generic term for a proprietary family of non-ionic detergents consisting of fatty acid esters of polyoxyethylene sorbitan

'Twentieth-century disease' see Environmental hypersensitivity

Twenty nail dystrophy A very rare disease of the finger- and toenails characterized by longitudinal ridging, fragility, notching and opalescent discoloration, associated with spongiosus and keratosis of the adjacent skin or as a variant of lichen planus

'Twigging' ACADEMIA Hyperspecialization in active branches of science as in computers and molecular biology or the fragmentation of specialties and subspecialties of medicine and natural sciences into subspecialties and sub-subspecialties, known as 'twigging', as the specialties themselves are 'branches' of the tree of knowledge

Twilight sleep A dream-like state of 'conscious sedation' induced by Versed, a drug that allows patients to undergo minimally invasive surgical procedures, eg colonoscopy or minor oral procedures, to be performed without subjecting a patient to general anesthesia, the agent recently associated by with a number of sudden deaths, possibly relateds to 'overshooting' of the therapeutic levels, and causing the patients to lapse into unconsciousness

'Twilight zone' MOLECULAR BIOLOGY A 'gray zone' that exists when base pairs of different DNA molecules, or amino acids from different proteins are compared to determine the degree of sequence similarity ('homology'); in the 'twilight zone', it cannot be said with certainty whether the molecules being compared are or are not related; the zone is broad and is a function of the length of the molecules being compared; molecules that share less than 5 to 10% of nucleotides or amino acids are usually regarded as devoid of sequence similarity, while a similarity of greater than 20 to 25% implies conservation of genomic motifs, among (seemingly unrelated) organisms, ie evolutionary homology, or conservation of structural motifs in proteins; the higher the number of matches between nucleotides in the DNA or amino acids in the proteins being compared, the greater is the likelihood that the sequences being compared are related; a 'match' of greater than 50% virtually confirms a relationship between two or more molecules and match of 80% or more percent are regarded as 'highly conserved'

Twin One of two gestational products that develop during a single intrauterine gestational period; monozygotic twins reared apart (MZA) are remarkably similar in temperament, personality, occupation, leisure-time interests and social attitutes; MZAs are as similar to each other as those reared together and these similarities are attributed to genetics on IQ, as the constraints in Western society are relatively loose and do not prevent the development of individual traits; the similarity of psychological traits due to their identical genomes make their effective environments similar (Science 1990; 250:233); see Higher multiples; Cf Siamese twins

'Twinkie® defense' FORENSIC PSYCHIATRY A legal tack that was used by the defense and supported by the defendant's psychiatric experts in the trial of a San Francisco supervisor, who in 1979 allegedly killed Mayor G Moscone and Harvey Milk; the contention was that the emotionally-strained defendant became unbalanced by eating 'junk food', citing the consumption of various carbohydrate-rich food products, including doughnuts, candy bars, soft drinks and a proprietary snack cake (Twinkies®) for his irrational behavior; the ploy reduced the defendant's conviction from that of first-degree murder to voluntary manslaughter, which carries a lesser sentence; see Television intoxication syndrome

'Twinkling star' sign A fanciful descriptor for the short linear radiations that extend from pulmonary vessels that parallel the long axis of the body on computed tomographic scans, most prominently seen at a 100-200HU window width; 'twinkling stars' help distinguish normal vessels from tumor masses that may have the same tomographic density

Twinning ORAL PATHOLOGY A dental malformation characterized by the adjoining of two teeth, most often seen in the mandibular incisors of the primary dentition, due to the processes of germination, fusion or concrescence

Twin-to-twin transfusion syndrome OBSTETRICS Intrauterine growth retardation in one twin due to an artery-to-artery vascular shunting, which may occur in a diamnionic-dichorionic placenta and be accompanied by hydramnios; the 'donor' twin is anemic, pale, lighter and smaller with organ hypoplasia; the recipient twin is plethoric, polycythemic and macrosomic

Twisting number MOLECULAR BIOLOGY A value that corresponds to the 'pitch' of the DNA molecule, or the number (T) of turns in its double helix, which is added to the writhe number (W) to yield a linking number (L); see Superhelicity

Two-dimensional echocardiography A technique for identifying end-diastolic intraventricular dimensions, septal and free wall thicknesses and depressed ventricular function

Two-dimensional gel electrophoresis LABORATORY TECHNOLOGY technique for characterizing a protein; in the firstdimension', a protein is separated according to charge by isoelectric focusing, in which a solution containing protein(s) that has not been denatured is placed in a gradient of pH and subjected to an electric charge, whereupon the protein migrates to the pH at which its total surface charge is neutral; the second dimension consists in rotating the gel 90°, layering it on a SDS-soaked gel and then electrophoretically separating the proteins based on size; the resulting pattern or 'fingerprint' is highly specific and constant

Two foot-one hand syndrome A clinical form of tinea pedis with diffuse, dry scaling and mild erythema of the plantar surface, extending to the sides of the feet, in a moccasin-like pattern, associated with dry scaling of one palm, an association of uncertain significance

Two-hit hypothesis see One-hit, two-hit model

Two-tiered billing HEALTH CARE INDUSTRY The charging of a larger fee for the same service, when the fee is expected to be paid by a 'third party' insurance carrier or by the settlement in a litigation; two-tiered billing is illegal in the US

Two-tiered system SOCIAL MEDICINE The existence of two levels of benefits and care, depending on whether the patient can afford to pay or not, an unfortunate reality that exists in the 'free market' form of medical reimbursement that is practiced in the US

Ty gene A retrotransposon; 'retro', ie like a retrovirus, it can reproduce itself via an RNA intermediary, using the enzyme reverse transcriptase; 'transposon', ie a piece of DNA that can insert itself in many different sites in a host genome

Tylectomy A dignified synonym for lumpectomy, see there

Tylosis An autosomal dominant condition characterized by palmo-plantar hyperkeratosis associated with oral leukoplakia and carcinoma of the lower third of the esophagus

Tympanostomy tube OTORHINOLARYNGOLOGY A small metal tube or grommet inserted in the tympanic membrane of patients (often young children) with recurring, antibiotic refractory otitis media; while the ventilating tube is in place, there is a significant decrease in episodes of otitis media; once removed, the surgically-treated ear has worse auditory discrimination, more otitis, tympanosclerosis, retraction and atrophy (Pediatr Infect Dis J 1991; 10:2)

Tyndall effect DERMATOLOGY The change that light undergoes as it passes through a turbid medium, eg skin, causing the colors of the spectrum to scatter; those colors with the longer wavelength (red, orange and yellow) tend to continue travelling forward while those with the shorter wavelength (blue, indigo and violet) scatter to the side and backward; thus explaining why a subcutaneous lesion that should have a red-brown hue due to hemorrhage or melanin deposition, has a blue tinge

Type A simple way of classifying practically anything is to divide it into two (or more) 'types'; in general, typing keeps the number of subgroups to a minimum, while satisfying those with obsessive-compulsive neuroses who are driven to classify diseases, objects, people and mechanisms; see Splitting, Twigging

Type I error α error STATISTICS Rejection of the null hypothesis when it is correct, or the error of falsely stating that two proportions are significantly different when they are the same; type I errors may occur when a sample is too small for true statistical power; the probability of such an error occurring is a value, designated α, set by the investigator, usually at .05; if the two proportions are significantly different, regardless of whether positive or negative, the α value is nondirectional or 'two-tailed', designated as $\alpha2$; a difference displayed in one direction, or one-tailed test is designated as $\alpha1$

Type II error β error STATISTICS Acceptance of the null hypothesis when it is incorrect, or the error of falsely stating that two proportions are not significantly different when they actually are; type II errors may occur when conclusions are based on the study of a small number of outcome events, ie misleading due to lack of statistical power; the probability of this occurring is designated as β and it is always unidirectional

Type A personality A relatively distinctive set of character traits (J Am Med Assoc 1959; 169:1286; ibid, 252:1385) that are commonly observed in individuals who are aggressive, hard-driving, 'work-aholics'; although 'type As' have been traditionally regarded as being at an increased risk for cardiovascular morbidity; it has been more recently postulated that a second component is required to place these people at risk for cardiovascular disease, which consists of of repressed hostilities towards others or hopelessly frustrating situations, inducing induce a 'toxic core' nidus, increasing the susceptibility for heart disease in type A persons; see 'Toxic core'

Type B ('C' and 'D') personality A characteristic set of personality traits described in individuals who tend to be relaxed and inclined to do things 'manana'); the simplistic Type A and B classification has critics who would add a cancer-prone type C personality and an anxiety and immunosuppression-prone type D personality

Type and screen TRANSFUSION MEDICINE A protocol that consists of determining the ABO and Rh of the red cells, (major crossmatch) and screening the serum for the presence of potentially hemolyzing antibodies; it is performed by using 'reagent' red cells, which have major blood group surface antigens; many transfusion services have a 'type and screen' policy for surgical procedures that are unlikely to require a transfusion Note: According to the AABB standards, the type and screen should be repeated every two days in pregnancy and if the subject has received any blood products or immunizing products within the last three months, given the potential for rapid formation of potentially harmful antibodies; see Cross-match, Immediate spin cross-match

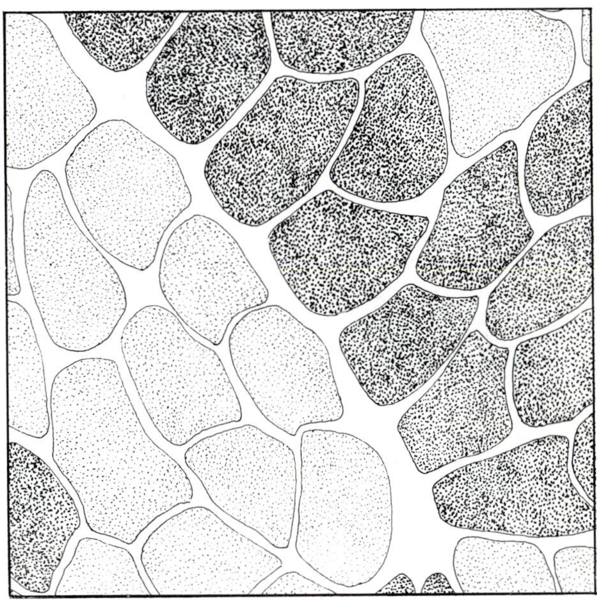

↑ Type grouping   Normal muscle ↓

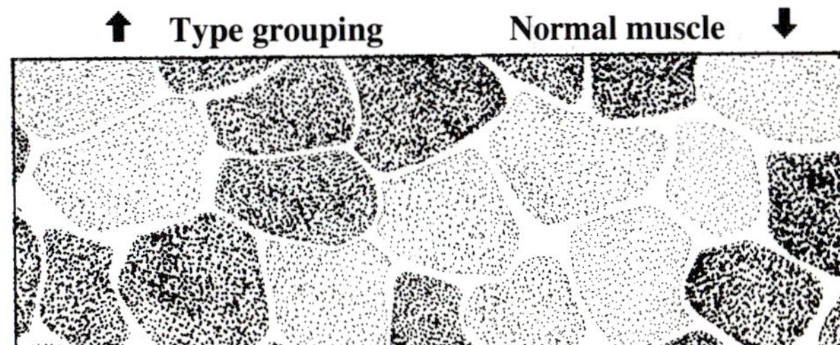

Type grouping A descriptor for the histopathologic changes in muscles affected by neurogenic atrophy, where the normal mosaic interspersion of light and dark (type I and II) muscle fibers (figure, above) is transformed into large fascicles of light or dark fibers with similar histochemistry (figure, above), due to limited reinnervation due to ingrowth of collateral sprouts from undamaged healthy axons; type grouping also refers to the presence of two populations of muscle cells: one atrophic and another relatively well-preserved and/or hyperplastic

'Typhoid Mary' A colloquial term for any person who is a carrier for a virulent strain of bacteria, eg salmonella or diphtheria or virus, eg hepatitis or HIV-1; Typhoid Mary Mallon (1870-1938), the 'most dangerous woman in America' was an itinerant cook and asymptomatic carrier of a highly virulent strain of *Salmonella typhi*;

she was held to be responsible for countless deaths in more than a dozen outbreaks of typhoid fever, one of which was the epidemic of Ithaca (1400 cases); she was temporarily quarantined in New York City (1906-1910), and released when she promised authorities she would find another occupation; when the epidemic in 1915 at Sloan Hospital for Women was traced to her, officials permanently retired her pots to Brother Island until her death; see High disseminator

Typhoid nodule A lesion seen in systemic dissemination of *Salmonella typhi*, classically located in the liver, which corresponds to scattered foci of trabecular necrosis with parenchymal replacement by phagocytosing mononuclear cell aggregates

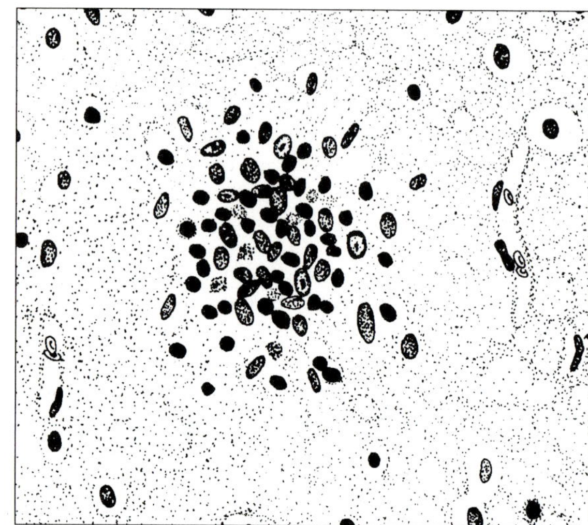

Typhus nodule

Typhus nodule A lesion of small blood vessels of the cerebral gray matter seen in Rocky mountain spotted fever, characterized by focal microglial proliferation, admixed with leukocytes (figure, above)

Tyramine hypertension Cheese disease A complication of monoamine oxidase inhibiting drugs (IMAO) that are used to treat depression and panic disorders; IMAO inhibits the metabolism of tyramines and catecholamines and ingestion of tyramine-rich food and/or beverages, eg Chianti wine, cheddar cheese, naturally fermented beer, chicken liver or drugs, eg ephedrine and amphetamines) evokes an acute hypertensive crisis due to the release of tissue catecholamines, which may be accompanied by sweating, tachycardia or arrhythmia

Tyrosine kinase receptor (TKR) A family of receptors that phosphorylate tyrosine residues of proteins, leading to various cell responses; TKRs may be integral transmembrane receptors, constituting a signal recognition site for growth factors, eg epidermal growth factor or platelet-derived growth factor, thereby regulating cellular proliferation and differentiation; TRKs may also be intracytoplasmic, including Abl, Fps and Src, the protein products of proto-oncogenes (Science 1991; 252:668)

Tyrosine phosphatase(s) A family of down-regulatory enzymes that have an inverse relation to the growth-promoting tyrosine kinases, acting to remove phosphates from tyrosine residues; tyrosine phosphatase closely resembles CD45, also known as leukocyte common antigen (Science 1991; 251:744)

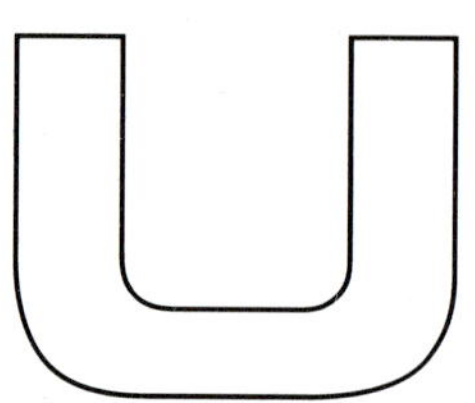

U Symbol for: International Unit of enzyme activity; uranium; uracil; uranium; uridine

u Symbol for: Atomic mass unit

U1-U6 A group of uridine-rich small nuclear ribonucleoproteins that has an essential role in processing pre-messenger RNA, splicing out the unwanted introns, which is involved in polyadenylation

U antigen TRANSFUSION MEDICINE A rare antigen of the MNSs red blood cell antigen group present on the erythrocytes of less than 1% of blacks and never in caucasians, which requires membrane sialoglycoproteins, glycophorin A and glycophorin B; in the absence of a U antigen, the s antigen is not expressed

UAS see Upstream activating sequence

Ubiquinone (CoQ) A protein that acts as a hydrogen carrier, which is intimately linked to the intramitochondrial electron transport cascade; the oxidized form, quinone accepts a single electron, forming semiquinone; acceptance of a second electron and two protons forms the fully reduced dihydroubiquinone

Ubiquitin A ubiquitous and highly conserved 7 kD protein found either free in the circulation or bound (through its -COOH terminal glycine residue) to various cytoplasmic, nuclear or integral membrane proteins, linked by isopeptide bonds to multiple lysine residues; ubiquitin attaches to the target protein as a multiubiquitin chain and 'tags' proteins for degradation (Science 1989; 243:1576); see Cyclin

'U-boat lesion' A fanciful synonym for an abdominal

aortic aneurysm which, like the Unterseeboot, is silent, deep, detected by reflecting sound waves, ie sonar or ultrasound and must be neutralized before it proves fatal (J Am Med Assoc 1987; 258:1732c); see Einstein sign

UCTS Undifferentiated connective tissue disease An early stage of collagen vascular disease in which the predominant organ of involvement or clinical form has yet to manifest itself; Cf Overlap syndrome, Palindromic rheumatism

UGH syndrome see PUGH 'syndrome'

'Ugly' A colloquial adjective for an aggressive disease or lesion INFECTIOUS DISEASE An 'ugly' infection is one that responds poorly to aggressive antibiotic therapy, most commonly seen in immunocompromised patients or those with terminal cancer ONCOLOGY An 'ugly' malignancy is characterized by fulminant deterioration, multiorgan failure, infection and poor response to therapy SURGICAL PATHOLOGY 'Ugly' usually refers to a malignancy with bizarre, poorly differentiated cells with marked nuclear atypia, pleomorphism and florid mitotic activity, eg giant cell tumor of the lung; the lineage of 'ugly' cells is often unclear, and may require the use of ancillary studies, eg special stains including immunoperoxidase staining for the presence of various intermediate filaments or molecular studies; 'ugly' tumors may be so anaplastic that even these studies do not elucidate the tumor's cell of origin

UIP see Usual interstitial pneumonia

Ulcer-carcinoma sequence see Stump carcinoma

Ulnar tunnel syndrome(s) A group of clinical complexes caused by ulnar nerve compression, most often due to a ganglion 'cyst', but which may also be occupation- or hobby-related or due to laceration, arteritis, fractures and inflammation Clinical Symptoms differ according to the site of nerve compression, and display varying degrees of motor defects and sensory loss of the medial aspect of the hand Treatment Physical therapy, occasionally surgery

Ultimate carcinogen A hypothetical molecule that reacts with DNA, causing the final step in the carcinogenic process; this agent is postulated to have an electrophilic component, eg a free radical, epoxide or carbonium ion, which reacts with susceptible electron-rich sites in theDNA; Cf Tumor initiator, Tumor promoter

Ultracentrifugation RESEARCH The spinning of cells, organelles and various molecules at high speeds (up to 60 000 rpm) with high gravitational force (up to 500 000 g), which allows separation of cell components, as in rate-zonal (differential velocity) centrifugation, in which the gravitational force is increased in a stepped fashion to allow removal of desired components; after filtration of a homogenate of tissue or cells from a culture medium, the sample is spun at 600 g for 10 minutes, which 'sediments' the nuclei; the fluid is then re-spun at 15 000 g for 5 minutes, which sediments cell organelles (mitochondria, lysosomes, peroxisomes); the fluid is then re-spun at 100 000 g for 1 hour, which sediments the plasma membrane, microsomal fraction, fragments of the endoplasmic reticulum and large polyribosomes; the fluid is re-spun at 300 000 g for 2 hours, which sediments the ribosomal subunits and small polyribosomes; the remaining fluid contains the soluble portion of the cytoplasm, the cytosol, which may be morphologically analyzed by the 'quick-freeze technique'; subcellular particles and molecules can also be separated by 'layering' the sample on a sucrose gradient, applying ultracentrifugation, then removing the desired 'zone' by pipette; ultracentrifugation also separates DNA fragments, as in equilibrium centrifugation; the DNA, RNA or proteins are radioactively labelled with either a lighter (eg ^{3}H) or a heavier (^{14}C) isotope, allowing the molecules to separate according to density; the sample may be then mixed with cesium chloride, which when combined with the molecules of interest, establishes a slight density gradient, allowing the molecules to migrate to a particular density equivalent; upon removal of the labeled molecules, a radioassay or electrophoretic gel pattern can be used to identify the fractions

Ultrasonography An imaging modality that generates diagnostic images based on the differences in the acoustic impedance of various tissues; electricity applied to a piezoelectric crystal or ceramic in the transducer, causes high-frequency (2.25-5.0 MHz/s) mechanical vibration, which emits ultrasound in the form of 'pressure waves'; these waves are transferred into tissues and organs, and at each tissue interface, a portion of the ultrasound wave is reflected, generating echoes; as the echoes return, there is a slight distortion or deformity of a piezoelectric crystal in the transducer, producing minute voltage pulses, which are then amplified and displayed in one of several 'modes' (the transducer is used to both generate the ultrasound beam and detect the returning echo; the number of pulses that may be generated in a second or pulse repetition frequency is inversely related to the tissue depth); the amplitude of the signal is recorded in scales of gray, where the whitest shades reflect the strongest signal, B-mode ultrasonography yields two-dimensional tissue 'slices' that are produced using different types of transducers, capable of scanning sequentially across a limited region or finite space Types **A-MODE DISPLAY ULTRASONOGRAPHY** An ultrasonographic modality that provides simple displays that are plotted as a series of peaks, the height of which represents the depth of the echoing structure from the transducer **B-MODE DISPLAY ULTRASONOGRAPHY** Brightness-modulated display An ultrasonographic modality with a wide range of applications including imaging of the fetus, kidneys, liver, gallbladder, uterus, cardiovascular structures, breast, prostate, in screening for early ovarian cancer (Br Med J 1989; 299:1363), in evaluating liver transplant recipients both preoperatively (a narrow or thrombosed portal vein precludes transplant) and postoperatively (used to assess various complications—rejection, infection thrombosis and patency of biliary tracts (Mayo Clin Proc 1990; 65:360) and identifying gall bladder calculi Note: The most common clinical use of B-mode ultrasonography is to evaluate fetal status, providing real-time two-dimensional evaluation of the fetus, presenting the images in rapid succession, likened to a motion picture; the 'biophysical profile' has a B-mode display, and measures the head (cephalometry), thorax, abdomen, estimates fetal maturation and identifies growth retardation and major congenital anomalies, including anencephaly, hydrocephaly, meningocele, congenital heart disease, dextrocardia, fetal tumors, diaphragmatic hernia, gastroschisis, omphalocele, polycystic kidneys, hydrops fetalis, gastrointestinal obstruction and death; B-mode helps localize the amniocentesis needle and is of use in identifying placental anomalies including hydatidiform mole or anomalous implantation, eg placenta previa Side effects of ultrasonography are minimal as the energy levels for diagnostic imaging are regarded as being too low to produce tissue destruction; leukocytes subjected to ultrasound demonstrate chromosomal defects, a finding of unknown clinical relevance **DUPLEX ULTRASONOGRAPHY** An ultrasonographic modality that combines the standard real-time B-mode display with pulsed Doppler signals, allowing analysis of frequency shifts in an ultrasonographic signal, reflecting motion within a tissue, eg blood flow and is thus useful in evaluating atherosclerosis of the carotid arteries, arteriovenous malformations and circulatory disturbances in the neonatal brain **M-MODE DISPLAY ULTRASONOGRAPHY** Time-motion display A modality in which the echo signal is recorded on a continuously moving strip of paper, with the transducer held in a fixed position over the aortic or mitral valves; each dot represents a moving structure has a sinewy path, while stationary structures are represented as straight lines; M-mode was the first display used and continues to be useful for precise timing of cardiac valve opening and correlating valve motion with EKG, phonocardiography and Doppler echocardiography (J Am Med Assoc 1991; 265:1155)

Ultrasonography angiographic catheterization A technique that uses a unique probe (1 mm diameter, 20-30 MHz energy emission versus the 10 cm diameter probe operating at 5 MHz used for fetal ultrasonography) to analyze the intensity of atherosclerotic plaque deposition (J Am Med Assoc 1990; 264:2046n)

Ultrastructure(s) Those organelles, structures, eg membranes, microtubules, microfilaments and molecules that are beyond the resolution of light microscopy; ultrastructural studies include scanning electron microscopy, of use for studying the surfaces of membranes and cells (magnifications of 2000x to 20 000x), transmission electron microscopy (resolution of structures from 2000x to 150 000x) and scanning tunnel electron microscopy, which has a magnification ceiling of up to 2 million x); see Electron microscopy, Microscopy

Ultraviolet radiation The segment of the electromagnetic spectrum lying between 200 and 400 nm, including photons emitted during electronic transition states; UV-C (200-290 nm) is damaging to DNA and amino acids, but is blocked by the stratospheric ozone layer, UV-B (290-320 nm) is partially blocked by the ozone layer; UV-A (320 to 400 nm) is the least dangerous but may be hazardous with photosensitizing medications (tetracyclines, thiazides), lupus erythematosus and light sensitivity disorders; UV-A suppresses delayed cutaneous hypersensitivity, causes photoaging and reduces serum carotenoid by 30%; the accelerating depletion of the stratospheric ozone is implicated in the increasing incidence of cataracts and malignant melanoma, and UV light causes a relative decrease in CD4 or helper T cells and an increase in CD8 (suppressor) T cells; pyrimidine dimer formation is a major consequence of UV light, affecting the DNA chain where adjacent thymine residues are joined by a cyclobutyl linkage; in bacteria and in yeasts, photolyase directly removes the cyclobutyl linkage in the presence of visible light (photoreactivation); in higher eukaryotes, UV light-induced damage to DNA is repaired by a helicase-like enzyme; UV light may also damage the less-sensitive purines, causing spontaneous depurination, leaving a bare deoxyribose residue in the DNA (apurinic sites); repair of UV light-induced DNA damage is defective in some 'chromosomal breakage syndromes', eg in xeroderma pigmentosa and Bloom syndrome Note: The mutational effect of UV light is not due to direct DNA damage, but rather occurs during the error-prone process of DNA repair; see CFCs, Greenhouse effect, Ozone layer, SOS repair, SPF rating Note: UVB considered by some workers to be a thousand-fold more carcinogenic than UVA; UVA increases free radical production, causing cell membrane damage and cross-linking of dermal proteins

Ulysses syndrome A complication of false positive patient tests that is responsible for a complete and aggressive diagnostic work-up to elucidate the nature of what is, in actual fact, a non-disease, before the patient is allowed to return to his original state of health (Can Med Assoc Journal 1973; 106:122) Ulysses, who fought in the Trojan war, required 20 years for the return leg of the journey, and all of the harrowing detours were probably unnecessary; various events may initiate a Ulysses syndrome or 'sequence', including *1) MISCHIEVOUS (UNNECESSARY) INVESTIGATION* That which is motivated by mass screening, eg 'blanket coverage' to pay for testing by an insurance company, house-staff 'overkill' to avoid criticism, laboratory request forms bearing the laboratory's entire menu *2) UNCRITICAL EXAMINATION* Lack of familiarity with a body region may mislead the examiner, especially if he encounters trivial anatomic variations of normal structures *3) SERPENTINO 'COMPLEX'* Two snakes consuming each other tail first A neurotic patient may succeed in making himself ill when there is unexpected interest in an otherwise trivial complaint *4) INVERTED SERENDIPITY* While Marie Curie's serendipitous dropping of a key on a pile of photographic film near radium was the founding event of radiology, 'discoveries' made while using an unfamiliar technique are usually 'red herrings' *5) NON-INVESTIGATIONAL INVESTIGATION* When a laboratory request form has a new test on it, the new box is checked off with disproportionate frequency Note: A review of statistical principles in laboratory medicine makes it surprising that the Ulysses syndrome doesn't occur with greater frequency, since results of certain laboratory tests are placed on a standard Gaussian curve of distribution and any value greater than two standard deviations (SD) above or below a mean is considered statistically abnormal (not biologically abnormal); this verification process is a function of daily fluctuations of machinery and other non-disease factors; thus 5%, ie, one in twenty of any normal population will be greater than two SD from the mean of a value, and therefore, abnormal; one in four hundred normal subjects will be statistically abnormal in two tests and so on

Umber codon UGA One of the three 'stop' codons that terminates protein production; an umber mutation is one in which a point mutation on DNA results in a nucleotide triplet ACT that is transcribed into a UGA stop codon

Umbrella CARDIOVASCULAR SURGERY The Mobin-Uddin umbrella was a stainless steel sieve placed intravenously below the renal arteries via the jugular vein that was designed to trap deep vein thrombi in the inferior vena cava; the device is of historic interest as it induced inferior vena cava thrombosis in 70% of cases, which occasionally detached, causing fatal thromboembolism

Umbrella cells CYTOLOGY A fanciful term for the multinucleated superficial cells of the bladder epithelium with vacuolated cytoplasm, which are thin but cover multiple underlying transitional cells in a parasol-like fashion

Umbrella effect IMMUNOLOGY The masking of low levels of immunoglobulin light chains in early clonal expansions of IgM macroglobulinemia and IgA myeloma, by the greater bulk of IgG, as seen in immunoelectrophoresis; this masking effect can be resolved by using immunofixation electrophoresis, which uses specific fluorescently-tagged anti-immunoglobulins

Umbrella growth pattern MICROBIOLOGY The characteristic growth pattern (figure, right) seen when *Listeria monocytogenes* is 'stab'-inoculated at 25°C in a tube filled with semisolid culture medium, fulfilling the organism's microaerophilic growth require-ment, displaying a 'head-over-heels' or tumbling pattern motility

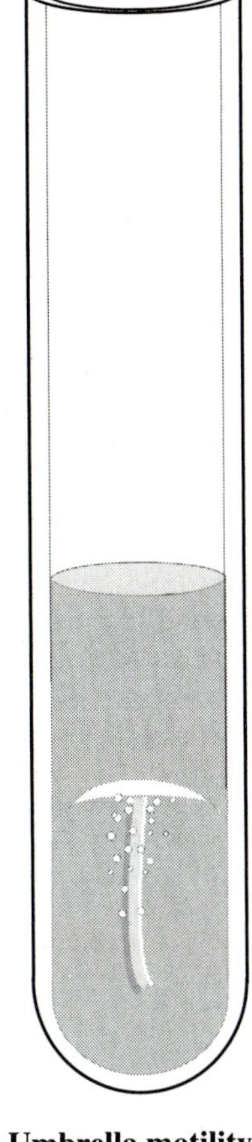

Umbrella motility

Unassigned reading frames see URFs

'Unbundling' HEALTH CARE INDUSTRY Separation of a group of health care services that are usually billed as one fee into separate components, resulting in a higher overall fee for those services, eg the 'unbundling' of a total abdominal hysterectomy and bilateral salpingo-oophorectomy with scar removal and the repair of a hernial sac into three separately-billed procedures

Uncinate fits NEUROLOGY Partial epileptic seizures that may begin with a patient's perception of an unpleasant odor, later generalizing into a clonic or tonic-clonic seizure, often the first manifestation of a temporal lobe tumor

Uncitedness index SCIENTIFIC JOURNALISM A measure of a manuscript's relative 'unworthiness'; if a publication in science is referred to in the bibliography of any subsequent publication, it has been 'cited', thus inferring that the first paper was thought to be of some merit and provide new information; 'uncitedness' implies that a paper was not considered important enough to be referred to by subsequent authors (and possibly had no merit in the first place); according to data collected by the Institute for Scientific Information, less than 20% of publications in physics are uncited, while 90% of papers in political science are uncited, with medicine and biological sciences falling between these extremes (Science 1991; 251:25); see Citation impact, CV-weighing

Unclear disease picture see Fehldiagnose

Uncoded amino acid An amino acid for which there is no codon; such amino acids arise from post-translational modification of an amino acid after it has been incorporated into a polypeptide chain, eg proline yielding hydroxyproline or lysine giving rise to hydroxylysine

Uncombable hair syndrome A condition characterized by the growth of scalp hair in directional 'anarchy', which may be idiopathic or associated with ectodermal dysplasia, progressive alopecia, atopic eczema, dental dysplasia and ichthyosis vulgaris Histopathology The hair shaft displays unilateral longitudinal canalicular depression (Arch Pathol Lab Med 1987; 111:754); see Kinky hair syndrome, Woolly hair syndrome

Uncompensated care Medical treatment of a patient provided in the US by a physician or other health care professional that is not paid by the patient, the government or an insurance carrier, divided into charity care, bad debt and discounted Medicaid care (J Am Med Assoc 1991; 265:2982); see Medicaid, 'Service' patient; Cf Pro bono

Unconventional cancer therapy see Unproven therapies for cancer

Unconventional 'virus' A group of infectious agents, formerly thought to be a type of slow virus, now known as prions, a small infectious particle, consisting entirely of subverted cell protein; prions cause degenerative encephalopathies in sheep and goats (scapie), cows (bovine spongiform encephalopathy) and humans (kuru and Creutzfeldt-Jakob disease); see Kuru, Prions, Slow viruses

Uncoupling PHYSIOLOGY 1) The separation of a metabolic process, eg the uncoupling of oxidative phosphorylation, so that one or more components, eg ATP synthesis, is dissociated from the electron transport chain at one or more phosphorylation sites in mitochondria 2) The separation of activities in receptor-ligand interactions, such that a ligand may bind its cognate receptor, but does not activate the usually coupled receptor

Undercall Underread A noun and a verb for an error in which a benign diagnosis was rendered on what ultimately proves to be a malignant lesion; misinterpretation of this nature may occur at any stage of patient evaluation by the clinician, from the time of physical examination for a mass or complaint to an endpoint of imaging analysis by the radiologist and histological examination by the surgical pathologist Note: There is a tendency to use 'undercall' for errors made in the early stages of patient evaluation, and 'underread' for errors made in the later stages of evaluation, since the radiologist and pathologist are trained in pattern recognition and must interpret or 'read' a pattern; see Misadventure, Overread

'Under general' A colloquial adverb for a surgical procedure performed under general anesthesia

Undergraduate education Background: In the USA, a four-year (or more) college or university education leading to a bacchalaureate degree is the minimum educational level required for admission to medical school; undergraduate medical education refers to the four years of medical school; graduate medical education refers to formal training programs, eg internship, residency and fellowship that follow completion of medical school, which are multiples of one year in duration and sponsored by teaching hospitals, many of which are affiliated with a university or medical school hospital; Cf CME (continuing medical education)

'Under local' A colloquial adverb for a surgical procedure performed under local anesthesia

Undifferentiated carcinoma A group that includes anaplastic carcinomas, 'monstrocellular' carcinomas, oat cell and small cell carcinomas, which may arise in the lungs, larynx, bronchus, esophagus, colon, urinary bladder, uterine cervix and salivary glands and lack epithelial differentiation; the epithelial nature may be subjectively inferred by the tumor pattern or confirmed by special studies including immunoperoxidase studies for cytokeratin and epithelial membrane antigen and ultrastructural studies for desmosomes; see Anaplastic carcinoma

Unethical medical research BIOMEDICAL ETHICS The performance of medical experiments on human subjectss against their will or knowledge of therapeutic options; these experiments range from the horrifying Nazi war-crimes including the Dachau hypothermia 'experiments' and other more bizarre quasi-research projects in which many of the participants died, to the withholding of therapy in order to determine the natural course of an infection as in the Tuskegee study of the evolution of untreated syphilis; there are viable arguments both for, but predominantly against the use of such data, not only regarding the ethical issues, but also that much of the data are flawed and the statistical methods inadequate (NY State J Med 1991; 91:54); see Helsinki Declaration, Nuremberg Code of Ethics

'Unhappy gut' Functional colitis A term that was introduced because 'irritable gut' had lost its specificity; 'unhappy gut' refers to dysfunctional gastrointestinal smooth muscle that is not 'in the mood' to function properly, while 'irritable gut' refers to a primarily colonic irritation due to unidentified intraluminal irritants (personal communication, RW McCullum)

Unique DNA Non-repetitive DNA DNA that is known to exist only once in a haploid genome; most structural DNA and introns are thought to be unique DNA sequences; Cf Repetitive DNA, Tandem repeats

Universal ancestor A phylogenetic term for organisms at or below the branching between progenotes (having rudimentary translation machinery) and genotes (modern translation machinery), based on the 'evolutionary clock', by which organisms are classified according to the evolution of the ribosomal RNA molecule; see Urkingdom; Cf Genote, Progenote

Universal code see Degenerate code

Universal donor TRANSFUSION MEDICINE A person with blood group O, whose red cells have neither A nor B antigens on the surface and therefore will not elicit a hemolytic transfusion reaction when the blood is transfused to a person with blood group A, B, AB or O Notes: 1) The production of anti-A, anti-B or anti-A,B antibodies occurs in everyone except those with blood group AB; this phenomenon that is poorly understood, and, being unrelated to previous exposure to specific antigens, is regarded as a 'natural' antibody 2) The term 'universal donor' requires the caveat that it is always preferable to transfuse type-specific blood, ie transfusion of group A blood to a group A recipient, since packed units of group O blood contains plasma with anti-A,B antibody, which may react with the recipient's blood 3) It is critical to note that a group O ('universal donor') may still have other blood group antigens on his red cells that are capable of causing hemolysis; Cf Universal recipient

Universal precautions INFECTIOUS DISEASE The constellation of safeguards for handling materials, tissues and fluids that may contain human pathogens; exposure to blood and body fluids is minimized by using isolation materials and removable and disposible barriers (latex and vinyl gloves, protective eyewear, masks and gowns and 'disposable sharps' containers), whenever there is contact or anticipated contact with hazardous body fluids or tissues that are potentially infected with hepatitis (HBV), human immunodeficiency virus (HIV, see MMWR 1987; 36(suppl 2S)1S-18S), Jakob-Creutzfeldt or any other highly virulent agent; these precautions serve to both protect the health care worker and prevent him from acting as an inadvertent vector for these pathogens; body fluids that require 'universal precautions' include blood (serum and plasma) and all body fluids containing visible blood, as well as maternal milk, semen, vaginal secretions and cerebrospinal, synovial, peritoneal, pleural, pericardial and amniotic fluids Note: Fluids that are thought by some to not require 'precautions' include feces, nasal secretions, saliva, sputum, sweat, urine and vomitus, unless they contain visible blood; the risk of transmission of human immunodeficiency virus and hepatitis B virus from these fluids is thought to be extremely low or nonexistent (Lab Med 1988; 19:667); implementation of 'universal precautions' is estimated to cost at least $\$336 \times 10^6$/year in the US, largely attributed to the increased use of disposable gloves (J Am Med Assoc 1990; 264:2083); universal precautions are reported to be effective in reducing contact with blood and body fluids (J Am Med Assoc 1991; 265:1123); see Precautions, Reverse precautions

Universal recipient TRANSFUSION MEDICINE A person with blood group AB, whose serum has no anti-A, anti-B and therefore can receive any ABO transfusion without suffering a hemolytic transfusion reaction when blood is transfused from a person with blood group A, B, AB or O Notes: 1) Although the term 'universal recipient' was coined in reference to the ABO blood group, such a recipient should ideally also be Rh-positive, ie have the Rh-D antigen (the so-called Rh factor) on the red cells, since the absense thereof, potentially sets the stage for development of a hemolyzing 2) It is critical to note that a group O ('universal recipient') may still have other blood group antigens on his red cells that are capable of causing hemolysis; Cf Universal donor

Unknown primary malignancy see Occult primary malignancy

Unmasking Biochemistry The conversion of a non-reactive site on a protein to a reactive one that is accessible to specific reagents capable of reacting with molecules of interest, eg an enzyme; unmasking reactions include conformational changes or proteolytic removal of a blocking molecule

UNOS United Network for Organ Sharing An organization dedicated to optimizing the use of transplantable organs; according to UNOS statistics, 4000 major organ transplantations are performed annually, while 1500 to 2000 die waiting for organs (J Am Med Assoc 1991; 265:1302); since successful survival of transplanted tissue is a function of the degree of histocompatibility matches, the larger the pool of donor and recipient haplotypes, the better the long-term survival of these organs (N Engl J Med 1988; 318:1289; 1329) ☎ 800.243.6667 (US) ☎ 804.330.8500 (Intl) 3001 Hungary Spring Rd, Richmond, Virginia 23228 USA; see Transplantation

Unpasteurized milk A product reported by self-proclaimed 'health advocates' to have a greater nutritive value than pasteurized cow's milk, which is alleged to reduce the incidence of caries, enhancing resistance to disease and containing beneficial enzymes and antibodies; no significant differences have been substantiated (J Am Med Assoc 1984; 252:2048); unpasteurized milk is associated with bacterial infection by ***Campylobacter jejuni, Salmonella*** species (***S dublin***, uncommon but serious, ***S typhimurium*** and ***S derby***), ***Brucella*** species, ***Escherichia coli***, ***Listeria monocytogenes, Mycobac-terium bovis, M tuberculosis, Corynebacterium pseudotuberculosis, Staphylococcus aureus, Streptococcus*** spp, ***Streptobacillus moniliformis*** and ***Yersinia enterocolitica,*** toxoplasmosis (goat's milk) and tick-born encephalitis (sheep's milk); see Holistic medicine; Cf Milk, White beverages

Unproven cancer therapy ALTERNATIVE MEDICINE A generic term for a wide variety of unorthodox therapeutic modalities of questionable benefit that are offered by some self-proclaimed cancer specialists (who often have no or little formal medical training); in a comparison study at similar stages of terminal malignancy between patients treated with conventional and unproven cancer therapies, those receiving convential therapy had better survival and quality-of-life scores than those receiving an unproven regimen, which consisted in a combination of autogenous immune-enhancing vaccines, bacille Calmette-Guérin (bCG), vegetarian diets and coffee enemas, although the difference does not reach statistical significance (N Engl J Med 1991; 324:1180); at least $4 x 10^9 are spent annually by US citizens on unproven cancer therapies

Unsaturated fatty acid An alkyl chain fatty acid that contains one or more double bonds between carbons; these fatty acids have lower melting points and most are liquid at room temperature; Cf Monounsaturated fatty acids, Polyunsaturated fatty acid

Unwinding protein A protein that binds to the single strands of DNA at the 'Y-fork' during DNA replication, maintaining the strands in an open position, preventing the unwound strands from reannealing before replication is completed; see Okazaki fragments

Uphill reaction BIOCHEMISTRY An endergonic reaction, ie one that requires energy for completion, eg the breaking of high-energy phosphate bonds in in vivo reactions

'Upper GI' A colloquial term for radiocontrast studies of the upper gastrointestinal tract, which allows examination of the esophagus, stomach and duodenum

Upside-down film(s) Wangensteen-Rice technique Radiologic studies that are performed on a child with a suspected imperforate anus, in which plain films are taken with the child's anus in the most superior position, in order to identify the level of atresia (Ann Surg 1930; 92:77)

Upside-down stomach A rare and extreme form of paraesophageal hiatal hernia, in which the entire stomach is within the thoracic cavity, having rotated on the organo-axial axis or cardiopyloric line Clinical Chronic occult blood loss with hypochromic anemia; in infants, recurrent vomiting and distended epigastrium Radiology Globular shadow with an air-fluid level superimposed on the cardiac shadow, seen in a plain chest film Treatment Reduction, gastropexy

'Upstairs-downstairs heart' see Crisscross heart

Upstream MOLECULAR BIOLOGY An adjective for a location or sequence of units that lies behind or previous to a reaction site, which is a function of the molecule or process being studied *PROTEIN* Upstream refers to the sequence of amino acids from the COOH-terminal to the NH_2-terminal *REPLICATION* Upstream refers to a location opposite that of the movement of the replicating fork *TRANSLATION* Upstream refers to a location or sequence of mRNA from the 3' to 5'-end *TRANSCRIPTION* Upstream refers to a location or sequence of DNA on the transcribed strand from the 5' to the 3' end; Cf Downstream

Upstream activating sequence (UAS) An oligonucleotide segment of DNA, located 50 to 300 base pairs in the 5' direction ('upstream') from the promoter site of a gene to be transcribed; the UAS is required for most, if not all transcriptional events and serves as a binding site for transcription factors

Urate milk see Tophus

Uremic frost A clinical finding in severe renal failure of long duration where the concentration of urea is markedly increased in the sweat, causing cutaneous precipitation of crystallized urea

Uremic 'syndromes' Clinical complexes caused by advanced chronic renal failure *UREMIC CARDIOPATHY* Congestive heart failure due to fluid retention by the kidney, which may be accompanied by moderate to severe hypertension *UREMIC NEUROMYOPATHY* Fatigue related to electrolytic imbalance with renal wasting of sodium and calcium, and retention of potassium and phosphate

URF Unassigned reading frame A large segment of DNA present in mitochondrial DNA that has an initiation codon and is not interrupted by stop codons; some URFs are within introns and may be involved in encoding intron-splicing proteins

Urgent care center HEALTH CARE INDUSTRY A (usually) free-standing mini-emergency center that is equipped to manage either non-life-threatening conditions requiring immediate primary care, or conditions that cannot be treated outside of hospital, but which require stabilization prior to being transferred; such facilities are usually staffed by salaried physicians, often have a 'stat' laboratory and on-site radiology equipment and are operated on a for-profit basis

URI Upper respiratory infection

Uric acid 'infarct(s)' Yellowish streaks seen in young children at the tips of the renal papillae, corresponding to normal collections of uric acid crystals

'Urinary ascites' The free flow of urine into the peritoneal cavity, in congenital urethral obstruction

'Urinoma' PEDIATRIC UROLOGY A tumor-like urine-filled cyst seen in the renal capsule of children, which arises secondary to congenital urethral obstruction, in which urine percolates into the subcapsular or perirenal spaces through ruptured calyceal fornices

Urkingdom EVOLUTIONARY BIOLOGY A conceptual 'superkingdom' lying at the root of the divergence between primitive organisms and bacteria from plants and animals (figure, below), in which the mother organism, recently graduated from the primordial ooze had a minimal complement of 'ur' genes essential for all organisms, including those genes encoding ribosomal RNA, ribosomal protein, enzymes and proteins required for DNA replication, DNA transcription and RNA translation; see Progenote

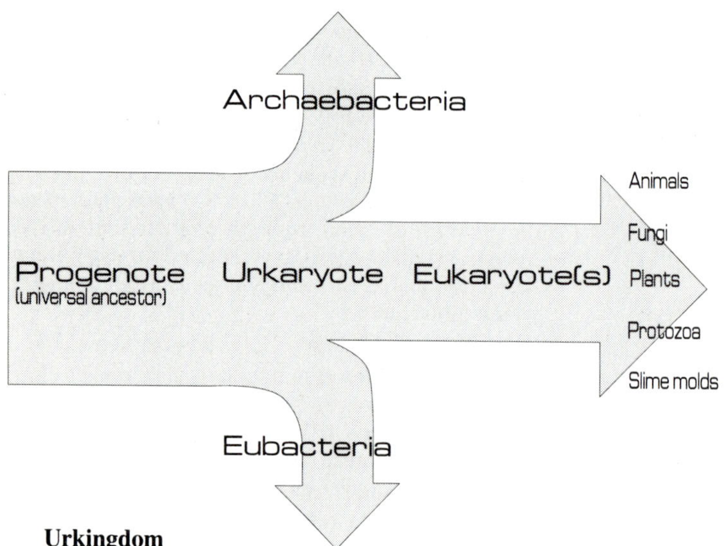

Urkingdom

Urogastrone see Epidermal growth factor

Urokinase A heterodimeric fibrinolytic enzyme composed of a 22 and 33 kD chain that derives from the prourokinase molecule; urokinase is involved in extracellular proteolysis and has increased activity during cell migration or tissue remodeling, cleaving fibronectin; urokinase has a connecting peptide, a kringle domain, a protease domain and a growth factor-like domain at the amino acid terminus, at which point urokinase binds to its receptor; see Kringle domain; Cf Streptokinase, tPA

Uromodulin Tamm-Horsfall protein, uromucoprotein, orosomucoid An 85 kD α_1 acid glycoprotein that is secreted by epithelial cells in Henle's ascending loop and distal convoluted tube; the kidneys produce up to 150 mg/d of protein of which 30-50 mg is uromodulin; it was first isolated from the urine of pregnant women and has potent immunosuppressive properties attributed to the N-linked carbohydrate residues, acting to inhibit antigen-induced T-cell proliferation and monocyte cytotoxicity Note: Since this 'activity' occurs only when the cytokines are denatured, the immunosuppression may be an artefact (FEBS Lett 1988; 226:314); uromodulin is a specific ligand for interleukins IL-1α, IL-1β and TNF, regulating the activity and the levels of these cytokines in the circulation; uromodulin has sequence similarity ('homology') with the lipoprotein lipase receptor and epithelial growth factor

Uropod Greek, uro tail; podos stalk, foot A distinct cytoplasmic process of lymphocytes that attaches to other cells and debris, which appears to play a role in lymphocyte function; see Hand mirror cell

Ursodiol Ursodeoxycholic acid A non-toxic hydrophilic bile acid that modifies the composition of the endogenous bile acid pool, ameliorating, or even partially reversing the clinicopathologic changes of primary biliary cirrhosis (PBC), a condition thought to be due to the toxic effects of bile acids (N Engl J Med 1991; 324:1548); PBC patients treated with ursodiol had statistically significant improvements in serum levels of bilirubin, alkaline phosphatase, cholesterol, IgM, alanine and aspartate aminotransferases, γ–glutamyl transferase, antimitochondrial antibodies and the Mayo risk score; see Primary biliary cirrhosis; ursodiol may be used alone or in combination with chenodiol to dissolve gallstones by extracorporeal shock-wave lithotripsy

Urushiol The generic name given to the four catechols in the ***Rhus*** genus that differ only in the saturation of their pentadecyl side chain, which induce delayed hypersensitivity; these 'poisonous' plants includes poison oak (***R diversiloba***), poison sumac (***R toxicodendron***) and poison ivy (***R radicans***); see Poison ivy

USFMG United States foreign medical graduate A North American who, for various reasons, often had a less than outstanding academic performance in college or university, and by extension, unable to obtain a seat in an American medical school, graduated from a foreign medical school; in general, USFMGs suffer from a wide array of discrimination and are often considered 'third-class' physicians in terms of abilities and knowledge Note: Malpractice lawsuits, used by some parties as a benchmark for determination of competence are no more common in foreign medical graduates than graduates of North American medical schools; see Foreign medical graduate

U-shaped scar A deep fibrotic depression on the cortical surface of the kidney, which is associated with arteriosclerosis and chronicpyelonephritis

U-shaped vertebrum An inverted U-shaped vertebrum (on an antero-posterior film), with marked flattening and central narrowing (lateral film), a characteristic deformity of the lumbar vertebra in thanatophoric dysplasia; see Cloverleaf skull, 'Telephone receiver' deformity

USOH Usual state of health

USP United States Pharmacopeia A compendium of drug standards that includes assays and tests for determining drug strength, purity and quality; the compendium is recognized by US federal law and published by the authorities of the United States Pharmacopeia convention; see National Formulary

Usual interstitial pneumonia (UIP) A disease that occurs in the middle-aged, often associated with connective tissue disease, characterized by insidious deterioration of respiratory function with dyspnea and tachypnea, right-sided cardiac failure, loss of lung capacity and decreased residual volume Radiology Early, 'ground-glass', linear or nodular markings, followed by coarsened shadows and cyst formation; the elevation of the diaphragm in end-stage UIP reflects the amount of tissue loss Pathology The lungs are heavy, rubbery, firm Histopathology Alveolar and septal breakdown is followed by 'hobnailing' of type II pneumocytes, loss of the flat type I alveolar lining cells and squamous metaplasia of the distal air spaces; end-stage UIP demonstrates chronic inflammation, hyaline membrane formation, 'honey-combing' with macroscopic cysts with a knobby pleural surface due to fibrosis, septal thickening and smooth muscle hyperplasia ('muscular cirrhosis') Treatment None has proven effective, although corticosteroids may be used to 'treat the physician'

Uterine apoplexy A uterus in which myometrial vessels have been stipped of protective endometrium, and are actively bleeding as occurs in abruptio placentae (Couvelaire uterus, uteroplacental apoplexy), or in placenta acreta or in massive cardiovascular collapse (apoplexia uteri)

UTI Urinary tract infection

Utilization gap The underutilization of an appropriate therapy, as in the inadvertent non-administration of Rh immune globulin in an Rh-negative woman, which may be required after abortion, ectopic pregnancy or in fetal death; Cf 'Skimping'

Utilization review A cost-containment process used in US health care in hospitals, health maintenance organizations and preferred provider organizations that includes pre-admission reviews, concurrent (while the patient is in the hospital) reviews, and reviews of procedures, levels of care and medical necessity (after the patient's discharge); the utilization review committee assesses the appropriateness of therapy and the efficiency of use of medical services, procedures and facilities

UV light see Ultraviolet radiation

Uvulopalatopharyngoplasty A procedure for treating obstructive sleep apnea that consists of resection of the uvula, the distal margin of the soft palate, palatine tonsils and any excessive lateral pharyngeal tissue; the procedure is successful in two-thirds of selected cases with obstructive sleep apnea in which there is focal airway collapse, which may cause the patients to snore (Mayo Clin Proc 1990; 65:1260); see Snore

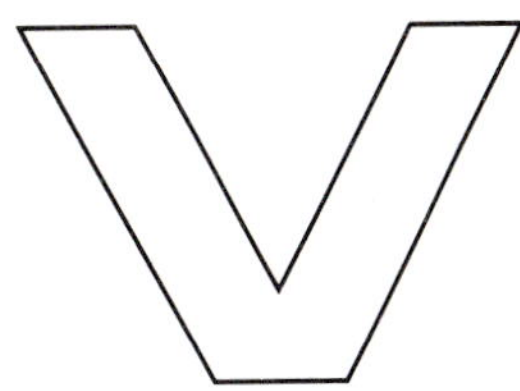

V Symbol for: valine; vanadium; vector; velocity; volt; volume

v Symbol for: Reaction rate; specific volume; velocity

V3 loop Principal neutralizing determinant A hypervariable 36 residue disulfide-linked polypeptide loop in the human immunodeficiency virus-1 (HIV-1) envelope protein; monoclonal antibodies raised against the V3 loop, bind to it and neutralize HIV-1 infectivity; V3 elicits the formation of HIV-neutralizing antibodies in vitro but not in vivo; when the peptide fragment is further dissected, a six-peptide subunit (Gly-Pro-Gly-Arg-Ala-Phe, abbreviated as GPGRAF) is sufficient to neutralize the divergent HIV-1 serotypes (Science 1990; 250:1590); see HIV vaccines

VA Veterans Administration Department of Veteran Affairs The hospital system sponsored by the US government for providing medical care directly to civilians, most of whom are related to veterans of the US military;

before a 1989 US government budget cut, all 30 million American veterans were eligible for VA benefits; the current rule allows benefits only for those with service-connected disabilities or veterans earning below the poverty levels (< $18 000 annual income); the 171 hospitals in the system are scattered throughout the USA, the locations having been dictated by historical precedent, political influence, demographic need and educational pressure Budget $11 x 10^9 (N Engl J Med 1990; 322:1851)

Vaccine A mixture of live, live-attenuated, killed, complete or incomplete microorganisms or products derived therefrom, which contains antigens capable of stimulating the production of specific protective antibodies against the microorganism; according to G Ada (Lancet 1990; 335:523), *A VACCINE* should meet certain immunological criteria; it *SHOULD A) CONTAIN A SUFFICIENT NUMBER OF DIFFERENT T CELL EPITOPES* that T cell responses will be achieved in all members of a genetically diverse outbred population *B) GENERATE A LARGE POOL OF MEMORY T (AND B) CELLS*; the greater the size of the pool, the more rapid is the appearance of effector T cell activity from the memory cells and *C) GENERATE PERSISTANT HIGH TITERS OF NEUTRALIZING ANTIBODIES*, such that the bulk of a challenge virus is prevented from infecting susceptible cells (Nature 1991; 349:369n&v); see Killed vaccine, Live attenuated vaccine

Vacor diabetes TOXICOLOGY A special form of 'brittle' diabetes mellitus, which is due to accidental or suicidal ingestion of the rodenticide Vacor (N-3-pyridyl-methyl-N'-nitrophenyl urea), a molecule that is structurally related to alloxan and streptozotocin, both of which induce experimental diabetes mellitus in laboratory animals Treatment Immediate gastric lavage and hyperdoses of nicotinamide

VACTERYL association Formerly, VATER or VACTER A clinical complex characterized by a multisystem association of vertebral defects, eg hemivertebra and scoliosis, anorectal atresia, cardiac malformations, eg ventricular septal defect, tracheoesophageal fistula, renal anomalies including agenesis, ureteropelvic junction obstruction, vesicoureteral reflux and crossed fused ectopia and radial upper limb anomalies, eg polydactyly (Am J Dis Child 1986; 140:386)

Vacuolar myelopathy A group of conditions characterized by spinal cord degeneration Histopathology Vacuolization of the white matter, accompanied by lipid-laden macrophages (resembling somewhat vitamin B_{12} and folic acid-related subacute combined degeneration of the spinal cord), which occurs in up to 20% of AIDS patients, which is most extensive in the lateral columns of the middle and lower thoracic segments; Cf Spongy degeneration

Vacuolar myopathy Cleared spaces within muscle cells are not uncommon True vacuoles are bound by membranes derived from the T tubules, sarcoplasmic reticulum or from the Golgi apparatus and perinuclear membranes; non-membrane-bound vacuoles are often mutiple and designated as 'hydropic degeneration' Necrotic vacuolated muscle may occur in anaerobic infections, eg *Clostridium* species or in absence of infection, polymyositis and may be a toxic effect of long-term chloroquine therapy for malaria, amebiasis, acid maltase deficiency, primary or secondary periodic paralysis or nemaline myopathy due to myophosphorylase deficiency

Vacuolization Cytoplasmic vacuolization is a non-specific finding described under various conditions CYTOLOGY 'Pap smears' of endocervical cells may be vacuolated in squamous metaplasia or when infected with *Chlamydia* or human papilloma virus HEMATOLOGY Vacuolization of lymphocytes occurs in either 1) Inborn errors of metabolism, including types II, III, V and VII glycogen storage diseases, GM1 gangliosidosis, Hurler-Hunter syndrome, neuronal ceroidlipofuscinosis (Batten's disease), Niemann-Pick disease, sea blue histiocytosis, Tay-Sachs disease, Wolman's disease or 2) Secondary to acquired conditions, eg Burkitt's lymphoma, chronic lymphocytic leukemia, infectious mononucleosis, as an in vitro artefact of EDTA anticoagulation in an aging specimen, normal lymphocytes and in Sézary lymphocytes HEPATOLOGY Vacuolization may affect circulating red cell normoblasts in alcoholic liver disease ONCOLOGY Vacuolization of plasma cells may occur in bone marrow afflicted by mu heavy chain disease RENAL PATHOLOGY Vacuolization of the glomerular basement membrane may be seen in the resolving phases of mild membranous glomerulonephritis

Vacuum phenomenon A linear or oval radiolucency corresponding to gas in the intervertebral space, most often seen in degenerative disk disease, which may also occur in vertebral osteomyelitis, Schmorl's nodes, spondylosis deformans and necrosis-induced vertebral collapse, often accompanied by loss of height and reactive osteosclerosis

Vacuum sign A normal radiologic finding seen when traction is applied to a joint, causing coalescence of gas within a joint, a sign that disappears in effusions

Vaginosis A vaginal infection without leukocyte infiltration Bacterial vaginosis is the most common vaginal infection of reproductive-aged women Etiology *Mobiluncus* species Clinical Range from asymptomatic to having a copious and malodorous milky discharge, which when mixed with 10% potassium hydroxide has a fishy odor

VAHS see Virus-associated hemophagocytic syndrome

Valley fever Desert rheumatism A clinical form of primary coccidioidomycosis, first described in the San Joaquin valley, California, most common in Caucasian women Clinical Fever, cough, pleuritic pain, arthralgia and erythema multiforme or nodosum Diagnosis Serologic detection of IgM antibody to the mycelial phase antigen, coccidioidin, elevated complement-fixing antibody and latex agglutination Treatment Ketoconazole (agent of choice), amphotericin B, miconazole

Valsalva maneuver Forced expiration against a closed glottis following full inspiration, described by Valsalva in 1704 to expulse pus from the middle ear; the 'Valsalva' increases the intrathoracic pressure for about ten seconds, eliciting a complex series of changes in the pulse rate and blood pressure involving both vagal and sympathetic responses

Valvular vegetation(s) CARDIOLOGY Variably-sized excrescences that are present on the heart valves, also known as vegetative endocarditis (table)

CARDIAC VALVE VEGETATIONS

Bacterial vegetations Friable, necrotic lesions measuring up to 1 cm in diameter that may perforate the underlying valve

Lupus erythematosus vegetations of Libmann-Sacks Lesions consisting of mucoid pools, fibrinoid degeneration and collagenous fibrosis occurring on both sides of the tricuspid and mitral valves

Non-bacterial thrombotic vegetations Relatively small foci of organizing thrombi that occur singly or multiply along the line of the leaflet's closure, or on either side of the ventricle

Rheumatic vegetations Small (1-2 mm) foci of friable fibrinoid necrosis located in the cardiac valve cusps along the lines of closure

Vampirism CLINICAL MEDICINE A 'vampire' is a clinician who requests excessive blood tests, potentially causing iatrogenic anemia, an event that is most common in young children with chronic, unusual or 'interesting' diseases PSYCHIATRY A form of deviancy in which blood is ingested, variably accompanied by necrophilic activity, occurring in a background of schizophrenia, psychosis, sadomasochism, cult, eg voodoo rituals, cannibalism, fetishism or drug intoxication

Vancouver group International Committee of Medical Journal Editors (J Am Med Assoc 1991; 265:2697); see Authorship

van Gogh 'syndrome' PSYCHIATRY Self-mutilation, eg amputation of an extremity, enucleation of an eye or castration, which may be associated with dysmorphic delusions, disturbances of the body image or psychosis, or a component of the congenital Lesch-Nyhan syndrome; see Self-mutilation

Vanishing bile duct syndrome, acute A poorly understood early complication of liver transplantation, in which there is irreversible destructive cholangitis and loss of bile ducts

Vanishing bone syndrome see Disappearing bone disease

Vanishing diabetes mellitus syndrome Houssay phenomenon A marked reduction in the requirement for exogenous insulin that occurs secondary to complete destruction of the pituitary gland, especially the anterior lobe; the phenomenon may rarely occur spontaneously in diabetes mellitus, since infarcts of the hypophysis are three times more common in diabetics; during the 1960s, hypophysectomies were performed to take advantage of this phenomenon, reducing the insulin requirements in these patients, at the considerable cost of making them hormonal 'cripples'; Cf Dawn phenomenon, 'Honeymoon period', Somogyi effect

Vanishing lung syndrome Giant bullous emphysema A disease affecting an estimated 1:1000 young, especially male subjects, which is characterized by multiple bullae of the apical portions of one or both lungs Clinical Increased resonance to percussion with radiologic disappearance of lung markings, hence, the term 'vanishing'; in absence of concomitant emphysema, the vital capacity is relatively normal; with extensive lesions, severe impairment of pulmonary function may occur Treatment Surgical excision of the afunctional bullae results in expansion of normally functioning pulmonary tissue and clinical improvement

'Vanishing twin' The spontaneous regression of a second gestational product, which occurs in 20% of twin pregnancies, detected by ultrasonography in the first trimester; Cf Twins

Variable region IMMUNOLOGY That region of the immunoglobulin molecule (antibody) that is shared by the variable domain of a (kappa or lambda) light chain and the variable domain of a (α, γ, μ, δ or ε) heavy chain; the variable region confers specificity to an antibody and is encoded by the V gene region(s); see Hot spot, Monoclonal antibody

Variance STATISTICS The variability in a Gaussian distribution of data that is markedly influenced by large outliers; the variance measures the dispersion of data about a mean of X

Variant angina Prinzmetal's angina Chest pain at rest that is associated with an ST segment deviation (usually an elevation) without a preceding increase in heart rate or blood pressure; this form of angina is caused by vasospasms of large caliber coronary arteries that oxygenate the entire thickness of myocardium Treatment Nitrates, nifedipine, or diltiazem with aspirin; slow calcium channel antagonists, eg verapamil are of use but may contribute to the atrioventricular block

Vascular integrity factor(s) Molecules or proteins that have been postulated to be produced by platelets, which are presumed to prevent spontaneous hemorrhage, although no candidate molecule has been identified

Vascular phase see Prevascular phase

Vascular sling A rare congenital malformation in which the left pulmonary artery arises from the right pulmonary artery, crossing to the left side, insinuating itself between the trachea and esophagus, forming a sling around the trachea, clinically characterized by tracheal stenosis (stridor, wheezing and choking) Treatment Surgery

Vasectomy A form of permanent contraception chosen by up to 500 000 males in USA/year; 10-20 ejaculates are required after the operation before there are no viable sperm; vasectomized subjects may experience long-term scrotal pain, possibly related to sperm granuloma formation, an event that is reported to occur in 1-10% of cases with congestive epididymitis; two-thirds of subjects develop circulating antibodies Note: SOme 'soft' data suggest a possible relation between vasectomy and atherosclerosis Histopathology Post-vasectomy testicles may demonstrate dysspermatogenesis, thickening of the tunica propria and seminiferous tubules, interstitial fibrosis, decreased Sertoli cells and spermatids, focal interstitial fibrosis (a predictor of reversal infertility) Failures In a large single-author series, 1.8% were failures (0.60% early overt, 1.14% technical and 0.08% late overt failures resulting in pregnancy J Am Med Assoc 1988; 259:3142) Reversal Vasectomies are difficult and expensive to reverse, but may be successful if done within 10 years of the operation; 40-70% fertility is achieved with reversal operations (normal fertility is 85%); pregnancy rate in banked frozen sperm, 5%, see in vitro fertilization Note: The (four-fold) increased incidence of testicular malignancy reported after the procedure may be an epidemiologic artefact related to increased testicular examination (Br J Med 1990: 300:370); there is also a reported increased incidence of prostate carcinoma (Am J Epidemiol 1990; 132:1051)

Vasoactive intestinal peptide see VIP

Vasoactive substances A group of circulating substances that regulate the vascular tone, causing either vasodilation (atrial natriuretic peptide, kinins and vasoactive intestinal peptide) or vasoconstriction (angiotensin II, epinephrine and norepinephrine and vasopressin)

Vasopermeability reaction PHYSIOLOGY An inflammatory response to a local increase in substances with vasomotor activity which are responsible for the egress of fluids and cells from the vascular compartment during inflamation, a response subdivided into *1) IMMEDIATE-TRANSIENT RESPONSE*, mediated by histamine, as well as leukotriene E_4, serotonin, bradykinin and others, a reaction affecting small (< 100 μm in diameter) venules, but not capillaries; during this phase, the endothelial cells contract, widening the interendothelial cell gaps *2) IMMEDIATE-SUSTAINED RESPONSE* that follows severe injury, eg burns and is associated with endothelial cell necrosis, affecting the small arterioles, capillaries and venules and *3) DELAYED-PROLONGED LEAKAGE* which begins after a delay of hours to days, representing a response to a vast array of environmental 'noxins', including burns, bacterial toxins, ultraviolet and X-rays and delayed hypersensitivity reactions, affecting venules and capillaries; see Slow-reactive substances of anaphylaxis, Triple response

'Vasopressin resistance' A therapeutic artefact seen in the treatment of diabetes insipidus with pitressin, due to inadequate mixing of the drug and injection only of the oily vehicle

VATER complex see VACTERYL

VBAC Vaginal birth after cesarian section

Vd see Volume of distribution

VDAC see Voltage-dependent anion-selective channel

VDCC see Voltage-dependent calcium channels

V(D)J recombinase MOLECULAR BIOLOGY An enzyme that has yet to be identified, which is capable of recognizing and splicing the V (variable), J (joining) and occasionally D (diversity) gene segments responsible for antibody diversity; one contender for V(D)J recombinase gene is RAG-1 (recombinase activating gene)

V(D)J recombination Class switching A process of exon combination by which developing lymphocytes are able to generate a vast array of binding specificities from a relatively limited 'palette' of genetic information comprised of gene segments designated as variable (V), joining (J) and sometimes diversity (D) gene segments at seven different loci (μ, κ and λ for the immunoglobulin genes of B cells and α, β, γ and δ genes for T cell receptors); this tightly regulated process occurs in chronologic sequence, mediated by recombination signal sequences that are conserved among different loci and species, suggesting the existence of a single 'V(D)J recombinase' Note: The experimental work that led to the understanding of V, D, and J gene splicing to produce antibody diversity netted S Tonegawa the 1987 Nobel prize; see RAG-1

VDRL Venereal Disease Research Laboratory test A reaginic screening test for syphilis Method Heat-inactivated serum is added to the VDRL antigen and agglutination is viewed by light microscopy at four minutes (the RPR or rapid plasma reagin test is a variant of the VDRL that is interpreted macroscopically at eight minutes); reaginic tests are useful screens in early syphilis, and are virtually always positive in secondary syphilis; VDRL test is highly variable in tertiary syphilis and is negative in 40-50% of cases of neurosyphilis; FTA-ABS is positive in the serum of 95% of those with late syphilis; reaginic tests may be biological false positives in malaria (up to 90% positive), acute infections (10-30%), lupus erythematosus (10-20%, the classic cause of a biological false positive VDRL test), viral hepatitis (10%), infectious mononucleosis (20%), rheumatoid arthritis (5-10%) and others including pneumococcal pneumonia, drug addiction and pregnancy

VDT see Video display terminal

Vector An 'inactive' vehicle of transport EPIDEMIOLOGY Vectors include any arthropod capable of transporting an infectous agent, in particular viruses and parasites MOLECULAR BIOLOGY A cloning vector is a segment of DNA capable of self-replication, which contains a selective marker, eg antibiotic resistance, and a site allowing cleavage by a restriction endonuclease; see Cosmid, Plasmid

Vegan PUBLIC HEALTH A strict vegetarian who ingests no proteins of animal origin, including meat, fish and dairy products; while all vegans are at risk for vitamin B_{12} deficiency, vegan adolescents are unlikely to meet energy requirements during the growth spurt and, in addition, may become deficient in vitamin B_6 and riboflavin; the high fiber vegan diet may furthermore chelate calcium, zinc and iron, reducing the absorption of essential cations and trace minerals; see Pareve; Cf Lacto-ovo vegetarian

'Vegetable' cell SURGICAL PATHOLOGY An enlarged cell with clear, lipid- and glycogen-laden cytoplasm, angulated borders and a small, hyperchromatic nucleus arranged in bundles and fascicles, which is highly characteristic of typical renal cell carcinomas (RCC), fancifully likened to the light microscopic appearance of vegetable cells; the other main cell type seen in RCCs is granular, organelle-rich with lesser amounts of glycogen and lipid, and is often arranged in papillary clusters; a variant cell, the mitochondria-rich oncocyte, is seen in very well-differentiated RCC, which have a very good prognosis; Cf Clear cell (multiple entries), Hobnail cells

Vehicle MOLECULAR BIOLOGY A self-replicating DNA molecule, eg a virus, plasmid or phage that serves as a vector for insertion of a segment of DNA into a host genome PHARMACOLOGY An inert carrier for a therapeutic agent, eg water, alcohol-containing elixirs or a sweetened syrup that solubilizes a drug, facilitating its deglution

Veiled appearance Dotted veil appearance A wispy, often punctate linear radiodensity that parallels the shaft and cortex of long bones, described as typical in myositis ossificans

Veiled cell IMMUNOLOGY An antigen-presenting cell of the mononuclear phagocytic system that is located in the marginal sinus of afferent lymphatics, which display IL-2 receptor when co-incubated with GM-CSF (Immunol 1989; 68:108); see Antigen-presenting cells, Dendritic reticular cells

'Venetian blind' artefact SURGICAL PATHOLOGY Parallel ridging and cracking with separation of tissues seen by light microscopy due to tissue brittleness; this artefact may be seen on frozen sections; making the differentiation between lymphoma and lymphoid hyperplasia by light microscopy a difficult task; Cf 'Cracking' artefact

Venezuelan equine encephalitis (VEE) An alphavirus infection first identified in a sick horse in Venezuela in 1938 that occurs as an epizootic infection in Central and northern South America; the equine mortality reaches 40%; most exposed humans develop flu-like symptoms; up to 4%, especially adolescents develop encephalitis with a mortality of up to 35% in younger subjects, in adults, less than 10% **Treatment** Supportive **Vaccine** Under development

Venous hum A low-pitched hum auscultated in the neck related to jugular vein turbulence, due to an altered or more intense flow pattern mimicking the machinery murmur of patent ductus arteriosus; the venous hum may be abolished by light lateral neck pressure and may be innocent or heard in younger patients with hyperthyroidism

Ventilating tubes see Tympanostomy tubes

Ventricular assist device CARDIOVASCULAR SURGERY A portable, battery-powered device that assists the flow of blood while a patient is awaiting heart transplantation; the device is connected at the apex of the left ventricle and pumps the blood past the effete ventricle and aortic valve directly into the aortic arch (J Am Med Assoc 1991; 265:2930n&v); Cf Artificial heart, Jarvik-7

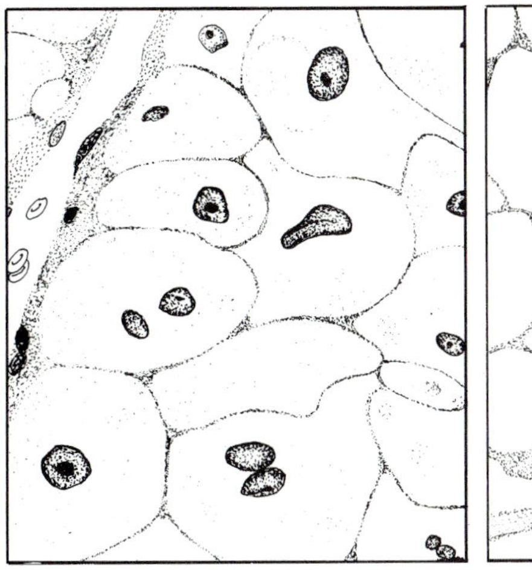

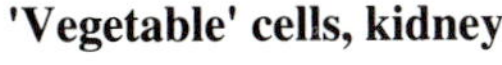

'Vegetable' cells, kidney

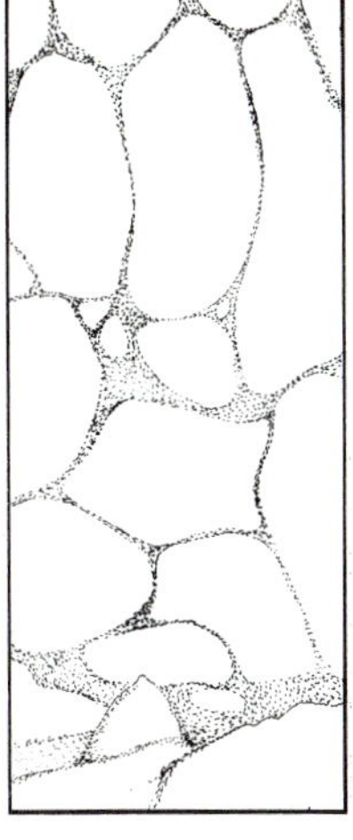

Vegetable cells

Verocytotoxin see VTEC

'Vero' toxin see Shiga neurotoxin

Verrucous carcinoma A variant of well-differentiated epidermoid carcinoma that is most common in the oral cavity, but also occurs in the larynx, nasal cavity, esophagus, penis, anorectal region, vulva, vagina, uterine cervix and skin, especially on the sole of the foot; most intraoral cases occur in elderly male abusers of 'smokeless' tobacco **Pathology** Exophytic and well-differentiated **Treatment** Surgical resection; radiotherapy is not indicated, as up to 30% of verrucous carcinomas treated with radiation become highly aggressive within six months; anorectal verrucous carcinoma may be similar to giant condyloma acuminatum of the penis, which is induced by human papilloma virus and comprises 5% of all penile carcinomas

Vertical transmission EPIDEMIOLOGY The transmission of an infection through the placenta to the fetus, as occurs in the 'TORCH' infections, including toxoplasmosis, rubella, cytomegalovirus, herpes, syphilis and human immunodeficiency virus Note: 30% of infants born to HIV-positive mothers are also infected; see Horizontal transmission; Cf Hereditary transmission

Very high density lipoprotein (VHDL) A plasma lipoprotein with a density of greater that 1.210 kg/L (US: 1.210 g/dl); VHDL is 57% protein (predominantly apolipoprotein A-I and A-II), 21% phospholipid, 17% cholesterol and 5% triglycerides and transports cholesterol from the intestine to the liver; the larger the HDL molecule, the more efficient the lipid transport and by extension, lipolysis Note: HDL levels are the single most important predictor of atherosclerosis-induced disease and are inversely related thereto; Cf HDL

Very low birth weight see Low birth weight

Very low-density lipoprotein see VLDL

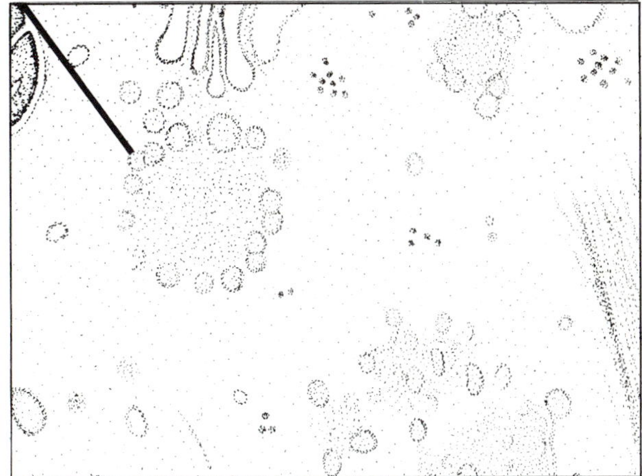

Vesicular rosettes

Vesicular rosettes A non-specific ultrastructural finding seen within lymphocytes (figure, above), which consists of circular clusters of vesicles of undetermined significance, possibly originating from the endoplasmic reticulum, first described as characteristic of AIDS, which has subsequently been seen in Hodgkin's disease, other lymphoproliferative disorders and various benign conditions; Cf Tubular complexes

Vesicular stomatitis virus see Foot and mouth disease

'Vest-over-pants' repair A method used in surgical correction of inguinal hernias, where the fascia above the hernia is brought down over the fascia from below, effecting a two-layer closure; there is little evidence that this repair is more effective than well-apposed approximation of the fascial margins

Veto cell An immune cell that suppresses the activity of T cells capable of reacting against self major histocompatibility complex (MHC) antigens, which derive from Thy lineage; these cells may 'veto' the activity of virtually any T cell that reacts to self surface determinants; veto activity can be found in the normal bone marrow, spleen, thymus and fetal liver, as well as in athymic nude mice; these cells provide specific suppressor activity, depressing host rejection; incubation of T-cell depleted bone marrow with IL-2 increases veto cell activity and enhances engraftment of MHC-mismatched T cell depleted marrow (Transplantation 1990; 49:931)

V factor Nicotinamide adenine dinucleotide MICROBIOLOGY A growth requirement for *Haemophilus* species (*H influenza, H parainfluenza, H aegyptiae*) that may be supplied by yeast extracts, *Staphylococcus*, *Pneumococcus* and *Neisseria* species; X factor is any of a group of tetrapyrrole compounds that are provided by iron-containing pigments, eg heme, used in the synthesis of catalases, peroxidases and in the cytochrome electron transport system

V gene Variability gene Two segments (exons) of DNA that encode the first 95-100 amino acids (the variable portion) of a light or heavy chain of immunoglobulin or β chain of the T cell receptor; the proteins encoded have the most extensive amino acid variability of the entire human genome allowing highly specific immune recognition, thus the greater the diversity of the recognition site, the more specific is the potential immune defense; see Variable region, 'Hot spot'

Vi antigen The capsular antigen of Salmonella species, especially S typhi, which is specifically associated with Salmonella virulence and which interferes with the serotyping of the 'O' antigen, the heat-stable lipopolysaccharide common to enterobacteriaceae

Vibration white finger syndrome An occupation-related, musculoskeletal disorder, in which vibrating hand-held tools, eg electric drills, jackhammers and grinders, evoke ischemia-inducing vasospasms that are virtually indistinguishable from Raynaud's phenomenon; plethysmographic studies reveal temperature-sensitive changes in blood flow, even in the absence of symptoms; with time, these subjects develop pain and numbness of the upper extremities suggestive of cervical, ulnar and median nerve entrapment (N Engl J Med 1990; 322:675)

Video display terminals (VDTs) A device containing a cathode ray tube generating a visual display, which emits both extremely low frequency (ELF, 45-60 Hz) and very low frequency (15 kHz) electromagnetic fields, the latter of which had been associated by some (very) 'soft' data with spontaneous abortion, which is either a statistical canard or due to another factor unrelated to VDTs (N Engl J Med 1991; 324:728) Note: The effects from prolonged exposure to liquid crystal display screens as used for laptop computers have not been formerly studied; 15% of the US workforce spends a large part of its day in front of a VDT; the potential adverse effects of VDTs are related to: 1) Irradiation by ultraviolet light and very low and extremely low frequency electromagnetic ELF radiation; four potential associations have been studied and not found to be significantly increased, including cataracts, reproductive disorders, facial dermatitis and epileptic reactions; for leukemia, see ELF 2) Ergonomic effects Visual (see McCullough effect) and musculoskeletal, due to posture required for typing Note: The 'Balans' type of backless chair is reported to significantly reduce lower back strain 3) Stress The psychological stress related to VDT use is thought by some workers to be more a function of the job per se than the VDT itself

'Vietnam syndrome' The psychosocial consequences of active participation in the Vietnam conflict; when compared with non-Vietnam veterans, active participants in the conflict were reported to have more depression-related complaints (4.5% vs 2.3%), anxiety (4.9% vs 3.2%) and alcohol-related problems (13.7% vs 9.2%); 15% had combat-related post-traumatic stress (2.2% had an 'event' in the month before examination), medical complaints including hearing loss and low sperm count (J Am Med Assoc 1988; 259:2701, 2708); see Burn-out syndrome, Post-traumatic stress disorder

Vigilance NEUROLOGY The conscious and semiconscious focusing and sustained attention to subtle sensory signals within a determined modality (eg auditory or visual), while eliminating distracting internal and external stimuli; positron emission tomography studies of humans localize the 'attention center' to the prefrontal and superior parietal cortex primarily in the right hemisphere, regardless of the modality or laterality of the stimulus (Nature 1991; 349:61)

Villin A 95 kD actin-binding protein of the microvilli of the small intestine, which in low calcium concentrations, cross-links actin filaments into bundles, forming a 'nucleation' center to accelerate actin polymerization

Vimentin A 55 kD protein that is one of the five major intermediate filaments, which is produced by normal mesenchymal cells, including vascular endothelial and smooth muscle cells, fibroblasts, histiocytes, lymphocytes, melanocytes, chondrocytes, osteocytes, astrocytes, rarely ependymal and glomerular cells; malignant cells tend to 'forget' their lineage and thus may display more than one intermediate filament, thus co-expression of cytokeratin and vimentin, as detected by immunoperoxidase staining, may occur in adenocarcinomas of the breast, lung, kidney, adrenal, endometrium and epithelioid sarcoma; see Brown stains, Intermediate filaments

VIN Vulvar intraepithelial neoplasm An umbrella term

encompassing two clinically distinct, but histologically similar lesions a) Carcinoma *in situ* (Bowen's disease) is an erythematous plaque-like lesion that may extend to the perineum and anus; most cases demonstrate human papilloma virus (HPV) type 16 by in situ hybridization, 10% of which evolve toward invasive carcinoma when untreated b) Bowenoid papulosis (bowenoid dysplasia) is characterized by solitary or multiple, often pigmented papules affecting young women, which clinically simulate verrucae and have cytologic atypia approaching that of Bowen's disease; although this lesion is also associated with HPV 16, it tends to resolve spontaneously or respond to therapies that might be considered 'homeopathic'; see Carcinoma in situ, CIN, Intraepithelial neoplasia

Vinblastine A chemotherapeutic alkaloid used to treat Hodgkin's disease, leukemia, other lymphoproliferative disorders and malignancies, which specifically interrupts the microtubules of the mitotic spindle, causing the lysis of rapidly-dividing cells

Vincristine A chemotherapeutic alkaloid used to treat leukemia disease and other malignancies, which like vinblastine, interrupts the mitotic spindle, causing lysis of proliferating cells

Vinculin A 130 kD phosphorylated fibrous protein that is present in the intercalated disks of cardiac muscle and membrane-associated plaques of smooth muscle, which binds α-actinin, uniting the actin cytoskeleton and plasma membrane at the adhesion plaques; increased vinculin production is associated with increased phosphotyrosine levels in transformed (malignant) cells, which may explain the hallmarks of these cells, eg altered morphology, reduced actin microfilaments, loss of anchorage dependence for growth, changed mobility of cell surface, changes that may be driven by the *src* and *abl* oncogenes; see Malignancy

Vinyl chloride see PVC (Polyvinyl chloride)

Violin band mark A distinct 'spot' on the dorsal cephalothorax of *Loxosceles reclusa*, a spider of the southern USA, the bite of which contains a cytotoxin causing painful blistering, necrosis and when severe, residual scarred ulcer; systemic manifestations of recluse spider bites include fever, nausea, vomiting, arthralgia and renal failure (hemoglobinuria and proteinuria), hemolysis and thrombocytopenia, which may be fatal in the very young

Violin string adhesions A descriptor for the taut fibrous bands present between the anterior parietal peritoneum and the anterior aspect of the liver, typically seen in *Neisseria gonorrhoeae*-induced perihepatitis, which may be accompanied by upper right quadrant pain, fever and a hepatic friction rub; violin string adhesions may also occur in the uterine adnexae in pelvic inflammatory disease due to *Chlamydia trachomatis* as well as in fibrinous mesothelial inflammation of the pericardium, pleura and peritoneum

VIP Vasoactive intestinal peptide A 28 residue neuropeptide of the secretin-glucagon family that is present in the nerve fibers of smooth muscle, blood vessels and in the glands of the upper respiratory tract; VIP stimulates adenylate cyclase, evoking potent vasodilation, pancreatic and intestinal secretion, inhibition of gastric acid secretion, increased cardiac output, glycogenolysis, bronchodilation and inhibition of macromolecule release from mucus-secreting glands; VIP deficiency may contribute to bronchial asthma, given its virtual absent in asthmatics (N Engl J Med 1989; 320:1271, 1244); VIP is markedly increased in VIPoma, a pancreatic islet G-cell tumor that is morphologically identical to G-cell tumors; see Watery diarrhea, hypokalemia, achlorhydria (WDHA) syndrome

V.I.P. 'syndrome' A very important person (V.I.P.) is anyone whose presence in a hospital, by virtue of fame, position or claim on the public interest, may substantially disrupt the normal course of patient care; often the V.I.P. wants to be treated as any other patient, but may in fact receive less than optimal emergency and critical care, as the patient management team may inappropriately alter its standard operating procedures (N Engl J Med 1988; 319:1421); see Chief 'syndrome'

Viral hemorrhagic fever syndrome(s) (VHFS) A group of clinical complexes caused by various viruses, including Filoviridae, eg Ebola and Marburg agents, Arenaviridae, eg Junin and Lassa agents, Togaviridae, including Flaviviridae, eg Dengue, Omsk and yellow fever agents and Bunyaviridae, Congo-Crimean, Hantaan virus and Rift Valley fever agents Vectors Arthropods, either ticks or mosquitoes, eg Dengue and Rift Valley and yellow fevers and environmental contaminants, eg Argentine, Bolivian, Ebola, Lassa and Marburg hemorrhagic fevers and hemorrhagic fever with renal syndrome **Clinical** Incubation 3 days to 3 weeks, followed by headache, myalgias, dysphagia, vomiting, diarrhea, abdominal and/or chest pain, pharyngitis, conjunctivitis, cervical lymphadenopathy, macular rashes and shock **Laboratory** Leukopenia and/or thrombocytopenia, proteinuria, disseminated intravascular coagulation

'Virgin birth' A term referring to a child who is born out of wedlock to a woman through artificial insemination by an often annonymous donor (Nature 1991; 350:96ed); see Artificial reproduction

Virilization Physical changes in the female resulting from androgen excess which include hirsutism, temporal balding, deepened voice, acne, enlarged clitoris and clitoral index (the ratio between the sagittal and transverse diameters of the clitoris) The androgen excess may be a) Adrenal, due to Cushing's syndrome, congenital enzyme deficiency, eg 11- or 21 hydroxylase deficiency or neoplasia, either benign or malignant or b) Ovarian, due to hyperplasia, eg polycystic ovaries or tumors, eg arrhenoblastoma, steroid cell tumors or gynandroblastoma; Cf Hermaphroditism, Intersex, Precocious puberty

Virion A complete virus, the genome of which is encapsulated in a protein coat

Virocytes Turk cells Atypical, enlarged lymphocytes with foamy cytoplasm filled with scattered small vacuoles in a moderately to deeply basophilic cytoplasm; the nuclear chromatin is coarse but less so than that of normal lymphocytes, with a sharp chromatin and parachromatin distinction and accelerated DNA synthesis; the term virocyte is appropriate when lymphocytes are reacting to viral infections (hepatitis, herpes zoster, herpes simplex, infectious mononucleosis, mumps, roseola infantum, rubeola, rubella and others) Note: Morphologically identical 'reactive' lymphocytes occur in other infections (diphtheria, malaria, rickettsial infections, scarlet fever, syphilis, tuberculosis, typhus), as a result of drugs and toxins (phenytoin, barbiturates, butazolidine, lead intoxication) and other causes (post-surgery, exposure to ionizing radiation, serum sickness, agranulocytosis, acute myocardial infarction, ulcerative colitis, dermatitis herpetiformis, pemphigus vulgaris)

Viroid Infectious RNA A 100 kD (circa 300 base pairs) subviral infectious particle composed of a small circular segment of single-stranded RNA that causes disease in higher plants; viroids are postulated to represent 'escaped' introns, with which they bear a degree of sequence 'homology'; Cf Prion

Virosome A semisynthetic complex homogenate derived from nucleic acid-free viral particles including membrane proteins and lipids that is prepared with lecithin and diacetyl phosphate and dialyzed

Virulence genes MOLECULAR BIOLOGY Genes that are thought to coordinate the expression of many other genes in response to environmental conditions (temperatures, osmolarity and pH), eg the ***toxR*** gene of ***Vibrio cholerae*** (which controls 14 other ***V cholerae*** genes); the agr gene of ***Staphylococcus aureus*** (controls expression of 12 different proteins) and the phoP regulatory locus in ***Salmonella typhi***

Virus A potentially infectious agent that ranges in size from 10^6 daltons for the small Parvoviridae to 200 x 10^6 for Poxviridae; viral nucleic acid is single- or double-stranded, either DNA or RNA (classification, table, right) and is closed in a circle or opened and linear; viral nucleic acid is packaged within a protein coat (capsid) composed of a few distinct types of protein, and most have a helical or icosahedral symmetry; some viruses have a lipid envelope which, as in the case of the influenzae virus may be 'studded' with viral proteins, including hemagglutinin and neuraminidase; viruses may be specifically identified by incubating them within specific 'host' cells and identifying the chacteristic cytopathic effects that each virus induces in the host cells; these cells include diploid fibroblasts (CMV, varicella-zoster, rhinoviridae), rhesus monkey kidney (influenza, parainfluenza, mumps, coxsackievirus and echovirus), human embryonic kidney (herpesvirus, varicella), human foreskin (CMV, HIV) and African green monkey kidney (for detecting rubella-induced 'interference' of cytopathic effects); inclusion bodies may occur in virally-infected cells; DNA viruses often induce cytoplasmic, while those of RNA viruses are often intranuclear **Mode of action** Viruses penetrate the host cells by using specific host receptors, including CMV binding to β_2-microglobulin, Epstein-Barr virus binding to C3d receptor (CR2), rabies to the acetylcholine receptor, vaccinia virus to the epidermal growth factor receptor and HIV-1 to CD4 with its gp120 glycoprotein; see Cytomegalovirus, Cytopathic effect, Epstein-Barr virus, Herpesvirus, HIV-1, HIV-2, HTLV-I, HTLV-II, Retrovirus; Cf Prion

Virus-associated hemophagocytic syndrome A florid reactive hemophagocytotic condition described in both immunocompromised (male:female ratio, 1:1) and in non-immunocompromised (male:female ratio, 4:1) subjects, most common in a background of herpetic infections, including CMV, EBV and Herpesvirus that may occur in infections by adenovirus, rubella, as well as brucellosis, candidiasis, leishmaniasis, tuberculosis, salmonellosis, and has been described in graft-versus-host disease and hemolytic anemia **Clinical** Hepatosplenomegaly, lymphadenopathy, pulmonary infiltrates, pancytopenia (with a depleted bone marrow) and a skin rash **Differential diagnosis** Lymphoma, malignant histiocytosis, sinus histiocytosis with massive lymphadenopathy, lymphomatoid granulomatosis

Virus-like particle (VLP) CLINICAL THERAPEUTICS A drug delivery system composed of self-assembling proteins encoded by the Ty gene of yeasts; when another gene is fused into the Ty gene, the transfected yeasts produce a hybrid protein that assembles itself into VLPs, bearing antigens on the surface that are encoded by the inserted gene; VLPs have potential for vaccine delivery and are in protocol for delivering HIV's p24 protein with the hope of eliciting protective anti-HIV antibodies (Science 1990; 249:626rn)

vis-a-tergo CARDIOLOGY The force driving venous return, which is supplied by the left ventricle; by the time the blood has passed through the capillary bed, its pressure, the vis-a-tergo, has been reduced to 15mm Hg

CLASSIFICATION OF VIRUSES

CLASS I Double-stranded DNA is transcribed into plus-stranded mRNA, then translated into a protein, a flow of genetic information identical to Watson and Crick's 'central dogma'

CLASS II Single, plus-stranded DNA generates double-stranded DNA, then transcribed into plus-stranded mRNA and translated into a protein

CLASS III Double-stranded RNA is transcribed into a plus-stranded mRNA, then translated into a protein

CLASS IV Single, plus-stranded RNA is transcribed into minus-stranded RNA, then transcribed into plus-stranded mRNA and translated into a protein

CLASS V Single, minus-stranded RNA is transcribed into a plus-stranded mRNA, then translated into a protein

CLASS VI Single, plus-stranded RNA is transcribed into minus-stranded DNA, which is transcribed to form a double-stranded DNA molecule that transcribes into a plus-stranded mRNA, then translated into a protein

Visual display terminal see Visual display unit

Vitamins Organic accessory factors present in foods in addition to the basic components of carbohydrates, fats, proteins, minerals, water and fiber, which are necessary in minimal or trace amounts (daily requirements of individual vitamins are measured in milligram to microgram quantities), as the body either does not produce them or does so in minute quantities; vitamins are the most commonly abused substances among the lay, vying with laxatives as a form of inappropriate self-medication; water-soluble vitamins are reasonably well-tolerated as they are easily excreted, while the lipid soluble vitamins accumulate in adipose tissue and have significant hepatotoxic potential Note: Lipid-soluble vitamins A, D, E and K and water-soluble vitamins B_1, B_2, B_6, B_{12} and C are valid and accepted terms; in contrast, a vast array of pseudovitamins have appeared on the shelves of 'health food' emporia that are delineated in this work under 'Vitamins'; Cf Chemoprevention, Pseudo-vitamin

'Vitamins' A family of substances or pseudovitamins that may be obtained in some 'natural food' stores, which are a) True vitamins, but not in humans b) Substances that were first described as vitamins, but no longer widely regarded as such and c) 'Factors' in the blood, exotic vegetables and fruits, or minerals that have been termed 'vitamins' by various persons Glossary (table, below); see also Pseudovitamins

'VITAMINS'

Vitamin B_3 Obsolete for pantothenic acid

Vitamin B_4 An ill-defined 'factor', of dubious validity, isolated from yeasts or liver, described as alleviating myasthenia in experimental animals; vitamin B_4 'deficiency' responds to a variety of agents, including adenine, arginine, cystine, glycine and thiamine

Vitamin B_5 Obsolete for nicotinic acid (niacin) and nicotinamide

Vitamin B_7 Carnitine (permeability factor)

Vitamin B_8 Adenylic acid (a nucleotide)

Vitamin B_{10} A growth and feathering promoter in chickens, considered a pseudovitamin, corresponding to a mixture of folic acid and vitamin B_{12}

Vitamin B_{11} A growth and feathering promotor of chickens, similar or identical to Vitamin B_{10} factor see Pseudovitamin

Vitamin B_{13} Orotic acid, an intermediate in pyrimidine metabolism and considered a pseudovitamin

Vitamin B_{15} Pangamate, a pseudovitamin with no known effects

Vitamin B_{17} A toxic substance claimed without substantial evidence to be effective in treating malignancy; see Laetrile

Vitamin B_c Folic acid

Vitamin B_p A factor that treats perosis in chicks that respond to a mixture of choline and manganese

Vitamin B_t A substance promoting insect growth corresponding to carnitine

Vitamin B_w Biotin

Vitamin B_x para-aminobenzoic acid

Vitamin C_2 Bioflavinoids, substances with activities that partially overlap those of true vitamin C

Vitamin F Obsolete for linoleic acid, an essential fatty acid

Vitamin G Obsolete for riboflavin

Vitamin GH_3 see Gerovital

Vitamin H Biotin A water-soluble factor with an uncertain role as a vitamin, which is a co-factor in enzymes catalyzing carboxylation reactions, eg pyruvate carboxylase and acetyl CoA carboxylase; biotin-deficiency is uncommon

Vitamin H_3 see Gerovital

Vitamin I Synonym for carnitine or vitamin B_7

Vitamin J Synonym for bioflavinoids or vitamin C_2

Vitamin L_1 Anthranilic acid, a liver 'factor' thought to be necessary for lactation

Vitamin L_2 Adenylthiomethylpentose, a yeast 'factor' thought to be necessary for lactation

Vitamin M Folic acid

Vitamin N A preparation from the brain or stomach, which was described as being anticarcinogenic

Vitamin P Synonym for bioflavinoids or vitamin C_2

Vitamin PP Obsolete for nicotinic acid

Vitamin P_4 Troxerutin, a pseudovitamin

Vitamin R A folic acid-related compound that promotes growth in bacteria

Vitamin S A streptogenin-related protein that promotes growth in chicks

Vitamin T A mixture of amino acids, DNA nucleotides, folacin and vitamin B_{12} that promotes growth and wound-healing in yeasts and insects

Vitamin U Methylsulfonium salts of methionine, derived from cabbage juice, claimed to heal peptic ulceration

Vitamin V A tissue 'factor' composed of NAD^+ and NADH, which promotes bacterial growth

Vitamin A Retinol, carotene A generic term for all β-ionone derivatives that exhibit the biological activity of trans-retinol; vitamin A is stored in the stellate cells of the liver, as well as the intestine, kidney, heart, blood vessels and gonads; after oxidation to retinoic acid, it diffuses into the nucleus, binds to a specific nuclear receptor and interacts with a 'responsive element', a DNA sequence that regulates the target genes (Sci 1990; 250:399); vitamin A is critical for fetal development, differentiation, cell proliferation and vision; empirical therapy in asymptomatic children results in two-fold decrease in childhood mortality from diarrhea, convulsions and infection-related symptoms

Vitamin A embryopathy A condition induced by in utero exposure to vitamin A analogs, which may be associated with cardiovascular (ventricular septal, aortic arch and conotruncal) defects, external ear deformity, cleft palate, micrognathia and central nervous system malformations; see Category X drugs, Isoretinoin

Vitamin B_1 Thiamine

Vitamin B_2 Riboflavin

Vitamin B_6 Pyridoxine

Vitamin B_6-dependency syndromes A group of functional or structural enzyme defects that respond to a massive excess (50-100-fold greater than minimum daily requirements) of pyridoxine; the vitamin B_6-dependency syndromes are heterogeneous in nature, and include vitamin B_6-dependent convulsions, vitamin B6-responsive anemia, xanthurenic aciduria, cystathioninuria, homocystinuria and may be due to a defective structure of the apoenzyme, its coenzyme binding site or some aspect of coenzyme synthesis **Clinical** Predominantly neurological disease including mental retardation, psychiatric symptoms, seizures, convulsions, ataxia, spasticity and peripheral neuropathy **Treatment** Neonates respond well to early therapy

Vitamin B_6-dependent streptococci MICROBIOLOGY Thiol-dependent, satelliting or nutritionally variant streptococci, which comprise 5-6% of all streptococci that may cause 'culture-negative' bacterial endocarditis; culture media supplemented with pyridoxal or L-cysteine support growth of these organisms and such special media when culturing blood from patients suspected of having a streptococcal endocarditis

Vitamin B_{12} Cobalamine; see Intrinsic factor

Vitamin C Ascorbic acid

Vitamin D A generic term for steroid vitamins with the biological activity of cholecalciferol **Vitamin D_1** A term that is not used, as the original vitamin D_1 was shown to consist of a mixture of vitamin D_2 and lumisterol **Vitamin D_2** Ergocalciferol **Vitamin D_3** Cholecalciferol; see Rickets, vitamin D-resistant

Vitamin E

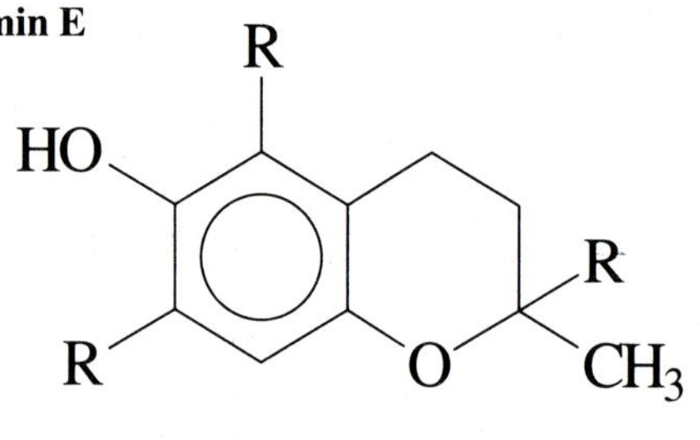

Vitamin E α-Tocopherol A family (basic structure, figure, above) of antioxidant that stabilizes unsaturated lipids, preventing autooxidation, eg peroxidative decomposition of membrane lipids and enzyme inactivation, as well as protecting against chemical toxins; vitamin E deficiency may be due to chronic fat malabsorption, as occurs in cystic fibrosis, but rarely causes clinical disease in humans, including spinocerebellar degeneration, progressive gait ataxia, loss of proprioception, incoordination, dysarthria, ophthalmoplegia, pigmentary retinopathy, generalized muscle weakness, superficial sensory loss, accompanied by chronic liver disease; pharmacologic doses of vitamin E in the elderly are reported to boost the immune system, increasing lymphokine and antibody production, mitogenic response and suppress prostaglandin production; dietary vitamin E supplementation is thought by some workers to reduce the risk for coronary artery disease, cancer and stress Note: Vitamin E deficiency was first associated with testicular atrophy in the male rat, leading to its intermittent abuse as a male 'sexual tonic'

Vitamin K A generic term for 2-methyl-1,4 naphthoquinone and its derivatives, which have antihemorrhagic activity

Vitamin K-dependent proteins A group of coagulation factor proenzymes (factors II, VII, IX and X) that are produced in the liver, which contain multiple residues of γ-carboxyglutamic acid, an amino acid produced by the post-translational action of a vitamin K-dependent γ-carboxylase on certain glutamyl residues; four other proteins bear γ-carboxyglutamic acid and have been designated proteins C, S, Z and M; while M is poorly characterized, proteins C, S, and Z have amino-terminal homology with prothrombin; vitamin K-dependent proteins also have another unusual amino acid, β aspartic acid, currently of unknown function

Vitronectin Epibolin, Protein S, Serum spreading factor A 65 kD glycoprotein with serum levels of 20 mg/L that mediates cell adhesion and interacts with proteins of the complement, coagulation and fibrinolytic cascade; vitronectin colocalizes with fibronectin in the basement membrane in proliferative vitreoretinopathy and may be etiologically linked thereto (J Biol Chem 1990; 265:9778)

Vivisection RESEARCH The cutting open of a living animal for the purposes of experimentation; see Autopsy; Cf Animal rights activism, Sacrifice

VLA proteins see Integrins

VLA receptors A group of cell-surface receptors which belong to the integrin receptor superfamily, characterized by heterodimeric α and β transmembrane chains with a VLA-binding region at the arginine-glycine-aspartamine binding region; the VLA receptors are found predominantly on T cells and bind to laminin and fibronectin

VLCD Very low calorie diet, see Diet

VLDL Very low-density lipoprotein A plasma lipoprotein that has a density of 0.950-1.006 kg/L (US: 0.950-1.006 g/dl); VLDL is 6-10% protein (apolipoprotein B-100 and apoC, with some apoE), 15-20% phospholipid, 20-30% cholesterol and 45-65% triglycerides; VLDL is composed of endogenous triglycerides of hepatic origin

VLIA Virus-like infectious agent A mycoplasma identified at the Armed Forces Institute of Pathology that may be synergistic with HIV-1, exacerbate immuno-deficiency; all four monkeys inoculated with VLIA developed low-grade fever and died in 9 months (Am J Trop Med Hyg 1989; 40:213); the agent has been designated '*Mycoplasma incognitus*', although it is probably a strain of *M fermentans*; if the early work survives the scrutiny of research in progress, it is possible that a percentage of AIDS patients may partially respond to antibiotics, a therapy that is effective for treating *Mycoplasma* infections (Science 1990; 248:682)

VLP see Virus-like particles

VNTR Variable number of tandem repeats MOLECULAR BIOLOGY Most of the 400 thus far identified polymorphic DNA markers have only two alleles and are thus uninformative for analysis of genetic linkage in families; some of these markers have loci that respond to restriction endonuclease cleavage by producing fragments of different lengths (restriction fragment length polymorphism, see RFLP); this polymorphism is due to tandem repeated segments of oligonucleotide sequences; Cf Lod score analysis

Void volume Outer volume INSTRUMENTATION The first quantity of fluid obtained in protein separation by gel filtration Note: In gel filtration chromatography, a column is packed with Sephadex or agarose beads that are rated according to pore size, which determines the size of the molecule that will pass through or be retained by a column; the void volume contains the first 'wash' through the column, usually the larger proteins that are not retained by the agarose beads

Volcano lesion see Mushroom lesion

Volitional collapse Loss of the 'will to live' or volition; Cf Todeserwartung

Voltage clamp experiment see Patch-clamp experiment

Voltage-dependent anion-selective channel A class of transmembrane proteins that form aqueous pores in cell membranes that open or close in response to changes in transmembrane voltage, changing the ionic permeability of the membrane; VDACs are present in membranes of neurons, muscle and other cells (Science 1990; 247:1233); see Porins

Voltage-dependent calcium channels (VDCC) PHYSIOLOGY Transmembrane proteins that act as ion channels and are present in all excitable cell membranes, which are closed at normal negative resting membrane potentials (completely closed at -70mV) and 'gated' by small changes in membrane potential (membrane depolarization) into open (completely opened at +20mV), calcium-permeable states of varying duration, a transition requiring 1-2 milliseconds that can be examined with the patch-clamp technique; VDCCs demonstrate tissue variability and different responses to ligands, eg conotoxins and nifedipine (Nature 1991; 350:398); VDCCs modulate synaptic plasticity, oscillatory behavior and rhythmic firing in certain brain regions, eg hippocampus, and are immobile as determined by photobleaching technique; selective regulation of VDCC immobilization may be critical in determining neuronal firing patterns(Science 1989; 244:1189); see Ion channel

Volume of distribution (V_d) CLINICAL PHARMACOLOGY A calculated value used to estimate the 'pull' that a storage tissue has on drugs in the circulation; lipotropic drugs have V_d of many liters, while high molecular weight substances stay within the blood vessels; the V_d is decreased with valproic acid, normal with lithium, phenobarbital and chloramphenicol and increased with lidocaine, procainamide and thiopental; see Apparent volume of distribution, Therapeutic drug monitoring

Voluntary sector The sum of all the organizations and agencies that are neither private (for profit) nor public (government-sponsored) sectors; this 'third' sector is comprised of non-profit and charitable organizations and philanthropies; see Howard Hughes Medical Institute, Imperial Cancer Research Fund

von Economo encephalitis Encephalitis lethargica A disease of historical interest, which caused a major global pandemic after World War I, most prominently affecting young adults, of presumed viral origin Clinical Ophthalmoplegia, headache, dizziness, fatigue, confusional psychosis, reversed sleep-wake pattern, hypersomnolence (a small subgroup experienced hyperactivity), focal rigidity evolving to complete parkinsonism Histopathology Congestion, perivascular mononuclear cell cuffing and degeneration of the nervous system

von Willebrand factor A large (> 20 x 10^6 daltons) multimeric molecule composed of multiple circa 200 kD monomers, which is synthesized by vascular endothelium, megakaryocytes and platelets; hemostatic efficiency is related to the size of the multimers; factor VIII:C is the classic hemophilia A protein Factor VIII:Ag is the antigen expressed in hemophilia A protein Factor VIII R:Ag is the antigenic expression of vW protein Factor VIII R:RCo is the ristocetin cofactor Note: von Willebrand's disease is an autosomal dominant condition, the defective proteins of which are defined by SDS gel electrophoresis; the relative rarity of von Willebrand's disease and the variability of the many multimeric proteins that may be deranged in this condition led one author to query whether this was merely a 'tempest in a teapot', potentially having little clinical significance; see Rocket electrophoresis

Voodoo death A precipitous death related to acute psychogenic stress, possibly due to an exaggerated autonomic nervous response to a frightening culturally-ingrained event(s), triggering a fatal dysrhythmia; the voodoo cult is practiced in Africa, Brazil and Haiti and a typical ceremony has two or more hours of pounding rhythms and incantations by the priests; this, in concert with the relevant cultural associations of the participant, act to produce hysterical trances, seizures or twilight states and chronic psychosomatic symptoms which may trigger fatal cardiac dysrhythmia; see Cultural psychosis, SUND

VOR Vestibulo-ocular reflex NEUROLOGY A reflex in which a movement of the eyes is produced that is equal and opposite to the movement of the head; loss of the VOR implies vestibular disease that may occur in aminoglycoside toxicity (Science 1988; 242:773)

VP16 A herpes simplex virus type 1 (HSV-1) protein that is a specific and potent activator of transcription of intermediate-to-early viral genes (Science 1991; 251:87); see Etoposide

VPI 'T4-1' A species of *Bacteroides*, recently dignified as *B merdae*, isolated from feces

V/Q scan Ventilation/perfusion scan A radioisotopic evaluation of the ratio of pulmonary ventilation (V) to pulmonary perfusion (Q), used to detect pulmonary embolism; quantitative V/Q may be obtained after inhalation of ^{133}Xe and intravenous injection of ^{99m}Tc; a V/Q 'mismatch' indicates preservation of ventilation with a defect in perfusion, a finding commonly associated with pulmonary embolism Note: The V/Q scan is falsely negative in up to 12% of 'low-probability' scans (PIOPED studies, J Am Med Assoc 1990; 263:2753, 2794); see Lung volumes, Pulmonary panel

V-shaped scar A sharply angulated fibrotic scar on the renal cortical surface, often due to bacterial infection and cortical abscess formation; Cf Rat-bitten kidneys

VTEC Verocytotoxin-producing ***Escherichia coli*** A serotype of ***E coli*** that produces verocytotoxin, a toxin similar to that produced by ***Shigella dysenteriae*** type 1; VTECs include ***E coli*** O157:H7, O4, O5, O26, O111, O125 and O145; two types of verocytotoxin have been isolated from ***E coli*** O157:H7, both of which are protein inhibitors; VT1 is homologous to the Shiga toxin except for a single acid substitution in the A subunit; VT2 is 60% homologous to Shiga toxin and shares the same intestinal cell receptor, globotriosylceramide

v wave CARDIOLOGY The wave in the normal jugular phlebogram corresponding to the atrial diastole

V-Y advance PLASTIC SURGERY A type of surgical advancement incision that allows lengthening of a contracted scar, where a 'Y'-shape is sewn into a V shaped incision

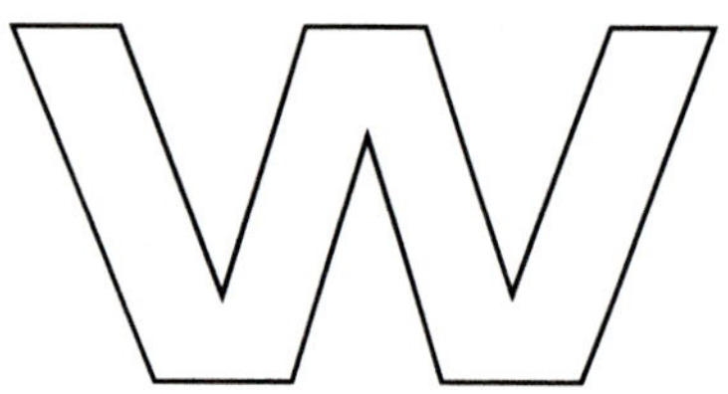

W symbol for: Tryptophan; tungsten; watt; work; writhing number

w symbol for: workshop (see there)

Wagon wheel fracture A fracture of historic interest, characterized by separation of the distal femoral epiphysis; this type of fracture was most common in children, whose legs were inadvertently caught in the western-bound wagon wheels

WAGR syndrome A clinical complex characterized by Wilm's tumor, aniridia, genitourinary abnormalities and retardation (mental); the association between Wilm's tumor (frequency: 1:10 000) and aniridia (frequency: 1:65-100 000) is strong; 1:50 of Wilm's children have aniridia and 1:3 of those with aniridia have Wilm's tumor; the defective gene complex has been localized to chromosome 11p13, near the H-*ras* 1 locus and flanked by the genes encoding catalase and the β subunit of FSH; the gene has a deletion with a balanced translocation which normally encodes a 'zinc-finger' protein; mRNA in situ hybridization analysis of the gene indicates it is well-expressed in developing human urogenital tissues, has a specific role in renal development and a wider role in mesenchymal-epithelial transitions (Nature 1990; 346:194), explaining the multi-system defects of the WAGR syndrome Note: A WAGR murine model was generated by an interspecies backcross between ***Mus musculus*** and ***M spretus*** (Science 1990; 250:823)

'Waiter accepting a tip' sign PEDIATRICS A deformity in which the arm hangs loosely at the side and the partially paralyzed hand is deviated posteriorly, a position fancifully likened to a waiter subtly accepting a pourboir, that may occur in the vaginal delivery of the after-coming head in breech delivery or by extreme lateral flexion of the infant's head in an effort to treat shoulder dystocia, which stretches the upper roots of the brachial plexus, especially C5 and C6 (Erb's palsy), either temporarily or permanently; the lower roots of the brachial plexus are less commonly involved, affecting the small hand muscles and the palmar grasp reflex, causing Klumpke's palsy

Waivered tests see POLs

Walk-in clinic see Ambulatory clinic

Walking, chromosomal see Chromosome walking

'Walking' pneumonia A descriptor for the clinical symptoms typical of the atypical pneumonia caused by ***Mycoplasma pneumoniae*** **Clinical** Usually mild with an insidious onset of malaise, headache and occasionally fever that is followed several days later by an intense, usually nonproductive cough, mixed with scant mucopurulent or hemorrhagic sputum. accompanied by chest tenderness on inspiration; auscultation may reveal wheezes, rhonchi and occasional moist râles; clinical and radiologic improvement of 'walking' bronchopneumonia with pleural effusions may require 2-6 weeks **Treatment** Tetracycline, erythromycin; a live attenuated vaccine is being developed

Walking-through phenomenon CARDIOLOGY Anginal pain that appears while the patient is walking and disappears if he 'walks through' the pain **Mechanism** Unknown

Wall effect LABORATORY MEDICINE The advanced movement of a substance adjacent to the wall of a chromatographic column, due to the increased rate of solvent migration; in contrast, a solvent migrates more slowly in the column's center as it interacts with the column's 'packing' material

Wallerian degeneration A neuropathologic event caused by transection of a peripheral nerve, in which there is axonal and myelin sheath disintegration and digestion by Schwann cells (which are facultative phagocytes) distal to the interruption, while proximal to the transection, the nerve degenerates to the nearest node of Ranvier; if the transection is very proximal, the neuronal cell body undergoes chromatolysis; wallerian degeneration occurs in the ophthalmic, spinocerebellar tracts and posterior columns

Walling-off reaction A tissue response to acute and subacute inflammation, in which the focus of infection or inflammation is 'isolated' and surrounded by fibrosis, serving to seal off the lesion, as occurs in the 'maturation' of an abscess

Wall sign Halo sign GYNECOLOGY A vague radiolucency imparted by the dense fibrous capsule of an ovarian dermoid cyst (mature teratoma), separating different sharply circumscribed tissue densities, often recognized by plain films of the lower abdomen

Walnut brain Narrowed cerebral gyri with widened sulci that occur in extreme atrophy of the frontal and temporal lobes, with relative sparing of the posterior brain, characteristic of Pick's disease; Alzheimer's disease is more globally atrophied, and is said to also affect the parietal lobe, and has been called 'knife blade atrophy'; as atrophy evolves, there is compensatory ventricular enlargement (hydrocephalus ex vacuo)

'Walt Disney' dwarf Geroderma osteoplastica Bamatter syndrome A rare inherited condition characterized by stunting of growth, marked senile changes of the skin with wrinkling, corneal opacification, osteoporosis with multiple bone fractures and deformities; see Progeria

Walter Reed staging A widely used system (table) for clinical staging of AIDS, which requires that the symptoms persist for more than three months, which is further characterized as to the presence of certain symptoms: Persistent constitutional symptoms (B), CNS involvement (C), Kaposi's sarcoma (K), neoplasia (N), and thrombocytopenia (T), N Engl J Med 1986; 314:131; ibid, 315:1357

WALTER REED STAGING

Stage	CD4+*	HIV-1†	CLA‡	Anergy	Thrush
WR 0	> 0.4 x 10^9/L	-	Asymptomatic-		
WR 1	> 0.4 x 10^9/L	+	-	-	-
WR 2	> 0.4 x 10^9/L	+	±	-	-
WR 3	< 0.4 x 10^9/L	+	±	-	-
WR 4	< 0.4 x 10^9/L	+	±	±	-
WR 5	< 0.4 x 10^9/L	+	±	+	-
WR 6	< 0.4 x 10^9/L	+	±	±	+

*CD4 T lymphocytes > 0.4 x 10^9/L (US: > 400/mm^3)
† HIV-1 antibody or antigen present
CLA‡ Chronic lymphadenopathy

Wandering spot technique MOLECULAR BIOLOGY A technique for sequencing synthetic nucleotides, in which the 5'-end of the oligonucleotides is labeled with ^{32}P and then partially digested by phosphodiesterase; the resulting fragments are fractionated by cellulose acetate electrophoresis, then chromatography and the sequence is determined by the patterns of mobility shift of the labeled fragments

Wandering pacemaker CARDIOLOGY An intermittent shift (or suppression) of one cardiac pacemaker, usually the sinus node to another, often the atrio-ventricular node; the contraction gradually increases in length of the cycle, most commonly occurring as an innocuous finding in infants, thought to reflect fluctuations in vagal tone; physical findings in a wandering pacemaker include bradycardia, variability of the first heart sound and size and shape of the 'P' wave

Warfarin An anticoagulant of the coumarin family that inhibits the synthesis of liver-dependent coagulation factors (the prothrombin complex, factors II, VII, IX and X that are formed by γ-carboxylation of the precursor proteins); warfarin is used for long-term prevention of uncomplicated distal deep vein thrombosis, prophylaxis and prevention of cardiogenic thrombo-emboli and for survivors of acute myocardial infarction; in one study, warfarin-treated patients had a 24% reduction in mortality, cerebrovascular accidents and re-infarction (N Engl J Med 1990; 323:147) Note: Coumarins are also effective rodenticides, and have intermittent currency as suicidal vehicles; warfarin therapy is monitored therapeutically by serial evaluation of the prothrombin time (two-to-four-fold the normal of 12 to 16 seconds); its activity is increased by phenylbutazone, clofibrate (by out-competing warfarin for plasma protein binding sites) and decreased by barbiturates, which stimulate hepatic metabolism Note: The agent's development was funded by the Wisconsin Alumni Research Foundation (WARF) in the 1940s (N Engl J Med 1991; 324:1865rv)

Warm agglutinin disease An autoimmune hemolytic syndrome caused by IgG antibodies, 40% of which are secondary to underlying conditions, including neoplasia, eg chronic lymphocytic leukemia, ovarian teratoma, collagen vascular disease, eg lupus erythematosus, progressive systemic sclerosis, rheumatoid arthritis, ulcerative colitis and others Clinical Brisk hemolysis is associated with symptoms of anemia, ie pallor, fatigue, exertional dyspnea, dizziness and palpitations with mild jaundice and splenomegaly Laboratory Moderate to severe anemia with a positive antiglobin (Coombs') test, spherocytes, schistocytes, erythrophagocytosis; bone marrow demonstrates erythroid hyperplasia and may reveal an underlying lymphoproliferative disorder Treatment Blood transfusions; glucocorticoids may ameliorate the hemolysis in two-thirds of patients and 20% may achieve complete remission when maintained with doses above 15-20 mg/day; two-thirds respond to splenectomy, but may relapse; other modalities with varying degrees of failure include immunosuppressive agents and plasmapheresis Prognosis 73% 10-year survival; Cold agglutinin disease

'Warm antibody' TRANSFUSION MEDICINE An antibody or agglutinin (usually IgG) that reacts optimally at 37°C and has an affinity for certain red cell antigens, eg Duffy, Kell, Kidd. MNSs and Rh, and if produced by a blood cell recipient, may cause an immune hemolytic response

'Warm' nodule Nuclear medicine A relatively circumscribed increase in radioisotope concentration seen by radionuclide imaging of the thyroid ('thyroid scan') in which functional thyroid lesions suppress TSH synthesis, but do not cause hyperthyroidism, the latter of which evokes 'hot' nodules; Cf Cold nodule

Warm shock syndrome A complex seen in early septic shock Clinical Normal cardiac activity, no fluid losses, enhanced peripheral perfusion and minimal catecholamine effect

Warning leak NEUROSURGERY A minor early hemorrhage that occurs in an evolving subarachnoid hematoma or hemorrhage, which is followed by the abrupt onset of an often severe headache, variably accompanied by nuchal stiffness; since significant subarachnoid hemorrhage is fatal if untreated; they must be recognized early, treated aggressively and the underlying pathology, eg angiomatous malformations, neoplasia and trauma addressed

Warts Verruciform lesions of mucocutaneous surfaces induced by papovaviruses that are the single most common reason for dermatologic consultation, most often affect children and adolescents and include the well-described benign 'usual' types, eg the common wart (verruca vulgaris), filiform wart, plantar wart and juvenile flat wart; the clinical course of warts ranges from spontaneous involution, not uncommon in flat warts to extreme recalcitrance, typical of periungual and moist plantar warts Histopathology Hyperplastic epithelium, koilocytosis, basophilic intranuclear inclusions (viral particles), parakeratosis, papillomatosis and eosinophilic cytoplasmic inclusions (keratohyalin) Treatment 'Benign neglect' and 'abracadabra therapy' are most effective in young children (implying a component of biofeedback control of the immune system), chemocautery (5-20% formalin, phenol-nitric acid-salicylic acid and podophyllin), electro-dissection, X-ray (narrow field, low dose) and DCNB immunotherapy Note: The human papilloma virus-induced and premalignant giant condyloma acuminatum of Buschke-Loewenstein are located on 'sexual' mucosae, most common on the uncircumcised penis and may betransmitted to females

Washboard scalp see Cutis verticis gyrata

Washed red cells TRANSFUSION MEDICINE Erythrocytes that have been washed in sterile saline (first with a 'light' spin to remove and/or salvage plasma, followed if desired, by 3 to 5 'heavy' spins) prior to transfusion, a process that removes most leukocytes, lytic mediators and non-self antigens; washed cells are most useful in IgA-deficient patients who have circulating anti-IgA antibodies, reducing the incidence of febrile, urticarial and anaphylactic reactions Note: Although washing of red cells reduces febrile, non-hemolytic transfusion reactions, because it is labor-intensive, 'exposes' the unit to air and pathogens, and if not transfused within 24 hours, the unit must be discarded, cells are only routinely washed in patients who have previously had a non-hemolytic transfusion reaction, an event that occurs in approximately 1:40 transfusions, which does not respond to the use of blood filters; see Blood filters

'Washerwoman' skin Superficial cutaneous rugosity, likened to those who have their hands immersed in water for prolonged periods, which later become dry and chapped, these latter known as 'dish-pan hands' FORENSIC PATHOLOGY Markedly rugose skin of the hands and feet seen in bodies recovered from water ('floaters'), the intensity of which is a function of the time immersed and water temperature, occurring as quickly as one-half hour at 15-20°C; the relatively loose skin may slough off in 'gloves' PEDIATRICS The skin of post-term infants that is loose and dry, has been likened to parchment or washer-woman's skin; alternatively, the loss of skin turgor caused by prolonged diarrhea of cholera may cause a similar appearance

Washington monument crystals A descriptor for the opaque red-brown, tetragonal rod-like hemoglobin crystals with rigid, parallel sides and tapered ends seen inside and outside of red cells in homozygous hemoglobinopathy C, best seen on a Wright-Giemsa-stained peripheral blood smear; similar crystals may also occur in heterozygous hemoglobin C, eg hemoglobin C-S, hemoglobin C-thalassemia and in hereditary persistence of Hemoglobin F

Wasp waist A descriptor for the body of a person affected by Löwenthal's disease, a familial condition with a thin waist, relatively enlarged pelvic and shoulder girdles, hyperextended and atonic extremities, muscular sclerosis and rhizomelic contractions

Wasserhellezellen see Water clear cells

Wastage, fetal Any loss of a gestational product, either voluntary or involuntary that occurs between the 20th week of pregnancy and the 28th day of life, a value known for epidemiological purposes, as 'total pregnancy wastage'

Waste see Biohazardous waste, Hazardous waste, Regulated waste

Wasting disease(s) see Runt disease, Kwashiorkor

'Wasting syndrome' A nonspecific clinical complex associated with chronic renal insufficiency, attributed to a combination of poor nutrition, endocrine dysfunction and catabolic stresses, including infection, uremia and dialysis

Water bath A water-filled vessel, usually large enough to hold one or more racks of test tubes, the temperature of which is stringently controlled by a thermostat, often set at a physiological temperature, eg 37°C for a biological system

Waterbed A bed with a water-filled mattress Therapeutic uses NEONATOLOGY Oscillating waterbeds in preterm infants provide compensatory movement stimulation, reducing uncomplicated apnea of prematurity, with increased periods of quiet sleep, decreased periods of crying/fussiness and enhanced growth; non-oscillating waterbeds are of use in treating narcotic-exposed neonates, one studied group had significantly lower central nervous system subscores, required less medication to control withdrawal symptoms and had an earlier onset of consistent weight gain (Am J Dis Child 1988; 142:186) GASTROENTEROLOGY Waterbed users are reported to be either five times more likely to suffer from reflux esophagitis (J Am Med Assoc 1987; 257:2033), or are at no increased risk for reflux (measured by pH monitors, Dig Dis Sci 1989; 34:1585)

Water-born infection see Tapwater infection

Water bottle heart A descriptor for the globose cardiac shadow typical of large pericardial effusions (effusions of less than 250 ml are radiologically 'silent'); pericardial effusions may be serous (due to congestive heart failure or decreased proteins in nephrotic syndrome, hepatic failure, malnutrition), sero-sanguinous (blunt chest trauma, cardiopulmonary resuscitation), chylous (lymphatic obstruction, one-half of which are caused by malignancy) and cholesterol ('pseudo-chylous' effusion, either idiopathic or related to myxedema)

Water brash Foam at the mouth Hypersalivation characteristic of reflux esophagitis (variably accompanied by chronic blood loss, anemia, aspiration, regurgitation and recurrent pneumonitis)

Water-clear cell Wasserhellezell A variant, glycogen-rich parathyroid chief cell (the glycogen may be lost in tissue processing) that is clear, large and may form distinct tubules

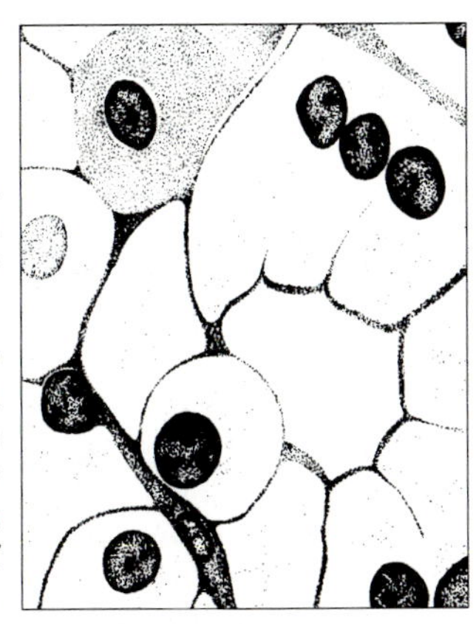

Water-clear cell

Water-clear cell hyperplasia Parathyroid gland A condition that has been less frequently diagnosed in recent years which, unlike chief cell hyperplasia, is neither familial nor associated with multiple endocrine adenomatosis; it is characterized by massive parathyroid gland enlargement, up to 100 g, associated with hyperparathyroidism and hypercalciuric hypercalcemia Pathology Combined hypertrophy and hyperplasia, coalescence of glands forming large brown cystic and hemorrhagic masses, and cells with 'water-clear' cytoplasm, minute scattered eosinophilic granules arranged in an 'alveolar' pattern

Watered silk appearance A pattern of wavy, glistening fascicles seen by gross examination of the surface of granulosa cell tumors of the ovary and uterine leiomyomata

Waterfall phenomenon Clinical toxicology The paralysis of a complex chain of enzymatic events at the beginning of the 'cascade' of reactions, eg intoxication of the cytochrome oxidase system by cyanide; by the time the respiratory paralysis first manifests itself, as occurs in nitroprusside poisoning, therapeutic attempts at removing the cyanide are fruitless

Water hammer pulse A booming, bounding or pistol-shot-like sound auscultated in a large patent ductus arteriosus (PDA) (smaller PDAs may be asymptomatic or have a 'machinery murmur'); the so-called 'small water hammer pulse' is due to a brisk rise in systemic arterial pulse pressure in the face of normal pulse pressure

Waterhouse-Friderichsen (WF) syndrome Massive hemorrhagic necrosis of the adrenal glands that may be confined to the zona reticularis or zona medularis or affect the entire gland and is most commonly caused by *Neisseria meningitidis*, but may occur with infections by *Streptococcus pneumoniae*, staphylococci, *Haemophilus influenzae*, or less commonly, result from hypoxia during a difficult labor and delivery

Watering-pot perineum Urology A descriptor for a complication of trauma to the urethra and covering structures (as may occur in urethral surgery), in which multiple fistulas associated with inflammatory strictures and diverticuli develop parallel to the urethra and penetrate tissues of the perineum and scrotum, forming draining sinuses; as the patient voids, infected urine is forced into these tracts, and the urine dribbles from multiple, watering-pot-like pores

Water intoxication Acute or chronic hyperhydration due to excess ingestion of water, causing dilutional hyponatremia; the condition is most common in patients with psychiatric or neurologic disease, and may be accompanied by impaired renal water excretion and increased secretion of antidiuretic hormone; acute water intoxication may also occur in normal subjects attempting to produce urine to elevate the bladder for pelvicultrasonography or for drug testing (J Am Med Assoc 1991; 265:84cr)

Water lily sign Radiology A cyst in the lung or liver with a laminated collapsed capsule and floating scolices outlined by air within the cyst, a finding typical of hydatid or echinococcal disease; see Hydatid sand

Watermelon stomach A pattern of tortuous vessels along the longitudinal folds of the stomach, radiating from the pylorus toward the antrum, fancifully likened to a watermelon's stripes, a finding characteristic of angiodysplasia of the gastric antrum, Cf 'Emperor's new clothes' syndrome

Watershed infarction Neurology An infarction of a region that is peripheral to two arteries and susceptible to ischemia; watershed infarctions occur in the brain after internal carotid artery occlusion, causing vascular 'steal' phenomena, or between the anterior and middle cerebral arteries that are compromised in circle of Willis occlusions, often in a background of generalized atherosclerosis and as a possible complication of directed therapeutic embolization (Arch Pathol Lab Med 1989; 13:1139); the cerebral perfusion may be impaired due to cardiac arrest, pericardial tamponade and exsanguination; these infarctions are often hemorrhagic, as restoration of the circulation allows blood to flow into damaged capillaries and 'leak' into cerebral tissue; watershed infarction may also occur in the large intestine at either the splenic flexure, the site of anastomosis between the inferior and superior mesenteric arteries, or at the rectum, a region supplied by peripheral irrigation from the inferior mesenteric artery and the hypogastric artery

Water softening The conversion of 'hard' (mineral ion-laden) water to soft water by ion exchange chromatography, which may be required for certain chemical reactions and for the optimal functioning of laboratory instruments

Water-soluble fibers Clinical nutrition Indigestible substances that are concentrated in certain foods, eg fruits, dried beans, legumes, guar gums, barley, psyllium and oat cereals, that increase the stool bulk and lower LDL-cholesterol; see Bran, Dietary fiber

Waters' position Radiology A position used to visualize the facio-maxillary bones and maxillary sinuses and determine the patency of the maxillary sinuses, in which the patient is placed at a 37° angle with the orbitomeatal line, perpendicular to the mid-sagittal plane

Water-suppressed nuclear magnetic resonance spectrum of plasma is predominantly a reflection of the resonances of plasma lipoprotein lipids (triglycerides), a spectrum which narrows in most malignancy and was initially reported as a potential screening assay formalignancy (N Engl J Med 1986; 315:1369)

Watery diarrhea-hypokalemia-achlorhydria syndrome see WDHA syndrome

Watson-Crick DNA The model of DNA, now known as B-DNA, proposed by James Watson and Francis Crick in their seminal paper, '*GENERAL IMPLICATIONS OF THE STRUCTURE OF DEOXYRIBONUCLEIC ACID*' in Nature (1953; 171:737), which was the founding event of molecular biology; see Central dogma, DNA, Human Genome Project

Wave front phenomenon CARDIOLOGY Thefinding that an increased time-span of coronary artery occlusion results in the expansion of a small subendocardial infarct into a larger transmural myocardial infarct, seemingly spreading in waves

Wavelet theory A mathematical model of universal phenomena Background: Fourier analysis, the current paradigm of data analysis, assumes that all data sets in the universe can be defined as sine and cosine curves, stretching to infinity and all subsets of data are miniature versions of the original sine/cosine curve; Fourier analysis is widely used to address such broadly divergent areas as weather prediction and computed tomographic (CT) imaging; there are two major disadvantages of Fourier transforms: 1) 'Peaks' and 'dips' of data (a normal event in an imperfect and chaotic universe), require that the entire data set be re-analyzed whenever these 'imperfections' are encountered and 2) Gaps in data cause the analytic algorithm to screech to a halt, requiring educated 'guesswork' to fill in the gaps; wavelet theory, instead of the sine/cosine curve stretching to infinity, uses a building block known as a 'mother wavelet', concentrated in an interval between 0 and 1; the daughter wavelets are created by moving the mother wavelet left or right in unit steps and dilating or compressing it by repeated factors of 2, an analogy that is extremely similar to musical notation; wavelet analysis, although in its infancy, is considered a theoretical advancement over the Fourier transform, potentially having applications for data compression of digitalized images, artificial intelligence, synthesis of speech and music and in improving computer tomography images (Science 1990; 249:858rn); Cf Chaos, Fourier analysis, Fractal analysis

Wavy changes Contraction bands CARDIAC PATHOLOGY The undulent kinking of cardiac muscle (figure, right) typical of early myocardial infarction, often seen within one hour of myocardial ischemia, involving random, focal individual myocytes, patches or extensive areas of the myo-cardium, usually at the border of the infarct, thought to be due to pulling of noncontracting dead fibers by adjacent viable myocytes; infarct borders are further characterized by vacuolar degeneration or myocytolysis, consisting of fine lipid droplets or large rounded cytoplasmic spaces (filled with water, scant glycogen and lipid) with a peripheral rim of sarcoplasm, seen in viable myocytes

Wax doll appearance see Porcelain doll appearance

Waxy casts NEPHROLOGY Homogeneous cylindrical structures seen in the urine by low-power light microscopy, which have a high refractile index (hyaline casts are morphologically similar but are not refractile) and correspond to the degenerated cellular casts typical of long-term oliguria and obstruction of the tubules, as occurs in chronic renal failure, acute and chronic renal rejection and amyloidosis; very broad waxy casts or 'renal failure' casts are typical of end-stage renal failure

Waxy degeneration Zenker's degeneration Acidophilic hyalinization of muscle, seen by light microscopy and considered the first step in segmental muscular necrosis; waxy degeneration may be induced by ischemia, trauma, temperature extremes, infections (scarlet fever, smallpox, typhoid fever, diphtheria, leptospirosis) and dehydration

Waxy exudates Retinitis pigmentosa Tapetoretinal degeneration OPHTHALMOLOGY A descriptor for the 'hard', yellow-white macular aggregates of fatty and proteinaceous material that leak into the retina through thinned and atrophied capillaries, seen in diabetes mellitus, causing decreased visual acuity

WC Fields nose A fanciful descriptor for end-stage acne rosacea, which affects middle-aged adults, characterized by proliferation of sebaceous glands and fibrous tissue, edema, erythema, telangiectasias, follicular and parafollicular abscessification, and eventually rhinophyma; it is cosmetically unesthetic with unpredictable flushing, which becomes especially prominent when eating spicy foods, coffee or when overindulging in alcohol (with which acne rosacea is classically associated) Treatment Topical metronidazole (J Am Med Assoc 1989; 261:2014), tetracycline, CO_2 laser, which in the defocused mode, bloodlessly vaporizes the skin Note: WC Fields was a vaudevillian artist cum legendary Hollywood comic actor of the 1930s and 1940s, famed for his inebriation and bulbous, pustular, bright pink bibulous proboscis

WDHA syndrome Watery diarrhea-hypokalemia-achlorhydria syndrome of Verner-Morrison, Pancreatic 'cholera' A disease complex due to increased serum VIP (vasoactive intestinal polypeptide), caused by a VIPoma, a pancreatic islet cell tumor, one-half of which are malignant, composed of clusters of insulinogenic B cells,

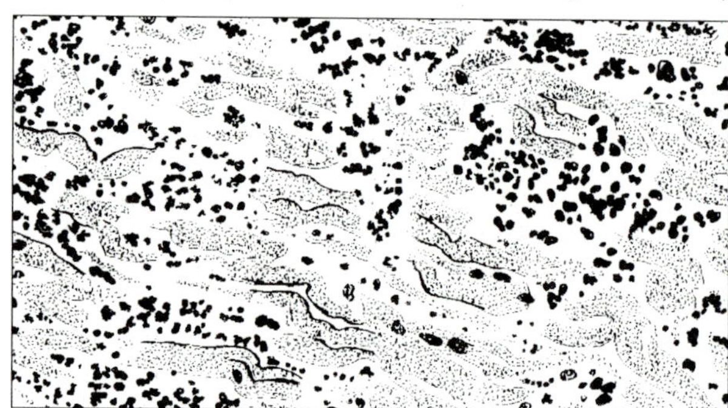

Wavy changes

glucagon-producing A-cells, somatostatin-producing D cells and pancreatic polypeptide-producing PP cells Clinical Profuse watery diarrhea, severe hypokalemia, achlorhydria, dehydration and shock, increased or decreased glucose, increased calcium, hypotension and episodic flushing; WDHA in children is associated with ganglioneuromas Note: 12% of VIPomas cause WDHA, an association that is not uncommon in the context of multiple endocrine neoplasia (MEN) type I

Weaning Wean, Old English, to accustom CRITICAL CARE MEDICINE The transferral of a patient's dependence on mechanical ventilation to spontaneous auto-regulated breathing, which requires that the indications for the use of mechanical ventilation no longer exist and the patient responds to verbal commands, is stable (circulation, normal chest films, no abdominal distension) and not be receiving muscle relaxants; the single best predictor of successful 'wean-ability ' is a low ratio of respiratory frequency to tidal volume (f/V_t); rapid shallow breathing after removal from mechanical supports accurately predicts failure (N Engl J Med 1991; 324:1445); see Pulmonary function tests, V/Q ratio

Weanling diarrhea Weaning diarrhea PEDIATRICS A condition occurring in a background of poor sanitation, commonly occurring in children in developing nations, affecting infants between 6-24 months of age, and a major cause of infant mortality in developing nations; weaning from maternal milk results in exposure of the infant to new organisms, deterioration of nutrition (a mechanism similar to kwashiorkor) and loss of the passively transferred IgA Clinical Acute, sporadic and watery diarrhea, low-grade fever and variable vomiting, most common in the summer months; in a well-nourished child, the process resolves in 2-3 days with adequate hydration, in the malnourished child, the diarrhea persists and may be associated with comorbidity Agents Enterotoxic ***Escherichia coli***, rotavirus and occasionally ***Shigella*** Diagnosis Ultrastructure of stool, counter-immunoelectrophoresis, enzyme-linked immunosorbent assay

Web Esophageal web A two-to-three mm in thickness stricture composed of mucosa and submucosa only (the term 'ring' is used when muscle is present, thus Schatzki's 'ring' is a misnomer), located anywhere along the length of the esophageal lumen; upper esophageal webs occur in the upper 2-4 cm of the esophagus, are lined by squamous epithelium, often associated with the Plummer-Vinson(-Paterson-Brown-Kelly) syndrome and after years may evolve into postcricoid carcinoma; webs in the body of the esophagus may be multiple, possibly representing embryonal remnants and may be associated with esophageal reflux; the lower esophageal web (or ring) of Schatzki is a thin membrane marking the squamocolumnar junction that is seen in about 10% of normal subjects; symptomatic subjects may suffer intermittent dysphagia and impaction of a bolus of bread or meat Treatment Intraluminal balloon dilation

Webbed neck Pterygium colli A sphinx-like neck characterized by a thick web of skin that extends from behind the ears to the distal clavicle and to the acromial process, classically described in Turner gonadal dysgenesis syndrome, but also seen in the fetal hydantoin, Noonan and trisomy 18 syndromes

Webster decision SOCIAL MEDICINE, OBSTETRICS A legal decision rendered in 1989 by the US Supreme Court (Webster *vs* Reproductive Health Services, 109 S Ct 3040, 1989) that represents a change in the 'officia'l position on a woman's right to have an abortion; the Court ruled on an abortion in the State of Missouri, and concluded that a state could constitutionally prohibit state-employed physicians from performing an abortion that is not necessary to save the mother's life, could prohibit the abortion from being performed in state-owned facilities and could require that the physicians attempt to determine fetal viability on or after the 20th week of gestation (N Engl J Med 1989; 321:1200); see Cf 'Gag rule', Mexico City policy

'Wedding ring' appearance CARDIAC PATHOLOGY A fanciful term for a regurgitating mitral valve deformity, where the valve ring and commissures are calcified, and 'frozen' in an opened position

Wedge fracture A sharply angulated post-traumatic fracture of the spine, most common in the thoracic vertebrae, usually with anterior wedging seen in a background of osteoporosis; Cf Teardrop fracture

Wedge pressure CARDIOLOGY A method for assessing cardiopulmonary pressure gradients; a Swan-Ganz catheter is inserted into a large systemic vein, 'threaded' through the right atrium under continuous pressure monitoring; the tip is then inflated and carried by the blood flow through the right ventricle and 'wedges' into a pulmonary arteriole, with the vessel being occluded by the balloon at the catheter tip, yielding close approximation of the left arterial or left ventricular filling pressures; the Swan-Ganz catheter also permits serial evaluation of cardiac output and access to the central oxygen supply

Wedge resection GYNECOLOGIC SURGERY A cuneiform section from an ovary which, by an unknown mechanism, may induce ovulation in polycystic ovaries, usually being performed after clomiphene and gonadotropic therapy have failed to correct infertility in women with Stein-Leventhal (polycystic ovary) syndrome

Wedge shadow RADIOLOGY A vaguely-defined radiopacity extending from the pulmonary hilum, which is thought to be characteristic of pulmonary edema

WEE see Western equine encephalitis

Weight-cycling hypothesis METABOLISM A hypothesis that holds that fluctuations in body weight have negative health consequences, including increased total mortality and increased mortality from coronary heart disease, independent of obesity and the trend of body weight over time (N Engl J Med 1991; 324:1839, 1887ed)

Weight-lifter's headache Severe headache and neck pain due to wrenching or tearing of cervical ligaments during the strain of exertion

Weil-Felix test LABORATORY MEDICINE A test in which agglutinins from non-motile strains (OX-19, OX-2 and OX-K) of ***Proteus vulgaris*** are used to serologically identify rickettsial organisms; Weil-Felix (W-F) reactions vary in sensitivity and are relatively non-specific;

false positivity is common and occurs in other infections, eg urinary tract infections, leptospirosis, borreliosis, hepatic or biliary tract; W-F agglutination occurs with the OX-2 and OX-19 strains in the spotted fever group (*R rickettsii, R conorii, R siberica* and *R australis*); the typhus group (*R prowasecki, R typhi*) agglutinates with OX-19 alone; *R tsutsugamushi* reacts with the OK-X antigen; *Rickettsia akari, Coxiella burnetii* and *Rochalimaea quintana* do not react with any OX antigens

Welding bodies OCCUPATIONAL MEDICINE Structures associated with asbestosis that are more common than asbestos bodies, and have a golden-brown, iron-rich coating and a central opaque core particle(s) composed of metal of carbon; unlike asbestos bodies, the iron coating is probably of exogenous origin, and is seen in digested samples of lung from welders; see Asbestos bodies

Well LABORATORY TECHNOLOGY A hole with sharp vertical margins that is cut into a 'slab' of gel, and into which an aliquot of a specimen, eg DNA, RNA or protein is placed at the beginning of electrophoresis

Wells *vs.* Ortho decision see Litogen

Wen Old English, a lump A protuberance anywhere on the body, commonly referring to a sebaceous cyst on the head

'Wendy dilemma' PSYCHIATRY A marital situation in which the wife is trapped into mothering the husband, although it reinforces his immature behavior, a term that derives from the children's story, Peter Pan, in which Wendy is the surrogate mother to the Lost Boys in the magical kingdom of Neverland; see Peter Pan and Wendy syndrome

Werther effect PUBLIC HEALTH An increased suicide rate that is alleged to occur after media coverage of suicide(s), or in individuals 'inspired' by reading about or having had a close personal relationship with a 'successful' suicide; the effect, if real, is most common in young males (suicide rate, ages 15-19, $14/10^5$ versus female $3.2/10^5$); the term derives from Goethe's The Sorrows of Young Werther, a story about a sentimental and daydreaming young man who fatally shoots himself; the story was blamed, when it was published in 1774 for a rash of young adult suicides and was banned in Milan, Leipzig and Copenhagen (N Engl J Med 1986; 315:705)

Westergren method A method for determining erythrocyte sedimentation rate (ESR), in which the blood is placed in EDTA in a tube measuring 30 cm in length X 2.5 cm in diameter Normal rate: 0-10 mm/hour in men; 0-20 mm/hour in women; since the Westergren method is inaccurate in renal failure and the values are increased in anemia, the zetacrit has become the ESR method of choice; see Zetacrit

Westermark sign An abrupt radiologic 'cutoff' in pulmonary vessels seen in a standard antero-posterior chest film in pulmonary embolism without infarction, often accompanied by dilation of vessels before the cutoff, eg the right descending pulmonary artery; the sign is also seen in other intravascular occlusions, most commonly in bronchogenic carcinoma, as well as in interstitial pulmonary fibrosis, histoplasmosis, pulmonary arteritis, parasitic embolism (*Schistosoma haematobium, S mansoni*), Swyer-Jones disease, or intravascular sarcoma (Acta Radiol 1938; 19:357)

Western blot Immunoblot MOLECULAR BIOLOGY A technique that identifies antibodies to proteins of specific molecular weights, of particular use for confirming HIV-1 antibody screening assays performed by the ELISA technique (Anal Biochem 1981; 112:195) Technique The proteins are separated by one- or two-dimensional electrophoresis, then transferred (blotted) to a nitrocellulose or nylon membrane that is then exposed to radioactively-labelled or biotinylated antibody; the antigen of interest is detected either by autoradiography or directly, by using a biotinylated antibody (Proc Natl Acad Sci 1979; 76:3116); see Blots; Cf Southern blotting

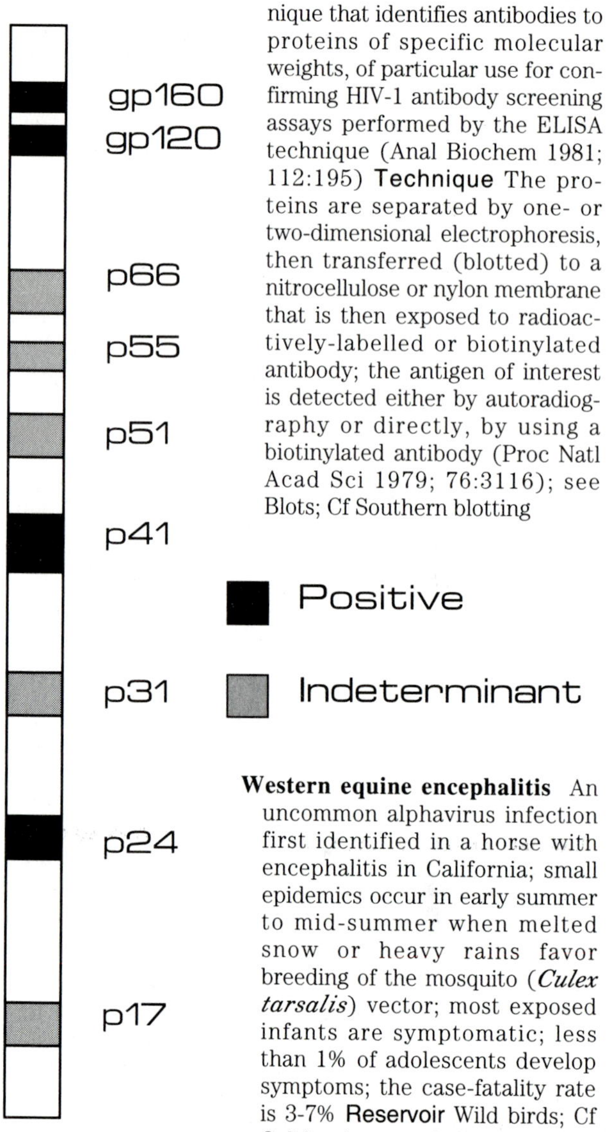

gp160
gp120
p66
p55
p51
p41
p31
p24
p17
Positive
Indeterminant

Western equine encephalitis An uncommon alphavirus infection first identified in a horse with encephalitis in California; small epidemics occur in early summer to mid-summer when melted snow or heavy rains favor breeding of the mosquito (*Culex tarsalis*) vector; most exposed infants are symptomatic; less than 1% of adolescents develop symptoms; the case-fatality rate is 3-7% Reservoir Wild birds; Cf California encephalitis, Eastern equine encephalitis, Japanese B encephalitis, St Louis encephalitis

Westgard's multirule LABORATORY MEDICINE A set of quality control guidelines for the clinical laboratory that act to ensure consistent and accurate results for analytes; see Multirule procedure, Quality control

West Indies ataxic syndrome see Tropical spastic paraparesis

West Nile fever An acute, mosquito (*Culex*)-borne flaviviral infection that is endemic (occasionally, epidemic) in regions of the Near East Clinical Following a 3-6 day incubation, children present with a non-specific febrile illness; older patients develop a dengue-like disease with fever, rash that clears without desquamation, frontal headaches, orbital pain, backaches, myalgia, anorexia, lymphadenopathy and leukopenia, sore throat and potentially meningoencephalitis in the elderly; usually it is self-limited, resolving in a week

Westphal-Leyden syndrome Acute ataxia An autosomal dominant disease of childhood that progesses to death within 10 years of onset Clinical Vertigo, vomiting, proximal muscular rigidity, convulsive seizures and mental defects

Westphal-Piltz reflex NEUROLOGY Neurotonic pupillary contraction following vigorous closing of the eyes with delayed reaction to light

Westphal sign NEUROLOGY Absence of knee jerk reflex in tabes dorsalis; see Neurosyphilis

West syndrome Massive myoclonus Infantile encephalopathy with arrest of psychomotor development, mental retardation, seizures and secondary generalized epilepsy, which may be accompanied by immune dysfunction and death at an early age due to bronchopneumonia; myoclonus may be an integral component of the Lennox-Gestaut syndrome; see Salaam convulsions

'West-to-east' phenomenon EPIDEMIOLOGY A poorly understood difference in the seasonal peaks in the annual rotavirus epidemic in North America; the epidemic reaches a maximum in Mexico and the Southwestern United States in late fall; the Midwestern US peaks in mid-winter and the incidence of rotavirus infections in Eastern US and Canada peaks in early spring (J Am Med Assoc 1990; 264:983)

Wet cerumen Earwax Cerumen may be 'dry' or 'wet', and the differences appear to be inherited; increased wet cerumen production is associated with breast carcinoma, a 'logical' association, as both are modified apocrine glands; Oriental women with wet cerumen are two-to-three times more likely to have proliferative breast disease or atypical hyperplasia, possibly related to an as-yet unidentified polymorphous trait that influences susceptibility (Breast Cancer Res 1990; 16:279)

Wet gangrene see Gangrene

Wet lung see Adult respiratory distress syndrome

'Wet shop' A 'hands-on' workshop designed to introduce a group of individuals to a technique, eg immunoperoxidase, in situ hybridization, polymerase chain reaction, with which they need to be familiar for research or diagnostic purposes; wet shops are sponsored by either academic institutions or companies interested in selling products related to the technique; Cf Workshop

Whalebone in a corset sign An arched configuration seen by barium studies in a semirigid, indurated superficial gastric carcinoma as it partially yields to outside pressure; in contrast, the classic ulcerating adenocarcinoma is rigid, see Meniscus sign of Carmen; Cf Quarter moon sign

Wheal-and-flare reaction IMMUNOLOGY A test for immediate hypersensitivity ('reaginic' or allergic reaction) to an antigen; the skin is scratched with the antigen and if reactive, reveals a characteristic erythema ('flare') and edema (wheal), a phenomenon seen in atopic individuals due to formation and release of IgE, a Gel and Coombs type I hypersensivity reaction; see P-K test

Wheat sheaves appearance A descriptor for the crystals seen in acid urine (pH < 5.0), which is most common in the face of dehydration, and concomitant sulfonamide, eg acetylsulfisoxazole, sulfadiazine, or less commonly, ampicillin therapy; the presence of sulfonamides is confirmed by diazotization of the free amino group, yielding a magenta color; a similar appearance is associated with hypertyrosinemia, in which there are fine silky needles, which may also form rosette or arrowhead structures

WHHL rabbit Watanabe hereditable hyperlipidemic rabbit An animal model for the study of atherosclerosis described by Watanabe (Kobe university, 1978); see Atherosclerosis, Cholesterol, LDL, Lipoprotein lipase

Whiff test GYNECOLOGY A clinical test in which vaginal secretions are mixed with 10% KOH, resulting in a fishy odor highly suggestive of bacterial vaginosis; see Vaginosis

Whiplash EMERGENCY MEDICINE Hyperextension injury to the neck, often the result of being struck from behind by a fast-moving vehicle, in an automobile accident; whiplash injuries have been markedly reduced by the high-backed headrests now standard in automobiles in the US; see Steering wheel syndrome

Whiplash shaken infant syndrome FORENSIC MEDICINE A form of severe child abuse that may be either fatal or leave its victim with permanent neurological sequelae; severe shaking of an infant who has virtually no neck muscle tone may cause bilateral subdural hematomas (resulting from laceration of the veins bridging the dura mater and cerebral cortex caused by rapid acceleration and deceleration as the chin strikes the chest and the occipital bone strikes the back), subarachnoid and retinal hemorrhage, cerebral edema and cortical contusions without signs of external cranial trauma Notes: 1) Skull fractures are uncommon given the relative softness of neonatal bone; the whiplash shaken infant injury occurs when an adult (often in a state of uncontrolled anger) holds the child by the upper body and violently shakes him 2) Similar lesions may occur when a parent 'rough-house' plays with the child and swings him in a circle or tosses him up and down; thus other signs of child abuse must be investigated (Am Fam Prac 1990; 41:1145); see Battered child syndrome, Bucket handle fracture; Cf Infanticide

Whipple's disease A malabsorption syndrome with rod-shaped bacteria-like forms, which is presumed to be infectious, although no organism has been consistently isolated from patient specimens Clinical Most common in middle-aged men; male:female ratio, 10:1, and accompanied by acropachyia digestiva, diarrhea, steatorrhea, arthritis, lymphadenopathy and central nervous system alterations (demyelination of the posterior columns may occur); the bacilliform inclusions occur in the skin, nervous system, joints, heart, vessels, kidney, lung, serosal membranes, lymph nodes spleen and liver Histopathology Histiocytes in Whipple's disease are similar to Gaucher's disease; definitive confirmation of the Whipple's disease particles requires high-power PAS-stained light microscopy or low-power electron microscopy Treatment Penicillin with streptomycin for two weeks, followed by tetracycline for one year; Cf

Pseudo-Whipple's disease

Whipworm *Trichuris trichiura* The nematode agent of the world's most common parasitic infection, which is transmitted by the oral-fecal route, occurring in a background of poor hygiene **Clinical** Vague abdominal complaints, colic, abdominal distension and when massive, mild anemia, bloody diarrhea and rectal prolapse **Treatment** Mebendazol

Whisker hair Short dark hair of the scalp that resembles pubic hair, first seen during puberty, often later developing into severe androgenic alopecia; whisker hair is a variant of acquired progressive kinky hair (Arch Dermatol 1985; 121;1031); see Kinky hair (Menke's) syndrome, Pili torti, Woolly hair syndrome

Whiskering appearance Short, linear spiculation seen by plain films of bone at the sites of muscle insertion and osseous stress, variably accompanied by osteosclerosis, cystic changes and dystrophic calcification, most common in the iliac, ischial and calcaneus bones, due to ankylosing spondylitis, DISH, in renal osteodystrophy

Whiskey test ENDOCRINOLOGY A stimulatory test for determining calcitonin levels; 50 ml of 'Scotch' is administered per os to patients with medullary thyroid carcinoma; within 15 minutes, calcitonin increases to levels comparable to those produced by calcium infusions; false negativity is uncommon **Side effects** Diarrhea and flushing, due to stimulation of hormonal release by alcohol

'Whistle-blowing' RESEARCH ETHICS The act of informing authorities of a person's alleged wrong-doings; 'whistle-blowing' in science is used in the context of research fraud, alleged fraud or blatant misinterpretation of data; the whistle-blower may take several levels of action ranging from the mere mention of an 'incident' to a colleague to the reporting of the improprieties to the individual's superiors, granting agency, academic institution or to a major peer-reviewed journal; junior people, eg post-doctorate fellows and graduate students in the academic hierarchy are in a position to recognize data manipulation at the 'bench' level (they also have the most to lose should they 'blow the whistle' on their superiors); a number of scientists at the National Institutes of Health (USA) have shifted their research interests and are actively examining cases of alleged fraud, embarking on so-called 'witch-hunts'; see Baltimore affair, 'Dingellization', Fraud in science, Qui tam suits

Whistling face syndrome of Freeman Craniocarpotarsal syndrome An autosomal dominant condition with a typical mask-like physiognomy (small 'pursed' lips, deep-set eyes, epicanthus, hypoplastic nasal alae, strabismus, blepharophimosis and ptosis), accompanied by failure to thrive, normal intelligence, short stature, scoliosis, 'windmill hands' and talipes equinovarus or clubfoot

White atrophy Milian syndrome Whitish scleroderma-like plaque(s) with ulceration present on the skin of the lower extremities of females, secondary to venous stasis

'White beverages' CLINICAL NUTRITION PEDIATRICS Imitation milks and nondairy milk substitutes, eg soy milk that are used in developed nations for children who are allergic to milk and milk products and are used in developing economies where animal fats are in short supply; see Breast milk, Unpasteurized milk

White blood cell differential (count) see 'Diff'

White coat hypertension A transient increase in blood pressure that occurs in apprehensive patients when faced with the 'white coat' of the physician, especially when the patient is female and the doctor male, possibly resulting in inappropriate anti-hypertensive therapy (J Am Med Assoc 1988; 259:225, 2847); this form of pseudohypertension may be prevented by either having a nurse or technician measure the pressure or by measuring the pressure after a physical examination; Cf Pseudohypertension, Small cuff syndrome

White eye reflex see Cat's eye reflex

White fat Usual adipose tissue, which contrasts with brown fat

White forelock Piebaldism A striking focal depigmentation of hair affecting the anterior scalp margin, which has no clinical significance of its own, but is typical of Klein-Waardenburg syndrome (an autosomal dominant condition characterized by leukoderma, a flattened nasal bridge and cochlear deafness), and may also be seen in tuberous sclerosis and Vogt-Koyanagi syndrome Note: piebaldism is a form of poliosis, localized depigmentation of the hair, especially of the scalp that may be due to alopecia areata, radiotherapy, severe localized dermatitis and vitiligo

'White' graft An anemic, ie 'white', transplantation tissue, eg skin or renal graft that is undergoing hyperacute rejection with overwhelming anoxia; vascularization is prevented from occurring since, although the host and graft vessels are successfully anastomosed, the arteries are immediately occluded by preformed antibodies, causing immediate infarction, necessitating a nephrectomy; see Rejection

Whitehead Closed comedo, milium Papular, millet seed-sized skin lesions in the 'sebaceous zones', characterized by aggregates of impacted keratin and sebaceous material, which may rupture 'spontaneously' when infected by ***Propionibacterium acnes***

Whitehead Institute RESEARCH A non-profit independent research and teaching affiliate of the Massachusetts Institute of Technology that was founded in 1982 by a gift from EC Whitehead **Research activities** at 'the Whitehead' encompass RNA polymerase II, protein folding, myosin, viral oncogenesis, sex chromosomes, adult diabetes mellitus, AIDS pathogenesis, AIDS vaccine and others **Director** GR Fink **Budget** (1990) $18.7 million Note: The Whitehead Institute has an enviably high citation impact in biomedical research, and thus is considered a 'high-power' institution; see Citation impact; Cf Howard Hughes Medical Institute

Whitehead's operation(s) Obsolete term for excision of tissue using scissors, eg glossectomy, hemorrhoidectomy

White infarct Anemic infarct A localized area of ischemic necrosis in a solid organ, due to abrupt arterial occlusion; while in the immediate post-insult period, blood may flow into the region yielding a false impression of a hemorrhagic infarct; by 1-2 days post-insult, the region is pale yellow-white and characteristic of occlusions in organs with one circulatory supply, eg kidney, spleen, heart; see 'White' graft

White leg Phlegmasia alba dolens

White lesions see Leukoplakia

White line response White dermatoglyphism A 5-20 minute-in-duration pallid line that is seen when the skin surface is firmly stroked with a blunt object, which corresponds to focal vasoconstriction or edema and is characteristic of atopic dermatitis

White line sign A flat white line seen by ultrasonography corresponding to mucosal thickening in the renal collecting system of renal transplant victims; this finding is not seen in the clinically similar minimal nephrosis (Urology 1990; 35:367)

White liver disease An autosomal recessive, rapidly fatal condition characterized by massive hepatic (and corporal) steatosis, characterized by progressive hypotonicity, lethargy, coagulopathy and jaundice Laboratory Increased triglycerides, chylomicrons, HDL-cholesterol, hypoglycemia, hypocalcemia

White lung The macroscopic morphology of a lung that has suffered repeated bouts of rheumatic pneumonitis, in which the anemic lung is scarred and pale in the lower lobes

White muscle A type of striated muscle that generates ATP by anaerobic metabolism of glucose and glycogen; white muscle or 'fast twitch' muscle, is capable of short and rapid activity that cannot be sustained over time; it has abundant sarcoplasmic reticulum, phosphorylase that utilizes intrinsic glycogen for energy, low oxidative enzyme activity and relatively fewer mitochondria than red muscle fibers; see Red muscle

White muscle disease Nutritional myopathy Degeneration of muscle most prominently affecting the 'fast twitch' muscle, which is secondary to various vitamin and nutritional defects, in particular, deficiencies of vitamin E and/or selenium

White nevus Nevus anemicus Sharply circumscribed, pale macules on the trunk, neck or limbs, attributed to a functional defect in the superficial dermal vessels, as these are not affected by vasodilators; the white nevus contrasts to achromic or depigmented nevi, eg Ito's nevus is due to a focal loss of melanin pigmentation

White noise That sound that has equal energy at every frequency and can be eliminated by raising the 'cut-off' of the detection device Note: Most early neonates fall asleep within 5 minutes in a background of white noise; one-quater of neonates fall asleep in the same time interval without white noise (Arch Dis Child 1990; 65:135); Cf Chaos

'White-out' SUBSTANCE ABUSE A generic term for commercial products, that are used to correct typed or written errors on paper documents by painting over the errors with an opaque white, rapidly-drying liquid; in their original formulations, these products contained trichloroethylene (TCE) and methylchloroform (1,1,1-trichloroethane); the latter substance has had some currency among pre-adolescents as a 'gateway' abuse substance, which is sniffed to induce a transient sensation of euphoria; the State of California's Proposition 65 regulations regarding human exposure to carcinogens forced a reformulation of 'white-outs', eliminating TCE; at the about the same time, allyl isothiocyanate (oil of mustard) was added to these products, the pungency of which discourages most casual abuse; see 'Gateway' drugs, Proposition 65, TCE; Cf Glue-sniffing

White plague Tuberculosis (TB) Infection of man by *Mycobacterium tuberculosis*, the 'robber of youth' has followed man through history, has been identified in the spine of Neolithic man and was first formally described by Homer in 900 BC; modern epidemics of tuberculosis began with the industrial revolution-related urban overcrowding in Britain, peaking in the mid-1800s, emigrated with the Europeans to the US and travelled with the settlers as they moved south and west, decimating the American aborigine; the incidence of TB reached a nadir in 1986 and has been increasing since that time due to its association with AIDS Note: More recently, press has been given to a new 'white plague', the epidemic of cocaine abuse; Cf Black plague

White pox Variola minor

White pulp A component of the normal splenic architecture, composed of peri-arteriolar lymphatic sheaths, surrounded by a mantle of small lymphocytes (predominantly T cell) surrounding germinal centers composed of B lymphocytes and B lymphoblasts; blood-born antigens contact the immune responsive cells in the germinal centers and within 24 hours, a primary response (IgM) occurs with immunoblastic proliferation and enlargement of germinal centers Cf Red pulp

White pulp disease Lymphoproliferative disorders that most prominently affect the white pulp of the spleen, including poorly differentiated lymphocytic leukemia, well-differentiated lymphocytic leukemia, histiocytic lymphoma and Hodgkin's disease

White's classification A system for categorizing gestational diabetes mellitus, designed to predict the maternal and fetal mortality and morbidity (table)

White's classification (modified)

Class	Duration	Lesions	Therapy
A	Any	None	Diet only
B	< 10 years	None	Insulin
C	10-19 years	None	Insulin
D	> 20 years	Benign retinopathy	Insulin
F	Any	Nephropathy	Insulin
H	Any	Heart disease	Insulin
R	Any	Proliferative retinopathy	Insulin

White's disease Generalized familial hyperkeratosis involving face, trunk, scalp and axilla crusted with warty excrescences

White's operation Castration for benign prostatic hypertrophy

White 'spider' FORENSIC PATHOLOGY An arachnoid skin lesion characterized by concentric geographic scarring and ulceration caused by fibrosis emanating centrifugally from the site of injection of illicit drugs, which is a typical post-mortem sign of subcutaneous heroin injection (skin 'popping')

White sponge nevus DERMATOLOGY A benign autosomal dominant disorder characterized by variably-sized, painless, albescent plaques, which by light microscopy display a 'basket-weave' epithelium, hyperparakeratosis and acanthosis of mucosae, especially of the nasopharynx (oral, nasal, esophagus, larynx), as well as vaginal and anal mucosae; the waxing and waning nature of the lesions may cause confusion with more serious white intralesions of the mouth, including leukoedema, leukoplakia, irritation, chewing tobacco dysplasia, lichen planus, Darier's disease, dyskeratosis congenita; although usually non-infectious, the skin lesions of white sponge nevus may respond to penicillin (J Am Dent Assoc 1988; 117:345)

White spot A generic term for any hypopigmented cutaneous macule that may appear in Addison's disease, alopecia areata, diabetes mellitus, halo nevus, hypomelanosis of Ito, amelanotic malignant melanoma, piebaldism, thyroid disease, tuberous sclerosis, vitamin B_{12} deficiency, vitiligo and Vogt-Koyanagi-Harada syndrome

'White spot disease' see Lichen sclerosis et atrophicus

White spot fundus Fundus albipunctatus An autosomal dominant recessive condition characterized by multiple macular lesions of the optic fundus which, with time, may progress to blindness

White stool diarrhea Hakuri Pseudocholera infantum A reovirus-induced acute gastroenteritis appearing in autumn and early winter in Japan (Lancet 1975; 1:918)

White strawberry tongue PEDIATRICS Red congested and edematous fungiform papillae in a whitish background of filiform papillae, a coating present between the second and fifth day of scarlet fever, which may also be seen in measles and in other febrile viral enanthemas

Whitlow A painful infectious dermatitis of the finger, seeded by contact exposure **HERPETIC WHITLOW** A herpes simplex-induced dermatopathy that may occur in occupationally-exposed health care workers, eg nurses on neurosurgical units, appearing as periungual blisters with a honeycombed appearance, later becoming purulent and accompanied by regional lymphadenopathy **MELANOTIC WHITLOW** A form of malignant melanoma that presents under or adjacent to the fingernail, which may extensively involve the finger Note: Felon and whitlow are regarded as synonymous by standard medical dictionaries, although in the surgical literature, felon connotes a deep, often purulent-ab-initio infection of a digit that may require active drainage

Whole blood TRANSFUSION MEDICINE A unit of blood that contains all the components (erythrocytes, leukocytes, platelets, plasma proteins and fluid); whole blood still has currency as a transfusion product as a) it isthe raw material from which other products are prepared and b) it may, under certain circucumstances, have some utility as a stand-alone product; under the usual circumstances, whole blood is almost invariably separated into components as this allows for more specific therapy while reducing the potential for infections and eliciting an immune response in the recipient to the extraneous transfused component; whole blood transfusion is acceptable (albeit not ideal) practice in the face of symptomatic anemia and hypovolemia, although packed red cells and 0.9% NaCl solution causes the patient less immune 'stress'; since patients may be asymptomatic despite a very low hematocrit, it is considered poor policy to transfuse blood products without addressing the underlying condition (Technical Manual, American Association of Blood Banks, Arlington, Virginia 1990)

Whooping cough The characteristic cough of pertussis, which infects circa 60 million worldwide and kills 1 million annually, caused by the gram-negative nonmotile ***Bordatella pertussis***; the 'whoop' occurs during the paroxysmal stage of infection (1-2 weeks after the onset, lasting for 2-4 weeks); a 'paroxysm' consists of 10-20 coughs of increasing intensity, a deep inspiration (the 'whoop') after which a thick, viscid plug of mucus is expelled, occasionally accompanied by vomiting; the paroxysms may occur every 1/2 hour, often accompanied by increased venous pressure, plethoric conjunctivae, periorbital edema, petechiae and epistaxis, infants may be cyanotic until relieved of the obstructing plug of mucus; see DTP; other 'whooping' infections of early infancy include adenovirus, ***Bordatella parapertussis, B bronchoseptica***

'Whore' see 'Hired gun'

Wicking INFECTIOUS DISEASE Enhanced penetration of liquids, and small infectious agents, through minute holes in latex membranes, eg surgical gloves that may occur when washed with surfactants, an effect that militates against the re-use of certain materials

Wild-type allele The allele for an inherited trait that is most frequent in a natural (wild) population

Wiggle see Squiggle

Willowbrook State School BIOMEDICAL ETHICS An extended-care facility in the United States, in which a group of mentally-retarded children were allegedly inoculated with live hepatitis virus during the 1950s; see Unethical medical research

Will Rogers phenomenon Stage migration EPIDEMIOLOGY The improved survival of patients with cancer (or other disease) due to either reclassification of patients into different prognostic groups through recognition of more subtle disease manifestations, or by using newer diagnostic modalities that allow the disease to be diagnosed at an earlier stage, which results in a 'zero-time shift' and 'improved' prognosis for a given disease; however when classified with symptom stages without new diagnostic procedures, survival for the same cancer has not changed (Ann Int Med 1983; 99:843, N Engl J Med 1985; 312:1604; ibid, 313:1291c); it is held by some pundits that the advances of diagnostic technology may have blinded physicians to the lack of progress in treating cancer Note: The eponym is dedicated to the cowboy-philosopher, Will Rogers (1879-1935), who often observed that truth was relative to one's vantage point

Wilm's nephritis A nephrotic syndrome seen in Wilm's tumor

Wilms tumor An embryonic tumor of the kidney that arises in aberrant mesenchymal renal stem cell lines, coupled with the loss of functioning tumor suppressor genes; Wilms' tumor comprises 92% of primary childhood renal malignancies (frequency: 1:10 000); the rest are sarcomas of various subtypes Etiology Four-to-eight-fold increased incidence if the father was an automobile mechanic, welder or auto body repairman, possibly related to occupational exposure to leaded gasoline or due to fumes from repairing automobile radiators with lead (Cancer Res 1990; 50:3212) Molecular biology A mutation in the Wilms' tumor locus abolishes the DNA-binding activity of a zinc finger domain that binds to a site of a growth factor inducible gene, suggesting that the loss of binding may be the critical tumorigenic event in Wilms' tumor formation (Science 1991; 250:1259) Clinical Wilms' tumor presents as a mass, often with hypertension 60%, hematuria 24%, nephritis (Wilms' nephritis) and serosal effusions (ascites, pleural effusions); 5% are bilateral and anaplasia connotes a poor prognosis Note: 20% of aniridia is associated with Wilms' tumor (see WAGR syndrome) Differential diagnosis Infants under 6 months of age may have a congenital mesoblastic nephroma, a histological mimic of Wilms' tumor that usually regresses spontaneously

Wimp allele MOLECULAR BIOLOGY A dominant maternal effect allele that reduces transcription of subsets of segmentation genes in Drosophila (Genes Dev 1991; 5:341) and has weak tyrosine phosphokinase activity

Windblown appearance A descriptor for the enlarged, crowded and hyperchromatic and irregular nuclei in the epithelium of Bowen's disease and bowenoid papulosis of the genitalia; the cells are pleomorphic, dyskeratotic and multinucleated with atypical mitotic figures, acanthosis and parakeratosis

Winding number Linkage number MOLECULAR BIOLOGY The number of times that the two strands of DNA cross through each other, an event requiring that the strands be nicked and rejoined; see Superhelix, Topoisomerase

Windmill hand A fanciful descriptor for a hand with ulnar deviation and induration of the flexor surface of the proximal phalanges, described in the whistling face syndrome

Window A commonly used term in various medical specialties referring to a space in time, eg Window period or to a position CYTOLOGY A 'window' is a narrow, slit-like clear space between two or more molded mesothelial cells, which may be joined to each other by 'articulations' PHYSIOLOGY An opening in a biological membrane, through which solutes may be transported RADIOLOGY An interval of photon energies used in a scintillation counter (γ-ray detector); the so-called 'pulse height analyzer' rejects any photon energy falling outside of the window (and is therefore not counted) SURGERY A region of an abscess in closest contact with the abdominal wall (or any accessible skin surface) without an intervening visceral organ, which can be opened for relatively safe drainage TOXICOLOGY The 'window period' corresponds to the time interval between ingestion of lethal quantities of a drug or toxin and the production of irreversible organ damage, eg a) Acetaminophen overdose in which there is a 2 to 3 day latency or window period, preceding irreversible liver damage b) Paraquat poisoning in which irreversible interstitial lung damage follows a three-to-five day window interval c) Phyllotoxin (*Amanita phylloides*) poisoning in which cardiac, renal and hepatic failure follows a 1 to 3 day latency period

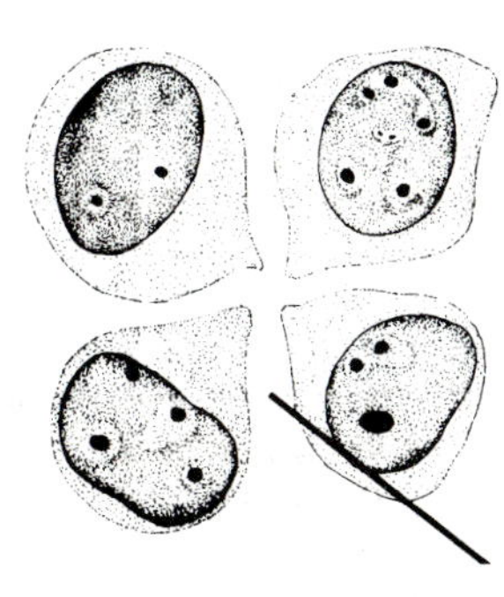

Window

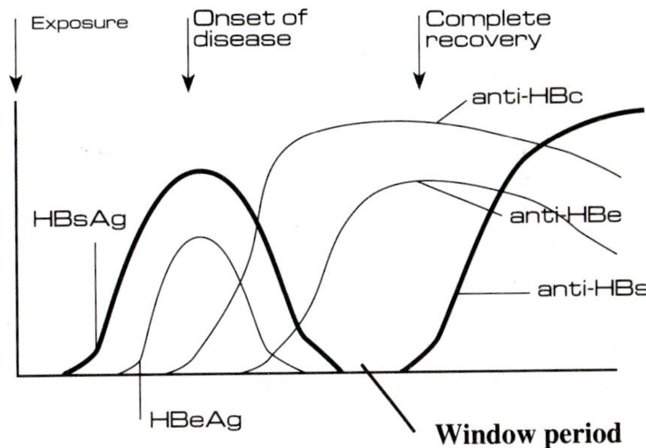

Window period

Window period IMMUNOLOGY An interval between the time of inoculation or exposure to a microorganism, usually viral and the ability to detect its presence by serological assays, ie by antigen-antibody reactions, occurring in a) Hepatitis B The hepatitis B 'core window' represents active but undetected hepatitis B infection, in which the circulating hepatitis B surface antigen (HBsAg) has fallen to undetectable levels and antibody to the hepatitis B surface antigen (anti-HB_S) has yet to rise to detectable levels; during the core window, the IgM antibodies to the hepatitis B core antigen (anti-HBc) are positive but not always included in the usual hepatitis screening battery b) HIV-1 window A time interval between the initial infection with HIV-1 (human immunodeficiency virus) that can be detected by the polymerase chain reaction or detection of the p24 antigen) and production of the anti-p24 and anti-p41 antibodies in quantities sufficient to be measured by the ELISA technique, the method most commonly used to screen for the presence of anti-HIV-1 antibodies; although usually the window period ranges from 3-9 months, it may be up to 36 months in duration Note: All units of blood donated in the US are screened for anti-HIV-1 p24 antibody and thus potentially in the 'window period' for HIV-1 infection

Windsock deformity CARDIOLOGY A descriptor for an aneurysm of the sinus of Valsalva, as seen by aortography, in which there is a wide base at the aortic origin and a nipple-like apex projecting into the right atrium, the usual site of rupture; the aneurysm is characterized by attenuation and separation of the aortic media within the sinus from the common fibrous junction of the aorta, the left ventricle and the aortic valve PEDIATRIC SURGERY A descriptive term for the characteristic balloon-like dilatation seen on a barium enema in neonates with membranous atresia of the colon, ileum or jejunum; when the deformity is colonic, the barium column reaches the membrane but is forced back by the fecal flow in the transverse colon, forming a cup-shaped or windsock-like radiolucency UROLOGY A descriptor for the soft redundant membrane that prolapses into the bulbous urethra, as seen on voiding urethrography in the rare, complete urethral obstruction, which affects boys, and is located in the urethra distal to the verumontanum, presenting in the neonatal period with severe obstruction and dysplastic kidneys; if the 'obstruction' is mild, the condition may present in later childhood with persistent nighttime bet-wetting and incontinence

Wind-swept cortex A fanciful descriptor for extreme gyral atrophy resulting from florid neurosyphilis that is accompanied by marked necrosis of cortical neurons, microglial (rod) cell proliferation and gliosis; Cf Knife-blade atrophy

'Wing beating' Rhythmic oscillating tremor of the upper extremities as they are outstretched, a characteristic neurologic sign of Wilson's disease, which is often accompanied by cerebellar ataxia and intention tremor

Winging of the scapula Elevation of the scapulae seen when the arm is abducted, a finding characteristic of limb-girdle dystrophy, due to paralysis of the long thoracic nerve (fifth, sixth and seventh nerve roots), but which also occurs in wrinkly skin syndrome and in heavy manual labor, especially affecting those who carry heavy, sharp-cornered objects on the shoulders, eg 'hod carrier's palsy

'Wintering tree' pattern A fanciful descriptor for the angiographic appearance of panacinar pulmonary emphysema, in which the vessels have an arborescent skeleton-like pattern, serving as a 'soft criterion' to differentiate this from bullous emphysema

Winter vomiting disease A one-to-three day, often parvovirus-induced intestinal 'flu' that is most common in the winter in temperate climates Clinical either mild, afebrile watery diarrhea or more severe, febrile with vomiting, headache and systemic complaints

Wire loop lesion RENAL PATHOLOGY A lesion characterized by capillary walls thickened with subendothelial immune complex deposits, located between the glomerular basement membrane and capillary endothelium, which are associated with proliferative glomerulonephritis; wire loops are typical of class IV lupus erythematosus (diffuse proliferative lupus nephritis), and may be seen in progressive systemic sclerosis and because they are often accompanied by necrosis, crescent formation and scarring, signal a poor prognosis

WISC Wechsler Intelligence Scale for Children A 10-category test that measures both verbal and performance intelligence quotient; see Psychological testing

Wisconsin solution Viaspan™ TRANSPLANTATION A hypothermic perfusate containing pentafraction, lactobionic acid, raffinose, glutathione, adenosine and other substances, which is gravity-fed into the vessels of organs destined for transplantation, after draining the blood from 'brain-dead' donors; see Procurement, Slush preparation, Transplantation

Wisdom teeth DENTISTRY A colloquial term for the third molars that usually erupt during late adolescence and which, given the physical confines of the jaw, often become impacted; wisdom teeth are so-called as their appearance coincides with the development, in later adolescence of some semblance of wisdom

Wish bias A systemic error that is due to the tendency on either the part of a patient, eg to underreport exposure to fatty foods, or the part of an investigator, eg to report only those trials with positive findings or to report results that support a particular vantage point (J Clin Epidemiol 1990; 43:619); see Placebo effect, Publication bias

Witch's milk PEDIATRICS A clear-to-lactescent discharge from the nipples of male and female neonates accompanied by breast hypertrophy, the result of transplacental hormonal effects, most commonly occurring in term infants

'Witch-hunting' see 'Whistleblowing'

Withdrawal emergent syndrome A tardive dyskinesia-like clinical complex that affects children and adolescents upon abrupt discontinuation of neuroleptic (antipsychotic) drugs, attributed to hypersensitivity of dopamine receptors, characterized by choreoathetosis and myoclonus Treatment Reintroduce the drug, taper the dose more slowly or await spontaneous resolution

Withdrawal, infantile syndrome see Neonatal withdrawal syndrome

Witzelsucht German, Joke addiction NEUROLOGY A manifestation of organic brain disease, eg tumors or atherosclerosis-induced lesions of the frontal cortex, in which the person compulsively tells jokes, often associated with childish behavior; witzelsucht represents a defense mechanism, as the person recognizes his memory defects and use the jocularity to deflect attention from them

***wnt*-1** Formerly, *int*-1 A proto-oncogene that may determine embryonic patterns through an unknown mechanism, encoding a 44 kD protein for which there are multiple receptors, that associates with the cell surface and extracellular matrix after secretion (Science 1991; 252:1173); when *int*-1 (*wnt*-1) is activated by insertion into the mouse mammary tumor virus (MMTV), it evokes histologic changes of malignant transformation in mammary epithelial cells

Wobble MOLECULAR BIOLOGY An instability in transfer RNA's affinity for the third base in a codon (at the 5'-end) ; this looseness allows the base of the anticodon to pair with an anti-codon other than that which would normally correspond to it; if perfect Watson-Crick base pairing were required between codon and anti-codon, 61 different transfer RNA (tRNA) species would be required; wobble (nonstandard) base pairing at the third nucleotide position of the codon allows most tRNAs to recognize more than one of the codons specifying for a given amino acid, serving to accelerate protein synthesis Note: The 'GU-wobble' is thought to be responsible for the difference in tRNAs (Science 1988; 240:793); the ability to recognize more than one codon is such that while the first and second nucleotides of the codon and their partners, the second and third of the anticodon bind by standard pairing, the binding of the third nucleotide of the codon and the first nucleotide of the anticodon is less restrictive and accepts a nonstandard pair, in this the so-called 'wobble' position, eg a single tRNA may bind to multiple codons, eg CUU, CUC, CUA and CUG; see Degenerate code, 'Second genetic code', tRNA

Wohlfahrtia A genus of flesh-eating flies, ***Sarcophagidae,*** that are associated with myiasis in living flesh

Wolf-Chaikoff effect ENDOCRINOLOGY An acute adaptive response to administration of high levels of iodine, in which increased intracellular levels of iodide block both the organic-binding and coupling reactions in the thyroid functionally 'turning off' the thyroid, an effect used to advantage in preparing the thyroid for surgery

Wolfe Classification A schema of four putatively distinct-mammographic patterns (Am J Radiol 1976; 126:1130), which were reported to allow detection of 'dysplastic' breasts at an increased risk for cancer; subsequent studies revealed that the initally-reported features were merely suggestive of malignancy (J Am Med Assoc 1985; 254:1050)

Wolffian duct Mesonephric duct An embryonal duct that forms from the 25-30th days of gestation in association with the rudimentary pronephros, later becoming the mesonephric excretory duct, the 'second embryonal kidney', giving rise to the male reproductive system (epididymis, vas deferens and seminal vesicles), largely regressing in the female at 10-11th week, a portion of which remains as embryonal 'rests' (Gartner's duct cysts, epoophoron and paroophoron), Cf Müllerian duct

Wolff-Parkinson-White (WPW) Pre-excitation syndrome CARDIOLOGY A conduction disorder with increased susceptibility to supraventricular paroxysmal tachyarrhythmias, in which the sinoatrial impulse travels directly to the atrioventricular (AV) node or anomalously via the bundle of Kent; this latter pathway is more rapid, resulting in premature ventricular contraction, with a short 'P-R' interval of less than 0.1 second and a 'delta wave'; common arrhythmias in the WPW syndrome include atrial tachycardia, atrial flutter and atrial fibrillation; the impulse may 'choose' either the normal route of conduction to the AV node (making the diagnosis of WPW difficult) or it may travel via an anomalous route, detected by a broader QRS with a delta wave; in the latter scenario, the 'physiologic' delay at the AV node is circumvented and the ventricular rate may exceed 200/min; WPW syndrome may occur in a normal heart (reverting to a normal rhythm with exercise or atropine) or be associated with premature atrial tachyarrhythmia, Ebstein anomaly and corrected transposition (ventricular 'reversal') and cardiomyopathy Treatment Cardioversion, intravenous procainamide and lidocaine or radiofrequency current ablation of the accessory AV pathway (N Engl J Med 1991; 324:1605, 1612)

Wolf-Hirschhorn 4p⁻ syndrome CLINICAL GENETICS A chromosomal deletion complex characterized by low birth weight, microcephaly, micrognathia, hypertelorism, epicanthus, beaked nose, redundant lateral nasal folds, cleft palate, inguinal hernia, cryptorchism, hypospadias and death before age three

Wolfram syndrome see DIDMOAD syndrome

Wombstone Stone mole A hydatidiform mole that has undergone extensive dystrophic calcification Note: Marked intrauterine calcification may occur in leiomyomas (fibroids), which have also been called wombstones

Women and disease Disease is unfair; in general, men die earlier and more often through the vicissitudes of war, homicide and suicide and die earlier from AIDS, alcohol, drugs of abuse, tobacco and most cancers; women live longer, better, and more disease-free; cancer mortality before age 20 is 22% lower in women and in certain tumors, eg sarcomas and carcinomas, women have longer survival; J Am Med Assoc 1990; 263:2189); certain diseases have a predilection for women; those with a female:male ratio of 10:1 lupus erythematosus; 9:1 Sjögren syndrome, chronic active hepatitis, primary biliary cirrhosis; 4:1 Idiopathic thrombocytopenic purpura; 3:1 Scleroderma, rheumatoid arthritis, myasthenia gravis, chronic fatigue syndrome

'Women who fall' see Factitial 'diseases', Psychogenic syndromes

'Wooden' sensation NEUROLOGY Tactile numbness of ten or more years duration, associated with limited cutaneous sclerosis, secondary to occupational use of vibrating machines; see Vibration white finger syndrome

Wood lamp DERMATOLOGY A lamp that transmits filtered ultraviolet light at 365 nm, which is used in darkened rooms by dermatologists to detect and evaluate autofluorescence of superficial fungal (dermatophytic) infections *ERYTHRASMA AGENT* ***Nocardia minutissima*** Color If present, bright coral-red *FAVUS AGENT* ***Trichophyton schoenleinii*** Color Dull olive-gray green *MICROSPOROSIS AGENT* ***Microsporum audoni, M canis*** Color Bright green 'black dot' *TINEA CAPITIS AGENT* ***Trichophyton violaceum***, Color Dull white *TINEA VERSICOLOR AGENT* ***Malassezia furfur*** Color Yellow to golden-brown Note: Some bacteria are also autofluorescent, eg *Pseudomonas aeruginosa* Color Blue

Woodruff's 'laws' A group of humorous variations of 'Murphy's law' broadly applicable to (laboratory) medicine 1) A specimen (or hospital chart) is lost only if it is important to a physician's credibility, if there is a lawsuit pending on the specimen, or if not lost, it will be switched with a specimen from a critically ill patient 2) Intense preparation for a conference ensures its cancellation and 3) Problems arise a) When the only person who can solve them is on vacation or b) When the party held responsible is due for contract renewal

Woolly hair disease Tight curly hair seen at birth in caucasians that is a) Sporadic, associated with the woolly hair nevus b) Autosomal recessive, in which the scalp hair is ash-white and the body hair is short and kinky or c) Autosomal dominant, in which the scalp hair is also ash-white, but with normal body hair; Cf Kinky hair disease, Uncombable hair syndrome

Wool-sorter's disease Inhalation anthrax An occupational infection by ***Brucella anthracis*** spores affecting those exposed to aerosols during the early stages of processing of goat hair Clinical The disease is biphasic, the early symptoms are influenza-like, lasting 2-3 days, then followed by severe hypoxia and dyspnea, and meningeal signs; 12/13 documented cases in the USA died Treatment Penicillin Note: The high mortality caused by aerosolized ***B anthracis*** has made it a popular experimental agent for biological warfare, although it has never been deployed

Word COMPUTERS A unit of data, consisting of two bytes of 8 bits (16 binary bits); one kilobyte is equal to 1024 (210 in binary computation); 1.0 megabyte of memory is approximately equal to 400 typewritten pages of manuscript

Word salad PSYCHIATRY A string of neologisms, words and phrases, in which there is a loosening of associations, shifting of topics that may progress to near incoherence, with a complete lack of logical connection; word salads are characteristic of disordered thought processes, typical of psychosis, eg schizophrenia; Cf Witzelsucht

Working diagnosis CLINICAL DECISION-MAKING A diagnosis based on experience, clinical epidemiology and some confirmatory evidence provided by ancillary studies, eg radiologic findings; working diagnoses allow early treatment of a disease while awaiting special or more definitive studies, eg immunoperoxidase stains or results from a reference laboratory

Working formulation A classification system for non-Hodgkin's lymphomas Background: By the late 1970s, six different histopathologic classifications of lymphomas were common use, which correlated poorly with clinical disease and did not translate well among pathologists; a group of experts convened and created a new system, the Working formulation (Cancer 1982; 49:2112), to facilitate communication among various 'lymphomaniacs' (those dedicated to creating new therapeutic modalities for lymphomas) and which has been increasingly accepted as it easily applied by pathologists and is relatively predictive of the future behavior of the lymphoma; in low-grade lymphomas, the affected lymph nodes are rubbery, mobile, not fixed to the skin, enlarge very slowly, may cause lymphedema, nerve compression or ureteral obstruction, but are painless; asymptomatic hepatosplenomegaly is common as are liver, spleen and marrow infiltration; extranodal disease may occur, but central nervous system and testicular involvement are relatively uncommon; intermediate and high-grade lymphomas share certain clinical and pathological features, including abrupt enlargement and 'matting' of lymph nodes, induration, fixation to skin with overlying erythema; bulky internal and midline lymph nodes may cause obstructive phenomena, including lymphedema, spinal cord compression, ureteral obstruction, thrombophlebitis, superior vena cava syndrome, hepatosplenomegaly, hepatic dysfunction and intrahepatic obstruction; marrow involvement is less common (table)

WORKING FORMULATION Malignant lymphomas (ML)

LOW-GRADE LYMPHOMA

ML, Small lymphocytic lymphoma(plasmacytoid, or CLL)

ML, Follicular small cleaved cell type, with diffuse zones (D) and sclerosis (S)

ML, Follicular mixed, small cleaved cells and large cell lymphoma+ D and S

INTERMEDIATE GRADE LYMPHOMA

ML, Follicular, predominantly large cell type+ D and S

ML, Diffuse, small cleaved + S

ML, Diffuse, mixed large and small cell + S + epithelioid cells (Lennert lymphoma)

ML, Diffuse large cell, cleaved and non-cleaved cell+ S

HIGH GRADE LYMPHOMAS

ML, Diffuse, large cell immunoblastic, with various predominating features

ML, Plasmacytoid cell, usually of B cell lineage

ML, Clear cell type usually of T cell lineage

ML, Polymorphous with epithelioid cells

ML, Lymphoblastic lymphomaConvoluted or non convoluted cell types

ML, Small non-cleaved, either Burkitt's or follicular (non-Burkitt's) type

OTHER LYMPHOMAS

Composite, Sezary syndrome/mycosis fungoides, true histiocytic, extramedullary plasmacytoma

Workshop ACADEMIA A specialized conference in which experts in a particular area of science or medicine, convene in order to compare data and establish or standardize criteria for a substance, disease or phenomenon; immunologists meet periodically to share information on newly identified human leukocyte antigen (HLA) groups and clusters of differentiation (CD) antigens on cell surfaces; those molecules that remain poorly characterized at the close of the workshop receive a 'w' prefix, eg HLA-DRw52, HLA-DRw53, CDw65, CDw70, to indicate that the experts have yet to fully establish the nature of the antigens; Cf 'Wetshop'

'Work-up' The combined activities of a physical examination, laboratory tests and imaging analyses that are required to arrive at a diagnosis Note: During the formative years of residency training, young physicians sail between 1) The Scylla of an excess 'work-up', in which they may establish the presence of 'disease(s)' that the patient may not have; see Diagnostic 'overkill', Ulysses syndrome and 2) The less common Charybdis of paucity, in which a diagnosis is not achieved, see Fehldiagnose (0.5-1.0% of those admitted to a hospital, leave or die without ever having a firmly established diagnosis)

Worm see Computer worm; Cf Computer virus

WORM Write-once/read-many COMPUTERS A form of permanent computer memory, eg CD/ROM, which allows the efficient permanent storage of data, including medical and laboratory records

Wormian bones see Mosaic bones, skull

'Worm project' see *Caenorhabditis elegans*

'Worn tennisball' appearance A fanciful descriptor for the 'fuzzy' margins surrounding a well-circumscribed peripheral adenocarcinoma of the lung seen in a plain chest film, an appearance that contrasts with the smooth margin considered by some to be more typical of a peripheral squamous cell carcinoma

Wound healing Repair of incisive insults to tissues may occur in one of two fashions; simple or 'clean' wounds with little loss of tissue heal by 'primary intention', while 'dirty' wounds heal by 'secondary intention' **WOUND HEALING BY PRIMARY INTENTION** (time required for each event) Filling-in of wound defects with inflammatory cells (24 hours) Epithelial response, basal cell proliferation (3 days) Infiltration by macrophages and deposition of collagen (5-7 days) Ingrowth of granulation tissue, maximum neo-vascularization, epidermal 'bridging' (2 weeks) Increased collagenization and proliferation of fibroblasts (2 months) **WOUND HEALING BY SECONDARY INTENTION** occurs when there is a massive tissue defect with an increase in fibrin, debris, more intense inflammation, large amounts of granulation tissue; massive wounds are prone to re-epithelialization defects and collagen deposition, including 'proud flesh' and/or keloid, which are more common in blacks; the wound-healing process is the result of a delicate interplay between a variety of growth factors, eg basic fibroblast growth factor, transforming growth factor-β and platelet-derived growth factor, cells, eg keratinocytes and the extracellular matrix which contains a variety of proteins, eg integrins, collagen, fibrinogen, fibronectin, heparin and others (Science 1991; 252:1064n) Note: Topical application of epidermal growth factor (EGF) stimulates regeneration of proliferation and migration of keratinocytes, binding and activating a tyrosine kinase receptor, although it is believed that proper wound healing requires a 'cocktail' of growth factors to optimize the process

WPW syndrome see Wolff-Parkinson-White syndrome

Wrap-around (policy) HEALTH CARE INDUSTRY A 'major medical' health insurance policy available in the US at a relatively high cost that provides full payment for fees charged by a hospital and/or physician(s), over the amount reimbursed by the 'basic carriers', eg Blue cross (for hospitals), and Blue shield (for physicians); Cf Blue Cross/Blue Shield, 'Major medical'

Wrap-around procedure SURGERY Any of the 'anti-reflux' operations, eg the Nissen, Belsey, and Hill procedures that restore the sphincter function to the lower esophagus; the Nissen procedure may afford the greatest long-term success; see 'Inkwell'

WRAT Wide Range Achievement Test An achievement-type of psychologic test that evaluates a child or adolescent's level in subject areas including reading, spelling and mathematics; see Psychological testing

Wreathed nucleus An annular, peripherally placed nucleus lying in pale eosinophilic cytoplasm that may be seen in the giant tumor cells of alveolar rhabdomyosarcoma, which lack the cross-striations required for the definitive diagnosis of rhabdomyosarcoma

'Wrecking ball' effect CARDIOLOGY That 'tethered ball'-like effect of a pedunculated tumor in the atrial or ventricular chambers, often due to a calcified myxoma, which may damage the mitral valve, rupture the chordae tendineae or cause severe mitral regurgitation, as it pounds against endocardial structures

Wringer injury An uncommon lesion formerly seen in children who, while feeding clothes into (or playing with) an electrically driven laundry wringer, literally got 'caught up' in their work; the injuries associated therewith include crushing of the hand and upper extremity, friction burns at points of increasing diameters, eg metacarpophalangeal joints, thenar and base of hand, elbow and shoulder, neurapraxia, edema, lacerations, hematoma formation, fractures and potentially complete avulsion of a hand or arm; similar injuries may occur in industrial accidents (eg in the hot rollers in a printing press) or in rotating farm equipment; in addition to the above morbidity, these accidents may add components of thermal injury, extensive crushing and soil-related infection, including *Clostridium* species contamination

Wrinkly skin syndrome An autosomal recessive condition characterized by decreased elasticity and wrinkling of the palmo-plantar and corporal skin, dwarfism, kyphosis, 'winging' of the scapulae, mental retardation, muscle hypotonia, myalgia and decreased visual acuity

Wrist drop NEUROLOGY A manifestation of peripheral neuropathy characterized by a loss of acral motor activity, which may be seen in a wide variety of conditions, including amyloidosis, Charcot-Marie-Tooth syndrome, collagen vascular diseases, diabetic mononeuropathy, lead poisoning and severe vitamin B_{12} deficiency; see Foot drop

Writer's cramp Conscious immobility PSYCHIATRY A transient occupational neurosis in which there is temporary loss of highly skilled motor sequences, considered to be a psychogenic conversion reaction

Writhe number MOLECULAR BIOLOGY The number of superhelical turns or times a double helix of DNA crosses over itself, corresponding to the concept of supercoiling, but which does not have the exact same value; in a completely relaxed molecule, the writhing number value is zero; see Superhelicity

Wrongful FORENSIC MEDICINE An adjective with considerable medico-legal currency that is used in several contexts **WRONGFUL BIRTH** An event resulting from the failure of a contraceptive or sterilization procedure, eg fallopian tube liagation, failure to diagnose pregnancy, or an unsuccessful attempt to abort a conceptus, see below, Wrongful life **Wrongful death** An event often falling under the rubric of negligence, see Negligence **Wrongful life** An event in which legal action may be taken by (or on behalf of) the baby suffering from a hereditary or congenital defect, eg Down syndrome or other disease, eg rubella, who would not have been born had the parents had the knowledge to opt for an abortion; wrongful life represents either the failure to a) diagnose in utero a condition that would lead to a major life-long handicap or b) recognize such a condition in a sibling, allowing a second, similarly afflicted child to be born; the child is the defendant named in a lawsuit initiated to defray the incurred and anticipated medical, nursing and related health expenses; in both wrongful birth and wrongful life, the defendent may be liable for support and care of the infant from 'cradle to grave'

Wry neck Congenital torticollis A defect consisting of one-sided contracture and palpable induration of the sternocleidomastoid muscle, causing the chin to turn towards the opposite side and the head to rotate towards the lesion; the wry neck deformity is accompanied by dysplasia of the facial muscles; the etiology of the congenital form is unclear, but may be due to in utero or peripartum trauma to the venous drainage, which may eventuate in asymmetrical development of the face and skull; the later it is recognized, the more likely surgical intervention is required

W syndrome An X-linked condition characterized by frontal bossing, hypertelorism, antimongolic palpebral fissures, broad flat nose, camptodactyly, mental retardation and seizures (Pallister PD, Birth Defects Orig Art Ser X 1974; 51-60)

WYSIWYG What you see is what you get; see Computers

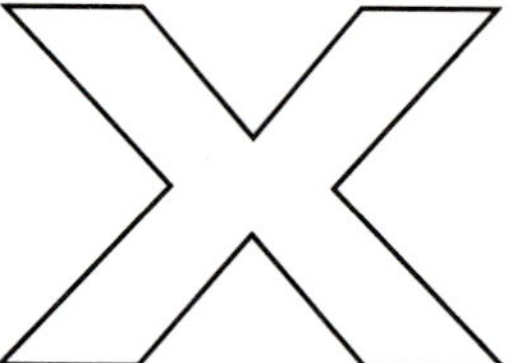

X Symbol for: Any unknown quantity; reactance; xanthine

x Symbol for: abscissa (horizontal axis); mean (statistics)

Xanthelasma A condition characterized by multiple xanthomas of the inner eyelid that are most common in normocholesterolemic elderly or hypercholesterolemic younger subjects Pathology Multiple soft, yellow plaques, seen by light microscopy as lipid-laden histiocytes surrounding blood vessels

Xanthogranulomatous pyelonephritis A malakoplakia-like lesion of the kidneys that lacks Michaelis-Gutmann bodies, which arises a background of *Escherichia coli* and *Proteus* infections, grossly appearing as yellowish lobulated masses that replace the renal architecture, potentially causing hydronephrosis, nephrolithiasis and giant cell formation

Xanthoma A yellow-orange lipid-filled papule or plaque located on the skin or tendons; not uncommon in the general population, markedly increased in various 'lipid' diseases, including lipoprotein lipase deficiency, a-β-lipoproteinemia, hypercholesterolemia or hypertriglyceridemia

Xanthomatosis Generalized, nonspecific increase in xanthomas that may occur in malignancy, eg lymphoma, multiple myeloma or be a component of other disease, eg familial hypercholesterolemia syndrome, Hand-Schüller-Christian and Wolman's diseases

X-body A morphological variant of Birbeck granules that is seen by electron microscopy in histiocytosis X; X-bodies represent incomplete 'tennis-racquet' forms lacking a terminal bulge, which have a constant thickness and vague internal striation

X cell see XYZ cell theory

X chromosome inactivation A chromosomal event that occurs during embryologic development of females; in a normal XX female, an inactive and active X chromosome is maintained in each somatic cell; determination of which X chromosome is active in peripheral B cells is based on three facets of the Lyon hypothesis 1) Only one X chromosome is active in a normal female somatic cell and that X chromosome is stably transferred to the progeny cells 2) The DNA methylation pattern differs on active cells (and can be monitored by using restriction endonucleases) and 3) Restriction fragment length polymorphisms (RFLPs) of the paternal and maternal genes allow identification of the parent of origin for each chromosome; X chromosome inactivation is thus the functional eliminationof all but one X chromosome in mammals and is a unique developmental regulatory event, proposed by Mary Lyon (Nature 1961; 190:372), which affects the expression of an entire chromosome (150 million base pairs of DNA and thousands of genes) in a *cis*-limited fashion, resulting in dosage equivalence between females who have two X chromosomes and males who have one X chromosome; the gene responsible for random inactivation of the X chromosome in females is designated XIST (X inactive-specific transcript) and is located to Xq13, within a larger 'X-inactivation center' region; XIST is only expressed in cell lines containing one or more inactive X chromosomes, ie it is female-specific in karyotypically normal individuals (Nature 1991; 349:38, 82, 15) and may play a role in establishing the phenotype of Klinefelter and Turner syndromes; see Methylation, Testis-determining factor

Xenobiotics Xeno, Greek, foreign IMMUNOLOGY Any compound that is foreign to a living system; alternatively, any natural or synthetic toxic, non-self substance, that may stimulate an immune or other form of defensive response

Xenodiagnosis PARASITOLOGY A method for diagnosing a disease in one animal by inoculating the putative causative organism in a second animal of a different species; xenodiagnosis allows detection of blood-borne hemoflagellates (*Trypanosoma cruzi* and *T spiralis*) when the peripheral blood smears are negative; insects are fed blood that is presumed to be positive for the hemoflagellate and 'incubated' for 10-30 days, after which the insects' feces are examined for the parasites (Am J Trop Med Hyg 1989; 41:521)

Xenograft A graft from an individual of one species to another individual of a different species

Xenopsylla Rat flea A genus of fleas that is a vector for dwarf and rat tapeworms (*Xenopsylla cheopis*), murine typhus (*X cheopis*) and plague (*X astia, X brasiliense, X cheopis*)

Xeroderma pigmentosa (XP) An autosomal recessive condition characterized by the inability to repair ultraviolet light-induced damage to pyrimidine nucleotide (cytosine, thymidine) dimers due to lack of one or more multigene products or complementation groups; XP may result from the absence of a nuclear factor responsible for binding and recognizing damaged DNA Molecular biology Of the nine genetic complementation groups (groups A-H and a variant group) of the autosomal recessive xeroderma pigmentosa, a defect of group A occurs on chromosome 9q34.1 and encodes a 273 residue protein with a zinc finger domain, which indicates that it has DNA-binding activity, possibly forming part of the enzyme complex making the excision near the damaged sites (Nature 1990; 348:73); the repair defect may occur in fibroblasts, epithelial cells and lymphocytes in XP and in the de Sanctis-Caccione syndrome (which also has microcephaly, mental retardation, dwarfism, hypogonadism, deafness, choreoathetosis and ataxia) Clinical Incidence $2/10^6$; the patients are normal at birth, freckling and xeroderma occur by age three, accompanied by telangiectasia, keratoacanthomas, keratoses, scarring and eventually cutaneous malignancy, in particular, basal cell carcinoma, as well as squamous cell carcinoma and malignant melanoma and internal malignancy (fibrosarcoma and angiosarcoma); see Photoactivation

Xerophthalmia A vitamin A deficiency-induced disorder causing dry, greasy, thickened and focally denuded cornea which may progress to keratomalacia, corneal ulceration, necrosis and secondary infections; xerophthalmia may also occur in Sjögren syndrome and in periorbital lymphoproliferative disorders

Xeroradiography A radiologic imaging technique in which aluminum plates coated with a semiconductor, eg selenium are used to record a latent image as a pattern of varying electrical charges, which is converted into a 'positive' image by a dry (xero-, Greek, dry) photoelectric process; xeromammography provides a relatively good image, since the entire breast is viewed at once and clearly delineates variability in tissue density, blood vessels, calcification and tumors; xeroradiography is on the decline as a major supplier of the technique withdrew from the market, the radiation dose is slightly higher that that used in modern high-resolution mammography, the equipment is prone to breakdown and the boundary between two differently charged areas is distorted, making potentially malignant ('borderline') lesions difficult to interpret

Xerostomia Dry mouth Dryness of the oropharyngeal mucosa, due to hyposecretion of the salivary glands is characteristic of Sjögren syndrome; the salivary glands become inflamed and are eventually replaced by fibrosis; xerostomia also occurs with HIV-1 and Candida species infections, malignancy and systemic sclerosis

X growth factor MICROBIOLOGY A group of heat-stable tetrapyrrole compounds that are provided by several iron-containing pigments, eg hemin and hematin, used in the synthesis of catalases, peroxidases and enzymes of the cytochrome electron transport system; organisms that depend on exogenous X factors for growth are incapable of synthesizing protoporphyrin from Δ-aminolevulinic acid; X factor is required by certain species of *Haemophilus (H influenza, H aegyptiae, H ducreyi, H aphrophilus*)

XIST X-inactivation-specific transcript see X chromosome inactivation

XLD agar Xylose-lysine-deoxycholate agar MICROBIOLOGY A highly selective bacterial growth medium used to isolate gastroenteric pathogens, which like the salmonella-shigella and Hektoen enteric agars contain substances that inhibit the growth of native coliform flora, allowing identification of ***Enterobacteriaceae*** (enteric gram-negative rods); 'lysine positive' XLD agar's normal pink color is converted to yellow by acid-producing bacteria, eg *Escherichia coli* and *Salmonella typhi,* the latter of which, in addition produces H_2S, as do some *Proteus* species, resulting in a black color on the culture plate

X-linked adrenoleukodystrophy An inherited peroxisomal disease due to a defective gene on chromosome Xq28, in which there is impaired degradation of saturated very long chain fatty acids (VLCFA) that accumulate with the cholesterol ester and gangliosides in the central nervous system, adrenal glands, plasma and leukocytes, causing multifocal demyelination of the central nervous system Clinical The phenotypic range of expression is broad and it is often first seen in childhood with major neurologic deterioration and death following within a few years Treatment Modifications in the lipid intake may normalize the serum levels of VLCFA (long-term effects are unknown), bone marrow transplantation (N Engl J Med 1990; 322:1860cr)

X-linked hypogammaglobulinemia X-linked agammaglobulinemia Bruton's disease A disease with defective humoral immunity due to an intrinsic B cell gene defect that 'maps' to chromosome Xq21.3-22 Clinical Recurrent pyogenic infections, affecting boys by 5-6 months of life, coincident with the fall in maternal IgG Laboratory Marked decrease in B lymphocytes and immunoglobulins, intact T cell function Treatment Antibiotics, monthly injections of gammaglobulins Prognosis Death is inevitable in early childhood, often secondary to fulminant pulmonary infection

X-linked lymphoproliferative disease A condition characterized by fatal or chronic infectious mononucleosis, aplastic anemia, agammaglobulinemia and lymphoma following Epstein-Barr virus infection, caused by a failure to make the heavy chain class switch from IgM and IgG after a second exposure to antigens

X-linked myotubular myopathy An often fatal, sex-linked form of centronuclear myotubular myopathy characterized by marked cellular hypertrophy, especially of type I fibers, and an ultrastructural appearance similar to that of fetal myotubules; the associated proliferation of sarcotubular organelles may be caused by impaired innervation (Hum Pathol 1984; 15:1107); the condition causes severe hypotonia that may be fatal to susceptible; adult survivors have minimal residual functional incapacity

X-rays A portion of the electromagnetic spectrum (wavelength 10^{-10} to 2.5×10^{-6}) named by Roentgen, which-corresponds to ionizing radiation resulting from high-energy (1 keV to 1 MeV or more) particles, eg electrons, colliding with target electrons, an event that raises the latter to higher energy levels, releasing high energy photons and a spectrum of characteristic radiation (X-rays) as the target electrons fall back to lower excitation levels; patient exposure levels to X-rays are divided into those that are an undesired side effect of a diagnostic procedure and those that are a necessary component of a therapeutic procedure Diagnostic X-rays impart 30-150 keV of energy and rare reports in the literature infer a possible relationship between exposure to low- (diagnostic-) level X-rays and an increased incidence of myeloproliferative disorders, recently associated (relative risk 1.14) with minimal increased risk for developing multiple myeloma (J Am Med Assoc 1991; 265:1290) Therapeutic X-rays can be in the form of 1) Low level radiation, eg 5-10 keV or 'grenz' radiation, which may be used to treat various recalcitrant skin conditions, eg psoriasis or 2) High level, eg mega-electron-volt (MeV) radiation, used to treat internal malignancy; X-rays may be detected by wavelength-dispersive spectrometry, energy-dispersive spectrometry and energy loss spectrometry; X-ray production requires 1) X-ray tube A vacuum tube with a cathode (tungsten filament, which when heated produces an electron cloud) and an anode (containing an angulated deflecting target), mounted within an electrically and radioactively insulated housing, the beam exits via an adjustable aperture (collimator) 2) High-voltage generator A device that generates power in the form of pulsating direct (or 'rectified' alternating) current, the X-rays hit the angulated tungsten target on the anode and useful wavelengths are emitted (90% of the energy is dissipated as heat) through the collimator 3) Control console The electronics which control the voltage, amperage and exposure time

X-ray crystallography X-ray diffraction A technique in which a beam of X rays is focused on a crystal, diffracted by the molecule(s) of interest and then recorded on film; the pattern of diffraction provides information on the amplitude of the crystal's Fourier transform; the phase information is deduced by comparing the diffraction patterns from related chemicals Note: Watson and Crick's model of DNA as a double-stranded molecule was deduced by X-ray crystallographic analysis of data via the Fourier transform; X-ray crystallographic images may be resolved by isomorphic replacement, solvent-flattening, model-building and various refinement methods

XTE syndrome A rare autosomal dominant condition characterized by xeroderma, talipes and enamel defect, accompanied by cleft palate, hypohidrosis and cutaneous bullae

XX male syndrome An uncommon sex chromosome anomaly that clinically mimics Klinefelter syndrome, characterized by male psychosexual orientation, masculine appearance, weak secondary sexual characteristics, azoospermia, low androgen levels and small testes; 70% of patients have a portion of the short arm of the Y chromosome translocated to the short arm of the X chromosome

XXX syndrome (47, XXX) The most common (1:1000) chromosomal abnormality of females Clinical Clinodactyly, epicanthal folds, ocular hypertelorism and an increased incidence of congenital defects in their children; most subjects with XXX syndrome have a normal IQ, they tend to be emotionally labile, have speech and learning defects

XXXX syndrome (48, XXXX) Superwoman A chromosomal defect associated with moderate mental retardation, behavioral problems, midfacial hypoplasia, clinodactyly, radial synostosis, hypertelorism, micrognathia, web neck and menstrual irregularity

XXXXX syndrome (49, XXXXX) Penta-X syndrome Females who may present in infancy with patent ductus arteriosus, mental and growth retardation, upward slanting of the eyes, carpal hypoplasia and clinodactyly of the fifth finger

XXY syndrome (47, XXY) Klinefelter syndrome

XXXY syndrome (48, XXXY) and XXXXY syndrome (49, XXXXY) A group of chromosomal defects characterized by multiple X chromosomes accompanied by one Y chromosome; the wide range of somatic defects overlap many of the somatic features of Klinefelter syndrome Clinical Small testes, hypoplastic penis, gynecomastia, mental retardation, wide-set eyes, ulnar and radial abnormalities; more than one-half of those with the 49, XXXXY syndrome present with low birth weight, muscle hypotonicity, profound mental and growth retardation, malformed ears, a short neck, hypertelorism with a mongoloid slant, a flattened nose, small undescended testes, hypoplastic external male genitalia, clinodactyly, radioulnar synostoses, coxa vara, genu varum, pes planus Treatment None, testosterone may improve secondary sexual characteristics

Xylose absorption test GASTROENTEROLOGY Administration of a pentose per os to determine intestinal absorptive capacity; 25 g of D-xylose is given orally and later measured in the urine; excretion of less than three grams in a five hour period is suggestive of enterogenous malabsorption, since pancreatic enzymes are not required for the absorption of D-xylose; high blood levels of D-xylose with low levels in the urine are typical of renal failure, and thus the test should not be used for patients with renal disease

XYY syndrome YY syndrome A media 'syndrome' that appeared when some scientific data suggested that males with an extra Y chromosome (47, XYY) tended to be more aggressive, antisocial and display criminal behavior; other components of this 'syndrome' included facial asymmetry, long ears, teeth and fingers, poor musculoskeletal development, cranial synostosis and a prolonged P-R interval on the electrocardiogram; it was subsequently shown that only a small percentage of subjects with XYY defects have the described anomalies

XYZ cell theory An obsolete postulate for antibody production, in which an 'X cell' was immune-competent and had yet to engage in a specific immune response, the 'Y cell' was immunologically activated or 'primed' by the interaction of the X cell and a target antigen, and a 'Z cell' produced antibodies after a second exposure to the antigen

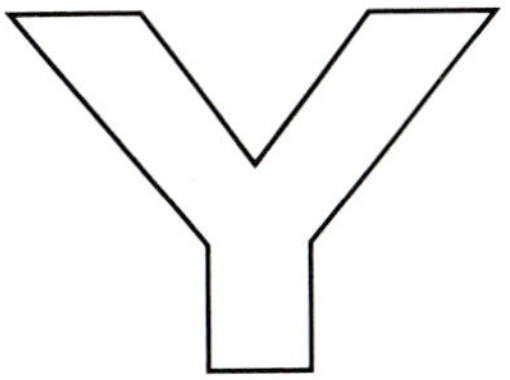

Y Symbol for: pyrimidine; tyrosine; yttrium

YAC cloning Yeast artificial chromosome cloning MOLECULAR BIOLOGY A cloning system based on the propagation of large 60-650 kilobase pair DNA molecules as linear, artificial chromosomes in the yeast *Saccharomyces cerevisiae*; YAC cloning is preferred to conventional closed-end cosmid cloning, since the DNA segments that can be manipulated by YAC cloning are up to ten-fold longer than segments cloned in cosmids, the yeast is a eukaryote (providing a different host environment for the DNA propagation) and the chromosomal DNA is more easily manipulated, offering the possibility of making specific changes in the large DNA molecules being YAC cloned (Science 1989; 244:1348)

YAG laser see Laser, Nd:YAG (neodymium:yttrium-aluminum-garnet) laser

Yaws TROPICAL MEDICINE An infection by a non-venereal spirochete (other non-venereal spirochetal diseases include bejel and pinta), *Treponema pertenue*, which is virtually identical to *T pallidum*, affecting rural children in the southern hemisphere, transmitted by direct contact, facilitated by poor personal hygiene and overcrowding; after a several week incubation, a primary granulomatous lesion, the 'mother yaw' appears at the site of inoculation, consisting of a maculopapular rash, usually on the leg, overlying a cluster of exudative nodules, later ulcerating and healing spontaneously; this is followed by secondary yaws (Yaws II), analogous to secondary syphilis and characterized by generalized granulomatous papulo-maculo-squamous coalescing eruptions that become purulent and are accompanied by malaise, lymphadenopathy and osteitis Note: Forest yaws, a localized leishmanial lesion of South America, characterized as a hyperkeratotic papillary lesion, mimics the second stage of yaws; after the second stage, yaws enters a long latency period, reappearing as a tertiary yaws (Yaws III) with painful nodulo-ulcerative papillomas of the hands and feet, gumma of the skin and bones, palmo-plantar hyperkeratosis and depigmentation Treatment Penicillin

Y body CYTOGENETICS A rounded mass corresponding to the Y chromosome, which is seen in fluorescently-stained metaphase and interphase nuclei of genotypic male (XY) cells—buccal mucosa epithelium, fibroblasts, amniotic cells and spermatozoa

Y cartilage A finding which when accompanied by stippled scimitar-shaped calcification of the inferior margin of the patella is characteristic of cerebrohepatorenal (Zellweger) syndrome that may be accompanied by calcification of the hyoid bone and thyroid cartilage, dolichocephaly, wormian bones, hand and foot deformities and bone immaturity, associated with seizures, flaccidity, facial dysmorphia, cataracts, flexion contractures, renal cortical cysts, liver fibrosis and death in early infancy

Y cell see XYZ cell theory

Yeast A unicellular spherical-to-oval organism measuring 3-5 μm, most of which reproduce by budding (some by binary fission), and which when adherent in end-to-end rows are termed pseudohyphae; most fungi are saprobes and used in the commercial production and fermentation of foods and beverages; seven genera of yeasts of the class Deuteromycetes (imperfect fungi) are pathogenic to humans, including ***Candida, Crytococcus, Geotrichum, Pityrosporum, Rhodo-torula, Torulopsis, Trichosporon***; the non-pathogenic 'beer-maker's yeast', ***Saccharomyces cerevisiae*** is of considerable use as a research organism in molecular biology, as like all fungi, it is a eukaryote, contains mitochondria and endoplasmic reticulum and contains a wide variety of structural and functional motifs in DNA and proteins; ***S cerevisiae*** is also of use in studying large segments of genes from other species, see YAC cloning

Yeast connection see Candidiasis hypersensitivity syndrome

'Yellow advertising' see Yellow professionalism

Yellow beeswax CLINICAL PHARMACOLOGY The purified wax from the honey comb of the honeybee, Apis mellifera, which is a mixture of myricin, cerin and cerolein, used as a stiffening agent in various pharmaceutical preparations and as an ingredient of many polishes; see Inert ingredients

'Yellow blood' TRANSFUSION MEDICINE A unit of packed red blood cells with a milky yellow-white discoloration, which implies bacterial contamination that must be discarded

Yellow creek ENVIRONMENT A Kentucky river that was used for illegal dumping of toxic chemicals (tannin and chromium) from a local factory, which was linked by some workers to a local epidemic of spontaneous abortions, nausea, rashes, diarrhea and glomerular disease; Cf Love canal

Yellow fat disease A vitamin E deficiency syndrome affecting various mammals fed excess n-3 polyunsaturated fatty acids, derived from fish oils Note: in humans, excess fish-oils cause pathologically-increased bleeding time, especially after aspirin ingestion, may play a role in cardiac necrosis and in increasing susceptibility to catecholamine-induced stress; see Fish oil

Yellow fever An acute mosquito (*Aedes aegypti*)-borne infection of tropical Africa and South America, by a flavivirus (a group B single-stranded 'negative'-sense RNA virus) Clinical The disease may be benign with a non-specific 'flu' syndrome to a pernicious disease characterized by an abrupt onset of high fever (with bradycardia, the Faget sign), headache, anorexia, myalgia, lumbosacral pain, nausea, vomiting that becomes blood-tinged up to 7-10 days post-onset, photophobia, flushing of face, a 'strawberry' tongue, insomnia, constipation, hypotension, jaundice ('yellow' fever) circa day four, generalized petechial hemorrhages and hematemesis, coagulation factor depletion, dilated cardiomyopathy, possibly coma; this is followed by a 'period of remission' of hours to several days in duration, after which the patient deteriorates and dies (up to 50% mortality) Laboratory Leukopenia, occasionally pronounced, disseminated intravascular coagulation, increased bilirubin, proteinuria, albuminuria with renal failure, rising titers in neutralizing antibodies, increased transaminase Histopathology Mid-zonal to complete lobular necrosis in a background of fatty degeneration

Yellow jacket venom A substance produced by hymenopteran insects, eg bees, wasps, ants that may prove fatal via a type I anaphylactic reaction with the release of vasoactive substances (leukotrienes, ECF-A and histamine), causing generalized urticaria, throat and chest tightness, stridor, fever, chills and cardiovascular collapse; toxic overload of hymenopteran venom may also be fatal to victims of 'swarmings'; see Swarming

Yellow mutant albinism Oculocutaneous (OCA) albinism, type IB, An autosomal recessive condition affecting the Amish, a genetically isolated group of German descent, living in Pennsylvania, USA (rare cases of OCA, type IB have been reported elsewhere in the USA, Sri Lanka and Africa) with white hair which later becomes yellow-red, hypopigmented skin, increased susceptibility for cutaneous malignancy, 'cartwheel' pigmentation in the ocular fundus; these patients do not form eumelanin, but rather a yellowish pigment (pheomelanin); pheomelanosomes mature to stage III melanosomes

Yellow nail syndrome A clinical complex characterized by a combination of slow-growing indurated flavescence of all or the distal part of the nail with the loss of the lunula, onycholysis, primary lymphedema of the extremities, idiopathic pleural effusions, lymphedema of the face and extremities, chronic bronchitis and chronic sinusitis; the nails are thickened without visible lunulae and have an exaggerated lateral curvature, in addition to slowed growth, which is thought to be due to primary stromal sclerosis, leading to lymphatic obstruction; although yellow nails are most commonly seen under 'physiologic' conditions on the fingers of heavy cigarette smokers with lung disease, eg chronic obstructive lung disease, the nails may also occur in malignancy, tetracycline therapy, thyroid disease, rheumatoid arthritis, diabetes mellitus, immunodeficiency, eg AIDS (J Am Acad Dermatol 1990; 22:608) Note: Although the yellow nail syndrome is relatively more common in smokers, it is not considered the same as the 'nicotine' nail of smokers; see Harlequin nail

Yellow ovary 'disease' An asymptomatic finding in which

the ovary demonstrates global luteinization, imparting a bright yellow-orange tinge to the organ

Yellow phosphorus White or elemental phosphorus A waxy solid used in fertilizers, water treatment, food products, beverages and in the synthesis of pesticides, eg rat and roach poisons; the vapors are highly irritating to the eyes and respiratory tract and cause deep thermal burns at sites of skin contact; prolonged exposure is associated with facial bone necrosis, abdominal pain, jaundice, 'garlic breath', anemia, cachexia, blepharospasm and photophobia **Histopathology** The liver is most severely affected with extensive 'large vacuole' fatty infiltration and necrosis (early periportal necrosis; late massive lobular necrosis); the central areas demonstrate 'fine vacuole' fatty infiltration, mid-zone demonstrates coagulation necrosis

'Yellow' professionalism Commercial advertising by health maintenance organizations (HMOs), and to a lesser extent, by private physicians in the Yellow Pages of telephone directories; competition for patients has traditionally been considered inappropriate in the medical profession; aside from the ethical dilemma, tsome physicians may not be certified specialists in the area of claimed expertise; the American Board of Medical Specialists maintains a list of physicians certified in one or more of 23 recognized medical and surgical specialties (☎ 800.776.2378, N Engl J Med 1987; 316:1315; ibid, 318:352)

Yellow rain ENVIRONMENT A fungal toxin (trichothecene T-2, produced by the mold, ***Fusarium***) that is an agent of biological warfare, allegedly supplied for use by the Communist troops in Kampuchea and Laos against the Hmong people of Thailand, so named for the yellow cloud that resulted from the exploding shells; the yellow 'rain' saga proved rather unclear as a similar cloud is said to be related to digested bee (***Apis dorsata***) pollen (Nature 1985; 315:284) **Clinical** Tricothecene, is a major radiomimetic that destroys bone marrow, causes immune compromise and gastrointestinal disease

Yellow salt OCCUPATIONAL MEDICINE A precipitated platinum salt, ammonium hexachloroplatinate that is the crude product from which highly purified platinum is produced; exposure to platinum fumes elicits a type IV hypersensitivity reaction in over half of the exposed workers, who complain of sneezing, runny nose, chest tightness, dyspnea, dry coughing and eventually interstitial pulmonary fibrosis

Yellow tag TRANSFUSION MEDICINE The color of the label used for blood group A (California standards); ABO blood group coding is not required by the US Food and Drug Administration

Yellow top tube LABORATORY MEDICINE A blood collection tube that may contain sodium polyanethol-sulfonate, used in microbiology for blood cultures, or thrombin for stat chemistries, ACD solution for processing specimens in the blood bank, or may contain no additives

Yellow urine A yellow-tinged urine, which in an acid pH urine, may be due to excretion of picric acid, dinitrophenol, phenacetin or chrysarobin or in alkaline pH urine, due to increased secretion of anthocyanin, or associated with ingestioin of beets or blackberries; pure yellow urine is associated with increased acriflavine and has a green fluorescence; yellow-orange urine may be highly concentrated or contain increased bilirubin-biliverdin

Yentl 'syndrome' A phenomenon in which once a woman shows herself to be equal to a man (in terms of risk factors), she receives equal medical treatment; the term was coined in an editorial regarding studies that revelaed that women despite similar risk factors for coronary artery disease and symptomatic disease, they were far less likely to receive the same diagnostic battery as a man; once cardiovascular disease was demonstrated, the women received the same treatment (N Engl J Med 1991; 325:274ed); Yentl is the 19th century heroine of Bashevis' story by the same name, who had to disguise herself as a man to be treated as one; Cf 'Yenta', a gossipy, scandal-spreading woman who cannot keep quiet

Y fork see Replicating fork

YIGSR A synthetic pentapeptide (Tyr-Ile-Gly-Ser-Arg) corresponding to the amino acids involved in binding native laminin by metastatic malignant cells; YIGSR inhibits tumor invasiveness when co-injected with malignant cells into mouse recipients and may have some currency in early therapy of cancer (Science 1987; 238:1132)

Yin-yang hypothesis PHYSIOLOGY A postulate that links cyclic AMP (cAMP) and cyclic GMP (cGMP) as opposing arms of a bidirectional intracellular control system, where an increased concentration of one is linked to a decreased concentration of the other, thus having a balanced relationship, likened to the Chinese yin and yang philosophy of universal balance

'Yin-yang tumor' see Gynandroblastoma

Yohimbine An agent that blocks the presynaptic α_2-adrenergic receptors, increasing cholinergic activity (increasing neuronal release of norepinephrine from the central and peripheral nervous systems), while decreasing sympathetic or adrenergic activity; yohimbine may be of use in treating a) Orthostatic hypotension and ischemic vascular disease caused by autonomonic dysfunction in diabetes mellitus (Hypertension 1990; 15:877) b) Narcotic overdose, possibly acting to increase the release of dopamine (Neuropharmacology 1990; 29:25) c) Psychogenic and organic impotence (Lancet 1987; 2:421), possibly acting to increase the inflow or decrease the outflow of blood to the penis Note: Yohimbine increases activity of the locus ceruleus, the site of the fear response in animals; low dose yohimbine has been used as a provocative test in those suffering from panic attacks

Yokohama asthma Tokyo-Yokohama asthma ENVIRONMENT A smog-induced asthmatiform complex described in Yokohama (Tokyo's port city), where nocturnal atmospheric conditions favor a dense buildup of industrial pollutants, eliciting wheezing and dyspnea in those with hyperirritable airways; the symptoms are worse when accompanied by chronic obstructive pulmonary disease; see Bhopal, Smog

Yolk sac tumor (YST) Endodermal sinus tumor A germ

cell tumor arising in the testis, ovary, other genitourinary regions, the mediastinum and sacrococcygeal region **FEMALE YST** A large (circa 15 cm in diameter) tumor of adolescents and young adults, which is associated with elevated circulating α-fetoprotein levels and reticulated or microcystic areas formed by a loose meshwork of pseudopapillary processes with a central vessel (Schiller-Duval bodies) Treatment Combination chemotherapy achieves a 50% rate in a formerly fatal lesion **MALE YST** A unilateral teratoma that mimics embryonal yolk sac tissue, that presents as a) Pure YST A tumor of male children under age two with an organoid cellular arrangement and an excellent prognosis or b) Mixed germ cell tumor of adults with poor differentiation, increased circulating α-fetoprotein and a poor prognosis similar to that of teratocarcinoma; Cf Sex cord-stroma tumors

Yom Kippur effect Spontaneous premature induction of labor occurring in pregnant Jewish women who observe Yom Kippur, the annual 24-hour religious fast of Judaism, in which there is total abstinence from food and water (J Am Med Assoc 1983;250:1317cr); Cf Judaism, practice of

Yo-yo effect UROLOGY A fanciful descriptor for an appearance caused by the disturbed peristalsis in an obstructed megaureter, where a bolus of contrast material cyclically regurgitates into the upper ureter after reaching the bottom of the dilated segment, with only a minute portion passing into the bladder

Yo-yo liver A liver characterized by an abrupt waxing and waning hepatomegaly, resulting from intermittent storage of a metabolic product, described in carnitine deficiency states (G Hug, U of Cincinnati) distinguishing this from other nonregressing metabolic hepatomegaly

YPLL Years of potential life lost PUBLIC HEALTH A statistic that is a measure of 'premature' death, ie that which occurs before age 65, calculated from the mortality data generated from the CDC's National Center for Health Statistics Causes of YPLL (1988) Accidents 19%, cancer, any site 15% (respiratory $279/10^5$, breast $206/10^5$, gastrointestinal tract $182/10^5$, oropharynx $28/10^5$), suicide and homicide 11% (black males $1669/10^5$; white females 99/100 000), congenital anomalies 5.5%; in 1988, AIDS became the sixth most common cause of YPLL, causing a 1.7% increase in the total YPLL (MMWR 1990; 39:20); magnitude of YPLL Cardiovascular disease $325/10^5$, malignancy $192/10^5$, cerebrovascular $64/10^5$; chronic obstructive pulmonary disease, $31/10^5$; pneumonia, $28/10^5$; suicide/homicide $20/10^5$, chronic liver disease, $11/10^5$ YPLL is increasing in AIDS (82%), diabetes mellitus (7%) and others; YPLL is decreasing in SIDS, cerebrovascular disese and prematurity; see 'Healthy people 2000'; Cf QALY

Y protein see Ligandin

Ypt1 protein A highly conserved 23 kD GTP-binding protein that is required for attachment and/or fusion of secretory vesicles from the endoplasmic reticulum with the acceptor compartment (the Golgi complex) during protein secretion (Science 1991; 252:1553)

Yucheng oil disease TOXICOLOGY An epidemic of congenital poisoning that occurred in Taiwan in 1979 due to the ingestion of cooking oil contaminated by polychlorinated biphenyls (PCBs) and dibenzofurans, eg 2,3,4,7,8-pentachlorodibenzofuran; congenital exposure resulted in lower birth weight, delayed growth, physical and mental retardation; defects in gingiva, skin, nails, teeth and lungs imply that the embryonal ectoderm is the most susceptible to the wiles of PCBs (Science 1988; 241:334); see PCBs, Toxic oil syndrome, Yusho disease

Yuppie disease see Chronic fatigue syndrome

Yusho disease Kanemi oil intoxication TOXICOLOGY A major episode of food poisoning that occurred in 1968 in Japan due to exposure to polychlorinated biphenyls (PCBs), eg 2,3,4,7,8-pentachlorodibenzofuran, which contaminated cooking oil, allegedly through faulty processing of rice bran oil; yusho afflicted an estimated 13 000 (official figure, 1614; 54 deaths) Clinical Nausea, vomiting, persistent adult respiratory distress syndrome, meibomian gland hyperplasia, chloroacne, cardiovascular and central nervous system disease, petechial and erythematous rashes with pulmonary hypertension (the latter features were not seen in the clinically similar Toxic-oil syndrome (N Engl J Med 1984; 310:1261c); see PCBs, Toxic oil syndrome, Yucheng disease

YY syndrome see XYY syndrome

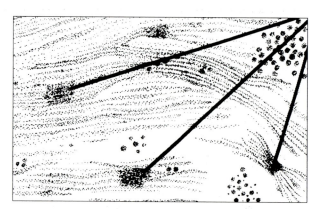

Z-band material

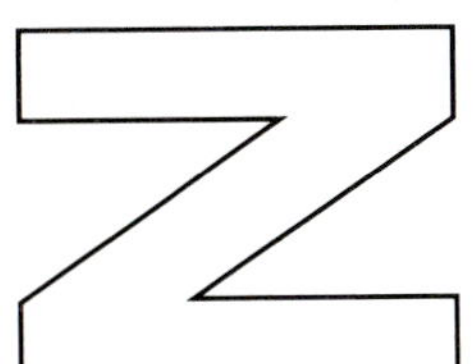

Z Symbol for: atomic number; total glutamic acid and glutamine; ionic number; net charge

Zagury, D An immunologist in Paris who developed a research protocol using a vaccinia virus that had been genetically engineered to express HIV on its surface (Science 1991; 252:1608n&v)

Z-band material An ultrastructural finding consisting of patches of disorganized myofilaments (figure, facing page), which is typical of rhabdomyosarcomas; other sarcomere-related structures seen by electron microscopy that support a diagnosis of rhabdomyosarcoma include thick and thin filaments in a hexagonal array, an A band with thick filaments and H and M bands or leptomeric structures; Z bands also occur in extracardiac rhabdomyoma, variably flanked by I bands

Z cell see XYZ cell theory

Z-DNA A variant configuration of DNA that is 'left-handed', 'antiparallel', has a deep single major groove with a zig-zag configuration, dinucleotide repeating units resulting from the alteration in the strand of sugar 'puckering' and torsional angles about a glycosidic bond; Z-DNA is a dramatic example of sequence-specific conformational change, where the major groove is more extreme and the minor groove is smaller than the 'usual' right-handed B-DNA; the base pairs are the same in each form; segments of Z-DNA occur in native DNA, require higher energy for maintenance than B-DNA, have a high content of guanine and cytosine and may have a role in signal recognition, possibly by initiating replication; see DNA

'Zebra' CLINICAL DECISION-MAKING A somewhat hackneyed aphorism often quoted to wide-eyed medical students during their clinical rotations is, '*WHEN YOU HEAR HOOF-BEATS, DON'T THINK OF ZEBRAS*'; this variation of 'Sutton's law' is designed to teach students a logical approach to achieving a diagnosis, since common things occur commonly and when one hears hoofbeats, one usually thinks of horses Note: In the Republic of South Africa, zebras are more abundant and the word 'canary' is substituted; Cf 'Red herring'

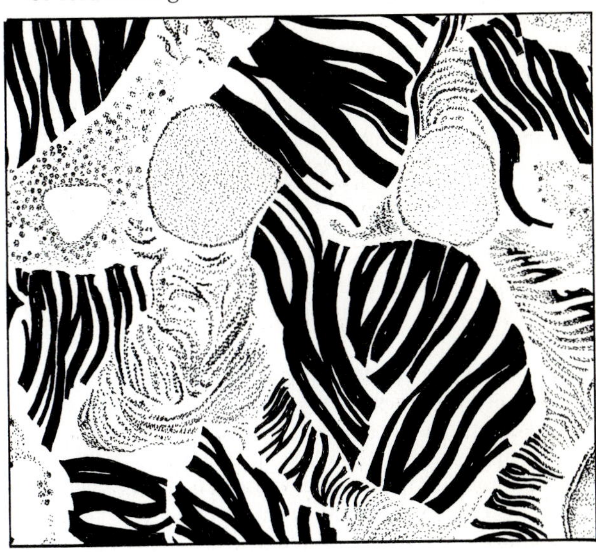

Zebra body

Zebra body A descriptor for a lysosome that contains broad transversely-stacked myelinoid membranes (figure, above), an ultrastructural finding typical of certain lysosomal storage diseases, found within neurons, Schwann cells, macrophages, smooth muscle cells, endothelial cells, pericytes, glomerular epithelial cells, hepatocytes and other cells; zebra bodies are classically seen in Fabry's disease, but are also well-described in Niemann-Pick, Landing's and Sandhoff's disease, some mucopolysaccharidoses, eg Hurler syndrome, myelinopathy, phenylketonuria and Tay-Sachs disease Note: 'Myelinosome' is the most correct term for any layered material within a lysosome; electron microscopists separate the myelinosomes into those with thick layering (zebra bodies) and thin layering, known as lamellar bodies ('myelin figures'), as each type is associated with certain diseases

Zebra body myopathy A congenital, non-progressive form of myopathy in which variably-sized muscle fibers have characteristic striped and rod-shaped bodies by electron microscopy (J Neurol Sci 1975; 24:437)

Zebrafish An experimental animal (*Brachydanio rerio*) that is useful in studying vertebrate development, which has transparent embryos, short (3 months) generation time and prolific egg production (Science 1990; 250:34); see *Caenorhabditis elegans*, *Drosophila melanogaster*, Guinea pig, Rat, *Saccharomyces cerevisiae*

ZEBRA gene A gene in the Epstein-Barr virus (EBV) genome that must be activated for the virus to replicate, thus serving as a switch between latency and replication; the gene is termed 'ZEBRA' as it is localized on the EBV Bam HI **Z** fragment that corresponds to the **EB**V **R**eplication **A**ctivator; the protein product of the ZEBRA gene is a transcriptional transactivator (G Miller, Yale)

Zebra pattern Alternating light and dark bands of the hair shaft seen by polarizing light microscopy in trichoschisis, an autosomal recessive condition caused by decreased sulfur content of the hair shaft that is further characterized by mental and growth retardation, ichthyosis and ectodermal dysplasia affecting the eyes, nails and teeth

Zeiosis A variant form of lymphocyte-mediated cytolysis, characterized by nuclear blebbing, disintegration of the nucleus and mitochondrial swelling

Zeitgeber German, time-keeper Any factor in the environment with periodicity, capable of synchronizing the endogenous circadian rhythm into a 24-hour cycle; without Zeitgebers, the free-running human clock is 25.3 hours; see Circadian rhythm, Jet lag, Shift work; Cf REM sleep

Zelen design CLINICAL TRIALS A design for a double-blinded study of experimental cancer chemotherapeutic agents that requires permission only from those patients receiving experimental drugs or therapy (N Engl J Med 1979; 300:1242); the patients are randomly assigned to one of two groups: the first receives the standard treatment, while the second group is allocated to the experimental group and then asked if they will participate; if they decline, they stay in the second group and are treated with the same protocol as the first group; any loss of statistical efficiency is compensated by increased numbers; the advantage is that the trial is truly randomized and the patients know whether they are being treated with an experimental regimen; see Leveno design (N Engl J Med 1986; 315:615)

Zellballen SURGICAL PATHOLOGY Nest-like clusters of uniform round-to-polygonal chief cells that are surrounded by delicate richly vascular tissue and sustentacular cells, a pattern characteristic of paraganglioma **Ultrastructure** 100-200 nm in diameter dense core granules, which are sites of norepinephrine production

Zero order kinetics THERAPEUTIC DRUG MONITORING The in vivo dynamics related to the rate of drug elimination, which is linear with time, and proportional to the concentration of the enzyme responsible for catabolism and independent of substrate concentration; see Michaelis-Menten equation; Cf First order kinetics

Zero population growth (ZPG) POPULATION The birth rate at which there is no net increase in a population (a goal targeted by birth control programs) and the number of births is equal to the number of deaths; the world population will stabilize at 8-14 billion by the middle of next century, but some modellers think that by the time stabilization occurs, it may be 'too late'; already, 15% of the world's population (800 million), live in a constant state of near-starvation; see Amsterdam protocol, Birth control, Greenhouse effect, Mexico City policy, Webster decision; Cf Title X

Zetacrit Zeta sedimentation rate A method for determining erythrocyte sedimentation rate, which is thought to be better than the Winthrobe or Westergren methods as it is not affected by hematocrit, it is linear with respect to fibrinogen and γ-globulin and has no male:female differences

Zeta potential The sum total of negative charges on red cell surfaces separating erythrocytes in a cationic medium; the cations in a medium can be divided into those that are firmly attached to the erythrocyte, moving as it moves and cations that are free in the medium; the boundary between these two planes of cations is known as the boundary of shear, a point at which the zeta potential may be measured as -mV; the optimal zeta potential for IgM antibodies is -22 to -17 mV and for IgG, -11 to -4.5 mV; the smaller the absolute mV values, the shorter the distance between cells; an increase of asymmetric proteins in the medium decreases the zeta potential, thereby increasing the erythrocyte sedimentation rate; the zeta potential can be artificially reduced by LISS, enzymes, albumin and polybrene

Zeugmatography A neo-Greek term for Magnetic resonance imaging

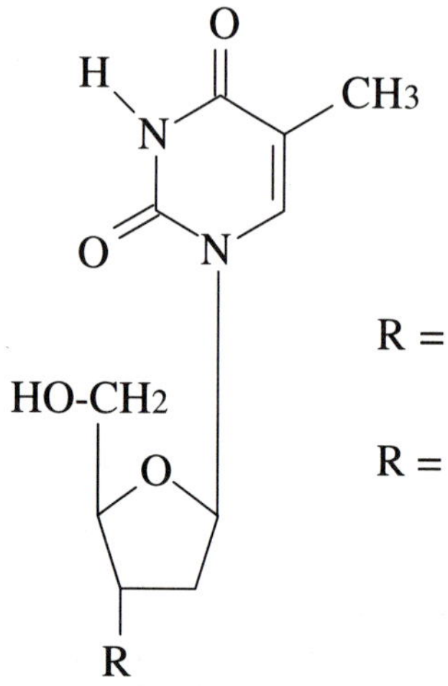

$R = NH_3$ Zidovudine

$R = OH$ Thymidine

Zidovudine AZT 3'-azido-3'-deoxythimidine A thymidine analog that slows the progression of AIDS, acting as an antimetabolite, terminating DNA chain growth of HIV-1; zidovudine is used in AIDS patients with *Pneumocystis carinii* and/or CD4+ T-helper cells less than 200/mm^3 and in HIV-1 infected children with neurodevelopmental abnormalities; AZT improves the survival of those with AIDS, 190 days without zidovudine, 770 days with zidovudine (N Engl J Med 1991; 324:1412); **Therapeutic effect** Increased sense of well-being, increased CD4+ T cells, fewer AIDS-related complications; patients may become refractory to AZT after 12-18 months due to development of multiple (three or more) mutations in HIV-1's reverse transcriptase (Science 1989; 246:1155) that are less susceptible to AZT, although the strains do not affect clinical disease (Science 1989; 243:1551, 1731) **Long-term complications** Mitochondrial myopathy, see Ragged red fiber disease; AIDS patients with profoundly decreased (< 100/mm^3) T cells who survive for long periods owing to AZT therapy, are at increased risk for high-grade B cell extranodal lymphoma, estimated to occur in 46% after 36 months of zidovudine therapy (Ann Intern Med 1990;113:276); the risk of non-Hodgkin's lymphoma is estimated at 1.6 per 100 patient years of zidovudine therapy (J Am Med Assoc 1991; 265:2208) **Side effects** Dose-limiting myelosuppression with granulocytopenia that may respond to lithium, anemia, headache, insomnia, mania, seizures, nausea, myalgia Note: Ribavirin antagonizes AZT's effect on HIV-1's replication; see AIDS therapy **Treatment guidelines Prophylactic** (500 mg/d) as CD4+ T cells fall below 0.5 x 10^9/L (US: 500 mm^3)(J Am Med Assoc 1990; 263:1606); in asymptomatic HIV patients with CD4+ T cells < 0.5 X 10^9/L (US: < 500/mm^3), 33/428 of the placebo group followed for one year developed clinical AIDS versus 11/453 of those receiving 500 mg/day of zidovudine (N Eng J Med 1990; 322:941) **Combination therapy** AZT (nausea, vomiting, anemia and marrow stem cell suppression) + a related drug 2', 3'-dideoxycitidine appear to prevent HIV replication within macrophages, requiring 1/5 usual AZT dose; alternatively AZT + amphotericin methyl ester (which increases the porosity of HIV's protein coat)

'Zigzag' QRS waves Sinusoidal QRS complexes seen by electrocardiography in ventricular flutter (240-280/min)

Zinc A trace mineral that is stored in synaptic vesicles and has a role as a synaptic neuromodulator, acting in the hippocampus to induce depolarizing synaptic potentials (Nature 1991; 349:521)

Zinc finger MOLECULAR BIOLOGY A tertiary protein structural motif of higher organisms consisting of a protein loop held together at both ends by a zinc ion, which is present in transcription factors (DNA-binding proteins that regulate gene expression by either suppressing or enhancing gene transcription), consisting of a 28-30 residue polypeptide with a consensus motif (see figure) that is folded around a zinc atom; the 'finger' is tetrahedrically coordinated by cysteine or lysine residues for proper folding and DNA binding (Science 1991; 252:809); the DNA-interacting 'fingertip' itself is composed of Lysine, His, Asn, Gln, Thr and Arg and contains an antiparallel β ribbon and an α helix; the zinc finger motif is present in many proteins that regulate the expression of eukaryotic genes, including proto-oncogenes, the Wilms' tumor gene and growth signal receptors

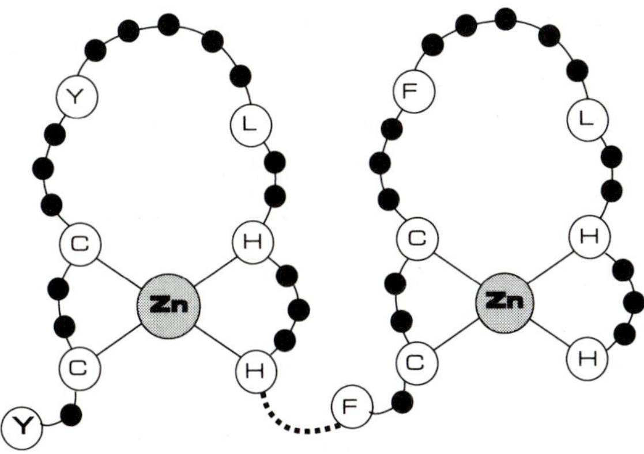

Zinc finger domains

Zinc finger proteins A superfamily of transactivating protein receptors that mediate the actions of steroids and steroid-like hormones; after a zinc finger receptor binds a hormone, it influences gene expression by associating with specific DNA elements, the HREs (hormone-responsive elements; zinc finger domains occur in the Wilm's gene product, protein kinase C proteins, glucocorticoid receptor DNA-binding domain (Science 1990; 249:157), HTLV-I and HTLV-II transformed cells (ibid 1990; 248:588) and the ZPY gene, which encodes a zinc-finger protein once considered a candidate for the testis-determining factor

'Zinc sandwich' A polypeptide hormone-receptor complex in which a hormone, eg growth hormone (hGH) binds to a another, not cognate receptor, eg prolactin receptor, forming a bridge between histidine and glycine residues and zinc, but not other divalent metal ions; a 'zinc sandwich' motif provides a molecular explanation of the broader effects of zinc deficiency (Science 1990; 250:1709)

Zippering MOLECULAR BIOLOGY Rapid annealment of two fully complementary strands of RNA and DNA into a double helix, which follows a short nucleation step PHYSIOLOGY The highly organized process of internalization of phagocytosed particles, which requires that the receptor ligands being internalized by the macrophage have multiple contacts with their cognate 'receptor'

Zipper-like junction An ultrastructural particle formed in vitro in hairy cell leukemia, as well as in monocytic leukemia grown in tissue culture when these cells phagocytose material from the surrounding culture medium

Zipper motif see Leucine zipper

Zipper proglottid A descriptor for the proglottid of *Taenia saginata* which have 15-20 lateral zipper-like branches, best seen when injected with safranin dye and India ink; in contrast, the proglottids of *T solium* have fewer than 13 lateral branches and have been fancifully likened to Rorschach bodies

Zollinger-Ellison syndrome A condition characterized by multiple duodenal ulcers and gastrin-secreting tumors, which causes recurrent and refractory upper gastrointestinal ulceration, diarrhea, steatorrhea and hypoglycemia due to 'little' gastrin, as well as pyrosis and dysphagia due to gastroesophageal reflux and increased gastric acid; 25% of cases have concomitant multiple endocrine neoplasm (MEN-I); malignant gastric carcinoid may be related to chronic gastrin hypersecretion **Diagnosis** Computed tomography, when positive, is reliable in the face of typical clinical findings **Pathology** Marked variation in tumor size, 60% are malignant, despite a 'bland' appearance **Laboratory** Hypergastrinemia, increased basal acid output (>15 mmol/hour), increased post-histamine stimulation acid production, a high ratio of basal acid output to maximum acid output (stimulation testing reveals fasting gastrin levels greater than 1000 pg/mL) and hypercalcemia **Differential diagnosis**, hypergastrinemia: Antral hyperplasia, retained antrum syndrome, chronic atrophic gastritis, pernicious anemia, short bowel syndrome, gastric outlet syndrome, gastric outlet obstruction, gastric carcinoma, pheochromocytoma, chronic renal failure **Treatment** Medical treatment with H_2 receptor antagonists, which with higher doses may be coadministered with antimuscarinic drugs that enhance the inhibition of gastric secretion by H_2 blockage; non-response to medical treatment may require total gastrectomy and or vagotomy

Zombie One of the 'living dead' of Haitian voodoo folklore; there is no scientific data to support their existence, although one ethnobiologist claimed to have identified Zombie powder from voodoo sorcerers (bokors) and concluded that the active ingredient was tetrodotoxin, which further required that the victim actually believed in zombies., a 'set and setting' event (Science 1988; 240:274); Cf Ethnomedicine, Voodoo death

'Zombie' effect A descriptor for the personality changes reported to be secondary to haloperidol's extrapyramidal effects, resulting in a syndrome virtually identical to idiopathic Parkinson's disease, with hypomimia, bradykinesia and flat affect

Zonal centrifugation MOLECULAR BIOLOGY A method for separating molecules by size, as a function of the time of centrifugation and the mass of the molecule; the level at which the molecules come to rest in an ultracentrifuge (60 000 rpm) can be stabilized by adding a fluid, eg sucrose solution, the density of which varies from top to bottom; see Ultracentrifugation

Zone electrophoresis A generic term for any electrophoretic technique in which components are separated into zones or bands in a buffer, and stabilized in solid, porous or any other support medium, including filter paper, agar gel or polyacrylamide gel

Zone of equivalence IMMUNOLOGY A region in an antigen-antibody reacting system where the ratio of antigen to antibody is equivalent; the in vivo correlate of a dynamic zone of equivalence is serum sickness, where antigen is excess in the first one to two weeks, and the patient is asymptomatic, as antibody production increases to a 1:1 ratio, immune complexes form, causing clinical disease, which resolves as the balance is tipped toward antibody excess

Zoning phenomenon HEMATOLOGY Layering of atypical platelets in the bone marrow in myelofibrosis SURGICAL PATHOLOGY Changes seen by low-power light microscopy in myositis ossificans, in which there are three zones of osteochondroma-like growth, the most immature of which has a fibroblast appearance, demarcating the lesion from the normal tissue

Zoo blot A technique used to determine DNA sequence homology among different species, in which a labelled probe of a gene of interest is allowed to hybridize with Southern blots from other organisms

Zoonoses Infections in which the microbe's infectious cycle is completed between man and mammal

Zosteriform Any band-like unilateral skin lesion located along the cutaneous distribution of a spinal or a branch of the trigeminal nerves, usually seen in the recrudescence of Herpes zoster but also (rarely) seen in metastatic breast carcinoma and hemangiomas of Sturge-Weber disease

ZPA Zone of polarizing activity EMBRYOLOGY A group of mesenchymal cells in developing vertebrates that is responsible for forming the limb bud, which is aided in its orientation by retinoic acid (Nature 1991; 350:81, 83, 15)

ZPG see Zero population growth

Z-plasty SURGERY A surgical incision that lengthens a zone of skin or a muscle, 'breaking up' a linear scar or repositioning an incision to a line of least tension; the classic 'Z' incision consists of two triangular incisions with equilateral sides and a 60 angle

Z protein A protein that is normally present in the Z band of striated muscle, which may be positive in rhabdomyosarcoma but, like α-actinin, titin and tropomyosin, is too non-specific a muscle 'marker' to have significant diagnostic utility; Cf Protein Z

Zuckergußdarm German, sugar-icing bowel Whitish induration of the serosal surface of the intestine in chronic fibrosing peritonitis, which may be accompanied by hyalinization

Zuckergußleber German, sugar-icing liver A markedly thickened and whitish hepatic capsule, which may be seen in chronic perihepatitis or in cardiac 'cirrhosis', due to congestive heart failure Histopathology Portal zone fibrosis and bile duct proliferation

Zuckerguß spleen German, sugar-icing spleen Perisplenitis, as above

Zung scale PSYCHIATRY An objective rating instrument that evaluates depression, anxiety, hostility, phobia, paranoid ideation, obsessive compulsiveness and others; use of this scale is declining as it is relatively insensitive to clinical improvement

Z value A statistical test for the hypothesis that a population's mean does not differ from the target value, ie assumes no inaccuracy; see One-tailed and two-tailed testing

Zyklon B The cyanide-tear gas combination formulated by the scientists of the Third Reich, and used for the 'efficient' wholescale massacre of the Jews and other 'undesirables' in concentration camps; see Chemical warfare; Cf Tabun, Unethical medical research

Zygomycetes A generic term for a group of fungi which grow in compromised hosts including ***Absidia, Cunninghamella, Mortierella, Mucor, Rhizopus***, which are pathogenic to humans; other organisms, eg ***Basiobolus, Conidiobolus*** and ***Rhizomucor***, which proliferate but are not regarded as pathogenic

ZZAP reagent TRANSFUSION MEDICINE A reagent used to dissociate IgG and C3d from the erythrocyte membrane, eliminating spontaneous agglutination and allowing for reliable typing of ABO, Rh-hr and Kidd blood groups; ZZAP is of use in detecting alloantibodies, which are potentially capable of causing a hemolytic transfusion reaction in the face of non-specific binding of autoantibody to erythrocytes, or for evaluation of patients with acquired immune hemolytic anemia Note: The name was originally SSAP, indicating a mixture of a sulfhydryl reagent (dithiothreitol, which reduces disulfide bonds, S-S) and the proteolytic enzyme, papain which dissociates IgG and C3d from red blood cells; ZZAP was substituted for euphony